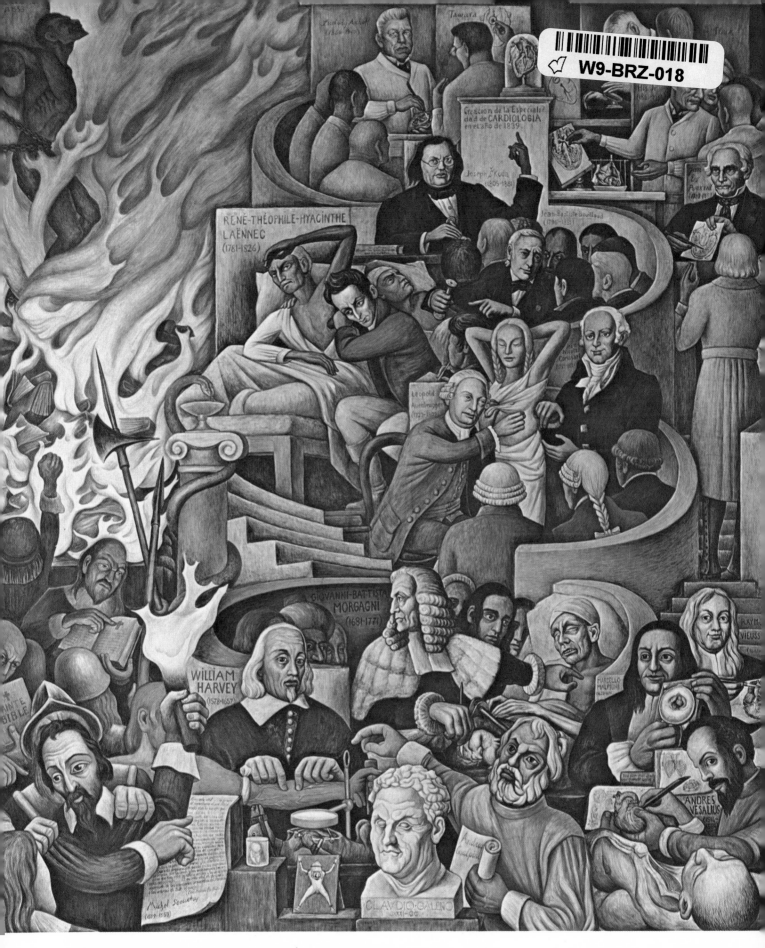

DIEGO RIVERA   "The History of Cardiological Doctrines" 1946

National Institute of Cardiology   Mexico D.F.

Jim Wellerson

THE HEART

ARTERIES AND VEINS

THE HEART

ARTERIES AND VEINS

Fourth Edition

J. Willis Hurst, M.D.
Professor of Medicine (Cardiology)
Chairman, Department of Medicine
Emory University School of Medicine
Atlanta, Georgia

R. Bruce Logue, M.D.
Professor of Medicine (Cardiology)
Emory University School of Medicine
Emory University Clinic
Atlanta, Georgia

Robert C. Schlant, M.D.
Professor of Medicine (Cardiology)
Director, Division of Cardiology, Department of Medicine
Emory University School of Medicine
Atlanta, Georgia

Nanette Kass Wenger, M.D.
Professor of Medicine (Cardiology)
Emory University School of Medicine
Director, Cardiac Clinics, Grady Memorial Hospital
Atlanta, Georgia

McGRAW-HILL BOOK COMPANY
A BLAKISTON PUBLICATION

*New York St. Louis San Francisco Auckland Bogotá Düsseldorf
Johannesburg London Madrid Mexico Montreal New Delhi Panama
Paris São Paulo Singapore Sydney Tokyo Toronto*

This book was set in Times Roman by Black Dot, Inc.
The editors were Joseph J. Brehm, J. Dereck Jeffers,
Richard S. Laufer, and Timothy Armstrong;
the designer was Barbara Ellwood;
the production supervisor was Robert C. Pedersen.
R. R. Donnelley & Sons Company was printer and binder.

THE HEART

ARTERIES AND VEINS

1234567890DODO783210987

Library of Congress Cataloging in Publication Data

Hurst, John Willis, date   ed.
    The heart, arteries, and veins.

    "A Blakiston publication."
    1. Cardiovascular system—Diseases. I. Title.
[DNLM: 1. Cardiovascular diseases. WG100 H436]
RC667.H85 1978   616.1   77-23537
ISBN 0-07-031472-1

LC CIP DATA (2 vol. ed.)

[RC667.H85 1978b]   616.1   77-23539
ISBN 0-07-031473-X (set)

LC CIP DATA (Special 2 vol. ed.)

RC667.H85 1978   616.1   77-015882
ISBN 0-07-031474-8

NOTICE

Medicine is an ever-changing science. As new research and clinical experience broaden our knowledge, changes in treatment and drug therapy are required. The editors and the publisher of this work have made every effort to ensure that the drug dosage schedules herein are accurate and in accord with the standards accepted at the time of publication. Readers are advised, however, to check the product information sheet included in the package of each drug they plan to administer to be certain that changes have not been made in the recommended dose or in the contraindications for administration. This recommendation is of particular importance in regard to new or infrequently used drugs.

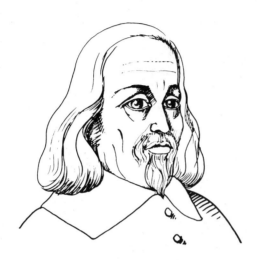

Dedicated to William Harvey (1578–1657) on his four-hundredth birthday.

He symbolizes all the pioneers—past, present, and future— who devote their lives to the study of cardiovascular disease and to the relief of patients who are afflicted with it.

CONTENTS

COLOR PLATES

JAMES K. ALEXANDER, M.D.
Professor of Medicine (Cardiology), Baylor College of Medicine, Houston, Texas

AARON H. ANTON, PH.D.
Professor of Anesthesiology and Pharmacology, Case Western Reserve University School of Medicine, Department of Anesthesiology, Cleveland, Ohio

MORTON F. ARNSDORF, M.D.
Assistant Professor of Medicine, Section of Cardiology, The Pritzker School of Medicine, The University of Chicago, Chicago, Illinois

ARTHUR C. BEALL, JR., M.D.
Professor of Surgery, Baylor College of Medicine, Houston, Texas

S. GILBERT BLOUNT, JR., M.D.
Professor of Medicine and Chief, Division of Cardiovascular Medicine, University of Colorado School of Medicine, Denver, Colorado

EUGENE BRAUNWALD, M.D.
Hersey Professor of the Theory and Practice of Physic (Medicine), Harvard Medical School; Physician-in-Chief, Peter Bent Brigham Hospital, Boston, Massachusetts

ALBERT N. BREST, M.D.
James C. Wilson Professor of Medicine, Director, Division of Cardiology, Jefferson Medical College, Philadelphia, Pennsylvania

DOROTHY E. BRINSFIELD, M.D.
Professor of Pediatrics (Cardiology); Executive Associate Dean, Emory University School of Medicine, Atlanta, Georgia

W. SCOTT BROOKS, JR., M.D.
Assistant Professor of Medicine, (Digestive Diseases), Emory University School of Medicine, Atlanta, Georgia

ROBERT A. BRUCE, M.D.
Professor of Medicine, Co-Director, Division of Cardiology, School of Medicine RG-20, University of Washington, Seattle, Washington

HOWARD B. BURCHELL, M.D.
Professor of Medicine Emeritus, University of Minnesota; Consultant in Medicine Emeritus, Mayo Clinic, Minneapolis, Minnesota

AGUSTIN CASTELLANOS, M.D.
Professor of Medicine, University of Miami School of Medicine; Director, Clinical Electrophysiology, Jackson Memorial Hospital, Miami, Florida

JAMES H. CHRISTY, M.D., F.A.C.P.
Professor of Medicine (Endocrinology), Emory University School of Medicine, Atlanta, Georgia

STEPHEN D. CLEMENTS, JR., M.D.
Associate Professor of Medicine (Cardiology), Emory University School of Medicine, Atlanta, Georgia

JAY N. COHN, M.D.
Professor of Medicine; Head, Cardiovascular Division, University of Minnesota School of Medicine, Minneapolis, Minnesota

ELIOT CORDAY, M.D.
Clinical Professor of Medicine, University of California, Los Angeles, School of Medicine; Senior Attending Physician, Cedars-Sinai Medical Center, Los Angeles, California

ERNEST CRAIGE, M.D.
Henry A. Foscue Distinguished Professor of Medicine, Professor of Cardiology, University of North Carolina School of Medicine, Chapel Hill, North Carolina

I. SYLVIA CRAWLEY, M.D.
Associate Professor of Medicine (Cardiology), Emory University School of Medicine; Chief, Cardiology Section, Atlanta Veterans Administration Hospital, Atlanta, Georgia

JAMES E. DALEN, M.D.
Professor and Chairman, Department of Cardiovascular Medicine, University of Massachusetts Medical School, Worcester, Massachusetts

MICHAEL E. DeBAKEY, M.D.
President, Chairman of the Cora and Webb Mading Department of Surgery; and Director of the National Heart and Blood Vessel Research and Demonstration Center, Baylor College of Medicine, Houston, Texas

ROBERT L. DeHAAN, PH.D.
W. P. Timmie Professor of Anatomy and Professor of Physiology, Emory University School of Medicine, Atlanta, Georgia

ANDREW L. DEUTSCH, M.D.
First Year House Officer, Department of Medicine, Emory University School of Medicine, Atlanta, Georgia

VICTOR G. deWOLFE, M.D.
Senior Physician, Department of Peripheral Vascular Disease, Cleveland Clinic Foundation, Cleveland, Ohio

LEWIS DEXTER, M.D.
Professor of Medicine Emeritus, Harvard Medical School and Peter Bent Brigham Hospital, Boston, Massachusetts

MARIO DiGIROLAMO, M.D.
Professor of Medicine (Endocrinology), and Associate Professor of Physiology, Co-Director, Division of Endocrinology, Department of Medicine, Emory University School of Medicine, Atlanta, Georgia

EDWARD R. DORNEY, M.D.
Professor of Medicine (Cardiology), Emory University School of Medicine, Atlanta, Georgia

JOHN S. DOUGLAS, JR., M.D.
Assistant Professor of Medicine (Cardiology) and Radiology (Cardiac Radiology); Co-Director of the Cardiovascular Laboratory, Emory University Hospital, Atlanta, Georgia

JOSEPH T. DOYLE, M.D.
Professor of Medicine and Head of the Division of
Cardiology; Director, Cardiovascular Health Center,
Albany Medical College, Albany, New York

E. E. EDDLEMAN, JR., M.D.
Professor of Medicine, University of Alabama School of
Medicine; Associate Chief of Staff for Research,
Veterans Administration Hospital, Birmingham, Alabama

JESSE E. EDWARDS, M.D.
Director of Laboratories, Miller Division-United
Hospital, St. Paul, Minnesota; Professor of Pathology,
University of Minnesota, Minneapolis, Minnesota

ROBERT S. ELIOT, M.D.
Professor of Medicine, Director of Cardio-
vascular Center and Division of Cardiovascular Medicine,
University of Nebraska Medical Center, Omaha,
Nebraska

NEIL T. FELDMAN, M.D.
Respiratory Division, Peter Bent Brigham Hospital;
Assistant Professor of Medicine, Harvard Medical
School, Boston, Massachusetts

JOEL M. FELNER, M.D., F.A.C.C.
Assistant Professor of Medicine (Cardiology), Emory
University School of Medicine; Director of Coronary
Care Unit and Director of Noninvasive Laboratory,
Grady Memorial Hospital, Atlanta, Georgia

SUSAN K. FELLNER, M.D.
Associate Professor of Medicine (Nephrology &
Inorganic Metabolism), Emory University School of
Medicine, Atlanta, Georgia

VICTOR J. FERRANS, M.D., PH.D.
Chief, Ultrastructure Section, Pathology Branch,
National Heart, Lung, and Blood Institute, National
Institutes of Health, Bethesda, Maryland

NOBLE O. FOWLER, M.D.
Professor of Medicine, Director, Division of Cardiology,
University of Cincinnati College of Medicine, Cincinnati,
Ohio

SAMUEL M. FOX III, M.D.
Professor of Medicine, Georgetown University School of
Medicine, Washington, D.C.

ROBERT H. FRANCH, M.D.
Professor of Medicine (Cardiology), Emory University
School of Medicine, Atlanta, Georgia

GOTTLIEB C. FRIESINGER, M.D.
Professor of Medicine; Director of the Division of
Cardiology, Vanderbilt University School of Medicine,
Nashville, Tennessee

V. F. FROELICHER, JR., M.D.
Assistant Professor of Medicine, Cardiology Department,
University of California, San Diego, California

JOHN J. GALLAGHER, M.D.
Director, Clinical Electrophysiology Laboratory;
Assistant Professor of Medicine, Department of
Medicine, Duke University Medical Center, Durham,
North Carolina

JOHN T. GALAMBOS, M.D.
Professor of Medicine; Director, Division of Digestive
Diseases, Emory University School of Medicine, Atlanta,
Georgia

BRIT B. GAY, JR., M.D.
Professor of Radiology and Director of Pediatric
Radiology, Emory University School of Medicine;
Radiologist, Henrietta Egleston Hospital for Children,
Atlanta, Georgia

PETER C. GAZES, M.D.
Professor of Medicine, Director, Cardiovascular Division,
Medical University of South Carolina, Charleston, South
Carolina

CHARLES A. GILBERT, M.D.
Professor of Medicine (Cardiology), Emory University
School of Medicine; Director of Cardiac Function
Laboratory, Grady Memorial Hospital, Atlanta, Georgia

LEON I. GOLDBERG, M.D., PH.D.
Professor of Medicine and Pharmacology, Chairman,
Committee of Clinical Pharmacology, University of
Chicago, Chicago, Illinois

JOHN F. GOODWIN, M.D., F.R.C.P., F.A.C.C.
Professor of Clinical Cardiology, Royal Postgraduate
Medical School, London, England; Consultant Physician
to Hammersmith Hospital, London, England; President,
International Society and Federation of Cardiology,
London, England

RICHARD GORLIN, M.D.
Murray M. Rosenberg Professor; Chairman, Department
of Medicine, Mount Sinai School of Medicine, Mount
Sinai Hospital, New York, New York

GILBERT D. GROSSMAN, M.D.
Associate Professor of Medicine (Pulmonary Disease),
Emory University School of Medicine, Atlanta, Georgia

ROBERT F. GROVER, PH.D., M.D.
Professor of Medicine, Director, Cardiovascular
Pulmonary Research Laboratory, Division of Cardiology,
University of Colorado Medical Center, Denver,
Colorado

J. CAULIE GUNNELLS, JR., M.D.
Professor of Medicine, Division of Nephrology,
Department of Medicine, Duke University Medical
Center, Durham, North Carolina

W. DALLAS HALL, M.D.
Professor of Medicine; Director, Division of
Hypertension, Emory University School of Medicine,
Atlanta, Georgia

W. PROCTOR HARVEY, M.D.
Professor of Medicine; Director, Division of Cardiology,
Georgetown University Medical Center, Washington,
D.C.

CHARLES R. HATCHER, JR., M.D.
Professor of Surgery and Chief, Division of Thoracic and
Cardiovascular Surgery, Emory University School of
Medicine; Director of Emory University Clinic, Atlanta,
Georgia

MICHAEL V. HERMAN, M.D.
Dr. Arthur M. and Hilda A. Master Professor of Medicine, Mount Sinai School of Medicine; Chief, Division of Cardiology, Mount Sinai Hospital, New York, New York

THEODORE HERSH, M.D.
Professor of Medicine; Co-Director of the Division of Digestive Diseases, Emory University School of Medicine, Atlanta, Georgia

YEN-YAU HSIEH, M.D.
Lecturer in Medicine (Cardiology and Clinical Pharmacology) College of Medicine, National Taiwan University Republic of China; Formerly, Research Associate Committee on Clinical Pharmacology, Departments of Pharmacological and Physiological Sciences and Medicine, The University of Chicago, Pritzker School of Medicine, Chicago, Illinois

REGINALD E. B. HUDSON, M.D. (LONDON),
F.R.C. Pathology, Hon. D. Sc. (Emory) Emeritus Professor of Pathology, Institute of Cardiology, University of London; Honorary Consultant Pathologist, National Heart Hospital, London, England

J. WILLIS HURST, M.D.
Professor of Medicine (Cardiology), Chairman, Department of Medicine, Emory University School of Medicine, Atlanta, Georgia

ROLAND H. INGRAM, JR., M.D.
Associate Professor of Medicine, Harvard Medical School; Director, Respiratory Division, Peter Bent Brigham Hospital, Boston, Massachusetts

JOHN B. IRVING, M.B., M.R.C.P.
Senior Registrar, Department of Cardiology, Royal Infirmary, Edinburgh, Scotland

THOMAS N. JAMES, M.D.
The Mary Gertrude Waters Professor of Cardiology and Chairman of the Department of Medicine; Physician-in-Chief, University of Alabama Hospitals, University of Alabama Medical Center, Birmingham, Alabama

MICHAEL L. JOHNSON, M.D.
Assistant Professor of Medicine and Radiology; Director-Division of Diagnostic Ultrasound, University of Colorado School of Medicine, Denver, Colorado

JOEL A. KAPLAN, M.D.
Associate Professor of Anesthesiology, Director, Division of Cardiothoracic Anesthesia, Emory University School of Medicine, Atlanta, Georgia

HERBERT R. KARP, M.D.
Professor and Chairman, Department of Neurology, Emory University School of Medicine, Atlanta, Georgia

ROBERT B. KARP, M.D.
Professor of Surgery, University of Alabama School of Medicine, Birmingham, Alabama

SPENCER B. KING III, M.D.
Associate Professor of Medicine (Cardiology) and Department of Radiology (Cardiac Radiology), Emory University School of Medicine; Director, Cardio-vascular Laboratory, Emory University Hospital, Atlanta, Georgia

JOHN W. KIRKLIN, M.D.
Fay Fletcher Kerner Professor and Chairman, Department of Surgery, School of Medicine and the Medical Center, University of Alabama, Birmingham, Alabama

NICHOLAS T. KOUCHOUKOS, M.D.
Professor of Surgery, Division of Cardiovascular and Thoracic Surgery, Department of Surgery, University of Alabama Medical Center, Birmingham, Alabama

TZU-WANG LANG, M.D.
Adjunct Associate Professor of Medicine, University of California, Los Angeles, School of Medicine; Senior Research Scientist, Cedars-Sinai Medical Center, Los Angeles, California

AUBREY LEATHAM, F.R.C.P.
Physician to St. George's Hospital and the National Heart Hospital; Formerly, Dean to the Institute of Cardiology, London, England

JOSEPH LINDSAY, JR., M.D.
Director of Noninvasive Laboratory, Department of Cardiology, Washington Hospital Center, Washington, D.C.

R. BRUCE LOGUE, M.D.
Professor of Medicine (Cardiology), Emory University School of Medicine, Atlanta, Georgia

THOMAS A. LOMBARDO, M.D.
Assistant Professor of Medicine, University of Texas Postgraduate School of Medicine; Director of Medical Education and Director of Electrocardiographic Laboratory, St. Elizabeth Hospital, Beaumont, Texas

RICHARD P. LYNCH, M.D.
Pathologist, Unity Hospital; Clinical Instructor, Department of Laboratory Medicine and Pathology, University of Minnesota Medical School, Minneapolis, Minnesota

MARVIN M. MCCALL III, M.D.
Associate Chairman, Department of Internal Medicine; Chief of Cardiology, Charlotte Memorial Hospital, Charlotte, North Carolina; Clinical Professor, University of North Carolina School of Medicine, Chapel Hill, North Carolina

WILLIAM L. MCGUFFIN, JR., M.D.
Assistant Professor of Medicine, Department of Medicine, Division of Nephrology, University of Alabama School of Medicine, Birmingham, Alabama

HENRY J. L. MARRIOTT, M.D.
Director of Clinical Research, The Rogers Heart Foundation, St. Petersburg, Florida; Clinical Professor of Medicine (Cardiology), Emory University School of Medicine, Atlanta, Georgia

KENNETH L. MATTOX, M.D., F.A.C.S.
Assistant Professor of Surgery, Baylor College of Medicine; Deputy Surgeon-In-Chief and Director of Emergency Surgical Services, Ben Taub General Hospital, Houston, Texas

JAMES METCALFE, M.D.
Professor of Medicine, Oregon Heart Association Chair of Cardiovascular Research, University of Oregon Health Sciences Center, Portland, Oregon

CANDACE L. MIKLOZEK, M.D.
Fellow in Medicine (Cardiology), Emory University School of Medicine, Atlanta, Georgia

DOUGLAS C. MORRIS, M.D.
Assistant Professor of Medicine (Cardiology), Emory University School of Medicine, Atlanta, Georgia

JOHN H. MOYER, M.D., D.SC.
Senior Vice President, Director of Professional and Educational Affairs, Conemaugh Valley Memorial Hospital; Regional Coordinator for Cambria-Somerset Council for Professional Education, Johnstown, Pennsylvania

ROBERT J. MYERBURG, M.D.
Professor of Medicine and Physiology, Director, Division of Cardiology, Department of Medicine, University of Miami School of Medicine, Miami, Florida

R. JOE NOBLE, M.D.
Associate Professor of Medicine, Director of Clinical Cardiology and Cardiovascular Training, Department of Medicine, Indiana University School of Medicine and Krannert Institute of Cardiology, Indianapolis, Indiana

ELIZABETH W. NUGENT, M.D.
Assistant Professor of Pediatrics (Cardiology), Emory University School of Medicine, Atlanta, Georgia

DONALD O. NUTTER, M.D.
Professor of Medicine (Cardiology) and Associate Professor of Physiology; Director of Cardiovascular Research Laboratory, Department of Medicine, Emory University School of Medicine, Atlanta, Georgia

RONAN O'RAHILLY, M.D.
Director, Carnegie Laboratories of Embryology, and Professor of Human Anatomy, University of California, Davis, California

EDWARD S. ORGAIN, M.D.
Professor (Emeritus) of Medicine, Consultant to the Medical Center, Duke University Medical Center, Durham, North Carolina

ALBERT D. PACIFICO, M.D.
Associate Professor of Surgery, School of Medicine and the Medical Center, University of Alabama in Birmingham, Alabama

LOREN F. PARMLEY, M.D.
Professor of Medicine, Director of Ambulatory Services, University of South Alabama Medical Center, Mobile, Alabama

OGLESBY PAUL, M.D.
J. Roscoe Miller Professor of Medicine, Northwestern University Medical School, Chicago, Illinois

JOSEPH K. PERLOFF, M.D.
Professor of Medicine and Pediatrics, University Hospital, University of California, Los Angeles, California

WILLIAM H. PLAUTH, JR., M.D.
Professor of Pediatrics; Director, Division of Pediatric Cardiology, Emory University School of Medicine, Atlanta, Georgia

CHARLES E. RACKLEY, M.D.
Professor of Medicine, Director of Specialized Center of Research for Ischemic Heart Disease, University of Alabama Medical Center, Birmingham, Alabama

C. THORPE RAY, M.D.
Professor and Chairman, Department of Medicine, Tulane University School of Medicine, New Orleans, Louisiana

T. JOSEPH REEVES, M.D.
Clinical Professor, Department of Medicine, University of Alabama in Birmingham, Birmingham, Alabama; Director of Cardiovascular Laboratory, St. Elizabeth Hospital, Beaumont, Texas

WILLIAM C. ROBERTS, M.D.
Chief, Pathology Branch, National Heart, Lung, and Blood Institute, National Institutes of Health, Bethesda, Maryland; Clinical Professor of Pathology and Medicine (Cardiology), Georgetown University, Washington, D.C.

MORTON ROBINS, M.S.P.H.
Public Health Consultant, Westat Research, Rockville, Maryland

PAUL H. ROBINSON, M.D.
Associate Professor of Medicine (Cardiology), Emory University School of Medicine, Atlanta, Georgia

ROYAL S. SCHAAF, M.D.
Medical Director, Prudential Insurance Company of America, Newark, New Jersey

ROBERT C. SCHLANT, M.D.
Professor of Medicine (Cardiology), Director, Division of Cardiology, Department of Medicine, Emory University School of Medicine, Atlanta, Georgia

DAVID V. SHEEHAN, M.D.
Instructor in Psychiatry, Harvard Medical School; Director, Psychosomatic Medicine and Hypnosis Clinic, Massachusetts General Hospital, Boston, Massachusetts

LIBI SHERF, M.D.
Associate Professor of Cardiology, Tel Aviv University Medical School; Associate Director, Heart Institute, Chaim Sheba Medical Center, Tel Hashomer, Israel

WADE H. SHUFORD, M.D.
Professor of Radiology, Emory University School of Medicine and Grady Memorial Hospital, Atlanta, Georgia

WAYNE SIEGEL, M.D.
Chief of Cardiology, The Stewart Medical Group, Miami, Florida

BARRY D. SILVERMAN, M.D.
Emory-Northside, Assistant Professor of Medicine (Cardiology), Emory University School of Medicine, Atlanta, Georgia

MARK E. SILVERMAN, M.D.
Associate Professor of Medicine (Cardiology), Emory University School of Medicine and Piedmont Hospital, Atlanta, Georgia

ERNEST G. SMITH, JR., M.D.
Clinical Associate Professor of Radiology, Emory
University School of Medicine; Director, Department of
Nuclear Medicine, Crawford W. Long Hospital of Emory
University, Atlanta, Georgia

ROBERT B. SMITH III, M.D.
Associate Professor of Surgery, Emory University
School of Medicine; Chief of Surgery, Veterans
Administration Hospital, Atlanta, Georgia

JAMES F. SPANN, M.D.
Professor of Medicine, Chief, Cardiology Section,
Temple University Health Sciences Center, Philadelphia,
Pennsylvania

SIDNEY F. STEIN, M.D.
Assistant Professor of Medicine (Hematology and
Oncology), Emory University School of Medicine,
Atlanta, Georgia

JOHN E. STEINHAUS, M.D., PH.D.
Professor and Chairman, Department of Anesthesiology,
Emory University School of Medicine, Atlanta, Georgia

GENE H. STOLLERMAN, M.D.
Goodman Professor and Chairman of the Department of
Medicine, University of Tennessee, Memphis, Tennessee

JOHN H. STONE III, M.D.
Professor of Medicine (Cardiology) Director, Division of
General Medicine, Director of Emergency Medicine
Residency, Grady Memorial Hospital, Emory University
School of Medicine, Atlanta, Georgia

HAROLD C. STRAUSS, M.D., C.M.
Assistant Professor of Medicine and Pharmacology,
Departments of Medicine and Physiology and
Pharmacology, Duke University Medical Center,
Durham, North Carolina

PANAGIOTIS N. SYMBAS, M.D.
Professor of Surgery, Thoracic and Cardiovascular
Surgery Division; Director, Daniel C. Elkin Surgical
Research Laboratory, Emory University School of
Medicine; Director, Thoracic and Cardiovascular Surgery
Department, Grady Memorial Hospital, Atlanta, Georgia

YAVUZ A. TARCAN, M.D.
Director and Professor in Nuclear Medicine; Assistant
Professor in Clinical Pathology, Emory University
School of Medicine, Atlanta, Georgia

W. JAPE TAYLOR, M.D.
Distinguished Service Professor of Medicine, Division of
Cardiology, University of Florida, Gainesville, Florida

ELBERT P. TUTTLE, JR., M.D.
Professor of Medicine; Director, Division of Nephrology
and Inorganic Metabolism, Emory University School of
Medicine, Atlanta, Georgia

KENT UELAND, M.D.
Professor of Obstetrics and Gynecology, Director of
Obstetrics, University Hospital, University of
Washington School of Medicine, Seattle, Washington

ANDREW G. WALLACE, M.D.
Professor of Medicine; Chief of Cardiology, Duke
University Medical Center, Durham, North Carolina

PAUL F. WALTER, M.D.
Associate Professor of Medicine (Cardiology), Emory
University School of Medicine; Chief of the Coronary
Care Unit, Cardiology Section, Veterans Administration
Hospital, Atlanta, Georgia

JAMES V. WARREN, M.D.
Professor and Chairman, Department of Medicine, Ohio
State University College of Medicine, Columbus, Ohio

WILLIAM C. WATERS III, M.D.
Clinical Associate Professor, Department of Medicine
(Nephrology), Emory University School of Medicine,
Atlanta, Georgia

H. STEPHEN WEENS, M.D.
Professor and Chairman, Department of Radiology,
Emory University School of Medicine; Chief of
Radiology, Grady Memorial Hospital, Atlanta, Georgia

ARNOLD M. WEISSLER, M.D.
Professor and Chairman, Department of Medicine,
Wayne State University; Chief of Medicine,
Harper-Grace Hospitals, Detroit, Michigan

NANETTE KASS WENGER, M.D.
Professor of Medicine (Cardiology), Emory University
School of Medicine; Director—Cardiac Clinics, Grady
Memorial Hospital, Atlanta, Georgia

EDWIN O. WHEELER, M.D.
Associate Clinical Professor of Medicine, Harvard
Medical School; Physician, Massachusetts General
Hospital, Boston, Massachusetts

CHARLES W. WICKLIFFE, M.D.
Clinical Assistant Professor of Medicine (Cardiology),
Emory University School of Medicine, Atlanta, Georgia

JOSEPH A. WILBER, M.D.
Clinical Associate Professor of Medicine, Emory
University School of Medicine, Atlanta, Georgia

A. CALHOUN WITHAM, M.D.
Professor of Medicine; Chief of Cardiology, Medical
College of Georgia; Talmadge Memorial Hospital,
Augusta, Georgia

J. EDWIN WOOD III, M.D.
Professor of Medicine, University of Pennsylvania
School of Medicine; Director, Department of Medicine,
Pennsylvania Hospital, Philadelphia, Pennsylvania

JESS R. YOUNG, M.D.
Head, Department of Peripheral Vascular Disease,
Cleveland Clinic Foundation, Cleveland, Ohio

DOUGLAS P. ZIPES, M.D.
Professor of Medicine; Director of Cardiovascular
Research, Division of Cardiology; Senior Research
Associate Krannert Institute of Cardiology, Indianapolis,
Indiana

Diego Rivera painted the murals that are shown inside the front and back covers of this edition of *The Heart*. These murals are housed in El Instituto Nacional de Cardiologia in Mexico City.* Dr. Ignacio Chávez guided Rivera's brush. Dr. Chávez wrote notes of instructions to Rivera in order that the artist might perceive the task that was before him. The following passage was written by Dr. Chávez and describes his notes to Rivera. The notes set the tone for this edition of *The Heart*.

In my notes I reminded the artist that "the men who forged cardiology are the most varied nationalities: Belgians and Frenchmen, Italians and Germans, Englishmen and Czechs, Spaniards and Americans—both of the Saxon and the Latin worlds—, Greco-Romans and Austrians, Dutchmen and Japanese. This single fact marks the spirit which should imprint itself upon the picture, which consists in emphasizing that scientific progress in our field, as in any other, has not been the patrimony of any race or of any tightly nationalistic culture. It is the genius of the man of every time and of every people which has developed universal culture. And it is this spirit of universality which you should embody in the two great frescoes."

The Notes also asked that the picture should indicate the ascending trend in knowledge and if possible should express "how slow and difficult has been the advance, how each of those men had to fight routine, prejudice, ignorance and fanaticism. If you could find the way, it would be beautiful to paint this group of men moving, striving in an upward march. . . .

DR. IGNACIO CHÁVEZ

This edition of *The Heart* pays tribute to the past, present, and future pioneers in cardiology. The new and dramatic concepts discussed in this book would not be possible without the elegant observations and clear writing of those who have preceded us. While we cannot thank them personally, we can honor them and continue to learn from them. Just as a magnificent painting becomes more remarkable each year, so do the observations of certain men. Their works should be read, pondered, and enjoyed by all of us.

This book is dedicated to William Harvey, who discovered the circulation of the blood. This edition of *The Heart* is published on his four-hundredth birthday. While he is singled out, he is representative of the army of men and women who have taught us what we know. Such men and women gave us more than medical knowledge. They also made our profession great by being men and women of integrity and compassion. The respect the public has for physicians on the day they graduate was earned by the excellent performance of the physicians who preceded them. Current physicians will pass on their knowledge and concern for patients to those who follow them, and many of them will be honored in the future as William Harvey is today.

This edition of *The Heart* emphasizes the following areas:

1 The book is dedicated to William Harvey, who symbolizes the many great observers and writers who made modern medicine possible. To further emphasize the contributions of those who went before us, the murals created by Diego Rivera are reproduced inside the front and back of the book. The portraits of the men who preceded and followed Harvey are shown in these murals.

Quotations of the medical masters of the past are reproduced in appropriate places throughout the book. Quotations from nonmedical men and women are also used.

2 This edition emphasizes, as did the preceding editions, the care of the patient with heart and blood vessel disease. The patient remains in the center of the stage and every effort is directed toward making him or her a nonpatient.

3 This edition continues to recognize that there should be an orderly sequence of learning and delivery of medical care. The sequence is: background information (a knowledge of anatomy, physiology, biochemistry, pathology, etc.) → information regarding disease process → the development of the skill required to collect information from a patient → the formulation of a set of medical problems based on the data collected → the creation of plans for the problems → the proper follow-up of the problems. Note that this edition defines and emphasizes the data to be collected on every patient who is thought to have heart disease and then discusses the additional data to be collected on selected patients. The indications for the procurement of additional data are discussed and the limitations of all the methods of data collection are highlighted.

4 There is a certain amount of duplication in the book. This duplication has been carefully planned for the convenience of the reader. There are times when an individual wishes to learn more about the physiology or anatomy of a subject. He or she will find detailed discussions on these subjects in *The Heart*. There are times when an individual wishes to learn more about the recognition and treatment of certain diseases. This is discussed in detail, but the proper amount of physiology and pathology may be laced through the discussion in order to assist one in using basic science information in the care of patients. Often a planned duplication is created simply to save the reader the valuable time it would take to refer to two or more places in the book. The amount and location of the duplication was determined by asking the following question: How would a reader look up a subject? With this as a guide the material has been organized to help the physician interested in physiology and the physician interested in the management of a patient. These could be different physicians or the same physician who may wish to look up different areas at different times, depending upon his or her interest at the time.

---

*Dr. Ignacio Chávez of El Instituto granted me permission to reproduce the murals and to use the quotation reproduced on this page. I am deeply grateful to him for his kindness and friendship.

5 Much has happened in the last four years. Accordingly, *The Heart* has been reorganized to some degree. All chapters have been updated and many new chapters have been added. Although all areas of cardiology have changed, the area that has changed most is the recognition and management of coronary atherosclerotic heart disease. Therefore, the discussion regarding this obstinate killer has been greatly expanded.

In our attempt to keep up-to-date we have for the most part used those abbreviations for units of measure recommended by the National Bureau of Standards, which recognizes the International System of Units (SI). Some of the more significant abbreviations are g for gram, s for second, ms for millisecond, and h for hour. We consider this an important effort to promote international scientific understanding through standardization of our tools of communication. Like the metric system, SI is here to stay, and let us hope that there is not too much confusion during the transition.

I wish to thank the authors of the various chapters. They are experts in their fields and many have grasped with great authority the baton that was passed on by their predecessors. Busy physicians are helpless without superb secretarial assistance. Therefore, I wish to thank all the secretaries who helped the authors. In my own office I thank Alex Nelson, who does everything and is loved by all; Carol Miller, who is the world's fastest typist and has a passion for accuracy; and Paula Noriega, who at the young age of 21 has the ability of many experts who are 40.

The staff of McGraw-Hill Book Company has been most helpful and creative. I thank them for their desire to help patients through the technique of communication to physicians who care for the patients. I especially thank Joe Brehm, Rich Laufer, Barbara Ellwood, and Bob Pedersen.

The preface to a book can be as personal as the author wishes it to be. Accordingly, for the first time I will write a personal note about the book. It is exciting to create *The Heart*. I like doing it. In fact, I would be unhappy not doing it. The act of creating *The Heart* requires daily work for 4 years. During the week I write for 1 to 2 hours every morning beginning at 4:45 A.M. On weekends the writing time expands to 3 to 4 hours on Saturday and Sunday. During the day I care for patients with heart disease and teach Emory medical students, house staff, and cardiac fellows. I am on the "firing line" of medicine everyday and get my best ideas in such a setting. I admire writers who gather up their notes and take off to an exotic and serene place to write. I cannot do that. My writing takes place in my home, in hotels in this country and abroad, in airplanes, etc. In a sense I must be bombarded by cardiovascular problems during the day and create solutions to them in the early morning. I test these ideas on my colleagues and trainees with whom I work during the day. Therefore, I thank them for their tolerance.

Now that the fourth edition of *The Heart* is completed the fifth edition is underway. The gestation period will be 3 or 4 years. The product of this gestation, the fifth edition, will be different from the first, second, third, and fourth editions. This is true because new information is being generated at such a rapid pace. I and the other authors who contribute to the book will evolve new views as new data dictate we should.

I wish to thank the readers here and abroad, without whom there would have been only one edition.

J. WILLIS HURST, M.D.

Rheumatic Heart Disease and Other Acquired Valvular Diseases

57
Etiology and Pathogenesis of Rheumatic Fever[1-11]

GENE H. STOLLERMAN, M.D.

ETIOLOGY

That the group A streptococcus is the sole agent causing initial and recurrent attacks of rheumatic fever rests firmly on four major lines of evidence: clinical, epidemiologic, immunologic, and prophylactic. All of these lines of evidence are of necessity indirect, because group A streptococci are not recoverable from the lesions of rheumatic fever, and no satisfactory experimental model of the disease has been demonstrated.

Clinical evidence

For at least 100 years clinicians have noted the frequency with which septic sore throat preceded acute rheumatic fever (ARF). The inconsistencies of this relationship, however, have been frequently pointed out. Almost a third of patients with acute rheumatic fever deny antecedent sore throat. Throat cultures and blood cultures in such patients show the former frequently negative and the latter virtually always sterile at the onset of the rheumatic attack. Recurrences of rheumatic fever appear even more mysterious clinically, particularly when the chronicity of a rheumatic attack and the hemodynamic complications of rheumatic heart disease make the issue of continued versus reactivated rheumatic carditis difficult to resolve. On clinical grounds alone, therefore, group A streptococci are difficult to establish as *the sole* etiologic agent.

Epidemiologic evidence

The environmental, bacterial, and host factors which appear to play a role in the development of rheumatic fever are important primarily because they are related to the incidence of preceding streptococcal infection. Thus, such factors as latitude, altitude, crowding, dampness, economic factors, and age all affect the incidence of rheumatic fever because they are related to the incidence and severity of streptococcal infections in general. Careful military epidemiologic studies over a period of 20 years show a clear sequential relationship of outbreaks of streptococcal

pharyngitis to rheumatic fever and, in turn, the virtually complete absence of ARF in the same population despite epidemics due to a variety of other respiratory pathogens when streptococcal infection is completely controlled by chemotherapy. Military recruits are extremely healthy young adults, optimally nourished, physically highly trained, and socially and ethnically very heterogeneous—yet rheumatic fever occurs among them in indiscriminate fashion except that it occurs more frequently in those with previous histories of ARF.

The modern confusion concerning the epidemiology of rheumatic fever has been caused by the declining prevalence and incidence of the disease in populations in which group A streptococcal sore throat still appears to be common. It is becoming increasingly clear that "group A streptococcal disease" may vary greatly as to (1) site of infection, (2) virulence and nature of infecting strains, and (3) the diagnosis of streptococcal pharyngitis—that is, the distinction between carriers of group A streptococci who sustain viral pharyngeal infections and patients with true primary streptococcal pharyngitis. Streptococcal disease in different socioeconomic groups and in different parts of the world has presented many confusing variables that demand more precise definition of the nature of the antecedent streptococcal infection required to trigger rheumatic fever.

Immunologic evidence

Initial (primary) or recurrent (secondary) rheumatic fever does not occur without a streptococcal antibody response. Furthermore, the magnitude of the antibody response is a major variable determining the attack rate of rheumatic fever following streptococcal pharyngitis. This is true for both primary and secondary attacks. Indeed, the streptococcal immune response is an important criterion for the diagnosis of rheumatic fever.

Prophylactic evidence

The final and perhaps most convincing evidence is the prevention of both initial and recurrent attacks of rheumatic fever by, in the former case, penicillin therapy, and in the latter, continuous chemoprophylaxis against streptococcal infections. The use of a single injection of benzathine penicillin G for the treatment and prevention of streptococcal infection cures streptococcal pharyngitis and at the same time protects against new infection for 1 month. This agent terminated epidemics of streptococcal pharyngitis and rheumatic fever in military recruits. Its monthly use in the prophylaxis of streptococcal infections in rheumatic subjects enables us to conclude that rheumatic fever cannot be activated by any other infection, illness, or trauma. Finally, the use of benzathine penicillin G intramuscularly coupled with careful immunologic and bacteriologic surveillance of rheumatic populations has helped the definition of the natural course of a single rheumatic attack without the confusion of intercurrent reactivations of the disease by clinically inapparent streptococcal infections.

PATHOGENESIS

A few absolute requirements are now known for the development of rheumatic fever: (1) the presence of the group A streptococcus, (2) a streptococcal antibody response indicative of actual recent infection, (3) persistence of the organism in the pharynx for a sufficient period of time, (4) location of the infection in the throat.

The site of infection and its severity

It is an old observation that ARF and acute glomerulonephritis rarely, if ever, occur in the same patient at the same time. It is also well established that ARF does not occur as a complication of streptococcal pyoderma. Several peculiarities of streptococcal impetigo may relate to failure of rheumatic fever to develop from this infection. "Skin strains" of group A streptococci belong to particular serotypes and have other special characteristics described below. Antistreptolysin-O titers in patients with skin infections are distinctly lower than those from patients with throat infections, and this is true also of anti-nicotinamide-adenine-dinucleotidase (anti-NADase) titers. In contrast, anti-deoxyribonuclease B (anti-DNAse B) and antihyaluronidase responses are quite vigorous in pyoderma. These differences illustrate the importance of the site of infection in the development of some immune responses, and such factors may be important in the pathogenesis of acute rheumatic fever.

Of particular interest is that pharyngeal carriage of skin strains is extremely common in patients with pyoderma. The streptococci appear first on normal skin where they can be isolated for at least a week before lesions appear, and these same strains then appear in the upper respiratory tract as long as 2 to 3 weeks later. Their localization in the throat rarely results in clinically apparent infection, and therefore the actual and potential virulence of these strains as primary pharyngeal pathogens is of interest.

In the southern United States the incidence of ARF is very low in summer among patients with sore throats from which group A streptococci are fre-

quently recovered. The relatively weak immune response in these infections has raised the question of whether the low rheumatic fever attack rate in such cases is due to *quantitatively* inadequate stimulus immunogenically or whether the strains are *qualitatively* different or "nonrheumatogenic."

Local factors

The possible role of lymphatic connections between the pharynx and the heart has been considered. The embryologic derivation of the heart links it structurally with the neck in its vascular, lymphatic, and nervous supply. There may be a direct route, therefore, for living streptococci, streptococcal L forms, or streptococcal antigens or toxins to pass freely from throat to heart. Streptococcal cultures or solutions of papaine injected into rabbit throats produce a very prompt myocarditis. Impressive connections between tonsils and the heart in human beings have been demonstrated by injections of lymphatic channels in cadavers. Such observations should stimulate further clinical and animal experimentation to elucidate the requirement for the pharyngeal route of infection in the pathogenesis of rheumatic fever.

The strain of group A streptococcus

There seems to be little doubt that the quantitative factor of severity of pharyngeal infection bears a general relationship to the attack rate of rheumatic fever. The greatest recorded attack rates have appeared in the most severe epidemics in military populations, and when freshly isolated strains from these epidemics are examined, certain bacteriologic features are striking: (1) They are very rich in M protein and highly resistant to phagocytosis; (2) very large hyaluronate capsules are present as is evident from the large mucoid colonies that form on blood agar; (3) such strains when freshly isolated are often mouse virulent or may be made so easily by a few passages through mice; (4) these strains are relatively easy to keep in the virulent phase by proper storage of cultures and occasional mouse passage; (5) strong anti-M antiserums can be produced readily against them in rabbits; and (6) they are "SOR negative"; that is, they lack the ability to produce a lipoprotein lipase called the "serum opacity factor" and thus fail to produce the "serum opacity reaction."

The strains that seem to be "nonrheumatogenic," and which come from pyoderma lesions and some pharyngeal M types, also contain M protein and may resist phagocytosis in human blood in vitro, but they rarely have large hyaluronate capsules, they are never mouse virulent even after repeated passages, they are very unstable with regard to their retention of M protein (they dissociate rapidly to avirulent strains on artificial media), and it is often difficult to prepare rabbit anti-M antibodies when the strains are no longer fresh and have been passed repeatedly on artificial media. Strains that produce lipoprotein lipase (SOR positive) do not appear to produce rheumatic fever, or if they do so, documented instances are not yet reported. It is of interest that SOR positive strains include many (but not all) skin serotypes but also some pharyngeal serotypes.

These differences reflect, perhaps, only relative degrees of virulence between "skin" and "throat" strains. Although a constant attack rate of rheumatic fever was shown to occur in military epidemics regardless of the M serotype of the infecting strain, these epidemics were caused by a relatively small number of M serotypes which are now well recognized as the most common and dangerous rheumatogenic pharyngeal strains. Several observers have commented on the rarity of rheumatic fever from some pharyngeal strains such as M types 2 and 4, and these latter two M types have not been associated with rheumatic fever despite their frequency as a cause of streptococcal pharyngitis. It is of interest that types 2 and 4 also resemble skin strains in some of the biologic properties discussed above, such as the production of the serum opacity factor. It seems increasingly likely that *qualitative* as well as *quantitative* differences exist in strains of group A streptococci that relate to their rheumatogenic potential.

Direct invasion by group A streptococci

The possibility that live streptococci may actually have reached the sites of rheumatic lesions, or that they may be present in an unidentifiable form, has always been intriguing. Because of the sterility of joint and cerebrospinal fluid (in chorea), most attention has been centered on a few reports of group A streptococci cultured from heart valves in acute rheumatic endocarditis. Although repetition and extension of this work was hampered by the discovery of penicillin, most invesitigators feel that these earlier reports were the results of either contamination at the time of autopsy or agonal or postmortem dissemination and proliferation of streptococci. One study on the factor of contamination, however, was completed in the preantibiotic years. Cultures of heart valves were positive at autopsy for group A streptococci in two of seven patients who died of rheumatic carditis, but no rigid precautions against contamination were taken. In the next four patients autopsied using surgical aseptic techniques, all were negative. Of interest is that in two of these last four cases, despite meticulous asepsis, streptococci were cultured from mediastinal lymph nodes.

Such observations, plus the more recent recognition of the role of bacterial L forms in microbial persistence, and the demonstration that group A streptococcal L forms can be produced in vitro and survive in vivo, have led to some uneasiness about the certainty that viable streptococci are absent from the lesions of rheumatic fever. To date, however, attempts to cure rheumatic fever by intensive antibiotic therapy have not been successful, nor have streptococal L forms in the pharynx of human beings so far appeared to show any relation to any disease process. Sporadic reports about transitional forms of cell wall–deficient variants of beta-hemolytic streptococci in the blood cultures of rheumatic fever pa-

tients require extensive confirmation due to the difficulties of interpreting the significance of retrieval of such variants from blood cultures in many diseases.

The role of toxins

Despite the popularity of the concepts of hyperimmunity and autoimmunity in the pathogenesis of rheumatic fever, none of the antibodies described to date, including those reactive with the heart, have been shown to be cytotoxic. Furthermore, one particular observation continues to challenge the hypersensitivity theory: the latent period between streptococcal infection and the onset of rheumatic fever does not shorten with rheumatic recurrences as one would expect in secondary immune responses. A direct toxic effect, therefore, of some streptococcal product, particularly on the heart, has not yet been ruled out as a pathogenetic mechanism. Several of the known components of the streptococcus have been studied for such an effect.

Streptolysin S has received considerable attention as a possible causative factor in rheumatic fever because the hemolytic moiety is not antigenic and thus is not neutralized by an immune response. Streptolysin S is inhibited by lipids, can be produced by resting streptococci (such as those lingering in the throat), and cause inflammation by rupture of phagocytic lysosomes, and has a cytotoxic effect on many cells, notably lymphocytes.

Streptolysin O is a potent cardiac toxin which also disrupts lysosomes in vitro. It is very antigenic, however, and its cytotoxic effect ought to be neutralized by repeated infections. Streptolysin O is bound by cholesterol and other lipids which inhibit toxicity.

Streptococcal proteinases have been shown to provoke myocarditis in rabbits after injection of the pharynx with these enzymes. Other papaine-like proteinases do the same.

Streptococcal endotoxin-like substances, such as mucopeptide-polysaccharide cell wall complexes produce remittent nodular lesions in dermal connective tissues of rabbits following a single injection of sonically disrupted group A streptococci. The granulomas produced contain prominent histiocytes and giant cells. Peritoneal injections into mice result in the development of such lesions in the myocardium and the valve cusps. The active endotoxic component is postulated to be the mucopeptide that is the basic building block of streptococcal cell walls. Streptococcal cell wall components can persist within human phagocytes and can be deposited in various human tissues. The immunology of mucopeptide has, therefore, received much attention. Streptococcal polysaccharide also interests investigators because it cross-reacts with glycoproteins extracted from mammalian heart valves. Furthermore, antibodies to group A polysaccharide persist longer in patients with rheumatic carditis than in those without cardiac involvement. Finally it has been shown that the injection of streptococcal products intravenously in rabbits causes necrotic lesions in the heart and liver, where macrophages laden with streptococci preferentially migrate and persist. Thus, cellular components of streptococci may be brought to damaged sites and may be capable of causing prolonged inflammatory reactions such as myocarditis in sites remote from the original infection.

Immunologic theories

Some type of hyperimmune reaction, due either to bacterial allergy or to autoimmunity, is the most popular pathogenic theory of rheumatic fever. This view is supported by strong evidence since rheumatic fever patients are, in general, the population that is most intensively hyperimmune to all streptococcal products.

ALLERGIC THEORIES

The latent period between streptococcal infection and the onset of rheumatic fever has been likened to serum sickness. The arthritis of serum sickness which resembles rheumatic fever closely is associated with circulating immune complexes, but, unlike rheumatic fever, it is also associated with angioneurotic edema and occasionally with acute glomerulonephritis. The latent period of ARF does not decrease, however, in rheumatic recurrences as one would expect with repeated bouts of serum sickness. Moreover, serum complement increases in ARF whereas when immune complexes are formed in large amounts in several serum sickness–like diseases, complement levels in the blood fall. Immune complex disease owing to a variety of causes results in serum sickness syndromes but ARF is unique to group A streptococcal infection alone. Fibrinoid degeneration of collagen and arteritis can occur in serum sickness as well as in ARF, but the former does not cause Aschoff bodies to appear in the myocardium.

One can still formulate the hypothesis that large amounts of streptococcal antigen are absorbed into the throat of a hyperimmune host following a particularly virulent pharyngeal infection and that a specific streptococcal product to which the host is very allergic is bound to the tissues affected by rheumatic fever. Immunologically damaged myocardium and particularly heart valves may then undergo the same slowly progressive changes that one sees following disruption of collagen due to a variety of causes. The localization of rheumatic lesions can be caused by specific binding of streptococcal products which are known to have close chemical similarities to human host tissues. Streptococcal antigens have not been found in rheumatic lesions, but this observation is difficult to interpret because immunologic cross-reactions between group A streptococci and host tissues may obscure the identity of streptococcal antigens.

AUTOIMMUNITY

For several decades investigators have pursued the theory that heart antibodies produced in rheumatic fever may cause carditis. Heart antibodies are gamma globulins with specificity for cardiac components reacting primarily with sarcolemma membranes. Their binding is also associated with deposition of large amounts of complement component C3. Heart antibodies occur more frequently in rheumatic fever patients who develop carditis than in those who escape it. The frequency of the appearance of such antibodies is very high in patients who have undergone mitral commissurotomy. These antibodies can be absorbed with the patient's own atrial tissue, and therefore are probably autoantibodies. Massive deposits of gamma globulin have also been identified in the hearts of children who died of rheumatic carditis. The role of such antibodies in the pathogenesis of rheumatic fever has been clouded by the growing understanding of autoantibody formation as a general response to tissue injury (such as occurs in burns). Cardiac damage by rheumatic, traumatic, or ischemic heart lesions leads to antigenic changes which are manifested by autoantibody production. Thus, myocardial infarction and postpericardiotomy syndromes have been associated with the production of heart antibodies. It is therefore possible that heart antibodies in rheumatic carditis are the *result* rather than the *cause* of tissue injury and that the myocardial damage is still due to some other toxic or immunologic event that liberates antigens or alters tissue substances to which the host is not immunologically tolerant. Indeed, such reactions may be a normal immunologic mechanism for attacking and clearing damaged tissues.

CROSS-REACTIONS BETWEEN STREPTOCOCCI AND HUMAN HEART

Rabbit antiserums against certain group A streptococci react with human heart preparations in the immunofluorescent test. Goat antiserums to human heart tissue precipitate streptococcal extracts. Some human serum precipitating antibodies against streptococcal extracts can be absorbed with human heart preparations. However, not all human autoantibodies to heart can be absorbed with streptococcal antigens. An intense search continues for the cross-reacting antigen(s) between group A streptococci and human myocardium. The antigen has been found to be closely associated with M protein. The antigen is not the type specific determinant of M protein but more likely is a part of the M-protein molecule common to most, if not all, M proteins of the streptococcus. This cross-reacting moiety is one to which human beings become intensely hyperimmune by repeated streptococcal infection. The same or a similar antigen appears to be present in protoplast membranes of the streptococcus and in streptococcal cell wall preparations. It is possible therefore that the cross-reacting antigen to the heart is on the fimbriae-like structures that project through the streptococcal cell wall and that contain M protein. In addition cross-reactions have been described between glycoproteins of the heart valves and group A polysaccharides.

The profusion of cross-reacting antigens between streptococci and heart tissue is augmented by studies of streptococcal antigens which cross-react with glomerular basement membranes, with skin tissues, and with striated and smooth muscle. There is not a clear relationship of heart antibodies in ARF to the development of rheumatic heart disease, and therefore there is no clear evidence for a causal relationship between such cross-reactions and the development of rheumatic carditis. One should bear in mind that cross-reactions of microbial agents with host tissues are very common phenomena in infections and may or may not bear on the production of tissue injury. The serologic test for syphilis is an example of a cardiolipin host antigen which reacts with a serum antibody in the host but does not produce myocardial damage. On the other hand, cold hemolysis in syphilis can be regarded as a true autoimmune disease.

One must conclude that so far autoimmunity is but an attractive hypothesis for the pathogenesis of rheumatic fever. Finally, most clinical and experimental observations of the immunology of streptococcal infections have been humoral rather than cellular. Although the methods for studying cell-mediated immunity are still relatively clumsy, many clinical investigations are underway to evaluate the intense delayed allergy to so many streptococcal antigens, so common in human beings, reactions which are even more intense and universal in ARF. Studies on cell-mediated immunity are spurred on further by the histologic appearance of the Aschoff nodule itself, which at least superficially has many morphologic features of a cell-mediated response.

The host

A peculiar paradox in the epidemiology of rheumatic fever is the frequent observation of strong familial histories of rheumatic fever in the face of the lack of evidence of clear genetic factors predisposing to the disease. Only a few adequate studies have been made of identical twins, and these have shown a relatively low concordance of rheumatic fever (less than 20 percent); actually considerably lower than that found in other infections, such as tuberculosis or poliomyelitis. Furthermore, the incidence of ARF is remarkably similar in every human race or ethnic group exposed to rheumatogenic streptococcal disease. It has not been possible, therefore, to define any clear genetic predisposition to the disease; and familial clustering may reflect the factor of infection rather than host predisposition.

Acquisition of host predisposition by repeated infection is, however, a very real issue in pathogenesis. The virtual absence of rheumatic fever in infancy and its rapidly increased frequency following the repeated streptococcal infections of childhood are noteworthy for the argument of hyperimmunity as a requirement for the disease. The heightened immune response to streptococci in rheumatic subjects and the gradual decline in the ARF attack rate with prolonged freedom from rheumatic attacks also suggest that host susceptibility may be acquired rather than genetic. On the other hand, the effect of other host variables, such as sex, in the frequency of certain complications of rheumatic fever undoubtedly play some part. The equal incidence of chorea among prepubescent boys and girls and the complete absence of chorea in the sexually mature male is such an example. Another example is the higher frequency of insidious isolated mitral stenosis in the female and of aortic stenosis in the male.

As in all infections and their complications, host factors invariably condition the features of disease. So far, however, ARF seems to threaten all people exposed to a pharyngeal infection with a rheumatogenic strain of group A streptococcus.

In conclusion, although the exact pathogenesis of ARF remains elusive, information is increasing concerning the special requirements for the production of a rheumatogenic group A streptococcal infection. At least the focus has now been narrowed to a pharyngeal infection with an appropriate strain whose characteristics are being ever more specifically defined.

REFERENCES

1 Stollerman, G. H.: "Rheumatic Fever and Streptococcal Infection," Grune & Stratton, Inc., New York, 1975.

2 Rammelkamp, C. H., Jr.: Epidemiology of streptococcal infections, *Harvey Lect.,* 51:113, 1955–1956.

3 Wannamaker, L. W., and Matsen, J. M. (eds.): "Streptococci and Streptococcal Diseases. Recognition, Understanding and Management," Academic Press, Inc., New York, 1972.

4 Lancefield, R. C.: Specific Relationship of Cell Composition to Biological Activity of Hemolytic Streptococci, *Harvey Lect.,* 36:251, 1940–1941.

5 Stollerman, G. H.: The Relative Rheumatogenicity of Strains of Group A Streptococci, *Mod. Concepts Cardiovasc. Dis.,* 44:35, 1975.

6 Wannamaker, L. W.: The Chain That Links the Heart to the Throat, *Circulation,* 48:9, 1973.

7 Bisno, A. L., Pearce, I. A., Wall, H. P., et al.: Contrasting Epidemiology of Acute Rheumatic Fever and Acute Glomerulonephritis. Nature of the Antecedent Streptococcal Infection, *N. Engl. J. Med.,* 283:561, 1970.

8 Widdowson, J. P., Maxted, W. R., Notley, C. M., et al.: The Antibody Responses in Man to Infection with Different Serotypes of Group A Streptococci, *J. Med. Microbiol.,* 7:483, 1974.

9 Dudding, B. A., and Ayoub, E. M.: Persistence of Streptococcal Group A Antibody in Patients with Rheumatic Valvular Disease, *J. Exp. Med.,* 128:1081, 1968.

10 Kaplan, M. H., and Frengley, J. D.: Autoimmunity to the Heart in Cardiac Disease. Current Concepts of the Relation of Autoimmunity to Rheumatic Fever, Post-Cardiotomy and Post-Infarction Syndromes and Cardiomyopathies, *Am. J. Cardiol.,* 24:459, 1969.

11 Zabriskie, J. B., Hsu, K. C., and Seegal, B. C.: Heart-reactive Antibody Associated with Rheumatic Fever: Characterization and Diagnostic Significance, *Clin. Exp. Immunol.,* 17:147, 1970.

58
Pathology of Rheumatic Fever and Chronic Valvular Disease

ROBERT S. ELIOT, M.D., and
JESSE E. EDWARDS, M.D.

Rheumatic carditis is the most common cause of chronic valvular stenosis and/or insufficiency.

While the dominant cause of mitral stenosis in adults is rheumatic in nature, mitral insufficiency and aortic insufficiency are each represented by a large number of possible causes. Aortic stenosis also is not always the result of rheumatic disease but may result from a congenitally deformed valve or, more commonly, calcification of the latter.

The following presentation is based on a consideration of rheumatic carditis and its late valvular effects. Conditions other than rheumatic in origin will be considered in sections following each of these major valvular diseases caused by rheumatic carditis.

Rheumatic involvement of the heart may be divided into two stages, acute and healed. Although characteristically, activity recurs in patients with healed lesions of earlier acute attacks, it is, nevertheless, convenient to consider the active and healed stages separately.

ACTIVE RHEUMATIC CARDITIS

Rheumatic fever has the potential for involving each layer of the heart, the endocardium, myocardium, and pericardium. Any one or all three of these layers may be involved in any given individual.

Endocardial involvement in acute rheumatic fever classically involves the valvular endocardium; the mural endocardium generally is spared. The primary process may be swelling of the valve leaflets, and an early secondary change is erosion along the lines of contact of the leaflets. At such sites elements of the blood, platelets and fibrin, are deposited as vegetations. Characteristically, the vegetations are small (usually less than 1 mm in diameter) beadlike deposits, uniformly distributed (Fig. 58-1). There is a strong tendency for the vegetations to be restricted to the line of closure, although, in the case of the atrioventricular valves, some vegetations may be deposited on the surfaces of the chordae. The mitral valve is most commonly affected; next most frequently involved is the aortic valve, and then the tricuspid. Only rarely is the pulmonary valve involved.

Histologically, the lesion of the valves is nonspecific. Beneath the vegetative material the cells of the leaflet, particularly macrophages and fibroblasts, are mobilized. Cells of the latter type tend to be arranged

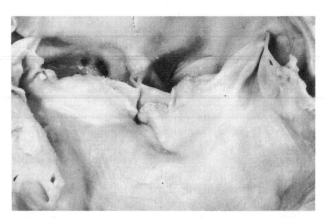

FIGURE 58-1 Acute rheumatic endocarditis of the aortic valve. The vegetations form a beadlike row of deposits which tends to conform to the line of closure.

at right angles to the surface of the leaflet, and together they yield a pattern of palisading. In the valvular endocardium Aschoff's bodies are uncommon, but they may be observed in the mural endocardium, particularly of the left atrium.

The myocardial lesions of acute rheumatic carditis are the basis on which histologic confirmation of this disorder depends. The specific lesion is Aschoff's body (Fig. 58-2). This is characterized primarily by swelling, eosinophilia, and fragmentation of interstitial collagen, particularly common in the perivascular supporting connective tissue. Cellular reaction to the altered collagen yields a nodule, the so-called Aschoff's body. The body contains a variety of cells, including the multinucleated Aschoff cells, the "owl-eyed" Anitschkow myocardial monocytes, and fibroblasts. As the lesion ages it becomes progressively less cellular and more fibrous. In a given patient with active rheumatic carditis, at any one time, Aschoff's bodies of varying age may be observed. It is to be emphasized that Aschoff's body is fundamentally a lesion of interstitial tissue and that there is only little evidence for loss of myocardial fibers, even in cases with extensive involvement of the myocardial layer.

Uncommonly, acute inflammation of intramyocardial branches of the coronary arteries may occur in acute rheumatic carditis. In involved arteries, luminal narrowing may result from cellular infiltration, from thrombosis, or from a combination of the two. Occlusive lesions so derived may be responsible for foci of acute myocardial infarction. These are, fortunately, uncommon and appear to be associated with cases of fulminating acute rheumatic carditis.

The pericardial lesion of acute rheumatic carditis by itself is not specific. It takes the form of a serofibrinous effusion. The amount of fluid compared to the amount of fibrin varies. The exterior of the heart has deposited upon it shaggy elements of fibrin, which has led to the unappetizing name of "bread-and-butter" heart.

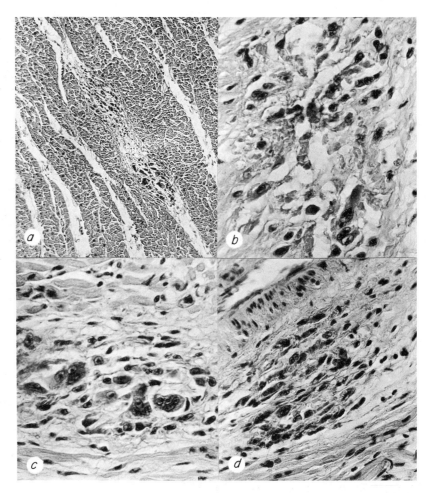

FIGURE 58-2 Myocardial Aschoff's bodies. *a.* Low-power view showing deposit of two Aschoff's bodies in the interstitial tissue between muscle bundles (H&E; × 120). *b.* High-power magnification of an early Aschoff's body showing eosinophilic necrosis of collagen and mobilization of tissue cells (H&E; × 460). *c.* A classic Aschoff's body with multinucleated giant cells (H&E; × 460). *d.* A late Aschoff's body lying in a perivascular position. A tendency for the cells to be predominantly fibroblastic is evidence of the healing stage (H&E; × 400).

HEALING OF RHEUMATIC CARDITIS

The lesions of acute rheumatic carditis heal in a way that is peculiar to the healing of acute lesions in other organs, i.e., by scar formation and/or by resolution.

In the endocardium and myocardium, healing by scar formation predominates. In the pericardium either resolution of the inflammatory process may occur, leaving a normal pericardium, or the fibrin may become organized, resulting in pericardial adhesions. As the two processes may occur simultaneously in some individuals, there are examples of healed rheumatic pericarditis in which part of the pericardium is normal while adhesions occur focally in other portions. Even in cases with diffuse adhesions or focal calcification of the pericardium as consequences of rheumatic pericarditis, constriction does not usually occur.

HEALED RHEUMATIC CARDITIS

One attack or a limited number of attacks of acute rheumatic carditis leaves relatively little residual change. In the valves, at the sites where vegetations had been present, there is a beadlike row of tiny fibrous elevations; removed from this zone, the leaf-

lets may exhibit slight degrees of fibrosis (Fig. 58-3). Vascularization of valve leaflets, particularly the anterior leaflet of the mitral valve, is still another minor residual effect. The chordae of the atrioven-

FIGURE 58-3 Photomicrograph of tricuspid valve in healed rheumatic endocarditis. There is nodular thickening at the "line of closure" by fibrous tissue, representing the site of vegetation during a preceding episode, or several preceding episodes, of acute rheumatic endocarditis. (Elastic tissue stain; × 10.)

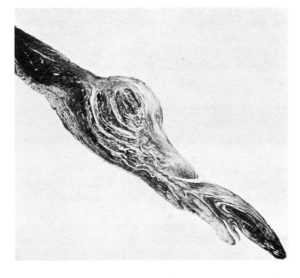

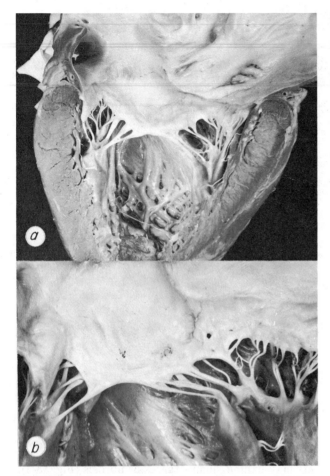

FIGURE 58-4 Two examples of minor residual changes of rheumatic endocarditis involving the mitral valve. *a*. Thickening of the valvular tissue, particularly in relation to the line of closure. Mild thickening of some chordae. Vascularization of the leaflet. *b*. Minor degree of thickening of the leaflets and of the chordae. There is minor fusion of the leaflets at the commissures.

tricular valves may exhibit minor degrees of thickening or may be normal (Fig. 58-4).

The myocardium may appear normal or show small perivascular scars as the only residua of previous Aschoff's bodies. The pericardial changes have been mentioned.

It is evident that the description just given does not conform to the cardiac changes of patients with clinical chronic rheumatic heart disease. The minor residua described are usually not associated with significant cardiac dysfunction except that the valves may be more susceptible to bacterial infection than are the valves of persons who have had no attacks of rheumatic carditis.

Clinical chronic rheumatic heart disease, commonly referred to pathologically as *healed rheumatic heart disease*, represents the compound effects of many recurrent attacks of active rheumatic carditis and of the associated healing. It is commonly recognized that clinically evident recurrent acute rheumatic carditis may follow known streptococcal infections of the respiratory tract. Less commonly

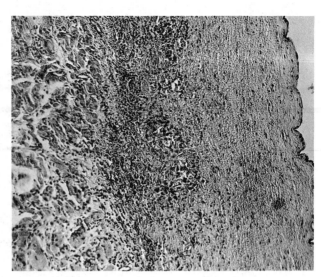

FIGURE 58-5 Aschoff's bodies at the junction of the base of the thickened endocardium and the myocardium of left atrium. From a patient with chronic, recurrent, acute rheumatic endocarditis and mitral stenosis.

appreciated is that episodes of recurrent active rheumatic carditis are without obvious clinical counterparts. The high incidence of histologically proved acute rheumatic carditis in subjects coming to necropsy with "healed" rheumatic heart disease was emphasized by Gross.[1]

The high incidence (average of about 40 percent) of Aschoff's bodies in amputated left atrial appendages from patients with mitral stenosis but without clinical evidence of active rheumatic carditis is additional evidence of the strong tendency for rheumatic patients to experience recurrent episodes of active carditis (Fig. 58-5).[2] It is the factor of recurrence that underlies the development of classic significant lesions of the valves.

HEALED RHEUMATIC CARDITIS OF SIGNIFICANT NATURE

Under this heading are considered those valvular lesions of rheumatic origin which cause significant alteration in the cardiac dynamics. The pulmonary valve, for practical purposes, may be considered immune from significant involvement and will not be considered further. Reference will now be made to each of the other valves according to the functional alteration that rheumatic endocarditis may cause in them.

Rheumatic mitral stenosis

The end result of recurrent rheumatic endocarditis is that the valvular leaflets and the chordae tendineae are affected by the addition of fibrous tissue, with concomitant contracture (Fig. 58-6). An additional feature is that at each of the two junctional areas (the commissures) between the two major leaflets there is interadhesion between the two leaflets. This process, along with concomitant shortening of the chordae,

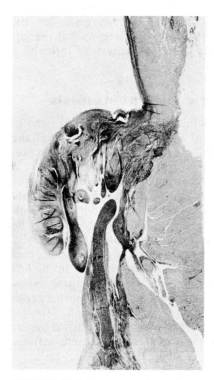

FIGURE 58-6 Low-power photomicrograph of left atrium, posterior wall of left ventricle, and posterior mitral leaflet and related chordae. As the result of recurrent rheumatic endocarditis, the valvular leaflet is thickened with fibrous tissue and shortened by contracture. Thickening by fibrous tissue of chordae, with a tendency of matting of chordae, is also evident. (Elastic tissue stain; × 5.)

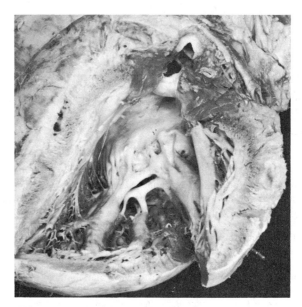

FIGURE 58-8 Mitral valve from below in a case of mitral stenosis. The valve is converted into a funnel-shaped structure, the apex of which is in the left ventricle and is narrow.

causes the two interadherent leaflets to be held downward. The entire process is manifested by the leaflets' forming a funnel-shaped structure (Figs. 58-7 and 58-8). The inlet to the funnel is at the level of the left atrial floor and is wider than the apex, which presents in the left ventricular cavity.

In the normal heart, blood flows freely through the mitral valve. It may flow through the principal "orifice," that part of the opening which lies between the papillary muscles. Also, it may flow through multiple "secondary orifices," which are the spaces between the chordae (Fig. 58-9A).[3]

In rheumatic mitral stenosis, because of interchordal fusion, the secondary orifices are obliterated and,

by virtue of commissural fusion, the principal orifice is reduced in size (Fig. 58-9B). As a consequence, obstruction to the flow of blood occurs. The left atrial pressure rises and the chamber dilates. As the pulmonary arterial pressure also rises, the right ventricle undergoes hypertrophy. The anterior leaflet of the stenotic mitral valve frequently exhibits an interesting deformity. Near its basal aspect the leaflet is convex toward the left atrium. It is possible that in early left ventricular diastole the deformity is buckled in the opposite direction and that this may account for the "opening snap" of mitral stenosis. Such movement does not affect the caliber of the effective orifice, which lies at a lower level. The deformity may contribute to closure of the valve as the prominence of the anterior leaflet is pressed against the base of the opposite leaflet during ventricular systole.

FIGURE 58-7 Mitral stenosis. a. Unopened mitral valve from above. The inlet to the funnel-like deformity which characterizes mitral stenosis is wider than the outlet, which lies in the left ventricle, below. b. The mitral valve from the left ventricular aspect. The valve has been converted into a funnel-shaped structure with a narrow orifice (containing probe).

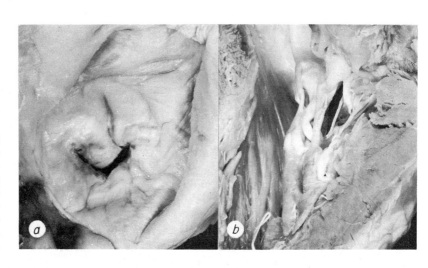

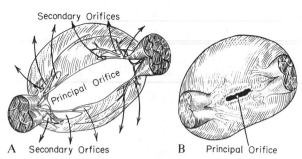

FIGURE 58-9 A. Diagrammatic portrayal of the normal mitral valve viewed from below. The principal orifice of the valve lies bounded by the anterior leaflet, anteriorly, the posterior leaflet, posteriorly, and each papillary muscle and its related chordae, laterally. Secondary orifices lie in the spaces between the chordae tendineae, and for the most part, blood flowing through these enters the left ventricle lateral to the respective papillary muscles. *B.* Diagrammatic portrayal of the stenotic mitral valve viewed from below. The principal orifice is narrow, and, on the basis of commissural and chordal fusion, the secondary orifices are obliterated. *(From Bonnabeau et al.,[3] with permission.)*

Certain observations may be made regarding the structure of the stenotic valve, as they pertain to present-day surgical procedures for relieving mitral stenosis.

It is to be realized in the first place that the structure of the stenotic mitral valve is such that a "successful" commissurotomy does not cure mitral stenosis. It simply opens the valve enough to make the stenosis less severe.

Two major factors in the alteration of the stenotic mitral valve contribute to "restenosis" following commissurotomy: (1) calcification of the leaflets and (2) short chordae. Calcified material, even if broken at the time of commissurotomy, tends to leave the leaflets fixed, allowing them to re-fuse. Short chordae also tend to keep the leaflets relatively immobile, favoring union of one with the other, following commissurotomy.

In mitral stenosis, thrombosis may occur in the left atrium and serve as a source for systemic arterial emboli. In about half these cases the thrombi are restricted to the left atrium. In the remainder, the thrombi are present against the free wall of the left atrium, either alone or in company with thrombi in the appendage.

Nonrheumatic mitral stenosis

In the majority of adults with mitral stenosis, whether or not a history of rheumatic fever is elicited, the consistent range of changes in the valve supports strongly a rheumatic origin.

In a rare adult, the stenosis may be on a basis of congenital deformity, the valve showing a parachute deformity.[4] This is characterized by only one papillary muscle being present. This type of valve may be part of the developmental complex described by Shone and associates.[5] In their fully developed complex, four obstructive lesions are present in the left side of the heart, namely, parachute mitral valve, supravalvular ring of the left atrium, subaortic stenosis, and coarctation of the aorta (see Chap. 53).

Myxoma of the left atrium or asymmetrical hypertrophic cardiomyopathy[6] may each present a functional state like mitral stenosis (see Chap. 86).

Rheumatic mitral insufficiency

The same fundamental processes which result in rheumatic mitral stenosis may cause mitral insufficiency. The differences depend, in part, on fortuitous differences in physical orientation of the leaflets. Changes which tend to maintain the valve in a closed position cause mitral stenosis; those which cause the valve to be held open are associated with incompetence of the valve. The following structural patterns are found among cases of mitral insufficiency of rheumatic origin: (1) calcification of commissures, (2) fibrous contracture of valvular tissue, and (3) minor intrinsic valvular shortening with secondary distortion of the valve.[7] That calcification which causes mitral insufficiency extends from one leaflet into the other across one or both of the commissures. The C-shaped plate of calcium is oriented across the commissure in such a way as to keep the two leaflets apart at the involved commissure (Fig. 58-10).

Fibrous contracture as a cause of mitral insufficiency is usually dominant at one commissure, with shortening of valvular tissue so great that the two

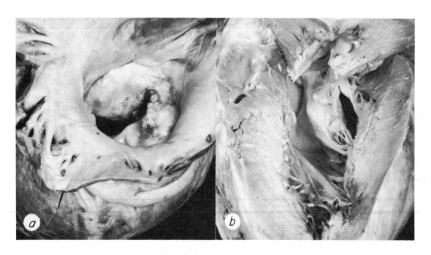

FIGURE 58-10 Mitral insufficiency resulting from shortening of leaflets and commissural calcification. *a.* Unopened mitral valve from above. At the posteromedial commissure is a plate of calcium which crosses from the anterior to the posterior leaflets. In the left side of the illustration the valvular tissue is short, making the two leaflets incapable of apposition. *b.* Mitral valve from below. The fixed orifice imparted by short valvular tissue and calcification of a commissure causes the valve orifice to be fixed in an open state, thus causing the valve to be incompetent.

leaflets cannot make contact. The shape of the deformity has been compared to a teardrop.

Perhaps the most interesting type of mitral insufficiency of rheumatic origin is that in which only minor scarring and shortening of the leaflets are present, while the valve is grossly incompetent. In such cases it is presumed that a series of circumstances is set into play.

The first step is intrisic shortening of the leaflets, which causes a mild degree of mitral insufficiency. The left atrium responds to this valvular dysfunction by dilating. As the left atrium dilates, it tends to pull the posterior leaflet of the mitral valve away from the anterior leaflet. As this process increases, the degree of mitral insufficiency increases, and the left atrium dilates further and causes ever-increasing tension on the posterior mitral leaflet. While this process is in operation, the posterior leaflet is restrained at the opposite extremity by the chordae which insert into it. In the final stage the posterior mitral leaflet is immobilized over the base of the left ventricular wall as it is pulled in a posterior direction by the large left atrium and concomitantly restrained by the chordae inserting into its opposite extremity.

The views expressed about the series of events in he third type of rheumatic mitral insufficiency conform to the concept that "mitral insufficiency begets mitral insufficiency."[8]

Nonrheumatic mitral regurgitation (insufficiency)

Anatomically, nonrheumatic types of mitral insufficiency are represented by a variety of changes including (1) loss of leaflet tissue, (2) restriction of motion of leaflets, (3) improper support of leaflets,

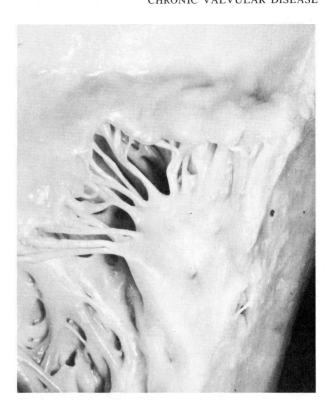

FIGURE 58-12 Loeffler's endocarditis with adhesion of posterior mitral leaflet to endocardial aspect of left ventricle.

allowing "overshooting," and (4) enlargement of the left ventricular cavity.

Loss of leaflet tissue resulting in mitral insufficiency results from bacterial endocarditis. The process is represented either by erosion in relation to the free aspect of leaflet tissue or perforation of the leaflet (Fig. 58-11). The latter is usually a complication of aortic valvular bacterial endocarditis, the anterior leaflet having been involved secondarily to infected aortic regurgitation.

Restriction of motion of leaflets has two main causes. The first is aortic valvular disease with enlargement of the left ventricle. In this process, the papillary muscles migrate downward as the ventricle enlarges, increasing the distance between the apexes of the papillary muscles and the mitral orifice. This process places undue tension on the chordae and leaflets, restricting the degree of upward excursion of the latter.

The second cause of restriction of motion is fibrous union with the left ventricular mural endocardium of either the posterior mitral leaflet or its chordae. Fusion of the leaflet itself may result from bacterial endocarditis or may be part of the process of fibroplastic parietal endocarditis as seen in Loeffler's endocarditis with eosinophilia (Fig. 58-12).[9] Rarely, calcification of the "mitral ring" may be extensive. The calcific mass may become adherent to the under aspect of the posterior leaflet, reducing its effective length as a flap (Fig. 58-13).[10]

Yet another change is that in which chordae

FIGURE 58-11 Healed bacterial endocarditis. Left side of heart shows major erosion of mitral valvular tissue and disappearance of many chordae.

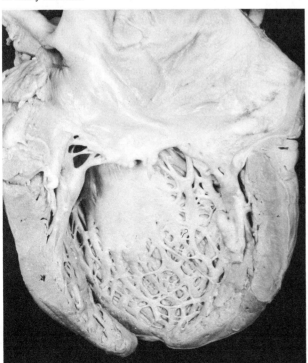

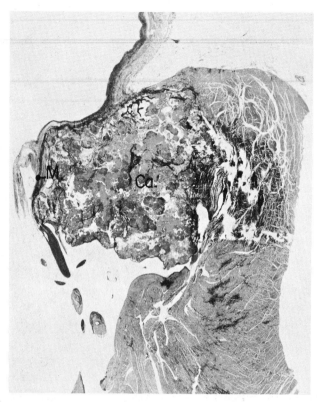

FIGURE 58-13 Calcification of mitral ring. Low-power photomicrograph showing calcific mass, Ca, at the junction of the left atrium and left ventricle. The posterior mitral leaflet, M, is in part adherent to the calcified mass, a process leading to its immobilization.

running to the posterior mitral leaflet become fused to the left ventricular wall. This process described by Salazar and Edwards[11] tends to be associated with myxomatous changes of the valve (see below).

"Overshooting" of mitral leaflets may result from alterations of papillary muscles, chordae, or leaflets.[12]

Disturbances of papillary muscles include rupture or healed infarction without rupture. While rupture of a papillary muscle (resulting from infarction or external or surgical trauma) is usually attended by overwhelming degrees of mitral insufficiency and early death, rarely a ruptured papillary muscle may be associated with chronic mitral insufficiency.[13]

Infarction of a nonruptured papillary muscle with mitral insufficiency is usually associated with infarction of the adjacent free wall of the left ventricle (Fig. 58-14). According to clinical and experimental evidence, incompetence of the valve depends not entirely upon intrinsic dysfunction of the papillary muscle but also upon distortion of the papillary muscular foundation by asynergic contraction of the related free wall.[14]

A condition which is of current interest is *myxomatous alteration* of the mitral valve. This condition goes by a variety of names, including the floppy, billowing,[15,16] or prolapsing mitral valve. Also, based upon auscultatory findings, this condition has been

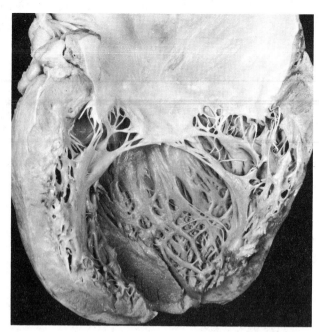

FIGURE 58-14 Healed myocardial infarction involving the inferior wall of the left ventricle and related papillary muscles. The latter are atrophic on the basis of coexistent infarction.

called the *mid-* or *mid-late systolic click syndrome.* The pathologic process may be seen either in subjects with Marfan's syndrome (arachnodactyly) or in subjects not displaying the physical characteristics of the Marfan syndrome.

The basic process is that of an increase in size of the normally present mucinous layer of the valve, the so-called spongiosa. The increase in the mucinous layer, which appears to be the primary structural alteration, tends to invade and interrupt the continuity of the supporting fibrous layer of the leaflet, the fibrosa (Fig. 58-15). As the latter is involved, there is

FIGURE 58-15 Photomicrograph of posterior mitral leaflet from a 29-year-old man with myxomatous mitral valve. The spongiosa layer (S) is increased in thickness and invades and interrupts the fibrosa (F). There is fibrous thickening on the atrial aspect of the leaflet (A), as well as a fibrous pad on the ventricular aspect under the fibrous layer. (Elastic tissue stain; × 15. *From Guthrie and Edwards;*[18] reproduced with permission.)

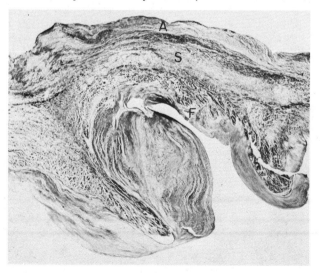

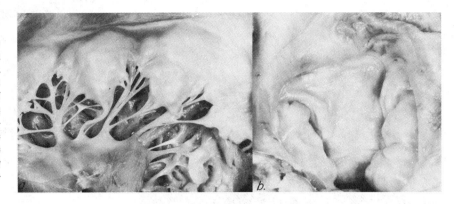

FIGURE 58-16 Photographs of the gross specimen from the case of which the photomicrograph is illustrated in Fig. 58-15. *a.* The opened mitral valve shows characteristic interchordal hooding of the leaflets. *b.* The unopened mitral valve viewed from above showing unusual degrees of scalloping characteristic of the myxomatously altered mitral valve, the so-called floppy valve. *(From Guthrie and Edwards;*[18] *reproduced with permission.)*

a corresponding weakness of the leaflet so that those segments of the valve which lie between chordal insertions prolapse or hood abnormally toward the left atrium during ventricular systole (Fig. 58-16). Part of the process of prolapse may result from weakness of chordae which are elongated.[17]

The hemodynamic stresses upon prolapsing segments result in secondary fibrotic changes in characteristic locations. The surfaces of prolapsed elements make faulty contact with opposite valvular elements, and this may cause denudation of the involved areas. Ultimately, fibroelastic thickening of the contact aspect of the leaflet occurs. On the under aspect of prolapsing segments, fibrous—mostly collagenous—tissue is deposited. The ultimate effect is that initially delicate, translucent leaflets may become opaque and thickened (Fig. 58-15).[18]

Any element of the mitral valve may be involved, although it is more common for the posterior leaflet, particularly its central part, to be involved.[19] In our experience, when the anterior leaflet is involved its medial half is more commonly affected than its lateral half.

Another effect of the process of prolapsing is that chordae tendineae which insert into the posterior leaflet may rub upon the related mural endocardium of the left ventricle. The response to this process is fibrous thickening both of the involved chordae and mural endocardium. In some cases the fibrotic process may be extensive and result in incorporation of chordae into the fibrous tissue of the mural endocardium, as described by Salazar and Edwards.[11] When this happens, the effective length of the chorda becomes reduced (Fig. 58-17).

Among the complications of the mucinous mitral valve are (1) calcification of leaflet tissue, (2) bacterial endocarditis,[20] and (3) rupture of chordae.[18,21] Chordal rupture most commonly involves those chordae which insert into the central segment of the posterior leaflet.

When chordal rupture occurs, the process of prolapse is accentuated in that segment of the valve that has lost its chordal support. The flail segment of the valve, acting as a baffle, tends to direct the regurgitant stream toward the atrial septum, and at the site of impact, jet lesions occur (Fig. 58-18).[22] As

the site of impact is behind the aortic valve, the murmur generated is located in the "aortic area" leading to confusion with aortic stenosis.[23]

In addition to myxomatous alteration of the mitral valve as a background for ruptured chordae, bacterial endocarditis should be numbered. The infection may be either primary in the mitral valve or secondary to aortic valvular endocarditis with aortic regurgitation.[24]

Chordal rupture is to be distinguished from rupture of a papillary muscle. The latter usually results from myocardial infarction and, less commonly, from trauma.

Enlargement of the left ventricular cavity is associated with enlargement of the mitral orifice and may be a cause for mitral insufficiency on this basis. Usually, there is an underlying myocardial disease such as extensive healed myocardial infarction or one of the cardiac myopathies.

FIGURE 58-17 Left atrium and left ventricle in a case of myxomatous alteration of the mitral valve in a patient with Marfan's syndrome. Friction lesions upon the left ventricular endocardium have caused incorporation and functional shortening of the related chordae of the posterior mitral leaflet. *(From Salazar and Edwards;*[11] *reproduced with permission.)*

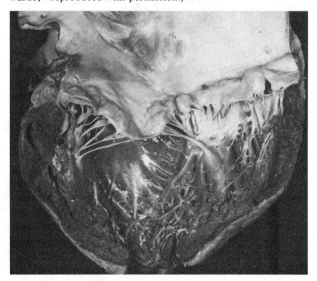

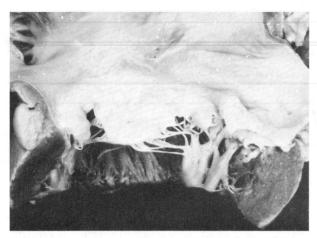

FIGURE 58-18 Left atrium, mitral valve, and a portion of the left ventricle in a case of ruptured chordae involving the posterior leaflet. In addition to this change, other segments of the valve show prolapse toward the left atrium. Upon the septal wall of the left atrium is a rough area representing jet lesions which characteristically form in this position when chordae of the posterior leaflets have ruptured.

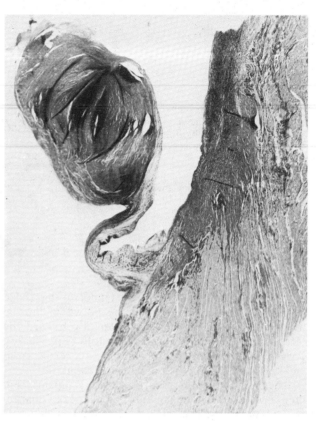

FIGURE 58-19 Low-power photomicrograph of an aortic cusp in chronic rheumatic aortic insufficiency. The distal one-half of the cusp is grossly thickened by fibrous tissue. (Elastic tissue stain; × 5.)

Rheumatic aortic insufficiency

Incompetence of the aortic valve of rheumatic origin is perhaps the simplest process to understand. In its pure form, there are scarring and contracture of the cusps, while no adhesions between the cusps at the commissures are present.

The normal aortic valve closes by virtue of the fact that each cusp is sufficiently long for its center to extend to the center of the aortic orifice during ventricular diastole. The cusps become shortened as a result of fibrous contracture (Fig. 58-19). Each is then incapable of extending to the center of the aortic orifice, and thus each lacks the ability to make full contact with the other two cusps. An illustration of this is the characteristic triangular defect at the center of the aortic orifice when the valve is in a "closed" position (Fig. 58-20).

In significant aortic valvular insufficiency the left ventricle undergoes enlargement of its chamber in a downward direction, giving the cavity a conical ap-

pearance. Absolute hypertrophy of the muscular wall is classically associated.

Frequently the impact of the regurgitant stream upon the wall of the left ventricular outflow tract will be responsible for a jet lesion.[22] Depending on the direction of the stream, the jet lesion may be present on the ventricular face of the anterior mitral leaflet or on the septal wall of the left ventricular outflow tract (Fig. 58-21).

Nonrheumatic aortic insufficiency

With the passage of time, the horizons have widened with respect to understanding the conditions that

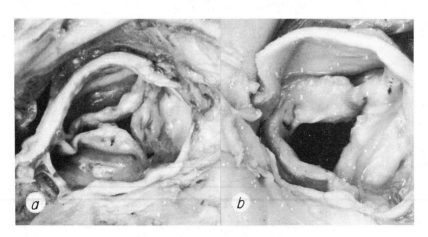

FIGURE 58-20 Two examples of rheumatic endocarditis with aortic insufficiency. a. The valve leaflets are thickened and shortened to a relatively minor degree. The shortening is responsible for a small triangular-shaped orifice being present in the center of the aortic valve during diastole. b. The aortic valve leaflets are significantly reduced in size, causing a wide triangular-shaped orifice to be present and the valve to be incompetent.

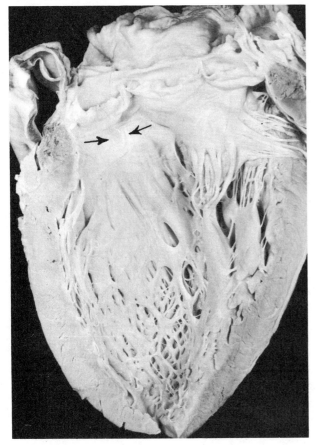

FIGURE 58-21 Left ventricle and aortic valve in a case of rheumatic aortic endocarditis with secondary aortic insufficiency. Enlargement of the left ventricular cavity in a downward direction. Beneath the right aortic cusp several endocardial pockets (between arrows) are present in the endocardium of the septal wall of the left ventricular outflow tract. These are considered to be jet lesions resulting from impact by the stream of regurgitant blood.

may cause aortic blood to regurgitate into the left ventricle.

In addition to destruction of aortic valvular tissue from bacterial endocarditis and the effects of syphilitic aortitis and other inflammatory diseases of the aorta (Fig. 58-22), a number of conditions primary in the ascending aorta may cause this functional disturbance. Such conditions were reviewed from our laboratory.[25] In general, some, such as cystic medial necrosis (Figs. 58-23 and 58-24) with or without Marfan's syndrome, myxomatous alteration of the aortic valve, aortitis of various varieties, dissecting aneurysm, and traumatic tears of the aorta (Fig. 58-25), allow regurgitation through the aortic valve.[26]

Other conditions primary in the aorta may allow blood to regurgitate through a channel which bypasses the aortic valve. Such conditions include mycotic aneurysm and congenital aortic–left ventricular tunnel (Fig. 58-26).[27]

The congenital bicuspid valve may be a basis for aortic insufficiency in adults. The process results from prolapse of the larger of the two cusps (Fig. 58-27).[25] While this condition is usually an isolated one, it may also be seen in association with coarctation of the aorta.

Rheumatic aortic stenosis

The crucial change of rheumatic endocarditis which leads to aortic stenosis is interadhesion between adjacent cusps at the commissures. As there are three aortic valvular commissures, the degree of obstruction caused primarily by the effects of rheumatic endocarditis depends on the number of commissures involved (Fig. 58-28).

When commissural adhesion occurs only at one commissure, the valve is converted into a bicuspid one (acquired bicuspid valve). In a valve so affected, the orifice is somewhat reduced, but usually not to such a degree that an obstructive effect may be demonstrated. Such valves, though not intrisically stenotic, offer (as do congenital bicuspid valves) the tendency for acquired calcification of the leaflets. This tendency in bicuspid aortic valves (whether congenital or acquired) is the usual basis for the appearance of calcific aortic stenosis.

At the opposite extreme in functional effect from rheumatic fusion of one aortic commissure is the situation in which there is fusion at each of the commissures. In such valves, each cusp is prevented from lateral excursion during ventricular systole and

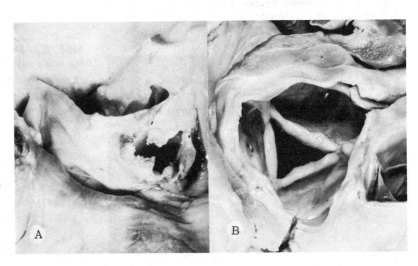

FIGURE 58-22 A. Healed bacterial endocarditis resulting in perforation of aortic cusp. B. Aortitis. Aortic valve viewed from above. Bowing of the cusps incident to dilatation of the aorta leaves a triangular defect through which regurgitation occurred.

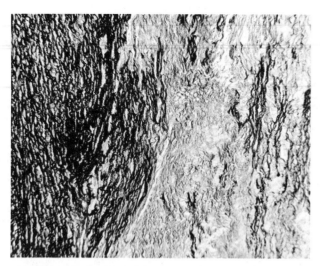

FIGURE 58-23 Cystic medial necrosis. Photomicrograph of aortic media showing a zone of extensive loss of continuity of aortic medial elements.

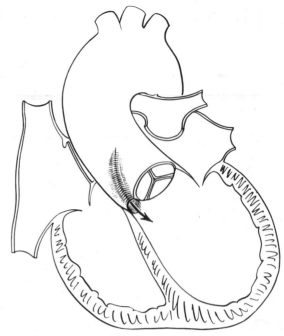

FIGURE 58-26 Diagrammatic portrayal of aorto-left ventricular tunnel. A channel from the aorta bypasses the aortic valve and leads to the left ventricle. Congenital or acquired disease, the latter secondary to bacterial infection, may be responsible for such a state.

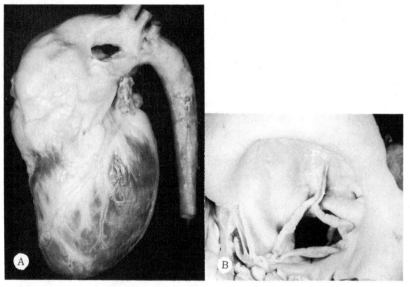

FIGURE 58-24 A. Cystic medial necrosis of aorta in Marfan's syndrome. Exterior view of heart and aorta viewed from the left side. Marked dilatation of the ascending aorta. B. Unopened aortic valve viewed from above in a case of extensive cystic medial necrosis. Major dilatation of aorta causes distortion of aortic cusps and the development of a triangular defect at the center of the aortic valve.

FIGURE 58-25 Traumatic ruptures of the ascending aorta. Each is located in relation to an aortic commissure. Loss of commissural support is responsible for prolapse of cusps and aortic insufficiency.

FIGURE 58-27 Congenital bicuspid aortic valve. The larger of the two cusps may prolapse and account for aortic insufficiency.

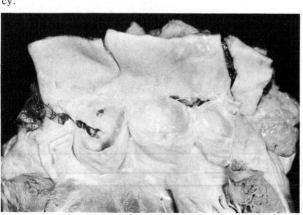

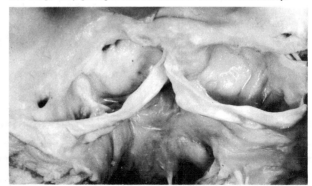

FIGURE 58-28 Aortic valve in rheumatic endocarditis. In each case, the unopened valve is viewed from above. *a.* Fusion between two adjacent leaflets at one commissure, creating an acquired bicuspid valve. Such valves are probably not stenotic but are subject to secondary calcification and also are susceptible to bacterial endocarditis. *b.* In this case there is fusion at two commissures, causing reduction in flexibility of the valve leaflets and an absolute reduction in size of the orifice during ventricular systole. *c.* Fusion at each of the three aortic commissures, causing an absolute reduction in size of the orifice. The orifice is now fixed and is both stenotic and incompetent.

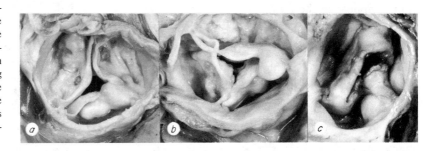

the valve is stenotic. In valves so affected, the presence of any opening in the valve is dependent on shortening of the cusps. When there is fusion at each of the three commissures, therefore, the valve has a restrictive orifice that cannot change its caliber. Incompetence of the valve accompanies this type of stenosis.

The stenosis may be called the fibrous type.[28] It is less common than the calcific type which is discussed in the next section.

Fusion at two commissures results in a variable effect, depending on the degree of shortening and the degree of rigidity of the valvular tissue. When the valvular tissue on each side of the one remaining normal commissure is pliable and but little shortened, incompetence of the valve may not be present, and though the orifice is reduced in size, a stenotic effect may not be measurable. Such valves present the same potential problems as the acquired bicuspid valve, i.e., tendencies for calcification with secondary stenosis or for bacterial endocarditis.

Most commonly, when fusion occurs at two commissures, the effects are fundamentally like those of fusion at each commissure, but the degree of stenosis may be less than when three commissures are fused.

The secondary effects of aortic stenosis include left ventricular hypertrophy and poststenotic dilatation of the ascending aorta. In aortic stenosis, as in aortic insufficiency, as the left ventricle enlarges downward, there may be undue restraint upon the mitral chordae, and secondary mitral insufficiency may result.[7]

Cystic medial necrosis of the aorta may occur, and dissecting aneurysm of the aorta may eventuate as a consequence.[29,30]

Although aortic stenosis has been claimed as protective against coronary atherosclerosis, current evidence indicates that the average degree of coronary atherosclerosis among patients with aortic stenosis is not materially different from that in persons with normal aortic valves.[31]

Nonrheumatic aortic stenosis

Obstruction in relation to the aortic valve of nonrheumatic origin may lie above the valve (supravalvular aortic stenosis), below the valve (subaortic stenosis) (see Chap. 53), or at the valve.[28] The most common type of aortic valvular stenosis is calcific. It usually involves a bicuspid valve which, of itself, is not stenotic, the rigidity of the calcific deposits being mainly responsible for the malfunction (Fig. 58-29A).[32] The two causes for the fundamental bicuspid nature are previous rheumatic disease and a congenital state. In all probability, a congenital bicuspid valve is a more common basis for calcific aortic stenosis than is a bicuspid valve acquired through rheumatic disease.[33]

The so-called unicuspid aortic valve is a congenital deformity characteristic of congenital aortic stenosis.[34] Most subjects with this condition manifest symptoms or succumb as infants because of the severity of the obstruction. Less commonly, the degree of obstruction may allow survival to adolescence or even adulthood. In such cases, symptoms may result from the intrinsic nature of the valve or from rigidity resulting from calcification (Fig. 58-29B). Then there are some cases of calcific aortic stenosis in valves which are so constructed as to be intrinsically stenotic to some degree.

At the opposite end of the age scale is the problem of calcification of tricuspid aortic valves in older

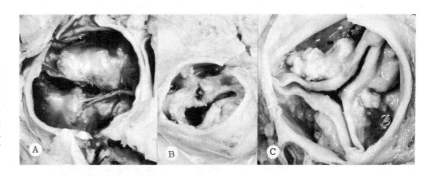

FIGURE 58-29 Varieties of nonrheumatic aortic stenosis. In each case, the unopened valve is viewed from above. *A.* Congenitally bicuspid aortic valve heavily calcified. *B.* Calcified unicommissural aortic valve. *C.* Senile calcific aortic stenosis. Three cusps are present. Each is rigid by virtue of acquisition of calcific deposits.

persons. It is common for some degree of calcification to appear in the normal aortic valves in persons 70 years and older. Usually, the calcification is inadequate to cause stenosis, although it may be responsible for a murmur. In exceptional cases, each of the three cusps is highly calcified, making the valve stenotic (Fig. 58-29C). This uncommon type of aortic stenosis may be called the *senile* type or *aortic valvular sclerosis*.

SECONDARY EFFECTS ON THE MITRAL VALVE IN AORTIC VALVULAR DISEASE

In the patient with aortic valvular disease in whom the mitral valve is incompetent, two pathologic processes are possible: (1) This valve may also be involved by changes of rheumatic origin and exhibit alterations like those already described. (It is significant that in aortic stenosis appearing upon a congenitally deformed valve, with or without calcification, the mitral valve is intrinsically normal.) (2) Enlargement of the left ventricle, on the basis of the aortic valvular disease, may have caused the mitral valve to become secondarily incompetent. Under such circumstances the mitral insufficiency appears to be dependent on displacement of the papillary muscles. In some cases, as the left ventricle elongates, the papillary muscles move downward, away from the mitral orifice. In such cases the chordae tendineae may show compensatory elongation. A stage may be reached beyond which chordal elongation is insufficient, and as the papillary muscles continue to be shifted downward with the enlarging ventricle, undue restraint is imposed on the mitral leaflets, and incompetence occurs.

The other process which may lead to secondary mitral insufficiency is left ventricular dilatation. This process causes the papillary muscles to shift away from one another. This results in loss of efficiency for restraint of the mitral leaflets by the chordae-papillary muscle systems. During ventricular systole the mitral leaflets may overshoot the level of optimal efficiency for closure of the valve, and mitral insufficiency results.

TRICUSPID INVOLVEMENT

In acquired conditions, tricuspid disease usually takes the form of incompetence. Stenosis, if present, is accompanied by incompetence. In most instances, tricuspid insufficiency is not associated with intrinsic disease, the malfunction being of secondary nature incident to conditions, including valvular disease, involving the left side of the heart with ultimate right ventricular enlargement. Intrinsic disease is usually of rheumatic origin and is probably always associ-

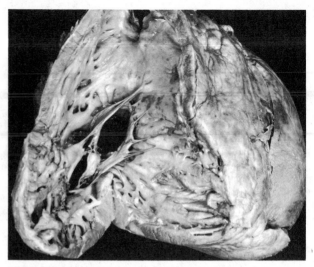

FIGURE 58-30 Tricuspid valve from below in chronic rheumatic endocarditis. Although the chordae are relatively uninvolved, there is fusion of the leaflets at the commissures, creating a narrowed and fixed orifice. The valve is both stenotic and incompetent.

ated with involvement of the mitral valve, either alone or with aortic valvular rheumatic disease.

Significant sequelae of rheumatic involvement of the tricuspid valve are rather uniform from case to case. The major change is obliteration of each of the commissures. In the valve so affected, the distinction between one leaflet and the adjacent one is lost, and separate flaps, characteristic of the normal, are no longer easily identifiable. Chordal shortening and contracture of valvular tissue are usually only of minor degree. The important change of commissural fusion results in a relatively fixed orifice which is more narrow than the original tricuspid orifice, and varying degrees of stenosis may be measurable (Fig. 58-30). Incompetence, because of fixation of the orifice, is inevitable.

REFERENCES

1 Gross, L.: Lesions of the Left Auricle in Rheumatic Fever, *Am. J. Pathol.,* 11:711, 1935.

2 McNeely, W. F., Ellis, L. B., and Harmen, D. E.: Rheumatic "Activity" as Judged by the Presence of Aschoff Bodies in Auricular Appendages with Mitral Stenosis: II. Clinical Aspects, *Circulation,* 8:337, 1953.

3 Bonnabeau, R. C., Jr., Stevenson, J. E., and Edwards, J. E.: Obliteration of the Principal Orifice of the Stenotic Mitral Valve: A Rare Form of "Restenosis," *J. Thorac. Cardiovasc. Surg.,* 49:264, 1965.

4 da Silva, C. L., and Edwards, J. E.: Parachute Mitral Valve in an Adult, *Arq. Bras. Cardiol.,* 26:149, 1973.

5 Shone, J. D., Sellers, R. D., Anderson, R. C., Adams, P., Jr., Lillehei, C. W., and Edwards, J. E.: The Developmental Complex of "Parachute Mitral Valve," Supravalvular Ring of Left Atrium, Subaortic Stenosis, and Coarctation of Aorta, *Am. J. Cardiol.,* 11:714, 1963.

6 Shebetai, R., and Davidson, S.: Asymmetrical Hypertrophic Cardiomyopathy Simulating Mitral Stenosis, *Circulation,* 45:37, 1972.

7 Levy, M. J., and Edwards, J. E.: Anatomy of Mitral Insufficiency, *Prog. Cardiovasc. Dis.,* 5:119, 1962.

8 Edwards, J. E., and Burchell, H. B.: Pathologic Anatomy of Mitral Insufficiency, *Proc. Staff Meet. Mayo Clin.,* 33:497, 1958.

9 Brink, A. J., and Weber, H. W.: Fibroplastic Parietal Endocarditis with Eosinophilia: Löffler's Endocarditis, *Am. J. Med.,* 34:52, 1963.

10 Korn, D., DeSanctis, R., and Sell, S.: Massive Calcification of the Mitral Annulus, *N. Engl. J. Med.,* 267:900, 1962.

11 Salazar, A. E., and Edwards, J. E.: Friction Lesions of Ventricular Endocardium: Relation to Chordae Tendineae of Mitral Valve, *Arch. Pathol.,* 90:364, 1970.

12 Edwards, J. E.: Mitral Insufficiency Resulting from "Overshooting" of Leaflets, *Circulation,* 43:606, 1971.

13 Lee, K. S., Johnson, T., Karnegis, J. N., Quattlebaum, F. W., and Edwards, J. E.: Acute Myocardial Infarction with Long-Term Survival Following Papillary Muscular Rupture, *Am. Heart J.,* 79:258, 1970.

14 Tsakiris, A. G., Rastelli, G. C., Amorim, D., Titus, J. L., and Wood, E. H.: Effect of Experimental Papillary Muscle Damage on Mitral Valve Closure in Intact Anesthetized Dogs, *Mayo Clin. Proc.,* 45:275, 1970.

15 Barlow, J. B., Bosman, C. K., Pocock, W. A., and Marchand, P.: Late Systolic Murmurs and Non-ejection ("Mid-Late") Systolic Clicks: An Analysis of 90 Patients, *Br. Heart J.,* 30:203, 1968.

16 Bittar, N., and Sosa, J. A.: The Billowing Mitral Valve Leaflet: Report on Fourteen Patients, *Circulation,* 38:763, 1968.

17 McCarthy, L. J., and Wolf, P. L.: Mucoid Degeneration of Heart Valves: "Blue Valve Syndrome," *Am. J. Clin. Pathol.,* 54:852, 1970.

18 Guthrie, R. B., and Edwards, J. E.: Pathology of the Myxomatous Mitral Valve: Nature, Secondary Changes and Complications, *Minn. Med.,* 59:637, 1976.

19 Trent, J. K., Adelman, A. G., Wigle, E. D., and Silver, M. D.: Morphology of a Prolapsed Posterior Mitral Valve Leaflet, *Am. Heart J.,* 79:539, 1970.

20 Roy, P., Tajik, A. J., Giuliani, E. R., Schattenberg, T. T., Gau, G. T., and Frye, R. L.: Spectrum of Echocardiographic Findings in Bacterial Endocarditis, *Circulation,* 53:474, 1976.

21 Goodman, D., Kimbiris, D., and Linhart, J. W.: Chordae Tendineae Rupture Complicating the Systolic Click–Late Systolic Murmur Syndrome, *Am. J. Cardiol.,* 33:681, 1974.

22 Edwards, J. E., and Burchell, H. B.: Endocardial and Intimal Lesions (Jet Impact) as Possible Sites of Origin of Murmurs, *Circulation,* 18:946, 1958.

23 Thomas, J. R.: Mitral Insufficiency due to Rupture of Chordae Tendineae Simulating Aortic Stenosis, *Am. Heart J.,* 71:112, 1966.

24 Edwards, J. E.: Mitral Insufficiency Secondary to Aortic Valvular Bacterial Endocarditis, *Circulation,* 46:623, 1972.

25 Eliot, R. S., Woodburn, R. L., and Edwards, J. E.: Conditions of the Ascending Aorta Simulating Aortic Valvular Incompetence, *Am. J. Cardiol.,* 14:679, 1964.

26 Carter, J. B., Sethi, S., Lee, G. B., and Edwards, J. E.: Prolapse of Semilunar Cusps as Causes of Aortic Insuffiency, *Circulation,* 43:922, 1971.

27 Levy, M. J., Lillehei, C. W., Anderson, R. C., Amplatz, K., and Edwards, J. E.: Aortico-Left Ventricular Tunnel, *Circulation,* 27:841, 1963.

28 Edwards, J. E.: Pathology of Left Ventricular Outflow Tract Obstruction, *Circulation,* 31:586, 1965.

29 McKusick, V. A., Logue, R. B., and Bahnson, H. T.: Association of Aortic Valvular Disease and Cystic Medial Necrosis of the Ascending Aorta, *Circulation,* 16:188, 1957.

30 Fukuda, T., Tadavarthy, S. M., and Edwards, J. E.: Dissecting Aneurysm of Aorta Complicating Aortic Valvular Stenosis, *Circulation,* 53:169, 1976.

31 Nakib, A., Lillehei, C. W., and Edwards, J. E.: The Degree of Coronary Atherosclerosis in Aortic Valvular Disease, *Arch. Pathol.,* 80:517, 1965.

32 Edwards, J. E.: On the Etiology of Calcific Aortic Stenosis, *Circulation,* 26:817, 1962.

33 Roberts, W. C.: The Structure of the Aortic Valve in Clinically Isolated Aortic Stenosis: An Autopsy Study of 162 Patients over 15 Years of Age, *Circulation,* 42:91, 1970.

34 Edwards, J. E.: Pathologic Aspects of Cardiac Valvular Insufficiences, *Arch. Surg.,* 77:634, 1958.

59

Altered Cardiovascular Function of Rheumatic Heart Disease and Other Acquired Valvular Disease

ROBERT C. SCHLANT, M.D.

This chapter will primarily consider the altered cardiovascular function of rheumatic heart disease. Other varieties of valvular heart disease are considered in Chaps. 54 and 55 (congenital lesions) and in Chap. 60 (miscellaneous acquired types of valvular disease). Detailed discussions of the evaluation of ventricular function and the and the adaptations have been presented in Chap. 41. The pathophysiology and natural history of valvular heart disease have been extensively reviewed.[1-3]

The changes in cardiovascular function in rheumatic heart disease may be divided into two types: the changes occurring during acute rheumatic fever and the chronic changes persisting and/or developing afterward. Often there is no sharp demarcation between the two categories, particularly in patients with "smoldering" rheumatic fever.

ACUTE RHEUMATIC FEVER

During acute rheumatic fever, there may be a pancarditis, with evidence of inflammation in virtually all of the heart, including the pericardium. The acute inflammatory process in the atria and ventricles interferes with their normal function. This alteration is reflected in their depressed "function curves." It may result in failure of either the right or left ventricle or both, although more frequently the left ventricle fails and produces pulmonary congestion. It is uncertain whether myocardial function is depressed by interference with cellular metabolic processes or by interference with the process of energy utilization and muscular contraction, or both. The depression of myocardial function is often apparent from the weak force of myocardial contraction of the ventricles, which may be extremely dilated, and from the cardiac output, which may be decreased despite elevation of left ventricular end-diastolic and atrial mean pressures. Patients with less severe depression of myocardial function may have normal cardiac output at rest[4] but frequently have an elevation of left ventricular end-diastolic pressure. These patients are often unable to increase their cardiac output during exercise despite further elevation of left ventricular end-diastolic pressure. Whenever there is an elevation of left atrial mean pressure, pulmonary venous and pulmonary capillary pressures are similarly elevated. If pulmonary capillary pressure exceeds the oncotic pressure of blood (normally 25 to 30 mm Hg), pulmonary transudation of fluid occurs. In addition to the myocardial element in acute rheumatic fever, there is usually valvular dysfunction, which further burdens the heart. Though some of the acute valvular dysfunction is caused by the acute valvulitis, mitral regurgitation may also be caused by the rather acute development of ventricular dilatation. This functional mitral regurgitation may be caused by several mechanisms. As a result of acute left ventricular dilatation, the mitral valve ring may be significantly dilated and may not be narrowed as much as normal during ventricular systole. Involvement of the mitral annulus and the adjacent myocardial fibers may also interfere with the normal narrowing of the mitral annulus during ventricular systole. Furthermore, acute left ventricular dilatation and myocardial dysfunction may interfere with the normal function of the papillary muscles and chordae tendineae in anchoring and maintaining normal valve function. Although murmurs associated with stenosis of the mitral or aortic valve may occur during acute rheumatic fever, hemodynamically significant valvular stenosis is rarely, if ever, present during the initial acute attack. The presence of the murmur of mitral stenosis during an initial attack of acute rheumatic fever is the consequence of several factors: a high flow across the mitral valve during diastole necessitated by the mitral regurgitation, a mitral valve deformed by rheumatic valvulitis, and a large, dilated left ventricle.

The moderate prolongation of AV conduction frequently present in acute rheumatic fever[5] probably does not, by itself, interfere significantly with cardiac performance. Very high degrees of first-degree block or second-degree block may decrease the efficiency of the atrial booster pump function. Complete heart block is rare during acute rheumatic fever.

Despite the frequent presence of large amounts of fluid in the pericardium associated with the pericarditis of acute rheumatic fever, it rarely, if ever, produces cardiac tamponade. It is thought that the relatively slow rate of accumulation of the fluid allows the pericardium to stretch without a significant elevation of pericardial pressure. Rheumatic pericarditis probably never produces chronic constrictive pericarditis.

CHRONIC RHEUMATIC HEART DISEASE

Myocardial dysfunction

Cardiac dysfunction in chronic rheumatic heart disease is principally the consequence of altered function of the cardiac valves. On the other hand, in some patients acute rheumatic fever results in chronic fibrotic changes in the myocardial musculature, connective tissue, or blood vessels[6–17] that contribute significantly to the derangement of function of the atria, the ventricles, or both. In addition, patients with chronic rheumatic heart disease may have significant coronary atherosclerosis.[18]

Valvular dysfunction

The normal valves of a human being offer minimal resistance to forward flow, yet they are able to close abruptly with minimal leakage and minimal displacement. Although there must be some pressure difference across the heart valves for blood to flow, the pressure difference across the valves of a normal heart is probably not greater than 1 to 3 mm Hg and is, therefore, usually too small to be measured accurately. With any form of significant obstruction to flow across a heart valve, there are three basic adjustments that may occur: (1) The pressure proximal to the obstruction may rise in an attempt to maintain the same quantity of flow; (2) the amount of flow may decrease and hence require less pressure difference across the obstruction; (3) the duration of flow past the obstruction may be prolonged, as systolic ejection is prolonged with aortic and pulmonary valve obstruction.

The basic relation between valve area, blood flow, and pressure difference across stenotic valves and orifices is shown by the Gorlin and Gorlin[19] modification of standard hydraulic formulas:

$$\text{Valve area} = \frac{\text{blood flow}}{K \times 44.5 \times \sqrt{P_1 - P_2}}$$

Valve area is in square centimeters; blood flow is in milliliters per second (for the mitral and tricuspid valves, milliliters per second of diastole; for the aortic and pulmonary valves, milliliters per second of systole); K is an empirical constant to correct for hydraulic losses through the valve orifice, for the conversion of milliliters of mercury to centimeters of water, and for errors introduced by the usual methods of measuring the periods of systole and of diastole; 44.5 equals $\sqrt{2g}$, where g equals the acceleration factor; and P_1 and P_2 represent the mean pressure in millimeters of mercury during the period of flow in the chambers or vessels on each side of the valve. As usually applied, K is 0.7 for the mitral valve and 1.0 for other stenotic valves and orifices. Estimations of valve area by this formula usually agree well with surgical and autopsy findings when the mitral orifice is less than 2.0 cm² or the aortic valve is less than 1.2 cm² and when there is a significant pressure difference across the valve. The presence of regurgitation makes it impossible to determine from routine measurements of cardiac output the total amount of blood flowing across the valve during forward flow, and therefore it is impossible to calculate valve area except by assuming various amounts of regurgitation. If the volume of regurgitation can be measured accurately angiographically to obtain the total volume of forward flow across the valve, a reasonably accurate effective valve area can be calculated.

Adjustments to valvular heart disease

The many adjustments to valvular heart disease are similar to the normal cardiovascular reserve mechanisms described in Chap. 7 and to the adjustments in heart failure described in Chap. 41. The acute, subacute, and chronic adjustments to valvular heart disease are summarized in Table 59-1. In general, most of the acute and subacute adjustments persist in subjects with chronic valvular disease. There is evidence that the myocardial hypertrophy that occurs in response to increased afterload or pressure

TABLE 59-1
General adjustments to valvular heart disease

I Acute adjustments
   A Decreased parasympathetic activity to heart
      1 Increased heart rate
   B Increased sympathetic activity
      1 Cardiac
         a Increased myocardial contractility
         b Increased heart rate
      2 Peripheral circulation
         a Arterial constriction
         b Venoconstriction
         c Increased venous return
   C Redistribution of blood flow
   D Increased oxygen extraction
   E Anaerobic metabolism by individual organs
II Subacute adjustments
   A Frank-Starling mechanism (increased preload)
      1 Fluid retention by kidneys
      2 Increased blood volume
      3 Increased ventricular end-diastolic volume (preload)
   B Alterations in the durations of systole and of diastole
   C Changes in the pulmonary circulation
      1 Redistribution of pulmonary blood flow
      2 Pulmonary lymphatic dilatation
   D Peripheral circulatory changes
      1 Increased arteriolar sodium and water ("stiffness")
   E Pericardial stretch
III Chronic adjustments
   A Ventricular hypertrophy and/or dilatation
      1 Altered myocardial contractility
      2 Altered ventricular compliance
      3 Altered ventricular relaxation, diastolic "suction"
      4 Ventriculosystemic reflexes
      5 Atrial hypertrophy and/or dilatation
   B Altered myocardial contractility
   C Alterations in hemoglobin-oxygen dissociation curve
      1 Decreased affinity of hemoglobin for oxygen
   D Altered activity in sympathetic-parasympathetic systems
      1 Depletion of myocardial norepinephrine
      2 Defective cardiac parasympathetic control

load is relatively early associated with a decrease in myocardial contractility per square millimeter of myocardium,[20–25] whereas when the hypertrophy occurs secondary to a chronic increase in preload or volume load, the myocardial contractility may not be diminished[23–29] until the later onset of dysdynamic myocardial failure. The cause of the decrease in myocardial contractility associated with hypertrophy secondary to increased afterload may be related to impaired excitation-contraction coupling, decreased myofibrillar ATPase, decreased efficiency of oxidative phosphorylation, or to the "wear and tear" mechanisms of Meerson[27,30] (see Chap. 41).

The alteration in the hemoglobin-oxygen dissociation curve which results in a decreased affinity of hemoglobin in chronic heart failure is associated with an increase in erythrocyte 2,3-diphosphoglycerate (2,3-DPG).[31] The depletion of myocardial norepinephrine (see Chap. 41) is of particular significance in chronic valvular heart disease in reference to the administration of β-adrenergic drugs such as propranolol, which may markedly decrease ventricular function, notably in severe aortic stenosis. Patients with congestive heart failure have elevated resting urinary norepinephrine excretion and an abnormal rise in plasma norepinephrine concentration during exercise. There is also evidence that patients with chronic heart disease have defective cardiac parasympathetic control.[32]

Evaluation of cardiac function in valvular heart disease[33–57]

The difficulties in evaluating overall cardiac function, ventricular function, and ventricular contractility are discussed in more detail in Chap. 41 and by Mason et al.[39] It is of particular significance that in the evaluation of ventricular function in valvular heart disease, the apparent "function" of one ventricle may be influenced by volume and pressure loading of the contralateral ventricle.[58–61]

AORTIC STENOSIS[1,62–81]

Hemodynamically significant aortic stenosis produces predominantly a resistance or pressure afterload on the left ventricle, which responds with marked *concentric hypertrophy* with relatively little or no dilatation. The tremendous concentric hypertrophy helps to maintain normal wall stress per unit area despite the elevated tension. Normally, the left ventricular pressure exceeds aortic pressure by 1 to 3 mm Hg during the initial third of ejection. With the development of aortic stenosis, the systolic pressure difference across the aortic valve changes relatively little until the valve area is markedly decreased. Although the effective cross-sectional area of the orifice of the aortic valve in the average adult is 2.6 to

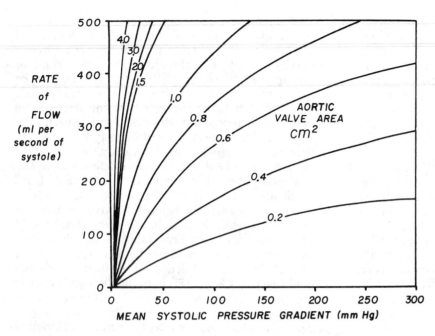

FIGURE 59-1 Chart illustrating the relation between mean systolic pressure gradient across the aortic valve and the rate of flow across the aortic valve per second of systole, as predicted by the Gorlin and Gorlin formula. Although the effective area of the aortic valve in the adult is about 2.6 to 3.5 cm², there is relatively little obstruction to blood flow until the area is markedly reduced. Below the "critical" valve area, about 0.5 to 0.7 cm², relatively little further increase in flow is achieved even with marked increases in mean systolic gradient.

3.5 cm², the "critical" aortic valve area at which patients with solitary aortic stenosis develop pulmonary congestion, angina pectoris, or syncope is only 0.5 to 0.7 cm². Figure 59-1 illustrates the basic relations between aortic valve area, blood flow, and mean systolic gradient across the aortic valve. Naturally, even mild aortic stenosis will contribute to ventricular dysfunction and clinical symptoms if there is associated disease, such as aortic regurgitation or coronary artery disease. Many patients with pure stenosis of the aortic valve will maintain a relatively normal cardiac output by means of left ventricular hypertrophy, even though this may be associated with a left ventricular systolic pressure of about 300 mm Hg, which is about the maximum the left ventricle can generate for any length of time. Actually, most patients with severe aortic stenosis seldom maintain left ventricular systolic pressure over 260 mm Hg for sustained periods. If the stenosis is severe, the cardiac output usually fails to increase normally during exercise, even though the left atrial and pulmonary capillary pressures rise. The thick, hypertrophied ventricle in aortic stenosis is less distensible than normal, and the diastolic pressure is frequently elevated even at rest. In this situation the elevated end-diastolic pressure reflects the decreased compliance of the hypertrophied ventricle rather than myocardial failure.[33] The final filling and the final increase in end-diastolic fiber length and pressure of the ventricle are normally accomplished by atrial contraction (see Fig. 54-2). In aortic stenosis, this forceful "atrial kick" is reflected in an increased amplitude of the left atrial *a* wave and from the marked increase in left ventricular end-diastolic pressure, just prior to ventricular contraction. This momentary increase in stretch and pressure produced by left atrial contraction increases the force of the subsequent ventricular contraction. Since the left atrial pressure is elevated for only a brief period, pulmonary edema may not be produced even though the height of the left atrial *a* wave may be 30 to 35 mm Hg. If, however, the *mean* pressure in the left atrium becomes elevated above 25 to 30 mm Hg, pulmonary edema is imminent. In severe aortic stenosis the loss of the atrial kick due to atrial fibrillation may result in a marked decrease in cardiac output and pulmonary edema.[82]

When left ventricular failure occurs in the late stages of aortic stenosis, the cardiac output may decrease, and there may be an increase in left ventricular pressure throughout diastole and in the pressures back through the left atrium to the right ventricle. Only rarely are pulmonary artery and right ventricular pressures more than moderately elevated in pure aortic stenosis. Rarely, aortic valve disease may result in a pressure gradient between the right ventricle and pulmonary artery.[83] This is sometimes referred to as the Bernheim phenomenon.

Arterial pulse changes

As a result of the obstruction at the aortic valve, the arterial pressure pulse is damped in most adult patients with aortic stenosis. Classically, the pulse wave is of low amplitude, with a slow rate of rise and a prominent anacrotic shoulder on the ascending limb, and has a low, rounded, delayed peak (see Fig. 14-4). The incisura and the dicrotic notch, which are delayed by the compensatory prolongation of the left ventricular ejection phase, are less prominent than normal or are absent, particularly with severe stenosis. This pulse wave is sometimes referred to as *parvus et tardus*. There is a tendency for the anacrotic shoulder, or notch, to occur earlier on the upstroke when the stenosis is more severe. Although the rate of rise of arterial pressure *(dp/dt)* is decreased, and the duration of systolic ejection and the period from the onset of the pulse wave to the peak pressure are prolonged in aortic stenosis, these measurements do not give an accurate estimation of the effective area of the stenotic aortic valve.

Patients with severe aortic stenosis may demonstrate *pulsus alternans*, with an alternation of the left ventricular systolic pressure and, to a lesser extent, the aterial systolic pressure.[84] In most instances the weak beat is initiated from a shorter end-diastolic fiber length than is the strong beat, whether the end-diastolic pressure is lower, the same, or higher. Pulsus alternans in itself is frequently evidence of ventricular myocardial failure.

Angina pectoris and syncope[74,76–78,78a,81,85,86]

In patients with significant aortic stenosis, ischemic heart pain is the result of many factors: increased myocardial requirement for oxygen associated with the high left ventricular tension-time index; relatively fewer capillaries per gram of myocardium as a result of hypertrophy; increased diffusion distance from capillary to the center of the hypertrophied myocardial fibers; relatively low pressure in the aorta during diastole, when most coronary flow to the left ventricle occurs, and during systole, when the high intramyocardial pressure may impede the small amount of coronary flow normally occurring during systole; relative shortening of diastole; and the frequent occurrence of associated coronary atherosclerosis. Although the mechanism of exertional syncope has been ascribed to a decrease in peripheral vascular resistance combined with a fixed cardiac output, producing a fall in arterial pressure, it is more often produced by the occurrence of asystole or transient ventricular dysrhythmias. Occasionally, it may also be produced by a reflex which originates in the left ventricle secondary to the marked increase in left ventricular systolic pressure and which produces a reflex decrease in peripheral resistance and pressure.[87]

Isolated calcific aortic stenosis most frequently results from calcification of a congenital bicuspid aortic valve.[88–90] In the very elderly, it may result from fibrosis and calcification due to chronic wear and tear.[89,90] Occasionally, this is associated with mild aortic regurgitation.

COMBINED MITRAL AND AORTIC STENOSIS[91–94]

Hemodynamically significant mitral stenosis and aortic stenosis may exist together in the same patient. In this situation, the cardiac output is limited by the mitral stenosis. As a result the left ventricle is spared or "protected" from much of the markedly excessive work and hypertrophy usually produced by aortic stenosis, since the low flow requires considerably less left ventricular systolic pressure. This is in contrast to pure aortic stenosis, in which the cardiac output is often normal or even slightly elevated until the terminal, decompensated phase of the disease is

reached. When a combination of aortic stenosis and mitral stenosis is suspected, it is imperative to obtain measurements of both pressure and flow and to calculate valve areas, since the mean systolic gradient across the aortic valve may be only 20 to 25 mm Hg even though the aortic valve is severely stenotic. In patients with both aortic and mitral stenosis, the hemodynamic changes across the mitral valve, in the left atrium, pulmonary circuit, and right side of the heart are similar to those in pure mitral stenosis. In most instances the left ventricle tolerates the limited increase in pressure work with only moderate elevation of its systolic pressure and without significant elevation of its diastolic pressure. If, however, the mitral stenosis is less severe and more blood enters the left ventricle, or if the left ventricle should "fail" from other causes, the diastolic as well as the systolic pressures may become elevated. In the presence of combined aortic and mitral stenosis any elevation of left ventricular diastolic pressures causes an increase in the left atrial and pulmonary capillary pressures. Similarly, if mitral regurgitation is present in addition to mitral and aortic stenosis, the elevation of left ventricular systolic pressure (produced by the aortic stenosis) results in more regurgitation back across the mitral valve during systole. In combined mitral and aortic stenosis the peripheral arterial pressure pulse wave is less likely to be distorted than in pure aortic stenosis. In most instances, however, it is still characterized by a small pulse wave having a prolonged systolic upstroke wave with an anacrotic shoulder, a delayed systolic peak, and a delayed incisura or dicrotic notch. The central incisura and peripheral dicrotic notch may be indistinct or even absent.

AORTIC REGURGITATION[1,29,95–105]

Both aortic regurgitation and mitral regurgitation impose a significant volume load on the left ventricle. The major response to the increased preload by the volume of aortic regurgitation is dilatation of the left ventricle and the development of *eccentric hypertrophy,* which is associated with an increase in cell size and length, possible "slippage" of myofibrils within the myocardial cells, and possibly an increase in the number of sarcomeres in series. In contrast to the hypertrophy that develops secondary to increased pressure "afterload," the ventricular hypertrophy produced by volume loading may be associated with the maintenance of normal myocardial contractility per cubic millimeter[23–29] and by the relatively normal performance of each sarcomere unit. In aortic regurgitation, as well as mitral regurgitation, the left ventricle is able to tolerate a high "volume work" reasonably well, since rapid left ventricular ejection is associated with a striking decrease in left ventricular diameter and wall tension during systole.[96] Such a rapid decrease in "instantaneous impedance" tends to increase the velocity and extent of myocardial fiber shortening, thereby helping to maintain or even increase the ejection fraction even with unchanged myocardial contractility. It thereby allows the ventricle to expend a greater proportion of its contractile energy in shortening than in tension development. For many years it has been known that "volume work" increases myocardial oxygen consumption less than "pressure work." As the left ventricle dilates and hypertrophies from aortic regurgitation, it also tends to become more spherical. An additional adaptation to aortic regurgitation and to mitral regurgitation is an increase in diastolic compliance, which enables the left ventricle to accommodate large volumes without a marked increase in pressure during diastole. Later, with either greater hypertrophy or dysdynamic myocardial "failure," the compliance of the left ventricle may decrease and the diastolic pressure may increase. An additional adjustment to the increased volume of left ventricular ejection necessitated by aortic regurgitation is a prolongation of the left ventricular ejection phase.[106]

The amount of blood regurgitated may be estimated by indicator-dilution techniques or by angiocardiography, but no simple, safe, and readily applicable and repeatable method has been proved to be quantitatively accurate in human beings. Clinically, a large regurgitant volume tends to be associated with an Austin Flint murmur and a wide pulse pressure. A very large amount of aortic regurgitation can occur through regurgitant areas of less than 1.0 cm^2, because of the relatively high pressure gradient between the aorta and the left ventricle during diastole. Initially, the ventricle accomplishes this increase in stroke volume with dilatation and an end-diastolic pressure that is within normal limits or only slightly elevated. Unless ventricular failure occurs, the pressure wave of the left ventricle is characterized by a very rapid rise of pressure during systole to an early peak that is frequently higher than normal and by a rapid decline in pressure late in systole, the "systolic collapse." Later, as ventricular myocardial "failure" occurs (see Chap. 41), the total output of the left ventricle may decrease, despite an elevation of left ventricular diastolic pressure and fiber length. The elevation of left ventricular diastolic pressure tends to close the mitral valve prematurely and to elevate the left atrial pressure. Patients with aortic regurgitation and prominent *a* waves on their apex cardiogram usually have elevated left ventricular end-diastolic pressure, although the converse is not true.[107] At times an elevation of ventricular diastolic pressure produced by left ventricular failure may decrease the diastolic (regurgitant) pressure difference across the aortic valve and therefore the amount of regurgitation.[108] Even the murmur of aortic regurgitation may disappear. When the aortic regurgitation is very severe, it may rapidly fill the left ventricle during diastole, increasing its pressure above that in the left atrium and prematurely closing the mitral valve.[109–112]

In the presence of aortic regurgitation, it is apparent that at the end of ventricular ejection, the relative amounts of blood passing to the periphery and passing back through the regurgitant valve during diastole will depend upon (1) the pressures in the aorta and left ventricle, (2) the relative resistance of the peripheral arterial system and of the regurgitant aortic valve and left ventricle, and (3) the duration of diastole. Thus, anything which increases peripheral vascular resistance tends to increase the amount of regurgitant flow.[103,113,114] In many patients with aortic regurgitation, there is apparent peripheral vasodilatation, which aids the rapid runoff of blood to the periphery and lessens the relative amount regurgitated into the left ventricle. The beneficial effect of mild tachycardia in aortic regurgitation is related to the associated shortening of the total period of diastole per minute.[115] When the left ventricle is markedly dilated because of aortic regurgitation, functional mitral regurgitation may occur because of interference with the function of the chordae tendineae and papillary muscles and because of dilatation of the mitral valve ring. Although the mitral valve may be prematurely closed by aortic regurgitation, the competence of the mitral valve tends to protect the left atrium from the pressure and volume effects of the aortic regurgitant flow. The development of mitral regurgitation is an important factor contributing to the rapid downhill course of patients with aortic regurgitation when left ventricular failure develops.

Arterial pulse changes

In aortic regurgitation, the typical arterial pressure pulse is characterized by a wide pulse pressure with a rapid rate of rise of pressure to a high systolic peak and by a low diastolic pressure (see Chaps. 14 and 17). At times coarse vibrations, which may be associated with a thrill, are present just prior to the peak. Following the early peak of the pulse wave, there is a rapid fall of pressure, much of which occurs during systole and continued ejection. The central incisura, or peripheral dicrotic notch, and the dicrotic wave are often lost completely. If they are present, they are usually less prominent and occur at lower levels than normal. Low arterial diastolic pressures in severe aortic regurgitation may surprisingly return toward normal, at times even to normal values, if there is severe left ventricular failure.

AORTIC STENOSIS AND AORTIC REGURGITATION

Aortic stenosis in association with aortic regurgitation is a vicious combination. In addition to the pressure work from the stenosis, the left ventricle has the added load of pumping an even greater volume of blood across the valve. From the basic relation of hydraulic flow across a stenotic valve, it is apparent that if the flow is to double, the mean pressure difference must increase fourfold. It should also be kept in mind that, as in mitral valvular disease, severe stenosis is hemodynamically impossible in the presence of severe regurgitation, although their contributory effects may be nearly balanced if both are moderate. The carotid or aortic pulse pressure tracing may often suggest which lesion predominates, although catheterization of the left side of the heart with measurement of the systolic gradient across the aortic valve and of the net cardiac output and estimation of aortic regurgitation by aortic angiography and/or special dilution techniques are frequently required. When a bisferiens carotid or arterial pressure tracing is encountered in mixed aortic stenosis and regurgitation, aortic regurgitation is usually the predominant lesion. This characteristic pulse consists of a rapid rise of pressure to an initial peak (the "percussion" wave), to a delayed second peak (the "tidal" wave), usually of about the same magnitude as the first peak or slightly lower. The central incisura and the peripheral dicrotic notch and wave tend to be less prominent than usual or may even be absent (see Chap. 14).

MITRAL STENOSIS[116-131]

After the initial acute attack of rheumatic fever, in childhood or adolescence, it is probable that the mitral valve becomes progressively narrowed over a period of time, usually 20 to 30 years, and rarely in only 5 to 10 years. As this occurs, the orifice of the mitral valve, which is normally 4 to 6 cm² in the adult, becomes smaller and smaller. During most of this time, however, the narrowing of the valve orifice produces no significant hemodynamic alterations. In fact, the effective valve area must be reduced very markedly before it seriously interferes with cardiovascular hemodynamics. The narrowing is probably insignificant down to 2.6 cm². Between 2.1 and 2.5 cm² the narrowing is usually responsible for symp-

toms only with extreme exertion. Between 1.6 and 2.0 cm² mitral stenosis may produce symptoms with moderate exertion but rarely produces severe interference with light physical activity unless it is complicated by other factors, such as mitral regurgitation, thyrotoxicosis, tachycardia, or pregnancy. The severity of the altered hemodynamics of pure stenosis of the mitral valve increases rapidly as the valve area becomes narrowed to 1.5 cm² or less. By the time the valve area is 1.0 cm², the patient will usually experience symptoms with very mild exertion. A mitral area of about 0.3 to 0.4 cm² is the minimal size compatible with life.

In most patients with significant mitral stenosis (i.e., with a valve orifice of 1.5 cm² or less), the flow across the valve is decreased and the left atrial pressure is increased. Occasionally, when the stenosis is not extreme, one of these factors may change proportionately much more than the other. Figure 59-2 illustrates the normal pressure and flow in the heart and the alterations present in severe mitral stenosis with and without severe pulmonary vascular disease. It is apparent that the rise in the left atrial mean pressure is accompanied by a rise in mean pressure in the pulmonary veins and capillaries and

FIGURE 59-2 Circulatory schemata of the pressures and flows in a normal person *(top)*, a patient with tight mitral stenosis without severe pulmonary vascular disease *(middle)*, and a patient with tight mitral stenosis with severe pulmonary vascular disease *(bottom)*. Note that patients with tight mitral stenosis complicated by severe pulmonary vascular disease have two areas of obstruction to blood flow. See text for details. *(Adapted from the publications of L. Dexter et al.)*

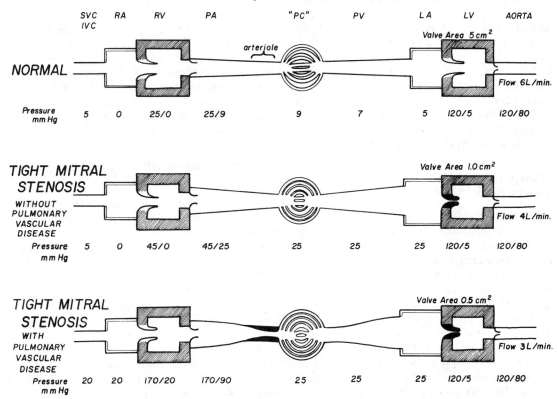

in the systolic pressure in the pulmonary artery. At a valve area of about 1.0 cm² the left atrial mean pressure, and hence pulmonary capillary pressure, is about 25 to 30 mm Hg at rest. This is about the level at which the oncotic pressure of blood is exceeded and pulmonary transudation occurs. If the rate of pulmonary transudation exceeds the rate of pulmonary lymphatic drainage, progressive pulmonary congestion will occur. In patients with milder degrees of stenosis, elevation of left atrial pressure and hence pulmonary edema may occur with exertion, emotion, or shortening of diastole with tachycardia. In patients with either low serum oncotic pressure from hypoalbuminemia or destruction of pulmonary lymphatics from chronic pulmonary fibrosis,[132] pulmonary edema may occur more readily and at a lower pulmonary capillary pressure.

The basic hemodynamic finding in mitral stenosis is a pressure difference between the left atrium and left ventricle during diastole. When the stenosis is severe, the pressure gradient persists throughout diastole, but in mild stenosis it may be present only during the initial phase of rapid ventricular filling and/or during the second phase of rapid flow in late diastole during atrial contraction. In addition to the measurement of diastolic pressure gradient, however, it is essential to measure the flow across the valve, since alterations in flow markedly influence the pressure difference across a stenotic valve. Some important relations between mitral valve area, flow, and pressure difference are shown in Fig. 59-3. It is apparent that with a severely stenotic mitral valve, the heart is unable to increase the forward flow significantly by elevation of the gradient across the mitral valve, since the pulmonary edema threshold of left atrial pressure is rapidly exceeded. It is also apparent that remarkable improvement in hemodynamics can be achieved by relatively slight increases in the mitral valve orifice. As noted previously, left ventricular function may be interfered with by rheumatic perivasculitis or by coronary artery disease. In addition, fibrosis of the mitral valve complex may extend into the endocardium and interfere with ventricular contraction in some patients.[133]

Response to exercise[1,117,118,121–124,126]

When patients with significant mitral stenosis exercise, their left atrial, pulmonary venous, pulmonary capillary, pulmonary artery, and right ventricular pressures increase. If the stenosis is relatively mild, the cardiac output may be normal at rest and may increase with exercise. If the stenosis is severe, however, the resting cardiac output is low, and exercise may produce no change or even a decrease in cardiac output, particularly if there is severe pulmonary vascular disease with right ventricular failure and tricuspid regurgitation. Since the stenotic valve area does not alter, the failure of the cardiac output to rise despite the elevation of left atrial

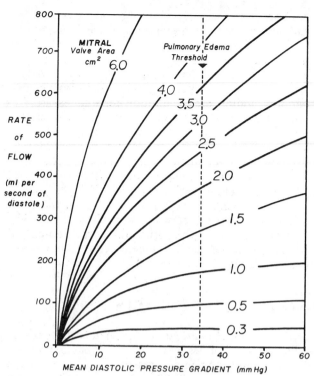

FIGURE 59-3 Chart illustrating the relation between mean diastolic gradient across the mitral valve and rate of flow across the mitral valve per second of diastole, as predicted by the Gorlin and Gorlin formula. Note that when the mitral valve area is 1.0 cm² or less, very little additional flow can be achieved by an increased pressure gradient. Transudation of fluid from the pulmonary capillaries and the development of pulmonary edema begin when pulmonary capillary pressure exceeds the oncotic pressure of plasma, which is about 25 to 35 mm Hg. It is also apparent that *severe* mitral regurgitation is incompatible with very tight mitral stenosis.

pressure is caused by the shortening of the total period of diastole available for flow across the mitral valve. Tachycardia from other causes may also result in a decreased cardiac output and/or elevation of left atrial pressure. Right ventricular failure and tricuspid regurgitation secondary to mitral stenosis with severe pulmonary vascular disease may also contriubte to the decrease in cardiac output during exercise in these patients.

Pulmonary vascular responses[134–137]

In patients with severe mitral stenosis, usually with a calculated mitral valve orifice of 1.0 cm² or less, pulmonary vascular changes often occur and markedly modify both the hemodynamics and the clinical symptoms. In the normal person large volumes of blood pass through the lung under low pressure and with little pressure difference across the lungs. In severe mitral stenosis, the resistance offered by the pulmonary vasculature may increase as a result both of structural changes in the arterioles and arteries and of vasoconstriction of the small arteries. This vasoconstriction has been said to function as a protective mechanism, preventing the pulmonary capillaries from being flooded by sudden surges of right ventricular output. The anatomic changes in the pulmonary vessels may markedly decrease the lumen of the vessels and thereby increase the vascular resistance. Further, vessels with medical muscular hypertrophy may respond with proportionately greater narrowing of the lumen to local hypoxic or other vasoconstrictive stimuli. As a result of the increase in pulmonary vascular resistance, which may be fifteen to twenty times normal and may be associated with a pulmonary artery pressure exceeding systemic pressure, the patient may have two areas of relatively fixed severe obstruction to flow: the mitral valve and the pulmonary vasculature. When patients develop extremely high pulmonary vascular resistance, they may have fewer respiratory complaints than previously. These patients also frequently have associated right ventricular failure with tricuspid regurgitation. Although severe external dyspnea may persist in these patients, attacks of acute pulmonary edema are often relatively uncommon, and many of their symptoms are related to the extremely low cardiac output and systemic venous congestion. At times patients with severe mitral stenosis and severe pulmonary vascular disease may even have lower left atrial pressures than patients with severe mitral stenosis but lower pulmonary vascular resistance.

In normal individuals at rest in the upright position, the upper portions of the lungs have significantly less perfusion than the basal portions because of the effect of gravity on the perfusing pressure of the upper and lower areas of the lungs.[138] This hydrostatic difference and the unequal distribution of blood flow are abolished when the person lies flat. In normal individuals in the vertical position, exercise is associated with a decrease in the normal difference between upper and lower lobe blood flow. Patients with moderately severe mitral stenosis and moderate pulmonary hypertension tend to have relatively greater perfusion of the upper areas of the lungs as compared with the lower areas.[138–140] If the pulmonary hypertension and pulmonary vascular resistance are extremely high, there may even be more perfusion of the upper zones than of the lower zones. This shift of blood flow to the upper lobes in severe mitral stenosis is in part related to the greater degree of pulmonary arterial vasoconstriction and pulmonary vascular disease, including arterial medial hypertrophy, present in the dependent portions. Patients in left ventricular failure from other causes may also reverse the normal distribution of pulmonary blood flow.

The mechanism of the pulmonary vasoconstriction in mitral stenosis is not clear, nor is it known why some patients have more marked vasoconstriction and more marked pulmonary vascular disease than other patients with similar hemodynamics.[1] The pulmonary vascular resistance in patients with mitral stenosis is often found to be chronically and markedly elevated in patients with a resting mean left atrial pressure of 20 to 25 mm Hg, which usually corresponds to a mitral valve area of about 1.0 cm². When the left atrial pressure is acutely elevated to similar levels in patients with milder degrees of mitral stenosis, increased pulmonary vascular resistance is usual-

ly much less apparent. The vasoconstriction, as well as the vascular disease changes in the pulmonary vasculature, in mitral stenosis is more marked in the dependent portions of the lungs. In these areas the vascular pressures are greater because of the effect of gravity, and there is a greater likelihood for transudation of fluid from the pulmonary capillaries into the interstitial spaces. The interstitial pericapillary edema, as well as edema of the blood vessels themselves, contributes to the increased resistance of these vessels as well as interfering with the diffusion of gases.[1,135,138] There is also probably more "reactive" hypertrophy of the arterial smooth muscle to these zones. Although it has been suggested that pulmonary vasoconstriction is produced by a reflex initiated by elevation of pressure in the left atrium, pulmonary veins, or pulmonary capillaries, it is perhaps more likely related to regional vasoconstriction produced by alveolar hypoventilation that occurs as the consequence of chronic excessive transudation of fluid from pulmonary capillaries.[1] The pulmonary arteries may also become more responsive and more effective vascular sphincters as a result of the medial hypertrophy secondary to chronic pulmonary arterial hypertension. In a significant number of patients with elevated pulmonary vascular resistance due to severe mitral stenosis, the resistance may drop rather dramatically toward normal soon after mitral valve replacement.[141–143]

Left atrial pressure pulse

In patients with significant mitral stenosis a characteristic left atrial pressure tracing (Fig. 59-4) has an elevated mean pressure level with a prominent, or even giant, a wave, usually a good x descent, and occasionally a prominent v wave, followed by a slow descent of the y wave with an absent diastasis. At times the c wave is also prominent. If atrial fibrillation is present, the a wave is absent, and the x descent is less pronounced whether or not stenosis is present. Unfortunately, the many variables affecting left atrial pressure tracings preclude accurate estimations of the degree of stenosis and/or regurgitation from the left atrial pressure tracing alone (see below).

Peripheral circulatory adjustments

Concurrently with the decreased cardiac output produced by mitral stenosis, major compensatory adjustments take place in the peripheral circulation. These adjustments are discussed in more detail in Chap. 41. Of particular value are a greater oxygen extraction per unit blood flow to tissues, resulting in a greater systemic arteriovenous oxygen difference; the utilization of anaerobic metabolism, particularly during exertion; an increase in total peripheral resistance; a redistribution of the available blood flow, which preserves flow to the brain and heart at the expense of the skin, skeletal muscles, abdominal

MITRAL STENOSIS

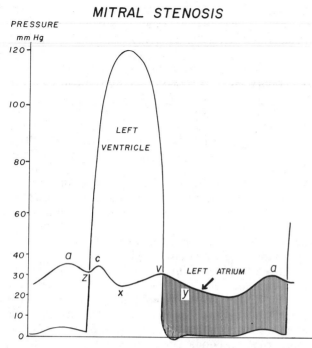

FIGURE 59-4 Simultaneous left atrial and left ventricular pressure tracings in mitral stenosis. The diastolic pressure gradient is indicated by the cross-hatched area. The left atrial pressure tracing has good *a* and *c* waves and a good *x* descent. The *y* descent following the opening of the mitral valve has a slow rate of descent. These findings are in contrast with the typical findings in "pure" mitral regurgitation (see Fig. 59-5).

viscera, and kidneys; and a decrease in the affinity of hemoglobin for oxygen, which makes it easier for oxyhemoglobin to give up its oxygen in relatively poorly perfused organs.[31]

MITRAL REGURGITATION[1,144-148]

Mitral regurgitation, when it is due to chronic rheumatic heart disease, usually coexists with some degree of narrowing of the mitral valve orifice. As a consequence, not only is the left ventricle burdened by the extra volume of blood regurgitated back across the mitral valve, but the left atrium is burdened to get this volume of blood across the mitral valve during diastole in addition to the volume which the ventricle pumps into the aorta. Both left atrium and left ventricle are therefore doing "high-volume" work. Consequently, both chambers are usually dilated and hypertrophied. The increased preload volume of the left ventricle results in dilatation and *eccentric hypertrophy.* As noted above, it appears likely that hypertrophy secondary to volume loading may be associated with normal myocardial contractility[23-29] until the onset of myocardial failure. The early, rapid decompression of the left ventricle

results in a rapidly decreasing "instantaneous impedance" to left ventricular emptying and a rapid decrease in left ventricular wall tension.[96] The decrease in wall tension tends to increase the velocity and extent of myocardial fiber shortening. These effects are more marked in mitral regurgitation than in aortic regurgitation, since left ventricular emptying commences sooner.[96] As in aortic regurgitation, the left ventricle usually accommodates the increased volume load with an increase in compliance, which enables it to increase its diastolic volume markedly with relatively slight, if any, elevation of diastolic pressure. The volume of blood ejected forward into the aorta may be normal if the regurgitation is mild or moderate, but it is usually decreased if the regurgitation is marked.[1,29,49,50,53-55,56] Since there are two orifices—the aortic valve and the regurgitant mitral valve—through which blood may flow as a result of ventricular systole, anything which increases resistance to flow out of the aortic valve (peripheral arterial vasoconstriction, aortic stenosis, etc.) will increase the relative amount of blood flowing backward across the mitral valve.[149-151] Conversely, drugs or procedures that decrease peripheral vascular resistance decrease the amount of mitral regurgitation and improve the function of the left ventricle.[148] The peripheral vasodilatation and decrease in peripheral resistance usually associated with exercise may help patients with mild or moderate mitral regurgitation to increase their peripheral output with exercise. Because of the large pressure gradient during systole between the left ventricle and left atrium, a very small mitral regurgitant orifice permits a large regurgitant flow, which may be three to five times the forward flow out of the aortic valve.[49,50,53,55,66]

In patients with combined mitral regurgitation and mitral stenosis causing a diastolic pressure gradient across the mitral valve, an elevation of left ventricular diastolic pressure caused by left ventricular failure will be reflected in an increase in left atrial, pulmonary venous, and pulmonary capillary pressures. As in pure mitral stenosis or other conditions with chronic elevation of pulmonary venous pressure, the pulmonary artery pressure also increases. Although some patients with severe mitral regurgitation have marked increases in pulmonary artery pressure and pulmonary vascular resistance, leading to right ventricular failure, this sequence is not so frequently encountered in the severe degree often found in "pure" mitral stenosis.

Left atrial pressure pulse

In patients with significant mitral regurgitation, the left atrial pressure tracing (Fig. 59-5) reveals no apparent distinct *c* wave since the *x* descent is absent and there is an early onset of a giant regurgitant *r* wave during ventricular systole. When the mitral valve opens very slightly after the peak of the *r* wave, there is a rapid *y* descent of the pressure tracing. When the regurgitant wave is very marked, the left atrial pressure pulse resembles the ventricular pressure tracing in form, referred to as "ventricularization" of the atrium. Occasionally, the giant regurgi-

PURE MITRAL REGURGITATION

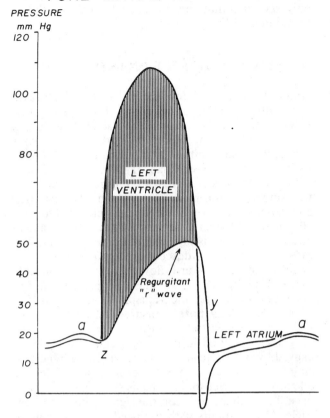

PRESSURE
mm Hg

FIGURE 59-5 Simultaneous left atrial and left ventricular pressure tracings in severe pure mitral regurgitation. The left atrial pressure tracing is characterized by a *regurgitant r wave* which begins in early systole, obscures the *c* wave, and obliterates the *x* descent. The regurgitant *r* wave is produced by the flow of blood into the left atrium from both the pulmonary veins and the left ventricle, in contrast to the normal *v* wave. (Some authors refer to the "abnormal" or "giant" *v* or *cv* wave.) In extremely severe mitral regurgitation, the regurgitant *r* wave resembles the ventricular systolic pressure tracing ("ventricularization" of the left atrium). The *y* descent of the left atrial pressure tracing following opening of the mitral valve shows a rapid fall in pressure, since the mitral valve offers relatively little resistance to the flow of blood into the left ventricle. These findings are in contrast with the typical findings in pure mitral stenosis (Fig. 59-4). Although little diastolic gradient between left atrium and left ventricle is present in this example, more commonly in patients with rheumatic mitral valve disease there is a moderate or high diastolic gradient. This is produced by a very high flow across a mitral valve which is only mildly or moderately stenotic.

tant *r* or *v* wave may be reflected back to the pulmonary artery pressure pulse, where it produces a notch—the "mitral insufficiency shoulder"—shortly after the peak systolic pressure.[152] In most patients with rheumatic mitral disease with predominant or even clinically pure mitral regurgitation, there is a pressure gradient between the left atrium and left ventricle during diastole. Because of the large flow during diastole, both the diastolic gradient and the left atrial mean pressure are often as high as in pure mitral stenosis of equal clinical severity. In patients with massive amounts of mitral regurgitation, the stenotic mitral valve area is usually over 1.8 cm². Patients with only mild to moderate mitral regurgita-

tion may have stenotic mitral valve areas as small as 0.9 to 1.6 cm²; however, hemodynamically severe mitral stenosis is incompatible with severe regurgitation. In pure mitral regurgitation, the left ventricular end-diastolic pressure may be normal at rest even with marked left ventricular dilatation, although the end-diastolic pressure usually increases abnormally with exercise. Rarely, patients with pure rheumatic mitral regurgitation may have significant symptoms with normal left ventricular diastolic and left atrial mean pressures at rest and with no pressure gradient across the mitral valve in diastole.[153,154] It should be emphasized that the compliance of the left atrium is a major determinant of how great an increase in left atrial pressure and in pulmonary congestion will occur with a given volume of mitral regurgitation. A large, capacious left atrium may accommodate very large volumes with little or no elevation of pressure and hence minimal symptoms of pulmonary congestion or edema. Conversely, a small, less compliant left atrium may have its pressure dramatically increased by a smaller regurgitant volume. The variation in this "reservoir" function or the compliance of the left atrium is, in part, responsible for some of the dramatic differences in symptoms and signs between patients with chronic mitral regurgitation and patients with acute mitral regurgitation.[130,155] These differences are discussed in more detail in Chap. 60B.

Estimation of regurgitant volume

Several methods of analysis of left atrial pressure tracings have also been used to estimate the severity of mitral regurgitation.[156,157] Because of the many variables affecting the atrial pressure tracing, particularly the compliance of the left atrium, these methods are of limited value in an individual patient except in an approximate, qualitative fashion. Estimations of regurgitation from "PC" or wedged pulmonary artery pressure tracings are of even less value in an individual patient. Clinically the most useful estimations of mitral regurgitation are obtained from left ventricular angiography[49,50,53] and from analysis of indicator-dilution curves.[157,158]

In some techniques, the indicator (dye, hydrogenated saline solution, ascorbic acid, saline solution, etc.) is introduced in the chamber immediately beyond the regurgitant valve (left ventricle), and indicator-dilution curves are obtained from the chamber proximal to the regurgitant valve (left atrium) as well as from a peripheral artery. Other techniques employ injection proximal to the regurgitant valve (pulmonary artery or left atrium) and analysis of the indicator-dilution curve obtained from a peripheral artery. Most of the techniques used have been of considerable clinical value in 90 to 95 percent of cases, but none of the available methods has been proved to provide an accurate measurement of the actual amount of blood regurgitated. Similarly, left angiography has not yet been proved to provide an absolute quantitative measurement of the amount of regurgitant flow actually present under normal conditions, although it is currently the most widely employed technique.

PULMONIC STENOSIS[1]

Although many types of lesions[159,160] may produce acquired pulmonic stenosis or obstruction to right ventricular outflow, it is most often congenital. Rheumatic involvement of the pulmonary valve is infrequent, although it may occur, especially in patients with severe rheumatic carditis involving all heart valves.[161] In general, pulmonic stenosis results in concentric hypertrophy of the right ventricle with relatively little dilatation or increase in diastolic volume.[162] The hypertrophy is reflected by the presence of prominent a waves in the right atrial and jugular venous pulse waves. As noted above, right ventricular pressure or volume loading may produce abnormalities of left ventricular end-diastolic pressure or compliance that are not related to left ventricular failure.[58–60] Although severe pulmonic stenosis may result in heart failure and death, recent studies have indicated that mild to moderate isolated pulmonic stenosis in adults is tolerated much better than was formerly thought.[163,164] Congenital stenosis is discussed in more detail in Chaps. 54 and 55.

PULMONARY REGURGITATION[165,166]

Pulmonary regurgitation most frequently occurs as a secondary valvular dysfunction in patients with chronic pulmonary hypertension due to chronic rheumatic mitral valve disease (producing the Graham Steell murmur) or with cor pulmonale or other causes of pulmonary hypertension. This "functional" pulmonic regurgitation is thought to be due to dilatation of the pulmonary valve ring. Pulmonary regurgitation may also occur as an isolated congenital lesion[167–169] or less frequently as the result of involvement of the valve by infective endocarditis (particularly in heroin addicts), or as the result of rheumatic fever. When pulmonary regurgitation is very severe, the pressures in the pulmonary artery and right ventricle may be equal or nearly equal at the end of diastole. Congenital isolated pulmonic regurgitation, which is usually not associated with pulmonary artery hypertension, is frequently associated with a low-pitched, diastolic crescendo-decrescendo diastolic murmur[167–169] in contrast to the usual high-pitched, diastolic "blowing" decrescendo murmur present in most patients with pulmonary regurgitation and pulmonary artery hypertension. Isolated pulmonary regurgitation is usually tolerated reasonably well by young patients or experimental animals without pulmonary hypertension, although the response to exercise may be decreased.[170,171] The vol-

ume of pulmonary regurgitation can be estimated only semiquantitatively by special indicator-dilution techniques.[172,173]

TRICUSPID STENOSIS[174–181]

Significant tricuspid stenosis due to rheumatic fever is usually found in association with severe mitral valvular disease. Occasionally tricuspid stenosis may be the predominant lesion; it may also occur as a congenital lesion, either isolated or in combination with other defects (see Chap. 55). The basic finding in tricuspid stenosis is a pressure difference across the tricuspid valve during diastole. The mean right atrial and venous pressures are frequently elevated to 10 to 20 mm Hg. If the atrial septum is intact, the a wave of atrial contraction is accentuated or even giant. The rate of fall of the y descent is slow because of the obstruction to forward flow across the tricuspid valve. Usually the mean diastolic pressure differences across the stenotic tricuspid valve are less (5 to 15 mm Hg) than those measured across the mitral valve in severe mitral stenosis. A very large a wave may also be found in right ventricular hypertrophy caused by pulmonic stenosis or pulmonary hypertension from any cause. It is therefore essential for the diagnosis of tricuspid stenosis to demonstrate a diastolic gradient between the right atrium and ventricle. Most patients with tricuspid stenosis begin to develop peripheral edema or even ascites when the mean right atrial pressure is above 10 mm Hg. The cardiac output tends to be low at rest, and it does not increase normally with exercise, particularly if the valve orifice is below 1.5 cm^2.

TRICUSPID REGURGITATION[182–186]

Tricuspid regurgitation is most commonly an acquired secondary dysfunction, although it may be congenital.[187–189] Most frequently, tricuspid regurgitation occurs because of right ventricular dilatation and failure secondary to chronic right ventricular hypertension resulting from (1) elevation of left ventricular diastolic or left atrial pressures from any cause, (2) pulmonary hypertension from cor pulmonale, or (3) pulmonic stenosis. At times, it is the result of infective endocarditis or of valvular damage from rheumatic fever, when it is often associated with some degree of tricuspid stenosis. "Functional" tricuspid regurgitation, like that of the mitral valve, is probably produced mainly by the inability of the papillary muscles and chordae tendineae to anchor the valve leaflets securely when the ventricular chamber is markedly dilated. The structure of the normal tricuspid valve is considerably less able to anchor the valve leaflets and to maintain competence in the presence of right ventricular hypertension than that of the mitral valve. Dilatation of the tricuspid valve ring itself may also contribute, though this mechanism is probably not as important as the papillary muscle-chordae tendineae dysfunction. The regurgitation into the right atrium produces a prominent "regurgitant" *r* wave in right atrial and internal jugular pulse recordings. (Fig. 15-6). When the regurgitation is marked, it causes a positive holosystolic wave in the right atrium beginning with ventricular systole, obliterating the *c* wave and the normal systolic *x* descent, and reaching a very high peak. The *y* descent following opening of the tricuspid valve is rapid if there is no associated tricuspid stenosis. The large atrial wave, which begins during early ventricular systole, is perhaps better referred to as a *regurgitant r wave* rather than a *v* wave, since much of its genesis is different from that of the normal *v* wave. (Traditionally, however, this wave is frequently referred to as a "giant" *v* or *cv* wave.) Like the murmur of tricuspid regurgitation, the right atrial regurgitant wave may be increased by inspiration. The size of the regurgitant wave is affected by many factors, particularly the volume of regurgitation and of venous inflow into the right atrium and the pressure-volume characteristics of the right atrium. At times, massive regurgitation into a flabby, giant right atrium may produce a relatively small regurgitant wave. Occasionally, tricuspid regurgitation may be present without a significant murmur. Rarely, tricuspid regurgitation may produce a protein-losing enteropathy, lymphocytopenia, and immunologic deficiency.[190] Although indicator-dilution techniques have been used to estimate the amount of tricuspid regurgitation,[172] the available methods do not give a consistently reliable and accurate measurement of the volume of regurgitation. Right ventricular angiography is also useful, particularly to rule out tricuspid regurgitation, but it has a moderately high incidence of false positive results.[191] False positive indicator-dilution or angiographic studies of regurgitation are probably related to the presence of the catheter across a cardiac valve, preventing complete closure, or to the presence of arrhythmias.[191,192]

REFERENCES

1 Schlant, R. C., and Nutter, D. O.: Heart Failure in Valvular Heart Disease, *Medicine (Baltimore)*, 50:421, 1971.

2 Werkö, L.: The Dynamics and Consequences of Stenosis of Insufficiency of the Cardiac Valves, in W. F. Hamilton and P. Dow (eds.), "Handbook of Physiology," sec. 2, "Circulation," vol. 1, American Physiological Society, Washington, 1962, p. 645.

3 Marshall, R. J., and Shepherd, J. T.: "Cardiac Function in Health and Disease," W. B. Saunders Company, Philadelphia, 1968.

4 Besterman, E. M. M.: The Cardiac Output in Acute Rheumatic Carditis, *Br. Heart J.*, 16:8, 1954.

5 Clark, M., and Keith, J. D.: Atrioventricular Conduction in Acute Rheumatic Fever, *Br. Heart J.*, 34:472, 1972.

6 Clawson, B. J.: Rheumatic Heart Disease: An Analysis of 796 Cases, *Am. Heart J.*, 20:454, 1940.

7 Murphy, G. E.: On Muscle Cells, Aschoff Bodies, and Cardiac Failure in Rheumatic Heart Disease, *Bull. N.Y. Acad. Med.*, 35:619, 1959.

8 Harvey, R. M., Ferrer, M. I., Samet, R., Bader, R. A., Bader, M. E., Cournand, A., and Richards, D. W.: Mechanical and Myocardial Factors in Rheumatic Heart Disease with Mitral Stenosis, *Circulation*, 11:531, 1955.

9 Soloff, L. A., Zatuchni, J., and Mark, G. E., Jr.: Myocardial and Valvular Factors in Rheumatic Heart Disease with Mitral Stenosis: An Analysis Based upon the Combined Techniques of Cardiac Catheterization and Sequential Venous Angiocardiography, *Am. J. Med. Sci.*, 233:518, 1957.

10 Fleming, H. A., and Wood, P.: The Myocardial Factor in Mitral Valve Disease, *Br. Heart J.*, 21:117, 1959.

11 Murphy, G. E.: The Characteristic Rheumatic Lesions of Striated and of Non-striated or Smooth Muscle Cells of the Heart, *Medicine (Baltimore)*, 42:73, 1963.

12 Miller, G. A. H., Kirklin, J. W., and Swan, H. J. C.: Myocardial Function and Left Ventricular Volumes in Acquired Valvular Insufficiency, *Circulation*, 31:374, 1965.

13 Feigenbaum, H., Campbell, R. W., Wunsch, C. M., and Steinmetz, E. F.: Evaluation of the Left Ventricle in Patients with Mitral Stenosis, *Circulation*, 34:462, 1966.

14 Grismer, J. T., Anderson, W. R., and Weiss, L.: Chronic Occlusive Rheumatic Coronary Vasculitis and Myocardial Dysfunction, *Am. J. Cardiol.*, 20:739, 1967.

15 Kasalicky, J., Hurycy, J., Widimsky, J., Dejdar, R., Metys, R., and Stanek, V.: Left Heart Haemodynamics at Rest and during Exercise in Patients with Mitral Stenosis, *Br. Heart J.*, 30:188, 1968.

16 Heller, S. J., and Carleton, R. A.: Abnormal Left Ventricular Contraction in Patients with Mitral Stenosis, *Circulation*, 42:1099, 1970.

17 Hildner, F. J., Javier, R. P., Cohen, L. S., Samet, P., Nathan, M. J., Yahr, W. Z., and Greenberg, J. J.: Myocardial Dysfunction Associated with Valvular Heart Disease, *Am. J. Cardiol.*, 30:319, 1972.

18 Befeler, B., Kamen, A. R., and MacLeod, C. A.: Coronary Artery Disease and Left Ventricular Function in Mitral Stenosis, *Chest*, 57:435, 1970.

19 Gorlin, R., and Gorlin, S. G.: Hydraulic Formula for Calculation of the Area of the Stenotic Mitral Valve, Other Cardiac Valves, and Central Circulatory Shunts: I, *Am. Heart J.*, 41:1, 1951.

20 Spann, J. F., Jr.: Heart Failure and Ventricular Hypertrophy: Altered Cardiac Contractility and Compensatory Mechanisms, *Am. J. Cardiol.*, 23:504, 1969.

21 Williams, J. F., Jr., and Potter, R. D.: Normal Contractile State of Hypertrophied Myocardium following Pulmonary Artery Constriction in the Cat, *J. Clin. Invest.*, 54:1266, 1974.

22 Sasayama, S., Theroux, P., Romero, M., Bishop, S., Bloor, C., Franklin, D., and Ross, J., Jr.: Adaptions of the Left Ventricle to Chronic Pressure Overload, *Am. J. Cardiol.*, 35:167, 1975.

23 Ross, J., Jr., Covell, J. W., and Mahler, F.: Contractile Responses of the Left Ventricle to Acute and Chronic Stress, *Eur. J. Cardiol.*, 1:325, 1974.

24 Alpert, N. R. (ed.): "Cardiac Hypertrophy," Academic Press, Inc., New York, 1971, p. 641.

25 Cohen, J., and Shah, P. M. (eds.): Cardiac Hypertrophy and Cardiomyopathy, *Circ. Res.*, 35(suppl. 2):I-223, 1974.

26 McCullagh, W. H., Covell, J. W., and Ross, J., Jr.: Left Ventricular Dilatation and Diastolic Compliance Changes during Chronic Volume Overloading, *Circulation*, 45:943, 1972.

27 Meerson, F. Z., and Kapelko, V. K.: The Contractile Function of the Myocardium in Two Types of Cardiac Adaptation to a Chronic Load, *Cardiology*, 57:183, 1972.

28 Cooper, G., Puga, F., Zujko, K. J., Harrison, C. E., and Coleman, H. N.: Normal Myocardial Function and Energetics in Volume-Overload Hypertrophy in the Cat, *Circ. Res.*, 32:140, 1973.

29 Ross, J., Jr.: Adaptations of the Left Ventricle to Chronic Volume Overload, *Circ. Res.*, 35(suppl. 2):II-64, 1974.

30 Meerson, F. Z.: Development of Modern Components of the

Mechanism of Cardiac Hypertrophy, *Circ. Res.,* 35(suppl. 2):II-58, 1974.

31 Woodson, R. D., Torrance, J., and Shappell, S. D.: The Effect of Cardiac Disease on Hemoglobin-Oxygen Binding, *J. Clin. Invest.,* 49:1349, 1970.

32 Eckberg, D. L., Drabinsky, M., and Braunwald, E.: Defective Cardiac Parasympathetic Control in Patients with Heart Disease, *N. Engl. J. Med.,* 285:877, 1971.

33 Braunwald, E., and Ross, J., Jr.: The Ventricular End-diastolic Pressure: Appraisal of Its Value in the Recognition of Ventricular Failure in Man, *Am. J. Med.,* 34:147, 1963.

34 Ross, J., Jr., Covell, J. W., Sonnenblick, E. H., and Braunwald, E.: Contractile State of the Heart Characterized by Force-Velocity Relations in Variably Afterloaded and Isovolumic Beats, *Circ. Res.,* 18:149, 1966.

35 Ross, J., Jr., Gault, J. S., Mason, D. T., Linhart, J. W., and Braunwald, E.: Left Ventricular Performance during Muscular Exercise in Patients with and without Cardiac Dysfunction, *Circulation,* 34:597, 1966.

36 Gault, J. H., Ross, J., Jr., and Braunwald, E.: Contractile State of the Left Ventricle in Man: Instantaneous Tension-Velocity-Length Relations in Patients with and without Disease of the Left Ventricular Myocardium, *Circ. Res.,* 22:451, 1968.

37 Mason, D. T.: Usefulness and Limitations of the Rate of Rise of Intraventricular Pressure (dp/dt) in the Evaluation of Myocardial Contractility in Man, *Am. J. Cardiol.,* 23:516, 1969.

38 Sonnenblick, E. H., Parmley, W. W., Urschel, C. W., and Brutsaert, D. L.: Ventricular Function: Evaluation of Myocardial Contractility in Health and Disease, *Prog. Cardiovasc. Dis.,* 12:449, 1970.

39 Mason, D. T., Spann, J. F., Jr., Zelis, R., and Amsterdam, E. A.: Alterations of Hemodynamics and Myocardial Mechanics in Patients with Congestive Heart Failure: Pathophysiologic Mechanisms and Assessment of Cardiac Function and Ventricular Contractility, *Prog. Cardiovasc. Dis.,* 12:507, 1970.

40 Paraskos, J. A., Grossman, W., Saltz, S., Dalen, J. E., and Dexter, J.: A Noninvasive Technique for the Determination of Velocity of Circumferential Fiber Shortening in Man, *Circ. Res.,* 29:610, 1971.

41 Noble, M. I. M.: Problems Concerning the Application of Concepts of Muscle Mechanics to the Determination of the Contractile State of the Heart, *Circulation,* 45:252, 1972.

42 Levine, H. J.: Compliance of the Left Ventricle, *Circulation,* 46:423, 1972.

43 Mirsky, I., Pasternac, A., and Ellsion, R. C.: General Index for the Assessment of Cardiac Function, *Am. J. Cardiol.,* 30:483, 1972.

44 Mitchell, J. H., Hefner, L. L., and Monroe, R. G.: Performance of the Left Ventricle, *Am. J. Med.,* 53:481, 1972.

45 Mason, D. T., Zelis, R., Amsterdam, E. A., and Massumi, R. A.: Clinical Determination of Left Ventricular Contractility by Hemodynamics and Myocardial Mechanics, in P. N. Yu and J. F. Goodwin (eds.), "Progress in Cardiology," Lea & Febiger, Philadelphia, 1972, p. 121.

46 Sonnenblick, E. H., and Brutsaert, D. L.: V_{max}: Its Relation to Contractility of Heart Muscle, *Cardiology,* 57:11, 1972.

47 Van den Bos, G. C., Elizinga, G., Westerhof, N., and Noble, M. I. M.: Problems in the Use of Indices of Myocardial Contractility, *Cardiovasc. Res.,* 7:834, 1973.

48 Ross, J., Jr., and Peterson, K. L.: On the Assessment of Cardiac Inotropic State, *Circulation,* 47:435, 1973.

49 Rackley, C. E., and Hood, W. P., Jr.: Quantitative Angiographic Evaluation and Pathophysiologic Mechanisms in Valvular Heart Disease, *Prog. Cardiovasc. Dis.,* 15:427, 1973.

50 Dodge, H. T., Kennedy, J. W., and Petersen, J. L.: Quantitative Angiocardiographic Methods in the Evaluation of Valvular Heart Disease, *Prog. Cardiovasc. Dis.,* 16:1, 1973.

51 Brutsaert, D. L., and Sonnenblick, E. H.: Cardiac Muscle Mechanics in the Evaluation of Myocardial Contractility and Pump Function: Problems, Concepts, and Directions, *Prog. Cardiovasc. Dis.,* 16:337, 1973.

52 Peterson, K. L. Skloven, D., Ludbrook, P., Uther, J. B., and Ross, J., Jr.: Comparison of Isovolumic and Ejection Phase Indices of Myocardial Performance in Man, *Circulation,* 49:1088, 1974.

53 Grossman, W. (ed.): "Cardiac Catheterization and Angiography," Lea & Febiger, Philadelphia, 1974, p. 339.

54 Dodge, H. T., Frimer, M., and Stewart, D. K.: Functional Evaluation of Hypertrophied Heart in Man, *Circ. Res.,* 35(suppl. 2):II-122, 1974.

55 Braunwald, E., Ross, J., Jr., and Sonnenblick, E. H.: "Mechanisms of Contraction of the Normal and Failing Heart," 2d ed., Little, Brown and Company, Boston, 1976, p. 417.

56 Naqvi, S. Z., Chisholm, A. W., Standen, J. R., and Shane, S. J.: Relative Insensitivity of Isovolumic Phase Indices in the Assessment of Left Ventricular Function. *Am. Heart J.,* 91:577, 1976.

57 Quinones, M. A., Gasseh, W. H., Alexander, J. K.: Influence of Acute Changes in Preload, Afterload, Contractile State and Heart Rate on Ejection and Isovolumic Indices of Myocardial Contractility in Man, *Circulation,* 53:293, 1976.

58 Taylor, R. R., Covell, J. W., Sonnenblick, E. H., and Ross, J., Jr.: Dependence of Ventricular Distensibility on Filling of Opposite Ventricle, *Am. J. Physiol.,* 213:711, 1967.

59 Herbert, W. H., and Yellin, E.: Left Ventricular Diastolic Pressure Elevation Consequent to Pulmonary Stenosis, *Circulation,* 40:887, 1969.

60 Kelly, D. T., Spotnitz, H. M., Beiser, G. D., Pierce, J. E., and Epstein, S. E.: Effects of Chronic Right Ventricular Volume and Pressure Loading on Left Ventricular Performance, *Circulation,* 44:403, 1971.

61 Bemis, C. E., Serur, J. R., Borkenhagen, D., Sonnenblick, E. H., and Urschel, C. W.: Influence of Right Ventricular Filling Pressure on Left Ventricular Pressure and Dimension, *Circ. Res.,* 34:498, 1974.

62 Mitchell, A. M., Sackett, C. H., Hunvicker, W. J. and Levine, S. A.: The Clinical Features of Aortic Stenosis, *Am. Heart J.,* 48:684, 1954.

63 Wood, P.: Aortic Stenosis, *Am. J. Cardiol.,* 1:553, 1958.

64 Hancock, E. W., and Fleming, P. R.: Aortic Stenosis, *Q. J. Med.,* 29:209, 1960.

65 Cullhed, I.: "Aortic Stenosis," Almqvist and Wiksells, Uppsala, Sweden, 1964.

66 Kennedy, J. W., Twiss, R. D., Blackmon, J. R., and Dodge, H. T.: Quantitative Angiocardiography: III. Relationships of Left Ventricular Pressure, Volume, and Mass in Aortic Valve Disease, *Circulation,* 38:838, 1968.

67 Anderson, F. L., Tsagaris, T. J., Tikoff, G., Thorne, J. L., Schmidt, A. M., and Kuida, H.: Hemodynamic Effects of Exercise in Patients with Aortic Stenosis, *Am. J. Med.,* 48:872, 1969.

68 Lee, S. J. K., Honsson, G., Bevegård, S., Karlöm, H.: Hemodynamic Changes at Rest and during Exercise in Patients with Aortic Stenosis of Varying Severity, *Am. Heart J.,* 79:318, 1970.

69 Levine, H. J., McIntyre, K. M., Lipana, J. G., and Bing, O. H.: Force-Velocity Relations in Failing and Nonfailing Hearts of Subjects with Aortic Stenosis, *Am. J. Med. Sci.,* 259:79, 1970.

70 Friedman, W. F., Modlinger, J., and Morgan, J. R.: Serial Hemodynamic Observations in Asymptomatic Children with Valvar Aortic Stenosis, *Circulation,* 43:91, 1971.

71 Bache, R. J., Wang, Y., and Jorgensen, C. R.: Hemodynamic Effects of Exercise in Isolated Valvular Aortic Stenosis, *Circulation,* 44:1003, 1971.

72 Frank, S., Johnson, A., and Ross, J., Jr.: Natural History of Valvular Aortic Stenosis, *Br. Heart J.*, 35:41, 1973.

73 Jelinek, V. M. J., McDonald, I. G., and Hale, G. S.: Haemodynamic Basis for Aortic Valve Replacement, *Br. Heart J.*, 36:69, 1974.

74 Vincent, W. R., Buckberg, G. D., and Hoffman, J. E.: Left Ventricular Subendocardial Ischemia in Severe Valvular and Supravalvular Aortic Stenosis: A Common Mechanism, *Circulation*, 49:326, 1974.

75 Hirshfeld, J. W., Jr., Epstein, S. E., Roberts, A. J., Glancy, D. L., and Morrow, A. G.: Indices Predicting Long-Term Survival after Valve Replacement in Patients with Aortic Regurgitation and Patients with Aortic Stenosis, *Circulation*, 50:1190, 1974.

76 Buckberg, G., Edber, L., Herman, M., Gorlin, R.: Ischemia in Aortic Stenosis: Hemodynamic Prediction, *Am. J. Cardiol.*, 35:778, 1975.

77 Brazier, J. R., Buckberg, G. D.: Effects of Tachycardia on the Adequacy of Subendocardial Oxygen Delivery in Experimental Aortic Stenosis, *Am. Heart J.*, 90:222, 1975.

78 Harris, C. N., Kaplan, M. A., Parker, D. P., Dunne, E. F., Cowell, H. S., and Ellestad, M. H.: Aortic Stenosis, Angina, and Coronary Artery Disease: Interrelations, *Br. Heart J.*, 37:656, 1975.

78a Hancock, E. W.: Aortic Stenosis, Angina Pectoris, and Coronary Artery Disease, *Am. Heart J.*, 93:382, 1977.

79 Anderson, J. A., Hansen, B. F., and Lyngborg, K.: Isolated Valvular Aortic Stenosis, *Acta Med. Scand.*, 197:61, 1975.

80 Liedtke, J. S., Gentzler, R. D., Babb, J. E., Hunter, A. S., and Gault, J. H.: Determinants of Cardiac Performance in Severe Aortic Stenosis, *Chest*, 69:192, 1976.

81 Trenouth, R. S., Phelps, N. C., Neill, W. A.: Determinants of Left Ventricular Hypertrophy and Oxygen Supply in Chronic Aortic Valve Disease, *Circulation*, 53:644, 1976.

82 Kroetz, F. W., Leonard, J. J., Shaver, J. A., Leon, D. F., Lancaster, J. F., and Beamer, V. L.: The Effect of Atrial Contraction of Left Ventricular Performance in Valvular Aortic Stenosis, *Circulation*, 35:852, 1967.

83 Epstein, E. J., Doukas, N. G., Coulshed, N., and Brown, A. K.: Right Ventricular Systolic Pressure Gradients in Aortic Valve Disease, *Br. Heart J.*, 29:490, 1967.

84 Cooper, T., Braunwald, E., and Morrow, A. G.: Pulsus Alternans in Aortic Stenosis: Hemodynamic Observations in 50 Patients Studied by Left Heart Catheterization, *Circulation*, 18:64, 1958.

85 Leak, D.: Effort Syncope in Aortic Stenosis, *Br. Heart J.*, 21:289, 1959.

86 Schwartz, L. S., Goldfischer, J., Sprague, G. J., and Schwartz, S. P.: Syncope and Sudden Death in Aortic Stenosis, *Am. J. Cardiol.*, 23:647, 1969.

87 Mark, A. L., Abboud, F. M., Schmid, P. G., and Heistad, D. D.: Reflex Vascular Responses to Left Ventricular Outflow Obstruction and Activation of Ventricular Baroreceptors in Dogs, *J. Clin. Invest.*, 52:1147, 1973.

88 Roberts, W. C.: The Structure of the Aortic Valve in Clinically Isolated Aortic Stenosis: An Autopsy Study of 162 Patients over 15 Years of Age, *Circulation*, 42:91, 1970.

89 Roberts, W. C., Perloff, J. K., and Constantino, T.: Severe Valvular Aortic Stenosis in Patients over 65 Years of Age: A Clinicopathologic Study, *Am. J. Cardiol.*, 27:497, 1971.

90 Schlant, R. C.: Calcific Aortic Stenosis, *Am. J. Cardiol.*, 27:581, 1971.

91 Katznelson, G., Hreissaty, R. M., Levinson, G. E., Stein, S. W., and Abelmann, W. H.: Combined Aortic and Mitral Stenosis: A Clinical and Physiological Study, *Am. J. Med.*, 29:242, 1960.

92 Honey, M.: Clinical and Haemodynamic Observations on Combined Mitral and Aortic Stenosis, *Br. Heart J.*, 23:545, 1961.

93 Morrow, A. G., Awe, W. C., and Braunwald, E.: Combined Mitral and Aortic Stenosis, *Br. Heart J.*, 24:606, 1962.

94 Zitnik, R. S., Piemme, T. E., Messer, R. J., Reed, D. P., Haynes, F. W., and Dexter, L.: The Masking of Aortic Stenosis by Mitral Stenosis, *Am. Heart J.*, 69:22, 1965.

95 Segal, J., Harvey, W. P., and Hufnagel, C.: A Clinical Study of One Hundred Cases of Severe Aortic Insufficiency, *Am. J. Med.*, 21:200, 1956.

96 Urschel, C. W., Covell, J. W., Sonnenblick, E. H., Ross, J., Jr., and Braunwald, E.: Myocardial Mechanics in Aortic and Mitral Valvular Regurgitation: The Concept of Instantaneous Impedance as a Determinant of the Performance of the Intact Heart, *J. Clin. Invest.*, 47:967, 1968.

97 Lewis, R. P., Bristow, J. D., and Griswold, H. E.: Exercise Hemodynamics in Aortic Regurgitation, *Am. Heart J.*, 80:171, 1970.

98 Gault, J. H., Covell, J. W., Braunwald, E., and Ross, J., Jr.: Left Ventricular Performance following Correction of Free Aortic Regurgitation, *Circulation*, 42:773, 1970.

99 Spagnuolo, M., Kloth, H., Taranta, A., Doyle, E., and Pasternack, B.: Natural History of Aortic Regurgitation: Criteria Predictive of Death, Congestive Heart Failure, and Angina in Young Patients, *Circulation*, 44:368, 1971.

100 Taylor, R. R., and Hopkins, B. E.: Left Ventricular Response to Experimentally Induced Chronic Aortic Regurgitation, *Cardiovasc. Res.*, 6:404, 1972.

101 Goldschlager, N., Pfeifer, J., Cohen, K., Popper, R., and Selzer A.: The Natural History of Aortic Regurgitation: A Clinical and Hemodynamic Study, *Am. J. Med.*, 54:577, 1973.

102 Griggs, D. M., Jr., and Chen, C. C.: Coronary Hemodynamics and Regional Myocardial Metabolism in Experimental Aortic Insufficiency, *J. Clin. Invest.*, 53:1599, 1974.

103 Bolen, J. L., Hollaway, E. R., Zener, J. C., Harrison, D. C., and Alderman, E. L.: Evaluation of Left Ventricular Function in Patients with Aortic Regurgitation Using Afterload Stress, *Circulation*, 53:132, 1976.

104 Bolen, J. L., and Alderman, E. L.: Hemodynamic Consequences of Afterload Reduction in Patients with Chronic Aortic Regurgitation, *Circulation*, 53:879, 1976.

105 Smith, H. J., Neutze, J. M., Roche, H. G., Agnew, T. M., and Barratt-Boyes, B. G.: The Natural History of Rheumatic Aortic Regurgitation and the Indications for Surgery, *Br. Heart J.*, 38:147, 1976.

106 Luomanmäki, K., and Heikkilä, J.: Estimation of the Severity of Aortic Incompetence from Prolongation of the Left Ventricular Ejection Time, *Acta Med. Scand.*, 188:107, 1970.

107 Parker, E., Craige, E., and Hood, W. P., Jr.: The Austin Flint Murmur and the a Wave of the Apexcardiogram in Aortic Regurgitation, *Circulation*, 43:349, 1971.

108 Gorlin, R., and Goodale, W. T.: Changing Blood Pressure in Aortic Insufficiency: Its Clinical Significance, *N. Engl. J. Med.*, 255:77, 1956.

109 Welch, G. H., Braunwald, E., and Sarnoff, S. J.: Hemodynamic Effects of Quantitatively Varied Experimental Aortic Regurgitation, *Circulation Res.*, 5:546, 1957.

110 Rees, J. R., Epstein, E. J., Criley, J. M., and Ross, R. S.: Hemodynamic Effects of Severe Aortic Regurgitation, *Br. Heart J.*, 26:412, 1964.

111 Oliver, G. C., Jr., Gazetopoulos, N., and Deuchar, D. C.: Reversed Mitral Diastolic Gradient in Aortic Incompetence, *Br. Heart J.*, 29:239, 1967.

112 Lochaya, S. Igarashi, M., and Shaffer, A. B.: Late Diastolic Mitral Regurgitation Secondary to Aortic Regurgitation: Its Relationship to the Austin Flint Murmur, *Am. Heart J.*, 74:161, 1967.

113 Regan, T. J., DeFazio, V., Binak, K., and Hellems, H. K.: Norepinephrine Induced Pulmonary Congestion in Patients

with Aortic Valve Regurgitation, *J. Clin. Invest.*, 38:1564, 1959.

114 Kloster, F. E., Bristow, J. D., Lewis, R. P., and Griswold, H. E.: Pharmacodynamic Studies in Aortic Regurgitation, *Am. J. Cardiol.*, 19:644, 1967.

115 Judge, T. P., Kennedy, J. W., Bennett, L. J., Wills, R. E., Murray, J. A., and Blackmon, J. R.: Quantiative Hemodynamic Effects of Heart Rate in Aortic Regurgitation, *Circulation*, 44:355, 1971.

116 Gorlin, R., Haynes, F. W., Goodale, W. T., Sawyer, C. G., Dow, J. W., and Dexter, L.: Studies of the Circulatory Dynamics in Mitral Stenosis: II. Altered Dyanmics at Rest, *Am. Heart J.*, 41:30, 1951.

117 Gorlin, R., Sawyer, C. G., Haynes, F. W., Goodale, W. T., and Dexter, L.: Effects of Exercise on Circulatory Dynamaics in Mitral Stenosis, *Am. Heart J.*, 41:192, 1951.

118 Gorlin, R., Lewis, B. M., Haynes, F. W., Spiegl, R. J., and Dexter, L.: Factors Regulating Pulmonary "Capillary" Pressure in Mitral Stenosis: IV, *Am. Heart J.*, 41:834, 1951.

119 Lewis, B. M., Gorlin, R., Houssay, H. E. H., Haynes, F. W., and Dexter, L.: Clinical and Physiological Correlation in Patients with Mitral Stenosis: V., *Am. Heart J.*, 43:2, 1952.

120 Dexter, L., McDonald, L., Rabinowitz, M., Saxton, G. A., Jr., and Haynes, F. W.: Medical Aspects of Patients Undergoing Surgery for Mitral Stenosis, *Circulation*, 9:758, 1954.

121 Wood, P.: An Appreciation of Mitral Stenosis: I. Clinical Features. II. Investigations and Results, *Br. Med. J.*, 1:1051, 113, 1954.

122 McDonald, L., Dealy, J. B., Jr., Rabinowitz, M., and Dexter, L.: Clinical Physiological and Pathological Findings in Mitral Stenosis and Regurgitation, *Medicine (Baltimore)*, 36:237, 1957.

123 Carman, G. H., and Lange, R. L.: Variant Hemodynamic Patterns in Mitral Stenosis, *Circulation*, 24:712, 1961.

124 Hugenholtz, P. G., Ryan, T. J., Stein, S. W., and Abelmann, W. H.: The Spectrum of Pure Mitral Stenosis: Hemodynamic Studies in Relation to Clinical Disability, *Am. J. Cardiol.*, 10:773, 1962.

125 Olesen, K. H.: The Natural History of 271 Patients with Mitral Stenosis under Medical Treatment, *Br. Heart J.*, 24:349, 1962.

126 Werkö, L.: "Mitral Valvular Disease: Hemodynamics Studies of the Consequences for the Circulation," The Williams & Wilkins Company, Baltimore, 1964.

127 Heidenreich, F. P., Thompson, M. E., Shaver, J. A., and Leonard, J. J.: Left Atrial Transport in Mitral Stenosis, *Circulation*, 40:545, 1969.

128 Dubin, A. A., March, H. W., Cohn, K., and Selzer, A.: Longitudinal Hemodynamic and Clinical Study of Mitral Stenosis, *Circulation*, 44:381, 1971.

129 Selzer, A., and Cohn, K. E.: Natural History of Mitral Stenosis: A Review, *Circulation*, 45:878, 1972.

130 Roberts, W. C., and Perloff, J. K.: Mitral Valvular Disease: A Clinicopathologic Survey of the Conditions Causing the Mitral Valve to Function Abnormally, *Ann. Intern. Med.*, 77:939, 1972.

131 Walston, A., Peter, R. H., Morris, J. J., Kong, Y., and Behar, V. S.: Clinical Implications of Pulmonary hypertension in Mitral Stenosis, *Am. J. Cardiol.*, 32:650, 1973.

132 Cross, C. E., Shaver, J. A., Wilson, R. J., and Robin, E. D.: Mitral Stenosis and Pulmonary Fibrosis: Special Reference to Pulmonary Edema and Lung Lymphatic Function, *Arch. Intern. Med.*, 125:248, 1970.

133 Heller, S. J., and Carlton, R. A.: Abnormal Left Ventricular Contraction in Patients with Mitral Stenosis, *Circulation*, 42:1099, 1970.

134 Parker, F., Jr., and Weiss, S.: The Nature and Significance of the Structural Changes in the Lungs in Mitral Stenosis, *Am. J. Pathol.*, 12:573, 1936.

135 Emanuel, R., and Ross, K.: Pulmonary Hypertension in Rheumatic Heart Disease, *Prog. Cardiovasc. Dis.*, 9:401, 1967.

136 Wilhelmsen, L.: Lung Mechanics in Rheumatic Valvular Disease, *Acta Med. Scand.*, 184(suppl.):489, 1968.

137 Ward, C., and Hancock, B. W.: Extreme Pulmonary Hypertension Caused by Mitral Valve Disease: Natural History and Results of Surgery, *Br. Heart J.*, 37:74, 1975.

138 West, J. B.: "Ventilation/Blood Flow and Gas Exchange," 2d ed., F. A. Davis Company, Philadelphia, 1970, p. 117.

139 Dollery, C. T., and West, J. B.: Regional Uptake of Radioactive Oxygen, Carbon Monoxide and Carbon Dioxide in the Lungs of Patients with Mitral Stenosis, *Circ. Res.*, 8:765, 1960.

140 Friedman, W. F., and Braunwald, E.: Alterations in Regional Pulmonary Blood Flow in Mitral Valve Disease Studied by Radioisotope Scanning: A Simple Nontraumatic Technique for Estimation of Left Atrial Pressure, *Circulation*, 34:363, 1966.

141 Dalen, J. E., Matloff, J. M., Evans, G. L., Hoppin, F. G., Jr., Bhardwaj, P., Harken, D. E., and Dexter, L.: Early Reduction of Pulmonary Vascular Resistance after Mitral-valve Replacement, *N. Engl. J. Med.*, 273:509, 1965.

142 Zerner, J. C., Hancock, E. W., Shumway, N. E., and Harrison, D. C.: Regression of Extreme Pulmonary Hypertension After Mitral Valve Surgery, *Am. J. Cardiol.*, 30:820, 1972.

143 Ward, C., and Hancock, B. W.: Extreme Pulmonary Hypertension Caused by Mitral Valve Disease: Natural History and Results of Surgery, *Br. Heart J.*, 37:74, 1975.

144 Gorlin, R., Lewis, B. M., Haynes, F. W., and Dexter, L.: Studies of the Circulatory Dynamics at Rest in Mitral Valvular Regurgitation with and without Stenosis, *Am. Heart J.*, 43:357, 1952.

145 Braunwald, E.: Mitral Regurgitation: Physiologic, Clinical and Surgical Considerations, *N. Engl. J. Med.*, 281:425, 1969.

146 Selzer, A., and Katayama, F.: Mitral Regurgitation: Clinical Patterns, Pathophysiology and Natural History, *Medicine (Baltimore)*, 51:337, 1972.

147 Eckberg, D. L., Gault, J. H., Bouchard, R. L., Karliner, J. S., and Ross, J., Jr.: Mechanics of Left Ventricular Contraction in Chronic Severe Mitral Regurgitation, *Circulation*, 47:1252, 1973.

148 Vokonas, P. S., Gorlin, R., Cohen, P. F., Herman, M. V., and Sonnenblick, E. H.: Dynamic Geometry of the Left Ventricle in Mitral Regurgitation, *Circulation*, 48:768, 1973.

149 Braunwald, E., Welch, G. H., Jr., and Morrow, A. G.: The Effects of Acutely Increased Systemic Resistance on the Left Atrial Pressure Pulse: A Method for the Clinical Detection of Mitral Insufficiency, *J. Clin. Invest.*, 37:35, 1958.

150 Jose, A. D., Taylor, R. R., and Bernstein, L.: The Influence of Atrial Pressure on Mitral Incompetence in Man, *J. Clin. Invest.*, 43:2094, 1964.

151 Goodman, D. J., Rossen, R. M., Holloway, E. L., Alderman, E. L., and Harrison, D. C.: Effect of Nitroprusside on Left Ventricular Dynamics in Mitral Regurgitation, *Circulation*, 50:1025, 1974.

152 Levinson, D. C., Wilburne, M., Meehan, J. P., Jr., and Shubin, H.: Evidence for Retrograde Transpulmonary Propagation of the V (or Regurgitant) Wave in Mitral Insufficiency, *Am. J. Cardiol.*, 2:159, 1958.

153 Braunwald, E., and Awe, W. C.: The Syndrome of Severe Mitral Regurgitation with Normal Left Atrial Pressure, *Circulation*, 27:29, 1963.

154 Gould, L., and Lyon, A. F.: Severe Mitral Regurgitation with Normal Pulmonary Artery Wedge Pressures, *Ann. Intern. Med.*, 66:748, 1967.

155 Ronan, J. A., Steelman, R. B., DeLeon, A. C., Waters, T. J., Perloff, J. K., and Harvey, W. P.: The Clinical Diagnosis of Acute Severe Mitral Insufficiency, *Am. J. Cardiol.*, 27:284, 1971.

156 Marshall, H. W., Woodward, E., Jr., and Wood, E. H.: Hemodynamic Methods for Differentiation of Mitral Stenosis and Regurgitation, *Am. J. Cardiol.*, 2:24, 1958.

157 Shillingford, J. P.: The Estimation of Severity of Mitral Incompetence, *Prog. Cardiovasc. Dis.*, 5:248, 1962.

158 Sinclair-Smith, B. C.: Measurement of Valvular Insufficiency, in D. A. Bloomfield (ed.), "Dye Curves: The Theory and Practice of Indicator Dilution," University Park Press, Baltimore, 1974, p. 145.

159 Seymour, J., Emanuel, R., and Pattinson, N.: Acquired Pulmonary Stenosis, *Br. Heart J.*, 30:776, 1968.

160 Alday, L. W., Moreyra, E.: Calcific Pulmonary Stenosis, *Br. Heart J.*, 35:887, 1973.

161 Vela, J. E., Contreras, R., and Sosa, F. R.: Rheumatic Pulmonary Valve Disease, *Am. J. Cardiol.*, 23:12, 1969.

162 Brodeur, M. T. H., Lees, M. H., Bristow, J. D., Kloster, F. E., and Griswold, H. E.: Right Ventricular Volumes in Pulmonic Valve Disease, *Am. J. Cardiol.*, 19:671, 1967.

163 Hoffmann, J. I. E.: The Natural History of Congenital Isolated Pulmonic and Aortic Stenosis, *Ann. Rev. Med.*, 20:15, 1969.

164 Johnson, L. W., Grossman, W., Dalen, J. E., and Dexter, L.: Pulmonic Stenosis in the Adult: Long-Term Follow-up Results, *N. Engl. J. Med.*, 287:1159, 1972.

165 Hamby, R. I., and Gulotta, S. J.: Pulmonic Valvular Insufficiency: Etiology, Recognition and Management, *Am. Heart J.*, 74:110, 1967.

166 Holmes, J. C., Fowler, N. D., and Kaplan, S.: Pulmonary Valve Insufficiency, *Am. J. Med.*, 44:851, 1968.

167 Criscitiello, M. G., and Harvey, W. P.: Clinical Recognition of Congenital Pulmonary Valve Insufficiency, *Am. J. Cardiol.*, 20:765, 1967.

168 Schloff, L. D., and Wang, Y.: Congenital Isolated Pulmonic Regurgitation, *Chest*, 55:254, 1969.

169 Rokseth, R.: Isolated Pulmonic Valvular Regurgitation: A Report on Nine New Cases, *Acta Med. Scand.*, 185:489, 1969.

170 Fowler, N. O., and Duchesne, E. R.: Effect of Experimental Pulmonary Valvular Insufficiency on the Circulation, *J. Thorac. Surg.*, 35:643, 1958.

171 Ellison, R. G., Brown, W. J., Jr., and Yeh, T. J.: Surgical Significance of Acute and Chronic Pulmonary Valvular Insufficiency, *J. Thorac. Cardiovasc. Surg.*, 60:549, 1970.

172 Collins, N. P., Braunwald, E., and Morrow, A. G.: Detection of Pulmonic and Tricuspid Valvular Regurgitation by Means of Indicator Solutions, *Circulation*, 20:561, 1959.

173 Wanzer, S. W., Cudkowicz, L., and Daley, R.: Diagnosis of Pulmonary Regurgitation by a Dye Method, *Br. Heart J.*, 22:720, 1960.

174 Smith, J. A., and Levine, S. A.: The Clinical Features of Tricuspid Stenosis, *Am. Heart J.*, 23:739, 1942.

175 Yu, P. N., Harken, D. E., Lovejoy, F. W., Jr., Nye, R. E., Jr., and Mahoney, E. B.: Clinical and Hemodynamic Studies of Tricuspid Stenosis, *Circulation*, 13:680, 1956.

176 Perloff, J. K., and Harvey, W. P.: Clinical Recognition of Tricuspid Stenosis, *Circulation*, 22:346, 1960.

177 Kitchin, A., and Turner, R.: Diagnosis and Treatment of Tricuspid Stenosis, *Br. Heart J.*, 26:354, 1964.

178 Keefe, J. F., Wolk, M. J., and Levine, H. J.: Isolated Tricuspid Valvular Stenosis, *Am. J. Cardiol.*, 25:252, 1970.

179 El-Sheriff, N.: Rheumatic Tricuspid Stenosis. A Haemodynamic Correlation, *Br. Heart J.*, 33:16, 1971.

180 Morgan, J. R., Forker, A. D., Coates, J. R., and Myers, W. S.: Isolated Tricuspid Stenosis, *Circulation*, 44:729, 1971.

181 Finnegan, P., and Abrams, L. D.: Isolated Tricuspid Stenosis, *Br. Heart J.*, 35:1207, 1973.

182 Sepulveda, G., and Lukas, D. A.: The Diagnosis of Tricuspid Insufficiency: Clinical Features in 60 Cases with Associated Mitral Valve Disease, *Circulation*, 11:552, 1955.

183 Osborn, K. R., Jones, R. C., and Jahnke, E. J.: Traumatic Tricuspid Insufficiency: Hemodynamic Data and Surgical Treatment, *Circulation*, 30:217, 1964.

184 Hansing, C. E., and Rowe, G. G.: Tricuspid Insufficiency: A Study of Hemodynamics and Pathogenesis, *Circulation*, 45:793, 1972.

185 Takabatake, Y., Iisuka, M.: Pathophysiology of Tricuspid Insufficiency: Clinical and Experimental Study, *Jap. Circ. J.*, 38:843, 1974.

186 Robin, E., Thoms, N. W., Arbulu, A., Ganguly, S. N., and Magnisalis, K.: Hemodynamic Consequences of Total Removal of the Tricuspid Valve without Prosthetic Replacement, *Am. J. Cardiol.*, 35:481, 1975.

187 Reisman, M., Hipona, F. A., Bloor, C. M., and Talner, N. S.: Congenital Tricuspid Insufficiency, *J. Pediatr.*, 66:869, 1965.

188 Ahn, A. J., and Segal, B. L.: Isolated Tricuspid Insufficiency: Clinical Features, Diagnosis, and Management, *Prog. Cardiovasc. Dis.*, 9:166, 1966.

189 Morgan, J. R., and Forker, A. D.: Isolated Tricuspid Insufficiency, *Circulation*, 43:559, 1971.

190 Storber, W., Cohen, L. S., Waldmann, T. A., and Braunwald, E.: Tricuspid Regurgitation: A Newly Recognized Case of Protein-losing Enteropathy, Lymphocytopenia and Immunologic Deficiency, *Am. J. Med.*, 44:842, 1968.

191 Cairns, K. B., Kloster, F. E., Bristow, J. D., Lees, M. H., and Griswold, H. E.: Problems in the Hemodynamic Diagnosis of Tricuspid Insufficiency, *Am. Heart J.*, 75:173, 1968.

192 Sobol, B. J., Bottex, G., Emirgil, C., and Gissen, H.: Valvular Insufficiency Occurring during Cardiac Catheterization, *Am. J. Cardiol.*, 14:533, 1964.

60
Clinical Recognition and Medical Management of Rheumatic Heart Disease and Other Acquired Valvular Disease

A
Acute Rheumatic Fever

ELIZABETH W. NUGENT, M.D.

Acute rheumatic fever is a diffuse inflammatory process which specifically affects the heart, joints, and subcutaneous tissues. Diagnosis may be difficult, since the clinical picture is variable, and there is no pathognomonic clinical manifestation or laboratory test. Although acute rheumatic fever and rheumatic heart disease are largely preventable, they continue to be common causes of death from cardiac disease in the United States and in many other countries. There are numerous comprehensive reviews of rheumatic fever and streptococcal infection which present details beyond the scope of this chapter (see Chap. 57 and references 1 and 2).

The association of rheumatic fever with a preceding streptococcal infection was noted as early as 1930.[3-5] Subsequently, epidemiologic evidence has clearly demonstrated that acute rheumatic fever is a sequel of an upper respiratory infection with group A beta-hemolytic streptococcus.[6-8] In general, the epidemiologic features of acute rheumatic fever closely reflect those of streptococcal infection itself. The processes involved during the latent period (1 to 3 weeks in the majority) are less clear.[9,10] The role of an immunologic process in the pathogenesis seems likely.[11-13] Other possibilities include the effect of a streptococcal toxin or of L forms of the streptococcus.[14] A virus may play a role as an additional etiologic agent.[15] The disease is familial, but does not follow a clear Mendelian pattern.[16,17] A combination of inherited and acquired host factors would help explain differences in individual susceptibility. Variations with climate and geography are predominantly due to differences in the socioeconomic factors which influence the attack rate of streptococcal infection itself, including overcrowding, poor nutrition, and inadequate health care.[18]

The incidence of acute rheumatic fever following untreated streptococcal infections is 3 percent during an epidemic in a closed population[8] and 0.3 percent after sporadic, endemic infections.[19] The absolute incidence of acute rheumatic fever is difficult to determine, but the prevalence of rheumatic heart disease reflects the magnitude of the problem. For several decades, rheumatic fever has been declining in prevalence and decreasing in severity in the United States. This trend began prior to the widespread use of penicillin. Although a change in the streptococcus itself may have played a role by alteration in virulence,[20] these trends have more closely paralleled socioeconomic changes.[1] In many of the countries and even in subpopulations of the United States where socioeconomic progress has not advanced to the same degree, the incidence of acute rheumatic fever and the prevalence of rheumatic heart disease appear to be much greater.[21,22]

Acute rheumatic fever and its sequel, rheumatic heart disease, remain major health problems throughout the world today in spite of the fact that prompt recognition and adequate treatment early in the course of streptococcal infections can prevent rheumatic fever. The problem of asymptomatic streptococcal infection still remains to be solved.

Acute rheumatic fever is largely an illness of children between 6 and 15 years of age, but does occur in adults[23] and rarely in children less than 3 years old.[24] There is no difference in incidence by sex and race when socioeconomic factors are considered in the latter.[1] The diagnosis is difficult to establish with certainty because of the variability of the clinical picture and lack of a diagnostic laboratory test. It is frequently a diagnosis of exclusion.

The risk of *recurrences* of acute rheumatic fever and the predisposing host factors are well known.[25,26] Recurrences can be prevented by prophylaxis against subsequent streptococcal infections. Recurrences tend to mimic the clinical pattern of the initial episode,[27] but carditis usually becomes more severe with each subsequent attack.

CLINICAL MANIFESTATIONS

The most common clinical presentation is that of polyarthritis with or without fever in a school-aged child. The incidence of the various manifestations appears to vary geographically and with age.

The *Jones criteria* (Table 60A-1), revised in 1965[28,29] to include evidence of a preceding streptococcal infection, continue to serve as a guide to diagnosis. Since no clinical manifestation or laboratory finding occurs exclusively in acute rheumatic fever, use of the Jones criteria yields a diagnosis based on statistical probabilities. The presence of two major or one major and two or more minor manifestations makes the diagnosis of acute rheumatic fever likely if there is evidence of preceding streptococcal infection. These criteria were designed for use only during the acute or early phase of the disease.

Laboratory studies giving evidence of inflammatory process and preceding streptococcal infection in the setting of compatible clinical manifestations form the basis of the diagnosis when other diagnoses have been excluded. The clinical course of the illness is frequently helpful in confirming the diagnosis of acute rheumatic fever and should not be prematurely altered by the use of anti-inflammatory drugs until the diagnosis is clear.

Arthritis

Inflammation of the joints is the most common clinical manifestation. *Arthralgia,* or joint pain alone, is less specific and therefore not a major manifestation of acute rheumatic fever. With arthritis, the joint pain is accompanied by the objective findings of swelling, erythema, and heat. Usually at least two of

TABLE 60A-1
Jones criteria (revised)

Major manifestations	Minor manifestations
Carditis	Previous rheumatic fever or rheumatic heart disease
Polyarthritis	Arthralgia
Chorea	Fever
Erythema marginatum	Acute phase reactions
Subcutaneous nodules	Prolongation of P-R interval

Plus evidence of preceding streptococcal infection

the large joints are involved, frequently the knees, ankles, elbows, and wrists. There is a typical migratory pattern. Untreated, the duration of involvement in each joint is a few days, with all joint symptoms usually subsiding in 2 to 4 weeks. The term *migratory polyarthritis* is appropriate. Although the pain is usually exquisite and out of proportion to the physical findings, prompt therapy with anti-inflammatory drugs is not indicated unless the diagnosis of acute rheumatic fever is clear. Symptomatic relief can be obtained with other analgesics without masking the migratory pattern of the joint manifestations which is very helpful in the diagnosis. The joint manifestations are self-limited without residual damage to the joint with the possible exception of an uncommon entity referred to as *Jaccoud's arthritis or arthropathy*.[30,31]

Carditis

As the term implies, there is an active inflammatory process involving the endocardium, myocardium, and/or pericardium. Carditis can lead to chronic rheumatic heart disease, especially if recurrences are not prevented. The mortality of rheumatic fever is the result of the carditis alone; death occurs both from problems related to chronic rheumatic heart disease and less commonly from events during the acute episode.

Most of those who are going to develop carditis do so early in the acute episode,[32] but the presenting complaint is usually not related to the cardiovascular system. Frequently a murmur is heard incidentally by the examining physician, and other manifestations of rheumatic fever are then sought when the diagnosis is suspected. Much less commonly, the patient presents with cardiovascular symptoms. Chest pain due to pericarditis is probably the most common. Rarely, the symptoms of congestive heart failure are the presenting complaint.

There is usually evidence of valvular involvement when the diagnosis is made. Mitral regurgitation alone is most common (70 percent), with combined aortic and mitral regurgitation second (22 percent) and aortic regurgitation alone third (7 percent).[32]

The physical findings of *mitral regurgitation* are characteristic. The murmur is holosystolic, loudest at the apex with radiation to the left axilla, and usually described as blowing or high-pitched in quality. The loudness of the murmur roughly corresponds to the degree of regurgitation. The intensity increases when the patient is placed in the left lateral position.

The *Carey-Coombs murmur* is an apical diastolic murmur that occurs during rapid ventricular filling. It is best heard at the apex with the bell of the stethoscope since it is low-frequency in character. This middiastolic murmur is particularly important, since it can occur in the absence of a definite murmur of mitral regurgitation but is evidence of active endocarditis. This murmur is usually transient, and careful, frequent auscultation is necessary for detection. A clinically indistinguishable diastolic murmur is also heard with hemodynamically significant mitral regurgitation due to the increased flow across the mitral valve. In this situation, there is commonly evidence of volume overload of the left atrium and left ventricle by chest roentgenogram and electrocardiogram.

The murmur of *aortic regurgitation* is early diastolic in timing. It begins with the second heart sound and is a decrescendo murmur. The length of the murmur roughly corresponds to the degree of regurgitation. It is a high-frequency murmur usually best heard at the left upper sternal border and magnified in intensity when the patient is sitting and leaning forward. The peripheral pulse pressure is increased with more severe aortic regurgitation, and an *Austin Flint murmur* may be heard. This murmur may be middiastolic and/or presystolic in timing and must be distinguished from the murmur of mitral stenosis.

Infrequently the *tricuspid valve* is involved and rarely the *pulmonary valve*. In certain geographic areas, right-sided valvular involvement is more common than in the United States, but this probably represents long-standing disease after recurrences in the face of predisposing socioeconomic factors.

The presence of *mitral or aortic stenosis* represents long-standing rheumatic heart disease and is not found with an initial episode of acute rheumatic fever. There are patients who present for the first time with severe mitral stenosis. In these patients there is usually no other evidence of an acute inflammatory process. The episode or episodes of acute rheumatic fever leading to mitral stenosis are frequently insidious and may go undetected clinically. When a patient presents initially with evidence of an active inflammatory process and a murmur of mitral stenosis, a recurrence of acute rheumatic fever with previous mitral stenosis is likely.

With *pericarditis*, a precordial friction rub is heard. This may be loud enough to obscure the murmurs of mitral and aortic regurgitation. The heart is usually enlarged to some degree by chest roentgenogram (Fig. 60A-1). The standard 12-lead electrocardiogram is helpful and may show diminished voltage, ST elevation, or T inversion with a marked shift in the T vector (Figs. 60A-2 and 60A-3). Serial electrocardiograms should be done frequently since these changes are transient. The presence of a pericardial effusion can be confirmed noninvasively by echocardiogram. Cardiac tamponade is rare with rheumatic pericarditis, presumably because fluid accumulation is slow. Chronic constrictive pericarditis results probably rarely, if at all.

Myocarditis is probably present to some degree in all patients with active carditis, although it is much more difficult to define myocardial involvement clinically. Cardiomegaly with only mild mitral regurgitation and no pericardial effusion is probably due mainly to the myocarditis. By electrocardiogram, premature beats or diffusely diminished QRS voltage (Fig. 60A-4) in the absence of a pericardial effusion probably indicate myocarditis. Prolongation of the *P-R interval* with respect to age and heart rate, or *first-degree atrioventricular block,* is common in

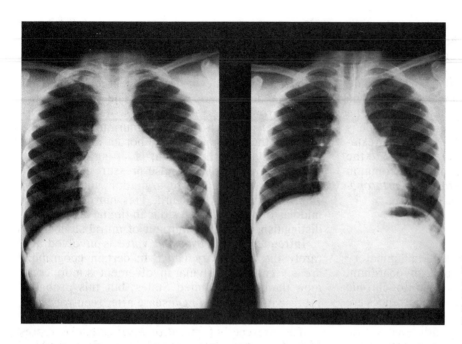

FIGURE 60A-1 Posteroanterior chest roentgenograms of a child with pericarditis initially (on the left) and 1 month later (on the right). The cardiothoracic ratio decreased from 0.63 to 0.51 with resolution of the pericardial effusion.

FIGURE 60A-2 Twelve-lead electrocardiogram of an 8-year-old child with pericarditis and moderate pericardial effusion. The ST segment is shifted with elevation most marked in leads V_5 and V_6. The QRS voltages in the standard limb leads are low normal. (All leads are full standard.)

FIGURE 60A-3 Twelve-lead electrocardiogram of a 12-year-old boy with pericarditis. Two weeks after onset, the T wave is abnormal with a vector that is superior and anterior. The QRS voltages have returned to normal. (Lead V_2 is $\frac{1}{2}$ standard.)

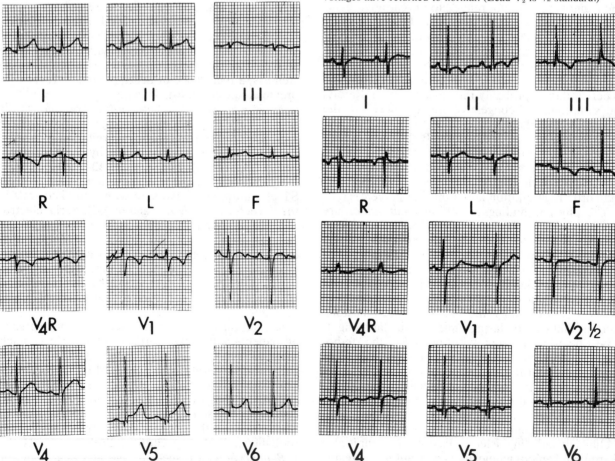

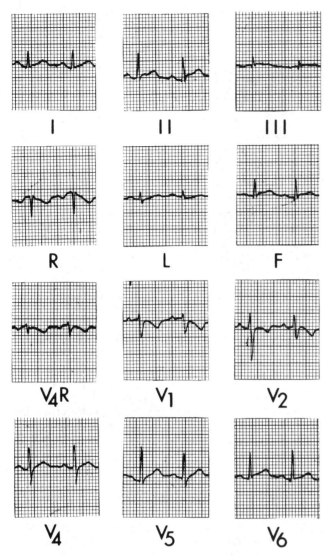

FIGURE 60A-4 Electrocardiogram of a 5-year-old boy with definite carditis but no clinical evidence of pericardial effusion. QRS voltages are low in all leads, particularly the standard limb leads. (All leads are full standard.)

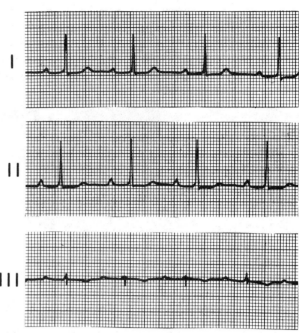

FIGURE 60A-5 Rhythm strips (leads I, II, and III) in a 14-year-old with acute rheumatic fever without carditis. There is a sinus arrhythmia with a rate of 60 to 75 and a markedly prolonged P-R interval of 0.26 s.

acute rheumatic fever and included as a minor manifestation in the Jones criteria (Fig. 60A-5). However, first- and second-degree block, usually of the *Wenckebach* type (Fig. 60A-6), are not evidence of active carditis, but are probably vagally mediated.[33,34]

Congestive heart failure can occur with acute rheumatic fever.[35–37] It is less likely to occur with the initial episode than with recurrences. Myocarditis usually plays a major role in the development of congestive heart failure. Mitral and/or aortic regurgitation impose a volume overload on the left heart and myocarditis depresses myocardial function, resulting in congestive heart failure (Fig. 60A-7). Other precipitating factors should be excluded. A *"chronic" form* of acute rheumatic fever with severe carditis and congestive heart failure has been described.[38]

The diagnosis of a *recurrence* of acute rheumatic fever in a patient with chronic rheumatic heart disease is more difficult. Active carditis is likely if

there is a new murmur, a significant change in a previous murmur, evidence of pericarditis, a significant increase in heart size, or congestive heart failure in a previously compensated patient. There should also be laboratory evidence of inflammation and a preceding streptococcal infection.

Erythema marginatum

Erythema marginatum is an evanescent, nonpruritic rash with sharp, erythematous borders that form a serpiginous pattern with a clear area in the center. The distribution is central rather than peripheral, and it frequently is migratory. Warmth tends to make the rash more obvious, but detection is difficult since it is very evanescent.

FIGURE 60A-6 Rhythm strip (lead II) in child with acute rheumatic fever without carditis: second-degree atrioventricular block of the Wenckebach type. The P-R interval progressively increases with block of every third atrial beat.

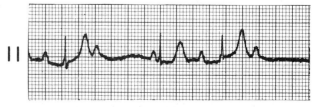

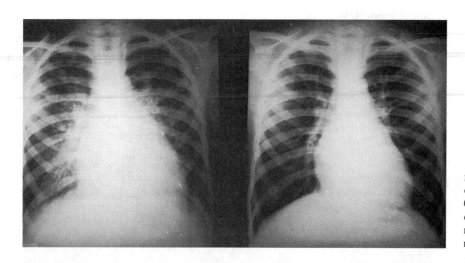

FIGURE 60A-7 Posteroanterior chest roentgenograms of a child with severe carditis. The cardiothoracic ratio was 0.60 initially (on the left) with pulmonary edema. After 3 weeks of therapy, the ratio diminished to 0.51 and the pulmonary edema cleared (on the right).

Subcutaneous nodules

Subcutaneous nodules are firm, nontender, and mobile. They are most commonly found over the extensor surfaces of joints and in the suboccipital region. They occur relatively late in the course of acute rheumatic fever and are most common with overt carditis.

Chorea

Sydenham's chorea is an even later manifestation with a latent period extending up to 6 months when all other manifestations of acute rheumatic fever may have subsided. Its rheumatic origin has been well documented.[39,40] Chorea is a self-limited disorder of the central nervous system characterized by emotional lability, weakness, and purposeless writhing movements which are involuntary. It may be manifested by clumsiness or facial grimacing alone. Frequently the presenting complaint is worsening of school performance. Handwriting is usually affected. Although no chronic neurologic sequelae occur, treatment may be indicated because of the duration and severity of motor impairment. The incidence of chorea has decreased over the past several decades.[1]

OTHER MANIFESTATIONS

Temperature is usually elevated above 38°C in acute rheumatic fever. The sleeping *pulse rate* is often greater than expected for a given age and temperature. *Abdominal pain* is occasionally the presenting symptom in acute rheumatic fever and may be severe with peritoneal signs mimicking appendicitis. Epistaxis and rheumatic "pneumonia" have become rare.

LABORATORY MANIFESTATIONS

The *erythrocyte sedimentation rate* (ESR) and *C-reactive protein* (CRP) test are nonspecific indicators of an inflammatory process. The ESR is almost always elevated early in the course of untreated acute rheumatic fever. It is increased with anemia. It may be decreased in the presence of congestive heart failure, but not usually to the normal range. Treatment with anti-inflammatory agents suppresses the ESR. The CRP test is frequently positive and is not influenced by anemia, but is frequently positive with congestive heart failure of any cause. Both tests may have returned to normal in the patient who presents with chorea.

Leukocytosis and mild to moderate *anemia* are frequently present early in acute rheumatic fever. The anemia is usually normochromic and normocytic and resolves without specific treatment. Increase in the globulin fraction of the *serum proteins* is also frequent and mainly due to an increase in immunoglobulins G and A. Abnormalities of *renal and hepatic function* have been noted,[23,41] but are less frequently reported.

Supporting evidence of preceding streptococcal infection is necessary to make the diagnosis of acute rheumatic fever. *Throat cultures* are positive in a minority of patients with acute rheumatic fever. This may be due to the relatively small number of organisms present, to antibiotic therapy, or to poor technique of obtaining the specimen for culture. Careful swabbing of the tonsillar tissue and posterior pharyngeal wall under direct vision and obtaining multiple throat and anterior nasal cultures may improve results. A positive throat culture for group A beta-hemolytic streptococcus does not indicate actual infection with the organism, since there is a carrier state in some individuals, particularly children.[2]

The *streptococcal antibody tests* offer more specific evidence of preceding streptococcal infection. The *antistreptolysin O titer* (ASO) is the most commonly used for this. An ASO titer of 250 Todd units in adults and 333 Todd units in children is considered diagnostic of preceding streptococcal infection. Serial titers are more helpful since an increase in titer of two tube dilutions gives more specific evidence of recent infection. The ASO titer will be elevated in the majority of patients during the first 3 months of acute rheumatic fever. If other streptococcal antibodies such an antihyaluronidase and antistreptokinase are also measured, almost all will show evidence of a recent streptococcal infection.[2] A rapid screening technique for multiple streptococcal antibodies (Streptozyme) has become available.[42,43] These antibody titers are not specific for streptococcal strains that cause rheumatic fever. They may remain elevated for a number of months and thus may not be indicative of a recent infection unless a significant change in titer is documented.

The well-documented history of *recent scarlet fever* is also evidence of preceding streptococcal infection.

PROBLEMS OF DIAGNOSIS INCLUDING DIFFERENTIAL DIAGNOSIS

The disease pattern of acute rheumatic fever is quite varied, and in the absence of a specific diagnostic test at present, the diagnosis is frequently difficult to establish with certainty. *Underdiagnosis* should be avoided since prophylaxis is effective in preventing recurrences. It is also desirable to prevent *overdiagnosis*. Former acute rheumatic fever patients frequently have problems in obtaining life insurance, employment, and military service. Much information has accumulated on the role of viruses in the etiology of acute and possibly chronic heart disease.[44] Careful diagnosis is a prerequisite to further understanding of the etiology and pathogenesis of these diseases.

Many diseases can cause arthritis and/or carditis. The most common in the *differential diagnosis* of acute rheumatic fever are rheumatoid arthritis and viral myopericarditis. Acute rheumatic fever can also mimic serum sickness, other collagen diseases such as systemic lupus erythematosis, and septic arthritis and pericarditis. Appropriate roentgenographic and laboratory studies should be done to exclude these diagnoses. Specifically, viral cultures and acute and convalescent antibody titers should be obtained. Septic arthritis is important to consider, particularly when a single joint is involved. In the appropriate clinical setting, joint fluid should be cultured and other laboratory studies done.

Occasionally a patient will present with only the murmur of mitral or aortic regurgitation. The diagnosis of acute rheumatic fever is unlikely in the absence of other manifestations. Not all mitral regurgitation is rheumatic in origin.[45] *Congenital mitral insufficiency* and *mitral valve prolapse* occur in the same age group. The late systolic click and T-wave abnormalities by electrocardiogram help distinguish mitral prolapse.[46] *Isolated aortic regurgitation* is probably more often related to a congenital abnormality of the aortic valve.[47] Studies of *antibody to streptococcal group A carbohydrate,* which is a cell wall component, have demonstrated detectable differences in patients with rheumatic heart disease both during the acute phase and for many years after.[48–50] Although the technique cannot be used for mass screening at present, it may become more simplified for use in the future.

Recurrence in a patient with a history of acute rheumatic fever or physical findings of rheumatic heart disease is a specific diagnostic problem that has been discussed in the foregoing. The Jones criteria for diagnosis are guidelines and do not substitute for the good judgment of the attending physician. They were not designed to diagnose rheumatic fever except in the acute, active phase. A recent critique of the diagnostic criteria for acute rheumatic fever clearly defines many of the difficulties.[51] The clinical pattern of the disease can be helpful, particularly the time course of events. Chances for correct diagnosis are best early in the course of the disease. Thus anti-inflammatory agents should not be given until the diagnosis is secure. Finally, use of the Jones criteria should be combined with proper laboratory and roentgenographic studies to exclude differential diagnoses.

TREATMENT

The treatment of acute rheumatic fever encompasses the following areas: (1) eradication of streptococcus, (2) control of the acute process, (3) prevention of chronic heart disease, and (4) prevention of recurrences including psychologic preparation for the institution of prophylaxis.

The drug of choice for *eradication of group A beta-hemolytic streptococcus* is penicillin. Fortunately penicillin-resistant strains have not developed. Dosage and duration of therapy are extremely important. Table 60A-2 gives the recommended regimens for treatment of streptococcal infections. For hospitalized patients, oral or intramuscular penicillin may be given. For those not hospitalized, benzathine penicillin is best to ensure that the entire dose is received for an adequate time. Erythromycin can be given to those who have a true penicillin allergy. Although useful for prophylaxis, sulfonamides do not eradicate an infection which is already present.

The *control of acute rheumatic carditis* and *prevention of chronic heart disease* continue to be controversial. Excellent reviews of various regimens recommended are available.[1,2] Treatment includes restriction of activity, anti-inflammatory agents, and specific measures for chorea and congestive heart failure.

The *severity of carditis* and *duration of preceding illness* are useful in establishing guidelines for treat-

TABLE 60A-2
Treatment of streptococcal infections

1 Benzathine penicillin, single intramuscular dose
　　small children　　600,000 units
　　adults　　　　　　1.2 million units
2 Penicillin G, orally for 10 days
　　250,000 units q. 6 h.
3 Erythromycin, orally for 10 days
　　250 mg q. 6 h.

TABLE 60A-3
Severity of carditis

Mild	*1* No cardiomegaly
	2 Carey-Coombs murmur *or* mitral insufficiency (grade 2/6 or less)
Moderate	*1* Greater than mild
	2 No congestive heart failure
Severe	*1* Cardiomegaly
	2 Congestive heart failure

TABLE 60A-4
Anti-inflammatory therapy

Aspirin (100 mg/kg/day)	No carditis
	Mild carditis
	Moderate carditis of > 3-week duration
Prednisone (2 mg/kg/day)	Pericarditis
	Moderate carditis of < 3-week duration
	Severe carditis

ment. It is frequently possible to date the onset of the illness from the time of onset of symptoms and signs of acute rheumatic fever when the onset has been abrupt. In those with more insidious onset, this is not reliable. Severity of the carditis can roughly be divided into mild, moderate, and severe. Mild carditis may be defined as the absence of cardiomegaly in the presence of a Carey-Coombs murmur or a murmur of mitral regurgitation of grade 2/6 or less in intensity. Severe carditis is associated with cardiomegaly and congestive heart failure. Moderate carditis is greater than mild but without congestive heart failure. By these definitions, which are summarized in Table 60A-3, the presence of aortic regurgitation or cardiomegaly without congestive heart failure would classify the carditis as moderate. Pericarditis has not been included since it is usually found with moderate or severe endocarditis as well and recommended treatment is rather uniform. These definitions are arbitrary but based to some extent on clinical correlations with long-term prognosis.

Bed rest should be individualized for each patient depending on the severity of carditis. Bed rest is recommended for all for the first 1 or 2 weeks. This is the period when carditis is most likely to be manifested.[32] Also the patients do not usually feel very well during this period. Progressive ambulation with bathroom privileges and passive wheelchair activities initially should always follow the period of bed rest. In most patients without carditis or with mild carditis, full activity can be resumed in 4 to 6 weeks. The benefits of more prolonged bed rest are not clear, and it is difficult to maintain bed rest in a child who feels well. Certainly the very long periods commonly used in the past are not indicated. In those with moderate or severe carditis, longer periods of bed rest must be tailored to the individual. Most school situations lend themselves to moderate activity restrictions, and thus children can often return to school before full activity is allowed.

Treatment of acute rheumatic fever with *anti-inflammatory drugs* is confusing because of the multiplicity of regimens. Adequate studies with a control group are lacking since clinicians are loathe to deny steroid therapy to very ill patients. Treatment on the basis of the experience of numerous clinicians is justified until studies clearly demonstrate the advantages of one regimen over another. It seems helpful to consider the aims of acute suppression and pre-

vention of chronic heart disease separately. Table 60A-4 summarizes the recommendations which follow.

Salicylates are superb for control of the fever and pain of arthritis of the acute process, but they have not been demonstrated to be of benefit for the acute manifestations of carditis. *For those without carditis,* aspirin is recommended. A serum salicylate level of 25 to 30 mg/dl is usually associated with optimal therapeutic results. A dose of 100 mg/kg/day given every 4 h will be adequate for this in most cases. This should be continued for 4 to 6 weeks, since this is the usual duration of fever and joint symptoms when untreated. Should symptoms recur when treatment is stopped *(rebound phenomenon),* the same dose of aspirin can be restarted and continued for another 2 to 4 weeks. Rebounds rarely occur beyond 6 to 8 weeks. Enteric coated aspirin should not be used, since absorption is poor. The signs of aspirin toxicity include nausea, vomiting, tinnitus, and hyperpnea. Bleeding due to the effect of aspirin on platelet function should be watched for. If antacids are also given, serum salicylate levels should be measured when the antacid is being given and again if the type of antacid is changed.[52] Fever and joint pain usually respond dramatically to aspirin in 24 to 72 h.

Prednisone is the other anti-inflammatory agent commonly used in acute rheumatic fever. It definitely suppresses the acute process (arthritis, fever, elevated ESR), but not necessarily the cardiac manifestations. There is no evidence that it reduces the duration of the illness. It is hoped that it might prevent chronic heart disease, but there has been no proof of this to date. All regimens proposed await more definitive, well-matched, and controlled studies.

Severity of the carditis and duration of illness should be considered when acute rheumatic fever is treated with prednisone. The rationale for this is as follows: It has been shown repeatedly that up to 95 percent of patients with mild carditis do not have evidence of chronic heart disease on follow-up as long as recurrences are prevented.[53] As might be expected, there is little evidence that steroids alter this figure significantly.[54] Some data suggest that steroids may significantly decrease the incidence and severity of chronic rheumatic heart disease in those with moderate carditis.[55] The duration of illness prior to treatment with steroids may also be a factor in this group. It might be expected that better results are possible in the group treated early in the course of the disease rather than later. Treatment has been arbitrarily defined as early if instituted less than 3 weeks after onset of symptoms.

For these reasons and the high incidence of significant side effects, steroid therapy *is not recommended for mild carditis or moderate carditis late in its course.* It *is recommended for treatment in moderate carditis when seen early* in the course of the acute illness.

The rationale for therapy in patients with *severe carditis* is quite different. Although the incidence of chronic heart disease is highest in this group, there is no evidence that steroids will affect this significantly. Steroids probably decrease acute morbidity and mortality in this group. It is for this reason, suppression of the acute process, that it is given to those with severe carditis. Steroids do not appear to alter the duration of the illness. In addition, these patients require vigorous *treatment for congestive heart failure,* including digitalis preparations, diuretics, and other supportive measures.

Pericarditis responds well symptomatically and clinically to the administration of steroids. Since pericarditis rarely occurs without significant endocarditis and probably myocarditis as well, steroids are also recommended for pericarditis.

Prednisone is the most frequently used steroid and may be given at a dose of 2 mg/kg/day. Prednisone can usually be stopped abruptly after 10 days in pericarditis or moderate carditis when there has been definite improvement in the cardiac manifestations and a decrease in the ESR. In more severe carditis, prednisone should be continued on an individual basis, but usually for a total of at least 4 to 6 weeks. It is then necessary to taper the dose gradually and monitor carefully for changes in the cardiac status. When prednisone is given less than 4 to 6 weeks, aspirin should be begun and continued for 4 to 6 weeks of combined therapy to prevent rebound of the symptoms of fever and arthritis. Longer periods of treatment may be necessary in some patients.

Although the problems of *valve replacement* in children are well recognized,[56] it is lifesaving for some and certainly improves many in terms of functional status. In the past, surgery has been thought to be contraindicated in the presence of acute rheumatic fever. However, there are a few patients with severe carditis who follow a rapid and relentless downhill course in spite of excellent medical management. This is particularly common in patients with multiple recurrences and with "chronic" acute rheumatic fever. When hemodynamically significant aortic or mitral regurgitation is demonstrable, valve replacement is indicated even *in the presence of acute rheumatic fever with severe myocarditis.* Mortality is less than in those managed medically, and functional status is almost uniformly improved.[57]

Although self-limited without neurologic sequelae, *chorea* may require specific treatment because of the duration and severity of motor impairment. When there is no evidence of inflammation, treatment with aspirin or prednisone is not necessary. A therapeutic course of penicillin should be given to eradicate streptococcus which may be present. Sedatives such as phenobarbital are traditionally used for symptomatic relief. Chlorpromazine[58] and haloperidol[59] have been used with some success more recently. The recommended initial dose of chlorpromazine is 25 mg every 6 to 8 h with increases of 10 to 25 mg/day until

improvement is noted.[58] Once symptoms have disappeared, the dose can be gradually tapered unless symptoms recur. Occasionally persistence of symptoms requires therapy for many months. Haloperidol is similar to the phenothiazines, but much more potent. It is thought to control the extrapyramidal movements by blocking dopamine receptors in the central nervous system.[59]

SECONDARY PREVENTION

Recurrences of acute rheumatic fever can be eliminated by the prevention of streptococcal infections. The report of the Inter-Society Commission for Heart Disease Resources is an excellent discussion of the prevention of rheumatic fever and rheumatic heart disease.[60] It is imperative that all individuals with acute rheumatic fever be started on a regimen of prophylaxis whether or not carditis was an initial manifestation. Since carditis probably increases in severity with each recurrence, many cases of severe carditis can be prevented by prophylaxis. About 70 percent of the murmurs of mitral regurgitation and 27 percent of the murmurs of aortic regurgitation will have disappeared in 10 years provided recurrences are prevented. With benzathine penicillin prophylaxis, no patients have developed mitral stenosis after 10 years.[61] Prior to the use of penicillin prophylaxis, the incidence was 28 percent after 10 years.[62] Thus prophylaxis is unequivocably recommended to prevent recurrences and long-term cardiac sequelae.

Before initiating such a regimen, it is important to make the patient and parents aware of the cause, nature, and prognosis of acute rheumatic fever. Teaching should be initiated during the acute illness and reinforced at each subsequent visit.

The recommended *regimens for prophylaxis* are given in Table 60A-5. Noncompliance with oral regimens for prophylaxis has been well demonstrated.[63] In addition, should streptococcal infection occur during periods of noncompliance, subsequent resumption of oral prophylaxis is not therapeutic. Intramuscular benzathine penicillin has been demonstrated to be superior to oral prophylaxis[54] with penicillin and sulfonamides for both of these reasons. Results of a 10-year follow-up with benzathine penicillin prophylaxis are encouraging.[61] Obviously the

TABLE 60A-5
Regimens for prophylaxis

1 Benzathine penicillin, intramuscular injection
   1.2 million units every 4 weeks
   (600,000 units in small children)
2 Penicillin G, orally
   250,000 units twice a day
3 Sulfadiazine, orally
   small children   500 mg daily
   adults   1 g daily
4 Erythromycin, orally
   250 mg twice a day

psychologic trauma of monthly injections occasionally will require special consideration. Erythromycin may be used when there are allergies to penicillin and sulfonamides, but the cost is greater and diagnosis of such allergies should be made carefully.

Regional clinics with trained personnel can promote better compliance. Programs such as those sponsored by the World Health Organization[21] are excellent examples of what can be done to control rheumatic fever and rheumatic heart disease throughout the world. Environmental factors will vary and should be considered individually.

Prophylaxis is obviously important in childhood but should be continued for life, since acute rheumatic fever occurs in adults as well. It is particularly important for individuals with frequent exposure to streptococcal infections, e.g., school teachers, and for those with severe rheumatic heart disease.

PRIMARY PREVENTION

Proper treatment of streptococcal infections can prevent rheumatic fever. Dosage and duration of therapy are important (see Table 60A-2). Detection is aided by routine use of good throat culture technique for all upper respiratory infections seen by a physician as well as proper attention to contacts of those with known infection. This obviously involves physician education. Education of the public to the proper indications for seeking medical attention also will help to decrease the incidence of acute rheumatic fever in any population. This of course requires adequate medical facilities for good health care. Since streptococcal respiratory infection is asymptomatic in many, primary prevention must also be aimed at the socioeconomic conditions which predispose to streptococcal infection.[21]

SUMMARY

Acute rheumatic fever is the sequel of infection with the group A beta-hemolytic streptococcus. The pathogenesis of acute rheumatic fever remains an intriguing mystery that has eluded many investigators. It persists as a major problem around the world. Hopefully continued interest and investigation have not been hampered by the decline in prevalence and severity in some areas.[64] The pathogenesis of rheumatic fever may hold the key to answers for many other diseases as well.

Proper diagnosis of acute rheumatic fever is important and methods for exclusion of differential diagnoses should be combined with thoughtful application of the guidelines offered by the revised Jones criteria. The limitations of laboratory studies in defining a preceding streptococcal infection should be considered. Once the diagnosis of acute rheumatic fever is made, eradication of streptococcal infection,

supportive treatment of the acute episode, and institution of prophylaxis are of primary importance. Use of anti-inflammatory agents is probably of lesser importance, particularly in view of the many unknowns in terms of the prevention of chronic rheumatic heart disease. A rational approach to the clinical recognition and management of acute rheumatic fever is possible in spite of the gaps in knowledge at the present time.

REFERENCES

1 Markowitz, M., and Gordis, L.: "Rheumatic Fever," W. B. Saunders Company, Philadelphia, 1972.

2 Stollerman, G. H.: "Rheumatic Fever and Streptococcal Infection," Grune & Stratton, Inc., New York, 1975.

3 Schlesinger, B.: The Relationship of Throat Infection to Acute Rheumatism in Childhood, *Arch. Dis. Child.*, 5:411, 1930.

4 Coburn, A. F.: "The Factor of Infection in the Rheumatic State," Williams & Wilkins Company, Baltimore, 1931.

5 Collis, W. R. F.: Acute Rheumatism and Haemolytic Streptococci, *Lancet*, 1:1341, 1931.

6 Denny, F. W., Wannamaker, L. W., Brink, W. R., Rammelkamp, C. H., and Custer, E. A.: Prevention of Rheumatic Fever: Treatment of the Preceding Streptococcic Infection, *JAMA*, 143:151, 1950.

7 Rammelkamp, C. H., Wannamaker, L. W., and Denny, F. W.: The Epidemiology and Prevention of Rheumatic Fever, *Bull. N.Y. Acad. Med.*, 28:321, 1952.

8 Rammelkamp, C. H., Denny, F. W., and Wannamaker, L. W.: Studies on the Epidemiology of Rheumatic Fever in the Armed Services, in L. Thomas (ed.), "Rheumatic Fever: A Symposium," University of Minnesota Press, Minneapolis, 1952.

9 Wannamaker, L. W.: The Chain that Links the Heart to the Throat, *Circulation*, 48:9, 1973.

10 Kaplan, E. L.: Epidemiology and Pathogenesis of Acute Rheumatic Fever: Recent Concepts, *Minn. Med.*, 58:592, 1975.

11 Kaplan, M. H., and Meyeserian, M.: An Immunological Cross-Reaction between Group-A Streptococcal Cells and Human Heart Tissue, *Lancet*, 1:706, 1962.

12 Read, S. E., Fischetti, V. A., Utermohlen, V., Falk, R. E., and Zabriskie, J. B.: Cellular Reactivity Studies to Streptococcal Antigens: Migration Inhibition Studies in Patients with Streptococcal Infections and Rheumatic Fever, *J. Clin. Invest.*, 54:439, 1974.

13 Lueker, R. D., Abdin, Z. H., and Williams, R. C.: Peripheral Blood T and B Lymphocytes during Acute Rheumatic Fever, *J. Clin. Invest.*, 55:975, 1975.

14 Mortimer, E. A., Jr.: Production of L Forms of Group A Streptococci in Mice, *Proc. Soc. Exp. Biol. Med.*, 119:159, 1965.

15 Burch, G. E., Giles, T. D., and Colcolough, H. L.: Pathogenesis of "Rheumatic" Heart Disease: Critique and Theory, *Am. Heart J.*, 80:556, 1970.

16 Stevenson, A. C., and Cheeseman, E. A.: Heredity and Rheumatic Fever: Some Later Information about Data Collected in 1950–51, *Ann. Hum. Genet.*, 21:139, 1956.

17 Taranta, A., Torosdag, S., Metrakos, J. D., Jegier, W., and Uchida, I.: Rheumatic Fever in Monozygotic and Dizygotic Twins, *Circulation*, 20:778, 1959 (abstract).

18 Shaper, A. G.: Cardiovascular Disease in the Tropics, I. Rheumatic Heart, *Br. Med. J.*, 3:683, 1972.

19 Siegel, A. C., Johnson, E. E., and Stollerman, G. H.: Controlled Studies of Streptococcal Pharyngitis in a Pediatric Population: Factors Related to the Attack Rate of Rheumatic Fever, *N. Engl. J. Med.*, 265:559, 1961.

20 Krause, R. M.: Prevention of Streptococcal Sequelae by

Penicillin Prophylaxis: A Reassessment, *J. Infect. Dis.,* 131: 592, 1975.

21 Strasser, R., and Rotta, J.: The Control of Rheumatic Fever and Rheumatic Heart Disease: An Outline of WHO Activities, *WHO Chron.,* 27:49, 1973.

22 Japan Heart Foundation: The First South-East Asia Rheumatic Fever and Rheumatic Heart Disease Prevention Conference, *Jpn. Circ. J.,* 39:151, 1975.

23 Barnert, A. L., Terry, E. E., and Persellin, R. H.: Acute Rheumatic Fever in Adults, *JAMA,* 232:925, 1975.

24 Rosenthal, A., Czoniczer, G., and Massell, B. F.: Rheumatic Fever under Three Years of Age: A Report of 10 Cases, *Pediatrics,* 41:612, 1968.

25 Spagnuolo, M., Pasternack, B., and Taranta, A.: Risk of Rheumatic-Fever Recurrences after Streptococcal Infections, *N. Engl. J. Med.,* 285:641, 1971.

26 Feinstein, A. R., Spagnuolo, M., and Taranta, A.: Host Factors in the Susceptibility of Rheumatic Patients to Streptococcal Infections, *Am. J. Epidemiol.,* 102:42, 1975.

27 Feinstein, A. R., Spagnuolo, M., Wood, H. F., Taranta, A., Tursky, E., and Kleinberg, E.: Rheumatic Fever in Children and Adolescents: A Long-Term Epidemiologic Study of Subsequent Prophylaxis, Streptococcal Infections, and Clinical Sequelae. VI. Clinical Features of Streptococcal Infections and Rheumatic Recurrences, *Ann. Intern. Med.,* 60(suppl. 5):68, 1964.

28 Jones, T. D.: Diagnosis of Rheumatic Fever, *JAMA,* 126:481, 1944.

29 American Heart Association, Council on Rheumatic Fever and Congenital Heart Disease: Jones Criteria (Revised) for Guidance in the Diagnosis of Rheumatic Fever, *Circulation,* 32:664, 1965.

30 Murphy, W. A., and Staple, T. W.: Jaccoud's Arthropathy Reviewed, *Am. J. Roentgenol. Radium Ther. Nucl. Med.,* 118:300, 1973.

31 Ignaczak, T., Espinoza, L. R., Kantor, O. S., and Osterland, C. K.: Jaccoud Arthritis, *Arch. Intern. Med.,* 135:577, 1975.

32 Massell, B. F., Fyler, D. C., and Roy, S. B.: The Clinical Picture of Rheumatic Fever: Diagnosis, Immediate Prognosis, Course, and Therapeutic Implications, *Am. J. Cardiol.,* 1:436, 1958.

33 Mirowski, M., Rosenstein, B. J., and Markowitz, M.: A Comparison of Atrioventricular Conduction in Normal Children and in Patients with Rheumatic Fever, Glomerulonephritis, and Acute Febrile Illnesses: A Quantitative Study with Determination of the P-R Index, *Pediatrics,* 33:334, 1964.

34 Clarke, M., and Keith, J. D.: Atrioventricular Conduction in Acute Rheumatic Fever, *Br. Heart J.,* 34:472, 1972.

35 Feinstein, A. R., and Arevalo, A. C.: Manifestations and Treatment of Congestive Heart Failure in Young Patients with Rheumatic Heart Disease, *Pediatrics,* 33:661, 1964.

36 Spagnuolo, M., and Feinstein, A. R.: Congestive Heart Failure and Rheumatic Activity in Young Patients with Rheumatic Heart Disease, *Pediatrics,* 33:653, 1964.

37 Abdin, Z. H., and Abul-Fadl, M. A. M.: Evaluation of Congestive Heart Failure in Children with Rheumatic Heart Disease as a Criterion of Activity, *Ann. Rheum. Dis.,* 31:134, 1972.

38 Taranta, A., Spagnuolo, M., and Feinstein, A. R.: "Chronic" Rheumatic Fever, *Ann. Intern. Med.,* 56:367, 1962.

39 Taranta, A., and Stollerman, G. H.: Relationship of Sydenham's Chorea to Infection with Group A Streptococci, *Am. J. Med.,* 20:170, 1956.

40 Taranta, A.: Relation of Isolated Recurrences of Sydenham's Chorea to Preceding Streptococcal Infections, *N. Engl. J. Med.,* 260:1204, 1959.

41 Cohen, S., Salomon, M., Grishman, E., Gribetz, D., and Churg, J.: The Kidney in Acute Rheumatic Fever: Clinicopathological Correlations, *Arch. Intern. Med.,* 127:245, 1971.

42 Klein, G. C., and Jones, W. L.: Comparison of the Streptozyme Test with the Antistreptolysin O, Antideoxyribonuclease B, and Antihyaluronidase Tests, *Appl. Microbiol.,* 21:257, 1971.

43 Bisno, A. L., and Ofek, I.: Serologic Diagnosis of Streptococcal Infection, *Am. J. Dis. Child.,* 127:676, 1974.

44 Burch, G. E., and Giles, T. D.: The Role of Viruses in the Production of Heart Disease, *Am. J. Cardiol.,* 29:231, 1972.

45 Blackman, N. S., and Kuskin, L.: Prophylaxis in Rheumatic and Nonrheumatic Mitral Insufficiency, *Clin. Pediatr.,* 14:261, 1975.

46 Steinfield, L., Dimich, I., Rappaport, H., and Baron, M.: Late Systolic Murmur of Rheumatic Mitral Insufficiency, *Am. J. Cardiol.,* 35:397, 1975.

47 Roberts, W. C.: Anatomically Isolated Aortic Valvular Disease: The Case Against Its Being of Rheumatic Etiology, *Am. J. Med.,* 49:151, 1970.

48 Dudding, B. A., and Ayoub, E. M.: Persistence of Streptococcal Group A Antibody in Patients with Rheumatic Valvular Disease, *J. Exp. Med.,* 128:1081, 1968.

49 Shulman, S. T., and Ayoub, E. M.: Qualitative and Quantitative Aspects of the Human Antibody Response to Streptococcal Group A Carbohydrate, *J. Clin. Invest.,* 54:990, 1974.

50 Shulman, S. T., Ayoub, E. M., Victorica, B. E., Gessner, I. H., Tamer, D. F., and Hernandez, F. A.: Differences in Antibody Response to Streptococcal Antigens in Children with Rheumatic and Non-rheumatic Mitral Valve Disease, *Circulation,* 50:1244, 1974.

51 Ward, C.: Observations on the Diagnosis of Isolated Rheumatic Carditis, *Am. Heart J.,* 91:545, 1976.

52 Levy, G., Lampman, T., Kamath, B. L., and Garrettson, L. K.: Decreased Serum Salicylate Concentrations in Children with Rheumatic Fever Treated with Antacid, *N. Engl. J. Med.,* 293:323, 1975.

53 U. K. and U. S. Joint Report: The Natural History of Rheumatic Fever and Rheumatic Heart Disease: Cooperative Clinical Trial of ACTH, Cortisone, and Aspirin, *Circulation,* 32:457, 1965.

54 Feinstein, A. R., Spagnuolo, M., Jonas, S., Kloth, H., Tursky, E., and Levitt, M.: Prophylaxis of Recurrent Rheumatic Fever, *JAMA,* 206:565, 1968.

55 Massell, B. F., Jhaveri, S., Czoniczer, G., and Barnet, R.: Treatment of Rheumatic Fever and Rheumatic Carditis: Observations Providing a Basis for the Selection of Aspirin or Adrenocortical Steroids, *Med. Clin. North Am.,* 45:1349, 1961.

56 Freed, M. D., and Bernhard, W. F.: Prosthetic Valve Replacement in Children, *Prog. Cardiovasc. Dis.,* 17:475, 1975.

57 Strauss, A. W., Goldring, D., Kissane, J., Hernandez, A., Hartmann, A. F., McKnight, C. R., and Weldon, C. S.: Valve Replacement in Acute Rheumatic Heart Disease, *J. Thorac. Cardiovasc. Surg.,* 67:659, 1974.

58 Tierney, R. C., and Kaplan, S.: Treatment of Sydenham's Chorea, *Am. J. Dis. Child.,* 109:408, 1965.

59 Shenker, D. M., Grossman, H. J., and Klawans, H. L.: Treatment of Sydenham's Chorea with Haloperidol, *Dev. Med. Child. Neurol.,* 15:19, 1973.

60 Rheumatic Fever and Rheumatic Heart Disease Study Group (A. Taranta, chairman, J. Fiedler, C. W. Frank, B. S. Gilson, L. Gordis, C. Hufnagel, M. Markowitz, and L. W. Wannamaker): Prevention of Rheumatic Fever and Rheumatic Heart Disease, *Circulation,* 41(suppl. A):1, 1970.

61 Tompkins, D. G., Boxerbaum, B., and Liebman, J.: Long-Term Prognosis of Rheumatic-Fever Patients Receiving Regular Intramuscular Benzathine Penicillin, *Circulation,* 45:543, 1972.

62 Walsh, B. J., Bland, E. F., and Jones, T. D.: Pure Mitral Stenosis in Young Persons, *Arch. Intern. Med.,* 65:321, 1940.

63 Gordis, L., Markowitz, M., and Lilienfeld, A. M.: Studies in the Epidemiology and Preventability of Rheumatic Fever. IV. A Quantitative Determination of Compliance in Children on Oral Penicillin Prophylaxis, *Pediatrics*, 43:173, 1969.
64 Taranta, A.: Rheumatic Fever: Its Public Relations and Private Life, *Minn. Med.*, 58:633, 1975.

B
Valvular Heart Disease

I. SYLVIA CRAWLEY, M.D.,
DOUGLAS C. MORRIS, M.D., and
BARRY D. SILVERMAN, M.D.

Of the four valves the mitral is the one most commonly diseased; it is damaged in well over half of the cases of valvular disease. Aortic valve disease is next in frequency, followed by lesions of the tricuspid valve which, though occasionally diseased, is but rarely deformed in any important extent. The pulmonary valve is very infrequently involved.[1]

PAUL DUDLEY WHITE, M.D., 1931

Valvular heart disease remains a common form of heart disease. However, our views about it have changed considerably since Paul White wrote the first edition of his classic book in 1931.[1] Since his annotation, rheumatic fever has decreased in incidence in the United States, and because of this valvular heart disease due to rheumatic fever has declined in frequency. (The disease is still common in many countries.) In addition to this we are now recognizing many different causes of valvular heart disease other than rheumatic fever. In this chapter rheumatic valvular heart disease and other acquired valvular diseases of the heart will be discussed.

MITRAL STENOSIS

Mitral stenosis may be defined as blockade at the level of the mitral valve as a result of abnormality in structure of the mitral leaflets preventing proper opening in diastole. By far the most common cause of structural abnormality of the mitral valve is rheumatic endocarditis. Congenital malformation of the mitral valve does occur but is rare. It is frequently associated with other congenital cardiovascular malformations, and signs and symptoms of mitral blockade occur in infancy or early childhood.[1a,2] Acute rheumatic fever with rheumatic endocarditis causes deformity of the mitral valve apparatus which can ultimately result in progressive sclerosis, fibrosis, and calcification.[3] These pathologic changes can prevent proper opening of the mitral valve which results in obstruction to blood flow. Signs and symptoms of this obstruction may occur in early adulthood or older age but occur most commonly in this country in the fourth or fifth decade of life.[4] Severe mitral stenosis during childhood or adolescence is more common in India, Africa, and Mexico.[5,6] Acute rheumatic endocarditis most commonly affects the mitral valve, and although insufficiency is the most likely predominant lesion, some degree of stenosis is frequently present.[7] In pure mitral stenosis a history of previous rheumatic fever can be obtained in only about half the cases.[7] Mitral stenosis is much more frequent in females.

Pathophysiology

The fundamental physiologic problem in mitral stenosis is impaired flow of blood through the mitral orifice. The scarring and fibrosis of the mitral leaflets and chordae tendineae, with or without calcification, and the commissural fusion produce a funnel-shaped mitral apparatus with reduction in the area of the mitral orifice.[8] A pressure gradient across the mitral valve is produced as determined by the degree of this reduction in mitral valve area and the maintenance of mitral valve flow, the latter determined by diastolic filling period and cardiac output. This mitral valve diastolic pressure gradient results in elevation of left atrial pressure and volume which is reflected into the pulmonary veins and capillaries. This begins the vicious pathophysiologic sequence of mitral stenosis. Distension, increased pressure, and volume of the pulmonary veins and capillaries can lead to pulmonary edema. When the pulmonary venous pressure exceeds plasma onchotic pressure, transudation of fluid into the alveoli and interstitial space occurs. This increased intravascular and interstitial fluid volume produces compliance changes in the lungs, increasing the work of breathing.[9] The elevation in pulmonary venous and capillary pressure is passively transmitted to the pulmonary arterial system. Reactive vasoconstriction, intimal hyperplasia, and medial hypertrophy in the pulmonary arterioles, especially in the lung bases, can further exaggerate pulmonary arterial hypertension. Right ventricular hypertrophy and dilatation follow. With the development of a markedly increased pulmonary vascular resistance and impaired right ventricular function a further reduction in cardiac output occurs, mitral valve flow decreases, and pulmonary congestion is lessened. Pulmonary blood volume is measurably lessened, but interstitial lung changes persist.[10]

Since the left atrial pressure is the instigator of this sequence, the factors determining this elevated pressure should be kept in mind. A mitral valve area of 1.5 to 2.0 cm^2 does not usually produce clinically significant changes unless there is an *increase* in mitral valve flow, as occurs with an increase in cardiac output during exercise, or a *decrease* in left atrial emptying, as occurs with abbreviated diastole during a rapid heart rate. With further reduction in mitral valve area, however, there are persistent hemodynamic changes, and a minimal change in either of these factors, mitral valve flow or left atrial emptying, can produce significant pulmonary congestion. More critical degrees of stenosis, 0.9 to 1.4 cm^2 and less than 0.9 cm^2, complete the hemodynamic

sequence.[4] There is then a general correlation of
symptoms with mitral valve area.[11] A few mildly
symptomatic patients are found to have a mitral
valve area of less than 1.5 cm².

Clinical recognition

The symptoms with which the patient presents, even
though related to mitral stenosis or its complications,
may be assumed to be related to other disease
processes. The patient may present with an entirely
different medical problem which occupies the physician's mind. There are, however, many clues to the
presence of mitral stenosis in the history, physical
examination, electrocardiogram (ECG), and chest
roentgenogram. Awareness of these findings provides ample opportunity for the clinical recognition
of mitral stenosis. In most cases the initial evaluation
of these subjective and objective findings forms a
firm data base for the diagnosis of mitral stenosis.
Echocardiography has provided a valuable diagnostic tool in difficult cases. Further assessment of the
significance of mitral stenosis in relation to the
patient's symptoms and future is provided by knowledge of hemodynamic and anatomic correlates. Thus,
proper medical and surgical management is offered
the patient for improved quality and quantity of life.

SYMPTOMS
Dyspnea is a prominent symptom in many patients
with mitral stenosis and is related to pulmonary
venous congestion.[12] Mild mitral stenosis produces
significant elevation of left atrial pressure only with
moderate to severe exertion, while more critical
mitral stenosis may produce prominent incapacitating dyspnea on minimal effort or at rest. The sudden
onset of other stressful situations may precipitate
pulmonary congestion even in those patients with
mild obstruction. Emotional stress, fever, and atrial
fibrillation with a rapid ventricular rate are common
offenders. With alleviation of these precipitating
factors a near-normal functional capacity may return
and remain for many years.[4] Pregnancy, especially
during the last trimester when cardiac output is
increased, may precipitate symptoms not previously
present.[13]

Enhancement of pulmonary venous congestion by
shifts in intravascular and/or extravascular volume
while the patient is in the recumbent position may
lead to *orthopnea* and *paroxysmal nocturnal dyspnea*
in patients with moderate to severe mitral blockade.
Again, these symptoms may be hastened by aggravating factors.

None of these pulmonary symptoms are specific
for mitral stenosis, nor is mitral stenosis the most
common cause of them. With evidence of some
degree of coexisting pulmonary disease, this may be
blamed for the dyspnea. This becomes a greater
pitfall when pulmonary disease is an obvious problem in a severely symptomatic patient. Orthopnea
and paroxysmal nocturnal dyspnea are more commonly attributed to left ventricular failure unless
other clues to mitral stenosis are sought.

With the development of increased fixed pulmonary vascular resistance, *fatigue* may be more incapacitating than the pulmonary symptoms. The enhancement of cardiac output during exercise is blunted, resulting in inadequate systemic perfusion and
less marked elevation of left atrial pressure for a
given level of exercise. As pulmonary hypertension
becomes more severe with right ventricular dysfunction, there are *symptoms of systemic venous congestion* with hepatic congestion and peripheral edema.
The unfortunate patient who initially presents at this
stage has prominent symptoms related to a depressed
resting cardiac output and systemic congestion, and
the symptoms of pulmonary venous hypertension
may be less evident.[11]

A few patients may progress through these stages
during the natural history of their illness as revealed
by retrospective analysis at the time of presentation
or by follow-up. In most cases, however, this sequence is not so obvious.[12] Clinical presentation may
occur at any of these stages, and in fact there may be
no history of prior significant dyspnea in some patients with severe congestive heart failure.[14]

Hemoptysis may occur in the course of mitral
stenosis and is related to the reflection of pulmonary
venous hypertension to the bronchial veins. Profuse
bleeding, pulmonary apoplexy of Wood,[12] is not seen
in mild cases. Milder degrees of hemoptysis associated with a transient sudden rise in pulmonary venous
pressure precipitated by vigorous exercise does not
necessarily imply serious mitral stenosis. Hemoptysis can occur as an early symptom prior to or at about
the same time as exertional dyspnea.[7] In patients
with pulmonary hypertension and pulmonary vascular disease it is much less common. It is rarely so
life-threatening as to require surgical intervention.[15,16]
Hemoptysis may occur as a result of pulmonary
infarction, especially in those patients with heart
failure.

The awareness of heartbeat irregularity, *palpitation,* is an individual variable. Many patients with
significant mitral stenosis have paroxysmal or sustained atrial fibrillation and may complain of palpitation. The presence of atrial fibrillation has more
significance in its relation to the exacerbation of
other symptoms.

Some patients with mitral stenosis have *chest
pain*. The approach to this problem should be the
same as in any other patient (see Chap. 62E). Coronary atherosclerotic heart disease should be suspected if the pain suggests myocardial ischemia. Pulmonary emboli should be considered with pleuritic chest
pain especially in patients with heart failure. Right
ventricular myocardial ischemia due to severe pulmonary hypertension has been postulated as a mechanism of chest pain in patients with mitral stenosis.[17]
Hoarseness, Ortner's syndrome,[18] may be a presenting complaint, and it is due to compression of the left
recurrent laryngeal nerve by a large pulmonary artery.[19] An increased incidence of *seizures* has been
reported and is probably related to cerebral emboli.[20]
Sudden death due to ball-thrombus occlusion of the
mitral orifice is a rare occurrence.[21]

PHYSICAL EXAMINATION

The *general appearance* is frequently normal. A malar flush has been described and attributed to peripheral cyanosis. This mitral stenosis facies is uncommon but is more likely seen in severe mitral stenosis with a low resting cardiac output.[12] Complications of mitral stenosis may alter the patient's appearance. Peripheral edema, abdominal distension or cardiac cachexia of severe heart failure, hemiparesis of a cerebral embolus, or an acutely ischemic extremity of a peripheral embolus may be readily apparent. The pulmonary manifestations of significant mitral blockade may be responsible for tachypnea or dyspnea at rest. The peripheral pulses are not significantly altered by mitral stenosis unless there is a marked reduction in cardiac output which can diminish pulse amplitude. The presence and equality of all peripheral pulses should be assessed not only for evidence of previous emboli but also for follow-up observations for this complication. The jugular veins may be normal in height and contour. With the development of right ventricular hypertrophy secondary to pulmonary hypertension prominent *a* waves reflecting loss of right ventricular compliance may be present. Prominent *v* waves of tricuspid regurgitation and elevated venous pressure reflect right ventricular dilatation and heart failure.

On *inspection* and *palpation* of the precordium the apex impulse is normal in size, location, and contour. Not infrequently the apex impulse is not easily palpated, in which case an extreme lateral decubitus position is helpful. An abnormal apex impulse implies some problem other than or in addition to pure mitral stenosis. With marked right ventricular dilatation an abnormal impulse of the right ventricle may be palpable laterally and mistaken for the left ventricular impulse. A sustained systolic parasternal lift of right ventricular hypertrophy may be present. With marked right ventricular dilatation and severe tricuspid regurgitation there may actually be systolic retraction at the apex with a systolic outward motion of the right side of the chest.[22] A first clue to mitral stenosis may be a palpable first heart sound over the precordium as well as a diastolic rumble at the apex (impulse). Occasionally an accentuated pulmonic component of the second heart sound or a loud opening snap (OS) is palpable.

Auscultation reveals the important physical findings of mitral stenosis: *accentuation of the first sound, opening snap,* and *diastolic rumble* (see Fig. 60B-1). The presence or absence of these findings and their auscultatory characteristics reflect some important pathophysiologic changes of mitral stenosis. The diastolic rumble is rarely absent in mitral stenosis,[19] but its presence is not diagnostic.[23] Likewise, there are other causes of an accentuated first heart sound and an opening snap.[23]

Accentuated first heart sound The mechanism of production of the first heart sound and its components is not completely understood.[24,25] The valvular

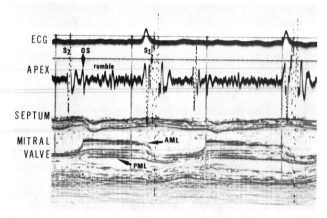

FIGURE 60B-1 Simultaneous phonocardiogram and echocardiogram of a patient with severe mitral stenosis. Accentuation of the first heart sound (S_1) and an opening snap (OS) as well as a diastolic rumble are present. Note the thickened anterior (AML) and posterior (PML) mitral leaflets and the abnormal anterior motion of the posterior leaflet during diastole. The opening snap occurs at the time of maximum anterior motion of the anterior mitral leaflet.

theory would propose that the major mitral component of the first heart sound is produced by vibrations of the valve leaflets and chordae as they are tensed, i.e., after coaptation of the leaflets and during early ventricular contraction.[25–27] Other investigators believe that the components of the first heart sound are produced by vibrations of the entire cardiohemic system[28–30] resulting from movement of the valve leaflets and chordae and/or from ventricular contraction.[31] Correlations of phonocardiography, cineangiography, echocardiography, and left ventricular–left atrial pressure events by most investigators have demonstrated that the "closure sound" of the mitral valve occurs not only after left ventricular–left atrial pressure crossover but also *after* actual coaptation of the leaflets.[25,28,32–35] The sudden cessation of motion of the leaflets toward and beyond the closed (or coapted) position seems to be responsible for the auditory vibrations. It follows, then, that any factor which influences the motion, whether excursion of motion or rate of motion, or any factor which affects the vibratility of the mitral leaflets can bring about changes in the time of occurrence or in the auditory characteristics of the mitral component(s) of the first heart sound. Leaflet mobility is the first obvious implication of an accentuated S_1. Any factor which keeps the position of the leaflets deeper in the left ventricular cavity at the onset of contraction requires a more rapid excursion of the leaflets to a closed position. The late diastolic left atrial–left ventricular pressure gradient of mitral stenosis which provides this change, coupled with changes in vibratory characteristics of the valve leaflets and chordae secondary to fibrosis and scarring, contributes to the accentuated S_1 of mitral stenosis. Since the proximity of atrial contraction to ventricular contraction influences the position of the leaflets at the time of ventricular contraction and contractility of the left ventricle influences rate of excursion of the leaflets, the first heart sound may be accentuated with tachycardia, fever, thyrotoxicosis, and short P-R interval.

In addition to accentuation of S_1 in mitral stenosis the mitral component may be delayed.[36] Although not appreciated on auscultation, the usefulness of this finding in assessing the severity of mitral stenosis has been studied by phonocardiography and found to be limited.[37,63]

Accentuation of S_1 is best appreciated by assessment of the relative intensity of S_1 to S_2 in the second right intercostal space. Normally S_2 is of greater intensity in this location, and a reversal of this relationship implies an accentuated S_1. This finding may be the first auscultatory clue to mitral stenosis. Its presence has no correlation with severity but does imply mitral valve mobility. The absence of an accentuated S_1 when there is evidence of significant mitral stenosis suggests immobility of the mitral leaflets or other factors which tend to reduce its intensity, i.e., mitral regurgitation, aortic regurgitation, or left ventricular dysfunction. Conversely, in a patient with obvious chronic aortic regurgitation or rheumatic mitral regurgitation in which S_1 is anticipated to be reduced in intensity, an accentuation demands careful search for evidence of coexisting mitral stenosis. With atrial fibrillation variation in intensity of S_1 with varying cycle interval also supports valve mobility.[37]

Opening snap Wood considered this the most important sign of mitral stenosis.[12] Sudden cessation of the opening motion of the mitral leaflets is thought by most investigators to be responsible for the opening snap, a postulate of Guttman and Sansom supported by work of Margolies and Wolferth in 1932.[38] Subsequent investigators have studied the usefulness of its presence and its occurrence in relation to S_2 (S_2-OS interval) as a predictor of the severity of mitral stenosis.[39] More recent work, utilizing not only phonocardiography, cineangiography, and intracardiac pressure events but also echocardiography, has confirmed its occurrence after left atrial–left ventricular pressure crossover, after the onset of mitral valve opening and flow, and at the time of maximum opening excursion of the anterior mitral leaflet.[28,33,40,41] Whether the sound produced is the result of vibrations of the leaflets or other cardiohemic structures[24] or of a subsequent closing motion[42] is not known. The time of its occurrence after S_2 is directly related to left atrial pressure. The higher the left atrial pressure, the shorter the S_2-OS interval. Since the left atrial pressure is determined in part by the degree of mitral obstruction, the interval is useful in assessing the severity of mitral stenosis.[43] Many formulas have been devised utilizing both S_2-OS and the QS_1 (by phonocardiography) for this purpose.[44–46] It is important to remember that other factors also influence the S_2-OS interval including cardiac output, heart rate, mobility of the valve, left ventricular systolic pressure, and rate of relaxation and compliance of the left ventricle.[47] Despite these many variables the S_2-OS interval does have some practical clinical significance since it can be determined at the bedside. The S_2-OS interval at normal heart rates is 0.03 to 0.14 s.[43] With critical mitral stenosis it is commonly less than 0.08 s. Occasionally it may be greater despite severe stenosis.[27] The presence of an opening snap implies mobility of the anterior mitral leaflet. With atrial fibrillation the S_2-OS interval generally varies directly with the preceding diastolic interval.[50] A constant S_2-OS interval despite variation in cycle length suggests less mobility of the mitral leaflets.[51] Simultaneous mitral valve flow and phonocardiographic studies[48,49] suggest that the time from S_2 to actual opening of the valve is related to severity while the delay from opening to the occurrence of the opening snap is related to leaflet mobility. This finding may explain some cases of a long S_2-OS interval despite severe stenosis.

The *normal* mitral valve can produce an audible opening sound in certain situations in which there is increased mitral valve flow. Mitral opening snaps have been described in mitral regurgitation,[52,53] ventricular septal defect, idiopathic second- and third-degree heart block, tricuspid atresia with a large atrial septal defect, and tetralogy of Fallot after a Blalock-Taussig procedure.[53] A left atrial myxoma may be associated with an early diastolic sound similar to an opening snap.[54] In addition an opening snap may be produced by the tricuspid valve in atrial septal defect,[55] Ebstein's anomaly,[56] and tricuspid stenosis[57] and must be differentiated from a mitral opening snap.

The mitral opening snap is best heard with a diaphragm and most often at or near the apex impulse or left lower sternal border. When loud, it may radiate to the base and be heard in the second right or left intercostal space. It must be differentiated from other heart sounds, most importantly the pulmonic component of S_2. A combination of two sounds around S_2 may be A_2 and P_2, S_2 and OS, or S_2 and S_3. If inspiratory splitting of the aortic and pulmonic components of S_2, in addition to the OS, can be heard, in the second left intercostal space (2 LICS), i.e., on inspiration A_2-P_2-OS and on expiration S_2-OS, then the OS can be confidently identified. The differentiation of S_2-OS versus A_2-P_2 without inspiratory splitting of S_2 is more difficult. Maneuvers known to vary the S_2-OS interval are helpful. Standing, by decreasing venous return and lowering left atrial pressure, can lengthen the S_2-OS interval unless it is abbreviated by an increase in heart rate, while an A_2-P_2 interval will decrease or remain constant.[58–60] Exercise will tend to shorten the S_2-OS interval depending on the severity of mitral stenosis[61] while it does not significantly influence splitting of A_2-P_2 except in acute thromboembolism[62] or acute cor pulmonale in which exercise may increase and fix the splitting of S_2. Both P_2 and OS may be heard at 2 LICS and apex. P_2 is usually louder at 2 LICS with radiation to apex when there is pulmonary hypertension or atrial septal defect. OS is best heard near apex or lower left sternal border (LLSB) with radiation to 2 LICS if it is very loud.

An opening snap is rarely confused with a ventricular gallop sound. The latter usually occurs later after S_2, 0.12 to 0.16 s, although the timing of an "early" S_3 may be the same as a "late" opening snap. Ventricular gallop sounds are usually of lower frequency with less radiation over the precordium. The left ventricular S_3 is localized at the apex impulse and the right ventricular S_3 at the left lower sternal border. Occasionally, however, ventricular gallop sounds may be heard at the second left or right intercostal space. The early diastolic sound of left atrial myxoma is usually of lower frequency and more often confused with a gallop sound.[54] A tricuspid opening snap is recognized by its localization of the left lower sternal border and associated findings of atrial septal defect, tricuspid stenosis, or Ebstein's anomaly.

The presence of an opening snap, like the accentuated S_1, implies valve mobility. It may be present in mild cases with or without other auscultatory features. In severe cases it may be absent due to a calcified immobile valve or coexisting mitral regurgitation. Associated aortic valve disease, especially aortic regurgitation or a dilated right ventricle,[12] may hinder its appreciation.

Since the S_2-OS interval is useful in assessing the severity of mitral stenosis, the ability to estimate this time interval at the bedside is important and can be mastered with a little practice. Cobbs has used ordinary speech rhythm for this purpose.[63]

As the examiner listens to the heart, he should silently pronounce each interval until he finds the proper fit. "Blah" equals approximately 0.03 sec; "b-t" equals 0.06 sec ("butter" pronounced silently and as quickly as possible); "d-t" equals 0.08 sec (the "d" and "t" sounds pronounced in quick sequence by moving the tip of the tongue as rapidly as possible back from behind the gum to the forepart of the palate); "pa-pa" equals 0.10 to 0.12 sec.

Diastolic rumble Mitral stenosis is almost always associated with a diastolic rumble. It is a low-frequency murmur which begins just after the opening snap with a subsequent decrescendo pattern forming a middiastolic component. Late diastolic may be clear, or there may be a crescendo-decrescendo or crescendo presystolic (late diastolic) component. The stenotic mitral orifice in middiastole with maintained valve flow and its exaggeration in late diastole by atrial contraction have been the classic explanation for the production of the noise. By simultaneous phonocardiographic and echocardiographic studies the middiastolic rumble occurs during movement of the mitral valve leaflets toward the closed position despite continued mitral valve flow produced by the persistent left atrial–left ventricular diastolic pressure gradient.[64,65] It is this closing motion of the mitral leaflets as well as the altered blood flow that are thought to contribute to the production of the middiastolic and presystolic rumble.[65] This concept may also explain the mechanism of diastolic rumbles associated with increased flow through a normal mitral valve. The presystolic rumble, contrary to original concepts, can occur in the presence of atrial fibrillation and even when the rumble is a function of increased flow through a

normal valve (see later discussion). The explanation for the presystolic murmur is quite controversial. Some investigators postulate it is due to continued mitral valve flow in the face of a narrowing orifice at the onset of ventricular contraction.[66,67] Others believe it is a ventricular event occurring during early ventricular systole and can be demonstrated with atrial fibrillation without mitral stenosis.[68,69]

The mitral diastolic rumble may be easily missed on auscultation. It is of low frequency with little radiation and is heard in a very localized area at the apex impulse. After the apex impulse is located, the bell of the stethoscope should be applied with just enough pressure to make contact with the skin. A slight left lateral decubitus position helps to bring the apex impulse closer to the chest wall. When the apex impulse cannot be located, and this is not unusual in pure mitral stenosis, "exploring" the area by auscultation to find the point of maximum intensity of S_1 to S_2 can locate the area of the rumble. Most often the rumble is heard only over the apex impulse but occasionally only *adjacent* to it; so it is wise to explore the area carefully. The most important point to remember in detection of the mitral stenosis rumble is that it may be heard *only* over an area *no larger than the diameter of the stethoscope bell*. Certain maneuvers at the bedside may aid in its detection. The rumble may be heard while the patient is turning from the supine to left lateral position or after enough exercise, sit-ups for example, to increase the heart rate. Auscultation after the patient coughs several times may be helpful.[23]

There is little correlation of the intensity of the diastolic rumble with the severity of stenosis. Severe mitral stenosis, for example, may be associated with a barely audible rumble or a rumble so loud as to be palpable. The duration and diastolic timing of the murmur, however, can provide clues to severity. A brief middiastolic rumble or a presystolic rumble suggests mild disease, while a middiastolic rumble which persists throughout diastole with presystolic accentuation, with a normal heart rate, suggests more significant stenosis. With atrial fibrillation the persistence of the rumble to S_1 even with long diastolic pauses has the same significance. However, with the development of severe pulmonary vascular disease and reduced cardiac output reducing mitral valve flow, the murmur may be brief and barely audible. This situation can be responsible for the "silent mitral stenosis" in which no rumble is easily audible. In these cases the rumble may be elicited by careful attention to auscultatory detail when other clues to the presence of mitral stenosis are appreciated.[19]

A mitral diastolic rumble is not diagnostic of mitral stenosis. Blockade to left atrial–left ventricular blood flow can result from left atrial myxoma,[54] cor triatriatum,[70] calcification of the mitral annulus,[71] or pericardial constriction localized to the left atrioventricular groove.[72] The Carey-Coombs murmur, a diastolic rumble which can be present during acute rheumatic fever, is transient, does not predict future mitral stenosis, and is probably due to distortion of the valve leaflets during the acute endocarditis. Other diastolic rumbles are a function of increased flow through a normal mitral valve as in mitral regurgitation, ventricular septal defect, patent ductus arteriosus, anemia, thyrotoxicosis, and complete heart block. Pure aortic regurgitation may produce a diastolic rumble (see later discussion). A pseudorumble produced by a summation gallop, when the atrial gallop so closely follows a ventricular gallop, must be recognized. Slowing of the heart rate by carotid sinus massage will usually separate the two gallop sounds.

A *Graham Steell murmur*[73a] of pulmonary regurgitation due to the severe pulmonary hypertension of mitral stenosis may be difficult to differentiate from that of aortic regurgitation. The latter is favored by the presence of peripheral signs; however, they are not always reliable indicators in the presence of severe mitral stenosis. Angiographic assessment for aortic regurgitation is indicated during cardiac catheterization.

ELECTROCARDIOGRAM

The electrocardiogram in mitral stenosis (1) provides clues to the presence of mitral stenosis, (2) is not reliably sensitive as an indicator of hemodynamic severity in isolated mitral stenosis, (3) can suggest the presence of coexisting disease in recognized mitral stenosis.

P wave changes of left atrial enlargement (see Chap. 23) include a broad notched P wave in lead II and a prominent negative terminal portion of the P wave in V_1 (Fig. 60B-2). The exact cause of this left atrial abnormality is not known.[73] It may be seen in many disease states[74] even without left atrial enlargement.[75] Even though it is not specific for mitral stenosis, it serves as a valuable *clue* to its presence.

Chronic atrial fibrillation can occur without other evidence of heart disease, but evidence for coronary atherosclerotic heart disease, hypertensive heart disease, rheumatic heart disease, or cor pulmonale is frequently present.[76] As many as 40 percent of patients with significant mitral stenosis will have atrial fibrillation.[12] Its occurrence has only slight correlation with severity[77,78] and is more frequent in patients over 40 years old.[78,79] The cause-and-effect relationship of left atrial enlargement and atrial fibrillation has not been clarified.[79]

With the development of pulmonary hypertension electrocardiographic evidence of right ventricular hypertrophy (RVH) would be anticipated. Unfortunately, the correlation of electrocardiographic evidence of RVH with the degree of pulmonary hypertension or mitral valve area has not been rewarding.[80–82] Computer multivariate analysis of the ECG may improve the correlation.[83] Severe mitral stenosis can be present despite a normal QRS.[84] The frontal-plane QRS axis is the most reliable of indicators: the more rightward the frontal axis, the more likely pulmonary hypertension and a significant reduction in mitral valve area. A frontal axis of greater than +60° predicts an 88 percent chance of a mitral valve area of less than 1.3 cm², and a frontal axis of +91° or greater reliably predicts a mean pulmonary artery pressure of 33 mm Hg or greater (normal less than 20 mm Hg).[77,84] This tendency toward rightward axis may serve as a clue to restenosis following a successful commissurotomy.[85] The higher the pulmonary artery pressure, the more likely RVH will be present on the ECG.[86] The presence of ECG evidence of RVH (Fig. 60B-3) is a reliable indicator of pulmonary hypertension. The electrocardiographic pattern in severe pulmonary hypertension is a rightward and anterior QRS axis with a clockwise horizontal loop as reflected in the QR pattern in V_1. Type C RVH,[87] more commonly associated with cor pulmonale, does occur with RVH of mitral stenosis.[82] The horizontal QRS loop is displaced to the right posterior quadrant and is reflected on the scalar leads as a smaller R and deeper S in V_6.

CHEST ROENTGENOGRAM

The roentgenographic findings of mitral stenosis reflect anatomic and physiologic changes of acute and chronic left atrial hypertension. Evidence for some degree of left atrial enlargement (Fig. 60B-4) is

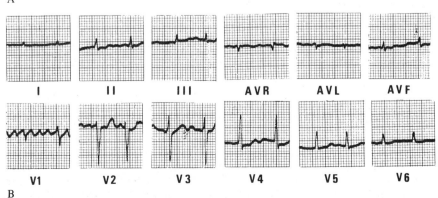

FIGURE 60B-2 Electrocardiograms of patient with mitral stenosis. The ECGs were made 7 years apart during which time the patient's symptoms and hemodynamic findings progressed. *A.* Left atrial abnormality and a +60° frontal QRS axis. *B.* Atrial fibrillation with coarse fibrillatory waves and a +85° frontal QRS axis.

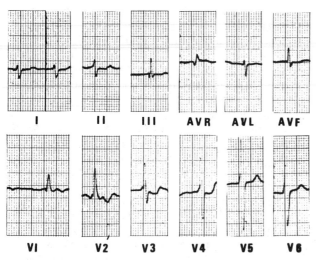

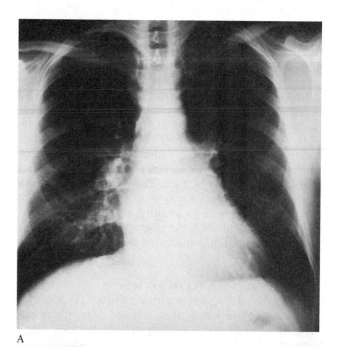

A

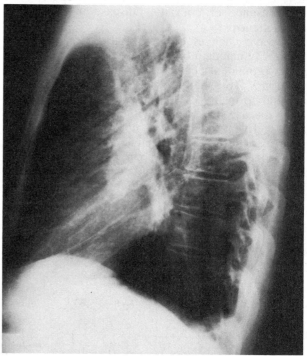

B

FIGURE 60B-3 ECG of severe right ventricular hypertrophy with a rightward and anterior frontal QRS axis. This patient had cardiac cachexia with severe mitral stenosis. A murmur of aortic regurgitation was present, and severe tricuspid regurgitation was obvious on examination of the jugular veins. At surgery the mitral, aortic, and tricuspid valves were replaced. The patient has had marked improvement in functional capacity as well as a 50-lb gain in lean body weight.

present in virtually all cases of symptomatic mitral stenosis[88–90,12] and in some with few symptoms.[90,77] On the posteroanterior view the left atrial appendage may be seen along the left heart border between the pulmonary artery segment and ventricle[7] forming the four bumps of mitral stenosis. A double density through the heart shadow to the right of the spine also suggests left atrial enlargement but can be seen in normal subjects.[91] Left atrial enlargement can also be appreciated on the lateral view, and since it displaces the middle one-third of the esophagus posteriorly, a barium-filled esophagus (Fig. 60B-5) improves detection.[88] The degree of left atrial enlargement does not correlate with left atrial pressure.[88,92,93] Marked enlargement does tend to be present in patients with severe mitral stenosis and atrial fibrillation.[88,89]

When pulmonary venous pressure approaches the plasma oncotic pressure (17 to 25 mm Hg), the capacity of lymphatic drainage is exceeded, and there is transudation of fluid into the interstitium of the lungs.[94] Accumulation of this fluid in the interlobular septa produces characteristic radiographic findings.[95] Linear shadows extending to the pleural surface in a perpendicular fashion, best seen in the costophrenic angles, 1 to 3 cm in length by 1 to 2 mm thick and ½ to 1 cm apart were originally labeled B lines by Kerley in 1933. Other interlobular septa in the upper lung fields, Kerley A lines, and in the bases, Kerley C lines, are less often appreciated.[91] The B lines are seen in one-third[96] to one-half[88] of surgical cases of mitral stenosis. Their absence does not necessarily imply a normal left atrial pressure. These septal lines may be seen in pulmonary venous hyper-

FIGURE 60B-4 Chest roentgenograms of a patient with calculated mitral valve area of 0.87 cm². Note prominent pulmonary arteries. Left atrial enlargement apparent on lateral view, and left atrial appendage seen on posteroanterior view.

tension due to other causes, left ventricular failure for example, as well as other causes of thickening of the septa as in pneumoconioses, lymphangitic metastasis, pneumonia, or pulmonary hemorrhage.[91] During the course of mitral stenosis B lines may occur transiently with an acute event raising left atrial pressure, for example atrial fibrillation with a rapid ventricular response, but eventually they persist with the development of chronic pulmonary venous hypertension. After surgical relief of the mitral blockade they may resolve or persist if hemosiderin depo-

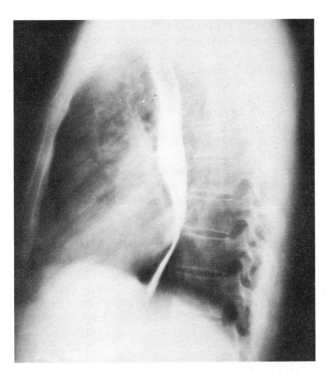

FIGURE 60B-5 Lateral roentgenogram with barium in esophagus demonstrating left atrial enlargement.

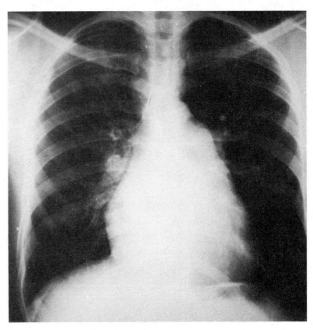

FIGURE 60B-6 Chest roentgenogram of a patient with a calculated mitral valve area of 0.7 cm² and moderate pulmonary hypertension. Tricuspid regurgitation was evident on physical examination. Note increase in cardiac silhouette due to right ventricular dilatation. Left atrial enlargement is evident by the double density of the heart shadow to the right of the spine and left atrial appendage on the left cardiac border.

sition has occurred.[96] Other roentgenographic findings of interstitial pulmonary edema include perivascular cuffing, peribronchial cuffing, subpleural thickening, perihilar haze, and a generalized loss of translucency.[98]

An acute elevation of pulmonary venous pressure is more likely to produce alveolar pulmonary edema with transudation of fluid into the alveolar spaces.[97] Patients with mitral stenosis, even those who ordinarily have few symptoms, may present with acute pulmonary edema and this radiographic appearance when tachycardia develops for any reason. Atrial tachycardia or atrial fibrillation with a rapid ventricular response are most common.

With pulmonary venous hypertension there is redistribution of pulmonary blood flow to the upper lobes.[98] This results in a characteristic radiographic pattern with attenuation of vascular markings in the lower lobes and prominent vasculature in the upper lobes. Most patients with significant mitral stenosis have this upper lobe shunting and enlarged pulmonary arteries.[88] Recent studies in the use of xenon radiospirometry are promising for more reliable correlations.[99]

Enlargement of the pulmonary arteries in mitral stenosis reflects the presence of pulmonary arterial hypertension. If the diameter of the proximal segment of the right descending pulmonary artery measures more than 15 to 17 mm, some degree of pulmonary hypertension can be predicted.[88] The size of the right pulmonary artery does not, however, increase linearly with progressive elevation of pressure, so that severity cannot be predicted. Another measurement using the ratio of the main pulmonary artery to the left hemithorax has slightly better correlation.[88]

These changes in the pulmonary vascular pattern and pulmonary artery size may occur as a result of

other problems. Any cause of an elevated pulmonary venous pressure can result in redistribution of blood flow, although mitral stenosis produces the most remarkable changes. Emphysema, with its loss of vasculature, may be localized to the lower lobes and produce this pattern. The pulmonary arteries may enlarge from many causes of pulmonary hypertension as well as from increased pulmonary flow without an increased pressure as in atrial septal defect.

The cardiac silhouette may be normal in size in mitral stenosis even when blockade is critical. Right ventricular enlargement may, however, produce considerable increase in heart size (Figs. 60B-6 and 60B-7) and be mistaken for left ventricular enlargement. Subtle changes in the posteroanterior and lateral views can aid in differentiation.[91]

Mitral valve calcification is frequently seen. It may be appreciated on the chest roentgenogram or more reliably on fluoroscopy. It is said to be more common in the male and in the older patient.[100,101]

This constellation of roentgenographic findings, (1) left atrial enlargement, (2) interstitial edema, (3) alveolar edema, (4) redistribution of blood flow to the upper lobes, (5) enlarged pulmonary arteries, and (6) right ventricular enlargement, although each individually is not specific for mitral stenosis, not only serves as a clue to its presence but also aids in assessment of severity. The computation of these findings in an individual case is influenced by other data, both subjective and objective.

ECHOCARDIOGRAM

The echocardiogram is an invaluable tool in the diagnosis or exclusion of mitral stenosis in questionable cases.[102] The characteristic echocardiographic features of mitral stenosis (Fig. 60B-1) include[103] (1) a decreased E to F slope of the anterior leaflet of the mitral valve with loss of the *a* wave, (2) decreased excursion of the mitral valve, (3) abnormal direction of motion of the posterior leaflet of the mitral valve, and (4) dense mitral valve echos of fibrosis or multiple mitral valve echos of calcification.[104] Left atrial enlargement, changes in pulmonary valve motion suggesting pulmonary hypertension, and right ventricular enlargement may be present. With pure mitral stenosis there is notable absence of left ventricular enlargement.[105] A decreased E to F slope may be present in other situations in which there is decreased mitral valve flow or impairment of left ventricular filling.[106–108] The posterior leaflet of the mitral valve normally moves posteriorly in a pattern that is mirror-image to the anterior leaflet. In mitral stenosis there is loss of this posterior motion, and the posterior leaflet may actually move anteriorly in a pattern parallel to the anterior leaflet.[109] This finding is specific for mitral stenosis, although mitral stenosis may be present without this finding.[110,111] Rarely, however, is posterior leaflet motion normal with significant mitral stenosis.[112] The decreased E to F slope and decreased excursion of the mitral valve have been used to predict the severity of mitral stenosis.[113] Recent reevaluation of this correlation questions its validity.[112,114] An E to F slope of less than 10 mm/s is a fair predictor of severe mitral stenosis. As a diagnostic tool, some degree of mitral stenosis is said to be present if the E to F slope is less than 35 mm/s (in the absence of other causes).[115,116] Echocardiographic findings in mitral stenosis may aid in planning the surgical approach.[115] The presence of a mobile valve favors commissurotomy, while an immobile calcified valve favors valve replacement.[117] The size of the left ventricular outflow tract assessed by the echocardiogram may aid the surgeon in the choice of the type of prosthetic valve when commissurotomy is not feasible.[118] The echocardiogram has also been used in the evaluation of the results of mitral commissurotomy.[119]

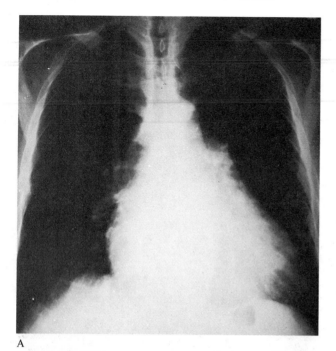

A

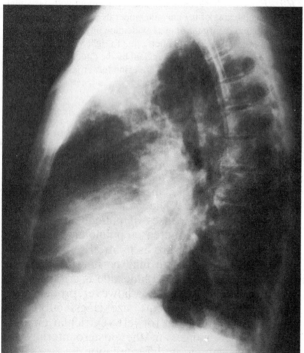

B

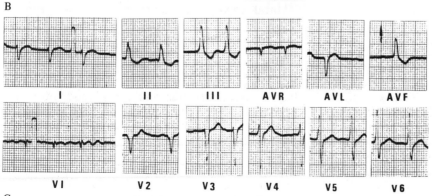

C

FIGURE 60B-7 Chest roentgenograms and ECG of a patient initially thought to have cardiomyopathy. Severe tricuspid regurgitation and peripheral edema as well as a systolic murmur of mitral regurgitation and a diastolic rumble were present. The roentgenograms demonstrate marked enlargement of the heart and pulmonary arteries. The ECG demonstrates atrial fibrillation and a mean QRS axis to the right and posterior compatible with right ventricular hypertrophy. The echocardiogram was compatible with severe mitral stenosis. Heavy mitral valve calcium was present on fluoroscopy. At surgery the mitral valve orifice was approximately 0.7 cm. There was no aortic valve or coronary artery disease.

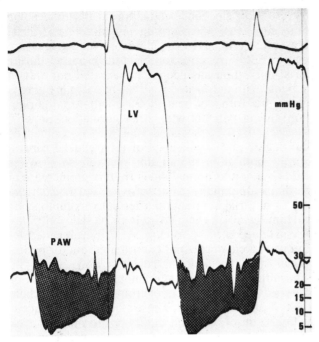

FIGURE 60B-8 Simultaneous pulmonary artery wedge (PAW) and left ventricular (LV) pressure recording in a patient with mitral stenosis. The shaded area represents the pressure gradient across the mitral valve during diastole. Note that the PAW pressure is approximately 30 mm Hg and the LV pressure at end diastole is 10 mm Hg.

CARDIAC CATHETERIZATION

Cardiac catheterization data in mitral stenosis demonstrate the mitral valve gradient in diastole. Normally left ventricular end-diastolic pressure equals mean left atrial pressure, but with a narrowed mitral valvular orifice a pressure gradient develops. The pulmonary capillary pressure, obtained by "wedging" an open-ended catheter into a peripheral pulmonary artery, is most often used as an indirect measure of left atrial pressure. This measurement made simultaneously with a direct left ventricular pressure provides the mitral gradient throughout diastole (Fig. 60B-8). Correlation of this pressure gradient with cardiac output, heart rate, and diastolic filling period provides the mitral valve area by the Gorlin and Gorlin formula[120] or its modification.[121] Most symptomatic patients have a calculated mitral valve area of less than 1.5 cm^2. There is a linear correlation of symptoms with mitral valve area. Some patients with few symptoms will have a mitral valve area of 1.0 cm or less.[77] Cardiac output at rest is most frequently in the low-normal range but can be significantly depressed especially with severe pulmonary hypertension. The pulmonary capillary pressure is usually over 15 to 18 mm Hg in the symptomatic patient.[77,12] Since the pulmonary capillary (indirect left atrial) pressure is influenced by cardiac output as well as mitral orifice size, a lower left atrial pressure may occur with significant mitral stenosis when the resting cardiac output is severely depressed. A rapid heart rate produced by decreasing diastolic filling period may enhance the mitral diastolic gradient. Thus to correlate the left atrial pressure with severity of mitral blockade the cardiac output and heart rate

must be considered. Some degree of pulmonary hypertension is present in most symptomatic cases, and occasionally it is severe. A reduced cardiac output and a mean pulmonary artery pressure that exceeds the mean left atrial pressure by greater than 25 mm Hg reliably predicts an elevated pulmonary vascular resistance.[12] This implies that the pulmonary artery pressure is more than passively elevated by the left atrial pressure. Regression of this abnormal pulmonary vascular resistance occurs after surgical intervention.[122]

A mild form of exercise significantly increases the left atrial pressure and mitral valve gradient.[123] An increase in heart rate and an increase in cardiac output are responsible for this augmentation of pressure gradient. The cardiac output does not, however, increase in a fashion normal for the degree of exercise.[124] The reduced resting cardiac output and the blunted increase with exercise are said to be the hemodynamic hallmark of mitral stenosis.[77]

Left ventricular dysfunction has been documented in mitral stenosis.[125] The exact mechanism is unclear.[126] Left ventricular angiography has demonstrated segmental and diffuse contraction abnormalities.[127–129] Left ventricular dysfunction has also been demonstrated by an abnormal response of the left ventricular diastolic pressure to atrial pacing.[130] Whether coexisting ischemic heart disease due to coronary artery disease, idiopathic cardiomyopathy, residual of rheumatic pancarditis, or other forms of heart disease are responsible has not been clarified by currently available studies. This left ventricular dysfunction has been implicated in the pathogenesis of the reduced cardiac output in mitral stenosis.[77] A significant degree of left ventricular dysfunction may explain the lack of symptomatic improvement postoperatively in some patients.

The assessment of mitral regurgitation by left ventricular angiography is an important aspect of catheterization in selected cases. The presence of significant mitral regurgitation mitigates against mitral commissurotomy. Left atrial angiography, either by selective left atrial injection or by levo-phase opacification after pulmonary artery injection,[131] can demonstrate filling defects of left atrial clot. These data are useful if closed commissurotomy is contemplated. The presence of clot on angiography makes this surgical approach inadvisable. The absence of an angiographically demonstrable left atrial filling defect, however, is not a reliable indication of the absence of left atrial clot.

Cardiac catheterization is not absolutely indicated in a young individual with isolated mitral stenosis in whom the symptoms, physical findings, electrocardiogram, chest roentgenogram, and echocardiogram corroborate significant mitral stenosis with a pliable mitral valve. Cardiac catheterization is indicated when (1) symptoms are disproportionate to objective evidence in the absence of other causes of the symptoms, (2) other forms of heart disease, valvular, myocardial, or coronary artery, are thought to coexist, (3) mitral regurgitation of uncertain degree is suspected, (4) findings are suggestive of myxoma and the echocardiogram is not confirmatory, and (5) "silent mitral stenosis" is suspected and an adequate echocardiogram cannot be obtained.

Coronary arteriography should be included in the catheterization study in patients with previous myocardial infarction, angina pectoris, or evidence (clinical or hemodynamic) of left ventricular dysfunction.

COMPLICATIONS

During the course of mitral stenosis the development of problems which are secondary to the pathophysiologic consequences of rheumatic heart disease and mitral blockade complicate the clinical picture. Atrial fibrillation is common and predisposes to further deterioration of hemodynamics and to the occurrence of systemic emboli. The development of severe pulmonary hypertension and the consequent right ventricular failure alter the subjective and objective manifestations and adversely influence outcome. An appreciation of their significance aids in early recognition and proper management.

Atrial fibrillation Forty[12] to fifty percent[132] of patients with symptomatic mitral stenosis have atrial fibrillation, although its presence has only slight correlation with severity.[77,78] The exact mechanisms of production are not known. The chronic pressure and volume overload of the left atrium leads to hypertrophy and dilatation. These structural changes alter electrophysiologic properties of the left atrium which predispose to atrial arrhythmias.[133] Fibrosis of the internodal tracts and damage to the sinoatrial node (loss of nodal muscle), the latter especially with associated fibrosis of the pericardium, are common pathologic findings in rheumatic heart disease with chronic atrial fibrillation.[76] These findings are not specific and may be found in other forms of heart disease with atrial fibrillation as well as in older patients with idiopathic atrial fibrillation. Atrial fibrillation is more common in patients with mitral stenosis who are over 40 years of age.[78] The cause-and-effect relationship of left atrial enlargement and atrial fibrillation has not been clarified. The greater degree of left atrial enlargement in patients with atrial fibrillation may be secondary to the development of the arrhythmia. It is postulated that the consequence of chronic pressure overload of the left atrium predisposes to the development of atrial fibrillation and, once the arrhythmia is established, further left atrial enlargement ensues and the arrhythmia is perpetuated.[79]

The hemodynamic consequences of atrial fibrillation in mitral stenosis are of considerable clinical importance.[134] The loss of atrial contribution to ventricular filling[135] and the abbreviated diastolic filling time with a rapid ventricular rate further impede an already compromised flow of blood from left atrium

to left ventricle. Since reduction in diastolic filling time correlates linearly with increase in left atrial pressure, a critical rise in pulmonary venous pressure may result.[136] A reduction of cardiac output during atrial fibrillation has been demonstrated not only in patients with mitral stenosis[135,137] but also in patients with other forms of heart disease with atrial fibrillation and in patients with atrial fibrillation alone.[138] The severity of associated heart disease influences the degree and significance of this reduced cardiac output both at rest and during exercise.[138] After cardioversion to normal sinus rhythm an increase in cardiac output may not occur for several days.[139] The return of atrial contraction after conversion to sinus rhythm may occur immediately or be delayed.[140]

Sustained atrial fibrillation may be preceded by frequent premature atrial contractions and/or paroxysmal atrial fibrillation. The latter may precipitate intermittent new onset pulmonary symptoms of dyspnea and orthopnea or transiently exacerbate them if already present. These symptoms may occur with the onset of atrial fibrillation in a patient who otherwise has few complaints. Paroxysmal as well as initial onset of sustained atrial fibrillation is amenable to therapy, and reversion to sinus rhythm with drugs and/or electroconversion is frequently successful.[141,142] Eventually atrial fibrillation becomes resistant to conversion. The exacerbated pulmonary symptoms may resolve with return to sinus rhythm and the patient remains nonprogressive. With chronic atrial fibrillation the control of the ventricular rate may also relieve symptoms. However, the already reduced resting cardiac output and blunted responses to exercise in mitral stenosis can be further exaggerated with the development of atrial fibrillation and account for worsened fatigue.

Systemic emboli Systemic embolization is a potentially serious complication of mitral stenosis. Most systemic emboli arise from the heart, and rheumatic heart disease is the cause in many. The majority, over 90 percent, of patients with rheumatic heart disease who have systemic emboli have mitral valve involvement, and some degree of mitral stenosis is prominent.[143] The exact incidence of systemic emboli in rheumatic mitral valve disease is obviously not known. Most series have reported from 9 to 20 percent.[144] Patient selection and methods of detection make comparisons difficult. Age and atrial fibrillation are independent variables associated with a high incidence.[144] Two-thirds of the patients with mitral stenosis and systemic emboli in Wood's series[12] had atrial fibrillation. Older patients even without atrial fibrillation tend to have a greater incidence of emboli.[144] The severity of mitral stenosis, left atrial size, or heart failure are not consistently related to the frequency of embolic events,[143,144] although some degree of left atrial enlargement is present in most cases.[143] Survival after the first embolus seems to increase chances of a subsequent embolus.[143,145] In one series 33 percent of patients with systemic emboli had clinically recognized multiple emboli.[145] The distribution of systemic emboli favors the brain but commonly includes extremities, aortic bifurcation, and abdominal viscera. The mortality of systemic emboli is greatest for a cerebral embolus, in which it approaches 50 percent. The average overall mortality for the first systemic embolus in patients with rheumatic heart disease is probably 15 percent with mortality increasing with subsequent emboli.[143]

Several important points emerge from this review: Systemic emboli may occur during *any state* in the natural history of mitral stenosis; *symptoms* related to the *embolus* may be the patient's presenting problem; *mitral valve disease* should always be considered as a possible cause of a *systemic embolus*. Thus the appreciation of the relation of mitral stenosis to the occurrence of systemic emboli affords a clinical clue to its presence and enhances proper management of the patient's problems.

Pulmonary hypertension and heart failure The development of pulmonary hypertension can modify the subjective and objective data in mitral stenosis. Severe elevation of pulmonary arterial pressure, approaching systemic levels, can occur. With the progression of pulmonary hypertension cardiac output is further reduced, and fatigue may terminate exercise prior to the development of dyspnea. Right ventricular hypertrophy and eventually dilatation follow. Severe systemic venous congestion can produce peripheral edema and symptoms of hepatic venous congestion. Cardiac cachexia may occur.[146] Elevation of the jugular venous pressure with prominent systolic *v* waves reflects tricuspid regurgitation frequently secondary to right ventricular dilatation and occasionally secondary to concomitant rheumatic tricuspid valve disease. On the contrary, if the jugular venous pulse in these patients with heart failure demonstrates prominent *a* waves, tricuspid stenosis of rheumatic origin is suggested. In the most severe form the patient may present with extreme fatigue, dyspnea, peripheral edema, ascites, and hepatomegaly. Liver function abnormalities associated with the hepatic congestion of heart failure may be prominent. The physical findings of pulmonary hypertension and right ventricular enlargement are present. The diastolic rumble may be of faint intensity and brief duration due to reduced mitral valve flow secondary to the extremely low cardiac output. The ECG will almost always show evidence of right ventricular hypertrophy and atrial fibrillation. The chest roentgenogram will show not only enlarged pulmonary arteries, upper lobe shunting, Kerley B lines, and left atrial enlargement but also some degree of cardiomegaly due to right ventricular dilatation. Mitral stenosis should always be considered as a possible cause in any patient who presents with obvious severe pulmonary hypertension. Echocardiology can be especially useful in these cases. Patients who reach this stage in the natural history have a very poor prognosis which may be improved with surgical intervention (see later discussion).

Endocarditis In isolated mitral stenosis, bacterial endocarditis is an uncommon complication. In the presence of fever, arthralgias, anemia, or systemic emboli in a patient with auscultatory findings suggestive of mitral stenosis, left atrial myxoma should be considered. (See later discussion of "Differential Diagnosis of Rheumatic Mitral Valve Disease.")

Medical management

There is no form of medical therapy directed specifically to the mitral blockade. In the asymptomatic patient who has no evidence by physical examination, ECG, roentgenogram, or echocardiogram of significant obstruction, no specific therapy is indicated. However, all patients with rheumatic heart disease regardless of hemodynamic severity must have appropriate rheumatic fever and endocarditis prophylaxis (see Chaps. 60A and 77). No specific limitations of activities are imposed. It is recommended, however, that even mild mitral stenosis preclude operation of an airplane.[147]

With the development of arrhythmias, specific therapy is indicated. Frequent premature atrial contractions or paroxysmal atrial fibrillation may herald the onset of sustained atrial fibrillation. The institution of antiarrhythmic therapy at this point, specifically with digitalis, may prevent the occurrence of atrial arrhythmias or control ventricular rate when they do develop. Sustained atrial fibrillation, whether or not it produces or aggravates symptoms, is an indication for specific therapy. Recent or acute onset of symptoms of pulmonary congestion may bring the patient to medical attention. There may be acute pulmonary edema or simply a recent decline in exercise tolerance. Bothersome palpitations may be the chief complaint. A systemic embolus may be associated with recent onset of atrial fibrillation.[143] The objective of therapy is to restore sinus rhythm, and if that cannot be done, then control of the ventricular rate is of importance. The urgency of the situation in part determines the therapeutic approach. Immediate electrical conversion is necessary only if there is significant hemodynamic impairment. Otherwise it is appropriate to institute digitalis therapy to control the ventricular rate and then add quinidine to the regimen to attempt pharmacologic conversion to sinus rhythm. Quinidine should not be administered prior to digitalis, since the former may enhance atrioventricular conduction and increase ventricular rate. If pharmacologic conversion is not successful, electrical synchronous dc cardioversion is attempted. Digitalis should be withheld for 24 to 48 h prior to cardioversion. The longer the atrial fibrillation has been present, the less likely sinus rhythm will be restored.[148] Anticoagulant therapy prior to attempts at conversion in all patients with mitral stenosis and atrial fibrillation is recommended by some. If there is evidence of an embolic event, recent or remote, the patient should have anticoagulant therapy for approximately 2 weeks prior to conversion. Neither the danger of precipitating a systemic embolus with cardioversion nor the efficacy of cardioversion or chronic anticoagulation in preventing recurrent emboli has been documented.[144,149] If surgical intervention is anticipated in the near future, cardioversion is best postponed until several weeks after surgery is performed. If chronic atrial fibrillation has to be accepted, control of ventricular rate is mandatory. Occasional patients will require more than the usual 0.25 mg digoxin daily. Since the abbreviation of diastole with tachycardia can increase pulmonary venous hypertension, the control of the ventricular rate not only at rest but also during mild exertion is important to minimize symptoms of exertional dyspnea. In the absence of specific contraindications, left ventricular dysfunction due to associated heart disease or severe lung disease for example, propranolol may be useful.[63] In pure mitral stenosis left ventricular dysfunction of clinical significance is unusual; therefore the use of propranolol is not deleterious [149a] and can be useful in the control of the ventricular response to atrial fibrillation. It may be useful to blunt exercise-induced increase in sinus rate.[149b] If cardioversion is successful, digitalis and quinidine should be continued in an attempt to prevent recurrent atrial fibrillation. Other antiarrhythmic combinations may be used for the same purpose. However, the ideal combination is not apparent. Quinidine is not indicated if chronic atrial fibrillation is to be accepted. See Chap. 46D for further discussion of the management of atrial fibrillation.

The occurrence of a systemic embolus necessitates the institution of chronic anticoagulant therapy in addition to any specific therapeutic interventions for the embolus itself. If there is cerebral embolus, anticoagulation is generally postponed for approximately 2 weeks. The early recognition of a mesenteric embolus or peripheral embolus is important in prompt and proper management. Systemic emboli may occur in patients with mild mitral stenosis and be the first presenting problem. Some physicians recommend mitral valve surgery when a systemic embolus has occurred (see Chap. 61), while others do not.[150] Patients who have had an embolus may not have demonstrable left atrial clot either by angiography or surgical exploration. Patients who have demonstrable left atrial clot by these techniques do not always have a history of emboli. Systemic emboli do occur after mitral commissurotomy.[151] Recurrent systemic emboli despite proper anticoagulation therapy, even in a patient with mild mitral stenosis is an indication for consideration of surgery.

Progressive symptoms of exertional dyspnea, orthopnea, and fatigue require not only the control or prevention of atrial arrhythmias with digitalis but also the use of salt restriction and diuretics. In the presence of heart failure pulmonary emboli are more likely, and this should be considered with symptoms of paroxysmal dyspnea, pleuritic chest pain, or suggestive roentgenographic findings.

The presence of other forms of heart disease—other valvular disease, coronary atherosclerotic heart disease, hypertensive cardiovascular disease, cardiomyopathy—can significantly alter both medical and surgical management.

Surgery (See Chap. 61)

The surgical treatment of mitral stenosis is considered a milestone in medicine.[152] Mitral stenosis was described by Vieussens in 1705, Morgagni in 1761, and Abernethy in 1806.[153] Experimental valvotomy was performed by Klebs in 1874 by the transcarotid approach to produce acute mitral regurgitation.[154] In 1902 Brunton suggested the surgical treatment of mitral stenosis.[155] The attempts of Cutler in 1923 and Souttar in 1925 to alleviate mitral stenosis surgically preceded the near-simultaneous work of Bailey and of Ellis and Harken in 1948.[156] By the mid-1950s the operative mortality for closed mitral commissurotomy was reported to be less than 3 percent in functional class II and III patients.[157] Symptomatic[158] and hemodynamic improvement[159,160] occurred. It was apparent, however, that the best results were obtained in patients with pliable noncalcified valves without regurgitation.[100] The development of cardiopulmonary bypass in the 1960s and the development of prosthetic valves afforded surgical treatment for those patients with a mitral valve not amenable to commissurotomy.[161,162] At present surgical mortality for closed commissurotomy is less than 1 percent and for mitral valve replacement less than 3 percent.[163] The presence of mitral regurgitation, of tricuspid regurgitation to require tricuspid valve replacement, or of an extremely low preoperative cardiac output increases mortality.[163] The effect of surgical intervention on long-term survival is thought to be quite favorable.[101] There are some reservations[150] due to limitations in methods of data collecting and comparison of medical and surgical series. With currently available methods of surgical techniques and perioperative care high-risk patients can be successfully operated on with an improved prognosis.[164]

The consideration of surgical intervention in a patient with mitral stenosis requires attention to (1) disability, (2) objective evidence of significant obstruction, (3) valve mobility, (4) presence or absence of mitral regurgitation, and (5) associated valvular or coronary artery disease as well as any associated medical problems. The time of intervention is determined by the assessment of potential benefit versus operative mortality and postoperative morbidity. At one end of the spectrum is the young female patient with mild to moderate disability, sinus rhythm, pliable mitral valve as evidenced by an accentuated first heart sound and an opening snap, no valve calcium on fluoroscopy, no mitral regurgitation, and no evidence for peripheral emboli. The risk of closed commissurotomy is less than 1 percent, there are no prosthetic valve complications, and improvement in symptoms is the rule.[163,165,166] The patient with lots of valve calcium (more frequently male)[100,101] and evidence of mitral regurgitation will likely require a mitral valve prosthesis and must run the risk of a slightly increased surgical mortality rate,[163,166] as well as the potential complications of a prosthetic valve. Thus more evidence of progressive and incapacitating symptoms despite medical management would be required to recommend surgery. The same reasoning applies if there is mitral stenosis amenable to commissurotomy but associated with other valvular disease that requires prosthetic valve replacement. However, postponement of surgery until class IV symptomatic state has been reached should be avoided, since it is in this state that the mortality rate is maximum.[163,167] A patient who initially presents with severe disease, class IV symptoms, and heart failure should not be denied surgery, since outlook at this stage is grave and surgical intervention can offer help.[164] Occasionally a patient will present with few symptoms despite objective evidence of severe mitral stenosis. It is important to carefully assess this "absence of symptoms." If cardiac catheterization documents critical mitral stenosis, a pliable mitral valve, and moderate to severe pulmonary hypertension without other complicating heart disease, surgery is recommended. Many patients with mitral stenosis are nonprogressive; i.e., they remain stable symptomatically for many years. An initial episode of atrial fibrillation even precipitating severe pulmonary symptoms may be followed, with proper medical management, by many years of nonprogressive disease.[142] Surgery is not hastily recommended in these individuals.

The presence of other valvular disease has an important influence on surgical consideration. When mitral stenosis is associated with significant aortic valve disease, especially aortic stenosis, surgical intervention may be determined by the latter (see later discussion). The presence of significant left ventricular dysfunction is a relative contraindication to surgical palliation of mitral stenosis unless the condition causing the dysfunction can be improved. Preoperative evaluation for the presence or absence of aortic valve disease, tricuspid valve disease, or coronary atherosclerosis is mandatory in suspicious cases to aid in the decision for surgery as well as in the surgical procedure.

Symptomatic and hemodynamic improvement in the majority of patients is reported in many series.[100,101,157,161,162,165–167] Hemodynamic measurements before and after surgery have also confirmed a decrease in left atrial pressure, a decrease in pulmonary artery pressure and pulmonary vascular resistance, and an increase in cardiac output. Symptomatic improvement correlates best with a postoperative increase of 1.0 cm^2 in mitral valve area.[168] Most patients with hemodynamic improvement have an increase in mitral valve area of at least 50 percent.[160] Postoperative reduction in pulmonary hypertension has been demonstrated by several studies.[169–171] This is thought to correlate with the reduced left atrial pressure by the relief of mitral blockade whether by commissurotomy or by prosthetic valve replacement. A concomitant rise in cardiac output implies a reduction in pulmonary vascular resistance. Gradual regression of pulmonary hypertension has been demonstrated,[169,172] and, as suggested by Wood, there may be not only an early postoperative decrease in pulmonary vascular resistance but also further improvement later. Severe pulmonary hypertension is not a contraindication to surgery.

Restenosis of the mitral valve after successful commissurotomy is said to occur in 5[173] to 30 percent[174] of patients within 5 years and as many as 60 percent after 9 years.[173] Early and late postoperative catheterization studies on patients with recurrent symptoms after a period of improvement following surgery have shown that the recurrence of symptoms is uncommonly due to restenosis.[175] Residual stenosis, mitral regurgitation, or other cardiac problems are more commonly responsible.[175–177] Assessment of objective evidence for the relief of mitral stenosis can be important in follow-up when symptoms recur. After successful commissurotomy the opening snap[37] and diastolic rumble may persist but with changes in characteristics suggesting less blockade. The S_2-OS interval is longer and the rumble of shorter diastolic duration and less intensity. The presence postoperatively of an apical systolic murmur may herald future mitral regurgitation. If cardiac enlargement by roentgenogram and right ventricular hypertrophy by ECG were present preoperatively, they will gradually regress after successful commissurotomy.

If atrial fibrillation is present after surgery, specific therapy is indicated. Attempts at conversion to sinus rhythm are best postponed for several weeks. The therapeutic approach would be the same as outlined previously. Successful conversion, either by drugs or electrical cardioversion, is likely to be successful if the atrial fibrillation developed in the postoperative period or if it was present for less than 1 year prior to surgery.[148]

RHEUMATIC MITRAL REGURGITATION

Rheumatic mitral regurgitation may be defined as reflux of blood from the left ventricle to the left atrium during systole due to incompetence of the mitral valve in its closure function, caused by residual rheumatic endocarditis. The mitral valve is the most frequently involved valve in rheumatic carditis.[12] Pure mitral regurgitation, however, seems to be an uncommon result. Pure mitral stenosis or mitral regurgitation with some degree of stenosis are more common.[12,178,179,180] During the nineteenth century all systolic murmurs were thought to represent severe mitral valve disease with a very poor prognosis. In the early twentieth century all systolic murmurs were considered benign. By the late 1920s the potentially serious nature of mitral regurgitation was recognized. The developments in noninvasive diagnostic techniques, cardiac catheterization, and cardiac surgery since that time have revealed the multiple causes and varied clinical spectrum of mitral regurgitation. Rheumatic mitral regurgitation is not the most common of all the causes of mitral regurgitation. It is, however, responsible for approximately one-half of fatal cases[8] or cases requiring surgery.[179]

Severe rheumatic mitral regurgitation may develop during acute rheumatic fever. More commonly, however, the systolic murmur of rheumatic mitral regurgitation is compatible with a long life.[181-183] In most cases symptoms do not develop until the fourth to sixth decades of life.[179] Most series show a female preponderance,[178,179,184-186] while others show a greater number of males.[187,12] A history of rheumatic fever is obtainable in about 75 percent of cases.[179,185,186]

Pathophysiology

During ventricular systole improper coaptation of the mitral leaflets results in ventricular emptying not only into the aorta but also into the left atrium. The gross pathologic study of the mitral valve in rheumatic mitral regurgitation reveals loss of leaflet tissue as a result of fibrosis and contracture. There is minimal commissural fusion.[188] Thickened, fused chordae tendineae are found infrequently.[8] Marked fibrosis and fusion of the posterior leaflet with little abnormality of the anterior leaflet can occur.[189] Depending on the volume of blood entering the left atrium, the left ventricle must compensate to maintain forward output. The left ventricle dilates to accommodate the increased volume introduced into it from the left atrium.[190] Thus the fraction of the total left ventricular output entering the aorta is maintained until marked mitral regurgitation develops or until left ventricular contractility is impaired. The regurgitant volume delivered into the left atrium is gradually progressive, and the left atrium can adjust to the increased volume by dilatation without an increase in mean left atrial pressure. This left atrial dilatation, however, contributes to the progression of the degree of mitral regurgitation. The posterior leaflet of the mitral valve is continuous with elements of the posterior left atrial wall. As the left atrium dilates, there is posterior and inferior displacement of the posterior mitral leaflet, and the mitral incompetence is enhanced.[188] Eventually left ventricular contractility is impaired, resulting in a reduction of forward flow and an increase in left ventricular end-diastolic pressure. Pulmonary venous hypertension passively raises pulmonary artery pressure. In addition reactive pulmonary hypertension similar to that in mitral stenosis occurs but is generally less frequent and less severe.[191] Severe pulmonary hypertension resulting in right ventricular hypertrophy and dilatation develops in some cases.

It is obvious from this slowly progressive process that abrupt rises in left atrial and pulmonary venous pressure, as is seen in mitral stenosis, are not a prominent feature. Acute pulmonary edema, for example, is less frequent in mitral regurgitation than in mitral stenosis. The onset of atrial fibrillation can exacerbate symptoms but usually not as severely as in mitral stenosis. It is important to remember that this gradually progressive profile is dependent on a gradual progression of the degree of mitral regurgitation which allows left atrial dilatation. The occurrence of a sudden worsening of the amount of mitral

regurgitation can significantly change the clinical picture. Patients with rheumatic mitral regurgitation are prone to rupture of the chordae tendineae and to bacterial endocarditis,[187] either of which may suddenly increase the volume of regurgitation. Without causes for sudden deterioration the average duration of symptoms before surgical intervention is 10 years.[179]

Clinical recognition

Many individuals with rheumatic mitral regurgitation are asymptomatic. It is important to remember that rheumatic heart disease can be the cause of a systolic murmur even though there are no symptoms, the physical examination is otherwise normal, and the ECG and chest roentgenogram have no specific abnormalities. Appropriate rheumatic fever and endocarditis prophylaxis must be instituted. At the other end of the spectrum is the patient who presents signs and symptoms of congestive heart failure. It is essential that mitral regurgitation, as well as other surgically amenable forms of valvular disease, be considered. In most cases the physical findings in significant mitral regurgitation are readily appreciated. However, difficult cases may require noninvasive and invasive techniques to clarify the contribution of mitral regurgitation to the patient's problem. On the other hand caution should be exercised in attributing a systolic murmur to rheumatic mitral regurgitation without careful analysis of all data.

SYMPTOMS

An asymptomatic patient who has evidence of rheumatic mitral regurgitation but no cardiac enlargement may remain so for many years.[183] Most frequently there is gradual progression of symptoms prior to overt incapacity.[43] Fatigue and dyspnea are the most common[185,186] and are the result of a reduced cardiac output and elevated pulmonary venous pressure. Orthopnea, paroxysmal nocturnal dyspnea, and peripheral edema are not infrequent. Atrial fibrillation occurs in about 75 percent[179,185] of cases and can exacerbate symptoms. Palpitation is a common complaint.[179,185]

Chest pain is uncommon in mitral regurgitation. If the patient has angina pectoris, coexisting aortic valve or coronary artery disease should be suspected. Hemoptysis occurs infrequently.[185,186] Systemic emboli do occur but are much less frequent than in patients with mitral stenosis.[186]

The occurrence of chordal rupture, endocarditis of the mitral valve, or the development of other forms of heart disease, especially those which increase the work of the left ventricle, may acutely or subacutely exacerbate symptoms. The patient with mild to moderate symptoms who develops systemic hypertension may have more problems until the hypertension is controlled. Rupture of the chordae tendineae is discussed under "Nonrheumatic Mitral Regurgitation."

Without appropriate medical treatment and surgical intervention severe pulmonary hypertension, right ventircular hypertrophy, and dilatation develop, and the patient may present with severe congestive heart failure. Symptoms of systemic venous congestion and peripheral edema as well as pulmonary symptoms are present.

PHYSICAL FINDINGS

The general appearance is usually normal. Stigmata of congestive heart failure may be apparent. On examination of the jugular venous pulsation a prominent *a* wave suggests right ventricular hypertrophy, while prominent systolic *v* waves suggest right ventricular dilatation with tricuspid regurgitation. The jugular venous pressure is usually elevated in the latter situation. The peripheral pulses may be smaller in amplitude but brisk in upstroke.[7,190] If there is left ventricular failure, pulsus alternans may be present.

Inspection and palpation of the precordium can provide very useful information in mitral regurgitation.[192] The apex impulse is frequently displaced laterally in relation to the midclavicular line and is larger than normal. On palpation it is sustained through systole, and an early diastolic filling wave is appreciated. A presystolic component, or *a* wave, the atrial contribution to ventricular filling, is infrequent in chronic rheumatic mitral regurgitation. Parasternal pulsations may be visible or palpable, and their timing by simultaneous palpation and auscultation is important. A left parasternal systolic pulsation in mitral regurgitation may be due to right ventricular hypertrophy or to the expansion of the left atrium by the regurgitant jet.[193] The pulsation of right ventricular hypertrophy begins and rises in early systole, is sustained, does not have great amplitude, and collapses slowly. In contrast the left parasternal pulsation of left atrial expansion begins in early systole but rises slowly with peak amplitude in late systole near the time of the second sound. It may have prominent maximum amplitude followed by a precipitous collapse.[194] This parasternal pulsation is not present in normal individuals, and its presence can aid in the differentiation of mitral regurgitation from other causes of systolic murmurs including ventricular septal defect and left ventricular outflow obstruction.[195] It is more common, however, in acute forms of mitral regurgitation, and the measurement of its amplitude by pulse recording may be useful in the assessment of the severity of the regurgitation.[195] This late systolic parasternal pulsation can be present without pulmonary hypertension and may be misleading[196] unless it is properly timed with the cardiac cycle.

Auscultation A systolic murmur is almost always present in rheumatic mitral regurgitation. A few cases of significant mitral regurgitation without a systolic murmur have been reported.[197–199] The murmur is typically holosystolic.[14] It begins with the first heart sound, and since left ventricular pressure exceeds left atrial pressure after aortic closure, the murmur continues to or through the aortic component of the second sound.[7] It is medium- to high-frequency and thus harsh or blowing but rarely coarse.[14] Typically it is of constant intensity throughout systole but occasionally has early, mid-, or late

systolic accentuation.[4,184] Although the intensity of the murmur does not correlate with the severity of regurgitation, in most symptomatic patients it is grade 3 (on a scale of six grades) or greater intensity.[179,184–186] The murmur of rheumatic mitral regurgitation most often radiates to the axilla, back, left infrascapular area, and by bone conduction along the spine from the cervical to lumbar vertebrae.[7,184] The murmur of mitral regurgitation may radiate anteriorly to the second right intercostal space and base of the neck and simulate aortic stenosis. This is more common, however, in acute forms of mitral regurgitation when the posterior mitral leaflet is primarily involved.

Unlike the systolic murmurs of left ventricular outflow obstruction the murmur of mitral regurgitation has little variation in intensity with the varying cycle interval of atrial fibrillation, and it does not increase in intensity in the first sinus beat after a premature atrial or ventricular beat.[184,200] A decrease in intensity on standing and increase in intensity on squatting is also characteristic of the murmur. Since tricuspid regurgitation can be associated with mitral valve disease, the differentiation of the murmurs of tricuspid and mitral regurgitation is important.[201] The murmur of tricuspid regurgitation is of maximum intensity along the left sternal border and frequently increases in intensity on inspiration. The murmur of rheumatic mitral regurgitation does not vary significantly with respiration and is of maximum intensity at the apex with radiation to the axilla. These bedside observations as well as other observations during pharmacologic maneuvers are useful in the differentiation of systolic murmurs.[202]

The first heart sound is normal or decreased in intensity in most cases.[184,185,203] Occasionally it is sharp and accentuated.[203] When the valve deformity primarily involves the posterior leaflet, the anterior leaflet has good mobility, and a loud first heart sound as well as an opening snap can occur.[189] The second heart sound may be normal. With abbreviation of ventricular systole due to the regurgitant volume the aortic component of the second sound can occur early and be responsible for persistent expiratory splitting of the aortic and pulmonic components.[184,204] When the intensity of the pulmonic component of the second sound equals or exceeds the intensity of the aortic component in the second left intercostal space, pulmonary hypertension is likely to be present.[205]

The presence of a ventricular gallop sound implies considerable mitral regurgitation and precludes significant mitral stenosis.[191,206,207] It occurs 0.12 to 0.24 s after S_2 and is coincident with the rapid filling wave of the apex pulse.[184,203] It frequently introduces a brief middiastolic rumble. A middiastolic pressure gradient across the mitral valve due to the regurgitant volume is responsible for the rumble.[184,203] Rapid closure of the mitral valve in the presence of increased mitral valve flow may contribute to the genesis of the rumble.[64] An atrial gallop sound is

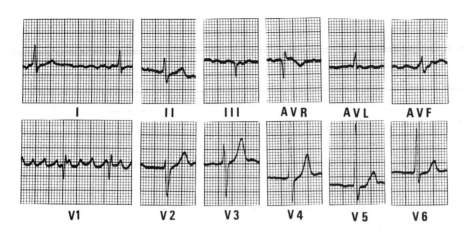

FIGURE 60B-9 ECG of a patient with systolic murmur of mitral regurgitation and a diastolic rumble introduced by a ventricular gallop sound suggesting predominant mitral regurgitation. The ECG shows atrial fibrillation and a frontal QRS axis of 0°, the latter being more compatible with mitral regurgitation than mitral stenosis.

uncommon in chronic mitral regurgitation. Powerful atrial contribution to ventricular filling is lost in the chronic state due to a fibrotic left atrial wall with loss of musculature.[190]

An opening snap may occur in pure mitral regurgitation.[52,179,184,189] A functioning mobile anterior leaflet is present. The first heart sound may be accentuated. The opening snap occurs prior to the ventricular gallop sound, and if the aortic component of the second sound is premature, the opening snap may be nearly coincident with the pulmonic closure sound.[189]

ELECTROCARDIOGRAM

Electrocardiographic changes may be of little help in the recognition or assessment of mitral regurgitation. The majority of symptomatic cases have atrial fibrillation[208] (Fig. 60B-9), and when sinus rhythm is present left atrial abnormality, P mitrale, is the rule. Obvious left ventricular hypertrophy is present in about one-half the cases[74] and is usually associated with a normal frontal plane QRS axis.[208] Right ventricular or biventricular hypertrophy is uncommon.

CHEST ROENTGENOGRAM

Left ventricular and left atrial enlargement are almost always present in symptomatic cases of chronic rheumatic mitral regurgitation.[179,185] Left ventricular dilatation is suggested by the enlarged cardiac silhouette on the posteroanterior view and by displacement of the ventricle toward the spine on the lateral view. On the posteroanterior view left atrial enlargement is represented by the left atrial appendage along the left heart border, a double density of the heart shadow to the right of the spine (Fig. 60B-10), and elevation of the left main stem bronchus increasing the normal angle of bifurcation of trachea to greater than 50°.[180] Posterior deviation of the esophagus by the left atrium is prominent and more diffuse than the localized displacement seen in pure mitral stenosis.[185] Massive left atrial enlargement filling both sides of the chest is seen occasionally.[14]

Changes in the roentgenographic appearance of the pulmonary vasculature are less striking in pure mitral regurgitation than in pure mitral stenosis. Severe mitral regurgitation of the gradually progressive variety may be associated with marked left ventricular and left atrial dilatation and normal pulmonary vessels.[185] However, when severe pulmonary venous and arterial hypertension do develop, upper lobe shunting and enlarged pulmonary arteries are likely to be present.

On cardiac fluoroscopy calcification of the mitral valve may be appreciated. In pure mitral regurgitation calcification is less frequent than in pure mitral stenosis or mixed mitral stenosis and regurgitation. Systolic expansion of the left atrium may be present but is helpful only when it is marked. It may be absent with severe mitral regurgitation.[180]

FIGURE 60B-10 Posteroanterior roentgenogram of a patient with severe mitral regurgitation. A commissurotomy for mitral stenosis had been done 8 years earlier. Note the absence of the left atrial appendage secondary to the prior surgical procedure. Left atrial enlargement is apparent from the double density of the cardiac silhouette to the right of the spine.

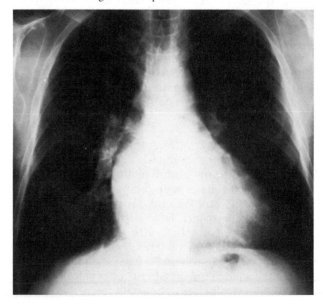

The diagnostic usefulness of the echocardiogram in rheumatic mitral regurgitation is limited.[115] Dense mitral valve echoes suggest rheumatic valvular disease but do not provide reliable information about the degree of mitral regurgitation. Other abnormalities of the mitral valve may suggest another cause of the mitral regurgitation, for example mitral valve prolapse or a flail valve,[103] but do not exclude the presence of rheumatic disease. Increased left atrial and left ventricular dimensions reflect the volume changes of these chambers. Exaggerated systolic expansion of the posterior left atrial wall is a useful diagnostic finding but is more common in acute mitral regurgitation.[116] The degree of mitral regurgitation cannot be determined by echocardiography.

CARDIAC CATHETERIZATION

Documentation of the degree of mitral regurgitation and an assessment of left ventricular function are important goals of cardiac catheterization in symptomatic patients. Quantitative angiography is the most accurate clinical method to assess the degree of mitral regurgitation.[209] The total left ventricular output per beat is determined by measurement of left ventricular end-diastolic and end-systolic volumes. The forward cardiac output as measured by the Fick method is subtracted from the total left ventricular output to give the regurgitant volume. In most symptomatic patients 50 percent or greater of the total left ventricular stroke volume enters the left atrium.[210] A reasonable estimate of the degree of mitral regurgitation can be obtained by subjective evaluation of left ventricular cineangiography. Left ventricular end-diastolic and end-systolic volumes are increased in chronic mitral regurgitation, but as long as left ventricular function is normal, the ejection fraction is not reduced.[209] Left ventricular end-diastolic pressure is frequently elevated but does not necessarily imply ventricular dysfunction.

Mild to moderate elevation of pulmonary capillary and pulmonary arterial pressures and an elevated pulmonary vascular resistance are usually present.[179,185,191] A normal left atrial pressure despite severe mitral regurgitation[211] is uncommon. The contour of the left atrial pulse may show a prominent *v* wave but is not a reliable indicator of the presence or the severity of regurgitation.[185,212] Simultaneous recording of left atrial and left ventricular pressures may demonstrate a middiastolic pressure gradient due to increased flow, but the pressures at end diastole are equal. Cardiac output is usually reduced in symptomatic cases of chronic mitral regurgitation.[179,191]

Angiography of the coronary arteries should be included in the catheterization study when mitral valve surgery is anticipated.

COMPLICATIONS

Atrial fibrillation is present in many of the patients. Its presence correlates with age,[208] duration of the disease,[185] and severity. There is a greater reduction of cardiac output when atrial fibrillation is present.[185]

Fatigue and dyspnea are more prominent. With the occurrence of a systemic embolus rheumatic mitral valve disease should be suspected. Systemic emboli do occur in patients with mitral regurgitation but less frequently than in patients with mitral stenosis.[186] Further discussion of this subject is included earlier in this chapter under "Mitral Stenosis."

Patients with rheumatic mitral valve disease are susceptible to bacterial endocarditis. Further destruction of mitral leaflet tissue can acutely enhance the clinical and hemodynamic findings. There may be an acute deterioration of symptoms to such a degree that acute pulmonary edema is the presenting problem. With sudden worsening of the regurgitant volume the physical examination, ECG, and roentgenogram may be more characteristic of acute mitral regurgitation. These changes are influenced by the degree of abnormality prior to the onset of acute deterioration. In a like manner rupture of chordae tendineae occurs in rheumatic mitral regurgitation and can be responsible for acute deterioration. The recognition of chordae rupture is discussed later in this chapter.

Severe congestive heart failure is a complication that should be avoided with proper medical management and surgical intervention. The development of severe left ventricular dysfunction may be due to the long-standing volume overload, rheumatic pancarditis, or other forms of heart disease. Severe pulmonary hypertension and a low cardiac output are responsible for the fatigue, dyspnea, and systemic congestion.

Medical management

Appropriate rheumatic fever and endocarditis prophylaxis is mandatory in all patients with rheumatic valvular disease (see Chaps. 60A and 77). Education of the patient regarding the importance of these measures improves compliance.

Symptoms of fatigue and dyspnea and roentgenographic evidence of cardiac enlargement are indications for digitalis therapy. The addition of diuretic therapy may provide further improvement in these symptoms and is especially useful when orthopnea and paroxysmal nocturnal dyspnea develop. Evidence of progressive fluid retention indicates the need for additional diuretics and sodium restriction.

Restoration of sinus rhythm should be attempted when atrial fibrillation is present unless it has been chronic for many years or surgery is anticipated in the near future. Pharmacologic or electrical conversion may be used. Two weeks of anticoagulation therapy should precede attempts at conversion if there is a history of systemic emboli. If atrial fibrillation is to be accepted, control of the ventricular rate with appropriate amounts of digitalis is imperative.

Vasodilator therapy[213] may be useful in the management of severe congestive heart failure as a temporary means of alleviating symptoms prior to surgical intervention. Digitalis and diuretic therapy should be continued.

Surgery (See Chap. 61)

Mitral valve replacement is the surgical procedure for rheumatic mitral regurgitation. Surgical mortality is less than 10 percent.[163,214] Surgical intervention is indicated prior to the development of New York Heart Association (NYHA) functional Class IV symptoms. Since prosthetic valve replacement is required, surgery is not indicated with minimal symptoms. Some patients deny significant symptoms despite objective evidence of severe mitral regurgitation associated with moderate cardiomegaly on medical therapy. Surgery should be considered in these individuals. Patients with mild to moderate symptoms may remain stable for years.[186] Clinical evidence of progressive deterioration is an indication for surgical intervention.

There is symptomatic improvement after mitral valve replacement in most patients.[162,215] The degree of this improvement as well as surgical mortality and long-term postoperative survival is influenced by the preoperative state. Patients in functional Class IV have a higher surgical mortality,[163] and their 5-year survival is 50 percent compared with the 70 percent 5-year survival of Class III patients.[162] The degree of symptomatic improvement and improved prognosis should be balanced against the surgical mortality and the complications of prosthetic valves in determining the appropriate time for surgery.

If atrial fibrillation is present after surgical intervention, synchronous dc cardioversion should be attempted. This is usually done several weeks after surgery (see earlier discussion).

MIXED MITRAL STENOSIS AND REGURGITATION

Pathophysiology

A mitral valve that is stenotic with fused commissures and shortened chordae tendineae but also has inadequate leaflet tissue to coapt properly in systole produces auscultatory findings of both mitral stenosis and regurgitation. In addition, pure or predominant mitral regurgitation produces some clinical findings that are present in pure mitral stenosis. The assessment of the predominant lesion is important in the total evaluation and management of the cardiac problem.

Three degrees of mixed mitral stenosis and regurgitation have been described.[141,206] When the mitral valve area is less than 1.0 to 1.5 cm², mitral stenosis is the predominant hemodynamic lesion, and there is no appreciable volume loading of the left ventricle. When the mitral orifice is greater than 2.0 cm, mitral regurgitation is the predominant lesion, and there is

volume loading of the ventricle with accentuation of ventricular filling during early and middiastole. The hemodynamics are similar to pure mitral regurgitation.[215] A *fixed*, i.e., fused and immobile, mitral orifice with an area of 1.5 to 2.0 cm² is relatively uncommon.[207] It produces some element of volume overload of the left ventricle as well as mitral blockade.

Clinical recognition

SYMPTOMS
Evaluation of symptoms is of limited usefulness in determining the predominant lesion. Both mitral regurgitation and mitral stenosis produce fatigue and dyspnea. Progressive pulmonary symptoms prior to the onset of symptoms of a reduced cardiac output are more characteristic of mitral stenosis. Cough, hemoptysis, and episodes of acute pulmonary edema favor mitral stenosis.

PHYSICAL FINDINGS
An apex impulse which is diffuse or sustained precludes pure mitral stenosis and favors significant mitral regurgitation. In addition, other forms of heart disease which affect the left ventricle must be considered. Coronary atherosclerotic heart disease, hypertensive cardiovascular disease, aortic valve disease, or idiopathic cardiomyopathy may coexist with rheumatic mitral valve disease and modify the subjective and objective data. A prominent rapid filling wave is produced by significant mitral regurgitation. A noncompliant ventricle due to myocardial hypertrophy or ischemia may produce a prominent presystolic a wave in response to atrial contribution to ventricular filling. Mixed or predominant mitral regurgitation is suggested by these abnormalities of the apex pulse. A left parasternal pulse of right ventricular hypertrophy may be present with either mitral stenosis or regurgitation. A parasternal pulsation which rises slowly and peaks late in systole is evidence for mitral regurgitation.

All the auscultatory findings of mitral stenosis may be present with pure or predominant mitral regurgitation or with mixed stenosis and regurgitation. The presence of an accentuated first heart sound or opening snap is of no aid in differentiation. A brief middiastolic rumble may represent mild stenosis, severe stenosis with a low cardiac output, or significant mitral regurgitation.[206] Unless there is tachycardia, the diastolic rumble of mitral regurgitation does not continue to end diastole.[207] With tachycardia or a short cycle interval in atrial fibrillation, stasis of ventricular filling may not occur, and the rumble will not end prior to S_1.[207] When the diastolic rumble is introduced by a loud ventricular gallop sound, mitral regurgitation is dominant. With mixed stenosis and regurgitation the gallop sound may not be very loud and may be difficult to distinguish from the onset of the rumble.

ELECTROCARDIOGRAM
Right ventricular hypertrophy is an uncommon electrocardiographic finding in chronic mitral regurgitation.[74] Its presence favors predominant mitral stenosis in patients with evidence of both regurgitation and

stenosis. Left ventricular hypertrophy favors considerable mitral regurgitation if other causes can be excluded. In mixed mitral stenosis and regurgitation the QRS may be normal or suggest right, left, or biventricular hypertrophy.[191]

CHEST ROENTGENOGRAM

Pure or predominant mitral regurgitation may produce massive enlargement of the left atrium. The most marked changes in pulmonary vasculature are produced by mitral stenosis. The presence of left ventricular enlargement is not compatible with pure mitral stenosis. Marked pulmonary vascular changes and an enlarged cardiac silhouette may be produced by pure mitral stenosis with right ventricular dilatation or by mitral regurgitation, with or without an element of stenosis, and its accompanying left ventricular enlargement. The separation of right versus left ventricular enlargement by chest roentgenograms is not always satisfactory.

ECHOCARDIOGRAM

The echocardiogram is of limited value in the assessment of mixed mitral stenosis and regurgitation. An E to F slope of less than 10 mm/s is compatible with severe stenosis but does not exclude some degree of regurgitation. Increased left ventricular dimensions and exaggerated wall motion suggest left ventricular volume overload and if present would imply significant regurgitation.

CARDIAC CATHETERIZATION

A normal left ventricular end-diastolic volume and pressure, a diastolic pressure gradient across the mitral valve in diastole, and no mitral regurgitation on left ventricular angiography are the features of pure mitral stenosis. With dominant mitral regurgitation there is left ventricular dilatation and frequently some elevation of end-diastolic pressure. The pressure gradient, however, may be present with pure mitral regurgitation. The magnitude of the gradient is most apparent in early diastole and with a normal heart rate disappears in middiastole.[215] Persistence of the pressure gradient throughout diastole supports some degree of stenosis. Thus elements of both obstruction and regurgitation are present in mixed stenosis and regurgitation.

Management

Some degree of mitral regurgitation, whether dominant or mixed, implies that surgical intervention will require a prosthetic valve. Thus, surgery is not as hastily recommended as in the patient with pure mitral stenosis and a pliable valve amenable to commissurotomy.

DIFFERENTIAL DIAGNOSIS OF RHEUMATIC MITRAL VALVE DISEASE

Other forms of heart disease may simulate rheumatic mitral valve disease. Conversely mitral stenosis, mitral regurgitation, or mixed stenosis and regurgitation may simulate other forms of heart disease. An appreciation of these mimicries is important in proper recognition. In addition, the association of pulmonary disease or other forms of heart disease with mitral valve disease may hinder the recognition of the latter.

The auscultatory findings of an *atrial septal defect* may be incorrectly attributed to mitral stenosis with or without mitral regurgitation. The fixed split of the aortic and pulmonic components of the second sound may be interpreted as S_2 and OS. The tricuspid rumble of an atrial septal defect may radiate from the left sternal border to the apex due to right ventricular dilatation and can be interpreted as a mitral rumble. The murmur of mitral regurgitation in a primum atrial septal defect can add further confusion. Important clues in the recognition of atrial septal defect include right bundle branch block without left atrial abnormality on the ECG, roentgenographic evidence of large pulmonary arteries without left atrial enlargement and prominent pulmonary artery pulsations and no mitral valve calcification on fluoroscopy. Echocardiographic findings compatible with an atrial septal defect and a normal mitral valve are most helpful. In the older patient with an atrial septal defect the simulation of mitral valve disease can be more striking with evidence of left atrial enlargement and the presence of atrial fibrillation.[216]

A *left atrial myxoma* (see Chap. 86) may simulate mitral stenosis or mitral regurgitation.[217] Symptoms of pulmonary venous hypertension indistinguishable from those of mitral stenosis can occur. An early diastolic third heart sound can mimic an opening snap or ventricular gallop sound. A mitral diastolic rumble is frequently present. A systolic murmur of mitral regurgitation has been reported as the predominant auscultatory finding.[218] Clues that the problem is myxoma and not mitral stenosis include apparent mitral stenosis with fever, arthralgias, anemia; marked variation in symptoms and auscultatory findings on repeat evaluation; symptoms out of proportion to findings of significant mitral stenosis, i.e., a long S_2-OS interval and minimal left atrial enlargement;[219] recurrent systemic emboli, espeically with sinus rhythm; an unusual "scraping noise" between S_2 and OS.[63] Echocardiography is useful in the differentiation but cannot be relied on entirely to exclude the presence of a myxoma. Angiography, either selective left ventricular or opacification of the left atrium after injection into the pulmonary artery, should be utilized in suspicious cases not confirmed by echocardiography.

Lutembacher's syndrome, the combination of mitral stenosis and atrial septal defect, is uncommon.[220] Proper surgical management is determined by the appreciation of their coexistence. Mitral stenosis may be associated with a left-to-right shunt at the atrial level due to an atrial septal defect, patent foramen ovale (opened due to a high left atrial pressure), or partial anomalous pulmonary venous return. The clinical presentation may be that of mitral stenosis or atrial septal defect. When mitral stenosis is apparent, clues that an atrial septal defect coexists include fewer pulmonary symptoms than anticipated, fixed splitting of S_2, systolic ejection murmur in the second intercostal space to the left of the sternum, presence of right bundle branch block, and absence of marked left atrial enlargement. When the atrial septal defect is apparent, clues that mitral stenosis coexists include history of rheumatic fever, left atrial abnormality on ECG, and Kerley B lines on the roentgenogram. In the young patient in whom an atrial septal defect is obvious, the presence of atrial fibrillation or left atrial enlargement would suggest coexisting mitral valve disease. Mitral stenosis and an atrial septal defect, congenital or acquired, may produce a continuous murmur at the left sternal border.[221,222] The presence of a systolic ejection murmur in the second intercostal space to the left of the sternum, incomplete expiratory closure of S_2, and roentgenographic evidence of plethora of one area of the lungs in a patient with recognized mitral stenosis would suggest coexisting partial anomalous pulmonary venous return.[223] The evaluation of these coexisting lesions by cardiac catheterization requires the documentation and quantitation of the left-to-right shunt at the atrial level and a diastolic mitral valve gradient. In addition a determination of the lesion responsible for the left-to-right shunt should be made.[224]

Cor triatriatum is a rare congenital cardiac anomaly[225] which can simulate mitral stenosis. It is a supravalvular mitral obstruction between the left atrium and an accessory chamber which receives the pulmonary venous return. Symptoms of pulmonary venous hypertension usually develop in childhood but occasionally not until early adult life.[226] Typical auscultatory findings of mitral stenosis are lacking. A diastolic rumble or continuous murmur may be present.[225]

Various forms of *cardiomyopathy* may simulate rheumatic mitral valve disease. The occurrence of an atrial gallop sound just after a ventricular gallop sound can mimic a diastolic rumble.[227] Asymmetric hypertrophic cardiomyopathy may produce a diastolic murmur suggesting mitral stenosis.[228,229] The presence of evidence for left ventricular disease by physical examination, ECG, or roentgenogram is helpful in recognition. The systolic murmur of obstruction cardiomyopathy (idiopathic hypertrophic subaortic stenosis) may be mistaken for mitral regurgitation. An increase in intensity of the murmur with standing and a decrease with squatting is an important observation for the recognition of obstructive cardiomyopathy. Important differences in management demand a proper differentiation of congestive cardiomyopathy and rheumatic mitral valve disease. Either may mimic the other in clinical presentation. A systolic murmur of mitral regurgitation and a ventricular gallop sound are common in congestive cardiomyopathy. In severe mitral regurgitation the systolic murmur may not be very loud, or a diastolic flow rumble is not appreciated. When cardiomyopathy is thought to be present, further evaluation for rheumatic mitral valve disease should be carried out when there is considerable left atrial enlargement, a diastolic rumble or opening snap is present, or the ECG suggests right ventricular hypertrophy. Echocardiography may substantiate suspicions of mitral valve disease and aid in differentiation. In some cases cardiac catheterization and selective left ventricular angiography are necessary for certainty of diagnosis.

The possibility of mitral stenosis should be considered when there is severe *pulmonary hypertension* of unknown cause. As discussed earlier in this chapter, the diastolic rumble of mitral stenosis may be brief and faint when severe pulmonary hypertension develops. Atrial fibrillation, left atrial enlargement, or mitral valve calcification are clues to mitral stenosis in a patient with pulmonary hypertension of unknown cause. Conversely primary pulmonary hypertension or that due to recurrent pulmonary emboli may simulate rheumatic heart disease especially when relative tricuspid and pulmonic insufficiency develops. The echocardiogram is quite useful in recognition or exclusion of mitral stenosis in these cases.

When there is severe *obstructive lung disease*, mitral stenosis is easily overlooked.[230] Attention is focused on the pulmonary problem, and exacerbations of pulmonary symptoms are attributed to acute bronchitis. Patients with mitral stenosis are less tolerant of pulmonary infections and are likely to present with symptoms related to acute bronchitis. Asthma may be incorrectly diagnosed on the basis of severe bronchospasm. The presence of atrial fibrillation, systemic emboli, or left atrial enlargement, or a history of hemoptysis in a patient with "lung disease" should alert the physician to a careful search for mitral stenosis by auscultation, echocardiography, cardiac fluoroscopy, and if necessary cardiac catheterization.

NONRHEUMATIC MITRAL REGURGITATION

Abnormality of anatomy or function of any element of the mitral apparatus can produce mitral regurgitation. Rheumatic heart disease is no longer considered the most common cause of mitral regurgitation. The systolic murmur of nonrheumatic forms of mitral regurgitation is not necessarily holosystolic, as is the case most frequently in rheumatic mitral regurgitation. This section of the chapter will deal with the nonrheumatic disease processes which produce mitral regurgitation (Fig. 60B-11). Highly distinctive clinical syndromes may result. Recognition and appreciation of the clinical implications of these nonrheumatic causes of mitral regurgitation are important to proper management of the patient's problem.

Functional anatomy of the mitral apparatus

The anatomy of the mitral valve is discussed in Chap. 3. For the purposes of this chapter, it is helpful to

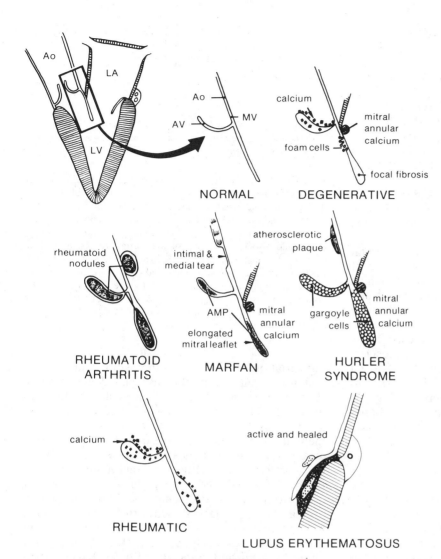

NORMAL   DEGENERATIVE

RHEUMATOID
ARTHRITIS   MARFAN   HURLER
SYNDROME

RHEUMATIC   LUPUS ERYTHEMATOSUS

FIGURE 60B-11 Diagrammatic representation of some of the conditions affecting the mitral and aortic leaflets. AO, aorta; LV, left ventricle; LA, left atrium; AV, aortic valve; MV, mitral valve; AMP, acid mucopolysaccharide. Lupus erythematosus has active lesions or verrucae, which are accumulations of fibrin and valvular debris, and healed lesions with fibrosis and scarring of valve tissue. (*Reproduced from Cardiovascular Clinics Series*[298] *with permission from William C. Roberts, M.D., Albert N. Brest, M.D., Editor in Chief, and F. A. Davis Company.*)

discuss current concepts of mitral apparatus function. Silverman and Hurst stressed that six elements are critical in the normal action of the mitral apparatus.[231] These are (1) the left atrium, (2) the mitral annulus, (3) the leaflets, (4) the chordae tendineae, (5) the papillary muscles, (6) the left ventricular wall. Dysfunction of any one or combination of these elements may result in mitral regurgitation. The exact mechanism for closure of the mitral valve is unknown. Current concepts suggest that valve closure is initiated by left atrial contraction. The force of left atrial contraction creates a jet stream across the mitral orifice and produces an area of negative pressure which exerts a suction effect pulling the valves together. Eddy currents created within the ventricle by the sudden movement of blood exert force on the ventricular surface of the leaflets, further aiding valve closure. The papillary muscles begin contraction just prior to ventricular systole, pulling the leaflets deeper into the ventricular cavity. Chordal attachments to both leaflets serve to tether the valve in early systole and bring the valves together.[231]

Cobbs[232] and Barlow[233] have stressed that the mitral apparatus is so designed that during normal function there is minimal stress on both chordae tendineae and papillary muscles. This is the result of two important factors named by Cobbs[232] as (1) the keystone effect and (2) the geometry of the mitral orifice. As the keystone of an arch supports the columns, so the mitral leaflets support one another as they coapt during systole. This phenomenon has been recognized at surgery, where the mitral leaflets are described as tightly sealed yet chordal and papillary muscle tension appears small.[234] Studies of chordal tension have indicated a fall in tension of the chordae tendineae after opening of the aortic valve.[235] These observations would suggest that the major emphasis to sealing the mitral valve is a cohesive force of the valves themselves. If this normal relationship is altered, simply by cutting chordae tendineae for example, there is increased force on the remaining chordae tendineae sustained throughout systole.[235] The anterior medial leaflet of the mitral valve is so positioned that the leaflets effectively divide the left ventricular chamber into a receiving and expelling chamber.[231] The anterior leaflet is tangential to systolic flow, so that there is reduced stress to the leaflet despite its large area.

Additional mechanical advantage may derive from the tilt of the mitral orifice, which is positioned perpendicular to the aortic valve.

Clinical studies have demonstrated posterior leaflets are particularly vulnerable to injury.[233,236-243] The anatomy of the posterior leaflet differs from the anterior leaflet in that the leaflet is broad with clefts or indentations along the free margin, giving it a scalloped appearance. It is protected by the anterior leaflet of the mitral valve and the orientation of the mitral orifice; however, the posterior leaflet is subject to greater tension than the anterior leaflet. This is related to both its configuration and its position, which is perpendicular to the flow of blood during systole.

"Mitral regurgitation begets mitral regurgitation."[244] When dysfunction occurs in any aspect of the mitral complex, a vicious cycle is initiated which may involve each element. Thus, as the left atrium enlarges, it may stretch the posterior leaflet and influence its coaptation with the anterior leaflet. The leaflets can disengage, producing an increase in the tension on chordae tendineae and papillary muscles. The volume overload to the left ventricle produced by mitral regurgitation will cause the left ventricle to dilate and alter the spatial relationship of the papillary muscles. The normal contribution of the papillary muscles to mitral leaflet closure is impaired, and further mitral regurgitation results.

Mitral valve prolapse

The auscultatory complex characterized by nonejection systolic click, a late systolic murmur, or a midsystolic click followed by a late systolic murmur has been intensively studied in the past decade. Important concepts concerning the etiology, pathophysiology, clinical characteristics, and prognosis have evolved. A hodgepodge of labels have been used to identify and characterize this syndrome, including billowing mitral valve syndrome, floppy mitral valve syndrome, prolapsing posterior mitral valve syndrome, midsystolic click–late systolic murmur syndrome, and Barlow's syndrome. We prefer the designation *mitral leaflet prolapse* in discussing this syndrome in general. This term reflects the single characteristic feature present in all patients with manifestations of this syndrome. We believe that it is worthwhile to further classify patients by using the eponym *Barlow's syndrome* when referring to patients with the typical clinical, auscultatory, and ECG findings and *Read's syndrome* when the pathologic process of the mitral valve is thought to be myxomatous degeneration and the clinical course is progressive. While eponyms are usually discouraged, in this case they avoid terms which may alarm or frighten the patient and recognize the complex and variable clinical spectrum present in this syndrome.[245]

Midsystolic clicks were first described by Cuffer and Barbillon[246] in 1887. Gallavardin[247] reported on a group of patients with systolic clicks in 1932, describ-

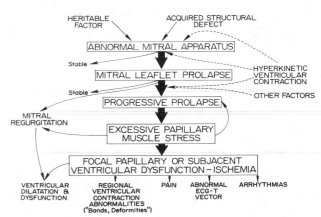

FIGURE 60B-12 "A proposed pathophysiologic mechanism for the development of the Idiopathic Mitral Valve Prolapse Syndrome, including most of the important clinical features. The heritable and acquired primary factors are unknown and might include myxomatous degeneration, although a myxomatous process could also be the result of long term stresses on leaflets, chordae, and papillary muscles. A hyperkinetic ventricular contraction pattern and other unidentified factors are considered to play a potentiating role. The tricuspid valve apparatus may be involved in a similar manner in an unknown number of these patients." (*Reprinted*[254] with permission of Don O. Nutter, M.D., and the American Heart Association.)

ing variation of the clicks with position and exertion and noting an intermittent associated late systolic murmur. He concluded that the auscultatory findings were the result of plural pericardial adhesions found at necropsy. Subsequent observations[248,249] commented on the benign course of patients with these auscultatory abnormalities and stressed the probable extracardiac origin. However, Paul White,[250] in his textbook in 1931, did suggest that the sounds may arise from the chordae tendineae, and Paul Wood, noting an association with rheumatic carditis, thought that the sound could be mitral valvular in origin. Our present concepts first evolved from a study by Reid and associates[251] in 1961 which proposed that systolic clicks and late systolic murmurs were mitral valvular in origin and associated with mxyomatous degeneration of the mitral valve. Barlow and colleagues[237] confirmed the presence of mitral regurgitation in patients with midsystolic clicks and late systolic murmurs. Subsequently, Ronan et al.[252] utilized intracardiac phonocardiography to demonstrate that the click and murmur arose from the mitral complex, and Criley et al.[241] demonstrated a relation between prolapse of the mitral valve and the systolic click.

Since Barlow's first description of the association of mitral valve prolapse and the characteristic syndrome of chest pain, auscultatory abnormalities, and typical ECG pattern, medical opinion about this disorder has changed from regarding it as an obscure curiosity to recognizing it as one of the principle pathologic anomalies affecting the mitral leaflets (Fig. 60B-12).

MECHANISM OF MITRAL VALVE PROLAPSE[231,246,250,252,253]

Three concepts have been proposed to account for the mechanism of mitral valve prolapse. They are (1) valvular origin, (2) myocardial origin, and (3) ischemic origin. The basis for each of these concepts is discussed below.

The valvular origin[232,233,237,238,254,255] The normal anatomy of mitral valve apparatus is described in Chap. 3. Several aspects of this anatomy deserve to be emphasized in relation to the mitral leaflet prolapse syndrome. The posterior leaflet comprises two-thirds of the circumference of the mitral orifice and during systole normally becomes inflated into a C-shaped gasket which engulfs the anterior leaflet. It is composed of three or more scallops. One, two, or all three of these scallops may be affected in pathologic deformities such as redundancy or myxomatous degeneration.[255] When there is prolapse of the posterior leaflet, the exaggerated inflation results in the leaflet's assuming the shape of an incomplete doughnut. A click appears to result from the abrupt deceleration of blood contained within the undersurface of the prolapsing leaflet. Multiple clicks may result from the asynchronous prolapse of the multiple scallops of the leaflet.[255] The chordae tendineae are attached to the posterior leaflet from both papillary muscles and directly to the leaflet from the posterior wall of the heart. The most important chordae in relation to prolapse of the valve appear to be those which support the belly, or middle sections, of the valve.

Pathologic abnormalities described within the mitral valve apparatus which produce mitral leaflet prolapse include myxomatous degeneration of the valve, elongation and thinning of the chordae tendineae, redundant and excessive valve tissue, and rheumatic endocarditis with leaflet or chordal involvement.[238,256]

Myxomatous degeneration is a degeneration of tissue within the spongiosis of the mitral valve. It is described as part of the normal aging process and is frequently seen at autopsy in patients over 50 years of age.[257] This is the principle pathologic derangement in patients with Marfan's syndrome and may occur sporadically in younger patients. The frequency of this anomaly cannot be determined because of the generally benign course of patients with this syndrome and the lack of pathologic material from patients in younger age groups. At present, it is felt that patients with myxomatous degeneration of the mitral valve represents only a small portion of those with mitral leaflet prolapse.

Patients with mitral leaflet prolapse frequently have a dilated mitral annulus, possibly representing an abnormality of the fibrous skeleton of the heart.[258,259] This condition may lead to premature calcification of the annulus. It does not appear to be secondary to ventricular dilatation or mitral regurgitation. Surgical and necropsy studies also describe thin, elongated chordae tendineae and marked redundancy of the mitral leaflet tissue.[260] The redundancy of valvular tissue typically involves the posterior leaflet to a greater extent. These changes may represent a congenital anomaly in the formation of the mitral valve complex or a biodegeneration of valvular tissue as a result of a collagen disorder.

A variance between left ventricular size, mitral leaflet area, and chordal length may result from the normal aging process. There is a reduction in left ventricular volume, mass, annular circumference, and long axis without a change in mitral leaflet or chordae tendineae. This results in a leaflet-chordae arrangement that is oversized for the left ventricle.[240] The preponderance of women with this abnormality may relate to postpubertal growth patterns. A female with less body growth has a relatively smaller left ventricular volume and mass, and hence may have a disproportion between valvular tissue and left ventricular size.[240] This would explain the apparent frequent occurrence of this syndrome in young females and a tendency for male incidence to increase with age.

Myocardial factors Asymmetric patterns of ventricular contraction are described in patients with mitral leaflet prolapse.[254,261–263] These abnormalities include marked posteroinferior bulging of the left ventricular wall encroaching into the left ventricular cavity, reduction in the extent and velocity of shortening in the region of the mitral valve ring and inflow tract area, and displacement of the posteromedial papillary muscle from its normal midventricular location with evidence of movement toward the mitral ring.[262] Although most patients with mitral leaflet prolapse have normal left ventricular function as assessed by left ventricular cineangiography, two variant patterns of left ventricular motion are described.[254] Both are unrelated to the severity of the mitral regurgitation. A hyperkinetic pattern of left ventricular contraction is seen and is usually associated with normal resting hemodynamics and normal left ventricular mass. The second pattern is one of diffuse hypokinetic ventricular contraction with ejection fractions below 55 percent. These patterns may have a reduced cardiac index and an increase in left ventricular end-diastolic pressure with left ventricular hypertrophy.

Several mechanisms are postulated for the resulting abnormalities in left ventricular contraction. There may be a primary dysfunction of the myocardium, a "cardiomyopathy," or the derangement may represent a malfunction of the papillary muscle or malposition of this muscle as a result of excessive chordal tug from the prolapsed mitral leaflet.[232] In accord with the Laplace principle, as the leaflet prolapses into the left atrium, increased tension is placed on the leaflet, papillary muscle, and chordae tendineae. The papillary muscle appears to have delayed or incomplete contraction. The contraction abnormality may be the result of regional ischemia induced by the excessive stress imposed by the tug of the mitral leaflet.

Ischemic factors Myocardial ischemia is a suspected abnormality because of the frequent triad of chest pain, ventricular premature contractions, and abnormalities in the resting and exercise ECG. There is no apparent relation to large vessel coronary artery disease.[254,264,265] It appears likely that regional myocardial ischemia is induced by the abnormal tug of the mitral leaflets and chordae tendineae on the papillary muscle and left ventricular wall.[236] Surgical and autopsy studies have demonstrated focal myocardial fibrosis in these regions.[266] Physiologic evidence suggesting regional myocardial ischemia is scant. Coronary lactate studies during atrial pacing have not demonstrated lactate production in these patients,[254] nor is there a correlation with exercise ECG abnormalities and chest pain complaints.[267–269] A study utilizing phenylephrine infusion in patients with mitral valve prolapse and chest pain was able to reproduce chest pain in these patients, suggesting that pain is associated with increased myocardial wall tension which may interfere with regional blood supply.[270] Patients in this study had normal coronary arteriograms and negative treadmill exercise tests.

Mitral leaflet prolapse is described as part of the spectrum of papillary muscle dysfunction in patients with ischemic heart disease from coronary atherosclerosis.[265] The prolapsed leaflet is felt to be from impaired contractility of ventricular myocardium and papillary muscles. However, there is no significant correlation between mitral leaflet prolapse and the distribution of coronary arterial obstructions or abnormal patterns of left ventricular contraction.[264] The presence of these two common disorders may represent a chance association, although in some cases there appears to be a causal relationship.

Mechanism of mitral leaflet prolapse remains unproved. Most data suggest that myocardial ischemia and primary abnormalities of the myocardial muscle are relatively uncommon and that the primary disorder is related to abnormalities of the mitral apparatus, usually the mitral leaflet or chordae tendineae.

CLINICAL RECOGNITION

The mitral leaflet prolapse syndrome is described in both sexes and in patients of all ages.[233,236,238,271] Adequate epidemiologic data are not available to determine the exact prevalence of this anomaly. The disorder is most commonly recognized in young females in the second to fourth decades. A study of females on a college campus revealed a 21 percent incidence of mitral leaflet prolapse, with a click or a click–late systolic murmur in 17 percent.[272] A study of both sexes between the ages of 17 and 39 found a 6 percent incidence of mitral leaflet prolapse in females and 0.5 percent in males.[273] A study of South African black school-aged children noted a 1.4 percent incidence of click–late systolic murmur or a combination of these auscultatory abnormalities,[233] and a study of 1,009 young females found a 0.33 percent incidence. The auscultatory abnormalities can be variable and occasionally completely disappear. Mitral leaflet prolapse can present as an auscultatory complex recognized on routine physical examination, as a symptomatic complex characterized by chest pains, palpitations, dyspnea, and fatigue, or as an anatomic anomaly recognized on echocardiography.

Symptoms Pain in this syndrome is atypical of angina pectoris.[256,238] It is rarely exercise-related but is substernal, prolonged, and described as sticky, knifelike, throbbing, or a pressure sensation. Symptoms rarely are reproducible on exercise testing and correlate poorly with changes in the ECG. Palpitation is a frequent symptom, but ambulatory monitoring has noted no correlation between the sensation of palpitation and the presence of arrhythmias.[267–269] Dyspnea and fatigue are very frequent.[238,240] There appears to be no decrease in exercise tolerance or associated orthopnea, nocturnal dyspnea, or objective signs of heart failure. Association of fatigue, atypical chest pain, and palpitations have led to the suggestion that psychic influences may be responsible for some manifestations of the patient's symptom complex.[233,238] At present, no definite psychic abnormalities or personality disorders can be related to the cardiac abnormality.

The syndrome may be familial[274,275] and has been said to occur in an autosomal dominant pattern.[276,277] An association is described of mitral leaflet prolapse with both myotonic dystrophy[278] and secundum atrial septal defect.[279,280]

Physical examination The physical examination in mitral leaflet prolapse syndrome is characterized by three features: (1) anomalies of the chest wall, (2) abnormal precordial impulse, and (3) an auscultatory complex of nonejection systolic clicks and late systolic murmurs.

The physical appearance is remarkable. The patients are frequently asthenic. There may be associated bony anomalies frequently of the palate and thoracic chest wall.[240,281] There appears to be an increase of pectus excavatum, pectus carinatum, scoliosis, and kyphosis. These anomalies, which are also common in connective tissue disorders, are felt to be related to abnormal development of collagen in supporting bone structure. Several investigators have described a relationship between mitral leaflet prolapse and bony thoracic chest wall deformities.[281,282] BonTempo et al.[281] have suggested that the same mesenchymal defect which affects the mitral valve may influence bony development of the thoracic cage. Embryologically, there is a temporal relationship in the development of these tissues.

An abnormal apical impulse is described in many patients with prolapse of the mitral leaflet.[283] The apex cardiogram records a systolic retraction, or "dip," occurring synchronously with the systolic click (Fig. 60B-13). An association is noted between the severity of the leaflet prolapse and the systolic retraction. The auscultatory complex of nonejection systolic clicks and a late systolic murmur is the characteristic feature in identification of mitral leaflet prolapse. These sounds are quite variable and appear to depend on the cause of the mitral apparatus deformity, left ventricular volume, and left ventricular function.[233,236,238,240,255] The nonejection systolic click may occur in early or late systole and will occasionally fuse with the first heart sound. The click may be single or multiple and is generally louder at the apex or along the left sternal border. Multiple

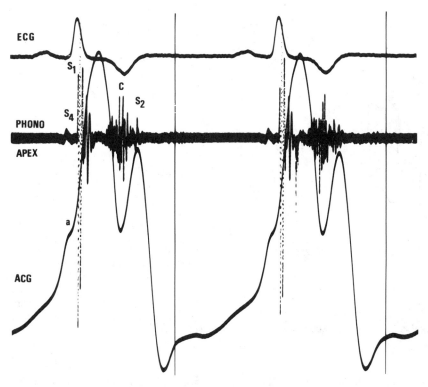

FIGURE 60B-13 Heart sounds (PHONO) at apex with electrocardiogram (ECG) and apex pulse (ACG) recording on a patient with mitral valve prolapse. Note systolic retraction of ACG coincident with click (C).

clicks may imitate a rubbing or scratchy sound along the apex. The click will vary with respiration or changes in position and increase in intensity with handgrip or phenylephrine. The position of the click is related to left ventricular volume and occurs at or near the maximal point of prolapse of the involved scallop of the mitral leaflets.

The systolic murmur is usually confined to late systole but has been described as pansystolic in approximately 10 percent of patients. The murmur is frequently associated with a click, commencing after the click in a crescendo pattern, extending to or just beyond the aortic second sound. The murmur can be crescendo-decrescendo, however, and occasionally an early systolic murmur is heard preceding the nonejection click. Origin of the early systolic murmur is unclear. Early systolic crescendo-decrescendo murmurs are common in patients who are thin or have chest wall deformities, both common traits in this syndrome. Also, mitral regurgitation has not been demonstrated by left ventricular cineangiograms during early systole in patients with this syndrome.

The auscultatory features of the mitral prolapse syndrome may be attenuated, augmented, or varied by physiologic, postural, or pharmacologic interventions.[255] An appreciation of these variables is necessary for proper recognition of the syndrome. In some patients, when examined in the supine position, both the systolic murmur and the nonejection click(s) are absent. The left lateral decubitus position or standing may be required for appreciation of the click(s) with

or without the midsystolic to late systolic murmur. Either alone may be heard supine, while both are present with the patient standing. The presence of a nonejection click with the systolic murmur is a helpful diagnostic observation. The clicks may occur near S_1 and be confused with an ejection click or near S_2 and be confused with an S_2-OS or S_2-S_3 combination. Bedside maneuvers which vary the systolic time of occurrence of the click as well as modify the presence of the systolic murmur are helpful in recognition of the syndrome. The click and onset of the murmur occur earlier in systole with any maneuver which decreases the size of the left ventricular cavity. Conversely their time of occurrence is later in systole when the left ventricular cavity size is increased.[284] The intensity of the murmur increases with maneuvers that elevate systolic blood pressure and decreases with maneuvers that lower systolic blood pressure. With standing the midsystolic to late systolic murmur can become holosystolic and the click fuse with S_1 (Fig. 60B-14). The intensity of the murmur may increase with standing.[256] Squatting results in a later onset of click and murmur with a decrease in intensity of the murmur.[283] The inhalation of amyl nitrite results in a smaller left ventricular volume and thus has an effect similar to standing: the click and onset of murmur occur earlier in systole, but the murmur more often decreases in intensity due to a decrease in left ventricular systolic pressure (Fig. 60B-15). The administration of phenylephrine results in an increase in intensity of the murmur with little change in configuration.[256] These maneuvers

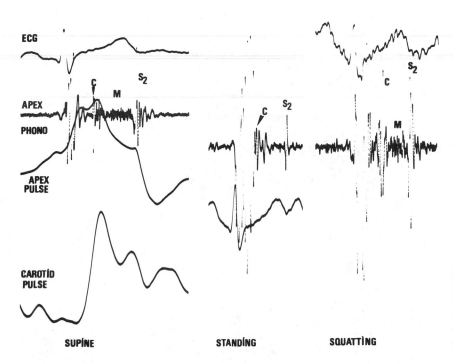

FIGURE 60B-14 Typical auscultatory findings in a patient with mitral valve prolapse. Midsystolic click (C) which introduces murmur (M) with patient supine fuses with first heart sound on standing and returns to midsystolic timing during squatting.

may aid in clarification of a holosystolic murmur or late systolic murmur by demonstration of the presence of clicks and the modification of the murmur configuration.

Cobbs has described a group of patients with a widely split second heart sound.[266] He feels this is a result of shortened ventricular systole. These patients displace a significant proportion of their stroke volume into the prolapsed leaflets. Prolapse may be so profound as to result in almost turning the ventricle inside out. These patients may be subject to ventricular arrhythmias and sudden death.

Electrocardiogram The electrocardiographic abnormalities noted in mitral leaflet prolapse syndrome are listed in Table 60B-1. The most common abnormality in the scalar ECG is an inverted or partially inverted T wave in leads II, III, and aV_F[285] (Fig. 60B-16). There is an abnormally wide mean frontal QRS-T vector angle. The ST segment is usually normal but may be slightly depressed. These changes are described in up to 40 percent of patients with mitral leaflet prolapse.[238,271] The T wave inversion may be more extensive and has been described in the precordial leads, particularly in leads V_4 to V_6. The T wave pattern can be variable and fluctuate with position or amyl nitrite inhalation.[238] Q-T prolongation is described, and one series noted 26 percent of patients with prolongation of the Q-T interval in relation to rate.[271] No relationship exists between this

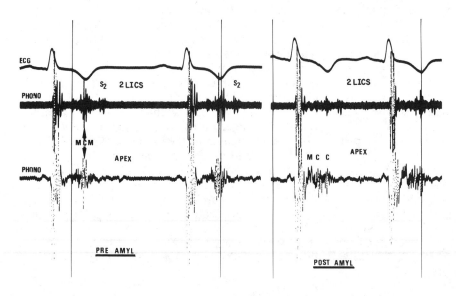

FIGURE 60B-15 Heart sounds recorded at second left intercostal space (2 LICS) and apex before and after administration of amyl nitrite in a patient with mitral valve prolapse. Note that there are multiple clicks (C) with a late systolic murmur (M). After amyl nitrite administration the murmur becomes holosystolic, and clicks persist.

TABLE 60B-1
ECG abnormalities in mitral leaflet prolapse

1 ST and T wave abnormalities in leads II, III, AVF, and V_4 to V_6
2 Q-T prolongation
3 Arrhythmias
   a Supraventricular
      (1) PAC (premature atrial contraction)
      (2) Atrial fibrillation
   b Ventricular
      (1) PVC (premature ventricular contraction)
      (2) Ventricular tachycardia
      (3) Ventricular fibrillation

prolongation of the Q-T interval and the syndrome of Q-T prolongation, congenital deafness, arrhythmias, and sudden death.

Arrhythmias[286] are frequently noted in association with mitral leaflet prolapse; sudden death is recognized as a complication of this syndrome.[261,268,269,287] Assessment by ambulatory monitoring has demonstrated premature ventricular contractions (PVCs) in approximately 60 percent of patients. Supraventricular tachyarrhythmias and bradyarrhythmias occur in approximately one-third. There is no relationship between the presence of arrhythmias and sex, age, severity of the valvular prolapse, mitral regurgitation, ST-T segment abnormalities, the presence of midsystolic clicks, or Q-T prolongation. Patients also

FIGURE 60B-16 ECG of a 50-year-old female with a 30-year history of a heart murmur and frequent palpitations. The echocardiogram demonstrated late systolic prolapse of both mitral leaflets. The ECG demonstrates typical ST-T wave changes of Barlow's syndrome, present in this patient in the inferior and lateral leads.

appear to have the subjective sensation of palpitations without concomitant arrhythmias when evaluated by ambulatory monitoring. One-third of the patients have arrhythmias detected on the resting ECG. The most sensitive method remains ambulatory ECG monitoring,[287] which is able to detect a higher frequency of arrhythmias than exercise stress testing. Arrhythmias which have been associated with this syndrome include marked sinus arrhythmia, sinus arrest, atrial fibrillation, ventricular premature beats, and ventricular tachycardia.

The origin of the electrocardiographic abnormalities in this syndrome is unknown. Studies of sinoatrial, atrioventricular nodal, His, Purkinje, and ventricular conduction are usually normal.[240] There is no correlation with coronary artery disease, nor is there an association with ventricular dysfunction. No association is noted with ST and T abnormalities either on the resting ECG or with the stress ECG. Most investigators believe that the ECG abnormalities are related to dysfunction of the mitral valvular apparatus. The mechanical stimulus to the left ventricle produced by excessive movement of the distended blood-laden valve tissue may interfere with continuous vascular supply to the papillary muscles. In addition, studies have demonstrated myocardial fibers within the leaflet which may be the site of ectopic impulse formation when stretched. Although several investigators have suggested that the arrhythmias are related to a cardiomyopathy, there is no

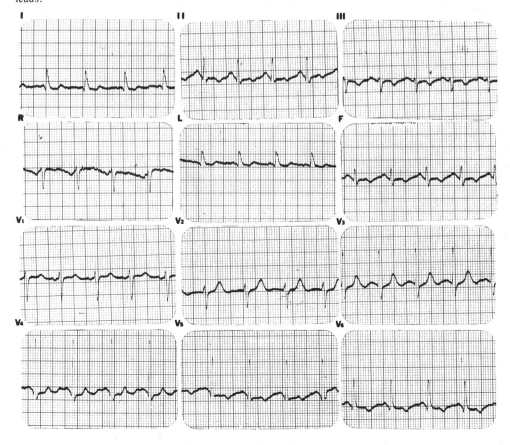

definite relationship between hemodynamics and abnormal ECG patterns.

Echocardiogram Echocardiography provides a relatively precise, atraumatic, noninvasive means for identification of mitral valve prolapse.[288-290] Echocardiographic abnormalities can be divided into two parts—those suggestive but not specific for mitral valve prolapse and those which are considered diagnostic of mitral leaflet prolapse. Features which are suggestive include (1) systolic sagging of the mitral leaflets, (2) a multiplicity of parallel mitral leaflet echoes, and (3) exaggerated mitral leaflet mobility during diastole, with diastolic contact between the leaflet and intraventricular septum. Specific or diagnostic features are (1) abrupt early systolic to midsystolic posterior motion of the mitral leaflet below a line connecting the C to D point of the mitral valve echo (Fig. 60B-17) and (2) holosystolic prolapse of the mitral leaflets below the C and D line of the mitral echo with an apparent "hammocking" of the echo (see Chap. 32C).

False positive interpretation of the echocardiogram can occur when improper transducer angulation is used.[272] If the ultrasound beam is angled inferiorly to the mitral ring and leaflets, they may move either perpendicular to or away from the transducer. The result is to register a false positive hammock-shaped posterior motion of the mitral leaflet. Best results are obtained when the transducer is perpendicular or pointing slightly upward to analyze the mitral valve. The third or fourth intercostal space appears to be the location of choice in most patients. A false positive result may also occur in patients with massive pericardial effusions and a free-swinging heart.[291] Apparent prolapse of the mitral leaflet is seen as the heart swings away from the transducer.

Failure to identify a prolapsing mitral leaflet in patients with known mitral leaflet prolapse is usually associated with incomplete echocardiographic scanning of the mitral valve or an inadequate "window" to fully visualize the mitral valve. Care must be taken to examine the patient in several positions and to utilize various positional and vasoactive maneuvers, such as sitting, handgrip, amyl nitrite inhalation, and phenylephrine administration to elicit abnormalities on the echocardiogram. Echocardiography has been especially useful in evaluating patients who have chest pain syndromes or arrhythmias of uncertain origin. Mitral leaflet prolapse in the absence of auscultatory abnormalities has been reported in approximately 10 percent of patients with this syndrome.

Roentgenographic findings Most patients with mitral leaflet prolapse syndrome have normal cardiac silhouettes on chest roentgenograms.[238,240,281,282] Roentgenographic abnormalities are usually related to coexistent thoracic chest bony abnormalities, concomitant disease processes of the mitral apparatus such as calcification of the mitral annulus or rheumatic valvular disease, or dilatation of the aorta as in Marfan's syndrome.

Cardiac catheterization Relatively few patients with mitral leaflet prolapse have been evaluated by cardiac catheterization, left ventricular cineangiography, and coronary arteriography. The relatively excellent prognosis and minimal symptoms negate invasive cardiovascular examination. In those studies which have been undertaken, hemodynamic evaluation is generally normal.[254,262] When abnormal, the abnormality appears related to the severity of the mitral regurgitation. In general, evaluations of left ventricular function and ejection fractions are within normal limits.[254,262]

Studies have commented on segmental wall abnormalities within the left ventricle.[254,262,263] Also frequently noted is reduced contraction of the mitral valve annulus, so that the ventricle has an overall appearance of a ballerina foot in the right anterior oblique projection. Controversy exists over whether wall contraction abnormalities are related to a myocardial defect or secondary to the mitral valve abnormality. A case of severe left ventricular contraction abnormality with marked indentation of the posterior medial wall is described which returned to normal after replacement of the mitral valve.[292] As discussed earlier, it appears that the abnormality of the mitral apparatus is responsible for abnormal contraction patterns within the left ventricle.

FIGURE 60B-17 Mitral valve echocardiogram of a 23-year-old asymptomatic female who was evaluated because of presence of midsystolic click–late systolic murmur. The echocardiogram demonstrates prolapse of the anterior leaflet (*A*) and posterior leaflet (*B*) in late systole.

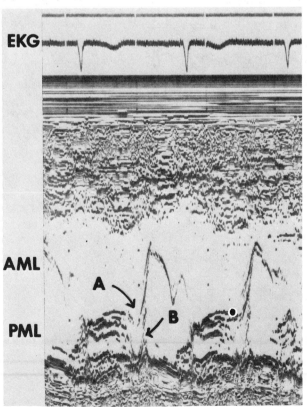

Complications It is important to recognize that most patients with mitral leaflet prolapse are asymptomatic. Although serious complications have been associated with this syndrome, for the vast majority the prognosis is excellent. Four major complications are associated with mitral leaflet prolapse: (1) sudden death, (2) active endocarditis, (3) rupture of the chordae tendineae, and (4) development of hemodynamically significant mitral regurgitation.

Even though sudden death has been reported numerous times,[236,238,268,287] it remains a relatively rare occurrence in patients with this syndrome. It is reasonable to assume that these deaths occur on the basis of an arrhythmia and that patients with frequent premature ventricular contractions or actual runs of ventricular tachycardia are at a higher risk. At present, we agree with the recommendations of O'Rourke and Crawford,[236] who suggest routine rhythm strips on patients with this syndrome and bedside exercise evaluation. Patients who demonstrate frequent premature ventricular contractions during this screening process are provided with ambulatory ECG monitoring. Those who are either symptomatic or have runs of ventricular tachycardia are treated with propranolol. In our experience and that of several other authors, this is usually an effective means for suppressing ventricular ectopy.

There is a definite association between mitral leaflet prolapse and infective endocarditis.[267,293] The value of antibiotic prophylaxis is unknown; however, because of the increased incidence of endocarditis in this syndrome, prophylaxis is presently recommended for all patients who have a holosystolic murmur or midsystolic click–late systolic murmur. At the present time, we also use antibiotic prophylaxis on all patients who have isolated nonejection systolic clicks or multiple nonejection systolic clicks. Barlow has recently suggested that patients with isolated systolic clicks have a reduced risk of endocarditis and questions the value of prophylaxis in these patients.

The complication of rupture of a chordae tendineae or progression of the mitral regurgitation is a relatively rare occurrence. A study of 62 patients with isolated late systolic murmur of whom 33 had an associated systolic click indicated that only 1 died from bacterial endocarditis; 1 died 11 years after the diagnosis at the age of 75 with increasing mitral regurgitation; in 1 patient chordal rupture necessitated valve replacement; and in 10 patients there was a slight progression in the hemodynamic significance of the murmur but no patients developed symptoms. Bacterial endocarditis occurred in 5 cases, and in 41 patients there was no deterioration at all over a period averaging 13.8 years.[267]

Four patients are described with mitral leaflet prolapse, myocardial infarction, and normal coronary arteries. The authors suggest that there is a causal relation between coronary spasm and mitral leaflet prolapse.[294]

MEDICAL MANAGEMENT
The majority of patients have no symptoms. It is important to educate and reassure the patient regarding the benign nature of the syndrome. Antibiotic prophylaxis for endocarditis is recommended. Propranolol is useful for the management of arrhythmias (see earlier discussion of complications). There are a few patients in whom the management of chest pain is extremely difficult. Nitroglycerin and propranolol are used with varying results. Coronary angiography is indicated in patients in whom chest pain cannot be clearly defined. Two errors may be avoided: The incorrect diagnosis of coronary atherosclerotic heart disease early in the course makes it more difficult later to rectify this error in the mind of the patient. Secondly, chest pain in a patient with mitral valve prolapse should not be too hastily attributed to the syndrome, since more than one form of heart disease can be present. The chest pain history should be carefully analyzed for features suggesting myocardial ischemia. Thus coronary angiography can aid in giving maximum reassurance to the patient and physician regarding the benign nature of the chest pain and can contribute to more appropriate management when the chest pain is not clearly nonischemic and significant coronary atherosclerosis is present.

SURGERY[260,295,296] (See Chap. 61)
Acute severe mitral regurgitation can result from chordal rupture, or hemodynamically significant mitral regurgitation can develop gradually over a period of years. In either situation the indications for surgery are based on hemodynamic severity. Although chordal rupture may occur spontaneously in these patients, its occurrence may be associated with infective endocarditis. Both mitral valvuloplasty and mitral valve replacement have been utilized in the surgical management of mitral regurgitation. Mitral valve replacement is considered to be the best approach. In those patients with extensive myxomatous degeneration surgical complications may be more frequent.[260] Dehiscence of the prosthetic valve has been reported.[297]

The precordial honk (See Chap. 18C)
The precordial honk is usually an intermittent loud, sonorous, musical murmur heard most frequently in late systole and best at the apex of the heart. This unique phenomenon was first described by Osler, who remarked on its being audible to the patient and audible at a considerable distance from the chest wall.[299] This murmur is a nonspecific indicator of mitral valvular dysfunction and correlates neither with the pathology nor physiology of myocardial lesion.[300,301] It is frequently associated with mitral leaflet prolapse and may occur in patients without cardiac symptoms. It has also been reported in patients with rheumatic heart disease with mitral regurgitation or mitral stenosis, ischemic heart disease, and cardiomyopathy.[300] Cardiac catheterization and left ventricular angiography may be normal or demonstrate severe mitral regurgitation and left ventricular dysfunction. No specific electrocardiographic or echocardiographic findings are noted in

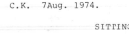

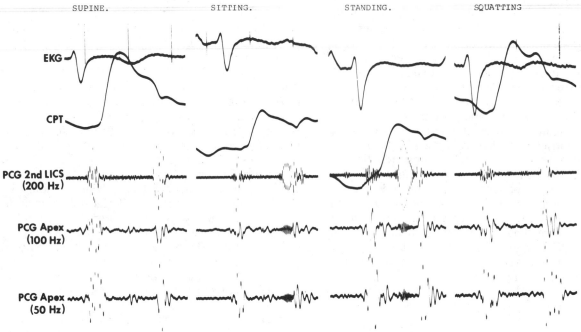

FIGURE 60B-18 This phonocardiogram demonstrates a mitral honk. The murmur is extremely variable and cannot be heard with the patient supine or squatting. The murmur is present in the sitting position and markedly accentuated by standing. (*Courtesy of Dr. Joel Felner.*)

patients with this syndrome. The mitral honk can best be elicited with the patient in the upright position (Fig. 60B-18) during expiration and may be brought on by effort or Isuprel infusion.[300] It generally diminishes or disappears with the Valsalva maneuver or amyl nitrite inhalation.[300] It is postulated that the murmur is related to left ventricular end-diastolic volume. The sounds are probably caused by tension along the edge of the mitral leaflets or chordae tendineae during systole.[302] The stretch induces a musical vibratory sound dimilar to plucking a string of a musical instrument. The honk is not solely a left-sided phenomenon and has been described as coming from the triscupid valve.[303]

Mitral regurgitation due to rupture of the chordae tendineae

Rupture of the chordae tendineae is responsible for a significant proportion of patients with acute mitral regurgitation.[304] In one series chordal rupture accounted for 19 percent of patients with mitral regurgitation. The condition is an infrequent complication of rheumatic[305] or bacterial endocarditis, left atrial myxoma,[306] or mitral valve prolapse syndrome, and can occur as an isolated spontaneous phenomenon in an otherwise normal heart.[234,307-309] New diagnostic techniques, particularly the echocardiogram, permit a more accurate diagnosis of this condition.

ETIOLOGY

Prior to the antibiotic era the most common cause of chordal rupture was active bacterial endocarditis. This is usually associated with significant destruction of the mitral leaflet; however, it may occur as a result of extension of endocarditis from the aortic valve with minimal involvement of both the mitral leaflet or left atrium.

While ruptured chordae tendineae are usually found in patients with infective endocarditis superimposed on rheumatic valvular disease, occasionally patients with rheumatic valvular disease alone suffer rupture of the chordae. In these patients, the chordae are generally thickened, contracted, irregular, calcified, and fused. Distortion of the normal anatomy of the mitral apparatus results in alteration of the normal stress relationships, and it is this tension that is felt to breed rupture.

Between 50 and 70 percent of patients with rupture of the chordae tendineae have no apparent heart disease.[307,308] Among these patients, there is a predominance of males, approximately 2:1, the onset most commonly occurring in the fourth to sixth decades. The increased prevalence of this disorder in males suggests that it is dissimilar to mitral leaflet prolapse syndrome in which chordal rupture is also a complication. The mitral leaflet prolapse syndrome is more common in females and is rarely associated with significant progression, chordal rupture being an uncommon complication. Chordal rupture has also been reported in patients with Ehlers-Danlos syndrome, idiopathic hypertrophic subaortic stenosis, trauma, nonbacterial endocarditis, achondroplasia with coexistent atrial septal defect, and aortic regurgitation.[304,307,308] Although occasionally reported as a complication of acute myocardial infarction, it is likely that such a development represents rupture of a head of a trabeculated papillary muscle rather than the rupture of the chordae tendineae. Finally, rupture of the chordae tendineae can be caused by trauma.

PATHOPHYSIOLOGY

Chordal rupture is a result of either abnormal stress on the chordae or a process producing dysplasia and necrosis.[234,304] Normal function of the mitral apparatus is described earlier under "Functional Anatomy of the Mitral Apparatus." The chordae tendineae normally act to tether the mitral valve in early sytole, preventing prolapse of the leaflet into the left atrium. Any change in the normal interrelationship of the components of the mitral apparatus may increase the duration and amount of tension of the chordae.[234] In addition, there are a number of disease processes which directly afflict the chordae, such as rheumatic endocarditis, which results in short, thick, irregular chordae; Marfan's syndrome, where the chordae are stretched, elongated, and thin; or idiopathic mitral valve prolapse, which has been associated with thinning and elongation of the chordae.

The pathology of isolated spontaneous chordal rupture is unclear. Several factors appear important: (1) Abnormalities in elastin and collagen are noted in patients with spontaneous chordal rupture.[310] (2) Chordae of the posterior leaflet are thinner and more susceptible to rupture.[304] Patients with chordal rupture secondary to specific disease processes have equal involvement of anterior and posterior leaflet chordae. However, in patients with spontaneous chordal rupture there is a significant increased incidence of involvement of the posterior leaflet.[234,304] It also appears likely that the posterior leaflet and its attachments are subject to greater stress than the anterior leaflet as a result of the position of the posterior leaflet in the mitral orifice.

CLINICAL RECOGNITION

Symptoms The clinical manifestation of chordal rupture are dependent on the number and location of chordae involved. If the patient ruptures critical supporting elements of the mitral valve, a highly distinctive syndrome may result.[307–309,311] Patients note the sudden onset of dyspnea, which is rapidly progressive. There may be fleeting chest pain suggestive of myocardial ischemia. The symptoms are usually of short duration with the patient rapidly progressing to severe intractable heart failure. When the syndrome occurs in a patient with preexisting mitral regurgitation, the only clue may be an abrupt change in symptomatology with sudden clinical deterioration.

Rupture of the chordae tendineae does not always produce acute severe mitral regurgitation. Patients with isolated chordal rupture may remain completely asymptomatic. Patients have described intermittent episodes of chest pain, sudden dyspnea, and mild pulmonary edema which are felt to represent isolated rupture of noncritical chordae tendineae. This syndrome may mimic pulmonary embolism or myocardi-

al infarction and is especially difficult to differentiate in patients who have chronic mitral regurgitation.

Physical examination in acute severe mitral regurgitation due to idiopathic chordal rupture With the development of acute severe mitral regurgitation some of the objective findings are quite different from those of chronic rheumatic mitral regurgitation.[307–309,311] Sinus rhythm is much more common in acute mitral regurgitation than in the chronic rheumatic form. The apex impulse is hyperactive with a nonsustained systolic component, a prominent presystolic atrial component, and an early diastolic rapid filling wave. A parasternal impulse may represent right ventricular hypertension or left atrial systolic expansion (see "Physical Findings," under "Rheumatic Mitral Regurgitation," earlier in this chapter). The systolic murmur of acute severe mitral regurgitation is usually pansystolic but may be early systolic to midsystolic. Unlike rheumatic mitral regurgitation it is frequently crescendo-decrescendo (ejection type) with a midsystolic to late systolic peak. In acute mitral regurgitation the murmur tends to be a function of left atrial compliance. With the rise of the v wave and increased left atrial pressure there is a decrease in regurgitant flow and a diminished intensity of the murmur in late systole. The murmur may extend beyond the aortic component of the second heart sound and render this sound inaudible. In addition to being crescendo-decrescendo, the murmur may mimic aortic stenosis by its radiation to the base of the heart. It may also radiate posteriorly to the thoracic spine and transmit to the top of the head and to the lumbar spine.[312,313] It has been observed that these divergent patterns of radiation may predict which mitral leaflet is involved, posterior radiation suggesting anterior leaflet involvement and anterior radiation suggesting posterior leaflet involvement. However, this interpretation is not always reliable.[314,315] In acute severe mitral regurgitation the intensity of the pulmonic component of the second sound is frequently accentuated and is a reflection of pulmonary arterial hypertension. In addition there is incomplete expiratory closure of the aortic and pulmonic components but with the normal inspiratory increase in splitting of the two components. The presence of an atrial gallop sound favors acute mitral regurgitation, being uncommon in gradually progressive rheumatic mitral regurgitation. A ventricular gallop (Fig. 60B-19) with or without an early diastolic rumble is also common in acute mitral regurgitation. If chordal rupture has involved the posterior mitral leaflet with a normal anterior leaflet remaining, an opening snap may be present.[208]

Patients with long-standing mitral regurgitation may rupture their chordae tendineae. The clinical picture includes a large heart including a large left atrium, atrial fibrillation, a ventricular gallop sound or a diastolic rumble at the apex, a change in the systolic murmur at the apex, and worsening of congestive heart failure.

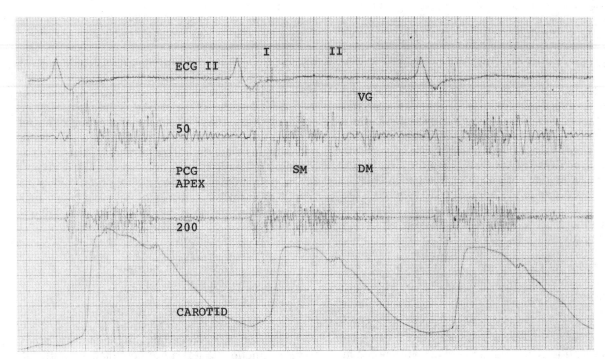

FIGURE 60B-19 Acute mitral regurgitation—phonocardiogram (PCG) recorded at the apex at 50 and 200 Hz. The recording demonstrates loud spindle-shaped apical systolic murmur, a ventricular gallop sound, and a diastolic flow rumble (DM) from the severe mitral regurgitation.

Chest roentgenogram The chest roentgenogram of a patient with chordal rupture and massive acute mitral regurgitation is characterized by acute pulmonary edema and a normal cardiac silhouette. Cardiac fluoroscopy may identify systolic expansion of the left atrium. Severe mitral regurgitation with a normal left atrial radiographic size is strongly suggestive of ruptured chordae tendineae.[307,316]

Electrographic features The ECG provides no diagnostic clues to the diagnosis of ruptured chordae tendineae. Patients are generally in normal sinus rhythm with a normal P wave axis.

Echocardiographic features of ruptured chordae tendineae[317] The echocardiogram (Fig. 60B-20) may demonstrate (1) increased motion of the interventricular septum and posterior wall, (2) increased diastolic excursion of the mitral valve often with contact of the interventricular septum, (3) redundant systolic echoes, (4) an abnormal echo in diastole at the level of the mitral valve representing the flail chordae, (5) a coarse, undulating motion in diastole of the flail mitral leaflets, (6) systolic atrial expansion, and (7) systolic prolapse of the mitral leaflets.

Cardiac catheterization The presence of giant *v* waves in the pulmonary artery wedge (Fig. 60B-21) or left atrial pressure recording suggests acute severe

mitral regurgitation. Selective left ventricular angiography documents severe mitral regurgitation. Left ventricular wall motion and coronary angiography are usually normal.

THERAPY
Patients with severe mitral regurgitation and symptoms of left ventricular failure who are unresponsive to medical therapy benefit from surgery. Valvuloplasty has been successful at some centers; however,

FIGURE 60B-20 Echocardiogram demonstrating a flail posterior leaflet. CW, chest wall; IVS, septum; EN, endocardium; E, epicardium; P, pericardium; A and B, systolic prolapse of the mitral leaflets; C and C', flail motion of the posterior leaflet in diastole. (*Reproduced*[615] *with permission of Joel Felner, M.D., and Grune & Stratton, Inc.*)

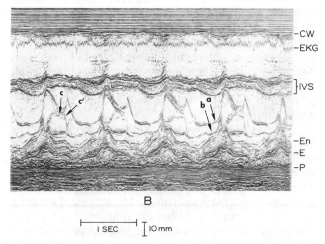

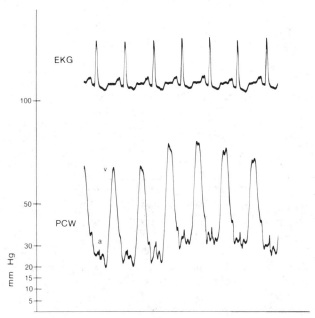

FIGURE 60B-21 Pulmonary capillary wedge pressure (PCW) of a patient with acute mitral regurgitation demonstrating giant *v* waves greater than 50 mm Hg.

TABLE 60B-2
Papillary muscle dysfunction

I Ischemic heart disease
  A Necrosis or fibrosis of the papillary muscle and adjacent left ventricular wall
  B Ischemic paralysis of the papillary muscle and adjacent left ventricular wall
  C Localized ventricular aneurysm
  D Papillary muscle rupture from infarction
  E Hypoxia without coronary obstruction
    1 Anemia
    2 Shock
II Primary papillary muscle disorders
  A Malposition
    1 Obstructive cardiomyopathy
    2 Congenital
      a Parachute mitral valve
      b Abnormal papillary muscle size or position
  B Infiltrative diseases
    1 Pyogenic abscess
    2 Neoplasm
    3 Sarcoid
    4 Calcium
    5 Syphilis
    6 Amyloidosis
  C Trauma
    1 Rupture
    2 Infarction
III Myocardial disorders
  A Left ventricular dilatation from any cause
  B Myocardial disease
    1 Progressive muscular dystrophy
    2 Myotonic muscular dystrophy
IV Endocardial disorders
  A Loeffler's endocarditis
  B Endomyocardial fibrosis
V Inflammatory diseases
  A Myocarditis
  B Polyarteritis
VI Disorder of activation and contraction

at Emory University valve replacement is the procedure of choice.

Papillary muscle dysfunction

The functional integrity of the mitral valve is dependent on the precise interaction and proper function of each component of the mitral apparatus.[231] Although ischemic malfunction of the papillary muscles was thought to be a cause of mitral regurgitation as early as 1935,[318] it was not until Burch and colleagues[319] in 1963 described the clinical syndrome of papillary muscle dysfunction that attention was focused on this problem. Burch and his associates recognized seven etiologic mechanisms for production of this syndrome.[320] These are (1) ischemia, (2) left ventricular dilatation, (3) atrophy of the papillary muscle, (4) defective development of the papillary muscle, (5) endomyocardial disease, (6) heart muscle disease, or cardiomyopathy, and (7) rupture of the papillary muscle.

In Table 60B-2 the syndrome is divided according to the most likely pathophysiologic mechanisms for production of papillary muscle dysfunction. The three principal mechanisms are (1) distortion of the normal spatial relationships of the papillary muscle, (2) transient papillary muscle abnormalities, and (3) asynchronous papillary muscle or left ventricular contraction.

FUNCTIONAL ANATOMY OF THE PAPILLARY MUSCLES[320-324]
Within the left ventricle lie two papillary muscle groups—the anterior lateral and the posterior medial. These muscles are not symmetric in position, number, size, or shape. They neither face one another at exactly 180° nor are in the same place. In diastole, the papillary muscles lie almost transverse at their maxi-

mal length; during systole, there is shortening of the anteroposterior diameter, and the ventricle moves in a wringing motion. Contraction of the papillary muscle is initiated just prior to ventricular contraction. By the end of systole, the papillary muscle lies perpendicular under the mitral valve.

The distortion of the normal spatial relationships of the papillary muscles results in a loss of the natural mechanical advantage and proper support for the mitral valve.[320] There is either retraction of the valve into the ventricle or prolapse of the valve into the atrium. Valvular cohesion is lost and mitral regurgitation results. This mechanism is the principal cause of the mitral regurgitation from ventricular dilatation and from akinesia or aneurysmal dilatation of the ventricle (Fig. 60B-22).

Experimental studies in dogs suggest that injury to the papillary muscle alone will not result in mitral regurgitation.[325,326] Regurgitation results from a combination of injuries to both the papillary muscle and the left ventricular wall.[327] Pathologic studies in

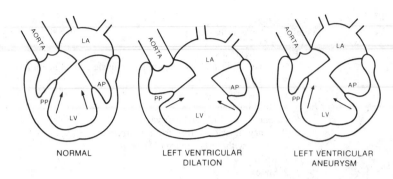

NORMAL LEFT VENTRICULAR DILATION LEFT VENTRICULAR ANEURYSM

FIGURE 60B-22 Diagrammatic representation of the mechanism of papillary muscle dysfunction. Normal papillary muscle (PM) position results in a force of contraction that brings the valves together within the left ventricle. Left ventricular dilatation of the papillary muscle position acts to pull the valves apart. In left ventricular aneurysm the malposition of the papillary muscle results in improper mitral valve closure (*Diagrams representative of illustrations by Burch et al., Arch. Intern. Med., 112:158, 1963, with permission from Dr. Burch.*)

human beings have also shown that marked atrophy and fibrosis of the papillary muscle alone will not cause mitral regurgitation.[328–330]

Ischemic injury to the papillary muscle is dependent upon coronary artery anatomy, collateral circulation, diastolic blood flow, and wall tension. The coronary vascular supply is variable.[322–324] The anterior lateral papillary muscle is supplied principally by the left circumflex coronary artery with branches from the left anterior descending and diagonal arteries. The posterior medial papillary muscle is supplied by the posterior descending branch of the right coronary artery with collateral branches from the left circumflex coronary artery. The subendocardial vascular supply is dependent on the linkage of the papillary muscle to the left ventricular wall. A papillary muscle that is sessile with a broad base or has multiple trabecular bridges has a richer blood supply than one which is a fingerlike extension into the left ventricular cavity. This papillary muscle generally has a long, penetrating central arterial radical without extensive anastomotic collateral blood supply present in the broad-based papillary muscle. The anatomy of the circulation produces an endocardium which is peculiarly sensitive and vulnerable to injury. Studies have demonstrated that the papillary muscle undergoes considerably more stress than the rest of the ventricular myocardium[331] and has a greater myocardial oxygen demand. The subendocardial position permits adequate coronary blood flow only during diastole,[332] and the muscle is particularly sensitive to those conditions which result in increased subendocardial tension or decreased subendocardial blood flow, such as hypertension or hemorrhagic shock. Injury to the papillary muscle can result from conditions other than ischemia. Vasculitis, syphilis, myocardial abscesses, trauma, and infiltrative cardiomyopathies such as amyloidosis have all been associated with papillary muscle injury and dysfunction.[323]

Burch has suggested that asynchronous contraction of the papillary muscle results in papillary muscle dysfunction. There is little direct evidence to support this mechanism. Papillary muscle dysfunction is uncommon in ventricular conduction disturbances. Mitral regurgitation which occurs with ventricular extrasystoles is felt to be related to contraction during diastole rather than to asynchronous papillary muscle contraction.[323]

PAPILLARY MUSCLE DYSFUNCTION IN CORONARY DISEASE

The most common cause of papillary muscle dysfunction is coronary atherosclerotic heart disease.[329] Studies have reported fibrosis and/or atrophy in one or more papillary muscles in up to 80 percent of random consecutive autopsies.[328] In fatal acute myocardial infarction necrosis in one or both papillary muscles is described in up to 50 percent of cases.[333] Mitral regurgitation is reported to occur in approximately 40 percent of posterior septal myocardial infarctions and 20 percent of anterior septal myocardial infarctions.[329] A consecutive case study of mitral regurgitation noted that approximately 11 percent of patients had papillary muscle dysfunction. Infarction of a posterior medial papillary muscle is associated with a greater percentage of papillary muscle rupture, and there is a higher incidence of death when myocardial infarction is associated with papillary muscle dysfunction.[329]

The sensitivity of the papillary muscles for ischemic injury is accounted for by the precarious position of the muscle within the left ventricular cavity. Oxygenation is threatened not only by myocardial ischemia but also by dysrhythmia, ventricular dilatation, or complications of myocardial infarction which increase myocardial oxygen demand, such as heart failure and shock. There appear to be certain changes within the coronary arteries related to aging which begin sooner in the papillary muscles, and the elderly have a proclivity for papillary muscle infarction.[322]

CLINICAL RECOGNITION

Symptoms The symptoms of papillary muscle dysfunction usually are those of the underlying heart disease.[323,334,335] Patients with coronary atherosclerotic heart disease may suffer angina pectoris or symptoms of left ventricular dysfunction, depending upon the extent of the ischemic disease and severity of the mitral regurgitation. There may be intermittent acute episodes of shortness of breath or chest discomfort related to the variable magnitude of the mitral regurgitation[336,337] and myocardial ischemia.

Physical examination The apical impulse is characterized by a late systolic bulge, a finding suggestive of a ventricular aneurysm.[195] In addition, a palpable presystolic component of the apical impulse can be appreciated. Patients who have considerable mitral regurgitation or papillary muscle rupture will have a broad, vigorous, displaced apical impulse from the increased volume load.[195]

The triad of an accentuated first heart sound, an early systolic to midsystolic crescendo-decrescendo murmur, and gallop rhythm[338] is felt to suggest papillary muscle dysfunction. The first heart sound is frequently accentuated but not necessarily so. The second heart sound is usually normal but has been reported to be widely split or paradoxic depending on the severity of the mitral regurgitation or left ventricular dysfunction. An atrial gallop is invariably present, and a ventricular gallop is not unusual. The ventricular gallop depends upon the severity of the mitral regurgitation and the extent of left ventricular dysfunction. An inspiratory increase in the intensity of the gallop sounds has been noted.[338]

The murmur is variable, reflecting the dynamic nature of the papillary muscle dysfunction. It can change from beat to beat and alter in timing, configuration, intensity, pitch, and duration.[329,339] The murmur is usually soft, high-pitched, crescendo-decrescendo in configuration, and associated with a slight pause after the first heart sound.[329,335,338] The murmur may be pansystolic or become so during heart failure or with angina pectoris.[336,340] The character of the murmur has a poor correlation with the functional significance of the mitral regurgitation.[339] However, persistent pansystolic murmurs are usually associated with the most significant hemodynamic lesion. A midsystolic click and occasionally a midsystolic click–late systolic murmur have been described[341,342] but are rare in our experience. A premature ventricular contraction is followed by a decrease in the intensity of the systolic murmur.[338] The effect of phenylephrine and amyl nitrite on established murmurs is less predictable than in rheumatic mitral regurgitation.[63] The use of phenylephrine may significantly accentuate the murmur and has been reported to produce acute pulmonary edema;[336] likewise the use of oral nitrites has been associated with a decrease in the intensity and duration of the systolic murmur. These findings suggest that maneuvers which increase myocardial oxygen consumption tend to accentuate the papillary muscle dysfunction and those which reduce myocardial oxygen consumption may diminish the severity of the papillary muscle dysfunction. We avoid the use of maneuvers which increase myocardial oxygen consumption such as handgrip or phenylephrine infusion in patients with recent myocardial infarction or unstable ischemic syndromes.

The electrocardiogram Electrocardiographic findings in papillary muscle dysfunction are variable and nonspecific. Three patterns of abnormal repolar-

ization are described which have a high correlation with papillary muscle dysfunction.[320] These are (1) moderate depression of the J junction with concave upward deformity of the ST segment, (2) slight to moderate depression of the J junction with convex upward deformity of the ST segment and terminal inversion of the T wave, and (3) marked J junction depression with either convex or concave upward deformity of the ST segment. These patterns are nonspecific and occur in many forms of subendocardial ischemia including left ventricular hypertrophy, intraventricular conduction defects, and digitalis effect. A more specific abnormality has been an acute shift in the terminal force of the P wave in the horizontal axis.[329,323] The posterior shift of this force reflects acute left atrial dilatation or strain. In contrast to the repolarization changes the P wave abnormalities are less frequent in patients without mitral regurgitation.

Roentgenographic findings The chest roentgenogram is usually unremarkable.[338] In most patients, heart size is normal, and there are no radiographic abnormalities in the lung fields. Presence of left atrial or left ventricular enlargement appears related to the severity of mitral regurgitation and myocardial disease. Patients with relatively recent onset of mitral regurgitation have normal chamber size, while those with mitral regurgitation of some duration generally have enlargement of the left ventricular and left atrial chambers. When mitral regurgitation is associated with an acute myocardial infarction, pulmonary edema is frequently present on the radiograph.[329,334]

Echocardiogram The echocardiogram may be helpful in identifying left atrial enlargement and abnormal contraction patterns of the left ventricle. No specific abnormalities of the mitral valve echo are recognized. There may be an increase in the E to F slope related to the severity of the mitral regurgitation or conversely a decrease in the E to F slope related to decreased left ventricular compliance from ischemic heart disease.[351a]

Gaited nuclear angiogram Gaited nuclear angiography has been a helpful noninvasive method for evaluating severity of left ventricular dysfunction in patients with mitral regurgitation and coronary artery disease.[343] This technique permits identification of ventricular aneurysms and assessment of ejection fraction in patients with asymmetric myocardial disease. The procedure is useful in evaluating a patient for surgical therapy.

Cardiac catheterization Pressures in the right and left sides of the heart are variable and are determined by the state of left ventricular function at that moment. Papillary muscle dysfunction can be dynamic, and with an acute transient episode of myocardial ischemia the left ventricular end-diastolic pressure (and pulmonary artery wedge pressure) may rise to alarming levels. Administration of nitroglycerin and resolution of the transient ischemia results in return of the left ventricular diastolic pressure to normal. This acute elevation of left atrial pressure may be associated with prominent *v* waves in the pulmonary artery wedge or left atrial pressure tracing, reflecting acute mitral regurgitation. When there is associated ventricular aneurysm and persistent left ventricular dysfunction, elevation of pressures may be present in the stable state.

Selective left ventricular angiography is the most sensitive test for the assessment of mitral regurgitation. The angiogram permits assessment of the mobility and appearance of the valve leaflets, the character of the regurgitant jet, left ventricular contractility, and left atrial size. The technique aids in the separation of rheumatic mitral regurgitation from nonrheumatic mitral regurgitation and is helpful in differentiating papillary muscle dysfunction from rupture of chordae tendineae.[304,344] Most importantly the technique permits evaluation of left ventricular function. Ventricular wall motion and ejection fraction are among the most important determinants of success in the surgical therapy. It is the left ventricular function which is the primary factor determining long-term survival. Ventricular contraction abnormalities are very common, and approximately one-half the patients will have a ventricular aneurysm.[338,339,345] Most patients have extensive coronary artery disease, frequently with three-vessel involvement.[338] There is an increased incidence of right coronary artery lesions.[339]

MANAGEMENT

Medical management may control clinical symptoms. Propranolol and nitrates are beneficial in the management of angina symptoms. Digitalis and diuretics may be helpful. In those patients in whom papillary muscle dysfunction dynamically manifests transient myocardial ischemia, management, both medical and surgical, is similar to that of the coronary atherosclerotic heart disease with angina pectoris. Vasodilator therapy may assist in the management of acute and chronic mitral regurgitation.[216,346,347] Surgery with mitral valve replacement may be necessary in the presence of severe mitral regurgitation and refractory heart failure. Surgical success is dependent upon the severity of the coronary artery disease and its amenability to revascularization, the presence of a ventricular aneurysm, and the function of the left ventricular myocardium. Patients with proximal obstructive large vessel coronary disease benefit from aortocoronary bypass during valve replacement. Surgical mortality is reported at approximately 20 percent in patients with chronic mitral regurgitation and 50 percent with acute mitral regurgitation.[348] Intraaortic balloon pumping has been utilized to achieve hemodynamic stability permitting angiographic evaluation and support through surgery.[349]

Papillary muscle rupture

Papillary muscle rupture occurs as a complication of myocardial infarction and is reported in 0.5 to 5 percent of these patients.[318,350] The papillary muscle can also rupture as a complication of chest trauma. Rupture of the belly of the papillary muscle is unusual; the most frequent pathologic condition is rupture of the trabeculated tip. Rupture of the belly of the papillary muscle is followed by a catastrophic course with rapid clinical deterioration and death. Patients with less severe injury usually have the abrupt onset of pulmonary edema with progressive clinical deterioration. About 35 percent die within the first 24 h and 75 percent within the first week of acute myocardial infarction. Rupture is more common in the posterior medial papillary muscle, compared with the anterior papillary muscle.[350] Patients suffering their first myocardial infarction, without an extensive collateral circulation, are most likely to develop this complication.

The onset is associated with severe dyspnea, verging on suffocation, with pulmonary edema and chest pain.[304] Hemoptysis may occur and syncope is frequent. Patients are usually refractory to medical therapy and rapidly progress to cardiogenic shock. Physical findings include a forceful hyperdynamic apical impulse, which may rapidly change as there is a decrease in cardiac output and progression of the profound left ventricular dysfunction. The first heart sound is soft, and the second heart sound is usually not remarkable. Atrial and ventricular gallop sounds are present. The murmur is pansystolic, constant, loud, and raspy, with wide radiation from the apex and usually not associated with a thrill. As the patient progresses into shock, the murmur becomes softer and may become barely audible.[304,323,334]

The diagnosis is facilitated by use of the Swan-Ganz catheter and recognition of large *v* waves in the pulmonary artery wedge tracing.[351] It is important to remember that in these patients there may be an oxygen step-up during catheterization that should not be confused with ventricular septal rupture.[352] The oxygen step-up is from severe mitral regurgitation with a permeable foramen ovale.[304] Cardiac catheterization and left ventricular angiography are usually necessary to confirm the diagnosis of acute mitral regurgitation with papillary muscle rupture. Intraaortic balloon pumping is frequently necessary prior to angiographic studies and surgical intervention. The diagnosis of ruptured papillary muscle cannot be made invariably at cardiac catheterization. It is essential that catheterization confirm the presence of acute mitral regurgitation, determine the extent of left ventricular dysfunction, and document the severity of coronary artery disease in order to plan the proper surgical management (see Chap. 62F).

Calcified mitral annulus

Calcification of the mitral annulus is frequently encountered at autopsy in persons over the age of 65.[298,353,354] The lesion is felt to represent a degenerative process involving the fibrotic skeleton of the heart. This may represent thrombosis in the mitral

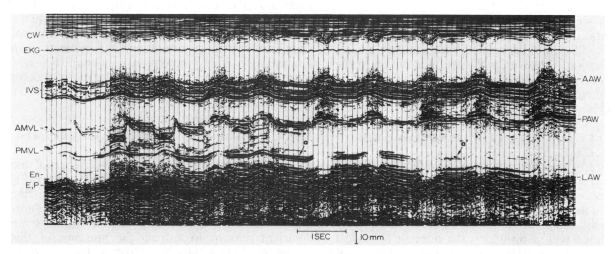

FIGURE 60B-23 Echocardiogram demonstrating calcified mitral annulus. CW, chest wall; ECG, electrocardiogram; IVS, intraventricular septum; AMVL, anterior mitral leaflet; PMVL, posterior mitral leaflet; EN, endocardium; EP, epi-pericardium; AAW, anterior aortic wall; PW, posterior aortic wall; LAW, left atrial wall; A and A', the heavy band of echoes from the calcified mitral annulus which disappear as the echo beam is scanned to the left atrium. (*Reproduced*[615] *with permission of Joel Felner, M.D., and Grune & Stratton, Inc.*)

subvalvular recess with subsequent organization.[298] The lesion occurs three times more frequently in women than in men and rarely involves the mitral valve, in contrast to calcific aortic sclerosis, which is more frequent in men and usually involves the aortic valve. The lesion is unusual in persons under the age of 40 but may occur in association with Marfan's syndrome, Hurler's syndrome, and metabolic disturbances producing hypercalcemia.[298] Diseases which accelerate arteriosclerosis such as hypertension or diabetes mellitus are associated with premature annular calcification.

Significant cardiac symptoms are 'unusual, and most cases are recognized either accidently by chest roentgenogram or during evaluation for cardiac murmurs. The calcific process is usually confined to the mitral annulus, most frequently along the posterior cusp;[298,253] it may, however, extend to the anterior cusp along the fibrosal layer or undersurface of the valve leaflet. If the process extends to the interventricular septum, it results in disturbances of the cardiac conduction system. The calcific process rarely extends into the leaflets but forms a shelf under the leaflets inhibiting their normal motion. The involvement of the leaflet may be so severe that the chordae tendineae are severely stretched as a result of impingement of the leaflets over the edge of the calcified ring; however, severe mitral regurgitation is rare. The murmur associated with a calcified annulus is an apical systolic murmur varying in intensity from grade 2 to 4 out of 6 grades. The murmur is generally crescendo-decrescendo in shape, is holosystolic, and radiates to the axilla. It may be musical. If not carefully auscultated, the murmur may be mistaken

for aortic stenosis. Auscultatory findings can be extremely variable; some patients will have no murmur, while at least one patient has been described with a thrill. Patients frequently have an additional murmur of aortic sclerosis. This makes evaluation of the murmur with amyl nitrite and phenylephrine difficult.[63] The diagnosis is generally made by chest roentgenogram and fluoroscopy. The hallmark is a thick line of calcification lying just to the left of the midline in the frontal projection and in the posterior third of the heart on the lateral projection. The density has a J, U, or oval shape.[298] Echocardiography identifies a heavy band of echoes at the level of mitral annulus with abrupt interruption of the echoes when scanning from the left ventricle to the left atrium[355] (Fig. 60B-23). The most important complication of calcification of the mitral annulus fibrosis is heart block.[253] This is noted frequently in patients with massive calcification of the mitral annulus, especially when the calcification extends into the interventricular septum.[298] Spontaneous calcific emboli from a calcified mitral annulus is reported with multiple brain infarcts.[356] Few patients with this syndrome are symptomatic; when symptoms are present, they are usually due to coexistent coronary disease and not to calcification of the mitral annulus.

Differential diagnosis of nonrheumatic causes of mitral regurgitation

PAPILLARY MUSCLE DYSFUNCTION

Papillary muscle dysfunction is differentiated from other types of mitral regurgitation by its distinctive historical, clinical, and laboratory findings. Patients with rheumatic regurgitation generally have a louder, pansystolic mitral murmur. An aortic systolic murmur may cause confusion, but careful auscultation generally indicates that the murmur is maximal to the left of the sternum and not in the aortic area. Palpitation of the carotid pulse also generally excludes significant aortic stenosis except in elderly patients. Idiopathic hypertrophic subaortic stenosis may be difficult to distinguish from papillary muscle dysfunction. However, with careful attention to the response of the murmur to various positional and vasoactive maneuvers diagnosis of this condition can be made.

RUPTURE OF THE PAPILLARY MUSCLE

Rupture of the papillary muscle is difficult to distinguish from rupture of the interventricular septum. Both occur as a result of acute myocardial infarction and are associated with sudden clinical deterioration and pulmonary edema. Septal rupture is frequently associated with a thrill, and the murmur is loudest along the left sternal border as opposed to rupture of the papillary muscle in which the murmur is generally louder at the apex and rarely has a thrill. Bedside evaluation with a Swan-Ganz catheter can be helpful by recognition of giant *v* waves in the pulmonary capillary wedge pressure in patients with ruptured papillary muscle and by measurement of an oxygen step-up in the right ventricle in patients with ruptured interventricular septum. Care must be taken in evaluating the oxygen step-up, since with acute mitral regurgitation an oxygen step-up can occur at the atrial level through a patent foramen ovale. The echocardiogram may be helpful. Patients with a ruptured interventricular septum may have paradoxic motion of the septum and an enlarged right ventricular cavity, while in patients with rupture of the papillary muscle a flail mitral leaflet can be recognized.

RUPTURE OF CHORDAE TENDINEAE

Chordal rupture may mimic valvular aortic stenosis. The diagnosis requires close evaluation of the carotid pulse and careful attention to the auscultatory findings. The carotid impulse is prolonged with a delayed peak in aortic stenosis in contrast to the quick, rapid upstroke of acute mitral regurgitation. The murmur of chordal rupture is distinguished by its location, loudest to the left of the sternum, and the aortic second heart sound is intact. Vasoactive maneuvers such as the use of amyl nitrite and phenylephrine further separates these entities. Papillary muscle dysfunction, rupture of the papillary muscle, and ruptured interventricular septum are differentiated by the absence of ischemic heart disease, which is common in the above syndromes and a rare cause of ruptured chordae tendineae.

CALCIFIED MITRAL ANNULUS

Calcification of the mitral annulus is frequently confused with aortic sclerosis and papillary muscle dysfunction. Both these disorders are commonly present in patients with a calcified mitral annulus. Aortic valve disease can generally be distinguished by careful attention to the auscultatory findings and

careful palpation of the pulse. As noted previously, the response to the vasoactive maneuvers is variable because of the presence of both aortic and mitral murmurs. The presence and severity of papillary muscle dysfunction is even more difficult to evaluate. Calcification of the mitral annulus is rarely a cause of significant mitral regurgitation, and patients with clinical signs and symptoms of moderate to severe mitral regurgitation are more likely to have other diseases involving the mitral apparatus.

BACTERIAL ENDOCARDITIS

Bacterial endocarditis may destroy any one of the four heart valves and produce serious valvular disease. The disease is usually superimposed on existing valvular disease but may occur in apparently "normal" hearts. Unexplained fever and murmurs are sufficient reasons to suspect the presence of this condition. Certain clinical syndromes should be highlighted; the abrupt development of aortic regurgitation, fever, and heart failure usually represents bacterial endocarditis on a bicuspid aortic valve, and this condition usually requires surgical intervention; the abrupt development of a loud systolic murmur in a patient with fever often represents a ruptured chordae tendineae due to endocarditis; and murmurs on the right side of the heart plus fever and pulmonary infiltrates suggest the possibility of right-sided endocarditis in a patient who may be "mainlining" drugs. See Chap. 77 for a detailed discussion of bacterial endocarditis.

INHERITED DISORDERS OF CONNECTIVE TISSUE AND VALVE DISEASE

The mucopolysaccharidoses

The mucopolysaccharidoses are autosomal recessive or X-linked recessive inherited disorders of lysosomal metabolism. This is an enzymatic disorder with involvement of many organ systems producing a characteristic phenotype. The mucopolysaccharide disorders which produce cardiac disease are Hurler's syndrome, Hunter's syndrome, Morquio's syndrome, and Scheie's syndrome.

Hurler's syndrome is an autosomal recessive disease with abnormal deposition of dermatan sulfate and heparitin sulfate. In this syndrome, virtually all patients have abnormal cardiac valves,[298,357] and necropsy studies disclose valvular thickening and coronary luminal narrowing. Within the valves and coronary arteries there are large cells with clear cytoplasm, the characteristic gargoyle cells; between these cells are deposits of fibrotic tissue. Mitral annular calcification, often occurring in childhood, is present, and many of these patients have premature angina pectoris, which has been reported to occur as early as at 4 years of age.

Hunter's syndrome is an X-linked recessive disorder with abnormalities in dermatan sulfate and heparitin sulfate. It is frequently associated with valvular and coronary artery disease. Death from heart failure frequently occurs before 20 years of age.[358] Morquio's syndrome and Scheie's syndrome are autosomal recessive disorders which have involvement of the aortic root and aortic valve.[358] Aortic regurgitation is a common sequela. These patients rarely reach their teens without the development of aortic valve disease.

Ehlers-Danlos syndrome

The Ehlers-Danlos syndrome is a heterogeneous inherited connective tissue disorder characterized by loose, fragile tissue, a bleeding diathesis, and hypermobile joints. Various cardiac defects are described, but no consistent anomaly is recognized. Patients have been noted with aortic regurgitation, mitral regurgitation, and systolic prolapse of the mitral valve with clicks and late systolic murmurs.[359,360]

Pseudoxanthoma elasticum

Pseudoxanthoma elasticum is a primary disorder of the elastic fiber which behaves as a bioatrophy. The most characteristic aspects of cardiovascular involvement include premature medial calcification of peripheral arteries and symptoms of coronary artery disease with angina pectoris and myocardial infarction.[358] Abnormalities of the mitral valve are described. Valvular heart disease is uncommon in this syndrome, and the extent and severity of valvular changes is unknown.

Marfan's syndrome

Marfan's syndrome is an inherited disorder of connective tissues characterized by tall, slender patients with high-arched palates, dislocated lenses, lax ligaments, and cardiovascular involvement.[358] Cardiovascular abnormalities are a frequent cause of death and most commonly involve the aortic and mitral valves. There is a weakness and degeneration of the tunica media of the aorta. There is dilatation of the aorta beginning at the aortic ring, and the dilatation is usually progressive.[298,358] Similar changes may occur within the pulmonary artery. Premature calcification of the annulus fibrosis occurs with myxomatous degeneration of the cardiac valves.[298] The mitral cusps and chordae tendineae may be redundant, stretched, and very thin. Nonejection midsystolic clicks and late systolic murmurs are common with this syndrome. In addition to the valvular defect, patients have bony chest wall defects, and cardiac disability may be contributed to by pectus excavatum.[358]

Treatment of cardiovascular complications in patients with Marfan's syndrome is aimed at reducing the probability of aortic dissection and decreasing the biodegradation of valvular tissue. In this regard, it is felt that use of propranolol may be beneficial therapy.[358] The beta blockade reduces the velocity and force of contraction, which it is hoped will produce less tension in the aortic root and less strain on the aortic and mitral valves. Surgical therapy in Marfan's syndrome has included aortic replacement with a Teflon prosthesis and replacement of the aortic and mitral valves by prosthetic valves.[361]

Unusual causes of mitral valvular disease

Systemic lupus erythematosus is a chronic disease of unknown cause characterized by an autoimmune phenomenon and a generalized systemic illness. Cardiac abnormalities include pericarditis, valvular lesions, and myocardial involvement. Atypical verrucous endocarditis has been reported at necropsy in up to 46 percent of patients with lupus erythematosus. The mitral valve is the most commonly involved,[362] but aortic valvular verrucae are also described.[298] Murmurs are very frequent in patients with this syndrome, but significant valvular disease is unusual.[298] The myocardial and pericardial lesions are generally the most likely to produce clinical manifestations.[362]

Radiation to the chest and mediastinum may produce morphologic changes within the heart.[363] Patients may develop myocardial fibrosis, pericardial thickening, and occasionally constrictive pericarditis. Pathologic changes have been described in the tricuspid, mitral, aortic, and pulmonary valves as well as the chordae tendineae. Valvular thickening is focal and does not produce dysfunction of the valves.

Trauma involving the heart may produce valvular damage with direct injury to the valve or result in injury to the papillary muscle, chordae tendineae, or aortic root, producing regurgitation across the mitral or aortic valve.[364] Methysergide maleate (Sansert) produces cardiac fibrosis and can involve the mitral and aortic valves.[365] Improvement may occur when the drug is discontinued. Silent mitral regurgitation is a rare condition and may be the result of factors such as obesity, emphysema, or chest deformity.[19] Most commonly it is found in association with other valvular disorders, especially aortic and mitral stenosis.

AORTIC STENOSIS

In 1846 James Hope[366] wrote:

> Contraction of the aortic valves must be very great to render the pulse small, weak, intermittent, and irregular . . . . Irregularity of the pulse is not necessarily or usually produced by contraction of the aortic valves, unless extreme; nor are the size and strength of the pulse materially diminished by moderate contraction.

The earliest description of aortic valvular stenosis is probably that of Carolus Rayger (1672) as recorded by Bonetus (1679) in his *Sepulchretum*. Rayger noted on postmortem examination of a middle-aged Parisian tailor who dropped dead in the street that the aortic valves had the consistency of bone.[367]

Many of the early physicians, beginning with Corvisart des Marets, recorded their impressions of the clinical manifestations of this disease. These recordings led to various misconceptions about the physical signs of aortic stenosis which were, to a large extent, corrected by Hope in his *A Treatise on the Diseases of the Heart and Great Vessels.*

Etiology

The etiology of aortic valvular stenosis (see Table 60B-3) presents one of the most confusing and disputed segments of cardiovascular pathology. Through the years the prevalence of the various causes has been altered due to the changing incidence of certain disease states (decreased incidence of rheumatic fever), a reinterpretation of pathologic findings (recognition of greater incidence of congenital bicuspid valves), and an increased longevity of the general population allowing for a wider manifestation of degenerative changes.

Monckeberg in 1904 ascribed aortic valvular stenosis to acute endocarditis or the gradual development of valvular sclerosis.[368] This dual causation, infective and degenerative, was generally accepted until the publication of Karsner and Koletsky in 1947. These investigators concluded that 196 of 200 patients with aortic stenosis had evidence of rheumatic valvulitis.[369] Supportive evidence from other reknowned cardiologists led to the general acceptance of rheumatic fever as the predominant cause of aortic valvular stenosis.[370–372] In 1953, however, Campbell and Kauntze described 40 cases of congenital valvular stenosis and suggested that this is a common cause.[367] Credence was given to this proposal in a review of bicuspid aortic valves from nine pathology museums by Bacon and Matthews.[373] While these investigators and subsequently others such as Hudson,[374] Roberts,[375] and Storstein[376] established the prevalence of the bicuspid valve as a cause of aortic stenosis, this association was recognized in 1858. In that year, Peacock pointed out that bicuspid valves could develop chronic inflammation "by which they are rendered thick and unyielding and often become extensively ossified, thus inducing, first obstruction to the flow of blood from the ventricle into the aorta, and then incompetency."[377]

TABLE 60B-3

Etiology of isolated aortic stenosis

Age, years	Disease prevalence, listed in decreasing frequency
0–30	Unicuspid valve
	Bicuspid valve
30–70	Bicuspid valve
	Rheumatic valvulitis
	Unicuspid valve
70+	Degenerative calcification
	Bicuspid valve
	Rheumatic valvulitis

While current opinion favors the bicuspid valve as the most common cause of aortic valvular stenosis,[374–378] the age at which significant aortic stenosis becomes clinically manifest is an important clue to the etiology. Significant valvular aortic stenosis developing in a person prior to age 30 is almost universally congenital, the majority having an aortic valve with one open commissure, a fused commissure attached to the opposite aortic wall, a congenital raphe, and an eccentric orifice.[379] Although these valves have usually been classified as bicuspid,[380] it is now believed that most are actually unicuspid, unicommissural valves with a false commissure rather than a fused commissure.[379] In the decades extending from age 30 to age 70, the most prevalent cause of isolated aortic stenosis is generally agreed to be the congenitally bicuspid valve.[374,378,381–384] It is during these same decades that rheumatic valvulitis gains significance as a cause of aortic stenosis, particularly in multivalvular disease. The most recent studies on the etiology of isolated aortic stenosis have found an incidence of rheumatic valvulitis of 6 to 27 percent.[376,378,381,384] These figures do not apply to combined aortic and mitral valve disease, in which the cause is generally rheumatic. Patients developing significant stenosis after age 70 usually manifest degenerative calcification of an otherwise normal tricuspid valve.[378,385] In these elderly patients with significant aortic stenosis, there is a slight predominance of women, while in the younger patients men predominate in a ratio of 2:1 to 4:1.[376,381,385]

Disease mechanisms

CONGENITAL AORTIC VALVE DISEASE

While a unicuspid, noncommissural aortic valve with an anatomic similarity to the congenital dome-shaped pulmonary valve has been described,[386] the unicuspid aortic valve is more frequently a unicommissural domed valve.[383,386,387] This malformation consists of a single leaflet which starts at the aortic wall, extends across the annulus without making contact with the aortic wall, bends on itself, and returns to reconnect to the aortic wall, forming a single commissure[386] (see Fig. 60B-24). The attachment of the unicommissural valve to the aortic wall at the site of the raphe is quite variable. The higher the attachment, the more the congenital raphe resembles a fused true commissure and the more the valve resembles a bicuspid valve. More importantly, the higher the attachment, the greater support afforded the cusp by the raphe and the greater the likelihood of successful valvotomy.[379]

The unicuspid aortic valve is inherently stenotic and is the only type of valve stenotic at birth.[388] These valves seem to develop calcification at an unusually young age (before age 30), which accentuates their inherent stenosis. Males predominate in a ratio of 3:1, and the murmur usually dates from birth.

BICUSPID AORTIC VALVE

The bicuspid aortic valve is the most common congenital malformation of the heart, occurring in 1 to 2

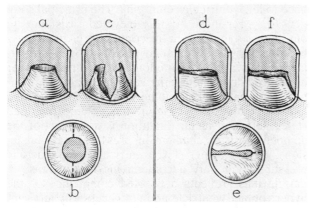

FIGURE 60B-24 A and *B.* Dome-shaped unicuspid, noncommissural aortic valve. *C.* Same valve postvalvulotomy. *D* and *E.* Unicuspid unicommissural aortic valve. *F.* Same valve postvalvotomy. (*Reprinted* [386] *with permission of Jesse E. Edwards, M.D., and A.M.A. specialty journals.*)

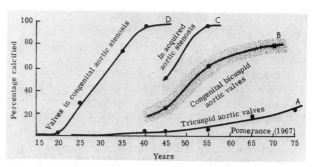

FIGURE 60B-25 Incidence of calcification with increasing age in various types of aortic valves. *A.* In normal aortic valves with three cusps. *B.* In congenital bicuspid aortic valves. *C.* In acquired aortic stenosis. *D.* In valves with congenital (unicuspid and/or bicuspid) aortic stenosis. (*Reprinted*[391] *with permission of The British Heart Journal.*)

percent of the general population.[375] In patients with coarctation of the aorta, the incidence of bicuspid valve has been reported to be as high as 80 percent.[386] As early as 1858, Peacock brought attention to the tendency of the bicuspid valve to develop stenosis by becoming "ossified."[377] Subsequently, in 1886, Osler described the abnormal propensity of the bicuspid valve for developing subacute bacterial endocarditis.[389]

Two basic configurations of the bicuspid valve occur with approximately the same frequency: In type I the two cusps are located anteriorly and posteriorly, the commissures are on the right and left, and both coronary arteries arise anterior to the anterior cusp. In type II the two cusps are located on the right and left, the commissures are located anteriorly and posteriorly, and a coronary artery arises from behind each cusp. Either the two cusps are equal in size or the conjoint cusp (cusp containing a raphe) is larger. The conjoint cusp is usually larger than one but smaller than two normal cusps.[375,383]

Unlike the unicuspid aortic valve, the bicuspid valve is not inherently stenotic. Stenosis, however, is the most frequent complication; regurgitation is next, usually as a consequence of endocarditis. Immobilization of the cusps by the deposition of calcium appears to be the most important factor in converting the bicuspid valve into a stenotic lesion. The exact explanation as to why these bicuspid valves become sclerotic and calcified has not been established but seems to lie with the fact that the bicuspid configuration causes the valve to open and close imperfectly. The process of collagenous degeneration, lipid deposition, and calcification occurring in the bicuspid valve is similar to that noted much later in life in some tricuspid valves [see "Degenerative Calcification of the Tricuspid Aortic Valve (Aortic Stenosis of the Elderly)"]. This similarity in pathologic findings suggests that stenosis in the bicuspid valve is a degenerative change accelerated by the abnormal mechanical stress imposed on the valvular tissue by its bicuspid arrangement.

The frequency of development of stenosis in a congenitally bicuspid valve is unknown. The best figures available in this regard were compiled by Campbell, who reported that the bicuspid valve occurred in 4 out of 1,000 live births with males predominating in a ratio of 4:1. The leaflets are often thickened by age 30, usually by age 40, and always by age 50. Calcium deposition rarely occurs before age 40 but is found in perhaps 25 percent of those patients aged 40 to 49 and in over half those aged 50 or more[388] (Fig. 60B-25). A stenotic congenital bicuspid aortic valve without calcification is extremely uncommon past the age of 30. Interestingly enough, development of infective endocarditis of a heavily calcified valve is rare.[375]

The congenital bicuspid aortic valve usually occurs as an isolated cardiovascular malformation. If a coexisting congenital condition is present, it is most commonly coarctation of the aorta, followed in frequency by a bicuspid pulmonic valve.[375]

RHEUMATIC AORTIC STENOSIS

The aortic valve is rendered stenotic by rheumatic valvulitis through either extensive fusion of commissures or by fusion of a single commissure with secondary calcium deposition. The latter mode of stenosis is the more common. Commissural fusion stems from healing of the active rheumatic endocarditis. The fusion which usually occurs between the right and left leaflets converts the aortic valve into a bicuspid configuration subject to the same abnormal stresses and degenerative changes as the congenital bicuspid valve.[388]

That this process of fusion followed by calcification is slow is evident in the natural history of rheumatic aortic stenosis. Patients presenting with hemodynamically significant aortic stenosis are some 10 to 15 years older than patients presenting with mitral stenosis.[376] Recognition that these figures are skewed by the almost certain inclusion of patients with nonrheumatic aortic stenosis does not negate the fact that aortic valvular obstruction secondary to rheumatic valvulitis is a very gradual process.

DEGENERATIVE CALCIFICATION OF THE TRICUSPID AORTIC VALVE (AORTIC STENOSIS OF THE ELDERLY)

Pomerance found that the three primary cardiac changes associated with aging were atheroma of the anterior mitral leaflet, calcification of the mitral annulus, and calcification of the aortic leaflets.[390] Approximately 5 percent of aortic tricuspid valves show some degree of calcification by age 55 with an added incidence of 1 percent per year up to 30 percent at age 85[391] (see Fig. 60B-25).

These degenerative valvular changes are those recognized by Monckeberg but are not due to atherosclerosis as he suggested. The early lesion of atherosclerosis includes fatty macrophages which are absent from the early stages of aortic valvular calcification. In the latter, the primary change is an alteration of connective tissue with extracellular droplets of neutral fat occurring within the collagen. This fatty material serves as a precursor for calcium deposition. The thickening and alteration of the valvular collagen begin at the bases of the cusps and extend toward the margins of the cusps as calcification develops. Usually the calcification is basal and entirely on the aortic side of the valve, the free margins remain mobile, and the commissures are not fused.[374,378,388,392] These changes are the same as those which occur earlier in many bicuspid valves. The basis for these changes is thought to be simple wear and tear, the connective tissue of the valve becoming traumatized by repetitive valve function. There is support for a traumatic basis in that the early fatty deposits within the collagenous tissue and secondary calcification have histologic counterparts in the supraspinatus tendon in cases of subdeltoid bursitis.[392]

A significant percentage of people develop a systolic murmur after age 60, and approximately 85 percent of these murmurs arise from the aortic valve.[393] Bruns and van der Hauwaert, in a study of 300 elderly patients, found that an aortic outflow murmur was audible in 37 percent between ages 50 and 59 and 69 percent at age 80 to 89.[394] Most of the aortic valves in these patients were not heavily calcified or stenotic, but the leaflets demonstrated a thickening and rigidity imparted by the precalcific and early calcific changes as described above. The clinical significance of this systolic murmur of the aged is discussed below under "Clinical Recognition."

Pathophysiology

The hemodynamic burden imposed by critical aortic stenosis (effective orifice area less than 0.7 cm²) is systolic ventricular overloading secondary to impedance to left ventricular emptying. The principal compensatory response to this elevated resistance to outflow is an increase in the contractile element mass by concentric ventricular hypertrophy. By distributing the increased pressure load over a larger number of contractile elements, the ventricle is able to maintain a normal stroke volume in the face of elevated tension. Unlike the case in the volume overload states, left ventricular dilatation is not a part of the compensatory mechanism in pressure overload lesions. The elevated left ventricular end-diastolic pressure commonly accompanying this increase in muscle mass reflects decreased compliance of the hypertrophied ventricle and not necessarily left ventricular failure.[395]

An important ancillary mechanism in the maintenance of cardiac output in severe aortic stenosis is the "atrial kick." Atrial contraction enhances left ventricular filling and produces an end-diastolic augmentation of pressure and fiber length which aids in left ventricular emptying through the Frank-Starling mechanism.[396] The importance of atrial contraction in aortic stenosis was clearly established by Stott et al. with the finding that 39 percent of the volume ejected during ventricular systole was contributed by the atrial stroke volume. In comparison, only 24 percent of the ventricular stroke volume in normal subjects was contributed by atrial contraction.[397] This augmentation of left ventricular performance is accomplished without undue elevation of mean left atrial pressure and its sequela, pulmonary edema.

The oxygen cost of this pressure work is high and may at times exceed the capacity of the oxygen delivery system (see "Angina Pectoris," below). If this discrepancy between oxygen supply and demand does not cause sudden death, the chronic pressure work will eventually lead to myocardial dysfunction. With impaired left ventricular performance, ventricular ejection is incomplete, and ventricular diastolic volume and pressure increase. The accompanying elevation of mean left atrial and pulmonary venous pressures are manifested by the symptoms of left ventricular failure.

Clinical recognition

HISTORY

The history is occasionally of value in determining the cause of aortic stenosis. If an aortic outflow murmur was present in the neonatal period and was heard consistently afterward, the cause is congenital valvular versus supravalvular stenosis or discrete subvalvular stenosis. The congenital valvular stenosis could reflect either a unicuspid or bicuspid valve with the former suggested by the early appearance (before age 30) of symptomatic aortic stenosis. The appearance of an aortic outflow murmur later in life (provided a competent observer previously failed to hear the murmur) suggests acquired valvular stenosis or idiopathic hypertrophic subaortic stenosis (IHSS). Coupling of the late appearance of the murmur with a history of rheumatic fever suggests both a rheumatic cause for the stenosis and accompanying anatomic changes in the mitral valve. These mitral valve changes may not be hemodynamically significant. On the other hand, severe clinically isolated aortic valvular stenosis with no history of rheumatic fever can be attributed to nonrheumatic disease with an accuracy approaching 90 percent. In turn, the very late appearance of a systolic murmur (after age 70) suggests degenerative calcification of either a bicuspid or, more likely, a tricuspid valve.

Unlike the case with mitral stenosis, the history in aortic stenosis cannot be relied upon to be the harbinger of significant disease. Symptoms appear later in the course of this condition; consequently, patients may have significant stenosis that remains unrecognized for years. During this asymptomatic period a small percentage (3 to 5 percent)[398,399] of the patients are subject to sudden death presumably on an arrhythmic basis (a figure that must be kept in mind when considering the advisability of surgery in a patient with severe but asymptomatic aortic stenosis). While physicians cannot rely upon symptoms to herald the onset of significant aortic stenosis, they can and must use the appearance of a triad of symptoms (angina pectoris, syncope, or symptoms of left ventricular failure) as indicators of critical (in both a hemodynamic and prognostic sense) obstruction. Mild aortic stenosis may be associated with quite severe symptoms in the presence of coronary artery disease, other cardiac lesions, or psychoneurosis; but in the absence of these conditions symptoms indicate hemodynamically significant stenosis. Furthermore, the appearance of any one of this triad of symptoms forecasts a life expectancy of less than 5 years[400] and a 15 to 20 percent incidence of sudden death.

Angina pectoris Angina pectoris is usually the initial and most common of the three symptoms with a reported incidence in symptomatic aortic stenosis of 50 to 70 percent.[370,401–405] The average life expectancy upon the appearance of this symptom is 5 years with a longer survival (10 to 20 years) noted in only 5 percent of the patients.[370]

While it has been suggested that the characteristics of the chest pain associated with aortic stenosis are not typical of angina pectoris,[402] this has not been the case in most studies[370,401,403–406] or in our experience. One slightly atypical feature of the chest pain of aortic stenosis alluded to in the past,[403] and occasionally noted in our clinical experience, is a delayed relation to exertion. The angina pectoris, in these few cases, developed immediately upon cessation of physical activity rather than during the activity. The typical character of the chest pain includes dramatic and quick relief with sublingual nitroglycerin. A higher incidence of nitroglycerin syncope in aortic stenosis as compared with coronary atherosclerotic heart disease, also previously alluded to, is not borne out in our experience or by a review of the literature.

Angina is generally considered to reflect a disparity between myocardial oxygen utilization and myocardial oxygen availability. Sarnoff et al. concluded that the primary determinant of myocardial oxygen utilization is the total tension developed by the myocardium, or the mean systolic pressure times the duration of systole.[407] In aortic stenosis, both the left

ventricular systolic mean pressure and the duration of systole are typically increased. Consequently, aortic stenosis must be accompanied by an increased myocardial oxygen requirement.[408] The appearance of angina would then reflect an inability of coronary blood flow to meet this demand. In approximately 50 percent of patients with aortic stenosis and angina pectoris, this inadequacy of myocardial oxygen availability is associated with significant coronary atherosclerotic disease.[108,401,404] Rarely the inadequate coronary blood flow may be due to calcific emboli from the aortic valve into a coronary artery[409] or, as in a single case report,[410] intermittent obstruction of a coronary ostium by a pedunculated calcific mass extending from the aortic valve. In the remainder of the patients (40 to 60 percent) there is no evidence of intrinsic disease of the coronary arteries to explain the inadequacy of coronary blood flow. This group of patients seems to have little or no reserve for increasing coronary flow to meet situations of augmented oxygen extraction.[401] Since these patients (those with angina without coronary atherosclerotic heart disease) tend to demonstrate the most severe stenosis,[404] it is conceivable that near-maximal (nonaugmentable) coronary blood flow exists in the basal state in patients with massive left ventricular hypertrophy.

Nitroglycerin is successful in alleviating the chest pain in these patients because it consistently decreases the total tension developed by the myocardium as reflected by the tension-time index. This reduction is due both to a fall in the left ventricular mean systolic pressure and a shortening of the duration of systole.[408] In addition, nitroglycerin reduces the end-diastolic and end-systolic dimensions of the left ventricle.[411] As predicted by the law of Laplace, this reduction in left ventricular dimension reduces transmural tension and, consequently, myocardial oxygen requirements.

Syncope The loss of consciousness characteristic of aortic stenosis either immediately follows exertion or interrupts it. This manifestation of aortic stenosis occurs much less often than angina pectoris, with a reported incidence of 15 to 30 percent of symptomatic patients.[370,398] In addition, the large majority of patients have previously manifested angina pectoris,[370,405] with a recurrent pattern of development of angina immediately preceding the loss of consciousness.

Another exertion-related symptom occasionally complained of by patients with aortic stenosis is variously described as "lightheadedness," "giddiness," or "going to faint." This symptom, generally referred to as *near-syncope,* is thought to portend the same poor prognosis as true syncope. The prognosis for survival of those patients manifesting either aberration of consciousness is usually 3 to 4 years.[398] Although there are reported incidences of patients manifesting recurrent episodes of syncope for 10 to 20 years,[109,398,405] these usually were instances of syncope as an isolated symptom in people with stenosis of questionable severity.[405]

The study of Flamm et al. suggests that effort syncope occurs in those patients who, at critical levels of exercise, develop left ventricular failure with an abrupt fall in cardiac output. The decline in cardiac output is accompanied by a marked decrease in arterial pressure because of an absence of an appropriate increase in systemic vascular resistance.[412] Schwartz et al. were able to divide the syncopal attacks into two distinct phases. The first phase, generally lasting 20 to 40 s and associated with a regular cardiac rhythm, was precipitated by a sudden drop in blood pressure. Pallor, absent heart sounds and murmur, loss of attention, and dizziness were the clinical manifestations of this stage.[413] It is interesting that Gallavardin in 1825 emphasized the extra feebleness of the ventricular contractions during syncope without stoppage of the heart. He attributed the syncope to an effort-related decrease in cardiac output and believed that an arrhythmia was only rarely responsible.[413] Schwartz et al. noted that arrhythmias developed only in the second stage of the syncopal attacks. This stage, occurring when the attack lasted longer than 40 s, was manifested by cyanosis, apnea or Cheyne-Stokes respirations, and occasionally convulsions.[413]

Left ventricular failure The significance of dyspnea varies among patients with aortic stenosis and seems dependent upon the age or, probably more importantly, the physical activity of the patient. In the younger, more active patients exertional dyspnea is an early symptom and is not associated with nocturnal dyspnea or cardiac enlargement.[405] While in the older, less active patients exertional dyspnea may be the first of the triad of symptoms to be manifest, it is usually associated with nocturnal dyspnea and has a much more sinister significance. The average survival with symptoms of left ventricular failure is 2 years.[398,405] While this average survival reflects the longer duration in younger patients and a much shorter course in older patients, it emphasizes the urgency of the situation in both groups.

Other symptoms Palpitation, particularly during exertion, is a significant complaint in some patients. Its appearance warrants careful evaluation to exclude mitral valve disease, coronary atherosclerotic heart disease, or left ventricular failure. Fatigue, particularly in children, may be the initial manifestation of this disease. Visual field defects, probably secondary to minute calcific emboli from the aortic valve, are an occasional occurrence with aortic stenosis.[405–409]

PHYSICAL EXAMINATION

Arterial pressure and pulse rate The pulse pressure in significant aortic stenosis is usually less than 50 mm Hg with an average of 30 to 40 mm Hg.[370,402]

This reduction in pulse pressure results primarily from a depression of the systolic pressure rather than elevation of the diastolic pressure. A systolic pressure over 200 mm Hg in significant aortic stenosis would be extremely unusual under any circumstances.[106,370,402] In the elderly, however, the systolic pressure may occasionally reach or exceed 180 mm Hg with a pulse pressure of 60 mm Hg or more.[414] Consequently, severity of the stenosis cannot be predicted from the amplitude of the pulse pressure alone.

The only noteworthy feature of the pulse rate is an occasional unexplained slow rate in association with significant aortic stenosis.[372]

Inspection The neck in the patient with valvular aortic stenosis is usually striking because of a complete absence of any visible arterial pulsations. Unless there are concomitant rigid atheromatous vessels or significant aortic regurgitation, visualization of carotid pulsations in the adult with critical valvular stenosis is unusual.[370–405]

Any visible abnormality of jugular venous pulsations should suggest coexisting mitral valve disease, as isolated aortic stenosis rarely causes pulmonary hypertension and tricuspid regurgitation. The single exception to this dictum is the presence of a prominent *a* wave. An increased amplitude of the jugular venous *a* wave is found most commonly in hypertrophic subaortic stenosis but occasionally in valvular or discrete subvalvular stenosis. It probably reflects reduced right ventricular compliance as a result of that chamber's sharing a common wall, the ventricular septum, with the hypertrophied left ventricle.[14,415,416]

Inspection of the chest should be directed toward confirming the presence of an atrial gallop by visualizing an atrial impulse, or toward delineating the thrust of a hypertrophied left ventricle. With the exception of young, thin-chest-walled patients, inspection of the chest is generally of little assistance.

Palpation Palpation of the carotid artery in aortic stenosis often reveals a pulsation of small amplitude, gradual upslope, and gradual downslope (pulsus parvus et tardus). The most characteristic and easiest feature to perceive is the slow rise of the pulsation. Assessment of this "rise time" is best accomplished by the simultaneous palpation of carotid pulsation and auscultation of the heart. In severe aortic stenosis, the peak of the carotid pulsation will occur late in systole, either immediately preceding or simultaneously with aortic closure. A complete absence of a carotid pulse contour and only systolic vibrations, or shudder, over the carotid artery may be perceived in the most severe cases of aortic stenosis. While the carotid pulsation will occasionally be the initial clue to aortic stenosis, it can also serve to obscure the diagnosis by being normal in patients with rigid atheromatous vessels or associated aortic regurgitation.

Indirect pulse tracings of the carotid artery often exhibit an anacrotic pulse. *Anacrotic* is an abbreviation of *anadicrotic* (twice beating on the upstroke). Through common use, it has come to mean a slow-rising pulse with a perceptible notch, hesitation, or shudder on the upstroke.[370] The more severe the stenosis, the earlier the notch tends to appear. The indirect tracings will also occasionally demonstrate vibrations termed *carotid shudder* at the height of the carotid pulse. However, these two features of indirect carotid tracing are not characteristic of the palpable carotid pulse.

Palpation of the chest will characteristically reveal a sustained, or "heaving," apical impulse. This prolonged outward movement persists up to or beyond the second heart sound. Simultaneous palpation and auscultation will allow this assessment. An increased amplitude of the apical impulse and displacement of the apex is not typically associated with aortic stenosis.[370,372,415] In addition to a heaving left ventricular impulse, there is often, but not invariably, a palpable presystolic pulsation.

A very important clue to the presence of significant aortic stenosis is palpation of a systolic thrill. Perception of the thrill is generally best in the second right intercostal space but occasionally is better over the manubrium or to the left of the sternum. The thrill may occasionally be palpated at the apex as well as the base and infrequently only at the apex.[403] Supravalvular aortic stenosis is suggested by a thrill that is disproportionately maximal below the right clavicle, while a thrill with maximum intensity along the left sternal border suggests hypertrophic subaortic stenosis.[416] Although a thrill is palpable in over three-fourths of the patients with significant aortic stenosis, it is not pathognomonic of critical stenosis, being frequently present in cases of combined stenosis and regurgitation in which the latter is dominant.[370]

Auscultation The four important auscultatory signs of aortic valve stenosis are the aortic ejection click, aortic ejection murmur, delayed aortic valve closure, and the aortic diastolic murmur.

The *aortic ejection sound* is discrete high-frequency vibrations occurring 0.04 to 0.08 s after the onset of the first sound.[370,417] The sound is of maximal amplitude at the apex but while less intense is usually also audible at the second right intercostal space. Since the click immediately precedes the systolic murmur, it will occasionally be distinct only in the axilla[417] or in the third right intercostal space[63] away from the areas of greatest intensity of the murmur. This sound occurs simultaneously with the systolic rise in the central aortic pulse and seems to originate from the aortic valve itself. While it is generally accepted that an ejection click is associated with mild stenosis, the sound is present because the valve is mobile, not because the stenosis is mild.[417] In children, severe aortic stenosis is almost universally accompanied by an ejection click, while in adults severe aortic stenosis is usually a consequence of leaflet calcification, and hence an ejection sound is heard in less than one-third.[370,417] The intensity of the ejection click generally is correlated closely with the intensity of the aortic component of the second sound (A_2). In those patients with a markedly reduced A_2 the ejection sound is usually absent, while all those with a normal A_2 have an ejection sound.

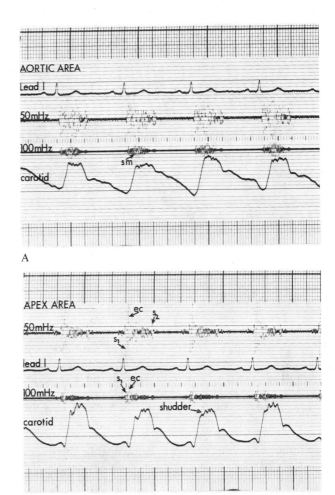

FIGURE 60B-26 Phonocardiogram recorded in a 33-year-old woman with congenital unicuspid aortic valve and transvalvular gradient of 95 mm Hg. *A.* Recorded at second right intercostal space and demonstrating spindle-shaped systolic murmur (SM). *B.* Recorded at apex and demonstrating loud ejection click in addition to murmur. Shudder on carotid pulse tracing is commonly recorded with severe aortic stenosis.

The presence of the ejection sound does localize the stenosis to the valve, as it is virtually always absent in supravalvular or subvalvular stenosis (Fig. 60B-26).

The most constant physical finding of aortic stenosis is a basal *systolic murmur*.[372] This typically harsh, grunting murmur is commonly loudest in the second right intercostal space with radiation into the carotids and to the apex. The intensity of the murmur at the apex is frequently equal to that at the base and, in some instances especially in the elderly, is greater at the apex.[372,403] The only invariable feature of this murmur is its diamond, spindle, or crescendo-decrescendo shape. The murmur begins a brief interval after the first sound (reflecting isometric contraction time), assumes its characteristic shape as a reflection of changing left ventricular ejection velocities, and ceases with protodiastole (onset of ventricular relaxation 0.20 to 0.04 s before closure of the

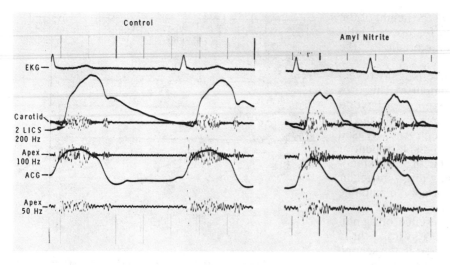

FIGURE 60B-27 Phonocardiogram from a patient with calcific aortic stenosis. Characteristic features include spindle-shaped systolic murmur at second left intercostal space (LICS) and apex delayed upstroke on carotid pulse training sustained impulse on apexcardiogram (ACG), and increase in intensity of murmur with amyl nitrite administration. Unlike the phonocardiogram in Fig. 60B-26, there is no ejection click.

aortic valve).[370,418,419] Although intensity, duration, and configuration of the murmur do not necessarily relate to the severity of the stenosis, some general conclusions can be drawn. The longer and louder the murmur and the later its systolic peak, the more likely the stenosis is severe. The shorter and softer the murmur and the earlier its systolic peak, the more likely the stenosis is mild.[415] This murmur may be misinterpreted as holosystolic if the aortic closure sound is inaudible or if, in the presence of reverse splitting, pulmonic closure is mistaken for aortic closure. In cases of doubt, augmentation of the murmur following administration of amyl nitrite or following an ectopic beat will point to an aortic outflow origin[420] (Fig. 60B-27).

A delay in aortic closure is the most common alteration of the *second sound* associated with significant aortic stenosis. This delayed closure is usually manifest (70 percent of cases) as a single second sound without inspiratory splitting.[370] In another significant proportion of the patients (perhaps as many as 25 percent), the delay will be even more marked, resulting in paradoxic splitting of the second sound.[109,370,405] While normal splitting is an uncommon occurrence with severe stenosis, such a finding cannot be used to exclude this diagnosis. As the aortic leaflets become calcified and immobile, the aortic component of the second sound (A_2) will also decrease in intensity.[367,403,405] Consequently the diminished A_2 would be a common feature of calcific aortic stenosis but would not be the case with congenital aortic stenosis. Like the changes in the ejection click, a decreasing intensity of second sound only indirectly and inconsistently reflects increasing stenosis while directly reflecting decreasing mobility of the leaflets.

One-third to one-half of the patients with essentially "pure" aortic valvular stenosis will have an early diastolic murmur audible at the base. Generally, this high-pitched decrescendo murmur reflects mild, insignificant valvular reflux as evidenced by a normal pulse pressure and absence of peripheral signs of aortic regurgitation.[367,370,403,409,421] Since this murmur may occur with discrete subvalvular stenosis but uncommonly with hypertrophic subaortic stenosis or supravalvular stenosis, its detection is good evidence that the stenosis is "fixed" and either valvular or subvalvular.

Physical examination in the elderly The evaluation of a systolic murmur in the elderly is frequently much more difficult than in younger age groups both with regard to determining the cause of the murmur and to assessing the severity of the lesion.

As discussed in the section on disease mechanisms, the aortic leaflets with degenerative sclerosis and calcification typically remain as separate (nonfused) units. Consequently, the ejection click is characteristically absent as the leaflets do not move abruptly as a single structure.[385] While the murmur may be the typical harsh, grunting, basal murmur of aortic stenosis, it will frequently masquerade as a pure-frequency, musical, cooing murmur, loudest at the apex.[393,414] The musical quality of the murmur is thought to arise from the nonfused but rigid aortic leaflets vibrating in the aortic root, while the reduced intensity of the murmur at the base is ascribed to altered thoracic dimension in the elderly and absence of the central high-velocity jet of blood associated with commissural fusion. Frequently the musical vibratory character of the murmur is so typical that (if recognized as such) an aortic valvular origin can be determined without hesitation. At other times the apical murmur is less typical, and the other primary cause of a systolic murmur in the elderly, mitral annulus calcification, must be considered.[422]

Even if the murmur is ascribed to an aortic valvular cause, significant aortic stenosis is not necessarily implied. The aortic leaflets might be rigid shelves of tissue protruding into the path of ejected blood and yet not offer significant obstruction to left ventricular outflow. Atrial sounds, which are useful in making this distinction in younger patients, are unreliable in this age group because of their essentially universal presence.[385,423] Moreover, the typical pulse contour of aortic stenosis is frequently "normalized" by the noncompliant vessels of the elderly. Even the classic symptoms of aortic stenosis (angina pectoris, syncope, and congestive heart failure) cannot be used as diagnostic of significant left ventricular obstruction, as they may be due to coronary atherosclerotic heart disease, cerebrovascular insufficiency, or one of the other conditions associated with old age. With the exception of the dictum that significant aortic stenosis can be excluded by a diastolic blood pressure consistently over 100,[63] we have found no reliable feature to distinguish the hemodynamically insignificant from the hemodynamically significant aortic systolic murmur in the elderly. If one of the classic symptoms of aortic stenosis is present, catheterization of the left side of the heart is necessary to make this critical distinction.[423]

ELECTROCARDIOGRAM

Sinus rhythm is the rule in isolated aortic valvular stenosis regardless of severity. With the exception of the elderly, atrial fibrillation suggests coexisting mitral valve disease. Although a normal P wave is the usual finding, a broad, deep terminal deflection of the P wave in V_1 is compatible with isolated aortic stenosis.[14] In fact, this single ECG feature, in the absence of another cause, would suggest severe stenosis.[424]

The sequential change in the QRS and T wave reflect the course and severity of aortic stenosis better than any single parameter obtained by noninvasive methods. In general, a perfectly normal ECG suggests that the obstruction is trivial.[370] Exceptions to this rule do occur, however, particularly in the child and young adult.[14,416] With moderate aortic stenosis, the ECG may be normal and have prominent QRS voltage alone or in combination with minimal ST and T wave changes. The typical ECG of severe aortic stenosis (in at least 90 percent of cases)[370,405,425] is characterized by increased voltage of the S waves in the right precordial leads and of the R waves in the left precordial leads. This pattern is accompanied by depression of the ST segment and deep inversion of the T waves in the leads with the most prominent R waves. This ECG pattern is commonly referred to as a *systolic overload* or a *left ventricular strain* pattern (Fig. 60B-28). In aortic stenosis, this pattern is typically associated with a normal, and even slightly vertical, QRS axis. With advancing age or increasing aortic regurgitation, the QRS axis will shift increasingly leftward. Vectorial interpretation of this ECG pattern would be a QRS vector of increased magnitude and normal, but slightly vertical, direction associated with a T wave vector of increased magnitude and directed at least 110° away from the QRS vector. The higher the gradient across the aortic valve, the more likely this systolic overload pattern is to be present.[413,426] In evaluating the ECG, consideration must be given to the limitations imposed by body build, age and age-related conditions, and the use of digitalis.

In addition to being a fairly reliable reflection of the presence and degree of hypertrophy, the ECG

FIGURE 60B-28 ECG from 65-year-old woman with 110 mm Hg gradient across the aortic valve. Prominent QRS voltage with associated ST depression and T wave inversion is typical for severe aortic stenosis. Left axis is not characteristic of aortic stenosis except in the elderly or with associated significant aortic regurgitation.

changes carry some prognostic significance. In approximately 70 percent of cases of sudden death there was left ventricular hypertrophy with "strain" indicated on the ECG, while in only 9 percent the patients had a normal ECG.[413] Progressive changes of left ventricular hypertrophy demonstrated on serial tracings indicate progression of the disease.

Conduction defects are not uncommon in aortic stenosis, first-degree atrioventricular block and left bundle branch block being the most frequently noted (incidence of each 5 to 14 percent).[370,372,414,425] Complete heart block is an infrequent but recognized finding associated with aortic stenosis.[370,372] Many of these conduction problems may be explained by the contiguous relationship of the specialized conducting fibers and the aortic annulus within the central fibrous body.

ROENTGENOGRAPHIC FINDINGS

In aortic stenosis, the heart is usually not enlarged.[367,405,416,427] In spite of this lack of enlargement, the cardiac silhouette has an abnormal configuration secondary to the concentric hypertrophy of the left ventricle. This concentric hypertrophy is manifested on chest roentgenogram by a convex bulging of the lower one-third of the left cardiac border.[405,427] Consequently, the most lateral point of the left border of the heart lies at a higher level above the diaphragm than in normal hearts. Elongation of the apex reflects left ventricular dilatation and is not a feature of aortic stenosis unless left ventricular failure has developed.[427] The other alteration in structural configuration commonly noted with aortic stenosis is dilatation of the ascending aorta. While this poststenotic dilatation is a common feature of aortic stenosis (75 to 85 percent),[370,405,427] the degree of dilatation does not reflect the severity of the stenosis. The poststenotic dilatation usually terminates at the brachiocephalic artery, and the aortic knob is normal or only minimally enlarged. This lack of significant enlargement of the aortic knob is useful in differentiating poststenotic dilatation from aortic ectasia seen in elderly patients[427] (Fig. 60B-29).

The final important roentgenographic manifesta-

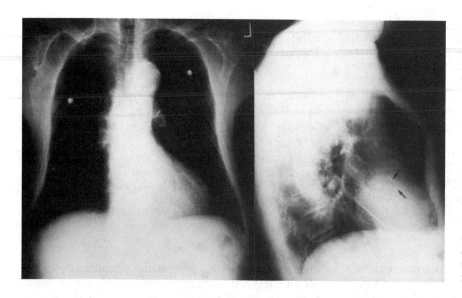

FIGURE 60B-29 Posteroanterior and lateral chest roentgenogram of a 62-year-old man with severe aortic stenosis. Typical features include convex bulging of lower one-third of left cardiac border, dilatation of ascending aorta, and calcified aortic valve (see arrows on lateral film).

tion of aortic stenosis is aortic valvular calcification, the presence of which should never be excluded without the use of fluoroscopy. In the left anterior oblique view, the aortic valvular calcification would be visualized in the upper one-half of the middle one-third of the heart. The posteroanterior view is seldom useful, since the aortic valve is superimposed on the spine. With only occasional exceptions, the absence of fluoroscopically visible calcification of the aortic valve in a patient over 40 years of age indicates that the stenosis is mild or not at the valve level.[405,416,427] The exceptions are usually women with coexisting mitral valve disease.[416]

The left atrium is frequently minimally enlarged in isolated valvular stenosis, but significant enlargement suggests mitral valve disease or hypertrophic subaortic stenosis.[416,427] In the absence of these two conditions, significant left atrial enlargement would suggest severe aortic stenosis.[407,428]

ECHOCARDIOGRAPHY

The three alterations in leaflet structure and function (thickening, calcification, and decreased mobility) characteristic of all types of acquired aortic stenosis may be reflected on the echocardiogram. The thickening of the leaflets would be manifest as absence of the fine vibratory motion on the leaflet echoes during systole.[116] Calcification of the leaflets is characterized by replacement of the one to three slender, delicate diastolic echoes of the normal leaflets with multiple dense echoes. These echoes have an intensity greater than the aortic wall echoes and occasionally persist uninterrupted through systole.[429] Decreased mobility is reflected by failure of the echo of either leaflet to open to the periphery of the aortic root during systole.[430] In our experience, the presence of all three of these findings in combination is diagnostic of significant calcific aortic stenosis (Fig. 60B-30). The absence of these findings, however, does not exclude severe aortic stenosis, as the congenitally domed valve may present with a normal

aortic valve echocardiogram (Fig. 60B-31). This echocardiographic appearance is explained by upward displacement of the domed orifice (Fig. 60B-32) out of reach of the ultrasound beam with the echo signals at the periphery of the root arising from the wide base of the dome.[431] Any echocardiographic evaluation should include left ventricular dimensions along with septal and wall thickness. These measurements will help to eliminate any misconception arising from the aortic root echoes. For example, a patient with the three echocardiographic features of calcific aortic stenosis but normal width to the septum and left ventricular posterior wall could not conceivably have severe aortic stenosis. Similarly, a patient with normal aortic valve echoes but a thick-

FIGURE 60B-30 Echocardiogram of a patient with calcific aortic stenosis demonstrating multiple linear echoes within the aortic root with a density greater than the anterior aortic wall (AAW) or posterior aortic wall (PAW) and decreased mobility of aortic leaflets in systole.

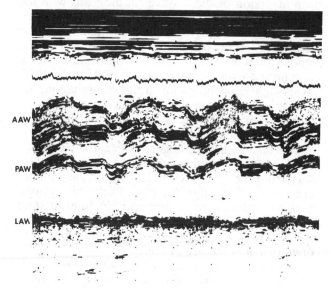

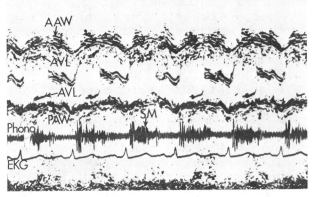

FIGURE 60B-31 Echocardiogram of a 33-year-old woman with unicuspid aortic valve with a 95 mm Hg transvalvular gradient. Significant feature is the location of the aortic valve leaflets (AVL) near the periphery of the aortic root during systole. The only suggestion of aortic valve abnormality is absence of fine fluttering in systole and increased density of aortic leaflet echoes in diastole. AAW, anterior aortic wall; PAW, posterior aortic wall; SM, systolic murmur. Compare echo with aortic root angiogram in Fig. 60B-32.

ened septum and left ventricular posterior wall must be considered to have some impedance to left ventricular outflow.

Echocardiography is also occasionally instrumental in diagnosing a bicuspid aortic valve. The feature common to many bicuspid valves that can be captured by ultrasound is the asymmetry of the two leaflets. This asymmetry is reflected by an eccentric diastolic position within the aortic root of the echoes of the closed leaflets. Measurements of the "eccentricity index" of the closed aortic valve leaflets is made at the onset of diastole. The eccentricity index is calculated as follows:

$$\text{E.I.} = \frac{\frac{1}{2}\text{ width of aortic lumen}}{\text{minimum distance of cusp echo to nearest aortic margin}}$$

FIGURE 60B-32 Supravalvular aortogram (60° LAO projection) in a 33-year-old woman with unicuspid noncommissural aortic valve. (Compare with echocardiogram in Fig. 60B-31.) Arrows indicate doming of aortic valve during systole.

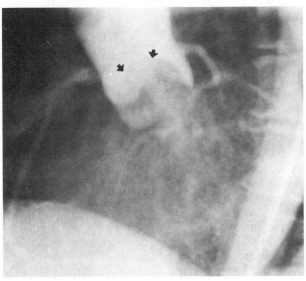

Depending on the study of reference, an index of 1.3[432] or 1.5[433] is diagnostic of a bicuspid valve. We have found that a tricuspid aortic valve with one abnormally small cusp can give a similar echocardiographic picture but otherwise suspect the diagnostic reliability of this eccentricity index is good.

CARDIAC CATHETERIZATION

Cardiac catheterization is indicated upon the development of angina pectoris, syncope or presyncope, or left ventricular dysfunction (exertional dyspnea, orthopnea, or paroxysmal nocturnal dyspnea) in the patient with aortic stenosis. The catheterization should be directed toward determining the gradient across the aortic valve and toward excluding other explanations (i.e., coronary atherosclerosis, mitral stenosis) for the complaints in question. There are pros and cons for either the retrograde catheterization across the stenotic valve or the transseptal approach, and the particular technique utilized must depend on the expertise and experience of the catheterization team. We do believe at least a brief attempt at the retrograde approach is appropriate before embarking on transseptal catheterization.

As demonstrated by Wiggers,[434] hemodynamically significant aortic stenosis implies a reduction of the aortic orifice to one-quarter its normal size. Since the normal aortic valve orifice area is approximately 3 cm², significant stenosis implies an orifice area of less than 0.75 cm² and, in association with a normal cardiac output, a mean systolic gradient of greater than 50 mm Hg.[370,435] Since the peak-to-peak systolic gradient usually closely approximates the mean systolic gradient, many laboratories,[436] including our own, use the peak-to-peak systolic gradient in determining the severity of stenosis. While a 50 mm Hg or greater transvalvular gradient implies critical stenosis, gradients of less than this may also reflect significant stenosis if associated with a reduced cardiac output. Consequently, in patients with gradients of less than 50 mm Hg the effective orifice area must be calculated in order to avoid underestimating significant stenosis.

The cardiac catheterization in cases of aortic stenosis generally includes left ventricular angiography. This maneuver is usually justified with the declaration that it is necessary to document the functional status of the left ventricle. The limited data available,[437] however, suggest that the parameters of left ventricular function are not as good as the functional status of the patient in predicting the operative results. Moreover, we would be reluctant to refuse aortic valve replacement to a patient with aortic stenosis because of discovery of left ventricular dysfunction on angiography. Perhaps a more important measurement to be gleaned from this study would be measurement of left ventricular muscle mass, but this has not been adequately investigated. Certainly, in congenital aortic stenosis left ventricular angiography is important in establishing the site of obstructon.

Despite early evidence to the contrary, there are now sufficient data[401,414,438] to refute the view that aortic stenosis serves a protective role for the coronary vasculature. Although the chances of a patient with severe aortic stenosis and no angina pectoris having significant coronary atherosclerosis are small,[438] we think the minimal risk of coronary angiography at our institution justifies our performing this study as part of a preoperative evaluation in any patient over age 45 years.

Management

Appropriate medical management of the patient with aortic stenosis should be based upon the recognition that this particular condition is unstable both in terms of its severity and its clinical course. In the adult, the severity of the stenosis is clearly intensified by the gradual deposition of calcium on the aortic leaflets; but even in children devoid of calcium, serial hemodynamic evaluations may reveal significant increases in the transvalvular gradient.[439] Accordingly, physicians must realize that their initial clinical assessment of the severity of the stenosis may require later modifications and plan for appropriate reexaminations. Moreover, in the setting of fixed severe stenosis, the adaptive responses will eventually fail to maintain adequate blood flow to the myocardial or peripheral tissues, following which the clinical course will pass from the asymptomatic to the symptomatic phase.

An awareness of the grave prognosis[400] (a rapidly progressive downhill course not responsive to medical therapy) attached to symptomatic aortic stenosis and the encouraging improvement in the immediate outlook afforded by valve replacement[214,398] makes recognition of symptoms in these patients imperative. The importance of immediate recognition of symptomatology is stressed by the 15 to 20 percent incidence of sudden death associated with symptomatic aortic stenosis[398] and the greater operative mortality accompanying the higher functional classes.[437]

A careful history will usually suffice as an adequate evaluation of a patient's functional status. In the patient who presents with clinically severe but apparently asymptomatic aortic stenosis, however, exercise electrocardiography may be a useful adjunct in making this assessment. While the wisdom of exercise electrocardiography in a patient with aortic stenosis has been questioned, we believe an exercise test monitored by the physician is a sound clinical method for determining a patient's functional classification. In spite of this provocative testing, some patients remain a therapeutic dilemma because of a questionable relation between their symptoms and the presence of severe aortic stenosis. In these patients, we would err in the direction of ascribing their symptomatology (angina-like chest pain, dyspnea, syncope, near-syncope) to the left ventricular outflow obstruction and proceed with valve replacement. If preoperative coronary angiography reveals a significant coronary artery obstruction in addition to a critically stenotic valve, we would recommend combined valve replacement and coronary artery bypass although either lesion in isolation may be the source of the patient's symptom.

The question of valve replacement in patients with severe but asymptomatic aortic stenosis remains unresolved. Proponents of this course of action emphasize the threat of sudden death.[440] While this possibility exists, the likelihood of sudden death is small (3 to 5 percent)[398] in asymptomatic patients. In children, however, the incidence is higher (range = 1 to 18 percent; average = 7.5 percent).[398] This increased incidence of sudden death in combination with the opportunity to reduce the obstruction by valvotomy convinces us that aortic valve surgery is indicated in children and young adults with severe stenosis regardless of the presence or absence of symptoms. On the other hand, we would apply the same operative criteria to those members of these age groups who preoperatively were recognized to require valve replacement (calcific valve, unicuspid valve) as we do to older age groups.

During the asymptomatic phase of their illness, we would interdict very strenuous exertion in patients with severe stenosis but would otherwise allow an active life-style. We do recommend bacterial endocarditis prophylaxis for all patients with stenotic valves including those with potentially (bicuspid) stenotic valves, but we do not suggest rheumatic fever prophylaxis in the absence of multivalvular disease or a history of rheumatic fever. We would prescribe nitroglycerin for the relief of angina but have little enthusiasm for the use of digitalis in patients with early symptoms of left ventricular failure. Digitalis seems to offer little benefit in obstructive valve disease and, in addition, renders the ECG less reliable as a diagnostic parameter of the severity of aortic stenosis. We would favor digitalis and diuretics prior to surgery in patients with advanced congestive heart failure or in patients with these symptoms who refuse surgery. The use of diuretics in these patients must be tempered by the realization that optimal left ventricular function may require an elevated left ventricular filling pressure.

AORTIC REGURGITATION

In 1832 Dominic Corrigan[441] wrote:

> The danger of the disease is in proportion to the quantity of blood that regurgitates, and the quantity that regurgitates will be large in proportion to the degree of inadequacy to the valves, and to the length of pause between the contractions of the ventricle during which the blood can be pouring back.

Although the valvular lesions of aortic regurgitation were first described in 1705 by Cowper, the classic clinical pathologic correlation of this condition was originally presented by Corrigan in 1832. Subsequently the myriad of physical findings accompanying this disease were individually noted and recorded by various physicians whose deeds were marked for posterity with eponyms. In a therapeutic sense, the greatest impact of this disease came in 1952 when the first prosthetic valve was implanted for amelioration of this particular condition.

Etiology

In recent years the etiology of aortic regurgitation has changed its clinical pattern. In the older literature virtually every occurrence of this condition was attributed to either rheumatic or syphilitic involvement. For example, Segal et al. in their 1956 review ascribed 83 percent of the cases of aortic regurgitation to rheumatic fever.[442] In a subsequent clinical analysis from the same institution a rheumatic cause was evident in only 54 percent,[443] and recent studies from other institutions have recorded an incidence of 39 percent (1971)[381] and 33 percent (1972)[444] (Table 60B-4). Although an even lower occurrence rate has been suggested,[445] the experience at Emory University Hospital seems to confirm that approximately one-third of the patients with clinically isolated aortic regurgitation have a rheumatic cause (Table 60B-4). In a similar fashion, the incidence of aortic regurgitation secondary to syphilis has decreased considerably during recent decades. Between 12 and 19 percent of the cases of aortic regurgitation in earlier reports were ascribed to syphilitic aortitis,[381,442] while current data indicate that syphilis accounts for no more than 2.5 to 7.0 percent[381,443,444] (Table 60B-4). With this decline in the incidence of these two diseases, the etiologic factors in aortic regurgitation have been more diversified.

Only recently, ankylosing spondylitis (Schilder et al., 1956)[446] and myxomatous degeneration of the aortic leaflets (Read et al., 1965)[447] have become recognized as specific causes of aortic regurgitation. Other conditions accepted as infrequent causes of significant aortic regurgitation include trauma, osteogenesis imperfecta, rheumatoid arthritis, Reiter's syndrome, Ehlers-Danlos syndrome, dissection of the aorta, Hurler's syndrome, and ventricular septal defect.

In addition to these entities, there are other, more common conditions which occasionally produce audible but rarely, if ever, hemodynamically significant aortic regurgitation. An early diastolic murmur in patients with severe anemia, without pathologic evidence of valvular heart disease, coupled with the disappearance of the murmur upon correcting the

anemia, was repeatedly documented in the older literature. The infrequency of such a murmur was also clearly established.[30,448] A faint, high-pitched, basal diastolic murmur has also been reported in hypertensive patients, one large study noting a 6 percent incidence in those with a diastolic blood pressure above 110 mm Hg.[449] The mechanism of this insignificant regurgitant lesion is probably dilatation of the aortic annulus.[450] A similar basilar diastolic murmur has been described in the pregnant female free of heart disease;[451] but a great deal of skepticism, including our own, remains as to the existence of such an association.

Disease mechanisms

RHEUMATIC

The mechanism by which the aortic valve is deformed with rheumatic valvulitis is discussed in Chap. 58, Pathology of Rheumatic Fever and Chronic Valvular Disease. In brief, the initial process is a thickening of the valve leaflets by edema and inflammatory cell infiltrates. The inflammatory exudate gradually becomes organized, resulting in scarring and further thickening of the leaflets. The leaflets shorten as the scar tissue contracts. The shortening is most marked in the central portion of each leaflet, resulting in a valve with a triangular defect at the center of the orifice.[386]

This particular disease process is characterized by a latent period of 7 to 10 years[442,452] between the occurrence of acute rheumatic fever and the development of "free" aortic regurgitation. ("Free" implies aortic regurgitation with definite peripheral signs of disease, such as wide pulse pressure, low diastolic pressure, and bounding peripheral pulses.) It would not be unusual for the diastolic murmur of aortic regurgitation to be first noted with the onset of rheumatic fever and to be audible throughout this latent period. Following the latent period is another 7 to 10 years before symptoms first appear.[442,452] Consequently, the majority of patients with rheumatic aortic regurgitation become symptomatic between ages 21 and 50 years.[381,442] An infrequent exception to the pattern of a prolonged latent period is the devel-

TABLE 60B-4
Most common causes of aortic regurgitation*

| Cause | Percentage incidence | | | | | |
	Rotman et al.[381]	Stapleton and Harvey[443]	Engloff[444]	Roberts[445]	Emory Univ.†	Average
Rheumatic	39	54	33	6?	42	34
Bacterial endocarditis	17	...	14	26	17	19
Cystic medial necrosis, myxomatous degeneration	8	...	3	15	25	13
Syphilitic	7	2	4	26	8	9
Ankylosing spondylitis	...	...	4	15	0	6

*Based on studies since 1969.
†Based on author's review of 2 years (1974–1976) experience at Emory University Hospital.

opment of "free" aortic regurgitation several months after an episode of rheumatic fever.[442]

SYPHILITIC

The disease mechanism of syphilitic aortitis and aortic insufficiency is discussed in detail in Chap. 85, Syphilitic Cardiovascular Disease. Basically, in syphilis the valvular changes are secondary to the primary changes in the aortic wall. Dilatation of the aortic annulus results in separation of the aortic valve commissures and prevents adequate coaptation of the leaflets at the center of the orifice. Subsequent intrinsic changes in the leaflets, such as rolling of the free edges, probably are secondary to the mechanical effects of stretching of the leaflets.[386]

In syphilis, significant aortic regurgitation usually develops between ages 35 and 50, some 15 to 25 years after initial infection. The subsequent course of the disease is thought to be more rapidly downhill than in rheumatic valvulitis.[442]

BACTERIAL ENDOCARDITIS

This condition is characterized by the deposition of bacterial vegetations and thrombus formation on the ventricular surface of the aortic valve. These friable vegetations are usually implanted on valves previously deformed by such processes as rheumatic valvulitis, myxomatous degeneration, valvular sclerosis, and syphilis. Distortion of the valve surface and endocardial injury seem to be important precursors to the development of platelet-fibrin thrombi in which bacteia are embedded.[453]

The mechanism by which this process increases aortic valvular incompetence can be either related directly to the destructive effect of the basic lesion, with rupture or perforation of the cusp, or contracture of the cusps during the process of healing.[454] The clinical course with valvular rupture or perforation, unless interrupted by valve replacement, is typically a rapid deterioration in cardiac status ending in death. Contractures of the cusps usually explain those cases characterized by slowly progressive congestive heart failure following an antibiotic cure of bacterial endocarditis. (For a more complete discussion see Chap. 77.)

MYXOMATOUS TRANSFORMATION OF THE AORTIC VALVE (FLOPPY VALVE, OR READ'S SYNDROME)

Although other investigators had previously noted aortic leaflets with the structural and histologic characteristics of this particular deformity, Read et al., in 1956, first categorized this connective tissue disorder as a distinct entity.[447] Myxomatous transformation consists of varying degrees of hyalinization, disruption, and loss of normal connective tissue architecture accompanied by an increase in ground substance, and in some cases, fibrosis.[447] This transformation may result in aortic valve incompetence in one of the following ways: (1) production of a floppy or weakened valve by a reduction of intrinsic rigidity resulting in stretching, rolling, wrinkling, inversion, and prolapse; (2) an actual loss of valve substance resulting in a defect in the leaflet; and (3) superimposed infection.[447,455]

This condition seems to be a progressive disorder of valvular tissue involving the mitral as well as the aortic valve. The aortic valvular incompetence occurs primarily in men and usually becomes manifest in the third to sixth decade of life, although the process may be hastened by development of bacterial endocarditis or by severe chest trauma. Cystic medial necrosis of the aorta has been found in all patients evaluated and some external stigmata of Marfan's syndrome in most.[447]

This condition appears to represent a forme fruste of Marfan's syndrome and is discussed as such under "Inherited Disorders of Connective Tissue and Valve Disease," as are the aortic valve changes associated with Marfan's syndrome.

ANKYLOSING SPONDYLITIS

The cardiovascular lesions in ankylosing spondylitis are limited primarily to the area immediately above and below the aortic valve. The aortic wall behind the sinuses of Valsalva is thickened by dense adventitial scarring which is relatively acellular except for perivascular infiltration around the partially obliterated vasa vasorum. Focal scarring and patchy degeneration of elastic fibers are found in the media of the involved segments. Proliferating fibrous tissue thickens the overlying intima but to a lesser degree than the adventitia.[298,456,457] With a few exceptions, these pathologic changes are identical to those of syphilis. In contrast to syphilis, the aortic wall changes in ankylosing spondylitis seldom extend more than a centimeter above the sinotubular junction. Secondly, only the distal margins of the aortic cusps are thickened in syphilis, while the basal portions of the cusps are thickened in ankylosing spondylitis. Finally, and most distinctively, in ankylosing spondylitis the dense adventitial scarring extends into the endocardium in the immediate subaortic region. This subaortic extension involves the base of the anterior mitral leaflet and the upper portion of the ventricular septum.[298,456,457]

Aortic regurgitation seems to be a consequence of a combination of thickening and shortening of the cusps, displacement of the cusps caudally by the mass of fibrous tissue behind the commissures, and dilatation of the aortic root.[457] Mitral regurgitation, usually infrequent and insignificant, results from dilatation of the left ventricle with resulting malalignment of the papillary muscles and fibrous thickening of the basal portion of the anterior mitral leaflet.[457] Rarely will the subaortic fibrosing process involve the entire anterior mitral leaflet and produce more severe mitral regurgitation.[456] The frequent conduction defects associated with this process are a consequence of the extension of the fibrous tissue into the muscular septum and destruction of the conduction fibers in the bundle of His and proximal bundle branches.[298,457]

While the aortic leaflets are anatomically involved in as many as 20 percent of patients with ankylosing spondylitis, clinical aortic regurgitation and/or heart block is present in only about 3 percent.[298,458] Symptoms of arthritis usually antedate the cardiac disease by 10 to 20 years with the frequency of aortic regurgitation directly related to the duration of arthritis. Occasionally the cardiac murmur appears within 1 to 2 years of onset of the arthritis,[298,457] and cardiac dysfunction may be manifest before signs of spondylitis are apparent.[457] Conduction defects, most commonly first-degree atrioventricular block but occasionally bundle branch block and complete atrioventricular block, are commonly associated with the valvular involvement.[298,459] The average life-span of patients with ankylosing spondylitis unassociated with aortic regurgitation is normal, while the life-span of those associated with severe aortic regurgitation averages about 45 years.[457]

Approximately 5 percent of the patients with *Reiter's syndrome* will develop aortic regurgitation. These patients typically manifest the most severe form of the syndrome with recurrent and prolonged disease and a high incidence of sacroiliac inflammation, iritis, and mucocutaneous manifestations.[460] The valvular involvement generally becomes manifest after some 15 years of disease and is frequently preceded by evidence of a conduction defect. While development of first-degree atrioventricular block may be considered early evidence of cardiac involvement, it does not necessarily forecast impending aortic regurgitation, since transient conduction defects have been reported.[460] The aortic regurgitation develops as a result of pathologic changes in the aortic root identical to those of ankylosing spondylitis.[460,461]

In *rheumatoid arthritis,* nodules identical to the subcutaneous nodules occur in the pericardium, myocardium, or endocardium in 1 to 3 percent of the cases.[462] The order of incidence of cardiac valvular involvement is mitral, aortic, tricuspid, and pulmonary. Usually the valvular lesions are focal and do not interfere with valve function, but occasionally with more diffuse involvement a regurgitant lesion is produced. The rheumatoid nodule begins as a reaction within the central portion of the valve leaflet, preserving the peripheral portions, in contrast to rheumatic valvular disease, which involves the entire leaflet.[462]

OSTEOGENESIS IMPERFECTA

Osteogenesis imperfecta belongs to that group of diseases classified as generalized heritable disorders of connective tissue. Other members of the group include Marfan's syndrome, Ehlers-Danlos syndrome, Hurler's syndrome, and pseudoxanthoma elasticum. The fundamental development defect in osteogenesis imperfecta is a failure of maturation of collagen beyond the reticulin fibril stage. The abnormalities in the skeleton (brittle, porotic bones), sclerae (blue), and ligament structures (hyperextensibility of joints) associated with this disease suggest that the defect in connective tissue is generalized. This defect in collagen tissue is thought to account for the aneurysmal dilatation of the aortic root which, in turn, accounts for the aortic regurgitation. Patients with the severe form of osteogenesis imperfecta (osteogenesis imperfecta congenita) succumb to bone injuries in early life prior to developing cardiovascular abnormalities. The aortic regurgitation tends to occur in the fifth and sixth decade in those patients with the milder form of the disease (osteogenesis imperfecta tarda).[463,464]

Pathophysiology

In aortic regurgitation, volume overload of the left ventricle is the basic hemodynamic abnormality. The magnitude of this volume overload is dependent upon the volume of the regurgitant blood flow, which, in turn, is determined by the area of the regurgitant orifice, the diastolic pressure gradient between the aorta and left ventricle, and the duration of diastole.[465]

Although the most critical determinant of the severity of reflux is the size of the regurgitant orifice, the absence of a direct relation between the regurgitant orifice area and the regurgitant flow points to the role of other physiologic factors. Perhaps the most striking feature with regard to the size of the regurgitant orifice is that extremely small orifices (0.13 to 0.44 cm^2/m^2) may allow profound regurgitation (63 to 75 percent of total forward stroke volume).[466] This profound reflux across these extremely small openings is made possible by the large diastolic pressure gradient between the aorta and left ventricle. The significant role played by this pressure gradient can be substantiated by inhalation of amyl nitrite. Peripheral vasodilatation and a decrease in total peripheral resistance with an ensuing facilitation of left ventricular ejection and reduction in the regurgitant volume result from this maneuver.[444] A decreased diastolic murmur is the clinical manifestation of this diminution in regurgitant flow. The reduction in regurgitation in association with decreased peripheral resistance is one of the factors in accounting for the surprising exercise capacity of some patients with aortic regurgitation.

The exact role of the other physiologic determinant of regurgitation, the duration of diastole, is controversial. The concept that the quantity of regurgitant flow is related to the length of the diastolic pause was first expounded by Corrigan in 1832 and has been propagated to the present time. Support for this concept came through studies such as those of Warner and Toronto, who found by a dye dilution method that the regurgitant flow per stroke was greater at slower heart rates.[467] The contrary opinion originated with Wiggers, who, from an analysis of canine aortic and left ventricular pressure curves, predicted that an increase in heart rate would have only minimal effect on the regurgitant volume. His prediction was based on recognition that increased heart rates eliminated only the last part of diastole, during which the regurgitant flow is least.[468] Confirmation of this prediction has been found in anesthetized patients by means of an electromagnet flowmeter and in catheterized patients by a combination of the Fick and angiographic methods of determining cardiac outputs.[469] Discovery in the latter study of a tachycardia-induced decrease in end-diastolic circumferential stress and end-diastolic load predicated upon a reduction in end-diastolic volume and pressure did suggest, however, a beneficial effect of increased heart rates. It must also be recognized that these studies based on pacemaker-induced tachycardia do not disprove the clinical observation that patients with aortic regurgitation tolerate exercise relatively well and conversely may develop pulmonary congestion at rest. With exercise, in addition to whatever benefit there is to increased heart rate, there are positive inotropic influences acting to increase stroke volume and a reduction in vascular resistance facilitating peripheral runoff of blood.[444]

The compensatory response of the left ventricle (as discussed in greater detail in Chap. 59, Altered Cardiovascular Function of Rheumatic Heart Disease and Other Acquired Valvular Disease) is dilatation and development of eccentric hypertrophy. Dilatation allows the left ventricle to maintain the large volume load by utilizing the Frank-Starling mechanism. The increased end-diastolic volume is accompanied by an increased stroke volume but not by a more complete emptying of the ventricle. Therefore, the ejection of the additional volume load is achieved by an increase in end-diastolic volume and not by increase in the proportion of end-diastolic volume ejected.[470] This left ventricular dilatation may occur without an increase in left ventricular end-diastolic pressure.[471] The explanation for this increased myocardial compliance remains undefined and the time course of these changes undetermined. The mechanism may be related to the phenomenon of stress relaxation[472] and be due to "slippage" of myocardial fibers or possibly myocardial filament disengagement.[473] In time, however, the hemodynamic burden imposed by volume overloading will result in depressed myocardial contractility and decreased compliance.[471] Once the myocardial function becomes impaired, there is a further increase in the end-diastolic volume without an additional increase in stroke volume.[470] The incomplete systolic ejection may, in turn, contribute further to the diastolic volume load.

An interesting circulatory phenomenon associated with chronic aortic regurgitation is peripheral vasodilatation. This phenomenon, though unexplained, accounts for the warm, flushed appearance of these patients and, in part, for the low diastolic blood pressure. With the development of myocardial failure, however, the augmented sympathetic vasoconstrictor tone in combination with an increase in intrinsic vascular stiffness results in peripheral vasoconstriction and, ultimately, in decreased cardiac output.

In sudden, severe aortic insufficiency the left ventricle is unprepared, possibly due to lack of stress relaxation, for the severe diastolic overload. As a consequence, there is increased resistance to diastolic filling, and markedly elevated end-diastolic left ventricular pressures develop. While these elevated pressures must be supported by increased left atrial and pulmonary venous pressures, a markedly elevated left ventricular diastolic pressure may serve some protective role. If the left ventricular pressure prematurely exceeds left atrial pressure, the mitral valve closure occurs early, protecting the lungs from high end-diastolic pressures. Furthermore, if the ventricular diastolic pressure rises to the level of the aortic pressure, the degree of aortic regurgitation is limited.[474] In a clinical setting, these so-called protective roles of excessive end-diastolic pressures are incapable of preventing the development of left atrial and pulmonary venous pressures sufficient to produce pulmonary edema.

Clinical recognition

HISTORY

Aortic regurgitation that develops *chronically and progressively* is generally characterized by a prolonged course with little disability for many years. The progress of the disease and disability is particularly slow if the aortic insufficiency is of slight or moderate hemodynamic significance at the time of its discovery. The 10-year mortality for this particular subset from the time of diagnosis is 5 to 16 percent, which is little different from that of the normal population.[452] We would take issue, however, with the idea that young patients with mild to moderate aortic regurgitation have a normal life expectancy. While this may frequently be the case, our reservations about the generalized applicability of such a statement are based on the following: (1) The available data demonstrating an uneventful course in such patients are based on 10-year follow-ups,[452,462] (2) all major causes of aortic regurgitation have the propensity for progressive valvular damage, and (3) all these patients are candidates for bacterial endocarditis. Cautious optimism would appear to be the attitude to adopt in advising these patients about their future.

Palpitations Those patients with severe aortic regurgitation will begin to experience symptoms a decade or more after recognition of their disease.[14] The onset of disability is usually insidious. In the more astute patients, the earliest symptoms are related to an awareness of the increased force of cardiac contraction as manifest by visible or palpable precordial or cervical pulsations.[442] The increased pulsations may prevent lying on the left side or produce annoying noises when the head is resting on a pillow. If there is associated ventricular ectopy, the hyperdynamic pulsations are even more disturbing. Some patients initially note these intense pulsations only with exertion.[444] Others will perceive the overactive cardiac pulsations as epigastric splashing sounds which occur upon lying down following a meal.[443]

Ventricular failure Further into the course of the disease, virtually all patients will begin to experience exertional dyspnea and easy fatigability. Upon the development of these symptoms, the clinical course is characterized by a gradual increase in their severity over the ensuing 5 to 10 years.[475] Once the exertional dyspnea becomes pronounced, other symptoms of left ventricular failure, such as orthopnea, paroxysmal nocturnal dyspnea, and excessive sweating, will have developed.[444] The excessive perspiration, often occurring at night, is thought to be a manifestation of congestive heart failure, since diaphoresis is more prevalent in the most advanced stages of the disease. The observation of Harvey et al. that following insertion of the Hufnagel prosthesis in the descending aorta the sweating was usually more severe above the prosthesis than below[476] challenges the validity of this assumption.

Angina pectoris Angina pectoris is noted in patients with severe aortic regurgitation, but it has a much different pattern than it shows in aortic stenosis. First, this symptom is much less common in aortic regurgitation with a reported incidence of 6 to 29 percent.[406,444] The exception to this reported incidence is a 50 percent occurrence in the study of Harvey et al.[476] Secondly, angina pectoris in aortic regurgitation is rarely the presenting symptom and is usually (approximately 70 percent of the cases) preceded by evidence of left ventricular failure. Finally, the pain has been noted to recur more often at rest, to last relatively longer, and to be frequently associated with vasomotor phenomenon and dyspnea.[406] A particularly intriguing pattern of angina seen occasionally in aortic regurgitation is nocturnal attacks of pain combined with palpitations, flushing, respiratory distress, sweating, and frequently nightmares.[444,476,477] In this symptom complex, the aforementioned symptoms usually precede the development of the angina.

Angina pectoris in patients with aortic regurgitation, without significant coronary atherosclerosis, is generally considered to be due to a reduced effective coronary blood flow secondary to low diastolic aortic pressure coupled with an increased requirement of blood by the hypertrophied left ventricle.[444,478] Much like the case with aortic stenosis, a reduced capacity for augmenting coronary blood flow to meet the demands of exercise seems to exist in some patients.[444]

Rest angina and nocturnal angina, both frequently associated with aortic regurgitation, are usually ascribed to the deleterious effects of bradycardia.[406] Patients with severe aortic regurgitation have a more effective stroke volume and significantly less regurgitation in response to the increase in heart rate associated with moderate exercise. The reduced regurgitant flow leads to a temporary decrease in left ventricular volume, wall tension, and oxygen consumption.[406]

Other symptoms Other symptoms which are rather uniquely associated with severe aortic regurgitation are neck pain, abdominal pain, and postural dizziness. The neck pain is usually acute in onset but persists from hours to as long as 5 to 6 days. It is generally bilateral and associated with tenderness over the carotids. Usually the pain is ascribed to stretching of the carotid sheaths but, in some instances, has almost certainly been secondary to a vigorously pulsating artery in the vicinity of inflamed

lymph nodes. The abdominal pain is usually a pounding or aching sensation in the epigastric region. Possible causes include constant stretching of the wall of the abdominal aorta or a vigorously pulsating aorta pounding against engorged viscera.[476] The dizziness is probably due to temporary cerebral ischemia caused by rapid, marked pressure changes in the cerebral vessels subject to a high pulse pressure. The fact that dizziness is usually found in patients with a pulse pressure greater than 100 mm Hg is compatible with this hypothesis.[444]

Clinical consequences of *acute aortic regurgitation* depend on the magnitude of the regurgitant flow and the suddenness of its onset.[475,479] The imposition of a severe diastolic overload on a relatively unprepared left ventricle by sudden severe aortic regurgitation can be catastrophic. These patients' survival often depends on immediate surgical intervention. Less severe regurgitation will result in lesser degrees of disability ranging from minimal exertional compliance to left ventricular decompensation managed only by intensive medical therapy. The subsequent course in these patients is similar to but more accelerated than that found with chronic aortic regurgitation.[475,479]

PHYSICAL EXAMINATION

Peripheral signs of aortic regurgitation Most of the peripheral evidence of aortic regurgitation is related to a wide pulse pressure. Since the pulse pressure is unaffected in mild to moderate disease, lesions of this severity are unaccompanied by peripheral stigmata. The widened pulse pressure associated with severe aortic regurgitation is secondary to a combination of increased stroke volume and diastolic aortic decompression. In determining the pulse pressure it must be recognized that while the Korotkoff sounds will frequently persist to zero in aortic regurgitation, true diastolic pressure correlates well with the pressure at which the sounds become muffled.[443] Instead of the normal 30 to 50 mm Hg pressure difference, the pulse pressure in aortic regurgitation usually exceeds 80 mm Hg and frequently is equal to or greater than 100 mm Hg.[442] The absence of a wide pulse pressure (pulse pressure greater than 50 percent of peak systolic pressure)[452] or a diastolic blood pressure greater than 70 in a patient without congestive heart failure will exclude severe aortic regurgitation.[480]

Palpation over the peripheral arteries will reveal a rapidly rising and collapsing pulse. The abrupt upstroke of the pulse is produced by the rapid ejection from the left ventricle of its increased end-diastolic volume. The swift collapse is attributed to the rapid loss of blood volume both across the incompetent aortic valve and into the dilated peripheral vessels. In addition, a double-peaked systolic impulse is occasionally perceived. This *bisferiens pulse* represents the palpable percussion wave of the arterial pulse followed by a palpable exaggerated tidal wave. The bisferiens pulse contour is frequently exaggerated peripherally and, consequently, more easily perceived over the brachial or femoral arteries.[14]

A host of peripheral manifestations of aortic regurgitation have been described and subsequently tagged with the describer's name. *Corrigan's pulse* refers to the abruptly rising and falling pulsation associated with aortic regurgitation.[481] While this pulse is characteristic of aortic regurgitation, it may also be associated with other high output states. Other signs attributed to the forcefulness of the arterial pulsations include *de Musset's sign* (a rhythmical nodding of the head synchronous with each heart beat) and *Müller's sign* (rhythmical pulsatory movements of the uvula). Transmission of these increased pulsations into the precapillary arterioles accounts for *Quincke's sign* (alternate reddening and blanching of the nail bed with each heartbeat). This phenomenon is elicited by observing the nail bed while the tip of the nail is compressed. *Duroziez's murmur* refers to the biphasic bruit detected by applying mild pressure with the stethoscope over the femoral artery. In normal subjects, compression of this vessel will elicit a systolic bruit as the blood passes the temporary obstruction. The additional diastolic bruit in aortic regurgitation reflects the rapid diastolic regurgitation toward the heart.[481] As with Quincke's pulse, this sign is not pathognomonic of aortic regurgitation since it can be detected in other high output states.[421] A phenomenon solely associated with aortic regurgitation is disproportionate femoral systolic hypertension, *Hill's sign*. Rather than the usual 10 to 20 mm Hg increase in systolic pressure in the femoral arteries over that in the brachial arteries, an increase of 60 to 100 mm Hg or more may be found.[482] This exaggerated systolic pressure in the femoral arteries is thought to reflect the direct flow of blood from the aorta into these vessels in contrast to the angulated route into the brachial arteries.

Inspection and palpation of the heart Visualization and palpation of the apical impulse in patients having aortic regurgitation, with the exception of those with a thick or deformed chest is very informative. Absence of an apical impulse implies mild disease, and a nondisplaced impulse suggests an early stage of the disease.[443] The apical impulse in chronic aortic regurgitation of at least moderate severity is displaced inferiorly and laterally. The displaced impulse tends to be diffuse (occupying more than one intercostal space) and is typically overacting (increased amplitude but normal contour).[14,46,483] This hyperdynamic systolic impulse is often followed by a palpable and, less frequently, visible rapid filling wave.[14]

Auscultation The first sound is usually normal but may be reduced in intensity in the presence of a prolonged P-R interval or bradycardia. The prolonged diastole associated with bradycardia may allow for sufficient regurgitation to increase left ventricular diastolic pressure above left atrial pressure and prematurely close the mitral valve.[14,442] The first sound is typically followed by an early systolic click in those patients with a combination of moderate to severe aortic regurgitation and good functional capacity of the left ventricle. As the left ventricle begins to decompensate, this sound usually disappears.[444] With phonocardiography the click is noted to occur slightly later (usually 0.10 s after S_1) than the ejection sound associated with aortic stenosis. In aortic regurgitation, the sound is probably not valvular in origin but is related instead to the rapid ejection of blood into the aorta.

Eighty-eight to one hundred percent of patients with moderate to severe aortic regurgitation will have a spindle- or diamond-shaped systolic murmur of grade 2 through 5 intensity.[442,444] Rapid ejection of an increased stroke volume across the aortic valve is thought to be the explanation for this finding, and its presence, even when accompanied by a thrill, does not necessarily imply coexisting aortic stenosis.[14]

The aortic component of the second sound is usually normal except in patients with very severe regurgitation. In these patients, the sound may be reduced in association with advanced left ventricular disease and marked cardiomegaly or may be accentuated in association with younger patients having good left ventricular function.[444]

A pure, high-frequency decrescendo diastolic murmur beginning with the second sound is the hallmark of aortic regurgitation. The contour of the murmur reflects the pattern of the regurgitant flow which is maximal in early diastole and decreases thereafter. Although the duration and intensity of the murmur reflect, to a degree, the amount of regurgitant flow, the severity of regurgitation correlates better with the murmur's duration.[14,444] Two features of the diastolic murmur which may serve as clues to the cause of the regurgitation are the site of maximal intensity and the musical quality. In patients having valvular lesions, the murmur is usually maximal at the left lower sternal or midsternal border but at times, particularly in the elderly, is loudest at the apex. If the regurgitation is related to dilatation of the ascending aorta, however, the murmur is commonly loudest along the right sternal border, usually in the second intercostal space.[444] A diastolic murmur with a very pure musical tone, the so-called sea gull, or cooing dove, murmur, indicates that the sound is arising from one of the following types of valve deformity: retroversion of the cusp edge, laceration or tearing of the cusp along its margin or line of attachment, or perforation of the cusp.[484] Valvular deformities of these types are found most often with myxomatous transformation, syphilis, trauma, and bacterial endocarditis. Frequently observed characteristics of this sea gull murmur are intense loudness and extensive radiation.[444,484]

A third heart sound, or diastolic gallop, is to be expected in severe aortic regurgitation. This sound reflects augmented left ventricular filling during the rapid diastolic filling phase and does not necessarily indicate left ventricular failure. Frequently, the third sound will initiate and enmesh with a diastolic rumble. Austin Flint initially described the rumble as presystolic, but the timing may be presystolic, mid-systolic, or both.[14,444] The presence of this rumble indicates severe aortic regurgitation.[443]

Opinions vary as to the origin of the Austin Flint murmur. Flint proposed that the rumble was related to functional mitral stenosis secondary to incomplete opening of the anterior mitral leaflet due to abnormal ventricular filling or impingement on this leaflet by the regurgitant blood flow.[485] Cineangiography suggests that the murmur might be due to vibrations of the anterior leaflet of the mitral valve as it is struck by two intersecting streams of flow.[41] The inconsistent correlation on echocardiography between the leaflet vibrations and the presence of a rumble, however, casts considerable doubt upon this proposal.[486] More recently, late diastolic mitral regurgitation in patients with severe aortic regurgitation has been noted, suggesting this as a possible mechanism for the murmur. Intracardiac phonocardiography, however, seems to disprove this explanation.[487] Phonocardiographic and echocardiographic correlations by Fortuin and Craige have offered a unifying mechanism for the various diastolic rumbles in aortic regurgitation.[485] These investigators found that most patients had a two-component murmur with both middiastolic and presystolic timing. The middiastolic component occurs as the mitral valve is quickly closing following the rapid ventricular filling phase. The closing movement of the mitral valve is unusually rapid because of abrupt rise in ventricular pressure resulting from filling via aorta and left atrium combined. As the mitral valve is closing, there is continued antegrade flow because of incomplete left atrial emptying. Turbulence set up in the antegrade stream accounts then for production of the murmur. A similar explanation could account for the presystolic component of the murmur. Excessively rapid closure of the mitral valve following atrial systole and secondary to a rapid rise in left ventricular diastolic pressure combined with continued antegrade flow produces increasing flow velocity and a crescendo murmur.[485] Furthermore, their results suggested a relation between the timing of the Austin Flint murmur and the hemodynamic severity of the aortic regurgitation. With mild to moderate regurgitation, no murmur is audible; moderately severe regurgitation produces a presystolic rumble; increasingly severe regurgitation results in a prolonged middiastolic-presystolic rumble; and the most severe chronic regurgitation and acute regurgitation are associated with only a middiastolic rumble as the mitral valve is completely closed after middiastole due to left ventricular pressures exceeding left atrial pressures.[485]

The hemodynamic feature specific for *acute, severe aortic regurgitation*, namely, premature closure of the mitral valve, accounts for certain clinical signs characteristic of this condition. A distinct first sound is rarely audible at the apex. Occasionally a faint single first sound, probably tricuspid closure, is audible along the lower left sternal border. Commonly, an early diastolic click, simultaneous with premature mitral closure, can be heard at the lower left sternal border or the apex. The manifestation of this premature closure on palpation is a *double diastolic apex beat*. This impulse contour is attributed to outward movement with the rapid filling wave followed by collapse with mitral closure. The outward movement then continues due to further filling of the ventricle by the regurgitant flow.[488] An additional clinical feature invariably associated with sudden severe aortic regurgitation is an unusually harsh diastolic murmur. The harshness of this murmur is often similar to that of the accompanying systolic murmur.[488]

ELECTROCARDIOGRAM

The typical ECG in "free" aortic regurgitation would include sinus rhythm, normal P waves, increased QRS amplitude, depressed ST segments, inverted T waves, and horizontal axis. The presence of atrial fibrillation should suggest concomitant mitral valve disease or myocardial failure. In the absence of mitral valve disease, atrial fibrillation suggests a poor prognosis.[425] While normal atrioventricular conduction is the usual finding, prolonged atrioventricular conduction is not uncommon and appears more frequent in the more advanced stages of disease.[442,444,489] Increased QRS amplitude is a common early electrocardiographic manifestation of aortic regurgitation. Occasionally in the early stages this change is accompanied by tall T waves in the left precordial leads and by prominent septal forces (deep, narrow Q waves in left precordial leads). This diastolic overload pattern, however, has been overemphasized, as it is seen only in the early stages of the disease and even then is merely an occasional finding.[444,490] The advanced stages of aortic regurgitation are typified by ST depression and negative T waves in association with the increased QRS voltage[444,491] (Fig. 60B-33). Another common electrocardiographic manifes-

FIGURE 60B-33 Serial ECGs recorded in 36-year-old man with chronic aortic regurgitation. The ECG in May 1972 is characteristic of diastolic overload pattern with increased QRS voltage and tall peaked T waves (V_5). The subsequent ECG demonstrates evolution of ST and T waves toward a "strain pattern" typical of long-standing severe aortic regurgitation. The patient was not taking digitalis on either date.

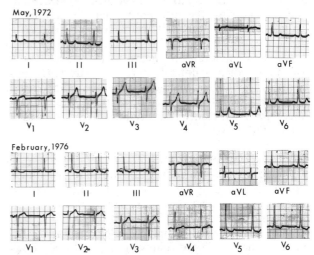

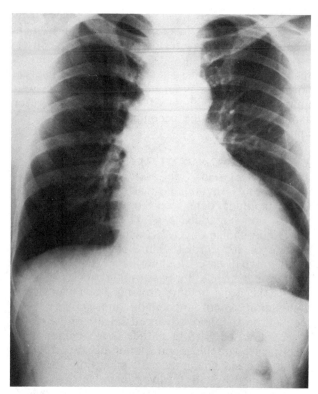

FIGURE 60B-34 Posteroanterior chest roentgenogram of a 26-year-old man with chronic aortic regurgitation. Characteristic features are the marked cardiomegaly with lateral and downward displacement of left ventricular border.

tation of aortic regurgitation is a horizontal QRS axis in contrast to the more vertical axis characteristic of aortic stenosis.

ROENTGENOGRAPHIC FINDINGS

The characteristic chest roentgenogram manifestation of aortic regurgitation is dilatation of the left ventricle with posterior and inferior elongation of the cardiac apex. Elongation of the apex seems to reflect left ventricular dilatation and is an important feature differentiating between aortic regurgitation and aortic stenosis[427] (Fig. 60B-34). Left atrial enlargement may accompany the left ventricular dilatation but usually reflects chronic left ventricular failure. With the exception of syphilitic aortitis and Marfan's syndrome, moderate to marked dilatation of the ascending aorta is not a feature of aortic regurgitation. Such dilatation should suggest coexisting aortic stenosis. Similarly, calcification of the aortic valve is uncommon with aortic regurgitation and implies a compound lesion[427].

ECHOCARDIOGRAPHY

Echocardiographic evidence for aortic regurgitation has been primarily reflected in alterations in the pattern of mitral valve motion during diastole. Abnormalities of mitral valve motion that have served as indirect echocardiographic evidence of aortic regurgitation include the following: (1) fast fine vibra-

tions or fluttering (frequency estimated to be 30 to 40 Hz and amplitude 4 mm) during diastole of the anterior mitral valve leaflet,[492] (2) an extremely rapid diastolic closure rate of the mitral valve leaflets,[493] (3) mitral valve closure occurring prior to the onset of the QRS complex,[494] and (4) thickening of the mitral valve leaflets.[493] Of these four features the only ones which have any degree of specificity is the rapid diastolic flutter of the anterior mitral valve leaflet seen in one-third to one-half of the patients with aortic regurgitation[492,493] and the premature closure of the mitral valve.[494] Fine diastolic fluttering of the anterior leaflet of the mitral valve may be accompanied by similar fluttering of the left ventricular surface of the septum[495] or of the posterior mitral leaflet. This echocardiographic finding is most commonly the result of aortic regurgitation but may also occur in other conditions.[615] There appears to be no good correlation between the presence of these vibrations and the severity of the aortic reflux[493] or with the presence of an Austin Flint murmur.[492] The echocardiographic appearance of premature mitral valve closure occurs only with severe, acute aortic regurgitation and demands consideration of immediate valve replacement.[494,496]

Additional echocardiographic features occasionally seen in association with aortic regurgitation are dilatation of the aortic root[497] and exaggerated amplitude of normally directed interventricular septal motion.[116] These echocardiographic patterns reflect the increased volume and flow in the left ventricle and aorta and, like the mitral valve abnormalities, are only indirect evidence of aortic regurgitation.

Generally, the echocardiographic appearance of the aortic leaflets do not offer a clue as to the existence of aortic regurgitation. An infrequent finding established by the study of Whipple et al. as diagnostic of a flail aortic leaflet with secondary aortic regurgitation is coarse diastolic oscillations in the aortic root or left ventricular outflow tract[498] (Fig. 60B-35). While this echocardiographic feature is quite specific and immediate recognition of its diagnostic significance is important, it is not a very

FIGURE 60B-35 Echocardiogram of aortic root and aortic leaflets from a 52-year-old man with aortic regurgitation secondary to myxomatous degeneration of the right aortic leaflet (RAVL). The second panel is an expanded view focused on the aortic root of the first panel. The RAVL evidences a coarse fluttering during diastole indicative of a prolapsing leaflet. AAW, anterior aortic wall; PAW, posterior aortic wall.

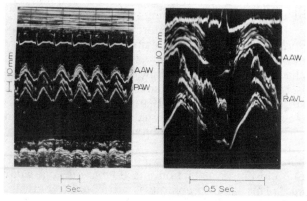

sensitive indicator of the existence of a flail leaflet. Another echocardiographic image of the aortic valve reported to suggest the presence of aortic regurgitation is a greater than 1-mm diastolic separation of the aortic leaflets.[499] In our hands, this finding is too insensitive and too nonspecific to be of any more value than to suggest a second careful cardiac auscultation of the patient.

In addition to the coarse diastolic oscillations suggestive of a flail leaflet and the premature mitral valve closure suggestive of acute severe regurgitation, bacterial endocarditis of the aortic valve may be diagnosed by one of the following echocardiographic features: irregular or shaggy thickening of the anterior or posterior aortic leaflets, disappearance of a cusp on sequential echocardiograms, or multiple linear or coalescent diastolic echoes within the aortic root.[500]

CARDIAC CATHETERIZATION

The preoperative hemodynamic status of the patient with aortic regurgitation is assessed to obtain one or all of the following: (1) more accurate index of the severity of regurgitation, (2) evaluation of left ventricular function, and (3) determination of any coexisting valvular or coronary pathologic condition.

Supravalvular cineaortography remains the most commonly utilized method for assessment of the severity of aortic regurgitation. While other more sophisticated, and perhaps more accurate, methods including indicator-dilution curves, volume quantitative angiography, and electromagnetic flowmeters are available, cineaortography is preferred because of technical simplicity and acceptable accuracy. This method depends upon a visual estimation of the quantity of opacified blood regurgitating into the left ventricle.[501] The quantity of reflux is generally graded on a scale of 1 to 4+, with 1+ reflecting small diastolic reflux cleared during the subsequent systole, 2+ denoting small reflux without clearing during systole, 3+ reflecting a progression to complete opacification of the left ventricle over several cycles, and 4+ denoting complete opacification at the end of the first diastole.[480]

Adherence to certain technical factors is important in achieving sufficient accuracy with this method. The catheter tip should be 1 to 3 cm above the aortic sinus. A lower catheter position can cause contrast leakage in even normal valves, and an inappropriately high position will minimize regurgitant flow. To achieve an adequate anatomic examination, injection of a relatively large amount of contrast medium over 2 s or less is advisable. Finally, a comparison of contrast medium density between the aorta and left ventricle is important in minimizing errors due to varying volumes of the ascending aorta.[444]

The ratio of the angiographic stroke volume to the end-diastolic volume, termed the *ejection fraction,* is generally considered the best single measurement of the functional status of the left ventricle.[395,502] In patients with chronic aortic regurgitation and normal myocardial function the increase in end-diastolic volume of the left ventricle directly reflects the amount of regurgitant flow.[503] As might be predicted

from the Frank-Starling mechanism, the total left ventricular stroke volume increases proportionally with the increase in the end-diastolic volume, while the ejection fraction remains normal.[395,502] Consequently, an increased end-diastolic volume accompanied by a reduced ejection fraction indicates disproportionate ventricular dilatation and suggests the presence of myocardial dysfunction.[395,504]

In recent years, another sensitive technique for evaluating left ventricular performance, applicable in any cardiac catheterization laboratory, has evolved. This technique is based on an angiographic determination of the mean velocity of circumferential fiber shortening (mean Vc_f). A comparative study concluded that this measurement was a more sensitive index of left ventricular dysfunction than the ejection fraction, but review of these data suggests that utilization of both indices would be the most sensitive method.[505]

Another parameter worth considering as an index of left ventricular function, but only as an adjunct to the more reliable indices, is the left ventricular end-diastolic pressure (LVEDP). The significance of this variable is based on the premise that a normally functioning, volume-overloaded left ventricle is characterized by increased compliance. Consequently, the increased left ventricular end-diastolic volume is accompanied by normal end-diastolic pressures. As the myocardium fails, the compliance is reduced and the end-diastolic pressure rises. As a result, left ventricular failure is usually reflected by an elevated end-diastolic pressure. However, correlative studies have revealed that this parameter, as an isolated variable, is not a reliable indicator of left ventricular function.[395]

The necessity for excluding any coexisting pathologic condition should be based on the clinical and noninvasive assessment of the patient. In the absence of any clinical or echocardiographic evidence of mitral stenosis, catheterization of the right side of the heart is not indicated. Furthermore, there are good data to suggest that in the absence of angina pectoris or ECG evidence of myocardial infarction coronary angiography is not necessary.[406,506] Since there are exceptions to this norm and since our complication rate with coronary angiography is minimal, we choose to perform coronary angiography on any patient over 45 years of age undergoing preoperative catheterization of the left side of the heart.

Treatment

In aortic regurgitation of all degrees of severity, a major responsibility of the examining physician is the institution of bacterial endocarditis prophylaxis and education. The single most important factor in producing a sudden deterioration in chronic aortic regurgitation is infection of the deformed aortic leaflets. The great tragedy of this frequently devastating condition is that it is usually preventable. Antibiotic prophylaxis is recommended with all dental procedures; surgery or instrumentation of the genitourinary tract, the lower gastrointestinal tract, and the gallbladder; obstetric complications such as septic abortions and complicated deliveries; cardiac surgery; surgery of infected tissues, including incision and drainage of abscesses; tonsillectomy and adenoidectomy; and bronchoscopy. Although no data are available from controlled clinical trials on the prevention of bacterial endocarditis, clinical experience is convincing as to the usefulness of prophylaxis. If the cause of the aortic regurgitation is possibly rheumatic, antistreptococcal prophylaxis should be prescribed until the patient is well into adulthood or no longer frequently associates with young children. The treatment of syphilitic aortic insufficiency should include a full course of penicillin therapy.

"The most important responsibility of the cardiologist is to decide when to refer the patient for surgery."[63] While the symptoms of left ventricular failure can often be substantially improved with digitalis, salt restriction, and diuretics and the associated angina may be relieved by nitroglycerin, the dilemma is whether the physician should allow these symptoms to develop before recommending surgery. There are some persuasive data suggesting that earlier surgery is advisable. Gault et al. found that while patients demonstrated clinical and hemodynamic improvement, neither the depressed myocardial inotropic state nor the reduced diastolic compliance were altered when valve replacement was performed after the development of myocardial dysfunction.[507] In addition, Hirshfield et al. noted a 43 percent 6-year survival in those patients with aortic regurgitation whose heart size on roentgenographic examination did not change over the first 6 months following valve replacement versus an 85 percent survival in those who experienced a postoperative decrease in heart size.[437] The assumption would be that those with an unchanging heart size preoperatively developed inappropriate left ventricular dilatation and myocardial dysfunction while their cohorts retained normal myocardial function.

Even the acknowledgment of these facts makes the problem no less difficult. We must next learn to recognize those patients who are on the verge of developing myocardial dysfunction. While the information in this regard is scanty, there are again some pertinent figures. Spagnuola et al. noted that patients with the triad of moderate to marked left ventricular enlargement, an abnormal blood pressure (systolic above 140 and diastolic below 40), and electrocardiographic evidence of left ventricular hypertrophy (including QRS voltage, increased ST depression, and T wave inversion) had an 87 percent likelihood of developing symptoms of congestive heart failure or of dying within 6 years.[491] Hirshfield et al. also discovered a significantly reduced survival in those patients with definite left ventricular hypertrophy as based on having 6 points on the scale of Romhilt and Estes[437,508] (only 1 point given for ST-T wave changes and 3 points given for left atrial enlargement).

Our approach based on these data is to submit to cardiac catheterization any patient with aortic regurgitation accompanied by moderate to marked left ventricular enlargement seen on chest roentgenogram and ECG evidence of left ventricular hypertrophy (prominent QRS voltage and oppositely directed ST and T vectors). For any of these patients who has evidence of left ventricular dysfunction on catheterization (determined as previously outlined) aortic valve replacement is recommended. Any patient with early symptoms of congestive heart failure without these significant roentgenographic or electrocardiographic changes is treated initially with digitalis and possibly diuretics, with any poor responder to this approach evaluated by catheterization. As noted by Spagnuolo et al., most patients demonstrate the roentgenographic and electrocardiographic changes previously alluded to prior to the development of failure.[491] We recognize this as a more aggressive approach than previously used but believe our operative mortality with valve replacement and the improvement in prosthetic valves makes it appropriate.

COMBINED AORTIC STENOSIS AND AORTIC REGURGITATION

A separation of aortic valvular disease into a third subset, in addition to aortic regurgitation and aortic stenosis, is rather artificial in that the majority of cases of aortic stenosis display at least minimal regurgitation and many cases of aortic regurgitation have a small transvalvular gradient. There are, however, a group of patients with aortic valvular disease whose hemodynamic burden is a combination of pressure overload and volume overload.[381] These patients have a transvalvular gradient greater than 25 mm Hg in combination with significant reflux across the valve. While the energy demands in combined valvular disease tend to be greater than that of either lesion in isolation, the clinical course for this condition is similar to that of isolated aortic stenosis. In both these conditions, a compensated state exists for a protracted interval before the development of angina, syncope, or left ventricular failure. The appearance of these symptoms denotes a poor prognosis in both groups.[381] In addition, the primary causes in both conditions are congenital and rheumatic, the only difference, a minor one, being a greater frequency of bicuspid valves in isolated aortic stenosis while rheumatic valvulitis is a more frequent cause in combined disease.[381]

The typical patient with combined aortic valvular disease will have prominent systolic and diastolic murmurs, including an Austin Flint rumble. The carotid pulse contour will likely be normal, and the apical impulse will be sustained, diffuse, and slightly displaced. The usual laboratory manifestations include the following: left ventricular hypertrophy with "strain" indicated on the ECG, moderate cardiomegaly and calcification of the aortic leaflets on roentgenographic studies, and multiple central linear echoes within the aortic root coupled with fine diastolic flutter of the anterior mitral leaflet on the echocardiogram.

One interesting fact arising from the study on aortic valvular disease by Rotman et al.[381] is that the long-term survival after valve replacement is better in combined valvular disease than in aortic stenosis. Perhaps the addition of a volume load in combined valvular disease leads to earlier development of symptoms and earlier, and more appropriate, timing of the surgery.

COMBINED AORTIC AND MITRAL VALVE DISEASE

The recognition and assessment of combined aortic and mitral valve disease can be difficult. The clinical features of involvement of one valve may be masked by the coexistent involvement of the other. The indications for surgery and the proper surgical procedure required are determined by the symptoms and hemodynamic significance of each. Clues to the presence of combined aortic and mitral valve disease will be discussed.

Aortic stenosis and mitral stenosis

This combination is not very common but is one of the most difficult to recognize. Symptoms of mitral stenosis are usually dominant. Compared with symptoms of isolated aortic stenosis, dyspnea, cough, and hemoptysis are more common while angina and syncope are less common.[509–513] Compared with symptoms of isolated mitral stenosis, angina and syncope are more common. Systemic emboli are more common in combined disease than in isolated aortic valve disease.[511,513]

The delayed carotid upstroke and the sustained apex impulse usually appreciated in isolated aortic stenosis are less frequent findings in combined mitral and aortic stenosis. The auscultatory findings of mitral stenosis are not as obvious as in isolated mitral stenosis. Accentuation of S_1 and an opening snap are less frequent[513] (Fig. 60B-36). Detection of the rumble may require special attention to auscultatory detail. A systolic ejection murmur may be the only

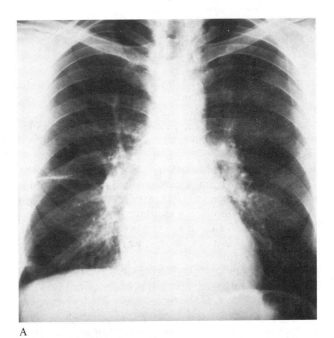

A

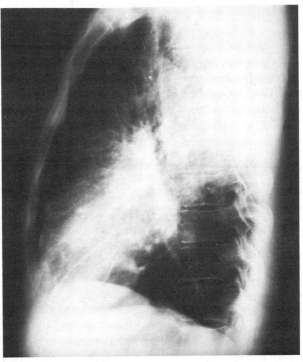

B

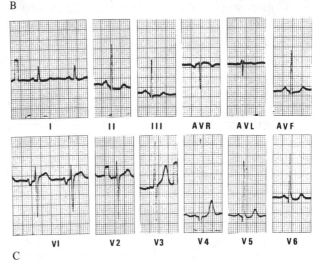

C

FIGURE 60B-36 Chest roentgenograms and ECG of a patient with mitral stenosis. *A.* Large pulmonary arteries and Kerley B lines are seen on the posteroanterior view. *B.* The lateral view shows left atrial enlargement and aortic, mitral, and pericardial calcification. The pericardial calcification is present retrosternally and posteriorly in the atrioventricular groove. *C.* The ECG shows sinus rhythm, left atrial abnormality, and increased QRS voltage in the mid- and lateral precordial leads. On physical examination carotid upstroke was slightly delayed, and there was a grade 3 (out of 6 grades) systolic ejection murmur, a grade 1 diastolic decrescendo murmur at left sternal border, and a grade 2 middiastolic rumble at the apex. The first heart sound was not increased, and there was no opening snap. Cardiac catheterization findings revealed a mitral valve area of 0.76 cm², aortic valve area of 0.89 cm², moderate pulmonary hypertension, and minimal aortic regurgitation. At surgery these findings were confirmed. The mitral and aortic valves were heavily calcified. There was adhesive pericarditis.

clue on physical examination to the presence of concomitant aortic stenosis,[514] and its intensity is less than is usual in isolated aortic stenosis.

Electrocardiographic evidence for left ventricular hypertrophy usually seen in significant aortic stenosis is not as apparent in combined aortic and mitral stenosis. Atrial fibrillation is common.[511–513] The chest roentgenogram is more typical for mitral stenosis with evidence of left atrial enlargement and changes in pulmonary vasculature. On fluoroscopy the presence of calcium in the aortic or mitral valve serves as a clue to coexisting valve disease. A significant mitral valve gradient is usually obvious at cardiac catheterization. The peak systolic gradient between the left ventricle and aorta may not be very impressive.[509–511,515] The presence of a low cardiac output in many of these cases will generate a relatively small gradient despite severe aortic stenosis.

In summary, the presence of prominent pulmonary symptoms, cough, hemoptysis, atrial fibrillation, or left atrial enlargement in a patient with obvious aortic stenosis requires a careful search for concomitant mitral stenosis. The presence of a systolic ejection murmur, angina, or syncope in a patient with obvious mitral stenosis requires a careful search for concomitant aortic stenosis. Echocardiographic findings as well as the presence of valve calcification on fluoroscopy may substantiate involvement of both valves, but catheterization is required in the symptomatic patient to clarify the degree of stenosis of each valve.

Aortic regurgitation and mitral valve disease

Aortic regurgitation and mitral regurgitation with or without some element of mitral stenosis is probably the most common combination.[516] Symptomatology is of little help in the recognition of the combination unless pulmonary symptoms are prominent or systemic emboli have occurred, both of which would favor the presence of mitral valve disease.

On physical examination hemodynamically significant aortic regurgitation is usually obvious. However, a mild to moderate degree may be overlooked when there is severe mitral valve disease. The intensity of the diastolic murmur and the peripheral signs of aortic regurgitation are not reliable indicators.[480] With obvious severe aortic regurgitation the presence of an accentuated first heart sound demands careful search for mitral stenosis. A diastolic rumble may represent the Austin Flint rumble of aortic regurgitation or the rumble of mitral stenosis. Bedside maneuvers may aid in the differentiation. The administration of amyl nitrite intensifies the murmur of mitral stenosis and attenuates the Austin Flint rumble. The presence of a holosystolic murmur at the apex with radiation to the axilla provides a clue to the presence of mitral regurgitation. Some degree of mitral regurgitation due to left ventricular dilatation and papillary muscle dysfunction may be present

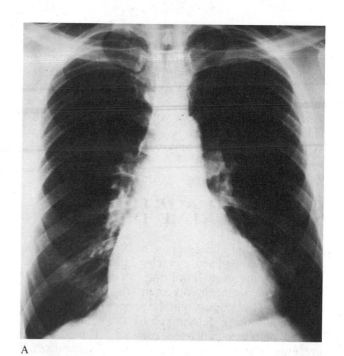

A

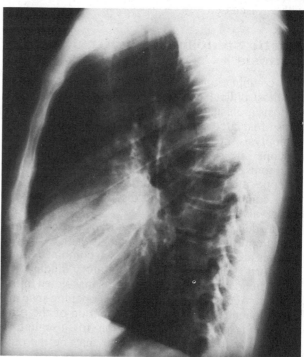

B

FIGURE 60B-37 Chest roentgenograms of a patient with moderately severe aortic regurgitation and mitral stenosis. There is left ventricular enlargement due to aortic regurgitation. Mitral stenosis would be suspected because of evidence for left atrial enlargement on the lateral view and the presence of the left atrial appendage on the posteroanterior view. The patient also had chronic atrial fibrillation.

with aortic regurgitation without intrinsic mitral valve disease.

With atrial fibrillation seen on the ECG, moderate left atrial enlargement on chest roentgenograms (Fig. 60B-37), and mitral valve calcium on fluoroscopy, mitral stenosis should be suspected.

An echocardiographic examination of the mitral valve in patients with aortic regurgitation can be quite helpful. The presence of a normal E to F slope and normal posterior mitral leaflet motion would exclude concomitant mitral stenosis.

In the presence of severe aortic regurgitation the assessment of catheterization data for mitral stenosis may be difficult. The left ventricular diastolic pressure may not reliably reflect the mitral valve gradient due to the aortic regurgitation. Preoperative angiographic assessment of the degree of aortic regurgitation, despite its limitations, should be performed in any patient with obvious mitral stenosis or regurgitation in whom a diastolic murmur of aortic regurgitation is present.[480]

In summary, the presence of atrial fibrillation, systemic emboli, accentuated S_1, an apical holosystolic murmur, or a diastolic rumble that does not attenuate with the administration of amyl nitrite in a patient with aortic regurgitation demands a careful search for concomitant mitral stenosis or regurgitation.

Aortic stenosis and mitral regurgitation

In the authors' experience the combination of severe aortic stenosis and significant mitral regurgitation requiring replacement of both valves is very uncommon. The systolic murmur of aortic stenosis, while harsh at the second right intercostal space, is frequently of higher frequency at the apex, and since S_1 and S_2 are not always easy to separate from the onset and termination of the murmur, a holosystolic murmur of mitral regurgitation is simulated. Radiation of the murmur to the left scapula would favor concomitant mitral regurgitation. The radiation of the murmur to the cervical and lumbar spine is used as a point in favor of mitral regurgitation. However, we have observed that the murmur of aortic stenosis may radiate in a similar pattern, presumably due to the direction of the poststenotic jet posteriorly toward the thoracic spine.

A history of systemic emboli, the presence of atrial fibrillation, or mitral valve calcium suggest the presence of mitral valve disease. Left ventricular angiography is an essential part of the preoperative evaluation to clarify the problem.

TRICUSPID STENOSIS

In 1930 Cabot[517] wrote: "I do not know how to diagnose tricuspid involvement . . . ."

This confession could be repeated by a large number of physicians as evidenced by the fact that tricuspid stenosis is clinically diagnosed in 2 to 3 percent of cases of multivalvular disease but detected at autopsy in 10 to 23 percent of these cases.[518] This deficiency in our diagnostic skills is not without serious consequences, as a failure to recognize the presence of this condition may result in an incorrect assessment of the severity of coexisting valvular disease or may explain a lack of improvement in a patient following mitral or aortic surgery.

While recognition of the existence of this particular valvular deformity occurred at approximately the time of the recognition of other valve disease, general awareness of its diagnostic clinical features has been a slow evolutionary process. Corvisart des Marets first recognized that stenosis of either atrioventricular valve could produce a precordial thrill but added that other signs of tricuspid stenosis were surrounded by obscurity. Subsequently, in 1824, Bertin described the diastolic murmur characteristic of tricuspid stenosis. In 1868, Duroziez presented 10 autopsy-proved cases of tricuspid stenosis and stressed the murmur's location at the inferior portion of the sternum.[518] It was not until 1950, however, that Carvallo reported the inspiratory augmentation of the murmur of tricuspid stenosis.[57]

Etiology

Tricuspid stenosis is secondary to rheumatic valvulitis in the vast majority of patients, but instances of the stenosis secondary to congenital heart disease, carcinoid, fibroelastosis, endomyocardial fibrosis, and systemic lupus erythematosus have been reported.[57,519]

Rheumatic valvulitis typically causes fusion of the adjacent free edges of the leaflets resulting in a shallow funnel-shaped structure. Fusion most often occurs at the anteroseptal commissure but may occur at any or all of the commissures. The cusps are only moderately thickened and remain pliable. Unlike the case with the mitral valve, the chordae are not severely deformed. Calcification of the tricuspid valve occurs rarely, if ever.[517,520]

Pathophysiology[521,522]

The major hemodynamic alterations of tricuspid stenosis are a decrease in cardiac output and an increase in right atrial pressures. Inability of the right atrium to propel blood across the stenotic tricuspid valve accounts for the reduction in cardiac output. The greater reduction in output associated with tricuspid stenosis in comparison with mitral stenosis is probably related to the relatively small force of contraction of the right atrium in comparison with that of the right ventricle. Blood flow across the stenotic mitral valve is maintained by elevated pressures primarily generated by the right ventricle, while the right atrium must exert this force in tricuspid stenosis. The degree of obstruction of the tricuspid valve which seriously impairs circulation has not been firmly established but is probably in the range of 1.5 cm² or less (normal tricuspid valve area greater than 7 cm²).

The level of right atrial pressure, which is influenced not only by the effective orifice area of the tricuspid valve but also by the level of right ventricular diastolic pressure, is a critical factor in the production of edema. Most patients begin to develop peripheral edema when the mean right atrial pressure reaches 10 mm Hg. In the setting of normal left ventricular end-diastolic pressures, this level of atrial pressure would be required to maintain a normal cardiac output across a valve area of 1.3 cm². The importance of atrial contraction in maintaining blood flow across the stenotic valve while preventing undue pressure elevation in the systemic venous system is evident in a comparison of patients with atrial fibrillation and those with sinus rhythm. As a group, patients with atrial fibrillation in association with tricuspid stenosis have a mean right atrial pressure nearly twice the pressure recorded in those patients with sinus rhythm. As would be expected, the patients with atrial fibrillation have a higher incidence of peripheral edema.

Clinical recognition[57,519,523]

HISTORY

The typical patient presenting with tricuspid stenosis is a woman, 20 to 48 years in age, with coexisting and usually dominant mitral stenosis. Tricuspid stenosis is associated with mitral regurgitation so infrequently that the presence of the latter makes the diagnosis of the former almost untenable. Perhaps the clinical pattern most suggestive of tricuspid stenosis is a patient with mitral stenosis and relatively little evidence of acute paroxysmal symptoms such as paroxysmal nocturnal dyspnea, pulmonary edema, or hemoptysis.

The symptoms most often attributed to the existence of tricuspid stenosis are effort intolerance and easy fatigability. These complaints are presumably secondary to the reduction in cardiac output. Exertional dyspnea, probably related to fatigue of respiratory muscles also secondary to the reduced output, is not an uncommon complaint. Fluttering in the neck due to perception of the giant jugular venous *a* waves is an occasional early complaint, while peripheral edema is always a very late development.

PHYSICAL EXAMINATION

The existence of tricuspid stenosis is more often suggested by recognition of its associated physical findings than by the presence or absence of any particular symptoms. In patients with sinus rhythm, the most striking physical finding is the "flicking" presystolic pulsations in the jugular veins. This *a* wave of significant magnitude in association with a small *v* wave and an imperceptible *y* descent could easily be mistaken for an arterial pulsation by a casual observer. Normally, the most prominent venous wave is a negative deflection, while in these patients a single positive, rather rapidly rising pulsation predominates. In the most severe diseases, the amplitude of the *a* wave may reach the angle of the mandible.[57,519] In the presence of atrial fibrillation, the characteristic *a* wave is lost, but the gentle *y* descent of the jugular venous pulsation persists. This finding falls into the category of those physical signs whose presence is established after a diagnosis is made, rather than one with any true diagnostic importance.

Palpation The characteristic palpatory evidence of tricuspid stenosis is the absence of a right ventricular lift.[523] The giant jugular venous *a* wave could reflect either pulmonary hypertension or pulmonic stenosis; however, either of these conditions, unlike tricuspid stenosis, would be invariably accompanied by the heaving lift of right ventricular hypertrophy.[57] The only positive finding on palpation would be the occasional perception along the left sternal border of a diastolic thrill which is accentuated by inspiration.

Auscultation Once suspicion of tricuspid stenosis has been raised, auscultation becomes the most important diagnostic maneuver. This evaluation is often made difficult by the presence of auscultatory evidence of the usually dominant mitral stenosis. In spite of this hindrance, careful auscultation will frequently yield several clues as to the presence of tricuspid involvement. The first sound (S_1) is often split as a result of simultaneous delay in both its mitral and tricuspid components (Fig. 60B-38). The delayed tricuspid component must be distinguished from the ejection sound associated with pulmonary hypertension. Important differentiating features of these sounds are their location and their respiratory variation in intensity. The tricuspid closing sound is loudest at the lower left sternal border and increases in intensity during inspiration. Conversely, the pulmonic ejection sound is heard best at or immediately below the pulmonic area and increases with expiration.[57]

Careful auscultation of the second sound (S_2) is important to exclude the loud pulmonic component associated with pulmonary hypertension. Attention to the splitting of the second sound is also of value, since inspiratory splitting is unusual in tricuspid stenosis. Probably tricuspid stenosis prohibits the inspiratory increase in right ventricular end-diastolic volume and stroke volume which accounts for the inspiratory splitting of S_2.[57]

The characteristic auscultatory feature of tricuspid stenosis is a middiastolic or presystolic murmur. Location of the murmur is at the left sternal border in the fourth or fifth intercostal space[57,517–519] and not over the sternum or to the right of the sternum as some texts report. Timing of the murmur is related to the cardiac rhythm. The murmur is presystolic in

FIGURE 60B-38 Phonocardiogram recorded on a patient with tricuspid stenosis. The striking features are the prominent tricuspid component of the first sound (t_1) in comparison to the mitral component (m) and the late diastole murmur which increases during inspiratory phase (ip) of respiration; ep, expiratory phase.

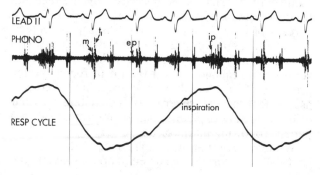

patients with a normal sinus rhythm because the gradient is small until the onset of atrial contraction. Since the gradient is maximal during early diastole and gradually diminishes in patients with atrial fibrillation, the murmur in these patients usually occurs during early diastole to middiastole.[517,518] The murmur is perhaps higher-pitched and closer to the ear than the mitral rumble, but the only certain way to distinguish between the two is to determine respiratory alteration in intensity (Fig. 60B-38).

The inspiratory increase in intensity of the diastolic murmur (Carvallo's sign) is the most valuable auscultatory sign in tricuspid stenosis.[57] Although Carvallo suggested auscultation during postinspiratory apnea, the preferable method is to listen while the patient breathes deeply, slowly, and continuously. The murmur will increase in intensity, by occasionally as much as two to three grades, during inspiration. This inspiratory augmentation in the intensity of the murmur is secondary to increased venous filling of the right atrium during inspiration due to lower intrathoracic, including intracardiac, pressures. The increased right atrial filling in combination with the reduced right ventricular pressures during inspiration establishes an increased transvalvular gradient, and consequently increased transvalvular flow.[57,517,523]

It is reported that inspiratory augmentation of the tricuspid diastolic murmur in association with a reduction in the intensity of the systolic murmur is useful in distinguishing dominant stenosis from dominant incompetence of the tricuspid valve.[519,522]

While this diastolic murmur may be preceded by an opening snap, the presence of the snap is usually difficult to substantiate. The usual circumstance is that the snap either cannot be clearly delineated or, if delineated, cannot be differentiated from mitral opening snap.[57,523]

ELECTROCARDIOGRAM

Tall peaked P waves in the absence of evidence of right ventricular hypertrophy are the most diagnostic electrocardiographic pattern for tricuspid stenosis.[57,517,523] The P waves, particularly in the right precordial leads, usually exceed 3 mm in height and frequently exceed 4 mm. A prolonged P-R interval is commonly associated. Unfortunately for diagnostic purposes, some of these patients have evidence for right ventricular hypertrophy,[519] and others develop atrial fibrillation which obscures the characteristic P wave changes. An electrocardiographic pattern unique for tricuspid stenosis is small QRS complexes of rsR' configuration in V_1 and V_2 associated with P waves of greater amplitudes than the QRS complex.[517]

ROENTGENOGRAPHIC FINDINGS

The most characteristic roentgenographic pattern of tricuspid stenosis is conspicuous dilatation of the right atrium without significant enlargement of the pulmonary arteries.[57,523]

ECHOCARDIOGRAPHY

A pattern of motion very similar to the mitral valve manifestations of mitral stenosis[421,524] is characteristic of the stenotic tricuspid valve on echocardiography. The diagnostic valve of this procedure is somewhat limited, however, by frequent failure to adequately visualize the tricuspid valve.

CATHETERIZATION

A definite diagnosis of tricuspid stenosis depends on establishment of an elevated mean transvalvular gradient at rest with widening of the gradient during exercise.[519,521] Simultaneous recording of the right atrial and right ventricular pressures with a double-lumen catheter are necessary in order to accurately calculate this gradient, which will fluctuate during the respiratory cycle.

The normal mean resting gradient across the tricuspid valve is usually less than 1 mm Hg and essentially always less than 1.9 mm Hg. While the end-diastolic gradient is a less sensitive parameter, more than 1.2 mm Hg for this measurement is unlikely in the absence of tricuspid stenosis.[521] A mean gradient of 3 mm Hg or more suggests significant tricuspid stenosis, and a gradient over 5 mm Hg suggests severe stenosis. Calculation of the effective orifice area is a more reliable method of determining the degree of valvular obstruction, valve area of less than 1.0 cm² reflecting severe tricuspid stenosis and between 1.0 and 1.5 cm² reflecting moderately severe stenosis.[519] In making these determinations, sufficient cardiac cycles should be analyzed to cover one complete respiratory cycle.[521]

Angiography provides useful confirmatory evidence for tricuspid stenosis by demonstrating prolonged opacification of an enlarged right atrium with a sharply defined atrioventricular border and by excluding a right atrial myxoma.[525]

Management

The usual management of a patient with tricuspid stenosis is determined by the more severely stenotic mitral valve. Prior to surgical intervention, the patient's management is unaltered by the addition of tricuspid stenosis. Furthermore, with a rare exception, the timing of surgery is determined by the mitral stenosis. The physician must avoid mistiming the surgery because of underestimating the degree of mitral stenosis due to the prevention of paroxysmal symptoms by the tricuspid stenosis. More importantly, the physician must not allow a stenotic tricuspid valve to go uncorrected and, as a result, hamper the expected improvement from successful mitral or aortic valve surgery. Moderately severe (1.0 to 1.5 cm² valve area) or severe tricuspid stenosis (1.0 cm² valve area) should be corrected by commissurotomy at the time of mitral or aortic valve surgery.

TRICUSPID REGURGITATION

Tricuspid regurgitation has been recognized clinically since 1836 when Benson described the jugular venous waves characteristic of this valvular abnormality.[526] In the following year, King published his hypothesis on the safety-valve action of the tricuspid valve and in doing so elucidated the beneficial effects of functional tricuspid regurgitation.[527] Later in the same century, Duroziez formulated the clinical picture of tricuspid regurgitation including the systolic murmur, distended neck veins, hepatic enlargement, and right atrial enlargement.[526]

Etiology

Clinically significant organic disease of the tricuspid valve in the absence of other cardiac abnormalities is extremely infrequent. The most common cause of organic tricuspid regurgitation is rheumatic valvulitis, but this cause is never anatomically and is rarely clinically isolated to the tricuspid valve. Other causes of organic tricuspid regurgitation include congenital anomalies (Ebstein's malformation, atrioventricular cushion defects), carcinoid heart disease, trauma, and infective endocarditis.[528,529] There is usually an associated cardiac abnormality in each of these conditions: atrial septal defect in congenital anomalies, pulmonary valve lesions in carcinoid heart disease, myocardial contusion or rupture in trauma, and infection of other valves in endocarditis.[528]

Disease mechanisms

Infective endocarditis is probably the most common cause of adult isolated tricuspid regurgitation.[528] In most large reviews on endocarditis, approximately 5 percent of the cases are limited to the right side of the heart, the tricuspid valve being the usual site of involvement. The incidence of tricuspid valve endocarditis is approximately three times that of the pulmonary valve.[530] Usually there is no underlying cardiac disease, and the vegetations occur on previously normal tricuspid leaflets. Septic pulmonary emboli resulting in pulmonary infarctions, pneumonitis, and abscesses usually dominate the clinical picture of tricuspid endocarditis, while the hemodynamic burden is relatively well tolerated.[528]

The predominant functional derangement of the tricuspid valve produced by carcinoid heart disease is regurgitation. The fibrous plaques characteristic of this disease primarily adhere to the ventricular aspect of the tricuspid leaflets, frequently fusing the leaflets to the underlying ventricular wall.[531] (This condition is discussed further in Chap. 86.)

Tricuspid regurgitation secondary to trauma is usually related to rupture of the papillary muscle or rupture of the chordae tendineae and/or leaflets.[520] Cases of the first condition tend to have a progressively downhill course, while those in the latter group usually follow a relatively benign course. The mechanism of rupture at either site is presumably due to violent compression of the heart during diastole associated with some obstruction to pulmonary outflow.[520]

A more frequent occurrence than organic tricuspid regurgitation is functional tricuspid regurgitation. Functional regurgitation presumably develops because the weak anatomic support structure cannot adequately anchor the tricuspid leaflets as the right ventricle dilates in response to primary or secondary pulmonary hypertension.

Pathophysiology

With the onset of tricuspid regurgitation, the normal decrease in right atrial pressure during ventricular contraction is replaced by an abrupt increase in pressure. This early rise in atrial pressure is secondary to regurgitation of a portion of the right ventricular stroke volume into the atrium. A right atrial pressure contour characterized by a sustained systolic elevation (peak-plateau contour) is indicative of tricuspid regurgitation and is referred to as *ventricularization* of the atrial pressure curve.[526]

This alteration of the right atrial pressure curve produces an increase in the mean right atrial pressure which is reflected in the systemic venous system. If the mean right atrial pressure reaches 10 mm Hg, the secondary elevation in systemic venous system is frequently sufficient to produce peripheral edema and ascites.[532]

Clinical recognition

HISTORY
The patient with organic tricuspid regurgitation is most often a young to middle-aged woman with severe mitral stenosis, followed in frequency by the narcotic addict presenting with fever. The clinical profile on the patient with functional tricuspid regurgitation is as varied as the causes of elevated right ventricular pressures.

The symptoms of tricuspid regurgitation are not distinctive but usually include fatigue and dyspnea related to reduced cardiac output. Probably as a group, patients with tricuspid regurgitation have less difficulty with symptoms such as paroxysmal nocturnal dyspnea and orthopnea than their counterparts without tricuspid regurgitation, but such a distinction is very difficult to make in the individual patient.

PHYSICAL EXAMINATION
Atrial fibrillation is present in 80 to 96 percent of patients with tricuspid regurgitation.[532–534] The high incidence of atrial fibrillation has led to the proposition that tricuspid regurgitation is dynamically related to atrial fibrillation because of poor valve closure consequent upon absence of atrial contraction just prior to ventricular systole.[533] An occasional patient has demonstrated no evidence of tricuspid regurgitation while in sinus rhythm, only to manifest tricuspid regurgitation upon developing atrial fibrillation. Conversion back to sinus rhythm would then be accompanied by disappearance of the tricuspid regurgitation.[534]

Inspection and palpation Probably the physical finding most widely recognized as evidence of tricuspid regurgitation is the prominent systolic venous pulsations in the neck. This finding is indicative of tricuspid regurgitation, but its absence does not exclude the condition.[520,532] The pulsations may be obscured by engorgement or distension of the neck veins. Occasionally scrutiny of the earlobes or eyeballs will reveal pulsatile movement of these structures reflecting venous pulsations not otherwise evident.

Palpation of the abdomen frequently reveals an enlarged liver which is occasionally pulsatile.

Auscultation A holosystolic murmur will usually, but not always, be audible to the left of the sternum in the fourth intercostal space. Inspiratory augmentation of the murmur indicates a tricuspid origin, but absence of this sign does not exclude such an origin. This inspiratory augmentation of the tricuspid regurgitant murmur (Carvallo's sign) is related to increased filling of the right ventricle due to lower intrathoracic pressures during inspiration. Whether this augmented ventricular volume intensifies the murmur by increasing the incompetence of the tricuspid valve or merely by increasing both forward and regurgitant flow is unsettled.[63] A low-pitched, early diastolic flow murmur is an additional auscultatory feature in many of these patients.

ELECTROCARDIOGRAM

As indicated previously, atrial fibrillation is the customary rhythm. A significant proportion of these patients (25 to 65 percent depending on which study is used)[532-534] have a right bundle branch block pattern (diastolic overload pattern). This incidence is in contrast to the low incidence of right bundle branch block in uncomplicated mitral valve disease.[533] Extremely small voltage of the QRS complex in V_1 with qr or qR pattern has also been reported to occur at an increased frequency with tricuspid regurgitation.

ROENTGENOGRAPHIC AND ECHOCARDIOGRAPHIC MANIFESTATIONS

Right atrial enlargement is usually suggested on chest roentgenogram. Overall cardiac enlargement is the rule due to the coexisting cardiac abnormalities.[532-534]

Direct echocardiographic manifestations of tricuspid regurgitation, as is the case with mitral regurgitation, are lacking. Indirect echocardiographic evidence includes diminished or paradoxic interventricular septal motion reflecting the volume overload of the right ventricle,[116] systolic prolapse of the tricuspid leaflets,[535] or shaggy irregular echoes attached to the tricuspid leaflet echoes during diastole suggesting bacterial vegetations.[536]

CATHETERIZATION

Investigation of patients with suspected tricuspid regurgitation should be directed toward confirming or denying the existence of the condition and toward determining whether the reflux is functional or organic. The presence of tricuspid regurgitation is best established by obtaining the characteristic ventricularized pressure curve in the right atrium (see "Pathophysiology"). The normal systolic decline in atrial pressure is obliterated or reversed by a positive systolic wave. In questionable cases, exercise will increase the true regurgitant wave.

Angiography has proved unreliable in demonstrating tricuspid regurgitation. The high-pressure delivery of contrast material into the right ventricle requently expels the catheter into the atrium or produces ventricular ectopy which provokes tricuspid incompetence. The only value of the procedure is exclusion of tricuspid regurgitation in those cases with adequate opacification of the right ventricle and no evidence of regurgitation.[526]

The differentiation between functional and organic regurgitation is also difficult. The two measurements helpful in making this distinction are the diastolic gradient across the tricuspid valve and the pulmonary artery systolic pressure. A diastolic gradient across the tricuspid valve suggests coexisting tricuspid stenosis and, consequently, organic disease.[526] Organic disease is also likely in those patients whose pulmonary artery systolic pressure is below 60 mm Hg.[533]

Management

The hemodynamic burden imposed by isolated tricuspid regurgitation is usually well tolerated for relatively long periods of time. Exceptions to this protracted course are apparent in those patients who die or require valve replacement surgery within 4 months of rupture of a right ventricular papillary muscle.[149,520] The usual approach in patients with isolated tricuspid regurgitation is to treat their initial symptoms, usually dyspnea and fatigue, with digitalis and diuretics and reserve surgery for the medical failures. While the development of irreversible right ventricular disease in some patients has led to the suggestion that earlier surgery might be appropriate,[529] more confirmatory data should be accumulated before endorsement of a more aggressive approach.

Our management of tricuspid regurgitation in multivalvular disease is also rather conservative and is based primarily on the data accumulated by Braunwald et al.[537] If the preoperative catheterization data suggest that the tricuspid regurgitation is functional and operative examination reveals intact delicate valve leaflets, we would favor no more than tricuspid annuloplasty. Even the benefit of annuloplasty remained unanswered in the Braunwald study[537] and remains questionable in our minds. On the other hand, we would recommend valve replacement for severe organic tricuspid regurgitation as part of a multivalvular procedure.

ACQUIRED LESIONS OF THE PULMONIC VALVE

Acquired lesions of the pulmonic valve are rare. Those disease processes which afflict this valve are listed in Table 60B-5.

TABLE 60B-5
Acquired lesions of the pulmonic valve

1 Malignant carcinoid syndrome
2 Inflammatory lesions
  a Rheumatic
  b Tuberculosis
  c Endocarditis
3 Primary tumors
  a Sarcoma
  b Myxoma
4 Marfan's syndrome
5 Surgical deformity secondary to correction of congenital lesions
6 Pulmonary hypertension with pulmonic regurgitation as a result of:
  a Chronic lung disease
  b Mitral stenosis
  c Pulmonary emboli
7 Syphilis

The carcinoid syndrome is a disease produced by malignant carcinoid tumors and characterized by the clinical manifestations of cutaneous flushes, telangiectasia, intestinal hypermotility, and bronchoconstriction. The pathophysiology and clinical manifestations of this disease are discussed in Chap. 86. Heart failure is the leading cause of death in metastatic carcinoid syndrome. In approximately one-half the patients, there is involvement of the right side of the heart. When the pulmonary valve is involved, there is usually a pearly white fibrous scarring with retraction which may produce both stenosis and regurgitation.

Inflammatory lesions which involve the pulmonary valve include rheumatic fever, bacterial endocarditis, and tuberculosis. Rheumatic involvement of the pulmonary valve is unusual. It occurs in patients with severe myocardial involvement and extensive, profound myocardial damage with involvement of the aortic and mitral valves and usually the tricuspid valve.[538] Involvement of the pulmonary valve may be aggravated by the presence of an elevated pulmonary artery pressure. A study of rheumatic pulmonary valve disease in Mexico City suggests that the high altitude and severity of the rheumatic disease may favor pulmonary valve involvement.[538]

Bacterial endocarditis involving the pulmonary valve occurs on congenitally deformed valves or spontaneously in association with opiate addiction or alcoholism.[539] The organisms are usually highly virulent, and staphylococcus is the most common.[539] Tuberculosis can involve the heart and result in a severe myocarditis. A tuberculoma has been described in the right ventricular outflow tract which obstructed intracardiac blood flow, simulating valvular obstruction.

Primary tumors of the pulmonary valve are described and include sarcoma and myxoma.[540] Patients with Marfan's syndrome may have involvement of the pulmonary valve with myxomatous degeneration and valvular regurgitation.[541] Surgical procedures for congenital deformities including tetralogy of Fallot and pulmonary valvular stenosis can result in further deformity of the valve and regurgitation.[541] Regurgitation across the valve may occur as a result of chronic pulmonary hypertension as seen in patients with chronic lung disease, mitral stenosis, and recurrent pulmonary emboli.[541]

Extrinsic lesions may compress or deform the pulmonary artery and simulate valvular stenosis. The most common causes of these lesions are mediastinal tumors, aneurysms of the ascending aorta, and sinus of Valsalva aneurysms.[540] Constrictive pericarditis can also produce obstruction in the right ventricular outflow tract.

Clinical manifestations depend upon the severity of the deformity and the etiology of the disease process. Severe hemodynamic changes as a result of injury to the pulmonary valve are unusual. Patients with severe obstruction may have syncope or symptoms of right ventricular failure. Pulmonary regurgitation is usually well tolerated but may contribute to cardiac decompensation when associated with other valvular lesions.[539]

The murmur of pulmonic stenosis is easily recognized. It may persist past the aortic second sound, and there is a correlation in congenital pulmonic stenosis between the peak of the crescendo-decrescendo murmur and the severity of the stenosis. Pulmonary regurgitation is more difficult to evaluate. The murmur may be confused with aortic regurgitation or middiastolic flow rumble. Its onset is generally delayed after the second heart sound, and duration is variable. Timing the murmur on the phonocardiogram may be helpful in diagnosis.[541]

QUADRIVALVULAR DISEASE

The simultaneous deformity of all four cardiac valves is extremely unusual. While multivalvular disease may be secondary to bacterial endocarditis, carcinoid syndrome, and calcific degenerative changes, the only condition which might simultaneously involve all four valves is rheumatic valvulitis. Even in rheumatic valvulitis quadrivalvular disease is unusual as evidenced by the single case of quadrivalvular involvement among 585 patients with chronic rheumatic valvular disease reviewed by Clawson[542] and the 1 among 400 catheterized at The New York Hospital.[543] The infrequent occurrence of quadrivalvular disease is primarily related to the very low incidence of rheumatic involvement (5.6 percent of 780 cases)[542] of the valves of the right side of the heart.

Another possible cause of quadrivalvular involvement is a combination of congenital and rheumatic disease, which is the only setting in which we have witnessed this entity. Quadrivalvular disease seems to be uniformly stenosis of all four valves, as our patient had congenital aortic and pulmonic stenosis in combination with rheumatic mitral and tricuspid stenosis while the previously reported cases were all rheumatic quadrivalvular stenosis.[542,543]

In the clinical evaluation of quadrivalvular disease, the most difficult component to diagnose is the pulmonic stenosis. The typical spindle-shaped murmur of pulmonic stenosis is obscured by the more prominent aortic stenotic murmur. The patients characteristically have a carotid pulse of very low amplitude with murmurs indicative of aortic and mitral stenosis. The tricuspid stenosis is suggested by a diastolic murmur augmented by inspiration or by prominent jugular venous *a* waves. Again, the pulmonic stenosis may well go unrecognized as there are no features which will distinguish this lesion in the presence of the other valve involvement. Fatigue and dyspnea, probably related to low cardiac output, seem to be the most prominent symptoms in those few patients with this condition.

PROSTHETIC CARDIAC VALVES

History

The era of prosthetic cardiac valves (Fig. 60B-39) opened in September 1952 with the implantation of a caged-ball prosthesis in the descending aorta by Hufnagel and his associates.[544] This prosthesis, composed of a Lucite ball valve in a long, solid Lucite cage, was implanted just distal to the left subclavian artery as treatment for aortic valvular regurgitation. The less than optimal site for valve insertion was selected to allow for prosthesis insertion without occlusion of total blood flow. Truly successful prosthetic valve surgery had to await the development of a technique of extracorporeal circulation and the refinement of the caged-ball principle by Harken and Starr.

In May 1960, Harken and associates reported on five cases of aortic valve replacement with a caged-ball prosthesis,[545] resulting in one survivor. Then, on September 21, 1960, Dr. Albert Starr first successfully implanted a caged-ball prosthesis in the mitral position.[546] The initial clinical success by Dr. Starr established the merit of both valve replacement surgery and the caged-ball prosthesis.

The subsequent history of prosthetic valves revolved around modification of this basic ball valve design, alteration of construction material, and introduction of new valve designs. Active investigation of new types of prostheses continued because of dissatisfaction with the hemodynamic characteristics, durability, or thrombogenicity of the previously available prostheses.

The first Starr-Edwards prostheses to be widely distributed were the 1000 series aortic valve and 6000 series mitral valve. These double-cage prosthetic valves were replaced in 1965 by a single-cage 1200 and 6200 series in an attempt to reduce the incidence of thromboembolism. Persistent problems with thromboembolism next led to a cloth covering of the seat in the 2160 and 6120 series. Covering the seat and cage with cloth (2300 aortic, 6300 mitral) followed because of the significant reduction in the thromboembolism (20 to 60 percent to 3 to 20 percent) noted with the reduction in exposed metal.[547] The 2300 and 6300 series prostheses were also first to incorporate the Stellite poppet. This design modification was stimulated by the recurring problem of ball variance, first reported by Krosnick in 1965.[548] Unacceptable postoperative gradients across the completely cloth-covered valve quickly led to the introduction of the composite-seat valve in the 6310 and 2310 series. Further refinement of the Starr-Edwards prosthesis with the 6320 and 2320 and later the 6400 and 2400 have been directed toward reducing strut-cloth wear.[549]

The caged-ball principle is also utilized in the Braunwald-Cutter[550] and the Smeloff-Cutter prostheses.[551] In addition, both these prostheses employ a silicone poppet which has not demonstrated ball variance since the curing process for the silicone elastomer was modified.[551] This nonmetallic poppet was selected for the Braunwald-Cutter prosthesis in an attempt to reduce strut-cloth wear.[550] Another problem associated with a cloth covering, the tendency to accumulate platelet fibrin deposits at the apex of the cage (potential source of emboli), was the impetus for the open-ended cage in this particular prosthesis.[550] While the Braunwald-Cutter prosthesis was designed to alleviate problems associated with a cloth covering, the Smeloff-Cutter prosthesis was designed to diminish the stenotic effect of ball valves. Its double-cage design allows the diameter of the valve orifice to be equal to or slightly larger than the ball diameter.[551]

Disk prostheses (Kay-Shiley, Kay-Suzuki, and Cross-Jones) were developed to overcome the problems of poppet inertia and ventricular-prosthetic

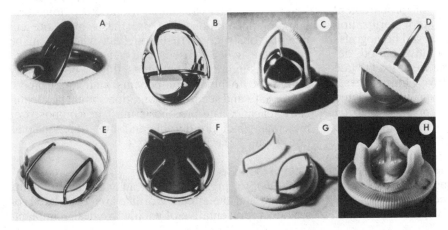

FIGURE 60B-39 Composite of the more widely utilized prosthetic valves. *A.* Bjork-Shiley aortic. *B.* Lillehei-Kaster aortic. *C.* Starr-Edwards 2320 aortic. *D.* Smeloff-Cutter. *E.* Kay-Shiley mitral. *F.* Cooley-Cutter. *G.* Beall. *H.* Hancock porcine mitral.

disproportion.[552,553] By employing a lightweight disk as an occluder, poppet inertia and the length of the cage were both reduced in these "low-profile" prostheses. However, the incidence of thromboembolism remained significant (14 to 38 percent)[554,555] and led to the development of a cloth-covered disk prosthesis, the Beall valve.[554] This prosthesis was first used clinically in February 1967.

In an effort to reduce postoperative pressure gradients associated with the central-occluder type of prosthesis, particularly in patients with a narrow aortic root, the eccentric monocusp central-flow prosthetic design was introduced. The first of these tilting disk valves, the Wada-Cutter prosthesis, was plagued by reports of intermittent fixation of the disk in an open position.[556] In 1969, the Bjork-Shiley model was introduced, with a free-floating and rotating disk designed to eliminate this problem.[557] A third pivoting disk valve, the Lillehei-Kaster prosthesis, was first used clinically in July 1970.[551] The disk, in this particular model, swings open to 80°, or 10° from the vertical axis, in contrast to the 60°-opening angle of both the Bjork-Shiley prosthesis and the Wada-Cutter prosthesis. This wider-opening angle is thought to decrease stagnation below the pivot point of the valve and consequently lessen the incidence of thromboembolism. The initial low incidence of thromboembolism with the Lillehei-Kaster prosthesis has induced some physicians to implant this prosthesis in the aortic position without the subsequent use of anticoagulants.[558]

The principal deficiency associated with the mechanical prosthesis is that none are free of thromboembolic complications (unless long-term data support the very preliminary studies with the Lillehei-Kaster prosthesis). This significant deficiency has been the stimulus for surgeons to attempt valve replacement with various types of tissue valves. Although these valves have seemingly overcome the problems of thromboembolism, they have been plagued by other problems such as difficulty of procurement and late valve failure due to deterioration of the tissue used.

In 1962 Ross[559] and Barratt-Boyes[560] began the clinical application of aortic valve homograft replacement in the subcoronary position. Initially fresh valves were used, but problems of procurement resulted in the use of various methods of sterilization and preservation. While these preserved homografts function well in the early postoperative period, degenerative changes in the nonviable cusps lead to late valve failure. Experience at the Mayo Clinic suggests that 25 to 30 percent of patients surviving isolated aortic valve replacement with a preserved aortic valve homograft will require reoperation during the ensuing 6 years.[561] Assessment of the data from the University of Alabama projects that 6.5 percent of patients surviving valve replacement with the aortic valve homograft will develop moderate or severe incompetence.[562] Those patients requiring tailoring of the aortic root at the time of valve replacement

develop a significantly higher incidence of homograft incompetence.[562] Homografts requiring replacement within the first 18 months after insertion usually had a prolapsed leaflet, while a tear or perforation of leaflet tissue is noted in those replaced later.[561] Reports from groups using fresh antibiotic-treated homografts (Angell et al.,[563] Barratt-Boyes et al.,[564] and Gonzalez-Lavin et al.[565]) suggest a reduced incidence of valve failure compared with that of chemically treated or irradiated valves.

Experience with and successful use of homografts for mitral valve replacement has been limited. Graham and associates found that only 50 percent of their patients receiving mounted aortic homografts for mitral valve replacement were alive with a well-functioning valve at 5 years.[566]

Difficulty in procuring homografts and the need for unusually precise surgical technique in their implantation have resulted in the use of bovine and porcine heterograft valves. The most widely utilized heterograft valve is the Hancock porcine prosthesis. This composite-tissue valve composed of porcine aortic leaflets mounted on a flexible stent and pretreated with a tanning agent, glutaraldehyde, was first clinically implanted in the mitral position in February 1969.[567] Drs. Charles Hatcher, Ellis Jones, Joseph Craver, and Joseph Miller at Emory University Hospital have utilized this prosthesis in the mitral position since June 1974 and the aortic position since July 1974 without a single incidence of valve failure.

Since 1967 Ross has utilized autologous pulmonary valves for aortic valve replacement.[568] The pulmonary valve is, in turn, replaced with a reconstructed aortic homograft or aortic heterograft. Ross uses this approach only in patients less than 40 years of age with isolated aortic valve disease. While two of these autografts examined 2 years after implantation were found to be living tissue with an intact structural and cellular content, a less than 4-year follow-up revealed that 27 percent of these patients manifested a diastolic murmur and approximately 3 percent demonstrated degenerative valve failure. However, these complications usually appeared within the first year following surgery with stabilization of the patient's course after this time.[569]

Clinical and hemodynamic assessment of valves

A prosthetic valve should satisfy certain design criteria in order to allow satisfactory long-term human implantation. The prosthesis must present minimal obstruction to blood flow when open, be competent when closed, and respond quickly to alterations in pressure gradients. It must be relatively atraumatic to blood components and nonthrombogenic. Safe and secure implantation should be technically feasible. The prosthesis must be composed of materials which are durable and must function so as not to annoy the patient.[570]

HEMODYNAMICS

Table 60B-6 presents the transvalvular gradients recorded and the effective orifice area calculated for a model representative of each valve design implant-

TABLE 60B-6
Prosthetic aortic valves: Postoperative hemodynamics

Valve type	No. of patients	Average gradient, mm Hg		Average valve area, cm²	Source
		Rest	Exercise		
Starr-Edwards 1000	10	21		1.5	Bristow et al.[574]
Starr-Edwards 2300	8	41*		0.92	Kloster et al.[608]
Starr-Edwards 2310	46	17.5	41	1.43	Rodriguez et al.[575]
Starr-Edwards 2310	15	15		1.5	Kloster et al.[609]
Smeloff-Cutter	7	19	29		McHenry et al.[610]
Kay-Shiley	28	28	37	1.36	Bjork et al.[611]
Bjork-Shiley	57	12.5	17	2.0	Bjork et al.[578]
Lillehei-Kaster	26	16.7		1.87	Starek et al.[572]
Hancock	20	23	37	1.25	Morris et al.[571]

*Numbers beneath bars represent average mean gradients; others represent average peak gradient.

ed in the aortic area. A comparison of the effective orifice areas indicates that the tilting disk valve offers less obstruction to left ventricular outflow. The ratio between total orifice area and tissue diameter of the prosthesis is significantly increased with the tilting disk valve. This feature, coupled with its central flow, results in the larger effective orifice area noted with this design. In addition to the variation in the degree of outflow obstruction depending on valve design, an obstructional difference dependent on valve size has been noted with the porcine heterograft valve[571] and the tilting disk valve.[572,573] The lessening of the degree of obstruction of left ventricular outflow with increasing valve size noted with these valves has not been consistently found with the central-occluder type of valve[574–576] (Table 60B-7). The larger effective orifice area for the tilting disk valve, relative to the other currently available prostheses, makes it the most appropriate prosthesis for a narrow aortic root. An alternative surgical approach to aortic valvular replacement in a narrow aortic root is to enlarge the annulus to permit implantation of a prosthesis with a greater annulus diameter.[38,577]

Table 60B-8 presents the published hemodynamic data for the various types of mitral prostheses currently employed. As is generally the case with the aortic prostheses, the gradient across the cloth-covered models tends to be higher than with the non-cloth-covered.

While minimal regurgitation is a feature of essentially all mechanical prostheses, significant valvular incompetence has not been characteristic of any valve design. In the Bjork-Shiley prosthesis this functional regurgitation is a consequence of its nono-verlapping occluder. Upon closing, the disk fits within the annulus, leaving a minimal space between the edge of the disk and the ring.[578] The minimal "physiologic" leakage through the ball valve occurs just before the ball is seated onto the annulus.[579]

ALTERATION OF BLOOD COMPONENTS

Increased destruction of red blood cells is the most common side effect following insertion of mechanical prostheses. Usually the hemolysis is slight and compensated by increased erythropoiesis, but in a few patients severe hemolytic anemia develops.[580] Hemolysis is more common and more severe after aortic valve replacement than after mitral valve replacement with a reported incidence of hemolytic anemia following aortic ball valve insertion of 5 to 15 percent.[547,581] The greater pressure and velocity of blood flow across the aortic valve probably accounts for this difference. In patients with multiple valve replacement, the incidence of hemolysis is similar to that of aortic valve replacement.[581,582] Valve design is also a critical factor in determining the incidence of hemolysis as evidenced by the lesser degree of hemolysis with the central-flow prostheses[572,573] when compared with the central-occluder prostheses.[580,581] Even the construction material plays a role in this complication with a lower reported incidence of hemolysis associated with the Silastic poppet than

TABLE 60B-7
Effective orifice area

Annulus diameter of prosthesis, mm	Effective orifice area, cm²		
	Bjork-Shiley[573]	Lillehei-Kaster[572]	Hancock[571]
21	1.30	1.30	1.05
23	1.70	1.40	1.29
25	2.20	1.90	1.42

TABLE 60B-8
Prosthetic mitral valves: Postoperative hemodynamics

| Valve type | No. of patients | Average gradient, mm Hg | | Average valve area, cm² | Source |
		Rest	Exercise		
Starr-Edwards 6100, 6120	30	5̄	9̄		Morrow et al.[612]
Starr-Edwards 6300	10	9.4		1.57	Kloster et al.[608]
Starr-Edwards 6310	8	4.9		2.6	Kloster et al.[609]
Smeloff-Cutter	8	6̄	15̄		McHenry et al.[610]
Kay-Shiley	9	10.0		1.7	Brown et al.[613]
Starr-Edwards disk	14	4.0		2.0	Brown et al.[613]
Beall	20	7.0	20.0		Linhart et al.[614]
Lillehei-Kaster	23	6.2		3.0	Starek et al.[572]
Reis-Hancock porcine	17	6.0		2.0	Brown et al.[613]

with the Stellite poppet[580] and significantly greater hemolysis noted with the cloth-covered valves than with their noncloth counterparts.[547,583] Red cell destruction is significantly increased by prosthetic malfunction, particularly paravalvular regurgitation and poppet variance.[547]

Much of the evolution of prosthetic valve design has been directed toward eliminating thromboembolism, another problem caused by the interaction between the foreign surface of the prosthesis and the constituents of blood. While the development of the cloth-covered prostheses and the central-flow tilting disk valves has lowered its incidence, none of the mechanical prostheses have completely eliminated this problem. The cloth-covered valves (Beall, Starr-Edwards 2310-2320) and the central-flow tilting disk valve (Bjork-Shiley) have reported an incidence of thromboembolism of less than 5 percent over 1 to 5 years of follow-up on anticoagulation.[549,576,584] Clearly, these design modifications have decreased the problem of thromboembolism; however, only with adequate anticoagulation is the incidence of thromboembolism in these prostheses insignificant. Bonchek and Starr had no occurrences of emboli among 116 patients with series 2310-2320 prostheses who received warfarin versus 23 thromboembolic episodes in 134 patients without anticoagulation.[549] Javier and associates found that embolization in their patients with Beall valves was four times more frequent when they were not given anticoagulants.[585] Reports of acute prosthesis malfunction due to thrombus formation in patients who are not on anticoagulants is the principal reason Bjork and Henze recommend anticoagulant use with the Bjork-Shiley prosthesis.[585a] While there are reports to the contrary, it appears that there is a higher incidence of embolism with mitral prostheses than with aortic prostheses.[586–588] Possibly the tissue valves represent a solution to the problem of thromboembolism, as there has been less than a 1 percent incidence at Emory University Hospital of thromboembolism with the porcine heterograft valve without anticoagulation regardless of valve site.

DURABILITY

Durability has been firmly established only for the non-cloth-covered ball valve. Strut-cloth wear has necessitated reoperation in some cloth-covered ball valves,[549] and the design modifications to reduce this problem are too recent to assess. Similarly, further follow-up is needed to determine the durability of the tilting disk valve and particularly the tissue valves.

PATIENT ACCEPTABILITY

Patient acceptability of the prosthesis is primarily dependent on the audibility of valve sounds and acceptance of long-term anticoagulation. While all mechanical prostheses are frequently audible to their recipients, the composite-seat Starr-Edwards seems to be the most noticeable.

Medical management of prosthetic valves

Effective long-term follow-up of patients with prosthetic valves is predicated upon careful, repeated auscultation of the prosthetic sounds and an unceasing quest for historical clues to the presence of valve dysfunction. While repeated phonocardiography, echocardiography, or cinefluoroscopy have been advocated as necessary for complete prosthetic follow-up, an approach limiting these expensive tests to a role of ancillary diagnostic procedures in appropriate patients seems more economical and just as effective. Careful observations through history and physical examination will isolate those patients requiring more complete evaluation to exclude prosthetic malfunction.

NORMAL PROSTHETIC VALVE SOUNDS

The opening and closing of mechanic prostheses are audible as sounds of high frequency and short duration. With the conventional ball and disk prostheses, the opening sound represents the impact of the occluder upon the cage, and the closing sound, the occluder striking the annulus of the apparatus. With the tilting disk valve, the closing sound is a metallic clank as the disk strikes the inferior restraining portion of the prosthesis. In the Bjork prosthesis, this restraining surface is the inferior strut, while in the Lillehei-Kaster prosthesis the restraining surface is a small protrusion located at the distal (outflow) edge of the annular housing called the *disk stop*. The opening sound of the Lillehei-Kaster prosthesis is usually inaudible, and this sound in the Bjork-Shiley valve (produced by the disk's striking the flexed portion of the inferior strut) is much less intense than the closing sound.

The closing click of the prosthetic mitral valve, best heard at the apex, is analogous to the mitral component of the first heart sound. The interval from the Q wave of the ECG to the closing click (Q-CC) varies from 0.06 to 0.09 s (average 0.075 s).[589–591] This slight delay in mitral closing as compared with that in normal subjects (0.06 s) probably reflects the small pressure gradient across most prostheses, but poppet inertia and loss of papillary muscle function have also been proposed as explanations.[589] The Q-CC interval may be prolonged further by the presence of atrial fibrillation, suggesting that atrial systole facilitates the closure of the mitral prosthesis.[589]

The opening click of the mitral prosthesis occurs 0.07 to 0.15 s (average 0.12 s) after the onset of aortic closure.[592,593] Conventional ball or disk prostheses are characterized by an opening sound with an intensity in the areas of maximal audibility (lower left sternal border and apex) of at least one-third that of the closing sound.[593] As previously indicated, the opening click of the tilting disk prostheses is much less intense than the closing sound regardless of location.

Patients with properly functioning mitral prostheses may have an early systolic to midsystolic murmur loudest at the apex.[590,591] This murmur probably reflects turbulence of blood as it flows around the prosthetic apparatus projecting into the aortic outflow tract.[590] The less intense and less frequent systolic murmurs associated with low-profile prostheses versus ball valve prostheses are compatible with this proposal.

Closing of the Hancock porcine valve is also defined by a loud, high-frequency sound. The most characteristic auscultatory feature of the Hancock valve in the mitral position, however, is the diastolic "grunt." This low-pitched sound more closely approximating the auscultatory features of a gallop than an opening sound probably represents the latter. This grunt occurs earlier in diastole than a gallop and begins with the 0 point of the apex cardiogram.

The opening click of an aortic prosthesis occurs an average of 0.07 s after the Q wave of the ECG but only 0.02 s after S_1.[590,594] Since the human ear usually perceives as distinct those sounds separated by 0.03 s or more, the aortic opening click may not be audibly separated from the first sound. Opening of the aortic prosthesis may be characterized by multiple clicks as the occluder bounces against the cage with prolonged ejection or decreased ventricular contraction.[594] While pulmonary valve closure can usually be separated from the closing of the aortic prosthesis on the phonocardiogram, the delay in aortic closure due to

poppet inertia may make these sounds indistinguishable to the human ear. All aortic prostheses have at least a grade 1 to 2 (on a scale of six grades) spindle-shaped systolic murmur audible at the second right intercostal space and apex.[590,594,595] The loudest systolic murmur, usually grade 3, is associated with the Hancock porcine prosthesis. Infrequently, a grade 1 early decrescendo diastolic murmur may be audible with a normally functioning mechanical prosthesis.[590] The systolic murmur reflects the turbulence in the blood flow across the prosthesis, while the diastolic murmur is secondary to "physiologic regurgitation."

ALTERATIONS OF PROSTHETIC SOUNDS[596]

While subtle alterations in the intensity and timing of these sounds might be documented by serial phonocardiography, the significance of these subtle changes is too ambiguous to dictate an alteration in the patient's management. Those gross changes which would dictate a change in management are obvious on careful auscultation.

PARAVALVULAR REGURGITATION

An early diastolic decrescendo murmur of grade 2 (out of 6) or greater intensity, particularly one developing 6 or more months after aortic valve replacement, demands evaluation for paravalvular regurgitation.[597] Paraprosthetic mitral regurgitation is characterized by a holosystolic murmur loudest at the apex. Severe mitral paravalvular regurgitation may be associated, however, with a soft, short murmur or even absence of a murmur.[593] A very short S_2-OC interval (0.04 to 0.07 s) is usually evident in these cases.[593]

Radiologic evaluation is particularly useful in cases of suspected paravalvular regurgitation. Prolonged exposure of a well-penetrating upright chest film (posteroanterior view for mitral prostheses and lateral for aortic prostheses) will usually distinguish between normal and abnormal prosthesis movement. This technique produces a double exposure of the prosthesis. The separation of images at the apex of the cage is normally no more than 3 to 5 mm with excessive movement suggesting a loose prosthesis[598] (Fig. 60B-40). Cineradiography can also be used to define the tilting motion for the prosthesis. However, the large degree of overlap between the tilting motion of normal and abnormal valves makes this procedure useful only for serial follow-up, a significant increase in the angle of tilt over a previous study in the same patient suggesting a loose valve.[599]

POPPET VARIANCE

Prosthetic valve dysfunction resulting from physical and chemical alterations in the poppets is termed *poppet* (ball or disk) *variance*. It has been documented most often in the Starr-Edwards 1000 series aortic valve (75 percent incidence in one group followed for 18 to 67 months)[597] but has also been detected in the

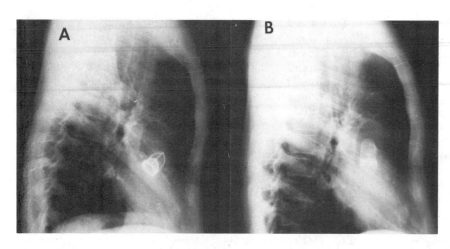

FIGURE 60B-40 Lateral chest roentgenograms taken on the same patient 6 months apart. *A.* A stable aortic ball valve prosthesis. *B.* A double image of the prosthesis indicative of a loose prosthesis with paravalvular regurgitation.

1200 Starr-Edwards valve, Magovern sutureless valve, Harken ball valve, and Hufnagel disk valve.[600]

Ball variance results from either lipid infiltration or abrasion injury. Lipid infiltration causes swelling of the poppet with an associated increase in weight, while the less common abrasion injury reduces the weight of the poppet. Both forms of ball variance occur much more frequently in the aortic position. Serum lipid levels do not seem to influence the development of ball variance. While a detection of very faint, absent, or low-pitched (thud rather than click) prosthetic opening sound (occurring in approximately 75 percent) is the best means of detecting ball variance, the following symptoms and signs should suggest this possibility: fatigue, exertional dyspnea, palpitations, dizzy spells, angina, syncope, emboli, hemolytic anemia, or late development of aortic regurgitation. In contrast to aortic ball variance, the patient with mitral ball dysfunction is usually symptomatic with signs of pulmonary congestion or emboli. A delayed and diminished opening sound is the auscultatory hallmark of this dilemma.[597] Mechanical malfunction related to the disk poppet differs from ball variance. In these prostheses, surface injury occurs at the edge of the poppet in the form of wearing and grooving. Wearing of the disk results in insufficiency due to incomplete occlusion of the inflow orifice, while grooving may lead to locking of the disk in a fixed position producing severe incompetence.[601] When the complication of poppet variance is suspected, phonocardiography, echocardiography, and cinefluoroscopy are indicated. Confirmation of this complication by any one of these procedures warrants immediate valve replacement.

THROMBOEMBOLISM

The clinical findings of thrombosis of prosthetic valves are identical to those of ball variance. For example, a diminished or absent prosthetic opening sound suggests thrombus of aortic ball prosthesis, while a diminished and delayed mitral opening sound (S_2-OC $\geq$ 0.15 s) suggests thrombus or tissue ingrowth.[602] Thrombus of the aortic Bjork-Shiley valve is characterized by absence of the closing click and increase in intensity of the systolic murmur and often an increased diastolic murmur.[603] As surgical intervention is indicated in either form of prosthesis malformation, a misdiagnosis of one problem in the presence of the other is acceptable. The reported incidence of mitral valve (disk or ball) thrombosis is greater than that of mitral variance or aortic valve thrombosis. Early mitral thrombosis is usually associated with a reduced cardiac output, while late thrombosis often accompanies endocarditis or discontinuation of anticoagulants. Previous discontinuation of anticoagulants is also frequently the case in aortic valve thrombosis.[601]

The thrombotic complications of prosthetic valves may be manifest as peripheral emboli. Approximately 65 percent of the clinically recognized emboli arising from the prosthetic valve are cerebral. The next most common site is coronary (15 to 25 percent). Other sites include renal, mesenteric and retinal sites, and the extremities.[588,604] As indicated earlier, we believe that all currently available mechanical prostheses require permanent anticoagulation to prevent these embolic episodes. Studies to date do not support the idea that anticoagulation can be discontinued after sufficient time has elapsed to allow for endothelialization of cloth-covered valves.[586] However, we do not believe anticoagulants are required with the porcine heterograft valve unless it is placed in the mitral position in a patient with chronic atrial fibrillation or a massive left atrium. Follow-up evaluation should include a search for transient or permanent neurologic deficits to exclude cerebral emboli and an ECG to exclude coronary emboli. Detection of an embolic episode should lead to evaluation of prosthesis malfunction and measurement of prothrombin time. In the absence of prosthesis malfunction, a single embolic episode is managed by closer control of anticoagulation and possibly the addition of dipyridamole. Repeated embolic episodes are generally managed by valve replacement even in the absence of prosthesis malfunction.

ENDOCARDITIS

Endocarditis of the prosthetic valve should also be considered following any embolic episode. Since fever is present in virtually all such patients, this complication can be excluded by the absence of fever or its associated symptoms, chills and night sweats.[582] In addition to fever and the evidence of systemic embolization, a new murmur of paravalvular regurgitation is the most common and helpful finding in the clinical recognition of this particular complication.[582] The paravalvular regurgitation develops as the sutures anchoring the prosthesis tear through the necrotic annulus which is the primary site of infection.[605]

The reported incidence of prosthetic endocarditis varies between 1 and 10 percent, most recent studies reporting less than 4 percent. Prosthetic endocarditis occurring within the first 60 days after surgery is usually secondary to contamination during surgery or to postoperative infections in noncardiac areas. *Staphylococcus epidermidis* or *S. aureus* is the infecting organism in about half of the cases, and fungal or gram-negative bacillary organisms are cultured in the others.[582] The mortality rate of 87 percent reported by Slaughter et al.[606] and 68 percent noted by Dismukes et al.[607] reflects the poor response to therapy with early prosthetic endocarditis. The response to therapy is significantly better in endocarditis developing more than 60 days after surgery. This improved prognosis is probably related to differences in the infecting organism. *Streptococcus* species are the most common implicated organisms, with *Staphylococcus* less common, and gram-negative and fungus organisms uncommon. The fact that the precipitating event is often a dental procedure, pyogenic skin infection, or genitourinary manipulation underlines the importance of prophylactic antibiotics in patients with prosthetic valves.[582] This aspect of the management of prosthetic valves as well as the antibiotic regimens used in treatment of endocarditis is outlined in Chap. 77.

HEMOLYSIS

Recognition that hemolysis may occur with a normally functioning mechanical prosthesis and is often an early harbinger of prosthetic malfunction dictates that follow-up evaluation includes a hematocrit and reticulocyte count. These two tests can effectively exclude significant hemolysis and hemolytic anemia. A suspicion of hemolysis arising from the results of these tests should be confirmed by the presence of schistocytes on peripheral smear, an elevated serum LDH (particularly fractions 1 and 2), and a decreased serum haptoglobin.[581,583] When confirmed, the hemolysis should be treated with oral iron and folic acid. A deficiency of these substances arises because of their increased utilization in the maintenance of accelerated erythropoiesis. The iron deficiency may be magnified by excessive urinary iron excretion. In chronic hemolysis, free hemoglobin passes through the glomerular filter into the proximal tubules where it is absorbed by the cells and converted to ferritin and hemosiderin. When these tubule cells desquamate, the iron is lost into the urine. Occasionally, hemolysis can be reduced by reduction of the patient's physical activity or by the use of Inderal (propranolol). Severe hemolysis which is not controlled by a combination of iron and folic acid plus reduced activity usually indicates valve dysfunction, either an abnormal transvalvular gradient or paravalvular regurgitation.

REFERENCES

1 White, P. D.: "Heart Disease," 1st ed., The Macmillan Company, New York, 1931, p. 480.

1a Van der Horst, R. L., and Hastreiter, A. R.: Congenital Mitral Stenosis, *Am. J. Cardiol.,* 20:773, 1967.

2 Khalil, K. G., Shapiro, I., and Kilman, J. W.: Congenital Mitral Stenosis, *J. Thorac. Cardiovasc. Surg.,* 70:40, 1975.

3 Rusted, I. E., Scheifley, C. H., and Edwards, J. E.: Studies of the Mitral Valve: II. Certain Anatomic Features of the Mitral Valve and Associated Structures in Mitral Stenosis, *Circulation,* 14:398, 1956.

4 Selzer, A., and Cohn, K. E.: Natural History of Mitral Stenosis: A Review, *Circulation,* 45:878, 1972.

5 White, P. D., and Donovan, H.: "Hearts: Their Long Follow-up," W. B. Saunders Company, Philadelphia, 1967.

6 John, S., Krishnaswami, S., Jairaj, P. S., Cherian, G., Muralidharan, S., Sukumar, I. P., and Cherian, G.: The Profile and Surgical Management of Mitral Stenosis in Young Patients, *J. Thorac. Cardiovasc. Surgery.,* 69(4):631, 1975.

7 Wood, P.: "Diseases of the Heart and Circulation," 2d ed., Eyre & Spottiswoode (Publishers), Ltd., London, 1957.

8 Roberts, W. C., and Perloff, J. K.: Mitral Valvular Disease: A Clinicopathologic Survey of the Conditions Causing the Mitral Valve to Function Abnormally, *Ann. Intern. Med.,* 77:939, 1972.

9 Wilhelmsen, L.: Lung Mechanics in Rheumatic Heart Disease, *Acta Med. Scand. Suppl.* 489, 1968.

10 Roy, S. B., Bherdwaj, P., and Bhatia, M. L.: Pulmonary Lung Volume in Mitral Stenosis, *Br. Med. J.,* 2:1466, 1965.

11 Gorlin, R.: The Mechanism of the Signs and Symptoms of Mitral Valve Disease, *Br. Heart J.,* 16:375, 1954.

12 Wood, P.: An Appreciation of Mitral Stenosis, *Br. Med. J.,* 1:1051, 1954.

13 Szekely, P., Turner, R., and Snaith, L.: Pregnancy and the Changing Pattern of Rheumatic Heart Disease, *Br. Heart J.,* 35:1293, 1973.

14 Reichek, N., Shelburne, J. C., and Perloff, J. K.: Clinical Aspects of Rheumatic Valvular Disease, *Prog. Cardiovasc. Dis.,* 15(5):491, 1973.

15 Schwartz, R., Meyerson, R. M., Lawrence, L. T., and Nichols, H. T.: Mitral Stenosis, Massive Pulmonary Hemorrhage and Emergency Valve Replacement, *N. Engl. J. Med.,* 275:755, 1966.

16 Ramsey, H. W., de la Torre, A., Bartley, T. D., and Linhart, J. W.: Intractable Hemoptysis in Mitral Stenosis Treated by Emergency Mitral Commissurotomy, *Ann. Intern. Med.,* 67:588, 1967.

17 Ross, R. S.: Right Ventricular Hypertension as a Cause of Precordial Pain, *Am. Heart J.,* 61:134, 1961.

18 Sharma, N. G. K., Kapoor, C. P., Mahambre, L., and Borkar, M. P.: Ortner's Syndrome, *J. Indian Med. Assoc.,* 60:427, 1973.

19 Harvey, W. P.: Silent Valvular Heart Disease, *Cardiovasc. Clin.,* 5(2):77, 1973.

20 Baker, C. G., and Finnegan, T. R. L.: Epilepsy and Mitral Stenosis, *Br. Heart J.,* 19:159, 1957.

21 Lie, J. T., and Entman, M. L.: "Hole-in-One: Sudden Death: Mitral Stenosis and Left Atrial Thrombus, *Am. Heart J.,* 91:798, 1976.

22 Mounsey, J. P. D.: Inspection and Palpation of the Cardiac Impulse, *Prog. Cardiovasc. Dis.,* 10:187, 1967.

23 Levine, S. A., and Harvey, W. P.: "Clinical Auscultation of the Heart," 2d ed., W. B. Saunders Company, Philadelphia, 1959.

24 Craige, E.: On the Genesis of Heart Sounds: Contributions Made by Echocardiography, *Circulation,* 53:207, 1976.

25 Lakier, J. B., Fritz, V. U., Pocock, W. A., and Barlow, J. B.: Mitral Components of the First Heart Sound, *Br. Heart J.,* 34:160, 1972.

26 Dock, W.: Mode of Production of the First Heart Sound, *Arch. Intern. Med.,* 51:737, 1933.

27 Criley, J. M., Chambers, R. D., and Friedman, N. J.: Departures from the Expected Auscultatory Events in Mitral Stenosis, *Cardiovasc. Clin.,* 5(2):191, 1973.

28 Thompson, M. E., Shaver, J. A., Heidenreich, F. P., Leon, D. F., and Leonard, J. J.: Sound, Pressure and Motion Correlates in Mitral Stenosis, *Am. J. Med.,* 49:436, 1970.

29 Rushmer, R. F.: "Cardiovascular Dynamics," 2d ed., W. B. Saunders Company, Philadelphia, 1961.

30 McKusick, V. A.: "Cardiovascular Sound in Health and Disease," The Williams & Wilkins Company, Baltimore, 1958.

31 Luisada, A. A., MacCanon, D. M., Kumar, S., and Feigen, L. P.: Changing Views on the Mechanism of the First and Second Heart Sounds, *Am. Heart J.,* 88:503, 1974.

32 Parisi, A. F., and Milton, B. G.: Relation of Mitral Valve Closure to the First Heart Sound in Man: Echocardiographic and Phonocardiographic Assessment, *Am. J. Cardiol.,* 32:779, 1973.

33 McCall, B. W., and Price, J. L.: Movement of Mitral Valve Cusps in Relation to First Heart Sound and Opening Snap in Patients with Mitral Stenosis, *Br. Heart J.,* 29:417, 1967.

34 Wooley, C. F., Klassen, K. P., Leighton, R. F., Goodwin, R. S., and Ryan, J. M.: Left Atrial and Left Ventricular Sound and Pressure in Mitral Stenosis, *Circulation,* 38:295, 1968.

35 DiBartolo, G., Nunez-Dey, D., and Bendezu, J.: Left Heart Studies in Mitral Stenosis with Special Reference to Intracardiac Phonocardiography, *Am. J. Cardiol.,* 10:93, 1962.

36 Waider, W., and Craige, E.: First Heart Sound and Ejection Sounds: Echocardiographic and Phonocardiographic Correlations with Valvular Events, *Am. J. Cardiol.,* 35:346, 1975.

37 Dack, S., Bleifer, S., Grishman, A., and Donoso, E.: Mitral Stenosis: Auscultatory and Phonocardiographic Findings, *Am. J. Cardiol.,* 5:815, 1960.

38 Margolies, A., and Wolferth, C. C.: The Opening Snap (*Claquement d'ouverture de la mitrale*) in Mitral Stenosis: Its Characteristics, Mechanism of Production and Diagnostic Importance, *Am. Heart J.,* 7:443, 1932.

39 Legler, J. F., Benchimol, A., and Diamond, E. G.: The Apex Cardiogram in the Study of The 2-OS Interval, *Br. Heart J.,* 25:246, 1963.

40 Friedman, N. J.: Echocardiographic Studies of Mitral Valve Motion: Genesis of the Opening Snap in Mitral Stenosis, *Am. Heart J.,* 80:177, 1970.

41 Ross, R. S., and Criley, J. M.: Cineangiographic Studies of the Origin of Cardiovascular Physical Signs, *Circulation,* 30:255, 261, 1964.

42 Robard, S.: The Mitral Closing Snap, *Am. Heart J.,* 83:19, 1972.

43 Mounsey, P.: The Opening Snap of Mitral Stenosis, *Br. Heart J.,* 15:135, 1953.

44 Wells, B.: The Assessment of Mitral Stenosis by Phonocardiography, *Br. Heart J.,* 16:261, 1954.

45 Davies, J. P. H.: A Simple Phonocardiographic Formula for Predicting Left Atrial Pressure in Mitral Stenosis, *Br. Heart J.,* 29:843, 1967.

46 Yigitbasi, O., Nalbantgil, I., Birand, A., and Terek, A.: O-I/II A-OS Formula for Predicting Left Atrial Pressure in Mitral Stenosis, *Br. Heart J.,* 32:547, 1970.

47 Ebringer, R., Pitt, A., and Anderson, S. T.: Haemodynamic Factors Influencing Opening Snap Interval in Mitral Stenosis, *Br. Heart J.,* 32:350, 1970.

48 Kalmanson, D., Veyrat, C., Bernier, A., Witchitz, S., and Chiche, P.: Opening Snap and Isovolumic Relaxation Period in Relation to Mitral Valve Flow in Patients with Mitral Stenosis: Significance of the A2-OS Interval, *Br. Heart J.,* 38:135, 1976.

49 Weisfeldt, M. L., Scully, H. E., Frederiksen, J., Rubenstein, J. J., Pohost, G. M., Beirholm, E., Bello, A. G., and Daggett, W. M.: Hemodynamic Determinants of Maximum Negative dp/dt and the Periods of Diastole, *Am. J. Physiol.,* 227:613, 1974.

50 Messer, A. L., Counihan, T. B., Rappaport, M. P., and Sprague, H. B.: The Effect of Cycle Length on the Time of Occurrence of the First Sound and O.S. in Mitral Stenosis, *Circulation,* 4:576, 1951.

51 Cheng, T. O.: Phonocardiographic Sign for Pliability of a Stenotic Mitral Valve, *Circulation,* 34(suppl. 3):72, 1966.

52 Nixon, P. G., Wooler, G. H., and Radigan, L. R.: The Opening Snap in Mitral Incompetence, *Br. Heart J.,* 22:395, 1960.

53 Millward, D. K., McLaurin, L. P., and Craige, E.: Echocardiographic Studies to Explain Opening Snaps in Presence of Non-stenotic Mitral Valves, *Am. J. Cardiol.,* 31:64, 1973.

54 Nasser, W. K., Davis, R. H., Dillon, J. C., Tavel, M. E., Helman, C. H., Feigenbaum, H., and Fisch, C.: Atrial Myxoma: II. Phonocardiographic, Echocardiographic Hemodynamic and Angiographic Features in Nine Cases, *Am. Heart J.,* 83:810, 1972.

55 Leatham, A., and Gray, I.: Auscultatory and Phonocardiographic Signs of Atrial Septal Defect, *Br. Heart J.,* 18:193, 1956.

56 Vacca, J. B., Bussman, D. W., and Mudd, J. G.: Ebstein's Anomaly: Complete Review of 108 Cases, *Am. J. Cardiol.,* 2:210, 1958.

57 Perloff, J. K., and Harvey, W. P.: Clinical Recognition of Tricuspid Stenosis, *Circulation,* 22:346, 1960.

58 Surawicz, B.: Effect of Respiration and Upright Position on the Interval between the Two Components of the Second Heart Sound and That between the Second Sound and Mitral Opening Snap, *Circulation,* 16:422, 1957.

59 Rodin, P., and Tabatznik, P.: The Effects of Posture on Added Heart Sounds, *Br. Heart J.,* 25:69, 1963.

60 Breen, W. J., and Rekate, A. C.: Effects of Posture on Splitting of the Second Heart Sound, *J.A.M.A.,* 173:1326, 1960.

61 Delman, A. J., Gordon, G. M., Stein, E., and Escher, D. J. W.: The Second Sound–Mitral Opening Snap (A2-OS) Interval during Exercise in the Evaluation of Mitral Stenosis, *Circulation,* 33:399, 1966.

62 Cobbs, W. B., Jr., Logue, R. B., and Dorney, E. R.: The Second Heart Sound in Pulmonary Embolism and Pulmonary Hypertension, *Am. Heart J.,* 71:6, 1966.

63 Cobbs, W. B., Jr.: in J. W. Hurst and R. B. Logue (eds.), "The Heart," 3d ed., McGraw-Hill Book Company, New York, 1974.

64 Fortuin, N. J., and Craige, E.: Echocardiographic Studies of Genesis of Mitral Diastolic Murmurs, *Br. Heart J.,* 35:75, 1973.

65 Toutouzas, P., Koidakis, A., Velimezis, A., and Avgoustakis, D.: Mechanism of Diastolic Rumble and Presystolic Murmur in Mitral Stenosis, *Br. Heart J.,* 36:1096, 1974.

66 Criley, J. M., and Hermer, A. J.: The Crescendo Presystolic Murmur of Mitral Stenosis with Atrial Fibrillation, *N. Engl. J. Med.,* 285:1284, 1971.

67 Lakier, J. B., Pocock, W. A., Gale, G. E., and Barlow, J. B.:

Haemodynamic and Sound Events Preceding First Heart Sound in Mitral Stenosis, *Br. Heart J.*, 34:1152, 1972.

68 Tavel, M. E., and Bonner, A. J., Jr.: Presystolic Murmur in Atrial Fibrillation: Fact or Fiction, *Circulation*, 54:167, 1976.

69 Bonner, A. J., Jr., Stewart, J., and Travel, M. E.: "Presystolic" Augmentation of Diastolic Heart Sounds in Atrial Fibrillation, *Am. J. Cardiol.*, 37:427, 1976.

70 McGuire, L. B., Nolan, T. B., Reeve, R., and Dammann, J. F., Jr.: Cor Triatriatum as a Problem of Heart Disease, *Circulation*, 31:263, 1965.

71 Korn, D., DeSanctis, R. W., and Sell, S.: Massive Calcification of the Mitral Annulus, *N. Engl. J. Med.*, 267:900, 1962.

72 Spodick, D. H.: Chronic and Constrictive Pericarditis, Grune & Stratton, Inc., New York, 1964.

73 Berkheit, S., Murtagh, G., Morton, P., and Fletcher, E.: His Bundle Electrogram in P Mitrale, *Br. Heart J.*, 34:1057, 1972.

73a McArthur, J. D., Sukumar, I. P., Munsi, S. C., Krishnaswami, S., and Cherian, G.: Reassessment of Graham Steell Murmur Using Platinum Electrode Technique, *Br. Heart J.*, 36:1023, 1974.

74 Rios, J. C., and Goo, W.: Electrocardiographic Correlates of Rheumatic Valvular Disease, *Cardiovasc. Clin.*, 5(2):247, 1973.

75 Saunders, J. L., Calatayud, J. B., Schulz, K. J., Maranhao, V., Gooch, A. S., and Goldberg, H.: Evaluation of E.C.G. Criteria for P-Wave Abnormalities, *Am. Heart J.*, 74:757, 1967.

76 Davies, M. J., and Pomerance, A.: Pathology of Atrial Fibrillation in Man, *Br. Heart J.*, 34:520, 1972.

77 Hugenholtz, P. G., Ryan, T. J., Stein, S. W., and Abelmann, W. H.: The Spectrum of Pure Mitral Stenosis: Hemodynamic Studies in Relation to Clinical Disability, *Am. J. Cardiol.*, 10:773, 1962.

78 Rowe, J. C., Bland, E. F., Sprague, H. B., and White, P. D.: The Course of Mitral Stenosis without Surgery: Ten and Twenty Year Perspectives, *Ann. Intern. Med.*, 52:741, 1960.

79 Probst, P., Goldschlager, N., and Selzer, A.: Left Atrial Size and Atrial Fibrillation in Mitral Stenosis: Factors Influencing Their Relationship, *Circulation*, 48:1282, 1973.

80 Trounce, J. R.: The Electrocardiogram in Mitral Stenosis, *Br. Heart J.*, 14:185, 1952.

81 Milnor, W. R.: Electrocardiogram and Vectorcardiogram in Right Ventricular Hypertrophy and Right Bundle Branch Block, *Circulation*, 16:348, 1957.

82 Lee, Y. C., Scherlis, L., and Singleton, R. T.: Mitral Stenosis: Hemodynamic, Electrocardiographic and Vector Cardiographic Studies, *Am. Heart J.*, 69:559, 1965.

83 Walston, A., Harley, A., and Pipberger, H. V.: Computer Analysis of the Orthogonal Electrocardiogram and Vectorcardiogram in Mitral Stenosis, *Circulation*, 50:472, 1974.

84 Semler, H. J., and Pruitt, R. D.: An Electrocardiographic Estimation of the Pulmonary Vascular Obstruction in 80 Patients with Mitral Stenosis, *Am. Heart J.*, 59:541, 1960.

85 Demerdash, H., and Goodwin, J. F.: The Cardiogram of Mitral Restinosis, *Br. Heart J.*, 25:474, 1963.

86 Cueto, J., Toshima, J., Armijo, G., Tuna, N., and Lillehei, W.: Vectorcardiographic Studies of Acquired Valvular Disease with Reference to the Diagnosis of Right Ventricular Hypertrophy, *Circulation*, 33:588, 1967.

87 Chou, T. C., Helm, R. A., and Kaplan, S.: "Clinical Vectorcardiology," 2d ed., Grune & Stratton, Inc., New York, 1974.

88 Chen, J. T. T., Behar, V. S., Morris, J. J., Jr., McIntosh, H. D., and Lester, R. G.: Correlation of Roentgen Findings with Hemodynamic Data in Pure Mitral Stenosis, *Am. J. Roentgenol. Radium Ther. Nucl. Med.*, 102:280, 1968.

89 Amplatz, K.: The Roentgenographic Diagnosis of Mitral and Aortic Valvular Disease, *Am. Heart J.*, 64:556, 1962.

90 Wade, G., Werko, L., Eliasch, H., Gidlund, A., and Lagerlof, H.: The Hemodynamic Basis of Symptoms and Signs in Mitral Valvular Disease. *Q. J. Med.*, 21:361, 1952.

91 Felson, B.: "Chest Roentgenology," W. B. Saunders Company, Philadelphia, 1973.

92 Melhem, R. E., Dunbar, J. D., and Booth, R. W.: "B" lines of Kerley and Left Atrial Size in Mitral Valve Disease: Their Correlation with Mean Left Atrial Pressure as Measured by Left Atrial Puncture, *Radiology*, 76:65, 1961.

93 Kennedy, J. W., Yarnall, S. R., Murray, J. A., and Figley, M. M.: Quantitative Angiography: IV. Relationships of Left Atrial and Ventricular Pressure and Volume in Mitral Valve Disease, *Circulation*, 41:817, 1970.

94 Grainger, R. G.: Interstitial Pulmonary Edema and Its Radiographic Diagnosis: Signs of Pulmonary Venous and Capillary Hypertension, *Br. J. Radiol.*, 31:201, 1958.

95 Fleischner, F. G., and Reiner, L.: Linear X-ray Shadows in Acquired Pulmonary Hemosiderosis and Congestion, *N. Engl. J. Med.*, 250:900, 1954.

96 Brewer, A. J., Ellis, F. H., and Kirklin, J. W.: Castophenic Septal Lines in Pulmonary Venous Hypertension, *Circulation*, 12:807, 1955.

97 Meszaros, W. T.: Lung Changes in Left Heart Failure, *Circulation*, 47:859, 1973.

98 Chait, A.: Interstitial Pulmonary Edema, *Circulation*, 45:1323, 1972.

99 Anderson, L. H., Johansen, J. K., and Hyldebrandt, N.: Regional Pulmonary Blood Flow in Mitral Disease Studied by Xenon Radiospirometry, *Br. Heart J.*, 38:573, 1976.

100 Ellis, L. B., and Harken, D. E.: Closed Valvuloplasty for Mitral Stenosis: A Twelve-Year Follow-up Study of 1571 Patients, *N. Engl. J. Med.*, 270:643, 1964.

101 Ellis, L. B., Singh, J. B., Morales, D. D., and Harken, D. E.: Fifteen to Twenty Year Study of One Thousand Patients Undergoing Closed Mitral Valvuloplasty, *Circulation*, 48:357, 1973.

102 Kruger, S., Starke, H., Miscia, V. F., and Forker, A. D.: Echocardiographic Diagnosis of Silent Mitral Stenosis, *Nebr. Med. J.*, 60(5):159, 1975.

103 Teicholz, L. E.: Echocardiography in Valvular Heart Disease, *Prog. Cardiovasc. Dis.*, 17(4):283, 1975.

104 Raj, M. V. J., Bennett, D. H., Stovin, P. G. I., and Evans, D. W.: Echocardiographic Assessment of Mitral Valve Calcification, *Br. Heart J.*, 38:81, 1976.

105 McDonald, I. G.: Echocardiographic Assessment of Left Ventricular Function in Mitral Valve Disease, *Circulation*, 53:865, 1976.

106 McLarin, L. P., Gibson, T. C., Waider, W., Grossman, W., and Craige, E.: An Appraisal of Mitral Valve Echocardiograms Mimicking Mitral Stenosis in Conditions with Right Ventricular Pressure Overload, *Circulation*, 48:801, 1973.

107 Quinones, M. A., Gaash, W. H., Waisser, E., and Alexander, J. K.: Reduction in the Rate of Diastolic Descent of the Mitral Valve Echogram in Patients with Altered Left Ventricular Diastolic Pressure-Volume Relations, *Circulation*, 49:246, 1974.

108 Wolfe, S. B., Popp, R. L., and Feigenbaum, H.: Diagnosis of Atrial Tumors by Ultrasound, *Circulation*, 39:615, 1969.

109 Duchak, J. M., Chang, S., and Feigenbaum, H.: The Posterior Mitral Valve Echo and the Echocardiographic Diagnosis of Mitral Stenosis, *Am. J. Cardiol.*, 29:628, 1972.

110 Levisman, J. A., Abassi, A. S., and Pearce, M. L.: Posterior Mitral Leaflet Motion in Mitral Stenosis, *Circulation*, 51:511, 1975.

111 Flaherty, J. T., Livengood, S., and Fortuin, N. J.: Atypical Posterior Leaflet Motion in Echocardiogram in Mitral Stenosis, *Am. J. Cardiol.*, 35:675, 1975.

112 Cope, G. D., Kisslo, J. A., Johnson, M. L., and Behar, V. S.: A

Reassessment of the Echocardiogram in Mitral Stenosis, *Circulation,* 52:664, 1975.

113 Winters, W. L., Riccetto, A., Gimenez, J., McDonough, M., and Soulen, R.: Reflected Ultrasound as a Diagnostic Instrument in Study of MVD. *Br. Heart J.,* 29:788, 1967.

114 Nanda, N. C., Gramiak, R., and Shah, P. M.: Echocardiographic Misdiagnosis of the Severity of Mitral Stenosis, *Clin. Res.,* 23:199A, 1975.

115 Gramiak, R., Nanda, N. C., in R. Gramiak and R. C. Waag (eds.), "Cardiac Ultrasound," The C. V. Mosby Company, St. Louis, 1975.

116 Feigenbaum, H.: Echocardiography, Lea & Febiger, Philadelphia, 1972.

117 Nanda, N. C., Gramiak, R., Shah, P. M., and DeWeese, J. A.: Mitral Commissurotomy versus Replacement: Preoperative Evaluation by Echocardiography, *Circulation,* 51:263, 1975.

118 Nanda, N. C., Gramiak, R., Shah, P. M., DeWeese, S. A., and Mahoney, E. G.: Echocardiographic Assessment of Left Ventricular Outflow Width in the Selection of Mitral Valve Prosthesis, *Circulation,* 48:1208, 1973.

119 Effert, S.: Pre and Post Operative Evaluation of Mitral Stenosis by Ultrasound, *Am. J. Cardiol.,* 19:59, 1967.

120 Gorlin, R., and Gorlin, S. G.: Hydraulic Formula for Calculation of the Area of the Stenotic Mitral Valve, Other Cardiac Valves and Central Circulatory Shunts, *Am. Heart J.,* 41:1, 1951.

121 Cohen, M. V., and Gorlin, R.: Modified Orifice Equation for the Calculation of Mitral Valve Area, *Am. Heart J.,* 84:839, 1972.

122 Selzer, A., and Malmborg, R. O.: Some Factors Influencing Changes in Pulmonary Vascular Resistance in Mitral Valve Disease, *Am. J. Med.,* 32:532, 1962.

123 Nakhjavan, F. K., Katz, M. R., Maranhao, V., and Goldberg, H.: Analysis of Influence of Catecholamine and Tachycardia during Supine Exercise in Patients with Mitral Stenosis and Sinus Rhythm, *Br. Heart J.,* 31:753, 1969.

124 Kasalicky, J., Huryck, J., Widimsky, R., Dejdar, R., Metys, R., and Stanek, V.: Left Heart Haemodynamics at Rest and during Exercise in Patients with Mitral Stenosis, *Br. Heart J.,* 30:188, 1968.

125 Bolen, J. L., Lopes, M. G., Harrison, D. C., and Alderman, E. L.: Analysis of Left Ventricular Function in Response to Afterload Changes in Patients with Mitral Stenosis, *Circulation,* 52:894, 1975.

126 Selzer, A., and Cohn, K.: The "Myocardial Factor" in Valvular Heart Disease, *Cardiovasc. Clin.,* 5(2):177, 1973.

127 Heller, S. J., and Carleton, R. A.: Abnormal Left Ventricular Contraction in Patients with Mitral Stenosis, *Circulation,* 42:1099, 1970.

128 Curry, G. C., Elliott, L. P., and Ramsey, H. W.: Quantitative Left Ventricular Angiocardiographic Finding in Mitral Stenosis, *Am. J. Cardiol.,* 29:621, 1972.

129 Hildner, F. J., Javier, R. P., Cohen, L. S., Samet, P., Nathan, M. J., Yahr, W. Z., and Greenberg, J. J.: Myocardial Dysfunction Associated with Valvular Heart Disease, *Am. J. Cardiol.,* 30:319, 1972.

130 Linhart, J. W.: Atrial Pacing in the Determination of Myocardial Function in Patients with Mitral Stenosis, *Chest,* 61:134, 1972.

131 Parker, B. M., Friedenberg, M. J., Templeton, A. W., and Burford, T. H.: Preoperative Angiocardiographic Diagnosis of Left Atrial Thrombi in Mitral Stenosis, *N. Engl. J. Med.,* 273:136, 1965.

132 Olesen, K.: The Natural History of 271 Patients with Mitral Stenosis under Medical Treatment, *Br. Heart J.,* 24:349, 1962.

133 Bailey, G. W. H., Braniff, B. A., Hancock, E. W., and Cohn, E. E.: Relation of Left Atrial Pathology to Atrial Fibrillation in Mitral Valvular Disease, *Ann. Intern. Med.,* 69:13, 1968.

134 Arani, D. T., and Carleton, R. A.: The Deleterious Role of Tachycardia in Mitral Stenosis, *Circulation,* 36:511, 1967.

135 Mitchell, J. H., and Shapiro, W.: Atrial Function and the Hemodynamic Consequences of Atrial Fibrillation in Man, *Am. J. Cardiol.,* 23:556, 1969.

136 Braunwald, E., Moscovitz, H. L., Amram, S. S., Lasser, R. P., Sapin, S. O., Himmelstein, A., Ravitch, M. M., and Gordon, A. J.: The Hemodynamics of the Left Side of the Heart as Studied by Simultaneous Left Atrial, Left Ventricular and Aortic Pressures: Particular Reference to Mitral Stenosis, *Circulation,* 12:77, 1955.

137 Selzer, A.: Effects of Atrial Fibrillation upon the Circulation in Patients with Mitral Stenosis, *Am. Heart J.,* 59:518, 1960.

138 Resnekov, L.: Hemodynamic Studies before and after Electrical Conversion of Atrial Fibrillation and Flutter to Sinus Rhythm, *Br. Heart J.,* 29:700, 1967.

139 Scott, M. E., and Patterson, G. C.: Cardiac Output after Direct Current Conversion of Atrial Fibrillation, *Br. Heart J.,* 31:87, 1969.

140 DeMaria, A. N., Lies, J. E., King, J. F., Miller, R. R., Amsterdam, E. A., and Mason, D. T.: Echocardiographic Assessment of Atrial Transport Mitral Movement, and Ventricular Performance following Electroversion of Supraventricular Arrhythmias, *Circulation,* 51:273, 1975.

141 Spann, J. E., Jr., and Sands, M. J., Jr.: The Incidence and Significance of Atrial Dysrhythmias in Rheumatic Valvular Disease, *Cardiovas. Clin.,* 5(2):115, 1973.

142 Selzer, A., and Cohn, K. K.: Natural History of Mitral Stenosis: A Review, *Circulation,* 45:878, 1972.

143 Daley, R., Mattingly, T. W., Holt, C. L., Bland, E. F., and White, P. D.: Systemic Arterial Embolism in Rheumatic Heart Disease, *Am. Heart J.,* 42:566, 1951.

144 Abernathy, W. S., and Willis, P. W., III: Thromboembolic Complications of Rheumatic Heart Disease, *Cardiovasc. Clin.,* 5(2):131, 1973.

145 Kellogg, F., Lui, C. K., Fishman, W., and Larson, R.: Systemic and Pulmonary Emboli Before and After Mitral Commissurotomy, *Circulation,* 24:263, 1961.

146 Pittman, J. G., and Cohen, P.: The Pathogenesis of Cardiac Cachexia, *N. Engl. J. Med.,* 271:403, 453, 1964.

147 Conference: Cardiovascular Problems Associated with Aviation Safety: Task Force VI. Valvular Heart Disease, *Am. J. Cardiol.,* 36:617, 1975.

148 Upton, A. R. M., and Honey, M.: Electroconversion of Atrial Fibrillation after Mitral Valvotomy, *Br. Heart J.,* 33:732, 1971.

149 Adams, G. F., Merrett, J. D., Hutchinson, W. M., and Pollock, A. M.: Cerebral Embolism and Mitral Stenosis: Survival with and without Anticoagulants, *J. Neurol. Neurosurg. Psychiatry,* 37:378, 1974.

149a Bhatia, M. L., Shrivastova, S., and Roy, S. B.: Immediate Haemodynamic Effects of a Beta Adrenergic Blocking Agent—Propranolol—in Mitral Stenosis at Fixed Heart Rates, *Br. Heart J.,* 34:638, 1972.

149b Feitosa, G. S., Engel, T. R., Helfant, R. H., Frankl, W. S., and Meister, S. G.: Potential Therapeutic Value of Propranolol in Mitral Stenosis during Sinus Rhythm, *Circulation,* 50(suppl. 3):III-225, 1974. (Abstract.)

150 Selzer, A.: Cardiac Valve Replacement: An Unanswered Question, *Am. J. Cardiol.,* 37:322, 1976. (Editorial.)

151 Deverall, P. B., Olley, P. M., and Smith, D. R.: Incidence of Systemic Emboli before and after Mitral Valvotomy, *Thorax,* 23:530, 1968.

152 Cohn, L. H., and Collins, J. J., Jr.: Surgical Treatment of Mitral Stenosis: A Medical Milestone, *N. Engl. J. Med.,* 289:1035, 1973. (Editorial.)

153 Kirsner, A. B., and Sheon, R. P.: Medico-Chirurgical Transactions, *Circulation,* 42:751, 1970.

154 Jarcho, S.: Historical Milestones: Edwin Klebs on Experimental Valvulotomy (1875), *Am. J. Cardiol.*, 19:572, 1967.

155 Brunton, L.: Preliminary Note on the Possibility of Treating Mitral Stenosis by Surgical Methods, *Lancet*, 1:352, 1902.

156 Harken, D. E., and Curtis, L. E.: Historical Milestones: Heart Surgery—Legend and a Long Look, *Am. J. Cardiol.*, 19:393, 1967.

157 Ellis, L. B., and Harken, D. E.: The Clinical Results in the First 500 Patients with Mitral Stenosis Undergoing Valvuloplasty, *Circulation*, 11:637, 1955.

158 Glover, R. P., Davilax, J. C., O'Neill, T. J. E., and Janton, O. H.: Does Mitral Stenosis Recur after Commissurotomy? *Am. J. Cardiol.*, 11:14, 1955.

159 Dickens, J., Villaca, L., Woldow, A., and Goldberg, H.: The Hemodynamics of Mitral Stenosis before and after Commissurotomy, *Br. Heart J.*, 19:419, 1957.

160 Gobel, F. L., Andrew, D. J., Witherspoon, J. M., Lillehei, R. C., Castandea, A., and Wang, Y.: The Hemodynamic Results of Instrumental and Digital Valvotomy in Patients with Mitral Stenosis, *Circulation*, 39:317, 1969.

161 Morrow, A. G., Oldham, H. N., Elkins, R. C., and Braunwald, E.: Prosthetic Replacement of the Mitral Valve: Preoperative and Postoperative Clinical and Hemodynamic Assessments in 100 Patients, *Circulation*, 35:962, 1967.

162 Levine, F. H., Copeland, J. G., and Morrow, A. G.: Prosthetic Replacement of the Mitral Valve: Continuing Assessments of the 100 Patients Operated upon During 1961–1965, *Circulation*, 47:518, 1973.

163 Appelbaum, A., Kouchoukos, N. T., Blackstone, E. H., and Kirklin, J. W.: Early Risks of Open Heart Surgery for Mitral Valve Disease, *Am. J. Cardiol.*, 37:201, 1976.

164 Ward, C., and Hancock, B. W.: Extreme Pulmonary Hypertension Caused by Mitral Valve Disease: Natural History and Results of Surgery, *Br. Heart J.*, 37:74, 1975.

165 Dahl, J. C., Winchell, P., and Borden, C. W.: Mitral Stenosis: A Long-Term Postoperative Follow-up, *Arch. Intern. Med.*, 119:92, 1967.

166 Mullin, E. M., Jr., Glancy, D. L., Higgs, L. M., Epstein, S. E., and Morrow, A. G.: Current Results of Operation for Mitral Stenosis: Clinical and Hemodynamic Assessments in 124 Consecutive Patients Treated by Closed Commissurotomy, Open Commissurotomy or Valve Replacement, *Circulation*, 46:298, 1972.

167 Barnhorst, D. A., Oxman, H. A., Connolly, D. C., Pluth, J. R., Danielson, G. K., Wallace, R. B., and McGoon, D. C.: Long-Term Follow-up of Isolated Replacement of the Aortic or Mitral Valve with the Starr-Edwards Prosthesis, *Am. J. Cardiol.*, 35:228, 1975.

168 Feigenbaum, H., Linback, R. E., and Nasser, W. K.: Hemodynamic Studies before and after Instrumental Mitral Commissurotomy: A Reappraisal of the Pathophysiology of Mitral Stenosis and the Efficacy of Mitral Valvotomy, *Circulation*, 38:261, 1968.

169 Braunwald, E., Braunwald, N. S., Ross, J., Jr., and Morrow, A. G.: Effects of Mitral-Valve Replacement on the Pulmonary Vascular Dynamics of Patients with Pulmonary Hypertension, *N. Engl. J. Med.*, 273:509, 1965.

170 Dalen, J. E., Matloff, J. M., Evans, G. L., Hoppin, F. G., Jr., Bhardwaj, P., Harken, D. E., and Dexter, L.: Early Reduction of Pulmonary Vascular Resistance after Mitral-Valve Replacement, *N. Engl. J. Med.*, 277:387, 1967.

171 Zener, J. C., Hancock, E. W., Shumway, N. E., and Harrison, D. C.: Regression of Extreme Pulmonary Hypertension after Mitral Valve Surgery, *Am. J. Cardiol.*, 30:820, 1972.

172 Donald, K. W., Bishop, J. M., Wade, O. L., and Wormald, P. N.: Cardiorespiratory Function Two Years after Mitral Valvotomy, *Clin. Sci.*, 16:325, 1957.

173 Logan, A., Lowther, C. P., and Turner, R. W. D.: Reoperation for Mitral Stenosis, *Lancet*, 1:443, 1962.

174 Dubost, C.: Evaluation of Surgery for Mitral Valve Disease, *Am. Heart J.*, 82:143, 1971. (Editorial.)

175 Higgs, L. M., Glancy, D. L., O'Brien, K. P., Epstein, S. E., and Morrow, A. G.: Mitral Restenosis: An Uncommon Cause of Recurrent Symptoms following Mitral Commissurotomy, *Am. J. Cardiol.*, 26:34, 1970.

176 Harken, D. E., and Ellis, L. B.: Recurrent Symptoms after Surgery for Mitral Stenosis, *Am. J. Cardiol.*, 26:219, 1970. (Editorial.)

177 Peterson, C. R., Herr, R., Crisera, R. V., Starr, A., Bristow, J. D., and Griswold, H. E.: The Failure of Hemodynamic Improvement after Valve Replacement Surgery, *Ann. Intern. Med.*, 66:1, 1967.

178 Ross, J., Jr., Braunwald, E., and Morrow, A. G.: Clinical and Hemodynamic Observations in Pure Mitral Insufficiency, *Am. J. Cardiol.*, 2:11, 1958.

179 Selzer, A., and Katayama, F.: Mitral Regurgitation: Clinical Patterns, Pathophysiology and Natural History, *Medicine (Baltimore)*, 51:337, 1972.

180 Priest, E. A., Finlayson, J. K., and Short, D. S.: The X-ray Manifestations in the Heart and Lungs of Mitral Regurgitation, *Prog. Cardiovasc. Dis.*, 5:219, 1962.

181 Tompkins, D. G., Boxerbaum, B., and Liebman, J.: Long Term Prognosis of Rheumatic Fever Patients Receiving Regular Intramuscular Benzathine Penicillin, *Circulation*, 45:543, 1972.

182 Magida, M. G., and Streitfeld, F. H.: The Natural History of Rheumatic Heart Disease in the Third, Fourth and Fifth Decades of Life: II. Prognosis and Special Reference to Morbidity, *Circulation*, 16:713, 1957.

183 Wilson, M. G.: The Life History of Systolic Murmurs in Rheumatic Heart Disease, *Prog. Cardiovasc. Dis.*, 5:145, 1962.

184 Perloff, J. K., and Harvey, W. P.: Auscultatory and Phonocardiographic Manifestations of Pure Mitral Regurgitation, *Prog. Cardiovasc. Dis.*, 5(2):172, 1962.

185 Bentivoglio, L., Urichio, J., and Goldberg, H.: Clinical and Hemodynamic Features of Advanced Rheumatic Mitral Regurgitation, *Am. J. Med.*, 30:372, 1961.

186 Ellis, L. B., and Ramirez, A.: The Clinical Course of Patients with Severe "Rheumatic" Mitral Insufficiency, *Am. Heart J.*, 78:406, 1969.

187 Brigden, W., and Leatham, A.: Mitral Incompetence, *Br. Heart J.*, 15:55, 1953.

188 Levy, M. J., and Edwards, J. E.: Anatomy of Mitral Insufficiency, *Prog. Cardiovasc. Dis.*, 5:119, 1962.

189 Nixon, P. G. F., Woller, G. H., and Radigan, L. R.: Mitral Incompetence Caused by Disease of the Mural Cusp, *Circulation*, 19:839, 1959.

190 Braunwald, E.: Mitral Regurgitation: Physiologic, Clinical and Surgical Considerations, *N. Engl. J. Med.*, 281:425, 1969.

191 McDonald, L., Dealy, J. B., Jr., Rabinowitz, M., and Dexter, L.: Clinical Physiological Findings in Mitral Stenosis and Regurgitation, *Medicine (Baltimore)*, 36:237, 1957.

192 Stapleton, J. F., and Groves, B. M.: Precordial Palpation, *Am. Heart J.*, 81:409, 1971.

193 Ewy, G. A., Gomex, L., and Marcus, F. I.: Left Parasternal Pulsations in Patients with Mitral Insufficiency, *Circulation*, 32(suppl. 2):II-83, 1965. (Abstract.)

194 Armstrong, T. G., Meeran, M. K., and Gotsman, M. S.: The Left Atrial Lift, *Am. Heart J.*, 82:764, 1971.

195 Basta, L. L., Wolfson, P., Eckberg, D. L., and Abboud, F. M.: The Value of Left Parasternal Impulse Recordings in the Assessment of Mitral Regurgitation, *Circulation*, 48:1055, 1973.

196 Manchester, G. H., Block, P., and Garlin, R.: Misleading Signs in Mitral Insufficiency, *J.A.M.A.*, 191:99, 1965.

197 Aravanis, C.: Silent Mitral Insufficiency, *Am. Heart J.,* 70:620, 1965.

198 Schrire, V., Vogelpoel, L., Nellen, M., Swanepoel, A., and Beck, A.: Silent Mitral Incompetence, *Am. Heart J.,* 61:723, 1961.

199 Fowler, N. O.: "Cardiac Diagnosis and Treatment," 2d ed., Harper & Row, Publishers, Incorporated, Hagerstown, Md., 1976.

200 Karliner, J. S., O'Rourke, R. A., Kearney, D. J., and Shabetai, R.: Haemodynamic Explanation of Why the Murmur of Mitral Regurgitation is Independent of Cycle Length, *Br. Heart J.,* 35:397, 1973.

201 Aravanis, C., and Michaelides, G.: Tricuspid Insufficiency Masquerading as Mitral Insufficiency in Patients with Severe Mitral Stenosis, *Am. J. Cardiol.,* 20:417, 1967.

202 deLeon, A. C., Jr., and Harvey, W. P.: Pharmacological Agents and Auscultation, *Mod. Concepts Cardiovasc. Dis.,* 44:23, 1975.

203 Bleifer, S., Dack, S., Grishman, A., and Donoso, E.: The Auscultatory and Phonocardiographic Findings in Mitral Regurgitation, *Am. J. Cardiol.,* 5:836, 1960.

204 Perloff, J. D., and Harvey, W. P.: Mechanisms of Fixed Splitting of the Second Heart Sound, *Circulation,* 18:998, 1958.

205 Sutton, G., Harris, A., and Leatham, A.: Second Heart Sound in Pulmonary Hypertension, *Br. Heart J.,* 30:743, 1968.

206 Nixon, P. G. F., and Wooler, G. H.: Clinical Assessment of Mitral Orifice in Patients with Regurgitation, *Br. Med. J.,* 2:1122, 1960.

207 Nixon, P. G. F., and Wooler, G. H.: Phases of Diastole in Mitral Valvular Disease. *Br. Heart J.,* 25:393, 1963.

208 Bentivoglis, L. G., Uricchio, J. F., Waldow, A., Likoff, W., and Goldberg, H.: An Electrocardiographic Analysis of Mitral Regurgitation, *Circulation,* 18:572, 1956.

209 Rackely, C. E., and Hood, W. P., Jr.: Quantitative Angiographic Evaluation and Pathophysiologic Mechanisms in Valvular Heart Disease, *Prog. Cardiovasc. Dis.,* 15:427, 1973.

210 Tyrrell, M. J., Ellison, R. C., Hugenholtz, P. G., and Nadas, A. S.: Correlation of Degree of Left Ventricular Volume Overload with Clinical Course in Aortic and Mitral Regurgitation, *Br. Heart J.,* 32:683, 1970.

211 Braunwald, E., and Awe, W. C.: The Syndrome of Severe Mitral Regurgitation with Normal Left Atrial Pressure, *Circulation,* 27:29, 1963.

212 Levinson, D. C., Wilburne, M., Meehand, J. R., Jr., and Shubin, H.: Evidence for Retrograde Transpulmonary Propagation of the V (or Regurgitant) Wave in Mitral Insufficiency, *Am. J. Cardiol.,* 2:159, 1958.

213 Goodman, D. J., Rossen, R. M., Holloway, E. L., Alderman, E. L., and Harrison, D. C.: Effect of Nitroprusside on Left Ventricular Dynamics in Mitral Regurgitation, *Circulation,* 50:1025, 1974.

214 Munoz, S., Gallardo, J., Diaz-Gorrin, Jr., and Medina, O.: Influence of Surgery on the Natural History of Rheumatic Mitral and Aortic Valve Disease, *Am. J. Cardiol.,* 35:234, 1975.

215 Nixon, P. G. F., and Wooler, G. H.: Left Ventricular Filling Pressure Gradient in Mitral Incompetence, *Br. Heart J.,* 25:382, 1963.

216 Kuzman, W. J., and Yuskis, A. S.: Atrial Septal Defects in the Older Patient Simulating Acquired Valvular Heart Disease, *Am. J. Cardiol.,* 15:303, 1965.

217 Nasser, W. K., Davis, R. H., Dillin, J. C., Tavel, M. E., Helmen, C. H., Feigenbaum, H., and Fisch, C.: Atrial Myxoma, *Am. Heart J.,* 83:694, 810, 1972.

218 Penny, J. L., Gregory, J. J., Ayres, S. M., Giannelli, S., Jr., and Rossi, P.: Calcified Left Atrial Myxoma Simulating Mitral Insufficiency, *Circulation,* 36:417, 1967.

219 Abbott, O. A., Warshawski, F. E., and Cobbs, B. W., Jr.: Primary Tumors and Pseudotumors of the Heart, *Ann. Surg.,* 155:855, 1962.

220 Steinbrunn, W., Cohn, K. E., and Selzer, A.: Atrial Septal Defect Associated with Mitral Stenosis: The Lutembacher Syndrome Revisited, *Am. J. Cardiol.,* 48:295, 1970.

221 Goldfarb, B., and Wang, Y.: Mitral Stenosis and Left to Right Shunt at the Atrial Level: A Broadened Concept of the Lutembacher Syndrome, *Am. J. Cardiol.,* 17:319, 1966.

222 Ross, J., Braunwald, E., Mason, D. T., Friedman, M., Braunwald, N. S., and Morrow, A. G.: Interatrial Communication and Left Atrial Hypertension: A Cause of Continuous Murmur, *Circulation,* 28:853, 1963.

223 Tandon, R., Manchanda, S. C., and Roy, S. B.: Mitral Stenosis with Left to Right Shunt at Atrial Level: A Diagnostic Challenge, *Br. Heart J.,* 33:773, 1971.

224 Singh, R., McGuire, L. B., Carpenter, M., and Dammann, J. F.: Mitral Stenosis Associated with Partial Anomalous Pulmonary Venous Return (with Intact Atrial Septum), *Am. J. Cardiol.,* 28:226, 1971.

225 Lucas, R. V., Jr., and Schmidt, R. E.: Anomalous Venous Connections, Pulmonary and Systemic, in A. J. Moss and F. H. Adams (eds.), "Heart Disease in Infants, Children and Adolescents," The Williams & Wilkins Company, Baltimore, 1968.

226 McGuire, L. B., Nolan, T. B., Reeve, R., and Dammann, J. F., Jr.: Cor Triatriatum as a Problem of Adult Heart Disease, *Circulation,* 31:263, 1965.

227 Segal, J. P., Harvey, W. P., and Stapleton, J. F.: Clinical Features and Natural History of Cardiomyopathy, in N. O. Fowler (ed.), "Myocardial Disease," Grune & Stratton, Inc., New York, 1973.

228 Shabetai, R., and Davidson, S.: Asymmetrical Hypertrophic Cardiomyopathy Simulating Mitral Stenosis, *Circulation,* 45: 37, 1972.

229 Smith, M. R., Agruss, N. S., Levenson, N. I., and Adoph, R. J.: Non-obstructive Hypertrophic Cardiomyopathy Mimicking Mitral Stenosis, *Am. J. Cardiol.,* 35:89, 1975.

230 Hurst, J. W., Lindsay, J., Jr., and Crawley, I. S.: Mitral Stenosis: How Not to Miss It, *Med. Times,* 97:163, 1969.

231 Silverman, M. E., and Hurst, J. W.: The Mitral Complex, *Am. Heart J.,* 76:399, 1968.

232 Cobbs, W. B., Jr., in J. W. Hurst and R. B. Logue (eds.), "The Heart," 2d ed., McGraw-Hill Book Company, New York, 1970.

233 Barlow, J. B., and Pocock, W. A.: The Problem of Nonejection Systolic Clicks and Associated Mitral Systolic Murmurs: Emphasis on the Billowing Mitral Leaflet Syndrome, *Am. Heart J.,* 90:636, 1975.

234 Marchand, P., Barlow, J. B., DuPlessis, L. A., and Webster, J.: Mitral Regurgitation with Rupture of Normal Chordae Tendineae, *Br. Heart J.,* 28:746, 1966.

235 Salisburg, P. F., Cross, C. E., and Richen, P. A.: Chordae Tendineae Tension, *Am. J. Physiol.,* 205:385, 1963.

236 O'Rourke, R. A., and Crawford, M. H.: The Systolic Click–Murmur Syndrome: Clinical Recognition and Management, *Curr. Probl. Cardiol.,* 1(1):1, 1976.

237 Barlow, J. B., Pocock, W. A., Marchand, P., and Denny, M.: The Significance of Late Systolic Murmurs and Mid-late Systolic Clicks, *Md. State Med. J.,* 12:76, 1963.

238 Jeresaty, R. M.: Mitral Valve Prolapse–Click Syndrome, *Prog. Cardiovasc. Dis.,* 15:623, 1973.

239 Aranda, J. M., Befeler, B., El-Sherif, N., Castellanos, A., and Lazzara, R.: Mitral Valve Prolapse, *Am. J. Med.,* 60:997, 1976.

240 Devereux, R. B., Perloff, J. K., Reichek, N., and Josephson, M. E.: Mitral Valve Prolapse, *Circulation,* 54:3, 1976.

241 Criley, J. M., Lewis, K. B., Humphries, J. O., and Ross, R. S.: Prolapse of the Mitral Valve: Clinical and Cine-angiocardiographic Findings, *Br. Heart J.*, 28:488, 1966.

242 Trent, J. K., Adelman, A. G., Wigle, E. D., and Silver, M. D.: Morphology of a Prolapsed Posterior Mitral Valve Leaflet, *Am. Heart J.*, 79:539, 1970.

243 Stannard, M., Sloman, J. G., Hare, W. S., and Goble, A. J.: Prolapse of the Posterior Leaflet of the Mitral Valve: A Clinical, Familial and Cineangiographic Study, *Br. Med. J.*, 3:71, 1967.

244 Edwards, J. E., and Burchell, H. B.: Pathologic Anatomy of Mitral Regurgitation, *Mayo Clin. Proc.*, 33:497, 1958.

245 Hurst, J. W.: The Mitral Valve Prolapse–Click Syndrome: II. *Am. J. Cardiol.*, 38:271, 1976.

246 Cuffer, P., and Barbillon, L.: Nouvelles recherches sur les bruits de galop, *Arch. Gen. Med.*, 1:129, 1887.

247 Gallavardin, L.: Nouvelle observation avec autopsied d'un pseudodeoublement du 2° bruit du coeur simulant le deoublement mitral par bruit extra-cardiaque télésystolique surajouté, *Prat Med. Franc.*, 13:19, 1932.

248 Leatham, A.: Auscultation of the Heart, *Lancet*, 2:703, 1958.

249 Humphries, J. O., and McKusick, V. A.: The Differentiation of Organic and "Innocent" Systolic Murmurs, *Prog. Cardiovasc. Dis.*, 5:152, 1962.

250 White, P. D.: "Heart Disease," chap. 13, The Macmillan Company, New York, 1931.

251 Reid, J. V.: Mid-systolic Clicks, *S. Afr. Med. J.*, 35:353, 1961.

252 Ronan, J. A., Perloff, J. K., and Harvey, W. P.: Systolic Clicks and Late Systolic Murmur: Intracardiac Phonocardiographic Evidence of Their Mitral Valve Origin, *Am. Heart J.*, 70:319, 1965.

253 Perloff, J. K., and Roberts, W. C.: The Mitral Apparatus: Functional Anatomy of Mitral Regurgitation, *Circulation*, 46:227, 1972.

254 Nutter, D. O., Wickliffe, C., Gilbert, C. A., Moody, C., and King, S. A.: The Pathophysiology of Idiopathic Mitral Valve Prolapse, *Circulation*, 52:297, 1975.

255 Fontana, M. E., Kissel, G. L., and Criley, J. M.: "Functional Anatomy of Mitral Valve Prolapse," American Heart Association Monograph 46, p. 126, 1975.

256 Barlow, J. B., Bosman, C. K., Pocock, W. A., and Marchand, P.: Late Systolic Murmurs and Non-ejection ("Mid-late") Systolic Clicks, *Br. Heart J.*, 30:203, 1968.

257 Pomerance, A., and Davies, M. J.: "The Pathology of the Heart," Blackwell Scientific Publications, Ltd., Oxford, 1975.

258 Bulkley, B. H., and Roberts, W. C.: Dilatation of the Mitral Annulus, *Am. J. Med.*, 59:457, 1975.

259 Leachman, R. D., DeFrancheschi, A., and Zamalloa, O.: Late Systolic Murmurs and Clicks Associated with Abnormal Mitral Valve Ring, *Am. J. Cardiol.*, 23:679, 1969.

260 McKay, R., and Yacoub, M. H.: Clinical and Pathological Findings in Patients with "Floppy" Valves Treated Surgically, *Circulation*, 48(suppl. 3):63, 1973.

261 Gooch, A. S., Vicencio, F., Maranchao, V., and Goldberg, H.: Arrhythmias and Left Ventricle Asynergy in the Prolapsing Mitral Leaflet, *Am. J. Cardiol.*, 29:611, 1972.

262 Scampardonis, G., Yang, S. S., Maranhao, V., Goldberg, H., and Gooch, A. S.: Left Ventricular Abnormalities in Prolapsed Mitral Leaflet Syndrome, *Circulation*, 48:287, 1973.

263 Engle, M. A.: The Syndrome of Apical Systolic Click, Late Systolic Murmur and Abnormal T Waves, *Circulation*, 39:1, 1969.

264 Verani, M. S., Carroll, R. J., and Falsetti, H. L.: Mitral Valve Prolapse in Coronary Disease, *Am. J. Cardiol.*, 37:1, 1976.

265 Aranda, J. M., Befeler, B., Lazzara, R., Embi, A., and Marchado, H.: Mitral Valve Prolapse and Coronary Artery Disease, *Circulation*, 52:245, 1975.

266 Cobbs, W. B., Jr.: Pathophysiological Basis for the Click-Murmur Syndrome (presentation at Frontiers in Cardiology, Atlanta, Ga., May 10–13, 1976).

267 Allen, H., Harris, A., and Leatham, A.: Significance and Prognosis of an Isolated Late Systolic Murmur: A 9 to 22-Year Follow-up, *Br. Heart J.*, 36:525, 1974.

268 Winkle, R. A., Lopes, M. G., Fitzgerald, J. W., et al.: Arrhythmias in Patients with Mitral Valve Prolapse, *Circulation*, 52:73, 1975.

269 Sloman, G., Wong, M., and Walker, J.: Arrhythmias on Exercise in Patients with Abnormalities of Posterior Leaflet of the Mitral Valve, *Am. Heart J.*, 83:312, 1972.

270 LeWinter, M. M., Hoffman, J. R., Shell, W. E., Karliner, S. S., and O'Rourke, R. A.: Phenylephrine-induced Atypical Chest Pain in Patients with Prolapsing Mitral Valve Leaflets, *Am. J. Cardiol.*, 34:12, 1974.

271 Malcolm, A. D., Bougher, D. R., Kostuk, W. J., and Ahuja, S. P.: Clinical Features and Investigative Findings in Presence of Mitral Leaflet Prolapse, *Br. Heart J.*, 38:244, 1976.

272 Markiewicz, W., Stoner, J., London, E., Hunt, S. A., and Popp, R. L.: Mitral Valve Prolapse in One Hundred Presumably Healthy Young Females, *Circulation*, 53:464, 1976.

273 Brown, O. R., Kloster, F., and DeMots, H.: Incidence of Mitral Valve Prolapse in the Asymptomatic Normal, *Circulation*, 52(suppl. 2):II-77, 1975.

274 Rizzon, P., Biasco, G., Brindicci, G., and Mauro, F.: Familial Syndrome of Mid-systolic Click and Late Systolic Murmur, *Br. Heart J.*, 35:245, 1973.

275 Hancock, E. W., and Cohn, K.: The Syndrome Associated with Midsystolic Click and Late Systolic Murmur, *Am. J. Med.*, 41:183, 1966.

276 Hunt, D., and Sloman, G.: Prolapse of the Posterior Leaflet of the Mitral Valve Occurring in Eleven Members of a Family, *Am. Heart J.*, 78:149, 1969.

277 Shell, W. E., Walton, J. A., Clifford, M. E., and Willis, P. W.: The Familial Occurrence of the Syndrome of Mid-late Systolic Click and Late Systolic Murmur, *Circulation*, 39:327, 1969.

278 Winters, S. J., Schreiner, B., Greggs, R. C., Rowley, P., and Nanda, N. C.: Familial Mitral Valve Prolapse and Myotonic Dystrophy, *Ann. Intern. Med.*, 85:19, 1976.

279 Keck, E. W., Henschel, W. G., and Gruhl, L.: Mitral Valve Prolapse in Children with Secundum Type Atrial Septal Defect (ASD II). *Eur. J. Pediatr.*, 121:89, 1976.

280 Murray, G. F., and Wilcox, B. R.: Secundum Atrial Septal Defect and Mitral Valve Incompetence, *Ann. Thorac. Surg.*, 20:136, 1975.

281 BonTempo, C. P., Ronan, J. A., DeLeon, A. C., and Twigg, H. L.: Radiographic Appearance of the Thorax in Systolic Click, Late Systolic Murmur Syndrome, *Am. J. Cardiol.*, 36:27, 1975.

282 Solomon, J., Shab, P. M., and Heinkle, R. A.: Thoracic Skeletal Abnormalities in Idiopathic Mitral Valve Prolapse, *Am. J. Cardiol.*, 36:32, 1975.

283 Epstein, E. J., and Coulshed, N.: Phonocardiogram and Apex Cardiogram in Systolic Click–Late Systolic Murmur Syndrome, *Br. Heart J.*, 35:260, 1973.

284 Fontana, M. E., Wooley, C. G., Leighton, R. F., and Lewis, R. P.: Postural Changes in Left Ventricular and Mitral Valvular Dynamics in the Systolic-Click–Late Systolic Murmur Syndrome, *Circulation*, 51:165, 1975.

285 Pocock, W. A., and Barlow, J. B.: Etiology and Electrocardiographic Features of the Billowing Posterior Mitral Leaflet Syndrome, *Am. J. Med.*, 51:731, 1971.

286 Pocock, W. A., and Barlow, J. B.: Postexercise Arrhythmias

in the Billowing Posterior Mitral Leaflet Syndrome, *Am. Heart J.,* 80:740, 1970.

287 DeMaria, A. N., Amsterdam, E. A., Vismara, L. A., Neumann, A., and Mason, D. T.: Arrhythmias in the Mitral Valve Prolapse Syndrome, *Ann. Intern. Med.,* 84:656, 1976.

288 Popp, R. L., Brown, O. R., Silverman, J. F., and Harrison, D. C.: Echocardiographic Abnormalities in the Mitral Valve Prolapse Syndrome, *Circulation,* 49:428, 1974.

289 Burgess, J., Clark, R., Kamigaki, M., and Cohen, K.: Echocardiographic Findings in Different Types of Mitral Regurgitation, *Circulation,* 48:97, 1973.

290 DeMaria, A. N., King, J. F., Bogren, H. G., Lies, J. E., Mason, D. T.: The Variable Spectrum of Echocardiographic Manifestations of the Mitral Valve Prolapse Syndrome, *Circulation,* 50:33, 1974.

291 Vignola, P. A., Pohost, G. M., Curfman, G. D., and Myers, G. S.: Correlation of Echocardiographic and Clinical Findings in Patients with Pericardial Effusion, *Am. J. Cardiol.,* 37:701, 1976.

292 Cobbs, B. W., Jr., and King, S. B., III: Mechanism of Abnormal Ventriculogram and ECG Associated with Prolapsing Mitral Valve, *Circulation,* 50(suppl. 3):III-7, 1974. (Abstract.)

293 Lachman, A. S., Bramwell-Jones, D. M., Lakier, J. B., Pocock, W. A., and Barlow, J. B.: Infective Endocarditis in the Billowing Mitral Leaflet Syndrome, *Br. Heart J.,* 37:326, 1975.

294 Chesler, E., Metesome, R. E., Lalsier, J. B., Pocock, W. A., Obel, I. W. P., and Barlow, J. B.: Acute Myocardial Infarction with Normal Coronary Arteries, *Circulation,* 54:203, 1976.

295 Bittar, N., and Sosa, J. A.: Billowing Mitral Valve Leaflet, *Circulation,* 38:763, 1968.

296 Hill, D. G., Davies, M. J., and Braimbridge, M. V.: The Natural History and Surgical Management of the Redundant Cusp Syndrome (Floppy Mitral Valve), *J. Thorac. Cardiovasc. Surg.,* 67:519, 1974.

297 Cooley, D. A., Gerami, S., Hallman, G. L., Wukasch, D. C., and Hall, R. J.: Mitral Insufficiency Due to Myxomatous Transformation: "Floppy Valve Syndrome," *J. Cardiovasc. Surg.,* 13:346, 1972.

298 Roberts, W. C., Dangel, J. C., and Bulkley, B. H.: Nonrheumatic Valvular Cardiac Disease: A Clinicopathologic Survey of 27 Different Conditions Causing Valvular Dysfunction, in W. Likoff (guest ed.), "Valvular Heart Disease," *Cardiovasc. Clin.,* 5(2):333, 1973.

299 Osler, W.: On a Remarkable Heart Murmur Heard at a Distance from the Chest Wall, *Med. Times Gazette,* 2:432, 1880.

300 Rizzon, P., Biasco, G., and Maselli-Campagna, G.: The Praecordial Honk, *Br. Heart J.,* 33:707, 1971.

301 Leon, D. F., Leonard, J. J., Kroetz, I. W., et al.: Late Systolic Murmurs, Clicks, Whoop Arising from the Mitral Valve, *Am. Heart J.,* 72:325, 1966.

302 Behar, V. S., Whalen, R. E., and McIntosh, H. D.: The Ballooning Mitral Valve in Patients with the "Precordial Honk" or "Whoop," *Am. J. Cardiol.,* 20:789, 1967.

303 Upshaw, C. B., Jr.: Precordial Honk Due to Tricuspid Regurgitation, *Am. J. Cardiol.,* 35:85, 1975.

304 Sanders, C. A., Armstrong, P. W., Willerson, J. T., and Dinsmore, R. E.: Etiology and Differential Diagnosis of Acute Mitral Regurgitation, *Prog. Cardiovasc. Dis.,* 14:129, 1971.

305 Hwang, W. S., and Lam, K. L.: Rupture of Chordae Tendineae during Acute Rheumatic Carditis, *Br. Heart J.,* 30:429, 1968.

306 Wise, J. R.: Mitral Regurgitation Due to Rupture of Chordae Tendineae by Calcified Atrial Myxoma, *Br. Med. J.,* 2:95, 1974.

307 Sanders, C. A., Austen, W. G., Harthorne, J. W., Dinsmore, R. E., and Scannell, J. G.: Diagnosis and Surgical Treatment of Mitral Regurgitation Secondary to Ruptured Chordae Tendineae, *N. Engl. J. Med.,* 276:943, 1967.

308 Luther, R. R., and Meyers, S. N.: Acute Mitral Insufficiency Secondary to Ruptured Chordae Tendineae, *Arch. Intern. Med.,* 134:568, 1974.

309 Selzer, A., Kelly, J. J., Jr., Vannitamby, M., Walker, P., Gerbode, F., and Kerth, W. J.: The Syndrome of Mitral Insufficiency Due to Isolated Rupture of the Chordae Tendineae, *Am. J. Med.,* 43:822, 1967.

310 Caulfield, J. B., Page, D. L., Kaster, J. A., and Sanders, C. A.: Dissolution of Connective Tissue in Ruptured Chordae Tendineae, *Circulation,* 40:57, 1969.

311 Sutton, G. C., Chatterjee, K., and Caves, P. K.: Diagnosis of Severe Mitral Regurgitation Due to Non-rheumatic Chordal Abnormalities, *Br. Heart J.,* 35:877, 1973.

312 Merendino, K. A., and Hessel, E. A.: The Murmur on Top of the Head in Acquired Mitral Insufficiency, *J.A.M.A.,* 199:392, 1967.

313 Giuliani, E. R.: Mitral Valve Incompetence Due to Flail Anterior Leaflet, *Am. J. Cardiol.,* 20:784, 1967.

314 Caves, P. K., Sutton, G. C., and Paneth, M.: Nonrheumatic Subvalvular Mitral Regurgitation: Etiology and Clinical Aspects, *Circulation,* 47:1242, 1973.

315 Ronan, J. A., Jr., Steelman, R. B., DeLeon, A. C., Jr., Waters, T. J., Perlokk, J. K., and Harvey, W. P.: The Clinical Diagnosis of Acute Severe Mitral Insufficiency, *Am. J. Cardiol.,* 27:284, 1971.

316 Lerona, P. T.: Acute Mitral Regurgitation Due to Rupture of the Chordae Tendineae: Status of the Left Atrium, *Radiology,* 113:593, 1974.

317 Sweatman, T., Selzer, A., Kamageki, M., and Cohn, K.: Echocardiographic Diagnosis of Mitral Regurgitation Due to Ruptured Chordae Tendineae, *Circulation,* 46:580, 1972.

318 Dusall, J. C., Pryor, R., and Blount, S. G.: Systolic Murmur following Myocardial Infarction, *Am. Heart J.,* 87:577, 1974.

319 Burch, G. E., DePasquale, N. P., and Phillips, J. H.: Clinical Manifestations of Papillary Muscle Dysfunction, *Arch. Intern. Med.,* 112:112, 1963.

320 Burch, G. E., DePasquale, N. P., and Phillips, J. H.: The Syndrome of Papillary Muscle Dysfunction, *Am. Heart J.,* 75:399, 1968.

321 Becker, A. E., and Anderson, R. H.: Mitral Insufficiency Complicating Acute Myocardial Infarction, *Eur. J. Cardiol.,* 2:351, 1975.

322 Schechter, D. C.: Cardiac Structural and Functional Changes after Myocardial Infarction, *N.Y. State J. Med.,* 74:1615, 1974.

323 Harrison, D. C., Isaeff, D. M., and DeBusk, R. F.: "Papillary Muscle Syndromes," *D.M.,* no. 3, 1972.

324 Estes, E. H., Jr., Dalton, F. M., Entman, M. L., et al.: The Anatomy and Blood Supply of the Papillary Muscle of the Left Ventricle, *Am. Heart J.,* 71:356, 1966.

325 Tsakiris, A., Rastelli, G. C., Amorim, D., Titus, J., and Wood, E.: Effect of Experimental Papillary Muscle Damage on Mitral Valve Closure in Intact Anesthetized Dogs, *Mayo Clin. Proc.,* 45:275, 1970.

326 Fischer, G. C., Wessel, H. U., and Sommers, H. M.: Mitral Insufficiency following Experimental Papillary Muscle Infarction, *Am. Heart J.,* 83:382, 1972.

327 Mittal, A. K., Langston, M., Jr., Cohn, K. E., Selzer, A., and Kerth, W. J.: Combined Papillary Muscle and Left Ventricular Wall Dysfunction as a Cause of Mitral Regurgitation: Experimental Study, *Circulation,* 44:174, 1971.

328 Brand, F. R., Brown, A. L., Jr., and Berge, K. G.: Histology of Papillary Muscles of the Left Ventricle in Myocardial Infarction, *Am. Heart J.,* 77:26, 1969.

329 Heikkila, J.: Mitral Incompetence Complicating Acute Myocardial Infarction, *Br. Heart J.,* 29:162, 1967.

330 DePasquale, N. P., and Burch, G. E.: The Necropsy Incidence

of Gross Scars on Acute Infarction of the Papillary Muscles of the Left Ventricle, *Am. J. Cardiol.,* 17:169, 1966.

331 Burch, G. E., and DePasquale, N. P.: Time Course of Tension in Papillary Muscles of the Heart: Theoretical Considerations, *J.A.M.A.,* 192:701, 1965.

332 Kirk, E. S., and Honig, C. R.: Non Uniform Distribution of Blood Flow and Gradients of O_2 Tension within the Heart, *Am. J. Physiol.,* 207:661, 1964.

333 Brand, F. R., Berge, G., and Brown, A. L.: Papillary Muscles in Myocardial Infarction, *Circulation,* 16:169, 1966.

334 DeBusk, R. F., and Harrison, D. C.: The Clinical Spectrum of Papillary-Muscle Disease, *N. Engl. J. Med.,* 281:1458, 1969.

335 Phillips, J. H., Burch, G. E., and DePasquale, N. P.: The Syndrome of Papillary Muscle Dysfunction, *Ann. Intern. Med.,* 59:508, 1963.

336 Markiewicz, W., Amikam, S., Roguin, N., and Riss, E.: Changing Haemodynamics in Patients with Papillary Muscle Dysfunction, *Br. Heart J.,* 37:445, 1975.

337 Brody, W., and Criley, J. M.: Intermittent Severe Mitral Regurgitation, *N. Engl. J. Med.,* 283:673, 1970.

338 Cheng, T. O.: Some New Observations on the Syndrome of Papillary Muscle Dysfunction, *Am. J. Med.,* 47:924, 1969.

339 Shelburne, J. C., Rubinstein, D., and Gorlin, R.: A Reappraisal of Papillary Muscle Dysfunction, *Am. J. Med.,* 46:862, 1969.

340 Holmes, A. M., Logan, W. F., and Winterbottom, T.: Transient Systolic Murmurs in Angina Pectoris, *Am. Heart J.,* 76:680, 1968.

341 Gould, L., Reddy, C. V. R., Vecchiotti, H. J., and Gomprecht, R. F.: Observations on Papillary Muscle Dysfunction, *Am. Heart J.,* 87:674, 1974.

342 Steelman, R., White, R., Hill, J., and Naple-Cheethm, M.: Mid-systolic Click in Arteriosclerotic Heart Disease, *Circulation,* 44:503, 1971.

343 Pitt, B., and Strauss, H. W.: Myocardial Imaging in the Non-invasive Evaluation of Patients with Suspected Ischemic Heart Disease, *Am. J. Cardiol.,* 37:797, 1976.

344 Wexler, L., Silverman, J. F., DeBusk, R. F., and Harrison, D. C.: Angiographic Features of Rheumatic and Nonrheumatic Mitral Regurgitation, *Circulation,* 44:1080, 1971.

345 Koide, T., Nakanishi, A., Ito, I., Yasuda, H., Takabatake, Y., Ueda, K., Sugishita, Y., Uchida, Y., Ozeki, K., Mechida, K., Morooka, S., Nakajima, K., and Kakihana, M.: Left Ventricular Asynergy in Mitral Valve Diseases, *Jap. Heart J.,* 16:221, 1975.

346 Sniderman, A. D., Marpole, D. G. F., Palmer, W. H., and Fallen, E. L.: Response of the Left Ventricle in Nitroglycerin in Patients with and without Mitral Regurgitation, *Br. Heart J.,* 36:357, 1974.

347 Harshaw, C. W., Grossman, W., Munro, A. B., and McCauren, L. P.: Reduced Systemic Vascular Resistance as Therapy for Severe Mitral Regurgitation of Valvular Origin, *Ann. Intern. Med.,* 83:312, 1975.

348 Wajafi, H., Javid, H., Hunter, J. A., Goldin, M. D., Serry, C., and Dye, W. S.: Mitral Insufficiency Secondary to Coronary Heart Disease, *Ann. Thorac. Surg.,* 20:529, 1975.

349 Lamberti, J., Cohn, L. H., and Collins, J. J.: Management of Papillary Muscle Dysfunction after Acute Myocardial Infarction, *J. Thorac. Cardiovasc. Surg.,* 67:349, 1974.

350 Sanders, R. J., Neubuerger, K. T., and Ravin, A.: Rupture of Papillary Muscles: Occurrence of Rupture of the Posterior Muscle in Posterior Myocardial Infarction, *Dis. Chest,* 31:316, 1957.

351 Meister, S. G., and Helfant, R. H.: Rapid Bedside Differentiation of Ruptured Intraventricular Septum from Acute Mitral Insufficiency, *N. Engl. J. Med.,* 287:1029, 1972.

351a Feigenbaum, H., Corya, B. C., Dillion, J. C., Weyman, A. E., Rosmussen, S., Black, M. J., and Chang, S.: Role of Echocardiography in Patients with Coronary Artery Disease, *Am. J. Cardiol.,* 37:775, 1976.

352 Fleming, H. A.: Ventricular Septal Defect and Mitral Regurgi-

tation Secondary to Myocardial Infarction, *Br. Heart J.,* 36:936, 1974.

353 Korn, D., DeSanctis, R. W., and Sell, S.: Massive Calcification of the Mitral Annulus, *N. Engl. J. Med.,* 267:900, 1962.

354 Rytand, D. A., and Lipsitch, L. S.: Clinical Aspects of Calcification of the Mitral Annulus Fibrosus, *Arch. Intern. Med.,* 78:544, 1946.

355 Hirschfeld, D. S., and Emilson, B. B.: Echocardiogram in Calcified Mitral Annulus, *Am. J. Cardiol.,* 36:354, 1975.

356 Ridolfi, R. L., and Hutchins, G. M.: Spontaneous Calcific Emboli from Calcific Mitral Annulus Fibrosus, *Arch. Pathol. Lab. Med.,* 100:117, 1976.

357 Krovetz, L. J., McLaughlin, T. G., and Silvebler, G. L.: Cardiovascular Manifestations of the Hurler Syndrome, *Circulation,* 31:132, 1965.

358 McKusick, V. A.: "Heritable Disorders of Connective Tissue," The C. V. Mosby Company, St. Louis, 1972.

359 Beighton, P.: Cardiac Abnormalities in the Ehlers-Danlos Syndrome, *Br. Heart J.,* 31:227, 1969.

360 Silverman, B. D., Fortuin, N. S., Pope, M., and McKusick, V. A.: Cardiac Auscultatory Findings in Ehlers-Danlos Syndrome. Unpublished.

361 Symbas, P. N., Baldwin, B. S., Silverman, M. E., and Galambas, S. T.: Marfan's Syndrome with Aneurysm of Ascending Aortic and Aortic Regurgitation, Surgical Treatment and New Histochemical Observations, *Am. J. Cardiol.,* 25:483, 1970.

362 Heftmanicik, M. R., Wright, J. C., Quint, R., and Jennings, I. C.: The Cardiovascular Manifestations of Systemic Lupus Erythematosus, *Am. Heart J.,* 68:119, 1964.

363 Stewart, J. R., Cohn, K. E., Fojardo, L. F., Hancock, E. W., and Kaplan, H. S.: Radiation-induced Heart Disease, *Radiology,* 89:302, 1967.

364 Ledthe, A. J., and DeMath, W. E.: Non-penetrating Cardiac Injuries: A Collective Review, *Am. Heart J.,* 86:687, 1973.

365 Bona, D. S., MacNeal, P. S., LaCompte, P. M., Shah, Y., and Graham, J. R.: Cardiac Murmurs and Endocardial Fibrosis Associated with Methysergide Therapy, *Am. Heart J.,* 88:640, 1974.

366 Hope, J.: "A Treatise on the Diseases of the Heart and Great Vessels," 2d American ed. from 3d London ed., Lea & Blanchard, Philadelphia, 1846.

367 Campbell, M., and Kauntze, R.: Congenital Aortic Valvular Stenosis, *Br. Heart J.,* 15:179, 1953.

368 Monckeberg, J. G.: Der normale histologische Bau und die sklerose der aortenklappen, *Virchows Arch. [Pathol. Anat.],* 176:472, 1904.

369 Karsner, H. T., and Koletsky, S.: "Calcific Disease of Aortic Valves," J. B. Lippincott, Philadelphia, 1947.

370 Wood, P.: Aortic Stenosis, *Am. J. Cardiol.,* 1:553, 1958.

371 White, P. W.: "Heart Disease," The Macmillan Company, New York, 1951.

372 Contratto, A. W., and Levine, S. A.: Aortic Stenosis with Special Reference to Angina Pectoris and Syncope, *Ann. Intern. Med.,* 10:1636, 1936.

373 Bacon, A. O., and Matthews, M. B.: Congenital Bicuspid Aortic Valves and the Aetiology of Isolated Aortic Valvular Stenosis, *Q. J. Med.,* 28:545, 1959.

374 Hudson, R. E.: "Cardiovascular Pathology: The Aortic Valve: Valvular, Subvalvular, and Supravalvular Lesions," vol. 3, Edward Arnold (Publishers) Ltd., London, 1965, pp. 581–584.

375 Roberts, W. C.: The Congenitally Bicuspid Aortic Valve: A Study of 85 Autopsy Cases, *Am. J. Cardiol.,* 26:72, 1970.

376 Storstein, O.: Etiology of Aortic Valvular Disease, *Acta Med. Scand.,* 185:17, 1969.

377 Peacock, T.: "On Malformations of the Human Heart," 2d ed., J. Churchill & Sons, Publishers, London, 1866.

378 Pomerance, A.: Pathogenesis of Aortic Stenosis and Its Relation to Age, *Br. Heart J.,* 34:569, 1972.

379 Glancy, D. L., and Epstein, S. E.: Differential Diagnosis of Type and Severity of Obstruction to Left Ventricular Outflow, *Prog. Cardiovasc. Dis.,* 14:153, 1971.

380 Ellis, H. F., Jr., and Kirklin, J. W.: Congenital Valvular Aortic Stenosis: Anatomic Findings and Surgical Technique, *J. Thorac. Cardiovasc. Surg.,* 43:199, 1962.

381 Rotman, M., Morris, J. J., Behar, V. S., Peter, R. H., and Kong, Y.: Aortic Valvular Disease: Comparison of Types and Their Medical and Surgical Management, *Am. J. Med.,* 51:241, 1971.

382 Cleland, W. P., Goodwin, J. F., Bentall, H. H., Oakley, C. M., Melrose, D. G., and Hollman, A.: A Decade of Open Heart Surgery, *Lancet,* 1:191, 1968.

383 Roberts, W. C.: The Structure of the Aortic Valve in Clinically Isolated Aortic Stenosis: An Autopsy Study of 162 Patients over 15 Years of Age, *Circulation,* 42:91, 1970.

384 Roberts, W. C.: Anatomically Isolated Aortic Valvular Disease: The Case against Its Being of Rheumatic Etiology, *Am. J. Med.,* 49:151, 1970.

385 Roberts, W. C., Perloff, J. K., and Costantino, T.: Severe Valvular Aortic Stenosis in Patients over 65 Years of Age: A Clinicopathologic Study, *Am. J. Cardiol.,* 27:497, 1971.

386 Edwards, J. E.: Pathologic Aspects of Cardiac Valvular Insufficiencies, *Arch. Surg.,* 77:634, 1958.

387 Roberts, W. C., and Morrow, A. G.: Congenital Aortic Stenosis Produced by a Unicommissural Valve, *Br. Heart J.,* 27:505, 1965.

388 Edwards, J. E.: Calcific Aortic Stenosis: Pathologic Features, *Mayo Clin. Proc.,* 36:444, 1961.

389 Osler, W.: The Biscuspid Condition of the Aortic Valves, *Trans. Assoc. Am. Physicians,* 2:185, 1886.

390 Pomerance, A.: Aging Changes in Human Heart Valves, *Br. Heart J.,* 29:222, 1967.

391 Campbell, M.: Calcific Aortic Stenosis and Congenital Bicuspid Aortic Valves, *Br. Heart J.,* 30:606, 1968.

392 Edwards, J. E.: On the Etiology of Calcific Aortic Stenosis, *Circulation,* 26:817, 1962.

393 Davison, E. T., and Friedman, S. A.: Significance of Systolic Murmurs in the Aged, *N. Engl. J. Med.,* 279:225, 1968.

394 Bruns, D. L., and van der Hauwaert, L. G.: Aortic Systolic Murmur Developing with Increasing Age, *Br. Heart J.,* 20:370, 1958.

395 Kennedy, J. W., Twiss, R. D., Blackmon, J. R., and Dodge, H. T.: Quantitative Angiocardiography: III. Relationships of Left Ventricular Pressure, Volume, and Mass in Aortic Valve Disease, *Circulation,* 38:838, 1968.

396 Braunwald, E., and Frahm, C. J.: Studies on Starling's Law of the Heart: IV. Observations on the Hemodynamic Functions of the Left Atrium in Man, *Circulation,* 24:633, 1961.

397 Stott, D. K., Marpole, D. G., Bristow, J. D., Kloster, F. E., and Griswold, H. E.: The Role of Left Atrial Transport in Aortic and Mitral Stenosis, *Circulation,* 41:1031, 1970.

398 Ross, J., Jr., and Braunwald, E.: Aortic Stenosis, *Circulation,* 38(suppl. 5):61, 1968.

399 Takeda, J., Warren, R., and Holzman, D.: Prognosis of Aortic Stenosis, *Arch. Surg.,* 87:931, 1963.

400 Frank, S., Johnson, A., and Ross, J., Jr.: Natural History of Valvular Aortic Stenosis, *Br. Heart J.,* 35:41, 1973.

401 Fallen, E. L., Elliott, W. C., and Gorlin, R.: Mechanisms of Angina in Aortic Stenosis, *Circulation,* 36:480, 1967.

402 Hancock, E. W., and Fleming, P. R.: Aortic Stenosis, *Q. J. Med.,* 29:209, 1960.

403 Kumpe, C. W., and Bean, W. B.: Aortic Stenosis: Study of the Clinical and Pathological Aspects of 107 Proved Cases, *Medicine (Baltimore),* 27:139, 1948.

404 Lewis, R. C., and Creus, A. B.: Angina Pectoris and Aortic Valve Disease, *Cardiovasc. Clin.,* 7:169, 1975.

405 Baker, C., and Somerville, J.: Clinical Features and Surgical Treatment of Fifty Patients with Severe Aortic Stenosis, *Guys Hosp. Rep.,* 108:101, 1959.

406 Basta, L. L., Raines, D., Najjar, S., and Kioschos, J. M.: Clinical, Hemodynamic, and Coronary Angiographic Correlates of Angina Pectoris in Patients with Severe Aortic Valve Disease, *Br. Heart J.,* 37:150, 1975.

407 Sarnoff, S. J., Braunwald, E., Welch, G. H., Case, R. B., Stainsby, W. N., and Marcruz, R.: Hemodynamic Determinants of Oxygen Consumption of the Heart with Special Reference to the Tension-Time Index, *Am. J. Physiol.,* 192:148, 1958.

408 Perloff, J. G., Ronan, J. A., Jr., de Leon, A. C., Jr.: The Effect of Nitroglycerin on Left Ventricular Wall Tension in Fixed Orifice Aortic Stenosis, *Circulation,* 32:204, 1965.

409 Holley, K. E., Bahn, R. C., McGoon, D. C., and Mankin, H. T.: Spontaneous Calcific Embolization Associated with Calcific Aortic Stenosis, *Circulation,* 27:197, 1963.

410 Smithen, C., Wilner, G., Baltaxe, H., Gay, W., Jr., and Killip, T.: Variant Angina Pectoris, *Am. Heart J.,* 89:87, 1975.

411 Williams, J. F., Glick, G., and Braunwald, E.: The Effect of Nitroglycerin on Ventricular Dimensions in Intact Unanesthetized Man, *Clin. Res.,* 12:195, 1964.

412 Flamm, M. D., Braiff, B. A., Kimball, R., and Hancock, E. W.: Mechanism of Effort Syncope in Aortic Stenosis, *Circulation,* 36(suppl. 2):II-109, 1967.

413 Schwartz, L. S., Goldfischer, J., Sprague, G. J., and Schwartz, S. P.: Syncope and Sudden Death in Aortic Stenosis, *Am. J. Cardiol.,* 23:647, 1969.

414 Andersen, J. A., Hansen, B. F., and Lyngborg, K.: Isolated Valvular Aortic Stenosis, *Acta Med. Scand.,* 197:61, 1975.

415 Perloff, J. K.: Clinical Recognition of Aortic Stenosis: The Physical Signs and Differential Diagnosis of the Various Forms of Obstruction to Left Ventricular Outflow, *Prog. Cardiovasc. Dis.,* 10:323, 1968.

416 Glancy, D. L., and Epstein, S. E.: Differential Diagnosis of Type and Severity of Obstruction of Left Ventricular Outflow, *Prog. Cardiovasc. Dis.,* 14:153, 1971.

417 Hancock, E. W.: The Ejection Sound in Aortic Stenosis, *Am. J. Med.,* 40:569, 1966.

418 Leatham, A.: Systolic Murmurs, *Circulation,* 17:601, 1958.

419 Spencer, M. P., and Greiss, F. C.: Dynamics of Ventricular Ejection, *Circ. Res.,* 10:274, 1962.

420 Tavel, M. E., "Clinical Phonocardiography and External Pulse Reading," 2d ed., Year Book Medical Publishers Inc., Chicago, 1973, pp. 149 and 155.

421 Friedberg, C. K.: Aortic Regurgitation, in "Diseases of the Heart," 3d ed., W. B. Saunders Company, Philadelphia, 1966, p. 1103.

422 Pomerance, A.: Cardiac Pathology of Systolic Murmurs in Elderly, *Br. Heart J.,* 30:687, 1968.

423 Finegan, R. E., Gianelly, R. E., and Harrison, D. C.: Aortic Stenosis in the Elderly: Relevance of Age to Diagnosis and Treatment, *N. Engl. J. Med.,* 281:1261, 1969.

424 Sutnick, A. I., and Soloff, L. A.: P-Wave Abnormalities as an Electrocardiographic Index of Hemodynamically Significant Aortic Stenosis, *Circulation,* 28:814, 1963.

425 Myler, R. K., and Sanders, C. A.: Aortic Valve Disease and Atrial Fibrillation: Report of 122 Patients with Electrographic, Radiographic and Hemodynamic Observations, *Arch. Intern. Med.,* 121:530, 1968.

426 Eddleman, E. E., Jr., Frommeyer, W. B., Jr., Lyle, D. P., Bancroft, W. H., Jr., and Turner, M. E., Jr.: Critical Analysis of Clinical Factors in Estimating Severity of Aortic Valve Disease, *Am. J. Cardiol.,* 31:687, 1973.

427 Klatte, E. C., Tampas, J. P., Campbell, J. A., and Lurie, P. R.: The Roentgenographic Manifestations of Aortic Stenosis and Aortic Valvular Insufficiency, *Am. J. Roentgenol. Radium Ther. Nucl. Med.,* 88:57, 1962.

428 Rockoff, S. D., Levine, N. D., and Austen, W. G.: Roentgenographic Clues to the Cardiac Hemodynamics of Aortic Stenosis, *Radiology,* 83:58, 1964.

429 Gramiak, R., and Shah, P. M.: Echocardiography of the Normal and Diseased Aortic Valve, *Radiology,* 96:1, 1970.

430 Johnson, M. L., Kisslo, J., Habersberger, P. G., and Wallace, A. G.: Echocardiographic Evaluation of Aortic Valvular Disease, *Circulation,* 47(suppl. 4):IV–46, 1973.

431 Feigi, O., Symons, C., and Yaroub, M.: Echocardiography of Aortic Valve: I. Studies of Normal Aortic Valve, Aortic Stenosis, Aortic Regurgitation, and Mixed Aortic Valve Disease, *Br. Heart J.,* 36:341, 1973.

432 Radford, D. J., Bloom, K. R., Izukawa, T., Moes, C. A. F., and Rowe, R. D.: Echocardiographic Assessment of Bicuspid Aortic Valves: Angiographic and Pathological Correlates, *Circulation,* 53:80, 1976.

433 Nanda, N. C., Gramiak, R., Manning, J., Mahoney, E. B., Lipchik, E. O., and DeWeese, J. A.: Echocardiographic Recognition of the Congenital Bicuspid Aortic Valve, *Circulation,* 49:870, 1974.

434 Wiggers, O. J.: "Physiology in Health and Disease," Lea & Febiger, Philadelphia, 1934.

435 Hancock, E. W., and Fleming, P. R.: Aortic Stenosis, *Q. J. Med.,* 29:209, 1960.

436 Braunwald, E., Goldblatt, A., Aygen, M. M., Rockoff, S. D., and Morrow, A. G.: Congenital Aortic Stenosis: I. Clinical and Hemodynamic Findings in 100 Patients; Morrow, A. G., Goldblatt, A., Braunwald, E.: Congenital Aortic Stenosis: II. Surgical Treatment and the Results of Operation, *Circulation,* 27:426, 1963.

437 Hirshfield, J. W., Jr., Epstein, S. E., Roberts, A. J., Glancy, D. L., and Morrow, A. G.: Indices Predicting Long-Term Survival after Valve Replacement in Patients with Aortic Regurgitation and Patients with Aortic Stenosis, *Circulation,* 50:1190, 1974.

438 Harris, C. N., Kaplan, M. A., Parker, D. P., Donne, E. F., Cowell, H. S., and Ellestad, M. H.: Aortic Stenosis, Angina, and Coronary Artery Disease: Interrelations, *Br. Heart J.,* 37:656, 1975.

439 Hohn, A. R., Van Praagh, S., and Moore, A. A.: Aortic Stenosis, *Circulation,* 31 and 32(suppl. 3):4, 1965.

440 Rapaport, E.: Natural History of Aortic and Mitral Valve Disease, *Am. J. Cardiol.,* 35:221, 1975.

441 Brawley, R. K., and Morrow, A. G.: Direct Determination of Aortic Blood Flow in Patients with Aortic Regurgitation: Effects of Alterations in Heart Rate, Increased Ventricular Preload or Afterload, and Isoproterenol, *Circulation,* 35:32, 1967.

442 Segal, J. Harvey, W. P., and Hufnagel, C. L.: A Clinical Study of One Hundred Cases of Severe Aortic Insufficiency, *Am. J. Med.,* 21:200, 1956.

443 Stapleton, J. F., and Harvey, W. P.: A Clinical Analysis of Aortic Incompetence, *Postgrad. Med.,* 46:156, 1969.

444 Engloff, E.: Aortic Incompetence: Clinical Haemodynamic and Angiocardiographic Evaluation, *Acta Med. Scand.,* 193(suppl. 538):3, 1972.

445 Roberts, W. C.: Anatomically Isolated Valvular Disease: The Case Against Its Being of Rheumatic Etiology, *Am. J. Med.,* 49:151, 1970.

446 Schilder, D. P., Harvey, W. P., and Hufnagel, C. A.: Rheumatoid Spondylitis and Aortic Insufficiency, *N. Engl. J. Med.,* 255:11, 1956.

447 Read, R. C., Thal, A. P., and Wendt, V. E.: Symptomatic Valvular Myxomatous Transformation (The Floppy Valve Syndrome): A Possible Forme Fruste of the Marfan Syndrome, *Circulation,* 32:897, 1965.

448 Hunter, A.: The Heart in Anaemia, *Q. J. Med.,* 15:107, 1946.

449 Puchner, T. C., Huston, J. H., and Hellmuth, G. A.: Aortic Valve Insufficiency in Arterial Hypertension, *Am. J. Cardiol.,* 5:758, 1960.

450 Darvill, F. R., Jr.: Aortic Insufficiency of Unusual Etiology, *J.A.M.A.,* 184:753, 1963.

451 Burch, G. E.: "A Primer of Cardiology," 4th ed., Lea & Febiger, Philadelphia, 1971, p. 31.

452 Hegglin, R., Scheu, H., and Rothlin, M.: Aortic Insufficiency, *Circulation,* 37(suppl. 5):77, 1968.

453 Lerner, P. I., and Weinstein, L.: Infective Endocarditis in the Antibiotic Era, *N. Engl. J. Med.,* 274:199, 1966.

454 Morgan, W. L., and Bland, E. F.: Bacterial Endocarditis in the Antibiotic Era, *Circulation,* 19:753, 1959.

455 Carter, J. B., Sethi, S., Lee, G. B., and Edward, J. E.: Prolapse of Semilunar Cusps as Causes of Aortic Insufficiency, *Circulation,* 43:922, 1971.

456 Roberts, W. C., Hollingsworth, J. F., Bulkley, B. H., Jaffe, R. B., Epstein, S. E., and Stinson, E. B.: Combined Mitral and Aortic Regurgitation in Ankylosing Spondylitis: Angiographic and Anatomic Features, *Am. J. Med.,* 56:237, 1974.

457 Bulkley, B. H., and Roberts, W. C.: Ankylosing Spondylitis and Aortic Regurgitation: Description of the Characteristic Cardiovascular Lesion from Study of Eight Necropsy Patients, *Circulation,* 48:1014, 1973.

458 Davidson, P., Baggenstoss, A. H., Slocumb, C. H., and Daugherty, G. W.: Cardiac and Aortic Lesions in Rheumatoid Spondylitis, *Mayo Clin. Proc.,* 38:427, 1963.

459 Toone, E. C., Pierce, E. L., and Hennigar, G. R.: Aortitis and Aortic Regurgitation Associated with Rheumatic Spondylitis, *Am. J. Med.,* 26:255, 1959.

460 Paulus, H. E., Pearson, C. M., and Pitts, W., Jr.: Aortic Insufficiency in Five Patients with Reiter's Syndrome: A Detailed Clinical and Pathologic Study, *Am. J. Med.,* 53:464, 1972.

461 Rodnan, G. P., Benedek, T. G., Shaves, J. A., and Fennel, R. H., Jr.: Reiter's Syndrome and Aortic Insufficiency, *J.A.M.A.,* 189:889, 1964.

462 Roberts, W. C., Kehoe, J. A., Carpenter, D. F., and Golden, A.: Cardiovascular Valvular Lesions in Rheumatoid Arthritis, *Arch. Intern. Med.,* 122:141, 1968.

463 Heppner, R. L., Babitt, H. I., Bianchine, J. W., and Warbasse, J. R.: Aortic Regurgitation and Aneurysm of Sinus of Valsalva Associated with Osteogenesis Imperfecta, *Am. J. Cardiol.,* 31:654, 1973.

464 Criscitiello, M. G., Ronan, J. A., Jr., Besterman, E. M., and Schoenwetter, W.: Cardiovascular Abnormalities in Osteogenesis Imperfecta, *Circulation,* 31:255, 1965.

465 Brawley, R. K., and Morrow, A. G.: Direct Determination of Aortic Blood Flow in Patients with Aortic Regurgitation: Effects of Alterations in Heart Rate, Increased Ventricular Preload and Afterload, and Isoproterenol, *Circulation,* 35:32, 1967.

466 Morrow, A. G., Brawley, R. K., and Braunwald, E.: Effects of Aortic Regurgitation on Left Ventricular Performance: Direct Determination of Aortic Blood Flow before and after Valve Replacement, *Circulation,* 31(suppl. 1):80, 1965.

467 Warner, H. R., and Toronto, A. F.: Effect of Heart Rate on Aortic Insufficiency as Measured by a Dye-Dilution Technique, *Circ. Res.,* 9:413, 1961.

468 Wiggers, C. J.: The Magnitude of Regurgitation with Aortic Leak of Different Sizes, *J.A.M.A.,* 97:1359, 1931.

469 Judge, T. P., Kennedy, J. W., Bennett, L. J., Willis, R. E., Murray, J. A., and Blackman, J. R.: Quantitative Hemodynamic Effects of Heart Rate in Aortic Regurgitation, *Circulation,* 44:355, 1971.

470 Miller, G. A., Kirklin, J. W., and Swan, H. J.: Myocardial Function and Left Ventricular Volumes in Acquired Valvular Insufficiency, *Circulation,* 31:374, 1965.

471 Gault, J. H., Covell, J. W., Braunwald, E., Gawt, J. H., and Ross, J., Jr.: Left Ventricular Performance following

Correction of Free Aortic Regurgitation, *Circulation*, 42:773, 1970.

472 Alexander, R. S.: Viscoelastic Determinants of Muscle Contractility and "Cardiac Tone," *Fed. Proc.*, 21:1001, 1962.

473 Lingbach, A. J.: Heart Failure from the Point of View of Quantitative Anatomy, *Am. J. Cardiol.*, 5:370, 1960.

474 Rees, J. R., Epstein, E. J., Criley, J. M., and Ross, R. S.: Haemodynamic Effects of Severe Aortic Regurgitation, *Br. Heart J.*, 26:412, 1964.

475 Goldschlager, N., Pfeifer, J., Cohn, K., Pepper, R., and Selzer, A.: The Natural History of Aortic Regurgitation: A Clinical and Hemodynamic Study, *Am. J. Med.*, 54:577, 1973.

476 Harvey, W. P., Segal, J. P., and Hufnagel, C. A.: Unusual Clinical Features Associated with Severe Aortic Insufficiency, *Ann. Intern. Med.*, 47:27, 1957.

477 Bland, E. F., and Wheeler, E. O.: Severe Aortic Regurgitation in Young People: A Long-Term Perspective with Reference to Prognosis and Prosthesis, *N. Engl. J. Med.*, 256:667, 1957.

478 Najafi, H.: Aortic Insufficiency: Clinical Manifestations and Surgical Treatment, *Am. Heart J.*, 82:120, 1971.

479 Wigle, E. D., and Labrosse, C. J.: Sudden, Severe Aortic Insufficiency, *Circulation*, 32:708, 1965.

480 Cohn, L. H., Mason, D. T., Ross, J., Jr., Morrow, A. G., and Braunwald, E.: Preoperative Assessment of Aortic Regurgitation in Patients with Mitral Valve Disease, *Am. J. Cardiol.*, 19:177, 1967.

481 Hudson, R. E.: "Cardiovascular Pathology: The Aortic Valve: Valvular, Subvalvular, and Supravalvular Lesions," vol. 1, Edward Arnold (Publishers) Ltd., London, 1965, pp. 1037–1054.

482 Hill, L., and Rowlands, R. A.: Systolic Blood Pressure: I. In Change of Posture: II. In Cases of Aortic Regurgitation, *Heart*, 3:219, 1911–1912.

483 Deliyannis, A. A., Gillam, P. M., Mounsey, J. P., and Steiner, R. E.: The Cardiac Impulse and the Motion of the Heart, *Br. Heart J.*, 26:396, 1964.

484 Groom, D., and Boone, J. A.: The Dove-Coo Murmur and Murmurs Heard at a Distance from the Chest Wall, *Ann. Intern. Med.*, 42:1214, 1955.

485 Fortuin, N. J., and Craige, E.: On the Mechanism of the Austin Flint Murmur, *Circulation*, 45:558, 1972.

486 Winsberg, F., Gabor, G. E., Hernberg, J. G., and Weiss, B.: Fluttering of the Mitral Valve in Aortic Insufficiency, *Circulation*, 41:225, 1970.

487 Reddy, P. S., Curtiss, E. I., Solerni, R., O'Toole, J. D., Griff, F. W., Leon, D. F., and Shaver, J. A.: Sound Pressure Correlates of the Austin Flint Murmur: An Intracardiac Sound Study, *Circulation*, 53:210, 1976.

488 Wigle, E. D., and Labrosse, C. J.: Sudden, Severe Aortic Insufficiency, *Circulation*, 32:708, 1965.

489 Herbert, W. A.: Prolonged Atrioventricular Conduction and Aortic Insufficiency, *Thorax*, 25:577, 1970.

490 Selzer, A., Naruse, D. Y., York, E., Kahn, K. A., and Matthew, H. B.: Electrocardiographic findings in Concentric and Eccentric Left Ventricular Hypertrophy, *Am. Heart J.*, 63:320, 1962.

491 Spagnuolo, M., Kloth, H., Taranta, A., Doyle, E., and Pasternack, B.: Natural History of Rheumatic Aortic Regurgitation: Criteria Predictive of Death, Congestive Heart Failure, and Angina in Young Patients, *Circulation*, 44:368, 1971.

492 Winsberg, F., Gabor, G. E., Hernberg, J. G., and Weiss, B.: Fluttering of the Mitral Valve in Aortic Insufficiency, *Circulation*, 41:225, 1970.

493 Pridie, R. B., Benham, M. B., and Oakley, C. M.: Echocardiography of the Mitral Valve in Aortic Valve Disease, *Br. Heart J.*, 33:296, 1971.

494 Pridie, R. B., Benham, M. B., and Oakley, C. M.: Recognition of Aortic Regurgitation of Recent Onset by Ultrasound Technique, *Am. J. Cardiol.*, 26:654, 1970. (Abstract.)

495 Cope, G. D., Kisslo, J. A., Johnson, M. L., and Myers, S.: Diastolic Vibration of the Interventricular Septum in Aortic Insufficiency, *Circulation*, 51:589, 1975.

496 Botvinick, E. H., Schiller, N. B., Wickramasekaran, R., Klausner, S. C., and Gertz, E.: Echocardiographic Demonstration of Early Mitral Valve Closure in Severe Aortic Insufficiency: Its Clinical Implications, *Circulation*, 51:836, 1975.

497 Gramiak, R., and Shah, P. M.: Echocardiography of the Normal and Diseased Aortic Valve, *Radiology*, 96:1, 1970.

498 Whipple, R. L., Morris, D. C., Felner, J. M., Merrill, A. J., and Miller, J. I.: Echocardiographic Manifestations of the Flail Aortic Valve Leaflet Syndrome, *J. Clin. Ultrasound*, in press.

499 Feizi, O., Symons, C., and Yacoub, M.: Echocardiography of the Aortic Valve: I. Studies of Normal Aortic Valve, Aortic Stenosis, Aortic Regurgitation, and Mixed Aortic Valve Disease, *Br. Heart J.*, 36:341, 1974.

500 Wray, T. M.: The Variable Echocardiographic Features in Aortic Valve Endocarditis, *Circulation*, 52:658, 1975.

501 Nelson, W. S., Molnar, W., Klassen, K. P., and Ryan, J. M.: Aortic Valvulography and Ascending Aortography, *Radiology*, 70:697, 1958.

502 Dodge, H. T., and Baxley, W. A.: Hemodynamic Aspects of Heart Failure, *Am. J. Cardiol.*, 22:24, 1968.

503 Jones, J. W., Rackley, C. E., Bruce, R. A., Dodge, H. T., Cobb, L. A., and Sandler, H.: Left Ventricular Volumes in Valvular Heart Disease, *Circulation*, 29:887, 1964.

504 Dodge, H. T., and Baxley, W. A.: Left Ventricular Volume and Mass and Their Significance in Heart Disease, *Am. J. Cardiol.*, 23:528, 1969.

505 Karliner, J. S., Gault, J. H., Eckberg, D., Mullins, C. B., and Ross, J., Jr.: Mean Velocity of Fiber Shortening: A Simplified Measure of Left Ventricular Myocardial Contractility, *Circulation*, 44:323, 1971.

506 Berndt, T. B., Hancock, E. W., Shumway, N. E., and Harrison, D. C.: Aortic Valve Replacement with and without Coronary Artery Bypass Surgery, *Circulation*, 50:967, 1974.

507 Gault, J. H., Covell, J. W., Braunwald, E., and Ross, J., Jr.: Left Ventricular Performance following Correction of Free Aortic Regurgitation, *Circulation*, 42:773, 1970.

508 Romhilt, D. W., and Estes, E. H., Jr.: A Point Score System for the ECG Diagnosis of Left Ventricular Hypertrophy, *Am. Heart J.*, 75:752, 1968.

509 Honey, M.: Clinical and Haemodynamic Observations on Combined Mitral and Aortic Stenosis, *Br. Heart J.*, 23:545, 1961.

510 Katznelson, G., Jreissaty, R. M., Levinson, G. E., Stein, S. W., and Abelmann, W. H.: Combined Aortic and Mitral Stenosis: A Clinical and Physiological Study, *Am. J. Med.*, 29:242, 1960.

511 Uricchio, J. F., Goldberg, H., Sinah, K. P., and Likoff, W.: Combined Mitral and Aortic Stenosis: Clinical and Physiologic Features and Results of Surgery, *Am. J. Cardiol.*, 4:479, 1959.

512 Schattenberg, T. T., Titus, J. L., and Parkin, T. W.: Clinical Findings in Acquired Aortic Valve Stenosis: Effect of Disease of Other Valves, *Am. Heart J.*, 73:322, 1967.

513 Uricchio, J. F., Sinha, K. P., Bentivoglio, L., and Goldberg, H.: A Study of Combined Mitral and Aortic Stenosis, *Ann. Intern. Med.*, 51:668, 1959.

514 Reid, J. M., Stevenson, J. G., Barclay, R. S., and Welsh, T. M.: Combined Aortic and Mitral Stenosis, *Br. Heart J.*, 24:509, 1962.

515 Terzaki, A. K., Cokkinos, D. V., Leachman, R. D., Meade, J. B., Hallman, G. L., and Cooley, D. A.: Combined Mitral and Aortic Valve Disease, *Am. J. Cardiol.*, 25:588, 1970.

516 Melvin, D. B., Tecklenberg, P. L., Holingsworth, J. F., Levine, F. H., Glancy, D. L., Epstein, S. E., and Morrow, A. G.: Computer-based Analysis of Preoperative and Postoperative Prognostic Factors in 100 Patients with Combined Aortic and Mitral Valve Replacement, *Circulation*, 48(suppl. 3):III-58, 1972.

517 Killip, T., and Lukas, D. S.: Tricuspid Stenosis: Clinical Features in Twelve Cases, *Am. J. Med.*, 24:836, 1958.

518 Bousvaros, G. A., and Stubinger, D.: Some Auscultatory and Phonocardiographic features of Tricuspid Stenosis, *Circulation*, 29:26, 1964.

519 Kitchin, A., and Turner, R.: Diagnosis and Treatment of Tricuspid Stenosis, *Br. Heart J.*, 26:354, 1964.

520 Morgan, J. R., and Forker, A. D.: Isolated Tricuspid Insufficiency, *Circulation*, 43:559, 1971.

521 Killip, T., and Lukas, D. S.: Tricuspid Stenosis: Physiologic Criteria for Diagnosis and Hemodynamic Abnormalities, *Circulation*, 16:3, 1957.

522 El-Sherif, N.: Rheumatic Tricuspid Stenosis: A Haemodynamic Correlation, *Br. Heart J.*, 33:16, 1971.

523 Gibson, R., and Wood, P.: The Diagnosis of Tricuspid Stenosis, *Br. Heart J.*, 17:552, 1955.

524 Joyner, C. R., Hey, E. B., Johnson, J., and Reid, J. M.: Reflected Ultrasound in the Diagnosis of Tricuspid Stenosis, *Am. J. Cardiol.*, 19:66, 1967.

525 Morgan, J. R., Forker, A. D., Coates, J. R., and Myers, W. S.: Isolated Tricuspid Stenosis, *Circulation*, 44:729, 1971.

526 Hansing, C. E., and Rowe, G. G.: Tricuspid Insufficiency: A Study of Hemodynamics and Pathogenesis, *Circulation*, 45:793, 1972.

527 McMichael, J., and Shillingford, J. P.: The Role of Valvular Incompetence in Heart Failure, *Br. Med. J.*, 1:537, 1957.

528 Glancy, D. L., Marcus, F. I., Cuadra, M., Ewy, G. A., and Roberts, W. C.: Isolated Organic Tricuspid Valvular Regurgitation, *Am. J. Med.*, 46:989, 1969.

529 Sbar, S., Daicoff, G., Nightgale, D., Ramsey, H. W., and Swanick, E. J.: Chronic Tricuspid Insufficiency, *South. Med. J.*, 66:917, 1973.

530 Bain, R. C., Edwards, J. E., Scheifley, C. H., and Geraci, J. E.: Right-sided Bacterial Endocarditis and Endoarteritis: A Clinical and Pathologic Study, *Am. J. Med.*, 24:98, 1958.

531 Roberts, W. C., and Sjoerdsma, A.: The Cardiac Disease Associated with the Carcinoid Syndrome (Carcinoid Heart Disease), *Am. J. Med.*, 36:5, 1964.

532 Sepulveda, G., and Lukas, D. S.: The Diagnosis of Tricuspid Insufficiency: Clinical Features in 60 Cases with Associated Mitral Valve Disease, *Circulation*, 11:552, 1955.

533 Salazar, E., and Levine, H. D.: Rheumatic Tricuspid Regurgitation: The Clinical Spectrum: *Am. J. Med.*, 33:111, 1962.

534 Muller, O., and Shillingford, J.: Tricuspid Incompetence, *Br. Heart J.*, 16:195, 1954.

535 Chandraratna, P. A., Lopez, J. M., Fernandez, J. J., and Cohen, L. S.: Echocardiographic Detection of Tricuspid Valve Prolapse, *Circulation*, 51:823, 1975.

536 Lee, C., Gangully, S. N., Magnisalis, K., and Robin, E.: Detection of Tricuspid Valve Vegetations by Echocardiography, *Chest*, 66:432, 1974.

537 Braunwald, N. S., Ross, J., Jr., and Morrow, A. G.: Conservative Management of Tricuspid Regurgitation in Patients Undergoing Mitral Valve Replacement, *Circulation*, 35(suppl. 1):I-63, 1966.

538 Espino Vela, J., Contreros, R., and Rustrian Sosa, F.: Rheumatic Pulmonary Valve Disease, *Am. J. Cardiol.*, 23:12, 1969.

539 Roberts, W. C., and Buchbinder, N. A.: Right Sided Valvular Infective Endocarditis, *Am. J. Med.*, 53:7, 1972.

540 Seymour, J., Emaneul, R., and Patterson, N.: Acquired Pulmonary Stenosis, *Br. Heart J.*, 30:776, 1968.

541 Holmes, J. C., Fowler, N. O., and Kaplan, S.: Pulmonary Valvular Insufficiency, *Am. J. Med.*, 44:851, 1968.

542 Clawson, B. J.: Rheumatic Heart Disease, *Am. Heart J.*, 20:454, 1940.

543 Ayres, S. M., Arditi, L. I., Lanbrew, C. T., and Lukas, D. S.: Quadrivalvular Rheumatic Heart Disease: Report of a Case with Marked Stenosis of All Valves, *Am. J. Med.*, 32:467, 1962.

544 Hufnagel, C. A., Harvey, W. P., Rabil, P. J., and McDermott, T. F.: Surgical Correction of Aortic Insufficiency, *Surgery*, 35:673, 1954.

545 Harken, D. E., Soroff, H. S., Taylor, W. J., Lefemine, A. A., Gupta, S. K., and Lunzer, S.: Partial and Complete Prostheses in Aortic Insufficiency, *J. Thorac. Cardiovasc. Surg.*, 40:744, 1960.

546 Starr, A., and Edwards, M. L.: Mitral Replacement: Clinical Experience with a Ball-Valve Prosthesis, *Ann. Surg.*, 154:727, 1961.

547 Behrendt, D. M., and Austen, W. G.: Current Status of Prosthetics for Heart Valve Replacement, *Prog. Cardiovasc. Dis.*, 15:369, 1973.

548 Krosnick, A.: Death Due to Migration of the Ball from an Aortic-Valve Prosthesis, *J.A.M.A.*, 191:1083, 1965.

549 Bonchek, L. I., and Starr, A.: Ball Valve Prostheses: Current Appraisal of Late Results, *Am. J. Cardiol.*, 35:843, 1975.

550 Braunwald, N. S., Tatooles, C., Turina, M., and Detmer, D.: New Developments in the Design of Fabric-covered Prosthetic Heart Valves, *J. Thorac. Cardiovasc. Surg.*, 62:673, 1971.

551 Brawley, R. K., Donahoo, J. S., and Gott, V. L.: Current Status of the Beall, Bjork-Shiley, Braunwald-Cutter, Lillehei-Kaster, and Smeloff-Cutter Cardiac Valve Prostheses, *Am. J. Cardiol.*, 35:855, 1975.

552 Kay, E. B., Suzuki, A., Demaney, M., and Zimmerman, H. A.: Comparison of Ball and Disc Valves for Mitral Valve Replacement, *Am. J. Cardiol.*, 18:504, 1966.

553 Cross, F. S., and Jones, R. D.: A Caged-Lens Prothesis for Replacement of the Aortic and Mitral Valves, *Ann. Thorac. Surg.*, 2:499, 1966.

554 Beall, A. C., Jr., Bloodwell, R. D., Liotta, D., Cooley, D. A., and DeBakey, M. E.: Clinical Experience with a Dacron-Velour-Covered Teflon-Disc Mitral-Valve Prosthesis, *Ann. Thorac. Surg.*, 5:402, 1968.

555 Vogel, J. H., Paton, B. C., Overy, H. R., Pappas, G., Davies, D. H., and Blount, S. G., Jr.: Advantages of the Beall Valve Prosthesis, *Chest*, 59:249, 1971.

556 Bjork, V. O.: Experience with the Wada-Cutter Valve Prosthesis in the Aortic Area: One-Year Follow-up, *J. Thorac. Cardiovasc. Surg.*, 60:26, 1970.

557 Bjork, V. O., and Olin, C. A.: A Hydrodynamic Comparison between the New Tilting Disc Aortic Valve Prosthesis (Bjork-Shiley) and the Corresponding Prosthesis of Starr-Edwards, Kay-Shiley, Smeloff-Cutter and Wada-Cutter in the Pulse Duplicator, *Scand. J. Thorac. Cardiovasc. Surg.*, 4:31, 1970.

558 Lillehei, C. W., Kaster, R. L., Coleman, M., and Block, J. H.: Heart-Valve Replacement with Lillehei-Kaster Pivoting Disc Prosthesis, *N.Y. State J. Med.*, 74:1426, 1974.

559 Ross, D. N.: Homograft Replacement of the Aortic Valve, *Lancet*, 2:487, 1962.

560 Barratt-Boyes, B. G.: Homograft Aortic Valve Replacement in Aortic Incompetence and Stenosis, *Thorax*, 19:131, 1964.

561 Wallace, R. B.: Tissue Valves, *Am. J. Cardiol.*, 35:866, 1975.

562 Pacifico, A. D., Karp, R. B., and Kirklin, J. W.: Homografts for Replacement of the Aortic Valve, *Circulation*, 45(suppl. 1):I-36, 1972.

563 Angell, W. W., Shumway, N. E., and Kosek, J. C.: A Five-Year Study of Viable Aortic Valve Homografts, *J. Thor. Cardiovasc. Surg.*, 64:329, 1972.

564 Barratt-Boyes, B., Roche, A., Agnew, T. M., Cole, D., Kerr, A., Monro, J. L., Lowe, J. B., and Brandt, P. W.: Homograft Valves, *Med. J. Aust.*, 2(suppl. 1):I-38, 1972.

565 Gonzalez-Levin, L., al-Janabi, N., and Ross, D. N.: Long-Term Results after Aortic Valve Replacement with Preserved Aortic Homografts, *Ann. Thorac. Surg.*, 31:594, 1972.

566 Graham, A. F., Schroeder, J. S., Daily, P. O., and Harrison, D. C.: Clinical and Hemodynamic Studies in Patients with Homograft Mitral Valve Replacement, *Circulation*, 44:334, 1971.

567 Personal communication from Hancock Laboratories.

568 Ross, D. N.: Replacement of Aortic and Mitral Valves with a Pulmonary Autograft, *Lancet*, 2:956, 1967.

569 Ross, D. N.: Biologic Valves: Their Performance and Prospects, *Circulation*, 45:1259, 1972.

570 Harken, D. E., Taylor, W. J., Lefemine, A. A., Lunzer, S., Low, H. B., Cohen, M. L., and Jacobey, J. A.: Aortic Valve Replacement with a Caged Ball Valve, *Am. J. Cardiol.*, 9:292, 1962.

571 Morris, D. C., Wickliffe, C. W., King, S., III, Douglas, J. S., Jr., and Jones, E. L.: Hemodynamic Evaluation of the Porcine Xenograft Aortic Valve, *Am. J. Cardiol.*, 37:157, 1976.

572 Starek, P. J., Wilcox, B. R., and Murray, G. F.: Hemodynamic Evaluation of the Lillehei-Kaster Pivoting Disc Valve in Patients, *J. Thorac. Cardiovasc. Surg.*, 71:123, 1976.

573 Bjork, V. O., Holmgren, A., Olin, C., and Ovenfors, C.: Clinical and Haemodynamic Results of Aortic Valve Replacement with the Bjork-Shiley Tilting Disc Valve Prosthesis, *Scand. J. Thorac. Cardiovasc. Surg.*, 5:177, 1971.

574 Bristow, J. D., McCord, C. W., Starr, A., Ritzman, L. W., and Griswold, H. E.: Clinical and Hemodynamic Results of Aortic Valvular Replacement with a Ball-Valve Prosthesis, *Circulation*, 29(suppl. 1):36, 1964.

575 Rodriguez, L.: Haemodynamic and Angiographic Findings in Patients with Isolated Aortic Valvular Disease before and after Insertion of a Starr-Edwards Aortic Ball-Valve Prosthesis, *Scand. J. Thorac. Cardiovasc. Surg.*, 4(suppl. 5):1, 1970.

576 Bjork, V. O., Olin, C., and Rodriguez, L.: Comparative Results of Aortic Valve Replacement with Different Prosthetic Heart Valves, *J. Cardiovasc. Surg.*, 13:268, 1972.

577 Blank, R. H., Pupello, D. F., Besson, L. N., Harrison, E. E., and Sbar, S.: Method of Managing the Small Aortic Annulus during Valve Replacement, *Ann. Thorac. Surg.*, 22:356, 1976.

578 Bjork, V. O., Henze, A., and Jereb, M.: Aortographic Follow-up in Patients with the Bjork-Shiley Aortic Disc Valve Prosthesis, *Scand. J. Thorac. Cardiovasc. Surg.*, 7:1, 1973.

579 Bjork, L., and Rodriguez, L.: Angiographic Follow-up Studies in Patients with Aortic Ball Valve Prosthesis, *Scand. J. Thorac. Cardiovasc. Surg.*, 1:57, 1967.

580 Myhre, E., Dale, J., and Rasmussen, K.: Erythrocyte Destruction in Different Types of Starr-Edwards Aortic Ball Valves, *Circulation*, 42:515, 1970.

581 Walsh, J. R., Starr, A., and Ritzmann, L. W.: Intravascular Hemolysis in Patients with Prosthetic Valves and Valvular Heart Disease, *Circulation*, 39(suppl. 1):I-135, 1969.

582 Kloster, F. E.: Diagnosis and Management of Complications of Prosthetic Heart Valves, *Am. J. Cardiol.*, 35:872, 1975.

583 Eyster, E., Rothchild, J., and Mychajliw, O.: Chronic Intravascular Hemolysis after Aortic Valve Replacement: Long-Term Study Comparing Different Types of Ball-Valve Prostheses, *Circulation*, 44:657, 1971.

584 Reid, J. A., Stevens, T. W., Sigwart, U., Fulweber, R. C., and Alexander, J. K.: Hemodynamic Evaluation of the Beall Mitral Valve Prosthesis, *Circulation*, 45(suppl. 1):I-1, 1972.

585 Javier, R. P., Hildner, F. J., Berry, W., Greenberg, J. J., and Somet, P.: Systemic Embolism and the Beall Mitral Valve Prosthesis, *Ann. Thorac. Surg.*, 10:20, 1970.

585a Bjork, V. O., and Henze, A.: Encapsulation of the Bjork-Shiley Aortic Disc Valve Prosthesis Caused by the Lack of Anticoagulation Treatment, *Scand. J. Thorac. Cardiovasc. Surg.*, 7:17, 1973.

586 Yeh, T. J., Anabtawi, I. N., and Cornett, V. E.: Influence of Rhythm and Anticoagulation upon the Incidence of Embolization Associated with Starr-Edwards Prostheses, *Circulation*, 35(suppl. 1):I-77, 1967.

587 Kloster, F. E., Bristow, J. D., and Griswold, H. E.: Medical Problems in Mitral and Multiple Valve Replacement, *Prog. Cardiovasc. Dis.*, 7:504, 1965.

588 Duvoisin, G. E., Brandenburg, R. O., and McGoon, D. C.: Factors Affecting Thromboembolism Associated with Prosthetic Heart Valves, *Circulation*, 35(suppl. 1):I-70, 1967.

589 Hultgren, H. N., and Hubis, H.: A Phonocardiographic Study of Patients with the Starr-Edwards Mitral Valve Prosthesis, *Am. Heart J.*, 69:306, 1965.

590 Njmi, M., and Segal, B. L.: Auscultatory and Phonocardiographic Findings in Patients with Prosthetic Ball-Valves, *Am. J. Cardiol.*, 16:794, 1965.

591 Gibson, T. C., Starek, P. J., Moos, S., and Craige, E.: Echocardiographic and Phonocardiographic Characteristics of the Lillehei-Kaster Mitral Valve Prosthesis, *Circulation*, 49:434, 1974.

592 Wise, J. R., Webb-Peploe, M., and Oakley, C. M.: Detection of Prosthetic Mitral Valve Obstruction by Phonocardiography, *Am. J. Cardiol.*, 28:107, 1971.

593 Willerson, J. T., Kaster, J. A., Dinsmore, R. E., Mundth, E., Buckley, M. J., Austen, W. G., and Sanders, C. A.: Noninvasive Assessment of Prosthetic Mitral Paravalvular and Intravalvular Regurgitation, *Br. Heart J.*, 34:561, 1972.

594 Dayem, M. K., and Raftery, E. B.: Phonocardiogram of the Ball-and-Cage Aortic Valve Prosthesis, *Br. Heart J.*, 29:446, 1967.

595 Boicourt, O. W., Bristow, J. D., Starr, A., and Griswold, H. E.: A Phonocardiographic Study of Patients with Multiple Starr-Edwards Prosthetic Valves, *Br. Heart J.*, 28:531, 1966.

596 Hylen, J. C., Kloster, F. E., Herr, R. H., Hull, P. Q., Amos, A. W., Starr, A., and Griswold, H. E.: Phonocardiographic Diagnosis of Aortic Ball Variance, *Circulation*, 38:90, 1968.

597 Hylen, J. C., Kloster, F. E., Starr, A., and Griswold, H. E.: Aortic Ball Variance: Diagnosis and Treatment, *Ann. Intern. Med.*, 72:1, 1970.

598 Lansing, A. M.: Unusual Radiologic Sign of Loose Mitral Valve Prosthesis, *Radiology*, 88:789, 1967.

599 White, A. F., Dinsmore, R. E., and Buckley, M. J.: Cineradiographic Evaluation of Prosthetic Cardiac Valves, *Circulation*, 48:882, 1973.

600 Hylen, J. C.: Durability of Prosthetic Heart Valves, *Am. Heart J.*, 81:299, 1971.

601 Hylen, J. C.: Mechanical Malfunction and Thrombosis of Prosthetic Heart Valves, *Am. J. Cardiol.*, 30:396, 1972.

602 Belenkie, I., Carr, M., Schlant, R. C., Nutter, D. O., and Symbas, P. N.: Malformation of a Cutter-Smeloff Mitral Ball Valve Prosthesis: Diagnosis by Phonocardiography and Echocardiography, *Am. Heart J.*, 86:399, 1973.

603 Ben-Zvi, J., Hildner, F. J., Chandraratna, P. A., and Samet, P.: Thrombosis on Bjork-Shiley Aortic Valve Prosthesis: Clinical, Arteriographic, Echocardiographic, and Therapeutic Observations in Seven Cases, *Am. J. Cardiol.*, 34:538, 1974.

604 Friedi, B., Aerichide, N., Grondin, P., and Campeau, L.:

Thromboembolic Complications of Heart Valve Prostheses, *Am. Heart J.,* 81:702, 1971.

605 Cohn, L. H., Roberts, W. C., Rockoff, S. D., and Morrow, A. G.: Bacterial Endocarditis following Aortic Valve Replacement: Clinical and Pathologic Correlations, *Circulation,* 33: 209, 1966.

606 Slaughter, L., Morris, J. F., and Starr, A.: Prosthetic Valvular Endocarditis, *Circulation,* 47:1319, 1973.

607 Dismukes, W. E., Karchmer, A. W., Buckley, M. J., Austen, W. G., and Swartz, M. N.: Prosthetic Valve Endocarditis: Analysis of 38 Cases, *Circulation,* 48:365, 1973.

608 Kloster, F. E., Herr, R. H., Starr, A., and Griswold, H. E.: Hemodynamic Evaluation of a Cloth-covered Starr-Edwards Valve Prosthesis, *Circulation,* 39(suppl. 1):I–119, 1969.

609 Kloster, F. E., Farrehi, C., Mourdjinis, A., Hodam, R. P., Starr, A., and Griswold, H. E.: Hemodynamic Studies in Patients with Cloth-covered Composite-Seat Starr-Edwards Valve Prostheses, *J. Thorac. Cardiovasc. Surg.,* 60:879, 1970.

610 McHenry, M. M., Smeloff, E. A., Davey, T. B., Kaufman, B., and Fong, W. Y.: Hemodynamic Results with Full-Flow Orifice Prosthetic Valves, *Circulation,* 35(suppl. 1):24, 1967.

611 Bjork, V. O., Olin, C., and Astrom, H.: Haemodynamic Results of Aortic Valve Replacement with the Kay-Shiley Disc Valve, *Scand. J. Thorac. Cardiovasc. Surg.,* 4:195, 1970.

612 Morrow, A. G., Oldham, H. N., Elkins, R. S., and Braunwald, E.: Prosthetic Replacement of the Mitral Valve: Preoperative and Postoperative Clinical and Hemodynamic Assessments in 100 Patients, *Circulation,* 35:962, 1967.

613 Brown, J. W., Myerowitz, P. D., Cann, M. S., Calvin, S. B., McIntosh, C. L., and Morrow, A. G.: Clinical and Hemodynamic Comparison of Kay-Shiley, Starr-Edwards No. 6520, and Reis-Hancock Porcine Xenograft Mitral Valves, *Surgery,* 76:983, 1974.

614 Linhart, J. W., Barold, S. S., Hildner, F. J., Samett, P., Piccinini, J. C., Marstein, J. L., and Greenberg, J. J.: Clinical and Hemodynamic Findings following Replacement of the Mitral Valve with a Beall Valve Prosthesis (Dacron-Velour-Covered Teflon-Disc Valve), *Circulation,* 39(suppl. 1):127, 1969.

615 Felner, J. M., and Schlant, R. C.: "Echocardiography: A Teaching Atlas," Grune & Stratton, Inc., New York, 1976.

61
Surgical Treatment of Acquired Valvular Heart Disease

JOHN W. KIRKLIN, M.D., and
ROBERT B. KARP, M.D.

MITRAL STENOSIS

Pathology and etiology

Rheumatic fever is considered the usual cause of mitral stenosis. A documented episode of it is apparent historically in 60 to 65 percent of cases.[1,2] The initial rheumatic involvement ordinarily occurs along

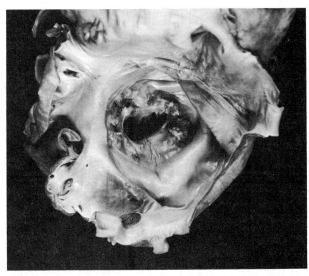

FIGURE 61-1 Extensive calcification of the anterior leaflet and both commissural areas. (Necropsy specimen of a calcified, stenotic, incompetent mitral valve.) Leaflets are immobile, and surgical correction obviously requires replacement of such a valve.

the free edges of the valve leaflets, where thickening and loss of pliability develop. Progressive scarring and deformity of the valve follow. Fusion at the anterolateral and posteromedial commissures causes narrowing of the valve orifice. Valve function frequently is further impaired by fusion and contraction of the chordae tendineae. Calcium deposits, either localized or generalized, are found in the valve leaflets in approximately 40 percent of operative cases (Fig. 61-1).[3]

Life history

Patients with mitral stenosis usually suffer gradual progression of disability, although temporary plateaus of remarkable exercise tolerance occur. Concomitant with advancing valvular obstruction, the end-diastolic pressure difference between left atrium and left ventricle increases and results in elevated left atrial and pulmonary venous pressure. Episodes of pulmonary edema occur, frequently initiated by the onset of atrial fibrillation. Later, pulmonary vascular disease develops in many patients, and resultant pulmonary artery hypertension increases the workload of the right ventricle. Right ventricular function may decrease, tricuspid valve incompetence develop, and fluid retention and hepatomegaly result. Left ventricular performance is decreased in some patients with long-standing mitral stenosis. For example, impaired contraction in the posterior basal portion of the left ventricle has been demonstrated.[4]

Olesen[2] reported that 20 percent of patients with mitral stenosis died within 1 year from the time that they were first seen. Sixty percent were dead within

10 years. In the survivors there was progressive cardiac disability.

Surgical treatment

The operation should usually be done, we believe, by an open technique with cardiopulmonary bypass. This is because the risk of mitral commissurotomy done in this way is low, less than 1 percent, and because a better commissurotomy, with splitting and freeing of the chordae and at times the papillary muscles, is possible than by closed techniques.[5] Also, the operation can easily be converted to one of valve replacement when this is indicated. Mitral commissurotomy, however, is the operation of choice. When existing or created mitral valvular incompetence is significant and not correctable by reparative measures or when immobility and calcification of leaflets prevent obtaining an adequate orifice by commissurotomy, valve replacement is done.

Operation

A median sternotomy incision is used routinely for the operation. The heart and the patient are cooled by the perfusate at the start of cardiopulmonary bypass, and the aorta is cross-clamped prior to opening the left atrium in order to avoid air embolization. An exception to this is made when ventricular fibrillation develops during cardiac cooling. Nearly all operations on the mitral valve can be completed within 30 min, which we consider to be a safe period of cardiac ischemia after thorough cooling of the heart in the manner described.

The mitral valve is studied for its suitability for mitral commissurotomy. If it is judged to be suitable, fine silk sutures are placed on the anterior and posterior leaflets for traction. With the knife an incision is made in the lateral commissure, usually to the edge of the valve ring. The chordae beneath the commissures go to both anterior and posterior leaflets and can be used as a guide to the commissures. When fused chordae exist beneath the commissure, these may be separated carefully by sharp dissection, in order to enlarge the orifice. A similar procedure is carried out at the medial commissure. At times when the chordae are short and the papillary muscles scarred, the muscle may be split between chordae to enlarge the orifice. Only if the leaflets are immobile or heavily calcified or if the valve is found to be incompetent after discontinuing cardiopulmonary bypass is valve replacement utilized. Any thrombi present within the left atrium are removed, taking precautions to avoid scattering them. The left atrial appendage is oversewn from within the left atrium or ligated externally before discontinuing cardiopulmonary bypass if it contains no thrombi. Strict precautions are taken to avoid air embolization as the heart is refilled with blood and cardiopulmonary bypass is discontinued.

Postoperative care

The postoperative course of patients undergoing open mitral commissurotomy is usually uncomplicated, and the care is similar to that given other patients undergoing intracardiac operations.[6] When cardiac performance is suboptimal, the infusion of blood is used to maintain the mean left atrial pressure at levels of about 14 mm Hg. If arterial blood pressure is higher than normal, reduction of left ventricular afterload is accomplished by the continuous intravenous infusion of nitroprusside. Efforts are made to maintain a sinus rhythm when possible, including the use of atrial pacing at a rate of about 110 beats per minute.

If the hemodynamic state is good, the patient is usually extubated a few hours after operation. When cardiac output is low, a nasotracheal tube is utilized, and the patient is maintained on intermittent mandatory ventilation with moderate positive end-expiratory pressure. In any event, extubation is usually possible 24 to 48 h after operation.

Urine flow is monitored, and when less than 15 mm/h, a diuretic such as furosemide is employed.

If thrombi have been found in the left atrium, anticoagulation with Coumadin is begun about 48 h postoperatively and maintained for about 10 days.

Hospital morbidity and mortality

The hospital mortality following open mitral commissurotomy is as low as that for closed commissurotomy and is approximately 1 percent. Morbidity is minimal. This low mortality and morbidity is in sharp contrast to that reported in earlier periods.[12]

Late results

The late results of open mitral commissurotomy are at least as good as those of closed mitral commissurotomy.[7] Therefore, good long-term results may be expected in 80 to 85 percent of the patients who survived the operation.[8] As has been demonstrated in the past for closed mitral commissurotomy, a tendency exists for restenosis to develop because of thickening and scarring of the mitral valve, or perhaps because of continuing rheumatic activity. Reoperation may be required 5 to 20 years after the operative procedure.[9,10] This deterioration has been estimated to be at the rate of about 5 percent of patients per year. Embolization occurs in the late follow-up period at a rate of about 0.5 to 0.7 percent of patients per year.

There is a striking hemodynamic correlation with the symptomatic improvement, as has been reported previously by Morrow and Braunwald.[11]

Present indications for operation

The development of symptoms which interfere with the patient's productivity and enjoyment of life is an indication for operation when a commissurotomy appears to be probably feasible. These symptoms are usually dyspnea and effort intolerance; later in the course of the disease they include fluid retention and weight loss. A history of systemic arterial embolization is an indication for operation. When the preoperative evaluation indicates that valve replacement will probably be required, more advanced disability [usually New York Heart Association (NYHA) Class III] is required before operation is advised. This is because of the somewhat greater long-term risks and imponderables of valve replacement, compared with commissurotomy.

MITRAL VALVULAR INCOMPETENCE

Etiology and pathology

Competence of the mitral valve depends on the integrity of the valve leaflets, chordae tendineae, and papillary muscles and the size of the valve ring. Inflammatory changes associated with rheumatic valvulitis may produce retraction of valve leaflets, particularly the posterior one, and fusion and contraction of the chordae tendineae, thus preventing apposition of the leaflets during systole. Dilatation of the valve ring may produce incompetence, there being a relative decrease in the amount of valve tissue. Calcification of the valve is present in 8 to 10 percent of cases in which the primary hemodynamic deficit is incompetence.[13] In such cases, the valve is usually somewhat stenotic as well.

Subacute bacterial endocarditis with chordal rupture and destruction of leaflet tissue may result in incompetence of the mitral valve. Myocardial infarction or ischemia involving the posterior wall and the anterolateral or posterior papillary muscles can lead to sudden development of incompetence of the mitral valve because of rupture of the papillary muscle or of the chordae tendineae.[14] Chordal rupture as an isolated lesion may occur in the absence of myocardial infarction or bacterial endocarditis and produce mitral regurgitation and a characteristic clinical syndrome. The syndrome of prolapsing mitral leaflet has become clearly defined, and this can lead to mitral incompetence. The leaflets may have mucoid degeneration in this condition. Incompetence also may follow surgical correction of mitral stenosis.

In recent years it has become clear that severe left ventricular failure from any cause may result in a significant degree of mitral regurgitation. The results of surgically treating the mitral regurgitation in this situation have been poor.

Life history

Pure rheumatic mitral valvular incompetence, mild to moderate in degree, may be well tolerated for a long time. Onset and progression of symptoms are often gradual. The acute onset of gross mitral regurgitation, which occurs on rupture of chordae tendineae or a papillary muscle, quickly produces severe symptoms, including dyspnea and weakness, and is tolerated poorly by some patients. Occasional individuals tolerate the lesion well for a long period of time. In the presence of incompetence of the mitral valve, congestive heart failure may be precipitated by the onset of atrial fibrillation, pulmonary embolism, or bronchopulmonary infection.

Surgical treatment

Surgical treatment consists either of repair or replacement.

A reparative procedure is done whenever the pathologic condition of the valve permits it. The advantage of reparative procedures is that they avoid the long-term risks and imponderables of devices used to replace the mitral valve, and the need for long-term anticoagulant therapy inherent in many of them. The disadvantages of a reparative procedure include some lack of certainty that total competence will be established and the difficulty in knowing before starting the repair whether sufficient valvular competence can be established to avoid valve replacement. We employ valve repair (rather than replacement) in about 20 percent of patients with pure incompetence.

Carpentier and his associates[15] have made major contributions to the treatment of mitral incompetence by reparative techniques by their careful study of the pathology of mitral incompetence and of the various procedures required for its repair. They, like Merindino,[16] Wooler,[17] Reed,[18] and Kay[19] and their associates, and others, have stressed that annuloplasty is a basic technique, required for most patients in whom mitral incompetence is repaired. Carpentier et al. have shown the advantages of performing this as a plastic, rather than narrowing procedure, using multiple-point fixation to a flexible ring. Procedures on the leaflets themselves are indicated in certain circumstances, particularly in ruptured chordae to the central portion of the posterior leaflet; here we follow the advice of Carpentier and his coworkers in making a quadrangular excision rather than a triangular one and in combining it with ring annuloplasty. Occasionally, a solitary perforation of the anterior leaflet from bacterial endocarditis can be simply repaired (Fig. 61-2).

When most of the chordae to the posterior leaflet are ruptured or more than one or two to the anterior leaflet, valve replacement is required. Calcification and immobility of the leaflets are an indication for replacement. In our experience, most patients with combined mitral stenosis and incompetence require valve replacement.

Postoperative care

This is the same as described for patients undergoing mitral commissurotomy.

Hospital morbidity and mortality

See also "Replacement of the Mitral Valve," below.

The risk of reconstructive operations on the mitral

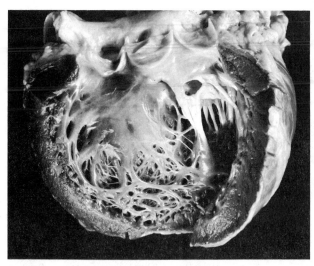

FIGURE 61-2 Solitary perforation of the anterior leaflet of the mitral valve. This could be repaired with a patch of pericardium.

valve is generally low. We and others have reported early mortality rates of less than 2 percent.[6]

The morbidity of reconstructive operations is low. Thromboembolism is rare.

Late results

The special situation of ruptured chordae to the central portion of the posterior leaflet has been documented to respond well to repair.[20-22] The results of annuloplasty, although not perfect, are good; 50 to 80 percent of the patients continue to have good results 5 to 10 years after the operation.[23-28]

Present indications for operation

Significant and progressing symptoms have been the traditional indications for surgical treatment for incompetence of the mitral valve. This was reasonable at a time when little information was available concerning the long-term results of replacement of the mitral valve. Today the prosthetic devices for replacement of the mitral valve are much improved over earlier models (see below), and a considerable amount is known about the long-term results of operation. Also there is growing awareness of myocardial mechanics in mitral regurgitation,[29] the high risk imposed by delaying operation until cardiac reserves have been lost,[30] and the irreversibility of some types of left ventricular failure. These all indicate the wisdom of advising operation for patients with mitral regurgitation when symptoms have become moderate or when left ventricular enlargement is progressive with or without symptoms. The presence of defects at other valves and presence of

chronic intractable heart failure increased the risk of operation but do *not* contraindicate it.

REPLACEMENT OF THE MITRAL VALVE

The device

A number of artificial and biologic valves have been used to replace the mitral valve. Since most of those presently in use have been in patients for less than 10 years, a final evaluation of each is not yet possible. Most of them have been durable and have given good long-term results.

At present, unless anticoagulants are strongly contraindicated for the patient in question, we use the Bjork-Shiley tilting disk valve prosthesis with a pyrolite occluder.[31] The sewing ring only is cloth-covered. Long-term anticoagulant therapy is required, but with it the incidence of thromboembolic complications is low. The orifice size is large in relation to its outside diameter. Mechanical failures have occurred only rarely. The proportion of patients who are long-term survivors is as good as that with any other device for mitral replacement.[32]

When anticoagulants are contraindicated or particularly undesirable, as in children, young adult females, patients over about 70 years of age, or persons with a history of bleeding peptic ulcer disease, we use the Hancock glutaraldehyde-preserved and stent-mounted porcine heterograft aortic valve.[33] Anticoagulant therapy is used for only 3 to 6 weeks postoperatively. Thromboembolic complications are rare. Although the follow-up period is only 8 years, the durability of the Hancock heterograft valve has been good. We believe it likely that eventually these valves will fail by low-grade rejection, but arguing by analogy with homografts inserted freehand in the aortic position, we believe the valve failure will be gradual and allow time for reintervention. We do not ordinarily use these valves when the external diameter that can be accepted is less than 25 mm Hg, because the ratio of internal diameter to external diameter of the stent-mounted heterograft is undesirably small, making them stenotic in the small sizes.

The cloth-covered composite-seat Starr-Edwards ball valve, series 6310-6320,[34] the Braunwald-Cutter cloth-covered valve,[35] the Starr-Edwards Silastic ball valve series 6300,[34] and the Lillehei-Kaster tilting disk valve[36] are reported to give good results in the mitral position, as are other valves, and are used by some surgeons.

Surgical technique

The general technique for the operation is the same as described for mitral commissurotomy. The mitral valve is excised after cooling the heart, cross-clamping the aorta, and opening the left atrium. We have in recent years employed a continuous suture technique using No. 2-0 monofilament suture and believe it superior to an interrupted technique. The left atrial appendage is oversewn from inside the left atrium or ligated from the outside.

Postoperative care

The care of patients after mitral valve replacement is similar to that for patients undergoing open mitral commissurotomy. However, the cardiac performance is apt to be not as good early after mitral valve replacement, and routine measurement of cardiac index is desirable in the immediate postoperative period. Maintenance of left atrial pressure at 14 mm Hg and reduction of left ventricular afterload by continuous infusion of nitroprusside when atrial blood pressure is above the normal value usually suffice to keep cardiac index above about 1.6 liters/(min)(m²). Special measures are indicated in the unusual circumstances of an index less than about 1.6 liters/(min)(m²) and a clinical state of the patient compatible with inadequate cardiac performance.[6] If this is thought to be transient, the continuous intravenous infusion of epinephrine in a dose of 0.05 to 0.1 mg/(kg)(min) is used. Otherwise, we have found the use of intraaortic balloon pulsation for 1 to 7 days to be the optimal form of treatment.

Hospital morbidity and mortality

The risk of mitral valve replacement is related to the clinical condition of the patient prior to operation. In our experience the risk of mitral valve replacement in patients with mitral incompetence has been 7 percent, but only 2.4 percent in patients with mitral stenosis.[6] In an experience with open operations in general for mitral valve disease, including replacement, the hospital risk has been 0 for patients in NYHA Class II, 1.3 percent in NYHA Class III, but 24.4 percent for patients with the advanced disability associated with NYHA Class IV.[6]

The morbidity in surviving patients is modest. Thromboembolic complications are rare. Pulmonary dysfunction can be significant, and about 80 percent of patients are best managed by ventilation and tracheal intubation for at least 24 h postoperatively.

Late results

Thromboembolic complications were common with the early models of prosthetic mitral valves but with currently used devices are much lower (Fig. 61-3). The survival rates for patients with presently available prosthetic or biologic valves in the mitral position are also considerably higher than with the devices that were initially available (Fig. 61-4 and 61-5). However, the results continue to be dependent on the degree of disability prior to operation (Fig. 61-6), nearly 90 percent of patients with Class III disability preoperatively having a good long-term result and only about 50 percent of patients with Class IV disability having good long-term results.[37] Again, this emphasizes the importance of advising operation before left ventricular dysfunction becomes advanced and irreversible.[38]

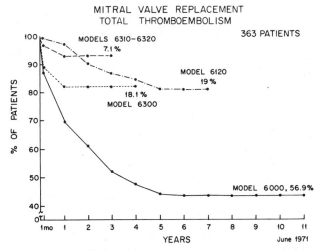

FIGURE 61-3 Percentage of patients suffering thromboembolism after mitral valve replacement with various models of the Starr-Edwards ball valve prosthesis, in the experience of Starr. Note the very low incidence with the model 6310-6320, whose nonmoving parts are totally cloth covered [*Reproduced with permission from A. Starr, Prosthetic Valve Replacement (presented at postgraduate course in cardiovascular surgery, American College of Surgeons, Chicago, October 1971.)*]

AORTIC STENOSIS

Surgical pathology

The appearance of the valve in adult patients with aortic stenosis may not permit distinction between congenital and acquired disease. However, most

FIGURE 61-4 Actuarial survival curves following the insertion of various ball valve prostheses. Note the improved results with the use of the model 6310-6320. (*Reproduced with permission from Kirklin and Pacifico.*[38])

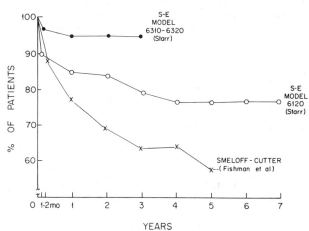

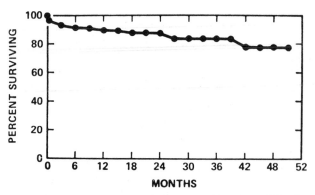

FIGURE 61-5 Actuarial survival curve of patients following isolated mitral valve replacement with Hancock stent-mounted porcine aortic valve heterograft (n = 87). The probability of survival is 90.0 percent (±2.76 SEM) at 1 year and 77.5 percent (±9.76) at 4 years. (*Reproduced with permission from Buch, Pipkin, Hancock, and Fogarty.*[33])

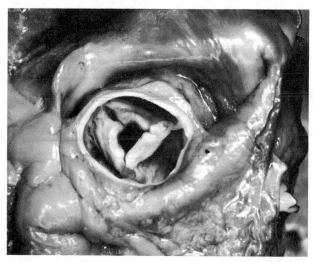

FIGURE 61-7 Stenotic aortic valve with thickened but noncalcified cusps. The commissures, now fused, are easily identified. This kind of pathologic condition suggests that rheumatic fever is causative of the lesion.

male patients with isolated aortic stenosis probably have a congenital bicuspid valve. A history of rheumatic fever in 51 percent of cases[39] and involvement of the mitral valve in approximately 50 percent of cases[40] suggest that rheumatic fever is frequently causative of aortic stenosis. Degeneration and calcification of an apparently originally normal tricuspid valve seems to be the cause of aortic stenosis in some elderly patients.

Calcification is present in a high percentage of male patients with aortic stenosis. In female patients

calcification occurs somewhat less frequently, and the basic architecture of the cusps is often preserved (Fig. 61-7). When the aortic valve is heavily calcified, the commissure between the left and right coronary cusps is usually unrecognizable, and there is only a slitlike orifice (Fig. 61-8). In the most advanced examples of the disease, the calcification involves and distorts all cusps and may extend down into the anterior leaflet of the mitral valve or into the ventricular septum. Complete heart block may result in the latter case. Because of the rigidity of the cusps, varying degrees of incompetence of the valve may be present.

Occlusive coronary artery disease is present in a significant number of patients with aortic stenosis and may complicate the therapeutic problem.[41] Calcific emboli dislodged spontaneously from the aortic valve may produce coronary artery obstruction. Such emboli may go also to the brain and kidney.[42]

FIGURE 61-6 Actuarial survival curve of patients following isolated mitral valve replacement with Starr-Edwards composite-seat cloth-covered prosthesis model No. 6310-6320 (n = 139). The survival is strikingly better (p < 0.05) for patients who were NYHA Class III preoperatively than for those who were NYHA Class IV. (*Reproduced with permission from Allen, Karp, and Kouchoukos.*[37])

FIGURE 61-8 Stenotic, calcified aortic valve in an adult male. This probably was a congenitally bicuspid valve which gradually became calcified, rigid, and stenotic.

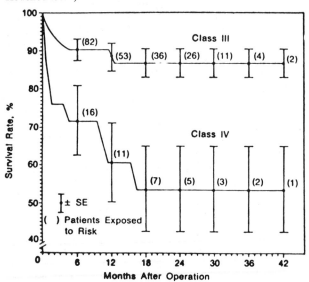

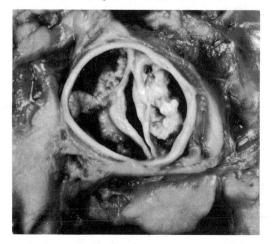

Life history

Aortic stenosis may be well tolerated for long periods without symptoms. Grant, Paul Wood, and Frank and Ross have reported data suggesting that at least 50 percent of patients identified as having severe aortic stenosis with or without symptoms, are dead in 5 years.[43–45] Sudden death, without significant preexisting symptoms, occurs in about 20 percent of untreated patients, presumably from cardiac arrhythmia resulting from myocardial ischemia. Angina develops in some patients as the first symptom.[46] Syncopal attacks are ominous. Symptoms of pulmonary venous hypertension (dyspnea, orthopnea, and paroxysmal nocturnal dyspnea) indicate reduction of left ventricular function and are often the prelude to death. Signs and symptoms of right ventricular dysfunction indicate that the end stage of the disease has been reached.

Surgical treatment

The pathologic alterations in the valve are such that a satisfactory result can rarely be obtained from incision of fused commissures and debridement of cusps. The operation of choice is usually excision and replacement of the valve (see below). The hospital mortality rate is less than 5 percent for most types of patients.[47]

Postoperative care

This is described under "Replacement of the Aortic Valve," below.

Hospital morbidity and mortality

These are described under "Replacement of the Aortic Valve," below.

Late results

These are described under "Replacement of the Aortic Valve," below.

Present indications for treatment

Asymptomatic patients with severe aortic stenosis and marked left ventricular hypertrophy (as evidenced by the chest roentgenogram and by electrocardiographic evidence of left ventricular hypertrophy with "strain pattern") should be advised to undergo operation. The risks and imponderables of the operation (see later) are presently fewer than those of the disease untreated. Patients with symptoms from pulmonary venous hypertension should be advised to undergo operation promptly, as should those with hepatomegaly and fluid retention. Patients with a history of repeated syncope or angina pectoris are also advised to have surgery.

When operation is being considered in a patient with aortic stenosis, the diagnosis can usually be based on the history and the presence of the characteristic murmur and of damped arterial pulses, the

radiologic identification of calcium in the valve, and the roentgenographic and electrocardiographic evidence of left ventricular hypertrophy. When the findings are not characteristic, the peak difference across the aortic valve is measured. Operation is ordinarily not advised when this gradient is less than 50 mm Hg. Coronary arteriography is advisable in all patients with aortic stenosis who are over about 40 years of age and are being considered for operation, because of possible coexisting coronary artery disease.[41] If surgically correctable occlusive coronary arterial disease is demonstrated, coronary bypass grafting should be carried out at the time of replacement of the aortic valve.

AORTIC VALVE INCOMPETENCE

Surgical pathology

Acquired incompetence of the aortic valve may result from deformity or loss of substance of the aortic cusp or from dilatation of the aortic annulus. The most common cause of cusp deformity is rheumatic fever. Bacterial endocarditis may result in loss of substance of a cusp (Fig. 61-9). Cases of traumatic rupture of aortic cusps, either from strenuous effort or from chest wall trauma, have been recorded.[48] Aneurysm of the ascending aorta from cystic medial necrosis can cause dilatation of the annulus and aortic valvular incompetence.[49] In this condition, the ascending aorta becomes dilated because of destruction of muscle and elastic fibers in the media. Dilata-

FIGURE 61-9 Ruptured aneurysm of an aortic cusp secondary to subacute bacterial endocarditis. Notice the rather discrete perforation in the noncoronary cusp with minimal distortion in the remainder of the cusps. (*Reproduced from J. E. Edwards, "An Atlas of Acquired Diseases of the Heart and Great Vessels: Diseases of the Valves and Pericardium," W. B. Saunders Company, Philadelphia, 1961, vol. 1, p. 331, with permission of author and publisher.*)

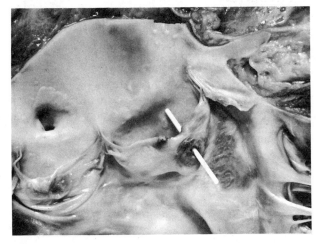

tion of the valve ring, shortening of the valve cusps, and widening of the commissures between the cusps produce valvular incompetence. Coronary blood flow may be impaired by involvement of the coronary ostiums. Rheumatic valvulitis, syphilitic aortitis, bacterial endocarditis, and aneurysms involving the ascending aorta may produce such deformities. The incidence of proximal aortic dilatation due to lesions of the medionecrosis cystica type appears to be increasing, perhaps only because greater awareness among physicians of the condition causes it to be reported more often.

Commonly, at operation for severe, noncalcific incompetence of the aortic valve, the cusps appear at first glance to be normal. Close inspection reveals that they are slightly thickened, the free edges are rolled, and the distance from the free margin to the aortic wall is shortened. Varying degrees of incompetence are found in patients with calcified, stenotic valves whose cusps are sometimes shortened and immobile.

Dissecting aneurysms of the ascending aorta may result in the sudden onset of incompetence of the aortic valve. The dissection proceeds down toward the sinuses of Valsalva, loosens the attachment of the cusps, and thus renders them deformed and incompetent.[50]

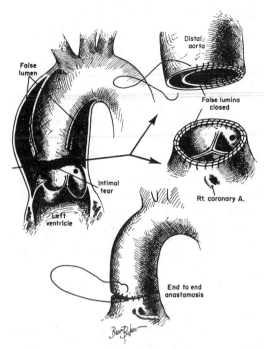

FIGURE 61-10 Incompetence of aortic valve due to dissecting aneurysm. Note the loss of attachment of the valve cusps. The aorta is transected just downstream of the aortic valve, and the false lumen is closed both proximally and distally. The aortic cusps are thereby resuspended and again are competent. End-to-end anastomosis then reestablishes continuity. (*Reproduced from Hufnagel and Conrad,*[53] *with permission of authors and publisher.*)

Life history

Spagnuolo, Koth, and associates have shown in a prospective study that patients with aortic regurgitation, moderate or marked left ventricular enlargement as determined radiologically, electrocardiographic evidence of left ventricular hypertrophy and S-T segment depression or T wave inversion in V_6, systolic blood pressure over 140 mm Hg, and diastolic blood pressure less than 40 mm Hg are at high risk of dying within 3 to 6 years, even though they were asymptomatic when first observed.[51] Symptoms of angina pectoris indicate an even shorter life expectancy. Symptoms of dyspnea, paroxysmal nocturnal dyspnea, and orthopnea indicate a life expectancy of less than 1 year.

Patients with aortic regurgitation, little widening of the pulse pressure, and only mild left ventricular hypertrophy have a long life expectancy, provided they do not develop the stigmata of high risk noted earlier.

In cases of acute onset of aortic regurgitation, as may occur with a dissecting aneurysm or rupture of a cusp, the course is rapid, and the response to medical management is poor.[52]

Surgical treatment and results

In most cases a deformed and incompetent aortic valve is best treated by excision and replacement (see farther on). In cases of dissecting aneurysm, competence can sometimes be restored by obliteration of the false channel, which relieves the deformity of the cusps resulting from their loss of proper suspension[53,54] (Fig. 61-10).

Postoperative care

This is described under "Replacement of the Aortic Valve," below.

Hospital morbidity and mortality

These are described under "Replacement of the Aortic Valve," below.

Late results

These are described under "Replacement of the Aortic Valve," below.

Present indications for treatment

Patients with chronic aortic valve incompetence are advised at present to undergo operation when symptoms are present. Asymptomatic patients with findings noted by Spagnuolo and colleagues to characterize the "cumulative high-risk category" are also advised to have operation. This is in hope of intervening before left ventricular hypertrophy becomes massive and cardiac reserves are lost. Gault and colleagues have shown that many patients continue to have, after operation, impaired cardiac performance and symptoms when this has happened.[55] When incompetence of the aortic valve develops suddenly, operation should be performed promptly because of the poor prognosis with medical treatment.

REPLACEMENT OF THE AORTIC VALVE

The device

As is the case in the mitral valve, a number of valve devices are available for the aortic position, both artificial and biologic.

In recent years, we have used the Bjork-Shiley tilting disk valve with the pyrolite occluder for most patients (Fig. 61-11).[56] It has the same characteristics as its counterpart for the mitral position described earlier. Long-term anticoagulation is required. As in the mitral position, we use Hancock glutaraldehyde-preserved, stent-mounted porcine heterografts in the aortic position in patients with an absolute or relatively strong contraindication for the use of anticoagulants. With the stent-mounted heterograft in the aortic position, anticoagulants are not used at all. The durability of this biologic device in the aortic position is presumed to be the same as described earlier for it in the mitral position.

Aortic valve homografts, fresh and sterilized with antibiotic solutions or irradiated for sterilization and stored up to 6 months at −70° (the former being preferable), have been used with satisfaction in many patients.[57] Long-term follow-up studies show that homograft valves in place 5 years have a significant tendency toward cusp rupture and incompetence which increases with time. This is believed to result from weakening of the cusps by a low-grade rejection process plus the mechanical stress on the cusps. We and nearly all surgeons therefore have aban-

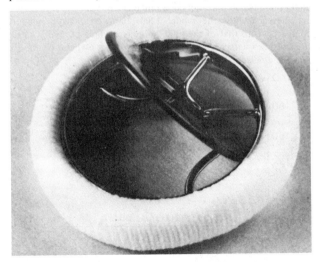

FIGURE 61-11 Bjork-Shiley tilting disk valve with pyrolite occluder, for replacement of the aortic valve. (*Reproduced with permission from Bjork, Henze, and Holmgren.[56]*)

doned the use in this way of homograft aortic valves. Dura mater is used for the leaflets of a stented valve by Zerbini, Jatene, and other surgeons, not only in the aortic position but also the mitral position. Anticoagulants are not required. Infection has been a problem with these valves, and eventually a rejection reaction seems likely to weaken the dura mater cusps.

The Starr-Edwards composite-seat cloth-covered prosthesis, No. 2310-2320, is used by some surgeons and performs well when long-term anticoagulant therapy is used. Some surgeons continue to favor the Starr-Edwards non-cloth-covered model 1200-1260 with the Silastic ball, which also requires long-term anticoagulation. The Lillehei-Kaster tilting disk valve, Smeloff-Cutter valve, and others have been used with success in the aortic position.

Surgical technique

The operation is done by us with cardiopulmonary bypass and profound cardiac cooling initially by the perfusate and continuously by bathing the heart in saline solution at 4°C. Our clinical investigations, an extensive clinical experience, and the work of others indicate to us that the early and late results of aortic valve replacement are as good with cold ischemic arrest of less than 60 min (preferably less than 45 min) as with direct coronary artery perfusion during the valve replacement.[58] Since less than about 45 min of aortic cross-clamping is usually required and more than 60 min very rarely required, we do not now use direct coronary artery perfusion for this operation.

The aorta is cross-clamped and the aortic root opened transversely. The aortic valve is excised, guarding meticulously and by special techniques against loss of any particles of calcium. The valve prosthesis is usually sewn in place with simple interrupted Dacron sutures. In some unusual circumstances, mattress sutures supported by small teflon pledgets are used. The aortic incision is closed with a continuous suture. As the aortic clamp is released and cardiac action resumes, a meticulous debubbling procedure is practiced for the removal of all air from the heart and ascending aorta.

Postoperative care

Postoperative care is similar in its general principles to that for patients undergoing operations on the mitral valve but is generally simple since nearly all patients have a good hemodynamic state after aortic valve replacement.

After aortic valve replacement by the techniques described, cardiac output is usually large [greater than 2.0 liters/(min)(m²)] and therefore is not measured unless the patient's peripheral pulses, skin temperature and color, arterial blood pressure, urine flow, or general appearance suggest that it is low. If the hemodynamic state is suboptimal and cardiac index is less than about 1.6, the intraventions and the order of their use are as described under "Replacement of the Mitral Valve."[59]

Many patients have atrial hypertension for 24 h or more after aortic valve replacement, which is of some hazard because of the stress it places on the aortotomy and aortic cannulation site and the increase it produces in left ventricular afterload.[60] We, therefore, under these circumstances start a continuous intravenous infusion of nitroprusside either in the operating room or in the intensive care unit, regulated so as to keep the mean arterial blood pressure between 90 and 100 mm Hg. A dose of 1 to 10 mg/(kg)(min) is usually required. It is gradually discontinued about 18 h after operation, and if the hypertensive tendency has not subsided, methyldopa is begun by mouth and continued as long as is necessary.

Most patients meet the criteria for cessation of ventilation and removal of the endotracheal tube within a few hours after operation. Urine flow is monitored but is usually greater than 15 ml/h, and special treatment is therefore usually not required.

Early and late results

The overall hospital mortality rate for aortic valve replacement as an isolated procedure or associated with coronary bypass grafting is about 5 percent. Most of the mortality, however, is in elderly patients, and the risk of uncomplicated cases with the techniques described is less than 2 percent.[61] Atrial arrhythmias, particularly atrial fibrillation, are common early postoperatively, and premature ventricular contractions may occur and require treatment. Myocardial necrosis of some degree occurs in about 10 percent of patients,[58] but usually is not clinically significant. Neurologic complications are rare.

Thromboembolic complications late postoperatively are much less frequent, in anticoagulated patients, with presently used artificial valves than with those used earlier (Fig. 61-12), and are rare when stent-mounted heterografts are used without anticoagulation.

The late survival of patients after aortic valve replacement is less than that of the population as a whole of similar age but is considerably greater than that of patients with surgically untreated aortic valve disease of the same stage (Fig. 61-13).[62,63] Late deaths are due to heart failure, complications of thromboembolism, myocardial infarction, and "sudden death." We do not yet know whether the concomitant bypassing of significant coronary artery stenoses when they are present will reduce the incidence of these last two late complications and thus whether they will improve still further the life expectancy of patients undergoing surgical treatment for aortic valve disease.

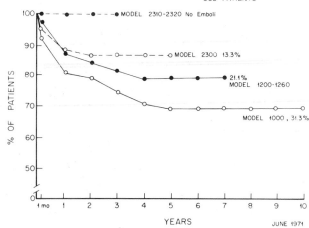

AORTIC VALVE REPLACEMENT
TOTAL THROMBOEMBOLISM

535 PATIENTS

FIGURE 61-12 Total thromboembolism (early and late) after aortic valve replacement with the various models of the Starr-Edwards ball valve prosthesis. Note the decreasing incidence of emboli with the newer models. [*Reproduced with permission from A. Starr, Prosthetic Valve Replacement (presented at postgraduate course in cardiovascular surgery, American College of Surgeons, Chicago, October 1971.)*]

COMBINED DOUBLE AND TRIPLE VALVE DISEASE

A number of patients with severe and progressing symptoms exhibit evidence of disease at both mitral and aortic valves. Our experience indicates that both valves can be replaced with a hospital mortality rate that is now about 10 percent, considerably less than the 22 percent reported for an earlier period.[64] There has been marked subjective and objective improvement in surviving patients. When tricuspid replacement has also been done, the risk of the operation has been higher (about 20 percent), but even here the long-term results are considerably better than the life history of surgically untreated patients with triple

FIGURE 61-13 Actuarial survival curve of patients (*n* = 962) undergoing isolated aortic valve replacement with Starr-Edwards prosthesis, mostly the model 1200-1260 with Silastic poppet, compared with that of the population as a whole of similar ages. (*Reproduced with permission from Barnhorst, Oxman, Connolly, Pluth, Danielson, Wallace, and McGoon.*[63])

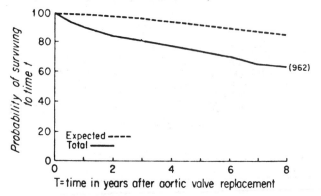

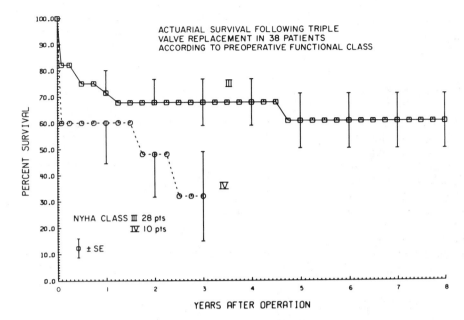

FIGURE 61-14 Actuarial survival following simultaneous aortic, mitral, and tricuspid valve replacement according to preoperative disability. The proportion of patients surviving for 3 or more years was significantly greater for patients in NYHA Class III preoperatively than for those in NYHA Class IV. (*Reproduced with permission from Stephenson, Kouchoukos, and Kirklin, Triple Valve Replacement: An Analysis of Eight Years Experience, Ann. Thorac. Surg., 23:327, 1977.*)

valve disease (Fig. 61-14). The increased use of tricuspid annuloplasty rather than replacement, when possible, has improved the early results of operation in this group of patients.

When hemodynamic derangement is significant at both valves, the decision to repair both is easily made, and the principles of surgical treatment are the same as when one valve alone requires attention. Median sternotomy is performed. Performance of the operation in an optimal manner, with present techniques, requires that both valves be replaced with a cardiac ischemic arrest of less than about 65 min, or that direct coronary artery perfusion be used throughout. We now rarely use the latter technique. On cardiopulmonary bypass, the heart is thoroughly cooled by the perfusate and by external cardiac cooling. The aorta is cross-clamped, the left atrium opened from the right side, and the mitral valve replaced. Leaving the left atrium open, the aortotomy incision is made, the aortic valve replaced, and the aortotomy incision closed. The aortic clamp is then released, the left atrium closed, and the usual procedures followed for removing all air from the heart and preventing its embolization as the heart begins to eject. If tricuspid valve disease is also present, the right atrium is opened and either annuloplasty or replacement is done.

When the aortic valve is severely diseased and only about Class II incompetence (on the basis of I to VI) is evident at the mitral valve, without stenosis, attention to the mitral valve seems unnecessary. This is true even if left atrial pressure is very high, since such pressure can result solely from severe pressure or volume overload of the left ventricle. After repair of the aortic valve disease, such incompetence of the mitral valve usually regresses.[65] When there is incompetence at the aortic valve of about Class II, in the presence of severe disease at the mitral valve, the aortic valve incompetence often appears to be of greater magnitude after repair of the mitral valve and may contribute to poor cardiac performance postoperatively. In these situations, therefore, repair of both mitral and aortic valves seems indicated.

TRICUSPID STENOSIS AND REGURGITATION

Intrinsic disease of the tricuspid valve, in association with involvement of the aortic or mitral valve, occurs in 10 to 15 percent of patients with chronic rheumatic heart disease.[66] The valve leaflets are thickened, and the commissures are fused and usually ill defined. The chordae may be fused and shortened. The tricuspid valve is usually rendered both stenotic and incompetent thereby.

Patients with disease of the mitral valve commonly exhibit signs and symptoms of tricuspid valve incompetence. In many such cases the leaflets of the tricuspid valve appear normal, and the incompetence is believed to be caused by malfunction of the valve due to severe right ventricular hypertension or dilatation of the right ventricle. When regurgitation at the tricuspid valve is mild, correction of the defect at the mitral valve usually produces a good result and regression of the malfunction at the tricuspid valve. When regurgitation is moderate or severe and the leaflet normal, the patient is usually far along in the course of this disease, and true reduction in myocardial function is often present. In this situation even temporary relief of the incompetence is helpful in the postoperative period, and annuloplasty is performed.[15,67,68] When there is some stenosis as well as incompetence, replacement of the tricuspid valve is indicated.

CARDIAC REPLACEMENT

Consideration has been given to total cardiac replacement in a few patients with far-advanced heart disease. Implantation of an artificial device seems the ideal type of replacement therapy, and progress is being made in the development of such devices. They have not yet been applied successfully to human beings. Human homotransplantation was first accomplished by Barnard.[69] The investigative studies of Shumway and associates[70] provided the basic information for these clinical applications. It is clear that cardiac transplantation as a surgical procedure can be accomplished by an experienced and well-disciplined surgical group. Palliation of the condition of some patients has already been achieved. The long-term physiologic and immunologic problems are not as yet clear. The place of this type of treatment for advanced heart disease has thus not been established at this time, and presently its use should be restricted to centers prepared for this type of clinical trial.

REFERENCES

1 Wood, Paul: An Appreciation of Mitral Stenosis: I. Clinical Features, *Br. Med. J.,* 1:1051, 1954.

2 Olesen, K. H.: "Mitral Stenosis: A Follow-up of 351 Patients," Ejnar Munksgaards Forlag, Copenhagen, 1958.

3 Baden, Helge: "Surgical Treatment of Mitral Stenosis," Store Nordiske Videnskabsboghandel, Copenhagen, 1958.

4 Heller, S. J., and Carleton, R. A.: Abnormal Left Ventricular Contraction in Patients with Mitral Stenosis, *Circulation,* 42:1099, 1970.

5 Nichols, H. T., Blanco, G., Morse, D. P., Adam, A., and Baltazar, N.: Open Mitral Commissurotomy: Experience with 200 Consecutive Cases, *J.A.M.A.,* 182:268, 1962.

6 Appelbaum, A., Kouchoukos, N. T., Blackstone, E. H., and Kirklin, J. W.: Early Risks of Open Heart Surgery for Mitral Valve Disease, *Am. J. Cardiol.,* 37:201, 1976.

7 Gerami, S., Messmer, B. J., Hallman, G. L., and Cooley, D. A.: Open Mitral Commissurotomy: Results of 100 Consecutive Cases, *J. Thorac. Cardiovasc. Surg.,* 62:366, 1971.

8 Ellis, L. B., Harken, D. E., and Black, H.: A Clinical Study of 1,000 Consecutive Cases of Mitral Stenosis Two to Nine Years after Mitral Valvuloplasty, *Circulation,* 19:803, 1959.

9 Ellis, F. H., Jr., Connolly, D. C., Kirklin, J. W., and Parker, R. L.: Results of Mitral Commissurotomy: Follow-up of Three and One-half to Seven Years, *Arch. Intern. Med.,* 102:928, 1958.

10 Baker, C., and Hancock, W. E.: Deterioration after Mitral Valvotomy, *Br. Heart J.,* 22:281, 1960.

11 Morrow, A. G., and Braunwald, N. S.: Transventricular Mitral Commissurotomy: Surgical Technique and a Hemodynamic Evaluation of the Method, *J. Thorac. Cardiovasc. Surg.,* 41:225, 1961.

12 Ellis, F. H., Jr.: "Surgery for Acquired Mitral Valve Disease," W. B. Saunders Company, Philadelphia, 1967.

13 Ross, J., Jr., Braunwald, E., and Morrow, A. G.: Clinical and Hemodynamic Observations in Pure Mitral Insufficiency, *Am. J. Cardiol.,* 2:11, 1958.

14 Edwards, J. E., and Burchell, H. B.: Pathologic Anatomy of Mitral Insufficiency, *Mayo Clin. Proc.,* 33:497, 1958.

15 Carpentier, A., Deloche, A., Dauptain, J., Soyer, R., Blondeau, P., Piwnica, A., and Dubost, C.: A New Reconstructive Operation for Correction of Mitral and Tricuspid Insufficiency, *J. Thorac. Cardiovasc. Surg.,* 61:1, 1971.

16 Merendino, K. A., Thomas, G. I., Jesseph, J. E., Herron, P. W., Winterscheid, L. C., and Vetto, R. R.: The Open Correction of Rheumatic Mitral Regurgitation and/or Stenosis, with Special Reference to Regurgitation Treated by Posteromedial Annuloplasty Utilizing a Pump-Oxygenator, *Ann. Surg.,* 150:5, 1959.

17 Wooler, G. H., Nixon, P. G. F., Grimshaw, V. A., and Watson, D. A.: Experiences with the Repair of the Mitral Valve in Mitral Incompetence, *Thorax,* 17:49, 1962.

18 Reed, G. E., Tice, D. A., Clauss, R. H.: Asymmetric Exaggerated Mitral Annuloplasty: Repair of Mitral Insufficiency with Hemodynamic Predictability, *J. Thorac. Cardiovasc. Surg.,* 49:752, 1965.

19 Kay, J. H., Magidson, O., and Meinaux, J. E.: The Surgical Treatment of Mitral Insufficiency and Combined Mitral Stenosis and Insufficiency Using the Heart-Lung Machine, *Am. J. Cardiol.,* 9:300, 1962.

20 McGoon, D. C.: Repair of Mitral Insufficiency due to Ruptured Chordae Tendineae, *J. Thorac. Cardiovasc. Surg.,* 39:357, 1960.

21 Ellis, F. H., Jr., Frye, R. L., and McGoon, D. C.: Results of Reconstructive Operations for Mitral Insufficiency Due to Ruptured Chordae Tendineae. *Surgery,* 59:165, 1966.

22 Selzer, A., Kelly, J. J., Jr., Kerth, W. J., and Gerbode, F.: Immediate and Long-Range Results of Valvuloplasty for Mitral Regurgitation Due to Ruptured Chordae Tendineae, *Circulation,* 45&46 (suppl. 1):I–52, 1972.

23 Stevenson, J. G., Kawabori, I., Morgan, B. C., Dillard, D. H., Merendino, K. A., and Guntheroth, W. G.: Rheumatic Mitral Regurgitation: The Case for Annuloplasty in the Pediatric Age Group, *Circulation,* 51&52 (suppl. 1):I–49, 1975.

24 Sulayman, R., Mathew, R., Thilenius, O. G., Replogle, R., and Arcilla, R. A.: Hemodynamics and Annuloplasty in Isolated Mitral Regurgitation in Children, *Circulation,* 52:1144, 1975.

25 Manhas, D. R., Rittenhouse, E. A., Hessel, E. A., II, and Merendino, K. A.: Reconstructive Surgery for the Treatment of Mitral Incompetence: Early and Late Results in 91 Patients, *J. Thorac. Cardiovasc. Surg.,* 62:781, 1971.

26 Pakrashi, B. C., Mary, D. A., Elmufti, M. E., Wooler, G. H., and Ionescu, M. I.: Clinical and Haemodynamic Results of Mitral Annuloplasty, *Br. Heart J.,* 36:768, 1974.

27 Reed, G. E.: Repair of Mitral Regurgitation: An 11 Year Experience, *Am. J. Cardiol.,* 31:494, 1973.

28 Reed, G. E., Kloth, H. H., Kiely, B., Danilowicz, D. A., Rader, B., and Doyle, E. F.: Long-Term Results of Mitral Annuloplasty in Children with Rheumatic Mitral Regurgitation, *Circulation,* 49&50 (suppl. 2):II–189, 1974.

29 Urschel, C. W., Covell, J. W., Sonnenblick, E. H., Ross, J., Jr., and Braunwald, E.: Myocardial Mechanics in Aortic and Mitral Valvular Regurgitation: The Concept of Instantaneous Impedance as a Determinant of the Performance of the Intact Heart, *J. Clin. Invest.,* 47:867, 1968.

30 Kirklin, J. W.: Replacement of the Mitral Valve for Mitral Incompetence, *Surgery,* 72:827, 1972.

31 Bjork, V. O.: The Central Flow Tilting Disc Valve Prosthesis (Bjork-Shiley) for Mitral Valve Replacement, *Scand. J. Thorac. Cardiovasc. Surg.,* 4:15, 1970.

32 Aris, A., Fast, A. J., Tector, A. J., Flemma, F. J., and Lepley, D.: A Comparative Study of Ball and Disc Prostheses in Mitral Valve Replacement, *J. Thorac. Cardiovasc. Surg.,* 68:335, 1974.

33 Buch, W. S., Pipkin, R. D., Hancock, W. D., and Fogarty, T. J.:

Mitral Valve Replacement with the Hancock Stabilized Glutaraldehyde Valve, *Arch. Surg.,* 110:148, 1975.

34 Starr, A.: Mitral Valve Replacement with Ball Valve Prostheses, *Br. Heart J.,* 33 (suppl.):47, 1971.

35 Braunwald, N. S., Tatooles, C., Turina, M., et al.: New Developments in the Design of Fabric-covered Prosthetic Heart Valves, *J. Thorac. Cardiovasc. Surg.,* 62:673, 1971.

36 Lillehei, C. W., Kaster, R. L., Starek, P. J., Bloch, J. H., and Rees, J. R.: A New Central Flow Pivoting Disc Aortic and Mitral Prosthesis: Initial Clinical Experience, *Am. J. Cardiol.,* 26:688, 1970.

37 Allen, W. B., Karp, R. B., and Kouchoukos, N. T.: Mitral Valve Replacement, *Arch. Surg.,* 109:642, 1974.

38 Kirklin, J. W., and Pacifico, A. D.: Surgery for Acquired Valvular Heart Disease, *N. Engl. J. Med.,* 288:133, 194, 1973.

39 Anderson, M. W.: The Clinical Course of Patients with Calcific Aortic Stenosis, *Mayo Clin. Proc.,* 36:439, 1961.

40 Mitchell, A. M., Sackett, C. H., Hunziker, W. J., and Levine, S. A.: The Clinical Features of Aortic Stenosis, *Am. Heart J.,* 48:684, 1954.

41 Linhart, J. W., de la Torre, A., Ramsey, H. W., and Wheat, M. W., Jr.: The Significance of Coronary Artery Disease in Aortic Valve Replacement, *J. Thorac. Cardiovasc. Surg.,* 55:811, 1968.

42 Holley, K. E., Bahn, R. C., McGoon, D. C., and Mankin, H. T.: Spontaneous Calcific Embolization Associated with Calcific Aortic Stenosis, *Circulation,* 27:197, 1963.

43 Grant, R. T.: After Histories for 10 Years of a Thousand Men Suffering from Heart Disease: A Study in Prognosis, *Heart,* 16:275, 1933.

44 Wood, P.: Aortic Stenosis, *Am. J. Cardiol.,* 1:553, 1958.

45 Frank, S., and Ross, J., Jr.: Natural History of Severe, Acquired Valvular Aortic Stenosis, *Am. J. Cardiol.,* 19:128, 1967. (Abstract.)

46 Ellis, L. B., and Hancock, E. W.: Evaluation of Surgical Treatment of Acquired and Congenital Aortic Stenosis, *Prog. Cardiovasc. Dis.,* 3:247, 1960.

47 Pacifico, A. D., Karp, R. B., and Kirklin, J. W.: Homografts for Replacement of the Aortic Valve, *Circulation,* 45 and 46 (suppl. 1):36, 1972.

48 Howard, C. P.: Aortic Insufficiency due to Rupture by Strain of a Normal Aortic Valve, *Can. Med. Assoc. J.,* 19:12, 1928.

49 Bahnson, H. T., and Spencer, F. C.: Excision of Aneurysm of the Ascending Aorta with Prosthetic Replacement during Cardiopulmonary Bypass, *Ann. Surg.,* 151:879, 1960.

50 Spencer, F. C., and Blake, H.: A Report of the Successful Surgical Treatment of Aortic Regurgitation from a Dissecting Aortic Aneurysm in a Patient with the Marfan Syndrome, *J. Thorac. Cardiovasc. Surg.,* 44:238, 1962.

51 Spagnuolo, M., Kloth, H., Taranta, A., Doyle, E., and Pasternack, B.: Natural History of Rheumatic Aortic Regurgitation: Criteria Predictive of Death, Congestive Heart Failure, and Angina in Young Patients, *Circulation,* 44:368, 1971.

52 Spurny, O. M., and Hara, M.: Rupture of the Aortic Valve Due to Strain, *Am. J. Cardiol.,* 8:125, 1961.

53 Hufnagel, C. A., and Conrad, P. W.: Dissecting Aneurysms of the Ascending Aorta: Direct Approach to Repair, *Surgery,* 51:84, 1962.

54 Morris, G. C., Jr., Henly, W. S., and DeBakey, M. E.: Correction of Acute Dissecting Aneurysm of Aorta with Valvular Insufficiency, *J.A.M.A.,* 184:63, 1963.

55 Gault, J. H., Covell, J. W., Braunwald, E., and Ross, J., Jr.: Left Ventricular Performance following Correction of Free Aortic Regurgitation, *Circulation,* 42:773, 1970.

56 Bjork, V. O., Henze, A., and Holmgren, A.: Five Years' Experience with the Bjork-Shiley Tilting-Disc Valve in Isolated Aortic Valvular Disease, *J. Thorac. Cardiovasc. Surg.,* 68:393, 1974.

57 Barratt-Boyes, B. G.: Long Term Follow-up of Aortic Valvular Grafts, *Br. Heart J.,* 33 (suppl.):60, 1971.

58 Sapsford, R. N., Blackstone, E. H., Kirklin, J. W., Karp, R. B., Kouchoukos, N. T., Pacifico, A. D., Roe, C. R., and Bradley, E. L.: Coronary Perfusion versus Cold Ischemic Arrest during Aortic Valve Surgery: A Randomized Study, *Circulation,* 49:1190, 1974.

59 Kouchoukos, N. T., Kirklin, J. W., Sheppard, L. C., and Roe, P. A.: Effect of Elevation of Left Atrial Pressure by Blood Infusion on Stroke Volume Early after Cardiac Operations, *Surg. Forum,* 22:126, 1971.

60 Kouchoukos, N. T., Sheppard, L. C., and Kirklin, J. W.: Effect of Alterations in Arterial Pressure on Cardiac Performance Early after Open Intracardiac Operations, *J. Thorac. Cardiovasc. Surg.,* 64:563, 1972.

61 Karp, R. B., and Lell, W.: Evaluating Techniques of Myocardial Preservation for Aortic Valve Replacement: Operative Risk, *J. Thorac. Cardiovasc. Surg.,* 72:206, 1976.

62 Barnhorst, D. A., Oxman, H. A., Connolly, D. C., Pluth, J. R., Danielson, G. K., Wallace, R. B., and McGoon, D. C.: Isolated Replacement of the Aortic Valve with the Starr-Edwards Prosthesis, *J. Thorac. Cardiovasc. Surg.,* 70:113, 1975.

63 Barnhorst, D. A., Oxman, H. A., Connolly, D. C., Pluth, J. R., Danielson, G. K., Wallace, R. B., and McGoon, D. C.: Long-Term Follow-up of Isolated Replacement of the Aortic or Mitral Valve with the Starr-Edwards Prosthesis, *Am. J. Cardiol.,* 35:228, 1975.

64 Duvoisin, G. E., Wallace, R. B., Ellis, F. H., Jr., Anderson, M. W., and McGoon, D. C.: Late Results of Cardiac Valve Replacement, *Circulation,* 37 & 38 (suppl. 2):75, 1968.

65 Austen, W. G., Kastor, J. A., and Sanders, C. A.: Resolution of Functional Mitral Regurgitation following Surgical Correction of Aortic Valvular Disease, *J. Thorac. Cardiovasc. Surg.,* 53:255, 1967.

66 Cooke, W. T., and White, P. S.: Tricuspid Stenosis: With Particular Reference to Diagnosis and Prognosis, *Br. Heart J.,* 3:147, 1941.

67 DeVega, N. G., deRabago, G., Castillon, L., Moreno, T., Fraile, J., and Batanero, J.: Immediate Results Six Months and One Year Later of the Surgical Treatment of Tricuspid Valvulopathy by Means of a New Original Technique, *Rev. Esp. Cardiol.,* 25:555, 1972.

68 Grondin, P., Meere, C., Limet, R., Lopez-Bescoc, L., Delcan, J. L., and Rivera, R.: Carpentier's Annulus and deVega's Annuloplasty, *J. Thorac. Cardiovasc. Surg.,* 70:852, 1975.

69 Barnard, C. N.: A Human Cardiac Transplant: An Interim Report of a Successful Operation Performed at Groote Schuur Hospital, Capetown, *S. Afr. Med. J.,* 41:1271, 1967.

70 Shumway, N. E., Angell, W. W., and Wuerflein, R. D.: Progress in Transplantation of the Heart, *Transplantation,* 5 (suppl.):900, 1967.

Coronary Artery Disease

62
Coronary Atherosclerotic Heart Disease

A
Definitions and Classification of Coronary Atherosclerotic Heart Disease

J. WILLIS HURST, M.D., and
SPENCER B. KING III, M.D.

The clinical manifestations of coronary obstruction will evidently vary, depending on the size, location and number of vessels occluded. The symptoms and end-results must also be influenced by blood-pressure, by the condition of the myocardium not immediately affected by the obstruction, and by the ability of the remaining vessels properly to carry on their work, as determined by their health or disease. *All attempts at dividing these clinical manifestations into groups must be artificial and more or less imperfect. Yet such an attempt is not without value, as it enables one the better to understand the gravity of an obstructive accident, to differentiate it from other conditions presenting somewhat similar symptoms, and to employ a more rational therapy that may, to a slight extent at least, be more efficient.*

JAMES HERRICK, M.D., 1912[1]

INTRODUCTION

Coronary artery disease will be discussed under two headings. *Coronary atherosclerosis,* the most common type of coronary artery disease, is discussed in Chaps. 62A through 62H, and *nonatherosclerotic coronary disease* is discussed in Chaps. 63A and 63B. In the past, various clinical syndromes were said to be due to coronary artery disease and little attempt was made to determine if the conditions were due to coronary atherosclerosis or to some other disease. Each edition of this book has emphasized that we should not use such a generic term as coronary artery disease to identify conditions when they can be more specifically labeled. In the past, even when the disease was identified as coronary atherosclerosis, the clinical subsets were not always specified. There-

fore, each edition of this book has further defined and emphasized the clinical subsets of coronary atherosclerotic heart disease. Over the years, it has become increasingly important to realize that we must use terms very carefully and be as specific and complete as the available data will permit. Now, it is imperative to do so. This is true because there are new methods of investigating and treating coronary artery disease (i.e., stress electrocardiography, echocardiography, coronary arteriography, ventriculography, new drugs, and coronary bypass surgery). If these procedures, drugs, and operations are to be used wisely, it is proper to link them to specific problems. It follows that the criteria required to formulate a specific problem must be carefully defined. Voltaire was pertinent when he said, "If you wish to converse with me define your terms." The next portion of this chapter emphasizes the definition of terms that are often used improperly or are used erroneously as being synonymous with other terms. The last portion of this chapter highlights our current taxonomy of clinical syndromes due to coronary atherosclerotic heart disease.

DEFINITIONS OF TERMS COMMONLY USED

The term *coronary artery disease* should be used in a generic sense because there are many different pathologic conditions that may involve the coronary arteries. When this term is used, it should imply that there is a reason to be deliberately nonspecific.

The term *coronary arteriosclerosis* is also nonspecific and in a sense is also a generic term. It implies the existence of a sclerotic abnormality of the coronary arteries without indicating the exact type of disease process.

The term *coronary atherosclerosis* is quite specific; it is used by the pathologist. It does not by itself imply that the heart muscle has been deprived of blood supply to the degree that the patient or doctor detects symptoms or signs of illness. Nor can the pathologist look at the coronary arteries and determine with certainty whether or not the patient had symptoms.

The term *coronary atherosclerotic heart disease* should be used to indicate that a specific form of heart disease—coronary atherosclerosis—is actually present. This term also indicates that either the clinician or the pathologist (or both) has evidence that the atherosclerotic process has reached a degree of severity that is sufficient to cause certain clinical syndromes or pathologic abnormalities which are the result of inadequate myocardial perfusion.

The term *coronary heart disease* implies that there is a disease of the coronary arteries (even though the term does not have the word "artery" in it) and that the disease is of sufficient severity to cause heart disease. The term is not specific and is not needed. Unfortunately, many surveys have used it. The use of the initials CHD to mean coronary heart disease is even worse, because confusion may arise if the initials are assumed to signify congenital heart disease.

The term *degenerative heart disease* has been used in the past by health statisticians. We now know the term is worthless and should not be used. Perhaps we cannot blame the statisticians entirely, since the clinicians of the era were not able to describe disease processes with the precision that is required for the work of the statistician. Therefore, they used a nonspecific term—degenerative heart disease—in their studies in order to include all cases. It is regrettable that this term was used as late as 1966.

The term *angina pectoris* belongs solely to the province of clinical taxonomy. Angina pectoris is a particular type of chest discomfort due to myocardial ischemia. (The clinical characteristics of angina pectoris are discussed in Chap. 62E.) The only way a diagnosis of angina pectoris can be made is for the physician to interpret the symptoms of the patient. Actually, angina pectoris may result from a number of diseases of the coronary arteries, including coronary atherosclerosis, coronary arteritis, fibromuscular hyperplasia of the coronary arteries, etc. Angina pectoris may also occur as a result of aortic valve disease (stenosis and regurgitation), cardiomyopathy, especially idiopathic hypertrophic subaortic stenosis, mitral valve prolapse, and mitral stenosis. Angina pectoris may be related to disease of the coronary arterioles and may possibly be related to peculiar reactivity (spasm) of the coronary arteries when there is no pathologic counterpart whatsoever. The purpose of this part of the discussion is to emphasize that angina pectoris is a clinical term and can be diagnosed only by the clinician talking with his patient. The most common cause of angina pectoris in most parts of the world is coronary atherosclerotic heart disease. There are other causes, however, and they must always be considered by the physician as he examines his patients. The mere identification of angina pectoris is not sufficient and the numerous subsets of this condition will be discussed later in this chapter.

The term *ischemic heart disease* has been used in the past, but since the term is nonspecific, it is now being abandoned. The words themselves indicate that a condition exists in which the myocardium has become ischemic. It is a physiologic term. Symptoms may or may not be present; e.g., angina pectoris can be considered to be ischemic heart disease, but not all patients with ischemic heart disease have angina pectoris. The term *ischemic heart disease* is so general that many types of disease may be placed in this category. For example, such diverse entities as

coronary atherosclerosis and aortic stenosis are considered to be ischemic heart disease. The term implies that the pathologic abnormality (which is not identified in the term) has attained a degree of severity which causes myocardial ischemia. It is essential to identify the exact cause of the ischemia in addition to identifying the presence of ischemia.

The term *preinfarction syndrome* was used a great deal a few years ago but is used less often today. The term was used when angina pectoris was unstable (initial angina pectoris, progressive angina pectoris, and angina decubitus) or when prolonged pain due to myocardial ischemia occurred without overt evidence of infarction. The term preinfarction syndrome is a poor one, because infarction may not actually take place in many such patients, or has already occurred, or is in the process of developing in others. It seems wiser to characterize the subsets that have composed this syndrome by using clinical terms rather than terms that forecast a pathologic entity (see later discussion).

The term *acute coronary insufficiency* was formerly used by Master to label patients who had experienced prolonged pain due to myocardial ischemia but who exhibited inadequate objective signs of infarction.[2] The term is a physiologic term rather than a clinical one and led to confusion, since in reality all of the clinical subsets of coronary atherosclerotic heart disease are due to acute coronary insufficiency. To add to the confusion, the pathologic counterpart of the clinical syndrome was focal disseminated necrosis of the subendocardium and papillary muscles without coronary occlusion. This was reflected in the electrocardiogram as depression of the ST-T segments and T-wave inversion, especially in leads I and II. These abnormalities usually returned to normal in a few days. Now it seems proper to describe the various subsets using clinical terms rather than a physiologic term (see later discussion).

The term *coronary occlusion* is often used synonymously with the term *coronary thrombosis*. A coronary artery may be occluded by the atherosclerotic process to the degree that infarction develops. Thrombosis of the vessel is not necessary for this to occur, but a clot in the artery may be found at autopsy. The question is whether or not the thrombosis comes before or after the infarction.

Myocardial infarction and *coronary thrombosis* are often used to imply the same condition. We now know that the two terms should not be used synonymously, since infarction may occur without coronary thrombosis, and thrombosis can occur without infarction.

The definition of *myocardial infarction* is the subject of much discussion. It is generally, but not universally, accepted that infarction may be said to be present if a patient exhibits *two* of the following three abnormalities: (1) chest pain typical of myocardial ischemia; (2) electrocardiographic abnormalities, including the development of new and abnormal Q waves or the development of ST- and T-wave changes consistent with myocardial ischemia or certain T-wave abnormalities; and (3) elevation of cardiac enzymes. In reality, infarction undoubtedly occurs in many patients with prolonged myocardial ischemia without QRS or ST-T changes in the electrocardiogram and without the elevation of the blood levels of cardiac enzymes. The fact that there are electrically silent areas in the heart and that infarctions of moderate size must take place in order to alter the electrocardiogram and enzymes (whereas small infarcts may not produce these changes) is not always remembered by the clinician. Ideally, it would be better to delineate the clinical event based on the abnormalities that are clearly evident rather than to infer that a pathologist might find a particular type of infarction. The term myocardial infarction is retained simply because it is deeply ingrained in medical thought.

Patients who experience *sudden death* are often said to have *myocardial infarction.* Actually, autopsy studies have revealed infarction in the minority cases of sudden death. Patients who die suddenly due to an acute coronary event die of an arrhythmia before infarction has time to develop.

REASONS FOR CREATING A CLASSIFICATION OF CORONARY SYNDROMES

There are three reasons why it is necessary to create a taxonomy of clinical syndromes caused by coronary atherosclerotic heart disease.

First, a review of the history related to the subject clearly shows the path on which we walk. Heberden, using purely *clinical* markers, described *angina pectoris.*[3] Herrick used clinical markers and *anatomic* terms to describe *"obstruction of the coronary arteries."*[1] This condition was subsequently called myocardial infarction. Later, the condition was further defined based on the abnormalities found in the electrocardiogram. Master used symptoms and the electrocardiogram to identify the syndrome he called *acute coronary insufficiency,* which was considered to be "in between" angina pectoris and "classical" myocardial infarction (although subendocardial necrosis was known to occur).[2] Note that he used a *physiologic* term to describe the condition. The emergence of these three terms, used to indicate three different clinical syndromes, indicates that it is valuable to identify the various subsets related to coronary atherosclerotic heart disease. Herrick saw the need. His magnificent statement regarding this subject is shown at the beginning of this chapter.[1]

Second, it is a human tendency to try to bring order out of chaos. This is especially true when the process of ordering makes it possible to attain a goal more easily. The expert carpenter will separate his nails according to their size and shape and place them into carefully labeled containers in order to be able to select the proper nail for a specific job. Ordering can, of course, be done in abstract and may, under such circumstances, have no real meaning except to the creator. The greatest value of ordering comes when the identification of a certain subset prompts a specific action that would not have occurred had the subset not been recognized. Therefore, a physician, whose goal it is to manage the problems of sick people, has the right to expect that a term which is used to identify a specific condition (a subset) can be linked to the type of action that should be taken in order to manage the patient.

Third, it is now possible to create more subsets than Heberden, Herrick, and Master did. This is true because of our new methods for studying the disease. New information concerning patients with symptoms due to coronary atherosclerosis is being generated daily. It is therefore helpful to organize the material into a system that is useful to the physician and to the patient.

The taxonomy presented here was created with the following three points in mind: First, practicing physicians have to make medical decisions when they first encounter patients who are ill. Very little medical information may be available at that point in time, yet physicians must act in such a way that the safety of their patient is assured. The formulation of the clinical problems determines what is then done for the patient and what additional diagnostic tests are ordered. Later, when new observations are made, the statement of the problem may need to be changed. The taxonomy presented here takes into account the difficulties of a physician in decision making at a time when all the desired information may not yet be available.

Second, the taxonomy presented here links the management of the patient to the clinical syndrome that is identified. An effort has been made in labeling a subset to use a term that implies few inferences of an anatomic or physiologic state. The objective is to characterize the subset by using the clinical data that is available to the physician at that point in time. For example, "coronary atherosclerotic heart disease with prolonged myocardial ischemia with T-wave change in the electrocardiogram" is more descriptive than the term "acute coronary insufficiency." The latter term is a physiologic definition and could be applied to a large number of conditions, while the former descriptive term is quite specific.

There are two major inferences retained in the taxonomy presented here. First of all, coronary atherosclerosis is assumed to be likely in a patient who has chest pain that has the characteristics of myocardial ischemia (see Chap. 62E). The statistical likelihood that this is true is increased when one excludes aortic valve disease, hypertrophic obstructive cardiomyopathy, other types of cardiomyopathy, prolapse of the mitral valve, mitral stenosis and other causes of pulmonary hypertension, coronary emboli, and dissection of the proximal portion of the aorta, etc. Secondly, and perhaps more importantly, is the inference that the abnormal physiologic condition—myocardial ischemia—is present because

Clinical syndromes due to coronary atherosclerotic heart disease

Clinical syndromes associated with "Chest Discomfort" subsets: see Tables 62A-3 to 62A-6

Clinical syndromes not associated with "Chest Discomfort" subsets: see table 62A-8

PHASES OF DECISION MAKING FOR PATIENTS WITH CHEST DISCOMFORT

The care of the patient who has chest discomfort due to myocardial ischemia related to coronary atherosclerotic heart disease can be divided into four phases (Table 62A-2). During each phase the physician is required to make diagnostic and therapeutic decisions.

Phase I

The first encounter the physician has with the patient is identified as Phase I. The physician must make diagnostic and therapeutic decisions based on the patient's symptoms, physical signs, and a single electrocardiogram.

The following subsets may be identified by physicians when they first encounter a patient with chest discomfort that has the characteristics of pain due to myocardial ischemia (Table 62A-3).

SYMPTOMS: CHARACTERIZATION BASED ON THE ANALYSIS OF THE PATIENT'S CHEST DISCOMFORT

The physician, having determined that the chest discomfort could be due to myocardial ischemia and having failed to detect noncoronary cardiac causes of the discomfort, should then determine if the chest discomfort is brief or prolonged, if it has occurred in the past, if a certain event provokes it, and if nitroglycerin relieves the discomfort promptly.

Brief chest discomfort implies that the discomfort lasts 1 to 10 min. Such discomfort is called *angina pectoris*.[3] The exact description of this type of discomfort is discussed in Chap. 62E. Angina pectoris can occasionally last up to 20 min when it is produced by emotional upheaval or if the patient continues the effort that produced it. Pain due to myocardial ischemia lasting longer than 20 min is referred to as *prolonged chest discomfort*. The characterization of this type of chest discomfort is discussed in Chap. 62E. It must not be confused with angina pectoris.

Eleven clinical syndromes (subsets) may be identified by analyzing the patient's chest discomfort (see Table 62A-3).

the patient has experienced a certain type of chest discomfort. Unfortunately, the positive correlation between chest discomfort and myocardial ischemia is not 100 percent. Despite this admonition, it is necessary for physicians to act responsibly with the data they have. Accordingly, we must accept the fact that an error can be made—especially when the patient is first encountered. The objective is not for physicians to be right or wrong but to act responsibly in our efforts to protect our patients and to keep an open mind. If a patient has chest discomfort that resembles the discomfort caused by myocardial ischemia, it is vital for the physician to act as if that is the case. It is during the follow-up that the true nature of the condition should be, and usually can be, clarified. This procedure is in sharp contrast to the attitudes expressed by a number of physicians two decades ago. Some diagnosed the presence of myocardial ischemia in most of their patients with chest pain because of the fear of missing it, while others considered it wise to "miss" a diagnosis of angina pectoris when one was not certain. Now, fortunately we have new diagnostic methods, such as coronary arteriography, to further delineate the problem.

Third, the taxonomy used here is teachable. We could present a shorter one, but that would not reflect the true state of the problem. We could easily present a longer one, but that would be so burdensome that the principles would be lost. A taxonomy must be teachable if it is to be useful to physicians and their patients.

The clinical syndromes due to coronary atherosclerotic heart disease may be divided into those which are associated with chest discomfort and those which are not (Table 62A-1). The majority of patients with coronary atherosclerotic heart disease enter the health care system because of chest discomfort, but we must not forget the minority who exhibit clues to coronary atherosclerotic heart disease other than chest discomfort (see Table 62A-8).

TABLE 62A-2
Phases of decision making in pain syndromes due to coronary atherosclerotic heart disease

Phase I	Phase II	Phase III	Phase IV
Decisions based on physician's first encounter. Classification based on symptoms, complications, and abnormalities (if any) found in the initial electrocardiogram (if available). (See Table 62A-3.)	Decisions based on subsequent encounters. Classification based on symptoms, complications, electrocardiographic findings, and level of cardiac enzymes.	Decisions based on results of submaximal exercise electrocardiogram test when test is indicated.	Decisions based on coronary arteriography and left ventriculography when study is indicated.

TABLE 62A-3
Clinical subsets identified in phase I (first encounter decision making)

Symptoms: Characterization based on analysis of patient's chest discomfort

1 Stable mild angina pectoris
2 Stable disabling angina pectoris
3 Recent onset angina pectoris without rest pain
4 Recent onset angina pectoris plus rest pain
5 Progressive angina pectoris without rest pain
6 Progressive angina pectoris with rest pain: not disabling
7 Progressive angina pectoris with rest pain: disabling
8 Any of the above in a patient with previous episodes of chest discomfort due to myocardial ischemia or with objective signs of previous coronary atherosclerotic heart disease
9 Prolonged chest discomfort attributed to myocardial ischemia in a patient without previous episodes of chest discomfort due to myocardial ischemia or objective signs of previous coronary atherosclerotic heart disease
10 Prolonged chest discomfort attributed to myocardial ischemia in a patient with previous episodes of chest discomfort due to myocardial ischemia or with objective signs of previous coronary atherosclerotic heart disease
11 Any of the above in a patient with previous coronary bypass surgery

Complications

1 No complications
2 Abnormal heart rhythm (state exact rhythm)
3 Heart failure (indicate degree)
4 Hypotension (indicate severity)

Initial electrocardiogram

1 Electrocardiogram not available
2 Normal
3 ST-segment displacement greater than 1 mm in leads I, II, III, aV_L, aV_F, and V_4–V_6 (subendocardial injury)
4 ST-segment elevation in leads II, III, and aV_F or leads I, aV_L, and V_1–V_6 (epicardial injury)
5 Tall, peaked T waves in leads I, aV_L, and V_4–V_6 (subendocardial ischemia)
6 T-wave inversion in leads II, III, and aV_F or leads I, aV_L, and V_1–V_6 (epicardial ischemia)
7 Abnormal Q waves with ST- and T-wave abnormality. State leads where abnormalities are found. (Dead zone effect, injury and ischemia.)

1 *Stable mild angina pectoris.* This term should be applied when the chest discomfort lasts a brief period of time (usually less than 10 min), and has the features which are characteristic of myocardial ischemia. The chest discomfort (angina pectoris) should not have changed in frequency, duration, time of appearance, and precipitating factors during the last 60 days and for these reasons is called stable. The chest discomfort should not interfere with the patient's desired life-style and is therefore not disabling. The chest discomfort is considered to be mild, since an ordinary day can be lived without the patient having the discomfort, and because more than usual effort is required to provoke the discomfort.

2 *Stable disabling angina pectoris.* This term should be used when the chest discomfort has not changed in frequency, duration, time of appearance, and precipitating factors during the last 60 days. It is therefore considered to be stable. The patient experiences the angina pectoris with less than his or her usual daily activity but does not have angina pectoris at rest. The chest discomfort interferes with the patient's desired life-style and is therefore considered to be disabling.

3 *Recent onset angina pectoris without rest pain.* This term should be used when the patient has developed angina pectoris within the last 60 days and when the angina pectoris does not occur at rest.

4 *Recent onset angina pectoris plus rest pain.* This term should be used when the patient has developed angina pectoris within the last 60 days and when angina pectoris occurs at rest as well as after effort.

5 *Progressive angina pectoris without rest pain.* This term should be used when angina pectoris has increased in frequency or severity or has been more easily provoked with less effort within the last 60 days but angina pectoris does not occur when the patient is at rest.

6 *Progressive angina pectoris with rest pain but not disabling.* This term is applied either when angina pectoris has increased in frequency or severity or when angina pectoris has been provoked with less than usual effort within the preceding 60 days and angina pectoris is also occurring at rest. The pain on effort and rest pain have not reached the degree that they interfere with the patient's desired life-style. This does not, however, imply that the situation is not dangerous to the patient.

7 *Progressive angina pectoris with rest pain which is disabling.* This term should be used when there has been an increase in frequency or severity of angina pectoris or when angina pectoris has been provoked with less effort within the preceding 60 days and when angina pectoris is occurring at rest. The discomfort produced by effort and the rest pain interfere with the patient's life-style, and the patient is considered to be disabled.

The syndromes described in categories 3 to 7 are often termed *unstable angina pectoris*. There are several subsets of unstable angina pectoris:

8 *Any of above in a patient with previous episodes of chest discomfort due to myocardial ischemia or with objective signs of previous coronary atherosclerotic heart disease.*

9 *Prolonged chest discomfort attributed to myocardial ischemia in a patient without previous episodes of chest discomfort due to myocardial ischemia or objective signs of coronary atherosclerotic heart disease.* This term should be used when the chest discomfort lasts longer than 20 min and when there is no history of previous episodes of chest discomfort and there have been no previous objective signs of coronary atherosclerotic heart disease.

10 *Prolonged chest discomfort attributed to myocardial ischemia in a patient with previous episodes of chest discomfort due to myocardial ischemia or with previous objective signs of coronary atherosclerotic heart disease.* This term should be used when the chest discomfort lasts longer than 20 min and the patient has a history of previous episodes of myocardial ischemia or when there is objective evidence of previous coronary atherosclerotic heart disease (such as evidence of old infarction in the electrocardiogram).

11 Any of the above in a patient with previous coronary bypass surgery.

The subsets labeled 3 to 11 have been designated in the past as belonging to the *preinfarction syndromes* when objective signs of fresh infarction are not apparent. We believe it more useful to describe the specific subset, as discussed in this chapter.

COMPLICATIONS: FURTHER CHARACTERIZATION BASED ON OTHER SYMPTOMS AND SIGNS

The general appearance of the patient is always important but the identification of (see Table 62A-3) (1) *no complications,* or (2) *abnormal heart rhythm,* (3) *heart failure,* and (4) *hypotension* is of great importance. Such observations permit a physician to identify two different types of patients: One type of patient has no complications, and the other type may have one or more of these abnormalities. The specific type of abnormality should be stated.

INITIAL ELECTROCARDIOGRAM: STILL FURTHER CHARACTERIZATION BASED ON THE FINDINGS IN THE ELECTROCARDIOGRAM

The findings should be characterized as follows: (1) Electrocardiogram is not available. If a single electrocardiogram is available, it may (2) be normal; or show (3) ST-segment displacement characteristic of subendocardial injury (ST-segment depression greater than 1 mm in leads I, II, III, aV_L, aV_F, and V_4 to V_6); (4) ST-segment elevation characteristic of epicardial injury (ST-segment elevation in leads II, III, and aV_F or leads I, aV_L, and V_1 to V_6); (5) tall, peaked T waves in leads I, aV_L, and V_4 to V_6 suggesting subendocardial ischemia; (6) T-wave inversion in leads II, III, and aV_F or leads I, aV_L, and V_1 to V_6 consistent with epicardial ischemia; or (7) Q-wave abnormalities with abnormal ST and T waves.

The particular electrocardiographic abnormality that is present enables one to further characterize the clinical subset.

Example of Phase I decision making: Date 4-8-78

Symptoms: Subset 9. Prolonged myocardial ischemia; no previous episodes of myocardial ischemia or objective signs of previous coronary atherosclerotic heart disease.

Complications: Subset 2. Uncontrolled atrial fibrillation.

Initial electrocardiogram: Subset 3. Subendocardial injury.

Phase II

The second phase of diagnostic and therapeutic decision making occurs when the physician has subsequent encounters with the patient (see Table 62A-4). During these encounters the physician notes the presence, absence, or change in chest discomfort;

TABLE 62A-4
Clinical studies identified in phase II (subsequent encounter decision making)

Symptoms: Characterization based on analysis of patient's chest discomfort

1 Chest discomfort no longer present
2 Chest discomfort improved (less severe or occurs less often)
3 Chest discomfort unchanged
4 Progressive chest discomfort (the chest discomfort has increased in frequency, becomes prolonged, or occurs at rest)

Complications: The development of complications must be identified and categorized

1 No complications
2 Normal rhythm
3 Abnormal heart rhythm (state exact rhythm)
4 Heart failure (indicate degree)
5 Hypotension (indicate severity)

Electrocardiogram

1 Electrocardiogram normal
2 No change since previous tracing
3 Further T-wave change of epicardial ischemia
4 Further ST-T change of subendocardial injury
5 Further ST-T change of epicardial injury
6 Development of abnormal Q waves (state where)
7 ST-segment abnormality of subendocardial injury occurring during chest discomfort
8 ST-segment abnormality of epicardial injury occurring during chest discomfort (Prinzmetal phenomenon)

Cardiac enzymes level

1 Enzyme blood levels not measured
2 No rise in blood level of cardiac enzymes
3 Slight rise in blood level of cardiac enzymes
4 Great rise in blood level of cardiac enzymes (CPK becoming four times normal value)

new symptoms or signs; changes in subsequent electrocardiograms; and changes in cardiac enzyme levels (when they have been obtained). Subsequent encounters may take place in minutes, hours, days, weeks, or months depending on the clinical situation as determined in Phase I. The diagnostic and therapeutic decisions based on the information gathered during the most recent encounter are described.

SYMPTOMS: CHARACTERIZATION BASED ON THE ANALYSIS OF THE PATIENT'S CHEST DISCOMFORT

Four categories can be identified (see Table 62A-4): (1) chest discomfort no longer present; (2) chest discomfort improved (less severe or occurs less often); (3) chest discomfort unchanged; and (4) progressive chest discomfort (the chest discomfort has increased in frequency, becomes more prolonged, or occurs at rest).

COMPLICATIONS: FURTHER CHARACTERIZATION BASED ON OTHER SYMPTOMS AND SIGNS

There may be (1) no complications; (2) normal rhythm (normal rhythm may persist or return if it was previously abnormal); (3) abnormal heart rhythm (state exact rhythm); (4) heart failure (indicates degree); or (5) hypotension (indicate severity).

ELECTROCARDIOGRAM AND CARDIAC ENZYMES LEVEL: STILL FURTHER CHARACTERIZATION BASED ON THE CHANGES IN THE ELECTROCARDIOGRAM AND RISE IN BLOOD LEVEL OF CARDIAC ENZYMES

(1) The electrocardiogram may remain normal. (2) The electrocardiogram may be unchanged as compared with the last electrocardiogram. The electrocardiogram may show (3) further T-wave abnormality representing epicardial ischemia; (4) further ST-T change consistent with more extensive subendocardial injury; (5) further ST-T change indicating additional epicardial injury; or (6) an initial QRS abnormality consistent with the development of dead zone. An attempt should be made to record an electrocardiogram during an episode of chest pain which can be classified as (7) ST-segment abnormality of subendocardial injury occurring during chest discomfort, or (8) ST-segment displacement due to epicardial injury occurring during chest discomfort—when this appears only while chest pain is experienced and returns to normal between such episodes, the process is identified as the *Prinzmetal phenomenon* (variant angina pectoris).

The blood level of cardiac enzymes need not be determined if the data on the initial encounter were indicative of infarction (see Chap. 62E). When cardiac enzyme levels are not measured, the label (1) is used. When the levels of cardiac enzymes are determined, the results may indicate that there is (2) no rise in the blood levels of enzymes; (3) a slight rise in the level of enzymes; or (4) a great increase in levels of enzymes, with the creatine phosphokinase (CPK) being four times normal value.

Example of Phase II decision making: Date 4-10-78

Symptoms: Subset 1. Chest discomfort no longer present.

Complications: Subset 2. Normal rhythm. Subset 4. Ventricular gallop at apex.

Electrocardiogram: Subset 6. Development of abnormal Q waves due to anterior infarction.

Cardiac enzyme blood levels: Subset 3. Slight rise in cardiac enzyme levels.

Phase III

The third phase of diagnostic and therapeutic decision making occurs when the physician determines if an electrocardiogram should be recorded during a submaximal exercise electrocardiogram test. Should such a test be done, how are the results to be categorized, and how will the new information alter the physician's view regarding the prognosis and management of the patient?

The indication for, and the interpretation of, the exercise electrocardiogram is discussed in Chaps. 28, 37, and 62E. One of the following should be recorded (Table 62A-5): (1) exercise electrocardiogram not done (state reason); (2) exercise electrocardiogram done but inadequate; (3) exercise electrocardiogram done and normal (record maximum heart rate and blood pressure achieved); (4) exercise electrocardiogram done with equivocal results (record maximum heart rate and blood pressure achieved); (5) exercise electrocardiogram done showing ST-segment depression of 1 to 1.9 mm occurring at stage 3 or 4 (record maximum heart rate and blood pressure achieved); (6) exercise electrocardiogram done showing ST-segment depression greater than 2 mm at stage 3 or 4 (record maximum heart rate and blood pressure achieved); (7) exercise electrocardiogram done showing ST segment greater than 2 mm at stage 1 or 2 (record maximum heart rate and blood pressure achieved); (8) angina pectoris developed at stage — (record stage and also record maximum heart rate and blood pressure achieved); (9) test stopped (state stage at which it was stopped and why; record maximum heart rate and blood pressure achieved); (10) arrhythmia (state type).

Example of Phase III decision making: Date 4-10-78

Exercise electrocardiogram: Subset 1. Not done because of recent infarct.

Suppose the patient has an uneventful recovery from

TABLE 62A-5
Clinical subsets identified in phase III (decision making based on exercise electrocardiogram)

1 Exercise electrocardiogram not done (state reason)
2 Exercise electrocardiogram done but inadequate
3 Exercise electrocardiogram done and normal (record maximum heart rate and blood pressure achieved)
4 Exercise electrocardiogram done with equivocal results (record maximum heart rate and blood pressure achieved)
5 Exercise electrocardiogram done showing ST-segment depression of 1–1.9 mm occurring at stage 3 or 4 (record maximum heart rate and blood pressure achieved)
6 Exercise electrocardiogram done showing ST-segment depression greater than 2 mm at stage 3 or 4 (record maximum heart rate and blood pressure achieved)
7 Exercise electrocardiogram done showing ST segment greater than 2 mm at stage 1 or 2 (record maximum heart rate and blood pressure achieved)
8 Angina pectoris developed at stage _____ (record stage and also record maximum heart rate and blood pressure achieved)
9 Test stopped (state stage in which it was stopped and why; record maximum heart rate and blood pressure achieved)
10 Arrhythmia (state type)

myocardial infarction and begins to develop additional chest discomfort thought to be due to progressive angina pectoris without rest pain (subset 4):

6-24-78 Phase II

Symptoms: Subset 4. Progressive chest discomfort.

Complications: Subset 1. No complications.

Electrocardiogram: Subset 2. No change since previous tracing.

Enzyme blood levels: Subset 1. Not done.

Phase III

Exercise electrocardiogram: Subset 1. Not done because of progressive chest discomfort.

A positive exercise stress test may be recorded in the electrocardiogram of asymptomatic patients. This condition is discussed in Chap. 62E.

Phase IV

The fourth phase of diagnostic and therapeutic decision making occurs when the physician determines if a coronary arteriogram and left ventriculogram should be done and if such an examination is done, how the new information alters the view regarding the prognosis and management of the patient (see Table 62A-6).

TABLE 62A-6
Clinical subsets identified in phase IV (decision making based on coronary arteriography and left ventriculography)

Coronary arteriography

1 Not done
2 Normal
3 Less than 75% proximal cross-sectional obstruction* of a major vessel (state name of vessel)
4 Greater than 75% cross-sectional obstruction of a single vessel (state name of vessel)
5 Greater than 75% cross-sectional obstruction of two vessels (state names of vessels)
6 Greater than 75% cross-sectional obstruction of three vessels (state name of vessels)
7 Greater than 75% cross-sectional obstruction of left main coronary artery
8 All vessels bypassable
9 Some obstructed vessels not bypassable (state which vessels are not bypassable)

Left ventriculography

1 Normal left ventricle
2 Single area of hypokinesia with ejection fraction greater than 40% (the area involved should be specified)
3 Two areas of hypokinesia with ejection fraction greater than 40% (the areas should be specified)
4 Two areas of hypokinesia with ejection fraction less than 40% (the areas should be specified)
5 Generalized hypokinesia with ejection fraction greater than 20%
6 Ejection fraction less than 20%
7 Large ventricular aneurysm

*75% cross-sectional obstruction is equivalent to 50% narrowing of the diameter of a vessel.

The indications for, and the interpretation of, the coronary arteriogram and left ventriculogram are discussed in Chaps. 29C and 62E. The following should be identified and recorded: Coronary arteriogram was (1) not done; (2) normal; or showed (3) less than 75 percent proximal obstruction (cross-sectional obstruction or, the equivalent, less than 50 percent narrowing of the diameter of the vessel) of a major vessel (state name of vessel); (4) greater than 75 percent obstruction (cross-sectional obstruction or greater than 50 percent narrowing of the diameter of the vessel) of a single vessel (state name of vessel); (5) greater than 75 percent obstruction of two vessels (state names of vessels); (6) greater than 75 percent obstruction of three vessels (state names of vessels); (7) greater than 75 percent obstruction of left main coronary artery; (8) all vessels bypassable; (9) some obstructed vessels not bypassable (state which vessels are not bypassable).

Left ventriculogram showed (1) normal left ventricle; (2) single area of hypokinesia (the area involved should be specified) with ejection fraction greater than 40 percent; (3) two areas of hypokinesia (the areas should be specified) with ejection fraction greater than 40 percent; (4) two areas of hypokinesia (the areas should be specified) with ejection fraction less than 40 percent; (5) generalized hypokinesia with ejection fraction greater than 20 percent; (6) ejection fraction less than 20 percent; (7) large ventricular aneurysm.

Example of Phase IV decision making: Date 6-26-78

Coronary arteriogram:

Subset 5. Greater than 75 percent obstruction of left anterior descending and circumflex arteries.

Subset 8. All vessels bypassable.

Left ventriculogram:

Subset 2. Hypokinesia of anterior portion of left ventricle with ejection fraction greater than 40 percent.

A FLOW SHEET

A flow sheet used to record follow-up information on patients with coronary atherosclerotic heart disease is shown in Table 62A-7. The example used in the preceding discussion of the four phases of decision making is also used in the flow sheet. Note how the characteristics of the subset can be shown in code form. Note, too, how by following the dates at the top of the flow sheet that it is possible to follow the changing status of the patient and determine at a glance the symptoms, complications, electrocardiographic abnormalities, enzymes abnormalities, results of exercise electrocardiogram if done, and results of the coronary arteriogram and left ventricu-

TABLE 62A-7
A flow sheet

Date	4/8/78	4/10/78	6/24/78	6/26/78
Phase I				
Symptoms	9			
Complications	2, atrial fibrillation			
Initial electrocardiogram	3			
Phase II				
Symptoms		1	4	
Complications		2; 4, ventricular gallops	1	
Electrocardiogram		6, anterior	2, anterior	
Enzymes		3	1	
Phase III				
Exercise				
Electrocardiogram		1, not done because of recent infarct	1, not done because of progressive chest discomfort	
Phase IV				
Coronary arteries				5, > 75% obstruction of LAD and circumflex 8, all vessels bypassable
Left ventriculogram				2, anterior hykinesia ejection fraction > 40%

logram. In actual practice the flow sheet shown in Table 62A-7 should be printed at the top of the page and the content of Tables 62A-3 to 62A-6 should be printed below it. In this way, the meaning of the code numbers can be easily determined. Furthermore, the system ensures that one is following and recording the proper items.

PROBLEMS IN PATIENTS WITH CORONARY ATHEROSCLEROTIC HEART DISEASE WHO HAVE NO CHEST DISCOMFORT

The majority of patients with coronary atherosclerotic heart disease are recognized because they have chest discomfort. This form of heart disease can, however, present itself in other ways. Patients who have (1) sudden death and syncope, (2) pulmonary edema, (3) chronic heart failure, (4) abnormal electrocardiogram, (5) certain cardiac arrhythmias, (6) profound fatigue, (7) an abnormal coronary arterio-

TABLE 62A-8
Clinical syndromes not associated with "chest discomfort"

1 Sudden death and syncope
2 Pulmonary edema
3 Chronic heart failure
4 Abnormal electrocardiogram
5 Certain cardiac arrhythmias
6 Profound fatigue
7 An abnormal coronary arteriogram
8 Abnormal x-ray of the heart
9 Abnormal physical findings

gram, (8) abnormal x-ray of the heart, and (9) abnormal physical findings may have coronary atherosclerotic heart disease as the basis for their problems (Table 62A-8). These conditions are discussed in Chap. 62E.

CONCLUSIONS

The purpose of this chapter is to emphasize that we have entered a new era in our efforts to recognize and manage coronary atherosclerotic heart disease. While the etiology of the disease remains obscure, the clinical recognition, natural history, and management of the condition are being clarified. A clinical taxonomy has been presented that emphasizes the four phases when a physician must make diagnostic and therapeutic decisions and links each clinical subset to specific medical and surgical management. This chapter is concluded with S. I. Hayakawa's admonition in mind: "Science seeks only the most generally useful systems of classification; these it regards for the time being, until more useful classifications are invented, as 'true.'"[4]

REFERENCES

1 Herrick, J. B.: Clinical Features of Sudden Obstruction of the Coronary Arteries, *JAMA*, 59:2015, 1912.
2 Master, A. M.: Coronary Heart Disease: Angina Pectoris, Acute Coronary Insufficiency, and Coronary Occlusion, *Ann. Intern. Med.*, 20:661, 1944.
3 Heberden, W.: "Commentaries on the History and Cure of Diseases," London, 1802.
4 Hayakawa, S. I.: "Language in Thought and Action," 2d ed., Harcourt, Brace & World, Inc., New York, 1964, p. 222.

B
Etiology of Coronary Atherosclerosis

MARIO DiGIROLAMO, M.D., and
ROBERT C. SCHLANT, M.D.

Tum penuria deinde cibi languentia leto membra dabat, contra nunc rerum copia mersat.

In earlier times, starvation consigned languishing bodies to death; now, on the other hand, prosperity plunges them to the grave.

LUCRETIUS, ca. 50 B.C.
De Rerum Natura, chap. 5, 1.1007

INTRODUCTION

The purpose of this chapter is to provide a brief review of the many factors that are considered contributory to the development of coronary atherosclerotic heart disease (CAHD). The etiologic factors include genetic and environmental factors, as well as factors related to the blood and the blood vessel wall. The interaction of these elements in the initiation of the atherosclerotic process will be discussed later in the chapter, under "Theories and Mechanisms Relating to the Pathogenesis of Atherosclerosis." In the last 25 years, epidemiologic and experimental studies have provided considerable evidence linking certain "risk factors" to the development of atherosclerotic lesions. Although our knowledge of the etiologic events and their pathologic sequence is still incomplete, this chapter will outline the available information and the prevailing concepts. The prevention of coronary atherosclerosis requires identification of the major contributing factors and a careful effort to correct or remove the modifiable risk elements involved. There is strongly suggestive evidence that a prudent approach to the primary prevention of coronary atherosclerosis is both feasible and beneficial. (See also Chap. 62H.) For more comprehensive reviews of the various components of coronary atherosclerosis, the reader is directed to references 1 to 11.

Definition of the problem

Coronary atherosclerosis is a pathologic condition of the coronary arteries characterized by abnormal lipid and fibrous tissue accumulation in the vessel wall with resulting disruption of the vessel architecture and function and variable reduction of blood flow to the myocardium.

Atherosclerosis (from the Greek *athērē,* mash or gruel, and *sklēros,* hardening) has been known for centuries, and until very recently the disease was considered a necessary component of the aging process. Epidemiologic studies of the last 40 years, however, have revealed wide regional differences in the incidence and prevalence rates of atherosclerosis

and have shown that *significant* atherosclerosis is not a necessary component of the aging process. The recognition of genetic, environmental, and other factors that can accelerate the atherosclerotic process has made aging an important, but not the only, determinant of the pathologic changes, which are influenced to different degrees by many factors, only some of which have been identified. All the evidence at present indicates that coronary atherosclerosis is a multifactorial disease.

The renewed interest in this disease and in the search for its etiologic factors stems from the fact that the incidence of coronary atherosclerotic heart disease has increased dramatically in the last 60 years and this disease is now recognized as the leading cause of death in the industrialized Western world. It is not clear what has produced such an apparent steep rise in coronary atherosclerotic heart disease in this century. Although the atherosclerotic disease has been causally linked to the development of "affluence" in some of the highly industrialized countries of the Western world, it is also likely that other factors, such as increased longevity, reduction of death due to other causes (perinatal mortality, infections, etc.), improved recognition and diagnosis, as well as a definite increase in incidence and prevalence of the atherosclerotic disease, have all contributed to the observed rise in morbidity and mortality in many countries throughout the world.

In some countries, including the United States and Finland, the incidence of clinically detected coronary atherosclerotic heart disease (myocardial infarction, angina pectoris, sudden death) has reached epidemic proportions.[12-14] In the United States coronary atherosclerotic heart disease has been estimated to be newly recognized in 1 out of 100 white male subjects every year (4 per 1,000 at ages 35 to 44, 10 per 1,000 at ages 45 to 54, and 20 per 1,000 at ages 55 to 64 years).[12] In these subjects the death rate in the first year was approximately 20 to 30 percent. In the general population of the United States in 1973, a total of 684,066 persons died from ischemic heart disease, and of these 246,440 were age 30 to 69 years. In other countries, including Japan, China,[15] and some in Central America, the incidence of coronary atherosclerotic heart disease and the death rate due to coronary atherosclerotic heart disease appear to be lower; again, it is difficult to identify all the reasons for this reduced incidence.[10,13] This will be discussed further in a later section.

Pathologic description[1-9,11,16-19]

The 1958 study group of the World Health Organization[15] has defined atherosclerosis as a "variable combination of changes of the intima of the arteries (as distinguished from arterioles) consisting of a focal accumulation of lipids, complex carbohydrates, blood and blood products, fibrous tissue and calcium deposits, and associated with medical changes."

Microscopic lesions appear to undergo progressive changes in the following recognized stages: (1) *fatty streaks or spots,* superficial yellow or yellowish gray intimal lesions, which are stained selectively by fat stains; (2) *fibrous plaques,* circumscribed, elevated intimal thickenings, which are firm and gray or pearly white; (3) *atherosclerotic plaques* (atheromata), which have smooth muscle cells (SMCs), abundant collagen, elastin, glycosaminoglycans (GAGs), and fatty softening produced by a necrotic center rich in cholesterol and cholesterol esters; a few monocytes or macrophages and a few fibroblasts are also observed in addition to fibrinogen or fibrin, and lipoproteins, both intact and partially altered; the cholesterol and lipid components are located both intracellularly and extracellularly; most of the intracellular lipid is in SMCs derived from the media; (4) *complicated lesions,* in which additional changes such as thrombosis, hemorrhage, ulceration, and calcareous deposits are present; there may be evidence of vascularization in advanced, complex lesions.

Figure 62B-1 illustrates schematically the appearance of such lesions on the clinical horizon. It should be noted, however, that fatty streaks do not necessarily progress to become fibrous plaques or atheromata. It is probable that many plaques develop and regress intermittently.[11]

Although no agreement has been reached on the precise progression of the various changes from the earliest recognizable lesions to the onset of clinically identifiable disease, the following histologic abnormalities are generally accepted[20] as being present at one time or another in the development of the atherosclerotic process: (1) patchy accumulation of lipid, mostly cholesterol and its esters, but also phospholipid and triglyceride, either intracellularly

(foam cells) or extracellularly in the intima and the inner media layers of affected arteries; (2) fibroplasia, largely confined to the subendothelial portion of the intima, in the form of mucopolysaccharides, reticulin, collagen fibers, and hyalinization; (3) fibrin-like film attached to the intimal surface or covered by endothelium; (4) accumulation of complex carbohydrates; (5) calcification in fine or coarse granules; (6) cholesterol crystals and fine, granular, amorphous glycoprotein material; (7) medial changes such as lipid infiltration, disintegration of smooth muscle fibers, disruption of elastic fibers, cellular infiltration around vasa vasorum, and mucoprotein accumulation; (8) secondary changes such as ulceration, thrombosis, or hemorrhage.

ETIOLOGIC FACTORS

The understanding of coronary atherosclerosis and its etiology has been enriched by studies directed toward three major lines of investigation: (1) epidemiologic studies attempting correlation between incidence and prevalence of coronary atherosclerosis at autopsy and in living populations, and various parameters such as geographic differences, race, age, sex, and nutrition; (2) experimental atherosclerosis in animals subjected to a variety of nutritional and other stimuli; and (3) physiopathologic studies attempting to relate observed early vascular changes with a variety of possible etiologic factors.

EPIDEMIOLOGIC STUDIES[2–6,10,13,14,21–30]

A great deal of information has been derived from epidemiologic studies in different countries of the world and in different strata of the population within the same country. Geographic differences in the occurrence of coronary atherosclerosis have been reported both from autopsy material and from living population studies.[6,31] Figure 62B-2 illustrates the mortality rates from arteriosclerotic heart disease and all other causes of death in males, aged 45 to 54 years, in 21 countries, reported for the year 1967. The limitations and imprecision inherent in such studies have to be kept in mind; nevertheless, certain important facts have been established: The lesions of coronary atherosclerosis are more frequent and more extensive in older individuals, in males more than in women of childbearing age, in individuals from more affluent countries, and in more affluent families within underdeveloped countries.

In an attempt to dissect the factors responsible for the higher prevalence rate in some of the more affected countries, a positive correlation has been found between mortality rates from coronary disease and per capita income, mode of life, and economic development. Additional evidence provided from studies comparing incidence of coronary atherosclerosis in different economic strata of population from the same country, in families where some members have emigrated from an underdeveloped country to a more developed one, and in European countries

FIGURE 62B-1 Schematic concept of the progression of coronary atherosclerosis. Fatty streaks are found as one of the earliest lesions of atherosclerosis. Many fatty streaks regress, whereas others progress to fibrous plaques and eventually to atheromata. These may then become complicated by hemorrhage, ulceration, calcification, or thrombosis and may produce myocardial infarction. (*Modified from McGill, Geer, and Strong.*[17])

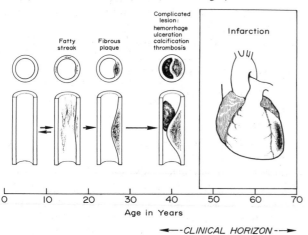

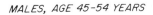

MORTALITY RATES FROM ARTERIOSCLEROTIC HEART DISEASE AND ALL OTHER CAUSES OF DEATH IN 21 COUNTRIES, 1967.

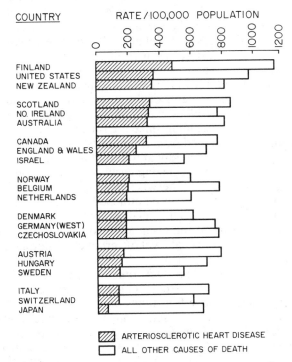

FIGURE 62B-2 Mortality rates from arteriosclerotic heart disease and from all other causes of death in 21 countries during 1967 in males aged 45 to 54 years.[12]

during and after drastic changes in nutrition and mode of life produced by World War II has also indicated that (1) the incidence rate of this disease varies directly with economic well-being and (2) the regional differences in occurrence of atherosclerotic coronary disease *cannot* be explained solely by differences due to race, ethnic origin, geography, or climate.

Nutrition is the one definite factor which has emerged from the epidemiologic studies and which forms the apparent link between affluence and increased risk of coronary atherosclerosis. In the last 30 years, numerous population surveys in many countries have reached the same basic conclusions: significant coronary atherosclerosis is prevalent in populations with habitual diets high in calories, total fat, saturated fat, cholesterol, and refined carbohydrates, whereas coronary atherosclerosis is rare or less frequent in populations whose diet is low in calories, total fat, and cholesterol.

Specific risk factors[1–13,23–37]

Additional elements have emerged from the epidemiologic studies. The information available on the association of certain factors with coronary atherosclerosis has led to the formulation of a number of "risk factors," some major, some minor, some reversible, and some irreversible. It should be empha-

sized that the concept of risk factors as applied to coronary atherosclerotic heart disease in highly industrialized countries requires special interpretation. The factors have been evolved from many types of studies to identify subjects at higher risk than others. It has to be recognized, however, that the presence of a risk factor in an individual patient gives no certainty of the presence or severity of coronary atherosclerosis. Neither should it be inferred from such studies that those individuals without an identified high-risk factor will be free of significant risk of developing coronary atherosclerotic heart disease. Indeed, in the United States, in individuals without such an identifiable risk factor the incidence of coronary atherosclerotic heart disease is unacceptably greater than that in many countries. This may be due either to poorly identified risk factors or to the fact that the "normal" serum cholesterol concentrations and the "normal" dietary content of saturated fats and cholesterol are abnormally high in the United States.

These high-risk factors, outlined in Table 62B-1, will now be considered in some detail.

NONMODIFIABLE RISK FACTORS

Age[14] The development of atherosclerosis and the emergence of the coronary lesions above the surface of clinical recognition are dependent on time. Therefore, it is expected, and it has been confirmed, that age has a strong and consistent association with atherosclerotic lesions. Other factors, such as mode of life, hyponutrition, or concomitant wasting disease, however, can significantly retard the atherogenic process or minimize its invasiveness. This argues in favor of the concept that a relation to age, although frequent, is not necessarily involved. Obviously, any risk factor or pathologic mechanism acting over a long period will result in more extensive disease.

TABLE 62B-1
Risk factors for coronary atherosclerotic heart disease (CAHD)

1 Nonmodifiable risk factors
  a Age
  b Sex
  c Familial history of premature CAHD
2 Modifiable risk factors
  a Major
    (1) Elevated serum lipid levels (cholesterol and triglyceride)
    (2) Habitual diet high in total calories, total fats, saturated fats, cholesterol, refined carbohydrates, and salt
    (3) Hypertension
    (4) Cigarette smoking
    (5) Carbohydrate intolerance
    (6) Obesity
  b Minor
    (1) Oral contraceptives
    (2) Sedentary living
    (3) Personality type
    (4) Psychosocial tensions
    (5) Others (see Table 62B-2 and text)

Sex[12–14,38] It is universally accepted that men are more prone to clinical manifestations of coronary atherosclerosis than are women of childbearing age. After the menopause, however, there is a rapid narrowing of sex difference in the incidence of angina pectoris or myocardial infarction. The sex difference appears to be more marked for the white than the black population.

Of the many reasons presented for a sex difference in susceptibility to atherosclerosis, a possible protective effect of estrogen, the differences in blood lipids and hematocrit, the reduced risk of cigarette smoking, and a more sheltered mode of life have been proposed. There is no conclusive evidence, however, for any of these; a modest effect of estrogen is observed on the β- and α-lipoproteins.

Familial history of premature coronary atherosclerotic heart disease[39–42] It has long been recognized that certain family groups have a predisposition for, or increased susceptibility to, premature coronary atherosclerotic heart disease. Recent studies have indeed confirmed that individuals with either parents or siblings affected by the disease prior to age 50 have a greater risk of developing coronary atherosclerosis at a younger age. In certain cases the relative risk may be as high as 5:1.[40] (See also Chap. 52.)

Even though the familial tendency may be influenced by genetic transmission, it is not completely clear to what extent the genetic elements act in combination with environmental factors such as nutritional, socioeconomic, and other risk factors.[41–51] In addition, information is lacking with regard to the mechanisms of genetic transmission and to whether a genetic tendency is modifiable. As noted below, it has been found that 1 out of 150 children at birth have a cholesterol concentration in the cord blood distinctly above normal, suggestive of type II hyperlipoproteinemia.[42,45] This abnormal elevation of the cholesterol level in the blood of infants and children appears to be amenable to partial correction by dietary and drug therapy.[45,48] Thus, the present state of knowledge does not allow the pessimistic conclusion that a coronary event will take place at a premature age in a subject whose parents or siblings were prematurely affected by the disease. Rather, the recently acquired evidence that many risk factors are amenable to correction should lead to a comprehensive approach in such patients to detect the elements that may mediate the genetic expression and to enforce early correcting measures when feasible.

MAJOR MODIFIABLE RISK FACTORS

Elevated serum lipid levels[5,11,22–34,52] In the last 20 to 30 years, both retrospective and prospective studies have shown a strong correlation between levels of circulating lipids and morbidity and mortality rates from coronary atherosclerotic heart disease. Among the serum lipids, cholesterol and low-density lipoproteins (LDL, or β-lipoproteins) have been found to have higher associative and predictive values than triglyceride.

Epidemiologic studies have shown greater morbidity and mortality rates due to coronary atherosclerotic heart disease in populations, such as those of the United States and Finland, with relatively higher values of cholesterol than in populations in Africa and Japan, in which ranges of blood cholesterol were 80 to 100 mg/dl lower. It has also become apparent that the older concepts of the range and upper limits of "normal" for blood cholesterol in a given population may be misleading since the ranges of "normal" were often obtained from measurements on individuals "apparently" healthy at different ages. In view of the difficulty in recognizing early or latent coronary atherosclerosis in otherwise healthy individuals, a limited significance can be attached to these relative "normal" values. The relation between level of serum cholesterol and disease is a continuous one, so that there is no critical level of serum cholesterol that clearly separates patients with low risk from patients with high risk. The fact remains, however, that patients with cholesterol level greater than 300 mg/dl were found to have four times more risk of coronary atherosclerotic heart disease than patients with levels of less than 200 mg/dl.[5] For all these reasons, it appears prudent to consider as normal or desirable that cholesterol level which is associated with the lower morbidity or mortality figures, whether taken from the United States population or from international studies on a variety of populations. Among epidemiologists, the upper limit of normal for serum cholesterol has usually been taken to be 220 to 240 mg/dl. According to Fredrickson, cholesterol concentrations above 220 mg/dl at any age should be considered suspicious, and efforts at clarification of the underlying disorder and correction of the abnormal cholesterol level appear indicated.[53] From the standpoint of lessening the development of coronary atherosclerosis, a cholesterol serum concentration of 140 to 160 mg/dl would be desirable, although somewhat difficult to attain.

Diet[2–15,21–37] A diet rich in total calories, total and saturated fats, cholesterol, refined sugars, and salt is a major coronary risk factor. A variety of studies in human populations and in experimental animals have given support to the link between diets rich in the above-listed constituents and the high incidence of, and high mortality rates from, premature coronary atherosclerotic heart disease. Conversely, populations consuming diets reduced in calories, total fats, saturated fats, and cholesterol have a lower mean serum cholesterol level and lower incidence of and mortality rates from premature coronary atherosclerotic heart disease.

Hypertension[5–12,21–37,54] Elevated blood pressure is a risk factor of prime importance and of established association with coronary atherosclerosis. Both retrospective and prospective studies have shown a definite association of hypertension with coronary atherosclerotic heart disease. The prevalence of coronary atherosclerotic heart disease is significantly higher in hypertensive individuals than in normotensive subjects. However, epidemiologic[55] and experimental studies[56] suggest that hypertension accelerates atherosclerosis only if hyperlipidemia is present, and that when hyperlipidemia is present, the effect of hypertension is related to the degree of lipid abnormality. Life insurance statistics have also shown that the expected mortality is several times higher than normal in the presence of hypertension. The beneficial effect of reducing blood pressure on coronary atherosclerotic heart disease remains to be established, although a Veterans Administration study[57] suggests a beneficial effect in regard to cerebral atherosclerosis.

Cigarette smoking[58–63] In a large number of prospective studies, the risk of coronary heart disease in relation to cigarette smoking has been estimated. Statistical evidence associating cigarette smoking with an increased risk of developing coronary atherosclerotic heart disease is impressive. In general, the risk of developing coronary atherosclerotic heart disease or the risk of death from coronary atherosclerotic heart disease is two to six times higher in smokers than nonsmokers, and the risk appears to be proportional to the number of cigarettes smoked per day. Pipe and cigar smoking are associated with surprisingly less added risk, possibly because less smoke is inhaled. There is good evidence that the cessation of smoking reduces the risk of developing coronary atherosclerotic heart disease.[58,63]

Abnormal glucose tolerance[5,17,21,64,65,65a] Patients with diabetes mellitus have been found in retrospective studies to have a greater prevalence of coronary atherosclerotic lesions, to have more extensive lesions, and to have evidence of coronary heart disease at an earlier age than nondiabetic patients. It is difficult, however, to isolate diabetes mellitus as a single factor, since it is well recognized that obesity, hypertension, and hyperlipidemia are also frequent in patients with impaired carbohydrate tolerance. There is some evidence that high levels of circulating insulin may have a role in the development of atherosclerosis and that the arterial wall is an insulin-sensitive tissue. Exposure of arterial tissue to insulin results in proliferation of smooth muscle cells, inhibition of glycolysis, and synthesis of cholesterol, phospholipid, and triglyceride.[65a]

Obesity[21,66–68] Obesity has been frequently mentioned as a significant coronary risk factor; insurance actuarial studies indicate a risk of dying from coronary atherosclerotic heart disease that appears to be related to the degree of overweight. Obese subjects are also significantly more prone to the development of hypertension, diabetes, and hyperlipidemia than lean subjects. These associated factors, rather than obesity per se, may provide the atherogenic link for the increased association of overweight with coronary atherosclerotic heart disease.

MINOR MODIFIABLE RISK FACTORS[2–6,21–31]

There is substantial evidence that women receiving oral contraceptives have a consistently higher risk of coronary heart disease than nonusers.[68a,b] In one study, the risk of death from myocardial infarction was increased 2.8 times in women 30 to 39 years and 4.7 times in women 40 to 44 years of age.[68b] In general, oral contraceptives are thought to act synergistically with other risk factors.

Sedentary living,[69–73] personality type, and psychosocial tensions[74–77] have been considered in investigations attempting to isolate these factors and to relate them to the incidence of coronary atherosclerotic heart disease in various groups. The results are less than final, but the current evidence suggests that each of these factors may enhance proneness to premature coronary atherosclerotic heart disease. The association of decreased vital capacity[78] or electrocardiographic abnormalities[79] with coronary atherosclerotic heart disease requires additional studies to be properly evaluated in atherogenesis.

Many other risk factors have been suggested, but the evidence for their participatory role in coronary atherosclerotic heart disease is not as convincing.

Possible contributing factors

Many other factors have been suggested as influencing atherosclerosis or its complications (Table 62B-2). Most have been found in at least one study to be associated with accelerated atherosclerosis, and some have been thought to be protective. At present, it is not possible to assess the relative importance, if any, of these individual factors upon the actual development of coronary atherosclerosis or its complications.

Combination of risk factors[4,5,10,11,13,21–30,32–37]

During the course of large-scale prospective epidemiologic studies, the observation was made that the risk of coronary event in an individual with two predisposing factors was not the simple sum of the two individual risks, but rather a much higher risk. For example, cigarette smoking is associated with a three- to fivefold increase in relative coronary risk and a cholesterol level above 275 mg/dl with a three- to fivefold greater risk than a cholesterol level lower than 225 mg/dl. When these two risk factors are present in the same individual, however, the coronary risk becomes fourteen to sixteen times (instead of six to nine times) greater than in an individual free from these two factors. The results of both the Gas Company Study reported by Stamler[21] and the Framingham study[22] showed the progressive and apparently synergistic effect of the presence of two, three, or four risk factors (hypertension, cigarette smoking, overweight, elevated cholesterol level).

TABLE 62B-2
Possible factors influencing the development of coronary atherosclerosis or its complications

Decreased physical activity
Decreased physical fitness
Type A personality
Psychosocial tensions
Hypoxia, carbon monoxide
Carboxyhemoglobin
Water softness
α-Radioactivity in water
Decreased stool roughage
Sucrose intake
Coffee intake
Alcohol intake
Deficiency: vitamin C or E, calcium, magnesium, chromium, manganese, vanadium, lithium, or fluoride
Relative or absolute deficiency of copper compared to zinc
Lack of pectin in diet
Abnormal methionine metabolism
Milk antibodies, homogenization
Immune reaction
Virus infection
Urban birthplace, residence
Social overcrowding
Income, living standards
Short stature
Heavy body frame
Respiratory impairment
Decreased vital capacity
Tachycardia at rest
Abnormal ECG at rest or during exercise
Abnormal cold pressor test
Abnormal ballistocardiogram
Blood group A
Coagulation disorders
Sticky platelets
Elevated hematocrit
Elevated erythrocyte sedimentation rate (in women in Sweden)
Leukocyte count
Axillary hair index
Increased ear canal hair (Gabriel's sign)
High levels of circulating insulin
Hyperuricemia
Hypothyroidism, latent
Hyperestrogenemia
Carbon disulfide exposure
Level of education
Birth order
Age of father at birth
Climate
Residence at low altitude
National energy consumption
Jewish ethnic background
Medical practice (British)

These observations indicate the complexity of the atherosclerotic process. It is quite clear that no single factor per se is responsible for the development of the atherosclerotic lesion, but that a multiplicity of factors contribute at various points and possibly by a variety of interacting mechanisms.

Modification of risk factors and reversibility of the atherosclerotic process

Once the relation between risk factors and the development of coronary atherosclerotic heart disease is accepted, the next logical question is: What evidence is there that avoiding or modifying one or more risk factors would result in reduction or modification of the atherosclerotic process? The evidence of the last few years, both in experimental animals and in the human being, although limited and still incomplete, is nevertheless encouraging. The reports of the Surgeon General have concluded that cessation of cigarette smoking is followed by a reduction in coronary atherosclerotic heart disease risk.[58,63] A report by the Veterans Administration Cooperative Study Group[57] has shown that the reduction of blood pressure by drug treatment in hypertensive patients results in a reduction in morbidity and mortality from the cardiovascular complications observed in untreated patients. It should be noted, however, that whereas treatment was statistically more effective in preventing stroke and congestive heart failure, there was little or no apparent benefit in preventing manifestations of coronary atherosclerosis.

In experimental animals, including primates, early atherosclerotic lesions are moderately reversed by dietary changes, even though a number of months or even years off the experimental diet may be required for the abnormal arterial lipids to regress.[80–89] Complex lesions with fibrosis, calcification, and other complications are, of course, more resistant to treatment and in some cases virtually irreversible. In the human subject there is now strongly suggestive evidence from many, but not all, published clinical studies that the introduction of preventive dietary measures can often be successful in the partial prevention of coronary events and in the reduction of the mortality from coronary atherosclerotic heart disease. This is true even in some elderly subjects, although the benefit is more apparent in younger subjects. These beneficial effects of diet have been shown in most "primary prevention" studies of high-risk subjects,[4,21,90–95] as well as in some, but not all, "secondary prevention" studies of subjects who had already sustained a myocardial infarction.[4,21,96–98] (See also Chap. 62H.) Unfortunately, none of the studies to date is completely satisfactory in regard to number of subjects, design, and execution. More evidence regarding the reversibility of the atherosclerotic process by modification of risk factors, as well as a prudent approach to the preventive aspect of this problem, is discussed in Chap. 62H. In summary, there is now reasonable evidence that certain manifestations of coronary atherosclerotic heart disease can be significantly altered by dietary and other measures, both in subjects who have never had evidence of coronary atherosclerotic heart disease and in patients who have. Further clarification of the extent of reversibility of coronary atherosclerosis in the human being must await the results of large clinical trials and of current studies.

Animal studies in primate and nonprimate species have paralleled the epidemiologic studies in the human being and have provided a wealth of useful information related to the pathophysiology of atherosclerosis and its inducibility by dietary and other manipulations. A detailed review of the animal studies available in the literature is beyond the scope of this chapter. Only certain aspects of experimental atherosclerosis will be emphasized. For more detailed information, the reader is referred to the comprehensive review of Constantinides.[81]

Contrary to earlier observations that animal species differed from the human species in that atherosclerotic lesions would rarely be seen, it is now well established that many animal species can develop spontaneous atherosclerosis and, in most species, appropriate techniques (such as use of diet rich in fat and cholesterol, production of hypothyroidism) can accelerate the development of atherosclerosis. It has been observed, however, that certain species (viz., rats) have a greater resistance than others (viz., rabbits) in the development of experimentally induced atherosclerotic lesions.

The experimental evidence has provided support for the following tentative conclusions: (1) In most species, high-cholesterol feeding leads to elevation of plasma cholesterol levels and development of premature atherosclerotic lesions if plasma cholesterol levels are high enough and if sufficient time is allowed for the lesions to develop; (2) studies of the initial stages of the arterial lesions have shown the accumulation of lipid, frequently with chemical characteristics similar to those of circulating lipids; (3) a variety of vessel injuries experimentally induced (by hypoxia, mechanical trauma, radiation, freezing, catecholamine injection, etc.) favor the formation of accelerated lesions at the site of the injury, and both local vessel reaction and lipid accumulation can be observed; (4) hypertension combined with hyperlipidemia leads to an accelerated formation and progression of atherosclerotic lesions.

Of great interest are the preliminary studies that suggest a degree of reversibility of the atherosclerotic lesions in animals in which the experimentally induced elevated lipid level in the plasma was corrected by a diet poor in cholesterol and/or by correction of the hypothyroid state.[16,19,81–88,99] This observation may offer some promise for attempts at both primary and secondary prevention of coronary atherosclerotic heart disease, but it must be emphasized that the improvement in the pathologic lesions produced was greater when the etiologic factors were removed relatively early. An encrusted, fibrotic, and calcified lesion has very little potential for reversibility.

It has been argued that the observations in the animal models provide information not entirely applicable to the studies of the atherosclerotic process in the human being. Even if this were so, it is

nevertheless comforting to find that the experimental observations conform to postulates derived from human pathologic and epidemiologic studies and that no major contradictory information has thus far been provided.[99]

PHYSIOPATHOLOGIC STUDIES[5,11]

It is now apparent that no *single* cause of coronary atherosclerosis has been or will be found. The understanding of the many facets of this complex disorder will be increased if we consider it a multifactorial disease. In this section, we shall focus on the normal physiology of the blood vessels, particularly the coronary arteries, the lipid constituents of plasma, and the main theories relating to the pathogenesis of atherosclerosis.

Broadly speaking, the coronary arteries serve the main function of providing blood flow to the myocardial cells for cardiac nerve conduction and cardiac muscle contraction to take place. The coronary vessels have to be patent, distensible to accommodate pulsatile pressure, and able to maintain adequate nutrition for effective myocardial function. It is well recognized that the intima and a significant portion of the media receive oxygen and nutrients directly from the bloodstream, whereas the outer portion of the media and the adventitia receive their nutrient supply from the vasa vasorum.

In normal vessels, a continuous flow of substances crosses the endothelial wall by complex mechanisms, including filtration and pinocytosis. These compounds undergo chemical reactions with the cellular elements of the vessel wall. The resulting products flow toward the outer portion of the vessel, where they are collected in the lymphatic and venous circulations in the adventitia and removed. Essential to this orderly nutritional flow is the hemodynamic driving pressure of the blood, which favors penetration of nutrients through and out of the coronary vessels. Before proceeding to the description of the theories relating to the pathogenesis of atherosclerosis, we shall review some aspects of lipid physiopathology in relation to atherogenesis.

LIPID CONSTITUENTS OF THE PLASMA[5,8,40,41,53,100–106]

Glossary

C Cholesterol, plasma concentration in mg/dl.

TG Triglycerides, plasma concentration in mg/dl.

PL Phospholipids, plasma concentration in mg/dl.

FFA Free fatty acids, plasma concentration in mEq/L.

hyperlipemia A milky appearance of plasma due to elevated TG concentration.

hyperlipidemia Excess C or TG, or both.

hyperlipoproteinemia An increase in plasma concentration of one or more lipoproteins.

chylomicron The least dense lipoprotein, containing particles of newly absorbed fat.

VLDL Very low-density lipoproteins, or pre-β-lipoproteins; transport TG synthesized mainly in liver.

LDL Low-density lipoproteins, or β-lipoproteins, containing most of the C.

HDL High-density lipoproteins, or α-lipoproteins, containing some C and most of the PL.

primary hyperlipoproteinemia Elevation of level of one or more lipoproteins; may be genetic or sporadic, not secondary to other diseases.

secondary hyperlipoproteinemia Elevation of level of one or more lipoproteins, secondary to other diseases and thus reversible if secondary cause is treatable.

The plasma lipids, composed mainly of cholesterol, triglyceride, phospholipid, and free fatty acids, are substances that are insoluble in water and, therefore, require a vehicle, or carrier, to circulate from one tissue to another. These vehicles are the lipoproteins which, as the term implies, are compounds formed of a protein and a lipid component. There are four major classes of lipoprotein: chylomicra, very low-density lipoproteins (VLDL, or pre-β-), low-density lipoproteins (LDL, or β-), and high-density lipoproteins (HDL, or α-). A fifth class is occasionally referred to as the free fatty acid–albumin complex. Each of the four major lipoprotein classes contains varying proportions of cholesterol, triglyceride, phospholipid, and protein, as illustrated in Fig. 62B-3. The lipoproteins also differ in their apoprotein content. Apoprotein A is mainly found in HDL, apoprotein B is mostly associated with LDL, and apoprotein C (made up of smaller peptides) is found in both the HDL and VLDL. The different chemical and physical composition of these protein-lipid aggregates has allowed separation and recognition of the different classes on the basis of lipoprotein density by ultracentrifugation and on the basis of different molecular changes by paper or agarose-gel electrophoresis.

It can be seen in Fig. 62B-3 that all four lipoproteins contain cholesterol, triglyceride, and phospholipid. Thus, in conditions in which abnormal elevations of lipid levels are observed, the increase in total cholesterol or triglycerides above "normal" limits could derive from the increase in concentration of one or more of the lipoproteins. Obviously, a marked hypercholesterolemia would derive more readily from an elevation of the level of LDL, which is richer in cholesterol.

There is one other advantage of applying the techniques to translate hypercholesterolemia or hypertriglyceridemia to a specific hyperlipoproteinemia. Recent studies have clarified the origin, metabolism, and fate of the lipoproteins. Thus, the classification of a lipid disorder in terms of the specific

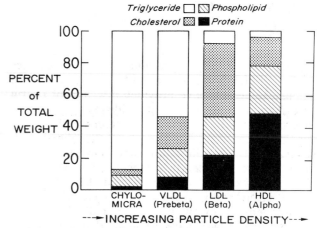

FIGURE 62B-3 Schematic bar graph illustrating the relative composition of the four major classes of circulating lipoproteins. Note the increased protein concentration as the particle density increases, the relatively high concentration of triglyceride in chylomicra and in very low-density lipoproteins (VLDL, or pre-β-lipoproteins), and the high cholesterol concentration in low-density lipoproteins (LDL, or β-lipoproteins).

abnormal lipoprotein types(s) may provide additional useful clues to understanding the underlying metabolic disorder, as well as valuable suggestions for prognosis and therapy. The clinical usefulness and indications for lipoprotein phenotyping are discussed in Chap. 62H.

Chylomicron is a lipoprotein of intestinal origin. Following hydrolysis and absorption of dietary lipid, chylomicra are formed with reconstituted triglyceride of dietary origin and small proportions of cholesterol, phospholipid, and protein. Chylomicra impart a visible milky, or lactescent, hue to the plasma for 1 to 5 h following a meal, as soon as they reach the peripheral circulation via the lymphatic system and the thoracic duct. Chylomicra carry the *exogenous triglycerides,* which are acted upon by a group of enzymes called *lipoprotein lipase* (LPL). Lipoprotein lipase, which can be activated by heparin, dissociates the triglyceride from the chylomicra, and the resulting free fatty acids are transferred to adipose tissue, heart and skeletal muscle, and other tissues, while the resulting glycerol is mainly removed by the liver.

The *VLDL* are synthesized in the liver. The triglyceride that makes up the bulk of the VLDL derives from precursors such as carbohydrate and from circulating free fatty acids mostly mobilized from adipose tissue. These *endogenous triglycerides* circulate in association with the other lipid and protein components of VLDL and undergo a fate similar to the exogenous triglyceride fo chylomicra.

The *LDL* carry the greatest portion of plasma cholesterol. This lipoprotein, which normally has a half-life of 3 days, appears to be the remnant of VLDL metabolism after this latter lipoprotein has unloaded the endogenous triglyceride. LDL has the greatest atherogenic potential.

The *HDL* carry a considerable amount of phospholipid, modest amounts of cholesterol, but the greatest proportion of protein. This lipoprotein as well as the chylomicra appears to have the least atherogenic potential. Several studies have suggested that there is a strong negative association between the plasma level of HDL cholesterol and the incidence of coronary heart disease.[100,100a,b] Experimentally, there is evidence that HDL apoproteins may act as receptors to carry cholesterol away from peripheral tissues, including atheromatous plaques.[101] Thus, it is possible that HDL cholesterol may actually be protective against the development of atherosclerosis. Some have recommended the routine determination of HDL cholesterol as a guide to diagnosis and therapy.[102]

Classification of hyperlipo- proteinemias[5,8,40,41,53,103–116]

Fredrickson and his associates proposed a classification of disorders of lipid metabolism based on the lipoprotein electrophoretic pattern.[103] According to this classification, depicted in Fig. 62H-2, one normal and five distinctly abnormal patterns can be seen. This classification is described in greater detail in Chap. 62H.

Phenotypic characterization of lipoproteins has been an effective tool in the elucidation of deranged lipid and lipoprotein metabolism and also in identifying recurrent manifestations of clinical abnormalities in affected populations. It has to be recognized, however, that numerous unresolved problems remain. Classification by electrophoretic phenotyping is to a large degree morphologic. A single phenotypic pattern may be produced by a variety of diseases or genetic mechanisms, and some patients have combined or mixed forms of hyperlipoproteinemias. Long-term follow-up studies of some patients with lipid disorders have revealed changes with time from one lipoprotein phenotype to another.[117] In addition, patients are occasionally seen with hyperlipidemias that do not fit any of the currently recognized patterns of lipoprotein abnormalities.[118–120] The precise mode of genetic transmission of these disorders as well as the mode of gene expression are still unclear. (See Chaps. 52 and 62H.)

Recently, the economy and necessity of routine lipoprotein phenotyping for treatment of patients with elevated cholesterol or triglyceride levels, or both, have been questioned.[121,122] In clinical practice, most patients can be adequately classified and managed on the basis of plasma levels of cholesterol and triglyceride without lipoprotein phenotyping. (See Chap. 62H.)

THEORIES AND MECHANISMS RELATING TO THE PATHOGENESIS OF ATHEROSCLEROSIS[1–11,16–19,81,123–125]

In our present state of knowledge, atherosclerosis must be viewed as a spectrum of arterial reactions that may result from many factors acting upon the vessel wall and producing their effects through different mechanisms in different subjects or even at different sites within the same subject. Thus, the relative importance of one mechanism or theory may, and probably does, vary significantly from one patient to another. We are very immature in our knowledge of the mechanisms of atherogenesis. Figure 62B-4 illustrates schematically the lumen and the different layers of the vessel wall. On the right-hand side are listed the many factors, both blood factors

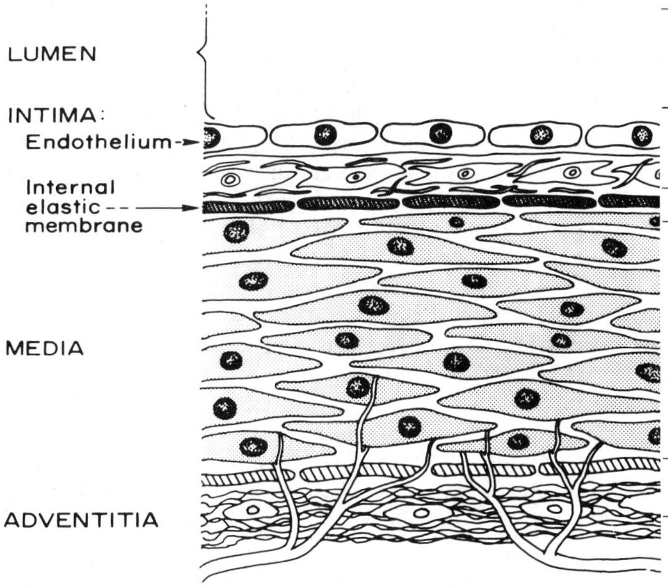

FIGURE 62B-4 Schematic cross section of the wall of an artery. The probable factors and mechanisms contributing to atherogenesis at different levels of the vessel wall are indicated on the right. See text for details. (*Modified from Getz, Vesselinovitch, and Wissler.*[16])

Increased intraluminal hydrostatic pressure.
Increased concentration of LDL and VLDL lipoproteins.
Increase in platelet agglutination and tendency to form platelet-fibrin clots.
Decrease in oxygen tension.

Increased intimal permeability due to hypertension, hemodynamic stress, stasis, hyperlipoproteinemia, hypoxia, carbon monoxide, vasoactive substances, injury, toxins, shock, or underlying fatty streak.

Fragmentation or plugging of internal elastic membrane.

Increased accumulation of lipoproteins, both extracellularly and intracellularly in smooth muscle cells (SMCs).
Proliferation and decreased metabolism of SMCs.
Altered activity of enzyme systems responsible for metabolism and removal of lipoprotein products.
Decrease in oxygen tension.
Increase in irritating or toxic products from lipoproteins leading to damage or necrosis of tissue cells.
Fibro-calcific tissue reaction.
Vascularization of advanced plaque.

Decrease in lymphatic drainage.
Decrease in vasa vasorum blood supply to outer media and adventitia.

LUMEN

INTIMA:
Endothelium→

Internal elastic -- membrane→

MEDIA

ADVENTITIA

and vessel factors, and mechanisms that are considered to play an important role in the formation of the atherosclerotic lesions.

Lipid infiltration mechanism[1-3,5-9,11,16,126,127]

This theory originated with R. Virchow, who in 1862 suggested that the lipids in atherosclerotic lesions were derived from the plasma by "imbibition" or "insudation."[128] Both Virchow and Rindfleisch in 1872 noted that any form of mechanical or inflammatory damage to the endothelium may result in increased imbibition of plasma lipids to the intima. The theory was supported by Ribbert in 1904 and in the same year by Marchand,[129] who introduced the term *atherosclerosis* to distinguish it from other forms of *arteriosclerosis*. Marchand favored the hypothesis of selective imbibition of lipids into the arterial intima with the formation of lipid pools and connective tissue reaction. In 1909 Ignatowski[130] published the results of his classic experiments in which he produced severe experimental atherosclerosis in rabbits by feeding them a diet of milk, meat extract, and egg yolk. His studies were soon confirmed by Starakadomsky and Ssobolew (1910) and by Fahr (1912). In 1913 Anitschkow and Chalatov[131] published the results of their classic experiment in which they fed rabbits pure cholesterol dissolved in vegetable oil and thereby established the importance of cholesterol in experimental atherosclerosis. In these studies, it was found that the first stage of their experimental atherosclerosis was a type of fatty infiltration, rather than a primary degeneration as had previously been thought. In 1928, Anitschkow described the regression of atherosclerotic lesions that had formed during previous periods of high cholesterol intake following removal of the atherogenic diet. This infiltration theory was also supported by Aschoff, who in 1914 noted that wear and tear with overstretching of the ground substance of the intima produced a reactive proliferation of elastic tissue and also permitted increased permeation of lipid from the lumen into the intima. In 1924, he expanded his theories and distinguished between the *atheromatosis* of youth, which is produced by lipid infiltration and is largely reversible, and the *atherosclerosis* of later life, which is characterized by secondary, complex degenerative changes.

According to the modern interpretation of this theory, plasma proteins, including the LDL and VLDL, are continuously entering the arterial wall through the endothelium (Fig. 62B-4).[132] The precise mechanism of entrance is uncertain and remains a central problem of atherogenesis. Although ultrastructural and physicochemical factors are important,[127] it is very unlikely that the process is a simple mechanical filtration. Parker[133] and others have identified by electron microscopy small vesicles on the intimal surface as well as within endothelial cells.

They suggested that these might represent the mechanism by which substances including lipoproteins are transported across the endothelial cell. Such a mechanism would be an active process, resembling phagocytosis or pinocytosis. Shimamoto has emphasized the contraction and swelling of endothelial cells as an important mechanism contributing to lipid accumulation and has suggested that lipoproteins enter through clefts or openings between endothelial cells.[134]

After the lipoprotein molecules pass through the internal elastic lamina into the inner media, they accumulate inside and outside smooth muscle cells (SMCs), which are the major cells involved in atherogenesis. SMCs also appear to have a strong tendency to migrate into developing atherosclerotic lesions and to proliferate there. BendITT and Bendit have suggested that the proliferating SMCs in an atherosclerotic plaque are of a clonally selected ("monoclonal") or mutant population, possibly transformed into somewhat autonomous behavior.[135,136,136a] In addition to being able to metabolize plasma lipoproteins, SMCs are able to decrease their own production of cholesterol in response to high tissue concentrations of LDL. Of great importance, Brown and Goldstein have found that fibroblasts from patients with type II hyperlipoproteinemia have a deficiency in specific cell membrane LDL receptors. This receptor normally binds LDL, regulates the transfer of cholesterol of LDL into the cell, stimulates cholesterol esterification, enhances the degradation of the apoprotein of LDL and suppresses cholesterol synthesis.[49,108-110] The major consequences of decreased LDL receptor function would be the accumulation of LDL and of cholesterol. Similar receptors have been found in arterial SMCs[137]; patients with type II hyperlipoproteinemia probably have defective LDL catabolism by their SMCs due to a similar receptor defect that may be important in the development of atherosclerosis.

When an excess of LDL accumulates within the arterial wall, the lipoproteins and their metabolic products are "trapped" and accumulate. Products of lipoprotein metabolism, particularly free cholesterol and cholesterol esters, when present in excess can result in a fibrocalcific reaction. In addition, hyperlipemic lymph and serum appear capable of stimulating the growth of both arterial SMCs and endothelial cells growing in intact animals[11,138] or in cell cultures.[11,139-141] This effect is not due to the increased concentration of total cholesterol but to a specific factor in LDL, particularly from patients with type II hyperlipoproteinemia.[142] Even mildly hyperlipemic serum from monkeys fed an average American table-prepared diet stimulates SMC division,[142] and the intimal proliferation of SMCs has been experimentally produced in monkeys by feeding small supplements of cholesterol for 18 months at a dosage insufficient to elevate serum cholesterol levels.[139] There is also evidence that the response of intimal cells and SMCs to lipoproteins varies significantly with the specific fatty acid composition of the lipoproteins.[16,143] LDL, LDL metabolic products, and glycosaminoglycans (GAGs) may also interact to form complex compounds that may have an important role in the initiation and growth of atheromatous plaques.[6,132,144–147]

It would appear that the early fatty streak, which is virtually universal in the aortae of children, is completely reversible. On the other hand, it is most probable that some, but not all, fatty streaks progress to become fibrous plaques, which may be raised and impinge upon the vessel lumen and which are no longer completely reversible.[2,5–9,11,16,17,148] These lesions eventually may progress to become an atheroma, which may then become a complicated lesion with hemorrhage, fibrosis, calcification, ulceration, or thrombosis. Such advanced lesions are obviously reversible only to a limited degree. The accumulation of lipid within the intima and media is often associated with evidence of scarring of the media and of fragmentation and damage to the internal elastic lamina.

The Virchow-Aschoff infiltration or imbibition theory is supported by abundant evidence including the following: the fact that the bulk of the cholesterol in atheromata appears to originate from circulating LDL from the vessel lumen[1–3,5–9,11,16,81,126,127,132]; the identification of radioactive albumin and radioactive cholesterol in concentration gradients from the intima to the adventitia of arteries[1,149]; the identification of LDL and VLDL in fatty streaks and in atheromata[7–9,150–153]; and the identification of isotopically labeled LDL, administered prior to death, within an atheromatous lesion in the aorta in greater concentration than in other organs.[8,9,153] The presence of LDL, which in general closely resemble the pattern in circulating blood, has been demonstrated by chemical extraction of LDL from atherosclerotic lesions, by histochemical stains, and by specific stains with fluorescent antibodies against LDL.[8,9,150–153] Smith and Slater[154] found a highly significant correlation between the amount of electrophoretically and immunologically intact lipoprotein in the aortic intima and the concentration in blood taken during the week before death. In contrast to LDL, HDL do not accumulate in human atherosclerotic lesions,[5–9,16–19,102,106,123,155] although HDL molecules appear to traverse the walls of peripheral vessels rather easily.[156] Interestingly, HDL apoproteins appear to be able to transport cholesterol away from aortic SMCs in culture.[157] Although most of the cholesterol in atheromatous lesions derives from circulating LDL, phospholipids accumulate predominantly by local synthesis.

There is evidence that the intima and perhaps the inner 1.0 mm of arteries receive oxygen and other metabolic requirements from the vessel lumen while the remaining media and adventitia receive their nutrition from the vasa vasorum. It is apparent that there is a "watershed" zone which lies at the junction of these two zones and which is very susceptible to any condition that might produce hypoxia and decrease the enzymatic metabolism and removal of lipoproteins.[1,8,158,159] There is substantial evidence indicating that both diminished oxygenation of the intima and internal medial and chronic exposure to carbon monoxide (CO) accelerate experimental atherosclerosis and SMC proliferation, whereas hyperoxia impedes the development of experimental atherosclerosis and significantly increases its regression.[16,160–165] There is also suggestive evidence that chronic hypoxia may promote elevated blood lipid levels.[11] Both hypoxia produced by high altitude and that produced by hyperlipidemia may lead to edema of the intima and opening of endothelial junctions, which would facilitate the passage of macromolecules such as lipoproteins into the artery wall.[11]

Intimal permeability and endothelial cell injury

Factors influencing the *permeability* of the intima to lipoprotein molecules are of great importance in atherogenesis, and *endothelial cell injury* is a very important factor in experimental atherosclerosis, and may also be important clinically. Experimentally, endothelial damage produced by heat, cold, or mechanical (catheter) injury markedly accelerates atherosclerosis in the presence of diet-induced hypercholesterolemia. Endothelial injury or permeability changes may also result from platelet agglutination with the release of vasoactive amines,[166,181,186] from areas of hemodynamic stress,[167–169] from hypertension,[170–172] from antigen-antibody complexes,[173] and by the "trapdoor" effect of angiotensin II.[174] The arterial intimal permeability to LDL also appears to be increased in areas of atheromata,[134,153,175] a change that would tend to promote a self-perpetuating cycle of atherogenesis.

Thrombogenic (encrustation) mechanisms[5,27,166,176–181]

This theory, which was initially propounded as the "encrustation" theory of Rokitansky in 1852, was revived by Clark in 1936 and later by Duguid,[176,177] Mustard and associates,[178] and others.[6,179] According to this theory, microthrombi with varying concentrations of fibrin, platelets, red blood cells, and serum lipids occur on the endothelial surface of arteries and eventually are incorporated into the intima. Earlier studies emphasized fibrin encrustation, but more recently the possible role of platelet aggregates has been proposed as an alternative mechanism.[7,8,166,181,186] By this mechanism, the accumulation of cholesterol and other lipids in atheromata might result from the lipids within platelets or blood cells, from trapped plasma lipids, from subsequent capillary hemorrhage, or even by filtration into the thrombus from the plasma.[81]

Although there is no question that both micro- and macrothrombosis are major complications of atheromata,[18,19,27] there is as yet inadequate evidence to establish that the thrombogenic mechanism is responsible for the earliest lesions of atherosclerosis or that the theory can account for most of the lipids in atherosclerotic plaques.[5,7–9,11,16,123,124] Most of the evidence for this mechanism has demonstrated mural thrombi occurring on top of older, more advanced atheromatous lesions.[81] Although small amounts of fibrin have been identified within fatty streaks by immunohistochemistry and electron microscopy,[182] this finding may represent the nonspecific filtration of plasma constituents, since fibrin may also be found in other inflammatory or granulomatous lesions.[1,8,81] It is well known that large thrombi in coronary arteries may become recanalized, much of the thrombus being incorporated into the wall of the atheromatous vessel.[18] Of great potential significance are studies strongly suggesting that hyperlipoproteinemia may accelerate or promote coagulation, increase platelet aggregation and adhesiveness, and inhibit fibrinolysis.[8,166,167,181,183] It is significant that platelets, when activated, may release enzymes that can directly alter the permeability characteristics of the endothelium.[181] There is evidence that platelets may contain a factor capable of stimulating SMCs.[125,181,183,184,186] Experimentally, platelets and high levels of LDL also act synergistically to promote arterial intimal cell proliferation and atherogenesis.[181,185,186]

In general, it does not appear that the thrombogenic or encrustation theory can be the sole cause of atherosclerosis or even that this mechanism is often responsible for the initial lesions of atherosclerosis. Both microscopic and macroscopic thrombi are well-recognized complications of atheromata and may result in death. On the other hand, if the thrombogenic theory were the primary mechanism of atherogenesis in human beings, one would expect a very low incidence of the disease in patients with coagulation deficiencies, whereas severe atherosclerosis has been noted in patients with hemophilia, Christmas disease, and von Willebrand's disease.

An important aspect of the relation between coronary atheromatosis and myocardial infarction is the concept that the fibrous cap of an atheromatous plaque may rupture, thereby exposing the passing blood to highly thrombogenic material within the plaque[187] and possibly also producing a downstream embolism of atheromatous debris. It appears very likely, though unproved, that some instances of sudden death in patients with coronary atherosclerotic heart disease, who often have no demonstrable thrombus at autopsy, result from the microscopic cracks or rupture of atheromatous plaques with the acute obstruction of vital coronary vessels or collaterals by platelet aggregation or fibrin thrombi, either of which may be difficult to detect several hours later at autopsy.[188] Abnormalities of platelet aggregation and survival may also play a role in producing ischemic coronary symptoms in some patients with normal or nearly normal coronary arteriograms.[189]

Hemodynamic mechanisms[190–198]

The importance of mechanical factors in contributing to the localization and genesis of atherosclerosis was recognized as early as 1856 by Virchow and 1872 by Rindfleisch. The strong correlation between arterial blood pressure and the development of atherosclerosis has been well recognized for many years, both epidemiologically and experimentally. The importance of mechanical factors in the localization of atherosclerosis accords with the Virchow-Aschoff "infiltration" theory of atherogenesis,[126,170,171,195] both by increasing the intraluminal pressure and by altering the intimal permeability to lipoproteins. The arteries of hypertensive patients and experimental animals appear to have increased permeability to large molecules including lipoproteins.[170,171] Mechanical factors may also induce changes in the intimal surface and induce platelet-fibrin microthrombi by the Rokitansky-Duguid (thrombogenic) hypothesis.

Localized atheromatous plaques are particularly likely to occur at sites of bifurcation or branching, in bends or curves, and in areas of arteries that are immobilized or that are subject to frequent bending and twisting. In addition to the important role of the pulsatile arterial blood pressure, many special types of local hemodynamic stress have been suggested to account for the localization of plaques. McDonald[196] concluded that the more important local stresses were turbulence and eddy currents, wave reflection, especially at areas of vessel branching, and viscous drag. In addition, he noted that each arterial pulse wave produces a longitudinal shearing strain between the layers of the arterial wall. Evans blue, which can demonstrate areas of increased arterial intimal permeability, preferentially localizes in such areas of hemodynamic stress.[168,197]

Although it is well known that arterial hypertension accelerates atherogenesis, Texon[190] has emphasized that many sites of predilection for atherosclerosis are sites of diminished local lateral pressure. Instances of low pressure that may predispose to atherosclerosis include the following: areas of vessel narrowing (narrowing produces increased velocity and decreased lateral or hydrostatic pressure), decreased pressure along the inner curve of a vessel such as the aortic arch, decreased lateral pressure with increased velocity at the medial walls of vessel branching or bifurcation, and relative decrease in lateral pressure at areas of external attachment. According to Texon, the localized decrease in lateral pressure produces a relative suction upon the intima, which is subjected to a lifting or pulling effect. This may induce a reactive intimal thickening, an alteration in endothelial permeability to lipoproteins, or injury to the intima inducing platelet or fibrin thrombi. In more advanced atheromata, the suction effect could even contribute to the rupture of the intimal surface, resulting in either distal embolization or a coronary thrombosis, or both.

Fox and Hugh[198] have demonstrated that zones of relative stasis may occur at areas of irregular flow or branching within the arterial system despite quite high velocities nearby, due to the process of boundary layer separation. They felt that static zones allow the interaction of platelets and fibrin to form a mesh in which lipid particles become entrapped and which becomes organized to form an atheromatous plaque as envisaged by the Rokitansky-Duguid mechanism.

In the coronary vessels, atheromata are more marked in the proximal portions of the three main epicardial coronary arteries and particularly at those locations that undergo marked kinking or twisting with each heartbeat. Of very great significance is the freedom from atherosclerosis in the penetrating branches of coronary arteries within the contracting myocardium, even though there may be extensive atherosclerosis in the epicardial vessels.

Capillary hemorrhage[199]

According to this theory, which was first formulated by Winternitz in 1938, the lipid in atherosclerotic lesions originates from repeated hemorrhages into the plaques due to rupture of capillaries originating either from the vessel lumen or from vasa vasorum. Although such a mechanism obviously does not account for the initial accumulation of lipid, it could contribute additional lipid accumulation and fibrosis once a plaque is present. Paterson[200] has emphasized the frequency and the role of capillary hemorrhages within plaques as a mechanism for the acute production of coronary artery obstruction.

Lipophage (macrophage) migration[201]

According to this theory, which was supported by Leary,[202] cholesterol accumulated in arteries by the intimal penetration of circulating lipophages (lipid-laden monocytes or macrophages), suggested to originate as Kupffer cells in the liver. These cells were thought either to penetrate the endothelium or to adhere to its surface and become covered by an overgrowth of endothelium. The lipophage (macrophage) migration mechanism would appear to be of significance only under severe experimental lipemia in some animals[203] and perhaps in the spontaneous atherosclerosis of the bluefin tuna.[99] At present, most investigators favor the alternative view that the foam cells of human lesions arise from lipid accumulation within SMCs of the arterial wall.[201,204]

SUMMARY OF POSSIBLE PATHOGENIC MECHANISMS OF MAJOR HIGH-RISK FACTORS

Although much remains unknown regarding the pathogenesis of atherosclerosis, available information permits the suggestion of several mechanisms by which high-risk factors may interact with the previously described pathogenetic mechanisms and thus contribute to the increased development of atherosclerosis.

Hypercholesterolemia

In the presence of hypercholesterolemia there is an increased penetration of LDL molecules by uncertain mechanisms across or between arterial intimal cells and into medial SMCs. In most studies the accumulation is exponentially proportional to the degree of elevation of LDL levels above the physiologic normal level of 140 to 160 mg/dl, and the regression of experimental lesions is significantly accelerated when elevated serum cholesterol levels are decreased from higher levels to 150 mg/dl.[82-87] Hypercholesterolemia may also promote stimulation and contraction of the endothelial cells, a process that would tend to increase the penetration of LDL through the intimal endothelium.[134] Hyperlipidemia may also promote platelet agglutination, especially in areas of increased hemodynamic stress or over fatty streaks.

Hypertension

Hypertension may accelerate the passage of LDL through or between intimal endothelial cells by increasing the stretch on the arterial wall or by the angiotensin (trapdoor) effect, especially in areas of increased hemodynamic stress or intimal damage. Hypertension may also increase platelet stickiness and the release of vasoactive amines in areas of endothelial damage.

Cigarette smoking

Chronic cigarette smoking, which may be associated with a blood concentration of carboxyhemoglobin of 20%, may alter endothelial permeability to LDL by means of carbon monoxide or other materials inhaled. The oxygen tension may be significantly decreased in the media, an effect which may decrease the normal degradation and removal of LDL. Carbon monoxide may also inhibit the cytochrome oxidase of the vessel wall, and nicotine may impair oxidative enzymes. Chronic cigarette smoking also tends to be associated with a higher serum cholesterol level, increased platelet stickiness and agglutination, and a shorter platelet half-life.

Diabetes mellitus

Diabetes mellitus tends to be associated with higher concentrations of serum cholesterol and especially VLDL. The serum of diabetic rabbits appears to contain a substance capable of stimulating SMCs, while the arteries of diabetic patients appears to have GAGs that tend to bind lipoproteins. Exposure of arterial tissue to insulin results in proliferation of SMCs, inhibition of lipolysis, and synthesis of cholesterol, phospholipid, and triglyceride. Chronic exposure to high concentrations of insulin results in the development of lipid-filled lesions similar to those of early atherosclerosis.[65a] The marked variations in serum glucose concentration and the occasional high levels of catecholamines may influence the endothelial penetration of LDL. A prescribed diet that restricts carbohydrate intake will usually result in an increased intake of fat, which would tend to promote hyperlipidemia.

SUMMARY AND CONCLUSIONS

It has been emphasized that the present state of knowledge of the atherosclerotic process indicates multiple etiologic factors in its pathogenesis. The atherosclerotic process may also be the common end result of multiple, different pathogenic mechanisms in different patients.

Epidemiologic studies have contributed greatly to the identification of the more influential factors. The high-risk factors outlined in Table 62B-1 and discussed in the text have been divided into two groups, (1) nonmodifiable and (2) modifiable. Among the latter, a rich diet, hyperlipidemia, hypertension, and cigarette smoking appear to carry a greater risk, whereas obesity and sedentary living appear to be associated with a lower risk.

Experimental studies in animals have provided valuable insights into the early changes in the arterial wall produced by maneuvers such as a hypercholesterolemic diet, which provides a definite atherogenic stimulus. The accumulation of lipid in the intima and in the SMCs of the media has been shown to be a very early event in the development of the atherosclerotic lesions.

The pathophysiologic studies have led to a basic change from the older concept of the "atheromatous plaque" resulting from a degenerative process associated with normal aging to the newer concept of a dynamic reaction of the arterial wall to a variety of stimuli and pathogenic influences.

Of the many theories and factors related to the pathogenesis of atherosclerosis, the *lipid infiltration* mechanism would appear to best explain the early development of the atherosclerotic process, whereas the *thrombogenetic* mechanism appears to be very important in the later progression or complications of the lesions.

From our current state of knowledge, it appears that many of the genetic and environmental factors channel their pathogenic influence through the production of distinct abnormalities of the plasma lipid components, which in turn combine with changes in the arterial endothelium and media and other dynamic factors (e.g., hypertension) in initiating, accelerating, and perpetuating the atherosclerotic lesion. Excessive elevations of LDL and VLDL levels (resulting in elevated plasma concentrations of cholesterol and triglyceride above the physiologic desirable levels) appear to be the cardinal factors, around which most of the others revolve.

Several studies have pointed to the reversible elements of the atherosclerotic process. The early fatty streaks and even the early uncomplicated atheromatous lesions appear to be potentially reversible in animals and human beings. On the other hand, advanced lesions with ulceration, severe fibrosis, and extensive calcification have little potential for significant reversal.

On the basis of the available evidence and data, it is suggested that a prudent approach to prevent, delay, or even decrease the atherosclerotic lesions should include reduction or exclusion of all or most of the modifiable high-risk factors in a particular individual as early as possible and certainly before the appearance of evident lesions on the clinical horizon (see also Chap. 62H). Much has been learned and much more needs to be learned about atherosclerosis. In the meantime, a careful and sound application of the knowledge already accumulated in studies of the etiology of atherosclerosis could have a beneficial influence in lessening the frightening consequences of uncontrolled coronary atherosclerotic heart disease.

REFERENCES

1 Adams, C. W. M.: "Vascular Histochemistry, in Relation to the Chemical and Structural Pathology of Cardiovascular Disease," Year Book Medical Publishers, Inc., Chicago, 1967.

2 Blumenthal, H. T. (ed.): "Cowdry's Arteriosclerosis: A Survey of the Problem," 2d ed., Charles C Thomas, Publisher, Springfield, Ill., 1967.

3 Jones, R. J. (ed.): "Atherosclerosis" (proceedings, second international symposium), Springer-Verlag OHG, Heidelberg, 1970.

4 "Arteriosclerosis: A Report by the National Heart and Lung Institute Task Force on Arteriosclerosis," vol. 2, DHEW Publication (NIH) 72-219, National Institutes of Health, Bethesda, Md., 1972.

5 Wissler, R. W., and Geer, J. C. (eds.): "The Pathogenesis of Atherosclerosis," The Williams & Wilkins Company, Baltimore, 1972.

6 Schettler, G., and Weizel, A. (eds.): "Atherosclerosis III" (proceedings, third international symposium), Springer-Verlag OHG, Berlin, 1974, p. 1034.

7 Friedman, M.: The Pathogenesis of Coronary Plaques, Thromboses, and Hemorrhages: An Evaluation Review, *Circulation,* 52(suppl. 3):34, 1975.

8 Walton, K. W.: Pathogenic Mechanisms in Atherosclerosis, *Am. J. Cardiol.,* 35:542, 1975.

9 Zilversmit, D. B.: Mechanisms of Cholesterol Accumulation in the Arterial Wall, *Am. J. Cardiol.,* 35:559, 1975.

10 Keys, A.: Coronary Heart Disease: The Global Picture, *Atherosclerosis,* 22:149, 1975.

11 Wissler, R. W., Vesselinovitch, D., and Getz, G. S.: Abnormalities of the Arterial Wall and Its Metabolism in Atherogenesis, *Prog. Cardiovasc. Dis.,* 18:341, 1976.

12 "World Health Statistics Annual, 1967," vol. 1, "Vital Statistics and Causes of Death," World Health Organization, Geneva, 1970.

13 Keys, A. (ed.): Coronary Heart Disease in Seven Countries, *Circulation,* 41(suppl. 1):211, 1970.

14 Moriyama, I. M., Krueger, D. E., and Stamler, J.: "Cardiovascular Diseases in the United States," Harvard University Press, Cambridge, Mass., 1971.

15 Cheng, T. O.: Changing Prevalence of Heart Disease in People's Republic of China, *Ann. Intern. Med.,* 80:108, 1974.

16 Getz, G. S., Vesselinovitch, D., and Wissler, R. W.: A Dynamic Pathology of Atherosclerosis, *Am. J. Med.,* 46:657, 1969.

17 McGill, H. C., Jr., Geer, J. C., and Strong, J. P.: Natural History of Human Atherosclerotic Lesions, in M. Sandler and G. H. Bourne (eds.), "Atherosclerosis and Its Origin," Academic Press, Inc., New York, 1963, p. 39.

18 Osborn, G. R.: "The Incubation Period of Coronary Thrombosis," Butterworth & Co. (Publishers), Ltd., London, 1963.

19 Jones, R. J. (ed.): "Evolution of the Atherosclerotic Plaque," The University of Chicago Press, Chicago, 1963.

20 "Classification of Atherosclerotic Lesions Report," World Health Organization Technical Report Series, no. 143, Geneva, 1958.

21 Stamler, J.: Atherosclerotic Coronary Heart Disease—Etiology and Pathogenesis: The Coronary Risk Factors, in J. Stamler, "Lectures on Preventive Cardiology," Grune & Stratton, Inc., New York, 1967, p. 107.

22 Kannel, W. B., Castelli, W. P., Gordon, T., and McNamara, P. M.: Serum Cholesterol, Lipoproteins, and the Risk of Coronary Heart Disease: The Framingham Study, *Ann. Intern. Med.,* 74:1, 1971.

23 Epstein, F. H.: International Trends in Coronary Heart Disease Epidemiology, *Ann. Clin. Res.,* 3:293, 1971.

24 Epstein, F. H., and Ostrander, L. D., Jr.: Detection of Individual Susceptibility toward Coronary Disease, *Prog. Cardiovasc. Dis.,* 13:324, 1971.

25 Keyes, A., Aravanis, C., Blackburn, H., Van Buchem, F. S. P., Buzina, R., Djordjevic, B. S., Fidanza, F., Karvonen, M. J., Menotti, A., Puddu, V., and Taylor, H. L.: Probability of Middle-aged Men Developing Coronary Heart Disease in Five Years, *Circulation,* 45:815, 1972.

26 Strasser, T.: Atherosclerosis and Coronary Heart Disease: The Contribution of Epidemiology, *WHO Chron.,* 26:7, 1972.

27 Roberts, W. C., Ferrans, V. J., Levy, R. I., and Fredrickson, D. S.: Cardiovascular Pathology in Hyperlipoproteinemia: Anatomic Observations in 42 Necropsy Patients with Normal or Abnormal Serum Lipoprotein Patterns, *Am. J. Cardiol.,* 31:557, 1973.

28 Stamler, J.: Epidemiology of Coronary Heart Disease, *Med. Clin. North Am.,* 57:5, 1973.

29 Hrubec, Z., and Zukel, W. J.: Epidemiology of Coronary Heart Disease Among Young Army Males of World War II, *Am. Heart J.,* 87:722, 1974.

30 Kannel, W. B.: Some Lessions in Cardiovascular Epidemiology from Framingham, *Am. J. Cardiol.,* 37:269, 1976.

31 McGill, H. C., Jr. (ed.): "The Geographic Pathology of Atherosclerosis," The Williams & Wilkins Company, Baltimore, 1968, reprinted from *Lab. Invest.,* 18:453, 1968.

32 Wilhelmsen, L., Wedel, H., and Tibblin, G.: Multivariate Analysis of Risk Factors for Coronary Heart Disease, *Circulation,* 48:950, 1973.

33 Hagerup, L. M.: Coronary Heart Disease Risk Factors in Men and Women: From the Population Study in Glostrup, Denmark, *Acta Med. Scand. Suppl.* 557, 1974.

34 Blackburn, H.: Progress in the Epidemiology and Prevention of Coronary Heart Disease, *Prog. Cardiol.,* 3:1, 1974.

35 Dolder, M. A., and Oliver, M. F.: Myocardial Infarction in Young Men: Study of Risk Factors in Nine Countries, *Br. Heart J.,* 37:493, 1975.

36 Ostrander, L. D., Jr., and Lamphiear, D. E.: Coronary Risk Factors in a Community: Findings in Tecumseh, Michigan, *Circulation,* 53:152, 1976.

37 Brand, R. J., Rosenman, R. H., Sholtz, R. I., and Friedman, M.: Multivariate Prediction of Coronary Heart Disease in the Western Collaborative Group Study Compared to the Findings of the Framingham Study, *Circulation,* 53:348, 1976.

38 Bentsson, C.: Ischaemic Heart Disease in Women: A Study Based on a Randomized Population Sample of Women and Women with Myocardial Infarction in Gotborg, Sweden, *Acta Med. Scand. Suppl.* 549, 1973, p. 128.

39 Epstein, F. H.: Hereditary Aspects of Coronary Heart Disease, *Am. Heart J.,* 67:445, 1964.

40 Fredrickson, D. S., and Levy, R. I.: Familial Hyperlipoproteinemia, in J. B. Stanbury, J. B. Wyngaarden, and D. S. Fredrickson (eds.), "The Metabolic Basis of Inherited Dis-

ease," 3d ed., McGraw-Hill Book Company, New York, 1972, p. 545.

41 Goldstein, J. L., Schrott, H. G., Hazzard, W. R., Bierman, E. L., and Motulsku, A. G.: Hyperlipidemia in Coronary Heart Disease: II. Genetic Analysis of Lipid Levels in 176 Families and Delineation of a New Inherited Disorder, Combined Hyperlipidemia, *J. Clin. Invest.,* 52:1544, 1973.

42 Goldstein, J. L., Albers, J. J., Schrott, H. G., Hazzard, W. R., Bierman, E. L., and Motulsky, A. G.: Plasma Lipid Levels and Coronary Heart Disease in Adult Relatives of Newborns with Normal and Elevated Cord Blood Lipids, *Am. J. Hum. Genet.,* 26:727, 1974.

43 Glueck, C. J., Heckman, F., Schoenfeld, M., Steiner, P., and Pearce, W.: Neonatal Familial Type II Hyperlipoproteinemia: Cord Blood Cholesterol in 1800 Births, *Metabolism,* 20:597, 1971.

44 Tamir, I., Bojanower, Y., Levtow, O., Heldenberg, D., Dickerman, Z., and Werbin, B.: Serum Lipids and Lipoproteins in Children from Families with Early Coronary Heart Disease, *Arch. Dis. Child.,* 47:808, 1972.

45 Glueck, C. J., and Tsang, R. C.: Pediatric Familial Type II Hyperlipoproteinemia: Effects of Diet on Plasma Cholesterol in the First Year of Life, *Am. J. Clin. Nutr.,* 25:224, 1972.

46 Kwiterovich, P. O., Levy, R. I., and Fredrickson, D. S.: Familial Hyperbetalipoproteinemia (Type II Hyperlipoproeinemia) in Children, *J. Clin. Invest.,* 52:49a, 1973. (Abstract.)

47 Goldstein, J. L., Albers, J. J., Hazzard, W. R., Schrott, H. R., Bierman, E. L., and Motulsky, A. G.: Genetic and Medical Significance of Neonatal Hyperlipidemia. *J. Clin. Invest.,* 52:35a, 1973. (Abstract.)

48 Fredrickson, D. S., and Breslow, J. L.: Primary Hyperlipoproteinemia in Infants, *Ann. Rev. Med.,* 24:315, 1973.

49 Brown, M. S., and Goldstein, J. L.: Familial Hypercholesterolemia: Genetic, Biochemical and Pathophysiologic Considerations, *Adv. Intern. Med.,* 20:273, 1975.

50 Breslow, J. L., Spaulding, D. R., Lux, S. E., Levy, R. I., and Lees, R. S.: Homozygous Familial Hypercholesterolemia: A Possible Biochemical Explanation of Clinical Heterogeneity, *N. Engl. J. Med.,* 293:900, 1975.

51 Motulsky, A. G.: Current Concepts in Genetics: The Genetic Hyperlipidemias, *N. Engl. J. Med.,* 294:823, 1976.

52 Albrink, M. J., Meigs, J. W., and Man, E. B.: Serum Lipids, Hypertension and Coronary Artery Disease, *Am. J. Med.,* 31:4, 1961.

53 Fredrickson, D. S.: A Physician's Guide to Hyperlipidemia, *Mod. Concepts Cardiovasc. Dis.,* 41:31, 1972.

54 Freis, E. D.: Hypertension and Atherosclerosis, *Am. J. Med.,* 46:735, 1969.

55 Jablon, S., Angerine, D. M., Matsumoto, Y. S., and Ishida, M.: On the Significance of Cause of Death as Recorded on Death Certificates in Hiroshima and Nagasaki, Japan, *Natl. Cancer Inst. Monogr.,* 19:445, 1966.

56 Pick, R., Johnson, P. J., and Glick, G.: Deleterious Effects of Hypertension on the Development of Aortic and Coronary Atherosclerosis in Stumptail Macaques (*Macaca speciosa*) on an Atherogenic Diet, *Circ. Res.,* 35:472, 1974.

57 Veterans Administration Cooperative Study Group on Antihypertensive Agents: Effects of Treatment on Morbidity in Hypertension: II. Results in Patients with Diastolic Blood Pressure Averaging 90 through 114 mm Hg, *J.A.M.A.,* 213:1143, 1970.

58 "The Health Consequences of Smoking: A Public Health Service Review, 1967," U.S. Public Health Service Publication 1696, Public Health Series, Washington, 1967.

58a "The Health Consequences of Smoking: A Public Health

Service Review, 1967, Supplement 1968," U.S. Public Health Service Publication 1969, Public Health Service, Washington, 1968.

59 Doyle, J. T.: Cigarette-smoking and Coronary Atherosclerosis, in W. Likoff, B. L. Segal, and W. Insull, Jr. (eds.), "Atherosclerosis and Coronary Heart Disease," The Twenty-fourth Hahnemann Symposium, Grune & Stratton, Inc., New York, 1972, p. 35.

60 Aronow, W. S.: Smoking, Carbon Monoxide, and Coronary Heart Disease, *Circulation,* 48:1169, 1973. (Editorial.)

61 Astrup, P.: Carbon Monoxide, Smoking, and Cardiovascular Disease, *Circulation,* 48:1167, 1973.

62 Wald, N., Howard, S., Smith, P. G., and Kjeldsen, K.: Association between Atherosclerotic Diseases and Carboxyhaemoglobin Levels in Tobacco Smokers, *Br. Med. J.,* 1:761, 1973.

63 Gordon, T., Kannel, W. B., and McGee, D.: Death and Coronary Attacks in Men after Giving Up Cigarette Smoking: A Report from the Framingham Study, *Lancet,* 2:1345, 1974.

64 Epstein, F. H.: Hyperglycemia, a Risk Factor in Coronary Heart Disease, *Circulation,* 36:609, 1967.

65 Roberts, W. B., and Strong, J. P.: Atherosclerosis in Persons with Hypertension and Diabetes Mellitus, *Lab. Invest.,* 18:538, 1968.

65a Stout, R. W.: The Relationship of Abnormal Circulating Insulin Levels to Atherosclerosis, *Atherosclerosis,* 27:1. 1977.

66 Roberts, J. C., Jr., Moses, C., and Wilkins, R. H.: Autopsy Studies in Atherosclerosis: I. Distribution and Severity of Atherosclerosis in Patients Dying without Morphologic Evidence of Atherosclerotic Catastrophe, *Circulation,* 20:511, 1959.

66a Roberts, J. C., Jr., Wilkins, R. H., and Moses, C.: Autopsy Studies in Atherosclerosis: II. Distribution and Severity of Atherosclerosis in Patients Dying with Morphologic Evidence of Atherosclerotic Catastrophe, *Circulation,* 20:520, 1959.

66b Wilkins, R. H., Roberts, J. C., Jr., and Moses, C.: Autopsy Studies in Atherosclerosis: III. Distribution and Severity of Atherosclerosis in the Presence of Obesity, Hypertension, Nephrosclerosis, and Rheumatic Heart Disease, *Circulation,* 20:527, 1959.

67 Keys, A., Aravanis, C., Blackburn, H., Van Buchem, F. S. P., Buzina, R., Djordjevic, B. S., Findanza, F., Karvonen, M. J., Menotti, A., Puddu, V., and Taylor, H. L.: Coronary Heart Disease: Overweight and Obesity as Risk Factors, *Ann. Intern. Med.,* 77:15, 1972.

68 Ashley, F. W., Jr., and Kannel, W. B.: Relation of Weight Change to Changes in Atherogenic Traits: The Framingham Study, *J. Chronic Dis.,* 27:103, 1974.

68a Beral, V.: Cardiovascular Disease Mortality Trends and Oral Contraceptive Use in Young Women, *Lancet,* 2:1047, 1976.

68b Mann, J. I., and Inman, W. H. W.: Oral Contraceptives and Death from Myocardial Infarction, *Br. Med. J.,* 2:245, 1975.

69 Larsen, O. A., and Malmborg, R. O.: "Coronary Heart Disease and Physical Fitness," University Park Press, Baltimore, 1971.

70 Fox, S. M., III, Naughton, J. P., and Haskell, W. L.: Physical Activity and the Prevention of Coronary Heart Disease, *Ann. Clin. Res.,* 3:404, 1971.

71 Froelicher, V. F., and Oberman, A.: Analysis of Epidemiologic Studies of Physical Inactivity as Risk Factor for Coronary Artery Disease, *Prog. Cardiovasc. Dis.,* 15:41, 1972.

72 Paffenbarger, R. S., Jr., and Hale, W. E.: Work Activity and Coronary Heart Mortality, *N. Engl. J. Med.,* 292:545, 1975.

73 Fox, S. M., III: Physical Activity and Coronary Heart Disease, in E. K. Chung (ed.), "Controversy in Cardiology: The Practical Clinical Approach," Springer-Verlag OHG, Heidelberg, 1976, p. 201.

74 Shekelle, R. B., Ostfeld, A. M., and Paul, O.: Social Status and Incidence of Coronary Heart, *J. Chronic Dis.,* 22:281, 1969.

75 Friedman, M., and Rosenman, R. H.: Type A Behavior Pattern: Its Association with Coronary Heart Disease, *Ann. Clin. Res.,* 3:300, 1971.

76 Syme, S. L.: Social and Psychological Risk Factors in Coronary Heart Disease, *Mod. Concepts Cardiovasc. Dis.,* 44:17, 1975.

77 Jenkins, C. D.: Recent Evidence Supporting Psychologic and Social Risk Factors for Coronary Disease, *N. Engl. J. Med.,* 294:987, 1976.

78 Friedman, G. D., Klatsky, A. L., and Siegelaub, A. B.: Lung Function and Risk of Myocardial Infarction and Sudden Cardiac Death, *N. Engl. J. Med.,* 294:1017, 1976.

79 Kannel, W. B., Gordon, T., Castelli, W. P., and Margolis, J. R.: Electrocardiographic Left Ventricular Hypertrophy and Risk of Coronary Heart Disease: The Framingham Study, *Ann. Intern. Med.,* 72:813, 1970.

80 Wilens, S. L.: The Resorption of Arteriol Atheromatous Deposits in Wasting Disease, *Am. J. Pathol.,* 23:793, 1947.

81 Constantinides, P.: "Experimental Atherosclerosis," Elsevier Publishing Company, Amsterdam, 1965.

82 Armstrong, M. L., Warner, E. D., and Connor, W. E.: Regression of Coronary Atheromatosis in Rhesus Monkeys, *Circ. Res.,* 27:59, 1970.

83 Tucker, C. F., Catsulis, C., Strong, J. P., and Eggen, D. A.: Regression of Early Cholesterol-induced Aortic Lesions in Rhesus Monkeys, *Am. J. Pathol.,* 65:493, 1971.

84 Armstrong, M. L., and Megan, M. B.: Lipid Depletion in Atheromatous Coronary Arteries in Rhesus Monkeys after Regression Diets, *Circ. Res.,* 30:675, 1972.

85 Vesselinovitch, D., Wissler, R. W., Fisher-Dzoga, K., Hughes, R., and Dubien, L.: Regression of Atherosclerosis in Rabbits: I. Treatment with Low-Fat Diet, Hyperoxia and Hypolipidemic Agents, *Atherosclerosis,* 19:259, 1974.

86 Kritchevsky, D., Davidson, L. M., Shaprio, I. L., Kim, H. K., Kitagawa, M., Malhotra, S., Nair, P. P., Clarkson, T. B., Bersohn, I., and Winter, P. A. D.: Lipid Metabolism and Experimental Atherosclerosis in Baboons: Influence of Cholesterol-free, Semi-synthetic Diets, *Am. J. Clin. Nutr.,* 27:29, 1974.

87 Vesselinovitch, D., Wissler, R. W., Hughes, R., and Borensztajn, J.: Reversal of Advanced Atherosclerosis in Rhesus Monkeys: I. Light-microscopic Studies, *Atherosclerosis,* 23:155, 1976.

88 Zelis, R., Mason, D. T., Braunwald, E., and Levy, R. I.: Effects of Hyperlipoproteinemias and Their Treatment on the Peripheral Circulation, *J. Clin. Invest.,* 49:1007, 1970.

89 Starzl, T. E., and Putnam, C. W.: Portal Diversion: Treatment for Glycogen Storage Disease and Hyperlipemia, *J.A.M.A.,* 233:955, 1975.

90 Rinzler, S. H.: Primary Prevention of Coronary Heart Disease by Diet, *Bull. N.Y. Acad. Med.,* 44:936, 1968.

91 Dayton, S., Pearce, M. L., Hashimoto, S., Dixon, W. J., and Tomiyasu, U.: A Controlled Clinical Trial of a Diet High in Unsaturated Fat in Preventing Complications of Atherosclerosis, *Circulation,* 40(suppl. 2):63, 1969.

92 Stamler, J.: Acute Myocardial Infarction: Progress in Primary Prevention, *Br. Heart J.,* 33(suppl.):145, 1971.

93 Turpeinen, O.: Primary Prevention of Coronary Heart Disease by Diet, *Ann. Clin. Res.,* 3:433, 1971.

94 Miettinen, M., Turpeinen, O., Karvonen, M. J., Elosuo, R., and Paavilainen, E.: Effect of Cholesterol-lowering Diet on Mortality from Coronary Heart-Disease and Other Causes: A Twelve-Year Clinical Trial in Men and Women, *Lancet,* 2:835, 1972.

95 Stamler, J.: Primary Prevention of Sudden Coronary Death, *Circulation,* 52(suppl. 3):258, 1975.

96 Research Committee: Low-Fat Diet in Myocardial Infarction: A Controlled Trial, *Lancet,* 2:501, 1965.

97 Leren, P.: The Oslo Diet-Heart Study: Eleven-Year Report, *Circulation,* 42:935, 1970.

98 Bierenbaum, M. L., Fleischman, A. I., Green, D. P., Raichelson, R. I., Hayton, T., Watson, P. B., and Caldwell, A. B.: The 5-Year Experience of Modified Fat Diets on Younger Men with Coronary Heart Disease, *Circulation,* 42:943, 1970.

99 Roberts, J. C., Jr., and Straus, R. (eds.): "Comparative Atherosclerosis: The Morphology of Spontaneous and Induced Atherosclerotic Lesions in Animals and Its Relation to Human Disease," Harper & Row, Publishers, Incorporated, New York, 1965.

100 Miller, G. J., and Miller, N. E.: Plasma High-Density-Lipoprotein Concentration and Development of Ischemic Heart Disease, *Lancet,* 1:16, 1975.

100a Castelli, W. P., Doyle, J. T., Gordon, T., Hames, C. G., Hjortland, M. C., Hulley, S. B., Kagan, A., and Zukel, W. J.: HDL Cholesterol and Other Lipids in Coronary Heart Disease: The Cooperative Lipoprotein Phenotyping Study, *Circulation,* 55:767, 1977.

100b Gordon, T., Castelli, W. P., Hjortland, M. C., Kannel, W. B., and Dawber, T. R.: High Density Lipoprotein as a Protective Factor against Coronary Heart Disease. The Framingham Study, *Am. J. Med.,* 62:707, 1977.

101 Stein, Y., Glangeaud, M. C., Fainaru, M., and Stein, O.: The Removal of Cholesterol from Aortic Smooth Muscle Cells in Culture and Landschutz Ascites Cells by Fractions of Human High-Density Apolipoproteins, *Biochim. Biophys. Acta,* 380:106, 1975.

102 Castelli, W. P.: Coronary Heart Disease Risk factors in the Elderly, *Hosp. Practice,* 11:113, 1976.

103 Fredrickson, D. S., Levy, R. I., and Lees, R. S.: Fat Transport in Lipoproteins: An Integrated Approach to Mechanisms and Disorders, *N. Engl. J. Med.,* 276:34, 1967.

104 Levy, R. I., and Fredrickson, D. S.: Diagnosis and Management of Hyperlipoproteinemia, *Am. J. Cardiol.,* 22:576, 1968.

105 Brown, D. F.: Blood Lipids and Lipoproteins in Atherogenesis, *Am. J. Med.,* 46:691, 1969.

106 Fredrickson, D. S.: An International Classification of Hyperlipidemias and Hyperlipoproteinemias, *Ann. Intern. Med.,* 75:471, 1971.

107 Castelli, W. P., and Moran, R. F.: Lipid Studies for Assessing the Risk of Cardiovascular Disease and Hyperlipidemia, *Hum. Pathol.,* 2:153, 1971.

108 Beaumont, J. L., Carlson, L. A., Cooper, G. R., Fejfar, Z., Fredrickson, D. S., and Strasser, T.: Classification of Hyperlipidemias and Hyperlipoproteinemias, *Circulation,* 45:501, 1972, reprinted from *Bull. WHO,* 43:891, 1970.

109 Jackson, R. L., Morrisett, J. D., and Gotto, A. M., Jr.: Lipoprotein Structure and Metabolism, *Physiol. Rev.,* 56:259, 1976.

110 Stone, N. J., Levy, R. I., Fredrickson, D. S., and Verter, J.: Coronary Artery Disease in 116 Kindred with Familial Type II Hyperlipoproteinemia, *Circulation,* 49:476, 1974.

111 Goldstein, J. L., and Brown, M. S.: Lipoprotein Receptors, Cholesterol Metabolism, and Atherosclerosis, *Arch. Pathol.,* 99:181, 1975.

112 Goldstein, J. L., and Brown, M. S.: Familial Hypercholesterolemia: A Genetic Regulatory Defect in Cholesterol Metabolism, *Am. J. Med.,* 58:147, 1975.

113 Brown, M. S., and Goldstein, J. L.: Expression of the Familial Hypercholesterolemia Gene in Heterozygotes: Mechanism for a Dominant Disorder in Man, *Science,* 185:61, 1974.

114 Hazzard, W. R., O'Donnell, T. F., and Lee, Y. L.: Broad-B Disease (Type III Hyperlipoproteinemia) in a Large Kindred: Evidence for a Monogenic Mechanism, *Ann. Intern. Med.,* 82:141, 1975.

115 Morganroth, J., Levy, R. I., and Fredrickson, D. S.: The Biochemical, Clinical, and Genetic Features of Type III Hyperlipoproteinemia, *Ann. Intern. Med.,* 82:158, 1975.

116 Wood, P. D. S., Stern, M. P., Silvers, A., Reaven, G. M., and Von de Groeben, J.: Prevalence of Plasma Lipoprotein Abnormalities in a Free-living Population of the Central Valley, California, *Circulation,* 45:114, 1972.

117 Khachadurian, A. K., and Uthman, S. M.: Experiences with the Homozygous Cases of Familial Hypercholesterolemia: A Report of 52 Patients, *Nutr. Metab.,* 15:132, 1973.

118 Goldstein, J. L., Schrott, H. G., Hazzard, W. R., Bierman, E. L., and Motulsky, A. G.: Hyperlipidemia in Coronary Heart Disease: II. Genetic Analysis of Lipid Levels in 176 Families and Delineation of a New Inherited Disorder, Combined Hyperlipidemia, *J. Clin. Invest.,* 52:1544, 1973.

119 Rose, H. G., Kranz, P., Weinstock, M., Juliano, J., and Haft, J. I.: Inheritance of Combined Hyperlipoproteinemia: Evidence for a New Lipoprotein Phenotype, *Am. J. Med.,* 54:148, 1973.

120 Rose, H. G., Kranz, P., Weinstock, M., Juliano, J., and Haft, J. I.: Combined Hyperlipoproteinemia: Evidence for a New Lipoprotein Phenotype, *Atherosclerosis,* 20:51, 1974.

121 Havel, R. J.: Hyperlipoproteinemia: Problems in Diagnosis and Challenges Posed by the "Type III" Disorder, *Ann. Intern. Med.,* 82:273, 1975.

122 Fredrickson, D. S.: It's Time to be Practical, *Circulation,* 51:209, 1975.

123 Porter, R., and Knight, J. (eds.): Atherogenesis: Initiating Factors, *Ciba Found. Symp.,* 12:233, 1973.

124 Adams, C. W. M.: The Pathogenesis of Atherosclerosis, *J. Clin. Pathol.,* 26(suppl. 5):38, 1973.

125 Ross, R., and Glomset, J. A.: Atherosclerosis and the Arterial Smooth Muscle Cell, *Science,* 180:1332, 1973.

126 Page, I. H.: Atherosclerosis: An Introduction, *Circulation,* 10:1, 1954.

127 Gofman, J. W., and Young, W.: The Filtration Concept of Atherosclerosis and Serum Lipids in the Diagnosis of Atherosclerosis, in M. Sandler and G. H. Bourne (eds.), "Atherosclerosis and Its Origin," Academic Press, Inc., New York, 1963, p. 197.

128 Virchow, R.: "Gesammelte Abhandlungen zur wissenschaftlichen Medicin," G. Grote, Hamm, 1862, pp. 458, 500, and 521.

129 Marchand, F.: Ueber Arteriosklerose, *Verh. Kongr. Inn. Med.,* 21:23, 1904.

130 Ignatowski, A.: Uber die Wirkung des Tierischen Eiweisses auf die Aorta und die parenchymatosen Organe der Kaninchen, *Virchows Arch. Pathol. Anat.,* 198, 1909.

131 Anitschkow, N., and Chalatov, S.: Ueber experimentelle Cholesterinsteatose und ihre Bedeutung für die Entstehung einiger pathologischer Prozesse, *Zentralbl. Allg. Pathol.,* 24:1, 1913.

132 Smith, E. B.: The Relationship between Plasma and Tissue Lipids in Human Atherosclerosis, *Adv. Lipid Res.,* 12:1, 1974.

133 Parker, F.: An Electron Microscope Study of Coronary Arteries, *Am. J. Anat.,* 103:247, 1958.

134 Shimamoto, T.: Hyperreactive Arterial Endothelial Cells in Atherogenesis and Cyclic AMP Phosphodiesterase Inhibitor in Prevention and Treatment of Atherosclerotic Disorders, *Jap. Heart J.,* 16:76, 1975.

135 Benditt, E. P., and Benditt, J. M.: Evidence for a Monoclonal Origin of Human Atherosclerotic Plaques, *Proc. Natl. Acad. Sci. U.S.A.,* 70:1753, 1973.

136 Benditt, E. P.: Evidence for a Monoclonal Origin of Human Atherosclerotic Plaques and Some Implications, *Circulation,* 50:650, 1974.

136a Benditt, E. P.: Implications of the Monoclonal Character of Human Atherosclerotic Plaques, *Am. J. Pathol.,* 86:693, 1977.

137 Bierman, E. L., and Albergs, J. J.: Lipoprotein Uptake by Cultered Human Arterial Smooth Muscle Cells, *Biochim. Biophys. Acta,* 388:198, 1975.

138 Fritz, K. E., Jarmolych, J., Daoud, A. S., and Peters, T., Jr.: Factors Influencing DNA Synthesis and Degradation Present in Swine Serum and Aortic Tissue, *Exp. Mol. Pathol.,* 16:54, 1972.

139 Armstrong, M. L., Megan, M. B., and Warner, E. D.: Intimal Thickening in Normocholesterolemic Rhesus Monkeys Fed Low Supplements of Dietary Cholesterol, *Circ. Res.,* 34:447, 1974.

140 Fisher-Dzoga, K., Chen, R., and Wissler, R. W.: Effects of Serum Lipoproteins on the Morphology, Growth, and Metabolism of Arterial Smooth Muscle Cells, *Adv. Exp. Med. Biol.,* 43:299, 1974.

141 Fisher-Dzoga, K., Wissler, R. W., and Scanu, A. M.: "The Lipoproteins and Arterial Smooth Muscle Cells: Cellular Proliferation and Morphology" (Proceedings of the International Workshop—Conference on Atherosclerosis, London, Ontario, Canada, 1975), in press.

142 Fisher-Dzoga, K., and Wissler, R. W.: Unpublished observations.

143 Enselme, J.: "Unsaturated Fatty Acids in Atherosclerosis," 2d ed., Pergamon Press, Oxford, 1969.

144 Iverius, P. H.: The Interaction between Human Plasma Lipoproteins and Connective Tissue Glycosaminoglycans, *J. Biol. Chem.,* 247:2607, 1972.

145 Berenson, G. S., Srinivasan, S. R., Radhakrishnamurthy, B., and Dalferes, E. R., Jr.: Mucopolysaccharide-Lipoprotein Complexes in Atherosclerotic Aorta, *Adv. Exp. Med. Biol.,* 43:141, 1974.

146 Bihari-Varga, M., Gergely, J., and Gero, S.: Further Investigations on Complex Formation In Vitro between Aortic Mucopolysaccharides and Beta-Lipoproteins, *Atherosclerosis,* 4:106, 1964.

147 Camejo, G., Lopez, A., Vegas, H., and Paoli, H.: The Participation of Aortic Proteins in the Formation of Complexes between Low Density Lipoproteins and Intima-Media Extracts, *Atherosclerosis,* 21:77, 1975.

148 Restrepo, C., and Tracy, R. E.: Variations in Human Aortic Fatty Streaks among Geographic Locations, *Atherosclerosis,* 21:179, 1975.

149 Schlant, R. C., and Galambos, J. T.: Autoradiographic Demonstration of Ingested Cholesterol-4-C^{14} in the Normal and Atheromatous Aorta, *Am. J. Pathol.,* 44:877, 1964.

150 Woolf, N., and Pilkington, T. R. E.: The Immunohistochemical Demonstration of Lipoproteins in Vessel Walls, *J. Pathol.,* 90:459, 1965.

151 Kao, V. C. Y., and Wissler, R. W.: A Study of the Immunohistochemical Localization of Serum Lipoproteins and Other Plasma Proteins in Human Atherosclerotic Lesions, *Exp. Mol. Pathol.,* 4:465, 1965.

152 Smith, E. B., and Slater, R.: The Chemical and Immunological Assay of Low Density Lipoproteins Extracted from Human Aortic Intima, *Atherosclerosis,* 11:417, 1970.

153 Scott, P. J., and Hurley, P. J.: The Distribution of Radioiodinated Serum Albumin and Low-Density Lipoprotein in Tissues and the Arterial Wall, *Atherosclerosis,* 11:77, 1970.

154 Smith, E. B., and Slater, R. S.: Relationship between Low-Density Lipoprotein in Aortic Intima and Serum-Lipid Levels, *Lancet,* 1:463, 1972.

155 Walton, K. W.: Immunological Studies on Atherogenesis, *Adv. Exp. Med. Biol.,* 38:221, 1973.

156 Reichl, D., Simons, L. A., Myant, N. B., Pflug, J. J., and Mills, G. L.: The Lipids and Lipoproteins of Human Peripheral Lymph, with Observations on the Transport of Cholesterol from Plasma and Tissues into Lymph, *Clin. Sci. Mol. Med.,* 45:313, 1973.

157 Stein, Y., Glangeaud, M. C., Fainara, M., and Stein, O.: The Removal of Cholesterol from Aortic Smooth Muscle Cells in Culture and Landschutz Ascites Cells by Fractions of Human High-Density Apolipoprotein, *Biochim. Biophys. Acta,* 380:106, 1975.

158 Robertson, A. L., Jr.: Oxygen Requirements of the Human Arterial Intima in Atherogenesis, *Prog. Biochem. Pharmacol.,* 4:305, 1968.

159 Wherate, A. F.: Is Atherosclerosis a Disorder of Intramitochondrial Respiration? *Ann. Intern. Med.,* 73:125, 1970.

160 Garbarsch, C., Matthiessen, M. E., Helin, P., and Lorenzen, I.: Arteriosclerosis and Hypoxia: I. Gross and Microscopic Changes in Rabbit Aorta Induced by Systemic Hypoxia: Histochemical Studies, *Atherosclerosis,* 9:283, 1969.

161 Kjeldsen, K., Astrup, P., and Wanstrup, J.: Reversal of Rabbit Atheromatosis by Hyperoxia, *Atherosclerosis,* 10:173, 1969.

162 Frith, C. H., McMurtry, I. F., Alexander, A. F., and Will, D. H.: Influence of Hypertension and Hypoxemia on Arterial Biochemistry and Morphology in Swine, *Atherosclerosis,* 20:189, 1974.

163 Vesselinovitch, D., Wissler, R. W., Fisher-Dzoga, K., Hughes, R., and Dubien, L.: Regression of Atherosclerosis in Rabbits: I. Treatment with Low-Fat Diet, Hyperoxia and Hypolipidemic Agents, *Atherosclerosis,* 19:259, 1974.

164 Wissler, R. W., Vesselinovitch, D.: Evidence for Prevention and Regression of Atherosclerosis in Man and Experimental Animals at the Arterial Level, in G. Schettler and A. Weizel (eds.), "Atherosclerosis III" (proceedings, third international symposium), Springer-Verlag OHG, Berlin, 1974, p. 747.

165 Wissler, R. W., and Vesselinovitch, D.: Regression of Atherosclerosis in Experimental Animals and Man, *Verh. Dtsch. Ges. Inn. Med.,* 81:857, 1975.

166 Mustard, J. F.: Platelets and Thrombosis, in E. Braunwald (ed.): "The Myocardium Failure and Infarction," HP Publishing Co., New York, 1974, p. 177.

167 Mustard, J. F., Glynn, M. F., Jorgensen, L., Nishizawa, E. E., Packhman, M. A., and Rowsell, H. C.: Recent Advances in Platelets, Blood Coagulation Factors and Thrombosis, *Prog. Biochem. Pharmacol.,* 4:508, 1968.

168 Somer, J. B., and Schwartz, C. J.: Focal [^{3}H]-Cholesterol Uptake in the Pig Aorta: II. Distribution of [^{3}H]-Cholesterol across the Aortic Wall in Areas of High and Low Uptake In Vivo, *Atherosclerosis,* 16:377, 1972.

169 Wissler, R. W.: Atherosclerosis: Its Pathogenesis in Perspective, *Adv. Cardiol.,* 13:10, 1974.

170 Esterly, J. A., and Glagov, S.: Altered Permeability of the Renal Artery of the Hypertensive Rat: An Electron Microscopic Study, *Am. J. Pathol.,* 43:619, 1963.

171 Glagov, S.: Hemodynamic Risk Factors: Mechanical Stress, Mural Architecture, Medical Nutrition and the Vulnerability of Arteries to Atherosclerosis, in R. W. Wissler, and J. C. Geer (eds.), "The Pathogenesis of Atherosclerosis," The Williams & Wilkins Company, Baltimore, 1972, p. 164.

172 Constantinides, P.: Endothelial Injury in the Pathogenesis of Arteriosclerosis, *Adv. Exp. Med. Biol.,* 16A:185, 1971.

173 Minick, C. R., and Murphy, G. E.: Experimental Induction of Atheroarteriosclerosis by the Synergy of Allergic Injury to Arteries and Lipid-rich Diet: II. Effect of Repeatedly Injected Foreign Protein in Rabbits Fed a Lipid-rich, Cholesterol-poor Diet, *Am. J. Pathol.,* 73:265, 1973.

174 Robertson, A. L., Jr., and Khairallah, P. A.: Arterial Endothelial Permeability and Vascular Disease: The "Trap-door" Effect, *Exp. Mol. Pathol.,* 18:241, 1973.

175 Adams, C. W. M., Morgan, R. S., and Bayliss, O. B.: The Differential Entry of [^{125}I]-albumin into Mildly and Severely Atheromatous Rabbit Aortas, *Atherosclerosis,* 11:119, 1970.

176 Duguid, J. B.: The Thrombogenic Hypothesis and Its Implications, *Postgrad. Med. J.,* 36:226, 1960.

177 Duguid, J. B.: The Thrombogenic Etiology and Its Mechanical Implications, in H. T. Blumenthal (ed.): "Cowdry's Arteriosclerosis: A Survey of the Problem," 2d ed., Charles C Thomas, Publisher, Springfield, Ill., 1967, p. 529.

178 Mustard, J. R., Murphy, E. A., Rowsell, H. C., and Downie, H. G.: Platelets and Atherosclerosis, *Atherosclerosis,* 4:1, 1964.

179 Schnetzer, G. W., III: Platelets and Thrombogenesis: Current Concepts, *Am. Heart J.,* 83:552, 1972.

180 Chandler, A. B.: Thrombosis in the Development of Coronary Atherosclerosis, in W. Likoff, B. L. Segal, and W. Insull, Jr. (eds.), "Atherosclerosis and Coronary Heart Disease" (twenty-fourth Hahnemann symposium), Grune & Stratton, Inc., New York, 1972, p. 28.

181 Ross, R., and Glomset, J. A.: The Pathogenesis of Atherosclerosis, *N. Engl. J. Med.,* 295:369, 420, 1976.

182 Haust, M. D., Wyllie, J. C., and More, R. H.: Electron Microscopy of Fibrin in Human Atherosclerotic Lesions: Immunohistochemical and Morphologic Identification, *Exp. Mol. Pathol.,* 4:205, 1965.

183 Carvalho, A. C. A., Colman, R. W., and Lees, R. S.: Platelet Function in Hyperlipoproteinemia, *N. Engl. J. Med.,* 290:434, 1974.

184 Ross, R., Glomset, J., Kariya, B., and Harker, L.: A Platelet-dependent Serum Factor that Stimulates the Proliferation of Arterial Smooth Muscle Cells In Vitro, *Proc. Natl. Acad. Sci. U.S.A.,* 71:1207, 1974.

185 Stemerman, M. B., and Ross, R.: Experimental Arteriosclerosis: I. Fibrous Plaque Formation in Primates: An Electron Microscope Study, *J. Exp. Med.,* 136:769, 1972.

186 Ross, R., Glomset, J., and Harker, L.: Response to Injury and Atherogenesis, *Am. J. Pathol.,* 86:675, 1977.

187 Lyford, C. L., Connor, W. E., Haok, J. C., and Warner, E. D.: The Coagulant and Thrombogenic Properties of Human Atheroma, *Circulation,* 36:284, 1967.

188 Haerem, J. W.: Sudden Coronary Death: The Occurrence of Platelet Aggregates in the Epicardial Arteries of Man, *Atherosclerosis,* 14:417, 1971.

189 Salky, N., and Dugdale, M.: Platelet Abnormalities in Ischemic Heart Disease, *Am. J. Cardiol.,* 32:612, 1973.

190 Texon, M.: The Hemodynamic Basis of Atherosclerosis: Further Observations: The Ostial Lesion, *Bull. N.Y. Acad. Med.,* 48:733, 1972.

191 Flaherty, J. T., Ferrans, V. J., Pierce, J. E., Carew, T. E., and Fry, D. L.: Localizing Factors in Experimental Atherosclerosis, in W. Likoff, B. L. Segal, and W. Insull, Jr. (eds.), "Atherosclerosis and Coronary Heart Disease" (twenty-fourth Hahnemann symposium), Grune & Stratton, Inc., New York, 1972, p. 40.

192 Fry, D. L.: Localizing Factors in Arteriosclerosis, in W. Likoff, B. L. Segal, and W. Insull, Jr. (eds.), "Atherosclerosis and Coronary Heart Disease" (twenty-fourth Hahnemann symposium), Grune & Stratton, Inc., New York, 1972, p. 85.

193 Friedman, M. H., O'Brien, V., and Ehrlich, L. W.: Calculations of Pulsatile Flow through a Branch: Implications for the Hemodynamics of Atherogenesis, *Circ. Res.,* 36:277, 1975.

194 Stehbens, W. E.: The Role of Hemodynamics in the Pathogenesis of Atherosclerosis, *Prog. Cardiovasc. Dis.,* 18:89, 1975.

194a Caro, C. G.: Mechanical Factors in Atherogenesis, in N. H. C. Hwang and N. A. Normann (eds.), "Cardiovascular Flow Dynamics and Measurements," University Park Press, Baltimore, 1977, p. 473.

195 Duncan, L. E., Jr., Cornfield, J., and Buck, K.: The Effect of Blood Pressure on the Passage of Labeled Plasma Albumin into Canine Aortic Wall, *J. Clin. Invest.,* 41:1537, 1962.

196 McDonald, D. A.: "Blood Flow in Arteries," 2d ed., The Williams & Wilkins Company, Baltimore, 1974, p. 496.

197 Fry, D. L.: Responses of the Arterial Wall to Certain Physical Factors, *Ciba Found. Symp.,* 12:93, 1973.

198 Fox, J. A., and Hugh, A. E.: Localization of Atheroma: A Theory Based on Boundary Layer Separation, *Br. Heart J.,* 28:388, 1966.

199 LeCompte, P. M.: Reactions of the Vasa Vasorum in Vascular Disease, in H. T. Blumenthal (ed.), "Cowdry's Arteriosclerosis: A Survey of the Problem," 2d ed., Charles C Thomas, Publisher, Springfield, Ill., 1967, p. 212.

200 Paterson, J. C.: Factors in the Production of Coronary Artery Disease, *Circulation,* 6:732, 1952.

201 Wurster, N. B., and Zilversmit, D. B.: The Role of Phagocytosis in the Development of Atherosclerotic Lesions in the Rabbit, *Atherosclerosis,* 14:309, 1971.

202 Leary, R.: The Genesis of Atherosclerosis, *Arch. Pathol.,* 32:507, 1941.

203 Balint, A., Veress, B., Nagy, Z., and Jellinek, H.: Role of Lipophages in the Development of Rat Atheroma, *Atherosclerosis,* 15:7, 1972.

204 Wissler, R. W., and Vesselinovitch, D.: Differences between Human and Animal Atherosclerosis, in G. Schettler and A. Weizel (eds.): "Atherosclerosis III" (proceedings, third international symposium), Springer-Verlag OHG, Berling, 1974, p. 319.

C
Pathology of Coronary Atherosclerosis and Its Complications

ROBERT S. ELIOT, M.D., and
JESSE E. EDWARDS, M.D.

Intrinsic disease of the coronary arteries is overwhelmingly atherosclerotic in nature. Uncommon forms of significant coronary disease include ostial stenosis from primary disease of the aorta, coronary embolism, coronary arterial involvement by inflammatory disease, of which periarteritis is the most common, and congenital states in which part of the coronary arterial system makes gross communication with the pulmonary trunk, a cardiac chamber, or a thoracic vein.

In this chapter we are concerned primarily with coronary atherosclerosis.

NATURE AND DISTRIBUTION

Controversy still exists as to the nature of the earliest change in atherosclerosis. A commonly held theory, based on histologic observations, is that first lipid-filled macrophages are localized in the arterial intima. The distribution is of interest in that often it does not follow a circumferential pattern. Rather, the lesion of atherosclerosis is focal. In cross section it is often apparent that one arc of the vessel is involved while the remainder is immune to the lesion. Variations in the cross-sectional distribution of lesions account for variations in the shape of the narrowed lumen (Fig. 62C-1). A circumferential lesion yields a *central lumen*. An eccentric atheroma yields an *eccentric lumen*. The latter may be further subdivided into *slitlike* and *polymorphous* in shape.[1] While the central lumen may show varying degrees of obstruction, the eccentric lumen is always narrowed. The importance of the eccentric slitlike lumen is that its greatest width may be as wide as the original lumen and in arteriograms obstruction may be overlooked. The eccentric polymorphous lumen may be either circular or odd in shape, sometimes stellate.

Atherosclerosis in the uncomplicated state always leaves some lumen, however narrow. From an anatomic point of view, total occlusion of the lumen is the result of a thrombus. In the chronic state, the organized thrombus is represented by vascular connective tissue. Total occlusion as seen arteriographically may be a manifestation of a thrombus, either acute or organized, or of severe obstruction by atherosclerosis. Embolism is another possibility and may be a complication of coronary arterial or left-sided catheterization. Development of collaterals is common in relation to obstructed foci, and these may allow flow in vessels beyond involved foci. The focal distribution lends support to the opinion that whatever the various factors are that stimulate atherogenesis, one of them is local and may represent localized hemodynamic forces. The tendency toward concentration of greatest atherogenic effect at bifurcations of arteries is also in support of local mechanical factors as playing roles either in stimulating or retarding atherogenesis.

Following the accumulation of lipid-laden macrophages, the intima is further thickened (at the expense of the lumen) by a fibrous reaction to the fatty material. The new fibrous tissue tends to encapsulate the foci of lipid-filled cells. Following the earliest stage, cells containing lipid disintegrate, and the lipid material is extruded into the extracellular areas of the intima. Crystallization and calcification of this material follow, as does progressive increase in the amount of encapsulating fibrous tissue. In the fibrous wall of the atheroma capillaries are formed. Medial atrophy and the presence of stainable neutral fat in he muscle cells beneath the atheroma are commonly observed.

Histologically, evidence for an episodic tendency toward atherogenesis may be observed. This evidence takes the following form: in arteries with "old" atheromata (i.e., extracellular lipids associated with crystallization and/or calcification) one may observe one or several more superficial accumulations of lipid-filled macrophages. These accumulations suggest an atheroma of more recent onset than the deeper "burned-out" lesion.

The distribution of lesions among the epicardial

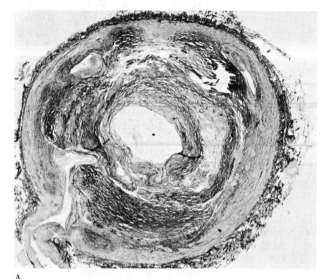

A

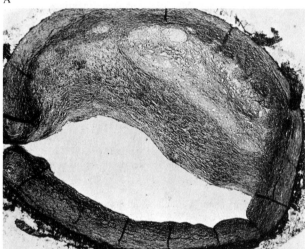

B

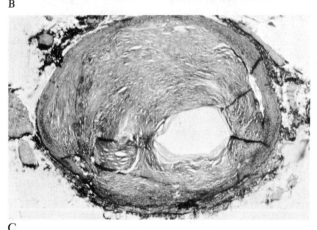

C

FIGURE 62C-1 Variations in shapes of lumens of coronary arteries harboring severe atherosclerosis as seen in cross sections. *A.* Central lumen. *B.* Eccentric slitlike lumen. *C.* Eccentric polymorphous lumen.

branches needs consideration. In the experience of Vlodaver and Edwards,[1] the segment of artery in which severe disease is most common is that segment of the right coronary artery which lies between the marginal and posterior descending branches of that artery ("intermediate segment"). Second to this segment, in their study, is the proximal one-half of the anterior descending artery. The third most common site for severe disease is the "anterior segment" of the right coronary artery, that segment which lies between the origin of the vessel and its marginal branch.

The observations mentioned with respect to anterior and intermediate segments of the right coronary artery strongly deny the concept of progressively less disease along the course of the artery. This concept gains some support from observations on the anterior descending artery, but specific cases do not conform. When the anterior descending artery was divided into proximal and distal halves, the lesions of obstructive nature were localized to the proximal segment in 76 percent of cases. In 17 percent, both the proximal and distal segments were involved, while in 7 percent only the distal segment harbored significant lesions.

The findings in the left circumflex artery, in general, conform to those in the anterior descending artery, again supporting the fact that in some cases a peripheral segment of a main coronary artery may be more severely involved than a proximal segment.

In a given patient with coronary heart disease it is characteristic that lesions are multiple and involvement of more than one artery is usual.

Diethrich and associates,[2] studying 313 selective coronary cinearteriograms in patients with angina pectoris, found that significant involvement of only one vessel occurred in 23 percent of the patients, while involvement of two vessels was seen in 40 percent, three vessels in 29 percent, and four vessels (including the main left coronary artery) in 9 percent of the subjects. The relatively high incidence of significant involvement of only one coronary artery in the arteriographic studies of Diethrich and associates should be tempered by the fact that pathologic examination tends to show more significantly obstructive lesions than are portrayed in the arteriogram.

While it has been claimed that diseases of intramyocardial branches may be the basis for clinical coronary disease, this is unusual. In classic states, atherosclerosis of the epicardial trunks represents the prevailing basis for myocardial ischemia and/or myocardial infarction.

INTRAARTERIAL COMPLICATIONS

The major intraarterial complications of atherosclerosis are (1) luminal narrowing by the fundamental process, (2) intramural hemorrhage, and (3) thrombosis. Embolism of atheromatous tissue and aneurysm formation are considered less common, although the incidence of embolism of material from an atheroma in one segment to a second segment of the same coronary artery is unknown.

Intramural (intimal) hemorrhage is a common phenomenon in well-established atheromata, as these lesions are supplied with capillaries. Opinions are not uniform as to the functional significance of such

hemorrhages. That they, per se, are common causes of acute coronary arterial occlusion seems doubtful. The basis for this opinion is the fact that even in instances of extensive intimal hemorrhage, the arterial lumen maintains a circular shape in cross section. One would expect flattening of the lumen were the hemorrhage directly responsible for narrowing of the lumen.

That intimal hemorrhages with associated rupture of the overlying tissue may be the cause of acute coronary arterial thrombosis must be accepted. That this process is not uncommonly observed in chance single sections of thrombosed coronary arteries suggests that it may indeed be a fairly common phenomenon in cases of acute coronary thrombosis. Hemorrhages with rupture of the lining may cause extrusion of atheromatous material into the lumen and set the stage for embolism of atheromatous material which is occasionally observed (Fig. 62C-2).

Yet another possible effect of intramural hemorrhage is that the hemorrhage is an irritant and sets into operation a reflex, the end result of which is spasm of collateral arteries.

Coronary thrombosis when present is usually observed in segments of arteries with established atherosclerotic lesions, supplying evidence for the opinion that atherosclerosis is the main underlying factor favoring thrombosis. It has already been mentioned that intramural hemorrhage with rupture of the intima may precipitate thrombosis. Thrombosis may occur over an atheroma in the absence of rupture of the atheroma. The classic thrombus within a coronary artery involves but a short length of the involved segment, usually less than 1 cm of the length of the vessel.

The usual appearance of the thrombus is uniform,

FIGURE 62C-2 Photomicrograph of an atherosclerotic coronary artery. At the left extreme of the illustration is a focus of hemorrhage within the atherosclerotic intima. There has been rupture of the overlying connective tissue, with extrusion of atheromatous material into the lumen of the vessel. Such material may embolize. Also, the process of the intimal hemorrhage with rupture of the overlying tissue may serve as a nucleus of thrombosis.

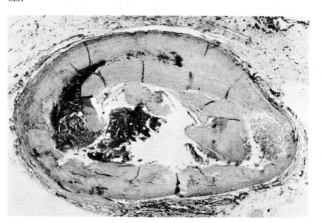

suggesting that the process which occludes the lumen occurs within a very short period of time. In some instances, however, one may observe only a mural thrombus, or if the lumen is occluded, the thrombotic material may suggest several ages, as though the initial stage was mural thrombosis followed by one or several additional episodes until the process of luminal occlusion was complete.

The reaction to a thrombus in a coronary artery is like that which occurs with thrombi in any vessel or cardiac chamber. Encapsulation and organization occur, but it is to be recognized that the process of organization of thrombi in atherosclerotic vessels proceeds at a considerably slower pace than organization of thrombi which occur, for one reason or another, in fundamentally normal arteries. So delayed may organization be in atherosclerotic coronary arteries that when there is an associated myocardial infarct, the latter may be completely healed while organization of the underlying arterial thrombus is far from complete. Such observations have suggested the theory that in some cases of myocardial infarction and coronary thrombosis the former precedes the latter.

The process by which a thrombus becomes replaced by fibrous and vascular tissue has been called *organization, recanalization,* or *organization and recanalization.* The term *recanalization* with regard to coronary arterial thrombi needs special consideration. Though the term may suggest that the original lumen is restored, this is far from reality. In arteries harboring "recanalized" thrombi, the vessels in the original lumen are usually narrow. Even if they communicate with the parent lumen, both proximal and distal to the thrombus, the channels are so narrow that they do not appear capable of carrying any significant volume of blood. Therefore, a segment of an artery at the level of a "recanalized" thrombus is, as a practical matter, an occluded segment (Fig. 62C-3A).

Occasionally an atheroma within a coronary artery may become dislodged, flow as an embolus peripherally, and become impacted at a distal point within the artery of origin. Here it may serve to cause myocardial ischemia, as the newly occluded segment may lie at a level distal to the level of entrance of collateral vessels that have bypassed the initially narrowed segment. Such emboli may also serve as nuclei upon which thrombosis occurs.

Atherosclerosis of coronary arteries commonly is associated with atrophy of the media underlying the intimal lesion. In spite of the common occurrence of medial atrophy and possibly because of splinting by the atheroma, aneurysms only rarely occur in atherosclerotic coronary arteries (Fig. 62C-3B). Such aneurysms are usually saccular, and laminated thrombi are present within them. Usually, however, an effective lumen for the flow of blood remains. The main complication of coronary aneurysms of atherosclerotic origin is that portions of the contained thrombus may become dislodged and embolize.

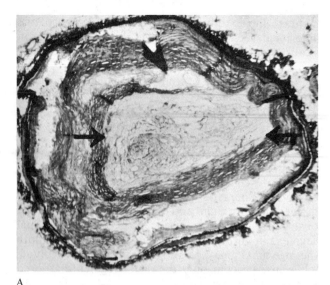

A

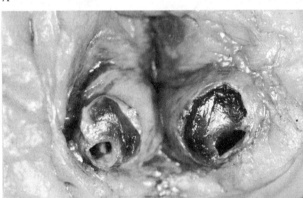

B

FIGURE 62C-3 A. Coronary atherosclerosis and organized thrombosis. Between the arrows the lumen, narrowed by fundamental atherosclerosis, is filled with loose vascular tissue representing organized (so-called recanalized) thrombosis. *B.* Cross sections of an atherosclerotic coronary artery with aneurysm formation.

MYOCARDIAL COMPLICATIONS

The main significance of coronary atherosclerosis is that the lesion, either alone or in association with acute coronary occlusion, is a cause of myocardial ischemia. Myocardial ischemia, in turn, is responsible for a variety of clinical states, including angina pectoris, sudden death, status anginosis, and acute myocardial infarction. In the material that follows the authors will consider these clinical states within the framework of the pathologic processes that underlie them. A new clinical classification is being developed (see Chaps. 62A and 62E), and new clinicopathologic correlations are now being investigated. In the meantime the following clinicopathologic relations can be emphasized.

Angina pectoris

It is firmly established that in angina pectoris, whether stable or unstable, organic coronary arterial disease is almost universally present.[3] In the overwhelming number of instances coronary atherosclerosis is widely distributed. Organized thrombi may also be present as causes of coronary arterial narrowing. At the same time, it is to be emphasized that in the patient with coronary atherosclerosis, angina is more common when hypertension is associated than when it is absent.

Zoll and associates[4] made a comprehensive comparison between the occurrence of angina and various factors studied pathologically, including postmortem coronary arteriography and dissection. In each of 177 patients in whom angina had been present for 1 month or longer, coronary atherosclerosis, arterial hypertension, or valvular heart disease, either alone or in combination, were present. In the majority (78 percent), two or more of the foregoing factors were found in individuals with a history of angina. The most common pattern was a combination of hypertension and coronary disease (61 percent), while the second most common pattern was isolated coronary disease in the absence of either valvular disease or hypertension, which was found in only 16 percent of their series.

In subjects with angina the myocardium may be normal, it may show evidence of a healed classic myocardial infarct, and/or there may be small scars which, from case to case, vary in number from a few to innumerable ones. These small scars have been considered by some investigators to be the lesions of *chronic infarction.* This term implies that chronic coronary arterial disease is responsible for "slow death" of muscle fibers with ultimate fibrous replacement. Such an explanation is not inviting to the authors. One would prefer to deny the concept of "slow death." Rather, the authors would consider that in the patient with clinical angina pectoris there occurs from time to time typical acute myocardial infarction which involves small areas of the myocardium. Such changes may be associated with unstable angina[3] or with episodes of acute myocardial infarction which are misinterpreted, denied, or even silent. The lesions characterized by acute myocardial necrosis go through the usual stages ending in scars.

Sudden death

Comprehensive consideration of the mechanisms of sudden coronary death has recently been given in a conference on that subject.[5] It is recognized that among patients who die while convalescing from acute myocardial infarction, sudden death is not uncommon. A more common circumstance among subjects with coronary atherosclerosis is sudden and unexpected death in the absence of acute myocardial infarction. This phenomenon has had relatively little emphasis in the literature dealing with the pathology of coronary arterial disease, as the latter is mostly derived from hospital experience. A broader view of the serious complications of coronary arterial disease should include data relating to deaths from coronary disease which occur outside the hospital. When this is done, as in the survey of one community by Spiekerman and associates,[6] sudden death in the absence of demonstrable acute myocardial infarction is the largest single type of death from coronary

disease and in fact is the largest single type of death from all causes.

Pathologic examination of subjects who die suddenly outside the hospital reveals several significant features: Acute coronary occlusion is uncommon, as is demonstrable acute myocardial infarction. Signs of earlier myocardial infarction, either that typical of an antecedent classic clinical attack or that characterized by small variously distributed scars, are common.[6]

Such observations suggest that the greatest single cause of death in coronary arterial disease is cardiac arrhythmia. Ventricular fibrillation is usually assumed to be the mechanism through which sudden death occurs under these circumstances.

In the minority of cases of sudden death without an antecedent suspicion of an acute coronary arterial problem, acute myocardial infarction is found. These are examples of silent or missed acute myocardial infarction.

Coronary insufficiency without myocardial infarction

Patients with chronic coronary disease may experience certain episodes which are indistinguishable from acute myocardial infarction. Electrocardiographically, signs of acute myocardial ischemia may be observed, but with this method of study necrosis of muscle cannot be established. Other laboratory studies do not indicate conclusive signs of acute myocardial infarction. Among such cases there are some in which circumstances permit a pathologic examination at such a time as to allow correlation with the clinical episodes. In some of these, the pathologic evidence is that focal subendocardial myocardial infarction had occurred when the patient presented with the clinical episode. In others, on the contrary, there are no signs of acute myocardial infarction having occurred at the time when the patient complained. In such cases a state of *coronary insufficiency without myocardial infarction* may be said to have been present. In those cases in which the episode of thoracic pain had been present over a protracted period, the term *status anginosis* may be applied.

There are cases with the clinical picture mentioned in which acute myocardial infarction is observed pathologically but in which the age of infarction clearly represents a shorter period between the time of its occurrence and death than between the onset of the clinical episode and death. Such cases are to be interpreted as examples of coronary insufficiency without infarction in which myocardial infarction represented a delayed complication of myocardial ischemia.

The pathologic evidence is that in most cases of those clinical states variously designated as coronary insufficiency without myocardial infarction, or status anginosis, there is no acute coronary arterial occlusion.

Acute myocardial infarction

PATHOLOGIC PROCESSES

Necrosis of cardiac muscle as a complication of ischemia is infarction. The ischemia may be precipitated by acute coronary occlusion (usually thrombotic in nature). Indeed, many hold to the concept that acute coronary occlusion is a prerequisite for acute myocardial infarction. That this is an untenable view is supported by the fact that in many cases (perhaps the majority) of acute myocardial infarction there is no acute arterial occlusion. In these, only old narrowing or occlusion, either by atherosclerosis or by atherosclerosis and organized thrombosis, is found in the coronary arteries. In some of these cases a basis for ischemia may be identified in a hypotensive episode or in demands upon the heart by unusual levels of work or emotional stress. In many instances, however, no immediate basis for ischemia can be identified.

Whether or not acute myocardial infarction is attended by acute coronary occlusion is related to the type of myocardial infarct present. In cases in which infarction involves the entire (or almost the entire) thickness of the muscle in the involved segment, so-called *transmural* infarction, there is a great tendency for acute coronary arterial occlusion to be present. When infarction is confined to a restricted segment of the myocardium (usually muscle in the endocardial half of the left ventricular wall), acute coronary occlusion is usually not present. In such infarcts, often termed *subendocardial infarcts,* there is a tendency for infarcted and noninfarcted muscle bundles to alternate.

The lack of consistency with which acute myocardial infarction is associated with acute coronary occlusion has raised the question as to whether myocardial infarction antedates coronary thrombosis when the latter is present. Spain and Bradess[7] and Baroldi[8] have supplied evidence which is in support of an affirmative answer to this question.

In the earliest stage of acute myocardial infarction both the gross and histologic appearances may reveal no change that may be considered abnormal, even though the electrocardiographic picture is specific and results of serum transaminase studies are incontrovertible. A stain recently introduced by Lie and associates[9] may aid in earlier histologic identification of acute myocardial infarction than has hitherto been possible.

At about 12 h the involved myocardium grossly may possess a bluish hue (Fig. 62C-4A). This appearance may lead to an erroneous impression of hemorrhage into the infarct. Hemorrhage is unusual in uncomplicated acute myocardial infarction. Histologically, at this stage, the myocardial fibers are somewhat more eosinophilic than are fibers in the uninvolved parts of the myocardium.

By 18 h, there may be some clumping of the cytoplasm of myocardial fibers. The capillaries tend to be dilated, and early interstitial exudation of

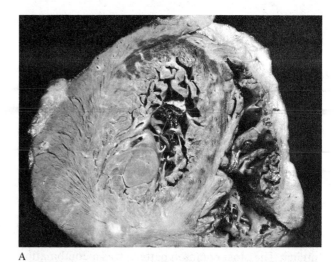

A

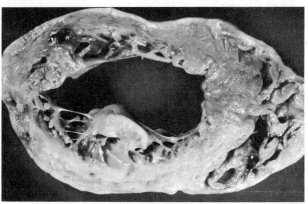

B

FIGURE 62C-4 A. Acute anteroseptal myocardial infarction in an early stage. The darker zone of the myocardium was purple in the fresh state and represents myocardial infarction of less than 1 day's duration. *B.* Acute myocardial infarction in the posterior wall of the left ventricle (lower part of illustration) and of the ventricular septum. The pallor of the muscle represents extensive acute myocardial infarction of several days' duration. In the fresh state this area was yellow. In the opposite wall focal thinning represents healed anterior subendocardial myocardial infarction.

leukocytes, predominantly neutrophils, takes place. Grossly, the myocardium has lost its bluish hue, and there is either no remarkable appearance or a shade of yellow.

After 24 h have elapsed, the stage of leukocytic infiltration is well established. The infiltration is derived mainly from the tissues around the infarcted zone and is, therefore, concentrated at the periphery of the infarct. Within the depths of the infarct lesser concentrations of leukocytic infiltration may occur around blood vessels. The corresponding picture grossly is that of an obvious yellow discoloration of the infarct. The demarcation between infarcted and noninfarcted muscle is fairly sharp (Fig. 62C-4B).

The appearances in the second and third days are elaborations of the leukocytic infiltrate of the first day. The nuclei of the myocardial fibers tend to become indistinct. Though the cross striations become altered, they do not disappear, contrary to common teaching. They become more coarse but continue to be demonstrable as long as infarcted fibers are demonstrable.

The stage of removal of muscle fibers follows the stage of leukocytic infiltration. First identifiable by the end of the third day, removal of fibers continues for days or weeks until usually all necrotic fibers are removed. The stage of removal dominates the picture during the second week. As the leukocytic infiltration begins at the periphery of the infarct, so does the removal of necrotic fibers. Here, there is fragmentation of muscle fibers and interstitial infiltration of macrophages and lymphocytes, while the stroma, composed of the capillaries and supporting connective tissue, remains. Deeper within the infarct the neutrophils, which infiltrated earlier, show various stages of disintegration.

As the removal starts at the periphery of the infarct, the gross characteristics of removal of muscle are noted in the same area. Here, between the yellow infarcted muscle on one side and the normal muscle more peripherally, there lies a band of reddish purple. On cut section of the myocardium this band is depressed.

The stage of removal of muscle fibers affords one an opportunity to appreciate the variation in effect of ischemia upon the myocardium. At the junction of the periphery of the zone of infarction with the intact muscle, even in large, seemingly well-demarcated infarcts, there is an irregular border between the necrotic and viable muscle. In this zone, even though elsewhere there may be conglomerate masses of infarcted muscle, characteristically small masses of viable muscle alternate with areas of infarction (Fig. 62C-5). This picture suggests that in the junctional zone ("the twilight zone") between obviously viable and obviously necrotic muscle, myocardial ischemia has a variable effect on the myocardium.[10]

Some affected muscles become necrotic while others survive. However, survival of fibers in this area is not necessarily to be taken as an ideal situation, when one recalls that though these fibers

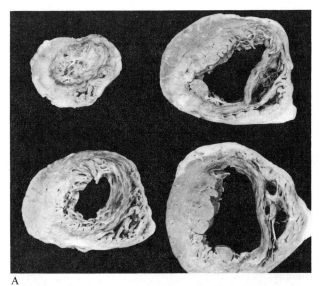

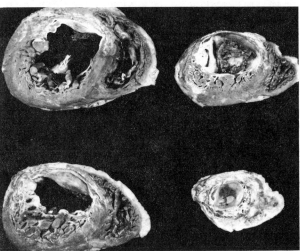

A

B

FIGURE 62C-5 Photomicrograph of healing acute myocardial infarction. In the lower portion of the illustration is intact muscle. In the upper portion is a zone of removal of muscle fibers peripheral to a large area of myocardial infarction. Between the facing arrows are collections of viable muscle fibers, demonstrating that at the periphery of a mass of infarcted myocardium, zones of intact muscle fibers alternate with infarcted ones.

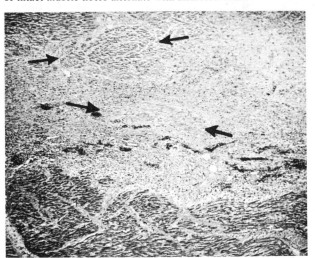

FIGURE 62C-6 A. Healing anterior and septal myocardial infarction. In the anterior and septal walls of the left ventricle, thinning represents myocardial infarction of extensive nature from which a considerable part of the necrotic muscle has been removed. In the two right-hand sections the pale area in the ventricular septum was yellow in the fresh state and represents necrotic, as yet unremoved muscle. The age of this infarct is about 3 weeks. *B.* Healed anterior and septal myocardial infarction. The main involvement is in the anteroseptal region, which is scarred and markedly thinned. The regional endocardium is thickened. Mural thrombosis is present over the infarct (particularly apparent in the right upper unit of this illustration).

survive, they are ischemic. During the early stages of infarction their ischemia may be reflected in certain of the electrocardiographic abnormalities of repolarization. Throughout the course of the clinical state of infarction and recovery, these fibers may be responsible for clinical episodes of myocardial ischemia and even for the initiation of ventricular fibrillation.

With the beginning of the third week, following infarction, the stage of scar formation becomes apparent (Fig. 62C-6A). At the periphery of the infarct where removal is proceeding and which is represented by a depressed red band during the second week, a change in color occurs. This is characterized by the appearance of a ground-glass gray hue to the depressed zone. Histologically, it is characterized by activity of fibroblasts and by the appearance of widening bundles of collagen. Some of the latter substance is undoubtedly of new origin, while some may simply represent consolidation of preexisting supporting collagenous fibers.

Removal of muscle is responsible, in part, for obvious thinning of the cardiac wall at the site of the infarct. It is to be emphasized, however, that thinning of the wall may occur early in myocardial infarction, before significant removal of muscle has taken place. The basis for this is that in large infarcts with paradoxic motion of the infarcted area the necrotic muscle is stretched, cannot recoil, and gradually becomes thin.

In most instances of myocardial infarction, regardless of the size of the lesion, the major portion of the necrotic muscle has been removed by the end of the fourth week. At the site of the previously necrotic muscle the process of scar formation proceeds so that in the case of large infarcts only a thin portion of the cardiac wall is represented, and this is formed principally by preexisting stroma and new connective tissue. Along with the healing that occurs within the infarct itself the overlying endocardium shows gradual increase in thickness, ultimately leading to obvious gray opaque thickening of the endocardium over the infarcted area (Fig. 62C-6*B*).

CAUSES OF DEATH

In patients who fail to survive from acute myocardial infarction, a number of pathologic states are evident.[11] Some may be related to known mechanisms; in other instances the exact mechanism of death is a matter of conjecture. It is to be emphasized that in many instances of acute myocardial infarction the death of the patient results not from a direct complication of the presence of necrotic muscle but rather from a complication which occurs within that muscle which survives. One of the common causes of death is considered to be acute coronary failure or acute coronary insufficiency wherein the mechanism of death is either ventricular fibrillation or cardiac arrest. In all probability, of the latter two rhythm disturbances ventricular fibrillation is the more common.

Pathologically, these cases are represented by myocardial infarction which conforms in appearance with the clinical age of the infarct, and no more recent infarction is identifiable, nor is there coronary thrombosis of any more recent age than the myocardial infarct. In many instances, as indicated earlier, a coronary occlusion is not even identifiable as related to the infarct that is present. In such cases there is usually a clinical history of recurrent episodes of

thoracic pain during the period of convalescence and often unexpected sudden death. The lungs show a variable appearance. In some instances there is no evidence of pulmonary edema, whereas in others pulmonary edema is present; such edema may develop rapidly during the terminal stages in patients who evidently die with rhythm disturbances.

Congestive cardiac failure with acute pulmonary edema is yet another cause of death in acute myocardial infarction. In some, the congestive cardiac failure is of the classic right-sided variety with accumulation of fluid in the serous cavities, edema, and hepatomegaly. This follows unrecognized left ventricular failure. In such cases coexistent hypertension is not infrequent, and often the myocardial infarct is large and/or associated with signs of preceding episodes of myocardial infarction.

Another major cause of death among patients dying with acute myocardial infarction is rupture of the heart. This type of death occurs decidedly more commonly among women than men. The prevalent type of rupture is that which occurs through the so-called free wall of the left ventricle leading to a fatal hemopericardium (Figs. 62C-7 and 62C-8). Less common types are rupture of the ventricular septum (Figs. 62C-9 and 62C-10) and rupture of a papillary muscle (Figs. 62C-11 and 62C-12), particularly the posteromedial muscle. The latter complication leads to acute and often massive mitral insufficiency. The anatomic site of the rupture of the papillary muscle is an important factor in determining the volume of regurgitant flow. Rupture of the main body of the muscle is not compatible with survival. Rupture of one of the heads of the muscle, however, may result in survival if the infarct of the left ventricular wall is of such a size that enough functioning ventricle remains to withstand the effects of the mitral insufficiency. Patients with such conditions then become candidates for surgical repair by prosthetic replacement of the mitral valve.[12-14]

It is significant that when rupture of the myocardium occurs as a complication of myocardial infarction, the rupture has a peculiar localization. It occurs in the periphery of the infarct near the healthy muscle. The basis for the rupture is probably that, during contraction, there is paradoxic motion of the infarcted area compared with the noninfarcted heart muscle. This motion causes a shearing action. With a tear of the endocardium and the endocardial aspect of the myocardium, there then follows a dissection of blood through the myocardium and ultimately through the epicardium into the pericardial sac. The channel which the rupture takes may undulate. In instances of rupture of the heart, histologic examination usually shows a heavy infiltration with leukocytes, and it is possible that uncommonly active proteolytic action on the cardiac muscle tends to underlie the factor of rupture. Rupture of the heart does not occur in so-called subendocardial myocardial infarcts but is restricted to those cases in which the infarct is of the transmural variety.

Contrary to earlier teaching, the peak of occurrence of rupture of the heart is not during the second

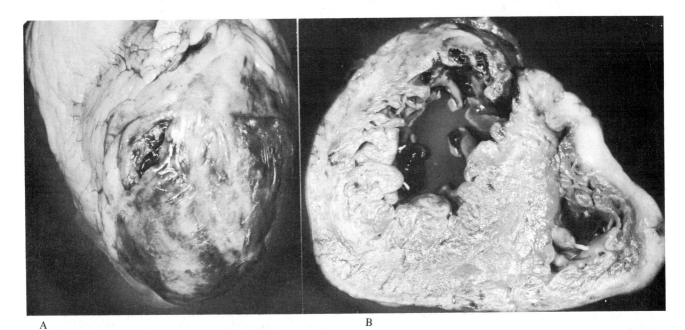

A

B

FIGURE 62C-7 Acute anterior myocardial infarction with rupture of the heart. *A.* Exterior of the heart viewed from in front. A laceration is present in the epicardium. *B.* Cross section of the ventricular portion of the heart. The rupture represents a laceration in the anterior wall at the periphery of the infarct (near the ventricular septum).

week following the onset of myocardial infarction but at an earlier period. In the majority of instances, rupture of the heart occurs in the third or fourth day after the onset of myocardial infarction. In exceptional cases rupture appears to be a complication of removal of tissue. This occurs in the individual in whom there is early formation of a ventricular aneu-

rysm. In such cases, rupture may occur through the thin part of the wall and occur about 2 weeks following the onset of acute myocardial infarction.[15]

Additional sequelae of acute myocardial infarction are the so-called thromboembolic complications. Two major sources for thrombosis occur in patients with acute myocardial infarction: (1) the left ventricular cavity and (2) the systemic veins. When left ventricular mural thrombosis occurs as a complication of myocardial infarction, the thrombus tends to involve the apical portion of the left ventricle, even though the infarct may be at a different location. In general, the larger the infarct, the more likely is left ventricular thrombosis to occur, and, indeed, in

FIGURE 62C-8 Cross sections of the ventricular portion of the heart in an example of acute lateral myocardial infarction (left side of each section) with rupture of the heart. The rupture site is seen in the right lower segment of the illustration. It is between the two papillary muscles and at the periphery of the infarct.

FIGURE 62C-9 Cross section of apex of ventricular portion of heart viewed from above, showing rupture of the ventricular septum (between arrows). Also, mural thrombus is present in the left ventricle.

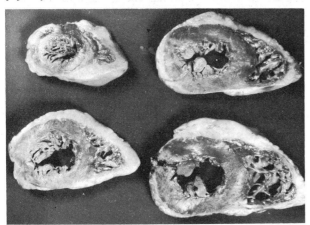

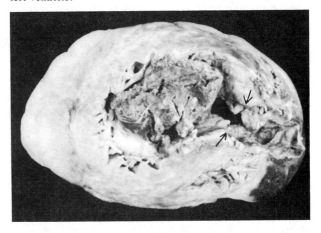

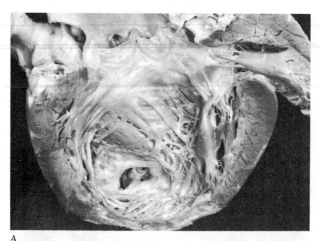

A

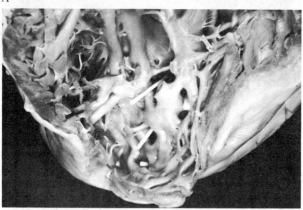

B

FIGURE 62C-10 Healed myocardial infarction with old rupture of the ventricular septum in a patient who had suffered an acute attack considered to have been that of acute myocardial infarction about 3 months before death from congestive cardiac failure. *A.* Left ventricular aspect. Near the apical region of the left ventricle is a large opening representing an old rupture of the ventricular septum. *B.* Right ventricle. In the apical region three probes lead from the single rupture seen in *A.* Muscle bundles of the right ventricle obscure the single rupture.

FIGURE 62C-11 Partial rupture of the posterior papillary muscle complicating acute posteromedial myocardial infarction. *A.* The posterior papillary muscle is lacerated (point of arrow). *B.* Between the arrows is a defect in the posterior papillary muscle, but continuity of this structure is still maintained. Beyond the point of the lower arrow, necrotic muscle, which was yellow in the fresh state, is identified. (*From Levy and Edwards, Prog. Cardiovasc. Dis., 5:119, 1962, with permission.*)

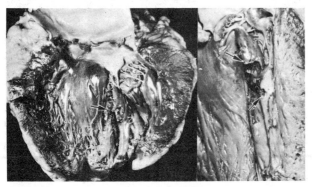

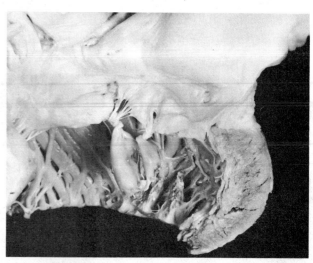

FIGURE 62C-12 Complete rupture of the posteromedial papillary muscle complicating acute myocardial infarction. The chordae tendineae to both mitral leaflets are twisted. The pale area in the subendocardial half of the myocardium represents the acutely infarcted muscle.

examples of transmural myocardial infarction, left ventricular mural thrombosis is more commonly present than not. Left ventricular mural thrombosis is a potential source for systemic arterial embolism to such important sites as the brain (Fig. 62C-13*A*), the coronary arterial system itself, and the mesenteric system, among others (Fig. 62C-14). It is significant that sudden death without any specific anatomic lesions is a much more common type of death than is that resulting from embolism.

In some instances of embolism the latter process may be the first objective abnormal clinical sign in a patient with a silent myocardial infarct (Fig. 62C-13).

Systemic venous thrombosis is important as a potential site for pulmonary embolism.

Pericarditis is a complication of acute myocardial infarction which is restricted to those cases in which the infarct is of the transmural variety. Usually the pericarditis is of passing interest and of no major functional significance. In a few cases, however, the pericarditis assumes importance. This occurs when during the stage of organization of the fibrinous pericarditis, hemorrhagic effusion occurs into the pericardium, with resulting cardiac tamponade. It is recognized that patients receiving anticoagulant therapy may have a greater risk of hemorrhage from coexistent pericarditis than those to whom no anticoagulants are administered. In the latter group, however, there is no absolute immunity from the hemorrhage of organizing pericarditis.

Healed myocardial infarction: prognosis of the patient

When a patient recovers from acute myocardial infarction, any of a wide variety of circumstances may ensue. Some persons continue without complications. The majority are subject to recurrent problems, either from considerable loss of muscle or from peculiar localization of the infarction in the papillary muscles (Fig. 62C-15), which causes mitral insuffi-

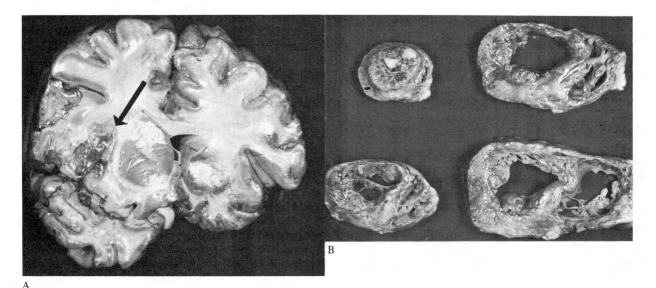

FIGURE 62C-13 Acute myocardial infarction with cerebral embolism and cerebral infarction. *A.* Brain. Recent cerebral infarction represented the primarily apparent medical problem of the patient who had suffered from a so-called acute silent myocardial infarction. *B.* Mural thrombus in the apical region of the left ventricle, the site of a healing acute myocardial infarct. The spleen also exhibited infarcts.

FIGURE 62C-14 Sites of systemic embolism with infarction representing complications of acute myocardial infarction. *A.* Small intestine. Discoloration of serosa is representative of changes in entire wall. *B.* Spleen. Multiple areas of discoloration represent acute infarction. *C.* Depressed areas on the surfaces of the kidneys are sites of infarction.

ciency. Others suffer from the effects of existing coronary arterial disease and experience either recurrent myocardial infarction or acute ischemic attacks which become complicated either by ventricular fibrillation or cardiac standstill.

The combined reviews of Achor and associates[16] and Juergens and associates[17] involved 329 patients with healed myocardial infarction observed at necropsy. Approximately one-third of these patients had died from noncardiac causes, and two-thirds had died of cardiac disease, usually a form of coronary disease but including embolism (Fig. 62C-16). Sudden death without recurrent acute myocardial infarction was the most common mode of death (38 percent) among those who died of cardiac disease. Of the other cardiac causes of death, congestive cardiac failure accounted for 27.5 percent and problems related to recurrent acute myocardial infarction for 34.5 percent.

In patients with healed myocardial infarction, congestive heart failure may be a combination of several coexisting conditions. In most instances loss of muscle in one way or another is a significantly contributing factor, but other conditions may also be associated to compound the effects of the loss of muscle incidence to the healed myocardial infarct. Such conditions are chronic pulmonary disease, valvular heart disease (particularly aortic stenosis), and hypertension, among others. For the moment, disregarding associated conditions which may contribute to healed myocardial infarction, there are certain features of healed infarction which have a positive effect in causing inadequate function of the left

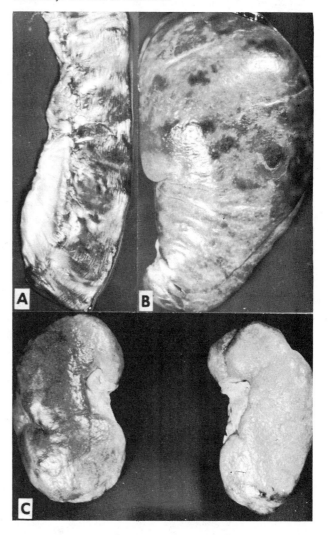

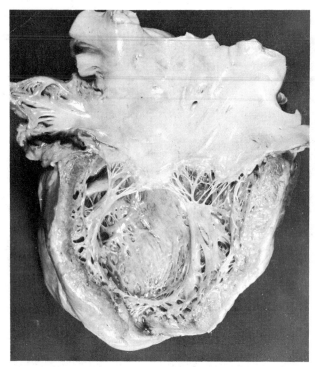

FIGURE 62C-15 Healed myocardial infarction with involvement of papillary muscles and mitral insufficiency. The left atrium is dilated. The two papillary muscles of the left ventricle are atrophic as a result of myocardial infarction, now healed. It is considered that mitral insufficiency had resulted from deficient action of the papillary muscles. Related free wall also scarred from infarction.

ventricle. These may be considered in three groups as follows: (1) extensive loss of muscle, (2) mitral insufficiency, and (3) asynchronous contraction or paradoxic motion of the ventricular wall. In certain situations extensive loss of muscle incident to several healed infarcts may represent the underlying cause of failure of the left ventricle, the latter resulting from inadequacy in the amount of the remaining muscle and malfunction of the scarred areas.[18]

Mitral insufficiency may appear either in an extensively scarred left ventricle or in a limited site of infarction. The latter involves the basal part of the inferior wall of the left ventricle and related posteromedial papillary muscle of the left ventricle. Concerning mitral insufficiency associated with an infarcted but intact papillary muscle, current experimental[19] and clinical[20] evidence indicates that, when infarction of a papillary muscle is associated with mitral insufficiency, there is also infarction of the related free wall of the left ventricle (Fig. 62C-15). The valvular disturbance is probably compounded of dysfunction both of the involved papillary muscle and the related infarcted free wall.

Yet another cause for congestive failure is loss of energy incident to asynchronous contraction or paradoxic motion of the left ventricular wall. The former is usually associated with a subendocardial scar, while the latter is associated with extensive loss of muscle as results from transmural infarction.[21,22]

In the latter situation, there may exist, but not necessarily, a left ventricular aneurysm (Fig. 62C-17). The aneurysm is characterized by extreme thinning of the cardiac wall, with a convex deformity of the external surface corresponding to the zone of infarction (Fig. 62C-17). Intraaneurysmal thrombosis is common, and the tendency toward systemic embolism is greater than average for all patients with healed myocardial infarction.

FIGURE 62C-16 Healed myocardial infarction and mural thrombosis. Cross sections of the ventricular portion of the heart. In these sections the anterior wall is toward the upper aspect of the illustration, the posterior wall toward the lower. There is healed infarction both of the septal and the lateral regions. A large mural thrombus present at the apical region represents a potential site for embolism. At the sites of healed infarction there is obvious thinning of the ventricular wall.

FIGURE 62C-17 Extensive healed anteroseptal myocardial infarction with early aneurysm formation. A mural thrombus is present in the apical region of the left ventricle. Thrombi in this location represent sites for systemic embolism.

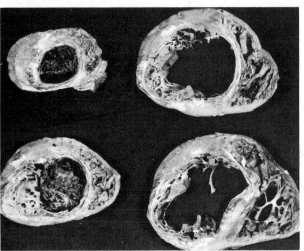

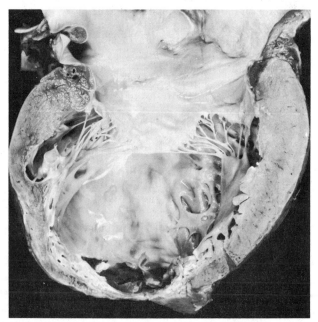

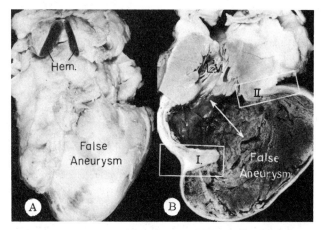

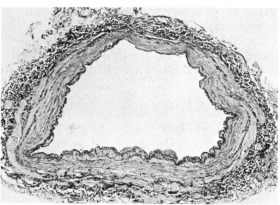

A

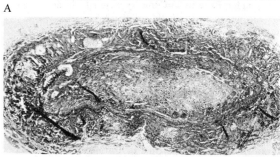

B

FIGURE 62C-18 False aneurysm of left ventricle. *A.* Exterior of heart viewed from in front. In addition to the false aneurysm, there is a localized pericardial hematoma, Hem. The localized effusion is considered to have resulted from ventricular rupture. *B.* Sagittal section through the heart showing the communication of the left ventricular cavity and the false aneurysm. (*From Chesler et al., Am. J. Cardiol., 23:76, 1969, with permission.*)

Calcification may be observed in the wall of some aneurysms, either in unremoved necrotic muscle or in unorganized thrombotic material near the wall of the aneurysm.

In the unusual instance of left ventricular aneurysm following myocardial infarction, the nature of the condition is that of a false aneurysm. This is an expression of the following pathogenic sequence: rupture of heart, confinement of resulting hematoma, and, finally, organization of the periphery of the hematoma (Fig. 62C-18).[23] While true aneurysms tend not to rupture, this tendency does occur in false aneurysm.[24]

POSTOPERATIVE CHANGES IN CORONARY BYPASS VEIN GRAFTS

The use of saphenous vein or certain arterial grafts to bypass obstructive zones in coronary arteries has become widespread. While the principle of the procedure is based firmly, one of the questions posed by this procedure concerns the long-range fate of these grafts. Not all grafts remain patent.

Two types of lesions may cause obliteration of the lumen of the graft, one thrombotic and the other proliferative in nature (so-called intimal fibrous proliferation) (Fig. 62C-19). Evidence suggests that if thrombosis is the basis for luminal obliteration, this process occurs in the early postoperative period. Fibrous intimal proliferation, on the contrary, is a late lesion which appears to take at least 3 months to develop.[25–27]

The thrombotic and the proliferative lesion which may occlude grafts may perhaps result, in part, from injury to the graft at the time of its handling and insertion.[28] Another factor may be the presence of undetected obstructive atherosclerosis downstream from the level of graft insertion.

Other complications that may occur following insertion of grafts are thrombosis of the recipient

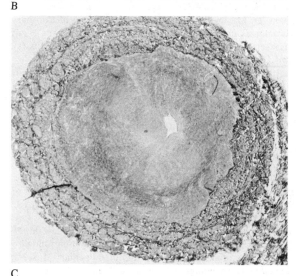

C

FIGURE 62C-19 Photomicrographs of saphenous veins used as grafts. *A.* Normal saphenous vein taken as a control at the time of insertion of the graft. Characteristically, the intima is thin and the lumen is wide. *B.* Lumen obliterated by vascular connective tissue representing an organized thrombus. Graft had been in place for 9 months. Elastic tissue stain; ×27. *C.* Lumen almost completely obliterated by intimal fibrous proliferation. Graft had been in place for 9 months. (*From Vlodaver and Edwards,*[28] *with permission.*)

artery proximal to the level of graft insertion and acute myocardial infarction.[29]

Acute myocardial infarction may be seen in over half of patients dying in the early postoperative period.[29] However, this figure is probably higher than average for the total population operated on. Either the infarction may involve a distinct segment of the left ventricle, or it may be represented by multifocal zones of necrosis. The latter type of lesion may be more closely related to the general problem of postoperative myocardial necrosis, as seen in valvular heart disease, than specifically to the presence of coronary disease.

REFERENCES

1 Vlodaver, Z., and Edwards, J. E.: Pathology of Coronary Atherosclerosis, *Prog. Cardiovasc. Dis.,* 14:256, 1971.

2 Diethrich, E. B., Liddicoat, J. E., Kinard, S. A., Garrett, E. E., Lewis, J. M., and DeBakey, M. E.: Surgical Significance of Angiographic Patterns in Coronary Arterial Disease, *Circulation,* 35&36(suppl. 1):155, 1967.

3 Guthrie, R. B., Vlodaver, Z., Nicoloff, D. M., and Edwards, J. E.: Pathology of Stable and Unstable Angina Pectoris, *Circulation,* 51:1059, 1975.

4 Zoll, P. M., Wessler, S., and Blumgart, H. L.: Angina Pectoris: Clinical and Pathologic Correlation, *Am. J. Med.,* 11:331, 1951.

5 Prineas, R. J., and Blackburn, H. (eds.): Sudden Coronary Death Outside Hospital, *Circulation,* 52(suppl. 3):1–287, 1975.

6 Spiekerman, R. E., Brandenburg, J. T., Achor, R. W. P., and Edwards, J. E.: The Spectrum of Coronary Heart Disease, *Circulation,* 25:57, 1962.

7 Spain, D. M., and Bradess, V. A.: Relationship of Coronary Thrombosis to Coronary Atherosclerosis and Ischemic Heart Disease (a Necropsy Study Covering a Period of 25 Years), *Am. J. Med. Sci.,* 240:701, 1970.

8 Baroldi, G.: Acute Coronary Occlusion as a Cause of Myocardial Infarct and Sudden Coronary Heart Death, *Am. J. Cardiol.,* 16:859, 1965.

9 Lie, J. T., Holley, K. E., Kampa, W. R., and Titus, J. L.: New Histochemical Method for Morphologic Diagnosis of Early Stages of Myocardial Ischemia, *Mayo Clin. Proc.,* 46:319, 1971.

10 Edwards, J. E.: What is Myocardial Infarction? *Circulation,* 39&40 (suppl. 4):5, 1969.

11 McQuay, N. W., Edwards, J. E., and Burchell, H. B.: Types of Death in Acute Myocardial Infarction, *Arch. Intern. Med.,* 96:1, 1955.

12 Morrow, A. G., Cohen, L. S., Roberts, W. C., Braunwald, N. S., and Braunwald, E.: Severe Mitral Regurgitation following Acute Myocardial Infarction and Ruptured Papillary Muscles: Hemodynamic Findings and Results of Operative Treatment in Four Patients, *Circulation,* 37(suppl. 2):124, 1968.

13 Austen, W. G., Sanders, C. A., Averill, J. H., and Friedlich, A. L.: Ruptured Papillary Muscle: Report of a Case with Successful Mitral Valve Replacement, *Circulation,* 32:597, 1965.

14 Lee, K. S., Johnson, T., Karnegis, J. N., Quattlebaum, F. W., and Edwards, J. E.: Acute Myocardial Infarction with Long-Term Survival following Papillary Muscular Rupture, *Am. Heart J.,* 79:258, 1970.

15 Van Tassel, R. A., and Edwards, J. E.: Rupture of Heart Complicating Myocardial Infarction: Analysis of Forty Cases Including Nine Examples of Left Ventricular False Aneurysm, *Chest,* 61:104, 1972.

16 Achor, R. W. P., Futch, W. D., Burchell, H. B., and Edwards, J. E.: The Fate of Patients Surviving Acute Myocardial Infarction, *Arch. Intern. Med.,* 98:162, 1956.

17 Juergens, J. L., Edwards, J. E., Achor, R. W. P., and Burchell, H. B.: Prognosis of Patients Surviving First Clinically Diagnosed Myocardial Infarction, *Arch. Intern. Med.,* 105:444, 1960.

18 Herman, M. V., and Gorlin, R.: Implications of Left Ventricular Asynergy, *Am. J. Cardiol.,* 23:538, 1969.

19 Tsakiris, A. G., Rastelli, G. C., Amorim, D. deS., Titus, J. L., and Wood, E. H.: Effect of Experimental Papillary Muscle Damage on Mitral Valve Closure in Intact Anesthetized Dogs, *Mayo Clin. Proc.,* 45:275, 1970.

20 Shelburne, J. C., Rubinstein, D., and Gorlin, R.: A Reappraisal of Papillary Muscle Dysfunction: Correlative Clinical and Angiographic Study, *Am. J. Med.,* 46:862, 1969.

21 Klein, M. D., Herman, M. V., and Gorlin, R.: A Hemodynamic Study of Left Ventricular Aneurysm, *Circulation,* 35:614, 1967.

22 Gorlin, R., Klein, M. D., and Sullivan, J. M.: Prospective Correlative Study of Ventricular Aneurysm, Mechanistic Concept and Clinical Recognition, *Am. J. Med.,* 42:512, 1967.

23 Ersek, R. A., Chesler, E., Korns, M. E., and Edwards, J. E.: Spontaneous Rupture of a False Left Ventricular Aneurysm following Myocardial Infarction, *Am. Heart J.,* 77:677, 1969.

24 Gobel, F. L., Visudh-Arom, K., and Edwards, J. E.: Pseudoaneurysm of the Left Ventricle Leading to Recurrent Pericardial Hemorrhage, *Chest,* 59:23, 1971.

25 Grondin, C. M., Meere, C., Castonguay, Y., Lepage, G., and Grondin, P.: Progressive and Late Obstruction of an Aorto-Coronary Venous Bypass Graft: A Case Report, *Circulation,* 43:698, 1971.

26 Marti, M. C., Bouchardy, B., and Cox, J. N.: Aorto-Coronary By-Pass with Autogenous Saphenous Vein Grafts: Histopathological Aspects, *Virchows Arch. [Pathol. Anat.],* 352:255, 1971.

27 Vlodaver, Z., and Edwards, J. E.: Pathologic Changes in Aortic-Coronary Arterial Saphenous Vein Grafts, *Circulation,* 44:719, 1971.

28 Vlodaver, Z., and Edwards J. E.: Occlusion of Coronary Grafts—Result of Injury? *Ann. Thorac. Surg.,* 20:719, 1975.

29 Vlodaver, Z., and Edwards, J. E.: Pathologic Analysis in Fatal Cases following Saphenous Vein Coronary Arterial Bypass, *Chest,* 64:555, 1973.

D
Altered Cardiovascular Physiology of Coronary Atherosclerotic Heart Disease

ROBERT C. SCHLANT, M.D.

> Besides, if the blood could permeate the substance of the septum, or could be imbibed from the ventricles, what use were there for the coronary artery and vein, branches of which proceed to the septum itself, to supply it with nourishments.
>
> **WILLIAM HARVEY, M.D., 1628**[1]

The purpose of this chapter is to review some of the physiologic and pathologic mechanisms responsible for many of the clinical manifestations of coronary artery disease. Although coronary atherosclerosis is the most common disease of the coronary arteries and this chapter is predominantly concerned with coronary atherosclerosis, many other diseases and conditions may also involve the coronary arteries (see Chaps. 63A and B). The altered physiology in many of the other diseases affecting the coronary arteries may be considerably different from that

ISCHEMIC MYOCARDIAL PAIN

Although not definitely proved, most current evidence favors the traditional concept, first proposed by Burns in 1809, that angina pectoris and other forms of cardiac pain or pain equivalents are the result of relative myocardial ischemia, due to an imbalance between oxygen supply and oxygen demand.[4]

Despite many years of study, the exact mechanisms or agent responsible for the stimulation of afferent sympathetic nerve fibers, which carry myocardial ischemic pain impulses, are unknown. The long search for a chemical nerve stimulant released by ischemia (the P factor of Sir Thomas Lewis) has thus far been unsuccessful, although it is still probable that such substances, perhaps a polypeptide of the type represented by kinins, are responsible for some ischemic pain. Tennant and Wiggers,[5] and later Harrison, suggested that an abnormal stretch of ischemic myocardium might be a second mechanism responsible for some episodes of ischemic pain. It would also appear theoretically possible that abnormal stretching or constriction of coronary blood vessels, which have an abundant nerve supply, within an ischemic area might produce ischemic pain in some patients. The possibility that some episodes of ischemic pain are related to mechanical or neural factors is perhaps strengthened by the clinical observations that angina pectoris may occasionally be promptly relieved by performing carotid sinus message,[6] performing a Valsalva maneuver,[7] or electrically stimulating the carotid sinus nerve.[8] These interventions may occasionally relieve the pain so promptly that the washout of a chemical stimulant from the heart may be less likely than a neuromechanical change in myocardial function. The afferent stimuli for myocardial pain appear to act upon sympathetic nerve endings which are distributed along coronary blood vessels and within the myocardium. The afferent impulses are carried by sympathetic nerves which enter the spinal cord from about the eighth cervical to the first four or five thoracic ganglions.

CORONARY BLOOD FLOW IN CORONARY ATHEROSCLEROTIC HEART DISEASE[9-20]

As noted in Chaps. 8 and 9, the normal heart extracts about 65 to 75 percent of the oxygen reaching it by the coronary arteries, leaving only 25 to 35 percent in the coronary sinus blood. Coronary vasodilatation in the normal heart is able to increase coronary blood flow four- or fivefold to meet increased oxygen requirements. Increased myocardial extraction of oxygen, which produces a lowering of coronary sinus oxygen content, is utilized by the normal heart to a much lesser extent than increased coronary flow and only when myocardial oxygen requirements ($M\dot{V}O_2$) are markedly increased. The major metabolic stimulus to coronary vasodilatation appears to be a local increase in adenosine produced by hypoxia,[17-19] although oxygen itself may directly influence coronary vascular tone.[21] Intrisic prostaglandin may also be released as a mediator of coronary artery vasodilation.[22-24b] The reports on the direct effects of epinephrine and norepinephrine on the coronary circulation under different experimental conditions are somewhat conflicting, in part because the coronary vessels appear to possess both α-adrenergic (vasoconstrictor) and β-adrenergic (vasodilator) receptor activity.[15-19] Most evidence indicates that stimulation of the sympathetic nerves to the heart and the infustion of norepinephrine produce transient coronary vasoconstriction of the coronary arteries.[12,15-19,25,26] Under normal conditions, this direct vasoconstrictive effect is soon overcome by vasodilatation, secondary to the increased myocardial mechanical and metabolic activity produced. In some patients with coronary atherosclerotic heart disease, it is very probable that myocardial ischemic pain sometimes results from a failure of the initial sympathetic vasoconstriction produced by emotion or exertion to be overcome by the normal vasodilator mechanisms. Such a delayed enhancement of the normal metabolic coronary vasodilatation could explain the clinical observation that patients with angina pectoris may experience pain when initially performing a given physical activity but not when the same activity is repeated. It might also explain how some patients are able to "walk through" an attack of angina pectoris.

In addition to being affected by changes in coronary vascular resistance, coronary blood flow is also directly related to the pressure difference between the aorta and the right atrium. This is especially important during hypotension after myocardial infarction, when the coronary bed may be maximally vasodilated and when the aortic driving (diastolic) pressure is of vital importance in maintaining coronary blood flow.[11,14,17-19] Clinically, however, this need for maintaining an adequate aortic pressure must be weighed against the increased left ventricular tension requirements and increased oxygen requirements produced by many of the drugs or procedures used to raise arterial blood pressure. A decrease in aortic pressure may also explain the occasional paradoxic production of angina pectoris by arrhythmias that produce arterial hypotension or by nitroglycerin, which can significantly decrease arterial pressure, especially in patients in the upright position. Anemia can also cause a significant depression of the ventricular function curve, particularly in the presence of coronary artery obstruction.

Coronary blood flow to the left ventricle occurs predominantly during diastole, because of the "throttle" action of left ventricular contraction,[10] which produces intramyocardial pressures that appear to be higher than the systolic pressure within the left ventricle and aorta.[10,20,27–29] Downey and Kirk[30] have suggested the inhibition of flow by a vascular waterfall mechanism as an alternate mechanism for the decrease in flow during systole. On the other hand, blood flow in the left circumflex artery during systole can equal 7 to 45 percent of diastolic flow, particularly after the initial phase of isovolumic contraction. During conditions of decreased systemic and coronary artery pressure, there may be very little systolic flow to the left ventricular endocardium.[14,20,31] In contrast, the rate of coronary flow to the right ventricle corresponds to the aortic pressure pulse, and even during systole it normally never approaches zero in the absence of right ventricular hypertrophy. Blood flow to the atria, which normally contract before the ventricles, may be considerably affected by an altered relation of atrial to ventricular contraction. The possible influence of an altered sequence of myocardial dyssynergy or asynergy upon local myocardial blood flow is still speculative, although James has suggested that such changes could significantly influence local coronary blood flow.[32]

In some patients, local coronary flow may also be significantly affected, particularly in the presence of coronary atherosclerotic heart disease, by compression of the arteries by myocardial bridges[33] or by intramyocardial pressure, especially in the subendocardial layers.[14,17,18,20,27–31,34] Coronary blood flow may also be somewhat impeded by markedly increased ventricular diastolic pressure.[14,31] There is a good correlation between the extent of angiographically demonstrated obstructive lesions and the ability of the coronary blood flow to increase during exercise or atrial pacing.[36] On the other hand, Proudfit et al.[35] found a relatively poor correlation between the clinical characteristics of angina pectoris and the extent of obstructive lesions demonstrated by selective coronary arteriography.

Coronary vasoconstriction (vasospasm)

Spasm of the large- or medium-sized coronary arteries is occasionally noted during coronary cineangiography. Often the spasm is not associated with pain or alteration of cardiac function, although it may be associated with severe angina pectoris. It is probable that coronary vasoconstriction of medium- or large-sized coronary arteries is a relatively rare cause of angina pectoris in the absence of coronary artery disease, although it is well documented, particularly in variant angina.[37–41,41a,98–109] It is well established that coronary flow and myocardial function and oxygen requirements are influenced by reflexes and by catecholamines, and numerous episodes of coronary spasm associated with angina pectoris have

been documented. Clinically, the concept of coronary arterial or arteriolar vasoconstriction as the mechanism for many episodes of angina pectoris is appealing, but the frequency is uncertain. It does appear to be relatively frequent in patients with variant (Printzmetal's) angina (see below). It should be noted that such vasoconstriction could involve either segments of the diseased vessels or collateral vessels to the ischemic areas. It is probable that coronary vasoconstriction is responsible for some instances of angina pectoris in patients with apparently normal coronary arteries demonstrated on angiography (see below and also Chap. 62E).

Subendocardial blood flow

The intramyocardial systolic pressure is highest in the inner half of the ventricle and appears to exceed ventricular pressure, particularly during the first half of systole.[10,14,17–20,27–31] Conversely, myocardial blood flow and oxygen tension are lowest in the inner layers and highest in the outer layers of theventricle.[14,17–20,27–31,42,43] These factors, plus the anatomy of the blood vessels to the endocardium,[44–46] contribute to the relatively increased susceptibility of the subendocardium to ischemia.[14,20,31,34,42,47,48] The decrease in coronary blood flow produced by an increase in ventricular diastolic pressure[14,31] probably has a greater effect upon subendocardial blood flow than upon other areas. This mechanism may explain some episodes of moderately prolonged ischemic pain that are not associated with significant increases in heart rate or systemic blood pressure. Clinically, this would be expected to occur most often in patients with hypertrophic cardiomyopathy, aortic stenosis, or coronary atherosclerotic heart disease.

Response to exercise

In patients with moderate coronary atherosclerotic heart disease, coronary blood flow and oxygen consumption per gram of tissue are usually normal at rest, but during exercise many such patients have an inadequate increase in coronary blood flow in association with the release of lactate, phosphate, and potassium from the myocardium (Chaps. 8 and 9) and with a significant decrease in the oxygen saturation of coronary sinus blood (an increased oxygen extraction ratio).[9–13,17–19]

DETERMINANTS OF MYOCARDIAL OXYGEN CONSUMPTION

The major determinants of myocardial oxygen consumption ($M\dot{V}O_2$) are (1) the mass of myocardium, (2) the heart rate, (3) the myocardial contractility, or inotropic state, and (4) the myocardial systolic wall stress. The latter is directly proportional to the ventricular systolic pressure and the ventricular radius and inversely proportional to the wall thickness. Three relatively minor determinants of myocardial oxygen consumption are (1) the external cardiac work, which is proportional to the arterial systolic pressure and the stroke volume, (2) the basal oxygen requirements of the heart, and (3) the activation energy requirements of the heart.[49-51] In patients with coronary artery disease, physical activity or emotional stress may increase myocardial oxygen requirements beyond the limited ability of the coronary circulation to increase flow. Clinically, the simple product of heart rate and systolic blood pressure is a useful index of changes in myocardial oxygen requirements.[52] Although this index obviously does not take into account all the determinants of $M\dot{V}O_2$, it is readily measured under standard clinical conditions.

Ventricular dilatation may significantly increase myocardial oxygen requirements according to the Laplace relationship (see Chap. 41), by which the force or tension that an average myocardial fiber must develop (in order to produce the same ventricular pressure) increases as the radius of the ventricle increases. Because of this relationship, the myocardial oxygen requirement of patients with ventricular dilatation may be significantly increased, a factor of major importance in patients with coronary atherosclerotic heart disease. During upright exercise, in patients with normal hearts, both heart size and the average ventricular radius decrease and the calculated ventricular efficiency increases (see Chap. 7). In contrast, patients with ventricular failure and dilatation during exercise may fail to decrease, or may actually increase, their ventricular end-diastolic and end-systolic volumes (radii), with a resultant increase in myocardial fiber tension and oxygen requirements (see Chap. 41). Moreover, areas of dyssynergy or asynergy can be responsible for a significant amount of "wasted work" and wasted oxygen consumption (see below).

ACUTE EFFECTS OF ISCHEMIA HYPOXIA ON MYOCARDIAL METABOLISM

The metabolic responses of the heart to ischemia hypoxia are discussed in more detail in Chap. 9 and will only be summarized in this chapter. An insufficiency of oxygen very rapidly impairs mitochondrial function, including oxidative phosphorylation and the citric acid cycle, causing the heart to shift to anaerobic glycolysis, which occurs predominately in cytoplasm, as its major source of energy.[53-62,62a] This results in increased glycogenolysis and increased uptake and utilization of glucose, with the eventual accumulation of pyruvate, much of which is reduced to lactate and released from the heart.

Phosphate and potassium may also be released from ischemic myocardium.[63] The anaerobic metabolism of glucose provides a net yield of only 2 high-energy phosphate bonds per molecule, whereas the complete metabolism of the same molecule of CO_2 and water theoretically could yield 36 high-energy phosphate bonds. Accordingly, ischemia is associated with an early depletion of myocardial

creatine phosphate (CP) and adenosine triphosphate (ATP), and with a decrease in the ratio of ATP to ADP (adenosine diphosphate). The balance between ATP and its breakdown products is important in regulating the rate of glycolysis and of glycogenolysis, both of which increased by ischemia.[53-62] Scheuer and Brachfeld have shown in the experimental dog that myocardial ischemia may produce accelerated anaerobic metabolism with the production of lactate prior to significant ST-segment alterations in the electrocardiogram; whenever the latter did occur, however, significant hemodynamic and metabolic changes were always present.[64] In the isolated ischemic rat heart, glycolysis and the production of high-energy phosphate by anaerobic metabolism are eventually inhibited by the accumulation of lactate.[65,66]

Patients with chronic ischemic heart disease at rest have greater than normal release of alanine from the myocardium, and the release remains unchanged during atrial pacing. Conversely, the uptake of glutamic acid is greater than normal at rest in ischemic heart disease, and the uptake persists during atrial pacing.[67]

The basic mechanism of early acute hypoxic myocardial failure is unknown.[68] The early hemodynamic manifestations of acute hypoxic myocardial failure are not thought to be entirely due to the depletion of myocardial high-energy phosphate stores (ATP and CP), since hemodynamic evidence of failure in hypoxia has been shown to occur before there is a significant decrease in total myocardial high-energy phosphate stores.[69] One possibility is that hypoxia initially produces a very rapid failure of the myocardial cell sodium pump, with a resultant decrease of the intracellular ratio of Ca^{2+} to Na^+ at special binding sites and a resultant decrease in the basic ability of the actin-myosin contractile sites to develop force or tension.[68,70] This might occur because of a localized depletion of ATP necessary for the sodium pump, even when total energy stores are still normal. When ischemia is more prolonged, there are marked depletions both of CP, which is the main reservoir of high-energy phosphate bonds, and of ATP, which is the immediate source of energy for the contraction of the actin and myosin filaments (see Chap. 9).

The stress of exercise, of tachycardia induced by pacing, or of isoproterenol infusion may bring out the inadequacy of the coronary circulation, which may be manifest by the release of lactate and potassium from the myocardium into the coronary sinus and by a decrease in coronary sinus oxygen content.[11-12,17-19,53-62] Herman, Elliott, and Gorlin[71] utilized the technique of selective coronary sinus sampling from different sites in the coronary venous system to determine zonal areas of lactate production and, therefore, of myocardial ischemia. In general, they found that the abnormalities in zonal myocardial lactate metabolism corresponded to the zones of myocardial asynergy seen on ventriculography or at surgery and to the zones of myocardial injury indicated by electrocardiography.

ACUTE EFFECTS OF MYOCARDIAL ISCHEMIA ON CARDIAC HEMODYNAMICS

Since the original observations of Porter,[72] of Orias,[73] and of Tennant and Wiggers,[5] many studies[1a,2,68] have confirmed that experimental myocardial ischemia produced by coronary artery occlusion or embolization produces, within a minute or two, a rapid decrease in contractility, which is soon followed by a passive, paradoxic outward bulging of the cyanotic, ischemic myocardium during systole. The decreased contractility is manifested by the following hemodynamic changes: a decrease in the force and velocity of contraction, a decreased maximal rate of change of left ventricular pressure (max dp/dt), decreased ventricular systolic pressure, decreased rate of ejection, decreased stroke volume despite an increase in end-diastolic volume, decreased ejection fraction with increased end-systolic volume, a delay in the development of peak myocardial force, a decreased rate of diastolic relaxation, and often an increase in left ventricular end-diastolic and left atrial pressures due to a decrease in diastolic compliance, or distensibility of the ventricle. Similar changes can occur during some episodes of angina pectoris.

HEMODYNAMICS OF ANGINA PECTORIS

In their review of the hemodynamics associated with angina pectoria, Roughgarden and Newman[74,75] concluded that prior to the onset of either spontaneous or exertional angina pectoris, patients frequently have systemic hypertension and/or increased pulse rate, often in association with elevation of pulmonary artery and pulmonary capillary pressures as a reflection of an increase in left ventricular diastolic pressure due to the acute decrease in ventricular compliance.[76–78] Similarly, in studies in which angina pectoris has been induced by exercise or electric pacing during cardiac catheterization, some patients have evidence of acute left ventricular failure preceding or during the pain, whereas other patients may experience pain without such changes.[76–78] The hemodynamic characteristics of this type of acute ischemic ventricular failure are the same as those listed above. In association with the pain or discomfort from myocardial ischemia, patients frequently experience dyspnea.[79] The dyspnea is most probably produced by an acute decrease in left ventricular compliance, with elevation of left atrial and pulmonary capillary pressures and early interstitial pulmonary edema and increased lung stiffness (decreased

pulmonary compliance). Some patients, especially those with severe coronary disease, may experience exertional hypotension or extreme fatigue. In such patients with atherosclerotic coronary artery disease, the episodes of exertional dyspnea or marked weakness are frequently the equivalent of classic angina pectoris. Although most episodes of angina pectoris occur in association with clinical situations or conditions that increase myocardial oxygen requirements (Chaps. 8 and 9), a substantial number occur in the absence of such conditions. In the latter circumstance, it is possible that the equilibrium between oxygen supply and demand is altered by changes in coronary vasomotion, which could be produced by active vasoconstriction or by failure of vasodilatation either of segments of the involved branches or of collateral vessels. In some patients, an increase in left ventricular diastolic pressure may decrease coronary blood flow enough to produce myocardial ischemic pain.[14,31] Recently, it has been suggested that the affinity of hemoglobin for oxygen in the coronary sinus is reduced in angina pectoris, an effect that would tend to assist the delivery of oxygen to the myocardium.[80,81]

Heart rate; atrial pacing

Tachycardia may produce angina pectoris by two mechanisms: (1) by increasing myocardial oxygen requirements and (2) by decreasing the time occupied by diastole, when most of the coronary blood flow to the left ventricle occurs. Clinically, tachycardia induced by right *atrial pacing* has been used to determine the threshold of angina pectoris.[82] In patients with coronary atherosclerotic heart disease, tachycardia induced by right atrial pacing can also produce evidence of myocardial anaerobic metabolism by an increase in the ratio of lactate to pyruvate in coronary venous blood and by lactate production by the heart. In some patients these changes were not associated with a decrease in coronary venous oxygen content despite the onset of angina pectoris. In those patients in whom the pain subsided despite continued pacing, it was noted that the evidence of anaerobic metabolism disappeared coincidentally with subsidence of the pain, suggesting that delayed vasodilatation of coronary collateral vessels occurred. Such a phenomenon or the release of vasoconstriction may explain "adaptation," or "second wind," angina pectoris, which may be manifest by the ability of some patients to "walk through" episodes of angina pectoris.

Emotional factors

Emotional stress and *excitement,* which can elicit a well-known strong sympathadrenal discharge, may produce significant changes in blood pressure, pulse, and coronary oxygen requirements.[17–19,83–86] During an attack of angina pectoris there is evidence of increased blood and urinary concentrations of catecholamines[87,88] although seldom to the degree found in association with myocardial infarction (see further on). Theoretically, emotional stress could also induce coronary artery spasm, although to date this has not been adequately documented (see above and Chap. 62E).

Prandial factors

Prandial or postprandial angina pectoris is probably caused either by the increased myocardial oxygen consumption secondary to tachycardia or by reflex coronary vasoconstriction.[89] It has also been suggested that the physical characteristics of lipemic blood may interfere with the delivery of oxygen to myocardial cells.[90]

Nocturnal angina pectoris

Nocturnal angina pectoris is particularly likely to occur during the periods of rapid eye movement (REM) associated with dreaming.[91] Though the mechanism is not clear, it is known that the pulse and blood pressure may increase during such periods, and it is likely that the level of sympathetic activity increases in general and particularly to the heart. If the initial coronary vasoconstriction produced by sympathetic stimulation is not overcome by vasodilatation from metabolic products, it might produce significant myocardial ischemia and pain. In other patients, nocturnal angina pectoris may be related either to an unusual decrease in aortic perfusion (diastolic) pressure during sleep or to the increased venous return produced by the reabsorption of fluid in the recumbent position with an increase in ventricular diameter and in myocardial oxygen requirements. Nocturnal angina pectoris may be an early symptom of left ventricular failure and is frequently relieved by therapy with digitalis. In this situation, and possibly in other situations in which hemodynamic failure precedes the occurrence of pain, angina pectoris may be the only symptom of heart failure. Most symptoms, of course, are related to dysfunction of other organ systems secondarily affected.

Effects of cold

The clinical relation of angina pectoris to cold air may be partially related to a reflex vasoconstriction of the systemic circulation and possibly of the pulmonary circulation.[92] In addition, extreme cold can cause an increase in catecholamine secretion. Patients with coronary artery disease have an abnormal increase in coronary vascular resistance while performing a cold pressor test, perhaps due to adrenergically mediated vasoconstriction.[93]

Physical manifestations of angina pectoris

During attacks of either spontaneous or exertional angina pectoris, evidence of the disordered ventricular performance may be detected by the development of ventricular filling or gallop (S_3) sounds or atrial gallop (S_4) sounds; by paradoxic splitting of the second heart sound; and by the development of an apical systolic (usually late systolic or holosystolic) murmur usually related to mitral regurgitation produced by papillary muscle ischemia and dysfunction; by the development of abnormal apexcardiograms or kinetocardiograms showing accentuated a waves, diminished inward motion during ejection, or early or late systolic ischemic bulges either at the apex impulse or medially in an ectopic area; and even by the development of increased pulmonary markings compatible with interstitial pulmonary edema often with a normal-sized heart seen on chest roentgenogram.[1a,94-97] The abnormal precordial impulses or systolic bulges may also be readily felt.[1a,94,97]

THE SYNDROME OF "VARIANT" ANGINA PECTORIS

This syndrome of angina pectoris differs from the usual type in that the pain is not brought on by increased cardiac work, it is usually more severe and of longer duration, it often waxes and wanes in cyclic fashion, it often occurs at about the same time each day, and it is not relieved by rest.[37-41a,98-109] Not infrequently, variant angina pectoris is associated with severe atherosclerosis or with vasospasm of a proximal major coronary artery. Occasionally, both are present.[37-41a,100,102-104,106-109] (See above and also Chap. 62E.)

THE SYNDROME OF ANGINA PECTORIS AND/OR MYOCARDIAL INFARCTION WITH NORMAL CORONARY ARTERIOGRAMS[110-116]

In recent years, reports from several centers have indicated that a significant number of patients with a typical history of angina pectoris have normal coronary arteriograms. Kemp, Elliott, and Gorlin[117] found that such individuals made up approximately 9 percent of patients with angina pectoris whom they studied. These patients frequently have an abnormal electrocardiogram after exercise, and a majority have abnormalities of either carbohydrate or lipid metabolism.[110,117] About two-thirds of these patients are female. Studies of the coronary circulation have indicated that these patients have normal coronary blood flow, myocardial oxygen extraction, and coronary sinus oxygen content, with a normal response to the infusion of isoproterenol.[110,117] Of great interest is the finding that about 30 percent of these patients have myocardial lactate production during isoproterenol infusion[110,117] or during tachycardia induced by right atrial pacing.

The mechanisms of this syndrome are not known. The findings of normal coronary flow and myocardial oxygen extraction at rest and during isoproterenol infusion or tachycardia are evidence against an abnormality of oxygen dissociation. Angina pectoris may occur in the absence of significant coronary atherosclerotic heart disease in patients with hypertension, valvular heart disease, especially aortic valve disease, or cardiomyopathy, with or without outflow tract obstruction. However, these conditions have not been clinically present in the reported patients with this syndrome. A few of the patients may ultimately be found to have disease of the small arteries (Chaps. 63A and 63B) beyond the resolution of coronary arteriography, although there is insufficient clinical evidence available at present to support this possibility. Kemp, Elliott, and Gorlin[117] suggested the possibilities of regional, functional arterial or arteriolar constriction or of unrecognized cardiomyopathy. Clinically, the mortality of patients with this interesting syndrome is much lower than that of other patients with angina pectoris, and relatively few necropsy studies have been performed. On the other hand, it is now clear that transmural myocardial infarction and even death can occur in such patients with apparently normal coronary arteries demonstrated angiographically or at autopsy.[112-117] Some of these patients may have mitral valve prolapse with the *billowing mitral valve leaflet syndrome.*[115a,193a] (See also Chaps. 60B and 62E.)

Platelet function, sudden death, and myocardial infarction

In most instances, it is not known exactly what initiates the onset of the usual episode of acute myocardial infarction. In many patients there is no preceding increase in heart rate or blood pressure, decrease in coronary perfusion pressure, or circumstance likely to induce reflex coronary vasoconstriction. Similarly, in many patients with coronary artery disease who die suddenly, there is often no coronary thrombosis or other cause of an acute imbalance between myocardial oxygen supply and demand found at autopsy. In both these clinical situations it is possible that a relatively small platelet thrombus forms in a coronary artery, initially perhaps on the surface of an atheromatous plaque, and releases thromboxane A_2, which is the most potent vasoconstrictor known to date.[118,119] Such a platelet thrombus may not be present when the usual autopsy examination is performed a number of hours later.

ALTERED CARDIOVASCULAR PHYSIOLOGY ASSOCIATED WITH MYOCARDIAL INFARCTION

The acute effects of myocardial infarction on left ventricular hemodynamics[2,120-133] are basically the same as those described above for ischemia and include a decrease in left ventricular systolic pressure and maximal rate of rise of pressure (*dp/dt* max), decreased stroke volume and cardiac output (often despite sinus tachycardia), decreased rate of left ventricular ejection, delay in the development of peak myocardial force, decreased ejection fraction, and decreased rate of left ventricular relaxation. There may be large areas of dyskinesia or akinesia of the left ventricle. The left ventricular compliance or distensibility is also usually decreased, and the left ventricular end-diastolic pressure may be significantly elevated if venous return is adequate. Left ventricular end-systolic and end-diastolic volumes both tend to increase. In human beings there is usually a significant decrease in left ventricular compliance after myocardial infarction[120-141] although experimentally compliance may transiently increase very briefly following myocardial infarction.[142] It is also significant that the distensibility of either ventricle may be influenced by the filling of the contralateral ventricle.[143,144]

Significant infarction of the right ventricle is much less frequent than infarction of the left ventricle or ventricular septum. Infarction of the right ventricle does occur, however,[132,144,145,146] and it has been suggested that it may be suspected from a syndrome of diaphragmatic wall infarction, distended neck veins, hypotension, heart block, and similarity between right atrial and pulmonary arterial diastolic pressure.[145] In our experience, most patients with this syndrome usually have severe right ventricular dysfunction without infarction, although a few have infarction.

In addition to the loss of mass of functioning myocardium by infarction or by severe ischemia and the development of areas of asynergy or dyssynergy,[147,148] several other factors contribute to the decreased pumping ability of the heart. These factors include a decrease in ventricular performance due to generalized myocardial ischemia; a decrease in coronary blood flow due to aortic hypotension, which may markedly decrease coronary blood flow even further; arterial and myocardial acidosis[149]; and arterial hypoxemia, which further limits the delivery of oxygen to the ischemic areas.[150,151] The development of ventricular dilatation further increases myocardial oxygen requirements by the Laplace relationship. In addition, overall cardiac function may be decreased by loss of atrial function with atrial fibrillation or improperly synchronized atrial and ventricular contractions, or by extreme bradycardia or tachycardia (Chap. 46B). As described farther on, some patients, particularly those with acute posterior or inferior myocardial infarction,[32,152,153] appear to have a strong vagal discharge, which may produce sinus bradycardia, increased atrioventricular block, and depressed atrial and ventricular function. Some of these patients may be considerably improved following the administration of atropine, although excessive tachycardia can also be produced.[153,154]

Systemic hemodynamic patterns associated with acute myocardial infarction

The systemic hemodynamic patterns associated with acute myocardial infarction are extremely complex and variable,[2,155-157,179-199] particularly in the presence of *cardiogenic shock*.[121,158-164] At one end of the spectrum are patients who initially have a transiently elevated systemic blood pressure and an elevated pulse rate with a normal or even increased cardiac output; similar findings have been reported following experimental coronary occlusion.[165,166] Patients with uncomplicated myocardial infarction with normal cardiac stroke volume and cardiac output may have a normal or only minimally elevated left ventricular end-diastolic pressure. The left ventricular angiogram may show the area of dysfunction, and there may be compensatory hyperfunction of other areas of the ventricle.

In patients with systemic hypotension or clinical shock, the most common hemodynamic pattern includes a decreased left ventricular stroke volume, a decreased cardiac output, decreased left ventricular systolic pressure, decreased maximal rate of rise of pressure (max dp/dt), decreased ejection fraction, and decreased mean rate of circumferential shortening. The left ventricular compliance is decreased; the end-diastolic pressure is usually significantly elevated unless the hypotension is due to inadequate preload (see below). The left ventricular angiogram shows markedly diminished motion of a significant amount of left ventricular myocardium, and the calculated systemic arterial resistance is significantly increased due to the generalized sympathetic response.

Many patients with mild or moderate hypotension following acute myocardial infarction are significantly improved by monitoring the pulmonary capillary (PC) or pulmonary artery wedge pressure and, if it is low or even normal, by cautiously expanding the blood volume until the hypotension is relieved or until the pulmonary artery wedge pressure, which normally reflects the left atrial pressure very well, reaches 18 to 22 mm Hg.[167]

A significant number of patients with mild to moderate decrease in blood pressure following an acute myocardial infarction have a relatively normal or mildly decreased cardiac output in association with a paradoxically normal or even *decreased* peripheral arterial resistance.[120-133,155-163,168] Thus, it appears that the variable response of the peripheral resistance vessels (mainly arterioles) is a major determinant of the systemic hemodynamic pattern following a myocardial infarction (see below). In some patients with acute myocardial infarction, it would appear that there is a "failure" of the normal peripheral arteriolar vasoconstriction following myocardial infarction. The reason for this failure is unknown, although there appears to be a strong possibility of reflexes originating from the heart. The decrease in peripheral resistance cannot usually be explained by the development of fever in these patients, although fever can contribute to a decreased peripheral resistance. The inappropriate peripheral vascular responses in these patients resemble somewhat the changes present during emotional or vasovagal syncope[169] and could result either from active vasodilatation or from decreased or inadequate vasoconstrictor impulses to certain vascular beds. The different patterns of peripheral vascular response in patients

following an acute myocardial infarction theoretically might be related to the particular areas of the heart which are ischemic or infarcted. The patterns might also be influenced by inherent, possibly genetic, differences in autonomic systems and reflexes, similar to the increased susceptibility of some patients to simple syncope and of other subjects to reflex bradycardia following immersion of the face in water, the oxygen-conserving, or "diving," reflex[170] (see below).

A knowledge of the peripheral vascular resistance is of obvious importance in the selection of drugs and techniques for the treatment of patients with hypotension or cardiogenic shock following myocardial infarction. It should be noted that in the presence of severe arterial vasoconstriction, sphygmomanometer blood pressure measurements may be significantly lower than simultaneous direct measurement of intraarterial pressure,[171] a situation which can lead to serious errors in treatment. Ideally, direct intraarterial measurement of blood pressure should be used to monitor patients with hypotension following acute myocardial infarction. The use of sonar or Doppler instruments to measure blood pressure in such patients is of very great value.

Autopsy studies of patients who died from acute myocardial infarction have indicated a reasonably good correlation between the mass of infarcted myocardium and the severity of the cardiogenic shock.[161,172,173] In patients with cardiogenic shock there is also some evidence for the presence of a *myocardial depressant factor* (MDF), which is thought to be produced by the activation of splanchnic lysosomes secondary to the severe reduction in cardiac output.[174,175]

In general, following an acute myocardial infarction, the body may utilize the same acute and subacute reserve mechanisms that it utilizes during other forms of heart failure. These mechanisms, which are described in more detail in Chap. 41, include the following: generalized arteriolar constriction and venoconstriction[176] with an increase in "venous tone"; redistribution of the cardiac output to maintain cerebral and coronary flow at the expense of less vital organs; increased extraction of oxygen from the available blood flow with an increased systemic arteriovenous oxygen difference; possible changes in red blood cell concentration of diphosphoglycerate (DPG), which may assist oxygen transport[177]; anaerobic metabolism; cardiac dilatation to maintain stroke volume by Starling's law; and retention of water and sodium by the kidneys.

Pulmonary edema in patients with acute myocardial infarction

Patients with acute myocardial infarction may develop acute pulmonary edema in the absence of preexisting heart failure and fluid retention[178-180] and in the absence of significant cardiac enlargement. It is produced by the elevated pulmonary capillary pressure secondary to left ventricular failure and acutely decreased left ventricular compliance,[134-141,156] which result in the transudation of fluid into the pulmonary perivascular space, interstitial space, and alveoli. To a limited degree, reflex peripheral vasoconstriction[176] may be considered beneficial by assisting in the maintenance of venous return to the right ventricle and detrimental by contributing to the development of pulmonary edema by allowing an acute shift of fluid from the systemic to the pulmonary circuit.

In the therapy of pulmonary edema secondary to acute myocardial infarction, one should be aware that early or interstitial pulmonary edema may be detected by roentgenologic examination before the development of rales and that evidence of pulmonary congestion may persist for a considerable period after the left atrial and left ventricular diastolic pressures have been decreased by acute diuretic therapy. When this situation exists in the presence of systemic hypotension, it is advisable to monitor the pulmonary capillary (or pulmonary artery wedge) and pulmonary artery pressures as the blood volume is cautiously reexpanded (see Chap. 62E).

Ventricular dyssynergy; ventricular aneurysm

Following myocardial infarction, ischemic areas of myocardium may form a true anatomic aneurysm or may have various degrees of abnormal motion (asynergy or dyssynergy). Herman et al.[147,148] have defined four types of local asynergy: *akinesis,* or total lack of motion of a portion of. the left ventricular wall; *dyskinesis,* or paradoxic systolic expansion of part of the wall; *asyneresis,* or diminished or inadequate motion of part of the wall; and *asynchrony,* or disturbed temporal sequence of contraction. Such areas of myocardium increase the burden on the rest of the ventricle by increasing ventricular volume and diameters; by acting as a "slack" area, thereby increasing the velocity of contraction necessary to generate tension during isovolumic systole; and by containing, or "wasting," a very substantial amount of the total left ventricular stroke volume and stroke work.[1a,145,147,181] It appears that either stroke volume must decrease or ventricular dilatation must occur whenever an area of akinesia (or ventricular aneurysm) approaches 20 to 25 percent of ventricular surface area, since above this percentage the extent of shortening required of the remaining heart begins to exceed physiologic limits.[181] In many patients with ventricular aneurysm or other forms of asynergy, isoproterenol improved the hemodynamic derangement, although it can also occasionally produce a significant deterioration of function.[147,148] The latter response is probably related to a much greater increase in contractility of the "normal" areas of myocardium than in the ischemic, asynergic areas. Rarely, postmyocardial infarction aneurysms may rupture.[182,183]

Clinically, either true or "functional" aneurysms may be detected by palpation,[12,97,184,185] by recording precordial pulsations (Chap. 16), by fluoroscopy or electrokymography (Chap. 29A), or by angiocardiography (Chap. 29C). The localization and function of areas of asynergy identified by left ventricular cine-angiography correlate reasonably well both with electrocardiographic studies and with biochemical studies indicating the regional production of lactate by ischemic myocardium.[225] The excision of ventricular aneurysms, either true or "functional," may produce dramatic clinical and hemodynamic improvement if there is an adequate amount of remaining ventricular myocardium with good function.[186-189]

Other causes of ventricular dyssnergy which may be important in special clinical situations include abnormal pathways of ventricular excitation, ventricular premature beats, ventricular tachycardia, and ventricular dilatation. Atrioventricular dyssynergy, produced by a failure of normal atrial contraction to occur at the appropriate time preceding ventricular contraction, may also contribute to decreased performance of the ventricles and of the heart (see Chaps. 41 and 46B).

Mitral regurgitation and papillary muscle dysfunction associated with myocardial infarction

In his elegant prospective study of 210 patients with acute myocardial infarction, Heikkilä[190] found that 55.7 percent developed a new mitral systolic murmur, usually within 5 days after admission. In most instances the murmur was faint, and in only one-third was it grade 3 or 4. He found that the murmur was most frequently holosystolic and also noted that midsystolic murmurs occasionally became holosystolic. The severity of mitral regurgitation is often poorly related to the loudness of the systolic murmur.[191] Occasionally, no murmur can be heard ("silent mitral regurgitation").[192] This phenomenon is probably related to markedly depressed left ventricular contractility. In addition, the left atrium initially may not be impressively dilated despite severe mitral regurgitation. Papillary muscle dysfunction or dysfunction of the ventricular myocardium adjacent to the origin of third-order chordae tendineae may also occasionally result in a characteristic syndrome with a midsystolic click and a midsystolic or late systolic murmur associated with mitral regurgitation in patients with myocardial infarction.[193] Overall, however, coronary heart disease is probably a relatively infrequent cause of the click-murmur or mitral valve prolapse syndrome.[115a,193,193a] (See also Chap. 60B.)

Papillary muscle infarction may produce moderate to massive mitral regurgitation[142,190-194] and rarely may lead to the rupture of chordae tendineae.[195] *Papillary muscle rupture* occurs in about 0.9 percent of patients with acute myocardial infarction[196]; it occurs more frequently in the posterior papillary muscle than in the anterior papillary muscle.

Rupture of a right ventricular papillary muscle

following acute myocardial infarction is rare.[190,197] The more frequent involvement of the left ventricular posteromedial papillary muscle[190,196] is related to its blood supply, which is principally from the posterior descending artery with some collaterals from the circumflex branch of the left coronary artery, whereas the anterolateral papillary muscle is supplied by one or more branches, from the left anterior descending coronary artery and by marginal tributaries from the circumflex.[62,63,198] The greater potential collateral circulation of the anterolateral papillary muscle would also imply that whenever infarction or severe ischemia of this muscle is present, significant obstruction either of the main left coronary artery or of both the anterior descending and the circumflex arteries is likely to be present. Often in this situation, massive infarction with rapid death may occur before anterolateral papillary muscle dysfunction or rupture is clinically or pathologically apparent. It should be noted that in experiments in dogs, isolated infarction of a left ventricular papillary muscle does not produce mitral regurgitation, whereas regurgitation is usually produced if the ventricular wall at the base of the papillary muscle is also infarcted.[199,200]

Mitral regurgitation may also occur after myocardial infarction due to ventricular dilatation, which can produce a realignment and a stretch of the papillary muscles and chordae tendineae so that they are no longer able to anchor the mitral valve leaflets without regurgitation. Theoretically, infarction of the mitral annulus might also produce mitral regurgitation, although this has not yet been proved.

Reflexes from the heart in association with acute myocardial infarction

Following an acute myocardial infarction, many patients respond to the emotional stress and pain and to the myocardial ischemia[251,252] with a significant sympathetic-adrenergic stimulation of central origin[201] (see below). In addition, reflexes initiated from the carotid sinus (decreased stretch or rate of stretch), from the carotid body (hypoxia), and from other reflexogenic areas of the cardiovascular system may participate in this reaction. The clinical importance of reflexes arising from the ischemic heart itself after myocardial infarction is unknown, but they may play a major role in the clinical course of some patients.

The *Bezold-Jarisch reflex*[202–204] refers to an experimental reflex which originates from unknown chemoreceptors in the heart, has both its afferent and efferent pathways in the vagus nerves, and results in sinus bradycardia, hypotension, and probably peripheral vasodilatation.[168,202–208] Vagal stimulation has been shown to depress pacemaker activity in the sinoatrial node, impulse transmission in the atrioventricular node, and the contractility of the atria and, to a lesser degree, the ventricles.[209] A wide variety of unrelated chemical substances, including veratrine, nicotine, ATP, and 5-hydroxytryptamine, may initiate this or a similar reflex in certain species when

injected intravenously or in the coronary artery,[204] or when applied directly to the epicardium.[204,210] Some of the same chemicals that can stimulate myocardial chemoreceptors also stimulate pulmonary chemoreceptors and produce reflex apnea.[204] As expected from its pathways, the reflex may be abolished by vagotomy, and the bradycardia may be abolished by atropine. The exact site of the cardiac receptors for the Bezold-Jarisch reflex is unknown,[202–207] though there is evidence that they are not located in the region of the sinoatrial node.[203,204] In addition to the classic Bezold-Jarisch reflex, there is evidence of similar reflexes originating from *chemoreceptors* in the heart that are stimulated by myocardial ischemia[168,207,211–218] or by left ventricular distension, or stretch.[208,219–223] It is uncertain whether or not the receptors of these reflexes are the same as for the Bezold-Jarisch type of reflex.

Although some workers previously concluded that reflexes of the Bezold-Jarisch type were not evident in patients with myocardial infarction, it would appear likely that a reflex corresponding to the Bezold-Jarisch reflex may be present in some patients, especially with acute posterior or inferior myocardial infarction. In these patients ischemia may result in stimulation of cholinergic ganglions and nerve endings lying in the lower posterior portion of the interatrial septum between the ostium of the coronary sinus and the posterior margin of the atrioventricular node.[152,224] The resulting vagal reflex may be responsible for the high incidence of intense sinus bradycardia, heart block, hypotension, sialorrhea, nausea, bronchospasm, and tracheal burning encountered in this group of patients, particularly when it can be shown that the symptoms are abolished by atropine.[32,152–154] In other patients with postinfarction sinus bradycardia, particularly when it is not reversed by atropine, the rhythm may be related to the negative chronotropic action of adenosine or related nucleotides on the sinus node.[32,152] As noted previously, adenosine and related nucleotides are released from myocardial cells by the stimulus of ischemia and may be important in the normal, metabolic autoregulation of coronary vasodilatation.[10–19]

It also appears quite possible from experimental data (although not yet proved by available clinical data) that reflex impulses originating from ischemic myocardium contribute to the apparent "failure" (or inhibition) in some patients of the peripheral vascular resistance to increase in response to the decrease in cardiac performance after an acute myocardial infarction, in addition to contributing to reflex cardiac depression.[168,223] Thus, the calculated total peripheral resistance in some patients with an acute myocardial infarction may be *normal* or *decreased* following myocardial infarction despite significant hypotension, which normally elicits reflex vasoconstriction. Accordingly, a type of peripheral vascular or autonomic nervous system "failure," perhaps related to reflexes originating in the heart itself, may be present in some patients who develop hypotension after an acute infarction but who do not increase their peripheral vascular resistance in the usual manner. If reflexes from the heart are, in part, responsible for this syndrome, the initiating stimulus in the heart could be related to ischemia (with the release or production of chemical substances which stimulate chemoreceptors, as in the Bezold-Jarisch reflex), to the stimulation of stretch receptors in the ischemic areas of the myocardium, or even to passive stretch of coronary vessels. In such a reflex arc efferent impulses might return to the heart in the vagus nerves and decrease both atrial and ventricular contractility,[209] as well as being transmitted in autonomic system fibers to the peripheral vascular system and either decreasing vasoconstriction or producing vasodilatation in some vascular beds.[168,202,212,223] It is also possible that the reflex fall in blood pressure represents a "protective" collapse mechanism similar to that produced by stimulation of visceral sensory nerves by a blow over the solar plexus or the testes, by irritation of the peritoneum, periosteum, or arterial walls, or by pressure on the eyeballs.[169,204] Such a reaction may act to decrease ventricular afterload, thereby tending to preserve ischemic myocardium.

Intercoronary reflex vasoconstriction (vasospasm)

There are conflicting data regarding the existence of intercoronary reflex vasospasm following acute obstruction of a major coronary artery. Although some earlier studies[225] indicated that such a reflex might exist and might produce additional myocardial ischemia by sympathetically mediated vasospasm, Joyce and Gregg[226] were unable to document the existence of this type of intercoronary reflex.

Systolic time intervals in acute myocardial infarction

The usual abnormalities of systolic time intervals (STI) noted in most types of chronic heart disease[227] are modified in patients with acute myocardial infarction.[227-229] In the early stages of acute infarction the durations of electromechanical systole (Q-A$_2$ interval) and of the left ventricular ejection time (LVET) are often both shortened simultaneously with an increase in urinary catecholamine excretion.[227-229] Although the *pre-ejection phase* (PEP) may be shortened in some patients with acute infarction, in other patients the PEP is prolonged. Serial studies have sometimes demonstrated a progressive lengthening of the PEP and shortening of LVET, both of which are maximal 3 to 5 days after the infarct. Similarly, some studies have indicated that the PEP/LVET ratio correlates well with the stroke index and has prognostic usefulness; however, most other studies have indicated that measurements of STI in patients with acute myocardial infarction have more limited value because of many variables.[227-229] In the presence of cardiogenic shock, measurements of STI are of even less value.[227-229]

Dysrhythmias in patients with acute myocardial infarction

The pathogenesis of arrhythmias in cases of sudden death or acute myocardial infarction is complex but related to myocardial ischemia.[32,152,230-235] In patients who die suddenly, ventricular fibrillation is the most probable rhythm disturbance. In patients with acute infarction, ventricular ectopic complexes are most frequently related to reentrant mechanisms (*focal* reexcitation, or *circus* reentry) or to enhanced automaticity. The reentry mechanism of dysrhythmias, which was proposed by Garrey,[236] is more likely to occur with the nonuniform recovery of excitability in ventricular muscle produced by ischemia.[237] (See Chaps. 46A to E and 49.)

Blood gas changes associated with acute infarction

Following an acute myocardial infarction, patients may develop arterial and tissue hypoxia and metabolic acidosis with a decrease in arterial pH and P_{O_2}, together with an increase in blood lactate concentration.[238-240] The major factors responsible for the acidosis appear to be the fall in cardiac output, arterial hypoxia, and peripheral vasoconstriction. The alveolar-arterial oxygen gradient is often increased in association with an overventilation that produces respiratory alkalosis. The arterial hypoxia may not be corrected by the administration of 98 to 99% oxygen,[238-241] probably because of functional pulmonary venoarterial shunting. Significantly better correction of the arterial hypoxemia can be achieved by using a well-fitting face mask rather than the more frequently employed nasal catheters or oxygen tents. Hemodynamically, oxygen breathing may result in a modest increase in systemic resistance and arterial pressure and in a decrease in cardiac output because of a decrease in both stroke volume and heart rate.[241-242] On the other hand, the benefits of the administration of oxygen in acute myocardial infarction to correct hypoxia and decrease myocardial ischemia probably outweigh any theoretical disadvantages.[243] The incidence of arrhythmias and the mortality rate are significantly greater in patients with severe acidosis, hypoxia, or lactacidemia. In addition to predisposing to arrhythmias[230-234,244] both acidosis and arterial hypoxia depress myocardial contractility.[149,245,246]

Catecholamines, corticosteroids, free fatty acids, and blood sugar in patients with acute infarction

Blood and urinary concentrations of norepinephrine and epinephrine may be elevated by physical or emotional stress, extreme exertion, surgery, hypoxia, or exposure to cold. There is also evidence for increased secretion of these catecholamines in association with angina pectoris.[87,88] Evidence for a sympathoadrenal response in association with acute myocardial infarction is found in the increased blood and urinary concentrations of norepinephrine, epinephrine, or their metabolic products[87,247–249] and in the elevated plasma hydrocortisone concentration and urinary excretion of 17-hydroxycorticosteroids.[201,250,251] The increased concentrations of plasma free fatty acids[247,252] and of blood glucose[201,253] following acute myocardial infarction may also be partially related to pituitary-sympathoadrenal stimulation. There is evidence which suggests that patients with higher plasma levels of catecholamines and free fatty acids have a higher incidence of severe arrhythmias, shock, and death than patients with lower levels.[247–252] The adrenal medulla can release circulating catecholamines as the result either of the generalized sympathetic stress reaction[87,88] or of arterial hypoxia. Sympathetic nerve endings throughout the body may also contribute important amounts of circulating norepinephrine, which is depleted from infarcted areas of myocardium.[254]

Although both norepinephrine and epinephrine increase myocardial contractility, they also significantly increase myocardial oxygen requirements. This increase is predominantly the result of the altered hemodynamics produced by the catecholamines, although there is also evidence of a relatively small, direct increase in myocardial oxygen consumption unrelated to the altered hemodynamic state.[255] The initial direct effect of norepinephrine or of stellate stimulation upon the coronary arterial system is vasoconstriction,[12,15,17,18,25,26] which is normally overcome by vasodilatation secondary to the increased myocardial metabolic and mechanical activity produced.

In general, the highest levels and most prolonged elevations of norepinephrine and epinephrine secretion and of free fatty acid concentration following myocardial infarction occur with extreme left ventricular failure and pulmonary edema, shock, severe arrhythmias, or death.[247–252] The occasional occurrence of peptic ulcer perforation or hemorrhage[256] is probably related to generalized stress reaction produced by the hemodynamic and emotional changes associated with acute myocardial infarction.

Patients with chronic congestive heart failure have a significant depletion of myocardial norepinephrine in association with augmented plasma levels of norepinephrine both at rest and during exercise (see Chap. 41). If such patients subsequently develop acute myocardial infarction, the depletion of myocardial norepinephrine may significantly decrease the reserve capacity and the function of the heart.

Cholesterol and triglyceride concentration in patients with acute infarction

Within hours after acute myocardial infarction, the plasma free fatty acid level often increases significantly,[257] whereas both plasma cholesterol and plasma triglyceride concentrations tend acutely to decrease.[258] Fyfe et al. found that measurements the morning after admission for acute infarction were close to measurements 3 months later and recommended that such measurements the morning after admission could be used for initial screening for abnormal lipid patterns, rather than waiting several months.[258] Although there is moderate variation in individual patients, the plasma cholesterol level, which reflects predominantly LDL cholesterol, tends slowly to decrease for a few weeks after acute myocardial infarction, whereas plasma triglyceride level tends to be moderately elevated for a few weeks following a brief decrease.[257]

Blood volume and hematocrit in patients with acute infarction

After acute myocardial infarction, circulating blood (plasma) volume may be decreased, together with a slight increase in hematocrit.[259] The decreased plasma volume is probably the result of reflex adrenergic discharge and vasoconstriction, pooling or tapping of blood, the administration of vasoconstrictive drugs, sweating, or the development of pulmonary edema. Patients with acute myocardial infarction may also have evidence of an increase in whole blood viscosity due to alterations in serum proteins during the acute phase of their illness.[260] There is also an epidemiologic relation between an elevated hematocrit and coronary atherosclerotic heart disease.[259,261]

Cardiovascular effects of morphine in patients with acute infarction

Morphine, which is frequently administered for the relief of pain associated with myocardial infarction, can produce respiratory depression and significant changes in the function of the cardiovascular system, including arterial hypotension, especially in the upright position; decrease in cardiac output; and depression of atrioventricular conduction, which can contribute to the production of significant heart block.[262–267] On the other hand, the decrease in venous and arterial tone produced by morphine can result in venous pooling with a decrease in venous return, a form of internal "pharmacologic phlebotomy" of great use in pulmonary edema, but potentially catastrophic in the setting of acute myocardial infarction. Recent studies have indicated that morphine produces little pooling of blood in the capacitance vessels of the limbs but rather produces a decrease in arterial resistance and an apparent opening up and enlarging of venous channels in the visceral circulations.[268–270] The decrease in ventricular afterload tends to improve ventricular function; however, if hypotension is produced, it could seriously decrease coronary blood flow and produce even more myocardial ischemia.

After the administration of morphine to experimental animals, myocardial contractility slowly increases and reaches its peak in about 30 min. This increased inotropism produced by morphine is the result of a sympathoadrenal discharge, and in experimental animals it is blocked by propranolol or by adrenalectomy.[271] It is uncertain whether or not this occurs in intact human beings.

Physical manifestations of myocardial infarction

Derangement of ventricular function in patients with acute myocardial infarction may be manifested by development of diminished and lower-pitched first heart sound (S_1),[272] ventricular filling or S_3 gallop sound, atrial (S_4) gallop sound, and paradoxical splitting of the second heart sound.[95,184-185,190,273,274] Occasionally, the first sound may be accentuated, particularly in association with an acute hypertensive response early after the onset of the infarction or in association with mitral regurgitation due to papillary muscle dysfunction. Palpation or the kinetocardiogram or apex cardiogram may demonstrate a prominent atrial *a* wave, an abnormal prolongation of the apical systolic impulse (late systolic bulge), or an ectopic systolic impulse.[97,184-185] The development of an apical systolic murmur, which may be holosystolic, midsystolic (ejection), or late systolic, and which is usually faint or transient, is frequent. It is probably caused by ischemia and dysfunction of the ventricular wall supporting a papillary muscle as well as by papillary muscle ischemia and dysfunction.[96,184-185,190,194]

Rupture of the ventricular septum and diastolic murmurs

Infarction of the interventricular septum may produce a ventricular septal defect and a loud systolic murmur.[184,191a,275,276] Rare causes of diastolic murmurs in ischemic heart disease are ventricular aneurysm[277,278] and stenosis of a coronary artery.[278,279]

Rupture of the heart[183,280-285]

This complication is usually manifest by the acute onset of severe shock which is often associated with marked increase in jugular venous pressure. Occasionally, various types of heart murmurs are heard, including systolic, systolic and diastolic, and continuous murmurs. Often the murmurs sound very close to the ear and/or have an unusual character. The electrocardiogram may show sinus bradycardia alternating with nodal bradycardia prior to the onset of electromechanical dissociation. Relief of the cardiac tamponade by pericardiocentesis may allow an attempt at surgical repair (see Chaps. 62E and F).

ALTERED CARDIOVASCULAR PHYSIOLOGY OF PATIENTS WITH CHRONIC ATHEROSCLEROTIC CORONARY HEART DISEASE

There is a wide spectrum of cardiovascular function in patients with chronic atherosclerotic heart disease.[1a,2,78,123,125,128-130,137-139,147,148,286-289] At one end are patients who experience mild angina pectoris only with extreme exertion. At the other end are patients who have sustained extensive infarction of the left ventricle and who have severe, chronic congestive failure even at rest. In between these extremes are many patients who have a slightly reduced left ventricular ejection fraction and reduced stroke volume index, cardiac index, and mean systolic ejection rate, with decreased left ventricular function (see Chap. 41). With extensive infarction and fibrosis, the compliance of the left ventricle may be significantly decreased, and there may be significant areas of dyssynergy with a markedly decreased ejection fraction.[78,129,130,134,135,138-141,147,148] Patients with chronic ischemic heart disease may respond to an increase in venous return (produced by a change in posture from a 20° feet-down position to the horizontal position with the legs elevated) with a *decrease* in stroke volume and an increase in heart rate, rather than with the normal increase in stroke volume and little change in the heart rate.[290,291] Many patients with chronic coronary atherosclerotic heart disease have nearly normal left ventricular function at rest but have striking abnormalities in ventricular function during exercise or atrial pacing.

Response to rhythmic (dynamic) exercise

Patients with coronary artery disease may not have the normal increase in coronary blood flow during rhythmic exercise but rather have an abnormal decrease in coronary sinus oxygen often with the release of lactate by the myocardium.[292] Similarly, nitroglycerin may fail to increase coronary blood flow in some patients with coronary artery disease. In such patients the relief of angina pectoris is presumably due to the decrease in cardiac work and oxygen requirements produced by nitroglycerin or to vasodilatation of collateral vessels to ischemic areas. Nitroglycerin has also been found to improve the hemodynamic response to exercise in patients with previous myocardial infarction, whether or not they have angina pectoris.[293,293a] The mechanisms for this action are unknown but may involve a decrease in afterload, a reduction in left ventricular volume with a reduction in left ventricular tension and oxygen requirements,[49-52] or an increase in coronary blood flow to ischemic areas. Nitroglycerin may produce beneficial effects upon abnormal wall motion both at rest and during exercise in patients with previous myocardial infarction.[293]

The mechanical efficiency of the heart of patients

with coronary atherosclerotic heart disease may fail to increase during exercise as in normal subjects,[9,292] perhaps because of wasted work spent in ischemic portions of the left ventricle that fail to contract normally, wasted work produced by mitral regurgitation due to papillary muscle ischemia, or increased oxygen requirements due to cardiac dilatation and the Laplace relationship. An abnormal increase in central venous pressure during exercise may also be found in some patients with chronic coronary atherosclerotic heart disease.[294] The hemodynamic response to exercise in patients with prior myocardial infarction appears to be improved following a period of physical exercise training.[295] Some patients with chronic coronary artery disease have exercise-induced ventricular premature beats.[296] The relationship of this phenomenon to sudden death is now under study.

Response to static (isometric) exercise

During sustained (static, or so-called isometric) exercise, there appears to be a reflex elevation of blood pressure and heart rate, which can reach quite high levels with relatively mild effort.[297-302] or with involvement of a small portion of the total body muscle mass. Clinically such forms of exercise can readily produce left ventricular ischemia and angina pectoris if performed injudiciously. In general, the cardiovascular effects of isometric exercise are additive when it is performed during simultaneous dynamic exercise.

Systolic time intervals in chronic coronary artery disease

In patients with chronic ischemic heart disease, Harrison and Reeves[1a] found that the duration of the *isovolumic contraction phase* is prolonged only when the duration of ventricular excitation is prolonged, although most of the other investigators have found that this phase may be prolonged without such electrical prolongation. In patients with milder degrees of ischemic heart disease, the duration of the LVET is within normal limits when corrected for rate, although patients with more severe disease may have a shortened LVET because of a decreased stroke volume.[227-229] Although a diminished stroke volume tends to shorten the PEP, the duration of systole and LVET tend to be prolonged by a decreased velocity of contraction and ejection secondary to decreased myocardial contractility and by the increased tension required in the presence of dilatation due to the Laplace relationship. These opposing tendencies, plus variations due to the speed of ventricular relaxation, heart rate, aortic compliance, and peripheral vascular factors, limit the value of the duration of the LVET. The duration of *isovolumic relaxation* is usually normal in chronic ischemic heart disease when corrected for age and heart rate.[1a]

Weissler et al.[227] have summarized the studies indicating that measurements of the STI, i.e., the

PEP, the LVET, and especially the PEP/LVET ratio, provide useful information regarding the overall performance of the left ventricle in patients with chronic coronary atherosclerotic heart disease, as in most other types of chronic heart disease. The decreased PEP/LVET ratio resulting from decreased left ventricular performance correlates well with the left ventricular stroke index[303] and may even be a more sensitive index of ventricular dysfunction than the stroke index or cardiac output. The PEP/LVET ratio also correlates well with the ejection fraction in patients with chronic heart disease of many types, including chronic ischemic heart disease.[304] In some patients with chronic coronary atherosclerotic heart disease who have minimal symptoms, the STI may be normal, presumably due to adequate compensatory hypertrophy. Patients who have angina pectoris with no history of myocardial infarction may have either normal or abnormal STI, the latter presumably due either to undetected myocardial disease or to transient myocardial ischemia.[94,227] Overall, measurement of STI, particularly the PEP/LVET ratio, provides highly useful information in assessing the adequacy of left ventricular mechanical function in chronic coronary atherosclerotic heart disease.[94,227,303]

Effects of sexual intercourse

During sexual intercourse, there are significant increases in arterial blood pressure and heart rate, which may also precipitate angina pectoris.[305-307] The changes may also precipitate a relatively pleasant sudden death, *la mort d'amour*,[308] which is presumably due to a cardiac arrhythmia. Following recovery from an acute myocardial infarction, the ability of patients to have satisfactory sexual intercourse without excessive tachycardia or pain can be considerably improved by a program of exercise rehabilitation and by a skillful, cooperative partner.

Cardiac hypertrophy

Cardiac hypertrophy, which probably results from a chronic increase of the mean systolic tension of the myocardial fibers,[309] has been reported to occur in coronary artery disease even in the absence of hypertension or failure.[310] The stimulus to hypertrophy in this situation is uncertain, but it may be related to ventricular dilatation, which increases the intramyocardial tension that is required to develop a given left ventricular systolic pressure, by the Laplace relationship, or to areas of dyssynergy, which increase the tension requirements of other areas of the heart that are not infarcted or ischemic.

In the hypertrophied myocardium there is conflicting evidence as to whether the ratio of capillaries to muscle fibers is decreased or is normal.[311] Even if this ratio is normal, however, the oxygen gradient between the capillaries and the inner aspects of the myocardial cells may be abnormally high because of distance and other physical factors.[312]

Ischemic cardiomyopathy[313–315]

In some patients, the clinical course of coronary atherosclerotic heart disease is manifest predominantly by the insidious, progressive damage to the myocardium with multiple small areas of infarction and/or fibrosis. In many instances, these patients have the clinical syndrome of congestive cardiomyopathy (see Chap. 81B), although they may occasionally present with the syndrome of constrictive cardiomyopathy.

Coronary collateral circulation[10–14,17–19,44,316–319a]

In patients with significant coronary artery disease, the capacity to develop an adequate coronary collateral circulation is a major determinant of how much myocardium will be ischemic or infarcted and of the functional capacity of the ventricular myocardium. The factors responsible for the development and growth of coronary collateral vessels are not completely understood. Hypoxia, which increases the local concentration of adenosine and produces vasodilatation, and intravascular coronary pressure differences, which alter the wall tension in the smaller, anastomotic vessels, appear to be major factors. Collateral vessel growth is also influenced by somatotropin (growth hormone). In general, the development of coronary vessels correlates reasonably well with the severity of the coronary obstructive lesions, and significant collateral circulation is seldom seen unless the diameter of a coronary artery is decreased by at least 50 percent.

REFERENCES

1 Harvey, W.: "Exercitatio Anatomica de Motu Cordis et Sanguinis in Animalibus," 1628, translated by C. D. Leake, Charles C Thomas, Publishers, Springfield, Ill., 1941.

1a Harrison, T. R., and Reeves, T. J.: "Principles and Problems of Ischemic Heart Disease," Year Book Medical Publishers, Inc., Chicago, 1968.

2 Braunwald, E. (ed.): "The Myocardium: Failure and Infarction," HP Publishing Co., New York, 1974, p. 409.

3 Gorlin, R. (ed.): "Coronary Artery Disease," W. B. Saunders Co., Philadelphia, 1976, p. 317.

4 Epstein, S. E., Redwood, D. R., Goldstein, R. E., Beiser, G. D., Rosing, D. R., Glancy, D. L., Reis, R. L., and Stinson, E. R. B.: Angina Pectoris: Pathophysiology, Evaluation and Treatment, Ann. Intern. Med., 75:263, 1971.

5 Tennant, R., and Wiggers, C. J.: The Effect of Coronary Occlusion on Myocardial Contraction, Am. J. Physiol., 112: 351, 1935.

6 Levine, S. A.: Carotid Sinus Massage: J.A.M.A., 182:1332, 1962.

7 Levine, H. J., McIntyre, K. M., and Glovsky, M. M.: Relief of Angina Pectoris by Valsalva Maneuver, N. Engl. J. Med., 275:487, 1966.

8 Epstein, S. E., Beiser, G. D., Goldstein, R. E., Redwood, D., Rosing, D. R., Glick, G., Wechsler, A. S., Stampfer, M., Cohen, L. S., Reis, R. L., Braunwald, N. S., and Braunwald E.: Treatment of Angina Pectoris by Electrical Stimulation of the Carotid-Sinus Nerves, N. Engl. J. Med., 280:971, 1969.

9 Messer, J. V., Wagman, R. J., Levine, H. J., Neill, W. A., Krasnow, N., and Gorlin, R.: Patterns of Human Myocardial Oxygen Extraction during Rest and Exercise, J. Clin. Invest., 41:725, 1962.

10 Gregg, D. E., and Fisher, L. C.: Blood Supply to the Heart, in W. F. Hamilton and P. Dow (eds.): "Handbook of Physiology," sec. 2, "Circulation," vol. 2, American Physiological Society, Washington, 1963, p. 1517.

11 Haddy, F. J.: Physiology and Pharmacology of the Coronary Circulation and Myocardium, Particularly in Relation to Coronary Artery Disease, Am. J. Med., 47:274, 1969.

12 Dempsey, P. J., and Cooper, T.: Pharmacology of the Coronary Circulation, Ann. Rev. Pharmacol., 12:99, 1972.

13 Mymin, D., and Sharma, G. P.: Total and Effective Coronary Blood Flow in Coronary and Noncoronary Heart Disease, J. Clin. Invest., 53:363, 1974.

14 Gordon, R. J.: A General Mathematical Model of the Coronary Circulation, Am. J. Physiol., 226:608, 1974.

15 Feigl, E. O.: Control of Myocardial Oxygen Tension by Sympathetic Coronary Vasoconstriction in the Dog, Circ. Res., 37:175, 1975.

16 Feigl, E. O.: Reflex Parasympathetic Coronary Vasodilation Elicited from Cardiac Receptors in the Dog, Circ. Res., 37:175, 1975.

17 Rubio, R., and Berne, R. M.: Regulation of Coronary Blood Flow, Prog. Cardiovasc. Dis., 18:105, 1975.

18 Klocke, F. J.: Coronary Blood Flow in Man, Prog. Cardiovasc. Dis., 19:117, 1976.

19 Klocke, F. J., Mates, R. E., Copley, D. P., and Orlick, A. E.: Physiology of the Coronary Circulation in Health and Coronary Artery Disease, Prog. Cardiol., 5:1, 1976.

20 Hoffman, J. I. E., and Buckberg, G. D.: Transmural Variations in Myocardial Perfusion, Prog. Cardiol., 5:37, 1976.

21 Gellai, M., Norton, J. M., and Detar, R.: Evidence for Direct Control of Coronary Vascular Tone by Oxygen, Circ. Res., 32:279, 1973.

22 Alexander, R. W., Kent, K. M., Pisano, J. J., Keiser, H. R., and Cooper, T.: Regulation of Post Occlusive Hyperemia by Endogenously Synthesized Prostaglandins in the Dog Heart, J. Clin. Invest., 55:1174, 1975.

23 Berger, H. J., Zaret, B. L., Speroff, L., Cohen, L. S., and Wolfson, S.: Regional Cardiac Prostaglandin Release during Myocardial Ischemia in Anesthetized Dogs, Circ. Res., 38: 566, 1976.

24 Kalsner, S.: Intrinsic Prostaglandin Release: A Mediator of Anoxia-induced Relaxation in an Isolated Coronary Artery Preparation, Blood Vessels, 13:155, 1976.

24a Berger, H. J., Zaret, B. L., Speroff, L., Cohen, L. S., and Wolfson, S.: Regional Cardiac Prostaglandin Release during Myocardial Ischemia in Anesthetized Dogs, Circ. Res., 38: 566, 1976.

24b Needleman, P.: The Synthesis and Function of Prostaglandins in the Heart, Fed. Proc., 35:2376, 1976.

25 Vatner, S. F., Higgins, C. B., and Braunwald, E.: Effects of Norepinephrine on Coronary Circulation and Left Ventricular Dynamics in the Conscious Dog, Circ. Res., 34:812, 1974.

26 Ross, G.: Adrenergic Responses of the Coronary Vessels, Circ. Res., 39:461, 1976.

27 Armour, J. A., and Randall, W. C.: Canine Left Ventricular Intramyocardial Pressures, Am. J. Physiol., 220:1833, 1971.

28 Downey, J. M., and Kirk, E. S.: Distribution of the Coronary Blood Flow across the Canine Heart Wall During Systole, *Circ. Res.,* 34:251, 1974.

29 Hess, D. S., and Bache, R. J.: Transmural Distribution of Myocardial Blood Flow during Systole in the Awake Dog, *Circ. Res.,* 38:5, 1976.

30 Downey, J. M., and Kirk, E. S.: Inhibition of Coronary Blood Flow by a Vascular Waterfall Mechanism, *Circ. Res.,* 36:753, 1975.

31 Archie, J. P.: Intramyocardial Pressure: Effect of Preload on Transmural Distribution of Systolic Coronary Blood Flow, *Am. J. Cardiol.,* 35:904, 1975.

32 James, T. N.: The Coronary Circulation and Conduction System in Acute Myocardial Infarction, *Prog. Cardiovasc. Dis.,* 10:410, 1968.

33 Polacek, P., and Zechmeister, A.: The Occurrence and Significance of Myocardial Bridges and Loops on Coronary Arteries, *Acta Facultatis Med. Univ. Brunensis (Brno),* no. 36, p. 101, 1968.

34 Brazier, J., Cooper, N., and Buckberg, G.: The Adequacy of Subendocardial Oxygen Delivery: The Interaction of Determinants of Flow, Arterial Oxygen Content and Myocardial Oxygen Need, *Circulation,* 49:968, 1974.

35 Proudfit, W. L., Shirey, E. K., Sheldon, W. C., and Sones, F. M., Jr.: Certain Clinical Characteristics Correlated with Extent of Obstructive Lesions Demonstrated by Selective Cinecoronary Arteriography, *Circulation,* 38:947, 1968.

36 Knoebel, S. B., Elliott, W. C., McHenry, P. L., and Ross, E.: Myocardial Blood Flow in Coronary Artery Disease, Correlation with Severity of Disease and Treadmill Exercise Response, *Am. J. Cardiol.,* 27:51, 1971.

37 Gensini, G. G.: Coronary Artery Spasm and Angina Pectoris, *Chest,* 68:709, 1975.

38 Chahine, R. A., Raizner, A. E., Ishimori, T., Luchi, R. J., and McIntosh, H. D.: The Incidence and Clinical Implications of Coronary Artery Spasm, *Circulation,* 52:972, 1975.

39 Yasue, H., Touyama, M., Kato, H., Tanaka, S., and Akiyama, F.: Prinzmetal's Coronary Artery Spasm: Documentation by Coronary Arteriography, *Am. Heart J.,* 91:148, 1976.

40 Engel, H. J., Page, H. L., and Campbell, W. B.: Coronary Artery Spasm as the Cause of Myocardial Infarction during Coronary Arteriography, *Am. Heart J.,* 91:501, 1976.

41 Kattus, A. A.: Coronary Artery Spasm: A New Appraisal, *Ann. Rev. Med.,* 27:69, 1976.

41a Maseri, A., L'Abbate, A., Pesola, A., Ballestra, A. M., Marzilli, M., Maltinti, G., Severi, S., DeNes, D. M., Parodi, O., and Biagini, A.: Coronary Vasospasm in Angina Pectoris, *Lancet,* 1:713, 1977.

42 Guy, C., and Eliot, R. S.: The Subendocardium of the Left Ventricle: A Physiologic Enigma, *Chest,* 58:555, 1970.

43 Moir, T. W.: Subendocardial Distribution of Coronary Blood Flow and the Effect of Antianginal Drugs, *Circ. Res.,* 30:621, 1972.

44 James, T. N.: "Anatomy of the Coronary Arteries," Paul B. Hoeber, Inc., Hagerstown, Md., 1961.

45 James, T. N.: Anatomy of the Coronary Arteries in Health and Disease, *Circulation,* 32:1020, 1965.

46 Estes, E. H., Jr., Entman, M. L., Dixon, H. B., II, and Hackel, D. B.: The Vascular Supply of the Left Ventricular Wall: Anatomic Observations, Plus a Hypothesis Regarding Acute Events in Coronary Artery Disease, *Am. Heart J.,* 71:58, 1966.

47 Neill, W. A., Oxendine, J., Phelps, N., and Anderson, R. P.: Subendocardial Ischemia Provoked by Tachycardia in Conscious Dogs with Coronary Stenosis, *Am. J. Cardiol.,* 35:30, 1975.

48 Domenech, R. J., and Goich, J.: Effect of Heart Rate on Regional Coronary Blood Flow, *Cardiovasc. Res.,* 10:224, 1976.

49 Sonnenblick, E. H., Ross, J., Jr., and Braunwald, E.: Oxygen Consumption of the Heart: Newer Concepts of Its Multifactoral Determination, *Am J. Cardiol.,* 22:328, 1968.

50 Braunwald, E.: Control of Myocardial Oxygen Consumption: Physiologic and Clinical Considerations, *Am. J. Cardiol.,* 27:416, 1971.

51 Parmley, W. W., and Tyberg, J. V.: Determinants of Myocardial Oxygen Demand, *Prog. Cardiol.,* 5:19, 1976.

52 Robinson, B. F.: Relation of Heart Rate and Systolic Blood Pressure to the Onset of Pain in Angina Pectoris, *Circulation,* 35:1073, 1967.

53 Opie, L. H.: Metabolism of the Heart in Health and Disease, p. 1–3, *Am. Heart J.,* 76:685, 1968; 77:100, 383, 1969.

54 Opie, L. H.: Metabolic Response during Impending Myocardial Infarction. I: Relevance of Studies of Glucose and Fatty Acid Metabolism in Animals, *Circulation,* 45:483, 1972.

55 Neely, J. R., Rovetto, M. J., and Oram, J. F.: Myocardial Utilization of Carbohydrate and Lipids, *Prog. Cardiovasc. Dis.,* 15:289, 1972.

56 Neely, J. R., Rovetto, M. J., Whitmer, J. T., and Morgan, H. E.: Effects of Ischemia on Function and Metabolism of the Isolated Working Rat Heart, *Am. J. Physiol.,* 225:651, 1973.

57 Rovetto, M. J., Whitmer, J. T., and Neely, J. R.: Comparison of the Effects of Anoxia and Whole Heart Ischemia on Carbohydrate Utilization in Isolated Working Rat Hearts, *Circ. Res.,* 32:699, 1973.

58 Braunwald, E. (ed.): Symposium on Myocardial Metabolism, *Circ. Res.,* 35(suppl. 3):III-1, 1974.

59 Lai, F., and Scheuer, J.: Early Changes in Myocardial Hypoxia: Relations between Mechanical Function, pH and Intracellular Compartmental Metabolites, *J. Mol. Cell. Cardiol.,* 7:289, 1975.

60 Wildenthal, K., Morgan, H. E., Opie, L. H., and Srere, P. A. (eds.): Regulation of Cardiac Metabolism, *Circ. Res.,* 38(suppl. 1):1, 1976.

61 Opie, L. H.: Effects of Regional Ischemia on Metabolism of Glucose and Fatty Acids: Relative Rates of Aerobic and Anaerobic Energy Production during Myocardial Infarction and Comparison with Effects of Anoxia, *Circ. Res.,* 38(suppl. 1):52, 1976.

62 Branchfeld, N.: Characterization of the Ischemic Process by Regional Metabolism, *Am. J. Cardiol.,* 37:467, 1976.

62a Hillis, L. D., and Braunwald, E.: Myocardial Ischemia, *N. Engl. J. Med.,* 296:971, 1034, 1093, 1977.

63 Parker, J. O., Chiong, M. A., West, R. O., and Case, R. B.: The Effect of Ischemia and Alterations of Heart Rate on Myocardial Potassium Balance in Man, *Circulation,* 42:205, 1970.

64 Scheuer, J., and Branchfeld, N.: Coronary Insufficiency: Relations between Hemodynamic, Electrical and Biochemical Parameters, *Circ. Res.,* 18:178, 1966.

65 Rovetto, M. J., Lamberton, W. F., and Neely, J. R.: Mechanisms of Glycolytic Inhibition in Ischemic Rat Hearts, *Circ. Res.,* 37:742, 1975.

66 Neely, J. R., Whitmer, J. T., and Rovetto, M. J.: Effect of Coronary Blood Flow on Glycolytic Flux and Intracellular pH in Isolated Rat Hearts, *Circ. Res.,* 37:733, 1975.

67 Mudge, G. H., Mills, R. M., Jr., Taegtmeyer, H., Gorlin, R., and Lesch, M.: Alterations of Myocardial Amino Acid Metabolism in Chronic Ischemic Heart Disease, *J. Clin. Invest.,* 58:1185, 1976.

68 Katz, A. M.: Effects of Ischemia on the Contractile Processes of Heart Muscle, in D. T. Mason (ed.): "Congestive Heart Failure: Mechanisms, Evaluation and Treatment," Yorke Medical Books, New York, 1976, p. 77.

69 Pool, P. E., Covell, J. W., Chidsey, C. A., and Braunwald, E.:

Myocardial High Energy Phosphate Stores in Acutely Induced Hypoxic Heart Failure, *Circ. Res.*, 19:221, 1966.

70 Langer, G. A.: Ion Fluxes in Cardiac Excitation and Contraction and Their Relation to Myocardial Contractility, *Physiol. Rev.*, 48:708, 1968.

71 Herman, M. V., Elliott, W. C., and Gorlin, R.: An Electrocardiographic, Anatomic, and Metabolic Study of Zonal Myocardial Ischemia in Coronary Heart Disease, *Circulation*, 35:834, 1967.

72 Porter, W. T.: On the Results of Ligation of the Coronary Arteries, *J. Physiol.*, 15:121, 1894.

73 Orias, O.: The Dynamic Changes in Ventricles following Ligation of the Ramus Descendens Anterior, *Am. J. Physiol.*, 100:629, 1932.

74 Roughgarden, J. W., and Newman, E. V.: Circulatory Changes during the Pain of Angina Pectoris: 1772–1965: A Critical Review, *Am. J. Med.*, 41:935, 1966.

75 Roughgarden, J. W.: Circulatory Changes Associated with Spontaneous Angina Pectoris, *Am. J. Med.*, 41:947, 1966.

76 Cannom, D. S., Harrison, D. C., and Schroeder, J. S.: Hemodynamic Observations in Patients with Unstable Angina Pectoris, *Am. J. Cardiol.*, 33:17, 1974.

77 Barry, W. H., Brooker, J. Z., Alderman, E. L., and Harrison, D. C.: Changes in Diastolic Stiffness and Tone of the Left Ventricle during Angina Pectoris, *Circulation*, 49:255, 1974.

77a Weisfeldt, M. L., Armstrong, P., Scully, H. E., Sanders, C. A., and Daggett, W. M.: Incomplete Relaxation between Beats after Myocardial Hypoxia and Ischemia, *J. Clin. Invest.*, 53:1626, 1974.

77b Mann, T., Brodie, B. R., Grossman, W., and McLaurin, L. P.: Effect of Angina on the Left Ventricular Diastolic Pressure-volume Relationship, *Circulation*, 55:761, 1977.

78 Rackley, C. E., and Russell, R. O., Jr.: Left Ventricular Function in Acute and Chronic Coronary Artery Disease, *Ann. Rev. Med.*, 26:105, 1975.

79 Pepine, C. J., and Wiener, L.: Relationship of Anginal Symptoms to Lung Mechanics during Myocardial Ischemia, *Circulation*, 46:863, 1972.

80 Shappell, S. D., Murray, J. A., Nasser, M. G., Wills, R. E., Torrance, J. D., and Lenfant, C. J. M.: Acute Change in Hemoglobin Affinity for Oxygen during Angina Pectoris, *N. Engl. J. Med.*, 282:1219, 1970.

81 Finch, C. A., and Lenfant, C.: Oxygen Transport in Man, *N. Engl. J. Med.*, 286:407, 1972.

82 Linhart, J. W.: Atrial Pacing in Coronary Artery Disease, *Am. J. Med.*, 53:64, 1972.

83 Adsett, C. A., Schottstaedt, W. W., and Wolf, S. G.: Changes in Coronary Blood Flow and Other Hemodynamic Indicators Induced by Stressful Interviews, *Psychosom. Med.*, 24:331, 1962.

84 Rayford, C. R., Khouri, E. M., and Gregg, D. E.: Effect of Excitement on Coronary and Systemic Energetics in Unanesthetized Dogs, *Am. J. Physiol.*, 209:680, 1965.

85 Lane, F. M.: Mental Mechanisms and the Pain of Angina Pectoris, *Am. Heart J.*, 85:563, 1973.

86 Bergamaschi, M., Caravaggi, A. M., Mandelli, V., and Shanks, R. G.: The Role of Beta Adrenoceptors in the Coronary and Systemic Hemodynamic Responses to Emotional Stress in Conscious Dogs, *Am. Heart J.*, 86:216, 1973.

87 Richardson, J. A.: Circulating Levels of Catecholamines in Acute Myocardial Infarction and Angina Pectoris, *Prog. Cardiovasc. Dis.*, 6:56, 1963.

88 Nestel, P. J., Verghese, A., and Lovell, R. R. H.: Catecholamine Secretion and Sympathetic Nervous Responses to Emotion in Men with and without Angina Pectoris, *Am. Heart J.*, 73:227, 1967.

89 Goldstein, R. E., Redwood, D. R., Rosing, D. R., Beiser, G. D., and Epstein, S. E.: Alterations in the Circulatory Response to Exercise following a Meal and Their Relationship to Postprandial Angina Pectoris, *Circulation*, 44:90, 1971.

90 Regan, T. J., Binak, K., Gordon, S., Defazio, V., and Hellems, H. K.: Myocardial Blood Flow and Oxygen Consumption during Postprandial Lipemia and Heparin Induced Lipolysis, *Circulation*, 23:55, 1961.

91 Nowlin, J. B., Troyer, W. G., Jr., Collins, W. S., Silverman, G., Nichols, C. R., McIntosh, H. D., Estes, E. H., Jr., and Bogdonoff, M. D.: The Association of Noctural Angina Pectoris with Dreaming, *Ann. Intern. Med.*, 63:1040, 1965.

92 Hattenhauer, M., and Neill, W. A.: The Effect of Cold Air Inhalation on Angina Pectoris and Myocardial Oxygen Supply, *Circulation*, 51:1053, 1975.

93 Mudge, G. H., Grossman, W., Mills, R. M., Jr., Lesch, M., and Braunwald, E.: Reflex Increase in Coronary Vascular Resistance in Patients with Ischemic Heart Disease, *N. Engl. J. Med.*, 295:1333, 1976.

94 Martin, C. E., Shaver, J. A., and Leonard, J. J.: Physical Signs, Apexcardiography, Phonocardiography, and Systolic Time Intervals in Angina Pectoris, *Circulation*, 46:1098, 1972.

95 Yurchak, P. M., and Gorlin, R.: Paradoxical Splitting of the Second Heart Sound in Coronary Heart Disease, *N. Engl. J. Med.*, 269:741, 1963.

96 De Pasquale, N. P., and Burch, G. E.: Papillary Muscle Dysfunction in Coronary (Ischemic) Heart Disease, *Ann. Rev. Med.*, 22:327, 1971.

97 Hurst, J. W., and Schlant, R. C.: "Inspection and Palpation of the Anterior Chest: Examination of the Heart, Part Three," American Heart Association, New York, 1972.

98 Prinzmetal, M., Kennamer, R., Merliss, R., Wada, T., and Bor, N.: Angina Pectoris: I. A Variant Form of Angina Pectoris: Preliminary Report, *Am. J. Med.*, 27:375, 1959.

99 Cosby, R. S., Giddings, J. A., See, J. R., and Mayo, M.: Variant Angina: Case Reports and Critique, *Am. J. Med.*, 53:739, 1972.

100 Oliva, P. B., Potts, D. E., and Pluss, R. G.: Coronary Arterial Spasm in Prinzmetal Angina: Documentation by Coronary Arteriography, *N. Engl. J. Med.*, 288:745, 1973.

101 Cheng, T. O., Bashour, T., Kelser, G. A., Jr., Weiss, L., and Bacos, J.: Variant Angina of Prinzmetal with Normal Coronary Arteriograms: A Variant of the Variant, *Circulation*, 47:476, 1973.

102 Scherf, D., and Cohen, J.: "Variant" Angina Pectoris, *Circulation*, 49:787, 1974.

103 Dhurandhar, R. W., Watt, D. L., Silver, M. D., Trimble, A. S., and Adelman, A. G.: Prinzmetal's Variant Form of Angina with Arteriographic Evidence of Coronary Arterial Spasm, *Am. J. Cardiol.*, 30:902, 1973.

104 Gaasch, W. H., Adyanthaya, A. V., Wang, V. H., Pickering, E., Quinones, M. A., and Alexander, J. K.: Prinzmetal's Variant Angina: Hemodynamic and Angiographic Observations during Pain, *Am. J. Cardiol.*, 35:683, 1975.

105 Meller, J., Conde, C. A., Donoso, E., and Dack, S.: Transient Q Waves in Prinzmetal's Angina, *Am. J. Cardiol.*, 35:691, 1975.

106 Shubrooks, S. J., Jr., Bete, J. M., Hutter, A. M., Jr., Block, P. C., Buckley, M. J., Daggett, W. M., and Mundth, E. D.: Variant Angina Pectoris: Clinical and Anatomic Spectrum and Results of Coronary Bypass Surgery, *Am. J. Cardiol.*, 36:142, 1975.

107 Owlia, D., Prabhu, R., Pierce, J. A., Stoughton, P. V., Shankar, K. R., and Nino, A.: Variant Angina Pectoris Due to Coronary Artery Spasm, *Chest*, 67:727, 1975.

108 Higgins, C. B., Wexler, L., Silverman, J. F., and Schroeder, J. S.: Clinical and Arteriographic Features of Prinzmetal's Variant Angina: Documentation of Etiologic Factors, *Am. J. Cardiol.*, 37:831, 1976.

109 Endo, M., Hirosawa, K., Kaneko, N., Hase, K., Inoue, Y.,

and Konno, S.: Prinzmetal's Variant Angina, *N. Engl. J. Med.,* 294:252, 1976.

110 Kemp, H. G., Jr., Vokonas, P. S., Cohn, P. F., and Gorlin, R.: The Anginal Syndrome Associated with Normal Coronary Arteriograms: Report of a Six Year Experience, *Am. J. Med.,* 54:735, 1973.

111 Bemiller, C. R., Pepine, C. J., and Rogers, A. K.: Long-Term Observations in Patients with Angina and Normal Coronary Arteriograms, *Circulation,* 47:36, 1973.

112 Schatz, I. J., Mizukami, H., Gallagher, J., and Greenslit, F. S.: Myocardial Infarction in a 14-year-old Boy with Normal Coronary Arteriograms, *Chest,* 63:963, 1973.

113 Brest, A. N., Wiener, L., Kasparian, H., Duca, P., and Rafter, J. J.: Myocardial Infarction without Obstructive Coronary Artery Disease, *Am. Heart J.,* 88:219, 1974.

114 Khan, A. H., and Haywood, L. J.: Myocardial Infarction in nine Patients with Radiologically Patent Coronary Arteries, *N. Engl. J. Med.,* 291:427, 1974.

115 Ciraulo, D. A.: Recurrent Myocardial Infarction and Angina in a Woman with Normal Coronary Angiograms, *Am. J. Cardiol.,* 35:923, 1975.

115a Chesler, E., Matisonn, R. E., Lakier, J. B., Pocock, W. A., Obel, I. W. P., and Barlow, J. B.: Acute Myocardial Infarction with Normal Coronary Arteries—Possible Manifestation of Billowing Mitral Leaflet Syndrome, *Circulation,* 54:203, 1976.

116 Arnett, E. N., and Roberts, W. C.: Acute Myocardial Infarction and Angiographically Normal Coronary Arteries: An Unproven Combination, *Circulation,* 53:395, 1976.

117 Kemp, H. G., Elliott, W. C., and Gorlin, R.: The Anginal Syndrome with Normal Coronary Arteriography, *Trans. Assoc. Am. Physicians,* 80:59, 1967.

118 Hamberg, M., Svensson, J., and Samuelsson, B.: Thromboxanes: A New Group of Biologically Active Compounds Derived from Prostaglandin Endoperoxides, *Proc. Natl. Acad. Sci. U.S.A.,* 72:2994, 1975.

119 Ellis, E. F., Oelz, O., Roberts, L. J., II, Payne, N. A., Sweetman, B. J., Nies, A. S., and Oates, J. A.: Coronary Arterial Smooth-Muscle Contraction by a Substance Released from Platelets: Evidence That It Is Thromboxane A_2, *Science,* 193:1135, 1976.

120 Ramo, B. W., Myers, N., Wallace, A. G., Starmer, F., Clark, D. O., and Whalen, R. E.: Hemodynamic Findings in 123 Patients with Acute Myocardial Infarction on Admission, *Circulation,* 42:567, 1970.

121 Swan, H. J. C., Forrester, J. S., Danzig, R., and Allen, H. N.: Power Failure in Acute Myocardial Infarction, *Prog. Cardiovasc. Dis.,* 12:568, 1970.

122 Karliner, J. S., and Ross, J., Jr.,: Left Ventricular Performance after Acute Myocardial Infarction, *Prog. Cardiovasc. Dis.,* 13:374, 1971.

123 Baxley, W. A., and Reeves, T. J.: Abnormal Regional Myocardial Performance in Coronary Artery Disease, *Prog. Cardiovasc. Dis.,* 13:405, 1971.

124 Wolk, M. J., Scheidt, S., and Killip, T.: Heart Failure Complicating Acute Myocardial Infarction, *Circulation,* 45:1125, 1972.

125 Broder, M. I., and Cohn, J. N.: Evolution of Abnormalities in Left Ventricular Function after Acute Myocardial Infarction, *Circulation,* 46:731, 1972.

126 Chatterjee, K., and Swan, H. J. C.: Hemodynamic Profile of Acute Myocardial Infarction, in E. Corday and H. J. C. Swan (eds.): "Myocardial Infarction," The Williams & Wilkins Company, Baltimore, 1973, p. 51.

127 Weber, K. T., Ratshin, R. A., Janicki, J. S., Rackley, C. E., and Russell, R. O.: Left Ventricular Dysfunction following Acute Myocardial Infarction, *Am. J. Med.,* 54:697, 1973.

128 Moraski, R. E., Russell, R. O., Jr., Smith, M., and Rackley, C. E.: Left Ventricular Function in Patients with and without Myocardial Infarction and One, Two or Three Vessel Coronary Artery Disease, *Am. J. Cardiol.,* 35:1, 1975.

129 Miller, R. R., Price, J., Amsterdam, E. A., and Mason, D. T.: Sequential Alterations of Left Ventricular Compliance following Myocardial Infarction: Comparison of Acute, Early and Late Recovery Periods in Patients with Similar Pump Dysfunction, *Am. J. Cardiol.,* 35:157, 1975.

130 Theroux, P., Sasayama, S., Massullo, V., Kemper, S. W., Bloor, C., Franklin, D., and Ross, J., Jr.: Regional Myocardial Function Early and during the Healing of Acute Myocardial Infarction, *Am. J. Cardiol.,* 35:173, 1975.

131 Rackley, C. E., and Russell, R. O., Jr.: Left Ventricular Function in Acute and Chronic Coronary Artery Disease, *Ann. Rev. Med.,* 26:105, 1975.

132 Russell, R. D., Dowling, J. T., Burdeshaw, J., Turner, M. E., and Rackley, C. E.: Comparison of Left and Right Ventricular Function in Acute Myocardial Infarction, *Cath. Cardiovasc. Diag.,* 2:253, 1976.

133 Rackley, C. E., Russell, R. O., Jr., Moraski, R. E., and Mantle, J. A.: Recent Advances in Hemodynamic Studies in Patients with Acute Myocardial Infarction, *Prog. Cardiol.,* 5:201, 1976.

134 Covell, J. W., and Ross, J., Jr.: Nature and Significance of Alterations in Myocardial Compliance, *Am. J. Cardiol.,* 32:449, 1973.

135 Mirsky, I., Cohn, P. F., Levine, J. A., Gorlin, R., Herman, M. V., Kreulen, T. H., and Sonnenblick, E. H.: Assessment of Left Ventricular Stiffness in Primary Myocardial Disease and Coronary Artery Disease, *Circulation,* 50:128, 1974.

136 Franklin, D., Theroux, P., and Ross, J., Jr.: Diastolic Properties and Regional Relaxation Abnormalities of the Left Ventricle during Acute Ischemia, *Circulation,* 50(suppl. 3):120, 1974.

137 Smith, M., Ratshin, R. A., Harrell, F. D., Jr., Russell, R. O., Jr., and Rackley, C. E.: Early Sequential Changes in Left Ventricular Dimensions and Filling Pressure in Patients after Myocardial Infarction, *Am. J. Cardiol.,* 33:363, 1974.

138 Gaasch, W. H., Quinones, M. A., Waisser, E. V., Thiel, H. G., and Alexander, J. K.: Diastolic Compliance of the Left Ventricle in Man, *Am. J. Cardiol.,* 36:193, 1975.

139 Bleifeld, W., Mathey, D., and Hanrath P.: Acute Myocardial Infarction: VI. Left Ventricular Wall Stiffness in the Acute Phase and in the Convalescent Phase, *Eur. J. Cardiol.,* 2:191, 1975.

140 Toyama, M., and Reis, R. L.: Effects of Myocardial Ischemia on Ventricular Compliance, *J. Thorac. Cardiovasc. Surg.,* 70:458, 1975.

141 Templeton, G. H., Wildenthal, K., Willerson, J. T., and Mitchell, J. H.: Influence of Acute Myocardial Depression on Left Ventricular Stiffness and Its Elastic and Viscous Components, *J. Clin. Invest.,* 56:278, 1975.

142 Forrester, J. S., Diamond, G., Parmley, W. W., and Swan, J. J. C.: Early Increase in Left Ventricular Compliance after Myocardial Infarction, *J. Clin. Invest.,* 51:598, 1972.

143 Taylor, R. R., Covell, J. W., Sonnenblick, E. H., and Ross, J., Jr.: Dependence of Ventricular Distensibility on Filling of the Opposite Ventricle, *Am. J. Physiol.,* 213:711, 1967.

144 Bemis, C. E., Serur, J. R., Borkenhagen, D., Sonnenblick, E. H., and Urschel, C. W.: Influence of Right Ventricular Filling Pressure on Left Ventricular Pressure and Dimension, *Circ. Res.,* 34:498, 1974.

145 Cohn, J. N., Guiha, N. H., Broder, M. I., and Limas, C. J.: Right Ventricular Infarction: Clinical and Hemodynamic Features, *Am. J. Cardiol.,* 33:209, 1974.

146 Ferlinz, J., Gorlin, R., Cohn, P. F., and Herman, M. V.: Right Ventricular Performance in Patients with Coronary Artery Disease, *Circulation,* 52:608, 1975.

147 Herman, M. V., Heinle, R. A., Klein, M. D., and Gorlin, R.:

Localized Disorders in Myocardial Contraction: Asynergy and Its Role in Congestive Heart Failure, *N. Engl. J. Med.,* 277:222, 1967.

148 Herman, M. V., and Gorlin, R.: Implications of Left Ventricular Asynergy, *Am. J. Cardiol.,* 23:538, 1969.

149 Regan, T. J., Effros, R. M., Haider, B., Oldewurtel, H. A., Ettinger, P. O., and Ahmed, S. S.: Myocardial Ischemia and Cell Acidosis: Modification by Alkali and the Effects on Ventricular Function and Cation Composition, *Am. J. Cardiol.,* 37:501, 1976.

150 Koerner, S. K.: Oxygen in Ischemic Heart Disease, *Am. Heart J.,* 82:269, 1971.

151 Radvany, P., Maroko, P. R., and Braunwald, E.: Effects of Hypoxemia on the Extent of Myocardial Necrosis after Experimental Coronary Occlusion, *Am. J. Cardiol.,* 35:795, 1975.

152 James, T. N.: Cardiac Innervation: Anatomic and Pharmacologic Relations, *Bull. N.Y. Acad. Med.,* 43:1041, 1967.

153 Webb, S. W., Adgey, A. A. J., and Pantridge, J. F.: Autonomic Disturbance at Onset of Acute Myocardial Infarction, *Br. Med. J.,* 3:89, 1972.

154 Thomas, M., and Woodgate, D.: The Effect of Atropine on Bradycardia and Hypotension in Acute Myocardial Infarction, *Br. Heart J.,* 28:409, 1966.

155 Russell, R. O., Jr., Hunt, D., and Rackley, C. E.: Left Ventricular Hemodynamics in Anterior and Inferior Myocardial Infarction, *Am. J. Cardiol.,* 32:8, 1973.

156 Russell, R. O., Jr., and Rackley, C. E.: "Hemodynamic Monitoring in a Coronary Intensive Care Unit," Futura Publishing Co., Mount Kisco, N.Y., 1974, p. 284.

157 Miller, R. R., Olson, H. G., Vismara, L. A., Bogren, H. G., Amsterdam, E. A., and Mason, D. T.: Pump Dysfunction after Myocardial Infarction: Importance of Location, Extent and Pattern of Abnormal Left Ventricular Segmental Contraction, *Am. J. Cardiol.,* 37:340, 1976.

158 Haddy, F. J.: Pathophysiology and Therapy of the Shock of Myocardial Infarction, *Ann. Intern. Med.,* 73:809, 1970.

159 Scheidt, S., Ascheim, R., and Killip, T., III: Shock after Acute Myocardial Infarction: A Clinical and Hemodynamic Profile, *Am. J. Cardiol.,* 26:556, 1970.

160 Cohn, J. N., and Franciosa, J. A.: Pathophysiology of Shock in Acute Myocardial Infarction, in P. N. Yu and J. F. Goodwin (eds.): "Progress in Cardiology," vol. 2, Lea & Febiger, Philadelphia, 1973, p. 207.

161 Kones, R. J.: Cardiogenic Shock: "Mechanism and Management," Futura Publishing Co., Mount Kisco, N.Y., 1974, p. 386.

162 Swan, H. J. C., Forrester, J. S., Diamond, G., Chatterjee, K., Parmley, W. W., and Mirsky, I: A Conceptual Model of Myocardial Infarction and Cardiogenic Shock, in I. Mirsky, D. N. Ghista, and H. Sandler (eds.): "Cardiac Mechanics," John Wiley & Sons, Inc., New York, 1974, p. 359.

163 O'Rourke, M. F. O., Chang, V. P., Windsor, H. M., Shanahan, M. X., Hickie, J. B., Morgan, J. J., Gunning, J. F., Seldon, A. W., Hall, G. V., Mitchell, G., Goldfarb, D., and Harrison, D. G.: Acute Severe Cardiac Failure Complicating Myocardial Infarction: Experience with 100 Patients Referred for Consideration of Mechanical Left Ventricular Assistance, *Br. Heart J.,* 37:169, 1975.

164 Daluz, P. L., Weil, M. H., and Shubin, H.: Current Concepts on Mechanisms and Treatment of Cardiogenic Shock, *Am. Heart J.,* 92:103, 1976.

165 Peterson, D. F., Kaspar, R. L., and Bishop, V. S.: Reflex Tachycardia Due to Temporary Coronary Occlusion in the Conscious Dog. *Circ. Res.,* 32:652, 1973.

166 Peterson, D. F., and Bishop, V. S.: Reflex Blood Pressure Control during Acute Myocardial Ischemia in the Conscious Dog, *Circ. Res.,* 34:226, 1974.

167 Russell, R. O., Jr., Rackley, C. E., Pombo, J., Hunt, D., Potanin, C., and Dodge, H. T.: Effects of Increasing Left Ventricular Filling Pressure in Patients with Acute Myocardial Infarction, *J. Clin. Invest.,* 49:1539, 1970.

168 Costantin, I. R.: Extracardiac Factors Contributing to Hypotension During Coronary Occlusion, *Am. J. Cardiol.,* 11:205, 1963.

169 Epstein, S. E., Stampfer, M., and Beiser, G. D.: Role of the Capacitance and Resistance Vessels in Vasovagal Syncope, *Circulation,* 37:524, 1960.

170 Andersen, H. T.: Physiological Adaptations in Diving Vertebrates, *Physiol. Rev.,* 46:212, 1966.

171 Cohn, J. N.: Blood Pressure Measurement in Shock, *J.A.M.A.,* 199:972, 1967.

172 Harnarayan, C., Bennett, M. A., Penetecost, B. L., and Brewer, D. B.: Quantitative Study of Infarcted Myocardium in Cardiogenic Shock, *Br. Heart J.,* 32:728, 1970.

173 Page, D. L., Caufield, J. B., Kastor, J. A., De Sanctis, R. W., and Sanders, C. A.: Myocardial Changes Associated with Cardiogenic Shock, *N. Engl. J. Med.,* 285:133, 1971.

174 Lefer, A. M.: Blood-borne Humoral Factors in the Pathophysiology of Circulatory Shock, *Circ. Res.,* 32:129, 1973.

175 Hosoho, K., and Okuda, M.: Myocardial Depressant Factor in Cardiogenic Shock, *Am. Heart J.,* 91:126, 1976.

176 Robinson, B. F., Collier, J., and Nachev, C.: Changes in Peripheral Venous Compliance after Myocardial Infarction, *Cardiovasc. Res.,* 6:67, 1972.

177 Kostuk, W. J., Suwa, K., Bernstein, E. F., and Sobel, B. E.: Altered Hemoglobin Oxygen Affinity in Patients with Acute Myocardial Infarction, *Am. J. Cardiol.,* 31:295, 1973.

178 Knutsen, B., and Broch, O. J.: Haemodynamics in Acute Pulmonary Oedema in Coronary Patients, *Acta Med. Scand.,* 183:531, 1968.

179 Dodek, A., Kassenbaum, D. G., and Bristow, J. D.: Pulmonary Edema in Coronary Artery Disease without Cardiomegaly: Paradox of the Stiff Heart, *N. Engl. J. Med.,* 286:1347, 1972.

180 McCredie, R. M., and Chia, B. L.: Measurement of Pulmonary Oedema in Ischaemic Heart Disease, *Br. Heart J.,* 35:1136, 1973.

181 Klein, M. D., Herman, M. V., and Gorlin, R.: A Hemodynamic Study of Left Ventricular Aneurysm, *Circulation,* 35:614, 1967.

182 Rosenthal, J. E., Daroca, P. J., Jr., and Cohen, L. S.: Rupture of Chronic Left Ventricular Aneurysm after Acute Coronary Thrombosis, *Am. J. Cardiol.,* 30:547, 1972.

183 Van Tassel, R. A., and Edwards, J. E.: Rupture of Heart Complicating Myocardial Infarction: Analysis of 40 Cases Including Nine Examples of Left Ventricular False Aneurysm, *Chest,* 61:104, 1972.

184 Harvey, W. P.: Some Pertinent Physical Findings in the Clinical Evaluation of Acute Myocardial Infarction, *Circulation,* 39-40(suppl. 4):175, 1969.

185 Heikkilä, J., Luomanmaki, K., and Pyörälä, K.: Serial Observations on Left Ventricular Dysfunction in Acute Myocardial Infarction: I. Gallop Sounds, Ventricular Asynergy and Radiological Signs, *Acta Med. Scand.,* 190:89, 1971.

186 Mundth, E. D., Buckley, M. J., Daggett, W. M., Sanders, C. A., and Austen, W. G.: Surgery for Complications of Acute Myocardial Infarction, *Circulation,* 45:1279, 1972.

187 Kouchoukos, N. T., Doty, D. B., Buettner, L. E., and Kirklin, J. W.: Treatment of Postinfarction Cardiac Failure by Myocardial Excision and Revascularization, *Circulation,* 45-46(suppl. 1):72, 1972.

188 Tesler, U. F., and Lemole, G. M.: The Surgical Treatment of Postinfarction Left Ventricular Aneurysm, *Eur. J. Cardiol.,* 2:407, 1975.

189 Cullhead, I., Delius, W., Björk, L., Hallen, A., and Nordgren,

L.: Resection of Left Ventricular Aneurysm: Late Results, *Acta Med. Scand.*, 197:241, 1975.

190 Heikkilä, J.: Mitral Incompetence as a Complication of Acute Myocardial Infarction, *Acta Med. Scand.*, 182 (suppl. 475):1, 1967.

191 Morrow, A. G., Cohen, L. S., Roberts, W. C., Braunwald, N. S., and Braunwald, E.: Severe Mitral Regurgitation following Acute Myocardial Infarction and Ruptured Papillary Muscle: Hemodynamic Findings and Results of Operative Treatment in Four Patients, *Circulation*, 37(suppl. 2):124, 1968.

191a Vlodaver, Z., and Edwards, E.: Rupture of Ventricular Septum or Papillary Muscle Complicating Myocardial Infarction, *Circulation*, 55:815, 1977.

192 Falcone, M. W., Ronan, J. A., Jr., and Roberts, W. C.: Silent Mitral Regurgitation Complicating Silent Myocardial Infarction: Hemodynamic and Morphologic Documentation, *Chest*, 62:226, 1972.

193 Barlow, J. B., Bosman, C. K., Pocock, W. A., and Marchand, P.: Late Systolic Murmurs and Nonejection ("Mid-late") Systolic Clicks: An Analysis of 90 Patients, *Br. Heart J.*, 30:203, 1968.

193a Barlow, J. B., and Pocock, W. A.: The Problem of Nonejection Systolic Clicks and Associated Mitral Systolic Murmurs: Emphasis on the Billowing Mitral Valve Leaflet Syndrome, *Am. Heart J.*, 90:636, 1975.

194 Heikkilä, J.: The Fate of Mitral Valve Complex in Acute Myocardial Infarction, *Ann. Clin, Res.*, 3:386, 1971.

195 Sanders, C. A., Austen, W. G., Harthorne, J. W., Dinsmore, R. E., and Scannell, J. G.: Diagnosis and Surgical Treatment of Mitral Regurgitation Secondary to Ruptured Chordae Tendineae, *N. Engl. J. Med.*, 276:943, 1967.

196 Cederqvist, L., and Söderström, J.: Papillary Muscle Rupture in Myocardial Infarction: A Study Based upon an Autopsy Material, *Acta Med. Scand.*, 176:287, 1964.

197 Eisenberg, S., and Suyemoto, J.: Rupture of a Papillary Muscle of the Tricuspid Valve following Acute Myocardial Infarction: Report of a Case, *Circulation*, 30:588, 1964.

198 Estes, E. H., Jr., Dalton, F. M., Entman, M. L., Dixon, H. B., II, and Hackel, D. B.: The Anatomy and Blood Supply of the Papillary Muscles of the Left Ventricle, *Am. Heart J.*, 71:356, 1966.

199 Symbas, P. N., Ferrier, F. L., Sybers, R. G., and Underwood, F. O.: Mitral Valve Function after Experimental Papillary or Left Ventricular Myocardial Infarction, *Curr. Top. Surg. Res.*, 2:451, 1970.

200 Mittal, A. K., Langston, M., Jr., Cohn, K. E., Selzer, A., and Kerth, W. J.: Combined Papillary Muscle and Left Ventricular Wall Dysfunction as a Cause of Mitral Regurgitation: An Experimental Study, *Circulation*, 44:174, 1971.

201 Bailey, R. R., Abernethy, M. H., and Beaven, D. W.: Adrenocortical Response to the Stress of an Acute Myocardial Infarction, *Lancet*, 1:970, 1967.

202 Jarisch, A., and Zotterman, Y.: Depressor Reflexes from the Heart, *Acta Physiol. Scand.*, 16:31, 1948.

203 Frink, R. J., and James, T. N.: Intracardiac Route of the Bezold-Jarisch Reflex, *Am. J. Physiol.*, 221:1464, 1971.

204 Dawes, G. S., and Comroe, J. J., Jr.: Chemoreflexes from the Heart and Lungs, *Physiol. Rev.*, 34:167, 1954.

205 Paintal, A. S.: A Study of Ventricular Pressure Receptors and Their Role in the Bezold Reflex, *Q. J. Exp. Physiol.*, 40:348, 1955.

206 Neil, E.: Afferent Impulse Activity in Cardiovascular Receptor Fibers, *Physiol. Rev.*, 40(suppl. 4):201, 1960.

207 Linden, R. J.: Reflexes from Receptors in the Heart, *Cardiology*, 61(suppl. 1):7, 1976.

208 Mancia, G., Lorenz, R. R., and Shepherd, J. T.: Reflex Control of Circulation by Heart and Lungs, in A. C. Guyton and A. W. Cowley, Jr. (eds.): "Cardiovascular Physiology II," vol. 9, University Park Press, Baltimore, Maryland, 1976, p. 111.

209 Harman, M. A., and Reeves, T. J.: Effects of Efferent Vagal Stimulation on Atrial and Ventricular Function, *Am. J. Physiol.*, 215:1210, 1968.

210 Bergel, D. H., and Makin, G. S.: Central and Peripheral Cardiovascular Changes following Chemical Stimulation of the Surface of the Dog Heart, *Cardiovasc. Res.*, 1:80, 1967.

211 Malliani, A., Peterson, D. F., Bishop, V. S., and Brown, A. M.: Spinal Sympathetic Cardiocardiac Reflexes, *Circ. Res.*, 30:158, 1972.

212 Hanley, H. G., Costin, J. C., and Skinner, N. S., Jr.: Differential Reflex Adjustments in Cutaneous and Muscle Vascular Beds during Experimental Coronary Artery Occlusion, *Am. J. Cardiol.*, 27:513, 1971.

213 Thoren, P.: Evidence for a Depressor Reflex Elicited from Left Ventricular Receptors during Occlusion of One Coronary Artery in the Cat, *Acta Physiol. Scand.*, 88:23, 1973.

214 Schwartz, P. J., Pagani, M., Lombardi, F., Malliani, A., and Brown, A. M.: A Cardiocardiac Sympathovagal Reflex in the Cat, *Circ. Res.*, 32:215, 1973.

215 Linden, R. J.: Function of Cardiac Receptors, *Circulation*, 48:463, 1973.

216 Kezdi, P., Kordenat, R. K., and Misra, S. N.: Reflex Inhibitory Effects of Vagal Afferents in Experimental Myocardial Infarction, *Am. J. Cardiol.*, 33:853, 1974.

217 Mark, A. L., Abboud, F. M., Heistad, D. D., Schmid, P. G., and Johannsen, U. J.: Evidence against the Presence of Ventricular Chemoreceptors Activated by Hypoxia and Hypercapnia, *Am. J. Physiol.*, 227:178, 1974.

218 Staszewska-Barczak, J., Ferreira, S. H., and Vane, J. R.: An Excitatory Nociceptive Cardiac Reflex Elicited by Bradykinin and Potentiated by Prostaglandins and Myocardial Ischaemia, *Cardiovasc. Res.*, 10:314, 1976.

219 Lloyd, T. C., Jr.: Control of Systemic Vascular Resistance by Pulmonary and Left Heart Baroreflexes, *Am. J. Physiol.*, 222:1511, 1972.

220 Shepherd, J. T.: Intrathoracic Baroreflexes, *Mayo Clin. Proc.*, 48:426, 1973.

221 Chevalier, P. A., Weber, K. C., Lyons, G. W., Nicoloff, D. M., and Fox, I. J.: Hemodynamic Changes from Stimulation of Left Ventricular Baroreceptors, *Am. J. Physiol.*, 227:719, 1974.

222 Mancia, G., and Donald, D. E.: Demonstration that the Atria, Ventricles, and Lungs Each Are Responsible for a Tonic Inhibition of the Vasomotor Center in the Dog, *Circ. Res.*, 36:310, 1975.

223 Mancia, G., Shepherd, J. T., and Donald, D. E.: Role of Cardiac, Pulmonary, and Carotid Mechanoreceptors in the Control of Hind-Limb and Renal Circulation in Dogs, *Circ. Res.*, 37:200, 1975.

224 Szentiványi, M., and Juhász-Nagy, A.: Two Types of Coronary Vasomotor Reflexes, *Q. J. Exp. Physiol.*, 47:289, 1962.

225 Grayson, J., Irvine, M., Parratt, J. R., and Cunningham, J.: Vasospastic Elements in Myocardial Infarction following Coronary Occlusion in the Dog, *Cardiovasc. Res.*, 2:54, 1968.

226 Joyce. E. E., and Gregg, D. E.: Coronary Artery Occlusion in the Intact Unanesthetized Dog: Intercoronary Reflexes, *Am. J. Physiol.*, 213:64, 1967.

227 Weissler, A. M., Lewis, R. P., and Leighton, R. F.: The Systolic Time Intervals as a Measure of Left Ventricular Performance in Man, in P. N. Yr and J. F. Goodwin (eds.): "Progress In Cardiology," vol. 1, Lea & Febiger, Philadephia, 1972, p. 155.

228 Lewis, R. P., Boudoulas, H., Forester, W. F., and Weissler, A. M.: Shortening of Electromechanical Systole as a Manifesta-

tion of Excessive Adrenergic Stimulation in Acute Myocardial Infarction, *Circulation*, 46:856, 1972.

229 Lewis, R. P., Boudoulas, H., Welch, T. G., and Forester, W. F.: Usefulness of Systolic Time Intervals in Coronary Artery Disease, *Am. J. Cardiol.*, 37:787, 1976.

230 Lown, B., Kosowsky, B. D., and Klein, M. D.: Pathogenesis, Prevention, and Treatment of Arrhythmias in Myocardial Infarction, *Circulation*, 39-40 (suppl. 4):261, 1969.

231 James, T. N.: Pathogenesis of Arrhythmias in Acute Myocardial Infarction, *Am. J. Cardiol.*, 24:791, 1969.

232 Han, J.: Mechanisms of Ventricular Arrhythmias Associated with Myocardial Infarction, *Am. J. Cardiol.*, 24:800, 1969.

233 Han, J.: Ventricular Vulnerability during Acute Coronary Occlusion, *Am. J. Cardiol.*, 24:857, 1969.

234 DeSanctis, R. W., Block, P., and Hutter, A. M., Jr.: Tachyarrhythmias in Myocardial Infarction, *Circulation*, 45:681, 1972.

235 Kent, K. M., and Epstein, S. E.: Neural Basis for the Genesis and Control of Arrhythmias Associated with Myocardial Infarction, *Cardiology*, 61:61, 1976.

236 Garrey, W. E.: The Nature of Fibrillary Contraction of the Heart: Its Relation to Tissue Mass and Form, *Am. J. Physiol.*, 33:397, 1914.

237 Han, J., and Moe, G. K.: Nonuniform Recovery of Excitability in Ventricular Muscle, *Circ. Res.*, 14:44, 1964.

238 Sukumalchantra, Y., Danzig, R., Levy, S. E., and Swan, H. J. C.: The Mechanism of Arterial Hypoxemia in Acute Myocardial Infarction, *Circulation*, 41:641, 1970.

239 Fillmore, S. J., Guimaraes, A. C., Scheidt, S. S., and Killip, T., III: Blood-Gas Changes and Pulmonary Hemodynamics following Acute Myocardial Infarction, *Circulation*, 45:583, 1972.

240 Helmers, C., Mogensen, L., Nordlander, R., Orinius, E., Sjogren, A., and Webster, P. O.: Acid-Base Disturbances in Patients with Acute Myocardial Infarction, *Acta Med. Scand.*, 194:421, 1973.

241 Davidson, R. M., Ramo, B. W., Wallace, A. G., Whalen, R. E., and Starmer, C. F.: Blood-Gas and Hemodynamic Responses to Oxygen in Acute Myocardial Infarction, *Circulation*, 47:704, 1973.

242 Buschmann, H. J., Dissmann, W., Siemon, G., Sonderkamp, H., and Schroder, R.: Die arterielle Hypoxamie bei akutem Myokardinfarkt, *Klin. Wochenschr.*, 45:113, 1967.

243 Harrison, D. C.: Potential Hazards and Benefits of Oxygen Therapy and Morphine in Acute Myocardial Infarction, in E. Corday and H. J. C. Swan (eds.): "Myocardial Infarction: New Perspectives in Diagnosis and Management," The Williams & Williams Company, Baltimore, 1973, p. 279.

244 Pilcher, J., and Nagle, R. E.: Acid Base Imbalance and Arrhythmias after Myocardial Infarction, *Br. Heart J.*, 33:526, 1971.

245 Ng, M. L., Levy, M. N., DeGeest, H., and Zieske, H.: Effects of Myocardial Hypoxia on Left Ventricular Performance, *Am. J. Physiol.*, 211:43, 1966.

246 Serur, J. R., Skelton, C. L., Bodem, R., and Sonnenblick, E. H.: Respiratory Acid-Base Changes and Myocardial Contractility: Interaction between Calcium and Hydrogen Ions, *J. Mol. Cell. Cardiol.*, 8:823, 1976.

247 Prakash, R., Parmley, W. W., Horvat, M., and Swan, H. J. C.: Serum Cortisol, Plasma Free Fatty Acids and Urinary Catecholamines as Indicators of Complications in Acute Myocardial Infarction, *Circulation*, 45:736, 1972.

248 Lukomsky, P. E., and Oganov, R. G.: Blood Plasma Catecholamines and Their Urinary Excretion in Patients with Acute Myocardial Infarction, *Am. Heart J.*, 83:182, 1972.

249 Videback, J., Christensen, N. J., and Sterndorff, B.: Serial Determination of Plasma Catecholamines in Myocardial Infarction, *Circulation*, 46:846, 1972.

250 Chopra, M. P., Thadani, U., Aber, C. P., Portal, R. W., and Parkes, J.: Plasma Cortisol, Urinary 17-Hydroxycorticoids, and Urinary Vanyl Mandelic Acid after Acute Myocardial Infarction, *Br. Heart J.*, 34:992, 1972.

251 Nitter-Hauge, S., Kirkeby, K., Alvsaker, J.-O., and Aakvaag, A.: Plasma II-Hydroxycorticosteroids in Acute Myocardial Infarction, *Acta Med. Scand.*, 192:535, 1972.

252 Kurien, V. A., and Oliver, M. F.: Free Fatty Acids during Acute Myocardial Infarction, *Prog. Cardiovasc. Dis.*, 13:361, 1971.

253 Datey, K. K., and Nanda, N. C.: Hyperglycemia after Acute Myocardial Infarction: Its Relation to Diabetes Mellitus, *N. Engl. J. Med.*, 276:262, 1967.

254 Barrera, F., Ascanio, G., Boutwell, J. H., Panis, M. P., and Oppenheimer, M. J.: Importance of Myocardial Catecholamines in Myocardial Infarction, *Am. J. Med. Sci.*, 252:177, 1966.

255 Klocke, F. J., Kaiser, G. A., Ross, J., Jr., and Braunwald, E.: Mechanism of Increase of Myocardial Oxygen Uptake Produced by Catecholamines, *Am. J. Physiol.*, 209:913, 1965.

256 Cassell, P., and Nicholson, R.: Perforation of Peptic Ulcer Complicating Myocardial Infarction, *Br. Heart J.*, 29:129, 1967.

257 Fredrickson, D. S.: The Role of Lipids in Acute Myocardial Infarction, *Circulation*, 39-40(suppl. 4):99, 1969.

258 Fyfe, T., Baxter, R. H., Cochran, K. M., and Booth, E. M.: Plasma-Lipid Changes after Myocardial Infarction, *Lancet*, 2:997, 1971.

259 Burch, G. E., and DePasquale, N. P.: The Hematocrit in Patients with Myocardial Infarction, *J.A.M.A.*, 180:62, 1962.

260 Jan, K.-M., Chien, S., and Bigger, J. T., Jr.: Observations on Blood Viscosity Changes after Acute Myocardial Infarction, *Circulation*, 51:1079, 1975.

261 Mayer, G. A.: Hemotocrit and Coronary Heart Disease, *Can. Med. Assoc. J.*, 93:1151, 1965.

262 Thomas, M., Malmcrona, R., Fillmore, S., and Shillingford, J. J.: Haemodynamic Effects of Morphine in Patients with Acute Myocardial Infarction, *Br. Heart J.*, 27:863, 1965.

263 Vasko, J. S., Henney, R. P., Oldham, H. N., Brawley, R. K., and Morrow, A. G.: Mechanisms of Action of Morphine in the Treatment of Experimental Pulmonary Edema, *Am. J. Cardiol.*, 18:876, 1966.

264 Henney, R. P., Vasko, J. S., Brawley, R. K., Oldham, H. N., and Morrow, A. G.: The Effects of Morphine on the Resistance and Capacitance Vessels of the Peripheral Circulation, *Am. Heart J.*, 72:242, 1966.

265 Pur-Shahriari, A. A., Mills, R. A., Hoppin, F. G., Jr., and Dexter, L.: Comparison of Chronic and Acute Effects of Morphine Sulfate on Cardiovascular Function, *Am. J. Cardiol.*, 20:654, 1967.

266 Hoel, B. L., and Refsum, H. E.: The Effect of Morphine on Arterial Blood Gases in Patients with Acute Myocardial Infarction, *Acta Med. Scand.*, 186:511, 1969.

267 Grendahl, H., and Hansteen, V.: The Effect of Morphine on Blood Pressure and Cardiac Output in Patients with Acute Myocardial Infarction, *Acta Med. Scand.*, 186:515, 1969.

268 Ward, J. M., McGrath, R. L., and Weil, J. V.: Effects of Morphine on the Peripheral Vascular Response to Sympathetic Stimulation, *Am. J. Cardiol.*, 29:659, 1972.

269 Zelis, R., Mansour, E. J., Capone, R. J., and Mason, D. T.: The Cardiovascular Effects of Morphine: The Peripheral Capacitance and Resistance Vessels in Human Subjects, *J. Clin. Invest.*, 54:1247, 1974.

270 Vismara, L. A., Leaman, D. M., and Zelis, R.: The Effects of Morphine on Venous Tone in Patients with Acute Pulmonary Edema, *Circulation*, 54:335, 1976.

271 Vasko, J. S., Henney, R. P., Brawley, R. K., Oldham, H. N., and Morrow, A. G.: The Effects of Morphine on Ventricular

Function and Myocardial Contractile Force, *Am. J. Physiol.,* 210:329, 1966.

272 Adolph, R. J., Stephens, J. F., and Tanaka, K.: The Clinical Value of Frequency Analysis of the First Heart Sound in Myocardial Infarction, *Circulation,* 41:1003, 1970.

273 Hill, J. C., O'Rourke, R. A., Lewis, R. P., and McGranahan, G. M.: The Diagnostic Value of the Atrial Gallop in Acute Myocardial Infarction, *Am. Heart J.,* 78:194, 1969.

274 Cohn, P. F., Vokonas, P. S., Williams, R. A., Herman, M. V., and Gorlin, R.: Diastolic Heart Sounds and Filling Waves in Coronary Artery Disease, *Circulation,* 44:196, 1971.

275 Selzer, A., Gerbode, F., and Kerth, W. J.: Clinical, Hemodynamic and Surgical Considerations of Rupture of the Ventricular Septum after Myocardial Infarction, *Am. Heart J.,* 78: 598, 1969.

276 Longo, E. A., and Cohen, L. S.: Rupture of Interventricular Septum in Acute Myocardial Infarction, *Am. Heart J.,* 92:81, 1976.

277 Fischer, T., and Oó, M.: Study of the Diastolic Murmur in Heart Aneurysm, *Cardiologia,* 50:56, 1967.

278 Fearon, R. E., Cohen, L. S., O'Hara, J. M., and Goodyer, A. V. N.: Diastolic Murmurs Due to Two Sequelae of Atherosclerotic Coronary Artery Disease: Ventricular Aneurysm and Coronary Artery Stenosis, *Am. Heart J.,* 76:252, 1968.

279 Cheng, T. O.: Diastolic Murmur Caused by Coronary Artery Stenosis, *Ann. Intern. Med.,* 72:543, 1970.

280 Lewis, A. J., Burchell, H. B., and Titus, J. L.: Clinical and Pathologic Features of Postinfarction Cardiac Rupture, *Am. J. Cardiol.,* 23:43, 1969.

281 Friedman, H. S., Kuhn, L. A., and Katz, A. M.: Clinical and Electrocardiographic Features of Cardiac Rupture following Acute Myocardial Infarction, *Am. J. Med.,* 50:709, 1971.

282 Biorck, G., Morgensen, L., Nyquist, O., Orinius, E., and Sjogren, A.: Studies in Myocardial Rupture with Cardiac Tamponade in Acute Myocardial Infarction: I. Clinical Features, *Chest,* 61:4, 1972.

283 Mogensen, L., Nyquist, O., Orinius, E., and Sjogren, A.: Studies of Myocardial Rupture with Cardiac Tamponade in Acute Myocardial Infarction: II. Electrocardiographic Changes, *Chest,* 61:6, 1972.

284 Naeim, F., de la Maza, L. M., and Robbins, S. L.: Cardiac Rupture during Myocardial Infarction: A Review of 44 Cases, *Circulation,* 45:1231, 1972.

285 Mundth, E. D.: Rupture of the Heart Complicating Myocardial Infarction, *Circulation,* 46:427, 1972.

285a Penther, P., Gerbaux, A., Blanc, J. J., Morin, J. F., and Julienne, J. L.: Myocardial Infarction and Rupture of Heart—Macroscopic Pathologic Study, *Am. Heart J.,* 93:302, 1977.

286 Bjork, L., Cullhed, I., and Buchholtz, B.: Left Ventricular Function in Ischemic Heart Disease: Angiocardiographic and Hemodynamic Studies, *Acta Med. Scand.,* 190:223, 1971.

287 Hamilton, G. W., Murray, J. A., and Kennedy, J. W.: Quantitative Angiocardiography in Ischemic Heart Disease: The Spectrum of Abnormal Left Ventricular Function and the Role of Abnormally Contracting Segments, *Circulation,* 45: 1065, 1972.

288 Rahimtoola, S. H., DiGilio, M. M., Ehsani, A., Loeb, H. S., Rosen, K. M., and Gunnar, R. M.: Changes in Left Ventricular Performance from Early after Acute Myocardial Infarction to the Convalescent Phase, *Circulation,* 46:770, 1972.

289 Feild, B. J., Russell, R. O., Jr., Moraski, R. E., Soto, B., Hood, W. P., Jr., Burdeshaw, J. A., Smith, M., Maurer, B. J., and Rackley, C. E.: Left Ventricular Size and Function and Heart Size in the Year following Myocardial Infarction, *Circulation,* 50:331, 1974.

290 Thomas, M., and Shillingford, J.: The Circulatory Response to a Standard Postural Change in Ischaemic Heart Disease, *Br. Heart J.,* 27:17, 1965.

291 Abelmann, W. H.: Alterations in Orthostatic Tolerance after

Myocardial Infarction and in Congestive Heart Failure, *Cardiology,* 61(suppl. 1):236, 1976.

292 Messer, J. V., Levine, H. J., Wagman, R. J., and Gorlin, R.: Effect of Exercise on Cardiac Performance in Human Subjects with Coronary Artery Disease, *Circulation,* 28:404, 1963.

293 Parker, J. O., West, R. O., and Di Giorgi, S.: The Hemodynamic Response to Exercise in Patients with Healed Myocardial Infarction without Angina: With Observations on the Effects of Nitroglycerin, *Circulation,* 36:734, 1967.

293a Henning, H., Crawford, M. H., Karliner, J. S., and O'Rourke, R. A.: Beneficial Effects of Nitroglycerin on Abnormal Ventricular Wall Motion at Rest and during Exercise in Patients with Previous Myocardial Infarction, *Am. J. Cardiol.,* 37:623, 1976.

294 Follath, F.: Central Venous Pressure and Cardiac Output during Exercise in Coronary Artery Disease, *Br. Heart J.,* 29:714, 1967.

295 Detry, J.-M. R., Rousseau, M., Vanderbroucke, G., Kusumi, F., Brasseur, L. A., and Bruce, R. A.: Increased Arteriovenous Oxygen Difference after Physical Training in Coronary Heart Disease, *Circulation,* 44:109, 1971.

296 McHenry, P. L., Morris, S. N., Kavalier, M., and Jordan, J. W.: Comparative Study of Exercise-induced Ventricular Arrhythmias in Normal Subjects and Patients with Documented Coronary Artery Disease, *Am. J. Cardiol.,* 37:609, 1976.

297 Donald, K. W., Lind, A. R., McNicol, G. W., Humphreys, P. W., Taylor, S. H., and Staunton, H. P.: Cardiovascular Responses to Sustained (Static) Contractions, *Circ. Res.,* 20(suppl. 1):15, 1967.

298 Lind, A. R., and McNicol, G. W.: Circulatory Responses to Sustained Hand-Grip Contractions Performed during Other Exercise, Both Rhythmic and Static, *J. Physiol.,* 192:595, 1967.

299 Nutter, D. O., Schlant, R. C., and Hurst, J. W.: Isometric Exercise and the Cardiovascular System, *Mod. Concepts Cardiovasc. Dis.,* 41:11, 1972.

300 Jackson, D. H., Reeves, T. J., Sheffield, L. T., and Burdeshaw, J.: Isometric Effects on Treadmill Exercise Response in Healthy Young Men, *Am. J. Cardiol.,* 31:344, 1973.

301 Quarry, V. M., and Spodick, D. H.: Cardiac Responses to Isometric Exercise: Comparative Effects with Different Postures and Levels of Exertion, *Circulation,* 48:905, 1974.

302 Quinones, M. A., Gaasch, W. H., Waisser, E., Thiel, H. G., and Alexander, J. K.: An Analysis of the Left Ventricular Response to Isometric Exercise, *Am. Heart J.,* 88:29, 1974.

303 Weissler, A. M., Harris, W. S., and Schoenfeld, C. D.: Bedside Technics for the Evaluation of Ventricular Function in Men, *Am. J. Cardiol.,* 23:577, 1969.

304 Garrard, C. L., Jr., Weissler, A. M., and Dodge, H. T.: The Relationship of Alterations in Systolic Time Intervals to Ejection Fraction in Patients with Cardiac Disease, *Circulation,* 42:455, 1970.

305 Masters, W. H., and Johnson, V. E.: "Human Sexual Response," Little, Brown and Company, Boston, 1966, p. 174.

306 Hellerstein, H. K., and Friedman, E. H.: Sexual Activity and the Postcoronary Patient, *Med. Aspects Hum. Sexuality,* 3:70, 1969.

307 Nemec, E. D., Mansfield, L., and Kennedy, J. W.: Heart Rate and Blood Pressure Responses during Sexual Activity in Normal Males, *Am. Heart J.,* 92:274, 1976.

308 Heggtveit, H. A.: La Mort d'amour, *Am. Heart J.,* 69:287, 1965.

309 Rabinowitz, M.: Overview on Pathogenesis of Cardiac Hypertrophy, *Circ. Res.,* 35:(suppl 2):3, 1974.

310 Zaino, E. C., and Tabor, S. H.: Cardiac Hypertrophy in Acute

Myocardial Infarction: A Study Based on 100 Autopsied Cases, *Circulation*, 28:1081, 1963,

311 Linzbach, A. J.: Heart Failure from the Point of View of Quantitative Anatomy, *Am. J. Cardiol.,* 5:370, 1960.

312 Forster, R. E.: Oxygenation of the Muscle Cell, *Circ. Res.,* 20-21 (suppl. 1):115, 1967.

313 Burch, G. E., Tsui, C. Y., and Harb, J. M.: Ischemic Cardiomyopathy, *Am. Heart J.,* 83:340, 1972.

314 Burch, G. E.: Ischemic Cardiomyopathy, *Am. Heart J.,* 86:276, 1973.

315 Yatteau, R. F., Peter, R. H., Behar, V. S., Bartel, A. G., Rosati, R. A., and Kong, Y.: Ischemic Cardiomyopathy: The Myopathy of Coronary Artery Disease: Natural History and Results of Medical Versus Surgical Treatment, *Am. J. Cardiol.,* 34:520, 1974.

316 Schaper, W.: Pathophysiology of Coronary Circulation, *Prog. Cardiovasc. Dis.,* 14:275, 1971.

317 Schaper, W.: "The Collateral Circulation of the Heart," American Elsevier Publishing Company, Inc., New York, 1971.

318 Knoebel, S. B., McHenry, P. L., Phillips, J. F., and Pauletto, F. J.: Coronary Collateral Circulation and Myocardial Blood Flow Reserve, *Circulation,* 46:84, 1972.

319 Cosby, R. S., Giddings, J. A., and See, J. R.: Coronary Collateral Circulation, *Chest,* 66:27, 1974.

319a Wechsler, A. S.: Development of Coronary Collateral Circulation, *Ann. Rev. Med.,* 28:341, 1977.

E
The Clinical Recognition and Management of Coronary Atherosclerotic Heart Disease[1-1c]

J. WILLIS HURST, M.D.,
R. BRUCE LOGUE, M.D., and
PAUL F. WALTER, M.D.

But there is a disorder of the breast marked with strong and peculiar symptoms, considerable for the kind of danger belonging to it, and not extremely rare, which deserves to be mentioned at length. The seat of it, and sense of strangling and anxiety with which it is attended, may make it not improperly be called angina pectoris.

WILLIAM HEBERDEN,* M.D. 1768[2]

Obstruction of a coronary artery or of any of its large branches has long been regarded as a serious accident. Several events contributed toward the prevalence of the view that this condition was almost always suddenly fatal. . . . But there are reasons for believing that even large branches of the coronary arteries may be occluded—at times acutely occluded—without resulting death, at least without death in the immediate future. Even the main trunk may at times be obstructed and the patient live. It is

*The original mention of angina pectoris was made by Heberden in a lecture before the Royal College of Physicians of London in July 1768 and published in their Medical Transactions in 1786 (II, 59) under the title "Some Account of a Disorder of the Breast,"[3]

the object of this paper to present a few facts along this line, and particularly to describe some of the clinical manifestations of sudden yet not immediately fatal cases of coronary obstruction.

JAMES HERRICK, M.D., 1912[4]

"Acute coronary insufficiency" is a syndrome of a more severe myocardial ischemia and is associated with myocardial damage. It is associated with a precipitating factor which decreases coronary flow or which increases the work of the heart and oxygen requirement of the heart muscle . . . -

ARTHUR M. MASTER, M.D., 1944[5]

INTRODUCTION

No field of medicine is changing more rapidly than the area related to coronary atherosclerotic heart disease. New information is being generated daily as a result of coronary arteriographic studies and coronary bypass surgery. Blumgart, Schlesinger, and Zoll taught us many new concepts as a result of their elegant postmortem injections of the coronary arteries.[6] The principles they taught us take on enormous meaning now that the anatomy of the coronary arteries can be delineated in a living patient. The technique of coronary arteriography was developed by Mason Sones in the late 1950s.[7] Innovative cardiac surgeons of the past attempted but failed in their efforts to "revascularize" the myocardium of patients with coronary atherosclerotic heart disease. Present-day surgeons have been remarkably successful in revascularization by coronary bypass surgery. Sabiston performed the first coronary bypass on April 4, 1962,[7a] using an end-to-end technique. Garrett and DeBakey were the first to use the end-to-side method of coronary bypass in 1965.[8] The technique was further developed by Favaloro, Effler, Johnson, Cooley, Kirklin, Austin, Spencer, and many others. Our own observations are based on the superb work of Hatcher, Jones, Craver, Miller, Symbas, and Williams of Emory University. Whereas in the past nitroglycerin was the only reliable drug available for the treatment of angina pectoris, we now have beta-blockers (for example, propranolol) that are extremely useful in the prevention of such attacks.[9] Isosorbide is more useful than the previously used "long-acting" nitrites in relieving angina pectoris. The treatment of myocardial infarction and its complications is changing rapidly because of new modes of medical and surgical therapy. The importance and need to classify the numerous clinical syndromes is now more generally understood. This effort, which has culminated in the taxonomy discussed in Chap. 62A, has been a major interest of one of us (J.W.H.) for the last 20 years. Now, new and fresh ideas regarding the recognition and management of certain aspects of coronary atherosclerosis are flowing more abundantly than they were 10 years ago. It is an exciting era.

Unfortunately, less progress has been made in the prevention of coronary atherosclerotic heart disease. The old ideas involving "risk factor" prevention are still being polished, but new ideas are sparse. Unfortunately, the current methods of prevention (Chap.

62H) have not gained universal popular acceptance, and the value of this approach is not absolutely proven. We need new ideas regarding the prevention of coronary atherosclerosis. In the meantime one can certainly defend the overall health value of not smoking, retaining a normal body weight, maintaining a normal blood pressure, being physically fit, and eating prudently (see Chap. 62H).

THE OBJECTIVE OF THIS CHAPTER AND HOW TO USE IT

The purpose of this chapter is to discuss the general principles of recognition and management of patients with coronary atherosclerotic heart disease and especially to highlight the approach to individual patients with specific clinical syndromes.

The etiology, pathology, and altered physiology of coronary atherosclerotic heart disease are considered in Chaps. 62B, 62C, and 62D. The definitions of various clinical syndromes are discussed in detail in Chap. 62A. The reader of this chapter should be familiar with, and should frequently refer to, Chap. 62A since the same "theme" will be continued in this chapter. The overriding principle is: The more precisely one states a problem, the more likely one is to solve it by linking it to specific management.

THE CLINICAL SETTING

There is abundant information to indicate that individuals who are in a certain age range; have hyperlipidemia; smoke tobacco; are hypertensive; are obese; have carbohydrate intolerance (diabetes); are inactive; have hyperuricemia; have certain electrocardiographic abnormalities; have a certain type of personality; have a family history of premature coronary atherosclerotic heart disease; or have xanthoma and hyperlipidemia have a greater chance of developing coronary atherosclerotic heart disease than have subjects who do not exhibit such abnormalities. The Framingham Study revealed that the combination of hypercholesterolemia, hypertension, and cigarette smoking increased the incidence of coronary atherosclerotic heart disease by eight times over that of men who had none of these factors (Chaps. 62B and 62H).

Although the preceding is true, it does not follow that the presence of "risk factors" makes it possible to attribute a vague clinical syndrome as being due to coronary atherosclerotic heart disease. Nor does the absence of risk factors allow one to exclude a clinical syndrome that would ordinarily be considered to be due to coronary atherosclerotic heart disease. This point is made here because of the errors we have seen when one assumes that the risk factors have absolute diagnostic value. For example, a few years ago coronary atherosclerotic heart disease would be excluded as a diagnostic possibility in a patient with chest pain simply because the patient was female. We are now recognizing the disease in women—even women under 40 years of age—with increasing frequency.[10-12] A few years ago coronary atheroscle-

rotic heart disease was considered to be unlikely in a patient with chest pain if the patient had normal blood pressure, normal cholesterol, was thin, and did not smoke. These errors are being made less often today because it is now clear that coronary atherosclerotic heart disease is common in the United States even in patients who show no risk factors (Chaps. 62B and 62H). The point is, the knowledge of risk factors is very important to the epidemiologist who is interested in the study of a population of subjects, but we as clinicians must not apply the result of their studies improperly to our individual patients. For example, it is true that a population of subjects who exhibit risk factors will also have a greater incidence of coronary atherosclerotic heart disease than will a population of subjects who have no risk factors. Such data does not, however, permit a physician to exclude coronary atherosclerosis in an individual patient who has no risk factors, since the population of subjects with no risk factors also has the disease—it simply has a lower incidence of the disease as compared with the population of subjects with risk factors.

CLINICAL METHODS USED TO RECOGNIZE AND MANAGE CORONARY ATHEROSCLEROTIC HEART DISEASE AND ITS COMPLICATIONS

The physician uses the medical history, the physical examination, and certain laboratory procedures to elicit the clues which permit the formulation of the problem—coronary atherosclerotic heart disease. It is not a question as to which of these three methods reveals the most information—we need all the methods, since each method makes its own contribution to the recognition of the problem. A single method may reveal pathognomonic clues or may reveal clues which are not individually pathognomonic but, when added to other clues obtained by the other methods, form a cluster of findings that may be diagnostic. While each method may reveal important information about coronary atherosclerosis, each method has its limitations. The physician can be led astray if he or she is not aware of the pitfalls that are inherent in each individual method.

Conditions other than atherosclerosis may affect the coronary arteries. The long list includes coronary artery spasm, dissection of a coronary artery, coronary ostial disease, coronary emboli, coronary thrombosis unrelated to atheroma, coronary arteritis, coronary trauma, and sickle-cell disease (see Chaps. 63A and 63B). In addition, conditions other than coronary disease can influence coronary blood flow, alter the oxygen transport system, or increase oxygen demand at the cellular level. For example, aortic stenosis, aortic regurgitation, hypertrophic cardiomyopathy, idiopathic hypertrophic subaortic stenosis, mitral stenosis, possibly some cases of click-murmur syndrome, anemia, or thyrotoxicosis may produce or contribute to the development of symptoms and signs which are secondary to myocardial hypoxia. Accordingly, it is necessary to search for such conditions by using the history, physical examination, and laboratory procedures, since their detection is necessary for proper understanding and management of the problem. Finally, we must never forget that two conditions may occur in the same heart and that the identification of one condition does not always exclude another.

The use and limitations of the history

The data base used to screen the cardiovascular system is discussed in Chap. 10. A portion of it is used to screen the patient for coronary atherosclerotic heart disease. The history may reveal symptoms such as chest discomfort, dyspnea, palpitation, and syncope that may be related to coronary atherosclerotic heart disease. A physician's skill can be assessed by his or her ability to elicit and to interpret these symptoms accurately. Time and time again coronary atherosclerotic heart disease is not identified because the history has been poorly taken or has been improperly interpreted (see Chap. 12). The symptoms associated with the specific clinical syndromes due to coronary atherosclerotic heart disease and the conditions from which they must be differentiated are discussed in detail in "The Recognition of Specific Clinical Syndromes" later in this chapter. The history of a past event, called a "heart attack" by the patient, should lead the physician to obtain the data from the previous physician, since the electrocardiogram may well have been abnormal at that time but may be normal when the second physician is evaluating the patient.

The limitations of the history as a diagnostic method needs to be highlighted. For centuries, the history has been considered to be the best arrow in the physician's diagnostic quiver and even to hint that it does not reveal everything borders on heresy. We ask the reader to forgive us when we point out that the history does not always reveal all of the answers. To begin with, we physicians are not equally skilled at history taking though all of us undoubtedly view ourselves as good historians. We may lead a patient to answer improperly or fail to listen when the "clues" are pouring out from the patient. Some patients with effort angina may walk more slowly and have fewer symptoms. In addition, some patients may deny symptoms even when the disease process is far advanced.

Denying symptoms, for some deep-seated emotional reason, is vastly different from withholding information. Many patients who withhold information about symptoms believe it is to their advantage (as they see it) to deny their existence. For example, an airline pilot may lose his license if he has symp-

toms of angina pectoris. On the other hand, some patients may exaggerate their symptoms for self gain in order to receive disability insurance or to win psychologic battles at home. Other patients, depending upon their cultural background and emotional maturity, deny symptoms because they are simply more stoic than others. Finally, some patients deny symptoms because they cannot cope with the consequences of recognizing the presence of a serious condition.

Everyone is aware of false positive and false negative laboratory tests, but few physicians have appreciated the false positive and false negative history. For example, an asymptomatic 40-year-old female may have a positive exercise electrocardiogram. The physician returns to the patient—as one should—to "go over the history" again. The physician often emerges with a history of angina pectoris. Is the new history accurate or created by "intimidation" of the patient? Was the first history a false negative history or the second history a false positive history? Symptoms depend upon a disease process and the sensitivity of the patient's nervous system, intellectual capacity, and psychologic makeup. The physician's ability to elicit and interpret the symptoms depends upon his or her skill and perception. It is a wonder that we do as well as we do with the analysis of symptoms. Even more alarming is the fact that diagnostic errors may be made even when the history-taking ability is excellent and a "clear-sounding" story is related by the patient. For example, when a patient gives a history of anterior chest discomfort produced by effort and relieved by rest and nitroglycerin, it is wise to think of angina pectoris. But the diagnostic error rate in this "classic" presentation is 6 percent.[13] When the story is difficult to obtain and the physician is less certain of all of the attributes of the symptoms, the diagnostic error rate is higher. When the anterior chest pain is prolonged and occurs intermittently at rest over a period of weeks, the ability of the physician to analyze the symptoms correctly is about 78 percent.[13] In the latter instance, if the prolonged pain *is* due to myocardial ischemia, it is quite serious, but there is a greater chance that it is not due to myocardial ischemia than when substernal pain is produced by effort.

Now that we can correlate symptoms with the results of coronary arteriography, we are all learning a great deal. We now see patients that we would have labeled as having coronary atherosclerotic heart disease a few years ago who have normal coronary arteriograms. We also see patients whose symptoms are not diagnostic but are sufficient to justify a coronary arteriogram. We are no longer surprised to find obstructive coronary disease delineated by coronary arteriography in some of these patients. Today the court of last appeal in the diagnosis of coronary atherosclerotic heart disease is the coronary arteriogram. The history is enormously important since, as a general rule, we do not perform coronary arteriography on asymptomatic patients. We do, however, listen to the history with the thought of coronary arteriography in mind. The questions are: Does the patient have symptoms that justify a coronary arteriogram? What is the diagnostic error rate in a patient with a certain history without a coronary arteriogram, and is the error rate acceptable? Does the patient with a history of myocardial ischemia have obstructive lesions in the coronary arteries that would compel one to proceed with bypass surgery even when no symptoms are currently present?

The use and limitations of the physical examination

The data base used to screen the cardiovascular system is discussed in Chap. 10. A portion of it is used to screen the patient for coronary atherosclerotic disease. The abnormalities of the cardiovascular system that can be found by physical examination are discussed in Chaps. 13 to 20. The abnormalities that are associated with the specific clinical syndromes associated with coronary atherosclerotic heart disease are discussed later in this chapter.

Coronary atherosclerotic heart disease may be associated with many abnormal physical signs. Few, if any, of the signs are pathognomonic, but they are quite useful in the overall assessment of the problem. First of all, one must establish that certain conditions are not present to account for angina pectoris. The presence of aortic stenosis, aortic regurgitation, mitral stenosis, hypertrophic cardiomyopathy, idiopathic hypertrophic subaortic stenosis, or mitral valve click-murmur syndrome (Barlow's syndrome) as a cause of angina pectoris can usually be accomplished by performing a careful physical examination (see Chaps. 60 and 81). There are many physical abnormalities associated with coronary atherosclerotic heart disease. For example, one must appreciate abnormal precordial movements, gallop sounds, new murmurs, abnormal neck veins, rales in the lungs, etc. (see Chaps. 13 to 20). One should study the precordial movements and auscultate the heart when the patient has an episode of chest pain, since certain abnormalities are heard during the episode but not between episodes.

The limitations of physical examination as a method of recognizing coronary atherosclerotic heart disease must be emphasized. First of all, certain physical signs are not teachable. The atrial gallop is an example of this. There is too much emphasis on this finding when many people have trouble learning to hear it and even more have trouble interpreting its significance. The patient with angina pectoris due to coronary atherosclerotic heart disease often exhibits no abnormalities on physical examination. Even the patient with prolonged myocardial ischemia and infarction may have a normal physical examination. The patient with heart failure secondary to myocardial infarction may not display physical abnormalities and the pulmonary congestion may be detected on the chest roentgenogram. Abnormal physical findings may be interpreted improperly. For example, a newly developed systolic murmur at the apex may be said to be due to myocardial infarction whereas it may really be due to rupture of a mitral valve chordae tendineae secondary to myxomatous change of the chordae.

Laboratory procedures

The laboratory tests used to identify the various clinical syndromes associated with coronary atherosclerotic heart disease include the electrocardiogram, the chest roentgenogram, certain cardiac enzymes, coronary arteriography, left ventriculography, blood lipids determination, echocardiography, radionuclide angiography (cardiac imaging), and a number of miscellaneous tests. The resting electrocardiogram and the chest x-ray are obtained on every patient (see Chap. 11), whereas other procedures such as cardiac fluoroscopy and exercise electrocardiography, certain cardiac enzyme determinations, coronary arteriography, cardiac catheterization, blood lipids measurement, etc., are not done on all patients but are obtained only when indicated.

Although the results of various laboratory procedures are discussed elsewhere in this book, certain aspects of these tests are discussed here for emphasis. Later in this chapter the discussion of the tests will be linked to the various clinical syndromes.

THE USE AND LIMITATIONS OF THE ELECTROCARDIOGRAM

The resting electrocardiogram may be normal in patients with coronary atherosclerotic heart disease. This fact has been difficult to teach. It must be appreciated since many of the most dangerous clinical syndromes are accompanied by a normal electrocardiogram. The electrocardiogram may reveal abnormal ST-T wave abnormalities after exercise. The electrocardiogram may reveal QRS, ST-T, or T-wave abnormalities, arrhythmias, and conduction disturbances as a result of coronary atherosclerotic heart disease, but many of these abnormalities may occur in other conditions. Electrocardiography is discussed in Chap. 23, and vectorcardiography is discussed in Chap. 28E. Exercise electrocardiography is discussed in Chap. 28A. A general textbook on heart disease cannot be used to discuss the details of electrocardiography. The reader is therefore referred to the texts *Introduction to Electrocardiography* by Hurst and Myerburg[14] and *Advances in Electrocardiography* by Schlant and Hurst.[15] The purpose of this discussion is to emphasize certain aspects of the use and limitations of electrocardiography.

Some of the problems associated with the use of the electrocardiogram in the identification of myocardial ischemia are as follows: Approximately 50 to 70 percent of patients with stable angina pectoris have normal electrocardiograms at rest when they are not experiencing angina pectoris.[16] When the electrocardiogram is abnormal, it may show nonspecific ST-T wave abnormalities, changes in atrioventricular or intraventricular conduction, and arrhythmias. Left ventricular hypertrophy, when present, is usually due to an associated condition such as aortic valve disease or hypertension. Less often there may be ST-segment displacement, which is characteristic, but not always pathognomonic, of myocardial ischemia (Fig. 62E-1).

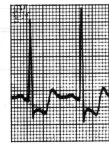

FIGURE 62E-1 The ST-segment displacement shown in this figure is characteristic of myocardial ischemia.

ST-segment displacement (see Fig. 62E-1) characteristic of myocardial ischemia may be recorded during a bout of angina pectoris in some patients.[17] Such ST-segment changes, although not pathognomonic, have a relatively high degree of specificity. The absence of such changes does not rule out coronary atherosclerotic heart disease even when maximal exercise tests are utilized. Prinzmetal changes are said to be present in the electrocardiogram when the mean vector representing the ST-segment displacement is directed toward a region of the left ventricular epicardium[18] rather than being directed away from the left ventricular endocardium (Fig. 62E-2). The electrocardiographic changes occur with the chest pain and disappear when the chest pain subsides. The electrocardiographic changes recur when the pain recurs. Infarction may ensue in patients with such changes, and the infarction is commonly located in the area identified by the ST-segment vector. The Prinzmetal phenomenon may be caused by obstructive coronary disease plus coronary artery spasm or by coronary artery spasm alone (see Chap. 62D).

Exercise electrocardiography has been developed in order to increase the yield of abnormalities in the electrocardiogram that may represent clues which are useful in the detection of coronary atherosclerotic heart disease.[19–19f] Exercise electrocardiography is discussed in Chap. 28A. The following statements are inserted here in order to caution the reader that many errors may be made in the interpretation of the electrocardiograms recorded during and after exercise (Fig. 62E-3). If one is to interpret exercise electrocardiograms properly, it is necessary to understand terms such as sensitivity, specificity, false positive, false negative, true positive, and true negative and to be familiar with Bayes' rule. Bayes' rule emphasizes that both the degree of sensitivity and the degree of specificity of a test are influenced by the prevalence of the disease in the population being studied. This is why a positive exercise test does not have the same meaning in an asymptomatic 40-year-old female as it does in a 50-year-old man with chest discomfort. (Bayes' rule is discussed at length in Chap. 29B in "Cinefluoroscopy of the Coronary Arteries.") The frequency of false positive and false negative tests vary with the population of patients being studied. For this reason, the results of the test must be considered in the light of all of the clinical data. A false positive test may occur when the patient is taking digitalis or when there is severe aortic or mitral valve disease, hypertension, cardiomyopathy, severe anemia, hypokalemia, cor pulmonale, vasoregulatory asthenia, and Wolff-Parkinson-White syndrome, and occasionally in the mitral valve prolapse (click-murmur) syndrome. Exercise tests should be done only in the presence of a physician plus at least one other trained person. As a general rule, the test should not be done if there has been a recent change in stable angina pectoris or if there has been a recent episode of discomfort compatible with prolonged myocardial ischemia.

Some of the problems associated with the use of the electrocardiogram in the identification of "myocardial infarction" are as follows: The majority of myocardial infarcts involve the left ventricle and septum. Some, but not all, myocardial infarcts produce an abnormality of the initial portion of the QRS complex, or QRS vector loop. The forces generated during the initial 0.02 and 0.04 s of ventricular depolarization tend to be directed away from the area of dead myocardial tissue. The ST segment may become displaced from the base line. When represented as a mean vector, it tends to be directed either toward the area of epicardial injury that surrounds the dead zone or away from an area of subendocardial injury. The T waves may become abnormal and when represented as a mean vector, tend to be directed away from the area of epicardial ischemia that surrounds the area of injury (see Chaps. 23 and 28E).

In order to understand how myocardial infarction alters the electrocardiogram and vectorcardiogram, it is necessary to appreciate the following:

1 The normal anatomic position of the left ventricle and septum in the chest
2 How the forces generated by the heart are projected onto and recorded from the body surface
3 The normal sequence of ventricular activation and how it is changed by myocardial infarction
4 The normal sequence of repolarization and how it is changed by myocardial infarction
5 How to recognize an abnormality of the first portion of the QRS that has been altered by myocardial infarction
6 How to recognize the new ST forces produced by myocardial injury
7 How to recognize the altered T waves produced by myocardial ischemia

When these are understood as a unified concept, it is possible to imagine an infarct occurring in any portion of the left ventricle and septum and to predict, within reasonable limits, what the electrocardiogram and vectorcardiogram would show. The thought process is carried out in reverse in practice when abnormalities of the first portion of the QRS, ST segment, and T waves are detected and one attempts to localize the site of infarction that would produce the abnormalities (Fig. 62E-4).

Although myocardial infarction is usually recog-

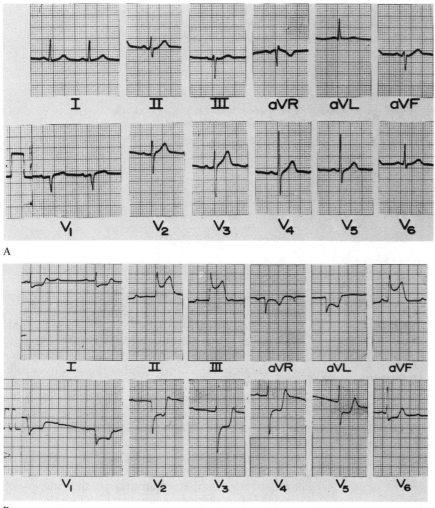

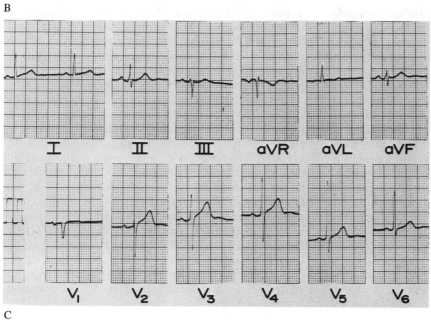

FIGURE 62E-2 Electrocardiogram recorded from a patient with Prinzmetal's angina pectoris. *A.* Electrocardiogram recorded at 10 A.M. on a 59-year-old male who was experiencing repeated bouts of anterior chest discomfort at rest. *B.* Electrocardiogram recorded at 5 P.M. during an episode of chest pain. Note the high degree of AV block and marked ST-segment displacement. The mean ST vector is directed inferiorly and posteriorly. *C.* Electrocardiogram recorded at 6:15 P.M. the same day. The tracing is similar to the one recorded at 10 A.M. (see panel *A*). Coronary arteriography revealed a discrete lesion (95 percent obstruction) in the right coronary artery.   Left ventricular function was normal. (*Courtesy of Dr. Don Nutter and Dr. Joel Felner of the Department of Medicine, Emory University School of Medicine and Grady Memorial Hospital.*)

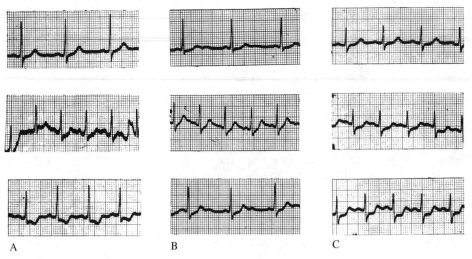

A   B   C

FIGURE 62E-3 All leads are V_4. The top row was taken at rest, the middle row immediately after exercise, and the lower row 5 min after exercise. *A.* Patient with classic angina pectoris. Note the junctional displacement immediately after exercise, whereas there is the downward-sloping segment characteristic of a positive response at 5 min. Note the difficulty of interpretation due to a wandering stylus immediately after exercise, i.e., ST elevation when the stylus is moving upward and ST depression when the stylus is moving downward. *B.* Patient with anxiety and functional chest pain and no evidence of coronary atherosclerotic heart disease. Note the displacement of the base line at the junction of the QRS with the ST segment (j point). The ST segment immediately slopes upward to the T wave. This may be because of repolarization of the atrium. This is a negative exercise test result. *C.* Patient with typical angina pectoris and a positive exercise test result, demonstrating the flat ischemic type of ST depression which extends horizontally for 0.12 s before joining the T wave.

nized by the history of chest pain, serial electrocardiographic changes, and cardiac enzyme changes indicative of muscle necrosis, the diagnosis is often imprecise. The limitations of the electrocardiogram in revealing infarction must be emphasized. A single normal electrocardiogram is worthless in ruling out acute myocardial infarction, since changes may never appear or may be delayed for hours or days. Abnormal Q waves may not occur if the infarct is small or located in certain anatomic sites within the heart. If abnormal Q waves develop, they generally do so within a few days, whereas the appearance of T-wave inversion may be delayed for a few days to several weeks. If there has been previous infarction, a new infarct that involves a diametrically opposite wall of the ventricle may cancel the effects of the first infarction and the tracing may return toward normal. Third and fourth infarcts rarely deform the QRS complex in a significant manner. When there is residual evidence of transmural infarction, or changes related to ventricular aneurysm with Q waves, ST-segment elevation, and inverted T waves, it may require properly placed extensive muscle necrosis to alter the tracing further. Left bundle branch block

often prevents the inscription of diagnostic Q waves unless a major portion of the septum is destroyed. A documented history or definite electrocardiographic evidence of prior infarction adds diagnostic weight to atypical symptoms or physical findings suggesting acute infarction. Unfortunately, the electrocardiographic evidence of old infarction may have disappeared, thereby removing an important diagnostic clue. Diagnostic Q waves due to myocardial infarction may disappear from the electrocardiogram within months or years. Kaplan and Berkson reported that abnormal Q waves had either disappeared or become of borderline significance in 30 percent of cases of myocardial infarction at the end of 18 months.[20] It is quite common for the ST-segment and T-wave abnormalities of myocardial infarction to return to normal. When the Q-wave, ST-segment, and T-wave abnormalities have returned to normal following a myocardial infarction, it may still be possible to detect a difference in the electrocardiogram if it is compared with a preinfarction tracing.

Careful studies of serial electrocardiographic changes correlated with pathologic findings indicate that the accuracy of diagnosis of acute infarction by electrocardiography is no greater than 80 percent.[21] Myocardial infarction may be found at autopsy, and the patient may never have had a diagnosis of infarction made during life. The detection of an old, healed myocardial infarction during life may be difficult, and it is likely that our diagnostic accuracy is far less than 80 percent. This means that (1) the symptoms (if any) of myocardial infarction may not have been deemed important by the patient or the physician and therefore appropriate studies were not made; (2) an insufficient number of electrocardiograms may have been made when the initial symptoms suggested infarction; (3) electrocardiographic changes may have developed but did not meet the physician's diagnostic criteria for infarction; (4)

FIGURE 62E-4 Most myocardial infarcts are located in the left ventricle and septum. (Right ventricular and atrial infarcts also occur.) This diagram shows the location of the left ventricle in the chest, the usual locations of infarcts that occur in this structure, and how the altered electrical forces are reflected on the electrocardiogram. *A.* The anatomic position of the left ventricle and septum viewed from the front. The normal mean QRS vector is located to the left and is directed inferiorly and slightly posteriorly. The normal mean T vector lies very near the mean QRS vector but slightly anterior to it. The forces generated during the first portion (initial 0.04 s) of the QRS, when represented as a mean vector, also lie very near the mean QRS vector but slightly anterior to it. *B* and *C.* Diagrams of myocardial infarction, zone of injury, and zone of ischemia. The mean dead-zone vector (initial QRS forces) points away from the infarct, the mean injury vector (ST-segment forces) points toward the area of epicardial injury, and the mean ischemia vector (T wave forces) points away from the area of epicardial ischemia. (1) Anteroseptal infarction.

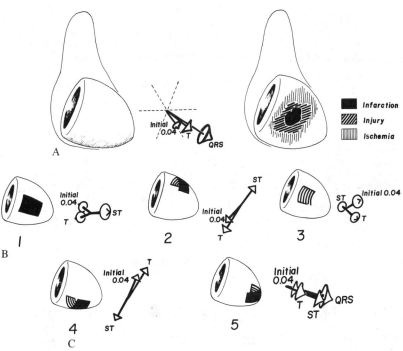

The electrocardiogram would show abnormal Q waves in leads I, aV_L, V_1, V_2, V_3, and V_4, abnormal ST-segment elevation in leads I, aV_L, and the anterior precordial leads, and abnormal T-wave inversion in leads I, aV_L, and the anterior precordial leads. (2) Lateral infarction. The electrocardiogram would show abnormal Q waves, abnormal ST-segment elevation, and abnormal T-wave inversion in leads I, aV_L, V_4, V_5, and V_6. (3) True posterior infarction. The electrocardiogram would show an abnormally tall R wave in lead V_1, and perhaps an abnormal Q wave in lead aV_F, abnormal ST-segment depression in leads V_1, V_2, and V_3, and tall T waves in leads V_1, V_2, and V_3. (4) Inferior infarction. The electrocardiogram would show abnormal Q waves in leads II, III, and aV_F, abnormal ST elevation in leads II, III, and aV_F, and abnormally inverted T waves in leads II, III, and aV_F. (5) Apical infarction. The dead-zone vector ("abnormal Q waves") may or may not appear. The mean ST and mean T vector may increase in size and point toward the apex. (The figures in this illustration are shown to illustrate a concept. They are not designed to illustrate all the variables that must be considered in the theory and practice of electrocardiography.)

undue reliance on the development of abnormalities in ancillary laboratory tests, such as change in the serum enzyme levels, may have prevented the diagnosis of myocardial infarction; or (5) serial electrocardiograms may have remained unchanged following an episode of chest pain because the area of infarction was small or the damage occurred in an electrically silent area of the myocardium.

The electrocardiograms shown in Figs. 62E-5 to 62E-8 have been chosen to dispel certain erroneous impressions that are held today. The legends which accompany the tracings make certain points that we believe to be important.

The limitations of the electrocardiogram in the diagnosis of myocardial infarction have just been emphasized. We now wish to stress that many disorders—some serious and some benign—may alter the electrocardiogram in such a way that myocardial infarction may be erroneously diagnosed. This discussion may be brought into focus by asking the following question: Which electrocardiographic abnormalities look like those produced by myocardial infarction but may be due to some other disease? A partial answer to this question is as follows: There are a large number of depolarization abnormalities

that suggest myocardial infarction. The electrocardiographic abnormality associated with the Wolff-Parkinson-White syndrome may simulate that of myocardial infarction. Patients with advanced pulmonary emphysema or pulmonary embolism may exhibit QRS abnormality that suggests myocardial infarction. Patients with left ventricle hypertrophy may have a posteriorly directed QRS loop which produces an absent R wave in leads V_1, V_2, V_3, and occasionally in lead V_4. The absence of R waves in these leads may be produced by infarction, but this finding is not as specific for infarction as when the R wave is absent in leads V_1 and V_2 and there is a QR pattern in lead V_3. In the latter situation the QRS loop is not smooth, and the initial forces are posterior to the subsequent QRS forces. Even when the latter abnormalities are identified, one cannot conclude the cause is always coronary atherosclerosis, even though the loop is characteristic of infarction. The depolarization abnormalities associated with the cardiomyopathies (especially asymmetric septal hypertrophy with or without subaortic stenosis) as well as those due to amyloid, sarcoid, neoplastic disease, etc., may mimic the QRS changes of infarction (Fig. 62E-9). Patients with neuromuscular disease, includ-

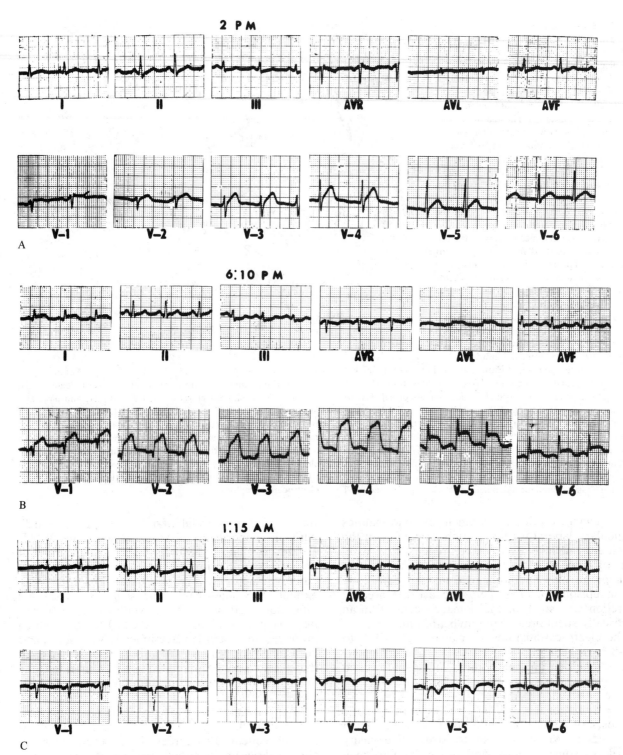

FIGURE 62E-5 A. One hour prior to the recording of this electrocardiogram the patient developed severe substernal "indigestion." The electrocardiogram shows slight ST and T-wave abnormalities, especially in V_2, V_3, V_4, V_5, and V_6. There appears to be slight ST-segment elevation, blending into a prominent T wave (note precordial leads). This type of abnormality is not infrequent in the early course of myocardial infarction, but it is often overlooked. *B.* The electrocardiogram 4 h and 10 min later shows extensive anterior epicardial injury with only slight QRS changes. *C.* Electrocardiogram 5 h and 5 min after *B* shows T-wave abnormality consistent with anterolateral ischemia and disappearance of the giant-sized ST-segment elevation. The QRS abnormality is now clearly seen, indicating anterior dead zone.

This series of tracings illustrates the difficulty in judging the age of an infarction by noting the configuration of QRS, ST, and T waves. (This one evolved in 12 h.)

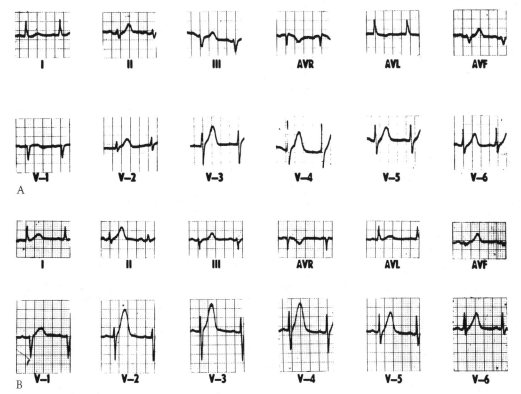

FIGURE 62E-6 An 84-year-old woman was admitted to the orthopedic service with a fractured hip. Five days after surgical treatment she had sudden collapse and hypotension and was transferred to the medical service with a diagnosis of massive pulmonary embolism. *A.* Electrocardiogram recorded several hours after symptoms began. The tracing shows prominent T waves. The QRS axis is rotated to the left because of terminal QRS force abnormality. *B.* Tracing recorded 4 days after *A* and 1 h prior to death. The T waves are more prominent, and the terminal QRS abnormality is less obvious.

Autopsy revealed a large apical myocardial infarction, but no evidence of pulmonary emboli. This tracing is shown to illustrate that large infarctions may be present in certain areas of the heart (the apex, in this case) without producing classic QRS, ST, or T-wave changes.

FIGURE 62E-7 A 54-year-old man 7 days prior to admission had severe substernal chest pain lasting 15 min and relieved by rest. Two days prior to admission the patient had a mild substernal discomfort radiating to the back and lasting 1 to 2 h. Thirty minutes prior to the above tracing the patient experienced sudden onset of severe chest pain, became dyspneic, and collapsed while climbing stairs. The electrocardiogram shows sinus tachycardia. The initial portion of the QRS complex is suggestive of an inferior dead zone. ST-segment displacement is consistent with subendocardial injury, and there are tall, peaked T waves in V_2, V_3, and V_4.

Autopsy revealed hemopericardium and rupture of the posterior wall of the left ventricle from massive inferoposterior myocardial infarction.

It would not be possible to diagnose myocardial rupture from this tracing.

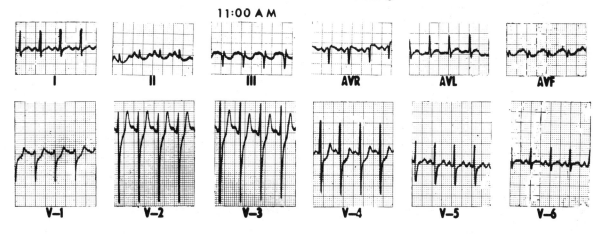

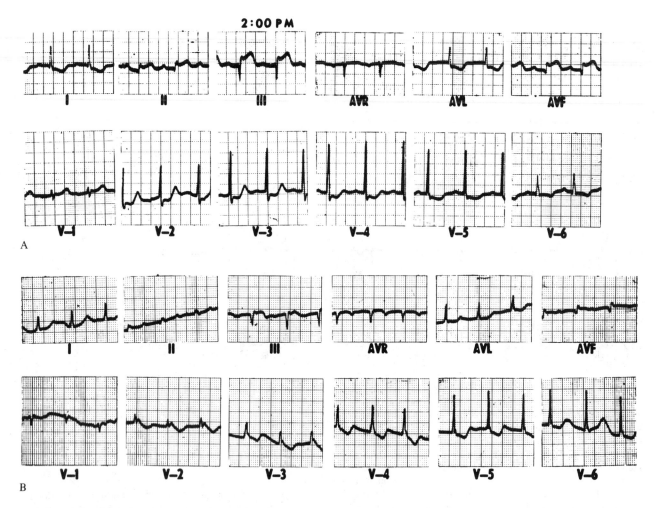

FIGURE 62E-8 A 64-year-old man with 2 h duration of severe substernal chest pain and moderate hypotension. *A.* Electrocardiogram reveals first-degree heart block and QRS, ST, and T-wave changes consistent with inferoposterior myocardial infarction. The P-Q interval is 0.24 s in lead II. Note the mean vector representing the ST-segment points inferiorly and posteriorly; the R waves are prominent in leads V_1, V_2, and V_3. *B.* One week later. A day before this tracing was recorded the patient developed complete heart block, and a catheter pacemaker was inserted; the heart block disappeared, and the catheter pacemaker was discontinued. This tracing shows nodal rhythm, inferior infarction, and a change in the T wave.

The patient died from ventricular fibrillation the day following the last tracing. Autopsy revealed a 7- to 8-day-old inferoposterior infarction of the left ventricle and a fresh hemorrhagic infarction of the entire right ventricle and right atrium.

This tracing illustrates that massive destruction of the right ventricle may occur without diagnostic electrocardiographic abnormalities.

ing progressive muscular dystrophy, Friedreich's ataxia, and myotonia atrophica, may have abnormal QRS complexes suggesting myocardial infarction. The initial portion of the QRS complex in patients with complex congenital heart disease may be deformed in such a way that infarction might be considered (Fig. 62E-10). The ST segments and T waves of the electrocardiogram may be altered by many disorders. These include the cardiomyopathies, pericarditis, pulmonary embolism, digitalis effect, anxiety with tachycardia, subarachnoid hemorrhage and other cerebral lesions, electrolyte disturbances, and numerous other conditions.

While the limitations of the electrocardiogram in the diagnosis of myocardial infarction just mentioned are of great importance, this issue is overshadowed by an even greater problem. The demand for Q waves to signify the presence of important and serious event called myocardial infarction has diverted the minds of many from the search for the numerous serious and dangerous syndromes due to myocardial ischemia that may occur without Q waves or even ST-T wave abnormalities. In fact, many such clinical syndromes due to myocardial ischemia are more dangerous than certain myocardial infarctions.

The value of electrocardiography in the diagnosis of myocardial infarction has been firmly established. We must not forget, however, that electrocardiography does not solve all problems and that many problems may be created by its use. Frank Wilson, who led us all to modern electrocardiography, expressed his views about the abuse of the technique he

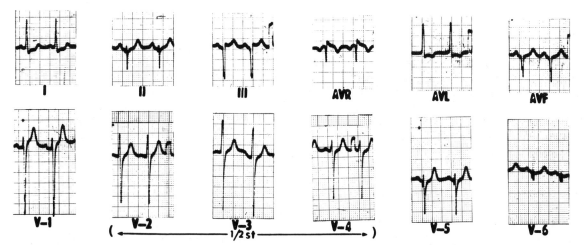

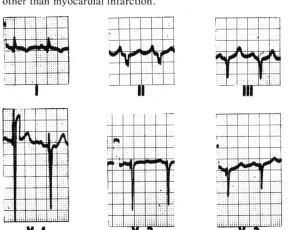

FIGURE 62E-9 Electrocardiogram of a 24-year-old woman with idiopathic hypertrophic subaortic and subpulmonic stenosis. Note the QRS complex abnormality suggesting lateral myocardial infarction. This type of abnormality is commonly observed in patients with idiopathic hypertrophic subaortic stenosis.

helped foster in the preface of his son-in-law's book in 1951.[22] He wrote:

> In the last two decades there has been a tremendous growth of interest in electrocardiographic diagnosis and in the number and variety of electrocardiographs in use. In 1914, there was only one instrument of this kind in the state of Michigan and this was not in operation; there were probably no more than a dozen electrocardiographs in the whole of the United States. Now there is one or more in almost every village of any size, and there are comparatively few people who are not in greater danger of having their peace and happiness destroyed by an erroneous diagnosis of cardiac abnormality based on a faulty interpretation of an electrocardiogram, than of being injured or killed by an atomic bomb.

FIGURE 62E-10 A 13-year-old boy with dextroversion and transposition of the great vessels. The QRS abnormality suggests an anterior dead zone, and the T-wave inversion in lead I might be interpreted as indicating ischemia. This tracing is shown to emphasize that "dead-zone effects" can be produced by heart disease other than myocardial infarction.

THE USE AND LIMITATIONS OF THE VECTORCARDIOGRAM

The use and limitations of the vectorcardiogram are discussed by Witham in Chap. 28E. He writes, "The recording of a vectorcardiogram requires more time and is more expensive than is the recording of an electrocardiogram. There is an unacceptably high cost-benefit ratio when it is used indiscriminately. There are, however, certain well defined situations in which it can supply critical data."

At present in day to day practice most cardiac problems are clarified by the use of the history, physical examination, electrocardiogram, and chest x-ray. If more information is needed, it is usually obtained by performing echocardiography and cardiac catheterization (including coronary arteriography and left ventriculography).

THE USE AND ABUSE OF CARDIAC ENZYMES IN DIAGNOSIS AND PROGNOSIS

When heart muscle cells undergo irreversible cellular damage, enzymes may be liberated into the bloodstream via the coronary lymphatic drainage.[23] The measurements of cardiac enzyme levels are used as a diagnostic test for myocardial necrosis and as a

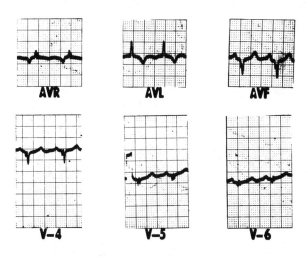

means of assessing prognosis following myocardial infarction. The correct interpretation of serum enzyme determinations is sometimes difficult, and problems may be created by their misuse.

The serum levels of many enzymes may increase following myocardial infarction. Since serum glutamic oxaloacetic transaminase (SGOT), lactic dehydrogenase (LDH), lactic dehydrogenase isoenzymes, creatine phosphokinase (CPK), and creatine phosphokinase isoenzymes determinations have become established requirements in the laboratory diagnosis of acute myocardial infarction in human beings, the material to follow will be concerned with these enzymes.

Each of these enzymes has its typical time course of appearance and of return to normal values following myocardial infarction. Knowledge of the typical time course of elevation for any enzyme is important because a pattern of enzyme elevation differing from that typically seen in patients with myocardial infarction may indicate a source of enzyme release from an organ other than the heart. After a patient sustains an acute myocardial infarction, the SGOT level becomes elevated above the normal value in 8 to 12 h. It usually reaches peak levels in 24 to 48 h and returns to normal in 3 to 4 days. The serum LDH activity reaches a peak elevation in 3 to 6 days and declines to the normal range within 8 to 14 days. Elevated levels of serum CPK activity appear in the serum within 6 h after a myocardial infarction, reach a peak within 24 h, and return to the normal range within 3 to 4 days.

Sensitivity of enzymes Myocardial ischemia is associated with different clinical syndromes and pathologic consequences. Elucidation of the relationships between each of these syndromes and changes in serum enzymes is difficult, but some generalizations can be made. A definite myocardial infarction with the appearance of new "Q" waves on the electrocardiogram will be accompanied by an elevation of cardiac enzymes in over 90 percent of cases.[24] Prolonged chest pain due to myocardial ischemia associated with transient ST-segment and T-wave changes in the electrocardiogram will be associated with elevation of the cardiac enzymes in only 50 to 60 percent of cases. When prolonged chest pain due to myocardial ischemia is not accompanied by electrocardiographic changes, the incidence of elevated enzymes declines further to approximately 25 percent. These data indicate that the sensitivity of serum enzymes is excellent when the electrocardiogram shows typical changes of myocardial infarction. Unfortunately, many myocardial infarctions are not accompanied by such diagnostic electrocardiographic changes, and the sensitivity of serum enzyme levels is less in those patients.

Specificity of enzymes Since the enzymes used in the diagnosis of myocardial infarction are found in organs of the body other than the heart, disease processes in other organs may produce elevations of any one or all of these enzymes. This lack of specificity is a major problem in the meaningful interpretation of serum enzymes. A complete listing of the disorders other than myocardial infarction that may produce elevations of cardiac enzymes is beyond the scope of this section. A brief discussion of the major causes of elevation for each enzyme will illustrate the magnitude of the problem.

Serum glutamic oxaloacetic transaminase (SGOT) Many disorders other than myocardial infarction may be associated with elevated SGOT levels. These include primary liver disease, liver congestion secondary to congestive heart failure, pulmonary infarction, biliary tract disease, pericarditis, and rapid tachyarrhythmias. Shock, direct current cardioversion, cardiac catheterization, and any surgical procedure may elevate the SGOT level as well as the CPK and LDH levels.

Lactic dehydrogenase (LDH) Total serum LDH activity may increase under the following conditions: hemolysis of red blood cells secondary to hemolytic anemia or trauma to the red blood cells during blood drawing, leukemia, acute and chronic liver disease, renal disease, pulmonary infarction, congestive heart failure, and neoplastic disease.

Lactic dehydrogenase (LDH) has been separated into five subgroups of isoenzymes by the use of electrophoretic techniques. Heart muscle contains primarily LDH_1 while liver or skeletal muscle contains mostly LDH_4 and LDH_5. Following myocardial infarction, LDH_1 may appear in the serum within a few hours and may persist up to 10 days. The LDH_1 fraction may be abnormally elevated when the total serum LDH is normal. LDH isoenzyme determinations have enhanced diagnostic accuracy remarkably. Many conditions in which the total LDH activity is increased, including liver disease, congestive heart failure, shock, and pulmonary infarction, are readily distinguishable from acute myocardial infarction because of a different isoenzyme profile. An elevated LDH_1 level is not, however, specific for myocardial infarction. An increase in LDH_1 levels can occur with hemolytic anemia, hemolysis of the blood specimen, renal disease, hyperthyroidism, and carcinoma of the stomach.

Creatine phosphokinase (CPK) Insufficient attention has been directed to the variables that affect the normal values of serum CPK. The CPK activity is generally greater in men than in women. It is greater in persons with a large skeletal muscle mass and in those engaged in vigorous physical activity. Serum CPK activity is increased in many patients with skeletal muscle disease, muscle injury, alcohol intoxication, convulsions, central nervous system disorders, and following intramuscular injections. CPK activity may be augmented by the administration of digitalis to patients with myocardial infarction.[24a] CPK elevation following an intramuscular injection creates a major problem because many patients with severe chest pain receive intramuscular injections of narcotics for analgesia, and such patients may be erroneously labeled as having undergone myocardial infarction.

A major advance in the laboratory diagnosis of

myocardial infarction is the development of tests measuring the isoenzymes of CPK. Extracts from human myocardium contain the MM isoenzyme and smaller quantities of the MB isoenzyme.[25] The only human tissue containing substantial amounts of MB CPK is cardiac muscle. Intramuscular injections, surgical trauma to skeletal muscles, surgery of the gastrointestinal tract, and injury to the brain are not associated with increased serum MB CPK activity despite marked elevations of total CPK.[26] Elevated serum MB CPK activity is the most specific enzymatic criterion of myocardial injury. An elevated MB CPK level does not necessarily indicate myocardial infarction[26a] because it may be increased following iatrogenic cardiac trauma. Also, MB CPK is present in skeletal muscle of patients with Duchenne's muscular dystrophy and other skeletal muscle diseases with regenerative skeletal muscle. It is likely that other conditions will be identified as potential causes of elevation of the MB CPK level. Unfortunately, quantification of serum MB CPK is a difficult laboratory procedure, and this has prevented widespread usage. Future technical advances should result in a reliable method for determination of CPK isoenzymes.

The poor specificity of the SGOT, total LDH, and total CPK levels for myocardial injury seriously limit their usefulness. It is hazardous to make the diagnosis of myocardial infarction on the basis of an elevation of the SGOT, total CPK, or total LDH in the absence of other evidence.[27] The enzyme determinations of greatest value are of the isoenzymes of the CPK and LDH. The serum MB CPK level is the most specific test if the patient is seen within 48 h after the onset of chest pain. The rapid return of MB CPK levels to the normal range make this enzyme particularly useful in the recognition of subsequent extensions of infarctions. The determination of LDH isoenzymes is most useful if the patient is seen more than 48 h after the onset of chest pain.

Use of enzymes in diagnosis When the symptoms of myocardial infarction are classic and the electrocardiographic abnormalities are definite, the determination of serum enzymes is not needed for diagnostic purposes. Conversely, serum enzyme determinations should be done and may provide objective evidence of myocardial necrosis in the patient with chest pain typical of myocardial ischemia but with an electrocardiogram that is normal or nonspecific.

The levels of serum enzyme activity may deceive the clinician in several ways. Elevated serum enzymes occurring in patients with atypical chest pain and nonspecific electrocardiographic alterations may lead to a false diagnosis of myocardial infarction. The enzyme changes may result from a variety of disorders other than myocardial infarction. False diagnoses of myocardial infarction based upon isolated enzyme elevations should become less common when isoenzyme determinations are substituted for total enzyme determinations. The finding of normal serum enzyme levels in patients with prolonged chest pain typical of myocardial ischemia and with nonspe-

cific electrocardiographic changes may produce the erroneous assumption that nothing new has happened to the heart. These patients can develop ventricular tachycardia, ventricular fibrillation, and conduction defects while in the hospital, and they are subject to high incidence of cardiac death following discharge from the hospital.[28]

Prognostic value of enzymes Recent studies suggest that the level of peak serum enzyme activity has prognostic value. When SGOT, LDH, or CPK activity increases more than tenfold, in-hospital mortality rises markedly. An elevation of serum enzyme activity of four to eight times normal has been shown to correlate positively with occurrence of complications such as ventricular arrhythmias, heart failure, or shock.[29]

Although the amplitude of peak serum enzyme elevation correlates with the various complications of myocardial infarction in a large group of patients, certain problems temper the application of this data to a single patient. The peak serum enzyme level may be missed if blood samples are drawn only once a day. Enzyme release from tissues other than the myocardium may contribute to the peak serum level. Peak serum enzyme activity often fails to correlate with the prognosis in patients with previous myocardial infarction. The enzyme level may suggest a "small" acute infarction, but when added to a previous myocardial infarction, the total loss of left ventricular mass may produce significant left ventricular dysfunction. Perhaps the greatest danger in using serum enzymes to assess prognosis comes from the pervasive clinical impression that patients having prolonged pain due to myocardial ischemia in the absence of diagnostic electrocardiographic changes or elevated serum enzyme activity have a good prognosis. These patients may develop serious arrhythmias and conduction disturbances in the hospital, and their risk of subsequent cardiac death following discharge from hospital is substantial.[28]

In many cases in which the serum enzyme activity is markedly elevated, it is readily apparent from other clinical parameters that the patient has sustained a large myocardial infarction. It is not certain that serum enzyme activity will reliably identify the patient destined to have serious complications at a time when the physical examination, chest x-ray, and electrocardiogram suggest that the patient is in a low-risk group. It also remains to be shown that the end result of patient care has been improved by the use of peak enzyme activity to predict impending complications.

THE USE AND LIMITATIONS OF THE CHEST ROENTGENOGRAM AND CARDIAC FLUOROSCOPY

The *roentgenogram of the chest* may reveal several important abnormalities that may be directly or indirectly related to coronary atherosclerotic heart disease and its complications. The heart size as determined by x-ray of the chest is normal in patients who have one of the varieties of angina pectoris due to coronary atherosclerosis. The heart size is usually normal in patients who have prolonged chest pain and objective evidence of muscle necrosis (myocardial infarction) even when acute heart failure is evident. The x-ray of the chest may reveal cardiac enlargement in patients with chronic heart failure due to coronary atherosclerotic heart disease. Signs of pulmonary congestion due to left ventricular dysfunction are commonly detected on the chest x-ray in patients with fresh myocardial infarction even when other signs of heart failure are absent (see Chap. 44). A portable x-ray cannot be used to determine heart size but may be used to assess the degree of pulmonary congestion. A myocardial bulge (aneurysm) secondary to myocardial infarction may be detected on x-ray of the heart. The size of a myocardial aneurysm is usually underestimated using this technique as compared to left ventriculography. Calcification of a myocardial infarction may be seen on the chest x-ray, and, rarely, calcification of the left main coronary artery may be detected.

Cardiac fluoroscopy may reveal pericardial fluid (poor cardiac pulsations and an epicardial fat line) or localized areas of abnormal cardiac movement that may be related to myocardial infarction (see Chap. 29A). An abnormal expansion of the left atrium due to mitral valve regurgitation secondary to papillary muscle dysfunction may be detected by cardiac fluoroscopy. Calcification of the coronary arteries may be detected on the chest x-ray, at fluoroscopy, or by cinefluoroscopy. The latter technique offers great advantages over the other techniques in detecting coronary calcification. Coronary calcification is virtually diagnostic of coronary atherosclerosis. This subject is discussed in detail in Chap. 29C.

THE USE AND ABUSE OF CARDIAC CATHETERIZATION AND ANGIOCARDIOGRAPHY

Cardiac catheterization and angiocardiography may occasionally be needed in order to evaluate coronary atherosclerotic heart disease (see Chaps. 29D and 33). For example, catheterization of the right side of the heart may be required to identify the presence of ruptured interventricular septum due to myocardial infarction. A Swan-Ganz catheter may be used for this particular purpose (see Chap. 36). As a rule, the physician hears a systolic murmur near the left lower sternal edge or at the cardiac apex in such patients. When such a murmur is heard in the setting of myocardial infarction and heart failure persists, it may be necessary to have cardiac catheterization of the right side of the heart in order to confirm or deny the presence of a left-to-right shunt at the ventricular level, since surgical correction may be required (see Chap. 62F). Catheterization and angiocardiography of the left side of the heart may be needed to ascertain the presence and degree of aortic and mitral valve disease. The left ventricular cineangiogram may be used to detect diffuse and localized areas of cardiac muscle dysfunction.

Coronary arteriography and left ventriculography (see Chap. 29D) are done for one of two reasons. (1) They are performed for diagnostic reasons when they are needed to clarify the cause of a syndrome, including heart failure due to ventricular aneurysm, that could be attributed to coronary atherosclerotic heart disease. The arteriogram is commonly done to clarify the cause of troublesome chest discomfort. It is well to remember that our diagnostic ability utilizing older methods has been imperfect and that many diagnostic mistakes have been made in the past. Coronary arteriography and left ventriculography will help clarify many diagnostic problems, but, of course, they will not solve all problems. For example, coronary artery spasm and infarct with a normal coronary arteriogram remain mysterious. The biplane left ventriculogram is an excellent method for detecting left ventricular dysfunction (especially localized areas of dysfunction). Ejection fractions calculated from left ventriculogram in one plane often underestimate the true ejection fraction. Frequently, there may be shocking disparity between the clinical evidences of ventricular dysfunction and what is evident in the left ventriculogram. It is common to have impairment of contractility of large segments of the ventricle with no clinical evidence of dysfunction. (2) Coronary arteriography and left ventriculography are used to delineate the anatomy of the coronary arteries and function of the left ventricle in order to determine if the proper anatomic and physiologic conditions are present in patients in whom an aorticocoronary bypass surgical procedure is being considered for one of the clinical syndromes (see Chap. 29D). The indications for coronary artery surgery are discussed later in this chapter and in Chap. 62F.

The work done in a modern cardiac catheterization laboratory is different from that which was done in the past. The time-consuming studies and the detailed calculation that were done in the past grew out of the research era and were carried over, sometimes unnecessarily, to the diagnostic work done on patients. Now the test is done more quickly, and the patient's comfort is considered to be extremely important, and only the pertinent information is sought. In the past it was even possible for "catheter men" to know a great deal about the catheter findings and know little about the patient. Many could not examine and evaluate the patient using the ordinary methods of examination and therefore could not correlate all aspects of clinical findings with findings in the laboratory. Now, in an excellent laboratory, the person who is performing the catheterization is a correlator and is skilled at examining the patient. Accordingly, he or she tends to do only what is needed for the complete diagnosis and care of the patient.

Errors in the interpretation of coronary arteriograms undoubtedly occur, and the technique will undoubtedly miss certain lesions. Modern equipment and techniques have decreased the error rate considerably, and interobserver differences are minimal in an excellent laboratory.

ECHOCARDIOGRAPHY (see Chaps. 32B, 32C, and 32E)

Echocardiography is a phenomenal diagnostic tool. The technique has not, however, at the time of this writing given us great insight into the diagnosis and management of the majority of patients with coronary atherosclerotic heart disease. Its chief use seems to be in the identification of certain cardiomyopathies that may closely mimic coronary atherosclerotic heart disease (see Chaps. 32B and 81); in the recognition of mitral valve abnormalities that could be related to coronary atherosclerotic heart disease; in the recognition of pericardial fluid that could be due to postmyocardial infarction syndrome (Dressler's syndrome) (see Chap. 32E); and in the determination of the left ventricular ejection fraction (see Chap. 32B). Unfortunately the measurement of the ejection fraction in patients with segmental disease by this technique is filled with error and can only be used as a gross index of the real ejection fraction. Real-time two-dimensional echocardiography may offer more help in visualizing more of the left ventricle.

Perhaps, with more research, the echocardiogram will be of great value in diagnosis and management of coronary atherosclerotic heart disease.

RADIONUCLIDE ANGIOCARDIOGRAPHY (CARDIAC IMAGING)[30-40b]

Radioisotopic imaging of the heart and great vessels is discussed in Chap. 30. Strauss and Pitt have emphasized that this noninvasive technique can be used to measure the regional distribution of myocardial perfusion, total and regional contractility, and the presence or absence of acute myocardial infarction.[32]

Tracers such as technetium-labeled red blood cells and technetium-labeled albumin have been used to study regional myocardial wall changes; to determine ventricular volume; and to estimate the ejection fraction. This is done by comparing the borders of the cardiac chamber as seen in end-systole with those seen in end-diastole.[32,33]

When thalium-201 is given to a patient at rest and again after exercise or cardiac pacing, it is possible to detect areas of decreased perfusion.[32,33] The development of new or enlarged areas of decreased concentration of the tracer after exercise suggests that myocardial ischemia has developed with stress. There is increasing evidence that this test is more sensitive than exercise electrocardiography in the identification of myocardial ischemia. Zones of decreased tracer concentration ("cold spots") at rest may be due to "fixed" or "transient" abnormalities of perfusion. When the zones of decreased tracer concentration found at rest do not change with stress, they are considered to be "fixed abnormalities." The site and size of myocardial infarction can be determined by the identification of a fixed "cold spot."[32,33]

Acute myocardial infarction can be separated from old infarction by using a tracer such as a ^{99m}Tc-pyrophosphate or -glycohepatomatic that is ordinarily excluded from the cells.[33] The tracer becomes bound to the damaged protein or to calcium within the cell (this is known as avid screening and the areas are known as "hot spots"). In this case a hot spot indicates poor perfusion and poor clearance of the isotope.

Limitations of the method Radioisotopic imaging of the heart will undoubtedly earn its place in medicine just as coronary arteriography has earned its place. More space will be devoted to a discussion of it in the next edition of *The Heart*. At present, the technique is still developing and the following limitations are currently apparent:

1 The technique is new and has not as yet been studied sufficiently long to permit the clinical correlations and inferences to be tested and retested.
2 The equipment and tracer substances are expensive. Currently very few hospitals possess the capability of radioisotopic imaging of the heart.
3 The ideal tracer substance has not yet been identified, and different tracers are needed to study different things.
4 All except the most severe coronary lesions will usually not be detected with tracer administered at rest because blood flow distal to the fixed orifice may be normal and equal to that found distal to nonobstructed vessels. Poor perfusion may be detected only after exercise.
5 The scan does not at this time substitute for a coronary arteriogram or left ventricular angiogram.

As stated earlier, with further development this technique will undoubtedly take its place in the evaluation of the patient with coronary atherosclerotic heart disease.

THE USE OF A SYSTEMIC ARTERIAL LINE AND THE SWAN-GANZ CATHETER

The use of a systemic arterial line and Swan-Ganz catheter is discussed in Chaps. 36, 44, and 48 in the section titled "The Use of Hemodynamic Measurements for the Management of the Patient with Acute Myocardial Infarction" later in this chapter. We do not routinely insert an intraarterial catheter and a Swan-Ganz catheter into all patients with "myocardial infarction." The vast majority of patients with myocardial infarction can be managed safely without the information that can be obtained from these procedures. Swan has not claimed that the procedures should be done on all patients, but he has pointed out to our satisfaction that the measurements obtained from such procedures are helpful in the management of certain patients. Patients with overt heart failure secondary to myocardial infarction who are not improving may be treated more physiologically with diuretics, nitroprusside, etc., with knowledge of these measurements. Cardiogenic shock is nearly always managed with greater precision if the measurements obtained from these procedures are known. The more skilled one is in eliciting pertinent clinical information from the patient, the less often the measurements derived from these procedures will be needed, but even the most skilled clinician occasionally needs to know the actual intraarterial pressure and the pulmonary wedge pressure (or pulmonary diastolic arterial pressure) in order to guide the therapy properly.

BLOOD GASES AND pH (see Chaps. 27 and 62D)

Serial determinations of arterial blood gases may be performed in patients with shock. Appropriate therapy to correct hypoxemia and significant deviations of arterial P_{CO_2} and pH may then be guided more carefully. When this procedure is not available to the physician, he or she must learn to assess the patient by monitoring skin color and temperature, urine flow, blood pressure, mental state, pulse rate, etc.

HOLTER MONITOR (see Chap. 28B)

Cardiac arrhythmias are common in patients with coronary atherosclerotic heart disease. One of the major reasons for creating coronary care units was to develop a system for the continuous monitoring of the heart rhythm. The patient who is in the hospital but not in the coronary care unit may be monitored by a system of telemetry. The Holter monitor may be used to record the heart rhythm of ambulatory patients. Monitoring the heart rhythm for long periods of time is discussed in Chap. 28B.

THE MEASUREMENT OF BLOOD LIPIDS (see Chaps. 62B and 62H)

There is evidence that hyperlipidemia plays a role in the etiology of coronary atherosclerosis. The hope has been that normalizing the blood lipids with diet and drugs might decelerate the atherosclerotic process. The value of this approach to the prevention of coronary atherosclerosis is now under study. If one is to use this approach to prevention, it is necessary to measure the blood lipids accurately and use the "lipid lowering" diet and drugs properly. (See suggestions outlined in Chap. 62H.) It is necessary to remember that the measurement of blood lipids in the setting of acute myocardial infarction often gives an improper picture of the situation since the level of individual blood lipids is often different at that particular time than when the patient is not under such stress (see Chap. 62H).

PERIPHERAL BLOOD CHANGES (see Chap. 27)

The *sedimentation rate* of red blood cells was formerly used as a laboratory sign of myocardial infarction, but it has little specific diagnostic value.[41] The *white blood cell count* may become elevated by the second or third day of infarction and usually reaches a maximum in a few more days, after which the count rapidly declines to normal. The peak white blood cell count is usually between 12,000 and 15,000 cells per cubic centimeter. On rare occasions the count may be as high as 20,000. The differential white blood cell count shows an increase of polymorphonuclear leukocytes, with an increase in young forms. Many investigators have reported that leukocytosis occurs in virtually all cases of myocardial infarction.[42] The authors believe that small infarcts occur without stimulating a significant increase in white blood cells. Certainly a normal white blood cell count should not be used as evidence against the diagnosis of myocardial infarction.

GLYCOSURIA AND HYPERGLYCEMIA (see Chaps. 27 and 62D)

When a myocardial infarction occurs in a patient with controlled diabetes mellitus, the blood sugar level may become elevated, and glycosuria may occur. Diabetic acidosis may be precipitated in such patients. Glycosuria and hyperglycemia may also occur in patients with myocardial infarction who are not obviously diabetic. This has been attributed to adrenal stimulation secondary to stress and shock. Some of these patients who have glycosuria and hyperglycemia have latent diabetes mellitus. Even though the findings may disappear shortly after the infarction, some of these patients will have abnormal glucose tolerance curves when checked some months later, and obvious diabetes mellitus may develop in a few.[43]

SERUM ELECTROLYTE DETERMINATION (see Chaps. 45 and 48)

It is necessary to monitor the serum potassium, sodium, chloride, and carbon dioxide levels in patients who are being treated for heart failure or shock. The frequency of the measurements is determined by status and treatment of the individual patient.

URINALYSIS (see Chaps. 26, 45, and 48)

Ordinarily the urinalysis offers little information that can be used in the diagnosis and management of heart disease. There are certain notable exceptions to this statement. There are times when an accurate 24-h fluid intake and 24-h urine output chart is important when one is managing a patient with congestive heart failure. The hourly urine output may be needed to follow the course of a patient in shock. The determination of the 24-h output of sodium, potassium, and chloride may assist one in the management of shock and heart failure and in the diagnosis of the certain types of hypertension. The performance of the renal clearance of creatinine assists in the identification of renal failure. The patient with tubular damage from shock may show abnormal casts in the urine, and the patient with endocarditis may have red blood cells in the urine.

BODY WEIGHT (see Chaps. 45 and 48)

The determination of body weight is fraught with difficulty. It is amazing that in this modern day of technology we cannot measure the body weight accurately and easily. The measurement of daily body weight is useful in the management of the patient with heart failure, and is necessary in a weight reduction program.

CLINICAL SYNDROMES DUE TO CORONARY ATHEROSCLEROTIC HEART DISEASE ASSOCIATED WITH CHEST DISCOMFORT

Myocardial ischemia due to coronary atherosclerosis is identified in most patients because it produces a rather specific type of chest discomfort. *Enormous skill on the part of the physician is needed to identify this particular variety of chest discomfort and, as emphasized earlier in this chapter, diagnostic errors are often made when chest discomfort is used as the single indicator of myocardial ischemia.* Myocardial ischemia (and its clinical counterpart, chest discomfort) may be due to conditions other than coronary atherosclerotic heart disease. These conditions include aortic valve disease (stenosis and regurgitation), cardiomyopathy (especially idiopathic hypertrophic cardiomyopathy), and the click-murmur "mitral valve leaflet prolapse" syndrome. As a rule these conditions can be suggested by physical examination. Other conditions, which are less common, such as nonatherosclerotic coronary disease can be identified by coronary arteriography. These include coronary ostial disease, coronary artery spasm, and dissection of the aorta and coronary arteries.

The chest discomfort associated with myocardial ischemia due to coronary atherosclerosis may be divided into two categories (Table 62A-1). *Brief chest "discomfort"* (which lasts for 2 to 15 min) and *prolonged chest "discomfort"* (which lasts longer than 15 min). Accordingly, the chest discomfort associated with myocardial ischemia will be discussed under these two headings. Some patients with coronary atherosclerotic heart disease do not have chest discomfort and are identified by an abnormality in the electrocardiogram, by coronary arteriography, and by symptoms other than chest discomfort (Table 62A-8). The recognition of these patients will be discussed under a separate heading.

The recognition of brief chest discomfort due to myocardial ischemia (angina pectoris)

THE HISTORY
The word brief implies that the chest discomfort lasts for 1 to 15 min. The word discomfort is used to describe the feeling the patient experiences. It is used in a generic sense, since it is less descriptive than the word pain. As will be discussed below, the patient may use any of a number of words to characterize his or her own unique chest discomfort. The brief chest "discomfort" associated with myocardial ischemia is called *angina pectoris* (see Heberden's quotation at beginning of chapter). It must be strongly emphasized that the mere identification of the presence of angina pectoris is not adequate. One must seek out every feature—every detail—of the symptoms so that the patient can be placed into the proper catego-

ry or subset of disease (see Chap. 62A). The placement of the patient into a clinical subset is necessary in order to develop the proper diagnostic, therapeutic, and educational plans for the patient. The characteristics of the symptoms that allow one to identify and classify patients with angina pectoris are described below. The conditions that mimic angina pectoris and must therefore be differentiated from it are discussed under the heading, *"Conditions Causing Chest Discomfort that Must Be Differentiated from Myocardial Ischemia."*

Angina pectoris (literally "strangling in the chest") is identified by analyzing the symptoms related by the patient. The physician must establish the *quality* of the discomfort, the *location* of the discomfort, the *duration* of the discomfort, what *provokes* the discomfort, what *relieves* the discomfort, and the *actions taken by the patient* during the episode.[44-50] It is also necessary to seek out *every detail* of the angina pectoris in order to classify the patient properly. Finally the degree of *disability* must be established.

QUALITY OF DISCOMFORT
It is always necessary to ascertain the quality or characteristics of the discomfort. Accordingly, the physician should not merely inquire about pain, since pain is often denied. The physician must ask about pain equivalents such as strangling, constriction, tightness, aching, squeezing, pressing, heaviness, expanding sensation, choking in the throat, indigestion, or burning. Our patients have even referred to the conditions as a "good feeling" or a "funny feeling." A patient of Dr. John Hurst referred to his discomfort as "only a faint, fuzzy, funny feeling—a softly spoken sternal word." The patient further advised us to pay attention to *"any* sternal feeling not normally there." Dyspnea on effort may be the complaint. In the past this complaint was thought to be due to the patient's difficulty in describing sensations to the physician. We now know that the transient myocardial ischemia associated with angina pectoris may produce heart failure. Accordingly, some patients with dyspnea on effort may have transient left ventricular failure (with acutely decreased left ventricular compliance) due to myocardial ischemia. A patient may be unable to put into words a description which the physician can recognize. The patient may simply say *"It bothers me here"* while pointing to the anterior portion of the chest. It is necessary to allow the patient to use his or her own words to describe the feeling. The terms that patients use are determined by their schooling, culture, occupation, and perceptiveness. The patient will often place the blame for the discomfort on the gastrointestinal tract. On the other hand, discomfort that is not due to heart disease may often be blamed on the heart.

LOCATION OF THE DISCOMFORT
The location of the discomfort, in the overwhelming majority of patients, is the retrosternal region. Al-

though the term angina pectoris originally referred only to sensations in the chest (pectoris), it is now used more generally to include sensations in the entire upper body and upper extremities. Thus, the discomfort may be confined to the chest, or there may be associated aching in one or both arms, more often the left. Many teeth are sacrificed on the altar of ignorance when pain due to myocardial ischemia is referred to the mandible or maxilla. Pain or burning sensation in the tongue or hard palate, induced by effort or emotional tension and relieved by rest or nitroglycerin, may be noted. Pain in the front or back of the neck may trip the unwary. Aching in the left interscapular region may occur. The distress may rarely be noted in the right side of the chest or axillary region. Aching confined to the shoulder, wrist, elbow, or forearm becomes significant when reproduced by effort which does not involve the shoulder or arm. Pain due to myocardial ischemia may also occur in these locations when the patient is at rest. In the natural history of coronary atherosclerotic heart disease, the location of angina pectoris may occasionally change. The reason for this is unknown, but it presumably has to do with ischemia of a new area of myocardium. The discomfort is occasionally accompanied by localized areas of tenderness in the chest wall, particularly in patients who have sustained a myocardial infarction. It is helpful to have the patient localize the site of distress by circumscribing the area with his or her finger. As a result of this action the size of the area of discomfort can be accurately determined. The size of the area is usually about the size of the hand when due to myocardial ischemia. Myocardial ischemia is seldom the cause of discomfort that describes an area no larger than a fingertip.

DURATION OF THE DISCOMFORT

The duration of the pain and the circumstances under which it occurs are as important as its location. Angina pectoris lasts only a short time, usually 2 to 5 min if the precipitating factor is relieved. Under certain circumstances it lasts 5 to 15 min. It rarely lasts 15 to 30 min. The patient may clench his fist over the sternum in an effort to graphically depict the constricting nature of the discomfort. This sign has been attributed to the late Dr. Samuel Levine.

PRECIPITATING FACTORS

The factors that precipitate angina pectoris are very important because they offer strong diagnostic clues. The attacks are commonly provoked *by effort* or *emotional distress*. The discomfort tends to occur during, rather than after, the exertion. A frequent story is that the discomfort first occurred while the patient was hurrying to catch a plane or bus or while he or she was carrying a bag to and from the plane. Parking a car in tight places, driving in heavy traffic, shaving, bathing, painful stimuli, sexual intercourse, micturition, or straining at stool may produce the

discomfort. There is a small group of patients who develop symptoms during effort whose distress disappears while activity is continued. This condition is called *second wind angina pectoris*. Curiously, work utilizing the arms above shoulder level may precipitate angina pectoris in patients in whom walking produces no discomfort. One or more episodes of angina pectoris may be associated with the *early morning activities* following a night's sleep. These activities include shaving, stooping over, drying oneself with a towel, etc. This early morning syndrome may surprise the patient and the physician, since the patient may be able to engage in more strenuous effort during the remainder of the day without symptoms. In a rare patient, talking or singing may induce angina pectoris, whereas physical effort may not. Angina pectoris may be precipitated when the patient *assumes the recumbent position*. When this occurs, the gastrointestinal system is often blamed for the discomfort. Occasionally *eating* or the post prandial state may induce angina pectoris (Chap. 62D). *Exertion following meals* is particularly likely to produce pain, and the sedentary individual may experience discomfort only after meals. When the chest, arm, neck, and jaw discomfort in question is precipitated by effort and relieved by rest, it is highly likely to be angina pectoris due to myocardial ischemia. When these characteristics can be clearly identified, the diagnostic accuracy is about 90 percent. Unfortunately a definite story is not always possible. Accordingly, the accuracy of diagnosis is diminished considerably when the history is difficult to obtain. When the chest discomfort occurs at rest, lasts longer than 3 to 5 min, and recurs frequently over weeks or months, the diagnostic accuracy is diminished to about 50 percent, but if the condition is truly due to myocardial ischemia, it is a serious type. Additional measures, such as coronary arteriography, are often needed to clarify the problem.

Of great importance is the intimate relationship of *emotional tension* and angina pectoris. Disturbing thoughts, stressful life situations, worry, anger, hurry, excitement, and nightmares commonly precipitate angina pectoris.

The tragic story of John Hunter, "the thunderbolt of surgery," makes the point. Hunter had said "that his life was in the hands of any rascal who chose to annoy and tease him." The following passage is reproduced in an effort to emphasize the role of emotional factors in the production of angina pectoris. It was written in 1796, by Everard Home, who was the brother-in-law of John Hunter.[51]

> Although evidently relieved from the violent attacks of spasm by the gout in his feet, yet he was far from being free from the disease, for he was still subject to the spasms, upon exercise or agitation of mind; the exercise that generally brought it on, was walking, especially on an ascent, either of stairs or rising ground, but never on going down either the one or the other; the affections of the mind that brought it on were principally anxiety or anger: it was not the cause of the anxiety, but the quantity that most affected him; the anxiety about the hiving of a swarm of bees brought it on; the anxiety lest an animal should make its escape before he could get a gun to shoot it, brought it on; even the hearing of a story in which the mind became so much engaged as to be interested in the event, although the

particulars were of no consequence to him, would bring it on; anger brought on the same complaint and he could conceive it possible for that passion to be carried so far as totally to deprive him of life; but what was very extraordinary, the more tender passions of the mind did not produce it; he could relate a story which called up all the finer feelings, as compassion, admiration for the actions of gratitude in others, so as to make him shed tears, yet the spasm was not excited; it is extraordinary that he eat and slept as well as ever, and his mind was in no degree depressed; the want of exercise made him grow unusually fat.

In the autumn 1790, and in the spring and autumn 1791, he had more severe attacks than during the other periods of the year, but of not more than a few hours duration: in the beginning of October, 1792, one at which I was present, was so violent that I thought he would have died. On October the 16th, 1793, when in his usual state of health, he went to St. George's Hospital, and meeting with some things which irritated his mind, and not being perfectly master of the circumstances, he withheld his sentiments, in which state of restraint he went into the next room, and turning round to Dr. Robertson, one of the physicians of the hospital, he gave a deep groan, and dropt down dead.

Exposure to cold weather, cold wind (especially on the face), cold bed sheets, or cold drinks may precipitate angina pectoris. The patient may walk less far in cold weather before angina pectoris occurs than he or she can in warm weather. Snow storms precipitate angina pectoris in climes where such occur. Shoveling snow, which combines effort and exposure to cold, is a common provoking action (see Chap. 62D).

Smoking tobacco may precipitate angina pectoris in an occasional patient (see Chap. 98).

THE RELIEF OF ANGINA PECTORIS

Angina pectoris which is provoked by effort will usually subside in 3 to 5 min if the patient discontinues the effort. Angina pectoris provoked by emotional tension will sometimes last longer than angina pectoris provoked by effort because one cannot control emotions as easily as one can control physical activity.

Nitroglycerin usually produces prompt and dramatic relief of angina pectoris within 1 to 2 min. The patient is able to walk further after using nitroglycerin in a prophylactic manner. Three points should be made if the relief offered by nitroglycerin is to be used as a diagnostic clue to the etiology of chest discomfort. A physician may be misled if he or she accepts too easily that the discomfort under discussion is truly relieved by nitroglycerin. The pain could be noncoronary in origin and might have lasted for only 2 min even if nitroglycerin had not been used. Occasionally angina pectoris due to idiopathic hypertrophic subaortic stenosis is made worse by the use of nitroglycerin. Finally, certain noncoronary causes of chest discomfort are actually relieved by nitroglycerin. The best example of this is esophageal spasm.

Carotid sinus massage applied during an attack of angina pectoris may give prompt relief of discomfort if the heart rate is slowed.[52] Levine pointed out that in order to evaluate the response properly, one should ask the patient if the pain is made worse by the maneuver, rather than asking whether the pain is lessened. We do not recommend this test because of the neurologic complications that may occasionally result from carotid sinus pressure.

The Valsalva maneuver may also relieve angina pectoris.

THE ACTION TAKEN BY A PATIENT DURING AN EPISODE

Some patients with angina pectoris produced by effort will merely slow their pace in order to achieve relief, while others will stop and act nonchalantly as if they are observing a building or to get the attention of those who are walking with them. The patient with prolonged discomfort may be restless and may walk the floor until relief comes from intravenous medication.

DETAILS SOUGHT IN DIAGNOSIS

The physician must seek out every detail of the angina pectoris. When did it begin? How often does it occur? How severe are the episodes? Is it getting worse? Does it occur with increasingly less effort? Does it occur at rest? Does the angina pectoris interfere with the patient's life-style and goals? These are the questions. Unless these questions are answered, it will not be possible to identify the subgroups of angina pectoris or to judge the degree of disability that is present (see Chap. 62A). One must not merely diagnose angina pectoris. One must also classify the patient.

DEGREE OF DISABILITY

The following variables are used to determine the degree of disability exhibited by a patient:

1 Determine the number of episodes of angina pectoris a patient has during the week. The severity of the episodes should also be estimated and graded by the patient as mild, moderate, or severe. It is important to remember that the severity of the episodes does not indicate the degree of danger that is present. Mild episodes occurring under certain circumstances may place the patient in a precarious category. The patient may find the use of a diary useful in his endeavor to keep an accurate record of his or her discomfort.

2 Determine the extent to which the angina pectoris interferes with the patient's life-style and goals. Some patients may have numerous episodes of angina pectoris each day but may manage to work and live as they wish with moderate happiness. Other patients may be disturbed by several episodes of angina pectoris each week and may feel it is interfering with their life to the point that they are quite unhappy. Even though the episodes are mild, the physician may determine that a serious state exists. For example, the development of angina pectoris at rest is often ominous. The physician understands this, but the patient may not. The establishment of the degree of disability is the result of the combined views of the physician and the patient. Fortunately, in

practice it is not difficult to establish the degree of disability if one keeps in mind the principles just stated.

3 It is important to determine the success of medical management in controlling the frequency of angina pectoris. In the past it was popular to judge the degree of disability in relation to what was called "optimum medical management." This made it possible to add all types of medication and use many dosage schedules before calling a patient "disabled" by angina pectoris. This permitted procrastination, since there is always an additional drug that can be tried. Today our recommendations are more specific. We suggest that propranolol (Inderal) be used until the heart rate is 50 to 60 beats per minute and that isosorbide dinitrate (Isordil, Sorbitrate) be used until flushing or mild headache occurs. One should then make a decision regarding the degree of disability of a patient with angina pectoris.

4 Finally, the problem of disability comes up most often in patients with long-standing, stable angina pectoris. The patients with one of the other syndromes of myocardial ischemia may be in a more precarious state and at times may have little discomfort. As will be pointed out later, descriptors other than angina pectoris are needed to classify some patients and to recommend specific therapy. The current New York Heart Association classification of *cardiac status* utilizes physiologic and anatomic markers in addition to symptoms to classify patients.[53] For example, a patient with 95 percent obstruction of the left main coronary artery and few symptoms is in great danger of sudden death.

THE PHYSICAL EXAMINATION

The physical examination of the cardiovascular system is usually normal in patients with angina pectoris due to coronary atherosclerosis. Evidence of hypertension, valve disease, cardiac enlargement, peripheral vascular disease, abdominal aneurysm, and retinal arterial abnormalities may be present, but these findings are not specific for coronary atherosclerosis. During an attack of angina pectoris, inspection of the patient may show either no alteration in appearance or the presence of pallor and cold, clammy skin. Other transient findings that may be detected during an attack include atrial or ventricular gallop sounds (see Chap. 18C), an apical systolic murmur due to papillary muscle dysfunction, paradoxic splitting of the second sound, pulsus alternans, and a precordial bulge due to myocardial ischemia. The abnormal precordial movement may be at the cardiac apex or in an ectopic position on the precordium (see Chap. 16). The pulse rate may accelerate and the blood pressure may rise just prior to or coincident with the onset of angina pectoris. These physical findings are seldom looked for, and we wish to emphasize their value. The search for them should be part of the exercise test.

THE LABORATORY EXAMINATION

The laboratory abnormalities associated with angina pectoris are useful when present but regrettably are often absent. The resting electrocardiogram may show ST-segment displacement or T-wave changes during an episode of angina pectoris (see earlier discussion). The exercise electrocardiogram may be abnormal (see Chap. 28A). The chest x-ray may be abnormal but does not assist in the recognition of angina pectoris. The serum cardiac enzyme levels are normal in patients with angina pectoris. Coronary arteriography is indicated in many of these patients (see later discussion).

The recognition of prolonged chest "discomfort" due to myocardial ischemia

THE HISTORY

The brief chest discomfort of angina pectoris usually lasts 3 to 5 minutes. The discomfort may last 15 to 20 min especially when the provoking effort is continued or when it is the result of an emotional upheaval. Myocardial ischemia in patients with coronary atherosclerosis lasting longer than 20 to 30 min is probably associated with the death of at least some myocardial cells. When certain specified objective findings develop in such a patient, a myocardial infarction is said to be present (see "Myocardial Infarction" later in this chapter). Since there are many dangerous syndromes associated with prolonged chest discomfort that do not have all of the objective features of infarction, it becomes necessary to identify the various conditions using more subtle objective clues and emphasizing the character of the chest discomfort due to myocardial ischemia.

Chest "discomfort" is the presenting symptom in the majority of patients with prolonged myocardial ischemia. The discomfort may occur anywhere in the anterior part of the chest, back, epigastrium, jaw, neck, shoulder, elbow, forearm, or wrist. The usual location is substernal. The patient may describe it as pain, heaviness, burning, indigestion, choking, constriction, tightness, pressure, aching, or expanding sensation. Expressions such as "It feels like a red hot poker," "like hot smoke," "like someone sitting on my chest," "like a belt tightening around my chest," "like an elephant stepped on me," or "feeling as if my forearms would break" may be used by the patient. Some patients describe a feeling of weakness or numbness of one or both arms. There may be minimal or absent discomfort in the anterior part of the chest, and the symptoms may be confined to one of the other areas listed above. In the majority of patients the duration of pain lasts from 20 min to several hours until it subsides spontaneously or is relieved by the administration of an opiate. Although the distress may progress in intensity during the early stages, it is constantly present and waxes and wanes very little until it goes away. Rarely, the discomfort may be aggravated slightly during inspiration or may be associated with hyperesthesia of the overlying skin. The pain may begin during the day while the patient is sitting at a desk or walking, or it may awaken him or her from sound sleep. Most patients are content to sit or lie quietly, but a few may be restive and may walk the floor clutching the chest. The patient may or may not give a history of prior angina pectoris or bouts of prolonged chest discomfort. Some patients may have experienced previous symptoms which they have ignored. Unaccountable weakness, an expression of impaired cardiac output, may precede other manifestations by several days or weeks.

It must be emphasized again that many patients give a history of prolonged chest discomfort that occurs repeatedly at rest over a long period of time. The chest discomfort may have many features thought to be characteristic of myocardial ischemia. Regrettably the specificity of this type of discomfort is not perfect. Many of the patients do not have coronary atherosclerosis, but it may be impossible to make an accurate diagnosis without a coronary arteriogram. On the other hand, such patients certainly might have coronary atherosclerotic heart disease, and if they do, they are in a particularly dangerous subset of patients. Other methods of study are often needed to clarify this situation. The identification of the subset to which such a patient belongs is determined not only by symptoms but by the abnormalities on physical examination, electrocardiography, and coronary arteriography (see Chap. 62A).

THE PHYSICAL EXAMINATION

The physical examination of patients with prolonged myocardial ischemia may be normal. These patients may have a normal appearance, a normal blood pressure, normal pulse rate, and normal heart sounds. On the other hand, there may be sweating, pallor, and hypotension. Ashen pallor may be described by the spouse. It is not generally appreciated that a good percentage of patients with prolonged myocardial ischemia may develop hypertension at the time of chest pain. Abnormal physical signs may be detected and may be particularly helpful when the symptoms are atypical and the initial electrocardiogram does not show diagnostic changes. Unfortunately, these important physical findings are commonly overlooked (see Chaps. 16, 18A to 18C, and 44). They include alteration in intensity of heart sounds, atrial gallop, ventricular gallop, paroxysmal splitting of the second sound, pulsus alternans, apical systolic murmur due to papillary muscle dysfunction, a systolic murmur near the lower end of the sternum due to septal rupture, pericardial friction rub, and an abnormal cardiac apex impulse or an ectopic precordial bulge due to an ischemic area of the myocardium.

THE LABORATORY EXAMINATION

The laboratory abnormalities associated with prolonged myocardial ischemia may be nil, subtle, or extensive. The initial electrocardiogram may be normal, show ST-T wave abnormalities, or show Q waves plus ST-T wave abnormalities. The measurement of cardiac enzymes is of no diagnostic value in the early stage of prolonged myocardial ischemia at a time when key decisions regarding management must be made. The diagnostic and prognostic values of the level of serum enzymes were discussed earlier in this chapter. The serum enzyme levels, especially the CPK, are of considerable value in determining if muscle necrosis is taking place in patients with recurrent prolonged chest discomfort who are under active consideration for coronary bypass surgery. As discussed in "Patients with Recurrent Myocardial Ischemia following Myocardial Infarction" later in this chapter, a rising level of serum enzymes (especially CPK) does not necessarily preclude surgical intervention in carefully selected patients. One must remember too, that a rise in CPK may occur after a bout of pain that lasts for 15 min and may not occur after an attack that lasts an hour. Coronary arteriography is indicated in many of these patients (see later discussion).

Conditions causing chest discomfort that must be differentiated from myocardial ischemia

There are many causes for chest discomfort. The work-up of a patient with chest discomfort is illustrated in the algorithm shown in Fig. 62E-11. It is reprinted here with the permission of the *Journal of the American Medical Association*.[54-70] The slight changes have been made by authors Hurst and King.

Note that the arrows [in Fig. 62E-11] are numbered and that the number assigned to the paragraph in the discussion relates to the number assigned to the arrow. The discussion of each arrow highlights some of the variables one needs to consider in order to move from one place in the algorithm to another.

1. The physician who analyzed the patient's history, physical examination, and laboratory work (including the chest roentgenogram and resting ECG) believes that the patient does not have myocardial ischemia but has another condition. Furthermore, the physician believes that further workup is not needed. Examples of this situation are anxiety and hyperventilation syndrome (neurocirculatory asthenia) or muscular pain of unknown cause requiring no further workup other than proper follow-up.

2. The physician believes the pain is noncoronary in origin and further workup is needed to clarify the cause or severity of the problem. An example of this situation is esophageal reflux, where the symptoms are definite but where gastric and esophageal abnormalities must be further delineated by appropriate workup.

3. The physician believes the pain to be coronary in origin. Furthermore, the physician sees no need for additional workup, since other data are sufficient to eliminate the need for exercise ECG or coronary arteriography. An example of this situation is the 75-year-old patient with typical angina pectoris that is produced by effort, that is not disabling, and has been present for several years.

4. The physician believes that the patient has chest pain caused by coronary atherosclerotic heart disease. The physician also believes that either an exercise ECG and/or coronary arteriogram is needed in order to make an appropriate decision regarding the management of the patient's condition. Patients with disabling angina pectoris, unstable angina pectoris, or recurrent episodes of prolonged pain thought to be caused by myocardial ischemia are in this group.

5. The physician is not certain as to the true nature of the

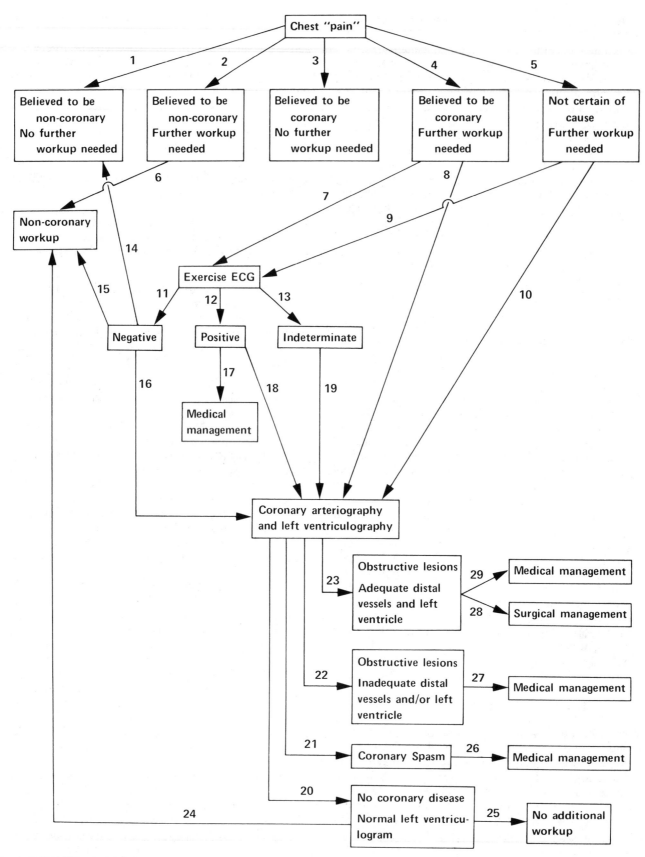

FIGURE 62E-11 Algorithm for the evaluation of chest pain.
Numbers correspond to discussion in text.

patient's chest pain. In such cases the physician is unwilling to dismiss the problem as unimportant and believes that further workup is needed in order to manage the patient's condition properly. The following are examples of this situation: (a) The chest discomfort has a few symptoms suggesting myocardial ischemia, but the real problem is that the physician is unable to get a reliable history related to the chest pain. The physician is shrewd enough to know that further questioning may simply create a false-positive history. (b) The history might be clear enough, but some features suggest symptoms caused by coronary atherosclerosis, and others do not. The physician remembers that classic angina pectoris with effort is misdiagnosed 10 percent of the time and that more prolonged chest discomfort occurring intermittently over a period of weeks is misdiagnosed 50 percent of the time. Knowing this, the physician turns to more definitive methods of study.

6. The physician, using the available data, has decided that the chest discomfort is not related to coronary atherosclerotic heart disease but is related to some other problem such as esophageal lesions.

7. The physician believes that the chest discomfort is caused by coronary atherosclerotic heart disease. Furthermore, the physician believes that an exercise ECG will be useful by adding support to the contention or by identifying certain features that indicate the severity of the problem.[55-63] The development of angina pectoris during the test often teaches the patient and physician a great deal. The stage of the exercise test in which the angina pectoris occurs is very important. The development of 2-mm ST segment displacement in the ECG during the test often signifies high-grade obstructive disease in the left main coronary artery or its equivalent (i.e., tight lesions in the proximal left anterior descending and circumflex or severe triple-vessel disease). We believe that this finding is even more meaningful if it occurs in stage 1 or 2 of the Bruce Exercise test.

Since the exercise test is dangerous in some patients, it is wise to think through in advance whether the results of the exercise test are going to be useful. For example, ST segment displacement during the stress test in patients with aortic stenosis, aortic regurgitation, hypertension, cardiomyopathy (especially obstructive cardiomyopathy), or the click-murmur syndrome. In some of these, myocardial ischemia may indeed be present but it may not be directly related to coronary atherosclerosis. The following conditions may invalidate the ECG changes during the stress test: digitalis medication, neurocirculatory asthenia, hypokalemia, WPW syndrome, and left and right bundle branch block. An exercise test may still be useful in patients with these conditions, since telltale symptoms may be identified during the test.

The physician must be familiar with incidence of false-positive and false-negative responses in various population groups else errors will be made in the use of the results of the test.

The exercise test is contraindicated in patients with recent myocardial infarction. The test is used in patients with chest pain when the symptoms do not contraindicate the test and when the results will assist the physician in clarifying the problem. The test may be used in patients with stable angina pectoris in order to assess the amount of work the patient can perform without symptoms or ECG evidence of myocardial ischemia. The test may be performed in certain carefully selected patients who are thought to have unstable angina pectoris or episodes of myocardial ischemia in order to determine if chest discomfort or ST segment displacement occurs

with exercise (see earlier discussion regarding the significance of greater than 2 mm of ST segment displacement). Considerable clinical judgment and experience is needed to select these patients, and if there is any concern for the safety of the patient it is proper to obtain a coronary arteriogram rather than require an exercise stress test. (See paragraph 8.)

8. The physician recognizes that the chest discomfort has been progressive and for this reason believes that the exercise stress test is dangerous to the patient and elects to obtain a coronary arteriogram as quickly as possible since coronary bypass surgery may be indicated. Patients with evidence of myocardial necrosis in the ECG or by serum enzymes are not usually candidates for coronary arteriography except when emergency surgery is required. Emergency surgery may be considered when the patient continues to have bouts of chest pain caused by myocardial ischemia following a myocardial infarction. This is an interesting subset of patients where there is evidence of step-by-step severe myocardial ischemia and necrosis.

9. The physician is not certain as to the cause of the chest discomfort. The chest pain has certain features that suggest myocardial ischemia and none of the features that contradict the performance of an exercise stress test. The result of the exercise stress test may be of value in such patients, but the clinician must be familiar with the frequency of false-positive and false-negative responses in the exercise ECG in different population groups. When this information is ignored, the stage is being set for confusion and misinterpretation of the significance of a positive or negative response in the stress ECG.

10. The physician is not certain as to the cause of the patient's discomfort but believes that myocardial ischemia caused by coronary atherosclerotic heart disease is a good possibility. Furthermore, the characterization (frequency and duration) of the discomfort supports the idea that if the discomfort is caused by to myocardial ischemia due to coronary atherosclerosis, that an exercise stress is contraindicated (see discussion in term seven). Therefore, it is necessary to have a coronary arteriogram performed in order to clarify the problem.

11. Results of the exercise stress test are normal. One must keep in mind that false-negative exercise stress test responses occur in 20 percent or more of certain population groups, else total reliance may be placed on the result of the test. Accordingly, a coronary arteriogram may be needed in some patients with a normal exercise ECG.

12. Results of the exercise stress test are abnormal. One must keep in mind that false-positive exercise test responses do occur. In fact, false-positive exercise test responses occur in more than one-third of women less than 40 years of age. Accordingly, by the time an exercise test is done for chest discomfort simulating myocardial ischemia, it is often necessary to perform a coronary arteriogram in order to clarify the clinical picture. When the exercise ECG is abnormal, it is necessary to decide if the patient's condition should be managed medically without a coronary arteriogram or move toward surgical management by obtaining a coronary arteriogram. Patients with chest pain who have a decidedly abnormal exercise ECG, stable disabling angina, or unstable angina should have coronary arteriography.

13. Results of the exercise test could not be interpreted.

There are many legitimate reasons why this occurs, including inadequate rate response and borderline or suggestive ST segment changes.

14. The physician believes that the normal results of the exercise test assist him in excluding coronary atherosclerotic heart disease and that the clinical features exhibited by the patient do not justify any additional workup.

15. The physician believes that the normal results of exercise test exclude coronary atherosclerotic heart disease, but the clinical features exhibited by the patient require that additional noncoronary workup be done.

16. The physician is still concerned that the clinical features exhibited by the patient may be caused by coronary atherosclerotic heart disease even though the exercise ECG is normal.

17. The physician believes that abnormal results of the exercise stress test support the contention that the chest pain is caused by coronary atherosclerotic heart disease but that medical management is the preferred method of treatment at that point in time.

18. A coronary arteriogram is needed to delineate the anatomy of the coronary arteries in order to determine whether coronary bypass surgery is feasible. Patients with stable disabling angina and unstable subsets of angina belong to this group. When 2-mm of ST segment displacement occurs in the exercise ECG there is an increased likelihood of a left main coronary obstruction or its equivalent. We believe this to especially be likely if the 2-mm displacement occurs during stage one or two of the Bruce test. This should stimulate one to move more rapidly to coronary arteriography in certain patients.

19. Results of the stress test cannot be interpreted, and a coronary arteriogram is needed in order to determine the presence or absence of obstructive coronary disease.

20. The coronary arteriogram shows no obstructive lesions, and the left ventriculogram is normal. Workup for a noncoronary etiology of chest pain may be indicated.

21. The coronary arteriogram shows abnormal coronary artery spasm that is accompanied by chest pain and Prinzmetal ST segment change in the ECG. Further plans are discussed in paragraph 26.

22. The coronary arteriogram shows obstructive lesions, inadequate distal vessels, or ventricular dysfunction. Coronary bypass surgery cannot be performed.

23. The coronary arteriogram shows obstructive lesions, distal arteries that are bypassable, and adequate left ventricular function for surgery. Coronary bypass surgery can be done if conditions justify the procedure.

24. No obstructive coronary disease was found, but the physician believes additional noncoronary workup is needed in order to clarify the cause of the chest pain.

25. The normal coronary arteriogram and normal left ventriculogram eliminate a diagnosis of coronary atherosclerotic heart disease, which was the only real concern the physician had about the patient. The other clinical features are such that no additional workup seems necessary.

26. Medical management is indicated for a patient who has been shown to have coronary artery spasm. Coronary bypass surgery has not proved to be effective in such patients.

27. Medical management is required because coronary artery surgery is not feasible, since the coronary arteries distal to the obstructive lesions do not permit the placement of a graft,

or left ventricular function is inadequate for surgical intervention.

28. Coronary bypass surgery is indicated.[64–70] While the indications will change as time passes, our current inclination is to operate on patients with disabling stable angina pectoris, certain patients with one of the numerous subsets of unstable angina pectoris, patients with episodes of prolonged myocardial ischemia, carefully selected patients with repeated bouts of myocardial ischemia after infarction has occurred, patients with left main coronary artery obstruction with minimal symptoms, patients with high grade obstruction of the proximal left anterior descending and circumflex arteries with minimal symptoms, patients with high grade obstruction of the proximal portion of the left anterior descending artery with minimal symptoms and decidedly abnormal exercise ECG, young patients with few symptoms who have a high grade obstruction in the left anterior descending artery and who have decidedly abnormal exercise ECG (2-mm ST segment displacement especially at low workload).

29. Medical management might be appropriate for certain patients with chest pain caused by myocardial ischemia secondary to coronary atherosclerotic heart disease. For example, a patient who has stable angina pectoris provoked by moderate exertion and an obstructive lesion in the right coronary artery would ordinarily be treated medically.

The noncoronary causes of chest discomfort may be divided into five groups. They are emotional causes; noncoronary cardiovascular causes; gastrointestinal causes; pulmonary causes; and neuromuscular-skeletal causes. Whereas the major purpose of this discussion is to describe the clinical features of the noncoronary causes of chest discomfort, the treatment of some of these syndromes is occasionally mentioned when it seems appropriate.

EMOTIONAL CAUSES OF CHEST DISCOMFORT (see Chap. 96)

Anxiety states The symptoms associated with anxiety states are commonly confused with angina pectoris (see Chap. 96). Patients with chest discomfort due to anxiety often have multiple complaints, such as weakness, giddiness, breathlessness, and palpitation. The chest discomfort associated with anxiety is of several types: (1) sharp, intermittent, lancinating, or stabbing pain located in the region of the left breast—the area of pain is often no larger than the tip of a finger and is often associated with a local area of hyperesthesia of the chest wall; (2) precordial aching pain which lasts hours or days and is unrelated to effort—the area of discomfort is often the size of the hand; (3) substernal tightness of variable duration which is unrelated to exercise. This type of discomfort may be associated with hyperventilation, but this is not always the case by any means. There may be choking sensation in the throat due to *globus hystericus,* which may be difficult to distinguish from the discomfort of myocardial ischemia.

Patients with anxiety may complain of palpitation, claustrophobia, and the occurrence of symptoms in crowded places. We have learned to ask the patient if he or she has to leave church. The quiet environment in a spiritual atmosphere commonly brings to the surface symptoms of anxiety such as the *hyperventi-*

lation syndrome.[71,72] Such patients have numbness and tingling of the hands and lips; feel as if they are going to "pass out"; have chest discomfort; and are convinced they are dying. The patients often complain that they cannot get a satisfying breath and are, therefore, short of breath. The physician may notice *deep sighing respiration* occurring several times each minute. The patient with anxiety may complain of persistent *weakness* and an *unpleasant awareness* of the heartbeat.

The patient with anxiety often feels certain that he or she has heart disease. Indeed, the symptoms from anxiety may be the major disabling symptoms in the patient with known coronary atherosclerotic heart disease—as, for example, following acute myocardial infarction. On the other hand, while symptoms due to anxiety may have brought the patient to the physician, a careful history may reveal true angina pectoris. It is often impossible to detect that a patient is chronically hyperventilating.[73] The exact reproduction of the patient's symptoms with forced hyperventilation may permit identification of the nature of the complaints. Hyperventilation for 2 min is usually sufficient, since many patients with chronic hyperventilation become troubled after a few deep breaths. One cannot invariably reproduce the symptoms by forced hyperventilation, perhaps because the physician's presence produces a sense of security, in contrast to the fear and terror engendered when the patient awakens at night with an attack. These patients often exhibit a junctional-type ST-segment displacement in the electrocardiogram taken at rest or during exercise, and this accentuates the problem of recognition. Furthermore, inversion of the T waves may be produced after 30 s of overbreathing. Friesinger et al. studied 14 patients with chest pain who were believed to have anxiety with false positive electrocardiograms.[74] The electrocardiograms actually showed classic "injury" changes, with "square wave" ST-segment depressions of 1.0 mm or more during the following exercise. On clinical grounds, none of the 14 patients had coronary heart disease. Eleven were subjected to coronary arteriography, and all were normal. One patient was given 5 mg propranolol orally which prevented the electrocardiographic changes when the tracing was repeated 1 h later. The clinical features associated with anxiety may, at times, simulate myocardial ischemia so closely that the physician may find it necessary to admit the patient to a coronary care unit. If the electrocardiogram shows ST-segment displacement or if the serum CPK level rises as a result of an intramuscular injection of opiate, a misdiagnosis of infarction is often made. This unfortunate coincidence occurs sufficiently often to recommend that every physician should be on the alert for it. A coronary arteriogram is often needed to clarify the problem.

Depression Patients with mental depression may have chest pain that simulates myocardial ischemia. In this setting, it is very difficult to diagnose heart disease with certainty. The chest discomfort may be prolonged, and the patient may have a feeling of despair, be agitated, be unable to concentrate, and

may have insomnia and loss of sexual interest and potency (see Chap. 96).

Self gain Informed persons who have various reasons for self gain, including those seeking sympathy or financial gain from pensions or insurance and narcotic addicts, can mislead the most experienced physicians. This is especially true of patients who have had previous well-documented myocardial infarctions, since in such patients even coronary arteriography cannot clarify the issue. Often the physician has a feeling that the patient's discomfort is not due to ischemia, but he or she may not be able to translate this impression into effective management in such an emotionally disturbed patient. Let us hope that radionuclide imaging will be useful in the diagnosis of such patients.

NONCORONARY CARDIOVASCULAR CAUSES OF CHEST DISCOMFORT

Extrasystoles or premature beats This arrhythmia may be accompanied by sharp, stabbing, or lancinating pain of brief duration. At times the complaint may be one of transient tightness or fullness. The uncomfortable feeling is usually felt in the precordial area. A choking sensation may be felt in the neck of patients with certain arrhythmias when the right atrium contracts against the closed tricuspid valve. A feeling of giddiness or faintness may occur. Extrasystoles commonly occur at rest, after meals, while reading the paper, or on retiring. Under these circumstances, activity may (1) accelerate the heart rate and eliminate the premature beats, or (2) accelerate the heart rate and decrease the premature beats only to result in a flurry of extrasystoles during deceleration of the pulse at the end of exercise. The anxiety engendered may produce dyspnea and hyperventilation. Accordingly, the patient may complain of pain and dyspnea related to exertion. If extrasystoles and symptoms occur fortuitously during the examination and during the recording of a routine electrocardiogram, recognition of the disorder may be simplified. At times an exercise electrocardiogram is needed in order to determine if extrasystoles or other arrhythmias are produced by exercise or occur after exercise. On rare occasions long-term monitoring of the heart rhythm with a Holter monitor is necessary to solve the problem (see Chap. 28B).

Some sensitive patients are so alarmed by the feeling produced by premature beats and other arrhythmias that they feel as though they are dying. The compensatory pause after a premature beat may cause a sensation as if the heart were stopping beating. This feeling may continue all of their lives despite their own experience of many years which should prove to them that their rhythm disturbance is benign. Other patients, of course, do not feel their premature beats or any other arrhythmia.

Acute pericarditis[75,76] This condition may produce precordial and substernal pain which is characteristically aggravated by deep inspiration, change of body position, and occasionally by swallowing (see Chap. 84). Pericarditis may be idiopathic in origin or may be due to viral or bacterial infection, rheumatic fever, collagen disease, neoplastic disease, trauma, uremia, or may be secondary to myocardial infarction, external trauma, or cardiac surgery. Stimulation of sensory fibers involving the pericardium and diaphragmatic pleura produces radiation of pain to the precordium, the trapezius muscle area, the back of the neck, or the upper part of the abdomen. Confusion occurs when the discomfort is confined to the neck, shoulder, right pectoral region, or abdomen, unless there is a clear relationship to breathing and turning. The pain of pericarditis may diminish if the breath is held. The pain tends to be sharp or cutting and may recur in intermittent bursts which are usually precipitated by a change of body position. At times the patient may become comfortable when he assumes the upright position and leans forward. The early appearance of fever and pericardial friction rub suggests pericarditis rather than myocardial ischemia and necrosis, in which these signs are usually delayed for several days. This rule is not always true since an occasional patient with myocardial infarction will have a silent infarct and experience the pain of pericarditis.

A pericardial friction rub due to pericarditis may be present without pain, and the typical pain of pericarditis may be present without a pericardial friction rub.

The electrocardiographic abnormalities are confined to the ST segment and T waves. Abnormalities of the QRS complex do not occur except for occasional lowering of amplitude due to pericardial effusion. In general, the mean ST-segment vector due to epicardial injury is located between $+30$ and $+90°$ in the frontal plane and is often directed slight posteriorly, so that the ST-segment change (elevation) is recorded in leads I, II, III, aV_F, and in V_4, V_5, and V_6. The T wave represented as a mean vector tends to point in a direction opposite to the direction of the mean ST vector. As a rule, the ST mean vector decreases in magnitude before the mean T vector reaches its greatest size. The ST-T abnormalities of apical infarction may simulate pericarditis when significant Q waves are absent. T-wave inversion of considerable magnitude may occur with infarction and is less likely to occur with pericarditis. Occasionally, acute pericarditis is first evident by isolated depression of the PR segment. Pericarditis may produce no alterations in the electrocardiogram, even when a precordial friction rub is present.

A small pleural effusion which obscures the left costophrenic angle may be detected in the roentgenogram of the chest in some patients with pericarditis. Modest elevation of serum transaminase (SGOT) level may occasionally occur as a result of pericarditis. This is especially likely to happen when pericardial effusion produces venous hypertension and hepatic congestion.

The clinical differentiation of pericarditis from infarction depends on the total synthesis of the history, physical findings, serial electrocardiographic changes, and echocardiographic changes.

Pericarditis following myocardial infarction is discussed in "Pericarditis" later in this chapter. Pericarditis following cardiac surgery is discussed in Chap. 95B. There are two conditions that should be emphasized. Mediasternal drainage tubes can stimulate the phrenic nerves and produce pain on the top of the shoulders and also produce a "pericardial rub."[77] The rub and the pain may subside when the tubes are removed. The aortic balloon pump produces a sound in the balloon when gas goes in and out of the balloon. This is heard over the entire chest and usually surprises the individual who first encounters the noise in such patients.

Dissecting aneurysm of the aorta Such a condition, although far less common than prolonged myocardial ischemia due to coronary atherosclerosis, is not rare (see Chap. 103). A past history of angina pectoris or prolonged myocardial ischemia due to coronary atherosclerosis always suggests that the most recent chest discomfort is more of the same, but such a history does not exclude dissecting aneurysm of the aorta.

The pain of dissecting aneurysm is usually maximum at the outset, whereas there is a gradual buildup of pain in most patients with prolonged myocardial ischemia. Although back pain may occur with prolonged myocardial ischemia, wide radiation of the pain to the back, flank, abdomen, or legs suggests dissecting aneurysm. A small percentage, perhaps 5 to 10 percent, of patients with dissection of the aorta have no chest pain. If the patient appears to be in shock, but hypertension is present, dissection should be considered. The diagnosis of dissecting aneurysm is suggested in a patient with chest pain who has any of the following signs and symptoms: syncope; weakness or transient paralysis of legs; hemiplegia; aortic regurgitation; pulsation of the sternoclavicular joint; wide differences in pulses or in blood pressure between arms, legs, or carotid arteries; left pleural effusion; and significant widening of the aortic shadow as seen on the roentgenogram. Pericarditis occurs with both myocardial infarction and dissecting aneurysm and is of little differential value.

Since systemic hypertension is frequently associated with dissecting aneurysm, the electrocardiogram commonly reveals the pattern of left ventricular hypertrophy. The demonstration of serial electrocardiographic changes assists in the diagnosis of myocardial infarction due to coronary atherosclerosis. It should be recalled, however, that on rare occasions myocardial infarction may be due to dissection of the coronary arteries.

The serum transaminase level is not helpful since modest elevations may occur in both dissection and infarction. Aortographic studies may be necessary to confirm the presence of dissecting aneurysm. The procedure should not be done simply because the electrocardiogram does not show abnormal Q waves or ST-T waves suggesting myocardial necrosis and ischemia, since myocardial infarction may occur without electrocardiographic changes. The decision to perform an aortogram should be based on the total clinical picture.

Superficial thrombophlebitis of the precordial veins Superficial thrombophlebitis of the veins of the precordial area may occur rarely and produce a confusing clinical picture (Mondor's syndrome).[78] The tender cordlike veins are often palpable in the precordial area and are the clue to the diagnosis.

Vasoregulatory asthenia This is a disturbance of the autonomic nervous system, and is characterized by marked asthenia. The patients may have difficulty in a physical training program. In the pure form there need be no chest discomfort. Many patients with vasoregulatory asthenia develop some of the same symptoms as patients with anxiety. This condition may be responsible for a false positive exercise test and should be suspected when there is lability of the T waves and ST segments of the electrocardiogram. The T waves may become inverted in the lateral precordial leads or in leads II, III, and aV_F. These abnormalities may develop on standing, with hyperventilation, or with the administration of amyl nitrite or other nitrite preparations. Junctional ST displacement commonly occurs after exercise, but at times a classic ischemic response may occur. The inversion of the T waves and ST-segment changes can be prevented in whole or in part by the Valsalva maneuver or by the administration of ergotamine tartrate or propranolol.[79-81] The symptoms and electrocardiographic abnormalities associated with anxiety (neurocirculatory asthenia), vasoregulatory asthenia, and mitral valve prolapse (click-murmur syndrome of Barlow) clearly overlap, and two of the conditions may be present in the same patient.

Paroxysmal hepatic engorgement Patients with heart failure may have pain in the right upper quadrant during exercise. This discomfort is due to paroxysmal hepatic engorgement and is rarely confused with angina pectoris.

GASTROINTESTINAL CAUSES OF CHEST DISCOMFORT
Theodore Hersh, M.D., Professor of Medicine (Digestive Diseases), Emory University School of Medicine, kindly prepared the following discussion on reflux esophagitis and hiatal hernia, diffuse esophageal spasm, esophageal rupture, and cholecystitis.

Reflux esophagitis and hiatal hernia[82-86] Reflux esophagitis is a result of failure of the lower esophageal sphincter to prevent the regurgitation of gastroduodenal secretions, with subsequent esophageal mucosal injury. The chronicity and the failure of the esophagus to clear the acid from its distal portion results in inflammation with consequent symptoms. The severity of the esophagitis depends on the concentration of the injurious agent such as acid and pepsin, or bile salts and pancreatic enzymes in patients with alkaline (bile) reflux esophagitis. The

aberration may be attributable to a loss of mechanical factors at the gastroesophageal junction or to an intrinsic incompetence of the lower esophageal sphincter. The former theory proposes that a sliding hiatal hernia plays a major role in the production of gastroesophageal reflux. This assumption, however, is based on the frequency of hiatal hernia documented in patients with reflux esophagitis. More likely, the physiologic sphincter in the gastroesophageal junction represents the main barrier preventing reflux. The lower esophageal sphincter maintains high pressures in the resting state and relaxes in response to swallowing. It also adapts to changing physiologic conditions maintaining favorable gastrosphincter pressure gradients which prevent reflux. Patients with reflux esophagitis have low or absent resting lower esophageal sphincter pressures when compared to normal subjects.

Heartburn and chest pain are the most prominent symptoms of reflux esophagitis. Heartburn is described as a substernal burning pain or discomfort noted by the patient as a quality moving from the xiphoid area to the suprasternal notch. Not infrequently, regurgitation of sour, bitter fluid and occasionally food is also described in association with the heartburn. Antacids and milk frequently relieve these symptoms. Belching may also alleviate this discomfort. The heartburn and the regurgitation often occur after meals or following postural changes; the patient is often awakened by heartburn due to free acid reflux in the recumbent position. Patients may also describe their esophagitis as a localized pressure or squeezing pain across the middle portion of the chest, and it may radiate to the back. Cases with long-standing symptoms may develop stricture with substernal pain following the ingestion of acid or hot liquids. Persistent dysphagia to solid foods also suggests development of a stricture.

The diagnosis is suggested by the patient history of heartburn, particularly in relation to meals and to posture and to relief by antacids. The esophagogram and upper gastrointestinal x-ray study may demonstrate hiatal hernia, but the important information regarding the lower esophageal sphincter is relayed by the fluoroscopist, who describes reflux of barium from the stomach into the esophagus. Cineesophagogram may more vividly record this abnormality. Esophagoscopy and esophageal biopsy may demonstrate mucosal lesions, including superficial ulceration, diffuse hemorrhagic lesions with exudate, deep esophageal ulcers, and stricture. The presence of a hiatus hernia on endoscopy alone is not sufficient to establish a diagnosis of esophagitis. The histology will show acute and chronic inflammatory changes. Sphincter incompetence may be further documented by use of esophageal manometry. Most normal subjects have resting lower esophageal sphincter pressure higher than 15 mm Hg, whereas patients with an incompetent sphincter with an excess of pressure to increments of gastric pressure induced by abdominal compression or leg raising, but the incompetent sphincter does not accommodate to these changes. In patients with severe esophagitis, the motility of the body of the esophagus may, in addition, show various degrees of motor incoordination and feeble contractions, contributing to the failure of acid clearance by the esophagus.

Determination of intraesophageal pH is another technique which demonstrates gastroesophageal reflux. The pH electrode, which is initially introduced into the stomach, is gradually pulled out, demonstrating the gastroesophageal pH gradient by this pull-through technique. The determination of acid reflux is performed with the electrode 5 cm above the lower esophageal sphincter. The *acid infusion (Bernstein) test* records a patient's esophageal sensitivity to perfusion with acid. It is performed with the patient in the sitting position and the tip of a nasogastric tub placed 30 cm from the nose; at different times normal saline and 0.1 *N* HC1 are dripped at a rate of 100 to 125 drops per minute. The patients with reflux esophagitis will experience substernal burning pain or reproduce their original chest pain during the acid drip.

Medical management of reflux esophagitis is directed to prevent the reflux of gastric contents into the esophagus as well as to bind the acid with antacids. The therapy of esophagitis also includes elevation of the head of the bed (15 to 20 cm), avoidance of bending over, weight reduction, and elimination of acid foods and excess fat from the diet, since the latter retards gastric emptying. Bethanechol chloride and metoclopramide may increase the lower esophageal pressure and prevent reflux. When medical treatment fails or when a stricture has formed, surgical repair may be necessary.

Diffuse esophageal spasm[83,84,87-89] Diffuse esophageal spasm is a neuromuscular motor disorder of the esophagus characterized by chest pain and difficulty in swallowing. It encompasses patients with various clinical, radiologic, and manometric findings. These patients may have thickened esophageal muscles, up to 2 cm in thickness, from the aortic arch to the distal end of the esophagus. Although there are no apparent defects in the ultrastructure of the esophageal smooth muscle, the adjacent vagal fibers exhibit degenerative changes. Diffuse spasm may be related to achalasia in that both conditions have positive methacholine tests indicating a sensitivity of denervated structures (Cannon's law), there are common manometric features, and case reports of transition from one to the other condition have been recorded. Vigorous achalasia combines the features of both entities—failure of relaxation of the lower sphincter, as in achalasia, and vigorous disordered contractions in the body of the esophagus, as in diffuse spasm.

Patients with diffuse spasm may present with symptoms most suggestive of coronary artery disease, and the chest pain in both conditions may respond to nitroglycerin. Of course, the two diseases may coexist. Esophageal spasm may occur in any age group but is more common in individuals in the fifth decade. Substernal chest pain with radiation to the back, arms, and jaw is the most frequent symptom. It can last minutes or persist for hours. The pain may be dull or sharp and squeezing in nature. It characteristically appears during or after a meal, particularly in association with the ingestion of cold liquids. Not infrequently, the painful swallow (odynophagia) is associated with difficulty in propelling the bolus of food to the stomach due to the spasm. Dysphagia without chest pain may also occur in diffuse spasm. Many of these patients experience severe nocturnal chest pain and are awakened from their sleep. Exertion less often initiates this pain, but anxiety and stress are common precipitating factors. Physical examination is unremarkable.

The diagnosis is based on the history, on the exclusion of cardiopulmonary and musculoskeletal causes of chest pain, plus the verification of esophageal spasm on radiologic and manometric studies. On esophagogram, a peristaltic wave is initiated by the swallow, but it only travels to the aortic arch. Isolated and incoordinated movements of the lower two-thirds of the esophagus are noted by the fluoroscopist and are described as curling, corkscrew esophagus, pesudodiverticula. When the lumen of the esophagus is full, the barium can be seen to be propelled by the contracting, spastic esophagus both orad and into the stomach. Esophageal manometric studies may confirm the radiologic observations. The peristaltic contractions of the normal esophagus are replaced after most swallows by simultaneous, repetitive contractions. Contractions may be not only of large amplitude but also of abnormal duration. Chest pain may be reported at this time. The methacholine test may be positive.

Symptoms of diffuse esophageal spasm may respond to sublingual nitroglycerin or isosorbide dinitrate, probably through their smooth-muscle relaxing effect. Nitroglycerin may be used before meals in patients with odynophagia or at the time of an episode of dysphagia. The beneficial symptomatic effect of nitroglycerin in both angina pectoris and diffuse esophageal spasm must alert the physician that other features must be present to make the appropriate diagnosis. Less often, diffuse esophageal spasm requires dilatation with bougies or pneumatic dilators. Occasionally, a long myotomy of the thickened muscle may afford symptomatic relief of the chest pain and dysphagia.

Esophageal rupture[90-92] Esophageal perforation or rupture is a serious and often rapidly lethal problem. The mortality has now been reduced to 30 percent after prompt surgical therapy. Spontaneous rupture was first described by Boerhaave in 1724; perforation is to be distinguished from esophageal mucosal tears *(Mallory-Weiss syndrome),* which presents as upper gastrointestinal bleeding following episodes of retching or vomiting. Today, esophageal instrumentation accounts for over 75 percent of the cases of esophageal rupture.

Spontaneous perforation of the esophagus may be the result of retching and vomiting following a heavy meal. This is associated with epigastric pain which may radiate between the shoulder blades. The patient then becomes dyspneic, diaphoretic, and cyanotic. The symptoms may vary in location depending on the site of perforation (cervical, thoracic, or abdominal). Pallor, tachycardia, and shock ensue, followed by signs of a presence of mediastinal air in the form of palpable crepitus in the chest wall, neck, or supraclavicular fossa. Auscultation over the heart reveals a mediastinal auscultatory crunch (*Hamman's sign*). There may be evidence of mediastinal air detected in the chest x-ray.

Iatrogenic instrumental perforations result from endoscopic procedures, from attempts at esophageal dilatation, or from balloon tamponade tubes. Perforations of either a diseased or of a normal esophagus may occur. Endoscopic perforations usually occur at the junction of the pharynx and esophagus, particularly in patients with osteoarthritic bony spurs. Bougies or pneumatic dilators usually perforate the lower esophagus. Esophageal ruptures may also follow pressure necrosis caused by foreign bodies or indwelling tubes, blunt or penetrating trauma, peptic ulcerations, carcinoma of the esophagus, and after devascularization procedures of the esophageal wall.

The diagnosis is established from a high index of suspicion of symptoms and signs following vomiting or from those ensuing from esophageal instrumentation. An upright chest x-ray will be helpful in the initial evaluation. Absence of free air under the diaphragm distinguishes esophageal rupture from a perforated intraabdominal viscus. The chest x-ray may reveal mediastinal air and pleural effusion. Confirmation of the rupture, however, can be accomplished by barium swallow roentgenologic study. The site of perforation may become evident on this x-ray study. Since the perforation may have sealed and is therefore not detected by the esophagogram, aspiration of fluid with an acid pH from the thorax may provide further evidence of rupture.

Treatment of esophageal perforation is usually surgical to repair the rent. Drainage of the mediastinum is also done. If the perforation occurs in a diseased esophagus (benign stricture or carcinoma), resection of the esophagus and bypass, such as with a segment of colon, may be necessary.

Cholecystitis and cholelithiasis[93][95] Cholecystitis is characterized by various degrees of inflammation of the gallbladder wall. In the majority of patients, cholelithiasis is a concomitant feature, although acalculous cholecystitis may indeed occur. The presence of gallstones manifests clinically by attacks of cholecystitis or by symptoms of obstruction of the common duct. Pigment stones (calcium bilirubinate) are usually radioopaque and are often associated with hemolytic anemias. In Japan, *Escherichia coli* is invariably grown from these stones. Cholesterol gallstones (radiolucent stones) are more common in the United States and result when bile contains high concentrations of cholesterol relative to the concentrations of bile acids and phospholipids. This phenomenon—lithogenic bile—has been shown to precede cholesterol crystal or stone formation.

Cholecystitis presents as discrete attacks of epigastric or right upper quadrant pain, associated with

nausea, vomiting, and fever and chills. The onset of the pain occurs abruptly and is either steady or intermittent and is associated with tenderness to palpation in the right upper quadrant. The pain may be referred to the back and right scapular area. Rarely, left upper quadrant and anterior chest pain occur. Dark urine and jaundice indicate that the stone has obstructed the common duct. Symptoms of dyspepsia, flatulence, indigestion, and intolerance to fatty and spicy foods often lead to the discovery of gallstones, yet the gallbladder is often not responsible for these symptoms.

Gallbladder disease is not uncommonly associated with coronary atherosclerotic heart disease; however, the demonstration of gallstones does not indicate whether or not they are symptomatic. Cholecystitis can precipitate angina pectoris in a patient with coronary atherosclerosis. Cholecystectomy may decrease the frequency and severity of attacks of angina pectoris.

The diagnosis is established from the clinical history and the presence of right subcostal tenderness. Radiologic examination of the gallbladder and biliary tract lead to the demonstration of cholelithiasis of choledocholithiasis. Calcified calculi are seen on supine films of the abdomen. Oral cholecystogram may reveal the presence of radiolucent gallstones, but not infrequently the diseased gallbladder will not concentrate the contrast agent; this nonvisualization also occurs when the calculus has obstructed the cystic duct. However, care must be taken in interpreting nonvisualization, for impaired absorption of the dye or disease of the liver may be responsible rather than a diseased gallbladder. Duodenal drainage may be undertaken for detection of cholesterol crystals or for determination of cholesterol, bile acid, and phospholipid concentrations in order to determine if lithogenic bile is present.

The recommended treatment of cholecystitis resulting from cholelithiasis is surgical, with cholecystectomy as the procedure of choice. There is less consensus in the therapy of the asymptomatic stone or that which is associated with nonspecific gastrointestinal symptoms without cholecystitis. Less than 3 percent of these gallstones may disappear, while more than 30 percent may become asymptomatic with attacks of cholecystitis within 5 years. Treatment with chenodeoxycholic acid will return cholesterol into solution in bile, and in 70 percent of cases with cholesterol (radiolucent) stones, dissolution of calculi will occur. Lithogenic bile, however, recurs on cessation of chenodeoxycholic acid therapy, suggesting long-term therapy may be required.

Peptic ulcer[96] The discomfort associated with a peptic ulcer is usually located in the epigastric region. The pain is relieved by food and is not produced by effort. It lasts longer than angina pectoris. The diagnosis is usually simple and is usually made by finding the ulcer by x-ray examination of the stomach and duodenum. At times, the discomfort of myocardial ischemia may be located a bit lower on the chest than usual or the pain of peptic ulcer may be felt a bit higher than usual, causing a diagnostic problem. The physician must be aware of this problem and obtain the proper x-rays at the proper time. One must remember, also, that both conditions may be present in the same patient.

Perforation of a peptic ulcer may occur without previous symptoms. The pain is usually confined to the epigastrium or upper abdominal region and is associated with tenderness and muscle spasm. X-ray of the abdomen made with the patient sitting will usually demonstrate air under the diaphragm.

Acute bleeding from a peptic ulcer may produce hypotension, syncope, or shock. Tachycardia is usually present, but some patients at the onset have a slow pulse which simulates that seen in occlusion of the right coronary artery. Depression of the ST segment in the electrocardiogram secondary to shock may cause confusion. The reduction of hematocrit, demonstration of blood in the stools, and abnormalities found in gastrointestinal roentgenograms identify the cause of the problem.

The long-term use of a diet containing large amounts of milk and cream by ulcer patients is associated with an increase in incidence of death due to coronary atherosclerosis.[97]

Acute pancreatitis[98] Acute pancreatitis may occasionally simulate myocardial infarction or dissecting aneurysm. This disease may be associated with biliary tract disease, alcohol intake, peptic ulcer, mumps, viral hepatitis, chlorothiazide intake, glucocorticoid intake, hypercalcemic states, hyperlipidemic states, and trauma, and may be a hereditary state. Pancreatitis is thought to occur when the proteolytic and lipolytic enzymes of the pancreas are activated with the pancreas.

Acute pancreatitis causes pain in the upper part of the abdomen which radiates to the back (at the level of tenth thoracic to second lumbar vertebrae) and may spread out over the lower chest. Severe pancreatitis may produce a shocklike state. Temperature may develop in a day or so. The degree of pain is out of proportion to the amount of abdominal tenderness. There may be a boardlike abdomen, and ileus may occur. Pleural fluid, pericarditis, and gastrointestinal bleeding may occur.

The white blood cell count may be as high as 20,000 to 50,000. The hematocrit rises because of hemoconcentration due to subcapsular, peripancreatic edema and "peritoneal burn" due to the enzymes. Hyperglycemia and jaundice may develop. The serum amylase level rises in 8 h in most cases and exceeds 280 Somogyi units. This elevation tends to return to normal in 48 h. The serum calcium level usually falls. Hyperlipidemia may be present and usually antedates the acute attack. The electrocardiogram may show ST-T depression and T-wave change. This may occur as the result of hypotension

and myocardial ischemia. The ST-T change of pericarditis may occur. On rare occasions the QRS changes of infarction may occur. This is probably due to hypotension in a patient with severe coronary atherosclerosis. An x-ray of the abdomen may show paralytic ileus, distended loops of intestine, calcification in the pancreas, and ascites. X-ray of the chest may show elevation of the left leaf of the diaphragm and pleural fluid, which, if tapped, has an amylase level higher than that found in the serum.

This serious disease is managed by treating the shock by maintaining an adequate blood volume, decreasing pancreatic secretion, and treating complications. Surgical drainage is no longer used. The mortality is high and ranges from 5 to 80 percent depending on the degree of pancreatic edema, necrosis, and hemorrhage.

The "cafe coronary" The dramatic and frightening occurrence of a *cafe coronary* must be recognized in order to execute specific treatment. When a person aspirates food, usually meat and sometimes peanut butter or bubble gum,[99] he may clutch his chest, become cyanotic, and die. Since these signs and symptoms may mimic an acute bout of myocardial ischemia, the event is referred to as a cafe coronary. The usual setting is that of a man eating steak at a restaurant. He has had a few drinks of alcohol and is enjoying the evening. He suddenly aspirates the meat and develops the symptoms. The victim is unable to talk and may rush to the restroom with food in his mouth. We have also observed the condition in psychotic patients who hold food in their mouths. If a victim is conscious but cannot talk and clutches his or her throat under the circumstances being discussed, one should consider the possibility of a cafe coronary. A blow over the back may produce expulsion of the bolus of food. Heimlich has devised a new treatment for this condition.[100] He recommends that the rescuer stand behind the victim; wrap his or her arms around the victim's waist; grasp one fist, with the other hand placing the thumb side of the fist against the victim's abdomen just above the navel and below the rib cage; press the fist into the victim's abdomen with a quick thrust; and repeat until the food is dislodged and expelled. The maneuver may not dislodge peanut butter.[101]

Distension of the splenic flexure of the colon[102] This condition may give rise to pain in the left hypochondrium and precordial region with referred pain to left arm. The lack of relation to effort, relief by bowel movements or passage of flatus, and reproduction of the pain by distension of the colon through use of a colon tube may clarify the nature of the symptoms. The splenic flexure syndrome is more common in patients who swallow air, have "irritable" colons, and are bowel-conscious.

PULMONARY CAUSES OF CHEST DISCOMFORT

Pulmonary hypertensive pain In the opinion of the authors, pulmonary hypertensive pain is not due to distension of the pulmonary artery, nor is it critically related to the height of the pulmonary arterial pressure. This pain may occur with lesions such as mitral stenosis, Eisenmenger's syndrome due to left-to-right shunt, primary pulmonary hypertension, pulmonary embolism, and cor pulmonale due to chronic lung disease. It may occur in the presence of low pulmonary arterial pressure, i.e., severe valvular pulmonic stenosis with right ventricular hypertension. The pain is believed to be caused by inadequate myocardial perfusion due to a limitation in cardiac output, reduced coronary flow during systole as a result of right ventricular systolic hypertension, and an increase in right ventricular oxygen demand. Therefore, the discomfort is due to nonatherosclerotic ischemic heart disease. It is not clear whether the ischemia is confined to the right or left ventricle, but logic dictates that the right ventricle may be more affected in some instances. Nitroglycerin produces a prompt reduction in pulmonary artery pressure, but the response to nitroglycerin is not as sharp as it is in angina pectoris due to coronary atherosclerosis. Since an attack of the discomfort may be self-limited and may disappear within a few minutes without therapy, the response to this drug may be difficult to evaluate. When pain can be reproduced by a given amount of exercise and can be prevented by the prophylactic administration of nitroglycerin, associated coronary atherosclerosis is the most likely cause. In contrast to the myocardial ischemia due to coronary atherosclerotic heart disease, this form of chest pain is almost invariably associated with dyspnea. In fact, dyspnea may be the dominant symptom. Many patients with this condition develop ST-segment displacement in the electrocardiogram during or after exercise.

A coronary arteriogram may be the only way to evaluate the coronary arteries in such patients and should be done if cardiac catheterization is performed to identify mitral stenosis, congenital shunt, primary pulmonary hypertension, or pulmonary emboli. Some patients with pulmonary emphysema who have chest discomfort should have a coronary arteriogram, since carefully selected patients may be candidates for coronary bypass surgery despite the lung disease.

Pulmonary embolism[103,104] The syndrome of massive pulmonary embolism without infarction of the lung may closely simulate myocardial ischemia due to coronary atherosclerosis, since impaired myocardial perfusion is present in both conditions. The diagnosis of pulmonary embolism is favored by the presence of intense cyanosis, profound dyspnea, and tachypnea which occurs simultaneously with the chest pain (see Chap. 75). Syncope may be the presenting or sole complaint of pulmonary embolism. Referred pain in the arms or jaw favors prolonged myocardial ischemia due to coronary atherosclerotic heart disease. The clinical setting of the patient may furnish a clue to the diagnosis. Pulmonary embolism is more likely to occur in the postoperative or postpartum period; after a long car or plane trip; following trauma, fractures, or amputation; in pa-

tients with congestive heart failure; and in the presence of thrombophlebitis. The development of acute tricuspid regurgitation, which may be recognized by observing a regurgitant systolic jugular venous pulse wave, in addition to prominent *a* waves, may be noted following a pulmonary embolism. The diagnosis of pulmonary embolism is favored by the following physical signs: fixed, wide splitting of the second heart sound; a new systolic murmur at the second and third left intercostal spaces; a contact sound in systole due to dilatation of the pulmonary artery simulating a pericardial friction rub; right atrial and ventricular gallop sounds; and, rarely, a systolic bruit which may be heard in the back or over the lateral thorax due to a partially obstructed pulmonary artery. A systolic impulse over the pulmonary artery area of a systolic lift of the sternum or parasternal area may occur.

Sinus tachycardia, atrial tachycardia, atrial fibrillation, or atrial flutter may develop in patients with pulmonary embolism. The electrocardiogram may exhibit evidence of myocardial ischemia and intraventricular conduction abnormalities. Sinus tachycardia with ST-segment displacement of variable degree is common. The terminal portion of the QRS complex may be altered as a result of acute cor pulmonale so that an S wave appears in leads I and V_6, and a terminal R wave appears in aV_R and V_1. Along with these changes, Q waves may appear in leads II, III, and V_F, suggesting inferior myocardial infarction. In other patients anterior myocardial ischemia with inverted T waves and transient loss of R waves in the right precordial leads may occur and simulate anterior myocardial infarction. On occasion myocardial infarction may actually be precipitated by pulmonary embolism.

The determination of SGOT levels will not routinely separate pulmonary embolism and infarction from myocardial infarction. The chest roentgenogram associated with pulmonary embolism may reveal the following: no abnormality; an increase in radiolucency in an area of the lung; dilatation of the proximal portion of the pulmonary artery with an abrupt decrease in size of a branch of the artery; or elevation of the hemidiaphragm. It should be reemphasized that less than 10 percent of pulmonary emboli produce infarction of the lung; however, the detection of an area of infarction by x-ray may clinch the diagnosis. Conventional pulmonary infarcts with pleuritic pain and pleural rub offer little diagnostic problem, but many do not have these features and therefore are difficult to identify. Selective pulmonary angiography or pulmonary scanning using radioactive substances may confirm the diagnosis (see Chaps. 30 and 75). An excellent sign that pulmonary embolism has occurred is the combination of a negative chest roentgenogram and an abnormal lung scan. Pulmonary embolism may produce an alteration in blood gases which includes a decrease in P_{O_2} and a normal-to-low P_{CO_2}.

Postmyocardial infarction syndrome (see discussion under "Complications")

Mediastinal emphysema (Hamman's disease)[105] Mediastinal emphysema due to rupture of the wall of the pulmonary alveoli causes dissection of air to occur along periarterial tissue spaces, which produces chest pain, mediastinal crepitation which is often noticed by the patient, air in the mediastinum and left pleural space, and occasionally subcutaneous emphysema of the neck and upper part of the thorax. The mediastinal crunch heard on auscultation is characteristic even to the uninitiated observer. The diagnosis may be established by detecting air in the mediastinum on the lateral chest roentgenogram.

Spontaneous pneumothorax[106] Pneumothorax may produce pain over the lateral portion of the thorax and is usually associated with dyspnea. The condition may or may not be suspected from physical findings but is confirmed by x-ray examination of the chest (if the observer looks carefully).

NEURO-MUSCULAR-SKELETAL CAUSES OF CHEST DISCOMFORT

Thoracic outlet syndrome[107–110] Robert B. Smith, M.D., Associate Professor of Surgery, Emory University School of Medicine, kindly prepared the discussion on thoracic outlet syndrome.

Thoracic outlet syndrome is a general term applied to compression of the neural and vascular structures that exit from, or pass over, the superior rim of the thoracic cage. A number of different names have been given to varieties of the condition in the past, including first thoracic rib, cervical rib, scalenus anticus, costoclavicular, and hyperabduction syndromes, according to the presumed site of major neurovascular compression. Pressure may occur at the interscalene triangle, in the costoclavicular space, or as the vessels pass under the pectoralis minor tendon at the coracoid process. Identifiable abnormalities of bone such as anomalous cervical ribs, bifid first rib, fusion of the first and second ribs, or clavicular deformities contribute to compression in 30 percent of the patients. Symptoms may be related to occupational activities, to poor posture, to sleeping with arms elevated over the head, or to acute injuries such as cervical whiplash. Most patients become symptomatic in the third or fourth decades; women are affected three times as often as men. The differential diagnosis includes any condition that can produce chronic, recurrent pain in the upper extremity: carpal tunnel syndrome, cervical arthritis, cervical disc syndrome, cervical cord lesions, superior sulcus tumor, peripheral neuropathy, causalgia, shoulder-hand syndrome, angina pectoris, arterial occlusive disease, and Raynaud's syndrome.

The majority of individuals with thoracic outlet syndrome experience pain in the upper extremity resulting from somatic nerve compression, usually in the distribution of the ulnar nerve. Paresthesias and hypesthesia are common, but anesthesia and motor weakness are reported in only 10 percent. While the pain almost always involves the hand and arm, it may also radiate into the neck, the shoulder region, the scapula, or the axilla. In a few individuals the pain is experienced mainly in the anterior chest wall and may occur in episodes suggestive of coronary heart disease. Vascular compression is thought to be responsible for symptoms in only a relatively few patients and is manifest as a more diffuse pain in the limb, with associated fatigue and weakness. With more severe arterial compromise the patient may describe coolness, pallor, cyanosis, or symptoms of Raynaud's phenomenon. Rarely the arterial impingement is sufficient to produce poststenotic dilatation of the subclavian artery with mural thrombus which may give rise to emboli and result in focal necrosis of the skin, or gangrene of a part. Venous compression symptoms infrequently result from thoracic outlet conditions but may present as episodic edema and plethora of the extremity; major venous thrombosis on this basis is rare.

The diagnosis of thoracic outlet syndrome can be confirmed in many patients by careful physical and neurologic examination. Palpation of the supraclavicular space may elicit tenderness or may define a prominence indicative of cervical rib syndrome; firm palpation at the root of the neck may reproduce the patient's symptoms. If nerve compression is suggested by the history, the examiner may detect confirmatory hypesthesia, anesthesia, paresis, or muscle atrophy in the appropriate distribution. Nerve conduction velocity studies should be obtained from the neck to the hand when neural pressure is suspected. A significant delay in nerve conduction at the thoracic outlet supports the diagnosis. This diagnostic test may also identify nerve compression at other sites in the arm, such as at the carpal tunnel, and thus allow surgical treatment at the correct level. Chest and cervical spine roentgenograms are obtained on all patients. Cervical myelography and neurologic consultation may be indicated if the diagnosis remains uncertain after the above studies have been completed. In patients with anterior chest pain as a major component, an exercise stress test and coronary arteriography should be considered as part of the complete work-up.

If the history indicates that compression of the subclavian artery is mainly responsible for the patient's discomfort, the examiner may find obliteration or significant diminution in the radial or the brachial pulses when the patient assumes a position that produces symptoms. The effect of *Adson's maneuver* (deep inspiration with the neck fully extended and the head rotated toward the side of symptoms), *the hyperabduction test* (arm extended overhead), and the *costoclavicular test* (exaggerated military attention posture) should be compared in both arms. Any changes in pulse amplitude should be confirmed by a decrease in blood pressure of that extremity as measured by a stethoscope or with a Doppler ultrasound instrument. A bruit also may be detectable along the course of the subclavian artery when the extremity is moved through the range of test positions. Interpretation of the results of these vascular studies, however, must include an awareness that false positive results occur with considerable frequency among asymptomatic, and presumably normal, individuals. If symptoms or physical findings suggest vascular involvement, it is desirable to obtain subclavian arteriograms, done with the extremity in both the neutral and the symptomatic positions. Venograms are useful only in the rare patient with evidence of impaired venous flow.

Although some forms of thoracic outlet syndrome have been recognized and treated surgically for more than 100 years, it is only in relatively recent times that the problem has been accurately diagnosed and appropriately treated. A trial of nonoperative therapy is desirable for several weeks in most patients and will be successful in many. The subject should be instructed to avoid the posture or activity known to provoke symptoms. Shoulder girdle exercises are prescribed along with the application of local heat, muscle relaxants and analgesic medications. Operative intervention should be recommended if conservative treatment fails, or if, at the time of initial evaluation, the patient has advanced physical signs such as motor weakness, muscle atrophy, or significant arterial ischemia. Successful operative management consists of elimination of all constricting forces on the neurovascular structures. This goal is achieved most reliably and with the least functional impairment by resection of the first rib via a transaxillary or supraclavicular approach. Removal of the first rib releases the floor of the interscalene triangle allowing the bracheal plexus and the subclavian artery to drop away from any impingements. During the same procedure, associated cervical ribs on constricting fibrous bands are excised and any necessary vascular repair or cervical sympathectomy accomplished. Operative morbidity and mortality should be quite low and the long-term results generally very satisfactory in properly selected patients. The few individuals who have poor results should be reevaluated carefully for the possibility of incorrect diagnosis, underlying psychogenic factors, or compensation-related malingering.

Tietze's syndrome[111,112] Local pain and swelling of costochondral or chondrosternal joints or of the xiphisternal joint may occur for unknown reasons (Tietze's syndrome). The second costocartilage on either side is the most common area of involvement, but any of the costochrondal articulations can be involved. Pain and tenderness may be reproduced by palpation of the local areas. The condition may persist for months without fever or systemic symptoms. The usual laboratory tests remain normal. The patient may not appreciate the superficial and local nature of the involvement and may wrongly attribute these sensations to the heart. The condition runs its course, but local procaine infiltration and local infiltration of corticosteroids may be needed for severe cases.

Herpes zoster[113] This condition may simulate myocardial ischemia. The pre-eruptive stage of herpes zoster is characterized by discomfort over one or more dermatomes. The skin is frequently sensitive over the involved area. The patient may complain of malaise, headache, and fever. The condition is commonly missed until the skin eruption develops, which may not occur for 4 to 5 days. The vesicles and pain are confined to the somatic distribution of one of the spinal nerves, and because of this distribution the condition may be confused with myocardial ischemia. Treatment should be directed toward the relief of pain.

Chest wall pain and tenderness[114] Chest wall pain and tenderness may occur for unknown reasons. The pain may be reproduced by palpating the area and by movements of the thoracic cage, such as bending, stooping, twisting, turning, or swinging the arms while walking. In contrast to angina pectoris, the pain may last for seconds or for hours, and prompt relief is not afforded by nitroglycerin. As a rule, no therapy is required. Salicylates may be needed on occasion.

Many types of chest discomfort occur after cardiac surgery. These include angina pectoris, pericarditis, and chest wall pain. The latter may be noted in the region of the incision. When there has been a sternal split, the patient may complain of discomfort at the superior portion of the incision and when the neck is hyperextended. The mediasternal tubes may stimulate the phrenic nerves and cause pain to be felt on top of the shoulders. Intercostal muscle pain is common following cardiac surgery. Cartilages or ribs may be fractured due to rib spreading at surgery, and pain associated with a "popping" sensation may be experienced by the patient.

CONDITIONS DUE TO CORONARY ATHEROSCLEROSIS NOT ASSOCIATED WITH CHEST DISCOMFORT

SUDDEN DEATH AND SYNCOPE[115–117i]
(see Chaps. 47 and 49)

There are many causes of sudden death in adults, but the most common cause is coronary atherosclerotic heart disease. The majority of these patients do not have acute myocardial infarction; however, a small percentage of the hearts will show evidence of an infarction that is several days old. Sudden death is common during the course of coronary atherosclerotic heart disease in both ambulatory and hospitalized patients. Many patients have syncope due to a cardiac arrhythmia secondary to coronary atherosclerotic heart disease. The episodes are due to ventricular fibrillation or cardiac standstill. If the arrhythmia lasts a short period, syncope occurs. If the arrhythmia lasts a long period of time, death ensues. The patient with syncope may or may not experience chest pain. Whereas sudden death or syncope may be due to an arrhythmia secondary to coronary atherosclerosis, one must remember that there are many causes of sudden death and syncope (see Chaps. 47 and 49). Dying *with* an arrhythmia is not the same thing as dying *as a result* of an arrhythmia. All people die with an arrhythmia. The group being discussed here die as the result of an arrhythmia. The therapeutic solution to the problem of sudden death and syncope due to coronary atherosclerotic heart disease lies in the following: (1) The prevention of coronary atherosclerosis, which is not yet possible in all patients. The elimination of risk factors beginning in early life seems prudent although the value has not been proven (see Chap. 62H). (2) The judicious use of bypass surgery in carefully selected patients. It is now clear that properly selected patients with coronary atherosclerotic heart disease live longer as a result of coronary bypass surgery. Obviously such patients live longer because the procedure decreases the incidence of sudden death and myocardial infarction.[117h,117i] (3) Patient education. The American Heart Association's endeavor to teach the American public the early warning signs of a "heart attack" is a step in the right direction. (4) Mastery by all health personnel and all teachable members of the public of the simple rules of modern cardiopulmonary resuscitation. (5) Continued research in the use of drugs such as propranolol in an effort to decrease the incidence of sudden death.

PULMONARY EDEMA (see Chap. 44)
Acute myocardial damage with muscle necrosis (myocardial infarction) due to coronary atherosclerosis may precipitate pulmonary edema. This may occur when the patient has no other cardiovascular disease. It may also occur in patients who have other types of heart disease, such as systemic hypertension, valve disease, cor pulmonale, etc. For example, the patient with systemic hypertension (or some other type of heart disease) who is active without symptoms or signs of heart failure may develop acute pulmonary edema. When this occurs, the physician must consider the possibility of myocardial infarction as a cause for the acute break in cardiac compensation. Acute pulmonary edema may be precipitated in patients with heart disease by a cardiac arrhythmia, pulmonary embolism, pulmonary infection, rupture of chordae tendineae of the mitral valve, abrupt damage of the aortic and mitral valve due to infective endocarditis, excessive salt intake, and, as discussed here, acute myocardial infarction due to coronary atherosclerotic heart disease.

Pulmonary edema may develop as a result of myocardial infarction, and the symptoms of breathlessness may dominate the clinical picture to the degree that a complaint of chest pain or discomfort may not be present. One might term this condition painless infarction but not a symptomless infarction. The examination of the heart may fail to reveal abnormalities because the loud rales secondary to pulmonary congestion may prevent auscultation of the heart. The heart size is usually normal unless it was large before the new infarction. The initial electrocardiogram may not be diagnostic of myocardial infarction. One reason why the electrocardiogram may fail to reveal a fresh myocardial infarction in the setting of acute pulmonary edema is that the base-line electrocardiogram already may be abnormal, showing infarction, bundle branch block, left ventricular hypertrophy, etc. When this is the case, a new infarction may be difficult to detect in the electrocardiogram. A portable chest roentgenogram reveals either alveolar or interstitial pulmonary edema. The cardiac enzyme levels are, of course, not available when an initial decision must be made.

Acute pulmonary edema may be the major clue that a myocardial infarction has occurred in a patient with or without additional heart disease. The physician must obtain follow-up electrocardiograms and cardiac enzyme level determinations and must examine the heart carefully on repeated occasions in an effort to identify additional diagnostic clues.

CHRONIC HEART FAILURE
(see Chaps. 44 and 81C)
Chronic heart failure and cardiac enlargement in the absence of angina pectoris, myocardial infarction, or some other sign of coronary atherosclerosis is occasionally seen. This condition is called ischemic cardiomyopathy (see Chaps. 62D and 81B). The usual idiopathic cardiomyopathy is sometimes difficult to distinguish from ischemic cardiomyopathy since cardiac enlargement, angina pectoris, heart failure, precordial abnormalities due to ventricular "bulges," left and right bundle branch block, depolarization defects in the electrocardiogram, various arrhythmias, and sudden death may occur in both conditions. A coronary arteriogram would be needed to clarify the diagnostic dilemma. However, when the heart is large and heart failure is chronic, it is not necessary to establish the exact status of the coronary arteries since coronary bypass surgery is not indicated in such patients unless the procedure is done in association with the removal of a ventricular aneurysm.

ABNORMAL ELECTROCARDIOGRAM (see Chaps. 23 and 28A)
The electrocardiogram may reveal the only clue to coronary atherosclerotic heart disease. The QRS, ST, and T waves may become abnormal in patients who have undergone surgery—such as surgery for abdominal aneurysm or surgery on the prostate—and the anesthesia and postoperative opiates may have masked the discomfort of myocardial infarction. Patients with diabetic ketoacidosis may experience prolonged myocardial ischemia with electrocardiographic signs of infarction. Such patients may not sense chest discomfort because of mental obtundation. We must recall, however, that abnormal Q waves or persistent and unchanging ST-T wave changes may occur in conditions other than myocardial infarction due to coronary atherosclerotic heart disease. A common example of this group of conditions is cardiomyopathy (see Chaps. 81B to 81D).

Right bundle branch block may be due to coronary atherosclerosis, but when this is the only abnormality present, it is more likely to be due to something else. Left bundle branch block may be caused by coronary atherosclerosis, but when this is the only finding, it is just as likely to be due to primary disease of the conduction system or sclerosis of the left ventricular skeleton.[118] Isolated left or right bundle branch block in a young person with no other evidence of heart disease is not sufficient evidence to indicate a poor prognosis. Complete heart block without other symptoms and signs was once thought to be due solely to coronary atherosclerosis, but it is now considered more likely to be due to primary disease of the conduction system or sclerosis of the left ventricular skeleton.

A positive response in the exercise electrocardiogram may be the only clue to coronary atherosclerotic heart disease. The problems of false positive and false negative responses have been discussed in Chap. 28 and in "The Use and Limitations of the Electrocardiogram" earlier in this chapter. One may have extensive coronary atherosclerosis with a normal exercise electrocardiogram, and one may have a positive exercise electrocardiogram with normal coronary arteries. Therefore, it is necessary for the physician to know all of the causes of a false positive response and to realize that in certain population groups (such as symptomatic patients) that a positive response to exercise may be far more specific than a positive response is in a different population of patients (such as young women).[19a,19b] Now that exercise electrocardiograms are made more often than in years past, it is not uncommon to encounter a positive test in asymptomatic patients. Circumstances will occasionally demand that a coronary arteriogram be made in some of these patients. The coronary arteriogram will be negative in some of these patients but will be positive in others. We have even seen high-grade left main coronary obstruction or severe triple-vessel disease in such patients. At the time of this writing it is not possible to give a rigid recommendation regarding the need for coronary arteriography in patients who have a positive exercise electrocardiogram who have no other evidence of disease. We are reluctant to recommend that coronary arteriography be performed in all patients who have positive exercise electrocardiograms; on the other hand, we have seen situations where this course of action revealed coronary disease that required coronary artery surgery. The greater the ST-segment displacement during the exercise test, the more we are prone to move on to coronary arteriography.

CARDIAC ARRHYTHMIAS
(see also Chap. 46D)
Certain cardiac arrhythmias may be caused by coronary atherosclerotic heart disease, and they may occur in patients who have not experienced chest discomfort. These same arrhythmias may be caused by many other forms of heart disease. Atrial arrhythmias are common and may occur in many conditions. Ventricular tachycardia, ventricular fibrillation, and complete heart block may be due to coronary atherosclerotic heart disease, but there are many other causes of such rhythms.

PROFOUND FATIGUE
Fatigue may be caused by coronary atherosclerotic heart disease. Not only may profound fatigue be the only symptom of myocardial infarction, it may precede infarction by days or weeks. There are many causes of fatigue, but coronary atherosclerotic heart disease must be considered when an individual complains of this symptom for the first time in the absence of anxiety and other conditions known to cause it.

Profound fatigue may occur in an abrupt fashion at the time angina pectoris is precipitated with effort. On rare occasions the fatigue may occur without the angina. This phenomenon may be observed and reproduced on the treadmill when the patient discontinues exercise because of fatigue and the electrocardiogram shows ST-segment change which is considered to be a positive response. The blood pressure falls during the test. This condition is probably due to transient ischemic paralysis of the left ventricle.

ABNORMAL CORONARY ARTERIOGRAM
A coronary arteriogram is always performed in adults who have cardiac catheterization for valvular heart disease. When this is done, it is not uncommon to discover high-grade obstructive lesions due to coronary atherosclerosis in patients with valve disease who have no symptoms due to myocardial ischemia. The association is especially common in adult patients with aortic stenosis who have angina pectoris. (See "Patients with Aortic Valve Disease Who Have Episodes of Myocardial Ischemia" later in this chapter.)

ABNORMAL X-RAY OF THE HEART
The x-ray of the heart may reveal the only abnormality due to coronary atherosclerotic heart disease. A ventricular aneurysm or ventricular wall calcification may rarely occur in the absence of a history of angina pectoris or myocardial infarction.

Calcification of the coronary arteries may be detected by x-ray examination or fluoroscopy. A superior method of detecting coronary calcification is cinefluoroscopy (see Chap. 29B). The patient may or may not have symptoms when the abnormality is detected.

ABNORMAL PHYSICAL FINDINGS
(see Chaps. 16 and 18)
The identification of a large apex impulse, atrial and ventricular gallop movements and sounds, signs of heart failure, and bundle branch block in the electrocardiogram, in the absence of hypertension, valve disease, or congenital heart disease should lead one to consider cardiomyopathy. One cause of congestive cardiomyopathy is coronary atherosclerotic heart disease in a patient without angina pectoris or episodes of prolonged myocardial ischemia, so-called ischemic cardiomyopathy.

High-grade obstruction in a coronary artery may produce an abnormal precordial murmur. The murmur may be heard only in diastole. It is surprising that this murmur does not occur more often.

The systolic murmur related to papillary muscle dysfunction may be heard in patients who never experienced chest discomfort.

PERIPHERAL ARTERIAL EMBOLISM (see Chaps. 103 to 105 and 107)

The first clue that myocardial infarction has occurred may be evidence of a peripheral arterial embolism. The embolus may obstruct the blood flow to a portion of the brain, the upper or lower extremities, spleen, intestine, kidney, or lower aorta. A cerebral vascular accident is the most commonly recognized sign of an embolus, and small renal infarctions are recognized less often. Mesenteric emboli are usually unrecognized. The evidence of myocardial infarction is often recognized when a patient with a rapidly resolving cerebral vascular accident has evidence of infarction displayed in the electrocardiogram.

THE RECOGNITION OF SPECIFIC CLINICAL SYNDROMES

The reader should be thoroughly familiar with the discussion in Chap. 62A, since the concepts stated there serve as background information for the discussion that follows here. The pertinent features of Chap. 62A are as follows: The variables used to identify the specific coronary syndromes or subsets are the variety of chest discomfort; abnormalities identified by physical examination; abnormalities detected in the initial and subsequent electrocardiograms; abnormalities found in the exercise electrocardiogram (when such a test is indicated); the level of serum cardiac enzymes; complications such as arrhythmias, shock, and heart failure; abnormalities found at coronary arteriography and left ventriculography (when such tests are indicated).

The discussion in Chap. 62A emphasized the problems that are related to the *time* a physician encounters a patient and described "The Four Phases of Decision Making." The objective of Chap. 62A was to create a clinical taxonomy that would enable the physician to categorize patients so that (1) specific medical and surgical treatment could be directly linked to a specific syndrome or subset, and (2) anyone would have a clear view regarding the patient's exact problem.

Since an infinite number of coronary syndromes or subsets can be identified, readers are asked to study the concepts promulgated in Chap. 62A and in Tables 62A-1 to 62A-8 and to create in their minds as many syndromes or subsets as possible. This mental exercise will enable one to "visualize" the numerous manifestations of this disease. This does not imply that each conceivable syndrome or subset has a different prognosis or requires a different treatment.

Fortunately, the same prognosis and treatment applies to groups of the syndromes or subsets. Accordingly, the more common syndromes or subsets can be grouped as follows:

1 THE PATIENT WITH CORONARY ATHEROSCLEROTIC HEART DISEASE WHO HAS NO CHEST DISCOMFORT[118]
(see Chap. 62A and Fig. 62A-8)

Angina pectoris and more prolonged chest discomfort are well-known manifestations of myocardial ischemia due to coronary atherosclerosis. Such discomfort is not the only manifestation of obstructive coronary disease. For example, coronary atherosclerotic heart disease may cause sudden death, syncope, acute pulmonary edema, chronic heart failure, an abnormal electrocardiogram, certain cardiac arrhythmias, profound fatigue, an abnormal coronary arteriogram, abnormal x-ray of the heart, and certain abnormal physical findings.

Three of these situations deserve emphasis. (1) *syncope* and *sudden death* (see sections which follow); (2) a positive exercise electrocardiogram test (The test may have been done as part of examination for life insurance or as part of an office visit. The positive exercise test may prompt the physician to obtain a coronary arteriogram, which may in turn lead to coronary bypass surgery.); (3) an advanced degree of coronary obstruction, which may be discovered when a coronary arteriogram is done for reasons other than chest discomfort. (For example, it is customary to perform a coronary arteriogram when an adult patient with aortic or mitral valve disease is undergoing cardiac catheterization. Coronary bypass surgery may be indicated at the time of valve surgery.)

The management of some of these conditions is discussed later in this chapter. See items 1, 9, and 10 in the section entitled "The Management of Specific Clinical Syndromes."

2 THE PATIENT WITH STABLE ANGINA PECTORIS

Stable angina pectoris is defined and discussed in Chap. 62A. In summary, the term stable angina pectoris implies that the discomfort has not changed in frequency, duration, and appearance time for at least 60 days. Stable angina pectoris is further divided into *mild* and *disabling*. Mild angina pectoris does not interfere with a patient's desired life-style, and disabling angina pectoris does interfere with a patient's life-style.

See item 2 in the section entitled "The Management of Specific Clinical Syndromes."

3 THE PATIENT WITH UNSTABLE ANGINA PECTORIS

Six varieties of angina pectoris belonging to the broader category of unstable angina pectoris are described in Chap. 62A. They are recent onset angina pectoris without rest pain; recent onset angina pectoris with rest pain; progressive angina pectoris without rest pain; progressive angina pectoris with rest pain but not disabling; progressive angina pectoris with rest pain which is disabling; and any of the varieties of angina pectoris just mentioned in a patient who has had previous episodes of chest discomfort due to myocardial ischemia or with objective signs of previous coronary atherosclerotic heart disease.

See item 3 in the section entitled "The Management of Specific Clinical Syndromes."

4 THE PATIENT WITH PROLONGED CHEST DISCOMFORT DUE TO MYOCARDIAL ISCHEMIA WHO HAS NO RECENT OBJECTIVE SIGNS OF INFARCTION (THE "PREINFARCTION SYNDROMES")

This group can be further subdivided into those patients who have had no previous evidence of myocardial ischemia and those patients who have had previous evidence of myocardial ischemia. These two categories of patients who have prolonged episodes of myocardial ischemia and the six categories of patients with unstable angina pectoris were formerly classified as belonging to the group designated as "preinfarction." The latter term is no longer used, but it does have the value of warning the physician that the patient may be in a precarious state.

See item 4 in the section entitled "The Management of Specific Clinical Syndromes."

5 THE PATIENT WITH PRINZMETAL'S SYNDROME[119-123a]
(see Chap. 62D and Table 62A-4)

The discussion of Prinzmetal's syndrome here and later in this chapter was written by Dr. Charles Wickliffe, Clinical Assistant Professor of Medicine, Emory University School of Medicine. The syndrome is discussed in detail here because of the mounting interest in it and because it is now being recognized more frequently.

Prinzmetal's syndrome (or variant angina) represents a form of chest pain due to myocardial ischemia which differs from classic angina pectoris in both clinical manifestations and underlying pathophysiology. This condition was first described by Prinzmetal[119] in 1959. He had collected a group of 20 patients with chest pain that did not demonstrate two of the major characteristics of the classic form of angina pectoris. These patients all had their chest pain either at rest or with ordinary exercise, but not with more vigorous exertion, and all showed transient ST elevation in the electrocardiogram during the pain, which returned to normal as soon as the pain subsided. Subsequently many investigators have confirmed and expanded, but not substantially altered, Prinzmetal's original description of what he called "a variant form of angina pectoris."[119]

The clinical recognition of Prinzmetal's syndrome depends upon a careful and detailed history and unique electrocardiographic abnormalities. Prinzmetal[18,119] described a constellation of symptoms, one or more of which is usually present.

The chest pain is usually similar in character and quality to that described by patients with classic angina pectoris, although it may be somewhat longer in duration. However, the pain is usually not brought on by increased cardiac work and therefore is not related to exercise and similarly may not be relieved by rest, although the same patients may also have typical exertional angina pectoris.[120,124] The discomfort is typically relieved promptly by nitroglycerin, though not always. The discomfort will often occur at the same time each day in a cyclic fashion, particularly on arising or in the early morning hours. The patient may notice palpitation or bradycardia or may have syncope at the peak of the pain. A small percentage of patients will have a history of prior myocardial infarction. Risk factors for coronary disease may be identified although this may be of no help in separating those patients with fixed lesions and those with coronary artery spasm as the underlying pathogenic mechanism for their chest pain.[125]

The electrocardiographic changes in Prinzmetal's syndrome are quite striking, with marked ST-segment elevation occurring during pain (see Fig. 62E-2). These ST changes are identical to those occurring during a typical transmural myocardial infarction, but resolve to normal as the pain subsides rather than evolving through the QRS and T-wave changes indicative of infarction. Prinzmetal[119] noted that an increase in R-wave voltage often accompanied the pain. Other reports have demonstrated loss of R-wave voltage[126] and even the development of "diagnostic" Q waves during pain with return to normal after the pain subsided.[127] One of the authors (J.W.H.) of this chapter has seen a similar patient. A recent report has even documented the appearance of typical ST elevations and hemodynamic changes characteristic of Prinzmetal's variant angina in the absence of any pain.[128] Prinzmetal first described the occurrence of ventricular arrhythmias during the pain of variant angina and also noted transient AV block in a small number of his patients.[119] These findings are now well accepted.[124,125]

The pathophysiology of Prinzmetal's variant angina has been partially elucidated with the widespread use of coronary arteriography and hemodynamic monitoring. There is no longer any doubt that coronary artery spasm plays a decisive role in producing pain in some of these patients.[129] Osler credited Allan Burns with the original description of coronary artery spasm. Osler wrote of "[the] theory of Allan Burns, revived by Potain and others, that the condition is one of transient ischemia of the heart-muscle in consequence of disease, or spasm, of the coronary arteries."[130] The original hypothesis of the role of coronary spasm as a cause of angina pectoris was probably made by Latham in 1876[131] and later by Osler,[130] although the first incontestable evidence for the occurrence of coronary spasm in Prinzmetal's angina was not available for almost 100 years[132-134] (see Chap. 62D). *It now appears that patients with Prinzmetal's variant angina fall into two major groups: those with significant, usually proximal ob-*

structive lesions and those with minimal or no coronary lesions.

Higgins,[125] Shubrooks,[124] Silverman,[135] Plotnick,[136] Prinzmetal,[119] MacAlpin,[137] King,[134] Maseri,[133] Oliva,[132] Betriv,[138] and Endo[139] have reported a group of patients with Prinzmetal syndrome. The results of their work indicate that about two-thirds of patients have fixed lesions of at least one major coronary artery, and the remaining one-third have essentially normal coronary anatomy. Of the latter group a few have been shown to have spontaneously occurring coronary artery spasm, associated with chest pain and ST changes in the anatomic area supplied by the vessel in spasm. Reversal of the spasm is associated with disappearance of the pain and return of the ST segments to normal.

In classic exertional angina pectoris, the onset of chest pain is associated with an increase in the left ventricular systolic pressure–time index (the triple product of left ventricular mean systolic pressure, heart rate, and the systolic ejection period).[140] This causes an increase in myocardial oxygen consumption ($M\dot{V}O_2$). The limited ability of the diseased coronary circulation to increase its delivery of oxygen results in myocardial ischemia.

In Prinzmetal's variant angina the onset of pain may not be associated with an increase in $M\dot{V}O_2$, suggesting that the problem is due to a primary decrease in the coronary blood flow.[141-144]

Numerous studies in recent years have confirmed the presence of coronary artery spasm in Prinzmetal's variant angina and have related the occurrence of spasm to the appearance of chest pain, and ST-segment elevation in the appropriate anatomic distribution. The resolution of these changes with disappearance of the spasm follows the administration of nitroglycerin.[125,132,134,138,139,141]

The underlying cause of coronary artery spasm remains unknown. Much attention has been directed toward an abnormal response of the large coronary arteries to alpha-adrenergic stimulation, either directly through increases in sympathetic nervous system activity or via an increase in circulating epinephrine, or both.[145] The increase in sympathetic activity may be secondary to an increase in parasympathetic tone. A recent study demonstrated provocable coronary artery spasm in response to the administration of a parasympathomimetic drug, methecholine, and the prevention of spasm by administration of atropine.[142] These data confirm observations made at Emory University Hospital that coronary artery spasm appears to be much less frequent when atropine is used prior to coronary arteriography.[146]

An increase in parasympathetic activity will result in a decrease in $M\dot{V}O_2$ through its effect on heart rate, myocardial contractility, and blood pressure. This effect may, directly or indirectly, produce a relative increase in alpha-adrenergic tone in the large coronary arteries leading to vasoconstriction and perhaps spasm producing significant coronary arteri-

al obstruction.[147] The exact interrelationship between the parasympathetic nervous system, the sympathetic nervous system, and neurohumoral factors on the coronary circulation in Prinzmetal's variant angina remains to be elucidated.

The search for a method of provoking coronary artery spasm during coronary arteriography in order to identify the contribution spasm makes to a clinical syndrome is now underway. Such a method must be safe and reliable. Some investigators have used ergonovine maleate for this purpose, but not much work is needed before the drug and technique can be recommended for wide usage.[148]

See item 5 in the section entitled "The Management of Specific Clinical Syndromes."

6 THE PATIENT WITH MYOCARDIAL INFARCTION DUE TO CORONARY ATHEROSCLEROTIC HEART DISEASE (see Chap. 62A)

The clinical and laboratory findings which are considered to be diagnostic of myocardial infarction include at least two of the following: (1) a history of pain consistant with myocardial ischemia, (2) electrocardiographic changes consistent with infarction (this includes appropriate changes in T waves, ST-T segments, or appropriate QRS, S-T and T change), and (3) a rise in the serum level of specific cardiac enzymes.[149] Small infarcts can occur unaccompanied by any of these changes.

By the fourth or fifth day of illness, specific criteria can be applied to assign certain patients to a subset with *"uncomplicated completed* acute myocardial infarction." These include the absence of evidence of continuing myocardial ischemia, left ventricular failure, shock, important cardiac arrhythmias, conduction disturbances, or other serious illnesses in patients with an established acute myocardial infarction.[149]

A patient with a fresh infarction who continues to have evidence of myocardial ischemia should be considered as having an *incompleted infarction.* A patient with fresh infarction who has heart failure, shock, arrhythmia, conduction disturbances, or other serious illnesses is considered to have *complications.*

See item 6 in the section entitled "The Management of Specific Clinical Syndromes."

7 THE PATIENT WITH CONTINUING OR RECURRENT MYOCARDIAL ISCHEMIA FOLLOWING MYOCARDIAL INFARCTION

Patients continuing to have evidence of myocardial ischemia soon after the infarction begins are said to have an incompleted infarction. When such occurs, the patient is destined to have additional infarction. This clinical situation is sometimes called "infarction on the installment plan." Recurrent episodes of ischemia may occur soon after the infarction begins or may develop weeks or months later.

See item 7 in the section entitled "The Management of Specific Clinical Syndromes."

8 THE PATIENT WITH MYOCARDIAL ISCHEMIA FOLLOWING BYPASS SURGERY

Patients who have evidence of myocardial ischemia a few days to a few months after bypass surgery may have closure of the grafts, whereas the reappearance of episodes of myocardial ischemia several years after bypass surgery may indicate progression of the atherosclerotic process.

See item 7 in the section entitled "The Management of Specific Clinical Syndromes."

9 THE PATIENT WITH SYNCOPE

(see Chap. 47)

On rare occasions it is possible to prove that syncope is due to ventricular tachycardia or fibrillation. Some of these patients should have coronary arteriography. When certain critical anatomic lesions are found, it is appropriate to consider bypass surgery for such patients.

See item 9 in the section entitled "The Management of Specific Clinical Syndromes."

10 SUDDEN DEATH[17a–17g]

(see Chaps. 49 and 62D)

Sudden death is usually caused by a cardiac arrhythmia secondary to abrupt ischemia due to coronary atherosclerotic heart disease. The difference between syncope and death in such patients is merely a matter of a few seconds—the rhythm spontaneously reverts to normal in patients with syncope and continues in patients who die. Occasionally a patient with sudden death will be resuscitated. Such a patient should have a coronary arteriogram performed unless a noncoronary cause can be identified.

See item 10 in the section "The Management of Specific Clinical Syndromes."

11 PATIENTS WITH AORTIC VALVE DISEASE WHO HAVE EPISODES OF MYOCARDIAL ISCHEMIA[150,150a]

Patients with aortic stenosis, aortic regurgitation, and combined aortic stenosis and regurgitation may have episodes of myocardial ischemia. Lewis observed that angina pectoris was present in 70 of 120 patients (58.4 percent) with pure or predominant stenosis.[151] Significant associated coronary artery disease (determined by coronary arteriography) was present in 40 (57.1 percent) of the 70 patients with angina pectoris. Angina pectoris was a prominent symptom in 14 or 76 patients (18.4 percent) with pure aortic regurgitation. Associated, significant coronary artery disease (determined by coronary arteriography) was present in 5 (35.7 percent) of the 14 patients with angina pectoris. Clinically, Lewis could not identify patients with associated coronary lesions without a coronary arteriogram. Therefore, a coronary arteriogram must be performed at the time of cardiac catheterization in order to delineate the anatomy of the coronary arteries.

Patients with aortic valve disease who do not have angina pectoris may have serious associated obstructive coronary atherosclerotic disease. Accordingly, it is proper to perform coronary arteriography in adult patients who are undergoing cardiac catheterization for aortic valve disease.

See item 11 in the section entitled "The Management of Specific Clinical Syndromes."

12 PATIENTS WITH MITRAL VALVE DISEASE WHO HAVE EPISODES OF MYOCARDIAL ISCHEMIA

Young women with mitral stenosis may have episodes of myocardial ischemia without associated obstructive coronary disease. Older patients, especially males, with mitral valve disease may have associated coronary lesions. It is wise to perform a coronary arteriogram in most adult patients who are undergoing cardiac catheterization for mitral valve disease in order to determine the status of the coronary arteries.

See item 12 in the section entitled "The Management of Specific Clinical Syndromes."

13 THE PATIENT WITH EPISODES OF MYOCARDIAL ISCHEMIA WHO ALSO HAS SIGNIFICANT EXTRACRANIAL ARTERIAL OCCLUSIVE DISEASE

Taylor has emphasized that some patients with episodes of myocardial ischemia also have significant extracranial arterial occlusive disease which is amenable to surgical treatment.[152] Symptoms of cerebrovascular insufficiency (such as transient ischemic attacks), a history of a cerebrovascular accident, or the presence of a significant carotid bruit indicate the need for careful neurologic evaluation and possibel carotid arteriography in patients who need coronary arteriography to clarify a particular coronary syndrome. See item 13 in the section entitled "The Management of Specific Clinical Syndromes."

RECOGNITION OF COMPLICATIONS OF CORONARY ATHEROSCLEROTIC HEART DISEASE

Certain medical events occur as a result of myocardial ischemia, injury, and necrosis secondary to obstructive coronary disease. These events are often called complications, which implies that they alter prognosis, demand treatment, or are troublesome to the patient. Patients with complications may be divided into three categories:

1 Sudden death may occur in individuals who have no previous symptoms. In such cases abrupt myocardial ischemia precipitates a lethal arrhythmia.

2 Patients who have symptoms characteristic of angina pectoris or have prolonged chest discomfort due to myocardial ischemia may also have cardiac arrhythmias and may experience sudden death or infarction. They may also experience emotional problems related to the recognition that they have a serious disease.

3 Patients who have myocardial ischemia, injury, and necrosis may have sudden death, cardiac arrhythmias, and a large number of cardiovascular and noncardiovascular complications. Myocardial infarction, the clinical counterpart of myocardial necrosis, is usually diagnosed when two of the following three items are present: prolonged chest discomfort which is characteristic of myocardial ischemia; the development of Q waves with characteristic ST-T wave change in the electrocardiogram or appropriate evolutionary change of the ST-T waves; and the elevation of certain serum enzyme levels. It is vital to remember that the methods used to recognize myocardial infarction are crude and that myocardial necrosis actually occurs with many of the clinical subsets or coronary atherosclerotic heart disease. Despite the difficulty in identifying all of the instances when myocardial necrosis actually occurs, it is important to realize that the larger the area of necrosis, the more likely it is for the patient to develop complications such as shock and heart failure.

Some of the complications discussed below are common to all three categories of patients, but the majority of the discussion deals with the complications of myocardial infarction. The recognition of these complications and, when appropriate, the method of monitoring their course will be discussed here, while the management is discussed in the section entitled "The Management of the Complications of Coronary Atherosclerotic Heart Disease" later in this chapter.

EMOTIONAL REACTIONS
There is almost always some degree of adverse emotional response on the part of the patient to the idea that he or she has coronary atherosclerotic heart disease. This may occur when the physician diagnoses the disease and explains his opinion to the patient. It may occur when a patient, on his own, determines he has heart disease because a friend or relative has the disease.

The exercise test, the coronary care unit, coronary arteriography, and coronary surgery have brought with them new opportunities for the development of emotional disturbances in patients. The family members of a patient who has been diagnosed as having one of the subsets of coronary atherosclerotic heart disease may develop emotional problems under the same circumstances.

Many patients go through the stages of denial, acceptance and fear, dependency, and depression before they enter the stage of realistic adaptation to their illness (see Chaps. 96 and 97). This may occur in patients with any one of the clinical subsets of coronary atherosclerotic heart disease, although it usually is identified in more dramatic form in patients with myocardial infarction. The sensitive physician must be constantly alert to these stages of emotional responses in order to rehabilitate the patient physically and mentally.

The clues that the patient denies the evidence that he or she has heart disease may be subtle. Denial may be detected because an intelligent patient does not follow simple orders (such as using nitroglycerin properly). The patient may articulate a good understanding of the problem but his or her actions can indicate a denial of their existence. On the other hand, the patient's denial may be obvious. The following example highlights this group of patients. Several years ago Dr. Charles Friedberg, Dr. T. Joseph Reeves, and one of the authors (J.W.H.) were in the same institution at the same time, and a resident asked us to help him with a problem in the emergency room. The patient, a young man in his forties, had pain that was characteristic of prolonged myocardial ischemia. All three of us felt the patient should remain in the hospital. He ignored us individually and collectively. He refused to accept that he might be having a "heart attack." He left the hospital despite our best efforts.

Most patients work through the stage of denial, and this is followed by acceptance and fear. An example of this is the middle-aged man who sustained a myocardial infarction 5 months earlier, at which time he experienced cardiac arrest requiring defibrillation. He had no other complications and could walk a mile twice a day without symptoms. He never returned to work for fear the event would recur. He verbalized, "I am living in terror and constant fear of dying" (fortunately he was rehabilitated and returned to his former occupation).

Today new hazards for the creation of fear exist in our offices and hospitals. For example, a 40-year-old woman had chest discomfort during the night. Her husband had died of a "heart attack." She had been diagnosed as having hyperventilation for 20 years, and she understood the condition. The physician performed an exercise test and it was "positive." The patient was told she had coronary atherosclerotic heart disease, and an exercise program was prescribed for her. Months later the asymptomatic patient had another exercise electrocardiogram. She felt she did beautifully, but the physician said to her, "You flunked, you have a time bomb in your chest. It can go off at any time." Arrangements were made for coronary arteriography to be done and coronary bypass to follow in a few days. The patient requested consultation. Whereas one could be virtually certain that she did not have coronary atherosclerotic heart disease, it was necessary to have a coronary arteriogram performed in order to clarify the situation. The coronary arteriogram was normal, and she was rehabilitated. The positive exercise test was a false positive test as it is in many 40-year-old women.

The following brief case report is included in order to emphasize how a family member can be terrorized as he observes his relative go through a diagnostic work-up and coronary bypass surgery. A 45-year-old, tennis-playing man applied for life insurance. An exercise electrocardiogram was made. He was found to have a markedly positive electrocardiogram after exercise. Furthermore, the test was markedly positive at the end of stage 2 of the Bruce test. Prior to the test the patient had a negative history of chest discomfort. After viewing the test the physicians were able to elicit a history of mild angina pectoris of recent onset. A coronary arteriogram showed high-grade obstructive lesions of the left coronary system, and coronary bypass surgery was successfully carried out. His young 35-year-old brother-in-law (and business partner), who had the Wolff-Parkinson-White syndrome, observed the course of events and developed fatigue, sighing respiration, sticks and stabs of pain over the left upper chest, and fear that left him in a state of panic. He demanded an exercise electrocardiogram. He was told none of his symptoms were due to coronary disease and that if he developed the W-P-W conduction during exercise (which he often did) it would be impossible to interpret the significance of the ST segment in the tracing. He was reassured as to his health and the cause of his symptoms was explained to him. This satisfied him for one week. An exercise test was then performed. He did not develop W-P-W conduction, and the ST segments remained normal. His anxiety then subsided.

When a patient works through the stage of acceptance and fear, he may enter the stage of dependency. In many respects this is the most harmful stage of all. The patient will not perform any new minor task without clearance from his physician. We as physicians must detect this dependency and realize that it is a harmful stage for the patient and assist the patient through it.

Some patients develop depression before they enter the stage of realistic adaptation to the illness (see Chap. 96). Mental depression is likely to occur several weeks after myocardial infarction. Patients may or may not verbalize their emotional feelings to their family and physician. If they do, the complaints may be dismissed as being due to anxiety, and the seriousness of the situation may not be recognized. Patients may state that they have trouble sleeping or "are worried" that something may happen. They may exhibit no interest in their work or in anything else and may speak of a fear of being disabled or that they "won't make it." Regrettably, on rare occasions a patient may commit suicide.

The coronary care unit undoubtedly saves the lives of patients with serious cardiac arrhythmias and makes it possible to deliver excellent nursing care to patients with heart failure and shock. The coronary unit may also create emotional problems for the patient and family. The patient and family may observe the problems of other patients, and this may precipitate new emotional problems. For example, if a patient sees or hears the activity surrounding the cardiac arrest of another patient, it may create an emotional response. The response may vary, with certain patients feeling "The staff did a good job" and that it is "comforting to know they are so efficient," and other patients experiencing a state of terror as they observe the action. An occasional patient may become disoriented as to time and place. The equipment is strange to the patient and this may disturb him or her. The family may be equally alarmed by the environment, and their alarm may be augmented as they talk with other families in the waiting room.

The patient and his or her family may be fright-

ened by an exercise stress test, especially if the patient has been frightened by the activity of the rehabilitation process. The procedure of coronary arteriography may frighten some patients unless it is explained to them carefully. Fortunately, the procedure is rarely painful. The needle stick in the skin and the hot flush produced by the contrast medium are all that is felt. It is important for the physician to have an open mind regarding the results of coronary arteriography. The physician should not play the predicting game with him(her)self, colleague, or patient. Both patient and physician must keep an open mind as to the results, since a surprise may be discovered as a result of the test.

A new syndrome has emerged. Patients who are discovered to have severe coronary disease or severe left ventricular dysfunction by coronary arteriography and left ventriculography may have placed their hopes in coronary bypass surgery. They may become extremely depressed because surgery cannot be done. It is necessary for the physician to be truthful in his or her explanations to patients, but the physician's duty does not demand that he or she be brutal. This is avoided by setting the stage properly before the coronary arteriogram. Patients should be told in advance that the test will assist the physician in determining if it would be better to treat them medically or surgically. The physician is then in a position to emphasize that medical management is preferred over surgical management when the coronary arteriogram reveals a condition that precludes surgery.

The patient who undergoes coronary surgery may encounter stressful situations. The patient may be placed in as many as four rooms within a few days. The patient may be admitted to one room; go to the operating room; spend several days in the cardiac surgical intensive care unit; and then be moved to another room where he or she may remain until discharged. This creates confusion and in some patients may precipitate disorientation. Hospital aides may create anxiety. For example, an aide said the following to a patient the day prior to surgery: "This is your last big meal." The patient pointed out that there was a vast difference between her statement and "This is your last big meal for a few days." Family members undergo enormous stress while surgery is being done. If the "waiting room" in the hospital is crowded with the family members of other patients, then great anxiety can develop as they discuss their problems with each other. Anxiety can be traced from one family to another as if it were labeled with a radioactive isotope. Specially designed "waiting rooms" and specially trained assistants who give appropriate information regarding the progress of the surgery decrease this anxiety considerably.

The purpose of this discussion on emotional reactions has been to point out the clinical situations that may create emotional stress and to highlight the fact that the progress of medicine has created several new situations where these can occur. Knowing that these emotional reactions occur is the first step in preventing the problem.

Emotional problems associated with recognition and management of coronary atherosclerotic heart disease are discussed later in this chapter.

CARDIAC ARRHYTHMIAS
(see Chap. 46D)

Although cardiac arrhythmias related to myocardial ischemia are usually discussed in the context of myocardial infarction, serious cardiac arrhythmias may occur in patients with any of the clinical syndromes due to coronary atherosclerotic heart disease. The following discussion will examine the problem of cardiac arrhythmias as it relates to some of the clinical syndromes associated with coronary atherosclerotic heart disease. The methods used to identify arrhythmias include Holter monitoring, monitoring in the coronary care units, and telemetry (see Chap. 28B and later in this chapter).

Arrhythmias as a cause of sudden death (see Chap. 49)

Stable angina pectoris The incidence and type of cardiac arrhythmias occurring in patients with stable angina pectoris have not been thoroughly studied. The frequency of arrhythmias will probably vary greatly among different groups of patients with stable angina pectoris. The number of diseased coronary arteries, presence of prior myocardial infarction, degree of myocardial ischemia during episodes of angina pectoris, and state of ventricular function are factors that may influence the incidence of cardiac arrhythmias associated with stable angina pectoris. It is known that patients with multiple-vessel disease and left ventricular wall motion abnormalities have a greater incidence of exercise-induced ventricular arrhythmias[153] (see Chap. 28A).

The occurrence of repeated syncopal attacks during episodes of classic angina pectoris is rare. Angina pectoris with syncope caused by transient atrioventricular block sinoatrial block or ventricular tachyarrhythmias has been reported.[154] These observations stress the important role of acute myocardial ischemia in the genesis of arrhythmias. The reason why syncopal attacks occurring as a result of cardiac arrhythmias are relatively rare during anginal episodes is not clear. The cause of syncope induced by angina pectoris may be difficult to establish. An ambulatory electrocardiogram may reveal the cause, or it may be necessary to induce an episode of angina pectoris with an exercise stress test in order to establish the mechanism for syncope. We have observed several patients with syncope during angina in whom transient sinoatrial block associated with angina could be demonstrated only during exercise stress testing. See discussion regarding treatment in Chap. 46D and "Treatment of Sinus Tachycardia" later in this chapter.

Prolonged chest discomfort without Q waves or enzyme changes This group of patients consists of those who have pain typical of myocardial ischemia that persists longer than 15 min; transient ST-segment and T-wave changes but no Q waves on the electrocardiogram; and no rise in serum enzyme levels. It has been thought that these patients have few hospital complications and enjoy a good prognosis for survival after discharge. However, important and potentially fatal arrhythmias are detected in patients with these syndromes.[155,156] The full spectrum of cardiac arrhythmias of infarction has been encountered in these patients: frequent premature ventricular beats, multiform ventricular beats, ventricular tachycardia, ventricular fibrillation, atrial fibrillation, and atrioventricular block.[155–157] Studies of the natural history of these patients indicate that they are at risk for sudden death or myocardial infarction in the next few months to a year.[157,158] In one study, 17 percent of patients had sudden death or myocardial infarction within 2 months following discharge from the hospital.[157]

Prinzmetal variant angina pectoris Tachyarrhythmias and conduction disturbances during attacks of variant angina pectoris are observed in about 40 percent of patients.[159] Ventricular premature beats and serious ventricular tachyarrhythmias are the most common arrhythmias associated with variant angina pectoris. Advanced atrioventricular block also occurs frequently and generally occurs in patients with disease of the posterior descending coronary artery. Impaired atrioventricular conduction results from severe ischemia to the atrioventricular node. A typical sequence is initiated by chest pain with ST-segment elevation in the inferior electrocardiographic leads followed by increasing degrees of atrioventricular block (Fig. 62E-2). Syncope is not uncommon during such episodes because of an inordinately slow junctional escape pacemaker rate or a low cardiac output produced by ischemia of a large portion of the left ventricle. The atrioventricular block subsides upon cessation of pain, and atrioventricular conduction is normal between attacks.[160,161]

Myocardial infarction (see Chap. 62A) It is often impossible to label a patient who is having chest discomfort as having an infarction when the patient is first seen. This is true because the electrocardiogram may not change until later and the level of serum enzymes may not be available. In such cases it is sufficient to know that the patient has chest discomfort characteristic of that due to myocardial ischemia.

Myocardial infarction is said to occur where two of the following exists: chest discomfort thought to be due to myocardial ischemia; QRS changes in the electrocardiogram or typical evolutionary changes of the ST-T waves; or a rise in serum enzyme levels.

The operation of mobile coronary care units has proved effective in the early treatment of acute myocardial infarction and in the resuscitation of patients from ventricular fibrillation. Experience gained from the use of the mobile coronary care unit has also resulted in a better understanding of events occurring within the first hour after the onset of acute myocardial infarction. This period is commonly called the *prehospital phase of myocardial infarction.* The spectrum of cardiac arrhythmias is not the same in the first hour after the onset of symptoms as it is in the hospital coronary care unit. Also, the effectiveness of some antiarrhythmic drugs may differ in the early and late stages of myocardial infarction.

Most patients seen within 30 min of chest pain have an abnormal heart rate or blood pressure.[162] Evidence of sympathetic nervous system overactivity (sinus tachycardia with or without transient hypertension) or parasympathetic overactivity (bradyarrhythmia with or without hypotension) may be seen in patients with either anterior or inferior infarction. However, sinus tachycardia is more common in patients with anterior infarction, whereas in patients with inferior infarction, sinus bradycardia is more common. The genesis and significance of sympathetic overactivity in patients with acute myocardial infarction is unknown. In experimental myocardial infarction, tachycardia may have an adverse effect on the ischemic area, and stimulation of cardiac sympathetic nerves lowers the ventricular fibrillation threshold. Various mechanisms have been proposed to explain the early bradyarrhythmias: stimulation of the vagal neuroreceptors in the region of the coronary sinus and atrioventricular node, ischemia of the sinoatrial and atrioventricular nodes, and interference with cholinesterase activity by the ischemic process.[163]

Ventricular fibrillation and bradyarrhythmias are more common in the first hour than at any time following myocardial infarction.[164] Pantridge and his colleagues found ventricular fibrillation in 10 percent of their patients, and it was the mechanism of death in most patients who died suddenly.[163] Bradyarrhythmias occur during the first hour in the majority of patients with acute inferior infarction.[163 164] There is considerable difference of opinion about the importance of bradycardia following acute myocardial infarction. Hospitalized patients who show sinus bradycardia have a good prognosis.[165] Bradycardia immediately after the onset of infarction may be of different import.[163–166] Bradyarrhythmias are not only more frequent but also are more serious at the very onset of myocardial infarction, because arterial hypotension is found in the majority of patients with bradycardia and the blood pressure is less than 80 mm Hg in nearly half of these patients.[163] The importance of bradycardia in the genesis of serious ventricular tachyarrhythmias during the first hour after myocardial infarction is controversial. Clinical evidence indicates that in some cases serious ventricular tachyarrhythmias, including ventricular fibrillation, appear when the heart rate slows, and that ventricular ectopic beats may be abolished by increasing a slow heart rate.[163–166]

Criteria for the accurate diagnosis of *subendocardial infarction* remain controversial. A commonly used definition includes (1) chest pain typical of myocardial ischemia lasting greater than 15 min, (2) ST-segment depression and/or T-wave inversion persisting for more than 48 h, (3) elevation of cardiac enzyme levels, and (4) no new Q waves. Patients with subendocardial infarction so defined make up a very nonhomogeneous group, some with and some without previous infarction. The "nontransmural infarction" may in fact be transmural, though new Q waves fail to appear in the electrocardiogram because of the QRS complex alterations from previous infarction, intraventricular conduction abnormalities, or infarction in an electrically "silent" area. Some patients with nontransmural infarction will develop recurrent chest pain and new Q waves later in their hospital course.[167] The incidence of pump failure is in large part determined by the presence of a previous myocardial infarction.[168] Despite these variables, it is important to note that several studies comparing the prevalence and type of arrhythmias occurring in patients with transmural and nontransmural infarction have shown no significant differences.[156,169,170]

Approximately one-third of hospital deaths from myocardial infarction occur after discharge from the coronary care unit, and one-half of these deaths are sudden. These have been labeled as *post-coronary care unit arrhythmias.* Most late hospital deaths occur within 12 days after discharge from the coronary care unit. Ventricular fibrillation is the arrhythmia detected most commonly at the scene of the cardiac arrest, but asystole or complete heart block may be found. Factors that enhance the possibility of late cardiac arrest are frequent ventricular premature beats, ventricular tachycardia, or ventricular fibrillation early in the course of the illness; persistent heart failure or hypotension; large anterior infarction; persistent sinus tachycardia, anterior infarction with bundle branch block; continued ST-segment displacement of 1 mm or more; delayed onset of atrial fibrillation; and recurrent ischemic chest pain.[171–173] Patients with anterior infarction and significant left ventricular dysfunction make up the largest group of patients subject to late hospital sudden death.

The relationship between ventricular arrhythmias and left ventricular function receives further support when patients are studied 2 to 4 weeks postinfarction. Frequent multiform or paired ventricular premature beats and ventricular tachycardia generally occur in patients with a decreased ejection fraction and more extensive left ventricular wall motion abnormalities.[174]

SPECIFIC ARRHYTHMIAS

Sinus tachycardia Sinus tachycardia complicating myocardial infarction is a nonspecific finding. Fever, anxiety, pericarditis, volume depletion, pulmonary embolus, and cardioaccelerator drugs may produce sinus tachycardia. Persistent sinus tachycardia, however, is an ominous sign, because it is commonly associated with severe left ventricular dysfunction.[165] In some cases, sinus tachycardia may precede other findings of left ventricular failure, such as ventricular gallop, rales, or radiographic evidence of interstitial edema. See discussion regarding treatment in Chap. 46D and in "The Treatment of Sinus Tachycardia" later in this chapter.

Sinus bradycardia The incidence of sinus bradycardia in monitored patients with myocardial infarction is approximately 20 percent.[165] The precise pathogenesis of sinus bradycardia is not known. Direct or reflex cholinergic suppression of the sinus node, ischemia or infarction of the sinus node, and the release of products of tissue breakdown are postulated mechanisms.[175] Drugs used in the treatment of patients with coronary atherosclerotic heart disease, morphine sulfate, propranolol, and digitalis, may cause sinus bradycardia in some patients. Sinus bradycardia portends a favorable outcome during the hospital phase of myocardial infarction.[165,171] The decreased inhospital mortality is explained, in part, by the lower incidence of pump failure in patients with sinus bradycardia.

Sinus bradycardia may cause or be accompanied by a reduction in cardiac output and may lead to an increase in myocardial ischemic injury. Systemic arterial hypotension accompanies sinus bradycardia more commonly in the prehospital phase of myocardial infarction than in the hospital phase. Patients having sinus bradycardia at a rate less than 40 beats per minute usually have evidence of decreased systemic arterial blood flow manifested by cool, clammy skin, hypotension, and lightheadedness.[165]

Although sinus bradycardia may be associated with an increased incidence of premature ventricular beats, the "malignant" potential of premature ventricular beats in patients with acute myocardial infarction and sinus bradycardia is unsettled. In the ischemic canine heart, studies have shown that bradycardia and vagal stimulation independently raise the threshold for electrically induced ventricular fibrillation.[176] In another study of experimental myocardial ischemia, ventricular fibrillation occurred at both rapid as well as slow heart rates, and there appeared to be an optimal intermediate rate for maximal suppression of ventricular ectopic beats.[177] The latter observations perhaps fit best the observations in patients, but conclusions based on animal models of myocardial ischemia must be applied with caution to human subjects. As a group, patients

monitored in a coronary care unit with sinus bradycardia do not experience a greater incidence of ventricular tachycardia or ventricular fibrillation.[165] However, sinus bradycardia may be associated with serious ventricular tachyarrhythmias which can be abolished by elevation of the heart rate. See discussion regarding treatment in Chap. 46D and in " The Treatment of Sinus Bradycardia" later in this chapter.

Sinus node dysfunction Sinus node dysfunction is a complication of myocardial infarction in approximately 5 percent of patients and occurs most commonly in patients with inferior infarction. The underlying abnormality may be the result of an arrest of sinus node impulse formation or impaired conduction from the sinus node to the atrium. The electrocardiogram reveals sinus pauses typical of sinoatrial Wenckebach or type II second-degree sinoatrial block, or sinus pauses greater than twice the sinus P-P interval (Fig. 62E-12)

Sinus node dysfunction following myocardial infarction has many of the features found in the chronic *sick sinus syndrome* (SSS).[175a] Atrial tachyarrhythmias alternating with periods of bradycardia are seen in one-third of the patients with sinus node dysfunction complicating myocardial infarction.[177] Atrioventricular nodal block is not uncommon. Dizziness or syncope are the most common symptoms and result from prolonged sinus node standstill associated with failure of the subsidiary pacemakers. A long sinus pause may follow the termination of an atrial tachyarrhythmia or the spontaneous appearance of advanced sinoatrial block. See discussion regarding treatment in Chap. 46D and in "The Treatment of Sinus Node Dysfunction" later in this chapter.

Atrial arrhythmias A number of mechanisms for atrial tachyarrhythmias in myocardial infarction have been proposed. Pathologic studies in some patients with infarction and atrial arrhythmias reveal evidence of ischemic injury to the sinoatrial node and the junction of the sinoatrial node with the right atrium.[178] Multiple factors are probably responsible for the arrhythmia in any single patient and include (1) depressed sinus node automaticity, (2) impaired sinus impulse transmission, (3) atrial wall infarction, (4) vagal reflexes, (5) pericarditis, (6) atrial distension, and (7) release of localized stores of myocardial catecholamines.[179]

Atrial premature beats are found in up to 50

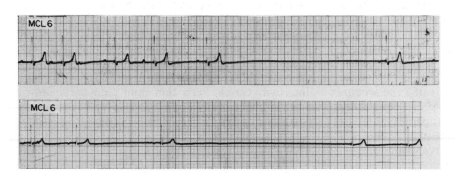

FIGURE 62E-12 Sinus pause in patient with acute inferior infarction. Top, sinus pause terminated by atrial escape beat. Bottom, atrial escape pacemaker with long pause.

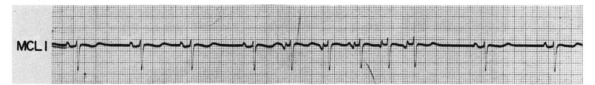

FIGURE 62E-13 Atrial tachycardia. Tachycardia begins with the fifth P wave, and the rate accelerates prior to spontaneous termination.

percent of monitored patients following myocardial infarction.[180] Atrial premature beats are not of consequence except that they sometimes initiate atrial tachyarrhythmias. See discussion regarding treatment in Chap. 46D and in "The Treatment of Atrial Premature Beats" later in this chapter.

Atrial tachycardia, defined as three or more consecutive ectopic P waves occurring at a rate greater than 100 beats per minute, is regarded as an uncommon arrhythmia following myocardial infarction. In our experience, the incidence of atrial tachycardia is substantially greater and is seen in up to 20 percent of patients. However, most episodes of atrial tachycardia are transient and self-limited and do not require treatment[181] (Fig. 62E-13). When the rate of the atrial tachycardia is rapid and the tachycardia is sustained, treatment is necessary (Fig. 62E-14). See discussion regarding treatment in Chap. 46D and in "The Treatment of Atrial Tachycardia" later in this chapter.

Atrial flutter is seen in less than 5 percent of patients with myocardial infarction, and it is less common than atrial fibrillation. Atrial flutter is usually associated with a 2:1 atrioventricular conduction ratio; therefore, the ventricular rate will be in the vicinity of 150 beats per minute. This rapid ventricular rate will increase myocardial oxygen requirement in all patients and will result in hemodynamic deterioration in many patients. The prompt restoration of a slow ventricular rate is imperative. See discussion regarding treatment in Chap. 46D and in "The Treatment of Atrial Flutter" later in this chapter.

Atrial fibrillation is the most common atrial tachyarrhythmiac complicating myocardial infarction. Atrial fibrillation may appear without warning, may be preceded by atrial premature beats, or may develop by increasing the atrial rate in atrial flutter. Atrial premature beats having a coupling index less than half the sinus P-P interval are somewhat more likely to initiate atrial fibrillation.[182] Atrial fibrillation usually appears during the first 4 days following myocardial infarction. It is often intermittent, and the spontaneous reversion to normal sinus rhythm is not uncommon.

Controversy continues regarding the prognostic significance of atrial fibrillation following myocardial infarction. Some investigators have found that there is no difference in mortality related to the presence or absence of atrial fibrillation.[181,183] Other studies have shown that atrial fibrillation is associated with a greater overall early mortality in patients with anterior infarction, but that it does not affect mortality with inferior infarction.[184] Signs of heart failure are present in the majority of patients with anterior infarction and atrial fibrillation, and heart failure usually precedes the onset of atrial fibrillation. Therefore, it appears that the major prognostic factor is the extent of myocardial damage and not the independent occurrence of atrial fibrillation. This does not mean that atrial fibrillation is a "benign" complication and that it cannot contribute to patient mortality. The loss of a synchronized atrial contraction and the rapid irregular ventricular rate may lead to further hemodynamic impairment, particularly in patients with extensive myocardial damage. See discussion regarding treatment in Chap. 46D and in "The Treatment of Atrial Fibrillation" later in this chapter.

Accelerated junctional rhythm (nonparoxysmal AV junctional tachycardia) Accelerated atrioventricular junctional rhythm (rate 60 to 100 beats per minute) and atrioventricular junctional tachycardia result from acceleration of impulse formation in the atrioventricular junction. Accelerated junctional rhythms are more commonly associated with inferior infarction than with anterior infarction. Junctional rhythms must be differentiated from accelerated idioventricular rhythm. In junctional rhythm, the QRS morphology is identical to the QRS morphology during sinus rhythm, or it shows slight aberration.

In general, the rate of the junctional rhythm and the clinical course vary with the site of infarction. With inferior infarction the junctional rate is only moderately accelerated, and the clinical course is usually benign unless the junctional rate exceeds 80 beats per minute.[185,186] Conversely, the junctional rate commonly exceeds 100 beats per minute, and the hospital mortality is greater than 60 percent in pa-

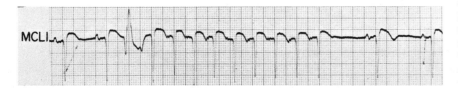

FIGURE 62E-14 Reentrant supraventricular tachycardia initiated by an interpolated ventricular premature beat. Rate of tachycardia was rapid, and many episodes were sustained. Supraventricular tachycardia was abolished by suppression of interpolated ventricular premature beats with lidocaine.

tients with anterior infarction.[185,186] Irrespective of the site of infarction, however, the faster the junctional rate, the greater the hospital mortality.[186] Most deaths are the result of severe pump failure. See discussion regarding treatment in Chap. 46D and in "The Treatment of Accelerated Functional Rhythm" later in this chapter.

Ventricular arrhythmias *Ventricular premature beats* (VPBs) occur in approximately 80 percent of constantly monitored patients with acute myocardial infarction.[179] Their greatest importance lies in the fact that they may precipitate ventricular tachycardia or ventricular fibrillation. Since the introduction of coronary care units, the generally accepted criteria for the suppression of VPBs have been based on the assumption that nearly all serious ventricular tachyarrhythmias are preceded by "warning VPBs." The warning arrhythmias include VPBs that interrupt the T wave of the previous beat, occur with a frequency of greater than 5 beats per minute, and are multiform or paired. Recent studies suggest that the guidelines do not accurately predict the malignant potential of any VPB in patients with acute myocardial infarction.[187,188] VPBs falling early or late in the cardiac cycle and VPBs arising from either the left or right ventricle may initiate ventricular fibrillation.[187,188] Although ventricular fibrillation may be preceded by warning arrhythmias in over half the cases, warning arrhythmias are common in patients who do not develop ventricular fibrillation.[188] Also, ventricular fibrillation may appear without warning ventricular ectopy.[189] Study of the relationship between VPBs and ventricular tachycardia shows a poor correlation between the coupling interval of the VPB and its ability to initiate ventricular tachycardia.[190] On the other hand, frequent multiform and paired VPBs are associated with a higher incidence of ventricular tachycardia.[190,191]

Studies of experimental acute myocardial ischemia show that in animals, as in human beings, VPBs with late diastolic coupling may precipitate serious ventricular arrhythmias.[192] In experimental myocardial ischemia, the malignancy of a VPB is related to slow, fragmented activation of the ischemic myocardium. The delay in activation of ischemic myocardium necessary to produce a ventricular tachyarrhythmia may occur with closely coupled VPBs. Closely coupled beats exhibit greater dispersion of activation of the ischemic zone than late coupled beats and are more likely to result in ventricular tachycardia.[192] The preceding discussion is not meant to negate the importance of closely coupled VPBs occurring in patients with acute myocardial infarction. Their potential for inciting serious ventricular arrhythmias surely exceeds that of late diastolic ventricular ectopic beats. However, it appears that the coupling index and QRS configuration of any VPB are not very reliable in predicting its malignant potential. See discussion regarding treatment later in "Treatment of Ventricular Premature Beats" and in Chap. 46D.

Ventricular tachycardia, defined as three or more successive beats of ventricular origin occurring at a rate greater than 120 beats per minute, is more common than formerly appreciated.[190] Attacks of ventricular tachycardia lasting longer than 15 min are relatively rare following acute myocardial infarction. Usually, ventricular tachycardia either stops spontaneously after a few seconds to minutes or degenerates into ventricular fibrillation. Persistent ventricular tachycardia may produce serious impairment of cardiac function. With rapid ventricular rates the cerebral blood flow may be reduced by as much as 40 percent. Although the exact electrophysiologic mechanisms for ventricular tachycardia complicating acute myocardial infarction cannot be established in human beings, the studies of Wellens and his colleagues suggest that long-lasting episodes may be due to enhanced automaticity.[193] Reentry may play a role in the short, more malignant runs of ventricular tachycardia, which seem more likely to deteriorate into ventricular fibrillation. See discussion regarding treatment in Chap. 46D and in "The Treatment of Ventricular Tachycardia" later in this chapter.

Resuscitation from primary *ventricular fibrillation* not associated with severe pump failure is highly successful. The outlook for patients successfully resuscitated from early ventricular fibrillation does not differ from that of other patients with myocardial infarction.[194] Ventricular fibrillation appearing more than 48 h after the onset of infarction is usually associated with persistent pump failure.[195] Resuscitative efforts in patients with late ventricular fibrillation may fail, and the hospital mortality exceeds 40 percent.[195] See discussion regarding treatment in Chaps. 46D and 50A to 50D and in "The Treatment of Ventricular Fibrillation" later in this chapter.

The incidence of *accelerated idioventricular rhythm* after myocardial infarction varies from 10 to 46 percent.[193,194] Accelerated idioventricular rhythm is defined as three or more ventricular beats in succession at a rate of 55 to 120 beats per minute (Fig. 62E-15). A clear distinction between accelerated idioventricular rhythm and ventricular tachycardia is sometimes impossible, because both rhythms may vary above and below 120 beats per minute. This variability of rate and intermittent appearance in brief paroxysms is characteristic of accelerated idioventricular rhythm. The paroxysm may begin as an escape rhythm following slowing of the sinus node, or following a postextrasystolic pause, but may appear also as an ectopic rhythm beginning in late diastole. When it appears, it may stop spontaneously after 3 to 30 beats, alternating with sinus rhythm, or it may be suppressed by acceleration of the dominant rhythm. Recent studies have suggested that patients with idioventricular rhythm have an increased incidence of ventricular tachycardia.[196–199] The association between idioventricular rhythm and ventricular tachycardia appears to be greater if the rate of the idioventricular rhythm exceeds 75 beats per minute.[199] The QRS morphology of the two rhythms is often similar, and extrasystoles of similar form may be present. In a few instances, the rate of the idioventricular rhythm will be exactly half or some other multiple of that of the ventricular tachycar-

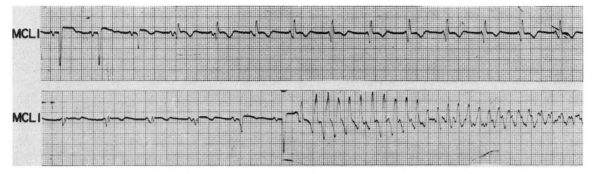

FIGURE 62E-15 Accelerated idioventricular rhythm. Top, run of accelerated idioventricular rhythm initiated by fusion beat (third QRS complex). Bottom, sixth QRS complex is first sinus beat following the run of idioventricular rhythm. T wave was interrupted by ventricular rhythm. Ventricular fibrillation ensues.

dia.[196,199] This suggests that some cases of idioventricular rhythm are caused by an ectopic focus with varying degrees of exit block. See discussion later regarding treatment in Chap. 46D and in "The Treatment of Accelerated Idioventricular Rhythm" later in this chapter.

Heart block The incidence of atrioventricular (AV) conduction disturbances varies between 12 and 25 percent and the incidence of complete AV block varies from 2 to 10 percent in patients with acute myocardial infarction.[175] AV conduction disturbances following inferior and anterior infarction differ in many respects, and they will be discussed separately. In rare patients AV block may not conform to such a clear distinction based upon the site of infarction.

AV conduction disturbances are two to three times more frequent in patients with *inferior infarction* than in those with anterior infarction. The site of block in most patients with inferior infarction is within the AV node or high in the bundle of His.[200] The pathogenesis of the AV nodal block following acute infarction is not fully understood, but increased vagal tone and ischemia play a role. Pathologic studies show only minor degrees of necrosis, if any, within the AV node and bundle of His.[175]

With inferior infarction, AV block usually begins with prolongation of the P-R interval followed by a progression to type I second-degree AV block (Wenckebach). A further progression to complete AV block may ensue. The recognition of complete heart block may be difficult if the rate of the junctional pacemaker is accelerated. When complete heart block occurs, the QRS morphology resulting from an escape pacemaker in the AV junction is usually normal, and the rate of the escape pacemaker is usually between 40 and 60 beats per minute. When AV block occurs lower in the bundle of His, the escape pacemaker rate may be slower. AV block is a common complication when an inferior infarction produces extensive infarction of the right ventricle.[201] On occasion, patients with inferior infarction will fail to conduct a P wave beyond the AV node because of a transient increase in vagal tone. This usually occurs during sleep or during bowel or bladder elimination. The electrocardiogram shows an increase in the P-P interval prior to the nonconducted P wave which is followed in a few seconds by a return to the base-line P-P interval and a normal P-R interval. Such episodes are of brief duration and generally require no treatment. See discussion regarding treatment in Chaps. 46D and 46E and in "The Treatment of Heart Block in Inferior Infarction" later in this chapter.

Heart block complicating *anterior infarction* results from extensive disease in the bundle branches. Necrosis involving the bundle branches and an extensive area of myocardium is found in most cases.[197] Localization of the conduction abnormality to the distal conducting system is further substantiated by intracardiac electrocardiograms. The AV interval is usually prolonged prior to the onset of complete heart block, and when complete block occurs, the site of block is distal to the bundle of His recording site.[200,202]

In contrast to AV block following inferior infarction, the only problem preceding AV block complicating anterior infarction may be an intraventricular conduction disturbance with or without minimal prolongation of the P-R interval. Progression to a high degree of block is often sudden, usually producing many consecutive nonconducted P waves, but occasionally resulting in a stable second-degree (2:1 or 3:1) pattern. If second-degree block is present, it is usually Mobitz type II block. The idioventricular escape rhythm is slow with a wide, bizarre morphology of the QRS complex indicating a lower site of origin. Idioventricular pacemakers are potentially unstable and may stop suddenly, producing asystole.

Since the progression to complete heart block is usually sudden, it is important to identify those patients in whom the risk of developing complete heart block is extraordinarily great. The conceptual division of the bundle branch system into three fascicles, right bundle branch, anterior division of the left bundle branch, and posterior division of left bundle branch, has produced electrocardiographic criteria for the diagnosis of block of one fascicle or any combination of fascicles. Although the three-fascicle concept is clinically useful, it is an oversimplification of the anatomy of the left bundle branch and only provides an approximation of the site of intraventricular block.

Patients with anterior infarction complicated by right bundle branch block, right bundle branch block with left anterior hemiblock, or right branch block with left posterior hemiblock have a particularly high risk of progression to complete heart block, especially if the P-R interval is also prolonged.[197,202–204] The progression of right bundle branch block to complete heart block is usually associated with either left anterior or posterior hemiblock, but the appearance of the hemiblock may be missed if scalar electrocardiograms are not recorded every few hours.[202] Bundle branch block that lasts less than 6 h or develops later than 24 h after the onset of symptoms may have a lower incidence of progression to complete heart block.[202] If the P-R interval is prolonged, the risk of subsequent complete heart block is greater, but a normal P-R interval offers no assurance that heart block will not occur. Left bundle branch block is a less common precursor of complete heart block in patients with anterior infarction. See later discussion regarding treatment in Chaps. 46D and 46E and in "The Treatment of Heart Block in Anterior Infarction" later in this chapter.

SHOCK (see Chap. 48)

At least two of the signs listed in Table 48-1 should be present before a diagnosis of shock is made. It is important to remember that cuff blood pressure determination may not give an accurate estimate of intraarterial pressure; that shock may proceed with a normal blood pressure; and that low arterial pressure may be well tolerated in certain clinical conditions. For example, the bradycardia-hypotensive syndrome sometimes seen with acute inferior infarction may exhibit none of the other features which are required to label the patient as having shock (see Table 48-1).

It is more important to recognize preshock than shock, since therapy should be instituted in an effort to prevent shock as defined in Table 48-1. The preshock state is recognized when a high-risk patient (such as a patient with myocardial infarction) exhibits an unexplained change in pulse rate, pulse volume, blood pressure, urine output, or skin temperature even though the findings do not fulfill the criteria listed in Table 48-1. The treatment of shock and preshock is discussed in Chap. 48 and later in this chapter.

CONGESTIVE HEART FAILURE
(see Chap. 44)

Patients with coronary atherosclerotic heart disease usually develop congestive heart failure under three circumstances: (1) Congestive heart failure may occur transiently during an episode of angina pectoris. When this occurs, the patient may complain of dyspnea on effort, and the chest discomfort of angina pectoris may not be appreciated if it is felt at all. Abnormal atrial and ventricular gallop sounds may be heard at the time. This is one of the reasons why it is important to listen to the heart after an exercise stress test. (2) Patients with acute myocardial infarction may develop pulmonary edema. The well-known signs of heart failure may be present, but the interstitial edema is best recognized on the portable chest roentgenogram (see Chap. 44). (3) Chronic heart failure due to coronary atherosclerosis, especially when it occurs in the absence of a history of angina pectoris or infarction, is often called ischemic cardiomyopathy (see Chaps. 44 and 81A). See discussion regarding treatment later in this chapter and in Chap. 45.

ELECTROMECHANICAL DISSOCIATION[205,206]

Electromechanical dissociation exists when the electric impulses to the heart are adequate (as determined by the electrocardiogram) but the mechanical force of the heart is either absent or grossly inadequate. The electrical impulse does not trigger the proper response. This phenomenon is seen in the following six situations:

1 Paroxysmal, ischemic paralysis of the left ventricle Abrupt paroxysmal myocardial ischemia may occur in patients with advanced obstructive coronary disease. This, of course, may produce angina pectoris, but it may also produce severe left ventricular dysfunction without angina pectoris. Left ventricular dysfunction may produce two different clinical syndromes. The patient may experience abrupt severe fatigue with or without dizziness related to effort or may have abrupt pulmonary edema. It is now well known that severe myocardial ischemia may produce severe fatigue. This is observed fairly often when the patient discontinues exercise because of severe fatigue during an exercise stress test that provokes no angina pectoris but does produce hypotension and marked displacement of the ST segment in the electrocardiogram. Such patients may have acutely decreased myocardial contractility without other evidence of heart failure. Rarely, patients with coronary atherosclerosis may develop paroxysmal episodes of severe left ventricular failure with alveolar *pulmonary edema*. Between the attacks the cardiac reserve may be surprisingly good, with no evidence of congestive heart failure. Roentgenograms of the heart and lungs may show no residual evidence of pulmonary venous hypertension or interstitial edema. There may be no residual evidence of ventricular dysfunction such as pulsus alternans, S_3 or S_4 gallop rhythm, or paradoxic splitting of the second sound. Such episodes of failure may or may not be associated with pain. The genesis of this condition is thought to be episodic ischemia of the left ventricle with impaired contractility or, rarely, transient severe mitral regurgitation.

2 Associated with angina pectoris On relatively rare occasions a patient with angina pectoris will experience syncope due to profound ischemia and electromechanical dissociation of the left ventricle. During the transient episode, the pulse is not palpable and there is no blood pressure, yet the electrocardiogram shows no arrhythmia but may show ST-segment abnormality. A small minority of these patients have hypertrophic subaortic stenosis, but the majority of patients have coronary atherosclerotic heart disease. The clinical event is called *syncope anginosus.*

3 Permanent electromechanical dissociation We have observed this phenomenon at the onset of cardiac arrest. The rhythm may be normal, but there is no pulse or blood pressure. Such patients are rarely resuscitated. The same phenomenon may also develop a few days after the original episode of myocardial ischemia, especially in older patients with massive anterior infarctions.

4 Rupture into pericardium Electromechanical dissociation may also occur when the heart ruptures into the pericardium. This condition is recognized when the neck veins become abruptly distended. The electrocardiogram may show tented T waves, ST-segment elevation or depression, and downward displacement of the cardiac pacemaker. One could argue that this condition is not true electromechanical dissociation since the intact heart muscle may continue to respond properly to an electrical stimulus. This is correct, but many patients with cardiac rupture have a great deal of myocardial ischemia and necrosis and undoubtedly have considerable electromechanical dissociation. For this reason the condition is included in this discussion.

5 Rupture of papillary muscle Electromechanical dissociation may develop in patients with acute massive mitral regurgitation due to rupture of a papillary muscle.

6 Cardiopulmonary bypass Electromechanical dissociation may occur at cardiac surgery after prolonged cardiopulmonary bypass, especially in patients with severe coronary atherosclerosis and/or marked hypertrophy. See discussion regarding treatment later in this chapter.

PERICARDITIS (see Chap. 84)
Pericarditis secondary to transmural myocardial infarction is much more common than the 15 percent incidence customarily quoted.[207] It is often unrecognized in spite of typical pain because the observer may demand the presence of a pericardial friction rub or typical changes in the electrocardiogram. Evidence of pericarditis is usually delayed for several days after myocardial infarction, and its peak incidence is within the first week. Occasionally it may be detected on the first day of admission to the hospital, suggesting that the onset of infarction antedated admission by several days, even when a history of prior pain is not obtained. At times it produces the dominant symptoms and findings preceding or associated with rupture of the heart. It may be a complication of catheter pacing from the right ventricle when perforation takes place. Fortunately, it is usually none of these serious conditions but represents the expected response of the heart to epicardial injury. The recognition of pericarditis is important, since the pain may be confused with extension of the

infarct, and the splinting and dyspnea seen at times may be misdiagnosed as congestive heart failure. Pericardial inflammation in the region of the sinus node may predispose to atrial arrhythmia or atrial fibrillation. Finally, unrecognized pericardial effusion may give a false impression of marked cardiac enlargement in the chest x-ray. The latter problem is more likely to arise when postmyocardial infarction (Dressler's) syndrome occurs than with acute infarction. Pleural fluid, especially on the left, may also occur with Dressler's syndrome.

While pericarditis may occur in the absence of pain, pain is usually the most prominent symptom. The pain may be precordial or may be confined to the trapezius area, neck, shoulders, and upper arm, particularly on the left side. Characteristically, the discomfort is aggravated by deep inspiration, change of position, swallowing, or coughing. On occasion it may be described as a sense of tightness; this serves to heighten the confusion with the distress of myocardial ischemia. Dyspnea with or without pain may be noted. Cough may be a complaint in the presence of significant pericardial effusion. Low-grade fever is often, but not invariably, present. Exceptionally, it may reach 103°F. The development of fever toward the end of the first week after infarction should arouse the suspicion of pericarditis.

A pericardial friction rub is often heard with or without accompanying symptoms. The frequency of the rub depends on how often the patient is examined and the expertise of the examiner. A pericardial rub may be detected in 5 to 10 percent of patients in a coronary care unit, and it usually appears within 4 days of the onset of myocardial infarction. The rub may be localized or diffuse. It can be heard maximally at various areas, including the cardiac apex, parasternal area, along the lower left sternal border, or over the region at the outflow tract of the right ventricle. Rarely, it may be heard to the right of the sternum. It is usually best heard in forced expiration while pressing firmly with the diaphragm of the stethoscope. The typical three-component rub poses no problem in recognition. When the rub is confined to atrial systole, ventricular systole, or ventricular diastole, serial observations noting a change or disappearance of the short, high-pitched vibrations may be needed. When the rub is scratchy or grating, it may simulate a systolic or diastolic murmur. The murmur of aortic regurgitation may be mimicked by a pericardial rub occurring in diastole. Similarly, the murmur of mitral or tricuspid insufficiency may be simulated by a rub occurring in systole. The atrial systolic component may be confused with an atrial or summation gallop. The rub is notoriously evanescent, being present one hour and gone the next; however, it may persist for days and occasionally for several weeks. A clue to pericarditis with effusion and tamponade may be abnormal distension of the external jugular veins or abnormal pulsation of the internal jugular veins when the head is elevated to 30° (see Chap. 15). This sign is especially suggestive of effusion in patients who show no interstitial pulmonary edema in the x-ray. Rarely, abnormal neck vein distension may be noted with right ventricular infarction and predominant right ventricular failure in the absence of pulmonary congestion. Abdominal discomfort due to hepatic congestion secondary to increased intrapericardial and systemic venous pressure may rarely be the initial complaint in patients with cardiac tamponade. Pericardial effusion related to infarction may be part of Dressler's syndrome.

The electrocardiogram may indicate pericarditis by the characteristic ST-segment elevation superimposed on the changes due to myocardial infarction. Unfortunately, the changes are obscured or absent in most instances of clinically recognized pericarditis, and the absence of ST-T changes in serial tracings should not be a deterrent to diagnosis and therapy.

In summary, pericarditis should be suspected when (1) there is recurrent chest pain a few days after infarction, particularly if the pain does not respond satisfactorily to opiates. The pain may be typically aggravated by inspiration or change of position. It may be described as a sense of tightness which serves to heighten the confusion with the distress of myocardial ischemia. A pericardial rub may not be heard. At times the pericardial origin of discomfort can be confirmed only in retrospect after a dramatic response to corticosteroid therapy. Relief may be obtained within 1 h of administration of 4 mg of Decadron intravenously. (2) The cardiac silhouette reveals cardiac enlargement which is out of proportion to that reasonably expected. (3) There is dyspnea in the absence of interstitial edema in the x-ray. (4) There is persistent fever or recurrent fever 3 to 4 days after an infarct. See discussion regarding treatment in Chap. 84 and later in this chapter.

PULMONARY EMBOLISM
(see also Chap. 75)

Pulmonary embolism may be a major complication of myocardial infarction and may precipitate sudden death, recurrent myocardial ischemia, congestive heart failure, or atrial arrhythmias. The frequency of pulmonary emboli is unknown, since the current techniques used for diagnosis are inadequate or are difficult to utilize in sick patients. Thrombi may form in the right ventricle at the site of endocardial infarction or in the right atrium incident to atrial fibrillation, but the overwhelming majority of emboli arise from the veins of the legs and pelvis.[207a] The astonishing frequency of deep venous thrombosis in the calf veins using ^{125}I radioactive fibrinogen assay is noteworthy. Maurer et al. noted that 37 percent of 90 patients with acute myocardial infarction showed evidence of venous thrombosis and that approximately one-half of thrombi developed within 72 h and less than 25 percent after the fifth day.[208] Thrombosis was more common in patients with preexisting varices and severe congestive heart failure or shock, and in those over the age of 70. There was no major

pulmonary embolism, and clinically detectable episodes were uncommon.

Recognition of pulmonary embolism without pulmonary infarction is difficult and must often be based on suspicion. If the chest x-ray is normal, the lung scan may be used if the patient's condition permits. Recurrent episodes of weakness, dyspnea, tachypnea, sweating, tachycardia, and arrhythmias in the absence of evidence of extension of myocardial infarction are highly suggestive. Often the diagnosis of repeated pulmonary emboli can be suggested from inspection of the graph of temperature, pulse rate, and respiratory rate.

Pulmonary infarction with pleural pain, friction rub, and shadows in the x-ray is readily recognized. The radiographic findings of pulmonary infarction may be confused with confluent areas of interstitial pulmonary edema or pleural effusion due to heart failure. Fixed splitting of the second heart sound in the absence of right bundle branch block may be noted at the onset of massive pulmonary embolism; however, this finding may occur in some patients with myocardial infarction. The pulmonic component of the second heart sound may be accentuated and the jugular venous *a* wave may be prominent following a pulmonary embolism. The electrocardiogram may occasionally show the nonspecific changes of pulmonary embolism, but commonly it is of little help (see Chap. 75). Many electrocardiographic changes attributable to pulmonary embolism are common accompaniments of myocardial infarction.

Rarely paradoxic embolism may occur. The occurrence of a stroke in close relation to clinical evidence of pulmonary embolism is highly suggestive of such an event. See discussion regarding treatment later in this chapter and in Chap. 75.

SYSTEMIC ARTERIAL EMBOLISM[209]
(see also Chaps. 103 to 105 and 107)

Mural thrombi may form at the site of endocardial injury as the result of infarction, and become the source of systemic emboli. The incidence of peripheral arterial emboli is less today than it was some years ago. The reason for this is not apparent. A favorite site for mural thrombus formation is the region of the cardiac apex. An embolus may produce an infarction of various organs, including the brain, spleen, liver, kidneys, or intestine. A clot lodged at the bifurcation of the aorta or in the arterial supply of an extremity may produce coldness, numbness, pain, and discoloration due to ischemia. When ischemia is persistent and severe, there is inability of the muscles to contract.

Patients may experience an embolism to a peripheral artery several days or weeks after the occurrence of myocardial infarction. On the other hand, a peripheral arterial embolus may be the first clue to the diagnosis of myocardial infarction. In such cases the myocardial infarction may have been painless (or nearly so), the symptoms may have been ignored, or the patient may have developed a "stroke" so that he was unable to relate the medical history.

See discussion regarding treatment later in this chapter and in Chaps. 104, 105, and 107.

PAPILLARY MUSCLE DYSFUNCTION (see Chaps. 60, 61, 62D, and 62F)

The integrity of the mitral valve apparatus is damaged when myocardial infarction injures either of the papillary muscles which anchor the mitral valve leaflets. The infarct that damages a papillary muscle usually damages the area of the left ventricular muscle wall which is adjacent to, and part of, the base of the papillary muscle. Mild, moderate, or severe mitral regurgitation may be produced when the papillary muscle fails to contract properly and/or when the ventricular wall at the base of the papillary muscle bulges outward during ventricular systole. The degree of mitral regurgitation is often underestimated when the patient is examined at rest. Isometric exercise produces a rise in systolic and diastolic blood pressure, and the mitral murmur increases in intensity as the mitral regurgitation increases.[210] The systolic mitral murmur may be delayed after the first sound, may be initiated with a systolic click, and may have a crescendic configuration. Some believe that myocardial infarction can produce the click-murmur syndrome due to mitral valve prolapse, while others believe the two occur by coincidence in the same patient. Actually, the configuration of the murmur is variable and is frequently nonspecific. When conditions such as heart failure or continued episodes of myocardial ischemia continue, it may be appropriate to perform left ventriculography and coronary arteriography in order to delineate the problem precisely, since surgical correction may be needed. See discussion regarding treatment later in this chapter.

RUPTURE OF THE PAPILLARY MUSCLE[211] (see Chaps. 60, 61, 62D, and 62F)

Rupture of the papillary muscle due to myocardial infarction usually produces profound heart failure, shock, and death.[211] Fortunately, the condition is rare. The physical findings include a systolic murmur at the apex due to mitral regurgitation and the clinical picture of electromechanical dissociation including hypotension, barely palpable pulses, and heart failure. We wish to stress that the systolic murmur at the apex may be grade 1 or 3, but we have seen patients with papillary muscle rupture who had no murmur, often in association with marked hypotension.

Tip necrosis of a papillary muscle creates a syndrome similar to that associated with rupture of the chordae tendineae, and the patient is characteristically not as ill as when there is rupture of the belly of the papillary muscle. Since the murmur of ventricular septal rupture may occasionally be heard loudest at the cardiac apex, it is necessary to have catheterization of the heart to rule out a left-to-right shunt at the ventricular level. This may be done by using a Swan-Ganz catheter. Left ventricular angiography and coronary arteriography are performed in order to determine the feasibility of surgical correction. See discussion regarding treatment later in this chapter and in Chap. 62H.

RUPTURE OF THE VENTRICULAR SEPTUM[212–213a] (see Chaps. 62D and 62F)

Rupture of the ventricular septum produces severe depression of the left ventricular function. Septal

rupture usually occurs several days after the onset of chest pain due to infarction. We have observed septal rupture during the first day on several occasions, presumably because the onset of infarction began earlier and was unrecognized by the patient. The recognition of septal rupture depends upon the discovery of a systolic murmur near the lower left sternal border. We wish to emphasize, however, that *the murmur may be louder at the apex* in some patients. When this occurs, it is not possible to separate this murmur from that due to papillary muscle rupture. Rupture is commonly associated with hypotension and heart failure of varying degrees. A left-to-right shunt into the right ventricle may be detected by using a Swan-Ganz catheter. See discussion regarding treatment later in this chapter and in Chap. 62F.

EXTERNAL RUPTURE OF THE HEART (see Chaps. 62D and 62F)

External rupture of the heart accounts for 10 to 15 percent of deaths due to acute myocardial infarction. In one series of 101 deaths, rupture occurred in 22 percent during the first 24 h, 69 percent during the first week, 21 percent during the second week, 6 percent at 2 to 3 weeks, and 1 percent at 6 weeks.[214] Rupture on the first day suggests that the infarction occurred a few days earlier. It is more common in the following circumstances: with the first myocardial infarction; with transmural infarction; where there is a history of preexisting hypertension; where hypertension has persisted after onset of infarction; and in the older patient. Delay in the diagnosis of myocardial infarction has been cited as a predisposing factor in some studies but not in others. It is rare under the age of 50, and the peak age incidence is the seventies. Cardiac rupture is more common in women than in men, since there is a similar incidence of rupture in males and females, even though myocardial infarction is approximately three times more common in the males. It has been suggested that the difference may be due to the increased frequency of hypertension, the older peak age, and possible delay in diagnosis of infarction in women. Rupture has been noted in relation to coughing and straining to have bowel movement. One might predict that any sustained isometric exercise might predispose to rupture at the time of acute rise in left ventricular pressure. The possible deterimental effect of continued physical activity after infarction has also been considered as a causal factor.

Most patients die suddenly without premonitory symptoms; others complain of new or recurrent pain due to myocardial ischemia. The typical pain of pericarditis may occur intermittently or may be persistent 1 or more days prior to terminal collapse. This may be associated with dissection of the myocardium through the epicardium with formation of a false aneurysm.

A pericardial friction rub may be noted in the minority of patients prior to rupture. Signs of congestive failure may be detected in some, but rupture is statistically more common in the absence of congestive failure. With final rupture and hemopericardium there may be no detectable peripheral pulse or blood pressure. The skin may be cool, clammy, or cyanotic. The neck veins may be distended, but the important clue to cardiac tamponade, pulsus paradoxus, may not be elicited because of absence of blood pressure. Pulsus paradoxus may be present when the blood pressure is maintained. Rare findings may include the recent appearance of a grating pericardial rub and a systolic murmur and thrill along the left sternal border simulating rupture of the ventricular septum. The pulse may be slow. Pathologic studies indicate that some patients with rupture have preceding unrecognized infarction, and the pain causing hospitalization may be related to the dissecting process incident to rupture. The final demise may be delayed be the formation of a false aneurysm. In one series this occurred in 9 of 40 instances, with rupture of the false aneurysm in 4 of 9.[215] External rupture is usually confined to the free wall of the left ventricle, but on rare occasions the rupture occurs in the right ventricle.

The electrocardiogram usually shows the unchanged pattern of transmural infarction in the face of an absent blood pressure. Sinus bradycardia followed by junctional rhythm may occur incident to intense vagal stimulation from stretching of the pericardial sac or from direct-pressure stimulation of the SA node. New ST-segment elevation, or less frequently ST-segment depression, may accompany the slowing of the rate. ST-segment elevation may be noted prior to rupture into a false aneurysm. Peaked T waves or reversal of previously inverted T waves may be noted in some patients. Leukocytosis and enzyme changes are those expected from the underlying infarction and give no diagnostic help. X-rays may show an unchanged cardiac silhouette or changes or pericardial effusion.

Death often occurs in a few minutes but prompt action may save a few patients. See discussion regarding treatment later in this chapter and in Chap. 62F.

VENTRICULAR ANEURYSM[216]
(see Chap. 62F)

A significant ventricular aneurysm is usually recognized by the following clues in a patient with a large myocardial infarction: heart failure; a palpable precordial pulsation in the region of the cardiac apex; an abnormal precordial pulsation located medially or superiorly to the cardiac apex; persistent ST-segment elevation in the precordial leads of the electrocardiogram; an abnormal contour of the left cardiac border on the posteroanterior (PA) roentgenogram of the chest; and an abnormal systolic bulge of the left ventricular wall as seen at fluoroscopy.

Aneurysms involve the left ventricle in 95 percent of cases and the right ventricle in 5 percent of cases. They are generally associated with transmural infarction and involve the anterior or apical area in 80 percent of cases. The electrocardiogram reveals persistent ST-segment elevation and inverted T waves with significant Q waves in the vast majority of patients. At times these electrocardiographic changes can be produced by exercise. Small aneurysms may not be associated with these electrocardiographic changes. Calcification may occur in the wall of the aneurysm or in mural thrombi within its pouch (see Chap. 24). Arterial embolism, impaired ventricular function with chronic congestive heart failure, and recurrent ventricular tachycardia are complications of aneurysm formation. Rupture virtually never occurs unless there is reinfarction at the border of the aneurysm where the tough fibrous sac adjoins viable muscle. Gorlin and associates have emphasized that when more than 20 to 25 percent of the surface area of the left ventricle is involved with a ventricular aneurysm, an adequate stroke volume and cardiac output cannot be attained.[217] If the aneurysm is not too large, the survival rate may be no different from that of patients without aneurysm formation. Dubnow and associates, however, noted a 5-year survival of only 27 percent in patients with ventricular aneurysm, as compared with 77 percent in those who had myocardial infarction without an aneurysm.[218]

Patients with refractory heart failure, recurrent arterial emboli, and recurrent ventricular tachycardia who have the clues mentioned above should have a left ventricular angiogram. The angiogram may reveal areas of poor contractility rather than a bulging aneurysm. The angiogram usually reveals more extensive damage than was suspected on x-ray, electrocardiogram, and physical examination. The angiogram allows one to assess the degree of mitral regurgitation and makes it possible for the cardiac surgeon to determine if surgical intervention is feasible. When possible, it is best to wait for several months after an infarction before considering surgery. A coronary arteriogram should also be done at the time of the left ventriculogram to determine the following: if coronary bypass surgery could be performed along with aneurysmectomy; if the removal of the aneurysm is possible or if it is too large to be removed; if the coronary arteries are so extensively diseased that surgical removal of the aneurysm will not be useful. See discussion regarding treatment later in this chapter and in Chap. 62H.

POSTMYOCARDIAL INFARCTION SYNDROME (DRESSLER'S SYNDROME) (see also Chap. 84)

The postmyocardial infarction syndrome, as emphasized by Dressler, occurs in a small percentage of patients.[219] The cause is unknown, but it has been attributed to a hypersensitivity reaction in which the antigen is necrotic cardiac muscle. The disorder usually occurs a few weeks or months after myocardial infarction. The syndrome is recognized by the pericardial type of pain, pericardial friction rub, and fever. At times there may be pneumonitis, left pleural effusion, leukocytosis, and pericardial effusion with cardiac tamponade. Kossowsky et al. believe that Dressler's syndrome can occur during the first week following myocardial infarction. It may last days to weeks. It must be differentiated from recurrent myocardial infarction, pulmonary infarction, and congestive heart failure.[220] See discussion regarding treatment later in this chapter and in Chap. 84.

CHEST WALL SYNDROMES[114]

Patients who have had a prolonged episode of myocardial ischemia with objective signs of myocardial damage have a variety of chest complaints. Some of the symptoms will be due to additional bouts of myocardial ischemia, but often the discomfort is due to anxiety or pericarditis. There is, however, a type of discomfort that is not explained by any of these possibilities. For lack of a better term, it is called the chest wall syndrome.

The clinical features of the chest wall syndrome include the following: The patient may complain of pain that comes and goes. The duration of discomfort ranges from a few seconds to several hours. The discomfort is located somewhere in the anterior position of the chest. For example, the discomfort may be noted in the right or left upper part of the chest, and there may be localized area of tenderness. Occasionally the discomfort is relieved by moving the arms or trunk as if the intercostal muscles were tense. See discussion regarding treatment later in this chapter.

"CEREBRAL SYNDROMES"[221]

Anxiety and depression are the most common of the cerebral syndromes. These have been discussed earlier. Patients with paroxysmal left ventricular paralysis due to abrupt myocardial ischemia which may or may not be associated with chest discomfort, may have dizziness and syncope as a result of this very special type of electromechanical dissociation (see discussion earlier in this chapter). Patients with transient arrhythmias may have intermittent cerebral symptoms (see Chap. 46B). Patients with angina pectoris may have dizziness, weakness, and syncope as a result of the use of nitroglycerin. Impairment of cerebral perfusion may produce a variety of cerebral disorders during the course of acute myocardial infarction. Hypoxia related to heart failure and shock may be associated with restlessness, confusion, and irritability.

In the presence of cerebral vascular disease, hypotension at the onset of myocardial infarction may produce transient cerebral ischemia or cerebral infarction. Fortunately, the latter complication is rare and is more prone to occur in the older patient with basilar-vertebral arterial disease. It may be the presenting complaint with painless myocardial infarction in the elderly, and the diagnosis may be overlooked unless serial electrocardiograms are taken. The development of cerebral infarction 24 h or more after myocardial infarction is more often due to cerebral embolism from mural thrombi that develop at the site of infarction of the endocardium in the region of the apex of the left ventricle (see Chap. 105). Dyskinetic or akinetic areas of the ventricle encourage thrombus formation. A discrete ventricular aneurysm serves as a nidus for thrombus formation and embolism long after recovery from myocardial infarction. It is surprising that cerebral embolism does not occur more frequently than it does.

Bradycardia and hypotension in the first hours following the clinical onset of infarction may produce dizziness and syncope if the patient is upright. Nitrites, large doses of antiarrhythmic drugs, or opiates may likewise induce postural hypotension and cerebral symptoms. Restlessness, anxiety, somnolence, and confusion may accompany bradycardia, many tachyarrhythmias, heart block, hypotension, or shock. However, these symptoms may also be noted with blood pressures in the normal range and are common accompaniments of pump failure. Hypoxia with a decrease in arterial P_{O_2} is common in this setting. There may be accompanying respiratory alkalosis or acidosis.

Metabolic acidosis due to excess lactate production, which may develop with shock syndromes or alveolar pulmonary edema, can produce mental confusion.

Drugs may intensify the symptoms associated with hypoxia. Cerebral syndromes may be due to drugs such as corticosteroids, lidocaine, diphenylhydantoin, sedatives, tranquilizers, nitrites, and insulin. Lidocaine may induce drowsiness, paresthesias, and convulsions. A dreaded cause of seizures in the coronary care unit is the "runaway lidocaine drip."

Following cardiac arrest there may be somnolence and confusion related to cerebral edema for days. Many such patients may have no memory of the events or even of the total period of hospitalization. Brain damage due to hypoxia may be permanent (see Chap. 50B). A hyperosmolar state may be induced by excessive administration of sodium bicarbonate after cardiac arrest, and this may induce confusion and coma.

Encephalopathy due to water intoxication is a rare complication and is usually due to excessive fluid administration when water is retained out of proportion to salt. Hypoglycemia following insulin administration may produce confusion, irrational behavior, or coma. When delirium or seizures occur, one should be certain that they are not due to withdrawal of alcohol, barbiturates, or tranquilizers.

Mental confusion may be associated with confinement in the coronary care unit. A past history of serious emotional problems often marks the patient as one who will experience such difficulty. See discussion regarding treatment later in this chapter.

BRONCHOPNEUMONIA

Bronchopneumonia may be a catastrophic complication of myocardial infarction. The diagnosis is difficult because fever, cough, leukocytosis, and signs of consolidation of the lung by physical examination and x-ray are common during the course of myocardial infarction in the absence of infection. The clinical picture is compounded further when the upper respiratory tract becomes irritated by the nasal administration of oxygen. Shaking chills are not encountered during the course of uncomplicated myocardial infarction, and their occurrence suggests bacteremia, often from pulmonary or genitourinary tract infection. Pleuritic pain, dyspnea, tachycardia, and blood-streaked sputum may alert the physician to the presence of bronchopneumonia or pulmonary embolism. Pericarditis with associated pleural effusion may simulate pneumonia. A common cause of bronchopneumonia in the patient with acute myocardial infarction is associated with cardiac arrest and resuscitation. Successful resuscitation is also frequently complicated by aspiration pneumonia.

The presence of purulent sputum may be the first definite clue to bronchopneumonia. The sputum smear and cultures may demonstrate the presence of pneumococci or other organisms. See discussion regarding treatment later in this chapter.

LATE CARDIAC ARREST
The patient with coronary atherosclerotic heart disease is at high risk of cardiac arrest due to ventricular fibrillation or ventricular standstill. The peak risk of ventricular fibrillation is within the first 8 h following the onset of myocardial infarction, but this catastrophe is a continuing threat to life during subsequent days and weeks (see earlier discussion). Thus, up to one-third or more of instances of cardiac arrest may occur later during the course of infarction. In one series of 273 patients there was an 8 percent incidence of sudden death after discharge from the coronary care unit.[192] The following factors enhance the possibility of late cardiac arrest: shock during the first week; frequent ventricular premature contractions, ventricular tachycardia, or ventricular fibrillation early in the course of the illness; persistent heart failure; complete AV block; anterior infarction with AV block, with right bundle branch block or left bundle branch block, or with right bundle branch block and left anterior hemiblock; recurrent pain; recurrent arrhythmia with frequent ventricular premature beats and ventricular tachycardia; cardiac enlargement; and persistent sinus tachycardia.

One should not forget that emotional factors may induce cardiac arrest in the patient with coronary atherosclerotic heart disease. For example, a 65-year-old patient with a transmural inferior myocardial infarction who had been discharged from the coronary care unit after 1 week became emotionally disturbed during a telephone conversation and dropped dead. The authors have observed that trivial upsets such as those related to venipuncture, changing the site of intravenous clysis, or fecal impaction can trigger arrhythmias such as atrial fibrillation,

ventricular tachycardia, and ventricular fibrillation. Adverse reactions to drugs such as morphine or tranquilizers may produce postural hypotension and syncope, thereby inciting recurrent ischemia, leading to cardiac arrest. See discussion regarding treatment later in this chapter.

GENITOURINARY SYNDROMES
Catheterization of the bladder may be necessary in patients who *cannot void* during the course of myocardial infarction. This problem occurs most often in male patients who have a large prostate. The problem is compounded by the use of opiates, atropine, sedatives, and lying in bed. A catheter is usually not needed after the first day or so, at which time nearly all male patients can stand, and narcotics are no longer needed. A few patients, however, may require a catheter for many days or weeks; rarely, it may be necessary for 2 to 3 months until a transurethral prostatectomy can be safely performed. Catheterization is also needed in the patient with shock in order to monitor the urine flow in response to fluid administration and to assess the effectiveness of pressor agents.

Urethral bleeding due to the indwelling catheter is an occasional problem, particularly when anticoagulant therapy is given. Trauma during catheterization, the presence of a urethral stricture, or the patient's pulling the catheter out may cause hemorrhage. Cystitis and pyelonephritis may develop and require antibiotic therapy. Such symptoms may develop days or weeks later. Bacteremia with gram-negative sepsis should be suspected when chills, fever, and hypotension occur during or following catheterization of the bladder. Pyuria and urine colony counts above 100,000 are often found in such patients.

Myocardial infarction with cardiogenic shock in the absence of other complicating diseases rarely results in acute renal failure. Azotemia and oliguria, however, are not uncommon functional derangements. Although glomerular filtration may be well preserved, congestive heart failure and cardiogenic shock stimulate avid tubular reabsorption of sodium and water, resulting in excessive reabsorption of urea and low urinary volume. The ratio of blood urea nitrogen (BUN) to creatinine in the serum is often greater than 20:1. The urine has a high osmolality, low sodium concentration, and a mild degree of proteinuria. Nonpigmented granular cases are frequently seen. See discussion regarding treatment later in this chapter.

SHOULDER-HAND SYNDROME[222,223]
The shoulder-hand syndrome occasionally occurs following myocardial infarction. It is much less common now than it was formerly, when it was said to occur in 15 percent of patients with myocardial infarction who were treated with strict bed rest. The condition may develop before the other signs of coronary atherosclerotic heart disease appear but usually occurs several months after infarction. Symptoms include tenderness, stiffness, and discom-

fort on abduction of the shoulder, usually on the left but occasionally bilaterally. The skin over the hands and fingers may be tense, shiny, and swollen. There may be swelling of the hands and fingers, with discoloration. Palmar nodules and Dupuytren's contracture are not infrequent. This neurotrophic disorder may persist for many months and may be mistaken by patients for recurrent angina pectoris or myocardial infarction. See discussion regarding treatment later in this chapter.

NONVASCULAR COMPLICATIONS
Both *gout* and *diabetes mellitus* may be precipitated by myocardial infarction and are occasionally brought to light by the administration of chlorothiazide drugs. See discussion regarding treatment later in this chapter.

HICCOUGHS, RETCHING, NAUSEA, AND VOMITING
These are occasionally troublesome complications. Hiccoughs are more often associated with diaphragmatic infarction. Hiccoughs may, on rare occasion, prevent the patient from resting. Nausea and vomiting may be due to the administration of opiates or related drugs but may occur as a result of infarction alone. Retching is an ominous sign and is associated with a high incidence of arrhythmia. See discussion regarding treatment later in this chapter.

GASTROINTESTINAL SYNDROMES
Severe gastric distension may produce hypotension, add to the respiratory difficulties, and induce poor ventilation and cardiac arrhythmias. Reflex ileus with abdominal distension and troublesome constipation and fecal impaction may be produced by opiates or potassium depletion following diuresis. Hemorrhagic disease of the bowel may follow prolonged shock. Gastrointestinal hemorrhage due to peptic ulcer may be precipitated by the stress reaction of myocardial infarction, and this may be complicated by the administration of anticoagulants. Occasionally, the onset of acute myocardial infarction may be associated with a very strong urge to defecate. Fecal impaction is serious and may induce recurrent myocardial ischemia and pain. It is more common in women. See discussion regarding treatment later in this chapter.

THERAPEUTIC MISADVENTURES
The treatment of coronary atherosclerotic disease includes the use of a diet, advice regarding activity, and the use of complex procedures and toxic drugs. This paragraph is added as a reminder that serious complications may result from the use of various drugs and procedures. This is not to say that they should not be used. It *is* to say that they should be used for the proper reasons and that their use should be monitored for their own unique complications. See discussion regarding treatment later in this chapter.

PROGNOSIS OF CORONARY ATHEROSCLEROTIC HEART DISEASE

The following discussion on prognosis was written by our friend Dr. Gottlieb C. Friesinger, Professor of Medicine and Director of the Division of Cardiology of Vanderbilt University School of Medicine in Nashville, Tennessee. Dr. Friesinger has had a special interest in the prognosis of patients with coronary atherosclerotic heart disease, and we greatly appreciate his contribution to this chapter.

In many areas of clinical medicine, confidently establishing prognosis is difficult. In coronary atherosclerotic heart disease, prognostication is particularly capricious. The principal contributors to problems in prognosis in this heart disease are the inherent complexity of the condition and the lack of adequate objective data. Fully satisfactory techniques to obtain objective data in many patients do not yet exist, although methods and information have considerably improved in the last several decades with the wide use of electrocardiography, the development of coronary care units, and the utilization of coronary arteriography. *A special liability in considering prognosis is the problem of sudden death.* The propensity for sudden death to occur in all groups of patients with coronary atherosclerotic heart disease provides a disconcerting element and adds an emotional element to prognoses not present in most other diseases.

The approach which is most useful and has provided recent additional insights into the prognosis of coronary atherosclerotic heart disease has been to place patients into subsets using multiple factors having independent importance (see Chap. 62A). This approach has been applied most extensively to the subset of patients with acute myocardial infarction, but considerable data have accumulated concerning other clinical subsets, especially patients with stable angina pectoris. This discussion will approach the problem of prognosis by considering the principal clinical subsets of ischemic heart disease, i.e., the asymptomatic group, those with stable angina pectoris, unstable angina pectoris and prolonged myocardial ischemia without objective signs of infarction, and myocardial infarction. The problem of sudden death will also be discussed. To consider the prognosis of coronary atherosclerotic heart disease on the basis of clinical presentation is appropriate since patients usually present to their physicians with a rather specific clinical syndrome. In addition, the clinical presentation per se contains considerable prognostic implication.

It must be emphasized that clinical presentations in coronary atherosclerotic heart disease are not always "clean and clear-cut." There may be "shading" from one clinical presentation to another. Patients often move from one clinical subset to another as their disease evolves. The movement is not usually orderly nor predictable; and movement from one subset to another obviously alters prognosis.

Despite these multiple problems critical clinical assessment coupled with appropriate laboratory studies, thoughtfully analyzed, ordinarily allows a reasonable estimate of prognosis. In each clinical subset, certain common determinants of prognosis, e.g., extent of atherosclerosis and degree of left ventricular scarring and dysfunction, are found; but in each clinical subset certain unique predictors exist. The paragraphs to follow approach prognosis by utilizing clinical subsets and emphasizing the multiple parameters of major importance in determining prognosis for each clinical group. It becomes obvious that each clinical subset consists of multiple subsets when additional objective data are obtained. *It is also apparent that the severity of the patient's complaints (e.g., chest discomfort due to myocardial ischemia) is not closely related to prognosis.*

The physician should always be aware that most patients with ischemic heart disease, even those patients who express no curiosity or concern (perhaps related to their fears and/or denial), are deeply concerned about their prognosis.

Patients will obtain information about prognosis from someone if not from their physician. The physician's willingness to discuss prognosis in a realistic and sympathetic manner, with as much optimism as is warranted, at the appropriate time and under proper circumstances, is an important part of the overall management of patients with ischemic heart disease.

Lastly, the physician must have a keen awareness of the importance of natural history and prognosis if he is to select the most rational therapy for his patient and if he is to make a realistic judgment about the factors involved in the outcome of his therapeutic decisions.

Asymptomatic group

The natural history of asymptomatic coronary atherosclerosis is unknown. The studies of Zoll, Blumgart, and Edwards, and their associates[224–226] made it evident that moderately severe or severe coronary atherosclerosis is common in our population and may not be associated with symptoms. It should be emphasized, however, that "asymptomatic" can be defined in a variety of ways. Patients whose histories do not disclose angina pectoris because they keep activity at a low level, but who develop angina with ischemic ST-segment shift if subjected to a heavier exercise load must be considered to have a different prognosis than patients who are asymptomatic by history and who develop neither angina nor electrocardiographic change with a heavy exercise load. Although this matter seems quite obvious, it complicates the evaluation of any data in "asymptomatic" populations. Hence, multiple subsets exist among the "asymptomatic" patients. Variable degrees of coronary atherosclerosis will be present, as well as vary-

ing degrees of left ventricular dysfunction—as in the symptomatic groups. Some patients will have had previous symptomatic ischemic heart disease and will have become totally free of symptoms without medication. Others will present with electrocardiographic changes, evidence of old myocardial infarction, or nonspecific ST-T changes. The only common feature in all groups that are truly asymptomatic is (assumed to be) adequate collateral vessel formation which prevents symptoms of angina and breathlessness. Since these multiple subsets of asymptomatic patients have not been characterized in any systematic way, no natural history data are available. It seems certain that the extent of coronary atherosclerosis and degree of left ventricular dysfunction will be important determinants of prognosis in this group. It is suspected that the prognosis is better in asymptomatic patients than in symptomatic patients for any similar degree of disease. The natural history of asymptomatic patients assumes increasing importance since the widespread use of coronary arteriography is disclosing many patients who have varying degrees of coronary atherosclerosis and angiographic abnormality who are truly asymptomatic.

Stable angina pectoris (Table 62E-1)

The distinctive and characteristic history of patients with typical angina pectoris has allowed physicians to be confident in their diagnosis long prior to the development and widespread use of modern diagnostic techniques. The history and resting electrocardiogram contain a surprising amount of prognostic information about stable angina pectoris. The studies of Block[227] and White[228] illustrate this point. Block analyzed 6,882 cases referred to the Mayo Clinic, and White personally followed a smaller group of patients for a long period of time, i.e., to death or for 25 years. In these studies mortality was higher for the first year following the initial consultation, over 10 percent, with a 6 to 9 percent annual mortality subsequently. It is likely that more severe cases would be referred for consultation, so it is suspected mortality rates would be higher in these patients than in the "average" patient with typical angina pectoris.

From these and other studies it can be concluded that the *severity and frequency of the angina per se does not hold much prognostic information.* This is understandable when it is realized that patients be-

TABLE 62E-1
**Stable angina pectoris:
prognostic determinants**

Angiographic findings:
  Coronary arteriographic anatomy
  Left ventricular abnormalities

Electrocardiographic findings:
  Resting abnormalities
  Exercise-induced abnormalities

Clinical features:
  Hypertension
  Male sex
  Congestive heart failure
  Ventricular arrhythmias (?)
  Etc.

come extremely "clever" at controlling their activity, using nitroglycerin prophylactically, and avoiding emotionally charged situations which might provoke episodes. Hence, they appear to have very "mild" (i.e., infrequent and not severe or prolonged) angina. However, it must be stated that among patients with very long-standing angina (more than 5 years) those who have frequent episodes with minimal activities, particularly at rest, generally have a poorer prognosis.

More recent studies in less selected patients in the Health Insurance Plan of New York[229] and the Framingham study[230] show a better prognosis, a 3 to 4 percent per year mortality. In fact, in patients who have neither hypertension nor an abnormal resting electrocardiogram, the mortality was extremely low, less than 2 percent per year for the 4.5 years of follow-up reported. If both hypertension and an abnormal resting electrocardiogram were present, however, the mortality was significantly higher, nearly 8 percent per year.

ELECTROCARDIOGRAPHIC DATA

The prognostic importance of abnormalities on the resting electrocardiogram is complex. The studies of Block (1952, probably utilizing only six leads!) are especially interesting and instructive (Fig. 62E-16).[227] The mortality for patients with a normal electrocardiogram at 10-year follow-up was 47 percent, a significantly lower mortality than for patients with electrocardiographic abnormalities. Patients with Q waves or T abnormalities had a 75 percent 10-year mortality; inverted TII and TIII (perhaps indicating inferior ischemia) had a 75 percent mortality; but inverted TI and TII (perhaps indicative of inferior and lateral and/or anterior ischemia) had a higher mortality of 90 percent and intraventricular conduction defects (which could be judged to be associated with the most extensive atherosclerosis and left ventricular dysfunction) also had a very high 10-year mortality, 87 percent. A recent study[231] of patients with ST-T changes whose arteriographic anatomy was known confirms the Block study. In 139 patients studied, mortality with patients in the ST-T abnormality

group was nearly four times that of the group with no ST-T abnormality. Sophisticated statistical analysis indicated the ST-T abnormalities were an independent prognostic factor.

A reasonable synopsis of these data might be that the resting electrocardiogram is helpful prognostically insofar as it reflects underlying disease, Q waves, and intraventricular conduction defects indicating past infarction and scarring, and ST-T abnormalities presumably reflecting ischemia. It must be recalled that a major proportion, often as high as 50 percent, of patients with stable angina pectoris have normal electrocardiograms; this group represents multiple hybrid subsets since many of the patients have far advanced disease and a poor prognosis. In addition, the prognostic implication of ST-T abnormalities are applicable only after it is ascertained with certainty that ischemic heart disease due to coronary atherosclerosis is present. Many patients with worrisome chest pain have ST-T abnormalities, and their prognosis is excellent if coronary atherosclerosis is not the cause of the problem.

Although the data are limited, exercise-induced ST-segment depression has been shown to have prognostic implications.[232–234] Virtually all studies utilize ST-segment changes in only a qualitative manner, i.e., the test is either negative or positive for ischemia. Quantitative data relating the time of onset of the ST-segment change, and the degree and duration of ST-segment depression to prognosis have not been systematically performed but probably would enhance the ability of the exercise electrocardiogram to be predictive. Limited semiquantitative data are available. Robb and Marks reported results of 2,224 individuals applying for life insurance. At a mean follow-up time of 5.6 years, the presence of and degree of ST-segment depression during exercise had great prognostic significance.[232] Even if the ST-segment depression was less than 1 mm, the mortality was increased two and one-half times over the population without such change. If the depression was 1 to 2 mm or more, there was a sixteenfold increase in the expected mortality over the group without any ST-segment shift. A more recent study by Ellestad using slightly different methodology has resulted in similar conclusions:[233] 2,700 patients were submitted to exercise testing and more than one-half of them were followed for 3 years; some were followed for as long as 8 years. In patients with no evidence of ST-depression during exercise, there was a 1.1 percent mortality over a 4-year period. In patients who were judged to have equivocal ST-segment depression due to ischemia, the mortality was increased to nearly 2.4 percent per year; and in those judged to have unequivocal ST-segment depression due to ischemia, the mortality was extremely high, approximately 10 percent per year. In studies where the ST-segment depression has been correlated with coronary arteriographic findings, it has usually been demonstrated that the most marked ST-segment depression (more than 2 mm) is often asso-

FIGURE 62E-16 The prognostic significance of the resting electrocardiogram.[227]

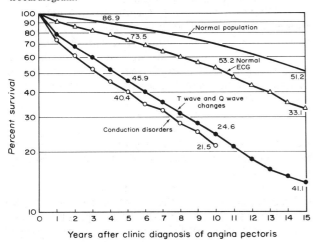

ciated with very far advanced disease, often involving all three major arteries or the left main coronary artery. Similarly, most studies have shown that the more extensive the coronary atherosclerosis is on arteriography, the more likely the exercise-induced ST-segment shift is to occur. Unfortunately, the absence of ST-segment depression does not necessarily denote a good prognosis in patients with stable angina pectoris. Exercise limitation by dyspnea and poor ventricular performance may carry at least as poor a prognosis as does ST-segment depression per se. Exercise-induced ST-segment changes are most useful when occurring in patients with normal resting electrocardiograms. Interpretation of exercise-induced electrocardiographic changes is fraught with many problems, especially if the resting tracing is abnormal (see discussion in Chap. 28A and in "The Use and Limitations of the Electrocardiogram" earlier in this chapter).

ARTERIOGRAPHIC DATA

Some of the most powerful prognostic data in patients with stable angina pectoris have been derived from studies utilizing angiographic techniques. Multiple studies have yielded remarkably similar data,[65,231,235-237] despite the variable circumstances of data collection and the considerable intraobserver variability in assessing arteriographic severity and ventriculographic abnormalities.[238,239] It is important to appreciate that arteriography is a gross method of estimating the degree of coronary atherosclerosis. Lesions judged to narrow the luminal diameter by more than 50 percent (75 percent cross-sectional area) are usually felt to be "clinically significant." However, any change on arteriography probably represents "significant disease." This is emphasized by studies in which the mortality at 5 to 7 year follow-up was less than 2 percent[235,236] when no lesions or trivial narrowings were visualized, but 12 percent if lesions of 30 to 50 percent narrowing (sometimes termed "significant") were present.[240]

The clinical course of 500 patients was studied by Dr. William Proudfit[241] at the Cleveland Clinic and followed for 5 years. There were 342 patients with entirely normal coronary arteriograms. There were only 2 (0.6 percent) who died of presumed cardiac deaths and 3 (0.9 percent) myocardial infarctions in 5 years. Both incidences are about half the expected rates in the average unselected population of the United States matched by age and sex. In 101 patients with lesions with less than 30 percent narrowing of the luminal diameter the prognosis was less good than in the normal group but still better than in the average population. In 57 patients with lesions that were from 30 percent to less than 50 percent narrowing of the luminal diameter there were 3 (5.3 percent) presumed cardiac deaths and 2 (3.5 percent) myocardial infarctions within 5 years. Both of these incidences are higher than in the average population. Serial arteriograms were done in 20 cases and showed progression of the lesions in the group with

moderate narrowing (30 percent to 50 percent), but progression or development of narrowing occurred in only one patient who had no lesions initially or who had lesions of less than 30 percent luminal narrowing initially.

Patients with arteriographic abnormalities localized to a single vessel have a low mortality (1 to 2 percent per year) for the first few years subsequent to arteriographic study, while those with severe narrowings in two or three trunks have a much poorer prognosis (6 to 10 percent per year).[235-237] The poorest prognosis of all involves patients who have disease in the left main coronary artery—which is usually accompanied by disease elsewhere. Most studies report greater than a 20 percent per year mortality in this group.[242,243] Left main coronary disease is found more frequently in patients with unstable angina pectoris than with stable disease.

Dr. William Proudfit made the following observation:[241] All of a group of 601 consecutive nonsurgical patients demonstrated arteriographically to have severely obstructed coronary disease when studied between January 1963 and July 1965 were followed for a minimum of 10 years or until death or termination of study because of operation for coronary disease. The overall 10-year survival was 44 percent. Those who had obstruction of single arteries had a 2.4 percent mortality per year for the first 4 years and 5.2 percent in the last 6 years; 10-year survival was 63 percent. Survival was lowest (54 percent) for left anterior descending artery obstruction. The survival of patients who had two arteries obstructed was 44 percent in 10 years. The survival of patients who had three arteries obstructed was 23 percent in 10 years. The survival of patients with left main coronary obstruction was the same as for patients with triple-vessel disease although the survival curve was lower for the left main coronary artery obstruction during the first 3 years than it was for triple-vessel disease. The 5-year mortality was about 50 percent for left main obstruction and for triple-vessel disease. Patients who would be candidates for bypass operation by present criteria had an annual mortality for survivors of 2.6 percent, 5.8 percent, 9.9 percent, and 10.7 percent for obstruction of one, two, three arteries, or left main artery.

A number of studies demonstrate that abnormalities on ventriculography worsen the prognosis for any coronary arteriographic abnormality. The additive effect of abnormal left ventricular function, as judged from the angiographic silhouette, was predictable on the basis of clinical observations since patients with ischemic heart disease and congestive failure, with or without angina, have a very grave prognosis; fewer than 20 percent are apt to be alive at the end of 5 years.

The data concerning prognostic implications of angiographic findings in stable angina pectoris may be summarized. The prognosis worsens as the extent of arteriographic abnormality increases. Single-vessel disease localized to the left anterior descending artery carries a worse prognosis than a similar degree localized to the right coronary artery. Double-vessel disease carries a worse prognosis than single-vessel disease. Triple-vessel disease has a very poor prognosis regardless of the precise configuration and extent of lesions. Left main coronary artery disease carries a very poor prognosis that is somewhat similar to that of severe triple-vessel disease in that 50 percent of patients are dead in 5 years and 80 percent of patients are dead in 10 years. The mortality of patients with left main obstruction is higher than triple-vessel disease during the first 3 years after discovery. Ventricular abnormalities on angiography are additive to arteriographic changes in worsening prognosis.

An oversimplified summary of this extensive body of angiographic data might be that *catastrophic complications, sudden death, and myocardial infarction are increasingly likely as the extent of arteriographic abnormality increases, and any ischemic and/or arrhythmic event is less well tolerated with increasing ventricular abnormality (as judged by angiography).*

Unstable angina and prolonged myocardial ischemia without objective signs of infarction
(Table 62E-2)

As discussed in Chap. 62A, unstable angina pectoris and prolonged myocardial ischemia without objective evidence of infarction are clinical entities which are located in between stable angina pectoris and established myocardial infarction. A large overlap exists between unstable angina pectoris, episodes of prolonged myocardial ischemia without objective signs of infarction, and myocardial infarction, as well as between stable and unstable angina pectoris. It is appropriate to speak of the unstable angina pectoris syndromes and not to consider this as a discrete clinical entity (see Chap. 62A).

As a corollary to this clinical observation, it is not surprising that multiple subsets exist when unstable angina is characterized by objective data. To date, there is no agreement on either descriptive terms or the most important aspects of objective characterization. As with all the other clinical subsets in coronary atherosclerotic heart disease, however, it seems certain that the extent of coronary atherosclerosis and the status of left ventricular function as determined by coronary arteriography and left ventriculography are very important determinants of prognosis. Since, by definition, this is an unstable phase of the disease, it is apparent that the degree of "unstableness" likely

TABLE 62E-2
Prognostic factors in unstable angina pectoris

Preexisting disease
  Myocardial infarction
  Angina pectoris

Severity and persistence of unstable complaints

Presence and character of ECG changes during pain
  ST-segment depression
  ST-segment elevation
  T-wave inversion
  None

Angiographic findings
  Arteriographic abnormalities
  Ventriculographic abnormalities

holds considerable prognostic information. Although data are inadequate, the systematic data which are available suggest that this is correct.

The elegant studies of Duncan et al.[244] in Edinburgh indicate that patients who have the onset of new or worsening angina not severe enough to require hospitalization have the following mortality following the onset of this unstable syndrome: In 251 patients, 4 percent had died and 12 percent had developed myocardial infarction at 6-month follow-up. At the 6-month follow-up 31 percent were free of angina. In these patients, who would be judged to have clinically "mild" unstable angina pectoris, no angiographic studies were performed. It is suspected that their 6-month mortality is significantly higher than patients with stable angina pectoris and comparable degrees of disease. Some would say that the mortality and morbidity in this group was not excessively high. *We would disagree.* We believe a mortality of 4 percent and an infarction rate of 12 percent at 6 months is unacceptably high and expect it to be even higher as the months and years pass for this group of patients.

In another clinical study, Gazes et al.[245] reported experience with 140 patients judged to have unstable angina severe enough to require hospitalization. The 1-year mortality was 18 percent and the 2-year mortality, 25 percent. This mortality is appreciably higher than that expected with stable angina pectoris. In addition, a subset within this hospitalized group was identified who had a very high risk. Patients with stable angina pectoris prior to the onset of the unstable phase, those with frequent episodes of ischemia after hospitalization, and patients who had ST changes accompanying the ischemia during the hospitalization had a higher mortality: 43 percent at 12 months and 53 percent at 24 months. These patients were studied clinically and not angiographically.

Multiple studies[246–249] have now included angiographic study of patients with unstable angina. As with all other clinical subsets of ischemic heart disease, a wide spectrum of arteriographic and ventriculographic abnormalities is seen. Many patients have extensive coronary atherosclerosis, especially if ischemic symptoms have been present prior to the onset of the unstable phase. In patients whose unstable angina is the first expression of their ischemic heart disease, lesser degrees of coronary atherosclerosis, even disease isolated to a single vessel, are sometimes present; however, in this group, *advanced lesions in all major trunks are present in a majority of patients.* Lesions of the left main coronary artery appear to be twice as frequent, in the range of 10 to 12 percent in patients requiring hospitalization for their unstable syndrome when compared with patients with stable pectoris.

Data are limited on the relationship between angiographic findings and prognosis in unstable angina pectoris, but it can be safely assumed that they will parallel the data seen in stable angina pectoris, although the early mortality (i.e., 1 year) is almost certainly higher for any given degree of disease in the unstable group. Medical and surgical therapy is being intensively utilized in the unstable syndromes, and it is doubtful that the exact natural history will ever be known.

Of particular interest is the fact that in each series, a small number of patients (usually in the range of 5 percent) have normal coronary arteriograms. This information is provocative and suggests that it may be difficult to be confident on clinical grounds alone that the patient has ischemic cardiac discomfort or that the discomfort is in fact due to myocardial ischemia but not related to anatomic abnormalities. Obviously, a combination of both these explanations may be correct. Insofar as the latter possibility is concerned, it is conceivable that coronary arterial spasm is present, that abnormalities in the clotting mechanism, such as platelet "stickiness," are occurring, or that there are other transient phenomena which can disturb the myocardial oxygen supply-demand relationship. This is a particularly provocative area of clinical investigation, since there is a strong suggestion that the unstable state is not always related primarily to a progression in the anatomic severity of the disease (see Chap. 63B).

The unstable state is a "transient phase" and after a few weeks, or perhaps several months, the patient moves to another phase. He or she may develop stable angina pectoris or become asymptomatic if sudden death or myocardial infarction has not intervened. The prognosis then becomes the prognosis of his or her new clinical subset.

Myocardial infarction

The prognosis of myocardial infarction is best considered by dividing the problem into three phases, "prehospitalization" (very early). in hospital, and "posthospital" (late). Figure 62E-17 illustrates the very high mortality in the first few hours following the onset of a "heart attack" and the subsequent lessened, but still high, mortality.

PREHOSPITALIZATION (VERY EARLY) PROGNOSIS

The term heart attack instead of myocardial infarction is used for the earliest phase since most patients who die in the first few minutes or several hours after the onset of an attack do not have myocardial necrosis demonstrable by current routine techniques. Most die of a catastrophic arrhythmia, primarily ventricular fibrillation, prior to the development of overt necrosis; some will die with overwhelming pulmonary edema and shock. Lethal arrhythmias due to ischemic heart disease are as much a cause of sudden death as is acute myocardial infarction (see Chap. 49). Studies in Seattle[250] and Miami[251] illustrate this point especially well. In their community-wide effort to resuscitate victims of sudden death, all of whom were demonstrated to have ventricular fibril-

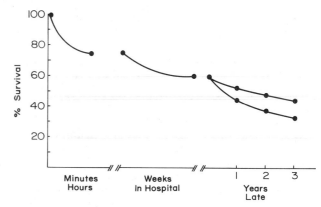

FIGURE 62E-17 Schematic illustration of mortality of acute myocardial infarction. The data are most applicable to first infarction. Subsequent infarctions are usually associated with a worsened prognosis. The late mortality depicted illustrates a "favorable" group and less favorable group. The latter would include patients who have such factors as chronic angina pectoris, significant hypertension, prominent residual electrocardiographic changes, cardiomegaly, etc.; these items would not be found in the "favorable" group.

lation, more than three-fourths of the successfully resuscitated patients did not manifest clinical or laboratory evidence of myocardial infarction.

Armstrong et al.[252] and Fulton et al.[253] have identified the following: Of all the patients who are destined to die within 30 days subsequent to an acute heart attack nearly 50 percent will do so in the first 1 to 2 h after onset of the episode, and 70 to 80 percent in the first 24 h. A conservative but reasonable mortality statistic is a 40 percent total mortality at 30 days. Hence, 20 of every 100 patients with an acute heart attack (myocardial infarction) have died in 1 to 2 h, often before reaching a medical facility.

This statistic and the pattern of mortality make it apparent that coronary care unit mortality statistics have little meaning and will vary widely unless the time between the onset of the patients' complaint and arrival at the coronary care unit is known. If admission to the coronary care unit is delayed for some hours, the highest mortality period is passed and hence the overall mortality in such a coronary care unit will be lower than in a unit whose location and/or admitting arrangements allow arrival of patients very early following the onset of symptoms.

INHOSPITAL PROGNOSIS

After arrival in the coronary care unit (and this can now include mobile units in which sophisticated emergency care can be given) the principal determinants of mortality are shown in Table 62E-3. It has become increasingly apparent on the basis of objective assessment of patients with acute infarction that the extent of myocardium involved in the infarct is a powerful determinant of outcome. Available clinical techniques are inadequate to estimate the extent of infarction precisely, but a combination of clinical and laboratory data which are routinely obtained can help in estimating prognosis. More precise techniques utilizing electrocardiographic, enzymatic, and radionuclide methods to assess infarct size are areas of intense clinical investigation at the present time.

TABLE 62E-3
Inhospital myocardial infarction prognostic determinants

Infarct size
  Clinical complications—especially left ventricular dysfunction
  Electrocardiographic changes—especially location of infarct
  Enzyme level elevations

Previous ischemia
  Angina pectoris
  Myocardial infarction

Age

Infarct extension

Heart size

Associated diseases (not strong factors)
  Diabetes
  Hypertension
  Pulmonary disease
  Etc.

Left ventricular dysfunction, assessed by clinical means, is of great importance in estimating prognosis. A simple clinical grading system (classes I to IV) as proposed by Killip[254] compares reasonably well with the hemodynamic objective estimates of left ventricular performance. A prognostic stratification of patients is possible from this approach as is illustrated in Table 62E-4. Postmortem correlative studies have been performed by multiple investigators since the initial quantitative postmortem studies reported by Page and others.[255,256,262] In patients who have profound left ventricular dysfunction (class IV, hemodynamic shock), massive left ventricular destruction—in the range of 40 percent of left ventricular mass—by current infarction and past scarring, can be anticipated. Lesser degrees of left ventricular destruction will be found in patients with congestive heart failure. Patients with less than 20 percent myocardium involved are not as apt to manifest significant left ventricular dysfunction.

Other clinical findings can be associated with poor prognosis.[257] A pericardial friction rub, leukocytosis greater than 20,000, and high fever (102 to 103° without complicating cause) are such items. However, such findings are nearly always accompanied by evidence of transmural infarction and/or congestive heart failure, features which indicate a large infarct. Hence, these items are accompaniments of a large infarct, but per se do not denote specific additive prognostic implications.

Serial electrocardiographic studies provide additional insight into the extent of myocardial necrosis, particularly if the changes are extensive. Numerous studies have indicated that electrocardiographic changes of transmural infarction denote larger areas of muscle necrosis than do the changes of subendocardial infarction. The degree of ST-segment elevation and the number of leads with ST-segment elevation in initial tracings give a crude estimate of the extent of necrosis and presage the development of Q waves and eventual scarring. Acute transmural anterior myocardial infarction tends, in general, to produce more muscle necrosis than transmural inferior myocardial infarction and is associated with a higher incidence of complications and mortality. Multiple investigators have utilized various electrocardiographic abnormalities, particularly ST-T changes in simple and sophisticated ("mapping" techniques) ways to estimate the extent of necrosis more precisely. However, readily applicable reliable methods for routine clinical use have not yet evolved. It should be noted that while the development of Q waves is used clinically to define transmural myocardial infarction, some patients with isolated subendocardial infarction may develop Q waves on their electrocardiogram.

As discussed earlier in this chapter, serum enzyme

TABLE 62E-4
Myocardial infarction prognosis and left ventricular function

	Clinical findings	LVFP	SWI	Mortality	Pathologic findings
Class I (uncomplicated)	No evidence of congestive failure	N	N	5–7%	No quantitative data
Class II (mild to moderate congestive failure)	Bibasilar rales* and/or S$_3$ gallop, tachycardia	↑	N	10–15%	Probably 20–30% LV mass destroyed
Class III (severe congestive failure or pulmonary edema)	Rales above the tip of the scapula,* S$_3$ gallop, tachycardia and/or frank pulmonary edema	↑	↓	20–50%	
Class IV (cardiogenic shock)	Markedly reduced peripheral perfusion (e.g., cool skin, diaphoresis, mental confusion, oliguria), tachycardia, hypotension (usually profound with systolic pressure <80 mm Hg)	usually ↑↑	↓↓	60–80%	30–40% of LV mass destroyed by current and past infarcts

*Data are more meaningful if confirmed by chest x-ray.
  N = normal, LVFP = left ventricular filling pressure equivalent to pulmonary wedge pressure,
  SWI = stroke work index (flow X pressure; q - M/M²)
  SOURCE: T. Killip, III and J. T. Kimball.[254] Reprinted with permission of author and publisher.

levels are virtually always abnormal in myocardial infarction if they are obtained at appropriate times. Multiple studies[24,258-260] have shown the level of peak elevation of enzymes are roughly correlated with the extent of necrotic myocardium. As a clinically useful prognostic feature, markedly elevated (five to six or more times normal) values indicate large infarcts and will be associated with more frequent complications and higher mortality. *On the other hand, lower values of enzymes do not necessarily guarantee a more favorable prognosis.* This is due to the fact that ancillary features (discussed below) also play an important role in prognosis. One additional feature when considering enzyme values is the fact that enzymes are relatively sensitive as predictors of myocardial necrosis but are very nonspecific. Isoenzymes, which are now becoming more widely used, may resolve this problem of specificity, at least in part. Studies by Sobel in animal models indicate serial enzyme values can be used to determine infarct size.[258] The mathematical treatment of the data is relatively sophisticated and whether such data can be regularly obtained and be useful in the management of infarction remains problematic.

The course of acute infarction is importantly influenced by the extent of previous myocardial damage.[257] The presence of angina pectoris and/or past myocardial infarction worsen the prognosis for a new infarction. Hence, it is the cumulative myocardial damage, not merely the necrosis related to the current episode, which is the determinant of left ventricular dysfunction and outcome. In this regard, electrocardiographic evidence of old myocardial infarction is a feature which is associated with worsening prognosis in a patient with a new infarction.

Increasing age has a definite adverse effect on prognosis. A variety of disease states are probably associated with a less favorable outcome, but it is difficult to prove independent importance for most of these associated disease conditions. Diabetes mellitus, principally in patients whose metabolic derangement is severe enough to require insulin; hypertension; and chronic pulmonary disease are three important and frequent diseases occurring in patients who suffer acute infarction. The effects operative in these diseases must be complex, but alteration in the metabolic processes, hypoxia, and increase in myocardial oxygen requirements would all worsen the ischemic and/or infarct state.

Several investigators[261-264] have attempted to simplify the multiplicity and complexity of features involved in estimating prognosis in acute infarction by developing a "prognostic index" which incorporates those factors which have greatest importance and which are additive. As this concept has evolved, the features "weighted" in prognosis have become more objective; *e.g., congestion on chest x-ray is utilized instead of rales,* and features which are "transient" and/or easily controlled in the coronary care unit, such as duration and severity of pain or arrhythmias, have been deleted from the prognostic

indexes such as the one devised by Norris and his colleagues.[263] Table 62E-5 lists the major prognostic features and is an example of the use of discriminant analysis in devising a prognostic index.[195a] Six factors obtained on admission to the coronary care unit were selected from many which had been recorded because they proved to be additive in establishing prognosis. Sophisticated analysis of the data gives a numerical weighting (X) from 0, absent, to 1. Each of the six items is further weighted according to the effect it has on mortality (Y). The prognostic index is arrived at by adding the values of the products XY, i.e., $X^1Y^1 + X^2Y^2 \pm ... = X^nY^n$ (prognostic index). Undoubtedly, better prognostic indexes will be devised, but it seems certain this approach will be used since it is so rational.

Physicians have long appreciated that a significant proportion of patients with acute myocardial infarction suffer a "recurrent" infarction or "extension" within a few hours or several days. Recent studies[265,266] utilizing careful serial enzyme and electrocardiographic methods in small numbers of patients indicate that "extension" is extremely common, possibly in the range of 50 percent of cases, in the first

TABLE 62E-5
Discriminant analysis in a prognostic index

Factor	X	Y
Age (yr) (X_1, Y_1)		
<50	0.2	
50–59	0.4	
60–69	0.6	3.9
70–79	0.8	
80–89	1.0	
Position of infarct (X_2, Y_2)		
Anterior transmural	1.0	
Left bundle branch block	1.0	
Posterior transmural	0.7	2.8
Anterior subendocardial	0.3	
Posterior subendocardial	0.3	
Admission systolic blood pressure (mm Hg) (X_3, Y_3)		
<55	1.0	
55–64	0.7	
65–74	0.6	
75–84	0.5	
85–94	0.4	10.0
95–104	0.3	
105–114	0.2	
115–124	0.1	
≥125	0	
Heart size (X_4, Y_4)		
Normal	0	
Doubtfully enlarged	0.5	1.5
Definitely enlarged	1.0	
Lung fields (X_5, Y_5)		
Normal	0	
Venous congestion	0.3	
Interstitial edema	0.6	3.3
Pulmonary edema	1.0	
Previous ischemia (X_6, Y_6)		
No ischemia	0	
Previous angina or infarction	1	0.4

NOTE: See explanation in text.
SOURCE: Norris et al.[263] Reprinted with permission of the author and publisher.

week following infarcts. This unexpectedly high incidence of infarct extension may be related to case selection. However, it is reasonable to suspect that extension is more common than casual clinical impressions suggest, and it can be assumed that infarct extension will worsen prognosis. This factor adds an element of uncertainty in reference to the initial prognostic impression with any infarction, particularly in patients who are judged to have "favorably" or "low-risk" outlooks.

The pain and/or discomfort of acute infarction has been accorded great emphasis in the diagnosis of acute myocardial infarction. This is appropriate, since misinterpretation of the widely varying spectrum of ischemic cardiac discomfort leads to grave management errors. In addition, persisting and recurring ischemic discomfort after infarction has often been judged to portend a poor prognosis. In fact, there is little evidence that ischemic discomfort per se is of major prognostic significance. Recall, at one extreme, many patients with extensive and even fatal infarction have little discomfort (sometimes none whatsoever), and other patients have persistent and recurring discomfort, which may be related to their "threshold for pain," not necessarily to the severity of the ischemia. In addition, multiple other common problems occur during the course of myocardial infarction and give rise to chest discomfort. Included in these complicating factors are pulmonary embolism, pericarditis, and upper gastrointestinal diseases, especially peptic ulcer problems. Pain and discomfort may be an important accompaniment of new and recurring ischemia, which will usually be documented by objective evidence of myocardial necrosis in the form of electrocardiographic or enzyme abnormalities. Hence, pain in the absence of other evidences of new ischemia and/or other complications should not be given undue emphasis in prognosis. This does not imply that recurrent pain after an infarction may not be utilized to indicate that bypass surgery should not be occasionally done, or that care should not be taken to identify objective signs of additional necrosis.

Arrhythmias constitute another feature in acute myocardial infarction where there is great uncertainty concerning the prognostic significance of the findings. The arrhythmias which occur in the setting of advanced left ventricular failure and associated with other evidences of extensive infarction, e.g., complete heart block with acute anterior infarction and intraventricular conduction defects, clearly do not have independent additional prognostic significance.[164,165] Similarly, so-called primary ventricular fibrillation, which occurs early in the course of infarction and has no associated left ventricular dysfunction and which responds promptly to defibrillation in the coronary care unit, does not measurably worsen the prognosis.[267-270] The arguments concerning arrhythmias as an independent prognostic factor or the relationship of arrhythmias to myocardial infarction size have recently been summarized by Cox et al.[271] It seems likely that for the inhospital mortality, arrhythmias per se are not an important prognostic feature. This relates to the fact that most of the arrhythmias are reasonably easily controlled

with current available therapy and that those which are not readily controlled have their genesis in a large infarct often associated with left ventricular dysfunction. In the latter situation, the patient's prognosis is more related to those factors than to the arrhythmia.

POSTHOSPITAL (LATE) PROGNOSIS (Table 62E-6)

The late, posthospital, prognosis of myocardial infarction is also dependent on multiple factors. Extensive studies have been reported, and data show moderate variability, but trends are remarkably similar.[257,271-275] During the first year subsequent to the convalescence from the myocardial infarction, the mortality is significantly higher, about 10 percent in all studies, than in the subsequent several years of follow-up when the mortality is 3 to 5 percent annually. Clinical features such as angina pectoris, hypertension, cardiomegaly, congestive heart failure, and residual electrocardiographic changes all tend to worsen prognosis. Age has an adverse effect on prognosis. Patients with persistent congestive heart failure due to ischemic heart disease with past myocardial infarction will survive about 5 years.

Arrhythmias as an independent predictor of late death are difficult to assess since they are extremely common.[276-278] Survivors of infarction monitored for more than 8 h usually have an arrhythmia incidence of 60 to 70 percent. These are usually ventricular premature contractions. There are some data to indicate that a classification of arrhythmias is important and that the more serious arrhythmias are related to more extensive disease as judged angiographically and that these arrhythmias have an increased incidence of sudden death. More serious ventricular arrhythmias are considered those which occur with greater frequency (more than 10 per minute), occur in couplets, or occur in bursts of ventricular tachycardia. More data are needed to determine the relationship between arrhythmias and other prognostic features.

TABLE 62E-6
**Prognostic determinants
myocardial infarction—late phase**

Age

Symptoms
  Angina pectoris
  Congestive heart failure

Extent of disease (as judged angiographically)
  Extent of coronary arteriosclerosis
  Extent of myocardial damage

Other
  Arrhythmias
  Hypertension
  Cardiomegaly
  Diabetes
  QRST abnormalities

Sudden death[117a,117b]

A discussion of sudden death is an integral part of any consideration of prognosis in ischemic heart disease since more than half the patients with known ischemic heart disease die suddenly and of all the patients presenting with ischemic heart disease, sudden cardiac death (SCD) is the initial and final event in nearly one-third. Although estimates vary, it is reasonable to suspect that at least 200,000 people a year in the United States are victims of sudden cardiac death. An extensive survey of this problem and résumé of the data available has recently been published.[279] The topic is an unusually complex one. Multiple diverse disciplines are important in providing a proper perspective on the issues involved. Disciplines as diverse as cellular electrophysiology and community-wide epidemiology are necessary to understand this problem. An enormous amount of data has been collected in the last few years, but information is still fragmentary.

The problems in defining sudden cardiac death are discussed in Chap. 49. Death occurring unexpectedly over a short period of time in an individual who has been functioning adequately at the time of the event is the usual definition. The time between collapse and death is the moot point in most definitions. Many would judge sudden cardiac death to occur within 1 or 2 h of the collapse while others would allow up to 24 h.

For those patients who have not yet manifested ischemic heart disease, multiple investigators have attempted to identify individuals at risk for SCD. The risk factors which have evolved prove to be virtually the same risk factors for the development of ischemic heart disease; e.g., male sex, hypertension, hypercholesteremia, heavy cigarette smoking, etc.

As with all subsets, utilizing objective data concerning the extent of abnormality on angiographic study, *it is apparent that major determinants of SCD are the extent and location of coronary atherosclerosis and the ventriculographic abnormalities.* The two items are additive. In one study, a follow-up of 536 medically managed patients disclosed 29 SCDs during a 4-year period. Only 1 of the 29 patients had evidence of slight coronary atherosclerosis on arteriography, and 80 percent had moderate to severe left ventricular functional impairment. Although this is obviously a highly selected group, the implication that SCD is much more likely in patients whose disease is anatomically far advanced seems clear.

For patients in clinical subsets with known ischemic heart disease, the factors involved in SCD are the same as in those with ischemic heart disease who do not die suddenly.

This conclusion would seem obvious from the information available on detailed postmortem studies of patients who have died suddenly. Several carefully done studies indicate that victims of SCD with or without preceding symptoms of ischemic heart disease virtually always have extensive coronary atherosclerosis, often with previous infarction, and not infrequently with hearts which are somewhat above normal weight. Conversely, it is very unusual in cases of SCD for the coronary atherosclerosis to be "mild" and to be localized to a single coronary vessel, although lesions of the left main coronary artery or the left anterior descending coronary artery may be the only lesions found.

Another major focus of interest in subjects already manifesting ischemic heart disease in reference to sudden cardiac death is cardiac arrhythmias, especially premature ventricular contractions (PVCs). Multiple studies[279] indicate that PVCs are an important risk factor in sudden cardiac death. In the widely cited coronary drug trial study,[280] the 3-year mortality for patients with PVCs on the routine 12-lead electrocardiogram was 21 percent, while it was only 11 percent in patients with none. Anatomic data from angiography were not available in this group of patients so it cannot be categorically assumed that PVCs are an additive and independent factor. Limited studies available support both points of view. Selecting patients with frequent or complex PVCs may enhance predictability for SCD.

The dilemma in assessing the independent predictive value of PVCs is related to several well-characterized problems. PVCs are quite frequent in patients with ischemic heart disease; nearly all studies find at least 10 percent incidence on the 12-lead electrocardiogram obtained at rest; the PVCs become extremely frequent, in more than 50 percent of cases, if monitoring is carried out for longer periods of time (8 to 24 h) or if the patients are exercised. A compounding problem is the fact that the normal population in the age group of the typical ischemic patient also has a relatively high incidence of PVCs. Since ventricular fibrillation is the ordinary mechanism of SCD, it is reasonable to assume that PVCs have an independent effect on this manifestation of ischemic heart disease, although the principal determinants may ultimately prove to be the anatomic severity of the disease and the extent of ischemia. Since only a minority of patients who are candidates for SCD will have anatomic characterization, careful attention to cardiac arrhythmias may be a major help in identifying and attempting to better control this most devastating manifestation of coronary atherosclerotic heart disease.

THE PATIENT'S RECORD

When appropriate data have been collected and the criteria required for problem formulation are known, it is then necessary to create a complete *problem list*. The complete problem list should reveal all of the patient's problems (see Table 62E-7).

Note that problem 1 shown in the problem list in Table 62E-7 is resolved to a very high level. The etiology of the condition is clearly stated. The specific subset of myocardial ischemia is also clearly stated. A complication, atrial fibrillation, is listed. The elements of the disorder that will require management are shown.

Problems 2 and 3 shown on the problem list (Table 62E-7) are stated at a low level of resolution. The cause of the hypertension is not known and, there-

TABLE 62E-7
Complete problem list

Date problem entered	Problem number	Active	Inactive
January 28, 1978	1	Coronary atherosclerotic heart disease (a) angina pectoris (stable) disabling (b) atrial fibrillation	
January 28, 1978	2	Systemic arterial hypertension ⟶	
January 28, 1978	3	Weight loss and intolerance to heat ⟶	

NOTE: For explanation of table, see text.

fore, is not stated. The cause of the weight loss and intolerance to heat is not known with certainty and, therefore, is not stated. The arrow after the problems indicates that they are at a low level of resolution. When the problems are solved, the new problem statements will be written at the end of the arrows. Dates will be written above the arrows indicating the date of the progress note that should state the data used to solve the problems.

It is extremely useful to study a properly constructed *complete problem list.* Note that it is possible to determine the following from the problem list in Table 62E-7: (1) that problem 1a must be managed with rest, nitroglycerin, long-acting nitrites, and propranolol and that the patient must be considered for coronary arteriography and possible bypass surgery. Problem 1b must be managed with digitalis and propranolol. (2) Note that problem 2 (hypertension) should be controlled. The propranolol used for problem 1 may be adequate, but if it is not, other antihypertensive drugs may be used. The control of the blood pressure and heart rate may assist in the control of the angina pectoris. A decision must be made as to whether or not it is necessary to pursue the etiology of the symptom complex listed as problem 3: Should diagnostic work be performed to identify thyrotoxicosis? Such a disease would have profound effect on problem 1. Propranolol given for problem 1a could actually influence problems 1b, 2, and 3.

This example illustrates the usefulness of the *complete problem list* in managing the "whole patient" and in determining how one problem may influence another problem. The more precisely one states a problem (based on the data available), the more likely it is that precise *initial plans* and meaningful *progress notes* will be conceived. The reader is referred to Chap. 10 for further discussion of the problem-oriented record.

The discussion that precedes this point in this chapter gives emphasis to the concept that certain defined data must be gathered; a problem list should be formulated; the prognosis of the problem should be known; and the patient's record should reveal all of these items. The discussion that follows will be concerned with the management of the various clinical syndromes due to coronary atherosclerotic heart disease. The fact that other noncardiac factors such as obesity, anemia, thyrotoxicosis, neoplastic disease, pulmonary disease, other diseases of other organs, emotional states, age, etc., influence the decisions that are made regarding the management of heart disease must not be forgotten. This is illustrated by problem 3 in the complete problem list shown in Table 62E-7. The record of the patient should reveal the logic and action of the physician who cares for the patient.

THE MANAGEMENT OF CLINICAL SYNDROMES DUE TO CORONARY ATHEROSCLEROTIC HEART DISEASE

The management of coronary atherosclerotic heart disease and its many complications will be divided into "General Considerations Regarding Management," "The Management of Specific Clinical Syndromes," and "The Management of Complications."

General considerations regarding management

FACILITIES, EQUIPMENT, PERSONNEL, LOGISTICS, AND EDUCATION

Introductory remarks As a general rule, patients with coronary atherosclerosis come to the attention of the physician for four reasons: (1) for advice regarding the prevention or deceleration of coronary atherosclerosis, (2) for the management of chest discomfort which may be mild and brief in some patients and severe and prolonged in others, (3) for the management of other complaints such as dyspnea or a fatigue that may be due to coronary atherosclerotic heart disease, and (4) because of "sudden death." The prevention and deceleration of coronary atherosclerosis, inadequate as it is, is discussed in Chap. 62H, and the management of sudden death is discussed in Chaps. 49 and 50.

The patient with chest discomfort due to myocardial ischemia may present to the physician in several ways. The physician may elicit a history of angina pectoris during an interview with a patient when the patient has little, if any, voluntary complaint or chest discomfort. The patient may note angina pectoris initiated by effort or excitement and may seek advice because of the symptoms. The patient may develop abrupt anterior chest discomfort without an obvious precipitating cause. The American Heart Association (AHA) addressed itself to the latter situation, since many such patients did not appreciate the early warning signals of a "heart attack" and since many deaths occurred because neither the patient nor his or her family knew what to do under such circumstances. The AHA has embarked upon a massive public education program to inform the public about the early warning signs of a "heart attack." Excerpts from one of the pamphlets are reprinted here with permission of the American Heart Association[218a]:

> If you feel an uncomfortable pressure, fullness, squeezing or pain in the center of your chest (which may spread to the shoulders, neck or arms) for more than two minutes, you could be having a heart attack.
>
> Severe pain, dizziness, fainting, sweating, nausea or shortness of breath may also occur. These signals, however, are not always present. Don't wait. Get help immediately.
>
> Call the emergency rescue service. If you can get to a hospital faster by car, have someone drive you. Find out which hospitals in your area offer 24-hour emergency cardiac care. Select in advance the facility nearest your home and office and tell your family and friends so that they will know what to do.

About 60 percent of the deaths among patients with myocardial infarction occur before they reach the hospital.[282] Therefore, it is important to move victims to the area of definitive care as quickly as possible. It is also essential for intelligent laymen to know how to manage cardiac arrest. Accordingly, the AHA has developed a large educational program in cardiopulmonary resuscitation for the public at large and for health care workers in an effort to prevent some of these sudden deaths.

The preceding discussion points out the problems of recognition, early action, and logistics. The solutions of these problems, along with the development of monitors, defibrillators, pacemakers, new drugs, and trained personnel, including highly skilled nurses and allied health workers, have led to a new era in patient care.

The medical care delivered to a patient with coronary atherosclerotic heart disease can be discussed in four parts: *ambulatory care or office and home care,* which ordinarily does not, but could, lead to immediate hospitalization; *prehospital care* for patients with an acute coronary attack, which, by definition, always leads to hospitalization; *hospital care,* which includes the care associated with the management of an acute attack in the emergency clinic, coronary care unit, and hospitalization outside the coronary care unit, and also includes the management associated with coronary arteriography and coronary artery surgery; and *posthospital care* and rehabilitation for patients who have had a period of hospitalization.

Ambulatory care or office and home care
Some individuals who visit the physician in the office have evidence of coronary atherosclerotic heart disease, while others want advice as to how to prevent it. The office should provide the individual with an appropriate questionnaire that should elicit among other things, the base information regarding the patient's profile, habits, and symptoms as they relate to coronary atherosclerosis. The physician should complete the history and perform the physical examination.

A resting electrocardiogram can be recorded in many physicians' offices. An exercise electrocardiogram is often needed in order to evaluate a patient who might have coronary atherosclerotic heart disease but should not be performed unless the physician is properly trained and skilled personnel and proper equipment for cardiopulmonary resuscitation are available should cardiopulmonary resuscitation be required. If this cannot be provided, the test should be done in another facility that can provide the expertise and protection for the patient.

It should be possible to obtain a chest x-ray either in the office or in another facility. Holter monitoring for the diagnosis of abnormal heart rhythm should be available either in the office or in another facility. Certain lab tests, such as the determination of levels of fasting blood sugar, cholesterol, triglycerides, etc., should be available either in the office or at some other facility. The point is, if certain items can't be obtained in the office, the indication for the procedures or tests should be known, and the logistics for obtaining them should be organized. After the predefined data on the patient have been collected, the physician creates a *complete problem list* of the patient's disorders; develops *initial plans* for each problem; and begins to follow the proper items and records the new observations and plans in carefully written *progress notes.*

Every physician's office should be an educational center for the patients who go there. The educational system should include the use of appropriate pamphlets, audiotapes, videotapes, and motion picture films. The material should include general subjects, such as the recognition of the symptoms due to coronary atherosclerosis, and specific subjects, such as the treatment of angina pectoris. When the physician sees an ambulatory patient in the office, it is necessary to determine if the diagnostic work-up and management can be safely implemented in the office. Most of the time, the patient continues to be cared for as an outpatient, but sooner or later the patient may need hospitalization in order to manage certain coronary syndromes or to clarify certain diagnostic problems with a coronary arteriogram and left ventriculogram. The logistics of accomplishing these ends must be organized so that the patient's safety is protected at all times.

The principles discussed here apply to the physician who works in a small village as well as to the physician who works in a medical center. The physician in the small village must be very skilled in history taking, physical examination, and interpretation of the chest x-ray and resting electrocardiogram. It may be necessary to arrange for another physician at another facility to do more (this is why we have emphasized the recognition of coronary syndromes based on the items collected in phases 1 and 2 of decision making) (Tables 62A-3 and 62A-4). The risk of doing "too little" for the patient plagues this physician. The physician at the medical center must be skilled in history taking, physical examination, interpretation of the chest x-ray and resting electrocardiogram, performing and interpreting the exercise electrocardiogram, and providing rapid access to excellent coronary arteriography and left ventriculography and cardiac surgery. The risk of doing "too much" for the patient plagues this physician. This can be worse than doing too little. *Therefore, common sense and concern for the whole patient must prevail.*

The home is an important facility for the ambulatory patient. This is obvious but two points should be made. (1) Conditions at home may be tranquil or emotionally traumatic. This can influence the well-being of anyone, but it especially influences the condition of the patient with one of the coronary syndromes (i.e., unstable angina pectoris). The same is true for the place of work. (2) Some clinicians have recommended that certain patients with myocardial infarction be treated at home and have data showing that they achieved the same survival rate with this approach as they did with hospital care. We hospitalize patients with myocardial infarction and most patients with unstable angina pectoris.

Prehospital care The following paragraphs were taken from the preface and chaps. 1 and 2 of the book *The Acute Coronary Attack,* by Pantridge et al., and is reproduced here with the permission of the author and publisher.[283]

Prehospital coronary deaths now constitute one of the major problems in medicine. It is salutary to remember that in his book *Observations on Some of the Most Frequent and Important Diseases of the Heart,* published in Edinburgh in 1809, Allan Burns wrote, 'where however, the cessation of vital action is very complete, and continues long, we ought to inflate the lungs, and pass electric shocks through the chest: the practitioner ought never, if the death has been sudden, and the person not very far advanced in life, to despair of success, till he has unequivocal signs of real death.' Nevertheless, 158 years were to elapse before the first successful resuscitation from ventricular fibrillation occurring outside hospital was reported by Pantridge and Geddes.

When cardiac resuscitation had become a practical proposition, Julian (1961) suggested that, 'all medical, nursing, and auxiliary staff should be trained in the techniques of closed-chest cardiac massage and mouth to mouth breathing . . . patients known to be at risk from ventricular fibrillation or asystole could have their cardiac rhythm constantly monitored'.[284] Reports of the establishment of coronary care units soon appeared (Day, 1963; Brown *et al.,* 1963; Julian *et al.,* 1964; Meltzer, 1964; Robinson *et al.,* 1964).[285-289] Within a few years the coronary care unit had become "an integral, essential part of customary hospital practice" (Meltzer, 1969). While the initial concept of the hospital coronary care unit involved the immediate detection and prompt correction of ventricular fibrillation, attention was soon directed to the possibility of preventing ventricular fibrillation by the administration of antiarrhythmic agents. However, since some two-thirds of the deaths occur outside hospital, the reduction of hospital deaths from 30 to 20 per cent had only a small impact on the community mortality. Indeed, even if all patients with coronary thrombosis were admitted to coronary care units it would be impossible to reduce the community mortality by more than 4.5 per cent (Pantridge, 1970).[290] The hospital coronary care unit did not influence the incidence of shock or pump failure nor did

it have a significant effect on the mortality from these complications.

The study of McNeilly and Pemberton (1968) showed that the majority of deaths from acute myocardial infarction occurred soon after the onset of symptoms.[291] The data of Yater *et al.* (1948) and those of Bainton and Peterson (1963) indicated that sudden coronary death was more likely to occur among the younger individuals.[292,293] It was found that among males 50 years and younger, 63 per cent of the deaths from acute myocardial infarction occurred within one hour of the onset of symptoms. That the majority of deaths occurred soon after the onset of symptoms was confirmed by the studies of Fulton *et al.* (1969) and those of Gordon and Kannel (1971).[294,295]

Since nearly two-thirds of premature deaths occur within one hour of the onset of symptoms and since the median delay in hospital admission may be eight hours or more (Mittra, 1965; McDonald, 1968; McNeilly and Pemberton, 1968), the majority of patients with acute myocardial infarction die unattended at or near the place where they are stricken.[291,296] Their predicament is somewhat similar to that of battle casualties in the eighteenth century. In 1792, Larrey, a young French army surgeon, noted the plight of the wounded. French army regulations at that time dictated that the medical personnel should remain one league (2.42 miles) behind the battle area. The wounded reached the surgical depots usually after a delay of some 24 hours and were frequently moribund or dead. Larrey devised a light vehicle that transported the surgeons and their equipment to the front line and thus revolutionised military surgery. Napoleon described the mobile unit as one of the finest conceptions of his time. One hundred and seventy-four years later, a mobile unit to deal with coronary casualties was initiated in Belfast.

The mobile coronary care unit enables personnel trained in coronary care to reach the patient at the site of the heart attack (at home or elsewhere) as soon as possible after the onset of symptoms to start emergency treatment immediately and to continue monitoring and therapy during transport to hospital.

Attempts had been made in the U.S.S.R. to provide prehospital coronary care (Moiseev, 1962).[298] These were limited to the treatment of shock and pump failure by a special team summoned after the personnel from the usual emergency service had reached the patient. This approach was clearly unrewarding.

Although the high incidence of early preventable deaths from acute myocardial infarction is one of the major problems in medicine in the Western World, there are still, unfortunately, many areas in which no attempt has been made to provide prehospital care.

Mittra found that in Belfast, in 1965, the hospital admission of a large proportion of patients with acute myocardial infarction was delayed more than twelve hours.[296] Many factors were concerned in the delay. Some patients did not seek medical help immediately. Others were unable to contact their family doctor. Practitioners were not all aware of the high risk of sudden and preventable death. The ambulance service was not always able to deal with the call immediately and patients with myocardial infarction were frequently unnecessarily delayed in casualty departments. It was reasoned that it should be possible to eliminate the causes of delay apart from that due to the patient's procrastination in seeking medical help (Pantridge and

Geddes, 1966, 1967).[299,300] It was hoped that public awareness might result in reduction in the patient delay.

The prototype mobile coronary care unit was initiated in Belfast in 1966. The Royal Victoria Hospital, the major teaching hospital, seemed geographically well situated for the operation of such a unit since it was near the centre of the city, the population of which was 550,000, of whom 100,000 lived within a one mile radius of the hospital. The ambulance depot for the city was in the hospital grounds some 300 yards from the coronary care unit. Thus, it was possible to integrate a mobile coronary care unit into the existing emergency service. The family doctors in Belfast were acquainted with the facts regarding the risk of unnecessary death immediately after the onset of symptoms suggesting acute myocardial infarction. A training scheme in the technique of resuscitation was arranged for medical practitioners, for some paramedical workers, and for appropriate lay individuals. The family doctors were given a special telephone number which enabled them to reach the coronary care unit directly. Delays at the hospital telephone exchange were thus avoided. The scheme initiated in 1966 continues to operate without significant modification.

A short-wave radio system enables the duty doctor in the coronary care unit to receive immediately the call for the mobile unit. A signalling system facilitates the rapid activation of ambulance control and an ambulance proceeds from the depot to the rendezvous point, where the coronary care unit personnel, a doctor and a nurse or medical student, are waiting. The team is on its way within two minutes of the receipt of the signal from the family doctor or member of the public. It proceeds with all possible speed to the patient.

The ambulance carries—

1 A battery-operated portable direct current defibrillator.

2 Oxygen, Ambu bags, endotracheal tubes, and suction apparatus.

3 A battery-operated monitoring oscilloscope and tape recorder.

4 Drugs and intravenous solutions normally available in a coronary care unit, including atropine and beta-blocking agents.

All the equipment is portable. The hardware is robust and, as far as possible, foolproof. Since the apparatus must, on occasions, be carried some distance and possibly in haste up several flights of stairs, the monitoring equipment and defibrillator are light and compact. It is unnecessary to use clumsy, expensive, and heavy defibrillators since small models are available.

When the team reaches the patient he will be under the same intensive care conditions as obtain in a hospital coronary care unit. Fifty per cent of the patients are reached within ten minutes of receipt of the call from the family doctor or lay individual and nearly three quarters are reached within fifteen minutes.

If the message the family doctor receives suggests a myocardial infarction, he will summon the mobile unit immediately and before he has seen the patient. A proportion of calls necessarily come from the general public, who dial "999" when unable to contact the general practitioner. Selected calls are referred to the coronary care unit personnel for screening. If the family doctor should, because of geographical proximity, reach the patient before the mobile unit, he may improve the patient's chance of survival by initiating immediately therapy for the relief of pain and for the control of autonomic distur-

bance or dysrhythmias. When the mobile team arrives, therapy is initiated or that of the general practitioner continued. Pain is relieved by intravenous heroin. Stabilisation of the rhythm may require antiarrhythmic agents, atropine, beta-blocking agents, or a combination of these drugs. Pain relief, stabilisation of the rhythm, and correction of the autonomic disturbances are considered mandatory before movement. Monitoring and therapy are continued during transport. Haste or fuss during transport is most carefully avoided. The patient is transferred directly from the ambulance to the hospital coronary care unit, monitoring continuing during this transfer.

Since the ambulance depot for the City of Belfast is in the grounds of the Royal Victoria Hospital and the mobile coronary unit operates through the ordinary emergency system, employment of ambulance drivers additional to the normal complement has been found unnecessary. No special ambulance is used but initially one of the 36 ambulances in the depot was slightly modified and now two have been modified.

A different scheme was required for that part of the Belfast population located east of the river and remote from the ambulance depot. Here, a mini-vehicle containing a battery-operated defibrillator and other necessary equipment, drugs, and intravenous solutions, is on standby proximal to the coronary care unit of the district hospital (Barber et al., 1970).[301] The mini-vehicle is linked by radio-telephone to ambulance control and to the hospital coronary care unit. When a call is received, a junior doctor and nurse from the coronary care unit travel to the patient in the mini-vehicle. If he proves to have an acute coronary episode monitoring is started, the necessary therapy is initiated, and an ambulance is summoned from the depot. Monitoring continues during the transfer to the ambulance. One of the personnel from the coronary care unit accompanies the patient to the district hospital, monitoring him on the way. The other drives the mini-vehicle back to its base. This scheme also avoids the necessity for employing additional ambulance drivers. The majority of the calls come from within a three mile radius of the district hospital for the east Belfast area (population approximately 250,000). A similar scheme operates in Dudley (Worcs) (Kubik et al., 1974).[302]

Mobile coronary care duty in both Belfast schemes is added to the other duties of the coronary care unit personnel. No individual is unemployed in the interval between calls. An important feature of the operation of the mobile units is that patients are admitted directly to the coronary care unit, thus bypassing the casualty or emergency department which may be, in many hospitals, the most dangerous place for the patient with acute myocardial infarction.

Results from the Royal Victoria Hospital mobile coronary care unit In the first five years of its operation (1966–1970) the unit had 3,882 calls, 21 patients refused hospitalisation, and 3,861 were managed by the unit (Table 62E-8). Of these 1,614 (42%) had evidence of acute myocardial infarction in that they showed: (a) indubitable electrocardiographic signs of recent infarction, or (b) sequential ST and T wave changes accompanied by significant and transient rise in S.G.O.T., or (c) left bundle branch block with similar enzyme changes. The diagnosis among 1,283 patients (33%) was acute coronary insufficiency. In 444 patients (12%) the emergency was not related to acute coronary disease: unjustified calls were 195 (5%).

Of the 1,614 with acute infarction, 41 (2.5%) were transferred from other hospitals, usually because of acute atrioventricular block requiring pacing. There was no arrhythmic death in transit during the five-year period.

TABLE 62E-8
Royal Victoria Hospital mobile coronary care unit:
1 January 1966 to 31 December 1970 (3882 calls—3861 managed)

	Ischemic pain		Noncoronary emergency		
Myocardial infarction	Abnormal ECG	Normal ECG	Cardiovascular	Non-cardiovascular	Unjustified calls
1,614 (T41)	1,121	162	289 (T12)	155	195
(42%)	(29%)	(4%)	(8%)	(4%)	(5%)

NOTE: Fatal arrest outside the hospital, probable myocardial infarction 242 (6 percent) which includes 18 arrests in other hospitals. Other pre-transport deaths (pump failure) 83 (2 percent). T = patients transferred from other hospitals.

When general practitioners became aware that the majority of coronary deaths were unnecessary and that a mobile unit was available, there was a progressive increase in the number of patients with acute infarction who came under intensive care soon after the onset of the coronary attack. Thus, in 1969, of the 447 patients with acute myocardial infarction managed by the mobile unit, 27.5 per cent came under intensive care within 1 hour (Adgey *et al.,* 1971) and the median delay was 1 hour 40 minutes.[303] This contrasts with a median delay of more than 8 hours in 1965 (McNeilly and Pemberton, 1968).[291] Most of the reduction has resulted from shortening of the administrative delay.

The work of Pantridge and others stimulated the development of schemes designed to quickly assist and transport a victim with an acute coronary attack to the coronary care unit. Many individuals, working in many cities all over the world, have developed their own local system. The objective is clear. The goal is to have personnel who are trained in cardiac resuscitation reach the stricken victim as quickly as possible and move the patient to the facility of definitive care (coronary care unit) as quickly as possible. The exact method used may vary with the size of the town, type of personnel, type of hospital, equipment, financial restraints, etc.

Hospital care The patient with coronary atherosclerotic heart disease may enter the hospital via the emergency clinic, may go directly to the coronary care unit, or may enter another part of the hospital where intensive care is not delivered. Where the patient goes initially depends upon the physician's perception of the problem and the organizational setup of the hospital. It is essential to cut the usual administrative red tape in order for the patient to be treated safely and humanely. For example, it is desirable for a patient with a suspected acute heart attack to go directly to the coronary care unit. When the patient is seen initially in the emergency room, it is vital for the physician to see and evaluate the condition of the patient as quickly as possible. In most instances the patient should be moved to the coronary care unit without delay. Patients who do not require the protection of a coronary care unit are admitted through the usual hospital mechanism but should not be asked to wait for hours in the admitting

area, which, in most hospitals, is not conducive to any degree of serenity. Most patients are moved from the coronary care unit to a room near it. A few patients may require additional telemetry outside the coronary care unit in order to detect rhythm disturbances. Some patients may be admitted to an ordinary room of the hospital and transferred back to the coronary care unit if the need arises. Many patients today are admitted to the hospital for coronary artery surgery. Regardless of where the patient enters the hospital, it is important to exert considerable effort in order to decrease confusion, to maintain quiet, and to plan for the next stage of management.

The architectural design of the hospital is quite important if one is to create the proper facilities for the care of patients with coronary atherosclerotic heart disease. At times it is necessary to work within the physical structure that exists. It may be possible to renovate areas of existing space in order to achieve what is needed. Occasionally it is possible to design a new facility.

The emergency clinic should be designed so that little time is wasted moving the patient with an acute heart attack to the coronary care unit in relation to the emergency clinic.

One of us (J.W.H.) designed the coronary care unit for Emory University Hospital (Fig. 62E-18). This unit was designed so that family members never enter the unit but have their own hallway with private alcoves "wrapped" around the coronary care unit. Each patient has an outside room "with a view." A physician's sleeping quarters is part of the unit, as is an x-ray room where pacemakers can be inserted. The inside of the unit has the usual equipment and personnel that are generally found in modern coronary care units.

The use of intermediate coronary care units is recommended by some.[303a,303b] A similar degree of protection can be offered the patient by utilizing telemetry with a readout at the nurses' station.

The consideration which should be given to the patient who is to undergo coronary arteriography and left ventriculography or coronary artery surgery deserves emphasis, for most hospitals have not prepared for it. The patient education aspects of this activity will be stressed subsequently. The cardiac

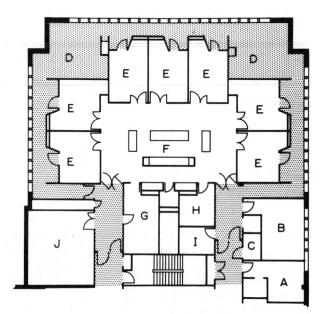

FIGURE 62E-18 Design of coronary care unit. *A.* Physician's room and sleeping quarters. *B.* Conference room. *C.* Dictating room. Shaded area shows where family wait. Note that each patient room (*E.*) has a small alcove designed for the family. *D* represents larger reception rooms. Family members do not enter the interior of the coronary unit (*F*) but enter the patient's room from the hallway (shaded area). *G.* Equipment area. *H.* Small conference room. *I.* Storage room. *J.* Fluoroscopy room. (This unit was designed by J. W. Hurst, M.D.)

catheterization laboratory must be a humane and safe place that patients appreciate. The family must be considered also, and the room where they wait during surgery must be pleasant. The responsible physician should be in contact with the family. The number of rooms a patient uses during a hospitalization for coronary artery surgery is astonishing. The patient may be admitted to the medical service; go to the operating room; be cared for in the intensive care unit; and be transferred to a room on the surgical service. While this may be necessary, it may confuse the patient. The operating suite itself must be carefully organized for safety. No patient should ever be left unattended and out of view of the personnel. The intensive care unit should be near the operating room and should be designed like the coronary care unit.

We have paid much attention to the "care of the family" of patients going to cardiac surgery. Special private waiting rooms are desirable. Several different families should not be crowded into one waiting room. The family room should be designed like the living room of a home. A telephone should be available. One of us (J.W.H.) utilizes a carefully trained nonmedical assistant to work with the family. The medical cardiologist or assistant gives appropriate messages to the family throughout the surgical procedure. This approach to the problems of the family has been quite successful.

Posthospital care The transportation from the hospital is almost always by automobile. Patients who live out of the state may travel by aeroplane. The number of patients who have acute heart attacks in a city other than their home town is increasing. As a rule, such patients are kept in the hospital a few days longer than are patients who are native to the city where they become ill. An ambulance may transport them to the airport, although in most instances a taxi is satisfactory. A family member, friend, or physician should be in attendance. Arrangements should be made for the patient to ride in a wheel chair once he or she is at the airport, since the halls of most airports are long and crowded. The patient should be transported in the wheelchair on the ramp to the first class section of the plane. The reverse is executed at the end of the flight.

Patients who have undergone coronary artery surgery usually go home on the seventh or eighth day. Those who live at a great distance may stay 4 or 5 days in a nearby motel and then fly home according to the plan discussed above.

The rehabilitation process that started in the hospital is continued at home. The home care is extremely important. The family and patient must be prepared for new problems. The excitement of returning home may give way to introspection and be followed by depression. Appropriate physical activity is a major tool in management at this stage (see Chap. 62G). Emotional crisis must be avoided. It is useful to set a date as to when the patient will return to work in order to have a definite goal and leave no doubt that total rehabilitation is expected. It is equally important to assist the patient and his or her family in facing the problem of retirement or disability when such is necessary.

Equipment Each facility needs a certain amount of equipment and drugs. The physician's office must be organized so that cardiac emergencies can be handled. The equipment and drugs usually found in every physician's office will suffice if in addition to this there is a portable defibrillator, oxygen, Ambubag, and an electrocardiograph machine.

The ambulance should have a portable battery-operated dc defibrillator, oxygen, Ambubags, endotracheal tubes, suction apparatus, a battery-operated oscilloscope and recorder, sphygmomanometers, drugs, and intravenous solutions usually available in the coronary care unit. The ambulance itself may have an oscilloscope that transmits the electrocardiogram to the hospital coronary care unit (or emergency clinic) with radio contact so that abnormal rhythms can be discussed with a physician.

The emergency clinic must have a dc defibrillator, oxygen, equipment for pulmonary resuscitation, drugs, and intravenous fluid.

The coronary care unit must have equipment for continuous monitoring of the heart rhythm, Ambubags, endotracheal tubes and a laryngoscope, equipment for the continuous monitoring of systemic arterial pressure, pulmonary artery pressure (Swan-Ganz technique), cardiac pacemakers, pericardiocentesis tray, oxygen, drugs such as atropine, propranolol, lidocaine, procainamide, digoxin, quinidine sulfate, Dilantin, nitroglycerin, nitroglycerin ointment, isosorbide dinitrate, nitroprusside, epinephrine, norepinephrine, dopamine, morphine sulfate, meperidine hydrochloride (Demerol), diazepam (Valium), sodium bicarbonate solution, and fluids for intravenous use.

The equipment and drugs required to protect patients who are not located inside the coronary care unit should be portable and stored on a cart that can be moved quickly to any portion of the hospital when an alert is sounded (such a "crash cart" should be available on the hospital floor area whenever the concentration of patients with heart disease can justify its presence). The equipment on the crash cart should include a portable dc defibrillator, Ambubag, oxygen, endotracheal tubes and laryngoscope, sphygmomanometer, and adequate supply of syringes and needles, atropine, propranolol, lidocaine, epinephrine, procainamide, digoxin, nitroglycerin, norepinephrine, dopamine, morphine sulfate, meperidine hydrochloride, diazepam, sodium bicarbonate solution, and fluids for intravenous use.

The equipment for the cardiac catheterization laboratory is discussed elsewhere in this book (Chaps. 29D and 33). The equipment used in the operating room unit is beyond the scope of this book. The equipment required in the surgical intensive care unit is similar to that used in the coronary care unit.

All units of the hospital must be able to obtain certain equipment, drugs, and solutions from central supply at a moment's notice, since they cannot be stored in all of the units. The emergency crash cart and trained personnel must be available (on signal) throughout the hospital 24 h every day.

Personnel The most important ingredient of any system of medical care is the personnel administering the care. The personnel must be knowledgeable and reliable, and must function in a humane way. These ideals must be met by the physicians, nurses, personnel who work with the mobile coronary care unit or ambulance, aides, technicians, etc. A continuous educational program is needed for all personnel.

Logistics The foregoing discussion emphasizes that each person and each facility has a role to play in the care of the multiple clinical syndromes associated with coronary atherosclerotic heart disease. The personnel range from a knowledgeable ambulance attendant to a highly skilled surgeon. A plan of action is obviously necessary if the skilled people and the sick patient are to be brought into proper relationship with each other. Logistics—the procurement, maintenance, and transportation of material, facilities, and personnel—will vary from locale to locale, but the objective remains the same. The objective is to manage and to move a sick patient from one location to another with maximum safety and minimum delay. Some places may use the fire department and others will use ambulances. Some places may use physician assistants, and others will use nurse clinicians. De-

spite the different vehicles, personnel, and equipment, the logistical objective remains the same.

Education Education was mentioned in most of the preceding sections. Continuous education is needed for all personnel in order that each member of the team may remain proficient. Patient education must be emphasized in the physician's office, the coronary care unit, and in the hospital prior to coronary arteriography and coronary artery surgery. Patient education is essential for good patient care.[304] It is very difficult to implement good medical or surgical management of a patient with coronary atherosclerotic heart disease unless the patient understands the problems.

PHYSICAL REST AND EXERCISE
There is some evidence that persons who are physically active all their lives are less likely to develop coronary atherosclerosis than their sedentary friends. This view has led to jogging clubs and many other group endeavors. The scientific benefit of exercise has not been settled. It is accepted that exercise creates a sense of well-being in the individual who exercises. It improves skeletal muscle strength and permits more physical work to be done with less cardiac work. Exercise assists in controlling weight. The pulse rate per minute may be less in the trained individual than in the untrained one. There is some evidence that exercise alters the blood lipid levels toward a more favorable pattern. It has not been proved that exercise encourages the development of new collateral vessels in the myocardium. There is suggestive evidence that the individual who has exercised for years has a better chance of surviving an acute coronary episode than a sedentary person.

On the other hand, many members of the public have been misled into believing that exercise will guarantee that they will not have coronary atherosclerosis. This clearly is not true. In addition, deaths have occurred in exercise programs. Regrettably, too, patients with mild heart failure or noncoronary disease (such as cardiomyopathy) may unwittingly be placed in exercise programs with disastrous results.

The proper management of the various syndromes that make up the full spectrum of coronary atherosclerosis demands the view that there is a time for rest and a time for exercise. The patient with stable angina pectoris requires a carefully tailored program for activity and rest. Patients with any of the subsets of unstable angina pectoris may require a period of carefully defined rest and possibly bypass surgery before activity is recommended. The patient with prolonged chest pain due to myocardial ischemia without objective signs of cardiac muscle necrosis requires a period of rest and possibly bypass surgery followed by rehabilitation. Patients with evidence of cardiac muscle necrosis require a period of rest before exercise can be recommended. Patients with complications such as heart failure due to infarction require more rest and less exercise than patients without such complications.

Patients with unstable angina pectoris or prolonged myocardial ischemia without objective signs of infarction and patients who have myocardial infarctions deserve special comment regarding the need for rest and ambulation. See discussion regarding exercise in the section "The Management of Specific Clinical Syndromes" later in this chapter.

MENTAL REST AND PATIENT PSYCHOLOGY

The role of emotional tension in the development of coronary atherosclerosis is still debated. There is no debate, however, regarding the deleterious effect of emotional tension in the precipitation of angina pectoris (see Chap. 96). There is strong belief that emotional tension can precipitate cardiac arrhythmias and perhaps sudden death in certain individuals. There is no doubt, either, that the onset of symptoms of coronary atherosclerotic heart disease can produce an emotional crisis in the life of many patients. Some of these individuals may become more disabled than their physical abnormalities justify. The problems of denial, fear, dependence, and depression occur in a surprising number of patients after myocardial infarction and to some extent go undetected.

The encouragement of emotional stability and the creation of mental rest require the time and talent of a sensitive physician. We can only highlight the importance of mental rest for patients with coronary atherosclerosis here. Regrettably, we do not have the ability to write a dissertation on the solution to the problem. The solution simply requires awareness on the part of the physician, the recognition that such matters are always important, the resistance on the part of the physician to try to solve all problems with tranquilizers or sedatives, and a willingness to listen and to serve as a sophisticated counselor.

The following discussion was prepared for the Coronary Care Committee of the Council of Clinical Cardiology and the Committee on Medical Education of the American Heart Association. This excellent discussion was written by Thomas P. Hackett, M.D., and Ned Cassem, M.D. It is reprinted here with the permission of the American Heart Association and the authors.[305–322]

Emergency ward Patients are rarely admitted directly to the coronary care unit (CCU). Usually the point of entry is the emergency ward (EW) or the hospital's receiving room. Psychologically, this initial point of contact is critical because it is the patient's introduction to the setting of care. His initial response often sets the tone for his pattern of adaptation to the hospital as a whole.

Most patients enter the receiving ward with apprehension. Waiting, even for a short time, intensifies anxiety and has caused patients to depart before meeting a physician. Fortunately, in most emergency wards a doctor examines the patient with chest pain quickly and waiting is rarely a problem. By and large the patients we interviewed were reassured by the speed with which they were processed through the admission ritual and were grateful to find themselves the center of undiluted attention within minutes after entering the hospital.

Patients often have an amnesia for part or all of their EW experience, a finding which may be explained by their rapid processing and medication as they pass through this facility. Although they forget the names of individual doctors and nurses, personality traits are recalled. Our research reveals two such traits most appreciated in physicians: compassion and forthrightness. One patient remembered a physician's saying to him, "You have had a heart attack, but it is not a large one. However, all heart attacks are serious and you will need our attention." The patient appreciated being told the truth directly and matter-of-factly. It is worth mentioning that of the hundreds of patients we examined not one complained of being told too much in the emergency ward. A possible rule of thumb then might be: when in doubt about how much to tell a patient, it is safer to err on the side of disclosing rather than withholding information. Patients commented favorably on the physician who began talking of a possible discharge date once admission from the EW to the CCU had been arranged. Although this discussion is rarely possible at such an early stage, a simple mention of discharge in the following weeks very often serves as a reassuring landmark for the patient who finds himself in an otherwise barren landscape.

Being left alone was regarded by most patients as the most distressing event of their EW experience. As one patient put it, "Within two minutes after walking through the front door I was surrounded by a dozen people. They examined me and gave me 'hypos.' I began to feel pretty good and closed my eyes. The next thing is I looked around and no one's there—like a vacuum cleaner sucked all the people out. I wanted to get up and run away. It was spooky as hell." Although being left alone is a rare occurrence, care should be taken to prevent it. A nurse, attendant, or relative should be in the room at all times.

It is often in the emergency ward that the sacrament of the sick or last rites are offered to Catholic patients. To the uninitiated this might seem to be one of the more stressful moments in the hospital experience. Most people associate the last rites with death. When the priest walked in with the oils some of our patients reported thinking "This is it, I've had it." However, in a study made some years ago,[306] we found that the religious significance of this ritual is apt to provide enough reassurance to outweigh the anxiety. For some patients the last rites appear to offer comfort. The critical variable seemed to be the manner in which the priest administered the sacrament. When the priest was self-possessed and comfortable in the presence of critically ill patients and explained the routine nature of the procedure, patients' responses tended to be more positive. When patients complained of being given last rites, it was almost invariably the manner of the priest that bore the brunt of their criticism. Women and older patients responded more positively than did others. As could be expected, individuals who maintained an active religious life were more receptive to the sacrament of the sick.

Preparing the patient for the CCU is one of the more important duties of EW personnel. The patient should be told whether he will have private or semiprivate accommodations. He should be prepared to experience 24-hour monitoring, the taking of hourly vital signs, and frequent "rounding" by physicians. The fact that his stay in the CCU will be limited to a given number of days should be explained. A physical description of the unit is helpful, especially if it is windowless or unusual in any other way.

Design of CCU The architecture or design of the CCU is a subject that needs discussion. In the course of visiting CCUs across the country we have been surprised at the relatively small number that are pleasant to the eye. Most are built as an afterthought, hastily constructed in obviously gerrymandered space. For the most part they are cramped, poorly lighted, and windowless. A study has been done to suggest that having windows in an intensive care unit (ICU) may result in less patient delirium.[307] Whether or not this would apply to the CCU remains to be demonstrated, but certainly a window with a view is a more attractive background for giving and receiving care than four blank walls.

There is some debate about whether single rooms are better than semiprivate accommodations in the CCU. Companionship is one argument for semiprivate rooms, while fear of witnessing cardiac arrest is used as an argument by proponents of private units. It has been our experience that patients in the CCU rarely complain about the presence or absence of roommates. Those who witnessed an arrest did, however, request a single room should they be readmitted. The only specific complaint about architecture we received was from patients who had been in a circular unit where the nursing station occupied the position of a hub and the rooms radiated off as spokes. All walls were of uncurtained glass. The patients disliked the feeling of being in a fishbowl.

Cardiac monitor Since being attached to a cardiac monotor is central to the experience of occupying a bed in a CCU, special attention must be paid to the manner in which this instrument is presented to the patient. In our early work we had expected that the experience of being monitored would produce discomfort and marked fear. The discomfort would stem from the limitation of movement due to the electrodes' wires. The fear would be engendered by a combination of the instruments' "bleeping" plus the sight of the luminous ECG tracing on the oscilloscope. Being hooked to such a contraption, we thought, could only serve to remind the patient of his potential for imminent demise. As our data accumulated, it came as a surprise that fear was a rare response.[308] Most patients were more reassured than scared by the cardiac monitor. Our error in prediction stemmed from our ignorance of the manner in which the instrument was presented. The nurse responsible for attaching the patient to the monitor introduced the latter as a "mechanical guardian angel." She went on to say, "As long as you are hooked up to this machine you couldn't die if you tried." This, of course, proved to be remarkably effective stratagem, particularly in a population that was predominantly Irish Catholic.

The nurse should explain the function of the monitor in a matter-of-fact fashion emphasizing its routine use in the CCU. One nurse succinctly summarized monitoring as "a modern method of taking a second-to-second pulse without the bedside presence of the nurse." Once the leads are attached, one should be removed to demonstrate how this can sound a false alarm. Anticipation of this kind is most valuable in reducing "startle" responses. It is particularly helpful to demonstrate circuit static and movement artifacts in order to show that they can arise from noncardiac causes. These irregularities upset only a small number of patients, most of whom are from a blue-collar background. Patients in this category should be given a more thorough explanation and then questioned to make sure they understand. The more the patient understands the purpose and function of mechanical devices in the unit, the less fearful the equipment is apt to make him. In general, our patients tended to worry less about mechanical breakdowns

than we had expected. Whether these breakdowns had to do with respirators, pacemakers, or monitoring systems, it was only the rare patient who needed reassurance about a mechanical failure. The American's penchant for mechanization may explain the trust in instruments.[309]

Witnessing cardiac arrest Physicians agree that the most distressing event in the experience of coronary care is to witness cardiac arrest. This event is, of course, obviated if the patient has a private room. Although there has been a steady trend in CCU design to provide more privacy, most of these units are double rooms or four-bed wards. As a consequence there is a real possibility that an arrest will be witnessed. In interviewing a series of patients who had witnessed an arrest we were surprised to find that only 20% of them were frightened by the scene.[310] Some patients were impressed with the speed with which the drill team responded to the alarm. Some were equally impressed with the amount of time spent on resuscitation. One individual said, "If they spent that much time on an 80-year-old woman, I thought to myself that they'd spend twice as long on me since I'm half her age."

Anger was commonly reported as a response by patients who witnessed the arrest and the ensuing resuscitation. This seemed a paradoxical response and yet, on closer examination, one can see its utility. If there is one emotion designed to diminish anxiety it is anger. If an anxious person can be made angry his apprehension declines or vanishes.

Another notable response was the lack of identification with the victim. Although empathy for the arresting patient was expressed by all, only the rare patient identified with him. In other words, they did not imagine themselves to be in the same position. They seemed able to erect between themselves and the victim a barricade which precluded any fantasied resemblance. Even when victim and observer were of the same age, sex and social background, some reason was always found to differentiate the onlooker's condition from that of the victim.

If death occurred, the staff, quite naturally, quickly reassured the survivor that the heart of the deceased was much worse than his own. No matter how obvious the excuse, patients were apt to accept it without question or reservation. The response of our patients to witnessing cardiac arrest offers a good example of how patients can grasp the most comforting meaning from an event while denying the more threatening aspects.

On the other hand, Bruhn et al. reported an increase in anxiety and in systolic pressure in patients who had viewed a fatal arrest.[311] We observed and were told by nurses that requests for tranquilizers, sedatives, and pain medication increase in the wake of an arrest. Another observation, made indirectly as part of a survey about room preference, disclosed that witnessing an arrest may be more traumatic than meets the eye. We asked all patients whether they would prefer to be in a single room or in a two-to-four-bed ward should they require another hospitalization. All of the patients chose a two- or a four-bed ward except those who had seen an arrest. The latter selected single rooms.

Lazarus complex Some years ago when the first reports were published describing the quality of life after surviving cardiac arrest, one could not help but question whether saving the patients was worth the trouble.[312] The victims were described as suffering what could best be called a traumatic neurosis. The incidence of depression, the occurrence of nightmares (mostly about being caught in fire), and the level of chronic anxiety were high. Furthermore, some survivors complained of "feeling different from other people," as though, like Lazarus, they had returned from the dead. Subsequent reports have not supported this earlier observation. Indeed, there appears to be a remarkable absence of psychopathology in the wake of surviving an arrest. The reason for the discrepancy between the early report and later ones may be the way the patient is told of the arrest. In the beginning there was no uniform policy of telling. Not infrequently the wife was the one who informed her husband that his heart had been revitalized. Doctors, unsure of how to interpret what had happened, usually remained silent. Since the experience was so unique to physician and patient alike, distortion, exaggerations and misinformation easily flourished. Whatever the reasons for the discrepancy, it now appears that chronic anxiety, depression, and emotional invalidism are not commonly found among those who survive cardiac arrest.

Dobson and his co-workers in Great Britain have followed a series of survivors for some years following arrest and report a uniformly good response.[313] He emphasizes the importance of informing the patient of what has happened. This need not be done within hours after the incident but should be done by the next day. It is helpful to stress the routine nature of the resuscitation and that it does not alter the prognosis. The fact that we now know that spontaneous ventricular fibrillation, in itself, does not influence the patient's chance for recovery makes it a good deal easier to reassure him. This information, of course, was lacking in earlier studies and may account for the sense of doom and foreboding—the Lazarus complex—experienced by the original survivors. The doctor, expecting another arrest momentarily, may have been uneasy in the patient's presence. The doctor's manner might well have been transmitted to the patient's spouse. All of this could have encouraged the Lazarus complex.[314] Fortunately, this complex has been laid to rest.

The experience of arrest itself, as it is subjectively recounted, is almost always clouded by amnesia. Nine out of ten patients do not remember anything specific about the event. One woman was unsure of whether she reported what had really happened or if it took place in a dream. "A funny experience . . . a hand down my throat squeezing my heart—I felt it was happening—but I don't know if it happened in a dream." The most complete account was given by a young teacher. He was brought into the emergency ward by his fiancée after having been stricken with severe chest pain. While being examined in the emergency ward, he arrested. After resuscitation he recounted a vivid dream. In it he found himself on a conveyor belt heading toward the checkout counter of a supermarket. He was trussed up like a package of meat. As he got closer to the cashier, he said to himself, and then aloud, "Oh no, oh no, they don't. They're not going to check me out." He awoke with a start after being defibrillated. Looking around and finding himself surrounded by men in white he exclaimed, "Christ, there are a lot of clerks in this market." Everyone laughed, and then his doctor explained what had happened. If he had not been told, this man would probably have had no clear recollection of the dream's signifi-

cance. He might have remembered it only as a nightmare. We had the impression that the passage of time caused most patients to forget that their heart had stopped and required assistance to regain its beat.

When the patient has undergone more than one resuscitation he is more apt to remember the event. Individuals who had multiple arrests often can recall the chest sensations prior to losing consciousness and also the pain of having a shock pass through the thorax. A small number remain alert and conscious throughout. Most of these individuals remember the event with anger about the amount of pain they withstood, but they complain of less anxiety than we might expect as a result of their harrowing experience.

Convalescent ward   There are three "rites de passage" in the hospital experience of patients with myocardial infarction (MI). The first, from the emergency ward to the CCU, has been described already. The second is from the CCU to the step-down unit or to the convalescent ward. The third is from the convalescent ward home.

The transition, from CCU to convalescent ward is usually viewed as a graduation exercise—a tangible, reassuring sign that progress has been made and the myocardium has healed sufficiently for the patient to be unhooked from his monitor. Departing from the CCU is not an unmixed blessing. The patient leaves a situation where he has been cared for not only intensively but often with great skill and compassion by his nurse. He leaves the security of having a doctor within calling distance. If there is no step-down unit and the patient goes directly to a convalescent ward, he often finds himself one of a dozen or more patients all serviced by two nurses. This comes as a shock to the patient after being accustomed to a far more favorable nurse/patient ratio. Furthermore, a number of patients miss being monitored and feel somehow more vulnerable without their "guardian angel." All of these factors may contribute to the incidence of insomnia, palpitations, anxiety reactions, arrhythmias and extended infarction which are apt to occur around the time of transition from the CCU. Klein *et al.* have found that these emotional changes correlated positively with elevated levels of urinary catecholamine.[315]

In order to decrease the negative effects of transfer, it is important to anticipate the anxiety the move may cause. The patient should be told about the prospect of moving a day before he is scheduled to go. In discussing the transfer we believe it is wise to warn the patient that he might feel anxious in this new surrounding because the nursing care will not be as intensive and he may be surprised to find himself missing the monitor. We suggest that tranquilizing medication be increased for the first day or two away from the CCU and that the nurses on the new floor give him special attention. The most obvious solution to the transition syndrome would be to have an intermediate or step-down ward for patients fresh from the CCU. In this setting, care would not be as intense as before, but neither could it be called lax by the newcomer.

Psychological problems   As can be seen from Fig. 62E-19, the three most common reasons for psychiatric consultations in the CCU are: anxiety, depression, and management problems. Delirium, which is the scourge of most ICU settings—especially surgical—is rare in the CCU. In Fig. 62E-20, the pattern of requests for psychiatric consultation follows a different distribution for each problem. Anxiety occurs early in the CCU experience, usually on the first or second day. Depression peaks on the third day and management problems

FIGURE 62E-19 Distribution of consultation requests according to the coronary care unit (CCU) day on which they were made.

have a bimodal distribution with a higher peak coming on the second day and a lower peak emerging on the fourth day.

Although anxiety is the most common problem for which psychiatric assistance is sought in the CCU, it is by no means as prevalent as might be thought. In a study of 100 patients, half white-collar and half blue-collar workers, 25 were rated as showing no anxiety; only five were found to be severely anxious. Forty were rated as moderate and 30 as mildly anxious. There was no relationship between anxiety and the seriousness of the illness or the patient's socioeconomic background. Anxiety usually stems from one of two sources: the prospect of sudden death, or the appearance of death's heralds—breathlessness, severe chest pain or complications (arrhythmias, cardioversion, pacemaker insertion).

One less obvious symptom that often evokes anxiety is the sensation of weakness. Particularly when the patient has been robust and hardy, being felled by an MI and feeling weak as a consequence frequently provoke marked anxiety. Patients often regard weakness as proof that their illness is irreversible or that heart damage is permanent. As a result it is wise to anticipate that the patient will feel weak and to explain that this is a normal occurrence after myocardial infarction. Sometimes the sense of weakness is increased by sedatives or tranquilizers. When this is the case, the latter can be reduced or discontinued. In the presence of the subjective complaint of weakness, one should always ask if the patient would prefer no tranquilizer.

We have observed that anxiety is difficult to identify in the CCU because patients consciously or unconsciously deny it. Furthermore, physicians do not have time on rounds to make an adequate judgment of the patient's mental condition. For this reason, we believe that mild-to-moderate anxiety is more common than the outward appearance of patients in the unit might suggest. As a consequence we think it advisable to regard every patient as anxious and to treat him accordingly even though supporting evidence may be lacking. Our suggestion is to order a minor tranquilizer for all patients with the promise that it can be discontinued or decreased. Since the CCU patient is commonly an undercomplainer, unlikely to make routine requests of the nurses, he is less apt to get medication on a p.r.n. basis than if it is regularly ordered. We make it a practice, therefore, to order a standard dose of a benzodiazepine upon entrance into the unit and to inform the patient that if he feels too drowsy for comfort, he should tell the nurse, who will either reduce the dose or withhold the

medication. Most patients prefer to be medicated, but there is a small percentage who respond poorly to sedation, and they should be allowed the privilege of having none if they desire. However, it is necessary to emphasize to each patient the importance of mental rest and to assure him that tranquilizers are a standard medication. Too many men equate the need for sedation with weakness, and this kind of thinking should be discouraged.

Depression is the second most common reason for psychiatric consultation in the CCU; it is reactive in nature and rarely assumes psychotic proportions. One would expect a patient with MI to be depressed. He has had a brush with death and has temporarily lost his autonomy and well-being. Loss is invariably followed by grieving which is, after all, a form of depression. The standard signs are a saddened face, disinterest or listlessness, pessimism or hopelessness, slowness of speech or movement, or weeping. Combined with this is the frustration of "Why did it happen to me? Why *now*? It's the time when I am most needed." In the series of 100 cases mentioned earlier, only six patients were severely depressed whereas 36 were moderately depressed and 33 were mildly depressed.[316] As with anxiety, 25 were rated as not depressed. The depression focuses around damaged self-esteem. Discouraging personal consequences of cardiac damage are foreseen. These include the specter of recurrence, reduced earning power, the inevitable restrictions of activity, sexual incompetence, invalidism, and premature old age.

The treatment of both anxiety and depression involves very simple principles which center chiefly around reassurance based upon explanation and education.[317] Explaining the nature of the infarction and the process of repair may seem a useless waste of the doctor's time, but such is not the case. We found, for example, that whereas both white-collar and blue-collar patients could define and describe infarction in terms of the damage done to the heart, the white-collar patient was far more aware of the process of repair and how the heart could mend. Some blue-collar patients knew nothing about scar formation and pictured the heart as permanently punctured. Providing information can do more to insure peace of mind than any type of medication.

FIGURE 62E-20 Hypothetical schedule of onset of emotional and behavioral reactions of a coronary unit (CCU) patient.

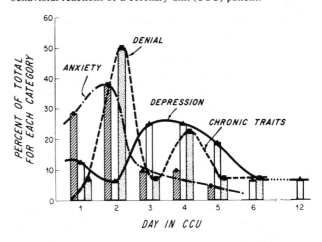

Much of the depression suffered by the post-coronary patient centers around the fear of not being able to resume work or lead an active life. Most patients have little or no idea of what they will face during convalescence and most are dogged by outmoded stereotypes which equate heart disease with automatic and permanent invalidism. Reminding them that many national and community leaders have sustained heart attacks and yet continue to function normally corrects their thinking. One should then go on to specify individuals known to the patient who have successfully completed convalescence and returned to work. The fact that Presidents Johnson and Eisenhower sustained coronaries without leaving the mainstream of life provides an encouraging framework for the future. The information that eight of the runners who completed a recent Boston Marathon had previously sustained an MI is heartening news for the man in the CCU who is mourning what he regards as the loss of his active life.

Aside from correcting misinformation and educating the patient, the best antidote for depression is, in our opinion, a program of physical conditioning.[318] Some hospitals start patients in such a program on the third CCU day.[319] Most reports to date indicate that both anxiety and depression are less troublesome when the patient is actively engaged in physical conditioning. These programs give the patient a sense of participating in his recovery as well as offering something to fill long stretches of vacant hours. They also restore confidence by demonstrating that activity is possible.

Tranquilizers, particularly the benzodiazepine group (chlordiazepoxide, diazepam and oxazepam) are important elements in the management of anxiety as well as providing for sleep. If one wants to avoid using barbiturates, doubling the dose of a benzodiazepine will often produce a night of sleep. The phenothiazines should not be used for sedation because conduction disturbances and sudden death have been reported in conjunction with their use.[320] Unfortunately the tricyclic antidepressants are less safe to use in acute coronary disease because of the high incidence of cardiac irregularities, including sudden death, reported with their use.[321] Since the MAO inhibitors can cause fatal hypertensive crisis unless a tyramine-free diet is adhered to rigidly, they are seldom used in patients with cardiovascular disease. Depression as mentioned earlier is best treated by starting the patient through inpatient physical conditioning. When programs of early mobilization, as described by Hutter et al.,[322] are more widely practiced, we will probably find less depression as a byproduct.

Of the two chief management problems, the threat to sign out is the more serious. This usually comes early in the hospital stay when the diagnosis of myocardial infarction is still uncertain. Most of these individuals can be persuaded to stay until the results of the tests have been returned. Should the ECG and enzymes reveal an infarction, it is our experience that most people are willing to remain in the hospital. When such is not the case and the patient is competent, we call in the key figures in his life—wife, children, friends, minister—in an attempt to induce him to stay. Should this fail, we do our best to provide care for him at home, always holding open the option of returning to the hospital.

Another common management problem is the male who makes either sexually provocative comments or physical advances to his nurses. On rare occasions, a man might repeatedly expose himself. The reason for these behavioral aberrations is the sense of threat to virility. Following infarction, men often feel impotent and sexually incompetent. The result is an attempt (often unconsciously motivated) to demonstrate their virility as a means of being reassured of their manhood by the nurses' response. Not infrequently patients do this without realizing the effect it has on the nurses. One patient was appalled when told by the psychiatrist that his "dirty jokes" were offending the nurses. He said, "My God! I thought they enjoyed them even more than I did." Other patients may deny making overtures or comments entirely. When this happens, and the behavior continues even after a psychiatric consultation, the best method of intervention is gentle and compassionate confrontation by individual nurses. On the few occasions we have employed this approach it has succeeded. Even when the individual insists on his innocence, as did one patient, his behavior improves.

Conclusion One might ask—What is the state of mind most conducive to surviving the coronary care unit experience? Are there psychological factors that appear to work for or against the patient? There is widespread belief that the stage of depression, for example, in preoperative patients increases postoperative mortality and morbidity. Similarly it has been our impression that depression hampers recovery in the CCU. Anxiety is so much more amenable to treatment through reassurance, tranquilization and encouragement that it seldom, of itself, constitutes a threat to well-being.

On the positive side our work has demonstrated what seems to be a significant relationship between the use of denial and survival in the CCU. Denial is defined as the conscious or unconscious repudiation of part or all of the total available meaning of an event to allay fear, anxiety or other unpleasant feelings. We divide denial into four categories based upon the extent to which it is used. The most extreme form is called major denial and is characterized by the complete disavowal of fear both in present as well as in past situations of danger. Minimal denial is at the opposite end of the scale and is used to describe patients who complain of anxiety and readily admit being frightened. In this group no consistent criteria for denial can be found. In between these two extremes are moderate and mild denial. In examining the data from an earlier study we found that not one single major denier died during the study period; two of the four deaths were from among minimal deniers and the other two were mild deniers. The minimal denier representing 8% of the total sample, contributed 50% of the mortality. Chi square analysis shows this relation to be significant beyond the 5% level. Follow-up data demonstrated that denial correlated with a lower mortality than was expected. Major deniers with Peel scores of 13 or below seemed to survive longer than individuals in the minimal, mild and moderate denial categories.

Although there are far too few cases involved for generalization, we can at least make an enlightened speculation. The patient who can effectively deny fear and anxiety, who can relax in the CCU may have a better chance for survival in both the short and the long run. The significance this has for clinical application is quite straightforward. No one is in a better position to enhance or reinforce denial than the physician. Most patients are predisposed to believe what the doctor tells them and the need to believe increases with the seriousness of the illness.

Enlightened optimism is therefore the keystone for our treatment program of patients in the CCU. The doctor can emphasize the hopeful and positive aspects of the patient's illness without minimizing the risks. It is largely a matter of emphasis. This will vary from case to case but the underlying principle will remain the same—accentuate the positive.

CHAPTER 62E **1233**
RECOGNITION AND MANAGEMENT OF CORONARY
ATHEROSCLEROTIC HEART DISEASE

PRINCIPLES OF REHABILITATION (THE USE OF REST AND EXERCISE)

Many patients with coronary atherosclerotic heart disease do too little physical work and avoid all mental problems, while other patients do too much physical work and take on too many mental problems. The physician must help each individual patient live an active, productive, and safe life within the constraints imposed by the disease process itself. Whereas most of the emphasis has been placed on the rehabilitation of the patient with myocardial infarction (see Chap. 62G), the same goals and principles apply to all patients with coronary atherosclerotic heart disease. With so many patients having coronary bypass surgery, we must include this group in our rehabilitation efforts.

The amount of physical and mental work that can be permitted patients with the various coronary syndromes is discussed later in this chapter in the section "The Management of Specific Clinical Syndromes." The approximate date of discharge from the hospital should be discussed as soon as the physician has sufficient information to do so, and the rehabilitation process should begin with the first encounter the physician has with a patient. For example, there is a vast difference between a physician saying "You must quit work because of your heart" and "You must stop work for a few weeks and then you must return to work. We have found that work is good for patients like you."

The rehabilitation of the patient with myocardial infarction is discussed in Chap. 62G. Two points will be emphasized here.

1 The use and abuse of bed rest for patients with myocardial infarction and the length of time a patient with myocardial infarction should remain in the hospital will be discussed later in the section dealing with the management of specific clinical syndromes.
2 The problems related to retirement have been discussed earlier. We wish to emphasize again that the act of retirement does not always achieve the goal one believes it will. Many patients become restless and depressed. The mental anguish that is created by retirement may provoke more angina pectoris.

DIET AND EATING

Obesity Obesity may be said to be present when the body weight increases 10 percent above the standard for individuals the same age, height, sex, and race (see Chap. 62H). This definition of obesity is not generally appreciated. It is difficult to accept that the average North American gains weight between the ages of 25 and 50. Just as the average person avoids scales, the same individual is likely to ignore the thick skinfold which surrounds his abdomen.

Obesity per se does not contribute directly to atherosclerosis. For example, in studies in which all other variables such as blood pressure, blood lipids, and carbohydrate tolerance are normal there is no increase in coronary atherosclerotic heart disease in individuals who are obese as compared to nonobese persons. There is, however, considerable evidence to indicate that individuals who are obese are more likely to have diabetes mellitus, abnormal blood lipid levels, and hypertension, which in turn increase the likelihood for atherosclerosis.

There is little doubt that the health of the citizens of the United States would be vastly improved if normal body weight could be achieved by each of them. Accordingly, a lean body weight should be achieved by limiting the caloric intake and, when appropriate, increasing the caloric expenditure. The obese patient may have less angina pectoris produced by effort when he reduces, because it requires less cardiac work when there is less weight to carry around.

The failure to accomplish weight reduction is often due to the physician's inability to translate the need for weight reduction into effective therapy. The mere giving of a diet form will not often accomplish the job. Instruction and follow-up with a dietician, where available, is the best means of ensuring weight reduction. This can be accomplished with due regard to the restriction of total calories, total fat, the use of unsaturated fat, and the restriction of carbohydrates (see Chap. 62H). A major deterrent to weight reduction is the use of alcohol and a lack of some form of exercise in conjunction with dietary measures. The patients whose appetite is enhanced because of the omission of smoking pose special problems requiring more intense treatment for smoking withdrawal and obesity.

Weight reduction is important because it creates an improved body image, enhances a sense of well-being, decreases the likelihood of diabetes, assists in the control of abnormal blood lipid levels, and decreases the work of the heart, thereby improving angina pectoris when it is present.

Eating and angina pectoris The patient with angina pectoris may detect the discomfort during or immediately after eating a meal. Some patients note that they can walk less after eating a meal before the onset of angina pectoris. Such patients should be advised to eat more slowly, to eat less, not to exercise soon after a meal, and to take nitroglycerin before eating.

Eating and "prolonged discomfort" due to myocardial ischemia The patient with prolonged pain due to myocardial ischemia should not be stressed with a regular diet that requires a moderate amount of chewing. Therefore, it is customary to prescribe a low calorie, liquid, and soft diet. Iced liquids should be avoided, since cold precipitates myocardial ischemia in some patients.

Diet to prevent and decelerate coronary atherosclerosis The prevention of coronary atherosclerotic heart disease is discussed in Chap. 62H. We strongly urge that obesity be controlled (see definition of obesity in preceding section of this chapter). The control of obesity by diet and carefully prescribed exercise will decrease the incidence of angina pectoris and may even alter blood lipids in a favorable manner.

The dietary approach to the treatment of coronary atherosclerotic heart disease is often applied in a most unscientific manner. For example, the obese patient may be obsessed with avoidance of eggs and have no interest in decreasing his caloric intake. This, of course, is absurd. It is equally absurd to insist that the patient with extensive coronary atherosclerosis with multiple infarctions and chronic heart failure adhere to a strict diet directed toward lowering the blood lipid levels (which may make the patient miserable and do no good) and to ignore the atrocious eating habits of children and teenagers (see Chap. 62H).

It is unfortunately true that additional problems are produced by the prescription of exacting diets. Overzealous family members who constantly insist that the patient follow the "orders" laid down by the physician and who follow the "rules" promulgated by lay and medical press may unwittingly create much unhappiness. One of us (J. W. H.) saw a patient many years after he had been told that he had a funny looking electrocardiogram and a cholesterol level of 260 mg/dl. He had been placed on a strict low fat, low cholesterol diet even though he was very thin. The patient had no heart disease except very slight aortic regurgitation of unknown cause. The wife refused to discuss any subject except the level of her husband's serum cholesterol and had no interest in discussing the prevention of bacterial endocarditis.

The prevention of coronary atherosclerosis by dietary means cannot be guaranteed at this time. The approach currently recommended by many individuals is discussed in Chap. 62H. We ask the reader to recognize that such an approach does not solve all of the problems, and if it is used, that common sense should prevail.

ADVICE REGARDING THE USE OF ALCOHOL[323,324]

Alcohol increases the caloric intake, alters blood lipid levels in some individuals, and depresses cardiac function. Alcohol may reduce exercise tolerance and decrease the interval between exercise and the onset of angina pectoris with concomitant increase in ST-segment depression when angina pectoris does occur. Susceptible patients may develop arrhythmia after ingestion of alcohol. Accordingly, alcohol cannot be recommended. Common sense dictates that one cannot be rigid in such views and prohibit the intake of alcohol in all patients. Some patients can use alcohol as a tranquilizer, but others misuse it. The physician who knows his patient can permit a reasonable amount of alcohol if its effect is not clearly deleterious and if important benefits are apparent.

ADVICE REGARDING THE USE OF TOBACCO

Smoking should be prohibited (see Chap. 98). The patient with angina pectoris should not smoke. An excellent time for the patient to stop smoking is at the time of myocardial infarction. The use of oxygen, sedation, etc., precludes smoking for several days, and after that period of time passes the patient is encouraged to continue to abstain.

Whereas most patients should be advised to stop the use of tobacco, it is unreasonable to insist that an elderly patient with severe disease discontinue all the things he enjoys.

DRUGS USED IN THE TREATMENT OF CORONARY ATHEROSCLEROTIC HEART DISEASE

The following discussion will emphasize the drugs that are commonly used in the treatment of certain aspects of coronary atherosclerotic heart disease. These and other drugs used in the treatment of patients with heart disease are discussed in "The Management of Specific Clinical Syndromes" later in this chapter and in Chap. 109.

Drugs used in the treatment of myocardial ischemia Nitroglycerin[325-343] The mainstay of treatment of angina pectoris for the last hundred years has been nitroglycerin.[325] It remains so today. This drug produces a favorable influence by an effect on the systemic circulation as well as the collateral circulation of the heart. The pharmacologic effects may be summarized as follows:[326,327] (1) It reduces the peripheral resistance or afterload of the heart; (2) it reduces the preload or filling pressure of the heart by its effect on dilatation of venous beds; (3) it secondarily increases the rate of pressure rise in the ventricle, dp/dt; (4) it increases the pulse rate; (5) it decreases the ventricular volume; (6) it increases ventricular compliance; (7) it dilates the large epicardial arteries; (8) it increases flow through collateral channels although the total coronary blood flow is unchanged; and (9) it decreases cardiac work and improves ventricular function (by a combination of the effects listed in 1, 2, and 5).

The education of the patient regarding the use of nitroglycerin is *extremely important.* When nitroglycerin is first used, one should use the smallest possible dose, such as 0.16 mg (1/400 gr) in order to minimize side effects such as headaches. If too large a dose is used initially, the patient may subsequently refuse to take the drug. The patient should be instructed to take the drug for substernal heaviness, tightness, pressure, burning, indigestion, constriction, dyspnea, aching, expanding sensation, or whatever characterizes the distress. Many have the mistaken impression that it should be used only for pain, and, of course, most individuals do not describe their discomfort as being painful. The physician must identify the varying sensations of angina for the patient, since many will not recognize ischemic distress; at times this can be done by using the treadmill exercise test. Reassurance is needed that the drug is not habit-forming and that it does not lose its effect with continued use. If it does not produce burning of the tongue or the characteristic nitrite effect of throbbing sensation in the head, it should be replenished; and it is a good general rule to replenish the supply of drug every 3 months. As angina pectoris worsens, one may need to increase the strength of the tablets to 0.40 mg (1/150 gr) or 0.64 mg (1/100 gr). The discomfort is characteristically relieved within 3 min unless there is severe myocardial ischemia or prolonged emotional tension. Lack of relief with nitroglycerin suggests (1) that the discomfort is of noncoronary origin, (2) that the distress is not simply angina pectoris but is due to more prolonged myocardial ischemia, (3) that the pain may be associated with conditions which are worsened by nitroglycerin administration, i.e., hypertrophic subaortic stenosis or Barlow's syndrome (prolapse of the mitral leaflets), or (4) that the drug has lost its potency. The patient should be educated to use the drug prior to an act that is known to precipitate angina pectoris. Thus, it should be used by some patients prior to meals or sexual intercourse, prior to lying down at night, on the first hole while playing golf, while towelling after a bath, and prior to any effort that is likely to induce the distress. One must remember that the drug may give transient or equivocal relief in esophageal spasm, pylorospasm, and gallstone colic.

Nitroglycerin has other effects. Fortunately, most of the effects are useful, but some are harmful. Nitrite-induced syncope may occur following the use of excessive amounts of the drug when the patient is in the upright position. Fortunately this occurs very rarely. The postural hypotension is more likely to occur when the patient is standing in a line, when he is overheated, with hyperventilation, when other drugs such as beta-blockers and antihypertensive drugs or phenothiazine derivatives have been administered and after excessive alcohol intake. Nitrite syncope is easily confused with acute myocardial infarction, since the patient may become transiently pulseless, cold, and clammy, and may sweat profusely. The patient may be admitted to the hospital with an erroneous diagnosis of acute myocardial infarction, but the history coupled with the lack of evidence of myocardial necrosis will usually clarify the issue. On the other hand, at the onset of acute myocardial infarction there may be increased sensitivity to the effects of nitroglycerin so that an alarming drop in blood pressure may occur. Nitrites given over a period of time may improve congestive failure after acute myocardial infarction.[328] Nitroglycerin may improve myocardial wall motion of hypokinetic and of some akinetic segments.[329,330] Intravenous nitroglycerin has been helpful in getting patients off cardiopulmonary bypass when coronary surgery has been performed.[331] Intravenous nitroglycerin may improve pump function and decrease the degree of myocardial ischemia as manifested by a reduction of the degree of ST elevation during acute myocardial infarction.[332] When it is used for this purpose the dose may be carefully titrated since the drop in blood

pressure and mean aortic flow may further compromise coronary blood flow. Nitroglycerin may reduce the fibrillation threshold in dogs.[333] Its effect in the human is yet to be shown. However sublingual nitroglycerin given at 4-h intervals during acute myocardial infarction has been reported to reduce premature ventricular contractions to approximately one-half the number occurring during control periods without nitroglycerin, suggesting improvement in myocardial ischemia. Intravenous nitroglycerin has also been used for the treatment of acute left ventricular failure following myocardial infarction.[334]

Long-acting nitrites[335–337b] It has been questioned whether long-acting nitrites are effective. Many observers have relegated an alleged benefit to a placebo effect. Current evidence suggests that certain long-acting nitrites produce an effect lasting a few hours. They improve the dynamics of the heart, and have direct and indirect effects on the coronary circulation. The filling pressures of the heart may be lowered for hours with oral forms of certain nitrites given in conventional dosage.[338] If the hemodynamics can be shown to be improved, it is reasonable to believe that the effects on ischemia can also be improved. Long-acting nitrites should be administered at a time when they could be effective, i.e., prior to the time when angina pectoris might be expected to occur.

Two percent *nitroglycerin ointment* applied to the skin has been used at night to reduce nocturnal angina but is also effective when applied every 4 h while awake.[339,340] Reicheck et al. noted significant increase in exercise capacity of patients for periods of up to 3 h after nitroglycerin ointment application.[341] Parker et al. and others reported that nitroglycerin ointment reduced the left ventricular end-diastolic pressure and systemic arterial pressure within 15 min and that the effect lasted 60 min.[343] The left ventricular stroke work, the time-tension index, and exercise tolerance were improved, suggesting that there was a reduction in myocardial oxygen requirements.

Mantle et al. noted a significant fall of the mean arterial pressure that persisted more than 4 h after either oral (20 to 50 mg) or sublingual *isosorbide dinitrate,* whereas the effect from sublingual nitroglycerin lasted only 15 to 30 min.[344] Sublingual isosorbide dinitrate was reported to reduce the left ventricular diastolic volume and pulmonary artery diastolic pressure up to 4 h.[345] Epstein et al. and Kattus et al. were able to demonstrate improved exercise tolerance for 1 to 2 h after sublingual isosorbide dinitrate.[346,347] Gensini demonstrated that vasodilatation of the large coronary arteries occurs after nitroglycerin and chewable isosorbide dinitrate but does not take place after oral isosorbide dinitrate.[348]

Beta-blockers Beta-adrenergic blocking agents such as propranolol have been the greatest advance in the treatment of angina pectoris since nitrites were introduced 100 years ago. We use propranolol whenever we diagnose angina pectoris or prolonged myocardial ischemia due to coronary atherosclerosis. We do not delay the use of the drug until nitrites have been tried. The effects of propranolol may be summarized as follows:[349,350] Propranolol (1) decreases the heart rate, (2) decreases myocardial contractility, (3) increases ventricular volume, (4) may increase left ventricular end-diastolic pressure, (5) decreases *dp/dt,* (6) increases coronary vascular resistance, (7) has a quinidine-like antiarrhythmic effect, (8) decreases myocardial oxygen consumption, (9) decreases renin secretion, (10) decreases essential tremor, and (11) occasionally improves migraine.

The side effects of propranolol are as follows:[349] The drug may produce (1) fatigue, (2) poor coordination, (3) mental depression, (4) amnesia, (5) hallucinations, (6) weakness, (7) bradycardia, (8) bronchospasm, (9) diarrhea, (10) heart failure, (11) a decrease in libido, (12) Raynaud's syndrome (or may aggravate it), (13) postural hypotension, (14) eosinophilia, and (15) problems for the diabetic since propranolol may prevent the symptoms of hypoglycemia.

The starting dose of propranolol is 10 mg four times daily. The dose may be increased every 3 to 4 days until a maximal effect is obtained or the heart rate is decreased to approximately 50 beats per minute. The average effective total daily dose is 80 to 160 mg, but some patients may require 240 to 320 mg. Remember that it is possible that angina pectoris may worsen with excessive dosage. Sudden omission of drug should be avoided in patients with severe disease since a rebound phenomenon may occur, increasing angina pectoris or precipitating infarction.[351–353]

The dosage of propranolol must be individualized since many patients feel exhausted and fatigued with even small doses. Mild symptoms of mental depression may develop. These effects are to a degree dose-related and may abate with continued use or decreased dose. The lessening of angina pectoris occurs predictably within a few days to a week.

Warren et al. treated 63 patients with angina pectoris with propranolol over a period of 5 to 8 years with a mean dose of 255 mg. They found that 84 percent of the patients had a 50 percent or greater reduction of angina pectoris. Heart failure occurred in 25 percent of the patients, often in relationship to acute or prior myocardial infarction.[354] The drug is almost completely absorbed from the gastrointestinal tract, but variability in absorption and metabolism may explain differences in dose responsiveness. The serum half-life is 3 to 6 h.[355,357] Secondary metabolites may result in persistent effects that may not be reflected in plasma levels. Although slowing of the heart rate is a major effect, a favorable influence may be noted with a heart rate of 60 beats per minute, while in other patients the heart rate may drop to 40 beats per minute with no additional benefit. Some patients with prior sinus bradycardia and shilling or latent sinus node dysfunction may not tolerate the drug without undue cardiac slowing. This is also influenced by the concomitant administration of other drugs such as digitalis or reserpine. Heart rates of 40 to 50 beats per minute may be well tolerated with benefit of angina pectoris.[354] Benefit occurs at 64 to 98 percent of total blockade, but in some cases coronary flow may be decreased more than the decrease in myocardial oxygen demands, thus decreasing delivery of oxygen to ischemic areas.[356,357]

Congestive heart failure may be induced in the patient with severe pump dysfunction, but it is surprising how well hearts with hypokinetic or akinetic areas at angiography tolerate propranolol. The drug should be used with caution in those patients with obvious S_3 gallop and a cardiothoracic ratio greater than 0.5, since many patients with such findings develop pulmonary congestion.[354] Oral propranolol may reduce the frequency of attacks of angina pectoris without improving exercise tolerance. The addition of digoxin may improve exercise performance, and the combination has been recommended for patients with abnormal ventricular function or large hearts.[358] Coexistent chronic lung disease associated with bronchospasm is a relative contraindication to the use of propranolol, and asthma may be produced in the susceptible individual. There is increasing evidence that the long-term use of propranolol after myocardial infarction may reduce the incidence of sudden death (see discussion later in this chapter). Propranolol is particularly useful in prevention of atrial arrhythmias, particularly when given in combination with quinidine preparations. Propranolol 20 to 40 mg four times daily with 300 mg quinidine gluconate two to three times daily is a commonly used regimen. Diarrhea is a major limiting factor in the use of propranolol in some patients.[359] It may be controlled by lessening the dose and by the concomitant administration of Lomotil. Raynaud's phenomenon may be produced or aggravated in susceptible individuals.[360] Some patients with essential tremor report improvement while on beta-blockers.

One important use of propranolol is in the prompt reduction of the pressure-rate product by giving small amounts such as 1 to 3 mg given intravenously in divided doses 3 min apart. This has particular usefulness in the catheterization laboratory when the pain of myocardial ischemia occurs. An acute elevation of the left ventricular end-diastolic pressure may be promptly reduced to normal along with slowing of the rate and decrease in the systolic blood pressure. This may be helpful in abolishing pain on admission to the coronary care unit when sinus tachycardia and elevated systolic pressure are present. It should not be used in the presence of bifascicular block, since complete heart block may be induced, or if there is systemic hypotension. The half-life of intravenous propranolol is 2 to 3 h.[361] While some authors have recommended 1 mg/min up to 10 mg intravenously, we have seen cardiac arrest occur with as little as 1 mg and therefore do not recommend the larger doses. Propranolol, combined with digoxin, is effective in managing atrial flutter or atrial fibrillation occurring in the first week after open heart surgery. Incremental doses of intravenous propranolol up to 3 to 5 mg are used.

Propranolol is helpful in the anxious patient with

extrasystoles as well as in those with thyrotoxicosis. It is not very effective in controlling ventricular premature beats that are not related to a reflex increase in sympathetic tone.

In preparing patients with severe ischemic symptoms for coronary bypass surgery, one must cautiously reduce the dose of propranolol, since angina pectoris may increase, and myocardial infarction may occur.[362,363] Our associates at Emory University Hospital concluded that there was no increase in operative risk by continuing propranolol up to the day prior to bypass surgery. We decrease the dose by one-half the day prior to surgery, and the last dose is given at 10 P.M. the night before surgery.[364] We increase the use of 2 percent nitroglycerin ointment and isosorbide during the day and night prior to surgery. In urgent situations requiring anesthesia and surgery, isoproterenol 1 to 2 mg/500 cc given slowly will counteract the slowing of the pulse rate and the decreased myocardial contractility produced by propranolol. Atropine may be given to counteract the bradycardia. Pain due to myocardial ischemia related to anxiety just prior to anesthesia and surgery can be relieved by 1 to 3 mg propranolol intravenously.

Some of the effects of nitrites (nitroglycerin and the long-acting nitrites) are diametrically opposite to propranolol, but they act synergistically.[365–367] The two acting together may increase the tendency toward postural hypotension. The decrease in pulse rate and the increase in coronary vascular resistance produced by propranolol may be counteracted to some extent by nitrites.

The hemodynamic effects of propranolol vary. In some patients the ejection fraction is reduced, and there is a decrease in segmental wall motion and accentuation of wall abnormalities. This may be due to inhibition of compensatory sympathetic mechanisms; and the ventricular diastolic volume may be increased for any given level of intraventricular pressure.[368]

The negative inotropic effect of beta-blockers such as propranolol demands caution in their use in patients with pump dysfunction, but occasionally paradoxic improvement has been noted by the authors in the treatment of ischemic cardiomyopathy. Waagstein et al. observed improvement in seven patients with congestive cardiomyopathy treated with Practolol and alprenolol.[369]

There are reports of an increase in incidence of heart failure and shock in patients who develop acute myocardial infarction while on beta-blockers.[370] The study by Warren et al. suggested a higher incidence of shock in patients admitted to the coronary care unit on propranolol.[354] Studies in dogs and human beings suggest that propranolol may have some effect in limiting infarct size by reduction of oxygen consumption.[371,372]

Double-blind studies of Tolamol, propranolol, Practolol, and placebo revealed that propranolol 80 mg three times a day was most effective in the treatment of angina pectoris, while Tolamol 200 mg three times daily was superior in reducing blood pressure. ST depression after exercise lessened after propranolol and Tolamol but not after Practolol.[373] Others report no difference between propranolol,

Practolol, oxprenolol, or alprenolol in the improvement of exercise tolerance of patients with angina pectoris. In those who do not respond to increased dosage of propranolol, however, a trial with another drug is recommended.[374]

Perhexiline maleate has been reported to be more effective than beta-blockers such as propranolol or Practolol in the treatment of angina, but side effects are more frequent.[375]

Oxprenolol is an effective beta-blocker that reaches a peak plasma level at 2 h with a gradual decline in levels over a period of 8 h. It has the advantage of being effective when given in a dose of 160 mg twice daily.[376]

Propranolol has been shown to reduce recurrent ventricular fibrillation.[377,378] Reduced incidence of sudden death, presumably due to ventricular fibrillation, was noted in the Multicenter International Study of patients on Practolol after anterior infarction. There were 47 cardiac deaths with 69 instances of reinfarction in those treated with Practolol versus 73 cardiac deaths and 89 nonfatal reinfarctions in the placebo group.[379] There was no significant difference between the treated and control groups in those with inferior infarction. Work in Sweden revealed reduced incidence in sudden death in patients treated with beta blockade after discharge from the hospital with myocardial infarction.[380]

Opiates Opiates are not needed for the relief of chronic angina pectoris. By definition angina pectoris is short-lived, usually lasting 3 to 5 min and occasionally 10 to 15 min. It is usually relieved by sublingual nitroglycerin. Opiates are usually required to relieve the pain associated with more prolonged myocardial ischemia, including acute myocardial infarction.

The prompt relief of pain due to acute myocardial infarction is essential.[382–386a] Some years ago we recommended the use of nitroglycerin for prolonged myocardial ischemia. We later reversed our view because its use delayed the use of an opiate which the patient usually needed. Epstein has recently suggested that nitroglycerin may be useful for prolonged myocardial ischemia (myocardial infarction) because experimentally it decreases the size of the ST segment; improves myocardial contractility in some situations; and might decrease the size of the "infarct."[387] Additional studies are now underway regarding this use for nitroglycerin (see discussion of the "Protection of Ischemic Myocardium" later in this chapter). *Pain due to myocardial infarction can be reliably relieved only by the administration of opiates.*[382] One should not make futile attempts to relieve prolonged discomfort by the continued use of nitroglycerin. The intravenous route of administration of an opiate affords quicker relief with smaller dosage as compared to the intramuscular injection of the drug. The intramuscular injection of the drug may cause a rise in creatine phosphokinase (CPK) which can cause one falsely to diagnose a myocardial infarction. In addition, if respiratory depression occurs secondary to intravenously injected narcotic, it can be promptly recognized and managed, whereas the delayed onset of hypoventilation following intramuscular injection may not be recognized. Morphine sulfate 10 mg may be diluted in 10 to 20 ml saline solution and given 2 ml at a time; one should pause several minutes between increments to be certain that respiratory depression does not occur. It is advisable to have a morphine antagonist such as naloxone hydrochloride (Narcan) available. Narcan is the preferred antagonist because it can reverse the respiratory depression of narcotic overdosage without the risk of augmenting or causing a depression of its own. Hypoxia is common during the early stages of myocardial infarction, and it may be sharply enhanced by the decreased alveolar ventilation that follows the administration of every opiate at any dosage level regardless of the route of administration. Respiratory depression may be enhanced when opiates are combined with other drugs such as phenothiazine derivatives, and the simultaneous administration of such drugs should be discouraged. It should be emphasized that the amplitude of respiratory excursions may be significantly diminished even though the respiratory rate remains normal. Pain must be relieved, but we must beware of the risk of creating hypoxia, In this setting, the hypoxia which occurs can predispose to ventricular fibrillation and cardiac standstill. Since morphine sulfate is vagotonic, atropine sulfate, 0.5 to 1.0 mg, is advised when morphine produces bradycardia, nausea, vomiting, AV block, nodal rhythm, or AV dissociation. These complications are especially likely to occur if the myocardial damage is posterior or inferior in location. Meperidene hydrochloride has an atropine-like effect, and on occasion it may increase the ventricular rate in patients with atrial flutter or fibrillation. This drug is preferred when there is inferior myocardial dead zone and injury and bradycardia. Meperidine hydrochloride is widely used because it is convenient to administer and is claimed to produce less nausea and respiratory depression than morphine. These possible advantages are not so apparent to us, and we generally prefer morphine sulfate for patients with anterior myocardial infarction because of its superior ability to relieve pain. All opiates and their derivatives may produce hypotension and shock by decreasing the peripheral arterial vascular resistance and increasing venous pooling.[383] Potent intravenous diuretics or nitrites may accentuate the hypotension. Opiates must be used with great care in patients with chronic pulmonary disease or myxedema.

Patients may have chest pain due to pericarditis and anxiety following myocardial infarction (see discussion on treatment later under the section "Complications"). Opiates are not needed and generally should not be used for many of the nonischemic causes of chest pain. Furthermore, after determining that the patient's discomfort is not due to ischemia, it is proper to explain to the patient that he is not having a "new heart attack."

Oxygen The administration of oxygen is recommended for the patient with chest pain due to myocardial ischemia who is treated in the home, office, or in the street. This has been suggested because in these settings the advantages outweigh the disadvantages. We must remember that it is difficult to make continuous and accurate observations during the transfer of a patient from the place where he is stricken to the facility where definitive care is to be given. When the patient is seen in the coronary care unit, one should make a more accurate assessment regarding the need for oxygen therapy. High concentrations of oxygen may increase the peripheral resistance and decrease (slightly) the cardiac output. The definite indication for oxygen is hypoxia. Patients with cyanosis, tachycardia, heart failure, shock, dyspnea, cough, wheezing, respiratory depression, and an increased respiratory rate should be given oxygen. When these conditions are present, the oxygen should be given at a high rate of flow via a rebreathing mask or if the patient has chronic obstructive pulmonary disease, via a Venturi mask. Other modalities of oxygen delivery are not as satisfactory. Nasal cannulas irritate the nasal passages and are not satisfactory for "mouth breathers" since they may cause gastric dilatation. An oxygen tent does not produce the desired effect. High flows of oxygen may precipitate respiratory failure in some patients with chronic lung disease.

Opinions differ as to whether oxygen therapy should be given to *every* patient with prolonged chest discomfort due to myocardial ischemia. There are insufficient data to give a definite answer to the question, but it is unlikely that harm could come from such a practice.

Rawles and Kenmure did a controlled study involving 200 consecutive patients with myocardial infarction with one group receiving oxygen by face masks and the other receiving room air by face masks.[388] There was no significant difference in the number of deaths, mean duration of hospital stay, use of narcotic analgesics, systolic time intervals, and various arrhythmias between the oxygen-treated and room air–treated patients. The mean P_{a,O_2}, the incidence of sinus tachycardia, and the rise in cardiac enzyme levels were higher in the oxygen-treated group. Oxygen given by intermittent positive pressure can on occasion terminate arrhythmias.

To date, hyperbaric oxygen treatment for prolonged myocardial ischemia has not been found to be consistently useful.

The use of digitalis in patients with angina pectoris and myocardial infarction[390–393] *Digitalis* has been used in patients with angina pectoris, but the results are conflicting. The often-expressed feeling that digitalis, through its effect of increasing the force of myocardial contraction and oxygen consumption, can induce or aggravate angina pectoris due to coronary atherosclerosis has not been observed to be warranted by the authors. Digitalis can undoubtedly produce any arrhythmia in toxic doses, particularly in the presence of hypokalemia or renal failure. On the other hand, it may protect against or convert atrial arrhythmias to normal rhythm and, to a lesser extent, may abolish certain ventricular arrhythmias. Digitalis in excess may induce ventricular premature beats, but in patients with cardiac dysfunction ventricular premature beats may lessen or disappear after the proper use of the drug.

Ventricular dysfunction is common during angina pectoris, and the pulmonary wedge pressure may or may not be elevated during an attack.[389] The majority of available studies indicate no benefit in angina pectoris, even though there may be improvement of the ventricular performance. Most of the studies have been carried out over a period of 1 to 2 h, using limited amounts of glycosides intravenously.[390] There are no data on the effects on angina pectoris by optimal use of digitalis over weeks or months. Clinical impressions of benefit cannot be substantiated, particularly since nitroglycerin, dinitrate isosorbide, and beta-blocking agents may be used in conjunction with digitalis. Some authors have expressed the fear that digitalis could aggravate angina pectoris in patients without left ventricular dilatation, but in practice this must be a rare occurrence.

The direct effect of digitalis upon the myocardium is to increase the force of myocardial contractions with subsequent increase in oxygen consumption. In many patients with angina pectoris, the left ventricular volume and end-diastolic pressure are increased in association with a decrease in the rate of rise of left ventricular pressure. The administration of digitalis to such patients tends to reverse those abnormalities. Thus, the net effect of digitalis may be reduction of oxygen consumption and lessening of angina pectoris. On the other hand, there may be an increased rate of rise of left ventricular pressure than can offset the decreased left ventricular volume and end-diastolic pressure, causing angina at a lower level of exercise. We have observed improvement following the administration of digitalis to occasional patients with complaints of easy fatigability in the absence of clinical evidence of ventricular dysfunction following digitalization.

A trial of digitalis is indicated in the management of angina pectoris when any of the following is present: nocturnal angina pectoris; progressive angina pectoris; angina decubitus; cardiomegaly; large doses of propranolol; significant mitral regurgitation; atrial arrhythmias; S_3 gallop; rales due to pulmonary congestion; or x-ray evidence of interstitial edema; and for the complaint of breathlessness or easy fatigability produced by effort or during the period prior to open heart surgery (but not immediately before it).

Digitalis should not be given routinely to patients who have an *acute myocardial infarction*. Some studies have shown that certain of the actions of digitalis might be harmful and presumably could increase the size of the infarct and precipitate cardiac arrhythmias.[391-393] We cannot substantiate these fears in the day-to-day use of digitalis in practice. Accordingly, we use digoxin, being careful not to give excess dosage, in patients with infarction who develop the following: persistent sinus tachycardia; atrial fibrillation or flutter; ventricular gallop rhythm; rales in the lungs; evidence of pulmonary congestion on chest roentgenogram; and elevated neck veins.

See discussion regarding "The Treatment of Heart Failure" later in this chapter.

A shocking amount of ventricular dysfunction can be demonstrated by ventriculography in some patients with coronary atherosclerotic heart disease. Many of these patients have had unrecognized myocardial infarction(s). Even those hearts with normal contraction patterns and normal ventricular volumes at rest may show abrupt rises in left ventricular end-diastolic pressure when contrast medium is injected or when the heart rate is increased by atrial pacing. This is true even when the heart size is normal and there has been no past or present evidence of a failing heart. The effects of digitalis have been studied with partial digitalizing doses over a limited period of several hours in patients at rest. It is not surprising that the results reported are variable and show no consistent improvement in hemodynamic parameters. The studies do not answer the problem of whether beneficial effects can be obtained over a more protracted period of time with the effects of many physical and emotional upsets that are placed upon an abnormal heart. There is a high incidence of ventricular dysfunction 3 weeks following myocardial infarction, and digitalis may improve hemodynamics by, among other actions, a reduction of the left ventricular end-diastolic pressure.

All experts agree that digitalization is indicated where there is "significant" heart failure due to acute myocardial infarction. Does this mean when the patient complains of dyspnea, when there is alveolar edema, when the pulmonary wedge pressure reaches a certain level, or when marked interstitial edema is present in the x-ray? There is some pump dysfunction in all patients with myocardial infarction. At what point does one introduce an agent that increases the force of myocardial contraction? We would prefer to use digitalis early, hoping that progressive heart failure might be prevented, even though there is no sure evidence that this can be accomplished. The improvement in dynamics must surely offset whatever increase in myocardial oxygen consumption is elicited. Current recommendations by some authorities have discouraged physicians from using digitalis, even when there is pronounced heart failure. The fact that we now have effective means of improving pump dysfunction by drug manipulation of preload and afterload does not negate the use of digitalis in the treatment of the failing heart.

The use of drugs that alter platelet function and anticoagulants There is current widespread interest in the use of *acetyl salicylic acid* (and other drugs such as indomethacin, Persantin, etc.) for the prevention of coronary events including myocardial infarction.[394] The theory behind the idea holds that platelet aggregation and release is involved in the development of atherosclerosis and its complications. Acetyl salicylic acid (aspirin), in doses of 300 to 1,000 mg daily, inhibits prostaglandin G_2 synthesis, which in turn prevents the aggregation and release of platelets. The effect persists for the life-span of the platelets.[395,396]

The National Heart, Lung, and Blood Institute (NHLBI) has initiated the Aspirin Myocardial Infarction Study, involving 4,500 patients between 30 and 69 years of age who have had one or more documented myocardial infarctions in the last 5 years who are otherwise free from major disease. The study will test the hypothesis that regular administration of aspirin will reduce the risk of new heart attacks. The program will last 3 years, unless results warrant early termination. The volunteers have been randomized into placebo and drug groups, the latter receiving 1 g of aspirin a day.[397] A specific recommendation regarding the use of aspirin (and other drugs) for the purpose being discussed cannot be made at this time, because the scientific studies regarding their use have not been completed. Despite the incompleteness of our knowledge there is a current tendency to employ the drugs on a long-term basis.

The role of *Coumadin* and *heparin* in the management of coronary atherosclerotic heart disease continues to be unresolved to everyone's satisfaction.[398] The fact that no clear decisions have been reached after more than 33 years of debate indicates (1) either that the drug does not affect the course of the disease, (2) that while helpful in selected cases, it is not always beneficial as routine therapy, or (3) that other forms of therapy of proven benefit are more important than wallowing in the why's and wherefore's of anticoagulation.

Dr. Alfred Soffer[398] has pointed out, "It was born in controversy, and anticoagulants for ischemic heart disease continues to be a subject that rouses vigorous debate." Dr. Soffer, as editor of the *Archives of Internal Medicine,* then published two articles in which the authors held diametrically opposite views regarding the value of anticoagulation in the management of coronary atherosclerotic heart disease.

Rocel and Basson surveyed the practice of the use or nonuse of anticoagulant therapy in 239 teaching hospitals located in the United States, Great Britain, and western Europe.[399] Answers to 84 percent of the questionnaires were received. Of the American hospitals surveyed 28 percent administer anticoagulants to most patients with myocardial infarction; 72 percent anticoagulate few or no patients, or only 5 to 15 percent of patients with high risk of thromboembolic complications. The British hospitals are similar, and only 11 percent anticoagulate most patients with acute myocardial ischemia. In Germany, Switzerland, Holland, and Scandinavia the situation is opposite, with 85 percent anticoagulating most patients. Only 3 percent of American hospitals use long-term anticoagulant therapy. Such therapy was used for patients who had suffered from a thromboembolic episode or who had severe heart failure or paroxysmal arrhythmia. The practice in British hospitals was the same as that of the United States, while 60 percent of the European hospitals surveyed routinely anticoagulate all patients following infarction. Of American hospitals 41 percent anticoagulate patients with "preinfarction" syndromes, while 61 percent of the British and 67 percent of the European hospitals do so. Oral agents were used for anticoagulation in the 67 hospitals that anticoagulated most of their patients, whereas heparin or heparin followed by oral agents was used in hospitals that did not anticoagulate most of the patients. Rocel and Basson used the results of their survey to suggest that the time has come for the profession to search for a form of therapy that is more promising!

Modan, Schor, and Modan are in favor of the use of anticoagulants in the treatment of myocardial infarction[400] and therefore disagree with the opinions of Rocel and Basson.[399] Modan et al. believe that anticoagulant therapy is justified even if only a 1 percent reduction in hospital mortality is achieved.

We do not recommend the use of anticoagulation for patients with stable angina pectoris, unstable angina pectoris, prolonged myocardial ischemia with little objective evidence of infarction, or for uncomplicated myocardial infarction. We do recommend its use in myocardial infarction when any of the following are present and when there are no contraindications: (1) cardiomegaly, (2) suspected or proven ventricular aneurysm, (3) congestive heart failure present prior to acute myocardial infarction, (4) chronic atrial fibrillation, (5) history of prior infarction, (6) history of prior thrombophlebitis or embolism, (7) history of a prior transient ischemic attack, (8) in the presence of calf tenderness or obvious phlebitis, and (9) in patients who are obese or who are too feeble to ambulate. We stop anticoagulants in the presence of pericarditis, particularly if the pericardial rub is diffuse or if it persists 24 h.

We use 3-(α-acetonylbenzyl)-4-hydroxycoumarin sodium warfarin (Coumadin), for the acute episode after ascertaining that there is no contraindication to the use of the drug. Caution in the use of Coumadin is needed in the presence of renal disease or hepatic disease, or when therapy is required with drugs that interfere with the metabolism of Coumadin. The drug should not be used when there is a possibility of dissecting aneurysm or gastrointestinal bleeding. The drug is discontinued at the end of the period of hospitalization. We rarely use anticoagulants for coronary atherosclerotic heart disease on a long-term basis. We do not use heparin routinely. Coumadin is started after the base-line prothrombin time has been determined to be normal. A large loading dose of Coumadin is no longer recommended. The drug should be given orally 10 mg/day until the therapeutic range is reached, usually in 4 to 5 days. The therapeutic range is considered to be 20 to 30 percent of the control prothrombin time. Thereafter, the drug dosage is increased or decreased in order to maintain the prothrombin time in this range.

The list of drugs that may interact with Coumadin is now too long to remember. It is a potential problem especially when Coumadin is used over a long period of time when the prothrombin time is measured less frequently. The physician must have ready access to an up-to-date list of drugs which interact with Coumadin. The barbiturates, chloral hydrate, chloramphenicol, quinidine, salicylates, clofibrate, etc., are among the long list. We usually observe no problem with drug interaction if Coumadin is not used on a long-term basis and a prothrombin time is done daily while the patient is in the hospital. (The problem of drug interaction is a real one when Coumadin is used continuously in an effort to prevent pulmonary emboli.) Anticoagulants should be continued for 2 to 3 weeks (the period of hospitalization).

There is still no conclusive evidence that heparin is superior to Coumadin in preventing the thrombotic complications of myocardial infarction. Common sense dictates that the lag in reaching therapeutic levels with current methods of Coumadin administration allows the most fertile time for laying down thrombi—i.e., during the period when shock, pump failure, arrhythmias, and heart block are more common. While minidoses of heparin (5,000 units subcutaneously every 8 h) have been shown to lessen thromboembolism following surgical procedures, there are few data to support its use in patients with myocardial infarction, in whom it can be shown by ^{131}I fibrinogen tests that leg thrombi occur in 76 h, but in whom the incidence of clinically detectable embolism or mortality related to embolism is rare.[401] The use of early ambulation and antiembolism stocking may have reduced the threat of embolism.

The value of potent fibrinolytic agents such as urokinase and streptokinase is being investigated in patients with myocardial infarction, but little can be said about their effect at the time of this writing.[402]

Drugs used to lower blood lipid levels Blood lipid levels are often measured improperly, and the drugs used to lower blood lipid levels are often used poorly. The value of such an endeavor is now under considerable scrutiny and is being criticized by many. For further discussion see Chap. 62H.

Drugs used to manage arrhythmias (and sudden death) associated with coronary atherosclerotic heart disease See Chaps. 46D, 49, and 109 and later in this chapter.

Drugs used to manage shock associated with coronary atherosclerotic heart disease See Chaps. 48 and 109 and later in this chapter.

Drugs used to manage heart failure associated with coronary atherosclerotic heart disease See Chaps. 49 and 109 and later in this chapter.

SURGICAL PROCEDURES USED IN THE TREATMENT OF CORONARY ATHEROSCLEROTIC HEART DISEASE

Coronary bypass surgery[403] (see Chap. 62H) The medical management of clinical syndromes due to coronary atherosclerotic heart disease has improved considerably over the last few years. This has been due to improved recognition of the various clinical states (subsets), to the management of cardiac arrhythmias in the coronary care units, and to the use of propranolol. Despite these significant and dramatic advances, many patients with coronary atheroscle-

rotic heart disease die suddenly, sustain massive myocardial infarction, or have disabling symptoms. Therefore, it can be stated emphatically that our best medical management has not solved the problems of coronary atherosclerotic heart disease. Coronary bypass surgery has been a welcome form of treatment for carefully selected patients. It has now earned a solid place in the care of patients with coronary atherosclerotic heart disease. The procedure is used frequently in most medical centers in the United States. For example, coronary artery bypass (CAB) surgery is the most commonly performed operation at Emory University Hospital in Atlanta.

There are three major reasons why coronary artery bypass surgery is used more frequently today than it was a few years ago:

First, coronary arteriography, when performed by a highly skilled team, has become safe, almost painless, and is no longer frightening to the patient.[404,404a] Interobserver variation in interpretation is no longer a serious problem. The refinement in technique has encouraged the more liberal use of the procedure. Accordingly, we subject our patients to coronary arteriography much more readily today than we did a few years ago.

Second, cardiac surgeons have developed their surgical techniques to the point where the operative risk ranges from 1 to 4 percent, contingent upon the individual patient's clinical problem.[405] The overall operative mortality at Emory University Hospital is 1.4 percent. The mortality for the last 500 patients is 1 percent. In selected patients the risk at surgery is less than 1 percent. Coronary bypass surgery carries a lower mortality than does surgery for mitral valve or aortic valve disease. Saphenous vein grafts remain patent 85 to 90 percent of the time. Internal mammary arterial grafts remain patent about the same percentage of time. Complications of surgery include hemorrhage requiring reoperation, pericarditis, and rarely mediasternal or sternal infections. Perioperative infarction occurs in 6 percent of patients but this does not slow rehabilitation. Serum hepatitis has been a problem in some centers but has been rare at Emory University Hospital, which uses no paid "donors." Patients often go home on the seventh or eighth postoperative day.

The vast majority of patients, perhaps 80 percent, are relieved of their angina pectoris and are much happier following surgery. *In addition, it is now clear that coronary bypass surgery not only relieves symptoms but prolongs life in carefully selected patients.*

Third, some years ago when coronary artery bypass surgery was in its developmental stage it was customary to reserve its use for patients who were disabled with angina despite medical management. The decision to operate was based almost exclusively on the severity of the patient's symptoms. Physicians were reluctant to promise that the operation would decrease the risk of sudden death or myocardial infarction or that it would prolong life. Now, with more experience and with more scientific data available, the procedure is recommended much more frequently than it was a few years ago. Experience and observation has taught us the following: Whereas bypass surgery is used for patients with disabling angina pectoris occurring despite optimum medical management, it has been necessary to more carefully define "disabled" and "optimum medical management" so that unwarranted and dangerous delays are not justified under such a plan. Even more important than this change in attitude is the newly appreciated view that the severity of angina pectoris does not always parallel the degree of danger associated with the condition. Now that we can delineate the anatomy of the coronary arteries by coronary arteriography, it has become apparent that symptoms can be misleading, even to an expert. Some patients thought to have coronary atherosclerotic heart disease do not have it, while others thought to have very little coronary atherosclerotic heart disease may have extensive obstruction in the coronary arteries. We have learned that the history of chest discomfort does not always reveal a true picture of the degree of obstructive coronary disease that is present. Since sudden death and massive muscle destruction (infarction) are unacceptable ways of identifying coronary atherosclerotic heart disease and since symptoms do not always reveal a clear picture of the seriousness of the problem, it is necessary to develop a new approach to the problem. Accordingly, the current approach is to utilize the patient's symptoms together with the results of the exercise stress test and the findings at coronary arteriography and left ventriculography to determine the need and feasibility for coronary bypass surgery. The 5- and 10-year follow-up of patients with matched coronary lesions as determined by coronary arteriography is now available, and the results are clear. *These studies show that the coronary arteriogram and left ventriculogram give anatomic information which is not available by other methods used to study such patients. Furthermore, and very importantly, certain anatomic lesions indicate a very poor prognosis, while other lesions indicate a relatively good prognosis. The best prognostic guide available today is the results of the coronary arteriogram and left ventriculogram. High-grade obstruction of certain parts of the coronary tree demand urgent surgery even if minimum symptoms—or under carefully selected circumstances, no symptoms—are present. Therefore, we are now in an era when the patient's symptoms do not always dictate the need for bypass surgery and when the results of the exercise stress test and the coronary arteriogram and left ventriculogram influence our recommendation regarding the need for surgical intervention.*

Since it has become evident that the results of coronary arteriography play a major role in determining the need and possibility of coronary bypass surgery, it is important to appreciate that coronary blood flow does not diminish until there is a decrease in luminal diameter of approximately 50 percent (this corresponds to 75 percent of the cross-sectional obstruction of the vessel). It is essential to identify the area of myocardium served by each of the coronary arteries. This is governed by the unique distribution of the vessels. For example, obstruction of the left main coronary artery will jeopardize a very large amount of the left ventricle (including the septum); the left anterior descending artery is unique in that the septal perforator arteries originate all along its course. Therefore, a large amount of the septum will be jeopardized when there is a proximal obstruction of this vessel compared with an obstruction further down its course. The circumflex coronary artery terminates in one, two, or more major divisions. Because of this, an obstruction of the circumflex prior to dividing will jeopardize more myocardium than will obstruction of one of its divisions; the right coronary artery is a long conduit. Accordingly, an obstruction anywhere along its course will jeopardize the posterior circulation of the left ventricle. Either the right coronary artery or circumflex coronary artery usually dominates the posterior left ventricular circulation. It is important to identify which of the two vessels supplies blood to this area of the left ventricle.

Anatomic lesions that compel us to consider coronary artery bypass surgery are

- High-grade obstruction of the left main coronary artery.
- High-grade obstruction of the proximal left anterior descending, proximal circumflex, and right coronary arteries.
- High-grade obstruction of the proximal left anterior descending and the proximal circumflex coronary arteries.
- High-grade obstruction of the proximal left anterior descending and right coronary arteries.
- High-grade obstruction of the proximal circumflex and right coronary arteries.
- High-grade obstruction of the proximal portion of the left anterior descending artery if symptoms are sufficient to justify surgical intervention. What to do about the asymptomatic patient has not been settled. We tend to go ahead with surgery if the patient is young and if the exercise test is clearly positive since our studies show that death and massive infarction can be caused by this lesion.
- High-grade obstruction of the mid or distal portion of the left anterior descending artery if symptoms are sufficient to justify surgical intervention.
- High-grade obstruction of the circumflex artery if symptoms are sufficient to justify surgical intervention.
- High-grade obstruction of the right coronary artery if symptoms are sufficient to justify surgical intervention.

Anatomic lesions that usually persuade us to use medical management rather than bypass surgery include:

- High-grade obstruction of the mid or distal portion of the left anterior descending artery in a patient with no symptoms or with mild stable angina pectoris.
- High-grade obstruction of the circumflex artery or its branches in a patient with no symptoms or with mild stable angina pectoris.

- High-grade obstruction of the right coronary artery in a patient with no symptoms or with mild stable angina pectoris.
- Inoperable distal coronary arteries where bypass surgery is not possible.
- Left ventricular disease that contradicts the use of bypass surgery.

A number of "controlled" studies will soon be released so that we may all analyze them. The studies will point out that modern medical management has improved and that modern medical or surgical treatment of coronary atherosclerotic heart disease has altered the natural history of the disease in a very favorable manner. The studies will show that bypass surgery clearly decreases the degree of angina pectoris in most patients who have not responded properly to medical management. Some studies will show that longevity is not altered by surgical intervention with the exception of obstruction of the left main coronary artery. It will be important to note the length of the follow-up period in these studies. The difference in longevity in a surgically treated group as compared to the longevity of a matched medically treated group may not be apparent until after 5 or more years. In addition, it will be important to note the initial operative mortality because some of the studies will reveal a very high (5 percent) hospital mortality. The whole story is not told in determining how long patients live. For example, a patient may have several infarcts and heart failure but live a number of years. Some of the studies will not emphasize this aspect of the problem.

Common sense dictates to us that proximal triple-vessel disease is nearly as bad as obstruction of the left main coronary artery. Obviously, obstruction may become critical in only one of these vessels at any one point in time but the prospect of sudden death or muscle destruction appears certain in such patients and a ten-year follow-up supports this view. Common sense also dictates that there is not 100 percent difference in the prognosis of a patient with left main or proximal triple-vessel coronary obstruction and proximal double-vessel disease when one of the vessels is the left anterior descending artery. This argument could be expanded but the principle is clear enough without further discussion.

We are liberal with coronary bypass surgery because the hospital mortality for bypass surgery at Emory University Hospital is 1 percent. The mortality in carefully selected patients is 0.2 to 0.6 percent. One of our surgeons has operated on 407 consecutive patients without a death. We would not be so liberal with our indications for surgery if there was an initial operative mortality of 5 percent.

We require more symptoms in the older age groups of patients (beyond 65 years of age) before we recommend bypass coronary artery surgery. The younger the patient, the fewer symptoms we demand and the more we depend on the type of coronary anatomy to determine if bypass surgery should be done. Surgery is done in the older age group to relieve symptoms. Surgery is done in the younger group to relieve symptoms but also to—we hope— group to relieve symptoms but also to—we hope—

prolong life over the next 10 years. In this group we hope to prevent sudden death and infarctions.

Finally, since bypass surgery can be performed with such incredibly low operative risk and since we also recommend the routine long-term use of propranolol along with long-acting nitrites when needed, we are in the position of offering the patient a combination of surgical *and* medical management rather than surgery *or* medical management.

As time passes new data will alter our views just as there is a difference in our recommendations in this edition of *The Heart* compared to the recommendations that we offered in the previous edition.

See Chap. 62H for further discussion of coronary bypass surgery.

Ileal bypass to lower blood lipid levels (see Chap. 62H) Ileal bypass has been used to alter blood lipid levels. The operation includes the surgical removal of the terminal third of the ileum and end-to-end anastomosis to the proximal portion of the cecum. It has been tolerated reasonably well and has not produced malabsorption, except of vitamin B_{12}, which can be replaced by parenteral injection. The serum level of cholesterol may fall a remarkable degree after this procedure. Levels below 200 mg/100 ml have been achieved in about half the patients. Despite the dramatic results of this procedure, it is unlikely that the operation will ever be used to any degree except in carefully selected patients.

THE MANAGEMENT OF SPECIFIC CLINICAL SYNDROMES

The general principles involved in the care of the patient with coronary atherosclerotic heart disease are discussed in the preceding section of this chapter. The reader should refer to that section for a general discussion regarding the facilities, equipment, personnel and logistics required to deliver care; mental rest and patient psychology; rehabilitation (rest and exercise); diet and eating; the use of alcohol and tobacco; drugs used to relieve and prevent myocardial ischemia, including nitroglycerin, nitrol ointment, isosorbide dinitrate, and propranolol; the use of opiates and oxygen; the use of anticoagulants; the control of hyperlipidemia; some simple procedures; the indications for coronary bypass surgery; and a discussion of the experimental procedure ileal bypass. The purpose of this chapter is to apply the principles discussed earlier to specific clinical syndromes. Accordingly, the thirteen clinical syndromes discussed earlier in the section entitled "The Recognition of Specific Clinical Syndromes" will be discussed here. Actual examples of patients will be utilized in order to make the presentation as realistic as possible. The material has been arranged so that the number used to designate the discussion of the *recognition* of the clinical syndrome is also used to designate the discussion of the *treatment* of the syndrome. The treatment of complications of coronary atherosclerotic heart disease is discussed at the end of this chapter.

1 THE TREATMENT OF PATIENTS WITH CORONARY ATHEROSCLEROTIC HEART DISEASE WHO HAVE NO CHEST DISCOMFORT

The recognition of patients with coronary atherosclerotic heart disease who have no chest discomfort is discussed earlier in this chapter in the section "The Patient with Coronary Atherosclerotic Heart Disease Who Has No Chest Discomfort." Patients who experience *sudden death* do not usually recover (see Chap. 49). *Some do, however, because the catastrophe occurs at a place where resuscitative measures can be successfully implemented.* Survivors should be admitted to the coronary care unit for futher observation and where the prompt treatment of cardiac arrhythmias is possible. Some of these patients develop evidence of myocardial infarction, but many do not. Should infarction become apparent, the patient is managed as such (see discussion later in this chapter). In any case, the treatment of cardiac arrhythmias with lidocaine, propranolol, digitalis, procainamide, or quinidine is indicated (see discussion later). Should infarction become apparent it is usually wise to wait several weeks before a coronary arteriogram is performed. If infarction is not apparent, it is appropriate to move quickly and perform a coronary arteriogram. The need for bypass surgery will be dictated by the findings in the coronary arteriogram and left ventriculogram in such patients. Surgery will be indicated for certain lesions and not indicated for others (see discussion in "Coronary Bypass Surgery" earlier in this chapter). Patients who are operated on are often placed on long-term propranolol, digoxin, and aspirin unless there is some contraindication to the use of these drugs. The value of propranolol can be defended by available data. Digoxin is used because the patient is on propranolol. The value of aspirin cannot be proven at this time. The same medication should be used in patients who are not subjected to bypass surgery.

Patients without symptoms who exhibit a positive "ischemia" response in the exercise electrocardiogram are being discovered by the hundreds. There are no data that clearly indicate the value of exercise testing of all patients beyond the age of 40. It is clear, however, that positive "ischemic" responses will be discovered when such is done. Accordingly, it is essential to be prepared to react to the discovery of a positive test. The question is, What does a positive response mean and what should be done about it? We need a great deal more information on this subject. We know that false positive responses occur in the

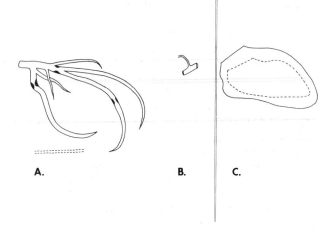

FIGURE 62E-21 Diagram of the coronary arteriogram and left ventriculogram of a 40-year-old man. Five years earlier he experienced anterior chest discomfort lasting 30 min while playing basketball. He denied chest discomfort or any other complaints even though he did manual labor. A recent exercise electrocardiogram revealed surprising and frightening abnormalities. The ST segment became displaced 3 mm, and a short bout of ventricular tachycardia developed after 20 s of exercise in stage 1 of the Bruce exercise test. Coronary bypass surgery was performed even though he had been asymptomatic for 5 years. He had no symptoms or arrhythmia following surgery. At the time of this writing the exercise test has not been repeated.

Pressures: Ao, 120/80; LVEDP pre angiogram, 10; LVEDP post angiogram, 15. (Ao=aortic; LVEDP=left ventricular end-diastolic pressure.)

A. Right anterior oblique view of left coronary artery. 99 percent of the proximal circumflex coronary artery with distal posterolateral obtuse marginal branch 2 mm in diameter. 75 percent stenosis of the left anterior descending coronary artery just distal to first septal perforator with distal vessel 2 mm in diameter; another 60 percent stenotic lesion in the mid left anterior descending artery. The posterior descending branch of the right coronary artery is visualized via collaterals and is less than 1 mm in diameter. *B.* Left anterior oblique view of right coronary artery. Total occlusion of proximal right coronary artery. *C.* Left ventriculogram shows severe inferior and mild anterior hypokinesia. (*This study was done in the cardiac catheterization laboratory at Emory University Hospital, Atlanta, Georgia. We wish to thank Dr. Spencer King, Dr. Ham McGill, Diane Anderson, and Steve Hudson for performing the test.*)

male population above 40 years of age, but that false positive responses occur with great frequency in the female population under 40 years of age. We know that false negative tests occur in all groups, but it is better to have a negative response than a positive one. We know that a coronary arteriogram gives more reliable information than does the exercise test. We are all plagued with the memory of asymptomatic patients who for one reason or another had an exercise test performed and that the positive response led us to obtain a coronary arteriogram which revealed severe, precarious, obstructive coronary disease (see Figs. 62E-21 and 62E-22). The problem is that we do not yet know how often this sequence of events occurs. It is possible that many patients in this group are the very patients who have sudden death—a catastrophe we must learn to prevent, since

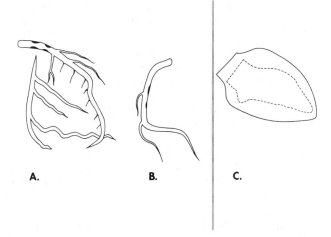

A.   **B.**   **C.**

FIGURE 62E-22 Diagram of the coronary arteriogram and left ventriculogram of a 46-year-old man. This patient was "asymptomatic" but was found to have 2.5 mm of ST-segment displacement during stage 1 of the Bruce test. The electrocardiogram was made as part of an insurance examination. After repeated questioning, the patient agreed that he had the slightest discomfort on vigorous effort such as playing tennis. (It is not known to this day if the initial history was a false negative response or if the later histories were taught and learned by the patient and were therefore false positive responses.) The positive stress test led to the coronary arteriogram, which revealed severe obstructive disease. He underwent successful coronary bypass surgery. He is now asymptomatic. Dr. William Waters kindly referred this patient to J.W.H.
Pressures: Ao, 120/75; LV, 120/80; LVEDP post angiogram, 12.
A. Right anterior oblique view of the left coronary artery. Two 75 percent cross-sectional stenoses are present in the proximal left anterior descending coronary artery. The distal left anterior descending artery is 2.5 mm in diameter, with mild lumen irregularity present. The circumflex coronary artery is totally occluded at its origin. The distal circumflex artery is opacified in a retrograde fashion via collaterals from the anterior descending artery. The obtuse marginal branches are over 2 mm in diameter distally and are angiographically normal. *B.* Approximately 60 percent cross-sectional narrowing is present in the proximal right coronary artery. The distal right coronary artery is 1.5 mm in diameter and suitable for coronary bypass. *C.* Left ventriculogram shows mild apical hypokinesia. (*This study was done in the cardiac catheterization laboratory at Emory University Hospital, Atlanta, Georgia. We wish to thank Dr. Spencer King, Dr. Ham McGill, Diane Anderson, and Steve Hudson for performing the test.*)

a large percent of deaths due to coronary disease occur in this manner.[117h,117i] We recommend the following plan at this time. As new information accrues, we may, of course, change our minds. We recommend that an exercise test be performed every 2 years on all males between 40 and 65 years of age and on all women who are 50 to 65 years of age. Those men and women who develop a positive response in the electrocardiogram of 2 mm or more during stage 1 or 2 of the Bruce exercise test or who develop angina pectoris or a serious arrhythmia during the exercise test should have a coronary arteriogram performed. The indications for bypass surgery will be dictated by the findings in the coronary arteriogram in such patients. Surgery will be indicated for certain lesions and not indicated for others (see "Coronary Bypass Surgery" earlier in

this chapter). Patients who develop more than 2 mm of ST-segment displacement or angina pectoris or an arrhythmia during stage 3 or 4 of the treadmill test should have a coronary arteriogram performed. Surgical treatment is then dictated by the findings in the coronary arteriogram (see "Coronary Bypass Surgery"). Patients who have 2 mm or less of ST-segment displacement during stage 3 or 4 of the exercise test would not have a coronary arteriogram performed. These latter patients should be followed carefully, and an exercise test should be repeated twice a year. The plan will, of course, permit one to miss occasional patients with high-grade lesions who have only a slightly positive exercise test at stage 3 and 4 of the Bruce test. This plan seems to be a practical screening procedure, for otherwise we would have to do coronary arteriograms on all asymptomatic adults—a plan that cannot be justified at this time.

Patients may experience *exhaustion* rather than chest discomfort as a manifestation of myocardial ischemia. The exhaustion may be felt continuously for several weeks, or the patient may feel abrupt exhaustion on effort with or without dyspnea (see discussion earlier in "The Patient with Coronary Atherosclerotic Heart Disease Who Has No Discomfort"). This sensation in a patient should prompt the physician to obtain an exercise stress test. If the test is positive, especially if the ST segment becomes displaced 2 mm or more during stage 1 or 2, a coronary arteriogram should be performed. The need for bypass surgery is determined by the findings in the arteriograms of such patients; surgery will be indicated for certain lesions and not indicated for others (see earlier discussion regarding "Coronary Bypass Surgery"). Figure 62E-23 illustrates a patient with this problem.

Adult patients with aortic and mitral valve disease who have no chest discomfort should have coronary arteriograms during the cardiac catheterization which is done for valve disease. The need for coronary bypass surgery is determined by the findings in the coronary arteriogram and left ventriculogram (see earlier section "Coronary Bypass Surgery" and items 11 and 12 later in this section).

The role cardiac radionuclide imaging will play in the evaluation of the patients that fall into the categories discussed above is not known at the present time, but the technique promises to be quite valuable. It may be especially useful in studying patients after coronary artery surgery has been performed (see "Radionuclide Angiography" which appeared earlier in this chapter).

2 THE MANAGEMENT OF THE PATIENTS WITH STABLE ANGINA PECTORIS

The recognition of stable angina is discussed earlier in "The Patient with Stable Angina Pectoris."

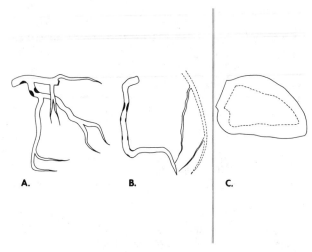

FIGURE 62E-23 Diagram of the coronary arteriogram and left ventriculogram of a 53-year-old man. The patient had complained of mild anterior chest discomfort produced by effort for 4 years. More troublesome to him, however, was the feeling of extreme weakness he had experienced for 9 months and the abrupt and transient exhaustion he felt when he walked a short distance. This feeling was reproduced on the treadmill at which time his blood pressure decreased and 2 to 3 mm of ST-segment displacement was noted on the electrocardiogram. Coronary bypass surgery relieved all of his symptoms. This is an example of transient left ventricular dysfunction produced by myocardial ischemia provoked by effort. Some patients have this syndrome and have weakness and dyspnea without angina pectoris. This patient had remarkable improvement after surgery. He could hunt for hours without angina or exhaustion. Dr. Jack Kaufman kindly referred this patient to J.W.H.

A. Right anterior oblique view of left coronary artery. Total occlusion of left anterior descending coronary artery just distal to first septal perforator. 90 percent stenosis of proximal circumflex coronary artery with distal anterolateral obtuse marginal branch 2.5 mm in diameter. 60 percent stenosis of left main coronary artery. *B*. 80 percent stenosis of proximal right coronary artery with distal posterior descending branch 2.5 mm in diameter. There is collateral filling of the distal left anterior descending coronary artery, which is 2 mm in diameter. *C*. Normal left ventriculogram. (*This study was done in the cardiac catheterization laboratory at Emory University Hospital, Atlanta, Georgia. We wish to thank Dr. Spencer King, Dr. Ham McGill, Diane Anderson, and Steve Hudson for performing the test.*)

Aggravating and precipitating factors   Always, it is important to search for factors that could precipitate or aggravate angina pectoris. These include anemia, thyrotoxicosis, etc. Such conditions must be treated and, in the case of anemia, the etiology must be identified.

Body weight and diet Patients with stable angina pectoris should achieve and maintain a normal body weight by eating the proper number of calories each day. The diet should be low in saturated fat, cholesterol, and refined carbohydrates (see Chap. 62H).

Activity The patient should be as active as the stable angina pectoris will permit. Walking is an excellent type of exercise because it is so controllable. Formal exercise programs are useful for some patients. Patients with mild angina pectoris usually continue their work. Many patients with disabling stable angina pectoris cannot work, and some, especially those with rest pain, are confined to rest in a chair.

Anxiety and stress Stressful situations should be avoided when possible.

Use of tobacco and alcohol Patients with stable angina pectoris should not use tobacco. Small amounts of alcohol may be permitted in selected patients.

Drugs Patients with stable angina pectoris should be given nitroglycerin for angina when it occurs and should use the drug to prevent episodes of angina pectoris when attacks can be anticipated. It is wise to begin with using 0.16 mg (1/400 gr) of nitroglycerin and later to increase the dosage to 0.32 mg (1/200 gr) and 0.64 mg (1/100 gr) in an effort to relieve angina pectoris without causing headache, since the development of the latter may cause the patient to avoid using the drug. The drug is discussed in detail in the section "Nitroglycerin" which appeared earlier in this chapter.

Nitrol ointment is usually not used for mild angina pectoris but is commonly used for disabling angina pectoris. One-half inch of 2 percent nitroglycerin ointment should be used two to four times a day at the outset. The drug dosage is then increased until the relief of angina pectoris occurs or until headache develops. The dosage is then adjusted until no headache develops.

Isosorbide dinitrate should be used every 3 to 4 h during waking hours. The drug is discussed in detail in "Long-acting Nitrites" earlier in this chapter. The chewable variety of the drug is recommended. The usual starting dose is 5 mg four to six times a day. It may be increased until a slight headache is noted, and then the dosage should be decreased.

As discussed in "Beta Blockers" earlier, almost all patients with angina pectoris should be given propranolol. When the diagnosis of angina pectoris is made, we do not wait to study the effect of isosorbide dinitrate before we start propranolol. It is wise to start with 10 mg four times a day and increase the dosage every 3 days until the heart rate is 50 to 60 beats per minute, or until satisfactory relief has been obtained.

We do not recommend that all types of drug regimens be tried to relieve angina pectoris. The preceding approach is quite satisfactory with specific endpoints to achieve. A system that permits procrastination must be avoided, since this may cause one to delay the performance of a coronary arteriogram and possible bypass surgery. Anticoagulants are not used in the treatment of patients with stable angina pectoris.

Exercise test The reader is referred to the discussion in Chap. 28A and to "The Use and Limitations of the Electrocardiogram" earlier in this chapter. An exercise test is carefully performed on most patients with stable angina pectoris. This is especially true for patients with mild angina pectoris who are active and working. It is done in an effort to determine how active the patient can be without danger signals appearing in the exercise electrocardiogram. In addition, a markedly positive test (2 to 3 mm ST-segment displacement) produced by a low workload (stage 1 or 2 of the Bruce test) is associated with a more serious prognosis and should prompt one to move more quickly to coronary arteriography.

Finally, it is useful to have an exercise electrocardiogram done prior to coronary artery bypass surgery to use as a control tracing for comparison with a postoperative exercise test in order to assess the effect of surgical intervention. Patients with stable but disabling angina pectoris should not be routinely exercised on the treadmill, since they are at greater risk from the procedure and because a sense of urgency already exists.

Coronary arteriography We now recommend that patients under the age of 65 with stable angina pectoris should have a coronary arteriogram performed. This is true even if nitroglycerin, isosorbide dinitrate, and propranolol have affected the angina in a favorable manner. Patients with stable but disabling angina pectoris should have a coronary arteriogram regardless of age unless other disease contradicts the wisdom of such a recommendation. In practice, it is rare that coronary arteriography is recommended beyond the age of 75. The reason a coronary arteriogram is needed in all patients is to delineate the anatomy of the coronary arteries, since such information assists one in determining the prognosis and the need for surgical interventions.

Cardiac radionuclide imaging As discussed earlier in "Cardiac Radionuclide Angiography," cardiac radionuclide imaging, especially before and after exercise, promises to give information that will be useful in the evaluation of patients with stable angina pectoris. The technique is not yet readily available in all locales. It may give useful information when done prior to and after coronary bypass surgery.

Coronary artery surgery The need for coronary bypass surgery will be dictated by the findings in the coronary arteriogram and left ventriculogram of patients with stable angina pectoris. Surgery will be indicated for certain lesions and not indicated for others (see discussion in "Coronary Bypass Surgery" earlier in this chapter). Figure 62E-24 illustrates a patient with this problem.

We commonly recommend surgery for patients under 65 years of age with mild stable angina pectoris if the coronary anatomy dictates the need and if we believe we can improve the prognosis of the patient. Coronary bypass surgery is offered to patients with stable angina pectoris beyond the age of 65 if the discomfort interferes with their life and if the coronary anatomy is favorable for surgery. In practice, it is uncommon to recommend the procedure for patients with stable angina pectoris beyond the age of 75, but it is not rare to recommend the procedure for patients who are 70 to 75 years of age (Fig. 62E-24).

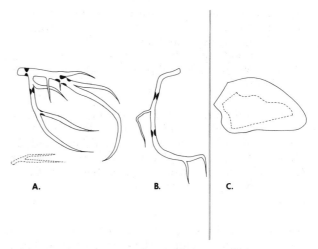

A. **B.** **C.**

FIGURE 62E-24 Diagram of the coronary arteriogram and left ventriculogram of a 74-year-old man. This patient had experienced angina pectoris produced by effort for several years. Because of his age, an attempt was made to control his angina pectoris with Inderal, isosorbide dinitrate, nitrol ointment, and nitroglycerin. The angina increased until it interfered with happiness to the degree that bypass surgery was performed. He is now active without symptoms and contributes significantly to the management of his community affairs. Dr. Irwin Leider kindly referred this patient to J.W.H.

Pressures; Ao 146/80; LVEDP pre angiogram, 10; LVEDP post angiogram, 36.

A. Right anterior oblique view of left coronary artery. 90 percent stenosis of left main coronary artery and 90 percent stenosis of left anterior descending coronary artery just distal to the first septal perforator, with distal left anterior descending artery 2.5 mm in diameter. 90 percent stenosis of proximal circumflex coronary artery and 90 percent stenosis of anterolateral obtuse marginal branch, with two distal obtuse marginal branches 2.5 mm in diameter. There is collateral filling of the distal right coronary artery. *B.* Left anterior oblique view of right coronary artery. 75 percent stenosis of proximal right coronary artery and 90 percent stenosis of the mid right coronary artery, with the distal vessel and posterior descending branch 2 mm in diameter. *C.* Left ventriculogram shows inferior wall hypokinesia. (*This study was done in the cardiac catheterization laboratory at Emory University Hospital, Atlanta, Georgia. We wish to thank Dr. Spencer King, Dr. Ham McGill, Diane Anderson, and Steve Hudson for performing the test.*)

Following surgery we commonly prescribe propranolol, digoxin, and aspirin even when the patient does not complain of angina. This action is based on the preliminary data that suggests that cardiac arrhythmias and sudden death are less common in patients with coronary atherosclerotic heart disease who are maintained on propranolol.[379] Digoxin is used because the patient is on propranolol. The value of aspirin cannot be proven at this time.

3 THE MANAGEMENT OF THE PATIENT WITH UNSTABLE ANGINA PECTORIS

The definition and recognition of unstable angina pectoris is discussed earlier in "The Patient with Unstable Angina Pectoris" and in Chap. 62A.

Aggravating and precipitating factors Such factors as anemia (usually from bleeding from the gastrointestinal system), thyrotoxicosis, etc., must be ruled out as a possible cause of unstable angina pectoris. When such factors are found, they must be treated promptly.

Body weight and diet The patient should attain and maintain lean body weight by limiting caloric intake and decreasing the intake of saturated fat, cholesterol, and refined carbohydrates (see Chap. 62H). The patient with frequent bouts of angina pectoris may profit from eating smaller portions of food.

Activity Activity should be curtailed in patients with unstable angina pectoris. The degree of curtailment depends upon the particular variety of unstable angina pectoris the patient exhibits. Certain patients may remain at home and be allowed activity within the house. An obvious example of this type of patient is the elderly patient with many problems in addition to angina pectoris. Most patients who have frequently recurring angina pectoris, especially occurring at rest, should be admitted to the hospital. The more severe cases should be admitted to the coronary care unit. Admission to the hospital serves four purposes. First, it permits some patients to escape a stressful emotional situation at home. Second, it is possible to make observations in the hospital that cannot be made at home. For example, it is useful to record an electrocardiogram during an episode of angina pectoris in order to identify Prinzmetal's angina and to observe the effect of medication on the angina pectoris. Third, hospitalization also makes it possible for the medical staff to identify complications such as arrhythmias and to treat them promptly. Finally, many patients with unstable angina should have a coronary arteriogram performed, and hospitalization permits careful planning of the procedure.

Patients with unstable angina pectoris who, for one reason or another, do not have coronary artery surgery should be rehabilitated like a patient with a small myocardial infarction (see discussion in item 6 later in this section).

Anxiety and stress Stressful situations should be avoided when possible. A mild sedative or tranquilizer, such as diazepam, may be used with success in some patients.

Use of tobacco and alcohol Patients with unstable angina pectoris should not use tobacco. Small amounts of alcohol may be permitted in selected patients.

Drugs Patients with unstable angina pectoris should receive nitroglycerin, isosorbide dinitrate, nitrol ointment, and propranolol in appropriate dosage (see

discussion regarding these drugs earlier in this chapter). Patients with unstable angina pectoris are not anticoagulated.

Exercise test As a general rule, it is not wise to perform an exercise stress test on patients with unstable angina pectoris. The only value an exercise test has in this group of patients is to have a control tracing prior to bypass surgery so that the exercise electrocardiogram made after surgery may be compared to it. While this information is useful, it is not of sufficient value to justify any risk to the patient that might occur during the exercise test. The exercise electrocardiogram is not needed for diagnostic reasons, since most of these patients will undergo coronary arteriography, and the decision regarding the need for surgery is usually based upon the extent and location of the obstructing lesions.

Coronary arteriography Most patients with unstable angina pectoris should have a coronary arteriogram performed. The delineation of the coronary artery anatomy is necessary in order to determine the feasibility of coronary bypass surgery and to determine prognosis. Coronary arteriography is not usually recommended in patients with unstable angina pectoris who are beyond 75 years of age, but it is not rare to recommend the procedure in patients who are 70 to 75 years of age.

Cardiac radionuclide imaging Myocardial perfusion can be estimated by cardiac radionuclide imaging. The role this technique will have in the study of patients with unstable angina pectoris has not yet been determined. It may give useful information if done prior to and after coronary bypass surgery.

Coronary artery surgery As stated above, most patients with unstable angina pectoris should have a coronary arteriogram. Coronary arteriography is not usually recommended for patients with unstable angina pectoris who are beyond 75 years of age. It follows that coronary artery surgery is usually not utilized for patients who are beyond 75 years of age. The feasibility of coronary bypass surgery is determined by the coronary anatomy revealed in the coronary arteriogram of patients with unstable angina pectoris. Coronary bypass surgery should be performed in such patients when the coronary arteriogram reveals high-grade lesions that are bypassable and when there are no contraindications to the procedure (Fig. 62E-25). See earlier section "Coronary Bypass Surgery" for further discussion of the coronary anatomy that compels one toward surgical treatment. Coronary artery surgery would not be recommended for patients with significant obstruction of the right coronary artery or circumflex artery (or a combination of each) unless the unstable angina pectoris showed no evidence of subsiding.

We commonly prescribe propranolol, digoxin, and aspirin following coronary artery surgery, hoping that cardiac arrhythmias will be significantly decreased. Current data support the use of propranolol,

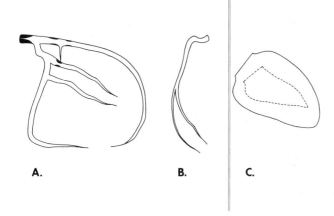

A.   **B.**   **C.**

FIGURE 62E-25 A diagram of the coronary arteriogram and left ventriculogram of a 58-year-old man. This patient had angina pectoris produced by effort for 4 months. The angina was increasing in frequency and occurred at rest. He was far more concerned about the pain associated with a kidney stone. The resting tracing showed ST-segment displacement, and an exercise test was not done. This patient illustrates that severe obstructive disease may produce mild symptoms. He had successful coronary bypass surgery. The patient had no angina pectoris after surgery. Dr. John Alley kindly referred this patient to J.W.H.

    A. Right anterior oblique view of left coronary artery. Greater than 95 percent cross-sectional stenosis of left main coronary artery with less than 50 percent narrowing of proximal left anterior descending. There is also a 60 percent stenotic lesion in a small anterolateral obtuse marginal branch. The distal left anterior descending, obtuse marginal, and posterior descending coronary arteries are 2 mm in diameter. *B.* Left anterior oblique view of right coronary artery. Small, nondominant right coronary artery which is free of disease. *C.* Normal left ventriculogram. (*This study was done in the cardiac catheterization laboratory at Emory University Hospital, Atlanta, Georgia. We wish to thank Dr. John Douglas, Dr. George Krisle, Gail Nelbach, and Rick Brown for performing the test.*)

and digoxin is given because the patient is on propranolol. The value of aspirin has not been proven.

4 THE MANAGEMENT OF THE PATIENT WITH PROLONGED CHEST DISCOMFORT DUE TO MYOCARDIAL ISCHEMIA WHO HAS NO RECENT SIGNS OF INFARCTION

The definition and recognition of prolonged chest discomfort due to myocardial ischemia is discussed earlier in "The Patient with Prolonged Chest Discomfort Who Has No Recent Objective Signs of Infarction" and in Chap. 62A. The approach to the management of the patient with prolonged chest discomfort due to myocardial ischemia who has no objective evidence of infarction is no different from the approach to the management of the patient with small infarction (see item 6 of this section for further discussion). These patients may have a single episode or may have repeated bouts of prolonged chest discomfort at rest. The electrocardiogram may show ST or T-wave change, but no QRS changes. The electrocardiogram may show subendocardial injury

during an episode of chest pain. The level of serum cardiac enzymes does not rise.

Aggravating and precipitating factors   Factors that influence the oxygen delivery system to the myocardium should be sought for and eliminated. These include anemia (often from blood loss), thyrotoxicosis, and cardiac arrhythmia, such as paroxysmal atrial tachycardia, etc.

Body weight and diet   Such patients should attain and maintain a normal body weight. This should be accomplished by reducing the daily intake of calories, saturated fat, cholesterol, and carbohydrates (see Chap. 62H).

Activity   Patients with this syndrome should, as a rule, be admitted to the coronary care unit where one has better control of the heart rhythm. The patient is usually comfortable within 3 days, but prognostication is more difficult than it is with a completed infarction. Recurrent pain following transfer out of the coronary unit is common and may require readmission to the coronary care unit. The patient may be permitted to sit in a comfortable chair during the hospital stay; and if for some reason coronary arteriography and coronary artery surgery are not performed, the patient is usually able to go to home care after 2 weeks.

Anxiety and stress   Anxiety and stress must be eliminated when possible. Admission to the hospital creates anxiety in many patients, but we have been equally impressed with the reduction of stress that occurs when certain patients are admitted to the hospital. A mild sedative or tranquilizer such as diazepam may be helpful.

Use of tobacco and alcohol   Patients with this syndrome should not use tobacco. Small amounts of alcohol may be permitted in selected patients.

Drugs   Patients who have episodes of prolonged chest discomfort yet show no objective signs of myocardial necrosis (though a small amount of necrosis is undoubtedly present) should receive nitroglycerin, isosorbide dinitrate, propranolol, nitrol ointment, and appropriate opiates in an effort to prevent or release the episodes of discomfort. The drugs must be given in proper dosage (see earlier discussion in this chapter). Antiarrhythmic drugs other than propranolol are not given routinely. Oxygen is not given routinely. Anticoagulants are not prescribed unless certain conditions are met (see earlier discussion and discussion in item 6).

Procedures   The patient's heart rhythm is continuously monitored. An indwelling catheter is inserted into an arm vein (usually at the wrist of the left hand for patients who are right-handed) in order to guarantee an open intravenous route and to enable one to avoid intramuscular injections that produce confusion in the interpretation of the serum creatine phosphokinase level. The determination of serum cardiac enzyme levels is much more important in this syndrome than it is in patients with "Q-wave infarcts." A plan for determining the serum level of cardiac enzymes, especially the creatine phosphokinase (CPK) and its isoenzyme (MB of CPK) must be implemented with precision (see discussion earlier in "The Use and Abuse of Cardiac Enzyme Levels"). A 12-lead electrocardiogram should be obtained during an episode of chest discomfort in order to study the ST-segment shift, since a small percentage of these patients have the variant angina (Prinzmetal) syndrome (see discussion in item 5 in this section).

Exercise test An exercise stress test is not recommended in these patients.

Coronary arteriography Unless there are compelling reasons not to perform a coronary arteriogram, it should be done as soon as it is feasible to do so. Patients with heart failure or other serious diseases and patients beyond age 75 should not, as a rule, be studied by coronary arteriography. Since the bulk of patients are not in such exceptional groups, we perform coronary arteriography in most patients with prolonged episodes of myocardial ischemia.

Cardiac radionuclide imaging The role of cardiac radionuclide imaging in patients with prolonged chest pain has not yet been established. It would seem to offer much promise since we need a new method of identifying areas of poor perfusion and infarction. It may yield useful information if done prior to and after coronary bypass surgery.

Coronary artery surgery We recommend coronary artery bypass surgery be performed in patients with bouts of prolonged myocardial ischemia who have no objective signs of myocardial infarction if the coronary arteriogram reveals the proper anatomy (Fig. 62E-26). This recommendation usually applies to patients who are under 75 years of age and have no other diseases that contraindicate surgical intervention. The indications for coronary bypass surgery are discussed earlier in "Coronary Bypass Surgery." Patients who have an obstruction in the right coronary artery alone or in the circumflex artery alone (or in combination) are not bypassed unless they have recurrent myocardial ischemia. Figure 62E-27 illustrates a patient with this problem.

Following surgery, patients are often placed on propranolol, digoxin, and aspirin in an effort to prevent the long range problems with arrhythmias. The use of propranolol can be defended by current data and digoxin is used because the patient is on propranolol. The value of aspirin has not been proven.

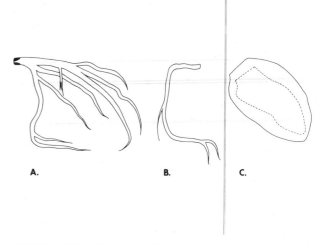

A. B. C.

FIGURE 62E-26 Diagram of the coronary arteriogram and left ventriculogram of a 51-year-old woman. She developed mild but prolonged upper chest and throat discomfort upon arising each morning for 3 days. The exercise electrocardiogram revealed 2 mm ST-segment displacement during the second stage of the Bruce test. She was placed in the coronary care unit. She was not inclined to have a coronary arteriogram and was discharged home for further rest. After 10 days she developed angina pectoris on effort and was readmitted for coronary arteriography. Coronary bypass surgery was successfully completed. This patient illustrated that some patients with mild episodes of prolonged chest discomfort have dangerous lesions in the coronary arteries. Note how clean the vessels are except for the severe obstruction of the left main coronary artery. The patient is now asymptomatic. Dr. John Stone kindly had one of us (J.W.H.) see this patient in consultation with him.

Pressure: Ao 180/90; LVEDP pre angiogram, 16; LVEDP post angiogram, 21.

A. Right anterior oblique view of left coronary artery. 80 percent stenosis of left main coronary artery with distal left anterior descending and obtuse marginal coronary arteries suitable for bypass graft. B. Left anterior oblique view of right coronary artery showing a normal artery. C. Anterior-apical hypokinesia. (*This study was done in the cardiac catheterization laboratory at Emory University Hospital, Atlanta, Georgia. We wish to thank Dr. John Douglas, Dr. George Krisle, Gail Nelbach, and Rick Brown for performing the test.*)

5 THE MANAGEMENT OF THE VARIANT ANGINA (PRINZMETAL'S SYNDROME)

The definition and recognition of variant angina or Prinzmetal syndrome are discussed in the earlier section "The Patient with Prinzmetal's Syndrome" and in Chap. 62A. The symptoms associated with Prinzmetal syndrome are similar to those discussed in items 3 and 4 of this section. The unique changes that occur in the electrocardiogram during an episode of chest discomfort enable one to diagnose this unusual condition.

The advice given the patient regarding body weight and diet, activity, anxiety and stress, and the use of tobacco and alcohol is the same as discussed in items 3 and 4.

Drugs The keystone of therapy for Prinzmetal's variant angina is nitroglycerin and other forms of vasodilator therapy, just as in classic angina pectoris. But the long-term management of Prinzmetal's variant angina is predicated upon whether there are fixed

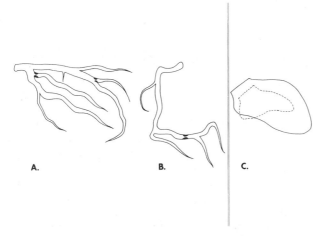

FIGURE 62E-27 Diagram of the coronary arteriogram and left ventriculogram of a 65-year-old man. He had numerous prolonged bouts of anterior chest pain in addition to angina pectoris produced by effort. The electrocardiogram showed no abnormality at rest or during spontaneous pain. He had coronary bypass surgery to the right coronary artery. This is an example of a patient with the major lesion in the right coronary artery. He has had occasional mild angina pectoris since surgery. Dr. Hugh Wells kindly referred this patient to J.W.H.

A. Right anterior oblique view of left coronary artery. 80 percent cross-sectional stenosis of anterolateral obtuse marginal branch of circumflex coronary artery with distal vessel 2 mm in diameter. 70 percent of a small diagonal branch with distal vessel 1 mm in diameter. B. Left anterior oblique view of right coronary artery. 80 percent stenosis of right coronary artery proximal to posterior descending branch with distal vessel 2 mm in diameter. C. Left ventriculogram showing posterior-basal dyskinesia. (*This study was done in the cardiac catheterization laboratory at Emory University Hospital, Atlanta, Georgia. We wish to thank Dr. John Douglas, Dr. George Krisle, Gail Nelbach, and Rick Brown for performing the test.*)

coronary artery lesions or coronary artery spasm as the basic pathogenic mechanism. For this reason, coronary arteriography is recommended early in the management of these patients. If coronary arteriography demonstrates spasm or only insignificant coronary lesions, only medical therapy is indicated, and surgical intervention should not be considered. Medical therapy should begin with nitroglycerin. In addition, a longer acting nitrate such as isosorbide dinitrate or nitroglycerin ointment should be administered. The use of propranolol is recommended in spite of the fact that there are theoretic reasons why beta blockade might be disadvantageous in this condition. It is known that propranolol results in a decrease in myocardial oxygen consumption, which might stimulate the development of coronary artery spasm. In addition, beta blockade will accentuate the alpha-adrenergic coronary vasoconstrictive effect of circulating catecholamines, and may prevent the indirect coronary vasodilatation effects of beta-adrenergic stimulation of the myocardium as well as the possible direct coronary vasodilatation of beta stimulation. In spite of this, several reports have shown that 25 to 50 percent of patients with Prinzmetal's variant angina without fixed coronary lesions will respond to a combination of nitrates and propranolol.[293,407]

Recent reports from Japan[139,408] have emphasized

outstanding results with the use of Nifedipine, which is a direct coronary vasodilator not yet available in the United States, and further studies of this drug are eagerly awaited.

Other drugs which have been used in an attempt to control the manifestations of Prinzmetal's variant angina are a variety of alpha-adrenergic blockers such as phenoxybenzamine or phentolamine, or epinephrine depleters such as guanethidine or reserpine, or parasympathetic blockers such as atropine or Pamine. There is little evidence that any of these drugs are clinically useful in the management of this disorder, though all have a good theoretic basis for their use.

Exercise test As a general rule it is not wise or necessary to perform an exercise electrocardiogram test in patients with known variant angina (Prinzmetal) syndrome.

Coronary arteriography Coronary arteriography should be performed as soon as is feasible in patients with Prinzmetal's syndrome, since it is imperative to learn if the syndrome is due to obstructive disease plus coronary artery spasm, or if it is due to coronary spasm alone, since management and prognosis depend upon which mechanism is present.

Cardiac radionuclide imaging The role of cardiac radionuclide imaging in patients with the Prinzmetal syndrome has not yet been established.

Coronary artery surgery Coronary artery bypass surgery is recommended if coronary arteriography demonstrates the presence of *obstructive* coronary lesions with good distal vessels. This includes patients with obstruction in a single artery (see earlier discussion in "Coronary Bypass Surgery" regarding the coronary anatomy that compels one to consider bypass surgery). The role of surgery in Prinzmetal's variant angina is still unclear. Conflicting reports range from no improvement[134,139,408] to excellent control of angina,[124] and the results of surgery will obviously depend upon whether coronary artery spasm occurs beyond the distal bypass site or in other, normal coronary arteries.

The role of provocative pharmacoangiography[143] in clearly delineating patients with spasm from those with fixed lesions is not yet defined, but continuing study seems indicated, although a recent editorial clearly pointed out the inherent dangers of this procedure and cautions against widespread use of such provocative methods.[409]

The role of coronary artery denervation is still experimental, and no clinical data are yet available. Coronary bypass surgery is contraindicated in patients with coronary artery spasm who have *no obstructive* lesions. Patients with AV block during pain have been successfully treated with permanent pacemakers,[410] though this does nothing for the underlying disease process.

Figure 62E-2 illustrates a patient with Prinzmetal's syndrome.

6 THE MANAGEMENT OF THE PATIENT WITH UNCOMPLICATED MYOCARDIAL INFARCTION DUE TO CORONARY ATHEROSCLEROTIC HEART DISEASE

The definition and recognition of myocardial infarction is discussed in "The Patient with Myocardial Infarction due to Coronary Atherosclerotic Heart Disease" and in Chap. 62A. The diagnosis of myocardial infarction requires two of the following:[149] (1) a history of pain consistent with myocardial ischemia, (2) the development of abnormal Q waves and ST and T waves in the electrocardiogram, or only ST-T wave abnormalities if they appear in the appropriate leads and evolve in the proper manner, and (3) a rise in the serum level of specific cardiac enzymes. As pointed out repeatedly in this book, the electrocardiogram and serum enzyme levels may not reveal information when the physician first sees the patient, and small infarcts may not alter the electrocardiogram or serum enzyme levels at all. It should also be remembered that cardiac arrhythmias and subsequent catastrophes are common in patients with prolonged myocardial ischemia without objective signs of infarction and in patients with myocardial infarction (see item 5). Therefore, the absence of objective signs of infarction does not imply that there is no danger ahead.

By the fourth or fifth day of the infarction, it is possible to assign certain patients to a subset of "uncomplicated completed acute myocardial infarction."[149] The criteria for this include the absence of (1) continuing myocardial ischemia, (2) left ventricular failure, (3) shock, (4) important cardiac arrhythmias, (5) conduction disturbances, and (6) other serious illnesses in patients with an established acute myocardial infarction. (The management of complications is discussed at the end of this chapter.)

Location of care The patient with myocardial infarction should be admitted to the coronary care unit. Rare exceptions to this plan do exist. For example, an elderly patient with cerebral disease may become so distraught and agitated in the hospital that it is preferable to leave the patient at home or in a nursing facility unless the complications are such that comfort cannot be assured outside the hospital. This statement is made because more and more patients attain the age at which this type of judgment must be exercised.

Aggravating or precipitating factors Myocardial infarction usually occurs spontaneously, but on occasion it is precipitated by hypotension, blood loss, or a cardiac arrhythmia. It is important to search for factors that could precipitate and perpetuate myocardial ischemia and infarction.

Diet and eating The patient with myocardial infarction should receive a liquid diet during the first 24 h or more after the onset of the illness. The liquids should not be cold, and sodium chloride should be restricted to less than 4 g daily. If the patient is nauseated, 2,000 ml of 5 percent glucose in one-half normal saline may be used during the first 24 h after the onset of the illness. A soft diet (one that requires no chewing) containing 4 h of sodium chloride may be started in 24 to 48 h and should be continued for 4 to 5 days. A week after the onset of illness the patient should be able to eat a regular diet.

The dietitian should be utilized to develop a diet of regular meals for the patient. The diet should contain the number of calories that will permit the patient to attain and maintain lean body weight. If the patient already has a normal body weight, we doubt if altering the diet will be very useful. If body weight is to be lost, then such should be done by decreasing the amount of saturated fat, cholesterol, and carbohydrates. The salt intake should be limited to 4 g daily. We do not use frequent determination of the level of serum cholesterol or triglycerides to guide dietary recommendation in most older patients who sustain a myocardial infarction (see Chap. 62H).

Every practitioner knows that each patient's preferences and happiness determine, to a large extent, the type of diet that is used after the first few days of the illness is over. Common sense also dictates that a rigid diet should not be prescribed routinely for patients who have already destroyed a large portion of their ventricle. Weight reduction can be defended in most patients, but excess dietary rigidity, such as strictly limiting the amount of cholesterol, is not indicated in most patients with heart failure due to a destroyed ventricle.

Activity The patient with acute infarction is usually placed in a coronary care unit where he or she remains under constant observation for 3 to 4 days, after which the patient is moved to a bed outside the unit, where he or she remains for 7 to 14 days or more depending upon the clinical problems.

The psychologic and physical rehabilitation of the patient must begin when the patient is first seen and continued throughout the hospitalization and at home afterwards.[410a] Although this is discussed in detail in Chap. 62G, certain aspects of rest, activity, and rehabilitation are discussed below. The abuse of bed rest was emphasized by Samuel Levine and Bernard Lown in 1951 when they wrote on the "chair" treatment of acute coronary thrombosis.[411] More than 25 years have passed since the publication of their observations and the following paragraph which is taken from their article makes excellent reading today.

The majority of patients were gotten out of bed during the first 2 days. They were helped out of bed and placed into a comfortable mobile chair with attention that no pressure was exerted on the popliteal spaces. They remained in a chair until they experienced fatigue. Our goal was to have these patients out of bed as much of the day as was comfortable. This was achieved in some who were up in the chair most of the day from the very beginning of their illness. In the majority, however, this usually meant that they were out of bed about one to two hours during the first day and increasing time intervals thereafter, so that by the end of the first week, they spent the larger portion of the day in a chair. The contraindications to the chair treatment were limited to patients with a continuing state of shock, those with marked debility and those with a concomitant cerebrovascular accident. High fever, severe pain, a friction rub, a diastolic gallop, heart block, cardiac arrhythmias, or the need for oxygen were not regarded as interdictions to the "chair" treatment. Nearly all patients fed themselves and were either permitted the use of the bedside commode or were granted toilet privileges . . .

One of us (J.W.H.) stated what, we hope, are "commonsense" rules for ambulation after infarction in an editorial in the *New England Journal of Medicine* (1975).[412] The following is quoted from that article, with permission by the publisher:

Common sense dictates that patient management should be individualized. Anyone who says he individualizes the management of patients should be able to enumerate the variables that he uses to make his decisions. Five major variables must be considered to individualize the amount of activity a patient with acute myocardial infarction is permitted: the emotional and physical status of the patient before the attack; the type and severity of additional noncardiac problems; the complications (carefully defined) of the myocardial infarction; the response of the patient to the physician's management (does sitting in the chair relieve dyspnea or produce an arrhythmia?); and the patient's home conditions.

Common sense also dictates that one cannot measure the beneficial or harmful effects of sitting in a chair for 30 minutes versus one hour or whether it is right or wrong to allow a patient to go home on the 10th, 11th, or 12th day. Accordingly, one should search for the principles that guide one's actions and leave the details to the physician who faces his patient day after day. The principles should emerge from carefully controlled studies, and the details should be determined by the individual physician, who should be prepared to indicate the variables he considers as he manages one patient one way and another patient another way.

Patients who were previously active and have no complications (shock, arrhythmia, or heart failure) are permitted to use the bedside commode or nearby toilet and to sit in a comfortable chair on the day after admission. Observations should be made to determine if postural hypotension and cardiac arrhythmias are produced by such maneuvers. If such complications occur, the plans should be altered; if such complications do not occur, the patient may sit in the chair as long as he does not perceive fatigue. Such patients are usually sitting up most of the day and walking in the room by the fifth day of hospitalization. As a rule, patients who have no complications (hypotension, arrhythmias, heart failure, recurrent myocardial ischemia, pulmonary emboli, etc.) on the fifth day of hospitalization may make plans to go home by about the 12th day, assuming that home conditions are proper. Therefore, to prepare patients for their home environment, it seems proper to permit them to walk 30 meters in the hallway (with supervision) three times a day on the ninth to 12th day.

Patients who have cardiogenic shock are in danger of dying and must remain in bed.

Patients with heart failure, recurrent chest pain, recurrent cardiac arrhythmias, etc., may be permitted the same privileges as those cited above. The appropriate observations must be made to be certain that postural hypotension does not occur

and that the chair management truly does rest the heart. Such patients usually remain in the hospital for about 19 days. Walking in the room may not be wise for some patients until the 12th day, and walking in the hallway may be delayed until about the 16th day.

After leaving the hospital the average patient should be able to go to the bathroom, eat at the table, and walk in the house. A week later the patient should be allowed to walk outside the house if the weather is nice for distances equivalent to those he or she walked in the house. After a week of this the patient can be permitted to walk a quarter of a mile (400 meters) twice a day. He or she should discontinue the effort if dyspnea, chest discomfort, or palpitation occurs. The walking may be increased gradually until the patient is walking a mile twice a day within a month. During this later period the patient may go for automobile rides but should not drive until 6 weeks have elapsed from the onset of the illness.

Sexual intercourse may produce a rise in the blood pressure and heart rate. Accordingly, sexual intercourse may precipitate angina pectoris and on rare occasions be responsible for sudden death. Recent studies have shown that the position of the partner does not matter. Males may be impotent because of fear and medication. A carefully planned physical activity program may reduce fear and improve sexual performance.

Patients usually return to work on a part-time basis in 6 weeks to 2 months and shortly afterwards work full time. As a rule, the patient should return to the same job.

The rehabilitation of the myocardial infarction patient is discussed in detail in Chap. 62G. Each individual physician can apply the principles set forth in that chapter.

Anxiety and stress It is essential for the physician to be sensitive to the patient's emotional status. The physician must recognize the stages of denial, acceptance, fear, dependence, and depression that may occur in patients with myocardial infarction (see Chap. 97). When the physician perceives the emotional problems, he or she is usually able to deal with them by use of common sense.

The reader should also review the earlier section of this chapter entitled "Mental Rest and Patient Psychology," a long portion of which was written by Hackett and Cassem and reprinted with permission of the authors and the American Heart Association. The discussion by Hackett and Cassem highlights the many stressful situations that patients face and emphasizes the principles the physician may employ to assist the patient in dealing with them.

Use of tobacco and alcohol Patients with myocardial infarction should discontinue the use of tobacco. In fact, confinement to the coronary care unit and hospital is an excellent time to accomplish this goal. Many patients with infarction receive opiates, sedatives, and tranquilizers and complain very little about the prohibition of cigarettes. The use of alcohol is usually denied during the hospitalization, but small amounts may be permitted carefully in selected patients. Once again, common sense dictates that some elderly patients and patients with advanced heart disease should be permitted more liberties with tobacco and alcohol.

Drugs and procedures The pain of myocardial infarction should be relieved with the intravenous injection of an opiate (see earlier discussion). As a rule 1 to 2 mg of morphine sulfate or 25 mg of Demerol given intravenously is sufficient. This should be accomplished by inserting an Intracath (heparin lock) into a vein of the wrist. This gives the physician and coronary care nurses ready access to a vein in order to treat arrhythmias, hypotension, and recurrent pain due to myocardial ischemia. An intravenous infusion of 1,000 ml of 5 percent glucose in one-half normal saline should be started and allowed to drip sufficiently fast to keep the vein open. Oxygen is not given in the uncomplicated case (see earlier discussion and discussion under "Complications"). Antiarrhythmic drugs are not used routinely (see discussion under "Complications" later in this chapter). Digitalis is not given routinely (see discussion). Anticoagulants are not given routinely (see discussion). A sedative or tranquilizer such as diazepam 2.5 mg given orally three or four times a day may allay anxiety in some patients. Vital signs such as blood pressure and respiration should be checked every hour while awake the first day, and the heart rhythm should be checked continuously. The bladder should not be catheterized unless the patient cannot void. Colace may be given in order to achieve gentle bowel actions. The diet and activity are discussed earlier in this section of this chapter.

The small number of drugs and procedures mentioned above are employed on every patient. There is currently a debate among experts regarding what else should be done. Those on one side of the argument believe that nothing else should be done. The proponents of this side of the argument would not insert a Swan-Ganz catheter in order to measure pulmonary artery wedge pressure or pulmonary artery pressure, or an intraarterial line in order to measure arterial pressure and blood gases. Those on the other side of the argument hold that a Swan-Ganz catheter and intraarterial line should be inserted in most patients with myocardial infarction. At the present time we recommend the following: The patient with uncomplicated myocardial infarction should not have and does not need a Swan-Ganz catheter and intraarterial line. This action implies that one is able to discover the clinical counterparts of hemodynamic alterations. Heart failure and shock and cardiac arrhythmias are the clinical consequences of hemodynamic alterations due to infarction. Accordingly, if more precise measurements are not done on every patient, it follows that the physician must be skilled at estimating the degree of heart failure and hypotension that is present and that one is able to insert the Swan-Ganz catheter and intraarterial line promptly when they are needed. These complications of myocardial infarction are discussed earlier in this chapter and are discussed later in the section dealing with complications. It seems appropriate to discuss the use of *hemodynamic monitoring* and how the results of it are used in therapy and to discuss the details of *clinical observations* that give a gross estimate of the hemodynamic state of the patient (see below).

Exercise test An exercise electrocardiogram test is contraindicated in patients with acute myocardial infarction. As stated in items 3, 4, and 5, the test is usually contraindicated in patients with unstable angina pectoris and is contraindicated in patients with prolonged chest discomfort that could be due to myocardial ischemia.

The exercise test may be performed *2 to 3 months after myocardial infarction* in patients under 65 years of age. It should not be done if there is unstable angina pectoris or bouts of prolonged chest discomfort due to myocardial ischemia. If there is right or left bundle branch block or ST-T wave abnormalities in the resting tracing, it will be difficult or impossible to properly interpret the ST-T wave abnormality after exercise. The value of the exercise test performed 2 to 3 months after acute infarction is (1) to determine if a patient has angina pectoris during effort. This would not apply to patients who give a definite history of angina pectoris with a defined amount of daily activity. In fact, the test is not needed in such a patient. There are patients, however, that cannot give a clear-cut history and others who have been physically active but have not been sufficiently active to provoke the occurrence of angina pectoris. (2) To determine the amount of ST-segment displacement that is produced by exercise (displacement of the ST segment during exercise can be accurately interpreted only when the resting tracing has an isoelectric ST segment). (3) To ascertain if rhythm disturbances occur which would lead one to curtail activity. (4) To determine if there is an abnormal rise or fall of systemic blood pressure. The result of the exercise test may be used as an additional source of information, though far from perfect, for determining the presence of angina pectoris, cardiac arrhythmia, and left ventricular function during exercise, and this information may, in turn, be used to guide the patient's therapy (including activity). A positive response may lead the physician to move more quickly to coronary arteriography. Certainly, the development of angina pectoris, a response of 2-mm ST-segment displacement during stage 1 or 2 of the Bruce test, or a fall in blood pressure during the test would lead one to obtain a coronary arteriography more promptly. In some patients, as discussed subsequently, the exercise test is done following the coronary arteriogram.

Cardiac radionuclide imaging The use of cardiac radionuclide imaging in the recognition of myocardial infarction is discussed earlier in this chapter. The technique is also used experimentally to estimate infarct size and the influence of treatment upon infarct size.

The use of hemodynamic measurements for the management of the patient with acute myocardial infarction[413-420] The use of precise hemodynamic monitoring emerged from the Myocardial Infarction Research Units (MIRU) that were established in this country in order to study the problem associated with myocardial infarction.

Dr. Charles Rackley, Professor of Medicine, University of Alabama School of Medicine, has kindly prepared the following discussion, which summarizes his current views on the use of hemodynamic measurements for the management of the patient with acute myocardial infarction.

The experience from several years of hemodynamic monitoring in patients with acute infarction has not only revealed that the measurements of pulmonary artery end-diastolic pressure (PAEDP) and cardiac index are useful in following the clinical course of the patient with acute infarction but also that management programs can be based on the initial hemodynamic measurements and the patient's clinical status. A management scheme is shown in Fig. 62E-28 for the clinical evaluation and potential interventions in patients who have initial measurements from the Swan-Ganz catheter during acute myocardial infarction.

The patients are divided into two groups based on the optimal range of the PAEDP and the mechanical performance of the infarcted left ventricle. The optimal range has been identified as 20 to 24 mm Hg, with the normal PAEDP being 12 mm Hg or less. In patients who present with acute infarction and have PAEDP less than 20 mm Hg, the additional measure-

ment of the cardiac index will provide several options and potential interventions in the patients. As shown in the diagram, patients with PAEDP less than 20 mm Hg and a cardiac index greater than 2.5 liters/min/m² who are clinically stable should be observed for several days during the acute infarction. If the hemodynamic measurements remain and rhythm disturbances do not occur, such patients may be candidates for early discharge from the hospital.

Group 1 In those patients presenting with a PAEDP less than 20 mm Hg and cardiac index greater than 2.5 liters/min/m² but who experience either recurrent ischemic pain or exhibit persistent hypertension, therapeutic interventions which reduce the stroke work index (SWI) of the ventricle should be considered.

Available pharmacologic agents include antihypertensives and vasodilators which can be given intravenously, sublingually, or orally. Occasionally, a hyperdynamic response with hypertension and tachycardia during the acute infarction will be encountered which is related to an increased release or response to circulating catecholamines. Such patients may possess a PAEDP less than 20 mm Hg and an elevated cardiac index above 4.0 liters/min/m² with persistent tachycardia. These individuals would be candidates for a reduction of the stroke work index of the ventricle by an agent such as propranolol.

Finally, a PAEDP less than 20 mm Hg and a cardiac index less than 2.5 liters/min/m², or a cardiac index greater than 2.5 liters/min/m² but associated with a tachycardia, will result in a reduced left

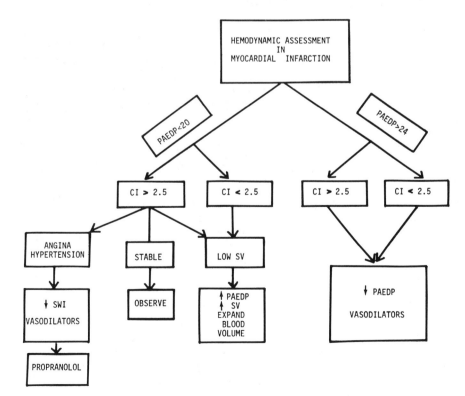

FIGURE 62E-28 An approach is illustrated for the management of the patient with acute myocardial infarction based on the hemodynamic measurements and clinical features. PAEDP = pulmonary artery end-diastolic pressure; CI = cardiac index; SWI = stroke work index; SV = stroke volume. (*Reproduced with permission.*)

ventricular stroke volume. These patients would be candidates for volume expansion and elevation of the filling pressure up to the optimal range of 20 to 24 mm Hg. Furthermore, the elevation in the filling pressure in these patients may increase the cardiac index with a compensatory reduction in the heart rate.

Group 2 In patients with a PAEDP greater than 24 mm Hg whether the cardiac index is above or below 2.5 liters/min/m², the hemodynamic goal is to reduce left ventricular filling pressure to the range of 20 to 24 mm Hg. Generally, symptoms relative to left ventricular failure, pulmonary congestion, or pulmonary edema will be present.

Currently available therapeutic interventions and the determinants of the mechanical performance of the infarcted left ventricle are listed in Fig. 62E-29. The determinants include afterload, the contractile state, preload, heart rate, metabolic state, and the infarct size. All of these determinants not only contribute to the mechanical performance of the left ventricle but also influence the myocardial oxygen requirements.

The afterload is calculated from left ventricular chamber dimensions, wall thickness, and pressure, but generally the arterial systolic blood pressure is measured for clinical purposes. Sodium nitroprusside, phentolamine, and long-acting nitrites can be effective in reducing the afterload. Nitroprusside and phentolamine must be monitored very attentively during the intravenous infusion, and it is usually preferable to have an indwelling arterial catheter for the direct measurement of blood pressure in these patients. The sublingual and oral long-acting nitrites can provide a smoother reduction in the afterload. Occasionally, the magnitude of the reduction after long-acting nitrites may be similar to that seen with the intravenous agents.

Although the contractile state has been difficult to

FIGURE 62E-29 The determinants of the mechanical performance of the infarcted left ventricle, available clinical interventions, and their effects are shown. Please see Table 62E-9. (*Reproduced with permission.*)

Determinants	Intervention	Effect
1 Afterload	Nitroprusside	↓
	Phentolamine	↓
2 Contractile state	Digitalis	↑
	Catecholamine	↑
	Propranolol	↓
3 Preload	Dextran	↑
	Diuretics	↓
	Phlebotomy	↓
	Nitrates	↓
4 Heart rate	Pacing	↑
	Atropine	↑
	Digoxin	↓
5 Metabolic state	Glucose-insulin-potassium	
6 Infarct size	Hyaluronidase	↓
	Glucose-insulin-potassium	↓

define in the intact human left ventricle, the PAEDP cardiac index and the slope of the ventricular function curve reflect the mechanical performance of the left ventricle. Digitalis and catecholamines are traditional agents that augment the vigor of myocardial contraction. In the hyperdynamic condition with a high cardiac output and a persistent tachycardia, a beta-adrenergic blocking agent such as propranolol can be cautiously infused to slow the heart rate and reduce the mechanical work of the ventricle.

The preload of the infarcted left ventricle is usually assessed by measurement of the PAEDP. The left ventricular filling pressure can either be elevated or reduced with several pharmacologic interventions. Dextran can expand the blood volume, raise the filling pressure, and increase the preload of the infarcted left ventricle. Diuretics, phlebotomy, and the long-acting nitrites can similarly lower the filling pressure by reducing the pulmonary blood volume. Diuretics and phlebotomy reduce total blood volume either by urinary loss or blood removal. The nitrites reduce the circulating blood volume by an increase in compliance of the veins and pooling in the peripheral venous system. This results in a decrease in venous return to the right and left ventricles with hemodynamic effects similar to diuresis and phlebotomy.

The heart rate in acute infarction can be altered either by pacing in those patients with bradyarrhythmias or by the administration of atropine. A rapid ventricular response to atrial fibrillation can be slowed by the use of digitalis. However, the acutely infarcted myocardium is sensitive to digitalis, and digitalis-induced arrhythmias may develop with usual clinical doses. When indicated for control of the ventricular response, approximately 50 to 70 percent of the usual digitalizing dose is recommended.

The metabolic state of both the body and the heart in acute myocardial infarction has recently been investigated clinically. One metabolic intervention has been the glucose-insulin-potassium (GIK) solution which can increase glucose availabilty and inhibit release of free fatty acids. Both glucose and free fatty acids are major substrates for the production of energy in the myocardium. An increase in glucose utilization through anaerobic pathways may be beneficial in ischemic tissue, and a reduction in the availability of circulating fatty acids may possibly influence arrhythmias or alter left ventricular mechanical performance. Infusion of the GIK should include hemodynamic monitoring so that blood volume overloading and excessive elevation of the PAEDP can be avoided.

Quantitation of the size of the myocardial infarction is of clinical interest, and several techniques have been developed to estimate the amount of damaged myocardium (see discussion "The Determination of Infarct Size" later in this chapter). Additional work in calibration will be required to determine whether techniques such as ST-segment mapping, cardiac enzymes, radionuclide scans, or possible hemodynamic measurements accurately reflect the amount of myocardium lost during the acute infarction. Additional investigation and clinical-pathologic correlations are required to evaluate these methods.

The clinical assessment of hemodynamic conditions If a Swan-Ganz catheter and intraarterial line are not placed in every patient with myocardial infarction, it implies that the physician uses clinical signals to recognize hemodynamic alterations and to determine the response to treatment.

Cardiac arrhythmias are recognized promptly in the coronary care unit and are treated according to the plans discussed in Chap. 46D and in "The Management of Cardiac Arrhythmias" later in this chapter. Certain arrhythmias may play a significant role in decreasing cardiac output.

Left ventricular dysfunction is recognized by breathlessness; sinus tachycardia; neck vein distension and pulsation; rales in the lungs; ventricular gallop sound; and, most importantly, signs of heart failure in the portable chest x-ray (see Chap. 44 and later in this chapter).

Shock and preshock can be recognized by a fall in systemic blood pressure and tachycardia; cold, clammy skin; a decreasing urine output; and mental confusion. See discussion later in this chapter.

The clinical signals just mentioned are sufficient to manage most patients with myocardial infarction. The extremely skilled physician can even use therapy such as sodium nitroprusside for heart failure and dopamine for preshock by following clinical signs, but more precise measurements of the arterial pressure and pulmonary artery diastolic pressure are usually needed to manage the patients that require such therapy. The point is that every patient with myocardial infarction does not fall into the latter category, but a few do.

The determination of infarct size Considerable research has been done in an effort to measure the size of infarction and to develop methods of decreasing the size of the infarcted area. The following principles underlie all attempts to preserve ischemic myocardium: (1) the mass of damaged myocardial tissue is a determinant of prognosis; (2) the mass of damaged myocardium can be measured quantitatively; and (3) ischemic myocardial damage may be modified by appropriate treatment. The discussion which follows will explore the basis for these assumptions.

The era for interventions to preserve ischemic myocardium did not begin until the older view of acute coronary occlusion and myocardial infarction was discarded. It had long been held that the myocardial tissue in the zone of distribution of a coronary vessel that had become occluded was destined to become irreversibly damaged. It is now clear that this is not the case. Recent work demonstrates that following coronary artery occlusion in experimental animals, substantial portions of the myocardium remain reversibly injured for a number of hours and may progress either to necrosis or to complete recovery. The myocardial tissue supplied by an occluded vessel shows a region of central necrosis surrounded in patchy fashion by jeopardized, but still viable,

ischemic myocardium. The ischemic zone may enlarge for some hours following coronary occlusion while the necrotic zone remains relatively small.[421] Later, the necrotic zone enlarges at the expense of the ischemic area. A similar sequence of progression presumably occurs in the human heart following coronary occlusion.

Relationship of infarct size and prognosis Severe left ventricular dysfunction is a major cause of death in patients with myocardial infarction. Severe left ventricular dysfunction is associated with necrosis of substantial portions of myocardium, and it may reflect destruction of a critical mass of functional heart muscle. Necrosis of between 40 to 50 percent of the left ventricular myocardium is commonly found in patients dying from cardiogenic shock. In patients with massive areas of necrosis (greater than 40 percent) the marginal ischemic zone is small, at least two epicardial coronary arteries are totally occluded, and little, if any, collateral flow can be seen in the area of infarction. Current forms of therapy are of little value for these patients. Not all patients dying from cardiogenic shock demonstrate such massive myocardial necrosis. Some have a smaller area of necrosis (20 to 30 percent), collateral blood flow into the noncontractile areas, and viable tissue in the noncontractile areas.[422] An intervention that could improve function in the ischemic, noncontractile areas might be of value for these patients.

The relationship between infarct size and ventricular dysrhythmias is complex and difficult to evaluate. In the first 20 h of hospitalization for acute myocardial infarction, Roberts et al. established a close correlation between enzymatic estimates of infarct size and the overall frequency and duration of ventricular dysrhythmias.[423] Several weeks following myocardial infarction, patients showing a greater depression of left ventricular function have more frequent and complicated ventricular dysrhythmias. Factors other than infarct size such as the heart rate, degree of sympathetic stimulation, and the state of the residual myocardium appear to have an important influence on the frequency and severity of arrhythmias. Myocardial ischemia frequently causes lethal arrhythmias in human beings even in the absence of death of substantial amounts of cardiac muscle. There is some evidence from animal studies that the incidence of ventricular fibrillation may be related to the amount of myocardium that is ischemic.

A number of studies have demonstrated a close correlation between early mortality and enzymatically estimated infarct size. Long-term survival does not appear to be directly dependent upon the extent of the initial infarction. Late mortality rates in patients with coronary atherosclerotic heart disease appear to depend more on the number of coronary arteries involved and the functional status of the left ventricle.

Assessment of myocardial injury and infarction Evaluation of interventions designed to protect ischemic myocardium and to reduce infarct size requires an accurate, easily used method for measuring the mass of ischemic and necrotic myocardium. This requirement has not been met. There is no effective, simple means for measuring myocardial infarct size in human beings. What should be measured? Should the mass of irreversibly damaged myocardium be measured? Should the amount of ischemic but viable myocardium be measured? Should both of these be measured? The development of a technique designed to measure the amount of myocardium that can potentially recover from ischemic injury should have high priority. The effect of therapeutic interventions on ischemic myocardium could be assessed if the amount of ischemic myocardium could be quantitated and if serial determinations could be done. Quantification of the extent of irreversibly damaged myocardium would be of value in determining the immediate prognosis, and it might detect the patient with massive myocardial necrosis in whom further aggressive treatment was not indicated.

A number of techniques have been used to characterize the extent and evolution of myocardial ischemic injury. Each technique focuses on selected aspects of myocardial ischemic injury. One method should not be espoused over another, because each characterizes a different aspect of myocardial injury. The following discussion will examine some of the strengths and weaknesses of each technique.

ST-segment analysis[424] The presence of ST-segment shifts in the electrocardiogram in both experimental and clinical myocardial ischemia and infarction have been noted for many years. Transient ST-segment changes may occur in the absence of anatomic evidence of myocardial infarction, and they are not a quantitative measure of myocardial necrosis. The mechanisms for ST-segment shifts during myocardial ischemia are not completely understood, but a resting current of injury rather than a primary ST-segment shift appears to be the dominant mechanism.

In dogs ST-segment shifts accompanying acute myocardial ischemia have been measured from intramyocardial, epicardial, and precordial sites. It is clear that intramyocardial ST-segment voltages provide a better index to myocardial ischemia than do epicardial or precordial ST-segment voltages. This is especially true when the ischemia is limited to the subendocardium, where reductions in blood flow correlate poorly with epicardial ST-segment change. Conversely, ST-segment elevation correlates well with reductions in subepicardial blood flow. A decrease in epicardial ST-segment elevation does not necessarily indicate a decrease in the extent of ischemic injury. In fact, just the opposite has been reported.

A reasonably good correlation is found between epicardial ST-segment elevation and precordial ST-segment elevation in closed-chest dogs. Precordial ST-segment mapping using many leads has been extended to the study of patients with acute anterior or anterolateral infarction. A number of patients have been studied using serial changes in summed

ST-segment elevation to assess therapy or to detect infarct extension. Serial measurements of the sum* of ST-segment elevation are of value in showing directional alterations in ischemic injury. The serial changes in the sum ST-segment elevation cannot be used to evaluate treatment in patients with intraventricular conduction defects, pericarditis, recurrent ischemic pain, or cardiac dysrhythmias. Spontaneous regression of the ST-segment during the first few hours following myocardial infarction is an additional problem. The technique is useful in detecting extensions of anterior or anterolateral infarctions.

Creatine phosphokinase (CPK) CPK release from myocardial cells appears to indicate cell death rather than nonspecific injury. In experimental animals, regional myocardial CPK depletion after coronary occlusion conforms closely to the extent of infarction recognized morphologically. A model in the dog relating serum CPK changes to myocardial CPK depletion has been developed to estimate the volume of infarcted myocardium, and it has been extrapolated to man.[316] The mathematical model is not, however, without its critics. In spite of this controversy and the limitations of the empirical approaches used, there is close correlation between infarct size determined from serial serum CPK level changes and prognosis.[425]

The correlations are less clear between enzymatically estimated infarct size and left ventricular hemodynamics. Some patients with a large infarct mass have only mild left ventricular dysfunction, while others with a small infarct may have severe hemodynamic impairment.[426] Many patients in the latter group have sustained a previous myocardial infarction. Only the recent infarction is discernible with CPK level changes, but the hemodynamics and ultimate prognosis are dependent on the additive effects of recent and remote muscle loss. Therefore, infarct size measured in conjunction with hemodynamic data should provide a more accurate assessment of prognosis than infarct size alone.

When serum CPK level changes are used to predict the final infarct size, additional problems arise. For the individual patient, infarct size predicted from serum CPK level changes observed during the first 7 h is subject to considerable error. When serum CPK level changes are measured for 14 h before predicting final infarct size, the agreement between predicted and actual infarct size as determined from the total CPK curve is quite good. The long delay required to obtain sufficient data for accurate projections of infarct size seriously limits the use of this technique to evaluate therapeutic interventions.

Radionuclide methods A number of radioindicators, including technetium-99m-tetracycline and technetium-99m-pyrophosphate, that are sequestered by irreversibly damaged myocardial cells provide a method to detect myocardial infarction.[427] These agents may offer the advantage of being able to

---

*The sum of the ST segments is arrived at by adding the ST-segment deflections that are recorded from multiple precordial sites. A precordial "grid" is created by the electrode placements sites and arranged so that it is reproducible.

distinguish between acute and chronic areas of infarction. Major disadvantages include (1) a delay of 12 to 24 h following infarction before the scan becomes positive; (2) the sequestration of ^{99m}Tc-pyrophosphate by ischemic as well as necrotic myocardium; (3) obscuration of the borders of the infarct by bone intake; (4) a long ^{99m}Tc half-life of 6 h. The long half-life of ^{99m}Tc precludes the use of serial myocardial scintigraphy in assessing acute changes in infarct size. The limitations of the scintillation camera also hinder the quantification of areas of infarction. The overlap of superimposed regions, the difficulty of distinguishing myocardium from contiguous tissues, and the attenuation of the gamma radiation in tissues between the heart and the detector allow only a qualitative estimate of infarct size. A promising new approach is positron-emission tomography used in combination with natural metabolites of myocardium, labeled with short-lived radionuclides. Preliminary studies suggest that this technique may be more useful in quantifying the extent of infarction.

Regional myocardial function Serial evaluation of regional myocardial dysfunction in experimental animals has provided information on changes in contractile function of marginally perfused and central ischemic zones.[428] The decrease in contractile activity coincides closely in time with the onset of ischemia. Persistent dysfunction in ischemic segments may correlate with the development of permanent damage. The contractile function of the marginal zone, composed of ischemic cells or a mixed population of normal and ischemic cells, is of particular interest. Following acute coronary occlusion, the marginal zone exhibits hypokinesis. Propranolol and nitroglycerin infusions may improve contractile functions in the marginal segment, but isoproterenol infusion may cause deterioration of active shortening in the ischemic zone. Since regional dysfunction occurs in areas of ischemia as well as in areas of necrosis, this technique is not ideally suited for prediction or quantitation of the extent of irreversible injury. There is currently no reliable noninvasive means for measuring serial changes in segmental left ventricular contractile function in human beings. Echocardiographic scanning of large regions of the left ventricle may be possible in the future.

Protection of ischemic myocardium A number of hemodynamic, pharmacologic, and metabolic interventions may reduce myocardial ischemia damage following experimental coronary artery occlusion. The final result of any intervention should depend primarily on its effect on the ischemic zone. However, many interventions affect nonischemic myocardium, the peripheral circulation, or the autonomic nervous system, and these actions could have an indirect influence on the ischemic zone. The critical factor for any intervention may be the adequacy of collateral blood flow to the ischemic area. Unless the drug can gain access to ischemic myocardium, therapeutic benefit cannot be expected. Another important factor is the amount of time available for a successful intervention. Although ischemic injury in experimental animals can be modified by interventions implemented some hours after onset, any intervention is

likely to be most effective if implemented as soon as possible after the onset of ischemia.

A variety of pharmacologic and hemodynamic interventions have been found to alter acute ischemic injury following coronary artery occlusion in experimental animals.[429] The reader is referred to Table 62E-9 for a listing on interventions that decrease ischemic injury in experimental animals. These results cannot be simply extrapolated to acute myocardial infarction in human beings because of differences in the extent of coronary vascular involvement, the number and size of coronary collateral vessels, the mechanism of infarct production, and the left ventricular hemodynamics.

The results from preliminary studies in human subjects suggest that some pharmacologic interventions may reduce myocardial ischemic injury. In patients with acute myocardial infarction complicated by left ventricular failure, the administration of nitroglycerin or sodium nitroprusside improves the hemodynamic abnormality. However, an improvement in left ventricular performance does not imply a reduction in ischemic injury. Nitroglycerin may reduce the summed ST-segment elevations in patients with left ventricular failure, but it may increase ST-segment elevation in some patients without left ventricular failure.[430] Sodium nitroprusside administered to patients with heart failure results in a decrease, no change, or an increase in ST-segment elevation. An increase in ST-segment elevation is accompanied by an increase in heart rate and the heart rate–mean arterial pressure product. The reason why nitroglycerin uniformly decreases ST-segment elevation in patients with heart failure while sodium nitroprusside does not is uncertain. It is possible that nitroglycerin has a greater effect on increasing coronary collateral blood flow to ischemic myocardium. Propranolol may reduce ST-segment elevation in patients with acute myocardial infarc-

TABLE 62E-9
Interventions that may reduce ischemic injury

Major mechanism	Intervention
1 Decreasing myocardial oxygen demands	Beta-adrenergic blockade
	Intraaortic balloon counter pulsation
	Reduction of excessive preload or afterload
2 Increasing coronary flow	Intraaortic balloon counter-pulsation
3 Redistribution of flow to ischemic area	Nitroglycerin
4 Reducing ischemic cell swelling	Hyperosmotic mannitol
5 Increasing energy supply—anaerobic glycolysis	Glucose-insulin-potassium
6 Increasing diffusion through extra-cellular space	Hyaluronidase
7 Increasing oxygen supply	Increasing inspiratory oxygen

*See Fig. 62E-29.

tion, and it may improve the metabolism of the ischemic heart as reflected by a shift from lactate production to lactate extraction. The administration of 100 percent oxygen and hyaluronidase have also been shown to reduce ST-segment elevation. Although these data suggest that ischemic injury can be modified in human beings, a cautious approach is advisable until the physiologic significance of a reduction in summed ST-segment elevation or a decrease in serum CPK level from predicted levels is demonstrated.

Before interventions designed to protect the ischemic myocardium are adopted as a standard form of practice, many problems must be solved. The efficacy of any intervention will not be resolved definitively until a technique is found to accurately measure and quantify the mass of jeopardized ischemic myocardium. This technique can then be applied to determine (1) the mass of ischemic myocardium preserved by a specific intervention, (2) the time limitations for effective therapy, (3) the effects of the intervention on immediate and late complications and on mortality.

Coronary arteriography and coronary artery surgery Coronary arteriography should not be done in patients with uncomplicated acute myocardial infarction unless coronary artery surgery is considered to be necessary. Accordingly, it is uncommon for coronary arteriography to be considered. The patient with Q waves in the electrocardiogram and elevated serum cardiac enzyme levels is not usually considered for coronary bypass surgery during the early stage of the illness because the risk of the procedures is considerable when it is done during this acute stage, and the value is small. In fact, some clinical investigators believe that increasing myocardial perfusion of an acutely infarcted area is harmful. The patient with myocardial infarction who continues to have episodes of myocardial ischemia is discussed in the next section of this chapter.

Patients with myocardial infarction may have no additional ischemic episodes during the acute phase of the illness, and convalescence may take place without complications. The question arises as to the indications for coronary arteriography in such asymptomatic patients who have "recovered" from an acute uncomplicated myocardial infarction, and when it should be done. At this time there are two approaches to this problem. One approach is to perform an exercise test on patients who are 65 years of age or under, 2 to 3 months after the infarction. Coronary arteriography is then done on those patients whose exercise test shows 2 mm of ST-segment displacement at a very low workload (grade I and II). Of course, if the ST segment is displaced considerably at rest as the result of the infarction, it is difficult to interpret the ST-segment displacement produced by exercise. Another approach is to perform a coronary arteriogram on all patients who are

under 65 years of age 2 to 3 months after the onset of the acute myocardial infarction.

The purpose of the coronary arteriogram is to gain new insight regarding the prognosis of the patient by identifying the extent and location of the obstructive lesions. The reader is referred to the earlier discussion of the indications for coronary bypass surgery. High-grade obstructive lesions in certain vessels are considered to be more important if the obstructed vessels supply the collateral channels to the area surrounding the infarction. The trend is to obtain a coronary arteriogram on younger patients even if the exercise test shows a negative response. The right coronary artery is often totally occluded in patients with inferior or posterior infarction and the left anterior descending artery is usually totally occluded in patients with a recent anterior infarction. When high-grade obstruction is found in an artery that provides collateral circulation to the area surrounding the infarct, it is proper to recommend bypass surgery. The objective is to prevent sudden death or further infarction.[117h,117i] Of course, patients who have had a myocardial infarction usually have an area of abnormal myocardial contractility demonstrated on the left ventriculogram. Surgery may be contraindicated because of it. Contractility may improve after nitroglycerin has been placed under the tongue, and we use this as evidence that ischemia is altering contractility although the patient feels no pain. Coronary artery bypass surgery may improve the poorly contractile segment in some of these patients.

7 THE PATIENTS WITH RECURRENT MYOCARDIAL ISCHEMIA FOLLOWING MYOCARDIAL INFARCTION

The recognition of myocardial ischemia following myocardial infarction is discussed earlier in "The Patient with Continuing or Recurrent Myocardial Ischemia Following Myocardial Infarction." As discussed in item 6, the patient with completed, uncomplicated acute myocardial infarction is not a candidate for an exercise test, coronary arteriography, or coronary bypass surgery. There are certain complications such as heart failure or shock that may lead the physician to recommend coronary arteriography and a surgical procedure; these are discussed in the subsequent section dealing with complications. Patients with acute myocardial infarction may have episodes of myocardial ischemia following the onset of the illness. When the episodes occur a few hours after the onset of the acute infarction, the patient is considered to have an incomplete infarct. When the episodes occur months or years after the infarction, it is wise to consider that obstruction has increased in the coronary arteries.

Coronary arteriography and coronary artery surgery are indicated in carefully selected cases that fall into one of the following categories:

1 Infarction is said to be present when there are two of the following present: characteristic chest discomfort; abnormal Q waves or evolving ST-T wave abnormalities;

or a rise in the serum level of specific cardiac enzymes. Again we wish to make four points: (1) that the electrocardiographic and enzyme abnormalities may not be present early in the illness; (2) that certain infarcts may not produce QRS changes in the electrocardiogram; (3) that many patients with infarction are also found in the group of patients with prolonged myocardial ischemia without objective signs of infarction; and (4) that the methods used to determine infarct size are not perfect. We need additional methods of examination in order to subclassify "infarctions."

At the present time it seems appropriate to consider coronary arteriography and coronary artery surgery for patients with acute infarctions who have recurrent pain due to myocardial ischemia that cannot be controlled with drugs. As a rule, such a decision cannot be made for several days, when it has become certain that the infarction is continuing. The procedure is not ordinarily considered during the early acute phase of the infarction for patients with Q waves; but if severe ischemic episodes continue, it may be necessary to have surgery performed if satisfactory coronary anatomy can be demonstrated by angiography. In such an instance, the potential benefit for surgery is to limit the size of the infarction. Obviously, the risk of surgery is higher during this stage of illness than it is at other times. The risk probably reaches the level of 5 percent rather than the usual 1 percent. Figure 62E-30 illustrates a patient with this problem.

2 Patients with characteristic pain of acute myocardial ischemia who exhibit an elevation in the serum level of specific cardiac enzymes, who may have a normal electrocardiogram or an electrocardiogram that shows ST-T or T-wave change (including hyperacute changes), and who continue to have ischemic episodes despite adequate drug therapy are considered to be candidates for coronary arteriography and surgery. The surgical risk of bypass of this group is probably less than when Q waves are present. Figure 62E-31 illustrates a patient with this problem.

3 Patients may become symptomatic for several weeks, months, or years after myocardial infarction. Such patients, unless excessively elderly, should have coronary arteriography if angina pectoris or prolonged myocardial ischemia occurs. An important point should be made again. It is naive to expect the heart to always notify the physician that it is in jeopardy by having just the "right amount" of chest discomfort. Unfortunately many patients die suddenly or have infarction (which when added to the old infarction may destroy the ventricle). It is for this reason that it seems proper to be more aggressive in patients with angina pectoris who have had a myocardial infarction. The unacceptable manifestations of coronary atherosclerotic heart disease—sudden death and myocardial infarction—may be prevented if dangerous lesions can be bypassed prior to the catastrophic events. Such an approach would not be necessary if patients always presented with just the "proper amount of safe angina." Certainly most patients with a history of remote infarction who develop episodes of chest discomfort should have a coronary arteriogram and, if high-grade obstructive lesions are found, should have coronary artery bypass surgery if the distal coronary vessels and myocardial function permit it.

Figures 62E-32 and 62E-33 illustrate patients with

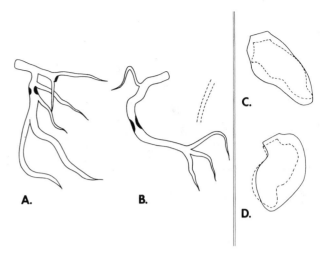

FIGURE 62E-30 A diagram of the coronary arteriogram and left ventriculogram of a 62-year-old man. He developed substernal pain while jogging. He had angina pectoris for 3 months. He developed increasing angina pectoris to the point that he had discomfort at rest. The exercise electrocardiogram was positive. His left ventriculogram showed anterior and apical hypokinesia. His surgery was delayed a few days since a recent infarction had undoubtedly occurred (changing T waves in the lateral precordial leads and moderate rise in CPK level). Recurrent chest pain lasting $1/2$ to $1^1/2$ h continued to occur, and coronary bypass surgery was performed even though he had a recent infarction.

This patient highlights the problem of recurrent myocardial ischemia following myocardial infarction and illustrates the necessity of urgent coronary bypass surgery in some cases. The patient was asymptomatic following surgery. Dr. Edwin Flournoy kindly referred this patient to J.W.H.

A. Right anterior oblique view of left coronary artery. Total occlusion of left anterior descending coronary artery just distal to the first septal perforator. 75 percent stenosis of proximal circumflex coronary artery, with distal anterolateral obtuse marginal branch 2.5 mm in diameter. B. Left anterior oblique view of right coronary artery showing 75 percent cross-sectional stenosis of mid right coronary artery, with distal vessel 2.5 mm in diameter. There is late collateral filling of the left anterior descending coronary artery, which is 2 mm in diameter. C. Right anterior oblique ventriculogram showing anterior and apical hypokinesia. D. Left anterior descending artery ventriculogram showing septal hypokinesia. (*This study was done in the cardiac catheterization laboratory at Emory University Hospital, Atlanta, Georgia. We wish to thank Dr. John Douglas, Dr. George Krisle, Gail Nelbach, and Rick Brown for performing the test.*)

this problem. The indications for coronary bypass surgery are discussed earlier in "Coronary Bypass Surgery."

8 THE PATIENT WITH MYOCARDIAL ISCHEMIA FOLLOWING BYPASS SURGERY

It is just as necessary to identify and classify the type of myocardial ischemia that occurs in a patient following bypass surgery as it is in the patient who has not had surgery (see discussion earlier in this chapter in "The Patient with Myocardial Ischemia following Bypass Surgery" and in Chap. 62A).

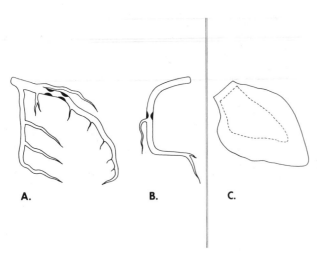

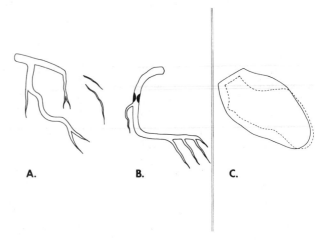

FIGURE 62E-31 Diagram of the coronary arteriogram and left ventriculogram of a 53-year-old man. He noted anterior chest pain playing tennis 1 month earlier. He then had several episodes of prolonged severe left shoulder and arm pain for no apparent reason. The electrocardiogram showed no abnormality, but the CPK level rose to 254μ. Because of recurrent pain and despite CPK level, he had coronary bypass surgery.

The patient highlights the need for coronary bypass surgery in patients with recurrent prolonged myocardial ischemia even when the CPK is rising. The patient is now asymptomatic. Dr. James Brawner kindly referred this patient to J.W.H.

Pressures; Ao, 100/62; LV, 100/13; LVEDP post angiogram, 24.

A. Right anterior oblique view of the left coronary artery. Two areas of 90 percent cross-sectional narrowing are present in the left anterior descending coronary artery distal to the first septal perforator. The distal left anterior descending artery was 2.5 mm in diameter and angiographically normal. B. Left anterior oblique view of the right coronary artery. 90 percent cross-sectional narrowing was present proximally. The distal vessel was 3 mm in diameter and angiographically normal. C. The left ventriculogram was normal. (*This study was done in the cardiac catheterization laboratory at Emory University Hospital, Atlanta, Georgia. We wish to thank Dr. Spencer King, Dr. John Hurst, Peggy May, and Steve Hudson for performing the test.*)

FIGURE 62E-32 Diagram of the coronary arteriogram and left ventriculogram of a 42-year-old man. He had an anterior infarction 2 years previously. The electrocardiogram showed persistently elevated ST segments and absent R waves in the precordial leads. Although he was asymptomatic, a decision was made to do a coronary arteriogram. Before the arteriogram could be done, he noted angina pectoris after walking uphill. The coronary arteriogram was done as soon as possible, and this was followed in a few days with coronary bypass surgery. The anterior infarction had been produced when the left anterior descending artery became totally occluded. His life was threatened when the right coronary artery became 99 percent obstructed. In this case a single bypass to the right coronary artery was extremely important. Mild angina pectoris continues after surgery. Dr. Tom Kitchens kindly referred this patient to J.W.H.

Pressures: Ao, 100/65: LV, 100/4; LVEDP post angiogram, 6.

A. Right anterior oblique view of the left coronary artery. The left anterior descending coronary artery is totally occluded after a large septal perforator. The distal anterior descending and diagonal branches are less than 1 mm in diameter and unsuitable for bypass. The circumflex artery is normal. B. Left anterior oblique view of the right coronary artery showing 99 percent cross-sectional stenosis proximally. The distal right coronary artery which was 3.5 mm in diameter and angiographically normal was opacified during right and left coronary injection. C. Left ventriculography demonstrated anterior apical and septal dyskinesia. The biplane ejection fraction was 0.34. (*This study was done in the cardiac catheterization laboratory at Emory University Hospital, Atlanta, Georgia. We wish to thank Dr. Spencer King, Dr. John Hurst, Peggy May, and Steve Hudson for performing the test.*)

Recommendations regarding the location of care, the identification of aggravating or precipitating factors, diet and eating activity, anxiety and stress, the use of tobacco and alcohol, and the use of various procedures and drugs are similar to those made for patients with myocardial ischemia who have not had bypass surgery (see items 2 to 4 and 6 of this section).

The evaluation of patients who have symptoms of myocardial ischemia following coronary bypass surgery is much more difficult than it is of patients who have not been submitted to surgery. The same is true for the management of such patients. This is true for three reasons:

1 Some patients develop chest discomfort after bypass surgery and the symptoms may be difficult to analyze. The patient may have pericarditis, chest wall discomfort, the pain of anxiety, or various types of chest pain due to myocardial ischemia.

2 Some patients are difficult to rehabilitate following bypass surgery. We have found that this correlates directly with the length of time the patient has been away from his or her professional activity prior to surgery. Patients who for one reason or another choose to give up their professional activity following bypass surgery and who were inactive in their occupation prior to surgery may be especially difficult to evaluate after surgery.

3 There is a natural resistance on the part of the patient and physician to seek further information from an exercise test or from coronary arteriography since the patient has "been through it all" before.

Myocardial revascularization relieves symptoms in 80 percent of patients and prolongs life in many patients. However, the operation does not "cure" patients because bypass surgery does not alter the progression of the atherosclerotic process. Symp-

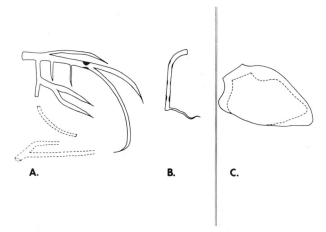

A.　　　　　B.　　　　C.

FIGURE 62E-33 Diagram of the coronary arteriogram and left ventriculogram of a 48-year-old man. The electrocardiogram showed evidence of old inferior infarction of undetermined age. He had progressive angina pectoris despite medical treatment. He underwent successful coronary bypass surgery. This patient illustrates the development of moderate symptoms following myocardial infarction and the need for coronary arteriography and coronary artery surgery. He was asymptomatic after surgery. Dr. Henry Threefoot kindly referred this patient to J.W.H.

Pressures: Ao, 95/60; LVEDP pre angiogram, 6; LVEDP post angiogram, 8.

A. Right anterior oblique view of the left coronary artery. 95 percent cross-sectional stenosis of left anterior descending coronary artery distal to first septal perforator, with distal left anterior descending and diagonal branch 2 mm in diameter. Total occlusion of mid circumflex coronary artery, with distal posterolateral obtuse marginal branch 1 mm in diameter. Collateral filling of distal right coronary artery and posterior descending branch, 1.5 mm in diameter. B. Left anterior oblique view of right coronary artery. Total occlusion of mid right coronary artery. C. Right anterior oblique ventriculogram. The inferior wall is akinetic. (*This study was done in the cardiac catheterization laboratory at Emory University Hospital, Atlanta, Georgia. We wish to thank Dr. Spencer King, Dr. John Hurst, Peggy May, and Steve Hudson for performing the test.*)

toms and signs of myocardial ischemia may appear months or years after successful bypass surgery. When this interval of time has elapsed, it is appropriate to consider that the atherosclerotic process has progressed in the native coronary arteries. When symptoms or signs of myocardial ischemia appear in the days or weeks immediately following the bypass surgery, it is wise to consider that the grafts have closed or that the initial revascularization was incomplete.

Because of the difficulties encountered in the evaluation of these patients (see preceding comments), it is customary to limit repeat coronary arteriography to those patients with troublesome symptoms that could be due to a recurrence of myocardial ischemia. An additional small group of patients might be investigated again because the result of the exercise electrocardiogram, which usually improves after successful surgery, has become worse than it was prior to surgery or early in the postoperative course.

Radioactive imaging (see Chap. 30) may yield useful information in patients who have had bypass surgery. If "cold spots" were found in the prebypass image and disappeared following surgery but reappeared later in the postoperative period, one could reason that certain symptoms and signs might be explained by their development. Mason and others concluded that the results of isotopic imaging before and after exercise is a more sensitive index of myocardial ischemia than is the exercise electrocardiogram.[431]

In summary, coronary arteriography is performed in patients who have had bypass surgery when their symptoms seem to be or could be due to myocardial ischemia. Arteriography may be done in a few patients whose exercise electrocardiogram has deteriorated. We predict that in the future arteriography will be done in some patients because of a change in the isotopic image of the myocardium.

The Cleveland Clinic reported on 200 consecutive patients who were reoperated between 1967 and 1975. The indication for surgery was "incapacitating angina pectoris." Of these patients 21 percent had symptoms due to obstruction of the grafts; 19 percent had symptoms due to progression of the atherosclerosis; 19 percent due to incomplete primary revascularization; and 41 percent because of a combination of these factors.

The operative mortality is higher in patients who have bypass surgery performed for a second time, being in the range of 3.7 percent.[432] The results of surgery are less gratifying in this group, but the effort is still justified in selected cases. If the patient is symptomatic because of incomplete revascularization or obstruction of the graft secondary to a technical problem or intrinsic disease of the graft, there is a good possibility that the reoperation will be successful. If the symptoms are due to obstruction of the graft because of poor runoff or extensive distal atherosclerosis, the reoperation is less likely to be successful. The indications for coronary bypass surgery are discussed earlier in "Coronary Bypass Surgery."

9 THE MANAGEMENT OF THE PATIENT WITH SYNCOPE

The definition and recognition of syncope is discussed in "The Patient with Syncope" earlier in this chapter and in Chap. 47. The point has been made that the difference in syncope and sudden death in a patient who is having a cardiac arrhythmia is only a matter of a few seconds and not a basic difference in mechanism. For example, if ventricular fibrillation lasts a few seconds it may produce syncope; if it lasts longer than that, death ensues.

It is not uncommon for patients with coronary atherosclerotic heart disease to have syncope. It may be due to a cardiac arrhythmia; angina pectoris when the cardiac output is markedly diminished (left ventricular paralysis or syncope anginosus); nitroglycerin taken for angina pectoris; or to any of the other causes of syncope.

It is not always easy to prove that syncope or near syncope due to a cardiac arrhythmia is occurring in a patient. Accordingly, it may be necessary to use a Holter monitor or some form of telemetry or to monitor the patient in the coronary care unit to demonstrate it. Even when a cardiac arrhythmia is discovered to be the cause of syncope, it does not automatically prove that the cause of the arrhythmia is due to coronary atherosclerotic heart disease. For example, patients with the sick sinus syndrome may or may not have associated coronary atherosclerotic disease; patients who develop abrupt high-grade AV block may have Lenegre's or Lev's disease and may or may not have associated coronary atherosclerosis; and patients with paroxysms of ventricular fibrillation may or may not have coronary atherosclerotic heart disease.

Exercise test An exercise test may be indicated in patients with syncope due to an arrhythmia in order to determine if syncope is precipitated by exercise and to determine the degree of ST-segment displacement related to exercise. Obviously, the test is dangerous in such patients and must not be done unless it is likely to produce useful information and adequate trained personnel are available should a catastrophe occur.

Coronary arteriography Coronary arteriography is not indicated in all patients with syncope because in many instances the mechanism of the syncope is not related to the heart. Coronary arteriography is indicated in patients who have syncope in the context of the following syndromes:

1 Syncope in the context of aortic valve disease dictates that cardiac catheterization be performed to study the aortic valve, but that coronary arteriography also be performed in order to identify the commonly associated coronary atherosclerosis.
2 Patients with syncope who give a history of angina pectoris—they may not seek medical advice because of the angina pectoris but may do so because of syncope.
3 Patients who have syncope associated with angina pectoris should be studied for idiopathic hypertrophic subaortic stenosis with echocardiography, but left ventriculography and coronary arteriography may also be needed to rule out associated coronary atherosclerosis.
4 Patients who develop a cardiac arrhythmia, a fall in blood pressure, or actual syncope during or after the exercise stress test should have coronary arteriography.
5 Most patients with proven episodes of ventricular fibrillation without appropriate cause should have a coronary arteriogram.
6 Patients who have an arrhythmia such as ventricular fibrillation and who faint and are defibrillated and resuscitated are discussed in item 10, which deals with sudden death. Such patients should have coronary arteriography.

Cardiac radionuclide imaging The role of cardiac radionuclide imaging in patients with syncope has not yet been established.

Coronary artery surgery The indications for coronary arteriography in patients with syncope are outlined above. The need for coronary bypass surgery in such patients is determined by the location and extent of the obstructive lesions (see "Coronary Bypass Surgery" earlier in the chapter). Patients with left main coronary artery obstruction or triple-vessel or double-vessel disease with syncope thought to be due to an arrhythmia due to ischemia may be considered for surgery. It is conceivable that it might be necessary to perform bypass surgery for right coronary artery disease or circumflex artery disease if the arrhythmia producing the syncope is clearly related to myocardial ischemia. The problem is that it is not easy to prove this point. If a patient has angina pectoris and syncope or a markedly positive exercise test and syncope, surgery should be performed for obstructive disease in a single coronary artery. It is hoped that isotopic imaging will assist in the solution of this problem.

The fact that coronary atherosclerotic obstructive disease can cause a cardiac arrhythmia and syncope does not permit one to assume that the arrhythmia and syncope are due to the coronary disease that is found by coronary arteriography. One is still obligated to determine if the arrhythmia is due to sick sinus node syndrome or Lenegre's or Lev's disease, which may not be due to coronary atherosclerosis. This is important since the sick sinus node syndrome or trifascicular block syndromes with arrhythmia and syncope may not be benefited by bypass surgery even if it is due to myocardial ischemia. Many of these patients need cardiac pacemakers as well as coronary artery bypass surgery.

10 THE MANAGEMENT OF SUDDEN DEATH

Sudden death is discussed in Chap. 49 and in the earlier section "Sudden Death." The purpose of this discussion is to emphasize the management of the patient who is successfully resuscitated.

Sudden death is usually due to a cardiac arrhythmia, and most often this is due to coronary atherosclerosis. The arrhythmia is usually ventricular fibrillation and occasionally asystole. On rare occasions electrical-mechanical dissociation may be the cause of sudden death. The resuscitation of such patients occurs more frequently now because there is more general knowledge of cardiopulmonary resuscitation, and there are emergency systems designed for the care of these patients.

A patient with sudden death who has been resuscitated should be placed in the coronary care unit for continued observation. Lidocaine should be administered as soon as possible for patients whose cardiac arrest was known to be due to ventricular fibrillation.

Cardiac "arrest" that has occurred once is likely to occur again. Accordingly, the hospital personnel must be prepared to act promptly to resuscitate the patient again. After the rhythm and other vital signs have become normal, it may be possible to elicit a history of recent angina pectoris or previous heart attack. Such a history is added evidence that the rhythm disturbance was due to coronary atherosclerotic heart disease. Patients with such a history and patients who have no evidence of a noncoronary cause of sudden death such as pulmonary embolism should be managed as if they have an acute myocardial infarction.

Drugs Most patients should have an arterial line and a Swan-Ganz catheter inserted in order to measure the intraarterial pressure and pulmonary artery diastolic pressure or wedge pressure. The electrocardiogram should be recorded daily for 3 days and then every 2 to 3 days in an effort to discover electrocardiographic clues of myocardial damage. It should be recalled, however, that the hypoxia of an agonal rhythm plus the process of cardiac "massage" (cardiac compression) may alter the electrocardiogram. The same can be said for the serum level of specific cardiac enzymes. The isoenzyme of creatine phosphokinase (MB) may be elevated as a result of cardiac contusion from resuscitation and cardiac hypoxia. Lidocaine is continued in doses necessary to suppress ventricular ectopic beats should they be present. Later, unless the nature of the rhythm dictates against it, the patient should be placed on propranolol. As a rule propranolol should be used for long-term treatment when coronary surgery cannot be performed. It should also be used after bypass surgery unless there are reasons not to do so.

Exercise test The exercise stress test is not performed in patients who have had sudden death and have been resuscitated.

Coronary arteriography Coronary arteriography should be performed on all patients who have been resuscitated from sudden death unless there is a compelling noncardiac reason not to do so. The test should be done in a few days after the event at a time when the patient's condition is stable. If an acute infarction evolves, the arteriogram should be delayed several weeks.

Cardiac radionuclide imaging Use of this technique should enable one to identify ischemic or infarcted areas in the myocardium. It should be useful in the careful study of patients with sudden death, though little is written about it at this time.

Coronary artery surgery Patients who have recovered from sudden death who have significant obstructive lesions in any coronary artery or combinations of arteries should have coronary bypass surgery. High-grade obstruction of the right coronary artery or circumflex artery should be bypassed since one would not wish to rely solely on the long-term

use of propranolol to prevent an ischemic area from triggering a lethal cardiac arrhythmia. Isotopic imaging may be of help in studying these patients. One should be able to determine if the coronary lesion seen in the arteriogram is indeed producing ischemia and if the bypass graft relieves it.

11 THE MANAGEMENT OF PATIENTS WITH AORTIC VALVE DISEASE WHO MAY OR MAY NOT HAVE EPISODES OF MYOCARDIAL ISCHEMIA[151]

The recognition of myocardial ischemia in patients with aortic valve disease is discussed earlier in this chapter in "Patients with Aortic Valve Disease Who Have Episodes of Myocardial Ischemia."

Aortic stenosis The majority of patients with valvular aortic stenosis who have angina pectoris or prolonged episodes of myocardial ischemia have associated obstructive coronary atherosclerotic heart disease. Therefore, a coronary arteriogram should be done at the time of cardiac catheterization to determine if the angina pectoris is due to aortic stenosis alone or to associated coronary atherosclerosis. The role of cardiac imaging in such patients has not been established. It should be recalled that angina pectoris is a definite signal to perform cardiac catheterization, including coronary arteriography, in patients with aortic stenosis. At the time of aortic valve surgery coronary bypass surgery should be performed in patients with high-grade obstructive lesions of the major coronary arteries.

The patient with aortic stenosis who has no angina pectoris or evidence of prolonged myocardial ischemia should also have coronary arteriography performed at the same time cardiac catheterization is performed for aortic stenosis. If such patients have high-grade obstructive lesions demonstrated in the coronary arteries, bypass surgery should be performed at the same time that aortic valve surgery is performed, even though the patient has no symptoms of ischemia. There are few data regarding this group of patients, but the plan seems reasonable.

Aortic regurgitation Patients with aortic regurgitation, with or without angina pectoris, probably have less associated coronary atherosclerosis than do patients with aortic stenosis. When angina pectoris or prolonged myocardial ischemia occurs in patients with aortic regurgitation, it is necessary to perform coronary arteriography at the time of cardiac catheterization in order to determine the cause of the ischemic episodes. Obviously, coronary arteriography should also be done in such patients even when there is no history of angina pectoris. The role of cardiac radionuclide imaging in such patients has not been established. Coronary bypass surgery should be performed in patients who have obstructive coronary disease who have aortic valve replacement performed for aortic regurgitation whether or not they have angina pectoris.

12 THE MANAGEMENT OF PATIENTS WITH MITRAL VALVE DISEASE WHO MAY OR MAY NOT HAVE EPISODES OF MYOCARDIAL ISCHEMIA

The recognition of myocardial ischemia in patients with mitral valve disease is discussed earlier in "Patients with Mitral Valve Disease Who Have Episodes of Myocardial Ischemia." Patients with tight mitral stenosis may have chest discomfort due to myocardial ischemia. The angina pectoris may be due to factors other than associated obstructive coronary atherosclerosis. Mitral stenosis is often seen in young women, and because of this the incidence of associated coronary atherosclerosis is low. It is proper, however, to have coronary arteriography performed at the time of cardiac catheterization in patients with mitral stenosis who are over 40 years of age regardless of the presence of angina pectoris in order to identify obstructive coronary disease. The role of cardiac radionuclide imaging in such patients has not been established. Coronary bypass surgery should be performed in patients with high-grade obstructive lesions in the coronary arteries at the same time surgery for mitral stenosis is performed even though the patient has no symptoms of ischemia.

Patients with mitral regurgitation over the age of 40 years who have sufficient signs and symptoms to justify surgery should have coronary arteriography when cardiac catheterization is performed for the mitral regurgitation. Coronary bypass surgery should be performed in patients with high-grade obstructive lesions in the coronary arteries at the same time surgery for mitral regurgitation takes place even though the patient has no symptoms of ischemia.

13 THE MANAGEMENT OF THE PATIENT WITH EPISODES OF MYOCARDIAL ISCHEMIA WHO ALSO HAS SIGNIFICANT EXTRACRANIAL ARTERIAL OCCLUSIVE DISEASE[152]

The recognition of myocardial ischemia in patients with extracranial arterial occlusive disease is discussed earlier in "The Patient with Episodes of Myocardial Ischemia Who Also Has Significant Extracranial Arterial Occlusive Disease." Patients who have evidence of obstructive coronary disease and obstructive extracranial arterial disease deserve special comment because their prognosis is poor, and medical and surgical management is poor. Taylor has emphasized the current trend to operate on the coronary arteries and carotid arteries during the same operation.[152] Earlier, carotid endarterectomy was done prior to the coronary bypass surgery. Patients with severe or unstable angina pectoris with critically obstructed coronaries and associated se-

vere carotid lesions particularly qualify for the combined approach, according to Taylor.[152]

Taylor studied 100 patients who had simultaneous carotid endarterectomy and coronary bypass or valve replacement.[152] The operative mortality was 5 percent. Postoperative cerebrovascular accidents occurred in 12 patients, 1 of whom died. Accordingly, the mortality and morbidity from surgery is four to five times higher in this group of patients than it is in patients who have bypass only.

Although data are incomplete, it seems reasonable to perform simultaneous surgery on patients who have evidence of severe obstruction in both the carotid arteries and the coronary arteries with full recognition of the high mortality and morbidity. Patients with stable angina pectoris and less critical coronary artery obstruction who have compelling and urgent reasons for carotid artery surgery should have the latter performed first. The decision regarding coronary bypass surgery should be postponed.

Note that in most instances both coronary and carotid arteriograms are required to make a decision. This is not always the case however. For example, a 75-year-old male with stable angina pectoris and a transient ischemic episode may have carotid arteriography and not have coronary arteriography. Certainly, all patients with carotid lesions do not require carotid artery surgery. Lesions in the carotid that are not obstructive may produce emboli, and antiplatelet medication may be tried, especially in older patients who have symptomatic coronary disease.

The role of cardiac radionuclide imaging in such patients has not yet been established.

THE MANAGEMENT OF THE COMPLICATIONS OF CORONARY ATHEROSCLEROTIC HEART DISEASE

A complication of coronary atherosclerotic heart disease may be defined as a condition that occurs as a consequence of a clinical event due to obstructive coronary disease. Any cardiac or noncardiac problem that alters prognosis, requires treatment, or concerns the patient is considered a *complication*.

THE MANAGEMENT OF EMOTIONAL REACTIONS

Any illness creates an emotional response in the afflicted person. Any serious illness, such as coronary atherosclerotic heart disease, will obviously provoke an emotional response in the patient more often than will a self-limited, benign disorder. The recognition of emotional reactions is discussed earlier in this chapter. The monograph by Hackett and Cassem was reprinted with the permission of the authors and the American Heart Association in order to emphasize the importance of this complication.

A commonsense approach to the patient is needed. The physician who is caring for the patient should be able to manage the emotional problems in almost all of his or her patients and should not require psychiatric consultation except on rare occasions. The physician must recognize the importance of the emotional reaction and not deal solely with the heart itself. He or she must be sensitive to the stages of emotional reaction through which a patient may go. They include denial of illness; acceptance of illness followed by fear; dependence; depression; and realistic adaptation to the disease. A positive attitude is preferable to one which dwells solely on the serious and terrible aspects of an illness. The physician can find something encouraging to say about most clinical conditions. For example, a patient with a heart attack should be told at the outset that he or she is expected to return to work. The virtues of modern treatment can be explained, and hope can be instilled into the patient with the most serious problems. When the prognosis is poor, it is the physician's job to lead the patient and the family to accept the inevitable.

A commonsense approach is usually successful in the management—and prevention—of emotional reactions in patients with coronary atherosclerotic heart disease if the preceding guidelines are followed. The rehabilitation process may require a formalized rehabilitation program following recovery from a heart attack and bypass surgery (see Chap. 62G). Emotional problems often diminish as a result of an active physical program. The physician may need the help of a psychiatrist when abnormal depression is detected in a patient with heart disease, but most emotional problems can be managed directly. All that is usually required is interest, commonsense, and time.

THE MANAGEMENT OF CARDIAC ARRHYTHMIAS

The recognition of cardiac arrhythmias associated with coronary atherosclerotic heart disease is discussed earlier in "Cardiac Arrhythmias." The general discussion of cardiac arrhythmias can be found in Chaps. 46D and 46E. Sudden death is discussed in Chap. 49.

The treatment of sinus tachycardia The recognition of sinus tachycardia is discussed in the earlier section "Sinus Tachycardia" and in Chap. 46D. The treatment of sinus tachycardia is directed at the underlying cause. Beta-adrenergic blocking drugs have been used to treat patients with evidence of sympathetic nervous system overactivity in the prehospital phase of myocardial infarction.[163] The rationale for such therapy is based upon recognition that heart rate is an important determinant of myocardial oxygen consumption and that sympathetic stimulation has an adverse effect on the ischemic zone in experimental myocardial infarction. The merit of this therapeutic approach in human beings remains to be established.

The treatment of sinus bradycardia The recognition of sinus bradycardia is discussed in the earlier section "Sinus Bradycardia" and in Chap. 46D. No treatment is required for many patients with sinus bradycardia following myocardial infarction. When sinus bradycardia is associated with hypotension or heart failure, increasing the heart rate may improve the hemodynamic state of the patient. Many patients with sinus bradycardia have a systolic blood pressure

of 90 to 100 mm Hg with good peripheral perfusion, and have a benign course without treatment. Sinus bradycardia is treated more frequently in the prehospital phase of myocardial infarction than in the coronary care unit because of the substantially greater incidence of accompanying hypotension in the first hour following the onset of symptoms.[163] When frequent premature ventricular beats or more complex ventricular arrhythmias are associated with sinus bradycardia, the heart rate should be cautiously increased.

The most effective means of increasing the heart rate in patients with sinus bradycardia is by the administration of atropine sulfate.[166] Atropine should be given slowly intravenously in a dose of 0.5 or 0.6 mg. Atropine dosages of 0.3 mg or less may cause further slowing of the sinus rate, and dosages of 0.8 mg or greater may produce sinus tachycardia.[174] Atropine will effect an increase in heart rate and blood pressure in most patients with sinus bradycardia and hypotension.[162,165] It is less likely to restore normal hemodynamics in patients with unusually severe bradycardia and hypotension.[155] Premature ventricular beats may decrease in number or be abolished by acceleration of the heart rate with intravenous atropine.[175]

The administration of atropine is not without risk. Sinus tachycardia, increasing numbers of premature ventricular beats, ventricular tachycardia, and ventricular fibrillation are potential adverse effects.[176,433] These serious arrhythmias are less likely to occur if smaller doses (0.5 mg or 0.6 mg) are used. Other troublesome side effects of atropine include urinary retention, increased intraocular tension, psychosis, and visual disturbances.

If the pulse rate response to atropine is not satisfactory, temporary atrial pacing may be used. Intravenous isoproterenol (0.5 to 2 μg/min) may increase the heart rate, but it has the disadvantage of increasing myocardial oxygen need because of its marked inotropic effects. In a few patients with sinus bradycardia and hypotension, atropine may increase the heart rate but the hypotension may persist. These patients are often hypovolemic and may benefit from the infusion of a colloid solution.

The treatment of sinus node dysfunction The recognition of sinus node dysfunction is discussed in Chap. 46D and in the section "Sinus Node Dysfunction" which appeared earlier in this chapter. Digitalis, propranolol, morphine sulfate, and lidocaine can cause sinus node dysfunction, and these drugs should be discontinued if sinus pauses are detected on the electrocardiogram. Sinus node dysfunction should be treated if there is accompanying dizziness, syncope, ventricular arrhythmias, paroxysmal atrial tachyarrhythmias, or hypotension. The intravenous administration of atropine will abolish the sinus pauses in some cases. The cautious administration of isoproterenol, 1 mg in 500 ml of saline given intravenously, may improve pacing function provided the rate of administration is sufficiently slow to avoid the precipitation of an arrhythmia. If atropine fails, temporary intracardiac pacing is the preferred treatment. Patients with symptomatic bradycardia syndrome are best treated with a temporary pacemaker for control of the bradycardia and drugs as needed to suppress the atrial tachycardia. If the bradycardia–tachycardia syndrome persists throughout the hospital stay, the insertion of a permanent pacemaker may be necessary.[434] In most cases, sinus node dysfunction following myocardial infarction is of short duration, and the long-term outlook as regards sinus node function is generally good.[173] However, long-term follow-up is justified because a chronic sick sinus syndrome occasionally appears later.[177]

The treatment of atrial premature beats   The recognition of atrial premature beats is discussed earlier in "Atrial Arrhythmias" and in Chap. 46D. In general, atrial premature beats do not require antiarrhythmic therapy. Treatment is reserved for atrial premature beats that repeatedly precipitate an atrial tachyarrhythmia, atrial bigeminy, and atrial premature beats with a short coupling interval. Digoxin 0.5 mg may be given intravenously or orally and followed by the administration of 0.25 mg every 4 to 6 h for a total of 1 to 1.5 mg. The use of digoxin may or may not be associated with a decrease in the atrial ectopy, but the ventricular rate may be slower if atrial fibrillation ensues. Propranolol given intravenously in increments of 0.5 mg every 3 to 5 min may be effective. If atrial premature beats increase in frequency despite the use of digoxin, quinidine sulfate 0.2 to 0.4 g may be given orally every 4 to 6 h. Procainamide (Pronestyl) 300 to 500 mg intravenously at a rate of 100 mg every 3 min often terminates atrial premature beats.

The treatment of atrial tachycardia   The recognition of atrial tachycardia is discussed earlier in "Atrial Arrhythmias" and in Chap. 46D. The choice of therapy is dictated by the urgency of converting the tachycardia. If the onset of atrial tachycardia is associated with hemodynamic deterioration or the tachycardia cannot be terminated with other forms of therapy, electrical cardioversion should be used. When the clinical situation is less urgent, other forms of therapy may be tried. In a patient not previously receiving digitalis, 0.5 mg digoxin may be given slowly intravenously followed by 0.25 mg every 2 h for two doses. Propranolol 1 to 5 mg given in small increments intravenously may be effective.

Other forms of therapy may abolish the tachycardia but may possess potentially undesirable effects. Carotid sinus stimulation may terminate atrial tachycardia but result in asystole because carotid sinus sensitivity is sometimes increased in patients with acute myocardial infarction. Sympathomimetic drugs such as phenylephrine (Neo-Synephrine) or metaraminol (Aramine) can be used intravenously if hypertension is not present, but the abrupt increase in afterload and myocardial oxygen requirement produced by these drugs can be deleterious. The parasympathomimetic effects of edrophonium hydrochloride (Tensilon) prohibit its use in patients with prior sinus bradycardia or hypotension. When sustained paroxysms of atrial tachycardia recur despite the administration of digoxin, quinidine sulfate 0.2 to 0.4 g may be given orally every 4 to 6 h in an attempt to suppress the inciting atrial premature beats. Occasionally, the combination of propranolol 10 to 20 mg every 6 h and quinidine sulfate will prevent the atrial tachycardia when either drug alone has failed. Atrial tachycardia with atrioventricular block may occur in digitalis toxicity.[179] This is especially likely to occur if hypokalemia is present as a result of diuretic therapy. Omission of digitalis and potassium replacement will generally control the arrhythmia.

The treatment of atrial flutter   The recognition of atrial flutter is discussed earlier in "Atrial Arrhythmias" and in Chap. 46D. Digoxin may be used to control the rapid ventricular rate associated with atrial flutter, but it is often difficult to achieve adequate control of the rate even with large doses of digitalis. Far too often, attempts to slow the ventricular rate with digitalis are continued for hours while a 2:1 atrioventricular conduction ratio persists, and the patient suffers from the deleterious effects of a heart rate of 150 beats per minute. Therefore synchronized dc cardioversion is often the preferred therapy for atrial flutter with a rapid ventricular response. Cardioversion will usually terminate atrial flutter, and successful reversion can frequently be achieved with low-energy shocks in the range of 25 to 50 J. We have, however, observed two incidences in which 400 w/s were ineffective but 1.0 mg of Neo-Synephrine given intravenously in the presence of hypotension reverted the rhythm to normal. Digitalis and propranolol may be used to slow the ventricular rate if atrial flutter is recurrent and cannot be suppressed. Lidocaine is contraindicated since it may produce 1:1 atrioventricular conduction and the development of shock, pulmonary edema, and death. Occasional patients with inferior infarction develop atrial flutter with a 3:1 or 4:1 atrioventricular conduction ratio because of ischemic injury to the atrioventricular node. Treatment of the atrial flutter is usually not necessary in these cases.

The treatment of atrial fibrillation[182–184]   The recognition of atrial fibrillation is discussed earlier in "Atrial Arrhythmias" and in Chap. 46D. In contrast to atrial flutter, the rapid ventricular rate associated with atrial fibrillation is more easily controlled by the administration of digoxin. If the patient has not received digitalis previously, 0.5 mg digoxin may be given intravenously, followed by 0.25 mg orally every 4 h until the ventricular rate is adequately controlled or 1.5 mg has been given. Occasionally the addition of propranolol, 1 to 3 mg given intravenously in the absence of significant left ventricular dysfunction, may aid in slowing the ventricular rate. Procainamide, 300 to 500 mg given intravenously, may on occasion terminate the arrhythmia. Prompt dc cardioversion is indicated when the onset of atrial fibrillation is associated with hypotension, heart failure, or a recurrence of ischemic chest pain. A few patients with myocardial infarction have atrial fibrillation related to chronic pulmonary disease, hypoxia, or pulmonary embolus. In these patients, treatment of the arrhythmia is directed to the underlying problem.

The treatment of accelerated junctional rhythm[185,186] The recognition of accelerated junctional rhythm is discussed earlier in "Accelerated Junctional Rhythm" and in Chap. 46D. Accelerated junctional rhythms at rates of less than 80 beats per minute rarely require treatment. Faster junctional rhythms, especially junctional tachycardia, pose a serious therapeutic problem. Many patients with faster junctional rhythms have severe left ventricular dysfunction, and the rapid ventricular rate and loss of atrial kick may further compromise left ventricular function. It is difficult to suppress junctional tachycardia complicating acute infarction. Major attention should be directed to treatment of the heart failure. Antiarrhythmic drugs, such as lidocaine, quinidine sulfate, or procainamide, deserve a trial, but they may not control the tachycardia. Digitalis intoxication is a common cause of accelerated junctional rhythms and should not be overlooked as being responsible for the arrhythmia.

The treatment of ventricular premature beats The recognition of ventricular premature beats is discussed earlier in "Ventricular Arrhythmias" and in Chap. 46D. Many factors may be considered in the development of a therapeutic plan for ventricular premature beats (VPBs) in patients with acute myocardial infarction. The risk of ventricular fibrillation during the first 4 h following the onset of chest pain is manyfold greater than between 4 and 12 h after.[163] Ventricular fibrillation may occur without warning ventricular arrhythmias. The administration of antiarrhythmic drugs does not invariably prevent primary ventricular fibrillation, and all antiarrhythmic drugs have important side effects.

Prehospital phase Experience obtained from the study of patients with acute myocardial infarction in a coronary care unit may not be directly applicable to the management of patients in the prehospital phase. For example, early studies suggest that lidocaine may be less effective in suppressing VPBs in the first hour after infarction than it is in the hospital phase.[163] In the first hour of infarction, lidocaine provides good suppression of ventricular premature beats when the heart rate is normal, but it is much less effective when sinus tachycardia is present. There is little information available concerning the value of antiarrhythmic therapy in the prevention of sudden death during the first hours following the onset of symptoms. The results from a single study suggest that the prophylactic administration of lidocaine (300 mg intramuscularly) may decrease the incidence of sudden death during the prehospital phase.[435] Guidelines for the proper management of VPBs occurring in the prehospital phase must await the results of further studies.

Hospital phase Since primary ventricular fibrillation may appear without warning, the question arises whether all hospitalized patients with acute myocardial infarction should receive prophylactic antiarrhythmic therapy if no contraindication exists. The effectiveness of lidocaine in the prevention of ventricular fibrillation and ventricular tachycardia is controversial. Lidocaine given as a loading dose of 75 to 100 mg followed by an intravenous infusion of 2 mg/min produced no significant reduction in the incidence of ventricular fibrillation or ventricular tachycardia.[436,437] Conversely, studies utilizing a continuous infusion rate of 2.5 or 3.0 mg/min have shown a significant reduction in the frequency of ventricular fibrillation and ventricular tachycardia.[438,439] The successful suppression of serious ventricular tachyarrhythmias found in the latter studies may in part be related to the higher infusion rate. When lidocaine is infused at a rate of 3 mg/min or greater the incidence of drug side effects is approximately 15 percent.[438]

Perhaps the most important criterion for the institution of prophylactic antiarrhythmic therapy is the patient's time of arrival at hospital. If the patient reaches the hospital within 4 h of the onset of symptoms, prophylactic antiarrhythmic therapy may be indicated. Routine lidocaine or procainamide prophylaxis should not be used for patients with hypotension, shock, severe heart failure, sinus bradycardia, or atrioventricular block. We do not routinely use lidocaine prophylactically because many patients arrive at the hospital more than 6 h after the onset of symptoms, and many patients have an increased risk of developing lidocaine toxicity due to old age or significant heart failure. VPBs that are multiform, paired, frequent, and short-coupled, and VPBs occurring in the bigeminal pattern should be treated because of their association with ventricular tachycardia and because they may occasionally impair cardiac function.[187] Ventricular parasystole is rare following myocardial infarction, and because of its benign course, treatment is rarely indicated.[440]

Lidocaine is the drug of choice for the treatment of VPBs. A loading dose of 1 mg/kg is given intravenously, followed by a continuous infusion of 1 to 4 mg/min. If the initial loading dose does not suppress the VPBs, additional intravenous injections of 50 mg can be given every 5 min until the arrhythmia is abolished or a total of 250 mg has been given. Occasionally toxic reactions necessitate stopping short of this total amount. Lidocaine is metabolized rapidly in the liver and should be used cautiously in the presence of primary liver disease or severe heart failure. Confusion, delirium, muscular irritability, slurred speech, and convulsions are important toxic central nervous system effects of lidocaine. Cardiac toxicity is manifested by hypotension, sinus node arrest, or atrioventricular block, but these manifestations are rare. Dangerous acceleration of the ventricular response to atrial flutter has been reported. In rare, highly selected patients who live significant travelling time from an emergency medical facility, one might consider use of an instrument to send an electrocardiogram by telephone in conjunction with a device which the patient uses to inject 300 mg of lidocaine intramuscularly. To date, however, there is little experience with this system.

For patients sensitive to lidocaine or exhibiting persistent ventricular arrhythmia, procainamide may be used. Procainamide 100 mg may be given intravenously every 5 min until the arrhythmia is abolished, 1 g of drug is given, or untoward drug effects appear.[441] The loading dose is followed by the oral administration of 250 to 500 mg every 3 to 4 h. Occasionally, better control of the ventricular arrhythmia is achieved with a continuous intravenous infusion of procainamide in a dose of 2 to 4 mg/min. Hypotension, atrioventricular or intraventricular conduction disturbances, or worsening of the arrhythmia are important side effects seen with short-term administration. Quinidine and propranolol may be useful in selected cases. Diphenylhydantoin has been used to treat refractory VPBs, but the results are disappointing unless the ectopy is due to digitalis intoxication. Occasionally patients have VPBs that are refractory to antiarrhythmic agents used singly or in combination. If ventricular tachycardia or ventricular fibrillation does not occur, it may be preferable to accept a certain degree of ectopy rather than risk serious toxicity with inordinately large doses of drugs. For a discussion of VPBs associated with bradycardia, see earlier "Treatment of Sinus Bradycardia."

The treatment of ventricular tachycardia The recognition of ventricular tachycardia is discussed earlier in "Ventricular Arrhythmias" and in Chap. 46D. The initial treatment of ventricular tachycardia is dictated by the patient's clinical status during the tachycardia. When the patient's clinical condition is stable, lidocaine or procainamide may be given intravenously as described previously. The trial of drug therapy should not continue beyond 15 to 20 min, because a sustained rapid ventricular tachycardia will result in hemodynamic impairment, and the tachycardia may deteriorate into ventricular fibrillation. Before ventricular tachycardia degenerates into fibrillation, shorter cycle ventricular ectopic beats may interrupt the regular tachycardia and serve as a warning that fibrillation may be imminent. Synchronized dc cardioversion is the preferred treatment when ventricular tachycardia produces serious hemodynamic impairment or when drug therapy is not quickly successful. Low energy, 10 to 25 J, will frequently terminate the ventricular tachycardia. Ventricular tachycardia secondary to digitalis intoxication may respond to the administration of potassium chloride, propranolol, or diphenylhydantoin. When hypotension is present, Neo-Synephrine 0.5 to 1.0 mg given intravenously may produce conversion of the rhythm. Follow-up antiarrhythmic therapy is indicated to lessen recurrences. Propranolol every 4 h along with other antiarrhythmic drugs may be beneficial.

The treatment of ventricular fibrillation[191–191b] The recognition of ventricular fibrillation is discussed earlier in "Ventricular Arrhythmias" and in Chap. 46D. The treatment of ventricular fibrillation is immediate dc cardioversion using 400 J. Patients who are very large or very obese may require even higher energy. The sooner the ventricular fibrillation is reverted, the greater the chances for a favorable outcome. The physical design and placement of dc cardioverters in a coronary care unit should be such that emergency defibrillation can be accomplished in less than 1 min. Following restoration of the normal rhythm, a lidocaine infusion should be used to help prevent further attacks. Repeated episodes of primary ventricular fibrillation refractory to lidocaine or procainamide may be suppressed by propranolol 1 to 3 mg intravenously followed by 20 mg orally every 4 h. If cardioversion fails to revert ventricular fibrillation, cardiac massage, intravenous sodium bicarbonate, and lidocaine should be used. Cardiac standstill is managed by external cardiac massage and the intravenous administration of sodium bicarbonate and isoproterenol or epinephrine. Only a few patients with cardiac standstill following myocardial infarction are successfully resuscitated, and the prospects for long-term survival are dismal because of the associated severe pump failure.[442]

Occasionally, ventricular tachyarrhythmias may be refractory to all pharmacologic measures. Ideally, an adequate blood level of an antiarrhythmic agent should be demonstrated before a therapeutic failure is declared. The first step in the management of refractory ventricular arrhythmia is to search for any possible precipitating causes. Severe left ventricular dysfunction is the problem most commonly associated with uncontrolled ventricular arrhythmias. Hypokalemia, respiratory alkalosis or acidosis, hypovolemia, and digitalis intoxication may be important factors in some patients. Correction of these abnormalities may abolish the arrhythmia.

In the presence of congestive heart failure, the administration of digitalis may lessen the occurrence of ventricular premature beats. Digitalis toxicity occurs with smaller-than-usual doses in experimental myocardial ischemia, and it is prudent to give less than the usual dose of digitalis to patients with heart failure. Digoxin 0.01 mg/kg given as a single dose does not appear to increase the occurrence of ventricular tachyarrhythmias in patients with acute infarction complicated by heart failure.[443] Ventricular arrhythmias associated with severe heart failure or shock may be difficult to suppress. Treatment should be directed primarily to the pump failure rather than to the ventricular arrhythmias. We have found that treatment of severe heart failure with intravenous sodium nitroprusside or phentolamine may result in the disappearance of ventricular ectopy during treatment and the recurrence of ectopy when vasodilator therapy is discontinued.

Suppression of ventricular arrhythmias employing agents that may decrease myocardial ischemia is an intriguing approach, but it has received scant attention. The occurrence of serious ventricular arrhythmias during episodes of variant angina pectoris is an example of the relationship between severe myocardial ischemia and serious ventricular arrhythmias. Relief of the myocardial ischemia by the use of nitroglycerin generally abolishes the ventricular ectopy that accompanies variant angina pectoris. Nitroglycerin may decrease the number of ventricular premature beats in patients with acute myocardial infarction, presumably by decreasing myocardial ischemia.

Refractory ventricular arrhythmias are sometimes controlled by overdrive cardiac pacing.[444] Pacing from the right atrium or left atrium via the coronary sinus is preferable when atrioventricular conduction is intact, because the atrial kick is maintained, and the risk of catheter-induced ventricular fibrillation is lessened. When atrioventricular conduction is impaired, right ventricular pacing is necessary. The pacing rate needed to suppress the ventricular arrhythmias may vary, and various pacing rates should be tried. Rates of 90 to 110 beats per minute are frequently required.

The role of surgery in the treatment of patients with acute infarction complicated by intractable ventricular arrhythmias is ill-defined. Resection of a ventricular aneurysm and revascularization of myocardium with saphenous vein bypass grafts have alleviated refractory ventricular arrhythmias in some patients with myocardial infarction. The surgical experience in treating recurrent ventricular tachycardia by resecting a ventricular aneurysm many months or years following a myocardial infarction is substantially greater. Recently, aortocoronary bypass with or without resection of a ventricular aneurysm has been used to control recurrent ventricular tachycardia.[433,445]

The treatment of accelerated idioventricular rhythm The recognition of accelerated idioventricular rhythm is discussed earlier in "Accelerated Idioventricular Rhythm" and in Chap. 46D. Despite the association between accelerated idioventricular rhythm and ventricular tachycardia, accelerated idioventricular rhythm is generally a benign complication of myocardial infarction. In our experience and that of others, most episodes of ventricular tachycardia that accompany accelerated idioventricular rhythm are unsustained and only rarely degenerate into ventricular fibrillation.[195] Accelerated idioventricular rhythm does not require treatment unless it is associated with rapid ventricular tachycardia, other forms of complex ventricular ectopy, or hypotension (Fig. 62E-15). When treatment is required, suppression of the idioventricular rhythm should be attempted by acceleration of the sinus rate with atropine or atrial pacing. Lidocaine may be used to treat idioventricular rhythm only when the sinus rate exceeds 75 beats per minute. Accelerated idioventricular rhythm may be seen with digitalis intoxication, and the omission of digitalis should always be considered when this rhythm is observed.

The treatment of heart block in inferior infarction[200] The recognition of heart block is discussed earlier in "Heart Block" and in Chap. 46D. The need for therapy is determined by the effective ventricular rate and by the presence or absence of associated complications. Therapeutic decisions based upon the degree of block may be misleading because excessively slow ventricular rates may occur with both second- and third-degree AV block and because an increase or decrease in atrial rate may alter the degree of block without any real change in AV conduction. If the AV block is associated with heart failure, hypotension, syncope, serious ventricular ectopy, or a ventricular rate less than 40 beats per minute, treatment is necessary. In the absence of these complications, however, there is no need for active therapy.

AV block occurring in the prehospital phase responds to the administration of atropine in the majority of cases.[163] Atropine may also increase the ventricular rate in hospitalized patients with inferior infarction complicated by AV block, but it is less effective when the block appears beyond the first day. The dose is 0.5 mg every 3 min for one to three doses. This suggests that cholinergic reflexes may have less influence on the genesis of AV block in the later stages of infarction. If the administration of atropine fails to improve AV conduction, a transvenous pacemaker should be inserted. Isoproterenol 0.5 to 2 mg/min may be used if cardiac pacing is not possible. The outlook for patients with inferior infarction and AV block and an escape pacemaker with a narrow QRS complex is generally favorable. If the AV block is associated with a wide QRS complex or severe heart failure, the mortality is high. The AV block following inferior infarction is usually transient, lasting hours to a few days, and permanent pacing is rarely necessary.

The treatment of heart block in anterior infarction The recognition of heart block is discussed earlier in "Heart Block" and in Chap. 46D. The presence of bundle branch block in the absence of complete heart block is associated with an increased mortality in patients with anterior infarction.[200,201] When complete heart block occurs, the mortality exceeds 75 percent, and most deaths are due to extensive myocardial damage rather than to the conduction disorder. Intracardiac pacing will be of benefit in only a small percentage of patients. The prophylactic insertion of a pacemaker is indicated for patients with right bundle branch block, with or without left anterior or posterior hemiblock, provided that signs of shock or pulmonary edema are absent at the time of appearance of the conduction disturbance. The occurrence of Mobitz type II AV block in a patient with bundle branch block requires the use of a pacemaker, because complete block will likely follow.[200] Despite the prevention of sudden cardiac standstill by the use of prophylactic pacing, however, most patients die because of severe, irreparable left ventricular dysfunction.

If complete AV block persists, a permanent pacemaker should be installed prior to the patient's discharge from hospital. When complete heart block is transient, the clinician faces a therapeutic dilemma. Several authors suggest that there is a high incidence of sudden death during the follow-up period in patients with anterior infarction and transient complete heart block. It is presumed that sudden heart block was the mode of death, but direct evidence for this is sparse. Until the issue is better resolved, it seems prudent to use permanent pacemakers in these patients unless there is severe left ventricular dysfunction.

THE TREATMENT OF SHOCK

Shock may develop as a consequence of myocardial infarction with or without an associated cardiac arrhythmia that may contribute to the problem. The definition and recognition of shock are discussed in Chap. 48 and earlier in this chapter. The treatment of shock is discussed in detail in Chap. 48.

We wish to make four points here:

1 The precise definitions of shock and preshock are often ignored. Any treatment plan must begin with a precise statement of the problem (see Chap. 48).

2 The clinical assessment of the patient in shock is very important. This method of evaluation is the only method available at most hospitals. It is now clear, however, that hemodynamic monitoring gives useful information that cannot be deduced clinically, just as the coronary arteriogram gives information that cannot be deduced clinically. Therefore, a patient in shock or preshock should have a catheter placed in a peripheral artery and a Swan-Ganz thermodilution catheter placed in the pulmonary artery in order to monitor the arterial pressure, pulmonary artery pressure, and cardiac output. If these are not available, one must depend on urine output, cuff blood pressure, skin characteristics, and heart rate to assess therapy. Finally, a catheter should be placed in the bladder in order to measure urine output.

3 Hypovolemia is often unrecognized in patients with shock following myocardial infarction. Hypovolemia—absolute or relative—may occur because of recurrent pain with profound sweating; vomiting related to cholinergic reflexes and opiates; prolonged use of catecholamines; and prior diuretic therapy. The patient is often said to be in "refractory shock," and more catecholamines are given. The patient's neck veins may be normal, and there may be no evidence of pulmonary congestion on chest x-ray. Hemodynamic monitoring may reveal a low cardiac output, and a normal or low left ventricular filling pressure (wedge pressure). The careful use of intravenous dextran or saline may correct the hypovolemia in such patients. The norepinephrine can be weaned gradually as the blood volume is corrected, and the shock may vanish.

4 The intraaortic balloon pump is currently used in the treatment of shock due to myocardial infarction (see Chap. 48). There may be prompt clinical improvement that may persist in a few patients. Unfortunately, the beneficial effect may be short-lived, and the patient may deteriorate as soon as the mechanical assistance is discontinued. When this occurs, it is assumed that the left ventricular damage is so severe that temporary support of the circulation is inadequate to reestablish adequate function. It may be wise to intervene with mechanical assistance earlier than has been the custom in an effort to prevent the irreversible organ damage that is the consequence of shock. Some patients who have exhibited temporary response to balloon counterpulsation have been salvaged when coronary bypass surgery is carried out during the period of mechanical assistance. This approach may permit the salvage of a few patients who are seen in the right place at the right time, but such an approach cannot solve the problem in every locale in the country.

THE TREATMENT OF HEART FAILURE

The recognition and management of heart failure is discussed in Chap. 45. The recognition of heart failure associated with coronary atherosclerotic heart disease is discussed earlier in this chapter. The patients with heart failure due to coronary atherosclerotic heart disease may be divided into those with mild and those with severe heart failure.

Mild heart failure This is recognized by dyspnea or exhaustion on effort, ventricular gallop rhythm, slight increase in pulsation of the neck veins, and slight pulmonary congestion noted on the chest x-ray.

This condition occurs transiently in patients with angina pectoris. In fact, a patient may not complain of angina pectoris but of dyspnea and exhaustion produced by effort. The treatment of this syndrome consists of curtailing activity so that the uncomfortable experience does not occur; controlling hypertension if it is present; decreasing salt intake; giving digoxin with careful observation as to improvement or lack of improvement; prescribing the use of nitroglycerin prior to effort; using isosorbide dinitrate or hydralazine for chronic vasodilation therapy (see discussion below); performing a coronary arteriogram to determine if bypassable lesions are present and if left ventricle function at rest is adequate; and undertaking coronary bypass surgery in suitable cases.

Mild heart failure due to coronary atherosclerosis also occurs in other clinical settings. Acute, mild heart failure may occur in the setting of acute myocardial infarction. Under these circumstances we use digoxin and diuretics with careful attention to unwanted side effects. Chronic vasodilator therapy with nitrol ointment and isosorbide dinitrate may be needed. As a rule, the presence of heart failure during the course of myocardial infarction often precludes coronary arteriography and bypass surgery unless a cardiac arrhythmia or some other noncardiac factor contributed to the failure.

Chronic mild heart failure may occur in patients with coronary atherosclerotic heart disease. As a rule the patients complain of angina pectoris, but they may not. The latter group of patients are said to have ischemic cardiomyopathy. Patients with chronic mild heart failure may well have had a recognized acute infarction in the past, and some of the patients have a ventricular aneurysm with or without recognizable papillary muscle dysfunction.

Patients with mild chronic heart failure should

receive digoxin with careful attention to toxicity. Diuretics should be used with caution, too, since the use of digoxin plus diuretics may precipitate arrhythmias. Occasionally chronic vasodilator therapy with isosorbide dinitrate may be needed. Coronary arteriography and left ventriculography may be needed to prove or disprove the presence of a ventricular aneurysm or papillary muscle dysfunction. Cardiac surgery may be needed to remove a ventricular aneurysm. When this is done, obstructed coronary arteries are bypassed when possible. Some patients with chronic heart failure who do not have a ventricular aneurysm may be salvaged by coronary bypass surgery. It is surprising that some of these patients improve. Unfortunately, it is not possible to predict the outcome in such patients, and the risk of bypass surgery is high. As a general rule, however, the presence of heart failure is a contraindication to bypass surgery unless it is done at the time a ventricular aneurysm is removed.

Severe heart failure This is recognized by severe dyspnea, gallop rhythm, abnormal neck vein pulsation, pulsus alternans, and severe congestion noted on chest x-ray (pulmonary edema).

Acute severe heart failure due to coronary atherosclerotic heart disease is often seen in the setting of acute myocardial infarction. The patient should be given a rapid-acting diuretic. Digoxin should be used, and the rhythm should be controlled. It is useful to place a Swan-Ganz catheter in the pulmonary artery in order to measure the pulmonary diastolic pressure and thermodilution cardiac output, and a line into a peripheral artery in order to measure the arterial pressure. Vasodilator therapy should be used (see later discussion in this chapter). The drugs used to decrease impedance to left ventricular ejection are nitroprusside and intravenous nitroglycerin. The more complex the clinical problem is, the greater the necessity of measuring the wedge pressure or pulmonary diastolic pressure, systemic pressure, and cardiac output.

The intraaortic balloon pump may be used in some patients with severe acute heart failure due to myocardial infarction, especially when shock or preshock is present. When it is used, it is employed as an adjunct to the therapy just mentioned.

Coronary arteriography and left ventriculography may be needed when a ruptured septum or muscle rupture is suspected. Cardiac surgery may be needed when there is a ruptured septum or rupture of the papillary muscle. Obviously the risk of surgery is great, but gratifying results can be achieved on occasion.

Rackley has discussed the value of hemodynamic monitoring of patients with myocardial infarction (see his discussion "The Use of Hemodynamic Measurements for the Management of the Patient with Acute Myocardial Infarction" earlier in this chapter). Obviously it is difficult to manipulate cardiac contractility, preload, and afterload without objective data. Whereas mild heart failure can be managed without a Swan-Ganz catheter or an arterial line, it is difficult to manage severe heart failure (often associated with preshock) occurring in the

setting of myocardial infarction without hemodynamic monitoring. Unfortunately, this approach cannot be used in every locale in this country. Accordingly, it is necessary for the physician to utilize clinical parameters to determine the need for and results of treatment. This is accomplished by (1) observing the general appearance of the patient; noting the heart rate; observing the neck veins; listening for rales; measuring the hourly urine output; determining the systemic blood pressure at frequent intervals (as often as every 15 min); and looking for congestion on the chest x-ray at frequent intervals, and (2) by understanding the action of digitalis, diuretics, dopamine and norepinephrine, morphine, intravenous nitroglycerin, nitroprusside, isosorbide dinitrate, and hydralazine—this makes it possible for the skilled physician to develop a strategy that is useful in the treatment of such patients.

Unfortunately, severe heart failure that occurs secondary to myocardial infarction is a sign of danger ahead. Most of the patients have severe left ventricular dysfunction and have a poor prognosis often measured in terms of months or a few years.

Chronic severe heart failure may occur in a patient who has had one or several infarctions or a ventricular aneurysm, or has end-stage ischemic cardiomyopathy. The treatment consists of decreasing the activity of the patient; decreasing the salt intake; the proper use of digoxin and diuretics; the use of chronic vasodilator therapy. Surgical removal of a ventricular aneurysm may occasionally produce an excellent result.

Comments regarding certain aspects of current therapy Digoxin There is experimental evidence suggesting that digitalis preparations may increase the myocardial demand for oxygen at a time when oxygen cannot be delivered to the myocardium and that this may increase the size of the infarction or precipitate cardiac arrhythmias. This has not been a problem for us although we admit that we cannot as yet *accurately* measure the size of an an infarct. We still use digoxin in patients who have heart failure as a result of acute myocardial infarction. There has been less controversy regarding the use of digitalis glycosides in patients with arrhythmias (such as atrial fibrillation) or chronic heart failure associated with coronary atherosclerotic heart disease. All efforts should be directed at avoiding digitalis toxicity when the drug is used during acute infarction for acute heart failure. The same admonition applies, however, to the use of digitalis for chronic heart failure.

Propranolol The action of propranolol is useful in that it clearly prevents angina pectoris by the actions mentioned earlier, but the price paid for this result is that it decreases myocardial contractility and may precipitate or aggravate heart failure. Propranolol has been used, as has practolol, during the acute phase of myocardial infarction with contradictory results. We use propranolol during acute infarction for cardiac arrhythmias and for persistent sinus tachycardia not caused by severe left ventricular dysfunction. Since heart failure of some degree is often present in patients with sinus tachycardia due to myocardial infarction, it follows that propranolol is often given to the patient with heart failure. Benefit may occur if the slowing of the heart rate overrides the harmful decrease in contractility that propranolol produces. Therefore, it is important to monitor the heart rate and relate it to the other signs of heart failure. If all parameters improve, the drug should be continued. If the heart rate slows and other signs of heart failure increase, the drug should be discontinued.

Diuretics These drugs are commonly used in patients with heart failure secondary to coronary atherosclerotic heart disease. Such drugs are extremely useful in most patients with chronic hypervolemia, and harmful hemodynamic consequences are seldom observed in such patients who receive diuretics.

There are two clinical situations where diuretics should be used with considerable caution. (1) Certain patients with severe chronic heart failure and large hearts do not tolerate diuresis to the point of dry weight. They may develop postural hypotension, weakness, and a reduced cardiac output with all of the consequences that go with it. These patients need a higher than normal ventricular filling pressure. (2) Patients with pulmonary edema who are normovolemic and have pulmonary edema with a normal size heart may occasionally react adversely to a vigorous diuresis. They may develop hypotension and subsequent oliguria. One reason this does not occur more often is that the oxygen exchange in the lung improves as the pulmonary edema subsides, and the improved oxygenation is beneficial to the heart and other organs.

Vasodilator therapy This new concept of treating heart failure is proving to be very useful.[445a] *Vasodilator therapy can be used for the treatment of acute severe heart failure* in patients with acute myocardial infarction. The usual therapy is instituted plus vasodilator therapy. The drugs used are usually intravenous nitroprusside (Nipride) or intravenous nitroglycerin. We suspect that intravenous nitroglycerin is superior to nitroprusside in this setting. Hydralazine may also be effective in selected patients. It is desirable to use hemodynamic monitoring when such therapy is employed (see earlier discussion by Rackley).

Vasodilator therapy is also used in patients with severe chronic heart failure.[328,446] Severe chronic heart failure may follow acute myocardial infarction or may occur in patients with coronary atherosclerotic heart disease who have considerable mitral regurgitation or "ischemic cardiomyopathy." The drugs generally used are sublingual isosorbide dinitrate, nitroglycerin ointment, and oral hydralazine. More experience has been gained with the first two of these drugs. Parmley and Chatterjee summarize their views as follows (reproduced with permission of the author and publisher):[446]

In general, the vasodilators produce a reduction in left ventricular filling pressure and an increase in forward cardiac output. Despite a slight fall in arterial pressure, heart rate does not change or may even fall slightly. Patients must have an elevated left ventricular filling pressure, however, to achieve beneficial hemodynamic results from vasodilator therapy. Given to patients with an initial low filling pressure, vasodilators tend to further lower this pressure, reduce stroke volume, and produce reflex tachycardia. Because the various forms of vasodilator have differing effects on venous capacitance and arteriolar resistance, it may be important to individualize therapy for a given patient. Hydralazine, for example, is primarily effective in reducing arteriolar resistance and increasing cardiac output. The nitrates, on the other hand, are most effective in reducing left ventricular filling pressure although they also produce an increase in cardiac output. In some patients, combination therapy may help to achieve both a reduction in filling pressure and an increase in cardiac output.

Results of Mantle et al. have been summarized as follows (reproduced with permission of the author and publisher):[447]

Severe congestive heart failure (CHF) secondary to myocardial infarction (MI) remains a difficult management problem. Although intravenous vasodilators and mechanical assist devices have been reported to improve the depressed hemodynamic function, they cannot be used for long-term management.

Sublingual administration of isosorbide dinitrate (Sorbitrate) (5 to 10 mg) in 7 patients with severe CHF following anterior wall MI was contrasted with the effects of sublingual nitroglycerin in patients with heart failure and with the effects of sublingual isosorbide dinitrate in patients without heart failure. Serial measurements of mean right atrial and pulmonary arterial end-diastolic pressure, heart rate, and cardiac output were obtained prior to and during the 4 hours after administration of isosorbide dinitrate.

Peak response occurred approximately 30 minutes after drug administration with an 83% reduction in mean right atrial pressure (from 6 to 1 mm. Hg, p< 0.02), a 36% reduction in pulmonary arterial end-diastolic pressure (from 25 to 16 mm. Hg, p<0.0001), and a 6% reduction mean blood pressure (from 94 to 88 mm. Hg, p<0.05). There were small increases in cardiac index (from 2.3 to 2.6 liters/minute/m.²) and stroke work index (from 26 to 32 Gm./beat/m.²). The total systemic vascular resistance was reduced by 5%, from 1605 to 1518 dynes sec. cm.$^{-5}$ (p<0.10). The baseline heart rate of 105 beats/minute was not significantly changed. The reduction in pulmonary arterial end-diastolic pressure remained significant for 3 to 4 hours, and was associated with relief of the patients' pulmonary symptoms.

The response to nitroglycerin (0.4 mg.) was similar in magnitude but of much shorter duration (approximately 15 minutes for nitroglycerin versus 4 hours for isosorbide dinitrate).

In left ventricular function curves, to compare the effects of isosorbide dinitrate in patients with and without CHF, the slope (calculated by dividing the change in cardiac index or stroke work index by the change in pulmonary arterial end-diastolic pressure) was significantly (p<0.05) depressed in patients with CHF.

Sublingual isosorbide dinitrate was also associated with a diuresis of 500 to 1000 ml. in patients who had been refractory to intravenous furosemide.

Apparently, symptomatic pulmonary venous hypertension

in patients with MI can be relieved effectively by isosorbide dinitrate without further compromising left ventricular function.

Miller et al. recommend the combined use of Dopamine and nitroprusside therapy in congestive heart failure. This unique approach utilizes inotropic stimulation with afterload reduction.[447a]

Intraaortic balloon pump The use of the intraaortic balloon pump in patients with heart failure is usually restricted to patients with acute myocardial infarction whose systemic pressure cannot be maintained at a satisfactory level.

Surgical treatment The surgical treatment of heart failure is limited to the removal of a myocardial aneurysm, the closure of a ruptured interventricular septum and the correction of severe mitral regurgitation.

THE TREATMENT OF ELECTROMECHANICAL DISSOCIATION

The *transient* variety of electromechanical dissociation is occasionally seen in patients with transient left ventricular ischemia. Syncope and ischemic paralysis of the left ventricle with or without associated angina pectoris may occur as a consequence of transient left ventricular ischemia. The treatment of this variety of electromechanical dissociation is directed to the correction of the myocardial ischemia with drugs such as nitroglycerin, isosorbide dinitrate, and coronary bypass surgery in suitable cases. Obviously, propranolol must be used carefully if at all in this group of patients.

Permanent electromechanical dissociation is a very serious complication of myocardial ischemia and myocardial infarction. Few patients recover from it. The prompt treatment of cardiac arrest (see Chap. 50) may reverse the condition in a few instances. The patient with electromechanical dissociation occurring after myocardial infarction rarely recovers.

The treatment of this variety of acute pump failure is poor, but it includes the use of digitalis; inotropic stimulation with isoproterenol or norepinephrine; and correction of the filling pressure of the left ventricle by giving intravenous fluid while monitoring the capillary wedge pressure with a Swan-Ganz catheter. When the latter is not possible, the fluid is given, and the urine flow and blood pressure are used as a guide to success. If the pressure goes up and pulmonary congestion does not increase, progress can be assumed. One should consider the use of mechanical circulatory assist where it is available. Coronary arteriography and emergency coronary bypass surgery have been successfully employed in a few patients.

THE TREATMENT OF PERICARDITIS[448]

The recognition of pericarditis is discussed earlier in this chapter and in Chap. 84. The treatment of pericarditis is discussed in detail in Chap. 84.

Pericarditis should be promptly recognized and treated. It may cause great anxiety and distress in the patient who may fear that another heart attack has occurred. The physician may be frustrated by the pain and dyspnea since there may be an incomplete response to opiate administration. There is danger of bleeding into the pericardial sac when pericarditis is unrecognized and anticoagulants are continued. *Therefore, anticoagulants must be omitted in the presence of persistent pericardial rub or a very loud diffuse pericardial rub.* If a rub is not apparent, the differential diagnosis presented is (1) further myocardial necrosis, (2) congestive heart failure, (3) pulmonary embolism, and (4) bronchopneumonia. Occasionally a therapeutic response to corticosteroids may indicate the pericardial origin of symptoms. Relief of pain and dyspnea may occur within several hours of administration of intravenous glucocorticosteroids such as 15 mg dexamethasone or 100 mg hydrocortisone. Oral dosage is then instituted with 40 mg prednisone daily with rapid tapering of the medication over a period of 1 week. Steroid suppression of inflammation may be accompanied occasionally by the reversion of atrial fibrillation or flutter to a normal sinus mechanism. Fever due to pericardial inflammation usually disappears within 24 h. Recurrence of symptoms following omission of steroids may require retreatment. Indomethacin, 100 to 200 mg daily, or salicylates may produce satisfactory remission in many patients, and in the authors' experience the "rebound phenomenon" is less prominent with these drugs. Recurrences may occur weeks or months later (Dressler's syndrome), but the likelihood of such cannot be predicted from the clinical findings observed during the initial stage of the illness. When significant pericardial fluid accompanies pericarditis, rapid resolution can be usually obtained by a combination of prednisone, 40 to 60 mg. and appropriate diuretic therapy such as 40 to 80 mg furosemide daily for 5 to 7 days. Precautions to avoid hypokalemia or hypovolemia should be taken. The blood pressure should be taken daily while the patient is in the standing position to detect postural hypotension, an important clue to hypovolemia. If hypovolemia occurs, diuretic therapy is stopped, and if indicated, fluid repletion by intravenous dextran is carried out.

The prognosis of patients with pericarditis complicating myocardial infarction is related to the size of the myocardial damage.

THE TREATMENT OF PULMONARY EMBOLISM

The recognition of pulmonary embolism is discussed earlier in this chapter and in Chap. 75. The treatment of pulmonary embolism is discussed in detail in Chaps. 75 and 108.

The threat of thromboembolism remains the major indication for anticoagulant therapy. (The indications for Coumadin therapy in patients with myocardial infarction are discussed earlier in this chapter). If the patient is not receiving anticoagulants, therapy with heparin is given for 1 week followed by sodium warfarin (Coumadin) for 2 to 3 months. If recurrent episodes occur in spite of adequate anticoagulation, insertion of a Mobin-Uddin umbrella in the inferior vena cava can be carried out with safety.

THE TREATMENT OF SYSTEMIC ARTERIAL EMBOLISM

The recognition of systemic arterial embolism is discussed earlier in this chapter and in Chap. 104. The treatment of peripheral arterial embolism is discussed in detail in Chap. 107.

The mortality rate due to arterial embolism to the bifurcation of the aorta, iliac arteries, and arteries of the extremities remains high but has been reduced significantly since the introduction of Fogarty's catheter-balloon technique. Using this technique, one may extract the clots under local anesthesia and save the limbs. When arterial embolism occurs, immediate intravenous heparin therapy is begun, using 75 to 100 mg. Some prefer to switch to subcutaneous heparin every 6 h, with clotting times being measured at 5 h and kept at two to three times the control value. Others prefer intermittent intravenous heparin at 6-h intervals, keeping the clotting time two to three times normal control values at 5 h.

THE TREATMENT OF PAPILLARY MUSCLE DYSFUNCTION

The recognition of papillary muscle dysfunction is discussed earlier in this chapter and in Chap. 60B. The treatment of papillary muscle dysfunction is discussed in Chaps. 60B and 62F.

Papillary muscle dysfunction may develop following myocardial infarction and is often associated with a dyskinetic segment of the left ventricle or ventricular aneurysm. There is no specific treatment for mild degrees of papillary muscle dysfunction except for the treatment of the myocardial ischemia with nitroglycerin, isosorbide dinitrate, and propranolol (used cautiously). Occasionally, the murmur of papillary muscle dysfunction may vanish after successful coronary bypass surgery done for angina pectoris or surgically compelling critical lesions of the coronary arteries. The murmur disappears because surgical revascularization of the myocardium may, at times, eliminate the dyskinetic area, and the papillary muscle dysfunction may decrease.

When severe, unrelenting heart failure seems to be related to the mitral regurgitation produced by papillary muscle dysfunction, it may be necessary to have surgical replacement of the mitral valve and at times resection of an associated ventricular aneurysm (see Chap. 62F). When possible, it is wise to delay surgical intervention for several weeks after acute infarction.

THE TREATMENT OF RUPTURE OF THE PAPILLARY MUSCLE

The recognition of papillary muscle rupture is discussed earlier in this chapter. The treatment of rupture of a papillary muscle is unsatisfactory and is purely surgical. The condition is always associated with heart failure and shock. Left ventriculography and coronary arteriography are necessary to reveal the degree of myocardial damage that is present; to identify the magnitude of mitral regurgitation; and to delineate the obstruction in the coronary arteries. The surgeon, using circulatory assist (the intraaortic balloon pump) prior to surgery and after surgery may successfully replace the mitral valve, remove a portion of the damaged and functionless left ventricular wall, and bypass several obstructed arteries.[449]

THE TREATMENT OF RUPTURE OF THE VENTRICULAR SEPTUM[449]

The recognition of rupture of the ventricular septum is discussed earlier in this chapter. The surgical treatment is discussed in detail in Chap. 62F.

This condition is usually associated with heart failure and shock. The treatment of these two conditions is discussed earlier in this section. The septal rupture is recognized by the presence of a murmur at the end of the sternum and less often at the apex. The condition is proven by detecting an increase in oxygen saturation by using the Swan-Ganz catheter. If the patient's condition is deteriorating and septal closure seems indicated, it is necessary to perform a left ventriculogram and a coronary arteriogram. The risk of these procedures is higher than when they are done for simpler conditions, but it is not prohibitive. The result of the study may reveal an inoperable situation. On the other hand, the condition is often operable. The problem becomes one of timing the surgical intervention properly. It is wise to delay surgical correction of a ruptured ventricular septum for several weeks if possible in order for the "rim" of the infarcted septum to become firm enough to hold the surgeon's sutures. The problem is that many patients will not live that length of time. Therefore, it is necessary to operate on some patients within days after the event occurs. Fortunately, the operative results have improved in the group of patients that require "early" surgery.

THE TREATMENT OF EXTERNAL RUPTURE OF THE HEART

The recognition of external rupture of the heart is discussed earlier in this chapter. The surgical treatment of the condition is discussed in Chap. 62E.

Death may occur within a few minutes, but survival may be sufficiently long to allow pericardiocentesis, constant drainage by intrapericardial catheter, and the rapid administration of dextran with norepinephrine. Temporary relief of tamponade and return of blood pressure may allow the institution of assisted circulation and removal to the surgical suite where corrective surgery can be instituted. Surgery is confined to closing the defect, using partial bypass–assisted circulation. The authors' associates at Emory University Hospital have performed this operation on three patients with two recoveries.[450]

THE TREATMENT OF VENTRICULAR ANEURYSM[451]

The recognition of a ventricular aneurysm is discussed earlier in this chapter. The surgical removal of a ventricular aneurysm is discussed in Chap. 62F.

Patients with a ventricular aneurysm following a myocardial infarction may have no difficulty. On the other hand, the aneurysm may produce heart failure, resistant cardiac arrhythmias, and peripheral arterial emboli. Chronic ventricular aneurysms rarely rupture. Heart failure and cardiac arrhythmias are treated according to the methods described earlier in this chapter. A left ventriculogram and a coronary arteriogram are performed in order to determine the amount of the ventricular wall and septum that are involved; to estimate the amount of mitral regurgitation that is present; and to delineate the obstruction in the coronary arteries. Surgical skill has improved so dramatically over the last decade that it is now possible to operate on many of these patients with an acceptable mortality.

THE TREATMENT OF POSTMYOCARDIAL INFARCTION SYNDROME (DRESSLER'S SYNDROME)

The recognition of Dressler's syndrome is discussed earlier in this chapter and in Chap. 84. The treatment is discussed in Chap. 84.

This condition is treated with corticosteroids, indomethacin, or aspirin. When cardiac tamponade occurs, and such is rare, it may be necessary to aspirate the pericardial fluid. Constrictive pericarditis is a rare complication. It may be necessary to remove the pericardium if pericardial pain is recurrent and disabling despite medical management, if cardiac tamponade recurs, or if constriction of the pericardium develops.

THE TREATMENT OF CHEST WALL SYNDROME

The recognition of chest wall discomfort is discussed earlier in this chapter. Little is known about this type of discomfort. The largest problem, however, is to identify the difficulty for what it is and to make certain the discomfort is not due to myocardial ischemia, pericarditis, anxiety, etc.

The management of chest wall discomfort includes reassurance to the patient that the discomfort is not serious and does not represent myocardial ischemia; the use of aspirin and indomethacin; and the use of physical therapy in the form of gentle arm and trunk exercises.

THE TREATMENT OF CEREBRAL SYNDROMES

The multiple causes of cerebral syndromes were enumerated earlier in this chapter. Certain of the cerebral syndromes may occur in the ambulatory patient, but as a rule they are recognized more frequently in the hospital (especially in the coronary care unit).

The patient may be anxious, restless, confused, delirious, and may have insomnia, weakness, and seizures. These may be due to "psychosis," hypoxia, drug reactions, etc. The treatment of the cerebral syndromes varies according to the cause. The treatment of intensive care psychosis includes moving the patient from the coronary care unit when it is safe to do so. The treatment of hypoxia includes managing heart failure, shock, cardiac arrhythmia, etc. The treatment of a metabolic disorder requires the control of electrolytes, pH, and blood gases. The treatment of associated renal failure may require specific therapy. Other diseases such as diabetes mellitus may make an appearance and require treatment. Cerebral vascular disease, including embolism, may require special treatment since it can be related to atrial fibrillation and the mural thrombus of an infarct. Many drugs lead to somnolence, confusion, and depression, and the withdrawal of certain drugs may produce delirium and seizures. In the former situation the drug is discontinued, and in the latter situation the drug may be restarted.

To restate, the treatment of cerebral syndromes requires the correction of mental stress, hypoxic, metabolic disorders, drug reactions and drug withdrawal, etc.

BRONCHOPNEUMONIA

The recognition of bronchopneumonia is discussed earlier in this chapter. The sputum smear and cultures may demonstrate the presence of pneumococci or other organisms. Leukocytosis is of little diagnostic help since it regularly occurs following myocardial infarction. X-ray examination of the chest may indicate areas of consolidation with an air bronchogram; however, differentiation must be made from confluent areas of edema and pulmonary infarction. A favorable site for interstitial edema is near the border of the right side of the heart, and bronchopneumonia or pneumonitis is commonly confused with congestion in this area.

Penicillin is given in the absence of a history of hypersensitivity to the drug. If pneumonia occurs as a result of aspiration, sodium cephalothin (Keflin) or ampicillin (Polycillin) combined with corticosteroid therapy is given. In all instances therapy is instituted promptly while awaiting cultures. When pulmonary embolism cannot be excluded, one must treat both for pneumonia and thromboembolism. When confluent areas of edema cannot be differentiated, treatment for congestive heart failure with digitalis and diuretics plus antibiotics may be required.

THE TREATMENT OF "LATE CARDIAC ARREST"

The treatment of cardiac arrest is discussed in Chap. 50, and the treatment of arrhythmias is discussed earlier in this chapter. Cardiac arrest associated with a heart attack usually occurs at the onset of the illness and may be the only manifestation of abrupt ischemia. Most arrests occur during the first 8 h of a heart attack. When cardiac arrest occurs several days or weeks after infarction, it is called "late cardiac arrest."

The prevention of late cardiac arrest must be considered.[452] Obviously we do not yet know how to prevent early or late cardiac arrest. This is the area where much research needs to be done, since it is a common way for the patient with coronary atherosclerotic heart disease to die.

One should not forget that emotional factors may induce cardiac arrest in the patient with coronary atherosclerotic heart disease. For example, a 65-year-old patient with a transmural inferior myocardial infarction, who had been discharged from the coronary care unit after 1 week, became emotionally disturbed during a telephone conversation and dropped dead. The authors have observed that trivial upsets such as those related to venipuncture, changing the site of intravenous clysis, or fecal impaction appear to trigger arrhythmias such as atrial fibrillation, ventricular tachycardia, and ventricular fibrillation. Adverse reactions to drugs may produce postural hypotension and syncope, thereby inciting recurrent ischemia leading to cardiac arrest. The Hopkins group have recently emphasized that ventricular premature beats increase the chances of sudden death during the year after myocardial infarction. Such is even more likely to occur when the ejection fraction is decreased.[452] Extended care in secondary coronary care units for patients with predisposing factors is currently being used in many hospitals, but the data are currently inadequate to assess their effectiveness.

Some physicians believe that the long-term use of beta-blocking agents such as propranolol may decrease the incidence of sudden death. We are currently using this approach in patients with angina pectoris, in asymptomatic patients after infarction, and after coronary bypass surgery unless there is a contraindication to the use of the drug such as sick sinus syndrome, AV block, inferior infarction, or evidence of left ventricular dysfunction. The results of a large-scale clinical trial of chronic propranolol therapy following acute myocardial infarction should be available by 1981.

Coronary bypass surgery prevents sudden death in selected patients. The prognosis of obstructive coronary disease is discussed earlier in this chapter. Prognosis is determined, to a large extent, on the degree and location of the obstruction. This information is obtained by performing a coronary arteriogram (see earlier discussion in this chapter and in Chap. 29D). It is now clear that certain carefully selected patients with coronary atherosclerotic heart disease live longer when coronary bypass surgery is performed than when they are treated medically. The patients live longer because they have less sudden death and infarction and heart failure. This is most likely to be true for patients with the following

findings at coronary arteriography: high-grade obstruction of the left main coronary artery; obstruction of the left anterior descending artery plus obstruction of the right and circumflex arteries; obstruction of the left anterior descending artery plus obstruction of either the right or circumflex arteries; or patients with high-grade obstruction of the proximal left anterior descending artery when angina is troublesome. Such patients should be considered for bypass surgery if there are no contraindications and if the surgical mortality at the institution where the surgery is to be done is 1 to 2 percent. In reality, the patient who has coronary bypass surgery derives both the benefit of surgery and the benefit of medical management.

THE TREATMENT OF GENITOURINARY SYNDROMES

The genitourinary complications of myocardial infarction are discussed earlier in this chapter. If an indwelling catheter is required, a slow constant drip of 0.25 percent acetic acid or dilute neomycin and polymycin solution has been shown to be capable of preventing bacteremia (40 mg neomycin in 1,000 ml isotonic saline solution, dripped into the bladder at a rate of 40 ml/h or 1 liter/day). Bleeding incident to catheterization or during the period the indwelling catheter is in place is an occasional problem, particularly when anticoagulant therapy is given. Trauma during catheterization or by the patient's pulling out the catheter may cause hemorrhage. Cystitis and pyelonephritis may develop and require antibiotic therapy. Such symptoms may develop days or weeks later. Bacteremia with gram-negative sepsis should be suspected when chills, fever, and hypotension occur during or following catheterization of the bladder. When this occurs, it is necessary to immediately institute treatment using ampicillin or sodium cephalothin and kanamycin while awaiting the report of blood cultures. Massive corticosteroid therapy using dexamethasone may be required in the presence of gram-negative bacteremia and shock. The therapy for acute renal failure is almost always directed toward the improvement of the underlying cardiovascular problem.

THE TREATMENT OF SHOULDER-HAND SYNDROME

The recognition of shoulder-hand syndrome is discussed earlier in this chapter. As stated there, the syndrome is less common now than it was in the era when patients with infarction were treated with prolonged bed rest. The condition is avoided if the patient is permitted to use his arms and shoulders for simple actions.

This syndrome is treated by physiotherapy, application of heat, and a program of gentle exercise of the shoulder. The course may be a protracted one, lasting many months. Some patients develop the rotator-cuff syndrome because of calcific tendonitis. In selected cases the intraarticular injection of hydrocortisone may give relief. Dupuytren's contracture and palmar nodules may occasionally require surgical treatment.

THE TREATMENT OF NONVASCULAR COMPLICATIONS

Gout and diabetes mellitus may be precipitated by myocardial infarction and by chlorothiazide and other diuretics such as furosemide and ethacrynic acid. The physician should be alert to the recognition of these two conditions.

Diabetes is usually recognized by the elevation of the blood sugar level and by the report of sugar in the urine. The condition is usually not severe, and no insulin is required. A weight reduction program is started since overt diabetes may appear months later if obesity is disregarded. Occasionally regular insulin may be needed. Silent myocardial infarction occasionally is the cause of a patient with stable diabetes mellitus going out of control for no apparent reason.

Gout should be suspected whenever joint pain occurs in the setting of myocardial infarction. Patients with a history of frequent attacks of gout should receive allopurine (allopurinol) as a prophylactic measure.

THE TREATMENT OF HICCOUGHS, RETCHING, NAUSEA, AND VOMITING

See discussion earlier in this chapter. Hiccoughs are troublesome to the patient with myocardial infarction and may prevent adequate rest. Sedation may help, but as a rule hiccoughs run their course, and drastic measures such as phrenic nerve crush are rarely, if ever, needed.

Retching, nausea, and vomiting may be part of the clinical picture of myocardial infarction but are often due to a drug reaction. When these worrisome symptoms occur, the physician should eliminate all drugs that can produce them. Certain drugs such as sedatives and tranquilizers may be tried. Compazine suppositories seem to be a favorite. Intravenous fluid such as 5 percent glucose in one-half normal saline with potassium chloride may be needed if the patient does not drink or if vomiting occurs.

THE TREATMENT OF CERTAIN GASTROINTESTINAL SYNDROMES

The gastrointestinal syndromes associated with the treatment of myocardial infarction are discussed earlier in this chapter. Gastric distension can usually be avoided if it is due to oxygen administration. An oxygen mask may decrease the amount of oxygen swallowed as compared to the use of intranasal prongs. Gastric distension occurring spontaneously is treated with a nasogastric suction.

Anticoagulants, corticosteroids, and indomethacin should be discontinued in patients who have evidence of a peptic ulcer manifested either by symptoms or by blood in the stool. Patients with a history of peptic ulcer who have a myocardial infarction should receive antacids prophylactically.

Straining at the stool and fecal impaction should be avoided in patients with myocardial infarction. Stool softeners or laxatives such as Ducolax, Colace, or milk of magnesia may be used to prevent this distressing complication.

THE TREATMENT OF THERAPEUTIC MISADVENTURES

See discussion earlier in this chapter. As stated earlier, the benefits accruing from the use of diet, drugs, and procedures are always balanced by the sobering realization that every drug that is used and every procedure that is performed may produce an unwanted or harmful side effect. Accordingly, it is necessary for us to be alert to the undesirable effects of all that we do.

Every time we order a drug or perform a procedure we must ask two questions: (1) Is the benefit to be gained from the drug or procedure worth the risk of unwanted side effects and dangers that sometimes occur as a result of the drug or procedure? and (2) Are all personnel aware of the side effects of the drugs and procedures, since they may occur at a time when the physician is not in attendance?

REFERENCES

1 Gorlin, R.: "Coronary Artery Disease," vol. XI, "Major Problems in Internal Medicine," W. B. Saunders Company, Philadelphia, 1976.

1a Hillis, L. D., and Braunwald, E.: Myocardial Ischemia (First of Three Parts), *N. Engl. J. Med.,* 296:1034, 1977.

1b Hillis, L. D., and Braunwald, E.: Myocardial Ischemia (Second of Three Parts), *N. Engl. J. Med.,* 196:1034, 1977.

1c Hillis, L. D., and Braunwald, E.: Myocardial Ischemia (Third of Three Parts), *N. Engl. J. Med.,* 296:1093, 1977.

2 Heberden, W.: Commentaries on the History and Cure of Diseases, chap. 70, in "Angina Pectoris," printed for T. Tayne, Mews-Gate, London, 1802.

3 Heberden, W.: Some Account of a Disorder of the Breast, *Med. Trans. R. Coll. Physicians,* II, London, 1786, p. 59 (The original mention of angina pectoris was made by Heberden in a lecture before the Royal College of Physicians in London in July 1768.)

4 Herrick, J. B.: Clinical Features of Sudden Obstruction of the Coronary Arteries, *J.A.M.A.,* 59:2015, 1912.

5 Master, A. M.: Coronary Heart Disease: Angina Pectoris, Acute Coronary Insufficiency and Coronary Occlusion, *Ann. Intern. Med.,* 20:661, 1944.

6 Blumgart, H. L., Schlesinger, M. J., and Zoll, P. M.: Angina Pectoris, Coronary Failure, and Acute Myocardial Infarction, *J.A.M.A.,* 116:91, 1941.

7 Sones, F. M., Jr., and Shirey, E. K.: Cine Coronary Arteriography, *Mod. Concepts Cardiovasc. Dis.,* 31:735, 1962.

7a Sabiston, D. C., Jr.: The Coronary Circulation, *Johns Hopkins Med. J.,* 134:314, 1974.

8 Garrett, H. E., Dennis, E. W., and DeBakey, M. E.: Aortocoronary Bypass with Saphenous Vein Graft. Seven-Year Follow-up, *J.A.M.A.,* 223:729, 1973.

9 Alderman, E. L., Davies, R. O., Crowley, J. J., Lopes, M. G., Brooker, J. Z., Friedman, J. P., Graham, A. F., Matlof, H. J., and Harrison, D. C.: Dose Response Effectiveness of Propranolol for the Treatment of Angina Pectoris, *Circulation,* 51:964, 1975.

10 Morris, D. C., Hurst, J. W., and Logue, R. B.: Myocardial Infarction in Young Women, *Am. J. Cardiol.,* 38:299, 1976.

11 Oliver, M. F.: Ischaemic Heart Disease in Young Women, *Br. Med. J.,* 2:253, 1974.

12 Engel, H. J., Page, H. L., and Campbell, W. B.: Coronary Artery Disease in Young Women, *J.A.M.A.,* 230:1531, 1974.

13 Proudfit, W. L., Shirey, E. K., and Sones, F. M., Jr.: Selective Cine Coronary Arteriography: Correlation with Clinical Findings in 1,000 Patients, *Circulation,* 33:901, 1966.

14 Hurst, J. W., and Myerburg, R. J.: "Introduction to Electrocardiography," 2d ed., McGraw-Hill Book Company, Inc., New York, 1973.

15 Schlant, R. C., and Hurst, J. W.: "Advances in Electrocardiography," vol. 2, Grune & Stratton, Inc., New York, 1976.

16 Robb, G. P., Mattingly, T. W., and Marks, H. H.: Stress Tests in the Detection of Coronary Disease, *Postgrad. Med.,* 24:419, 1958.

17 Wood, P. W., McGregor, M., Magidson, O., and Whittaker, W.: The Effort Test in Angina Pectoris, *Br. Heart J.,* 12:363, 1950.

18 Prinzmetal, M., Ekmekci, A., Kennamer, R., Kwoczynski, J. K., Shubin, H., and Toyoshima, H.: Variant Form of Angina Pectoris: Previously Undelineated Syndrome, *J.A.M.A.,* 174:1794, 1960.

19 McHenry, P. L., and Morris, S. N.: Exercise Electrocardiography—Current State of the Art, in R. C. Schlant and J. W. Hurst (eds.), "Advances in Electrocardiography," Grune & Stratton, Inc., New York, 1976, vol. 2, p. 265.

19a McHenry, P. L.: The Actual Prevalence of False Positive ST-segment Responses to Exercise in Clinically Normal Subjects Remains Undefined, *Circulation,* 55:683, 1977.

19b Sheffield, L. T., Reeves, T. J., Blackburn, H., Ellestad, M. H., Froelicher, V. F., Roitman, D., and Kansal, S.: The Exercise Test in Perspective, *Circulation,* 55:681, 1977.

19c McHenry, P. L.: Risks of Graded Exercise Testing, *Am. J. Cardiol.,* 39:935, 1977.

19d Irving, J. B., and Bruce, R. A.: Exertional Hypotension and Postexertional Ventricular Fibrillation in Stress Testing, *Am. J. Cardiol.,* 39:849, 1977.

19e Irving, J. B., Bruce, R. A., and DeRouen, T. A.: Variations in and Significance of Systolic Pressure during Maximal Treadmill Testing: Relation to Severity of Coronary Artery Disease and Cardiac Mortality, *Am. J. Cardiol.,* 39:841, 1977.

19f Bruce, R. A., DeRouen, T. A., Peterson, D. R., Irving, J. B., Chinn, N., Blake, B., and Hofer, V.: Noninvasive Predictors of Sudden Death in Men with Coronary Heart Disease: Predictive Value of Maximal Stress Testing, *Am. J. Cardiol.,* 39:833, 1977.

20 Kaplan, B. M., and Berkson, D. M.: Serial Electrocardiograms after Myocardial Infarction, *Ann. Intern. Med.,* 60:430, 1964.

21 Levine, H. D., and Phillips, E.: Appraisal of the Newer Electrocardiography Correlations in One Hundred and Fifty Consecutive Cases, *N. Engl. J. Med.,* 245:833, 1951.

22 Wilson, F.: Foreword, in E. Lepeschkin, "Modern Electrocardiography," The Williams & Wilkins Company, Baltimore, 1951, vol. 1, p. v.

23 Shell, W. E., and Sobel, B. E.: Biochemical Markers of Ischemic Injury, *Circulation,* 53(suppl. 1):98, 1976.

24 Sobel, B. E., and Shell, W. E.: Serum Enzyme Determinations in the Diagnosis and Assessment of Myocardial Infarction, *Circulation,* 45:471, 1972.

24a Varonkov, Y., Shell, W. E., Smirnov, V., Gukovsky, D., and Chazov, E. I.: Augmentation of Serum CPK Activity by Digitalis in Patients with Acute Myocardial Infarction, *Circulation,* 55:719, 1977.

25 Konttinen, A., and Somer, H.: Determination of Serum Creatine Kinase Isoenzymes in Myocardial Infarction, *Am. J. Cardiol.,* 29:817, 1972.

26 Roberts, R., Gowda, K. S., Ludbrook, P. A., and Sobel, B. E.: Specificity of Elevated Serum MB Creatine Phosphokinase Activity in the Diagnosis of Acute Myocardial Infarction, *Am. J. Cardiol.,* 36:433, 1975.

26a Tonkin, A. M., Lester, R. M., Guthrow, C. E., Roe, C. R., Hackel, D. B., and Wagner, G. S.: Persistence of MB Isoenzyme of Creatine Phosphokinase in the Serum after Minor Iatrogenic Cardiac Trauma, *Circulation,* 51:627, 1975.

27 Goldberg, D. M., and Winfield, D. A.: Diagnostic Accuracy of Serum Enzyme Assays for Myocardial Infarction in a General Hospital Population, *Br. Heart J.,* 34:597, 1972.

28 Lopes, M. B., Spivack, A. P., Harrison, D. C., and Schroeder, J. S.: Prognosis in Coronary Care Unit—Noninfarction Cases, *J.A.M.A.,* 228:1558, 1974.

29 Coodley, E. L.: Prognostic Value of Enzymes in Myocardial Infarction, *J.A.M.A.,* 225:597, 1973.

30 Wagner, H. N., Jr.: The Quiet Revolution in Cardiovascular Nuclear Medicine, *Appl. Radiat. Nuclear Med.,* May–June, 1975, p. 145.

31 Strauss, H. W., Pitt, B., and Everette, J. A., Jr. (eds.): "Cardiovascular Nuclear Medicine," The C. V. Mosby Company, St. Louis, 1974.

32 Strauss, H. W., and Pitt, B.: Common Procedures for the Noninvasive Determination of Regional Myocardial Perfusion, Evaluation of Regional Wall Motion and Detection of Acute Infarction, *Am. J. Cardiol.,* 38:731, 1976.

33 Pitt, B., and Strauss, H. W.: Myocardial Perfusion Imaging and Gated Cardiac Blood Pool Scanning: Clinical Application, *Am. J. Cardiol.,* 38:739, 1976.

34 Salel, A. F., Berman, D. S., DeVardo, G. L., and Mason, D. T.: Radionuclide Assessment of Nitroglycerin Influence on Abnormal Left Ventricular Segmental Contraction in Patients with Coronary Heart Disease, *Circulation,* 53:975, 1976.

35 Gould, L. A., Perez, L. A., Hayt, D. B., Reedy, C. V. R., Blatt, C., and Gomprecht, R. F.: Clinical Experience with Technetium-99m Stannous Polyphosphate for Myocardial Imaging, *Br. Heart J.,* 38:744, 1976.

36 Ahmad, M., Dubiel, J. P., Logan, K. W., Verdon, T. A., and Martin, R. H.: Limited Clinical Diagnostic Specificity of Technetium-99m Stannous Pyrophosphate Myocardial Imaging in Acute Myocardial Infarction, *Am. J. Cardiol.,* 39:50, 1977.

37 Coleman, R. E., Klein, M. S., Ahmed, S. A., Weiss, E. S., Buchholz, W. M., and Sobel, B. E.: Mechanisms Contributing to Myocardial Accumulation of Technetium-99 Stannous Pyrophosphate after Coronary Arterial Occlusion, *Am. J. Cardiol.,* 39:55, 1977.

38 McLaughlin, P. R., Doherty, P. W., Martin, R. P., Goris, M. L., and Harrison, D. C.: Myocardial Imaging in a Patient with Reprducible Variant Angina, *Am. J. Cardiol.,* 39:126, 1977.

39 Bailey, I. K., Griffith, L. S. C., Rouleau, J., Strauss, H. W., and Pitt, B.: Thallium-201 Myocardial Perfusion Imaging at Rest and during Exercise: Comparative Sensitivity to Electrocardiography in Coronary Artery Disease, *Circulation,* 55:79, 1977.

40 Prasquier, R., Taradash, M. R., Botvinick, E. H., Shames, D. M., and Parmley, W. W.: The Specificity of the Diffuse Pattern of Cardiac Uptake in Myocardial Infarction Imaging with Technetium-99m Stannous Pyrophosphate, *Circulation,* 55:61, 1977.

40a Ritchie, J. L., Hamilton, G. W., Trobaugh, G. B., Weaver, W. D., Williams, D. L., and Cobb, L. A.: Myocardial Imaging and Radionuclide Angiography in Survivors of Sudden Cardiac Death due to Ventricular Fibrillation: Preliminary Report, *Am. J. Cardiol.,* 39:852, 1977.

40b Rothschild, M. A., and Fisher, V. J.: Myocardial Imaging, *Prac. Cardiol.,* 3:55, 1977.

41 Plotz, M.: Sedimentation Rate in Myocardial Infarction, *Am. J. Med. Sci.,* 224:23, 1952.

42 Shillito, F. H., Chamberlain, F. L., and Levy, R. L.: Cardiac Infarction: The Incidence and Correlation of Various Signs, with Remarks on Prognosis, *J.A.M.A.*, 118:779, 1942.

43 Goldberger, E., Alesio, J., and Woll, F.: Significance of Hyperglycemia in Myocardial Infarction, *N.Y. State J. Med.*, 45:391, 1945.

44 Osler, W.: Lecture on Angina Pectoris and Allied States, Lecture One, D. Appleton & Company, Inc., New York, 1897, pp. 8 and 9.

45 Mackenzie, J.: "Angina Pectoris," Oxford Medical Publications, London, 1923, chap. 18.

46 White, P. D., "Heart Disease," 3d ed., The Macmillan Company, New York, 1944, chap. 31.

47 Levine, S. A.: Angina Pectoris and Coronary Thrombosis, chap. 6, "Clinical Heart Disease," 5th ed., W. B. Saunders Company, Philadelphia and London, 1958.

48 Wood, P.: "Diseases of the Heart and Circulation," J. B. Lippincott Company, Philadelphia, 1956, chap. 15.

49 Friedberg, C. K.: Angina Pectoris—Clinical Features, Etiology and Pathogenesis, in C. K. Friedberg (ed.), "Diseases of the Heart," W. B. Saunders Company, Philadelphia and London, 1966.

50 Short, D., and Stowers, M.: Earliest Symptoms of Coronary Heart Disease and Their Recognition, *Br. Med. J.*, 2:387, 1972.

51 Home, E.: "A Treatise on the Blood, Inflammation, and *Gun Shot* Wounds by the Late John Hunter. To which is prefixed an account of the authors life by his brother-in-law, Everard Home," Thomas Bradford, No. 8, South Front Street, Philadelphia, 1796. (An earlier edition was published in England in 1794.)

52 Levine, S. A.: Carotid Sinus Massage: A New Diagnostic Test for Angina Pectoris, *J.A.M.A.*, 182:1332, 1962.

53 "Nomenclature and Criteria for Diagnoses of Diseases of the Heart and Great Vessels," 7th ed., The Criteria Committee of the New York Heart Association, Little, Brown and Company, Boston, 1973.

54 Hurst, J. W., and King, S. B., III.: The Problem of Chest "Pain": Emphasis on the Workup of Myocardial Ischemia, *J.A.M.A.*, 236:2100, 1976.

55 Blackburn, H., Taylor, H. L., and Keys, A.: The Electrocardiogram in Prediction of Five-Year Coronary Heart Disease Incidence among Men Aged 40 Through 59, *Circulation*, 41(suppl. 1):154, 1970.

56 Cohen, M. V., Cohn, P. F., Herman, M. V., and Gorlin, R.: Diagnosis and Prognosis of Main Left Coronary Artery Obstruction, *Circulation*, 45(suppl. 8):57, 1972.

57 Profant, G. R., Early, R. G., Nilson, K. L., Kusumi, F., Hofer, V., and Bruce, R. A.: Responses to Maximal Exercise in Healthy Middle-aged Women, *J. Appl. Physiol.*, 33:595, 1972.

58 Redwood, D. R., and Epstein, S. E.: Uses and Limitations of Stress Testing in the Evaluation of Ischemic Heart Disease, *Circulation*, 46:1115, 1972.

59 Barnard, R. J., MacAlpin, R., Kattus, A. A., and Buckberg, G. D.: Ischemic Response to Sudden Strenuous Exercise in Healthy Men, *Circulation*, 48:936, 1973.

60 Cumming, G. R., Dufresne, C., and Samm, J.: Exercise ECG Changes in Normal Women, *Can. Med. Assoc. J.*, 109:108, 1973.

61 Cheitlin, M. D., Davia, J. E., de Castro, C. M., Barrow, E. A., and Anderson, W. T.: Correlation of "Critical" Left Coronary Artery Lesions with Positive Submaximal Exercise Tests in Patients with Chest Pain, *Am. Heart J.*, 89:305, 1975.

62 Siegel, W., Lim, J. S., Proudfit, W. L., Sheldon, W. C., and Loop, F. D.: The Spectrum of Exercise Test and Angiographic Correlations in Myocardial Revascularization Surgery, *Circulation*, 51(suppl. 1):156, 1975.

63 Froelicher, V. F., Thompson, A. J., Longo, M. R., Jr., Triebwasser, J. H., and Lancaster, M. C.: Value of Exercise Testing for Screening Asymptomatic Men for Latent Coronary Artery Disease, *Prog. Cardiovasc. Dis.*, 18:265, 1976.

64 Krauss, K. R., Hutter, A. M., Jr., and DeSanctis, R. W.: Acute Coronary Insufficiency, Course and Follow-up, *Circulation*, 45(suppl. 1):66, 1972.

65 Bruschke, A. V. G., Proudfit, W. L., and Sones, F. M.: Progress Study of 590 Consecutive Nonsurgical Cases of Coronary Disease Followed Five to Nine Years: I. Arteriographic Correlations, *Circulation*, 47:1147, 1973.

66 Bruschke, A. V. G., Proudfit, W. L., and Sones, F. M., Jr.: Progress Study of 590 Consecutive Nonsurgical Cases of Coronary Disease Followed 5–9 Years: II. Ventriculographic and Other Correlations, *Circulation*, 47:1154, 1973.

67 Cheanvechai, C., Effler, D. B., Loop, F. D., Groves, L. K., Sheldon, W. C., and Sones, F. M., Jr.: Aortocoronary Artery Graft during Early and Late Phases of Acute Myocardial Infarction, *Ann. Thorac. Surg.*, 16:249, 1973.

68 Spencer, F. C., Isom, O. W., Glassman, E., Boyd, A. D., Engelman, R. M., Reed, G. E., Pasternack, B. S., and Dembrow, J. M.: The Long-Term Influence of Coronary Bypass Grafts on Myocardial Infarction and Survival, *Ann. Surg.*, 180:439, 1974.

69 Reul, G. J., Jr., Cooley, D. A., Wukasch, D. C., Kyger, E. R., III, Sandiford, F. M., Hallman, G. L., and Norman, J. C.: Long-Term Survival Following Coronary Artery Bypass, *Arch. Surg.*, 110:1419, 1975.

70 Sheldon, W. C., Rincon, G., Pichard, A. D., Razavi, M., Cheanvechai, C., and Loop, F. D.: Surgical Treatment of Coronary Artery Disease: Pure Graft Operations, with a Study of 741 Patients Followed 3–7 Years, *Prog. Cardiovasc. Dis.*, 18:237, 1975.

71 Evans, D. W., and Lum, L. C.: Hyperventilation: An Important Cause of Pseudoangina, *Lancet*, 1:155, 1977.

72 Lum, L. C.: Hyperventilation: A Bad Breathing Habit, *Mod. Med.*, 44:91, 1976.

73 Okel, B. B., and Hurst, J. W.: Prolonged Hyperventilation in Man, *Arch. Intern. Med.*, 108:757, 1961.

74 Friesinger, G. C., Likas, I., Beirn, R., and Mason, R. E.: Vasoregulatory Asthenia: A Cause for False Positive Electrocardiograms, *Circulation*, 32(suppl. 2):90, 1965. (Abstract)

75 Shabetai, R. (ed.): Symposium on Pericardial Disease, *Am. J. Cardiol.*, 26:445, 1970.

76 Spodick, B. H.: Acoustic Phenomena in Pericardial Disease, *Am. Heart H.*, 81:114, 1971.

77 Hurst, J. W.: Personal observations.

78 Mondor, H.: Tronculite sous-cutanée subaiguë de la paroi thoracique antéro-latérale, *Mem. Acad. Chir., Paris*, 65:1271, 1939.

79 Wendkos, M. H., and Logue, R. B.: Unstable T Waves in Leads II and III in Persons with Neurocirculatory Asthenia, *Am. Heart J.*, 31:711, 1946.

80 Nordenfelt, O.: Orthostatic ECG Changes and the Adrenergic Beta-Receptor Blocking Agent, Propranolol (Inderal), *Acta Med. Scand.*, 178:393, 1965.

81 Furberg, C.: Adrenergic Beta-Blocking and Electrocardiographical ST-T Changes, *Acta Med. Scand.*, 181:21, 1967.

82 Dodds, W. J., Hogan, W. J., and Miller, W. N.: Reflux Esophagitis, *Am. J. Dig. Dis.*, 21:49, 1976.

83 Bennett, J. R., and Atkinson, M.: The Differentiation between Oesphageal and Cardiac Pain, *Lancet*, 2:1123, 1966.

84 Hersh, J., and Jinich, H.: Esophageal Rupture: A Dramatic Instance of Chest Pain, *Chest Pain*, 2:1, 1976. (Marion Laboratories, Kansas City, Mo.)

85 Behar, J.: Reflux Esophagitis: Pathogensis, Diagnosis, and Management, *Arch. Intern. Med.*, 136:560, 1976.

86 Bernstein, L. M., Fruin, R. C., and Pacini, R.: Differentiation

of Esophageal Pain from Angina Pectoris: Role of Esophageal Acid Perfusion Test, *Medicine,* 41:143, 1962.

87 Castell, D. O.: Achalasia and Diffuse Esophageal Spasm, *Arch. Intern. Med.,* 136:571, 1976.

88 Orlando, R. C., and Bozymski, E. M.: Clinical and Manometric Effects of Nitroglycerin in Diffuse Esophageal Spasm, *N. Engl. J. Med.,* 289:23, 1973.

89 DiMarino, A. J., Jr., and Cohen, S.: Characteristics of Lower Esophageal Sphincter Function in Symptomatic Diffuse Esophageal Spasm, *Gastroenterology,* 66:1, 1974.

90 Youngs, J., and Nicoloff, D.: Management of Esophageal Perforation, *Surgery,* 65:264, 1969.

91 O'Connell, N. D.: Spontaneous Rupture of the Esophagus, *Am. J. Roentgenol.,* 99:186, 1967.

92 Foster, J. H.: Esophageal Perforation, in T. M. Bayless (ed.), "Management of Esophageal Disease," Harper & Row, Publishers, Incorporated, New York, 1970.

93 Spiro, H. M.: Structural Disorders, chap. 43, and Inflammatory Disorders, chap. 44, in "Clinical Gastroenterology," The Macmillan Company, London, 1970, pp. 734–758.

94 Becker, W. F., Powell, J. L., and Turner, R. J.: A Clinical Study of 1,060 Patients with Acute Cholecystitis, *Surg. Gynecol. Obstet.,* 104:491, 1957.

95 Thistle, J. L., and Hofmann, A. F.: Efficacy and Specificity of Chenodeoxycholic Acid Therapy for Dissolving Gallstones, *N. Engl. J. Med.,* 289:655, 1973.

96 Silen, W.: Peptic Ulcer, in G. W. Thorn, R. D. Adams, E. Braunwald, K. J. Isselbacher, and R. G. Petersdorf (eds.), "Harrison's Principles of Internal Medicine," 8th ed., McGraw-Hill Book Company, New York, 1977, p. 1494.

97 Briggs, R. D., Rubenberg, M. L., O'Neal, R. M., Thomas, W. A., and Hartroft, W. S.: Myocardial Infarction in Patients Treated with Sippy and Other High-Milk Diets: An Autopsy Study of Fifteen Hospitals in the U.S.A. and Great Britian, *Circulation,* 21:538, 1960.

98 Crentzfeldt, W., and Schmidt, H.: Aetiology and Pathogenesis of Pancreatitis (Current Concepts), *Scand. J. Gastroenterol., [Suppl.],* 6:47, 1970.

99 Flowers, N.: Personal observations.

100 Heimlich, H. J.: A Life-saving Maneuver to Prevent Food-Choking, *J.A.M.A.,* 234:398, 1975.

101 Atlas, D. H.: "Cafe Coronary" from Peanut Butter, *N. Engl. J. Med.,* 296:399, 1977.

102 Isselbacher, K. J.: Indigestion, in G. W. Thorn, R. D. Adams, E. Braunwald, K. J. Isselbacher, and R. G. Petersdorf (eds.), "Harrison's Principles of Internal Medicine," McGraw-Hill Book Company, New York, 1977, p. 207.

103 Sasahara, A. A.: Current Problems in Pulmonary Embolism: Introduction, *Prog. Cardiovasc. Dis.,* 17:161, 1974.

104 Wilhelmsen, L., Hagman, M., and Werko, L.: Recurrent Pulmonary Embolism-Incidence, Predisposing Factors and Prognosis, *Acat Med. Scand.,* 192:565, 1972.

105 Hammon, L.: Spontaneous Mediastinal Emphysema, *Bull. Johns Hopkins Hosp.,* 64:1, 1939.

106 Inouye, W. Y., Berggren, R. B., and Johnson, J.: Spontaneous Pneumothorax: Treatment and Mortality, *Dis. Chest,* 51:67, 1967.

107 Dale, W. A., and Lewis, M. R.: Management of Thoracic Outlet Syndrome, *Ann. Surg.,* 181:575, 1975.

108 Lord, J. W., Jr., and Rosati, L. M.: Thoracic-Outlet Syndromes, *Clin. Symposia,* Ciba, 23:3, 1971.

109 Urschel, H. C., Jr., and Razzuk, M. A.: Management of the Thoracic-Outlet Syndrome, *N. Engl. J. Med.,* 286:1140, 1972.

110 Urschel, H. C., Jr., Razzuk, M. A., Hyland, J. W., Matson, J. L., Solis, R. M., Wood, R. E., Paulson, D. L., and Galbraith, N. F.: Thoracic Outlet Syndrome Masquerading as Coronary Artery Disease (Pseudoangina), *Ann. Thorac. Surg.,* 16:239, 1973.

111 Tietze, A.: Ueber eine eigenartige Haufung von Fallen mit Dystrophie der Rippenknorpel, *Berl. Klin. Wochenschr.,* 58: 829, 1921.

112 Karon, E. H., Achor, R. W. P., and Janes, J. M.: Painful Nonsuperative Swelling of Costochondral Cartilages (Tietze's Syndrome), *Proc. Staff Meetings Mayo Clinic,* 33:45, 1958.

113 Ray, C. G.: Chickenpox (Varicella) and Herpes Zoster, in G. W. Thorn, R. D. Adams, E. Braunwald, K. J. Isselbacher, and R. G. Petersdorf (eds.), "Harrison's Principles of Internal Medicine," 8th ed., McGraw-Hill Book Company, New York, 1977, p. 1020.

114 Silverman, M. E., and Hurst, J. W.: Chest Wall Pain: The Great Masquerader, *Chest Pain,* 1:1, 1976. (Marion Laboratories, Kansas City, Mo.)

115 Doyle, J. T.: Mechanisms and Prevention of Sudden Death, *Mod. Concepts Cardiovasc. Dis.,* 45:111, 1976.

116 Lassen, N. A.: Cerebral Blood Flow and Oxygen Consumption in Man, *Physiol. Rev.,* 39:183, 1959.

117 Patterson, J. L., Jr.: Circulation through the Brain, in T. C. Ruch, J. R. Fulton (eds.), "Medical Physiology and Biophysics," 18th ed., W. B. Saunders Company, Philadelphia, 1960.

117a Lown, B., Verrier, R. L., and Rabinowitz, S. H.: "Neural and Psychologic Mechanisms and the Problem of Sudden Cardiac Death, *Am. J. Cardiol.,* 39:890, 1977.

117b Hinkle, L. E., Jr., Argyros, D. C., Hayes, J. C., and Robinson, T. A.: Pathogenesis of an Unexpected Sudden Death: Role of Early Cycle Ventricular Premature Contractions, *Am. J. Cardiol.,* 39:873, 1977.

117c Talbott, E., Kuller, L. H., Detre, K., and Perper, J.: Biologic and Psychosocial Risk Factors of Sudden Death from Coronary Disease in White Women, *Am. J. Cardiol.,* 39:858, 1977.

117d Vismara, L. A., Zakauddin, V., Foerster, J. M., Amsterdam, E. A., and Mason, D. T.: Identification of Sudden Death Risk Factors in Acute and Chronic Coronary Artery Disease, *Am. J. Cardiol.,* 39:821, 1977.

117e Reichenbach, D. D., Moss, N. S., and Meyer, E.: Pathology of the Heart in Sudden Cardiac Death, *Am. J. Cardiol.,* 39:865, 1977.

117f Schroeder, J. S., Lamb, I. H., and Harrison, D. C.: Patients Admitted to the Coronary Care Unit for Chest Pain: High Risk Subgroup for Subsequent Cardiovascular Death, *Am. J. Cardiol.,* 39:829, 1977.

117g Moss, A. J., DeCamilla, J., and Davis, H.: Cardiac Death in the First 6 Months After Myocardial Infarction: Potential for Mortality Reduction in the Early Posthospital Period, *Am. J. Cardiol.,* 39:816, 1977.

117h Hammermeister, K. E., DeRouen, T. A., Murray, J. A., and Dodge, H. T.: Effect of Aortocoronary Saphenous Vein Bypass Grafting on Death and Sudden Death: Comparison of Nonrandomized Medically and Surgically Treated Cohorts with Comparable Coronary Disease and Left Ventricular Function, *Am. J. Cardiol.,* 39:925, 1977.

117i Vismara, L. A., Miller, R. R., Price, J. E., Karem, R., DeMaria, A. N., and Mason, D. T.: Improved Longevity Due to Reduction of Sudden Death by Aortoconary Bypass in Coronary Atherosclerosis: Prospective Evaluation of Medical Versus Surgical Therapy in Matched Patients with Multivessel Disease, *Am. J. Cardiol.,* 39:919, 1977.

118 Cohn, P. F.: Severe Asymptomatic Coronary Artery Disease: A Diagnostic, Prognostic and Therapeutic Puzzle, *Am. J. Med.,* 62:565, 1977.

119 Prinzmetal, M., Kennamer, R., Merliss, R., Wada, T., and Bor, N.: Angina Pectoris: I. A Variant Form of Angina Pectoris: Preliminary Report, *Am. J. Med.,* 27:375, 1959.

120 Hurst, J. W.: Personal observations.

121 Cheng, T. O., Bashour, T., Kelser, G. A., Jr., Weiss, L., and Bacos, J.: Variant Angina of Prinzmetal with Normal Coronary Arteriograms: A Variant of the Variant, *Circulation,* 47:476, 1973.

122 Gensini, G. G.: Coronary Artery Spasm and Angina Pectoris, *Chest*, 68:709, 1975.

123 Weiner, L., Kasparian, H., Duca, P. R., Walinsky, P., Gottlieb, R. S., Hanckel, F., and Brest, A. N.: Spectrum of Coronary Arterial Spasm. Clinical, Angiographic and Myocardial Metabolic Experience in 29 Cases, *Am. J. Cardiol.*, 38:945, 1976.

123a Johnson, A. D., and Detwiler, J. H.: Coronary Spasm, Variant Angina, and Recurrent Myocardial Infarctions, *Circulation*, 55:947, 1977.

124 Shubrooks, S. J., Bete, J. M., Hutter, A. M., Block, P. C., Buckley, M. J., Daggett, W. M., and Mundth, E. D.: Variant Angina Pectoris: Clinical and Anatomic Spectrum and Results of Coronary Bypass Surgery, *Am. J. Cardiol.*, 36:142, 1975.

125 Higgins, C. B., Wexler, L., Silverman, J. F., and Schroeder, J. S.: Clinical and Arteriographic Features of Prinzmetal's Variant Angina: Documentation of Etiologic Factors, *Am. J. Cardiol.*, 37:831, 1976.

126 Roesler, H., and Dressler, W.: Transient Electrocardiographic Changes Identical with Those of Acute Myocardial Infarction Accompanying Attacks of Angina Pectoris, *Am. Heart J.*, 47:520, 1954.

127 Meller, J., Conde, C. A., Donoso, E., and Dack, S.: Transient Q Waves in Prinzmetal's Angina, *Am. J. Cardiol.*, 35:691, 1975.

128 Guazzi, M., Olivari, J. T., Polese, A., Fiorentini, C., and Magrini, F.: Repetitive Myocardial Ischemia of Prinzmetal Type without Angina Pectoris, *Am. J. Cardiol.*, 37:923, 1976.

129 King, S. B. III: Personal observations.

130 Osler, W.: "The Principles and Practice of Medicine," 3d ed., D. Appleton & Company, Inc., New York, 1899, p. 763.

131 Latham, P. M.: "Collected Works," vol. 1, London New Syndenham Society, 1876, p. 445. Quoted by C. K. Friedberg, "Diseases of the Heart," 3d ed., W. B. Saunders Company, Philadelphia, 1966.

132 Oliva, P. B., Potts, D. E., and Pluss, R. G.: Coronary Arterial Spasm in Prinzmetal Angina: Documentation by Coronary Arteriography, *N. Engl. J. Med.*, 288:745, 1973.

133 Maseri, A., Mimmo, R., Chierchia, S., Marchesi, C., Pesola, A., and L'Abbate, A.: Coronary Artery Spasm as a Cause of Acute Myocardial Ischemia in Man, *Chest*, 68:625, 1975.

134 King, S. B., Mansour, K. A., Hatcher, C. R., Silverman, M. E., and Hart, N. C.: Coronary Artery Spasm Producing Prinzmetal's Angina and Myocardial Infarction in the Absence of Coronary Atherosclerosis, *Ann. Thorac. Surg.*, 16:337, 1973.

135 Silverman, M. E., and Flamm, M. D., Jr.: Variant Angina Pectoris, Anatomic Findings and Prognostic Implications, *Ann. Intern. Med.*, 75:339, 1971.

136 Plotnick, G. D., and Conti, C. R.: Transient ST-Segment Elevation in Unstable Angina—Clinical and Hemodynamic Significance, *Circulation*, 51:1015, 1975.

137 MacAlpin, R.: Variant Angina Pectoris, *N. Engl. J. Med.*, 282:1491, 1970. (Letter)

138 Betriu, A., Solignac, A., and Bourassa, M. G.: The Variant Form of Angina: Diagnostic and Therapeutic Implications, *Am. Heart J.*, 87:272, 1974.

139 Endo, M., Kanda, I., Hosoda, S., Hayashi, H., Hirosawa, K., and Konno, S.: Prinzmetal's Variant Form of Angina Pectoris: Re-evaluation of Mechanism, *Circulation*, 52:33, 1975.

140 Cohn, P. F., and Gorlin, R.: Abnormalities of Left Ventricular Function Associated with the Anginal State, *Circulation*, 46:1065, 1972.

141 Maseri, A., Pesola, A., Mimmo, R., Chierchia, S., and L'Abbate, A.: Pathogenetic Mechanisms of Angina at Rest, *Circulation*, 52(suppl. 2):89, 1975. (Abstract)

142 Gaasch, W. H., Adyanthaya, A. V., Wang, V. H., Pickering, E., Quinones, M. A., and Alexander, J. K.: Prinzmetal's Variant Angina: Hemodynamic and Angiographic Observations during Pain, *Am. J. Cardiol.*, 35:683, 1975.

143 Whiting, R. B., Klein, M. D., Vander Veer, J., and Lown, B.: Variant Angina Pectoris, *N. Engl. J. Med.*, 282:609, 1970.

144 Guazzi, M., Polese, A., Fiorentini, C., Magrini, F., and Bartorelli, C.: Left Ventricular Performance and Related Haemodynamic Changes in Prinzmetal's Variant Angina Pectoris, *Br. Heart J.*, 33:84, 1971.

145 Yasue, H., Touyama, M., Kato, H., Tanaka, S., and Akiyama, F.: Prinzmetal's Variant Form of Angina as a Manifestation of Alpha-adrenergic Receptor-mediated Coronary Artery Spasm: Documentation by Coronary Arteriography, *Am. Heart J.*, 91:148, 1976.

146 King, S. B.: Unpublished observations.

147 Yasue, H., Touyama, M., Shimamoto, M., Kato, H., Tanaka, S., and Akiyama, F.: Role of Autonomic Nervous System in the Pathogenesis of Prinzmetal's Variant Form of Angina, *Circulation*, 50:534, 1974.

148 Heupler, F., Proudfit, W., Siegel, W., Shirey, E., Razavi, M., and Sones, F. M.: The Erognovine Maleate Test for the Diagnosis of Coronary Artery Spasm, *Circulation*, 52(suppl. 2):11, 1974–75.

149 Swan, H. J. C., Blackburn, H. W., DeSanctis, R., Frommer, P. L., Hurst, J. W., Paul, O., Rapaport, E., Wallace, A., and Weinberg, S.: Duration of Hospitalization in "Uncomplicated Completed Acute Myocardial Infarction," *Am. J. Cardiol.*, 37:413, 1976.

150 Hancock, E. W.: Aortic Stenosis, Angina Pectoris, and Coronary Artery Disease, *Am. Heart J.*, 93:382, 1977.

150a Graboys, T. B., and Cohn, P. F.: The Prevalence of Angina Pectoris and Abnormal Coronary Arteriograms in Severe Aortic Valvular Disease, *Am. Heart J.*, 93:683, 1977.

151 Lewis, R. C.: Personal communication, Cleveland Clinic Foundation, Cleveland, Ohio, 1976.

152 Taylor, P. C.: Personal communication, Cleveland Clinic Foundation, Cleveland, Ohio, 1976.

153 McHenry, P. L., Morris, S. N., Kavalier, M., and Jordan, J. W.: Comparative Study of Exercise-induced Ventricular Arrhythmias in Normal Subjects and Patients with Documented Coronary Artery Disease, *Am. J. Cardiol.*, 37:609, 1976.

154 Chiche, P., Haiat, R., and Steff, P.: Angina Pectoris with Syncope due to Paroxysmal Atrioventricular Block: Role of Ischaemia: Report of Two Cases, *Br. Heart J.*, 36:577, 1974.

155 Skjaeggestad, O.: Arrhythmias in Different Types of Acute Coronary Heart Disease, *Acta Med. Scand.*, 193:299, 1973.

156 Scheinman, M. M., and Abbott, J. A.: Clinical Significance of Transmural Versus Nontransmural Electrocardiographic Changes in Patients with Acute Myocardial Infarction, *Am. J. Med.*, 55:602, 1973.

157 Skjaeggestad, O.: The Natural History of Intermediate Coronary Syndrome, *Acta Med. Scand.*, 193:533, 1973.

158 Gorfinkel, H. J., Inglesby, T. V., Lansing, A. M., and Goodin, R. R.: ST-segment Elevation, Transient Left-Posterior Hemiblock, and Recurrent Ventricular Arrhythmias Unassociated with Pain. A Variant of Prinzmetal's Anginal Syndrome, *Ann. Intern. Med.*, 79:795, 1973.

159 MacAlpin, R. N., Kattus, A. A., and Alvaro, A. B.: Angina Pectoris at Rest with Preservation of Exercise Capacity. Prinzmetal's Variant Angina, *Circulation*, 47:946, 1973.

160 Botti, R. E.: A Variant Form of Angina Pectoris with Recurrent Transient Complete Heart Block, *Am. J. Cardiol.*, 17:443, 1966.

161 Harper, R., Peter, R., and Hunt, D.: Syncope in Association with Prinzmetal Variant Angina, *Br. Heart J.*, 37:771, 1975.

162 Webb, S. W., Adgey, A. A. J., and Pantridge, J. F.: Autonomic Disturbances at Onset of Acute Myocardial Infarction, *Br. Med. J.*, 3:89, 1972.

163 Pantridge, J. F., Webb, S. W., Adgey, A. A. J., and Geddes, J. S.: The First Hour after the Onset of Acute Myocardial Infarction, "Progress in Cardiology," Lea & Febiger, Philadelphia, 1974, vol. 3.

164 Adgey, A. A. J., Geddes, J. S., Webb, S. W., Allen, J. D., James, R. G. G., Zaidi, S. A., and Pantridge, J. F.: Acute Phase of Myocardial Infarction, *Lancet*, 2:501, 1971.

165 Norris, R. M., Mercer, C. J., and Yeates, S. E.: Sinus Rate in Acute Myocardial Infarction, *Br. Heart J.*, 34:901, 1972.

166 Warren, J. V., and Lewis, R. P.: Beneficial Effects of Atropine in the Pre-Hospital Phase of Coronary Care, *Am. J. Cardiol.*, 37:68, 1976.

167 Kossowsky, W. A., Mohr, B. D., Rafii, S., and Lyon, A. F.: Superimposition of Transmural Infarction following Acute Subendocardial Infarction: How Frequent? *Chest*, 69:758, 1976.

168 Madigan, N. P., Rutherford, B. D., and Frye, R. L.: The Clinical Course, Early Prognosis and Coronary Anatomy of Subendocardial Infarction, *Am. J. Med.*, 60:634, 1976.

169 Madias, J. E., Chahine, R. A., Gorlin, R., and Blacklow, D. J.: A Comparison of Transmural and Nontransmural Acute Myocardial Infarction, *Circulation*, 49:498, 1974.

170 Rigo, P., Murray, M., Taylor, D. R., Weisfeldt, M. L., Strauss, H. W., and Pitt, B.: Hemodynamic and Prognostic Findings in Patients with Transmural and Nontransmural Infarction, *Circulation*, 51:1064, 1975.

171 Wilson, C., and Pantridge, J. F.: ST-Segment Displacement and Early Hospital Discharge in Acute Myocardial Infarction, *Lancet*, 2:1284, 1973.

172 Thompson, P., and Sloman, G.: Sudden Death in Hospital after Discharge from Coronary Care Unit, *Br. Med. J.*, 4:136, 1971.

173 Bornheimer, J., de Guzman, M., and Haywood, L. J.: Analysis of Inhospital Deaths from Myocardial Infarction after Coronary Care Unit Discharge, *Arch. Intern. Med.*, 135:1035, 1975.

174 Schulze, R. A., Jr., Rouleau, J., Rigo, P., Bowers, S., Strauss, H. W., and Pitt, B.: Ventricular Arrhythmias in the Late Hospital Phase of Acute Myocardial Infarction, *Circulation*, 52:1006, 1975.

175 Rotman, M., Wagner, G. S., and Wallace, A. G. P.: Bradyarrhythmias in Acute Myocardial Infarction, *Circulation*, 45:703, 1972.

175a Bigger, J. T., Jr.: Arrhythmia Clinic: The Sick Sinus Syndrome, *Prac. Cardiol.*, 3:66, 1977.

176 Kent, K. M., Smith, E. R., Redwood, D. R., and Epstein, S. E.: Electrical Stability of Acutely Ischemic Myocardium. Influences of Heart Rate and Vagal Stimulation, *Circulation*, 47:291, 1973.

177 Hatle, L., Bathen, J., and Rokseth, R.: Sinoatrial Disease in Acute Myocardial Infarction. Long-Term Prognosis, *Br. Heart J.*, 38:410, 1976.

178 James, T. N.: Myocardial Infarction and Atrial Arrhythmias, *Circulation*, 24:761, 1961.

179 DeSanctis, R. W., Block, P., and Hutter, A. M., Jr.: Tachyarrhythmias in Myocardial Infarction, *Circulation*, 45:681, 1972.

180 Harrison, D. C.: "Management of Acute Myocardial Infarction," Medcom, Inc., New York, 1972.

181 Liberthson, R. R., Salisbury, K. W., Hutter, A. M., and DeSanctis, R. W.: Atrial Tachyarrhythmias in Acute Myocardial Infarction, *Am. J. Med.*, 60:956, 1976.

182 Killip, T., and Gault, J. H.: Mode of Onset of Atrial Fibrillation in Man, *Am. Heart J.*, 70:172, 1965.

183 Julian, D. G., Valentine, P. A., and Miller, G. G.: Disturbances of Rate, Rhythm and Conduction in Acute Myocardial Infarction, *Am. J. Med.*, 37:915, 1964.

184 Cristal, N., Peterburg, I., and Azwarcberg, J.: Atrial Fibrillation Developing in the Acute Phase of Myocardial Infarction: Prognostic Implications, *Chest*, 70:8, 1976.

185 Fishenfeld, J., Desser, K. B., and Benchimol, A.: Non-

186 Konecke, L. L., and Knoebel, S. B.: Nonparoxysmal Junctional Tachycardia Complicating Acute Myocardial Infarction, *Circulation*, 45:367, 1972.

187 Lie, K. I., Wellens, H. J. J., Downar, E., and Durrer, D.: Observations on Patients with Primary Ventricular Fibrillation Complicating Acute Myocardial Infarction, *Circulation*, 52:755, 1975.

188 El-Sherif, N., Myerburg, R. J., Scherlag, B. J., Befeler, B., Aranda, J. M., Castellanos, A., and Lazzara, R.: Electrocardiographic Antecedents of Primary Ventricular Fibrillation. Value of the R-on-T Phenomenon in Myocardial Infarction, *Br. Heart J.*, 38:415, 1976.

189 Dhurandhar, R. W., MacMillan, R. L., and Brown, K. W. G.: Primary Ventricular Fibrillation Complicating Acute Myocardial Infarction, *Am. J. Cardiol.*, 27:347, 1971.

190 De Soyza, N., Bissett, J. K., Kane, J. J., Murphy, M. L., and Doherty, J. E.: Ectopic Ventricular Prematurity and Its Relationship to Ventricular Tachycardia in Acute Myocardial Infarction in Man, *Circulation*, 50:529, 1974.

191 Mogensen, L.: Ventricular Tachyarrhythmias and Lignocaine Prophylaxis in Acute Myocardial Infarction, *Acta Med. Scand.*, 168(suppl. 513):30, 1970.

191a Fasola, A. F., Noble, R. J., and Zipes, D. P.: Treatment of Recurrent Ventricular Tachycardia and Fibrillation with Aprindine, *Am. J. Cardiol.*, 39:903, 1977.

191b Lown, B., and Graboys, T. B.: Management of Patients with Malignant Ventricular Arrhythmias, *Am. J. Cardiol.*, 39:910, 1977.

192 Williams, D. O., Scherlag, B. J., Hope, R. R., El-Sherif, N., and Lazzara, R.: The Pathophysiology of Malignant Ventricular Arrhythmias during Acute Myocardial Ischemia, *Circulation*, 50:1163, 1974.

193 Wellens, H. J. J., Lie, K. I., and Durrer, D.: Further Observations on Ventricular Tachycardia as Studied by Electrical Stimulation of the Heart. Chronic Recurrent Ventricular Tachycardia and Ventricular Tachycardia during Acute Myocardial Infarction, *Circulation*, 49:647, 1974.

194 Kushnir, B., Fox, K. M., Tomlinson, I. W., Portal, R. W., and Aber, C. P.: Primary Ventricular Fibrillation and Resumption of Work, Sexual Activity, and Driving after First Acute Myocardial Infarction, *Br. Med. J.*, 4:609, 1975.

195 Wilson, C., and Adgey, A. A. J.: Survival of Patients with Late Ventricular Fibrillation after Acute Myocardial Infarction, *Lancet*, 2:124, 1974.

196 de Soyza, N., Bissett, J. K., Kane, J. J., Murphy, M. L., and Doherty, J. E.: Association of Accelerated Idioventricular Rhythm and Paroxysmal Ventricular Tachycardia in Acute Myocardial Infarction, *Am. J. Cardiol.*, 34:667, 1974.

197 Norris, R. M., and Mercer, C. J.: Significance of Idioventricular Rhythms in Acute Myocardial Infarction, *Prog. Cardiovasc. Dis.*, 16:455, 1974.

198 Talbot, S., and Greaves, M.: Association of Ventricular Extrasystoles and Ventricular Tachycardia with Idioventricular Rhythm, *Br. Heart J.*, 38:457, 1976.

199 Lichstein, E., Ribas-Meneclier, C., Gupta, P. K., and Chadda, K. D.: Incidence and Description of Accelerated Ventricular Rhythm Complicating Acute Myocardial Infarction, *Am. J. Med.*, 58:192, 1975.

200 Rosen, K. M., Loeb, H. S., Chuquimia, R., Sinno, M. Z., Rahimtoola, S. H., and Gunnar, R. M.: Site of Heart Block in Acute Myocardial Infarction, *Circulation*, 42:925, 1970.

201 Cohn, J. N., Guiha, N. H., Broder, M. I., and Limas, C. J.: Right Ventricular Infarction. Clinical and Hemodynamic Features, *Am. J. Cardiol.*, 33:209, 1974.

202 Lie, K. I., Wellens, H. J., Schuilenburg, R. M., Becker, A. E., and Durrer, D.: Factors Influencing Prognosis of Bundle Branch Block Complicating Acute Antero-septal Infarction. The Value of His Bundle Recordings, *Circulation*, 50:935, 1974.

203 Atkins, J. M., Leshin, S. J., Blomqvist, G., and Mullins, C. B.:

Ventricular Conduction Blocks and Sudden Death in Acute Myocardial Infarction, *N. Engl. J. Med.,* 288:281, 1973.

204 Godman, M. J., Alpert, B. A., and Julian, D. G.: Bilateral Bundle-Branch Block Complicating Acute Myocardial Infarction, *Lancet,* 2:345, 1971.

205 Friedman, H. S.: Diagnostic Considerations in Electromechanical Dissociation, *Am. J. Cardiol.,* 38:268, 1976.

206 Raizes, G., Wagner, G. S., and Hackel, D. B.: Instantaneous Nonarrhythmic Cardiac Death in Acute Myocardial Infarction. Role of Electromechanical Dissociation, *Am. J. Cardiol.,* 39:1, 1977.

207 Hurst, J. W.: Personal observations.

207a Moser, K. M., Brach, B. B., Dolan, G. F.: Clinically Suspected Deep Venous Thrombosis of the Lower Extremities, *J.A.M.A.,* 237:2195, 1977.

208 Maurer, B. J., Wray, R., and Shillingford, J. P.: Frequency of Venous Thrombosis after Myocardial Infarction, *Lancet,* 2:1385, 1971.

209 Thompson, J. E.: Acute Peripheral Arterial Occlusions, *N. Engl. J. Med.,* 290:950, 1974.

210 Nutter, D. O., Schlant, R. C., and Hurst, J. W.: Isometric Exercise and the Cardiovascular System, *Mod. Concepts Cardiovasc. Dis.,* 44:11, 1972.

211 Morrow, A., Cohen, L., Roberts, W., Braunwald N., and Braunwald, E.: Severe Mitral Regurgitation following Acute Myocardial Infarction and Ruptured Papillary Muscle, *Circulation,* 37 & 38(suppl. 2):124, 1968.

212 Selzer, A., Gerbode, F., and Kerth, W. J.: Clinical, Hemodynamic and Surgical Considerations of Rupture of the Ventricular Septum after Myocardial Infarction, *Am. Heart J.,* 78:598, 1969.

213 Longo, E. A., and Cohen, L. S.: Rupture of Interventricular Septum in Acute Myocardial Infarction, *Am. Heart J.,* 92:81, 1976.

213a James, T. N.: De Subitaneis Mortibus. XXIV: Ruptured Interventricular Septum and Heart Block, *Circulation,* 55:934, 1977.

214 O'Rourke, M. F.: Subacute Heart Rupture following Myocardial Infarction: Clinical Features of a Correctable Condition, *Lancet,* 2:123, 1973.

215 VanTassel, R. A., and Edwards, J. E.: Rupture of Heart Complicating Myocardial Infarction. Analysis of 40 Cases Including Nine Examples of Left Ventricular False Aneurysm, *Chest,* 61:104, 1972.

216 Loop, F. D., Effler, D. B., Navia, J. A., Sheldon, W. C., and Groves, L. K.: Aneurysms of the Left Ventricle: Survival and Results of a Ten-Year Surgical Experience, *Ann. Surg.,* 178:399, 1973.

217 Herman, M. V., Heinle, R. A., Klein, M. D., and Gorlin, R.: Localized Disorders in Myocardial Contraction, *N. Engl. J. Med.,* 272:222, 1967.

218 Dubnow, M. H., Burchell, H. B., and Titus, J. L.: Postinfarction Ventricular Aneurysm: Clincopathologic and Electrocardiographic Study of 80 Cases, *Am. Heart J.,* 70:753, 1965.

219 Dressler, W.: A Post-myocardial Infarction Syndrome, *J.A.M.A.,* 160:1379, 1956.

220 Kossowsky, W. A., Epstein, P. J., and Levine, R. S.: Post Myocardial Infarction Syndrome: An Early Complication of Acute Myocardial Infarction, *Chest,* 63:35, 1973.

221 Hurst, J. W.: Personal observations.

222 Russek, H. I.: Shoulder-Hand Syndrome following Myocardial Infarction, *Med. Clin. North Am.,* 42:1555, 1958.

223 Johnson, A. C.: Disabling Changes in the Hands Resembling Sclerodactylia following Myocardial Infarction, *Ann. Intern. Med.,* 19:433, 1943.

224 Zoll, P. M., Wessler, S., and Blumgart, H. L.: Angina Pectoris, Clinical and Pathologic Correlations, *Am. J. Med.,* 11:331, 1951.

225 White, N. K., Edwards, J. E., and Dry, T. J.: The Relationship of the Degree of Coronary Atherosclerosis with Age, in Men, *Circulation,* 1:645, 1950.

226 Ackerman, R. F., Dry, T. J., and Edwards, J. E.: The

Relationship of the Degree of Coronary Atherosclerosis with Age, in Women, *Circulation,* 1:1345, 1950.

227 Block, W. J., Jr., Crumpacker, E. L., Dry, T. J., and Gage, R. P.: Prognosis of Angina Pectoris: Observations in 6,882 Cases, *J.A.M.A.,* 150:259, 1952.

228 Richards, D. W., Bland, E. F., and White, P. D.: A Completed 25-Year Follow-up Study of 456 Patients with Angina Pectoris, *J. Chronic Dis.,* 4:423, 1956.

229 Frank, C. W., Weinblatt, E., and Shapiro, S.: Angina Pectoris in Men: Prognostic Significance of Selected Medical Factors, *Circulation,* 47:509, 1973.

230 Kannel, W. B., and Feinleib, M.: Natural History of Angina Pectoris in the Framingham Study. Prognosis and Survival, *Am. J. Cardiol.,* 29:154, 1972.

231 Humphries, J. O., Kuller, L., Ross, R. S., Friesinger, G. C., and Page, E. E.: Natural History of Ischemic Heart Disease in Relation to Arteriographic Findings: A Twelve-Year Study of 224 Patients, *Circulation,* 49:489, 1974.

232 Robb, G. P., and Marks, H. H.: Postexercise Electrocardiogram in Arteriosclerotic Heart Disease: Its Value in Diagnosis and Prognosis, *J.A.M.A.,* 200:918, 1967.

233 Ellestad, M. H., and Wan, M. K. C.: Predictive Implications of Stress Follow-up of 2700 Subjects after Maximum Treadmill Stress Testing, *Circulation,* 51:363, 1975.

234 Doyle, J. T., and Kinch, S. H.: The Prognosis of An Abnormal Electrocardiographic Stress Test, *Circulation,* 41:545, 1970.

235 Friesinger, G. C., Page, E. E., and Ross, R. S.: Prognostic Significance of Coronary Arteriography, *Trans. Assoc. Am. Physicians,* 83:78, 1970.

236 Proudfit, W. L.: Personal communication, Cleveland Clinic Foundation, Cleveland, Ohio, 1976.

237 Burggraf, G. W., and Parker, J. O.: Prognosis in Coronary Artery Disease, Angiographic, Hemodynamic, and Clinical Factors, *Circulation,* 51:146, 1975.

238 Zir, L. M., Miller, S. W., Dinsmore, R. E., Gilbert, J. P., and Harthorne, J. W.: Interobserver Variability in Coronary Arteriography, *Circulation,* 53:627, 1976.

239 Detre, K. M., Wright, E., Murphy, M. L., and Takaro, T. T.: Observer Agreement in Evaluating Coronary Angiograms, *Circulation,* 52:979, 1975.

240 Bruschke, A. V. G., Proudfit, W. L., and Sones, F. M., Jr.: Clinical Course of Patients with Normal, and Slightly or Moderately Abnormal Coronary Arteriograms, A Follow-up Study on 500 Patients, *Circulation,* 47:936, 1973.

241 Proudfit, W. L.: Personal communication, Cleveland Clinic, Cleveland, Ohio, October 1976.

242 Cohen, M. V., and Gorlin, R.: Main Left Coronary Artery Disease: Clinical Experience from 1964–1974, *Circulation,* 52:275, 1975.

243 Zeft, H. J., Manley, J. C., Huston, J. H., Tector, A. J., Auer, J. E., and Johnson, W. D.: Left Main Coronary Artery Stenosis: Results of Coronary Bypass Surgery, *Circulation,* 49:68, 1974.

244 Duncan, B., Fulton, M., Morrison, S. L., Lutz, W., Donald, K. W., Kerr, F., Kirby, B. J., Julian, D. G., and Oliver, M. F.: Prognosis of New and Worsening Angina Pectoris, *Br. Med. J.,* 1:981, 1976.

245 Gazes, P. C., Mobley, E. M., Faris, H. M., Jr., Duncan, R. C., and Humphries, G. B.: Preinfarctional (Unstable) Angina—A Prospective Study—Ten-Year Follow-up, *Circulation,* 48:331, 1973.

246 Unstable Angina Pectoris: National Cooperative Study Group to Compare Medical and Surgical Therapy, 1. Report of Protocol—Patient Population, *Am. J. Cardiol.,* 37:896, 1976.

247 Bonchek, L. I., Rahimtoola, S. H., Anderson, R. P., McAnulty, J. A., Rosch, J., Bristow, J. D., and Starr, A.: Late Results

following Emergency Saphenous Vein Bypass Grafting for Unstable Angina, *Circulation,* 50:972, 1974.

248 Scanlon, P. J., Nemickas, R., Moran, J. F., Talano, J. V., Amirparviz, F., and Pifarre, R.: Accelerated Angina Pectoris. Clinical, Hemodynamic, Arteriographic, and Therapeutic Experience in 85 Patients, *Circulation,* 47:19, 1973.

249 Friesinger, G. C., Perry, J. M., and Smith, R. F.: Unstable Angina Pectoris: Clinical and Angiographic Findings in 154 Patients Prospectively Evaluated. (In preparation)

250 Baum, R. S., Alvarez, H., and Cobb, L. A.: Survival after Resuscitation from Out-of-Hospital Ventricular Defibrillation, *Circulation,* 50:1231, 1974.

251 Liberthson, R. R., Nagel, E. L., Hirschman, J. C., and Nusserfeld, S. R.: Prehospital Ventricular Fibrillation, *N. Engl. J. Med.,* 291:317, 1974.

252 Armstrong, A., Duncan, B., Oliver, M. F., Julian, D. G., Donald, K. W., Fulton, M., Lutz, W., and Morrison, S. L.: Natural History of Acute Coronary Heart Attacks: A Community Study, *Br. Heart J.,* 34:67, 1972.

253 Fulton, M., Julian, D. G., and Oliver, M. F.: Sudden Death and Myocardial Infarction, AHA Monograph no. 27, Research in Acute Myocardial Infarction, *Circulation,* 40(suppl. 4):182, 1969.

254 Killip, T., III, and Kimball, J. T.: Treatment of Myocardial Infarction in a Coronary Care Unit, *Am. J. Cardiol.,* 20:457, 1967.

255 Page, D. L., Caulfield, J. B., Kastor, J. A., DeSanctis, R. W., and Sanders, C. A.: Myocardial Changes Associated with Cardiogenic Shock, *N. Engl. J. Med.,* 285:133, 1971.

256 Alonso, D. R., Scheidt, S., Post, M., and Killip, T.: Pathophysiology of Cardiogenic Shock: Quantification of Myocardial Necrosis, Clinical, Pathologic, and Electrocardiographic Correlations, *Circulation,* 48:588, 1973.

257 Sievers, J.: Myocardial Infarction: Clinical Features and Outcome in Three Thousand Thirty-Six Cases, *Acta Med. Scand.,* 175(suppl. 406):1964.

258 Sobel, B. E., Markham, J., and Roberts, R.: Factors Influencing Enzymatic Estimates of Infarct Size, *Am. J. Cardiol.,* 39:130, 1977. (Editorial)

259 Chapman, B. L.: Correlation of Mortality Rate and Serum Enzymes in Myocardial Infarction: Test of Efficiency of Coronary Care, *Br. Heart J.,* 33:643, 1971.

260 Kibe, O., and Nilsson, N. J.: Observations on the Diagnostic and Prognostic Value of Some Enzyme Tests in Myocardial Infarction, *Acta Med. Scand.,* 182:597, 1967.

261 Peel, A. A. F., Semple, T., Wang, I., Lancaster, W. M., and Dall, J. L. G.: A Coronary Prognostic Index for Grading the Severity of Infarction, *Br. Heart J.,* 24:745, 1962.

262 Hughes, W. L., Kalbfleisch, J. M., Brandt, E. N., and Costiloe, J. P.: Myocardial Infarction Prognosis by Discriminant Analysis, *Arch. Intern. Med.,* 111:338, 1963.

263 Norris, R. M., Brandt, P. W. T., Caughey, D. E., Lee, A. J., and Scott, P. J.: A New Coronary Prognostic Index, *Lancet,* 1:274, 1969.

264 Helmers, C.: Short- and Long-Term Prognostic Indices in Acute Myocardial Infarction, *Acta Med. Scand.,* 195(suppl. 555):1973.

265 Reid, P. R., Taylor, D. R., Kelly, D. T., Weisfeldt, M. L., Humphries, J. O., Ross, R. S., and Pitt, B.: Myocardial-Infarct Extension Detected by Precordial ST-Segment Mapping, *N. Engl. J. Med.,* 290:123, 1974.

266 Madias, J.: Precordial Mapping in Acute Anterior Myocardial Infarction, *Clin. Res.,* 23:194A, 1975. (Abstract)

267 Epstein, S. E., Besser, G. D., Rosing, D. R., Talano, J. V., and Karsh, R. B.: Experimental Acute Infarction: Characterization and Treatment of the Malignant Premature Ventricular Contraction, *Circulation,* 47:446, 1973.

268 Burgess, M. J., Abildskov, J. A., Millar, K., Gesses, J. S., and Green, L. S.: Time Course of Vulnerability to Fibrillation after Experimental Coronary Occlusion, *Am. J. Cardiol.,* 27:617, 1971.

269 Han, J.: Mechanisms of Ventricular Arrhythmias Associated with Myocardial Infarction, *Am. J. Cardiol.,* 24:800, 1969.

270 McNamee, B. T., Robinson, T. J., Adgey, A. A. J., Scott, M. E., Geddes, J. S., and Pantridge, J. F.: Long-Term Prognosis following Ventricular Fibrillation in Acute Ischemic Heart Disease, *Br. Med. J.,* 4:204, 1970.

271 Cox, J. R., Jr., Roberts, R., Ambros, H. D., Oliver, G. C., and Sobel, B. E.: Relations between Enzymatically Estimated Myocardial Infarct Size and Early Ventricular Dysrhythmia, *Circulation,* 53(suppl. 1):50, 1976. See also M. F. Oliver, p. 55, and H. A. Fozzard, p. 158.

272 Beard, O. W., Hipp, H. R., Robins, M., and Verzolini, V. R.: Initial Myocardial Infarction among Veterans: Ten-Year Survival, *Am. Heart J.,* 73:317, 1967.

273 Thygesen, K., Dalsgaard, P., and Nielsen, B. L.: Prognosis after First Myocardial Infarction, *Acta Med. Scand.,* 195:253, 1974.

274 Norris, R. M., Caughey, D. E., Mercer, C. J., and Scott, P. J.: Prognosis after Myocardial Infarction: Six-Year Follow-up, *Br. Heart J.,* 36:786, 1974.

275 Weinblatt, E., Shapiro, S., Frank, C. W., and Sagen, R. V.: Prognosis of Men after First Myocardial Infarction: Mortality and First Recurrence in Relation to Selected Parameters, *Am. J. Public Health,* 58:1329, 1968.

276 Vismara, L. A., DeMaria, A. N., Hughes, J. L., Mason, D. T., and Amsterdam, E. A.: Evaluation of Arrhythmias in the Late Hospital Phase of Acute Myocardial Infarction Compared to Coronary Care Unit Ectopy, *Br. Heart J.,* 37:598, 1975.

277 Vismara, L. A., Amsterdam, E. A., and Mason, D. T.: Relation of Ventricular Arrhythmias in the Late Hospital Phase of Acute Myocardial Infarction to Sudden Death after Hospital Discharge, *Am. J. Cardiol.,* 59:6, 1975.

278 Kotler, M. N., Tabatznik, B., Mower, M. M., and Tominaga, S.: Prognostic Significance of Ventricular Ectopic Beats with Respect to Sudden Death in the Late Postinfarction Period, *Circulation,* 47:959, 1973.

279 Prineas, R. J., and Blackburn, H.: Sudden Coronary Death outside Hospital, *Circulation,* 52(suppl. 3):1, 1975.

280 The Coronary Drug Project Research Group: Prognostic Importance of Premature Beats following Myocardial Infarction: Experience in the Coronary Drug Project, *J.A.M.A.,* 223:1116, 1973.

281 "How It Feels to Have a Heart Attack," American Heart Association, Dallas, Texas, 1977.

282 Feinleib, M., and Davidson, M. J.: Coronary Heart Disease Mortality: A Community Perspective, *J.A.M.A.,* 222:1129, 1972.

283 Pantridge, J. F., Adgey, A. A. J., Geddes, J. S., and Webb, S. W.: "The Acute Coronary Attack," Grune & Stratton, Inc., New York, 1975.

284 Julian, D. G.: Treatment of Cardiac Arrest in Acute Myocardial Ischaemia and Infarction, *Lancet,* 2:840, 1961.

285 Day, H. W.: Preliminary Studies of an Acute Coronary Care Area, *Lancet,* 83:53, 1963.

286 Brown, K. W. G., Macmillan, R. L., Forbath, N., Mel'grano, F., and Scott, J. W.: Coronary Unit: An Intensive-Care Centre for Acute Myocardial Infarction, *Lancet,* 2:349, 1963.

287 Julian, D. G., Valentine, P. A., and Miller, G. G.: Routine Electrocardiographic Monitoring in Acute Myocardial Infarction, *Med. J. Aust.,* 1:433, 1964.

288 Meltzer, L. E.: The Concept and System for Intensive Coronary Care, *Bull. Acad. Med. New Jersey,* 10:304, 1964.

289 Robinson, J. S., Sloman, G., and McRae, C.: Continuous Electrocardiographic Monitoring in the Early Stages after Acute Myocardial Infarction, *Med. J. Aust.,* 1:427, 1964.

290 Pantridge, J. F.: Mobile Coronary Care, *Chest,* 58:229, 1970.

291 McNeilly, R. H., and Pemberton, J.: Duration of Last Attack

in 998 Fatal Cases of Coronary Artery Disease and Its Relation to Possible Cardiac Resuscitation, *Br. Med. J.,* 3:139, 1968.

292 Yater, W. M., Traum, A. H., Brown, W. G., Fitzgerald, R. P., Geisler, M. A., and Wilcox, B. B.: Coronary Artery Disease in Men Eighteen to Thirty-nine Years of Age: Report of 866 Cases, 450 with Necropsy Examinations, *Am. Heart J.,* 36:334, 481, 683, 1948.

293 Bainton, C. R., and Peterson, D. R.: Deaths from Coronary Heart Disease in Persons 60 Years of Age and Younger, *N. Engl. J. Med.,* 268:569, 1963.

294 Fulton, M., Julian, D. G., and Oliver, M. F.: Sudden Death and Myocardial Infarction, *Circulation,* 40(suppl. 4):182, 1969.

295 Gordon, T., and Kannel, W. B.: Premature Mortality from Coronary Heart Disease, *J.A.M.A.,* 215:1617, 1971.

296 Mittra, B.: Potassium, Glucose and Insulin in Treatment of Myocardial Infarction, *Lancet,* 2:607, 1965.

297 McDonald, L.: The London Hospital, in D. G. Julian and M. F. Oliver, (eds.), "Acute Myocardial Infarction," proceedings of a symposium, E. and S. Livingstone, Edinburgh, 1968, p. 29.

298 Moiseev, S. G.: The Experience of Rendering First Aid to Myocardial Infarction Patients in Moscow, *Sov. Med.,* 26:30, 1962.

299 Pantridge, J. F., and Geddes, J. S.: Cardiac Arrest after Myocardial Infarction, *Lancet,* 1:807, 1966.

300 Pantridge, J. F., and Geddes, J. S.: A Mobile Intensive-Care Unit in the Management of Myocardial Infarction, *Lancet,* 2:271, 1967.

301 Barber, J. M., Boyle, D. McC., Chaturvedi, N. C., Gamble, J., Groves, D. H. M., Millar, D. S., Shivalingappa, G., Walsh, M. J., and Wilson, H. K.: Mobile Coronary Care, *Lancet,* 2:133, 1970.

302 Kubik, M. M., Bhowmich, B. K., Stokes, T., and Joshi, M.: Mobile Cardiac Unit: Experience from a West Midland Town, *Br. Heart J.,* 36:238, 1974.

303 Adgey, A. A. J., Allen, J. D., Geddes, J. S., James, R. G. G., Webb, S. W., Zaidi, S. A., and Pantridge, J. F.: Acute Phase of Myocardial Infarction, *Lancet,* 2:501, 1971.

303a Resnekov, L.: Intermediate Coronary Care Units, *J.A.M.A.,* 237:1697, 1977.

303b Resnekov, L.: Invited Article: The Intermediate Coronary Care Unit. A Stage in Continued Coronary Care, *Br. Heart J.,* 39:357, 1977.

304 Hurst, J. W.: "Four Hats," Year Book Medical Publishers, Inc., Chicago, 1970, p. 55.

305 Hackett, T. P., and Cassem, N. H.: Coronary Care: Patient Psychology, American Heart Association, Inc., New York, 1975.

306 Cassem, N. H., Wishnie, H. A., and Hackett, T. P.: How Coronary Patients Respond to Last Rites, *Postgrad. Med.,* 45:147, 1969.

307 Wilson, L. M.: Intensive Care Delirium, *Arch. Intern. Med.,* 130:225, 1972.

308 Browne, I. W., and Hackett, T. P.: Emotional Reactions to the Threat of Impending Death. Study of Patients on Monitor Cardiac Pacemaker, *Ir. J. Med. Sci.,* 6:177, 1967.

309 Hackett, T. P., and Cassem, N. H.: Psychological Effects of Acute Coronary Care, in L. E. Meltzer and A. J. Dunning (eds.), "Textbook of Coronary Care," The Charles Press, Philadelphia, 1972, p. 443.

310 Hackett, T. P., Cassem, N. H., and Wishnie, H. A.: The Coronary Care Unit: An Appraisal of Its Psychological Hazards, *N. Engl. J. Med.,* 279:1365, 1968.

311 Bruhn, J. G., Thurman, A. E., Jr., Chandler, B. C., and Bruce, T. A.: Patients' Reactions to Death in a Coronary Care Unit, *J. Psychosom. Res.,* 14:65, 1970.

312 Druss, R. G., and Kornfeld, D. S.: Survivors of Cardiac Arrest: Psychiatric Study, *J.A.M.A.,* 201:291, 1967.

313 Dobson, M., Tattersfield, A. E., Adler, M. M., and McNicol,

M. W.: Attitudes and Long-Term Adjustment of Patients Surviving Cardiac Arrest, *Br. Med. J.,* 3:207, 1971.

314 Hackett, T. P.: The Lazarus Complex Revisited, *Ann. Intern. Med.,* 76:135, 1972.

315 Klein, R. F., Kliner, V. A., Zipes, D. P., Troyer, W. G., Jr., and Wallace, A. G.: Transfer from a Coronary Care Unit, *Arch. Intern. Med.,* 122:104, 1968.

316 Hackett, T. P., and Cassem, N. H.: White- and Blue-Collar Responses to a Heart Attack, paper presented at the American Psychosomatic Society National Meeting, Boston, 1971.

317 Hackett, T. P., and Cassem, N. H.: Detection and Treatment of Anxiety in the Coronary Care Unit, *Am. Heart J.,* 78:727, 1969.

318 Cassem, N. H., and Hackett, T. P.: Psychological Rehabilitation of Myocardial Infarction Patients in the Acute Phase, *Heart and Lung,* 2:382, 1973.

319 Naughton, J. P., and Hellerstein, H. K. (eds.): "Exercise Testing and Exercise Training in Coronary Heart Disease," Academic Press, Inc., New York, 1973, p. 311.

320 Lesstma, J. E., and Loenig, K. L.: Sudden Death and Phenothiazines, *Arch. Gen. Psychiatry,* 18:137, 1968.

321 Coull, D. C., Crooks, J., Dingwall-Fordyce, I., Scott, A. M., and Weir, R. D.: Amitriptyline and Cardiac Disease: Risk of Sudden Death Identified by Monitoring System, *Lancet,* 2:590, 1970.

322 Hutter, A. M., Sidel, V. W., Shine, K. I., and DeSanctis, R. W.: Early Hospital Discharge after Myocardial Infarction, *N. Engl. J. Med.,* 288:1141, 1973.

323 Regan, T. J., Haider, B., Ahmed, S. S., Lyons, M. M., Oldewurtel, H. A., and Ettinger, P. O.: Whiskey and the Heart, *Cardiovasc. Med.,* 2:165, 1977.

324 Orlando, J., Aronow, W. S., Cassidy, J., and Prakayh, R.: Effect of Ethanol on Angina Pectoris, *Ann. Intern. Med.,* 84:652, 1976.

325 Brunton, T. L.: On the Use of Nitrite of Amyl in Angina Pectoris, *Lancet,* 2:97, 1867.

326 Nickerson, N.: Vasodilator Drugs, in L. S. Goodman and A. Gilman (eds.) "The Pharmacological Basis of Therapeutics," 5th ed., The Macmillan Company, Inc., New York, 1975, chap. 34, p. 734.

327 Aronow, W. S.: The Medical Treatment of Angina Pectoris. IV. Nitroglycerin as an Antianginal Drug, *Am. Heart J.,* 84:415, 1972.

328 Chatterjee, K., and Parmley, W. W.: The Role of Vasodilator Therapy in Heart Failure, *Prog. Cardiovasc. Dis.,* 19:301, 1977.

329 Kent, K. W., Smith, E. R., Redwood, D. R., and Epstein, S. E.: Beneficial Electrophysiologic Effects of Nitroglycerin during Acute Myocardial Infarction, *Am J. Cardiol.,* 33:513, 1974.

330 Helfant, R. H., Pine, R., Meister, S. G., Feldman, M. S., Trout, R. G., and Banka, V. S.: Nitroglycerin to Unmask Reversible Asynergy: Correlation with Post Coronary Bypass Ventriculography, *Circulation,* 50:108, 1974.

331 Kaplan, J. A., Dunbar, R. W., and Jones, E. L.: Nitroglycerin Infusion during Coronary-Artery Surgery, *Anesthesiology,* 45:14, 1976.

332 Williams, D. O., Amsterdam, E. A., and Mason, D. T.: Hemodynamic Effects of Nitroglycerin in Acute Myocardial Infarction: Decrease in Ventricular Preload at the Expense of Cardiac Output, *Circulation,* 51:421, 1975.

333 Borer, J. S., Kent, K. M., Goldstein, R. E., and Epstein, S. E.: Nitroglycerin-induced Reduction in the Incidence of Spontaneous Ventricular Fibrillation during Coronary Occlusion in Dogs, *Am. J. Cardiol.,* 33:517, 1974.

334 Armstrong, P. W., Walker, D. C., Burton, J. R., and Parker, J.

O.: Vasodilator Therapy in Acute Myocardial Infarction. A Comparison of Sodium Nitroprusside and Nitroglycerin, *Circulation*, 52:1118, 1975.

335 Kasparian, H., Wiener, L., Duca, P. R., Gottlieb, R. S., and Brest, A. N.: Comparative Hemodynamic Effects of Placebo and Oral Isosorbide Dinitrate in Patients with Significant Coronary Artery Disease, *Am. Heart J.*, 90:68, 1975.

336 Goldstein, R. E., Rosing, D. R., Redwood, D. R., Beiser, G. D., and Epstein, S. E.: Clinical and Circulatory Effects of Isosorbide Dinitrate: Comparison with Nitroglycerin, *Circulation*, 43:629, 1971.

337 Zelis, R., and Mason, D. T.: Isosorbide Dinitrate: Effect on the Vasodilator Response to Nitroglycerin, *J.A.M.A.*, 234:166, 1975.

337a Abrams, J.: Current Status of Long-Acting Nitrates in Clinical Medicine, *Prac. Cardiol.*, 3:17, 1977.

337b Cohn, P. F., Maddox, D., Holman, B. L., Markis, J. E., Adams, D. F., and See, J. R.: Effect of Sublingually Administered Nitroglycerin on Regional Myocardial Blood Flow in Patients with Coronary Artery Disease, *Am. J. Cardiol.*, 39:672, 1977.

338 Sweatman, T., Strauss, G., Selzer, A., and Cohn, K. E.: The Long-acting Hemodynamic Effects of Isosorbide Dinitrate, *Am. J. Cardiol.*, Monograph on Angina Pectoris, 1973.

339 Davis, J. A., and Wiesel, B. H.: The Treatment of Angina Pectoris with a Nitroglycerin Ointment, *Am. J. Med. Sci.*, 230:259, 1955.

340 Meister, S. G., Engel, T. R., Guiha, N., Furr, C. M., Feitosa, G. S., Hart, K., and Frankl, W. S.: Sustained Haemodynamic Action of Nitroglycerin Ointment, *Br. Heart J.*, 38:1031, 1976.

341 Reichek, N., Goldstein, R. E., Redwood, D. R., and Epstein, S. E.: Sustained Effects of Nitroglycerin Ointment in Patients with Angina Pectoris, *Circulation*, 50:348, 1974.

342 Parker, J. O., Augustine, R. J., Burton, J. R., West, R. O., and Armstrong, P. W.: Effect of Nitroglycerin Ointment on the Clinical and Hemodynamic Response to Exercise, *Am. J. Cardiol.*, 38:162, 1976.

343 Taylor, W. R., Forrester, J. S., Magnusson, P., Takano, T., Chatterjee, K., and Swan, H. J. C.: Hemodynamic Effects of Nitroglycerin Ointment in Congestive Heart Failure, *Am. J. Cardiol.*, 38:469, 1976.

344 Mantel, J. A., Russell, R. O., Moraski, R. E., and Rackley, C. E.: Isosorbide Dinitrite for Relief of Severe Heart Failure after Myocardial Infarction, *Am. J. Cardial.*, 37:263, 1976.

345 Willis, W. H., Russel, R. O., Mantle, J. A., Ratshin, R. A., and Rackley, C. E.: Hemodynamic Effects of Isosorbide Dinitrate vs Nitroglycerin in Patients with Unstable Angina, *Chest*, 69:15, 1976.

346 Epstein, S. E., Redwood, D. R., Goldstein, R. E., Beiser, G. D., Rosing, D. R., Glancy, D. L., Reis, R. L., and Stinson, E. B.: Angina Pectoris: Pathophysiology, Evaluation, and Treatment, *Ann. Intern. Med.*, 75:263, 1971.

347 Kattus, A. A., Alvaro, A. B., and Coulson, A.: Effectiveness of Isosorbide Dinitrate and Nitroglycerin in Relieving Angina Pectoris during Uninterrupted Exercise, *Chest*, 67:640, 1975.

348 Gensini, G. G., Kelly, A. E., DaCosta, B. C. B., and Huntington, P.: Quantitative Angiography: The Measurement of Coronary Vasomotility in the Intact Animal and Man, *Chest*, 60:522, 1971.

349 Dollery, C. T., and George, C.: Propranolol—Ten Years from Introduction, *Cardiovasc. Clin.*, 6:255, 1974.

350 Alderman, E. L., Davies, R. O., Crowley, J. J., Lopes, M. G., Brooker, J. Z., Friedman, J. P., Graham, A. F., Matlof, H. J., and Harrison, D. C.: Dose Response Effectiveness of Propranolol for the Treatment of Angina Pectoris, *Circulation*, 51:964, 1975.

351 Panatano, J. A., and Lee, Y. C.: Abrupt Propranolol With-drawal and Myocardial Contractility, *Arch. Intern. Med.*, 136:867, 1976.

352 Alderman, E. L., Coltart, D. J., Wettach, G. E., and Harrison, D. C.: Coronary Artery Syndromes after Sudden Propranolol Withdrawal, *Ann. Intern. Med.*, 81:625, 1974.

353 Slome, R.: Withdrawal of Propranolol and Myocardial Infarction, *Lancet*, 1:156, 1973.

354 Warren, S. G., Brewer, D. L., and Orgain, E. S.: Long-Term Propranolol Therapy for Angina Pectoris, *Am. J. Cardiol.*, 37:420, 1976.

355 Wolfson, S., and Gorlin, R.: Cardiovascular Pharmacology of Propranolol in Man, *Circulation*, 40:501, 1969.

356 Becker, L., and Pitt, B.: Regional Myocardial Blood Flow, Ischemia and Antianginal Drugs, *Ann. Clin. Res.*, 3:353, 1971.

357 Pine, M., Favrot, L., Smith, S., McDonald, K., and Chisdey, C. A.: Correlation of Plasma Propranolol Concentration with Therapeutic Response in Patients with Angina Pectoris, *Circulation*, 52:886, 1975.

358 Crawford, M. H., LeWinter, M. M., O'Rourke, R. A., Karliner, J. S., and Ross, J.: Combined Propranolol and Digoxin Therapy in Angina Pectoris, *Ann. Intern. Med.*, 83:449, 1975.

359 Amsterdam, E. A., Gorlin, R., and Wolfson, S.: Evaluation of Long-Term Use of Propranolol in Angina Pectoris, *J.A.M.A.*, 210:103, 1969.

360 Hurst, J. W.: Personal observation.

361 Conolly, M. E., Kersting, F., and Dollery, C. T.: The Clinical Pharmacology of Beta-Adrenoceptor-Blocking Agents, *Prog. Cardiovasc. Dis.*, 19:203, 1976.

362 Miller, R. R., Olson, H. G., Amsterdam, E. A., and Mason, D. T.: Propranolol-Withdrawal Rebound Phenomenon: Exacerbation of Coronary Events after Abrupt Cessation of Antianginal Therapy, *N. Engl. J. Med.*, 293:416, 1975.

363 Alderman, E. L., Coltart, D. J., Wettach, G. E., and Harrison, D. C.: Coronary Artery Syndromes after Sudden Propranolol Withdrawal, *Ann. Intern. Med.*, 81:625, 1974.

364 Jones, E. L., Dorney, E. R., King, S. B., Gray, B. L., and Hatcher, C. R.: Propranolol Therapy in Patients Undergoing Myocardial Revascularization, *Circulation*, 50:112, 1974.

365 Lesch, M., and Gorlin, R.: Pharmacological Therapy of Angina Pectoris, *Mod. Concepts Cardiovasc. Dis.*, 42:5, 1973.

366 Goldbarg, A. N., Moran, J. F., Butterfield, T. K. Nemickas, R., and Bermudez, G. A.: Therapy of Angina Pectoris with Propranolol and Long-acting Nitrates, *Circulation*, 40:847, 1969.

367 Aronow, W. S., and Kaplan, M. A.: Propranolol and Isosorbide Dinitrate Versus Placebo in Angina Pectoris, *N. Engl. J. Med.*, 280:847, 1969.

368 Coltart, D. J., Alderman, E. L., Robinson, S. C., and Harrison, D. C.: Effect of Propranolol on Left Ventricular Function, Segmental Wall Motion, and Diastolic Pressure-Volume Relation in Man, *Br. Heart J.*, 37:357, 1975.

369 Waagstein, F., Hjalmarson, A., Varnauska, E., and Wallentin, I.: Effect of Chronic Beta-adrenergic Receptor Blockade in Congestive Cardiomyopathy, *Br. Heart J.*, 37:1022, 1975.

370 Bloch, A., Beller, G. A., and DeSanctis, R. W.: Chronic Propranolol Administration and Acute Myocardial Infarction, *Am. Heart J.*, 92;121, 1976.

371 Reimer, K. A., Rasmussen, M. M., and Jennings, R. B.: On the Nature of Protection of Propranolol against Myocardial Necrosis after Temporary Coronary Occlusion in Dogs, *Am. J. Cardiol.*, 37:520, 1976.

372 Pitt, B., Weiss, G. L., Schulze, R. A., Taylor, D. A., Kennedy, H. L., and Caralis, D.: Reduction of Myocardial Infarct Extension in Man by Propranolol, *Circulation*, 53 & 54(suppl. 2):29, 1976.

373 Jackson, G., Atkinson, L., and Oram, S.: Double Blind Comparison of Tolamolol, Propranolol, Practolol, and Placebo in the Treatment of Angina Pectoris, *Br. Med. J.*, 1:708, 1975.

374 Sowton, E., Das Guyster, D. S., and Baker, I.: Comparative Effects of Beta Adrenergic Blocking Drugs, *Thorax,* 30:9, 1975.

375 Morgans, C. M., and Rees, J. R.: The Action of Perhexiline Maleate in Patients with Angina, *Am. Heart J.,* 86:329, 1973.

376 Taylor, S. H., and Thodain, U.: Oxprenolol in Angina Pectoris, Abstract VI, Asian-Pacific Congress of Cardiology, 1976.

377 Sloman, G., Robinson, J. S., and McLean, K.: Propranolol (Inderal) in Persistent Ventricular Fibrillation, *Br. Med. J.,* 1:895, 1965.

378 Rothfeld, E. L., Lipowitz, M., Zucker, I. R., Parsonnet, V., and Bernstein, A.: Management of Persistently Recurring Ventricular Fibrillation with Propranolol Hydrochloride, *J. A.M.A.,* 204:546, 1968.

379 Multicentre Study: Improvement in Prognosis of Myocardial Infarction by Long-Term B-Adrenoceptor Blockade Using Practolol, *Br. Med. J.,* 3:735, 1975.

380 Wilhelmsson, C., Vedin, J. A., Wilhelmsen, L., Tibblin, G., and Werko, L.: Reduction of Sudden Deaths after Myocardial Infarction by Treatment with Alprenolol, *Lancet,* 2:1157, 1974.

381 Ahlmark, G., and Saetre, H.: Position of Myocardial Infarction and Result of Alprenolol Treatment, *Br. Heart J.,* 1:837, 1976.

382 Modell, W.: Narcotic Analgesics in Heart Disease, *Am. Heart J.,* 65:709, 1963.

383 Vasko, J. S., Henney, R. P., Oldham, H. N., Brawley, R. K., and Morrow, A. G.: Mechanisms of Action of Morphine in the Treatment of Experimental Pulmonary Edema, *Am. J. Cardiol.,* 18:876, 1966.

384 Thomas, M., Malmcrona, R., Fillmore, S., and Shillingford, J.: Haemodynamic Effects of Morphine in Patients with Acute Myocardial Infarction, *Br. Heart J.,* 27:863, 1965.

385 Kerr, F., Irving, J. B., Ewing, D. J., and Kirby, B. J.: Nitrous oxide Analgesia in Myocardial Infarction, *Lancet,* 1:63, 1972.

386 Moon, A. J., Williams, K. G., and Hopkinson, W. I.: A Patient with Coronary Thrombosis Treated with Hyperbaric Oxygen, *Lancet,* 1:18, 1964.

386a Lee, G., DeMaria, A. N., Amsterdam, E. A., Henderson, G. L., and Mason, D. T.: Analgesic Agents in Acute Myocardial Infarction: Clinical Pharmacology and Therapeutics, *Prac. Cardiol.,* 3:31, 1977.

387 Epstein, S. E.: Hypotension, Nitroglycerin, and Acute Myocardial Infarction, *Circulation,* 47:217, 1973.

388 Rawles, J. M., and Kenmure, A. C. F.: Controlled Trial of Oxygen in Uncomplicated Myocardial Infarction, *Br. Med. J.,* 1:1121, 1976.

389 Mullar, O., and Rornik, K.: Hemodynamic Consequences of Coronary Heart Disease with Observations during Anginal Pain and on the Effect of Nitroglycerin, *Br. Heart J.,* 20:302, 1958.

390 Glancy, D. L., Higgs, L. M., O'Brien, K. P., and Epstein, S. E.: Effects of Ouabain on Left Ventricular Response to Exercise in Patients with Angina Pectoris, *Circulation,* 43:45, 1971.

391 Rahimtoola, S. H., and Gunnar, R. M.: Digitalis in Acute Myocardial Infarction: Help or Hazard? *Ann. Intern. Med.,* 82:234, 1975.

392 Hodges, M., Friesmyer, G. C., and Riggins, R. C. K.: Effects of Intravenously Administered Digoxin on Mild Left Ventricular Failure in Acute Myocardial Infarction in Man, *Am. J. Cardiol.,* 29:749, 1972.

393 Cohn, J. N., Fristani, F. E., and Kholn, I. M.: Cardiac and Peripheral Effects of Digitalis in Clinical Cardiogenic Shock, *Am. Heart J.,* 78:318, 1969.

394 Magenis, P. W.: Why Aspirin? *Circulation,* 54:357, 1976.

395 Vane, J. R.: Inhibition of Prostaglandin Synthesis as a Mechanism for Action for Aspirin-like Drug, *Nature [New Biol.],* 231:232, 1971.

396 Hamberg, M., Svensson, J., Wakaboyoski, T., and Samuelsson, B.: Prostaglandin Endoperoxides. Novel Transformation of Arachidonic Acid in Human Platelets, *Proc. Natl. Acad. Sci. USA,* 71:3400, 1974.

397 Cardiovascular Studies: *Arch. Intern. Med.,* 136:1213, 1976.

398 Soffer, A.: *Arch. Intern. Med.,* 136:1229, 1976. (Editorial Comment.)

399 Rogel, S., and Bassan, M. M.: Anticoagulants in Ischemic Heart Disease, *Arch Intern. Med.,* 136:1229, 1976.

400 Modan, B., Schor, S. S., and Modan, M.: The Case for Anticoagulants in Acute Myocardial Infarction: How Do You Know You Cannot Do It Better? *Arch. Intern. Med.,* 136: 1231, 1976.

401 Wessler, S.: Prevention of Venous Thromboembolism by Low-Dose Heparin, *Mod. Concepts Cardiovasc. Dis.,* 45:105, 1976.

402 Fratantoni, J. C.: Thrombolytic Therapy, *Am. Heart J.,* 93:271, 1977.

403 Gorlin, R.: Revascularization of the Myocardium, in R. Gorlin (ed.), "Coronary Artery Disease," W. B. Saunders Company, Philadelphia, 1976.

404 Conti, R.: Coronary Arteriography, *Circulation,* 55:227, 1977.

404a Bristow, J. D., Burchell, H. B., Campbell, R. W., Ebert, P. A., Hall, R. J., Leonard, J. J., and Reeves, T. J.: A.H.A. Special Report: Report of the Ad Hoc Committee on the Indications for Coronary Arteriography, *Circulation,* 55: 969A, 1977.

405 Mundth, E. D., and Austen, W. G.: Surgical Measures for Coronary Heart Disease, *N. Engl. J. Med.,* 293:13, 75, 124, 1975.

406 MacAlpin, R. N., Kattus, A. A., and Alvara, A. B.: Angina Pectoris at Rest with Preservation of Exercise Capacity: Prinzmetal's Variant Angina, *Circulation,* 47:946, 1973.

407 Guazzi, M., Magrini, F., Fiorentini, C., and Polese, A.: Clinical, Electrocardiographic, and Haemodynamic Effects of Long-Term Use of Propranolol in Prinzmetal's Variant Angina Pectoris, *Br. Heart J.,* 33:889, 1971.

408 Endo, M., Hirosawa, K., Kaneko, N., Hase, K., Inoue, Y., and Konno, S.: Prinzmetal's Variant Angina: Coronary Arteriogram and Left Ventriculogram during Angina Attack Induced by Methacholine, *N. Engl. J. Med.,* 294:252, 1976.

409 MacAlpin, R.: Provoking Variant Angina, *N. Engl. J. Med.,* 294:277, 1976. (Editorial)

410 Lasser, R. P., and de la Paz, N. S.: Repetitive Transient Myocardial Ischemia, Prinzmetal Type, without Angina Pectoris, Presenting with Stokes-Adams Attacks, *Chest,* 64:350, 1973.

410a Thornley, P. E., and Turner, R. W. D.: Rapid Mobilisation After Acute Myocardial Infarction: First Step in Rehabilitation and Secondary Prevention, *Br. Heart J.,* 39:471, 1977.

411 Levine, S. A., and Lown, B.: The "Chair" Treatment of Coronary Thrombosis, *Trans. Assoc. Am. Physicians,* 64:316, 1951.

412 Hurst, J. W.: "Ambulation" after Myocardial Infarction, *N. Engl. J. Med.,* 292:746, 1975. (Editorial)

413 Gorlin, R.: Current Concepts in Cardiology: Practical Cardiac Hemodynamics, *N. Engl. J. Med.,* 296:203, 1977.

414 Rackley, C. E., Russel, R. O., Jr., Moraski, R. E., and Mantle, J. A.: Recent Advances in Hemodynamic Studies in Patients with Acute Myocardial Infarction, *Prog. Cardiol.,* 5:201, 1976.

415 Rackley, C. E., Russell, R. O., Jr., Moraski, R. E., and Mantle, J. A.: Recent Advances in Hemodynamic Studies in Patients with Acute Myocardial Infarction, in P. N. Yu and J. F. Goodwin (eds.), "Progress in Cardiology," Lea & Febiger, Philadelphia, 1976, vol. 5, pp. 201–226.

416 Russell, R. O., Jr., Rackley, C. E., Pombo, J., Hunt, D., Potanin, C., and Dodge, H. T.: Effects of Increasing Left

Ventricular Filling Pressure in Patients with Acute Myocardial Infarction, *J. Clin. Invest.,* 49:1539, 1970.

417 Franciosa, J. A., Guiha, N. H., Limas, C. J., Rodriguera, E., and Cohn, J. N.: Improved Left Ventricular Function during Nitroprusside Infusion in Acute Infarction, *Lancet,* 1:650, 1972.

418 Mantle, J. A., Russell, R. O., Jr., Moraski, R. E., and Rackley, C. E.: Isosorbide Dinitrate for the Relief of Severe Heart Failure following Myocardial Infarction, *Am. J. Cardiol.,* 37:263, 1976.

419 Rogers, W. J., Stanley, A. W., Jr., Breinig, J. B., Prather, J. W., McDaniel, H. G., Moraski, R. E., Mantle, J. A., Russell, R. O., Jr., and Rackley, C. E.: Reduction of Hospital Mortality of Acute Myocardial Infarction with Glucose-Insulin-Potassium, *Am. Heart J.,* vol. 92:441, 1976.

420 Maroko, P. R., Davidson, D. M., Libby, P., Hagan, A. D., and Braunwald, E.: Effects of Hyaluronidase Administration on Myocardial Ischemic Injury: A Preliminary Study in 24 Patients, *Ann. Intern. Med.,* 82:516, 1975.

421 Cox, J. L., McLaughlin, V. W., Flowers, N. C., and Horan, L. G.: The Ischemic Zone Surrounding Acute Myocardial Infarction. Its Morphology as Detected by Dehydrogenase Staining, *Am. Heart J.,* 76:650, 1968.

422 Caulfield, J. B., Leinbach, R., and Gold, H.: The Relationship of Myocardial Infarct Size and Prognosis, *Circulation,* 53(suppl. 1):141, 1976.

423 Roberts, R., Husain, A., Ambos, D., Oliver, G. C., Cox, J. R., and Sobel, B. E.: Relation between Infarct Size and Ventricular Arrhythmia, *Br. Heart J.,* 37:1169, 1975.

424 Ross, J., Jr.: Electrocardiographic ST-Segment Analysis in the Characterization of Myocardial Ischemia and Infarction, *Circulation,* 53(suppl. 1):73, 1976.

425 Sobel, B. E., Bresnahan, G. F., Shell, W. E., and Yoder, R. D.: Estimation of Infarct Size in Man and Its Relation to Prognosis, *Circulation,* 46:640, 1972.

426 Bleifeld, W. H., Hanrath, P., and Mathey, D.: Serial CPK Determinations for Estimation of Size and Development of Acute Myocardial Infarction, *Circulation,* 53(suppl. 1):108, 1976.

427 Holman, B. L.: Radionuclide Methods in the Evaluation of Myocardial Ischemia and Infarction, *Circulation,* 53(suppl. 1):112, 1976.

428 Theroux, P., Ross, J., Jr., Franklin, D. Kemper, W. S., and Sasayama, S.: Regional Myocardial Function in the Conscious Dog during Acute Coronary Occlusion and Responses to Morphine, Propranolol, Nitroglycerin, and Lidocaine, *Circulation,* 53:302, 1976.

429 Maroko, P. R., and Braunwald, E.: Modification of Myocardial Infarction Size after Coronary Occlusion, *Ann. Intern. Med.,* 79:720, 1973.

430 Epstein, S. E., Borer, J. S., Kent, K. M., Redwood, D. R., Goldstein, R. E., and Levitt, B.: Protection of Ischemic Myocardium by Nitroglycerin: Experimental and Clinical Results, *Circulation,* 53(suppl. 1):191, 1976.

431 Mason, D. T.: Personal communication.

432 Proudfit, W. L: Cleveland Clinic Foundation, Cleveland, Ohio.

433 Graham, A. F., Miller, D. C., Stinson, E. B., Daily, P. O., Fogarty, T. J., and Harrison, D. C.: Surgical Treatment of Refractory Life-Threatening Ventricular Tachycardia, *Am. J. Cardiol.,* 32:909. 1973.

434 Ferrer, M. I.: "The Sick Sinus Syndrome," Futura Publishing Company, Mount Kisco, New York, 1974.

435 Valentine, P. A., Frew, J. L., Mashford, M. L., and Sloman, J. G.: Lidocaine in the Prevention of Sudden Death in the Pre-hospital Phase of Acute Infarction, *N. Engl. J. Med.,* 291:1327, 1974.

436 Chopra, M. P., Thandani, U., Portal, R. W., and Aber, C. P.: Lignocaine Therapy for Ventricular Ectopic Activity after Acute Myocardial Infarction, A Double-Blind Trial, *Br. Med. J.,* 3:668, 1971.

437 Darby, S., Bennett, M. A., Cruickshank, J. C., and Pentecost, B. L.: Trial at Combined Intramuscular and Intravenous Lignocaine in Prophylaxis of Ventricular Tachyarrhythmias, *Lancet,* 1:817, 1972.

438 Lie, K. I., Wellens, H. J., van Capelle, F. J., and Durrer, D.: Lidocaine in the Prevention of Primary Ventricular Fibrillation, *N. Engl. J. Med.,* 291:1324, 1974.

439 Pitt, A., Lipp, H., and Anderson, S. T.: Lignocaine Given Prophylactically to Patients with Acute Myocardial Infarction, *Lancet,* 1:612, 1971.

440 Baxter, R. H., and McGuinness, J. B.: Comparison of Ventricular Parasystole with Other Dysrhythmias after Acute Myocardial Infarction, *Am. Heart J.,* 88:443, 1974.

441 Giardina, E. G., Heissenbuttel, R. H., and Bigger, J. T., Jr.: Intermittent Intravenous Procaine Amide to Treat Ventricular Arrhythmias, *Ann. Intern. Med.,* 78:183, 1973.

442 Robinson, J. S., Sloman, G., Mathew, T. H., and Goble, A. J.: Survival after Resuscitation from Cardiac Arrest in Acute Myocardial Infarction, *Am. Heart J.,* 69:740, 1965.

443 Reicansky, I., Conradson, T., Holmberg, S., Ryden, L., Waldenstrom, A., and Wennerblom, B.: The Effect of Intravenous Digoxin on the Occurrence of Ventricular Tachyarrhythmias in Acute Myocardial Infarction in Man, *Am. Heart J.,* 91:705, 1976.

444 Bennett, M. A., and Pentecost, B. L.: Suppression of Ventricular Tachyarrhythmias by Transvenous Intracardiac Pacing after Acute Myocardial Infarction, *Br. Med. J.,* 4:468, 1970.

445 Sami, M., Charpin, D., Chabot, M., and Bourassa, M. G.: Long-Term Follow-up Aneurysmectomy for Recurrent Ventricular Tachycardia or Fibrillation, *Am. J. Cardiol.,* 39:269, 1977. (Abstract)

445a Cohn, J. N., and Franciosa, J. A.: Medical Intelligence: Drug Therapy–Vasodilator Therapy for Cardiac Failure, *N. Engl. J. Med.,* 297:27, 1977.

446 Parmley, W. W., and Chatterjee, K.: Vasodilator Therapy for Chronic Heart Failure, *Cardiovasc. Med.,* vol. 1:1, September, 1976, p. 17.

447 Mantle, J. A., Russell, R. O., Jr., Moraski, R. E., and Rackley, C. E.: Isosorbide Dinitrate for Relief of Severe Heart Failure after Myocardial Infarction, *Cardiology Digest,* December, 1976.

447a Miller, R. R., Awan, N. A., Joye, J. A., Maxwell, K. S., DeMaria, A. N., Amsterdam, E. A., and Mason, D. T.: Combined Dopamine and Nitroprusside Therapy in Congestive Heart Failure: Greater Augmentation of Cardiac Performance by Addition of Inotropic Stimulation of Afterload Reduction, *Circulation,* 55:881, 1977.

448 Spodick, D. H.: "Pericardial Diseases," F. A. Davis, Company, Philadelphia, 1976.

449 Buckley, M. J., Mundth, E. D., Daggett, W. M., DeSanctis, R. W., Sanders, C. A., and Austen, W. G.: Surgical Therapy for Early Complications of Myocardial Infarction, *Surgery,* 70:814, 1971.

450 Cobbs, B. W., Jr., Hatcher, C. R., Jr., and Robinson, P. H.: Cardiac Rupture: Three Operations with Two Long-Term Survivals, *J.A.M.A.,* 223:532, 1973.

451 Cullhed, I., Delius, W., Bjork, L., Hallen, A., and Nordgren, L.: Resection of Left Ventricular Aneurysms Late Results, *Acta Med. Scand.,* 197:241, 1975.

452 Schulze, R. A., Jr., Strauss, H. W., and Pitt, B.: Sudden Death in the Year following Myocardial Infarction. Relation to Ventricular Premature Contractions in the Late Hospital Phase and Left Ventricular Ejection Fraction, *Am. J. Med.,* 62:192, 1977.

F
Surgical Treatment of Coronary Atherosclerotic Heart Disease

NICHOLAS T. KOUCHOUKOS, M.D., and
JOHN W. KIRKLIN, M.D.

Bypass grafting of obstructing lesions of the coronary arteries, using free grafts of autogenous saphenous vein or the internal thoracic artery, has been applied to large numbers of patients in recent years. Indirect myocardial revascularization using the internal thoracic artery is now seldom used. Surgical treatment of complications resulting from myocardial infarction has also received increasing attention. In the last several years, information on the long-term results of these surgical procedures has become available, as well as data on the natural history of coronary atherosclerotic heart disease in patients managed without operation. Comparison of patients with similar symptoms, degrees of coronary atherosclerosis, and left ventricular dysfunction treated with and without operation provides the basis for most of the current patient management programs. These, no doubt, will require modification as new information becomes available.

PREOPERATIVE EVALUATION

In patients being considered for operation, the frequency and severity of symptoms (angina pectoris, congestive cardiac failure), the extent of coronary atherosclerosis, the functional status of the left ventricle, and the presence of associated lesions should be carefully evaluated.

For patients with chest pain as their only complaint, objective as well as subjective evaluation of the presence and severity of coronary occlusive disease is desirable. Our preference for objective testing is the submaximal graded exercise test, which allows evaluation of the severity of angina and other symptoms under controlled conditions, as well as evaluation of the electrocardiographic changes resulting from myocardial ischemia produced by exertion.[1] This test is relatively reproducible and can be performed at intervals following operation. A standard electrocardiogram is obtained to determine the presence of significant areas of transmural infarction in the distribution of the three major coronary arterial systems (right, left anterior descending, and circumflex), and as a base line for comparison with electrocardiograms taken postoperatively. Serum enzymes [serum glutamic oxaloacetic transaminase (SGOT), lactic dehydrogenase (LDH), and creatinine phosphokinase (CPK)] are obtained to exclude the presence of myocardial necrosis preoperatively and for comparison with values following operation. The isoenzymes of LDH and CPK, in particular, are useful in determining the presence of myocardial necrosis. Myocardial scanning using technetium pyrophosphate may demonstrate areas of acute necrosis in the absence of previous infarction, and may be useful in the evaluation of patients with unstable angina pectoris who are considered for operation (see below). Roentgenography of the chest and cardiac fluoroscopy are performed to determine heart size, signs of pulmonary congestion secondary to left ventricular dysfunction, and atherosclerotic changes in the thoracic aorta. Cardiac fluoroscopy may indicate areas of abnormal left ventricular wall motion and abnormal expansion of the left atrium if mitral regurgitation is present.

Coronary arteriography, using either the Judkins' or Sones' technique, is performed to determine the location and severity of the obstructive lesions, the extent of development of the collateral circulation around them, and the suitability of the arteries distal to the obstructions for grafting. Assessment of left ventricular function is necessary since the risk of operation and the likelihood of obtaining an optimal result following operation correlate most closely with the severity of left ventricular dysfunction present preoperatively. Measurements of left ventricular end-diastolic pressure, end-diastolic volume, and ejection fraction are useful in this regard. Left ventriculography allows identification of areas of akinesia, hypokinesia, or dyskinesia and of aneurysms or scars which may require excision. In addition, the presence of a ventricular septal defect secondary to rupture of the ventricular septum or of mitral regurgitation due to rupture or dysfunction of a papillary muscle can be determined.

SURGICAL TECHNIQUES

Coronary artery bypass grafting

Coronary artery bypass grafting consists of direct anastomosis of reversed segments of saphenous vein to the ascending aorta and to a patent segment of one or more of the three major coronary arteries and their primary branches, or anastomosis of the divided internal thoracic artery to the anterior descending or circumflex coronary artery beyond the major obstruction. Cardiopulmonary bypass is generally required. We utilize mild hypothermia (28 to 32°C) and hemodilution with a buffered electrolyte solution to a hematocrit of 25 to 30 percent. A quiet, dry operative field is essential for performance of the small distal anastomoses. This can be achieved by allowing the heart to fibrillate or with anoxic arrest induced by intermittently clamping the ascending aorta. Use of fine suture material combined with low-power magnification allows precise approximation of the intima of the venous or arterial graft to that of the recipient artery. The veins are sutured end to side to the major coronary arteries and individually to the aorta (Fig. 62F-1). When two or more branches of the three major arterial segments require grafting, we prefer sequential grafts with the distal anastomosis constructed end to side and the middle anastomosis side

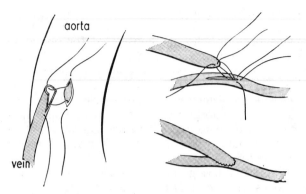

FIGURE 62F-1 All veins are sutured end to side to the coronary artery. The tip is carefully rounded so that it immediately flares out with proper angulation after the two or three crucial corner sutures are placed. *(Reproduced with permission from W. D. Johnson, R. J. Flemma, D. Lepley, Jr., and E. H. Ellison, Extended Treatment of Severe Coronary Artery Disease: A Total Surgical Approach, Ann. Surg., 170:460, 1969.)*

to side. The latter technique reduces the duration of cardiopulmonary bypass and, because of greater flow through the grafts, may result in patency of small branches which would not be large enough to support individual grafts.[2] If the artery is totally occluded at the site selected for anastomosis, endarterectomy of the distal arterial segment can be performed manually or using carbon dioxide to develop a plane of dissection.

As in all surgical procedures, the early and late results following operation are related significantly to events in the operating room. Proper management of anesthesia and supportive treatment by the anesthesiologist, employing interventions to minimize myocardial oxygen requirements while at the same time maintaining adequate coronary flow, are essential if low operative mortality and cardiac morbidity rates are to be achieved. The saphenous vein or internal thoracic artery must be meticulously prepared. Cardiopulmonary bypass should be as optimal as present techniques allow. Prevention of ischemic myocardial injury during the procedure is a major consideration. We avoid ventricular fibrillation and prefer ischemic cardiac arrest for periods of 10 to 15 min at 28 to 32°C. If longer periods of arrest are required, the myocardium is cooled by the perfusate and externally with iced saline solution to temperatures of 18 to 24°C for periods not exceeding 30 to 40 min.

Resection of ventricular aneurysms, areas of dyskinesia or akinesia

The majority of ventricular aneurysms and areas of dyskinesia or akinesia amenable to surgical excision are located on the anterolateral and apical aspects of the left ventricular wall. These scars generally result from transmural myocardial necrosis following occlusion of the anterior descending coronary artery or

its major branches. Less often, noncontracting areas are located posteriorly or inferiorly, and these result from occlusion of the branches of the circumflex or right coronary arteries.

Excision of left ventricular aneurysms or dyskinetic or akinetic areas also requires the use of cardiopulmonary bypass. Exclusion of the scar by plication is not advisable, since thrombotic material which is often adherent to the surface of the scar may be dislodged and embolize. The area to be excised is best identified by venting the left ventricle, allowing it to collapse. This causes the thinned, scarred areas to become more apparent. An incision is made into the aneurysm or scar, and excision up to relatively normal-appearing myocardium is carried out (Fig. 62F-2*A*). When the tissue to be removed is in the distribution of the anterior descending coronary artery, the excision usually extends to the level of the ventricular septum and to the edge of the anterior papillary muscle in the lateral directions, and to the apex inferiorly. Care must be taken to remove the mural thrombotic material which may be dislodged from the ventricular wall when the heart is opened. The papillary muscles, chordae tendineae, and mitral valve leaflets should be examined for any gross abnormalities. The edges of the defect are then approximated using horizontal heavy silk mattress sutures reinforced with a continuous suture (Fig. 62F-2*B*). Posterior aneurysms or scars requiring excision are usually located between the ventricular septum and the posterior papillary muscle and are similarly excised. Air is evacuated from the left ventricular chamber and left atrium before closure, and cardiopulmonary bypass is discontinued. When indicated, coronary artery bypass grafting is combined with the resective procedure.

Ventricular septal defect

Ventricular septal defects occur as a result of rupture of the ventricular septum following myocardial infarction. They usually involve the inferior portion of the muscular septum and are often contiguous with areas of necrosis of either the anterior or posterior left ventricular wall. Because of the difficulty in achieving adequate visualization of such defects through a right ventriculotomy, and the usual presence of associated areas of scarring of the adjacent left ventricular wall, the defects are best approached from the left ventricle through the anterior or posterior area of scarring using cardiopulmonary bypass.[3] If the defect is small, it can be closed directly with heavy mattress sutures. If it is large, it is closed with a patch of synthetic cloth (Fig. 62F-3). If the adjacent area of left ventricular scar is extensive, it should be excised as outlined above. Coronary artery bypass grafting may also be indicated in some patients.

Mitral valvular incompetence

Mitral valvular incompetence may occur following myocardial infarction as a result of rupture of a papillary muscle or of the chordae tendineae, or from papillary muscle dysfunction. Although reconstructive procedures on the mitral valve are occasionally

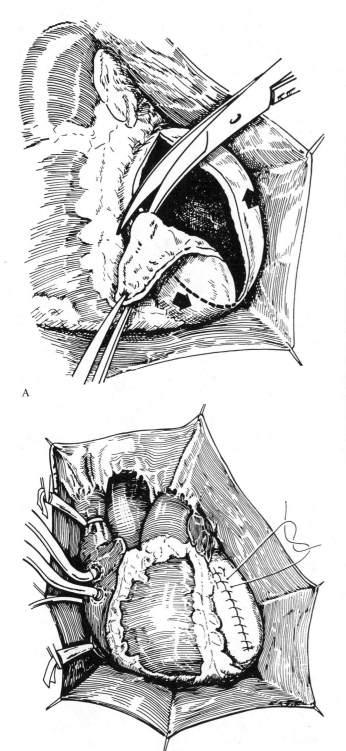

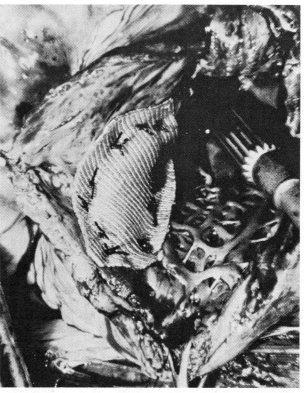

FIGURE 62F-3 Left ventricular chamber exposed through an incision in anterior scar. A 4- by 5-cm woven plastic patch has been sutured over a ventricular septal defect 2- by 3-cm in diameter. Anterior scar is then excised and closure of the ventricle carried out as in Fig. 62F-2*B. (Reproduced with permission of the American Heart Association from J. A. DeWeese, A. J. Moss, and P. N. Yu, Infarctectomy and Closure of Ventricular Septal Defect Rupture following Myocardial Infarction, Circulation, 45, 46(suppl. 1):1–97, 1972.)*

FIGURE 62F-2 A. The entire ventricular aneurysm should be resected, leaving a rim of scar tissue at the edges for support of the sutures. *B.* Reconstruction of the left ventricle is done by a continuous running suture; initial closure is reinforced by interrupted horizontal sutures. *(Reproduced with permission from R. G. Favaloro, D. B. Effler, L. K. Groves, R. N. Westcott, E. Suarez, and J. Lozada, Ventricular Aneurysm: Clinical Experience, Ann. Thorac. Surg., 6:227, 1968.)*

successful, mitral valve replacement is generally required if the incompetence is severe. The technique for mitral valve replacement is that described in Chap. 61. Occasionally, there are areas of noncontracting left ventricular myocardium that require excision in combination with mitral valve replacement. In this situation, the mitral valve can be replaced through the opened ventricle.[4]

Saphenous vein or internal thoracic artery bypass grafts may be utilized in conjunction with valve replacement if preoperative coronary arteriograms demonstrate high-grade stenotic lesions of the proximal portions of the main coronary arteries.[5]

POSTOPERATIVE MANAGEMENT

The postoperative management of patients having the above surgical procedures is similar to that for patients undergoing other types of cardiac surgery (see the discussion in Chap. 95B). Cardiac output is usually normal or near normal following coronary bypass grafting in patients without significant impairment of left ventricular function. Low cardiac output with its attendant problems may complicate the postoperative course of patients undergoing aneurysmectomy, septal defect repair, or mitral valve replacement, and of some patients having only coronary bypass grafting. The latter usually have symptoms of congestive failure or other evidence of significant impairment of left ventricular function preoperatively.

With current techniques and broad operative experience, electrocardiographic evidence of acute myocardial infarction following elective coronary artery bypass grafting occurs in 5 to 15 percent of patients.[6–8] The majority of these infarctions occur without hemodynamic difficulties, although they may occasionally be fatal.[8] Ventricular arrhythmias occurring with or without myocardial infarction can also result in death. Most arrhythmias occurring postoperatively, either ventricular, junctional, or supraventricular, are transient and are not associated with overt infarction. They can be successfully managed with pacing or appropriate drug therapy.[9]

Postoperative cardiac failure is generally manifested by clinical and hemodynamic evidence of low cardiac output, elevated left ventricular filling pressure, and ventricular arrhythmias. It usually results from insufficient myocardial reserves in patients who have severely impaired left ventricular function preoperatively. These patients have myocardial fibrosis involving significant portions of the left ventricular wall, and there may be superimposed acute myocardial necrosis as well.[10] Treatment consists of avoidance of excessively low or high left ventricular filling pressures, maintenance of systemic mean arterial pressure above 80 to 90 mm Hg with epinephrine and/or norepinephrine, use of afterload-reducing agents such as sodium nitroprusside or trimethaphan camsylate when indicated, and aggressive treatment of ventricular arrhythmias.[9] The intraaortic balloon assist device has been used in patients in whom cardiopulmonary bypass could not be discontinued without hemodynamic deterioration, and in patients who deteriorated later in the postoperative period.[11,12] Intraaortic balloon counterpulsation reduces left ventricular work and oxygen consumption and may improve coronary perfusion.[13] The indications for its use are not completely defined, but it has generally been used when there is evidence for significant hemodynamic deterioration (mean aortic pressure less than 80 mm Hg, mean left atrial pressure greater than 25 mm Hg, and low cardiac output despite maximal pharmacologic support). Hospital mortality for patients requiring intraaortic balloon counterpulsation postoperatively has ranged between 40 and 50 percent, and approximately 40 percent of the patients have been long-term survivors. Although these results are not optimal, the majority of these patients would have died without the period of circulatory support.

Postoperative bleeding, significant pulmonary, renal, or neurological dysfunction, and problems related to removal of the saphenous vein (edema or phlebitis of the lower extremity) occur in only a small percentage of patients and generally respond to appropriate therapeutic measures. Anticoagulation with warfarin derivatives is advisable for 7 to 10 days following operation to minimize the likelihood of venous thrombosis in the lower extremities and pulmonary embolism. Patients having excision of ventricular scars should receive anticoagulant therapy for 4 to 6 weeks if mural thrombus is present at the time of operation. Patients having replacement of the mitral valve are placed on permanent anticoagulant therapy.

INDICATIONS FOR OPERATION AND RESULTS IN THE CLINICAL SYNDROMES OF CORONARY ATHEROSCLEROTIC HEART DISEASE

Until recently, the major indication for direct coronary revascularization has been the presence of disabling angina pectoris, refractory to medical therapy, in patients with angiographically demonstrated high-grade obstructions in the proximal segments of the major coronary arterial segments but without severe left ventricular dysfunction. *Studies of the natural history of coronary atherosclerotic disease using coronary arteriography alone[14–18] or in combination with some assessment of left ventricular function[14,18,19] have now defined subsets of patients who are at varying degrees of risk of death from coronary atherosclerosis, so that other indications for operation (i.e., prolongation of life, reduction in the incidence of myocardial infarction) have emerged.* The severity of the coronary atherosclerotic process and of left ventricular dysfunction are the most important determinants of survival in patients with coronary atherosclerosis managed nonoperatively (Figs. 62F-4 and 62F-5). These data and knowledge of the current risk of operation for patients in the various subsets noted above must be carefully evaluated when deciding for or against operation in a particular patient. Prospective, controlled trials of medical and surgical therapy should provide definitive answers as to the relative effectiveness of these two methods of treatment, and information of this type will be available in the next few years.

Stable angina pectoris (See Chap. 62E)

The *risk* of coronary artery bypass grafting for patients with stable angina pectoris is more directly related to the degree of left ventricular dysfunction present preoperatively than to the number of diseased vessels present, number of grafts inserted, age of the patients, severity of symptoms, or previous myocardial infarction. In patients without significant left ventricular dysfunction, revascularization procedures can currently be carried out at centers with experienced surgical teams with hospital mortality rates of between 1 and 3 percent.[20–22] For patients with symptoms of congestive failure with or without

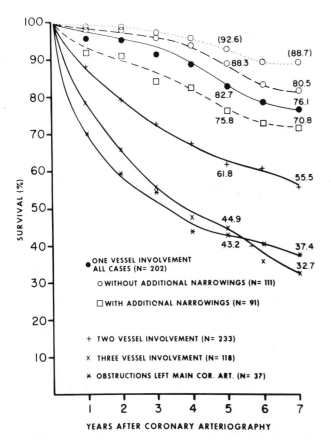

FIGURE 62F-4 Survival curves for individual arteriographic categories. Cases with one-vessel involvement were divided into cases with and without additional moderate (>30 and <50 percent) narrowings. For cases with one-vessel disease without additional narrowings the survival curve for cardiac death only is also given (interrupted line); in the other cases the influence of noncardiac deaths was virtually negligible. *(Reproduced with permission from Bruschke et al.[15])*

LEFT VENTRICULAR ANGIOGRAM

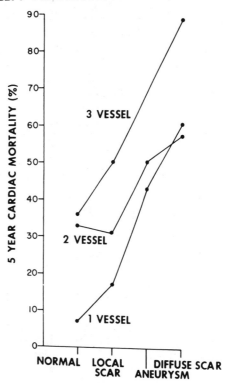

FIGURE 62F-5 Five-year cardiac mortality related to left ventricular angiogram and coronary arteriogram (divided into cases with one-, two-, and three-vessel involvement). Within each arteriographic category the left ventricular angiogram retains a high predictive value. *(Reproduced with permission from Bruschke et al.[19])*

angina, or with other evidence for significant impairment of ventricular function, hospital mortality has ranged from 10 to 50 percent.[23–26] Patients with cardiomegaly, predominant symptoms of cardiac failure, diffuse contractile abnormalities, elevated end-diastolic pressure, and depressed ejection fraction (< 0.20 to 0.25) are at greatest risk for the procedures.[10,27] With improved intraoperative and postoperative management including the use of the intraaortic balloon, however, the hospital mortality rates for these patients have steadily declined.[27a]

As noted above, between 5 and 15 percent of patients sustain *myocardial infarction* as a result of the surgical procedure. The effects of nonfatal perioperative infarction on relief of angina pectoris, ventricular function and survival are not clearly established at the present time. It appears unlikely that necrosis of previously ischemic myocardium is the cause of relief of angina in the majority of patients who are symptomatically improved following operation (see below). Perioperative infarction has been correlated with a higher frequency of late deaths and reinfarction, and onset of congestive failure,[28,29] and must be considered as the major complication of bypass grafting.

Relief of angina pectoris following coronary bypass grafting has been noted in approximately 70 to

90 percent of patients in the early years following operation.[21,25,30,31] Fifty to seventy percent of these patients are totally free of pain, and the remainder are considered improved. The completeness of revascularization appears to influence the degree of symptomatic improvement. Sheldon et al.,[31] reporting on 476 patients evaluated by repeat coronary arteriography a mean of 16 months postoperatively, noted total relief of symptoms in 87 percent of patients with complete revascularization (all grafts patent, no lesions in excess of 75 percent of the luminal diameter in arteries distal to the grafts or in ungrafted arteries), in 56 percent of patients with incomplete revascularization, and in 42 percent in whom no grafts were functioning. With continued follow-up, the percentage of patients totally free of angina has declined.[22,32] This may be the result of graft failure, progression of coronary atherosclerosis, or both.

Among 100 patients with stable angina and comparable severity of coronary atherosclerotic heart disease randomly allocated to medical or surgical therapy reported by Mathur et al.,[33] 70 percent of the surgically treated patients were asymptomatic in the follow-up period, which averaged 2 years, as compared with only 8 percent of the medically treated group, and fewer of the surgical patients required cardiac medications. Similar findings have been observed in retrospective studies comparing medical and surgical therapy.[34,35] Thus, coronary bypass grafting appears to be more effective than current medical therapy in controlling angina pectoris in the early years after arteriographic diagnosis.

Objective assessment of the results of operation with *exercise testing* has demonstrated improvement in the majority of patients, although the percentage is less than the number experiencing symptomatic improvement.[35–37] In the randomized study of Mathur et al.,[33] more surgically than medically treated patients demonstrated increased exercise tolerance time (+89 versus +42 percent), and more did not develop angina during testing (70 versus 20 percent). These differences were statistically significant. A correlation between graft patency and improvement in exercise testing has also been observed.[22,36]

Data demonstrating improvement in *left ventricular function* and in *symptoms of cardiac failure* following bypass grafting remain inconclusive. In general, minimal or no improvement in resting ventricular function has been noted following bypass grafting.[38,39] This is particularly true for patients with moderate or severe impairment of ventricular function preoperatively. Improvement in symptoms of cardiac failure has been noted in the majority of the survivors of coronary bypass grafting. The best results have generally occurred in patients with associated angina pectoris, intermittent symptoms of cardiac failure, and dyskinesia limited to one or two areas of the left ventricle.[10,40] While improvement in ventricular performance has not been consistently demonstrated, prevention of further deterioration following bypass grafting has been observed,[41] and may represent a major indication for operation in patients with extensive coronary atherosclerosis.

The long-term function of bypass grafts to the coronary arteries is unknown at present. Approximately 80 to 85 percent of grafts are patent 1 year following operation.[22,23,31] Only an additional 5 percent of venous grafts have become occluded between 1 and 3 years,[42] and in the majority of these stenoses were present at an earlier study. Whether additional grafts will occlude in the later years after operation, either as a result of progression of atherosclerotic disease distal to the grafts or of degenerative changes occurring in the grafts, is unknown. Whether the internal thoracic artery will be a more effective long-term conduit than the saphenous vein is also not established at present.

In assessing the effects of surgical therapy on *survival,* it is essential that comparison, either retrospective or prospective, be made between comparable groups of patients. As previously mentioned, the major determinants of survival are the severity of the coronary atherosclerosis determined by coronary arteriography and the degree of left ventricular dysfunction. (See the discussion that follows.)

LEFT MAIN CORONARY ARTERY DISEASE

Studies of the natural history of patients with atherosclerotic disease of the left main coronary artery have documented the relatively unfavorable prognosis of this subgroup (Fig. 62F-4).[15,43] The 5-year mortality rates were high (> 40 percent) in patients with more than two other vessels involved (the majority of patients) and even in the presence of normal ventriculograms (45 percent).[43] Recent studies comparing surgical and nonsurgical therapy in comparable patients with greater than 50 percent stenosis of the left main coronary artery have consistently demonstrated improved survival in the surgically treated patients.[44–45a] The study of Takaro et al.[45] represents a prospective, randomized trial of these two forms of therapy. The other two studies are retrospective, comparing surgically treated patients with patients considered candidates for operation who were managed nonoperatively. Statistically significant differences in survival have been demonstrated in all three studies in the first 2 years following diagnosis (Fig. 62F-6).

TRIPLE-VESSEL DISEASE

Patients with high-grade occlusive lesions in the three major coronary arterial systems also have a relatively unfavorable prognosis (Fig. 62F-4). This risk is greater when there is angiographic evidence of local scar, diffuse scar, or aneurysm (Fig. 62F-5). In comparing patients with triple-vessel disease and similar degrees of left ventricular dysfunction managed with and without operation, significant differences in survival have been observed[46] (Fig. 62F-7). These patients were also similar with regard to age, sex, and coronary risk factors. Comparable survival data in surgically treated patients have been observed in other studies.[31,47] Thus, surgical treatment does appear to improve survival in this subgroup in the early years after diagnosis.

DOUBLE-VESSEL DISEASE

The survival of patients with significant occlusive disease in two of the three major coronary systems is greater than for patients with triple-vessel disease but is also influenced by the extent of left ventricular scarring (Figs. 62F-4 and 62F-5). Data demonstrating a beneficial effect of surgical therapy on survival have recently become available.[31,46] In our own experience with 403 comparable patients managed with and without operation, a statistically significant difference in survival has been demonstrated with increasing follow-up (Fig. 62F-8).[46]

SINGLE-VESSEL DISEASE

With the possible exception of patients with lesions of the proximal anterior descending coronary artery, bypass grafting has not been shown to enhance survival in patients with occlusive disease confined to one of the major coronary arterial systems in the early years after diagnosis.[31] Data from the Cleveland Clinic Foundation suggest greater survival with surgical than with medical therapy in patients with predominant anterior descending involvement, al-

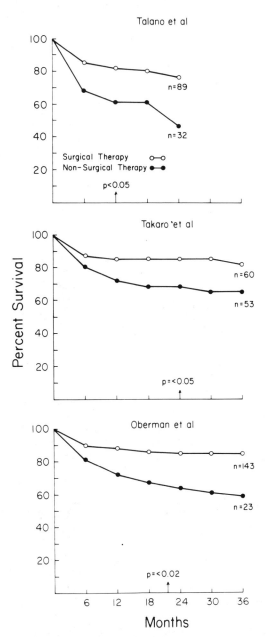

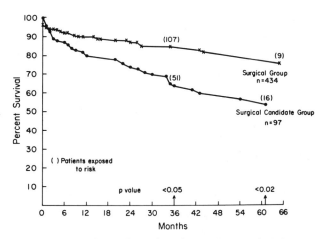

FIGURE 62F-7 Comparison of surgical and nonsurgical therapy in patients with triple-vessel disease. Patients in the surgical candidate group met anatomic and hemodynamic criteria for bypass grafting. The differences in survival at 36 and 61 months, when the last death occurred in the surgical candidate group, were statistically significant. *(Modified from Oberman et al.[46])*

FIGURE 62F-6 Comparison of surgical and nonsurgical therapy in comparable patients with greater than 50 percent stenosis of the left main coronary artery. *(Data of Talano et al.[44] and Oberman et al.[45a] are from retrospective studies; data of Takaro et al.[45] from a prospective randomized study.)*

though the comparability of the two groups is not clearly established.[31] In our own experience with comparable patients with stable angina and occlusive disease of the proximal anterior descending artery managed with and without operation, survival in the two groups has been similar.[35]

INDICATIONS FOR OPERATION
On the basis of the above information, operation is advised for *all* patients with severe and disabling angina who do not respond to adequate medical therapy and who do not have evidence of severe impairment of ventricular function, regardless of the extent of disease. Asymptomatic or minimally symptomatic patients with lesions of the left main coro-

nary artery or triple-vessel disease without severe impairment of ventricular function should also be advised to undergo operation because of the beneficial effect of bypass grafting on survival in these subgroups. In patients with double-vessel disease, bypass grafting is advisable if there are no major contraindications to operation, since longevity appears to be improved in this subgroup as well. Asymptomatic or minimally symptomatic patients with lesions in only one of the three major coronary systems are not advised to undergo operation at the present time.

Unstable angina pectoris and prolonged episodes of myocardial ischemia

Unstable angina pectoris includes initial angina pectoris, progressive angina pectoris, and angina decubitus. Patients who have one of these subgroups of angina pectoris or who have prolonged pain due to myocardial ischemia usually associated with transient electrocardiographic changes of ischemia but with no electrocardiographic or enzymatic changes indicative of myocardial necrosis ("acute coronary insufficiency," "intermediate syndrome") are said to have one of the "preinfarction" syndromes (see Chap. 62A). Coronary artery bypass grafting has been advised for such patients to prevent or reduce the possibility of sustaining a myocardial infarction, as well as to relieve pain. Results from several surgical series indicate that operation is associated with a generally higher operative mortality and incidence of perioperative myocardial infarction than for patients with stable angina pectoris treated in the same institutions.[48–51] The results of randomized trials comparing medical and surgical therapy in pa-

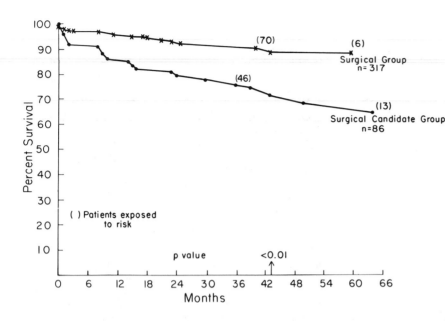

FIGURE 62F-8 Comparison of surgical and nonsurgical therapy in patients with double-vessel disease. Patients in the surgical candidate group met anatomic and hemodynamic criteria for bypass grafting. The difference in survival at 43 months, when the last death occurred in the surgical group, was statistically significant. *(Modified from Oberman et al.[46])*

tients with unstable angina pectoris have demonstrated comparable early mortality rates[52–54] and early infarction rates that are comparable[54] or somewhat higher[53] in the surgically treated group. Symptomatic improvement has been significantly greater in the surgically treated patients within the first year following diagnosis in all three of these studies. Thus, surgical therapy has not been shown to date to reduce the incidence of myocardial infarction early after the diagnosis of unstable angina is made. As with stable angina pectoris, subsets of patients exist in whom long-term survival appears to be enhanced by bypass grafting. These include patients with left main coronary stenosis and with triple-vessel disease. Optimal medical therapy, including the use of propranolol, has minimized the incidence of myocardial infarction and death even in patients with the "intermediate coronary syndrome."[54,55] In view of this and the higher hospital mortality and infarction rates in surgically treated patients with unstable as compared with stable angina pectoris, intensive medical therapy, allowing stabilization, followed by bypass grafting on a semiurgent basis, usually during the same hospitalization, provides, in our opinion, the most rational approach to managing the majority of patients with unstable angina pectoris.[50,54] Patients with prolonged episodes of chest pain which persist despite intensive medical therapy and who have distal vessels suitable for grafting are advised to have immediate operation.

Acute myocardial infarction without left ventricular failure

Coronary artery bypass grafting has been employed in a few centers for patients with acute myocardial infarction but without significant impairment of left ventricular function and cardiogenic shock.[56,57] The rationale for immediate revascularization in patients of this type is the assumption that while irreversible myocardial necrosis may have occurred, improvement in oxygen delivery to the myocardium adjacent to the area of infarction will prevent or minimize subsequent necrosis in this area and further impairment of left ventricular performance. Salvage of myocardial tissue[58] and improvement in ventricular wall motion[59] have been demonstrated in the dog after acute occlusion of the anterior descending coronary artery if reperfusion of the artery is established 3 h after occlusion.

In the limited experience with coronary artery bypass grafting in patients with documented acute myocardial infarction but without significant hemodynamic abnormalities, operative mortality has been under 5 percent.[56,57] The majority of these patients were operated upon following infarction occurring during or early after coronary arteriography, and the operations were generally performed within hours after onset of symptoms. The results have been generally good, although electrocardiographic evidence of infarction and abnormalities of left ventricular wall motion have persisted in a number of patients.[56,57] Whether surgical therapy is more effective than medical therapy in reducing the extent of myocardial necrosis in patients with comparable degrees of coronary atherosclerosis and ischemic myocardium is not established at the present time. Development of techniques for adequate estimation of infarct size may permit more meaningful comparisons of the two methods of treatment.

The results of coronary artery bypass grafting in patients who sustain myocardial infarction while hospitalized cannot be extrapolated to patients with acute myocardial infarction admitted to coronary care units with acute infarction and chest pain of longer duration (over 6 to 8 h). Myocardial revascularization in such patients has been associated with an operative mortality of 38 percent if operation is

performed within 7 days, 16 percent between 8 and
30 days, and 6 percent between 31 and 60 days after
the infarction.[60]

CHAPTER 62F **1299**
SURGICAL TREATMENT OF CORONARY
ATHEROSCLEROTIC HEART DISEASE

On the basis of this information, we
like to defer revascularization for a minimum of 4
weeks in patients who have an uncomplicated myocardial infarction. The role of early infarctectomy
alone or in combination with coronary bypass grafting in patients with acute infarction without cardiogenic shock has not been established.

Acute myocardial infarction with left ventricular failure and cardiogenic shock without associated lesions

Coronary bypass grafting combined on occasion with
infarctectomy has been utilized in a small number of
patients with cardiogenic shock complicating myocardial infarction in the absence of associated mechanical complications such as rupture of the ventricular septum or of a papillary muscle. Operation
has usually been carried out following a period of
circulatory support with intraaortic balloon pumping.
Of 15 patients treated in this manner by Dunkman et
al.,[61] there have been 4 long-term survivors. Survival
after this form of treatment appears to be directly
related to the size of the infarction, and this may be
difficult to precisely quantitate preoperatively. Patients with cardiogenic shock and necrosis of greater
than 40 percent of the left ventricular mass or
irreparable, severe triple-vessel disease will not likely benefit from coronary bypass grafting after periods of circulatory support.[61] Whether this combined
method of treatment will improve survival and reduce the extent of myocardial necrosis in patients
with lesser degrees of necrosis is not established at
the present time.

Acute myocardial infarction with left ventricular failure and cardiogenic shock with associated lesions

RUPTURE OF THE VENTRICULAR SEPTUM

Repair of rupture of the ventricular septum is generally advisable, since less than 15 percent of patients
with this condition survive more than 2 months with
conservative management.[62] If the hemodynamic
state permits, operation should be delayed for 4 to 6
weeks following infarction to allow fibrous healing of
the septum adjacent to the defect and to minimize the
possibility of incomplete closure or recurrence of the
defect.[63] Successful closure of septal defects early
after infarction in patients with cardiogenic shock or
intractable left ventricular failure has been accomplished, but the risk of operation is approximately 50
percent.[64,65] Use of the intraaortic balloon pump
preoperatively in such patients has resulted in significant hemodynamic and clinical improvement and has
allowed uncomplicated coronary arteriography and
left ventriculography.[64] The long-term results following operation will be affected by the severity of the
underlying coronary atherosclerosis and left ventricular scarring. Of 65 patients reviewed by Kitamura et
al.,[66] 38 (58 percent) survived longer than 2 months,
and 12 of 37 (32 percent) were alive 1 year following
operation. These survival figures are distinctly superior to those in patients managed without operation.

As mentioned previously, a number of patients
with rupture of the ventricular septum will have
associated left ventricular aneurysms or scars that
should be excised at the time of repair of the septal
defect. Left ventricular angiography should be performed preoperatively to delineate these areas and
coronary arteriography as well, if the condition of the
patient permits. The value of concomitant coronary
artery bypass grafting has not been established. In
our own experience, bypass grafting can be performed at the time of repair of the septal defect with
no increased operative risk.

PAPILLARY MUSCLE RUPTURE OR DYSFUNCTION

Rupture of a papillary muscle generally results in
severe mitral regurgitation, acute left ventricular
failure, and even cardiogenic shock. Operation is
advisable, since less than 20 percent of patients with
this complication of acute infarction survive for
more than a few weeks.[67] Papillary muscle dysfunction following acute infarction may occasionally produce severe mitral regurgitation, cardiac failure, and
shock.[68] Cardiac catheterization is generally required
to differentiate mitral regurgitation from rupture of
the ventricular septum. Buckley et al.[69] reported nine
patients with severe mitral regurgitation who had
intraaortic balloon assist followed by cardiac catheterization and operation within 18 days following
infarction. Eight had concomitant bypass grafting of
at least one coronary artery, and three had infarctectomy as well. The four patients with rupture of a
papillary muscle survived. Three of the five patients
with papillary muscle dysfunction had extensive
areas of infarction and died early postoperatively,
and two were long-term survivors. Of 18 patients
with mitral regurgitation (10 with rupture of a papillary muscle and 8 with papillary muscle dysfunction)
having mitral valve replacement from 3 to 7 months
after operation, there were 15 long-term survivors.

Congestive cardiac failure

Coronary bypass grafting has been employed in
patients with chronic congestive cardiac failure as
the predominant manifestation of their coronary
atherosclerotic disease, often in association with
excision of noncontracting areas of left ventricular
myocardium and occasionally with mitral valve
replacement or annuloplasty for papillary muscle dysfunction. The results in patients with severe impairment of left ventricular function have been disappointing.[10,70] Although the majority of the bypass
grafts remained patent in the patients reported by
Spencer et al.,[71] little or no improvement in ventricular contractility or in the elevated left ventricular
end-diastolic pressure or decreased cardiac output

present before operation was demonstrated postoperatively. Of 23 patients with severe or intractable failure, 57 percent died within a year after operation, and a good result was obtained in only 2 patients (9 percent). Postmortem studies in six patients with severe congestive failure, cardiomegaly, elevated left ventricular end-diastolic pressures (18 to 35 mm Hg) and volumes (153 to 324 ml/m²), and depressed ejection fractions (0.10 to 0.22) who died following coronary bypass grafting and excision of left ventricular scars reported by us[10] showed extensive residual scarring comprising 25 to 45 percent of the left ventricular myocardium and diffuse atherosclerotic involvement of all three major coronary arterial systems. Operation is currently not advised for patients of this type.

The results of operative treatment in patients with lesser degrees of left ventricular dysfunction are somewhat better. With improved intraoperative techniques and postoperative management, including use of the intraaortic balloon, patients with moderately depressed left ventricular function (ejection fraction 0.2 to 0.4) can be operated upon with a hospital mortality of 10 to 15 percent.[26,72,73] Although left ventricular hemodynamics are not restored to normal, improvement in many parameters of left ventricular function has been noted in the majority of hospital survivors and is correlated with improvement in symptoms.[72] Follow-up of these patients suggests that survival may be improved when compared with that of similar patients managed without operation.[73,74] A major consideration in patients of this type is that although overall left ventricular performance may not be appreciably improved following operation, further deterioration may be prevented or delayed by operation,[41] and this may prove to be the strongest argument for surgical intervention in this group. Operation is currently advised for patients in this category who are severely symptomatic (particularly with angina pectoris) despite optimal medical therapy, recognizing a slightly increased operative risk.

Left ventricular aneurysm

The major indications for resection of left ventricular aneurysms are progressive left ventricular failure and angina pectoris with coexisting multiple vessel disease. Less common indications include ventricular arrhythmias and systemic embolization from mural thrombus. As noted previously, the majority of such aneurysms involve the anterior and apical areas of the left ventricular wall and are associated with complete occlusion or severe stenosis of the anterior descending coronary artery. Of 102 patients with left ventricular aneurysms followed by Schlicter et al.,[75] 73 percent died within 3 years and 88 percent within 5 years after diagnosis, chiefly from congestive failure, recurrent myocardial infarction, or arterial embolization.

Resection of left ventricular aneurysms can be

accomplished with a hospital mortality of approximately 10 percent. Addition of bypass grafts to the aneurysmectomy increases the risk to about 15 percent.[76] Of 392 patients having ventricular aneurysmectomy with or without associated procedures reported by Loop et al.,[76] 76 percent were alive 4 years after operation. Symptomatic improvement was noted in 83 percent of the survivors who had presented with congestive failure, in 91 percent of those with angina pectoris, and in 77 percent of those with recurrent ventricular arrhythmias. The results were generally better if the coronary atherosclerosis was confined to the anterior descending artery.

Ventricular arrhythmias

Life-threatening ventricular arrhythmias refractory to medical therapy can be eliminated by surgical treatment in some patients. In those with ventricular tachycardia and fibrillation induced by exercise testing, coronary bypass grafting has been successful in abolishing the arrhythmias.[77] Ventricular tachyarrhythmias occurring early after acute myocardial infarction have also been successfully treated with bypass grafting, usually in association with infarctectomy or resection of a left ventricular aneurysm.[78] Intraaortic balloon pumping has been a useful adjunct in these patients. Ventricular arrhythmias occurring more than 4 to 6 weeks following myocardial infarction and refractory to medical therapy have also been eliminated by bypass grafting with or without concomitant aneurysmectomy.[79] As noted above, ventricular aneurysmectomy alone has been successful in abolishing ventricular arrhythmias in some patients. In general, bypass grafting of all severely stenosed major coronary arteries should be performed with the ventricular excision. Surgical treatment of ventricular arrhythmias should be considered in all patients who remain refractory to medical therapy and in whom there are no major contraindications to operation.

REFERENCES

1 Roitman, D., Jones, W. B., and Sheffield, L. T.: Comparison of Submaximal Exercise ECG Test with Coronary Cineangiocardiogram, *Ann. Intern. Med.*, 72:641, 1970.

2 Cheanvechai, C., Groves, L. K., Surakiatchanukul, S., Tanaka, N., Effler, D. B., Shirey, E. K., and Sones, F. M., Jr.: Bridge Saphenous Vein Graft, *J. Thorac. Cardiovasc. Surg.*, 70:63, 1975.

3 Collis, J. L., MacKinnon, J., Raison, J. C. A., and Whittaker, S. R. F.: Repair of Acquired Ventricular Septal Defect following Myocardial Infarction, *Lancet*, 2:172, 1962.

4 Schimert, G., Lajos, T. Z., Bunnell, I. L., Greene, D. G., Falsetti, H. L., Gage, A. A., Dean, D. C., and Bernstein, M.: Operation for Cardiac Complications following Myocardial Infarction, *Surgery*, 67:129, 1970.

5 Berger, T. J., Karp, R. B., and Kouchoukos, N. T.: Valve Replacement and Myocardial Revascularization: Results of Combined Operation in 59 Patients, *Circulation*, 51-52(suppl. 1):126, 1975.

6 Manley, J. C. and Johnson, W. D.: Effects of Surgery on Angina (Pre- and Postinfarction) and Myocardial Function (Failure), *Circulation*, 46:1208, 1972.

7 Cooley, D. A., Dawson, J. T., Hallman, G. L., Sandiford, F. M.,

Wukasch, D. C., Garcia, E., and Hall, R. J.: Aortocoronary Saphenous Vein Bypass: Results in 1,492 Patients with Particular Reference to Patients with Complicating Factors, *Ann. Thorac. Surg.,* 16:380, 1973.

8 Kansal, S., Roitman, D., Kouchoukos, N. T., and Sheffield, L. T.: Ischemic Myocardial Injury following Aortocoronary Bypass Surgery, *Chest,* 67:20, 1975.

9 Kouchoukos, N. T., and Karp, R. B.: Management of the Postoperative Cardiovascular Surgical Patient, *Am. Heart J.,* 92:513, 1976.

10 Kouchoukos, N. T., Doty, D. B., Buettner, L. E., and Kirklin, J. W.: Treatment of Postinfarction Cardiac Failure by Myocardial Excision and Revascularization, *Circulation 45-46*(suppl. 1):72, 1972.

11 Buckley, M. J., Craver, J. M., Gold, H. K., Mundth, E. D., Daggett, W. M., and Austen, W. G.: Intraaortic Balloon Pump Assist for Cardiogenic Shock after Cardiopulmonary Bypass, *Circulation,* 47-48(suppl 3):90, 1973.

12 Lamberti, J. J., Jr., Cohn, L. H., Lesch, M., and Collins, J. J., Jr.: Intraaortic Balloon Counterpulsation: Indications and Long-Term Results in Postoperative Left Ventricular Power Failure, *Arch. Surg.,* 109:766, 1974.

13 Weber, K. T., and Janicki, J. S.: Intraaortic Balloon Counterpulsation: A Review of Physiological, Clinical Results, and Device Safety, *Ann. Thorac. Surg.,* 17:602, 1974.

14 Oberman, A., Jones, W. B., Riley, C. P., Reeves, T. J., Sheffield, L. T., and Turner, M. E.: Natural History of Coronary Artery Disease, *Bull. N.Y. Acad. Med.,* 48:1109, 1972.

15 Bruschke, A. V. G., Proudfit, W. L., and Sones, F. M., Jr.: Progress Study of 590 Consecutive Nonsurgical Cases of Coronary Disease Followed 5-9 Years: I. Arteriographic Correlations, *Circulation,* 47:1147, 1973.

16 Webster, J. S., Moberg, C., and Rincon, G.: Natural History of Severe Proximal Coronary Artery Disease as Documented by Coronary Cineangiography, *Am. J. Cardiol.,* 33:195, 1974.

17 Humphries, J. O., Kuller, L., Ross, R. S., Friesinger, G. C., and Page, E. E.: Natural History of Ischemic Heart Disease in Relation to Arteriographic Findings: A Twelve Year Study of 224 Patients, *Circulation,* 49:489, 1974.

18 Burggraf, G. W., and Parker, J. O.: Prognosis in Coronary Artery Disease: Angiographic, Hemodynamic, and Clinical Factors, *Circulation,* 51:146, 1975.

19 Bruschke, A. V. G., Proudfit, W. L., and Sones, F. M., Jr.: Progress Study of 590 Consecutive Nonsurgical Cases of Coronary Disease Followed 5-9 Years. II. Ventriculographic and Other Correlations, *Circulation,* 47:1154, 1973.

20 Bennett, D. J., Loop, G. D., Sheldon, W. C., and Effler, D. B.: Direct Myocardial Revascularization: Operative Mortality in the Cleveland Clinic Experience, *Cleve. Clin. Q.,* 41:51, 1974.

21 Hutchinson, J. E., III, Green, G. E., Mekhjian, H. A., Gallozzi, E., Cameron, A., and Kemp, H. G.: Coronary Bypass Grafting in 476 Patients Consecutively Operated On, *Chest,* 64:706, 1973.

22 Kouchoukos, N. T., Oberman, A., and Karp, R. B.: Results of Surgery for Disabling Angina Pectoris, in S. H. Rahimtoola and A. N. Brest (eds.),"Cardiovascular Clinics Coronary Bypass Surgery," F. A. Davis Company, Philadelphia, in press.

23 Morris, G. C., Jr., Howell, J. F., Crawford, E. S., Reul, G. J., and Stelter, W.: Operability of End State Coronary Artery Disease, *Ann. Surg.,* 175:1024, 1972.

24 Oldham, H. N., Kong, Y., Bartel, A. G., Morris, J. J., Jr., Behar, V. S., Peter, R. H., Rosati, R. A., Young, G., Jr., and Sabiston, D. C., Jr.: Risk Factors in Coronary Artery Bypass Surgery, *Arch. Surg.,* 105:918, 1972.

25 Kouchoukos, N. T., Kirklin, J. W., and Oberman, A.: An Appraisal of Coronary Artery Bypass Grafting (Sixth Annual George C. Griffith Lecture), *Circulation,* 50:11, 1974.

26 Mitchel, B. F., Jr., Alivizatos, P. A., Adam, M., Geisler, G. F., Thiele, J. P., and Lambert, C. J.: Myocardial Revascularization in Patients with Poor Ventricular Function, *J. Thorac. Cardiovasc. Surg.,* 69:52, 1975.

27 Loop, F. D., Berrettoni, J. N., Pichard, A., Siegel, W., Razavi, M., and Effler, D. B.: Selection of the Candidate for Myocardial Revascularization: A Profile of High Risk Based on Multivariate Analysis, *J. Thorac. Cardiovasc. Surg.,* 69:40, 1975.

27a Kouchoukos, N. T., Oberman, A., Karp, R. B., and Russell, R. O., Jr.: Coronary Bypass Surgery: Assessment of Current Operative Risk, *Am. J. Cardiol.,* 39:285, 1977.

28 Brewer, D. L., Bilbro, R. H., and Bartel, A. G.: Myocardial Infarction as a Complication of Coronary Bypass Surgery, *Circulation,* 47:58, 1973.

29 Schrank, J. P., Slabaugh, T. K., and Beckwith, J. R.: The Incidence and Clinical Significant of ECG-VCG Changes of Myocardial Infarction following Aortocoronary Saphenous Vein Bypass Surgery, *Am. Heart J.,* 87:46, 1974.

30 Hall, R. J., Dawson, J. T., Cooley, D. A., Hallman, G. L., Wukasch, D. C., and Garcia, E.: Coronary Artery Bypass, *Circulation,* 47-48(suppl. 3):146, 1973.

31 Sheldon, W. C., Rincon, G., Pichard, A. D., Razavi, M., Cheanvechai, C., and Loop, F. D.: Surgical Treatment of Coronary Artery Disease: Pure Graft Operations, with a Study of 741 Patients Followed 3-7 Yr., *Progr. Cardiovasc. Dis.,* 18:237, 1975.

32 Adam, M., Mitchel, B. F., Lambert, C. I., and Geisler, G. F.: Long-Term Results with Aorta-to-Coronary Artery Bypass Vein Grafts, *Ann. Thorac. Surg.,* 14:1, 1972.

33 Mathur, V. S., and Guinn, G. A.: Prospective Randomized Study of Coronary Bypass Surgery in Stable Angina: The First 100 Patients, *Circulation,* 51-52(suppl. 1):133, 1975.

34 Aronow, W. S., and Stemmer, E. A.: Bypass Graft Surgery versus Medical Therapy of Angina Pectoris, *Am. J. Cardiol.,* 33:415, 1974.

35 Kouchoukos, N. T., Oberman, A., Russell, R. O., Jr., and Jones, W. B.: Surgical versus Medical Treatment of Occlusive Disease Confined to the Left Anterior Descending Coronary Artery, *Am. J. Cardiol.,* 35:836, 1975.

36 Lapin, E. S., Murray, J. A., Bruce, R. A., and Winterscheid, L.: Changes in Maximal Exercise Performance in the Evaluation of Saphenous Vein Bypass Surgery, *Circulation,* 47:1164, 1973.

37 Guiney, T. E., Rubenstein, J. J., Sanders, C. A., and Mundth, E. D.: Functional Evaluation of Coronary Bypass Surgery by Exercise Testing and Oxygen Consumption, *Circulation,* 47-48(suppl. 3):141, 1973.

38 Arbogast, R., Solignac, A., and Bourassa, M. G.: Influence of Aortocoronary Saphenous Vein Bypass Surgery on Left Ventricular Volumes and Ejection Fraction, *Am. J. Med.,* 54:290, 1973.

39 Hammermeister, K. E., Kennedy, J. W., Hamilton, G. W., Stewart, D. K., Gould, K. L., Lopscomb, K., and Murray, J. A.: Aortocoronary Saphenous-Vein Bypass: Failure of Successful Grafting to Improve Resting Left Ventricular Function in Chronic Angina, *N. Engl. J. Med.* 290:186, 1974.

40 Mundth, E. D., Harthorne, J. W., Buckley, M. J., Dinsmore, R., and Austen, W. G.: Direct Coronary Arterial Revascularization: Treatment of Cardiac Failure Associated with Coronary Artery Disease, *Arch. Surg.,* 103:529, 1971.

41 Gaarder, T. D., and Sanmarco, M. E.: Preservation of Ventricular Function as an Indication for Coronary Artery Bypass Surgery in Severe Coronary Disease, *Am. J. Cardiol.,* 37:137, 1976.

42 Grondin, C. M., Lespérance, J., Bourassa, M. G., Pasternac, A., Campeau, L., and Grondin, P.: Serial Angiographic Evaluation in 60 Consecutive Patients with Aortocoronary Artery Vein Grafts 2 Weeks, 1 Year, and 3 Years after Operation, *J. Thorac. Cardiovasc. Surg.,* 67:1, 1974.

43 Lim, J. S., Proudfit, W. L., and Sones, F. M., Jr.: Left Main

Coronary Arterial Obstruction: Long-Term Follow-up of 141 Nonsurgical Cases, *Am. J. Cardiol.,* 36:131, 1975.

44 Talano, J. V., Scanlon, P. J., Meadows, W. R., Kahn, M., Pifarre, R., and Gunnar, R. M.: Influence of Surgery on Survival in 145 Patients with Left Main Coronary Artery Disease, *Circulation,* 51-52(suppl. 1):105, 1975.

45 Takaro, T., Hultgren, H. N., Lipton, M. J., and Detre, K. M., and Participants in the Study Group: The VA Cooperative Randomized Study of Surgery for Coronary Arterial Occlusive Disease: II. Subgroup with Significant Left Main Lesions, *Circulation,* 54(supp. III):107, 1976.

45a Oberman, A., Kouchoukos, N. T., Harrell, R. R., Holt, J. H., Jr., Russell, R. O., Jr., and Rackley, C. E.: Surgical versus Medical Treatment in Disease of the Left Main Coronary Artery, *Lancet,* 2:591, 1976.

46 Oberman, A., Kouchoukos, N. T., Russell, R. O., Jr., Holt, J. H., Jr., Turner, M. E., and Soto, B.: "Coronary Artery Surgery: Long-Term Results at the University of Alabama Medical Center" (proceedings, second Henry Ford Hospital International Symposium on Cardiac Surgery), in press.

47 Anderson, R. P., Rahimtoola, S. H., Bonchek, L. I., and Starr, A.: The Prognosis of Patients with Coronary Artery Disease after Coronary Bypass Operations: Time-related Progress of 532 Patients with Disabling Angina Pectoris, *Circulation,* 50:274, 1974.

48 Scanlon, P. J., Nemickas, R., Moran, J. F., Talano, J. V., Amirparviz, F., and Pifarre, R.: Accelerated Angina Pectoris: Clinical, Hemodynamic, Arteriographic, and Therapeutic Experience in 85 Patients, *Circulation,* 47:19, 1973.

49 Bonchek, L. I., Rahimtoola, S. H., Anderson, R. P., McAnulty, J. A., Rosch, J., Bristow, J. D., and Starr, A.: Late Results following Emergency Saphenous Vein Bypass Grafting for Unstable Angina, *Circulation,* 50:972, 1974.

50 Kouchoukos, N. T., Russell, R. O., Jr., Moraski, R. E., Karp, R. B., Oberman, A., and Rackley, C. E.: Surgical Treatment of Unstable Angina Pectoris: Results in 65 Patients, *Am. J. Cardiol.,* 35:149, 1975.

51 Berndt, T. B., Miller, D. C., Silverman, J. F., Stinson, E. B., Harrison, D. C., and Schroeder, J. S.: Coronary Bypass Surgery for Unstable Angina Pectoris: Clinical Follow-up and Results of Postoperative Treadmill Electrocardiograms, *Am. J. Med.,* 58:171, 1975.

52 Bertrolasi, C. A., Trongé, Carreño, C. A., Jalon, J., and Vega, M. R.: Unstable Angina: Prospective and Randomized Study of Its Evolution, with and without Surgery, *Am. J. Cardiol.,* 33:201, 1974.

53 Conti, C. R., Gilbert, J. B., Hodges, M., Hutter, A. M., Jr., Kaplan, E. M., Newell, J. B., Resnekov, L., Rosati, R. A., Ross, R. S., Russell, R. O., Jr., Schroeder, J. S., and Wolk, M.: Unstable Angina Pectoris: Randomized Study of Surgery vs. Medical Therapy, National Cooperative Unstable Angina Pectoris Study Group, *Am. J. Cardiol.,* 35:129, 1975.

54 Selden, R., Neill, W. A., Ritzmann, L. W., Okies, J. E., and Anderson, R. P.: Medical versus Surgical Therapy for Acute Coronary Insufficiency: A Randomized Study, *N. Engl. J. Med.,* 293:1329, 1975.

55 Fischl, S. J., Herman, M. V., and Gorlin, R.: The Intermediate Coronary Syndrome: Clinical, Angiographic and Therapeutic Aspects, *N. Engl. J. Med.,* 288:1193, 1973.

56 Scanlon, P. J., Nemickas, R., Robin, J. R., Jr., Anderson, W., Montoya, A., and Pifarre, R.: Myocardial Revascularization during Acute Phase of Myocardial Infarction, *J.A.M.A.,* 218:207, 1971.

57 Loop, F. D., Cheanvechai, C., Sheldon, W. C., Taylor, P. C., and Effler, D. B.: Early Myocardial Revascularization during Acute Myocardial Infarction, *Chest,* 66:478, 1974.

58 Ginks, W. R., Sybers, H. D., Maroko, P. R., Covell, J. W.,

Sobel, B. E., and Ross, J., Jr.: Coronary Artery Reperfusion: II. Reduction of Myocardial Infarct Size at One Week after the Coronary Occlusion, *J. Clin. Invest.,* 51:2717, 1972.

59 Maroko, P. R., Libby, P., Ginks, W. R., Bloor, C. M., Shell, W. E., Sobel, B. E., and Ross, J., Jr.: Coronary Artery Reperfusion: I. Early Effects on Local Myocardial Function and the Extent of Myocardial Necrosis, *J. Clin. Invest.,* 51:2710, 1972.

60 Dawson, J. T., Hall, R. J., Hallman, G. L., and Cooley, D. A.: Mortality in Patients Undergoing Coronary Artery Bypass Surgery after Myocardial Infarction, *Am. J. Cardiol.,* 33:483, 1974.

61 Dunkman, W. B., Leinbach, R. C., Buckley, M. J., Mundth, E. D., Kantrowitz, A. R., Austen, W. G., and Sanders, C. A.: Clinical and Hemodynamic Results of Intraaortic Balloon Pumping and Surgery for Cardiogenic Shock, *Circulation,* 46:465, 1972.

62 Sanders, R. J., Kern, W. H., and Blount, S. G., Jr.: Perforation of the Interventricular Septum Complicating Myocardial Infarction: A Report of Eight Cases, One with Cardiac Catheterization, *Am. Heart J.,* 51:736, 1956.

63 Giuliani, E. R., Danielson, G. K., Pluth, J. R., Odyniec, N. A., and Wallace, R. B.: Postinfarction Ventricular Septal Rupture: Surgical Considerations and Results, *Circulation,* 49:455, 1974.

64 Gold, H. K., Leinbach, R. C., Sanders, C. A., Buckley, M. J., Mundth, E. D., and Austen, W. G.: Intraaortic Balloon Pumping for Ventricular Septal Defect of Mitral Regurgitation Complicating Acute Myocardial Infarction, *Circulation,* 47:1191, 1973.

65 Graham, A. F., Stinson, E. B., Daily, P. O., and Harrison, D. C.: Ventricular Septal Defects after Myocardial Infarction: Early Operative Treatment, *J.A.M.A.,* 225:708, 1973.

66 Kitamura, S., Mendez, A., and Kay, J. H.: Ventricular Septal Defect following Myocardial Infarction: Experience with Surgical Repair through a Left Ventriculotomy and Review of Literature, *J. Thorac. Cardiovasc. Surg.,* 61:186, 1971.

67 Sanders, R. J., Neubuerger, K. T., and Ravin, A.: Rupture of Papillary Muscles: Occurrence of Rupture of the Posterior Muscle in Posterior Myocardial Infarction, *Dis. Chest.,* 31:316, 1957.

68 Phillips, J. H., Burch, G. E., and De Pasquale, N. P.: The Syndrome of Papillary Muscle Dysfunction: Its Clinical Recognition, *Ann. Intern. Med.,* 59:508, 1963.

69 Buckley, M. J., Mundth, E. D., Daggett, W. M., Gold, H. K., Leinbach, R. C., and Austen, W. G.: Surgical Management of Ventricular Septal Defects and Mitral Regurgitation Complicating Acute Myocardial Infarction, *Ann. Thorac. Surg.,* 16:598, 1973.

70 Buckley, M. J., Mundth, E. D., Daggett, W. M., DeSanctis, R. W., and Austen, W. G.: Surgical Therapy for Early Complications of Myocardial Infarction, *Surgery,* 70:814, 1971.

71 Spencer, F. C., Green, G. E., Tice, D. A., Wallsh, E., Mills, N. L., and Glassman, E.: Coronary Artery Bypass Grafts for Congestive Heart Failure: A Report of Experiences with 40 Patients, *J. Thorac. Cardiovasc. Surg.,* 62:529, 1971.

72 Lefemine, A. A., Moon, H. S., Flessas, A., Ryan, T. J., and Ramaswamy, K.: Myocardial Resection and Coronary Artery Bypass for Left Ventricular Failure following Myocardial Infarction, *Ann. Thorac. Surg.,* 17:1, 1974.

73 Manley, J. C., King, J. F., Zeft, H. J., and Johnson, W. D.: The Bad Left Ventricle: Results of Coronary Surgery and Effect on Late Survival, *J. Thorac. Cardiovasc. Surg.,* 72:841, 1976.

74 Isom, O. W., Spencer, F. C., Glassman, E., Dembrow, J. M., and Pasternack, B. S.: Long-Term Survival following Coronary Bypass Surgery in Patients with Significant Impairment of Left Ventricular Function, *Circulation,* 51-52(suppl. 1):141, 1975.

75 Schlichter, J., Hellerstein, H. K., and Katz, L. N.: Aneurysm of the Heart: A Correlative Study of One Hundred and Two Proved Cases, *Medicine (Baltimore),* 33:43, 1954.

76 Loop, F. D., Effler, D. B., Navia, J. A., Sheldon, W. C., and

Groves, L. K.: Aneurysms of the Left Ventricle: Survival and Results of a Ten-Year Surgical Experience, *Ann. Surg.*, 178: 399, 1973.

77 Bryson, A. L., Parisi, A. F., Schechter, E., and Wolfson, S.: Life-threatening Ventricular Arrhythmias Induced by Exercise, *Am. J. Cardiol.*, 32:995, 1973.

78 Mundth, E. D., Buckley, M. J., DeSanctis, R. W., Daggett, W. M., and Austen, W. G.: Surgical Treatment of Ventricular Irritability, *J. Thorac. Cardiovasc. Surg.*, 66:943, 1973.

79 Graham, A. F., Miller, D. C., Stinson, E. B., Daily, P. O., Fogarty, T. J., and Harrison, D. C.: Surgical Treatment of Refractory Life-threatening Ventricular Tachycardia, *Am. J. Cardiol.*, 32:909, 1973.

G
Rehabilitation of the Myocardial Infarction Patient

NANETTE KASS WENGER, M.D., and
CHARLES A. GILBERT, M.D.

Rehabilitation is a component of the plan of care for the patient with myocardial infarction—or, indeed, with any acute coronary episode—and has diagnostic, therapeutic, and educational aspects. The rehabilitation approach is equally applicable to and indicated for the patient who has had myocardial revascularization surgery.

INTRODUCTION

The concept that many patients with symptomatic coronary atherosclerotic heart disease—both angina pectoris and myocardial infarction—can and should return to normal living is the basis of the rehabilitation effort. The responsibility for the restoration of the coronary patient to productive or to independent living rests with the primary physician, who may utilize and coordinate the knowledge, skills, and techniques of many disciplines and individuals in this process.

While rehabilitation includes disease prevention, diagnosis, and medical and surgical care, its emphasis is on assessment of function (physical, emotional, social, educational, and vocational) and the provision of medical services, education, training, and other means needed to enhance function. It includes the institution of measures to prevent the progression of disease; it aims to help the patient achieve self-sufficiency and be able to cope with his or her problems. Rehabilitation is inseparable from both the philosophy and the programming of comprehensive, continuing health care.[1] The vocational objective, i.e., remunerative employment, is neither the sole justification nor the only criterion of success of a rehabilitation program. While job-oriented features are important in any rehabilitation effort, the return of the patient to complete independence is not always possible. At times, particularly for the older patient, a more realistic objective may be the attain-

ment of meaningful retirement or home-environment activities, or perhaps only a level of partial self-care.

Much of the capacity to effect rehabilitation should be available in the office of the primary physician or within the local community, using the community hospital and public and voluntary health care agencies and facilities. Patients with special problems may require referral to regional cardiac centers for consultative services.

ECONOMIC ASPECTS

An important consideration for health care planners, physicians, patients, and the general public concerns the economic feasibility of cardiac rehabilitation. What is the cost/benefit ratio? Do the results justify the expenditure of manpower and funds? For example, although it increased the cost of acute care, the coronary care unit effected a 5 to 15 percent increase in the survival of patients hospitalized for acute myocardial infarction. The costs of rehabilitation programming appear to result in an improved quality of life for the survivors of myocardial infarction and in their earlier return to work.[2] The earnings of patients who were rehabilitated after myocardial infarction and the savings of the disability or pension funds *not* expended for them far exceeded the costs of rehabilitation services.[3,4] In recent years, over 80 percent of cardiac patients referred to work evaluation units or special rehabilitation centers,[5] at times with complex medical, psychological, or vocational problems, were returned to work; the actual monetary value of their employment varied with their prior training and the availability of jobs. A British report[6] recommends that all patients who have not returned to work at 3 months after myocardial infarction be referred for detailed assessment of physical and psychosocial status and for appropriate rehabilitative services.

A 1970–1971 survey of U.S. physicians[7] designed to assess current practice in the management of patients with myocardial infarction indicated that over 85 percent of previously employed patients under age 65 had returned to work within 2 to 4 months after an uncomplicated myocardial infarction; the time period varied with the physical requirements of the job. Over three-fourths of these patients had resumed work at the same level of physical activity as prior to their myocardial infarction. Over 400,000 survivors of myocardial infarction are discharged from U.S. hospitals each year; using these statistics, the 15 percent of myocardial infarction survivors under age 65 who do not return to work each year constitute a significant number of individuals, perhaps as many as 60,000 patients. These patients may have special need for rehabilitation services, possibly because of increased impairment—physical, emotional, or educational. In general, "blue collar" workers appear to require more rehabilitative support services.[2] In addition, older patients, those not in the work force, may require special training to enhance function or to learn the work simplification techniques which will permit them to continue independent living.

PROGRAM COMPONENTS: AN OVERVIEW

Rehabilitation programs for the patient with myocardial infarction are best discussed in relation to the phase of the illness (see Table 62G-1). At each phase, the physician formulates a plan to assess and manage the patient's illness; the plan is then modified according to the patient's response to therapy. The plan includes evaluation of function (the severity of the disease, the complications, the emotional response to illness), monitoring of the desired and the adverse effects of therapeutic maneuvers, and periodic reassessment of function as it is changed by therapy.

Phases I and II involve the acute illness; phase I includes the time in the coronary care unit, and phase II the remainder of the hospital stay. Currently, the average duration of hospitalization in the United States for the patient with an uncomplicated myocardial infarction is 14 to 21 days. Nearly half of all myocardial infarction survivors have a mild, uncomplicated illness without significant residual physiologic cardiovascular disability.[2,6]

Phase III is the period of convalescence, generally at home, and usually 2 to 5 weeks in duration. Most patients return to work by 8 to 12 weeks after an uncomplicated acute myocardial infarction.[7] Phase IV can be designated as the recovery and maintenance phase; its particular concerns include efforts to enhance function, to decrease coronary risk factors, and to prevent the recurrence or progression of the disease.

The needs of the myocardial infarction patient for care by various members of the health team vary with the phase of the illness. In the coronary care unit, phase I, physicians and nurses with specialized training in intensive medical care have the greatest responsibility; emphasis is on the control of arrhythmia, shock, and heart failure. However, major emotional reactions also characteristically occur in this phase; the threat of dying produces anxiety, and the patient responds to his or her anticipated restrictions and invalidism and to loss of self-esteem by depression.[8] During the latter part of the hospital stay, phase II, there is an increasing role for the nurse and nurse-educator, nutritionist, social worker, occupational and physical therapists, and vocational counselor. The role of family members and the importance of cultural differences in the patient's reaction to illness should not be underrated at any phase.[9] The convalescent period, phase III, is characterized by a lessening role for the physician and nurse, and by greater involvement of the family, friends, public health nurse, social worker, vocational counselor, employer, and a variety of individuals involved in efforts to enhance function and self-sufficiency. When the patient returns to work, phase IV, the scope of rehabilitation programming becomes even more diverse, and the vocational counselor, the employer, and the industrial physician and industrial nurse assume preeminent roles. This health maintenance phase also emphasizes dominant roles for individuals concerned with community programming, including exercise training programs and educational and recreational programs.

The concepts and procedures to be discussed for the specific phases of myocardial infarction are derived in large part from the Cardiac Rehabilitation Program conducted at Grady Memorial Hospital and the Emory University School of Medicine in Atlanta, Georgia, since 1966–1967[10] (Table 62G-2). Comparable programs are now in operation in many cardiac centers and community hospitals.

Phase I: The coronary care unit

A hospital with facilities for continuous electrocardiographic monitoring and with appropriately trained personnel provides the accepted standard of care for patients with acute myocardial infarction. It is the responsibility of the primary physician to arrange immediate admission of his or her patient with a myocardial infarction to a coronary or intensive care unit. All hospitals admitting patients with myocardial infarction should also have the personnel and facilities to assist the primary physician in providing or implementing a rehabilitation program for these patients. The program should include[11] gradually progressive physical activity, *with the increases in the level of activity specified by the patient's primary physician.* The rehabilitation program should also include patient and family education regarding the coronary care unit—its purposes and the reasons for its regulations and procedures; coronary atherosclerotic heart disease and myocardial infarction—the characteristics of the disease and their relation to

TABLE 62G-1
Phases of myocardial infarction rehabilitation

Phase	Description	Time after myocardial infarction	Location
I	Acute illness	3–5 days	Coronary or intensive care unit
II	Acute illness	Remainder of hospital stay	General hospital care
III	Convalescence	3–8 weeks	Home
IV	Recovery-maintenance	After week 8	Return to work or prior activity

TABLE 62G-2
Fourteen-step myocardial infarction rehabilitation program

Step	Exercise	Ward activity	Educational and craft activity
1	Passive ROM* to all extremities (5 × ea); patient to do *active* plantar and dorsiflexion of ankles several times/day	Feeding self, sitting with bed rolled up to 45°, trunk and arms supported by over-bed table.	Initial interview and brief orientation to program.
2	Repeat exercises of Step 1.	1. Feed self. 2. Partial A.M. care (wash hands, face, brush teeth) in bed. 3. Dangle legs on side of bed (1×).	Light recreational activity, such as reading.
3	Active assistive exercise in shoulder flexion; elbow flexion and extension; hip flexion, extension, and rotation: knee flexion and extension: rotation of feet (4× ea).	1. Begin sitting in chair for short periods as tolerated, 2×/day. 2. Bathing whole body. 3. Use of bedside commode.	More detailed explanation of program. Continue light recreation.
4	Minimal resistance, lying in bed in above ROM, 5× ea. Stiffen all muscles to the count of 2 (3×).	1. Increase sitting 3×/day. 2. Change gown.	Begin explanation of what is an MI.* Give patient pamphlets to read. Begin craft activity: 1. Leather lacing. 2. Link belt. 3. Hand sewing, embroidery. 4. Copper tooling.
5	Moderate resistance in bed at 45° above ROM exercises; hands on shoulder, elbow circling (5× ea arm).	1. Sitting ad lib. 2. Sitting in chair at bedside for meals. 3. Dressing, shaving, combing hair—*sitting down*. 4. Walking in room, 2×/day.	Continue education about healing of heart, reasons for early restrictions in activity.
6	1. Further resistive exercises sitting on side of bed, manual resistance of knee extension and flexion (7× ea). 2. Walk to bathroom and back (note if patient needs help).	1. Walk to bathroom, ad lib if patient can tolerate. 2. Stand at sink to shave.	Continue craft activity or supply patient with another one. Patient may attend group meetings in a wheelchair for no more than 1 h.
7	1. Standing warm-up exercises: a. Arms in extension and shoulder abduction, rotate arms together in circles (circumduction), 5× ea arm. b. Stand on toes, 10×. c. May substitute abduction, 5× ea leg. 2. Walk length of hall (50 ft) and back at average pace.	1. Bathe in tub. 2. Walk to telephone or sit in waiting room (1×/day).	May walk to group meetings on the same floor.
8	1. Warm-up exercises: a. Lateral side bending 5× ea side. b. Trunk twisting, 5× ea side. 2. Walk 1½ lengths of hall, down 1 fl stairs, elevator up.	1. Walk to waiting room, 2×/day. 2. Stay sitting up most of the day.	Continue all previous craft and educational activities.
9	1. Warm-up exercises: a. Lateral side bending, 10× ea side. b. Slight knee bends, 10× with hands on hips. 2. Increase walking distance, walk down one flight of stairs.	Continue above activities.	Discussion of work simplification techniques and pacing of activities.
10	1. Warm-up exercises: a. Lateral side bending with 1-lb weight (10×). b. Standing—leg raising leaning against wall, 5× ea. 2. Walk two lengths of hall and downstairs, take elevator up.	Continue all previous ward activities.	1. Patient may walk to OT* clinic and work on craft proj. for ½ h. a. Copper tooling; b. woodworking; c. ceramics; d. small weaving proj. e. metal hammering; f. mosaic tile. 2. Discussion of patient's home exercises.
11	1. Warm-up exercises: a. Lateral side bending with 1-lb weight, leaning against wall, 10× ea side. b. Standing, leg raising, 5× ea. c. Trunk twisting with 1-lb weight, 5× ea. side. 2. Repeat part 2 of Step 10.	Continue all previous ward activities.	Increase time in OT clinic to 1 h.
12	1. Warm-up exercises: a. Lateral side bending with 2-lb weight, 10×. b. Standing—leg raising, leaning against wall, 10× ea. c. Trunk twisting with 2-lb weight, 10×. 2. Walk down two flights of stairs.	Continue all previous ward activities.	Continue craft activity with increased resistance.
13	Repeat all exercises of Step 12.	Continue all previous ward activities.	Complete all projects.
14	1. Warm-up exercises: a. Lateral side bending with 2-lb weight, 10× ea. side. b. Trunk twisting with 2-lb weight, 10× ea. side. c. Touch toes from sitting position, 10×. 2. Walk up flight of 10 stairs and down.	Continue all previous ward activities.	Final instructions about home procedures and activities.

*ROM = range of motion, MI = myocardial infarction, OT = occupational therapy.

therapy; and the patient's responsibility or role in the care of the illness—particularly regarding response to symptoms and adherence to prescribed therapy. Although most of this education is planned for phase II, the concepts are introduced while the patient is in the coronary or intensive care unit. It is of major importance to focus on the temporary character of most restrictions, which are designed to allow healing of the myocardium.

There is extensive documentation of the deleterious effects of prolonged bed rest,[12,13] and these must be considered in the patient with an uncomplicated myocardial infarction. Evidence of "deconditioning" may be seen as early as phase I and includes a decrease in physical work capacity, an increase in the heart rate response to effort, a decreased adaptability to change in posture which is manifest primarily as orthostatic hypotension, a decrease in the circulating blood volume (with plasma volume decreasing to a greater extent than red blood cell mass), decreased lung volume and vital capacity, decreased serum protein concentration, negative nitrogen and calcium balance, and a decrease in muscular contractile strength. The increased blood viscosity and leg circulatory stasis, due to lessened use of the leg muscle pump, predispose to thromboembolic complications.[14] Emotional complications include increased anxiety, hostility, and depression.[15]

There is increasing acceptance of the safety and advantages of bedside chair treatment and early ambulation for the patient with uncomplicated myocardial infarction;[16-21] and a number of cardiac centers have developed guidelines and programs for carefully supervised, gradually progressive physical activity for these patients.[5,22] Systematic provision of information and education to the patient and a progressive ambulation program afford the patient tangible and realistic reassurance; they decrease the anxiety commonly encountered during the first day or two of hospitalization, when physical activity restriction evokes feelings of helplessness and vulnerability. Structured plans for return toward normal living help allay the depression which characteristically appears during the third or fourth day after myocardial infarction and which may persist for days or weeks.[23-25] The association of depression with recurrent myocardial infarction and sudden cardiac death further emphasizes the importance of recognizing the emotional concomitants of myocardial infarction.

Phase I activities may begin within the day after hospitalization if the patient's clinical condition is stable and there are no complications of myocardial infarction: heart failure, shock, intractable or recurrent pain, or uncontrolled arrhythmia. These life-threatening complications are indications for bed rest and for specific therapeutic intervention. For the patient with an uncomplicated myocardial infarction, low-energy-level physical activities may be begun in the coronary care unit; these include self-care (feeding, shaving, and the use of a bedside commode or the bathroom with assistance); supervised active and passive extremity movements, designed primarily to decrease venous stasis and to maintain muscle tone and flexibility; and progression to sitting in a bedside chair. An apparent increase in physical activity, as seen by the patient, may actually involve decreased oxygen cost; for example, the myocardial work is less when sitting in a chair than when recumbent in bed and the use of a bedside commode involves less caloric expenditure than the use of a bedpan. The primary physician is responsible for prescribing this low-level physical activity and its serial progression, but the performance of the activity may be implemented by a nurse, therapist, physician assistant, or even family members if properly instructed and supervised. The coronary care unit electrocardiographic monitor affords optimal documentation of the patient's cardiovascular response to any particular level of activity. A disproportionate response to the effort, requiring a decrease in the level of physical activity for the patient, is indicated by (1) the appearance of chest pain or dyspnea, (2) an increase in the heart rate to over 120 per minute, (3) increased ST-segment displacement on the electrocardiogram or monitor, (4) the occurrence of significant arrhythmias, or (5) a fall in systolic blood pressure greater than 20 mm Hg (as the expected response to physical activity is a slight increase in the systolic blood pressure).

A structured rehabilitation program and the rehabilitation team personnel help provide the needed continuity of care when the patient is transferred out of the coronary care unit.

Phase II: The remainder of the hospitalization

The goal of gradually increasing physical activity during the remainder of the hospital stay, phase II, is to enable the patient to reach the activity level required for self-care by the time he returns home; this is generally at 14 to 21 days. With even earlier safe discharge from the hospital appearing to be feasible for selected patients with uncomplicated myocardial infarction,[26,26a] early ambulation assumes even more importance.

The activities allowed include self-care, sitting in a bedside chair for gradually increasing periods of time, and body motion and rhythmic exercises. The patient progresses to ambulation, in the room and in the hospital corridor, and then to stair climbing. Physical activities are interspersed with rest periods, and physical activity is avoided immediately after meals when the patient is not in a near basal state. Isometric exercises are avoided because of the increased workload they impose on the left ventricle, and the potential danger of provoking arrhythmias. Similar criteria as in phase I are employed to identify an excessive or disproportionate response to a particular level of activity and to indicate a need to decrease the level of activity.

Using these guidelines[27] over 3,000 patients with a coronary incident or definite acute myocardial infarction have participated in a progressive physical activity program at Grady Memorial Hospital and the Emory University School of Medicine since 1966.

There has been no episode of cardiac arrest, sudden death, recurrent myocardial infarction, or life-threatening arrhythmia immediately associated with the physical activity program except for one episode of ventricular fibrillation which was promptly reverted by defibrillation; episodes of angina pectoris have been controlled by the administration of nitroglycerin.

A "homecoming depression" has been described as common in post-myocardial infarction patients;[25] it is often triggered by the patient's awareness of weakness and fatigue upon returning home. These manifestations of the "deconditioning" effects of prolonged bed rest can be minimized or averted by an inhospital physical conditioning program.[28] Additionally, the patient's response to the inhospital rehabilitation program can guide the physician in recommendations for physical activity levels during convalescence at home.

Recent well-designed, controlled studies have documented the desirability, feasibility, safety, and cost effectiveness of this approach. Hospital stay has been abbreviated;[28a] patients' self-image and ability to perform self-care has been enhanced; and the requirements for program personnel and facilities have been modest. Of major importance is that there was no difference in hospital or follow-up mortality, recurrent myocardial infarction, dysrhythmias, heart failure, angina pectoris, ventricular aneurysm, or cardiac rupture between the early mobilization and traditional hospital regimen groups;[29,30] however, significantly greater disability was demonstrable in the control than in the early ambulation groups at follow-up examination.[31]

There has been considerable recent interest in predischarge submaximal exercise stress testing. Its safety, its role in altering the plan of medical and/or surgical management, and its prognostic value all require further evaluation.

The latter part of the hospitalization also provides the ideal opportunity, facilities, and personnel for patient and family education.[9,32] The patient's understanding and acceptance of his or her illness help in the understanding of the plan of therapy and in the acceptance of the prescribed changes in behavior: in diet, activity, and smoking. The patient education curriculum should include, at a minimum, the following prescriptive items: (1) nutrition—dietary modification of calories, fat, or sodium as needed and the reasons for recommended changes; (2) physical activity—the basis for the recommendations,[33] the magnitude and type of exercise prescribed and its relation to the patient's prior level of activity and job requirements, and resumption of sexual activity (this should be discussed with the patient and spouse; since the physiologic cost of conjugal sexual activity in middle-aged individuals is modest, participation in sexual activity is generally recommended when the patient returns to his or her other usual daily-life activities);[34] (3) prescription for cessation of smoking and its rationale; (4) immediate and long-term plans for management—understanding the character of the illness enables the patient to have a more realistic expectation of his or her future pattern of living and requirements for health care; (5) control of associat-

ed diseases, particularly hypertension and diabetes mellitus, and of other coronary risk factors; (6) prescription for the patient's response to new or recurrent symptoms, particularly chest pain; intensive education of the patient and family to seek immediate medical care is mandatory to decrease the risk of sudden death from recurrent myocardial infarction; (7) information about actual medications prescribed—their name, dosage, desired effects, and possible adverse effects; and (8) counseling regarding psychosocial problems which may confront the patient after discharge. Many patients anticipate encountering psychosocial problems at home, at work, or in the community; and, indeed, psychosocial problems may be as disabling as or more disabling than the physical illness.[35] Frequently, the delay in return to work does not correlate with either the severity of the original illness or the current cardiovascular symptoms and impairment.[36] Patients and their families should be counseled regarding problems of return to work, to sexual activity, to recreational activity; in regard to family life adjustment, the physician should attempt to avert the family's overprotection of the myocardial infarction patient.

An educational algorithm[37] (Table 62G-3) has been formulated for the problem of coronary atherosclerotic heart disease and myocardial infarction as part of the Grady-Emory Cardiac Rehabilitation Program. This enables automatic, systematic implementation of a predetermined core curriculum for each patient; general group and individual instruction is supplemented by specific instruction for individual patient problems. Documentation in the patient's record of the information presented and an evaluation of the patient's comprehension enables communication among the health care personnel involved in patient education; this results in better patient instruction, both during and after the hospitalization. Advantages gained in a hospital rehabilitation program, however, may be lost if posthospital rehabilitation does not ensue.

Phase III: Convalescence

When the patient returns home, phase III, the goal of progressive increase in physical activity is to achieve a level of function which will permit return to work by the eighth to twelfth week. Supervised progressive ambulation during the hospitalization helps to allay the patient's and family's fear of recurrent myocardial infarction or of sudden death resulting from physical exertion;[8] these psychologic barriers to rehabilitation may be greater than the physical limitations. Perhaps both the physician's and the patient's fear of reinfarction and/or sudden cardiac death present the main stumbling blocks to early return to work and to normal living.[38]

Most usual household activities are permitted, including complete self-care. Women are allowed to do light housework, specifically avoiding bed-making, washing and hanging clothes, and floor

TABLE 62G-3
Patient education program components*

Problem: myocardial infarction

I Adjustment to coronary care unit
  A Purpose of coronary care unit
  B Regulations of unit (visiting, smoking, flowers)
  C Monitor (sounds and leads)
  D Intravenous infusions and medications
  E Oxygen
  F Activity (leg exercise, etc.)
  G ECG, blood tests, x-rays
  H Diet
  I Personal emergencies (e.g., financial, job)
II Adjustment to transfer from unit
  A Constant observation no longer necessary
  B Activity as prescribed
  C Plan for education program (see III)
III Information needed for adaptation to disease
  A Normal anatomy and function of heart
  B Development of coronary atherosclerotic heart disease
  C Heart attack
    1 Risk factors
      (a) General discussion
      (b) Emphasis on risk factors of individual patient
    2 Warning signs of heart attack
    3 Healing relation to physical activity
  D Personal response to myocardial infarction
    1 Group discussion
    2 Individual conference with patient, family
IV Plans for care after discharge from hospital
  A Diet
    1 Group discussion
    2 Individual conference with patient, family
  B Discharge medications (each medication, its dosage, is listed for teaching to patient)
  C Activity
    1 General
    2 Sexual
    3 Work simplification
  D Symptoms which should be reported
  E Rehabilitation exercises
  F Clinic or physician appointments
  G Community resources
V Other areas for teaching (e.g., pacemaker, diabetes)
VI Educational materials given to patient (a basic pamphlet list is checked and additional educational materials are recorded)
VII Outpatient (clinic) education
  A Review of IV in class and individual instruction
  B Patient self-learning tapes and slide-tapes

*For each item listed, the date of teaching and instructor's name are recorded, as is the need for further patient education on that topic and the instructor's comments regarding the patient's comprehension.

scrubbing. Men may perform desk or paper work or minor household tasks. The physical activity of the last days in the hospital is maintained; progressive activity consists primarily of walking and involves a gradual increase in the distance walked and the speed of walking. By the end of the sixth week, the average patient may walk 1 or 2 mi each day, divided into two or three activity periods. Specific, structured physical conditioning programs increase the patient's confidence and sense of well-being; they have the added advantage of enabling the convalescent myocardial infarction patient to schedule and organize his or her daily activities.[32]

The physician's evaluation of the patient during phase III should include assessment of the patient's response to the prescribed level of physical activity prior to increasing the activity level. At least once during convalescence the patient should have a resting electrocardiogram and a test of cardiac function of a magnitude at least equal to the prescribed physical activity level. If there is no disproportionate response to the magnitude of effort, the patient is directed to increase the speed and duration of walking. This type of physical activity program is designed to increase endurance. The patient who can walk without symptoms at a speed of about $3\frac{1}{2}$ mi/h at the end of phase III has attained a level of function somewhat in excess of that required for most desk or bench jobs; this functional capacity is adequate to permit most patients to return to work.

Phase IV: Recovery-maintenance

Phase IV for the myocardial infarction patient, the recovery-maintenance phase, assumes that the patient's cardiovascular status has improved sufficiently for return to his or her prior occupational or daily living activity level. Alternatively, the patient has been retrained for a more suitable occupational or activity level. In this phase, enhancement of physical function can be attained by participation in individual or supervised community physical conditioning programs.[5,39] Before beginning exercise at these higher levels of physical activity, formal multistage exercise testing is required both for safety and for accuracy of exercise prescription.[33,40] Additionally, for patients whose occupations require high-level physical activity, data obtained from exercise testing can be correlated with known job energy requirement measurements, furnishing an objective basis for recommendations regarding safe return of the patient to work.[41]

As with any other therapeutic modality, the physician who prescribes physical activity should know its indications and contraindications; the recommended intensity, frequency, and duration needed to produce and maintain a "training effect"; the desired and adverse effects; the requisite emergency care measures and equipment; and the recommended guidelines for the design of an exercise program.[33] Indeed the concept of prescriptive exercise[38] is central to the recommended plan of care. Exercise "dosage," to maintain a training effect in patients after myocardial infarction, involves (1) an intensity of 75 to 85 percent of the maximum heart rate safely achieved at prior exercise stress testing (in general, the 75 percent level is used for unsupervised home programs and the 85 percent level for supervised gymnasium programs), (2) a duration of about 30 min per session including warm-up and cool-down periods, and (3) a frequency of two to three times weekly, preferably on nonsuccessive days.[22,33,40,42] It is not known whether similar benefit can be obtained with a less prolonged or less intense exercise training program. Dynamic exercise, rhythmic repetitive movements involving large muscle groups, is recommended. Training may be continuous or intermittent during an exercise session, with continuous exercise accelerating the development of a "training effect," but with an intermittent exercise protocol more applicable to the more impaired patient.

Continued medical management and, when appropriate, surgical intervention, such as myocardial revascularization or aneurysmectomy, constitute the cornerstone of efforts to enhance cardiac function. The total rehabilitation program as presented is equally applicable to the patient who undergoes myocardial revascularization and should be instituted early in the postoperative period.

Systematic physical activity rehabilitation programs[39] after hospitalization for myocardial infarction can enhance the functional capacity of cardiac patients.[33,43,44] However, these high-level exercise training programs (as well as high-level exercise testing) are contraindicated for patients with very recent myocardial infarction, new or unstable angina pectoris, many cardiac arrhythmias, high-degree atrioventricular block, a fixed-rate cardiac pacemaker, uncompensated congestive heart failure, significant obstructive valvular disease, uncontrolled diabetes mellitus or hypertension, etc.

The energy costs for various physical activities appear comparable for apparently normal individuals and for patients with coronary atherosclerotic disease after myocardial infarction; this information can serve as a guide for introducing progressively more difficult and demanding physical activities in exercise training programs. Exercises must be designed to train both arms and legs, as leg training does not alter the cardiovascular response to arm work and vice versa, and in our society most individuals earn their living using their arms.

Patients must be taught to adhere to their exercise prescription during the exercise training program, not to become competitive, and not to exercise when unduly fatigued or when subjected to increased or excessive stress; patients must be instructed to report chest pain, dyspnea, palpitations, dizziness, or any other new symptoms which might signal a temporary contraindication to exercise training or a need for reduction in the intensity of physical activity. Exercise, to become a lifetime habit, must be designed to be enjoyable to the participant.

After training, the patient's cardiovascular response to the same workload is characterized by a lesser increase in heart rate and in systolic blood pressure, and a lesser increase in cardiac output; the classic posttraining bradycardia in patients with coronary atherosclerotic heart disease appears to be compensated for by an increase in the arteriovenous oxygen difference rather than by an increased stroke volume, as occurs in normal individuals.[45] The "training effect" is further characterized by decreased or absent angina pectoris and decreased ST-T changes on the electrocardiogram for the same amount of external work.[45a] The improved symptomatic and electrocardiographic responses to exercise after physical training are not related to an increase in the coronary collateral circulation, but rather to an improvement in the heart-rate and blood pressure

response to exercise; myocardial oxygen delivery may also be enhanced.[42,45a] The development of a coronary collateral circulation (as measured angiographically) appears related only to progression of the underlying coronary obstructive disease, and an exercise training program seems to have little if any effect on the progression of the atherosclerosis.[46] Physical training does not appear to alter the relation of the magnitude of ST-segment changes to their hemodynamic determinants, as ST-segment abnormalities appear at the same level of heart-rate and pressure-rate product as prior to training.[44]

The crucial question regarding the effect of exercise on the long-term prognosis after myocardial infarction—does it alter morbidity and mortality?—has not yet been definitively answered. Sanne's data suggest an improvement in long-term mortality without an effect on reinfarction rate.[47] Randomized studies, now in progress, may provide needed information. Nevertheless, there is improvement in the anxiety and depression scores on standard psychologic tests[28] and improvement in the patient's sense of "well-being," self-confidence, assertiveness and self-esteem.[43] Patients who had been physically active prior to their myocardial infarction had a more favorable prognosis for return to work.

SUMMARY

Inhospital progressive physical activity rehabilitation programs may help to reduce the duration of hospitalization for the myocardial infarction patient. It has been estimated that if the hospital stay for each myocardial infarction patient could safely be reduced by just 1 day, the annual saving in the cost of medical care in the United States would be at least $40 million. More coronary patients now return to work than was the case one or two decades ago; in a recent study, the employment status of men surviving their first myocardial infarction was similar to that of men clinically free of coronary atherosclerotic heart disease.[48] This increased return to work is related partly to improved patient, community, and employer education about myocardial infarction; partly to lesser job energy requirements with increasing mechanization; and partly to the efforts of work classification or evaluation units in matching the level of a patient's impairment and the job energy requirements.

The end points or criteria for a successful rehabilitation program for patients[2,6,38] after myocardial infarction include (1) a return to gainful employment or to independent living (successful retirement or self-care); (2) a reduction of the economic burden of myocardial infarction on the patient, his or her family, and the community through a shortened hospital stay, a decreased need for convalescent care, and an increased and more rapid and successful return to work;[18,19] (3) reduction of the risk of recurrent myocardial infarction, premature death, or complications of myocardial infarction,[49] i.e., implementation of a secondary prevention program; and (4) improvement of the quality of life for the increasing number of patients who now survive myocardial infarction.

REFERENCES

1 Naughton, J., Bruhn, J., Lategola, M. T., and Whitsett, T.: Rehabilitation Following Myocardial Infarction, *Am. J. Med.,* 46:725, 1969.

2 Report of the Task Force on Cardiovascular Rehabilitation, National Heart and Lung Institute: "Needs and Opportunities for Rehabilitating the Coronary Heart Disease Patient," December 15, 1974, Washington, D.C., Department of Health, Education, and Welfare Publication (NIH) 75-750.

3 Helander, E.: Economic Aspects of the Rehabilitation of Patients with Cardiovascular and Cerebrovascular Diseases, *Acta Cardiol. Suppl.,* 14:53, 1970.

4 Wigle, R. D., Symington, D. C., Lewis, M., Connell, W. F., and Parker, J. O.: Return to Work after Myocardial Infarction, *Can. Med. Assoc. J.,* 104:210, 1971.

5 Kellerman, J. J., and Kariv, I.: "Rehabilitation of Coronary Patients," Segal Press, Tel Aviv, Israel, 1971.

6 Report of a Joint Working Party of the Royal College of Physicians of London and The British Cardiac Society on Rehabilitation after Cardiac Illness: Cardiac Rehabilitation 1975, *J. R. Coll. Physicians Lond.,* 9:281, 1975.

7 Wenger, N. K., Hellerstein, H. K., Blackburn, H., and Castranova, S. J.: Uncomplicated Myocardial Infarction. Current Physician Practice in Patient Management, *JAMA,* 224:511, 1973.

8 Fisher, S.: International Survey on the Psychological Aspects of Cardiac Rehabilitation, *Scand. J. Rehabil. Med.,* 2–3:71, 1970.

9 Croog, S. H., Levine, S., and Lurie, Z.: The Heart Patient and the Recovery Process: A Review of the Directions of Research on Social and Psychological Factors, *Soc. Sci. Med.,* 2:111, 1968.

10 Wenger, N. K., Gilbert, C. A., and Skorapa, M. Z.: Cardiac Conditioning after Myocardial Infarction: An Early Intervention Program, *Cardiac Rehabil.,* 2:17, 1971.

11 Mulcahy, R., and Hickey, N.: The Rehabilitation of Patients with Coronary Heart Disease: A Comparison of the Return to Work Experience of National Health Insurance Patients with Coronary Heart Disease and of a Group of Coronary Patients Subjected to a Specific Rehabilitation Programme, *J. Ir. Med. Assoc.,* 64:541, 1971.

12 Saltin, B., Blomqvist, G., Mitchell, J. H., Johnson, R. L., Wildenthal, K., and Chapman, C. B.: Response to Exercise after Bed Rest and Training, *Circulation,* 37–38(suppl. 7):1, 1968.

13 Chobanian, A. V., Lille, R. D., Tercyak, A., and Blevins, P.: The Metabolic and Hemodynamic Effects of Prolonged Bed Rest in Normal Subjects, *Circulation,* 49:551, 1974.

14 Broustet, J. P., Dubecq, M., Bouloumie, J., and Baron, P.: Rehabilitation of the Coronary Patients: Mobilization Program in the Acute Phase, *Schweiz. Med. Wochenschr.,* 103:57, 1973.

15 Ryback, R. S., Lewis, O. F., and Lessard, C. S.: Psychobiologic Effects of Prolonged Bed Rest (Weightless) in Young, Healthy Volunteers (Study II), *Aerosp. Med.,* 42:529, 1971.

16 Takkunen, J., Huhti, E., Oilinki, O., Vuopala, U., and Kaipainen, W. J.: Early Ambulation in Myocardial Infarction, *Acta Med. Scand.,* 188:103, 1970.

17 Duke, M.: Bed Rest in Acute Myocardial Infarction: A Study of Physician Practices, *Am. Heart J.,* 82:486, 1971.

18 Groden, B. M.: The Management of Myocardial Infarction: A Controlled Study of the Effects of Early Mobilization, *Cardiac Rehabil.,* 1:13, 1971.

19 Harpur, J. E., Kellett, R. J., Conner, W. T., Galbraith, H. J. B., Hamilton, M., Murray, J. J., Swallow, J. H., and Rose, G. A.: Controlled Trial of Early Mobilization and Discharge from Hospital in Uncomplicated Myocardial Infarction, *Lancet,* 2:1331, 1971.

20 Lamers, H. J., Drost, W. S. J., Kroon, B. J. M., van Es, L. A., Meilink-Hoedemaker, L. J., and Birkenhager, W. H.: Early Mobilization after Myocardial Infarction: A Controlled Study, *Br. Med. J.,* 1:257, 1973.

21 Rose, G.: Early Mobilization and Discharge after Myocardial Infarction, *Mod. Concepts Cardiovasc. Dis.,* 41:59, 1972.

22 Zohman, L. R., and Tobis, J. S.: "Cardiac Rehabilitation," Grune & Stratton, Inc., New York, 1970.

23 McPherson, B. D., Paivio, A., Yuhasz, M. S., Rechnitzer, P. A., Pickard, H. A., and Lefcoe, N. M.: Psychological Effects of an Exercise Program for Post-infarct and Normal Adult Men, *J. Sports Med. Phys. Fitness,* 7:95, 1967.

24 Cassem, N. H., and Hackett, T. P.: Psychiatric Consultation in a Coronary Care Unit, *Ann. Intern. Med.,* 75:9, 1971.

25 Hackett, T. P., and Cassem, N. H.: Psychological Adaptation to Convalescence in Myocardial Infarction Patients, in J. P. Naughton and H. Hellerstein (eds.), "Exercise Testing and Exercise Training in Coronary Heart Disease," Academic Press, Inc., New York, 1973.

26 McNeer, J. F., Wallace, A. G., Wagner, G. S., Starmer, C. F., and Rosati, R. A.: The Course of Acute Myocardial Infarction: Feasibility of Early Discharge of the Uncomplicated Patient, *Circulation,* 51:410, 1975.

27 Wenger, N. K., Gilbert, C. A., and Siegel, W.: Symposium: The Use of Physical Activity in the Rehabilitation of Patients after Myocardial Infarction, *South. Med. J.,* 63:891, 1970.

28 Wishnie, H. A., Hackett, T. P., and Cassem, N. H.: Psychological Hazards of Convalescence Following Myocardial Infarction, *JAMA,* 215:1292, 1971.

28a Swan, H. J. C., Blackburn, H. W., DeSanctis, R., Frommer, P. L., Hurst, J. W., Paul, O., Rapaport, E., Wallace, A., and Weinberg, S.: Duration of Hospitalization in "Uncomplicated Completed Acute Myocardial Infarction," An Ad Hoc Committee Review, *Am. J. Cardiol.,* 37:413, 1976.

29 Boyle, J. A., and Lorimer, A. R.: Early Mobilization after Uncomplicated Myocardial Infarction: Prospective Study of 538 Patients, *Lancet,* 2:346, 1973.

30 Hayes, M. J., Morris, G. K., and Hamptom, J. R.: Comparison of Mobilization after Two and Nine Days in Uncomplicated Myocardial Infarction, *Br. Med. J.,* 3:10, 1974.

31 Bloch, A., Maeder, J.-P., Haissly, J.-C., Felix, J., and Blackburn, H.: Early Mobilization after Myocardial Infarction: A Controlled Study, *Am. J. Cardiol.,* 34:152, 1974.

32 Groden, B. M., Semple, T., and Shaw, G. B.: Cardiac Rehabilitation, *Br. Heart J.,* 33:425, 1971.

33 Fox, S. M., III, Naughton, J. P., and Gorman, P. A.: Physical Activity and Cardiovascular Health: I. Potential for Prevention of Coronary Heart Disease and Possible Mechanisms; II. The Exercise Prescription: Intensity and Duration; III. The Exercise Prescription: Frequency and Type of Activity, *Mod. Concepts Cardiovasc. Dis.,* 41:17, 1972.

34 Hellerstein, H. K., and Friedman, E. H.: Sexual Activity and the Post-coronary Patient, *Arch. Intern. Med.,* 125:987, 1970.

35 Cay, E. L., Vetter, N., Philip, A. E., and Dugard, P.: Psychological Status during Recovery from an Acute Heart Attack, *J. Psychosom. Res.,* 16:425, 1972.

36 Hay, D. R., and Turbott, S.: Rehabilitation after Myocardial Infarction and Acute Coronary Insufficiency, *N. Z. Med. J.,* 71:267, 1970.

37 Wenger, N. K., and Mount, F.: An Educational Algorithm for Myocardial Infarction, *Cardiovasc. Nursing,* 10:11, 1974.

38 Wenger, N. K.: Cardiac Rehabilitation: The United Kingdom and the United States, *Ann. Intern. Med.,* 84:214, 1976 (editorial).

39 Fletcher, G. F., and Cantwell, J. D.: "Exercise in the Management of Coronary Heart Disease: A Guide for the Practicing Physician," Charles C Thomas, Publisher, Springfield, Ill., 1971.

40 Prepared for the Central Committee for Medical and Community Program, Committee on Exercise: "Exercise Testing and Training of Individuals with Heart Disease or at High Risk for Its Development: A Handbook for Physicians," American Heart Association, Dallas, Tex., no. 70-008B, 1975.

41 Blomqvist, C. G.: Use of Exercise Testing for Diagnostic and Functional Evaluation of Patients with Arteriosclerotic Heart Disease, *Circulation,* 44:1120, 1971.

42 Redwood, D. R., Rosing, D. R., and Epstein, S. E.: Circulatory and Symptomatic Effects of Physical Training in Patients with Coronary-Artery Disease and Angina Pectoris, *N. Engl. J. Med.,* 286:959, 1972.

43 Kellerman, J. J., Modan, B., Levy, M., Feldman, S., and Kariv, I.: Return to Work after Myocardial Infarction: Comparative Study of Rehabilitated and Nonrehabilitated Patients, *Geriatrics,* 25:151, 1968.

44 Detry, J.-M., and Bruce, R. A.: Effects of Physical Training on Exertional S-T Segment Depression in Coronary Heart Disease, *Circulation,* 44:390, 1971.

45 Detry, J.-M. R., Rousseau, M., Vandenbroucke, G., Kusumi, F., Brasseur, L. A., and Bruce, R. A.: Increased Arteriovenous Oxygen Difference after Physical Training in Coronary Heart Disease, *Circulation,* 44:109, 1971.

45a Clausen, J. P.: Circulatory Adjustments to Dynamic Exercise and Effect of Physical Training in Normal Subjects and in Patients with Coronary Artery Disease, *Prog. Cardiovasc. Dis.,* 18:459, 1976.

46 Mitchell, J. H.: Exercise Training in the Treatment of Coronary Heart Disease, *Adv. Intern. Med.,* 20:249, 1975.

47 Sanne, H.: Exercise Tolerance and Physical Training of Nonselected Patients after Myocardial Infarction, *Acta Med. Scand. [Suppl.],* 551, 1973.

48 Shapiro, S., Weinblatt, E., and Frank, C. W.: Return to Work after First Myocardial Infarction, *Arch. Environ. Health,* 24:17, 1972.

49 Rechnitzer, P. A., Pickard, H. A., Paivio, A. U., Yuhasz, M. S., and Cunningham, D.: Long-Term Follow-up Study of Survival and Recurrence Rates Following Myocardial Infarction in Exercising and Control Subjects, *Circulation,* 45:853, 1972.

H
Modification of Risk Factors in the Prevention and Management of Coronary Atherosclerotic Heart Disease

ROBERT C. SCHLANT, M.D., and
MARIO DIGIROLAMO, M.D.

INTRODUCTION

The purpose of this chapter is to review briefly the evidence indicating that the development of coronary atherosclerosis in human beings is not the ineluctable

concomitant of aging and that the disease process can be modified or even to a degree prevented, and to present a simple algorithm for the recognition of risk factors and for the classification and management of patients with lipids disorders. The practical therapeutic recommendations presented here are based upon both basic information and developing knowledge.

There are considerable epidemiologic, clinical, and experimental data indicating a strong association between certain "risk" factors and an increased incidence of coronary atherosclerotic heart disease[1-45] (see also Chap. 62B). On that basis, it would seem logical to recommend removal or correction of the known risk factors to decelerate or prevent the atherosclerotic process and its complications. On the other hand, coronary atherosclerosis is a multifactorial disease, and many important pathogenetic factors and mechanisms may not as yet have been finally identified. In addition, final proof of therapeutic benefits deriving from strict application of available measures is not available, although many encouraging results have been obtained. For these and other reasons, both physicians and lay people have been exposed to a barrage of information and counseling which is, at times, contradictory. In response to these data, two extreme reactions are sometimes seen. One type of reaction states that absolute, final proof of the beneficial effects of intervention is not yet available and that, therefore, no recommendations are appropriate. The opposite reaction may be seen in an immediate reliance upon drug treatment in all patients with a lipid disorder, without having properly identified all the risk factors involved and without having initially attempted more physiologic interventions such as weight reduction and diet modification. In between these two extremes, there seems to be a reasonable, prudent approach. This approach recognizes the severe epidemic of coronary heart disease in the United States and many other industrialized nations and recognizes the difficulty of changing human behavior, while considering the benefit-hardship ratio of any recommendation for each individual patient. Certain recommendations appear to us to be justified and indicated at present, even though no final, unequivocal evidence of benefit is yet available. It should be emphasized that the magnificent achievements in recent years in the fields of acute coronary care, emergency medical care, or coronary artery surgery have not and cannot bring about a major reduction in the overall burden of coronary heart disease.[46] Such a reduction can only come from preventive measures.

In this chapter we will review the following: (1) pertinent background information; (2) the "desirable" ranges of major health parameters involved; (3) office screening and the assessment of the deviation from "desirable" or "optimal" levels of various risk factors; (4) the general principles to be kept in mind when preventive and therapeutic intervention is considered; (5) a "prudent" set of recommendations to decrease the rate of progression of coronary atherosclerosis, both for the general population and for certain sets of individual patients; (6) recognition and treatment of specific hyperlipidemias; (7) the pharmacology of drugs used in the management of hyperlipidemia; and (8) some clinical examples of the spectrum of therapeutic intervention. The mechanisms of the atherogenesis are reviewed in Chap. 62B and elsewhere.[4,7,15,19,24,30,43]

BACKGROUND INFORMATION

Epidemiologic evidence

Extensive epidemiologic evidence,[1–45,47,48] reviewed in Chap. 62B, strongly establishes an association between many population characteristics and the incidence of coronary atherosclerotic heart disease (CAHD). Certain important identified characteristics such as sex, age, and family history of early atherosclerotic disease are not generally amenable to modification. On the other hand, a number of other "risk factors" bearing a high association with CAHD have been identified, and some of these are amenable to change or modification. The three "cardinal" risk factors identified to date are hypercholesterolemia (frequently associated in the general population with a diet higher than ideal in cholesterol and saturated fatty acids, mostly deriving from excessive consumption of eggs and animal fat), systemic arterial hypertension, and cigarette smoking.[1–48] As noted in Chap. 62B, the epidemiologic studies have clearly shown that, when two or more major risk factors are present, their effects are more than simply additive.[8,15,39,41] The epidemiologic data on hypercholesterolemia also indicate that there is a progressive continuity of risk and that there is no clear-cut, physiologic "normal" level of serum cholesterol. Several studies have actually suggested that the incidence of clinical coronary atherosclerotic heart disease increases exponentially (serum cholesterol[2.66]) with the serum cholesterol concentration.[49] On the basis of epidemiologic and experimental data, it would appear that the "desirable" or "optimal" serum cholesterol level is probably in the range of 140 to 180 mg/dl, a figure considerably lower than the usual epidemiologic "normal" value observed in the population of the United States in which cholesterol levels of 220 to 260 mg/dl are frequently observed.[2,3,6,8,16,17,20,22,23,31,34,37–42,50–54] If this is true, it implies that a considerable percentage of adults in the United States and many other industrialized nations have moderate, mostly dietary-induced hypercholesterolemia.[6,27,31,34,41,50,55] Although the statistical association between the level of plasma cholesterol and the development of coronary heart disease or coronary incidents decreases with age, the relationship is still valid both in the elderly[56] and in patients who have already sustained a myocardial infarction.[57]

The plasma cholesterol level is affected by the dietary intake of both cholesterol and saturated fatty acids.[31,55,58–67a] Epidemiologic studies of populations in countries with markedly different dietary intakes of cholesterol and saturated fat have shown similar effects.[1–6,9,15,20,50] During World War II, there was a noticeable decrease in plasma cholesterol as well as mortality from coronary heart disease in those countries that had a marked decrease in dietary cholesterol and saturated fat intake.[15,31] Furthermore, different types of dietary fats have significant effects upon platelet function and the formation of arterial thrombosis. In general, saturated fats tend to increase platelet adhesiveness and platelet accumulation.[68–71] Besides contributing directly to plasma lipid elevation, such effects of dietary fats may be of primary importance in both the pathogenesis of atherosclerosis and in the development of complications (see Chap. 62B).

The influence of hypertension on the development of coronary atherosclerosis is also continuous, and there is no single systolic or diastolic blood pressure level above which it does occur and below which it does not occur. The association with CAHD is highly significant for both systolic and diastolic blood pressure[8,31,38–41,72–74] (see also Chap. 62B.

In addition to these "cardinal" risk factors, other important risk factors that have been identified include diabetes mellitus[3,47,75–78] and obesity.[79–82] Obesity appears to be important primarily because of the frequent association with hypertension, diabetes mellitus, and hyperlipidemia.[31,41,80,82] Many other characteristics have been suggested as being associated with the development of coronary atherosclerosis (see Chap. 62B and Table 62B-2), but the relationship is less clear for these additional "minor factors."

Primary prevention

The term *primary prevention* implies the prevention of coronary atherosclerosis or at least a slowing in its progression so that clinically detectable lesions are postponed, minimized, or absent. A number of studies of the primary prevention of atherosclerotic coronary heart disease have provided data strongly suggesting that modifications of life-style are both feasible and of benefit in decreasing the incidence of clinical events due to CAHD.[3,16,20,28,31,34,41,83–98a] Although none of the studies to date is completely satisfactory, particularly due to the limited number of subjects studied and the duration of study, the data are highly encouraging. The four most important studies of primary prevention are the New York Anti-Coronary Club,[88–90] the Finnish Mental Hospital Study,[91–93] the Los Angeles Veterans Administration Domiciliary Study,[94,95] and the Chicago Coronary Prevention Evaluation Program.[96–98] All these studies suggest that changes in living habits, particularly diet, can be accomplished with relative ease and can contribute to a decreased morbidity and/or mortality from CAHD. As expected, there appears to be significantly more benefit when the modifications are introduced in younger individuals. For example, studies in two boarding schools for boys have demonstrated that reducing saturated fatty acids and cholesterol and increasing polyunsaturated fatty acids in ordinary school diets produced a prompt reduction of 10 to 15 percent in mean cholesterol levels.[296,297] Even though these studies could not show (in view of the subjects' ages) major reductions in morbidity due to CAHD, they nevertheless showed how a simple and harmless dietary intervention could promptly affect a partial correction of the elevated lipid levels.

Currently, there are several ongoing studies of primary prevention of CAHD. The Multiple Risk Factor Intervention Trials (MRFIT) has as its goal the prevention of first heart attacks among 12,000 men, aged 35 to 37 years, predicted to be in the upper decile of risk of death from coronary heart disease but without clinically apparent coronary heart disease. The Lipid Research Clinical Coronary Primary Prevention Trial (LRC-CPPT) is a 7-year study to determine whether or not lowering plasma cholesterol in 4,000 men with hypercholesterolemia (type IIa) will reduce the development of premature coronary heart disease. The national Hypertension Detection and Follow-up Program (HDFP) will follow approximately 11,000 men and women and should provide additional data regarding the effects of the control of hypertension upon the incidence of clinical coronary atherosclerotic heart disease.

A number of primary prevention studies have been or are being conducted utilizing the drug clofibrate alone without concomitant dietary therapy.[16,28,31,34,41,45,99,100] To date, none of these has convincingly shown definite beneficial long-term effects upon coronary atherosclerosis or its complications, even though minor reduction in blood lipids has occurred in some studies. An unblinded primary prevention study of clofibrate in United Air Lines personnel[101] resulted in a reduction in new coronary events in the treatment group, but the design of the trial has been vigorously criticized.[102] A 5-year primary prevention study utilizing clofibrate (the World Health Organization Cooperative Trial) was restricted to men with hypercholesterolemia. This study, completed in 1977, failed to demonstrate a statistically significant benefit,[99] but it has to be emphasized that this study employed the use of this drug (which may not be the drug of choice in this condition) along with minimal changes in diet and no correction of other risk factors. The negative results of purely drug trials are not surprising in view of the relatively inadequate control of diet, body weight, and other risk factors, as well as the limited duration of these studies. In general, the studies to date have not adequately tested the lipid hypothesis (i.e., a reduction in lipid levels will reduce or reverse the atherosclerotic process) in the primary prevention of coronary atherosclerosis.[103] It should be kept in mind that the ongoing studies may only provide additional

"suggestive" data, since it is not now economically feasible to conduct the types of trials that would provide absolute proof based on hard data.[103,103a] Nevertheless, it is very encouraging that in the last few years, possibly due to dissemination of information and improved health habits, there has been an apparent real decrease in the overall mortality from coronary heart disease in the United States.[104,105]

Secondary prevention

The term *secondary prevention* implies that preventive measures are used after symptoms and signs of CAHD have appeared so that subsequent extension of the lesions may be postponed, minimized, or prevented. Significant regression of advanced lesions is theoretically possible, but difficult to achieve in human beings.

The evidence for a beneficial influence of moderate diet alterations in secondary prevention studies of patients who have angina pectoris or who have already sustained an acute myocardial infarction, and therefore have advanced coronary atherosclerosis, is strongly suggestive but not absolutely convincing.[3,16,20,28,29,31,34,41,45,106,107] Again, the beneficial effect appears to be greatest in younger subjects.

In general, the benefits of secondary prevention are less than those of primary prevention.

The Coronary Drug Project (CDP) was a 5-year study of 8,431 male patients who had sustained one or more confirmed myocardial infarctions.[108] Three treatment regimens (high estrogen, low estrogen, and *d*-thyroxine) were discontinued early in the study because patients in these groups displayed adverse effects without increasing survival rates. Patients in the high-estrogen group had more serious, nonfatal cardiovascular events than the controls; the low-estrogen group had an increased incidence of thromboembolism; and the *d*-thyroxine group had a decreased survival rate, particularly among high risk patients. Patients receiving clofibrate or nicotinic acid had slight lowering of blood lipids (6.5 to 9.9 percent decrease in serum cholesterol), but neither group had an appreciable improvement in survival rate.[108] Diet modification was not emphasized to the participants in this study. It should be noted that all the patients in this study had advanced atherosclerosis evident by a myocardial infarction, and no conclusions can be made from this study regarding the efficacy of lipid-lowering therapy in preventing a first myocardial infarction in patients at high risk.

The data from the CDP also supported previous studies indicating that the adverse influence of serum cholesterol upon cardiovascular mortality was still apparent in men following myocardial infarction.[57] There is evidence suggesting that the progression of coronary atherosclerosis estimated by coronary angiography is also positively related to the plasma cholesterol concentration.[109]

Several other studies of clofibrate therapy in the secondary prevention of coronary heart disease in men and women have either failed to demonstrate a convincing reduction in mortality or have had serious weaknesses in the design of the study.[110,111]

The Aspirin Myocardial Infarction Study (AMIS) is an ongoing, double-blind, randomized study of approximately 4,200 men and women with documented myocardial infarction.[112] It will test the hypothesis that aspirin (1 g/day) decreases the mortality and the recurrence of myocardial infarction. An additional ongoing secondary prevention trial utilizes ileal bypass in patients with hypercholesterolemia and previous myocardial infarction.[113,114]

Animal experiments

A large number of animal experiments since 1910 has established that it is possible to produce atherosclerosis in most mammalian species by adequate elevation of serum cholesterol[115] (see Chap. 62B). These studies have also demonstrated significant differences in the susceptibility to experimental atherosclerosis between different species and between individual members of the same species. The very strong accelerating influence of hypertension upon atherosclerosis has been readily demonstrated in experimental animals, but only in the presence of an elevated serum cholesterol concentration. Recent studies have demonstrated significant regression of atherosclerotic lesions in several species, including primates.[4,7,16,19,43,116–125a] This regression has included not only the lipid components of the atherosclerotic lesion but also some regression of the accumulated collagen and calcium (see also Chap. 62B). Even though animal studies may not be entirely applicable to human beings, no information has been collected in animals that would contradict the hypothesis that the atherosclerotic process can be influenced negatively by the presence and severity of the recognized major risk factors and positively by the removal or correction of the same factors.

ALGORITHM FOR THE RECOGNITION, DIAGNOSIS, AND MANAGEMENT OF PATIENTS AT RISK FOR CAHD

Figure 62H-1 shows how clinical information on a patient or relative can be channeled into a management algorithm. This offers a simple and practical way to direct the physician through his task of identifying patients at risk, determining the severity of the risk, and selecting the appropriate management measures. This algorithm should be utilized with specific sections of this chapter as indicated.

EVALUATION OF MAJOR RISK FACTORS: PROGRESSION FROM THE OPTIMAL TO THE ABNORMAL

Introduction

One of the more difficult problems in medicine is the definition of *normality* or *desirable limits* for a given population. This is particularly difficult for the United States population in which conditions such as coronary atherosclerosis, dietary hypercholesterolemia, and obesity are common and thus contribute to the "average" values for that population.

The problem of defining normality, which implies a clear-cut separation of *normal* from *abnormal*, is compounded by the observation that, for many risk factors, the relationship between the level of parameter measured (e.g., cholesterol, blood pressure) and the CAHD risk is a continuous one and that no meaningful cutoff points can be established. On the basis of epidemiologic and experimental evidence reviewed earlier in this chapter and in Chap. 62B, it is possible to indicate three stages or ranges for many parameters which could provide a practical means of relating the abnormal levels to the CAHD risk. A first stage is the physiologically "optimal" or "desirable" level; a second stage includes "suspicious" and "possible abnormal" values; and a third stage which many experts would consider to be definitely abnormal and to contribute to the pathogenesis of CAHD. It is our contention and that of some epidemiologists that, even though values in the second range or stage may be quite common in a given population, these values may already provide an added risk of CAHD, both by themselves and particularly in association with other risk factors (e.g., cholesterol of 260 mg/dl and diastolic blood pressure of 105).

Plasma lipids

Table 62H-1 presents three ranges for plasma cholesterol and triglyceride concentrations. The first range is that which would be physiologically "optimal" or "desirable" on the basis of epidemiologic and experimental data (even though it might be somewhat difficult for some individuals to achieve at present); the second range, which identifies values considered suspicious and possibly abnormal; and the third range, which is considered to be definitely abnormal and usually requires treatment, particularly in younger patients. It appears likely that future studies may provide confirmation that the upper level of desirable or optimal serum cholesterol is about 180 to 190 mg/dl for all ages.

Blood pressure

For a more detailed discussion, see Chaps. 64 to 73. For present purposes the limits for blood pressure at rest in Table 62H-2 may be used.

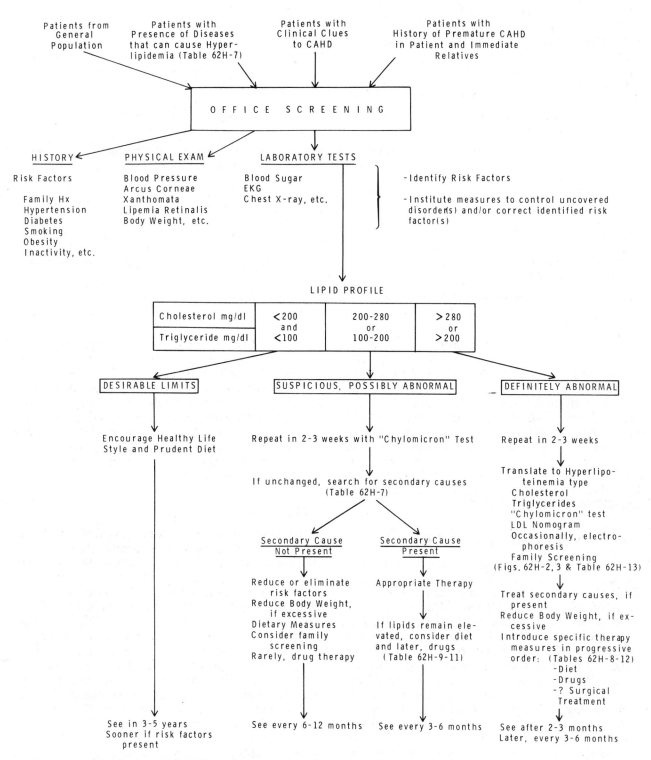

FIGURE 62H-1 Showing how clinical information on a patient or relative can be channeled into an algorithm. This offers a simple and practical way to direct the physician through his task of identifying patients at risk, determining the severity of the risk, and selecting the appropriate management measures.

Smoking

Smoking, of any type and to any degree, should be considered abnormal. It should be noted that cigarette smoking appears to be associated with greater morbidity and mortality than either cigar smoking or pipe smoking.[126–131] There is evidence that those who discontinue smoking have decreased risk of developing coronary heart disease if this change occurs before age 65.[132]

Diabetes

Carbohydrate intolerance (e.g., a fasting plasma glucose exceeding 130 mg/dl, or an inability to handle normally a glucose load reflected in elevated blood glucose levels at 1, 2, or 3 h, of >195, >140, or >130

TABLE 62H-1
Plasma cholesterol and triglyceride levels

	Plasma cholesterol level, mg/dl*			Plasma triglyceride level, mg/dl		
	Desirable or optimal	Possibly abnormal	Abnormal	Desirable or optimal	Possibly abnormal	Abnormal
Men						
Age: 20–40	140–200	200–260	> 260	10–100	100–200	> 200
40–60	150–200	200–270	> 270	20–120	120–220	> 220
60+	150-200	200–280	> 280	30–140	130–240	> 240
Women						
Age: 20–40	140–200	200–260	> 260	10–100	100–200	> 200
40–60	160–200	200–280	> 280	20–120	120–220	> 220
60+	160–200	200–300	> 300	30–140	130–240	> 240

*Cholesterol mol wt = 386.66: 100 mg/dl = 2.59 mmol/liter, 200 mg/dl = 5.17 mmol/liter, 300 mg/dl = 7.76 mmol/liter, 400 mg/dl = 10.35 mmol/liter.

mg/dl, respectively) can be considered evidence of diabetes mellitus.[133] The strong association of diabetes mellitus with the acceleration of atherosclerosis in the coronary, cerebral, and peripheral vessels has been recognized for many years, although the precise mechanisms responsible are not known. A possible link is the level of blood lipids which are frequently elevated in diabetes mellitus. The obesity that frequently precedes and accompanies maturity-onset diabetes may also be a contributing factor, since elevation of plasma lipids and hypertension are frequently concomitants of obesity.

Body weight, body build

The Metropolitan Life Insurance Company has provided tabular material (Table 62H-3) which indicates desirable body weights for adult men and women 25 years of age or older.[134] These tables were derived from observations linking body weights to the *least* degree of morbidity and mortality. Allowance is introduced for body frame (small, medium, and large), although a precise definition of body frame is lacking. In recent years, it has been recognized that body weight may give an incomplete measure of body fatness. Ideally, measurements of skin-fold thickness[135] with standard calipers should be made to provide a simple and reliable estimate of body fat percentage in men and women. Such measurements can be obtained in a few minutes by a physician's assistant. Clinically, obesity has often been defined as body weight exceeding 120 percent of desirable weight.[136] Definition of obesity by skin-fold thickness in excess of "normal" values[137] has the added advantage of separating overweight individuals from obese ones. When measurement of body fatness becomes more readily available, it may be possible to further refine the criteria of obesity (e.g., body fat exceeding 20 to 22 percent of total body weight in men and 30 to 32 percent in women).

Diet

A definition of *desirable* diet is very difficult in view of incomplete information, personal preferences, and the infinite variety of food types available. Desirable elements of a general diet can be summarized as follows: (1) adjustment of total calories to achieve and maintain ideal body weight; (2) limitation in fat to < 35 percent of total calories; (3) limited use of refined sugar with greater use of complex natural carbohydrates; (4) avoidance of excessive salt intake (e.g., > 6 g/day); (5) greater use of fish, poultry, vegetables, grains, legumes, cereals, and fruit; (6) variable composition to assure introduction of essential components and vitamins; and (7) for most individuals, some limitation of cholesterol intake, i.e., no more than an average of 300 mg/day. For most patients, who do not have a specific type of hyperlipoproteinemia as usually defined, it is better to emphasize an alteration in *general* eating habits rather than the necessity for adhering to a specific diet.[138]

Physical activity

Daily physical work and physical activity vary considerably from one individual to the next. It is recognized, however, that modern affluence and life-style in the United States have reduced the average level of exercise in daily activities. This may have contributed to the increasing prevalence of obesity. A minimum desirable level of physical activ-

TABLE 62H-2
Blood pressure limits

	Desirable	Possibly abnormal	Abnormal
Men			
Systolic	110–135	135-160	> 160
Diastolic	60–85	85–95	> 95
Women			
Systolic	110–130	130–150	> 150
Diastolic	55–80	80–95	> 95

TABLE 62H-3
Desirable (not "average" or "standard") weights

For men 25 years of age or older

Height (with shoes, 1-in. heels)		Weight in pounds (as ordinarily dressed)		
		Small frame	Medium frame	Large frame
Feet	Inches			
5	2	112–120	118–129	126–141
5	3	115–123	121–133	129–144
5	4	118–126	124–136	132–148
5	5	121–129	127–139	135–152
5	6	124–133	130–143	138–156
5	7	128–137	134–147	142–161
5	8	132–141	138–152	147–166
5	9	136–145	142–156	151–170
5	10	140–150	146–160	155–174
5	11	144–154	150–165	159–179
6	0	148–158	154–170	164–184
6	1	152–162	158–175	168–189
6	2	156–167	162–180	173–194
6	3	160–171	167–185	178–199
6	4	164–175	172–190	182–204

For women 25 years of age or older

Height (with shoes, 2-in. heels)		Weight in pounds (as ordinarily dressed)		
		Small frame	Medium frame	Large frame
Feet	Inches			
4	10	92–98	96–107	104–119
4	11	94–101	98–110	106–122
5	0	96–104	101–113	109–125
5	1	99–107	104–116	112–128
5	2	102–110	107–119	115–131
5	3	105–113	110–122	118–134
5	4	108–116	113–126	121–138
5	5	111–119	116–130	125–142
5	6	114–123	120–135	129–146
5	7	118–127	124–139	133–150
5	8	122–131	128–143	137–154
5	9	126–135	132–147	141–158
5	10	130–140	136–151	145–163
5	11	134–144	140–155	149–168
6	0	138–148	144–159	153–173

SOURCE: *Metropolitan Life Insurance Company, Statistical Bulletin, 40:11–12, 1959.

ity for persons with no heart disease can be defined as active participation in a relaxed environment, in one or more forms of exercise, for a minimal duration of about 30 min, three to five times a week, of sufficient exertion to increase the pulse rate by approximately 30 to 50 beats per minute. Walking at a fast pace, jogging, bicycle riding, tennis, gymnastics, and swimming are all good examples of enjoyable activities that can provide a good level of physical work. It should be emphasized that moderate, regular exercise may produce a feeling of well-being and may improve exercise tolerance in addition to helping maintain proper body weight. To date, however, there are inadequate data to support other beneficial claims of exercise programs, either in primary pre-

vention or in secondary prevention for patients with known coronary artery disease.

RECOMMENDED OFFICE SCREENING TO DETECT ABNORMALITIES RELATED TO CAHD

This section is not intended to provide complete recommendations as to which individuals in the general population should be seen in the doctor's office or how frequently they should be seen or which elements of the complete history, physical examination, and laboratory tests should be collected. Rather, this section intends to emphasize important clues to abnormalities, related to presence of risk factors and atherosclerotic cardiovascular disease, that can be detected in the office of a physician alert to subtle manifestations of the atherosclerotic process and interested in the preventive aspects of treatment for this disease. In this manner, patients and offspring of patients with CAHD or at serious risk for CAHD may be identified and therapeutic measures initiated, if appropriate. Other essential aspects of the physician's office screening not related to coronary atherosclerosis will not be mentioned.

History

All patients seen in the physician's office should be questioned about a family history of premature CAHD (e.g., immediate relatives having suffered from myocardial infarction or angina pectoris prior to age 55 to 60; age and cause of death of parents, parents' siblings and grandparents, etc.). A family history of hypertension, diabetes mellitus, thyroid disorders, renal diseases, and hematologic diseases should be sought. Similarly, elements of the patient's life-style (diet, activity, stress, smoking habits, weight history) should be collected. It is particularly important to screen family members of patients with type II hyperlipoproteinemia or manifest coronary artery disease prior to age 60[142] for clinical clues of lipid disorders, such as abdominal pain, arcus corneae, lipemia retinalis, xanthelasma or xanthomata, etc. (see Chap. 12).

In women, the use of oral contraceptives should be recorded, together with possible side effects. Since oral contraceptives are associated with an increased risk of myocardial infarction[139–139b] (see Chap. 62B) and hypertension, they should not be used in patients with a positive family history, with hypertension or other major risk factors, or in patients over 40 years of age.

Physical examination

The general physical examination should include the following elements: measurements of patient's height and weight (ideally, with measurement of skin-fold thickness in four locations); measurement of blood pressure (initially in both arms and, if blood pressure is elevated, in at least one leg) both in sitting and standing positions; search for xanthelasma, xanthomata (tendinous, tuberous, palmar, eruptive), and arcus corneae; funduscopic examination for evidence of hypertensive retinopathy, diabetes mellitus, or lipemia retinalis; and routine complete cardiovascular examination (see Chaps. 13 to 20).

Routine laboratory tests

The laboratory evaluation of a new patient being screened for risk factors associated with coronary atherosclerosis includes the following: urinalysis, hematocrit, white blood cell count, fasting blood sugar, creatinine, uric acid, plasma cholesterol (C) and triglyceride (TG). If the plasma appears "milky" or lipemic, an aliquot is stored in the refrigerator (at 4°C) for 12 to 24 h and observed for layering of lipid ("chylomicron test").

Blood samples for lipid analysis should be obtained under standard conditions, as noted in Table 62H-4: habitual diet, steady weight, 14 to 16 h fasting, free from acute stress or infection, and at least 3 months following acute myocardial infarction. If a test is abnormal, it should be repeated in 1 to 3 weeks. If there is no family history of CAHD, we recommend measurement of these lipid levels at about age 10 to 15 years and approximately every 5 years afterwards. If there is a family history of premature coronary heart disease, it would be reasonable initially to screen the children between 1 and 4 years of age. If the family history is suggestive for type II hyperlipoproteinemia, however, C and TG should be measured as soon as possible after birth and about every 6 to 12 months thereafter.[140–142] It should be noted that the plasma cholesterol may decrease up to 9 percent after 30 min recumbancy due to hemodilution[143] and that the plasma cholesterol tends to decrease in summer and to rise in winter.[134] Several autonomic drugs may produce neurogenic hypercholesterolemia.[144]

A chest roentgenogram (posteroanterior and lateral) should be obtained every 5 years and more often if there is a history of smoking. We recommend that an electrocardiogram be obtained by at least 40 years of age and repeated every 5 years if patient is asymptomatic for CAHD and if no obvious risk

TABLE 62H-4
Recommended conditions for screening for hyperlipidemia

1. Habitual diet
2. Steady weight
3. 14- to 16-h fast prior to sampling
4. No acute illness or stress—sample at least 3 months after acute myocardial infarction
5. No lipid-influencing drugs (except insulin in patients with diabetes mellitus)
6. No alcoholic beverages for 48 h.

factors exist. If a considerable number of risk factors are present and/or the patient is symptomatic, an electrocardiogram should be obtained at least every 2 to 3 years. In patients with homozygous type II hyperlipoproteinemia or familial hypercholesterolemia, it would be well to obtain a base line electrocardiogram at whatever age the condition is identified and every 2 years thereafter.

It should be emphasized that these are subjective impressions of what would be both feasible and effective in detecting individuals at increased risk. Such guidelines must be modified appropriately by the individual physician for his patients and practice.

Special laboratory tests

The great majority of patients with elevated cholesterol and/or triglyceride levels do not require lipoprotein electrophoresis.[145,249] In general, we would perform this test only if there is a strong suspicion of a familial hyperlipidemia or if secondary causes of hyperlipidemia are ruled out, and if, on repeated measurements, the plasma cholesterol level is over 280 mg/dl and/or the plasma triglyceride level is over 200 mg/dl. Even then, most patients can be well managed and followed without necessarily obtaining lipoprotein electrophoresis. Special ultracentrifuge studies are usually reserved for the unusual patient with type III hyperlipoproteinemia.

There is increasing evidence suggesting that elevated levels of high-density lipoproteins (HDL) may protect against the development of atherosclerosis,[43,146–146d] and some workers have advocated its routine measurement.[56] As yet, measurement of HDL is not widely utilized, and there are not adequate data to recommend it routinely, although it would appear to be very useful.

CLASSIFICATION OF HYPERLIPOPROTEINEMIAS[13,18,29,45,147–160]

The classification of disorders of lipid metabolism proposed by Fredrickson and Lees[147] based on the lipoprotein electrophoretic pattern has been widely accepted. According to this classification, depicted in Fig. 62H-2, one normal and at least five distinctly abnormal patterns can be seen. Normal subjects who have fasted for at least 14 h have both α- and β-lipoprotein bands. At times a faint pre-β band is present, but chylomicra are absent. Each of the five major lipoprotein phenotypes can occur as a primary disorder (either familial or sporadic) or secondary to other disorders, as noted below.

Type I hyperlipoproteinemia is characterized by an increased level of chylomicra even though the patient has not ingested food for at least 14 h. This form of exogenous hypertriglyceridemia is due to reduced lipoprotein lipase activity. This rare condition is usually familial and is easily recognized if fasting plasma is examined. It is rapidly corrected by a reduction of the dietary fat content.

Type II hyperlipoproteinemia is characterized by an increase in β-lipoproteins (low-density lipopro-

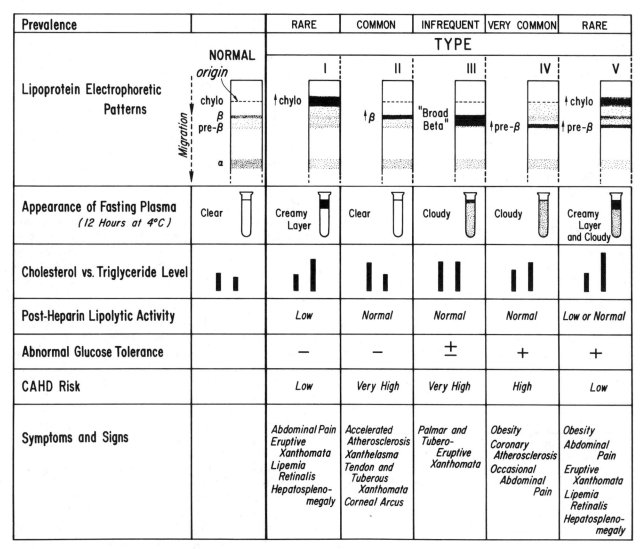

Prevalence			RARE	COMMON	INFREQUENT	VERY COMMON	RARE
			TYPE				
Lipoprotein Electrophoretic Patterns	NORMAL		I	II	III	IV	V
	↑chylo		↑chylo	↑β	"Broad Beta"	↑pre-β	↑chylo ↑pre-β
Appearance of Fasting Plasma (12 Hours at 4°C)	Clear		Creamy Layer	Clear	Cloudy	Cloudy	Creamy Layer and Cloudy
Cholesterol vs. Triglyceride Level							
Post-Heparin Lipolytic Activity			Low	Normal	Normal	Normal	Low or Normal
Abnormal Glucose Tolerance			−	−	±	+	+
CAHD Risk			Low	Very High	Very High	High	Low
Symptoms and Signs			Abdominal Pain Eruptive Xanthomata Lipemia Retinalis Hepatospleno-megaly	Accelerated Atherosclerosis Xanthelasma Tendon and Tuberous Xanthomata Corneal Arcus	Palmar and Tubero-Eruptive Xanthomata	Obesity Coronary Atherosclerosis Occasional Abdominal Pain	Obesity Abdominal Pain Eruptive Xanthomata Lipemia Retinalis Hepatospleno-megaly

FIGURE 62H-2 Chart of the principal laboratory and clinical characteristics of the five major types of hyperlipoproteinemias. See text for details.

teins, LDL) clearly visible on electrophoresis. Since LDL carry both cholesterol and, to a lesser degree, triglyceride, there is usually a marked elevation of plasma cholesterol and a modest elevation of plasma triglyceride. Type II has been subdivided into type IIa, in which the cholesterol level is elevated but the triglyceride level is normal, and type IIb, in which both lipid fractions are elevated.[154-157,159,160] Some investigators have considered this latter type an example of combined or mixed hyperlipoproteinemia. Type II hyperlipoproteinemia has been recognized in families, and the cord blood of afflicted newborn babies shows an elevated level of cholesterol.[29,45,148,159,161-167] Type II may also occur secondary to numerous other conditions, as noted in Table 62H-8.

Type III hyperlipoproteinemia is characterized by a "broad-β" band on electrophoresis[29,45,148,156,159,160,168-170] and marked elevation of both cholesterol and triglyceride. Precise identifica-

tion of this rare disorder may require ultracentrifuge studies (see below).

Type IV hyperlipoproteinemia, a very common form of hyperlipoproteinemia in the United States,[37,81,171-175] is characterized by an increase of very low-density lipoproteins (VLDL) or pre-β-lipoproteins. The VLDL originate in the liver and contain large quantities of endogenous triglyceride, which is largely derived from carbohydrate and free fatty acid (FFA) precursors. The secondary form of type IV is found in patients with many other conditions listed below. Frequently, no external manifestations of the hypertriglyceridemia are present. Since ingestion of large amounts of carbohydrate can lead over a period of time to a transient increase in synthesis and release of VLDL, the disorder has in the past been referred to as carbohydrate-induced hypertriglyceridemia.[176] It has to be noted, however, that in most individuals the rise in plasma triglyceride is of minor degree and is transient.

Type V hyperlipoproteinemia is characterized by marked elevations of chylomicra and VLDL. The secondary forms frequently present with abdominal pain, lipemia retinalis, and eruptive xanthomata in patients with uncontrolled diabetes mellitus, acute pancreatitis, nephrosis, or alcoholic liver disease (see below). An increased synthesis and release of VLDL is usually considered responsible for the type V pattern; lipoprotein lipase activity in these patients is relatively normal.[156]

GENERAL PREVENTIVE AND THERAPEUTIC MEASURES[18,29,41,45,148,156–160,177,178]

General principles

It is appropriate to propose general recommendations for the population at large. The recommendations that are listed in Table 62H-5 may contribute to the maintenance of health and, especially, cardiovascular health.

Ideally, each physician's office and each health clinic should be the source of health material regarding the maintenance of health and the prevention of disease, in addition to information about disease states. The local affiliates of the American Heart Association have extensive patient education materials (see below).

In most situations, patients should be educated to the extent considered appropriate by the physician and to the ability of patients to understand the nature of their health problems. Similarly, patients should be apprised, when appropriate, of the nature and significance of findings that indicate an increased likelihood of the development of CAHD in the future. At the same time the physician should consider all of the factors in Table 62H-6 in planning a program for each individual patient. For example, the finding of a serum cholesterol of 290 mg/dl and a history of heavy cigarette smoking in an intelligent 20-year-old male whose father died at age 43 of a myocardial infarction would usually indicate a different approach than the same blood chemistry found in a 73-year-old woman.

Each of the specific types of hyperlipoproteinemia can occur secondary to other primary medical disorders. These are listed below in Table 62H-8. In these patients, proper treatment should be at first directed

TABLE 62H-5
General health recommendations

---

1 Eat a prudent diet with caloric intake to achieve or maintain ideal body weight.
2 Avoid smoking.
3 Have a periodic measurement of blood pressure; control blood pressure, if necessary.
4 Have periodic health examinations, including screening for carbohydrate intolerance and hyperlipidemia. Treat, if appropriate.
5 Avoid excessive use of alcoholic beverages.
6 Participate in regular physical activity.

TABLE 62H-6
General considerations relative to possible therapeutic interventions

Patient age and sex
Family history of premature atherosclerosis, associated conditions, or risk factors
Concomitant diseases
Presence and severity of coronary atherosclerotic heart disease, cardiac status
Dietary habits: personal and family
Personal characteristics, personality, habits, emotional needs, life-style
Physical activity history and usual habits
Emotional support from family
Financial resources
Personal potential for education and cooperation
Availability of medical resources

at the primary disorder rather than at the hyperlipidemia. In patients who present with hyperlipidemia but do not have a recognized disease process, one should consider whether or not it is secondary to diet. Frequently, this can be determined only after a trial diet selected on the basis of the patient's plasma cholesterol and triglyceride levels. Attainment of proper weight may also be necessary. If the lipid disorder still persists, it would strongly suggest a primary hyperlipidemia. At this point, one should consider recommending that family members have measurements of their plasma lipid made under standard conditions. It should be kept in mind that some recent studies have suggested that an apparent single genetic trait for a specific hyperlipidemia may be expressed by different lipoprotein phenotypes in different family members[45,156,158–160,179–186] (see below and Table 62H-14).

It should be noted that correction of existing risk factors is indicated for the majority of patients for many other reasons in addition to atherosclerosis. Thus, there are many reasons to achieve and maintain ideal body weight, to correct hypertension, and to stop smoking (e.g., prevention of diabetes, lung cancer, etc.). In addition, the importance of a given risk factor is much greater if other concomitant risk factors are present. It is also apparent that the importance of all risk factors tends to decrease with age.

Diet therapy[29,41,45,109,148,156–160,177,187,188]

Dietary therapy is the keystone to the management of all types of hyperlipidemia. In virtually all patients, diet therapy should be utilized prior to drug therapy. A primary principle of diet therapy is the attainment and maintenance of ideal weight. A second important principle is to introduce qualitative changes. In general, drug therapy is reserved for patients who fail to respond satisfactorily to diet therapy (or patients with a very poor chance of having a good response to dietary therapy, i.e., type III hyperlipoproteinemia or homozygous type IIa hyperlipoproteinemia). Most patients respond better to diet therapy that is carried out as a combination of individual and group therapy and that includes frequent contact with a dietitian or nutritionist. Diet therapy is much less likely to be successful in patients with psychiatric disorders, alcoholism, or tobacco addiction.

GENERAL POPULATION

For the general population above infancy, we would recommend the following dietary guidelines, which are very similar to those of the American Heart Association[189] and of the Atherosclerosis Study Group of the Intersociety Commission for Heart Disease Resources:[16] calories sufficient to achieve and maintain weight close to ideal weight; restriction of total fats to less than 30 to 35 percent of total calories, with no more than about 10 percent from saturated fatty acids and about 10 percent from polyunsaturated fatty acids; average cholesterol intake limited to about 300 mg/day; decreased use of purified sugars and sweets (including bakery products, candy, other sweets, and beverages); increased use of poultry, fish, vegetables, legumes, cereals, whole grain breads, and fruits; limited intake of salt (< 6 g/day), and use of other condiments in its place; and ingestion of a wide variety of foods. We recognize, however, that there is controversy regarding general dietary recommendations, particularly in childhood.[103,190]

PATIENTS WITH HYPERLIPIDEMIA

In patients with hyperlipidemia, the determination of cholesterol and triglyceride levels is often sufficient to characterize the lipid disorder and to provide therapeutic guidelines. Occasionally, translation of hyperlipoproteinemic disorder (see also Figs. 62H-1 and 62H-2) is helpful to clarify the underlying pathophysiologic disorder. It may be possible to prescribe a diet for the specific hyperlipoproteinemia. A number of educational dietary guides for both general and specific types of hyperlipidemia are available from the local affiliates of the American Heart Association and from the National Heart and Lung Institute. Several of these are listed in Table 62H-7. A number of excellent cookbooks are also available.[191-195]

Drug therapy

As a general principle, drug therapy should not be initiated until an earnest trial with diet alone has been conducted. Drug therapy is necessary in most patients with type III hyperlipoproteinemia or homozygous type II hyperlipoproteinemia. In patients with type V or heterozygous type II, drug therapy may also be indicated if diet therapy is not satisfactory. In the frequent type IV hyperlipoproteinemia, however, it is not at all clear when it is appropriate to treat asymptomatic hypertriglyceridemia that fails to respond to diet therapy and weight reduction with a decrease in triglyceride concentration to desirable levels. It has been demonstrated that a very large majority of subjects with type IV hyperlipoproteinemia in a working population can be readily identified and effectively treated either in a clinic or by a private physician.[196] In general, the influence of elevated plasma triglyceride level upon the risk of developing coronary heart disease as an isolated

TABLE 62H-7
Dietary material

Local affiliates, American Heart Association:
 "Diet and Coronary Heart Disease" (EM 379)
 "Planning Fat-Controlled Meals for 1200–1800 Calories" (EM 288)
 "Planning Fat-Controlled Meals for 2000–2600 Calories" (EM 288A)
 "A Maximal Approach to the Dietary Treatment of the Hyperlipidemias" (EM 585)
 "Diet A: The Low Cholesterol (100 mg), Moderately Low Fat Diet" (EM 585A)
 "Diet B: The Low Cholesterol (200 mg), Moderately Low Fat Diet" (EM 585B)
 "Diet C: The Low Cholesterol, High Polyunsaturated Fat Diet" (EM 585C)
 "Diet D: The Extremely Low Fat Diet" (EM 585D)

Public Inquiries and Reports Branch, National Heart and Lung Institute, National Institutes of Health, Bethesda, Md.
 "The Dietary Management of Hyperlipoproteinemia: A Handbook for Physicians and Dieticians" (DHEW Pub. 73-110)
 "Diet 1 (Type I Hyperlipoproteinemia)" (DHEW Pub. 73-111)
 "Diet 2 (Type IIa Hyperlipoproteinemia)" (DHEW Pub. 73-112)
 "Diet 3 (Type III Hyperlipoproteinemia)" (DHEW Pub. 73-113)
 "Diet 4 (Type IV Hyperlipoproteinemia)" (DHEW Pub. 73-114)
 "Diet 5 (Type V Hyperlipoproteinemia)" (DHEW Pub. 73-115)

factor is controversial.[6,9,20,31,197] Most studies have concluded that the cholesterol level accounted for most of the increased risk,[3,6,8,10,15,19,45,256] although Carlson and Bottiger[198,252] found that the triglyceride level seemed to have an independent influence in older women. In view of the side effects of all drugs currently available, it is important to consider the cost-benefit/toxicity ratios carefully for each patient.

RECOGNITION, PATHOPHYSIOLOGY, AND TREATMENT OF SPECIFIC TYPES OF HYPERLIPIDEMIAS[29,45,65,96,97,142,148,149,156-160]

Introduction

Both the recognition and the classification of hyperlipidemia have undergone remarkable developments within the last two decades. In the next few years, there almost certainly will be newer, even more precise, techniques for the classification of hyperlipidemias. The introduction by Fredrickson and associates of the concept of classifying hyperlipidemias by specific lipoprotein phenotypes has been a major advance,[147-156] even though it was recognized from the beginning that some patients may not fit into one of the major phenotypes and that phenotypes in some patients may vary depending upon many variables, including their recent diet and weight change. Recently, it has been suggested that patients with hyperlipidemia may also be classified into specific categories of hyperlipidemia on the basis of combined genetic and biochemical considerations (see below).[179-186,199] The Fredrickson classification, however, remains a valid effort to foster dialogue and research in the field and is still widely used both for classification and for therapy of individual patients. Table 62H-8 lists the many causes of secondary hyperlipoproteinemia.

In general, the lipid abnormality can be recognized and managed satisfactorily in over 95 percent of patients on the basis of two base-line measurements of serum cholesterol and triglyceride without obtaining a lipoprotein electrophoresis.[29,145,150,159,249] In the majority of patients with types IIa, IIb, or IV hyperlipoproteinemia the effects of diet and drug therapy can also be satisfactorily followed by measurements of total cholesterol and triglyceride. LDL-cholesterol can be estimated from the nomogram in Fig. 62H-3. Some have recommended the routine measurement of high-density lipoproteins (HDL) by the relatively simple heparin-manganese precipitation technique.[56,200] Detailed studies of serum lipoproteins by electrophoresis or ultracentrifugation are currently reserved for selected patients with either plasma cholesterol or triglyceride levels that are "definitely abnormal" by Table 63H-1 or with findings suggestive of a type I, III, or V hyperlipoproteinemia that need to be further identified and documented.

Conversion of hyperlipidemia to hyperlipoproteinemia

For most patients, the serial determination of cholesterol (C) and triglyceride (TG) levels permits an initial accurate determination of the type of hyperlipoproteinemia which can be either primary or secondary. The following combinations are frequently encountered:

Elevated cholesterol but normal triglyceride is type IIa. There is no chylomicron layer in the plasma.

TABLE 62H-8

Secondary causes of hyperlipoproteinemias

Secondary type I
  Insulinopenic diabetes mellitus
  Dysglobulinemia
  Lupus erythematosus

Secondary type II
  Diet habitually high in cholesterol and saturated fatty acids
  Myxedema, hypothyroidism
  Nephrotic syndrome
  Dysgammaglobulinemia, multiple myeloma
  Obstructive liver disease
  Acute porphyria
  Androgenic steroids (high dosage)
  Ketogenic diet
  Autonomic drugs (mild)

Secondary type III
  Myxedema
  Dysgammaglobulinemia

Secondary type IV
  Obesity
  Excessive dietary alcohol without "alcoholism"
  Alcoholism
  Poorly controlled diabetes mellitus
  Oral contraceptives
  Estrogens
  Pregnancy
  Corticosteroids
  Stress
  Acute myocardial infarction (transient)
  Nephrotic syndrome
  Uremia
  Pancreatitis, usually alcoholic
  Hypothyroidism
  Dysproteinemias, lupus erythematosus
  Glycogen storage disease
  Storage diseases [Gaucher, Neimann-Pick, lecithin-cholesterol acyltranferase (LCAT) deficiency]

Secondary type V
  Alcoholism
  Poorly controlled diabetes mellitus, especially insulinopenic
  Oral contraceptives (in women with primary type IV)
  Estrogens (in women with primary type IV)
  Nephrotic syndrome
  Hypothyroidism (rare)
  Myeloma
  Dysproteinemias, lupus erythematosus
  Pancreatitis, usually alcoholic
  Glycogen storage disease

FIGURE 62H-3 Nomogram for the estimation of plasma low-density lipoprotein (LDL) concentration from the plasma concentrations of cholesterol (C) and triglyceride (TG). The nomogram is derived from the equation LDL = C − (TG/5 + HDL) (Friedwald, Levy, and Fredrickson[218]), in which HDL is assumed to be 45. A line connecting the known cholesterol (C) and triglyceride (TG) concentrations crosses the LDL line at the estimated concentration.

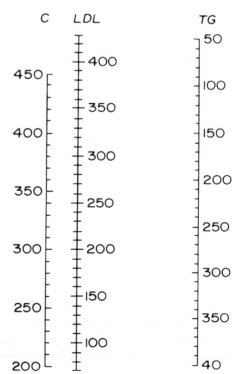

Elevated cholesterol, triglycerides 150 to 400 mg/dl usually signifies type IIb or IV. The nomogram in Fig. 62H-3 may be used to estimate LDL to separate these types. In general, LDL above 180 mean type II. In some instances, the distinction between types IIb and IV is not clear. The unusual type III may have similar C and TG levels but will usually have a slight creamy supernate due to chylomicra and often a broad, continuous β and pre-β band on electrophoresis. If type III is suspected on the basis of marked fluctuations in the C and TG levels from week to week that stay close to a 1:1 ratio, unusual palmar or elbow deposits, diabetes, or premature peripheral vascular disease, confirmatory analysis of lipoprotein composition should be performed by a special laboratory.

Elevated cholesterol, triglycerides 400 to 1,000 mg/dl usually signifies type IV or type V. The chylomicron test will reveal a creamy supernate in type V but not in type IV. Some type III patients may also present in this group.

Elevated cholesterol, triglycerides over 1,000 mg/dl usually signifies type V or type I. The chylomicron test in type V reveals a creamy layer over a turbid infranate, whereas the infranate is clear in the very rare type I. A lipoprotein lipase assay should be used to confirm type I, which is associated with severe deficiency of this enzyme.

Normal cholesterol, elevated triglyceride level usually signifies type IV, although rarely type III may be associated with this combination.

Incidence of abnormalities

As noted above, a plasma cholesterol concentration above the physiologic "optimal" or desirable upper level of 180 to 190 mg/dl is perhaps the most common type of secondary hyperlipoproteinemia, being presently found in a very high proportion of adults and even children in westernized, industrialized countries. It is probably due to excessive dietary intake of cholesterol and saturated fatty acids, although some genetic predisposition cannot be excluded.[3,6,20,27–31,34,41,51–55,87,159,201–203b] Of specific hyperlipoproteinemia phenotypes generally recognized, however, most frequent in the general population in the United States and Europe is usually said to be type IV or IIa and b.[23,25,31,34,37,38,50,51,55,81,171–175,204,205] Types I, III, and V are relatively rare. In a free-living population of nearly 1,000 men and women in California, type IV was the most frequent phenotype identified, being present in 13 percent of men and 4.8 percent of women. In contrast, type II was present in 4.6 percent of women and 2.8 percent of men.[174]

Lipid studies of patients with coronary atherosclerotic heart disease and of their families have indicated a significantly higher incidence (16 to 44 percent) of elevated plasma cholesterol and/or triglyceride levels, usually classified as type II or type IV.[34,165,171,172,179,181,183,204,206–216] Unfortunately, different studies have used different levels of cholesterol or triglyceride for classification, and it is not always possible accurately to determine the incidence of some of these disorders.

Type I hyperlipoproteinemia[29,45,156,217]

The primary form of this rare disorder of lipid metabolism, which is also known as *familial hyperchylomicronemia*, is usually inherited as a recessive trait. Secondary forms may occur in patients with insulinopenic diabetes, dysglobulinemia, or lupus erythematosus (Table 62H-8). The basic defect appears to be a deficiency of one of the lipoprotein lipase enzymes that results in an inability to clear the plasma of chylomicra which transport exogenous triglyceride from the intestines. Plasma triglyceride levels are markedly elevated while cholesterol levels are only slightly to moderately increased, and the triglyceride/cholesterol ratio may be from 10 to 20:1. When the blood sample is stored overnight at 4°C in a "chylomicron test," a creamy layer of chylomicra layers over a clear infranate.

Clinically, type I usually appears in childhood with recurrent episodes of abdominal pain, with or without pancreatitis. It is interesting that accelerated atherosclerosis is not a usual feature, although the patients develop eruptive xanthomata, lipemia retinalis, and hepatosplenomegaly (Table 62H-9).

DIET THERAPY
Total calories should be adjusted to achieve and maintain ideal weight. A low fat diet with no more than 20 percent of total calories from fat is recommended. Alcohol is generally not recommended, and average daily cholesterol intake should probably be limited to about 300 mg.

Type II hyperlipoproteinemia

There are two patterns of type II hyperlipoproteinemia: type IIa, which is characterized by an isolated elevation of LDL (reflected in an elevation of total plasma cholesterol), and type IIb, which is characterized by elevations of both LDL and VLDL (reflected in elevations of both plasma cholesterol and plasma triglyceride levels). Patients with primary familial type II hyperlipoproteinemia have plasma cholesterol levels that are often 300 to 600 mg/dl and have a high incidence of severe, premature coronary atherosclerosis.[165] As discussed under "Familial Hypercholesterolemia" below, it may be possible to diagnose genetic forms by the analysis of cord blood at the

TABLE 62H-9
Therapeutic regimen for type I hyperlipoproteinemia

1 Assess for secondary hyperlipidemia and treat the primary disease state (Table 62H-8).

2 Diet: Low fat (25–35 g/day in adults, 10–15 g/day in children); medium-chain triglycerides (MCT) may be added to make diet more palatable. Carbohydrates may be increased to maintain body weight.

3 Drugs: Currently available agents are not effective.

birth of children of a parent with known type II,[140–142,164] as well as later in life from family studies.[163–165]

In patients with elevation of both plasma cholesterol and triglyceride (so-called mixed hyperlipidemia), it may be necessary to quantify levels of LDL cholesterol in order to differentiate between types IIb, III, and IV. While LDL-cholesterol levels are best determined using an ultracentrifuge, they can be approximated using the Friedewald formula: LDL-cholesterol = total cholesterol − (triglyceride/5 + HDL-cholesterol).[218] This estimation is reasonably accurate when the triglyceride level is less than 400 mg/dl and requires only the additional measurement of HDL (high-density lipoprotein or α-lipoprotein) by heparin-manganese precipitation.[143,194] The formula is not accurate for the estimation of LDL when chylomicra are present or in type III, which requires both electrophoresis and ultracentrifugation studies for proper identification. If it is not possible to measure HDL, one may use an assumed level of 45 mg/dl and the nomogram in Fig. 62H-3 to obtain the LDL-cholesterol level. In general, increased VLDL levels produce plasma turbidity, whereas if only LDL is elevated, the infranate is clear.

Familial or primary type II hyperlipoproteinemia (see "Familial Hypercholesterolemia" below) is probably the most common of the currently recognized primary types of hyperlipoproteinemia. Secondary forms of type II may occur in patients with many conditions listed in Table 62H-8. A very frequent secondary form of type II hypercholesterolemia is seen in patients who habitually consume a diet high in cholesterol and saturated fatty acids. This variety of dietary, secondary hypercholesterolemia, which may cause the serum cholesterol to be only moderately elevated above "optimal levels" (and within many published ranges of "normal" plasma cholesterol), is probably very widespread in westernized, industrialized countries. The incidence of this form obviously varies with the plasma cholesterol level used to define "hypercholesterolemia." For example, if one uses the upper levels of "desirable or optimal" cholesterol in Table 62H-1, the frequency is much greater than if one used the upper level of the suspicious or "possibly abnormal" range. Although an arbitrary upper level that includes 95 percent of the population is sometimes used in clinical studies to define the upper limits of normal, such a level is obviously much too high if many subjects in the population under study have a form of dietary hypercholesterolemia.

Recent studies with cultured fibroblasts and other cells from patients homozygous for familial hypercholesterolemia (type II hyperlipoproteinemia) have revealed a defect in the capacity of cell surface receptors to bind LDL, whereas fibroblasts from heterozygous patients had a less marked reduction in receptor activity.[182–185,199,219] Since this receptor regulates cholesterol metabolism by suppressing cholesterol synthesis and increasing LDL degradation, the identification of this genetic regulatory defect may be important in the elucidation of pathogenetic mechanisms and in the design of corrective measures (see also Chaps. 52 and 62B).

Clinically, corneal arcus, xanthelasma, and xanthomata (usually tendinous in location) are seen. The high incidence of atherosclerosis in patients with type II hyperlipoproteinemia[165] has been attributed to the high cholesterol content and to the capacity of the excess plasma LDL to penetrate and accumulate in the arterial wall.

DIET THERAPY

Total calories should be adjusted to achieve and maintain ideal body weight, especially in type IIb. Cholesterol intake should be as low as possible and definitely less than 300 mg/day. Total calories from fat should be less than 40 to 45 percent of total daily calories, and polyunsaturated fats should be used in preference to saturated fats. Carbohydrate intake is not restricted except to control calories, but the intake of purified sugars and concentrated sweets should be decreased, especially in type IIb. Protein intake is not limited except as a source of cholesterol; egg yolks are not allowed. Alcohol may be used only with discretion (Table 62H-10).

DRUG THERAPY

Most patients with secondary type II hyperlipoproteinemia due to diet have a substantial decrease (approximately 15 to 25 percent) in plasma cholesterol after 8 to 12 weeks of a diet low in cholesterol (< 300 mg/day) and with a ratio of at least 2:1 in the relative amounts of polyunsaturated and saturated fatty acids. If the response is not satisfactory, however, one may consider drug therapy.

In patients with heterozygous or homozygous type IIa and IIb (or familial hypercholesterolemia), the response to diet therapy is seldom adequate by itself. In these patients, one should usually institute therapy with cholestyramine.[220] The initial dose of 16 mg/day is increased by 4 g each month, until a daily dose of 32 g/day is reached. Most patients find it easier to take two to four divided doses. Some patients with familial homozygous type II have a further decrease in plasma cholesterol if nicotinic acid is given in addition to cholestyramine.[29,156,159,160,221–225] Some investigators have used cholestyramine in combination with clofibrate, sitosterol, or neomycin, but the results to date are too limited to make recommenda-

TABLE 62H-10
Therapeutic regimen for type II hyperlipoproteinemia

1 Assess for secondary hyperlipidemia and treat the primary disease state (Table 62H-8).

2 Diet: Calories to achieve and maintain ideal weight; low cholesterol (< 300 mg/day); fats, reduced intake of saturated fatty acids, increased intake of polyunsaturated fatty acids; alcohol with discretion.

3 Drugs: Most primary and some secondary types require drug supplement to normalize LDL cholesterol:

  a Cholestyramine (Questran), 12–32 g/day.

  b Clofibrate (Atromid-S), 1–2 g/day, useful adjunct with cholestyramine in type IIb patients with elevated triglyceride level.

  c Nicotinic acid, 3 to 9 g/day, useful adjunct with cholestyramine, especially in type IIb.

tions.[226] Preliminary results of therapy with colestipol[227] or para-aminosalicylic acid[228] have been moderately encouraging. Patients receiving digitalis or other drugs that may be affected in their absorption by cholestyramine should be instructed to ingest these drugs 1 to 2 h prior to the ingestion of the cholestyramine.

In infants of parents with primary type II hyperlipoproteinemia who are identified as having familial hypercholesterolemia, it is uncertain at present how early to begin therapy and how strict the dietary recommendations should be. Some of the concerns are that the long-term effects of cholesterol restriction and of an increase in polyunsaturated fatty acids begun in infancy are unknown, that there is a very remote chance that moderate exogenous cholesterol is necessary for proper myelin formation in the central nervous system, or that early cholesterol feeding may be necessary to induce cholesterol catabolic enzyme systems. To date none of these concerns are satisfactorily documented in human beings when the usual dietary recommendations have been followed. In general, however, neonates with familial hypercholesterolemia can be maintained at relatively normal plasma cholesterol levels with moderate reduction of intake of cholesterol and saturated fat.[202,229,230] Over the age of 2 years, the diet should contain less than 200 mg cholesterol per day with a ratio of polyunsaturated to saturated fat of 0.9:1. Eggs are limited to one per week, and organ meats are eliminated. Foods rich in iron, such as lean meats, fruits, peas, beans, and iron-enriched bread and cereal, are encouraged. Milk with 2 percent butterfat is encouraged for calcium and vitamins A and D.[229]

In children at least 5 years of age, a modified NIH-NHLI type II diet is used. Cholesterol intake is limited to less than 200 mg/day, and saturated fat intake is decreased with elimination of egg yolks, organ meats, and dairy fat; fat-free milk is used, and fish and poultry are encouraged to reach a polyunsaturated/saturate ratio of 2:1. If the plasma cholesterol remains significantly elevated at 3 and 6 months, cholestyramine therapy in dosages appropriately related to the patient's weight, given in three to four doses, should then be added,[202,230] together with multivitamin supplementation.

Treatment of children with type IIb phenotype and familial hypercholesterolemia should be with the same diet but with stricter control of body weight and carbohydrate intake, particularly purified sugars.[202,230] Long-term drug therapy with clofibrate or nicotinic acid in children should be reserved for the most extreme cases.

EXPERIMENTAL PROCEDURES IN THE MANAGEMENT OF TYPE II HYPERLIPOPROTEINEMIA

Partial ileal bypass[113,114,231–237] Ileal bypass has produced a decrease in plasma cholesterol (41 percent) in patients with type II, as well as types III and IV. The results in patients with homozygous type II were less dramatic. It can also produce transient diarrhea, weight loss, and vitamin deficiency. At present, ileal bypass should probably be reserved for patients with type II who are unable to adhere to proper dietary and drug regimens.

Portacaval shunt[238–242] Portacaval shunt has been utilized in only a few patients to date. In one 12-year-old girl it resulted in a marked decrease in plasma cholesterol with improvement in angina pectoris and congestive heart failure. There also appeared to be some regression of the coronary artery obstruction on repeat coronary angiography.[238] Portacaval shunt is considered experimental at present and is perhaps best restricted to patients with severe homozygous familial hypercholesterolemia or type IIa hyperlipoproteinemia.

Plasma exchange[243–245] To date, only a few patients with familial hypercholesterolemia with a type IIa hyperlipoproteinemia pattern have been treated by plasma exchange, which is a relatively simple procedure but which requires periodic repetition. It does produce a prompt decrease in plasma cholesterol levels. It may hold promise for some patients with type II hyperlipidemia, particularly those who are homozygous. A similar technique that employs affinity chromatography has been used in two patients and has the advantage of avoiding homologous plasma transfusions.[246]

Type III hyperlipoproteinemia

Type III hyperlipoproteinemia (or broad-β disease) is characterized by elevation of plasma levels of both cholesterol and triglyceride and by a "floating-β lipoprotein" on electrophoresis. Often, there is an increase in plasma chylomicra. The VLDL in type III may have a characteristic abnormally low triglyceride/cholesterol ratio of 1:1. The diagnosis can be confirmed by ultracentrifugation studies. The demonstration of floating-β lipoprotein in the D (density) < 1.006 fraction is strongly suggestive, but the diagnosis is best confirmed by the ratio of VLDL-cholesterol to the plasma triglyceride concentration ($C_{VLDL}/TG = r$). When the TG concentration is between 150 and 1,000 mg/dl, an r value not less than 0.25 is suggestive and an r value not less than 0.30 is diagnostic.[170,247–249]

Type III hyperlipoproteinemia is almost always familial, unlike the more common types II, IV, and V. Type III can be inherited as either an autosomal recessive or autosomal dominant trait; type IV, however, is frequent in family members. Secondary type III can also occur (Table 62H-8). The primary, familial type III usually appears in the second or third decade in men and about 10 to 15 years later in women. The finding of orange-yellow xanthomatosis in the palmar creases (xanthoma striatum palmaris) is nearly pathognomonic, and there may also be eruptive xanthomatosis, tuberous xanthoma, or tendon xanthomata. Many type III patients tend to be obese and to have glucose intolerance. There is a very strong association between type III and severe cardiovascular, cerebrovascular, and peripheral vascular disease.[170,247-249] On the other hand, the response and apparent regression of lesions is perhaps more dramatic with type III than most other types.[250] The biochemical defect is not clear, but may be either a failure of conversion of VLDL to LDL or an overproduction of VLDL.

DIET THERAPY

The total caloric intake should be adjusted to achieve and maintain ideal body weight. The recommended calorie distribution is as follows: protein, 20 percent; carbohydrate, 40 percent (most purified sugars and concentrated sweets are eliminated); and fat, 40 percent (approximately 10 percent polyunsaturated, 20 percent monosaturated, and 10 percent saturated fatty acids). Average daily cholesterol intake should be less than 300 mg, and alcohol is limited to two servings, substituted for carbohydrate calories (Table 62H-11).

DRUG THERAPY

The combination of ideal weight, diet therapy, and clofibrate is very effective.[223] Nicotinic acid used in place of clofibrate is also effective, but it usually has more side effects.

Type IV hyperlipoproteinemia

The characteristic lipid abnormality in type IV is an increase in plasma triglyceride and VLDL-cholesterol levels. The total plasma cholesterol concentration is usually found to be epidemiologically "normal" or only moderately elevated. If determined (or estimated from the nomogram in Fig. 62H-3), plasma LDL-cholesterol is usually normal (< 170 mg/dl) and there is no floating LDL. Type V is similar to type IV except for the additional presence of elevated chylomicra, which represent dietary or exogenous triglycerides. In some patients, a type IV pattern can be converted to a type V pattern by a succession of high fat meals, poorly controlled diabetes mellitus, alcoholic excess, oral contraceptives, or estrogens.[159]

TABLE 62H-11

Therapeutic regimen for type III hyperlipoproteinemia

1 Assess for secondary hyperlipidemia and treat the primary disease state (Table 62H-8).

2 Diet: Calories to achieve and maintain ideal weight; cholesterol (< 300 mg/day); fat, 40% of total calories (polyunsaturated fatty acids in preference to saturated fatty acids); carbohydrates, 40% of total calories (eliminate most concentrated sugars and sweets); protein, 20% of total calories (limited to saturated fat and cholesterol); alcohol moderately restricted (maximum of two servings per day).

3 Drugs:

  a Clofibrate (Atromid-S), 2 g/day.

  b Nicotinic acid, 3 to 9 g/day.

Secondary type IV is currently considered to be one of the more common lipid abnormalities in the United States.[171] Both types IV and V can occur secondary to a wide variety of diseases, drugs, and dietary habits.[159] The more frequently recognized causes of secondary type IV and type V are listed in Table 62H-8. Since plasma triglycerides may fall acutely during weight and calorie reduction, it is important to obtain samples for diagnosis when the patient is consuming his habitual diet and his weight is steady. A type IV pattern shortly after acute myocardial infarction may not indicate a preexisting condition, since plasma triglycerides may be transiently elevated after acute myocardial infarction.[251] If indicated, resampling may be repeated at 3-month intervals after myocardial infarction to define any lipid abnormality. The diagnosis of primary familial type IV requires both the absence of disorders that can cause secondary hypertriglyceridemia (see Table 62H-8) and the study of blood lipids in family members.

Primary type IV (familial hyperpre-β-lipoproteinemia) has been ascribed to both overproduction and decreased rates of clearance of VLDL. It may occur in families with types I, II, and III;[156] and some families have both types IV and V.[160]

The clinical characteristics of type IV may at times not be evident, although there is often evidence of one of the conditions listed in Table 62H-8. Patients with familial type IV may have xanthelasma and rarely arcus corneae. If the VLDL level is markedly elevated, there may be eruptive xanthomata. Glucose intolerance is present in about half the patients with primary type IV, frequently in association with hyperuricemia. To date, there is no conclusive proof that isolated type IV is associated with premature atherosclerosis, although the data more and more strongly suggest that there may be an increased risk of developing coronary heart disease for these patients.[159,160,175,252,253]

DIET THERAPY

Weight control is the keystone of diet therapy in type IV.[196] Patients should be placed on a reducing diet to achieve ideal body weight, which should then be maintained. Carbohydrates should be limited to 40 to 45 percent of total calories. Purified sugars should be limited in preference to grains and complex carbohydrates. Total fat is limited primarily to control weight, and polyunsaturated fats are to be preferred to saturated fats. Cholesterol is moderately limited to an average of 300 mg/day. Protein intake is not limited, except for weight control and its content of saturated fat and cholesterol. Ideally, alcohol intake should be limited as much as possible.[254-256] Frequently, the hypertriglyceridemia will persist until the alcohol intake is markedly decreased. In patients with diabetes mellitus, it is particularly important to control blood sugar (Table 62H-12).

Patients with type IV hyperlipidemia may have an elevated plasma cholesterol, both before treatment and even after clofibrate therapy, which reduces triglyceride levels by increasing the catabolism of VLDL or very low-density (pre-β) lipoproteins to

Therapeutic regimen for type IV hyperlipoproteinemia

1 Assess for secondary hyperlipoproteinemia and treat the primary cause of disease state (see Table 62H-8).

2 Diet: Achieve and maintain ideal weight; carbohydrates, 40 to 45% of total calories (restrict purified sugars and sweets); fats, limited by weight control (polyunsaturated fatty acids preferred to saturated fatty acids); cholesterol moderately restricted (300 mg/day); alcohol, limited to two servings (may be necessary to eliminate).

3 Drugs:

   a Clofibrate (Atromid-S), 2 g/day.

   b Nicotinic acid, 3 to 9 g/day.

LDL or low-density (β) lipoproteins. This tendency toward an increase in cholesterol should be managed by greater restriction of cholesterol intake and restriction of saturated fatty acid intake.

DRUG THERAPY

Drug therapy should be used only after the effects of diet therapy have been monitored, and drug therapy should be used only *in addition* to diet therapy, not in place of diet therapy. The effects of each drug should be evaluated before another drug is used to supplement or replace the first drug. In general, chronic drug therapy is not indicated unless it can be documented that the drug produces a maintained decrease in the lipid level of at least 15 percent. All patients should be appropriately informed and followed regarding side effects and potential toxicity of the drug used.

If the plasma triglyceride level remains significantly elevated despite diet therapy, clofibrate (Atromid-S) from 1.5 to 2 g/day in divided doses may be considered.[196,257,258] Nicotinic acid, 3 to 9 g/day, can be used if clofibrate is not successful, but it is frequently associated with significant side effects (see below). Clofibrate therapy can lower plasma triglyceride level in patients with type IV who cannot or will not follow an appropriate diet, although such therapy is not recommended.[257]

Type V hyperlipoproteinemia

The relatively uncommon type V phenotype is characterized by a combined increase in chylomicra and in very low-density lipoproteins (VLDL). Plasma triglycerides are increased while plasma total cholesterol is normal or moderately elevated. After storage for 12 h at 4°C, the plasma has a characteristic creamy layer with turbid infranate due to the chylomicronemia. There is also an increased pre-β band on electrophoresis. The basic defect in lipid metabolism is uncertain, but lipoprotein lipase activity is usually less abnormal than in type I. It is currently thought to be transmitted as a dominant trait with either type IV or type V in affected family members.

The familial form most often appears in the second decade. There are many causes of the more common secondary form (Table 62H-9). In familial type V, especially with plasma triglyceride levels from 1,000 to 6,000 mg/dl, many clinical features resemble type I, including recurrent abdominal pain

and pancreatitis, eruptive xanthomata, lipemia retinalis, hepatosplenomegaly, and foam cells in the bone marrow. Patients with either type V or type IV frequently have hyperuricemia, gouty arthritis, or essential hypertension. Both type IV and type V may be exacerbated by dietary or alcoholic excesses, and some type IV patients may be transiently converted to type V.[158] Type V is not definitely associated with an increased risk of premature atherosclerotic heart disease.

DIET THERAPY

Total calories are restricted to achieve and maintain ideal body weight. Total fat is restricted to 30 percent of total calories, and saturated fat calories should be limited to 10 percent of total calories. Carbohydrate calories are limited to 50 percent of total calories, and purified or concentrated sweets are to be avoided. Alcohol is not recommended. Cholesterol intake is restricted to an average of 300 mg/day. Protein intake is limited only by the total calories allowed and the content of saturated fat and cholesterol. Unfortunately the diet, which is restricted in fat and carbohydrate but high in protein (NIH-NHLI type V diet), is relatively difficult to follow and somewhat expensive (Table 62H-13).

DRUG THERAPY

If plasma triglyceride levels cannot be reduced to normal by weight control and diet, the diet should be maintained and consideration given to the addition of nicotinic acid, 3 to 9 g/day, which is probably the most effective drug in type V, although it may exacerbate diabetes mellitus. Clofibrate, 1 g b.i.d., may also be tried, but is often of little benefit. In men unresponsive to either of these agents, one may consider the use of oxandrolone (Anavar), 7.5 mg/day, a synthetic anabolic steroid, whereas in women one may consider the use of the progestational agent, norethindrone acetate (Norlutate), 2.5 mg/day.[224,259,260] At present, the use of the latter two drugs in the treatment of patients with the type V phenotype is *not approved* by the Food and Drug Administration.

Therapeutic regimen for type V hyperlipoproteinemia

1 Assess for secondary hyperlipoproteinemia and treat primary cause of disease state (see Table 62H-8).

2 Diet: Achieve and maintain ideal body weight; fat restricted to 30% of total calories (polyunsaturated fatty acids preferred to saturated fatty acids); carbohydrates, 50% of total calories (purified sugars and concentrated sugars eliminated); protein intake, 20% of total calories; cholesterol moderately restricted (300 mg/day); alcohol not recommended.

3 Drugs:

   a Nicotinic acid, 3 to 9 g/day.

   b Clofibrate (Atromid-S), 2 g/day.

   c Oxandrolone (Anavar), 7.5 mg/day (men only).

   d Norethindrone acetate (Norlutate), 2.5 mg/day (women only).

COMBINED GENETIC AND BIOCHEMICAL CLASSIFICATION OF HYPERLIPIDEMIAS

Although the classification of hyperlipidemia based primarily on lipoprotein phenotyping has been widely adopted and is the most widely utilized throughout the world, it has also been proposed that the detailed study of lipid abnormalities within families permits a more accurate identification and classification of familial hyperlipidemias that differs somewhat from the usual classification. It should be kept in mind, however, that therapy is ordinarily selected on the basis of the cholesterol and triglyceride levels and of the lipoprotein pattern. In addition, the genetic classification (Table 62H-14) requires detailed study of family lipids, and this is seldom practical in clinical practice.

Goldstein et al.[179] studied 2,520 relatives and spouses of 176 survivors of myocardial infarction. They concluded that there are five distinct lipid disorders which they feel do not correspond exactly with the usual hyperlipoprotein phenotypes as proposed by Fredrickson. Of these, three disorders (*familial hypercholesterolemia, familial hypertriglyceridemia,* and *familial combined hyperlipidemia*), which occurred in 20 percent of survivors below 60 years of age and in 7 percent of older survivors, appeared to represent the dominant expression of three different and distinct autosomal gene mechanisms. The other two disorders (*polygenic hypercholesterolemia* and *sporadic hypertriglyceridemia*) each affected about 6 percent of survivors in both age groups. In their study, the most common genetic form of hyperlipidemia was the familial combined hyperlipidemia, in which both cholesterol and triglyceride were characteristically elevated, although frequently only one was elevated. These individuals may have any one of the following lipoprotein phenotypes: IIa, IIb, IV, and V. On the basis of their genetic and familial studies, Goldstein et al.[179] concluded that this disorder was distinct from both familial hypercholesterolemia (type II) or familial hypertriglyceridemia (type IV).

The three lipid disorders they defined and the estimates of frequency in the general population were as follows: familial hypercholesterolemia (0.1 to 0.2 percent), familial hypertriglyceridemia (0.2 to 0.3 percent), and familial combined hyperlipidemia (0.3 to 0.5 percent). The combined incidence of these three disorders in the general population is estimated at 0.6 to 1.0 percent. Since these estimates include a number of assumptions, however, they are minimal and probably too low.

Goldstein et al.[179] concluded that the general population without manifest coronary heart disease frequently possesses heterozygosity for one of the three lipid-elevating genes identified. They found that the most common types are probably the *polygenic* and *sporadic* forms of hyperlipidemia, which may affect as much as 4 percent of the population. This study and the studies of Rose et al.[180] emphasize the necessity for studying family members in many types of lipid disorders in order to determine accurately both the genetic and the biochemical expression of the various types of lipid disorders. In patients with apparent primary hyperlipoproteinemia, perhaps one-third will not have familial hyperlipidemia upon study of the immediate family; presumably, these patients have *sporadic hyperlipoproteinemia*, which can manifest itself with any of the common phenotypes.[156-160]

Familial hypercholesterolemia (FH)[184]

Familial hypercholesterolemia (FH), which is transmitted by an autosomal dominant gene, is one of several genetic causes of familial type IIa or IIb hyperlipoproteinemia, the others being familial combined hyperlipidemia (FCH) and polygenic hyper-

TABLE 62H-14
Genetic classification of hyperlipidemia

	Lipoprotein phenotype	Cholesterol	Triglyceride	LDL	Presumptive kinetic defect	Diagnostic criteria
Familial hyperchylomicronemia	I	Normal or high	Very high	Low	Impaired chlyomicron removal	Absent lipoprotein lipase
Familial hypercholesterolemia	IIa, IIb	High	Normal or high	High	Impaired LDL removal	Deficient LDL receptor
Polygenic hypercholesterolemia	IIa, IIb	High	Normal or high	High	Impaired LDL removal	Family data
Familial combined hyperlipidemia	IIa, IIb, IV, V	Normal or high	Normal or high	High	Unknown	Family data
Broad-β disease	III, IV	High	High	Normal	Faulty conversion of VLDL to LDL	Palmar xanthomata, VLDL analysis
Familial hypertriglyceridemia	IV, V	Normal	High	Normal	Impaired VLDL removal	Family data

cholesterolemia. In addition, dietary and nongenetic causes of type II hyperlipoproteinemia probably are very common.

Heterozygotes for FH have hypercholesterolemia at birth, but are usually asymptomatic until age 15 to 20 years when they begin to develop arcus corneae, tendinous xanthomata, or painful Achilles tendonitis. By the third decade, these are present in about one-half of heterozygotes. The mean age at onset of coronary heart disease is 43 years in men and 53 in women.[5,261] The plasma cholesterol is usually between 270 and 550 mg/dl and rarely over 600 mg/dl. In individuals without tendinous xanthomata, it is difficult to rule out other causes of elevated levels of LDL cholesterol.[179,209,211] It actually appears that most individuals with hypercholesterolemia and a type IIa and IIb lipoprotein pattern due to a familial form of hyperlipidemia do not have FH.[156,179,229,262]

Homozygotes for FH also have hypercholesterolemia at birth. By the age of 4, they all develop unique yellow-orange cutaneous xanthomata on the buttocks, in the creases of the hands, and over the kneecaps. They all also develop arcus corneae and tendinous xanthomata in childhood. The finding of profound hypercholesterolemia (650 to 1,000 mg/dl) in a nonjaundiced child is pathognomonic of this disorder. Death from myocardial infarction may occur as early as 18 months of age and very often occurs before 20 years of age. In addition to coronary, cerebral, and peripheral atherosclerosis, they may develop significant valvular and supravalvular aortic stenosis from xanthomatous infiltration.[263,264]

In contrast to the genes related to familial hypertriglyceridemia or familial combined hyperlipidemia, FH does not appear to predispose to carbohydrate intolerance, hyperuricemia, or obesity. Three studies of survivors of myocardial infarction suggest the frequency of FH to be 3 to 6 percent.[179,209,211] In London the hererozygote frequency was estimated to be 1 in 200;[262] and in North America the minimal frequency in Caucasians was 1 in 500.[179] The theoretical frequency of homozygotes in the general population in the United States has been estimated to be about 1 in 1 million (see also Chap. 52).

If a parent is known to carry the FH gene, it is possible to detect the children who are heterozygotes at birth;[141] on the other hand, the majority of newborns with hypercholesterolemia appear not to have FH.[140–142,162,164,166,167,265,266] In general, the earliest age at which FH heterozygotes can be accurately identified by routine screening of unselected infants is about 1 year; even then, a family analysis is necessary to determine that it is due to FH.[166,167,266] The cholesterol elevation in FH is localized to the LDL. The basic abnormality of FH appears to be an abnormality in a high-affinity cell surface receptor that binds LDL and mediates the feedback suppression of HMG CoA reductase and cholesterol synthesis.[267] Cholestyramine treatment markedly increases the excretion of bile acids, although there may be little change in the plasma level of cholesterol.[180,268] Several different groups concluded that combined hyperlipidemia was different from either familial hypercholesterolemia or familial hypertriglyceridemia[211,269,270] (see also Chap. 52).

Familial combined hyperlipidemia (FCH)

This condition is thought to be the most common cause of a familial elevation of the LDL-cholesterol level; and in patients with coronary heart disease, it is about three times more common than familial hypercholesterolemia. FCH is distinguished by the variability in expression of lipid levels among affected members of the same family.[181] Most patients with FCH have a type IIb phenotype with elevated of both LDL-cholesterol and VLDL-triglyceride levels; other patients within the family may have only an increased level of cholesterol (type IIa) or of triglyceride alone (type IV or V). Accordingly, in a patient with a type II lipoprotein pattern with tendinous xanthomata it may be difficult to distinguish between heterozygous familial hypercholesterolemia (FH) and the more common FCH. In general, heterozygotes with FH tend to have higher cholesterol levels (350 ± 40 mg/dl) than subjects with FCH (300 ± 40 mg/dl).

Familial hypertriglyceridemia

Primary familial hypertriglyceridemia is thought to be usually transmitted as a dominant gene but with delayed expression in childhood. Accordingly, it may be necessary to examine the plasma lipids of children of parents with primary hypertriglyceridemia (primary type IV) every 5 years up to the age of 30 to avoid overlooking the condition.[202,230,239,271] The *sine qua non* for management of familial hypertriglyceridemia, both in children and in adults, is weight reduction to ideal body weight and restriction of carbohydrate intake, with a sharp reduction in starches and elimination of sweets. Other dietary principles are noted above. In children, clofibrate and nicotinic acid should be used only in extreme, symptomatic hypertriglyceridemia.

Broad-β disease

This unusual condition is discussed above under "Type III Hyperlipoproteinemia."

Familial hyperchylomicronemia

This rare condition is discussed above under "Type I Hyperlipoproteinemia."

Treatment of specific genetic types of hyperlipoproteinemias

As noted above, diet is the basis for treatment for both familial and primary disorders of lipid metabolism.[187,188] A hypocaloric diet is necessary for patients with excessive body weight (and body fat), since at least a partial reduction in both cholesterol and triglyceride levels is achieved by the return of the body weight to desirable limits. As a rule, diet should be tried before any hypolipidemic drug is used. When the effect of the diet on lipid levels is unsatisfactory and drug therapy is introduced, dietary therapy should be continued in view of the additive effect of both diet and drugs.

The dietary instruction, prescribed by the physician or by a specialized dietitian or nutritionist, should be tailored to the type of lipid abnormality as classified above and to the individual patient's habits and needs.[187,188] Although adherence to the diet should be strict to provide the expected benefits, flexibility on the part of the physician or dietitian is necessary to allow palatability. Recognition of personal or ethnic preferences and periodic reinforcements are also necessary to maintain adherence. The National Heart and Lung Institute, Public Inquires and Reports Branch, National Institutes of Health, and the local affiliates of the American Heart Association have available on request a series of handbooks for both physicians and patients, containing dietary guidelines for specific types of hyperlipoproteinemias (Table 62H-7). In the future, it is probable that more general, widely applied dietary recommendations will be made that will combine several groups of patients.

PHARMACOLOGY OF DRUGS USED IN THE MANAGEMENT OF HYPERLIPIDEMIA[106,156–160,222–224,260,272–281]

Introduction

In the last decade, several powerful drugs have become available for use in the treatment of hyperlipoproteinemias. Since all of these agents possess sizable side effects, it is important to *reserve* the use of these drugs for those patients in whom dietary therapy has not produced the expected lowering of the lipid levels. *Hypolipidemic agents should be* introduced only after diet therapy has failed. Both diet and drugs should be continued concomitantly. Substitution of one drug for another or addition of a second drug should be made only when frequent blood lipid controls have determined that a given drug is ineffective, i.e., reduction in blood lipids of less than 15 percent after 6 to 8 weeks of drug treatment. There is little purpose in administering a drug unless a clear-cut benefit can be established after 6 to 8 weeks.

It has been recognized that certain hypolipidemic drugs appear more effective in certain types of lipid disorder. Examples of this are (1) the effect of clofibrate in type III hyperlipoproteinemia, and (2) the effect of cholestyramine in type II hypercholesterolemia. The effect of a given drug on a particular type of lipid disorder may be due to its mode of action (e.g., certain drugs restrict lipoprotein production whereas certain others increase lipoprotein re-

moval) and to the underlying pathologic disorder. The physician, however, after selecting the most appropriate drug and a suitable trial period for his patient, has to realize that at times his therapeutic strategy may require changing to another drug or adding another one to potentiate the hypolipidemic effect. In addition to the agents described below, other investigational drugs which may become available include inositol, lecithin, pyridinolcarbamate, and phosphatidylcholine. Very large doses of ascorbic acid and methionine have also been investigated.

Cholestyramine (Questran)

Cholestyramine resin is the quaternary ammonium chloride salt of a high-molecular weight copolymer composed of a 2 percent divinyl benzene skeleton. It is insoluble in water and nearly completely unabsorbed in the gastrointestinal tract. In the small intestine the chloride ion is exchanged for bile acids. The binding of bile acids interrupts the enterohepatic circulation and results in an increased conversion of cholesterol to bile acids and also in an increased synthesis of cholesterol. The plasma level of LDL decreases secondary to the increase in removal rate from the circulating plasma. The effects of cholestyramine upon plasma triglyceride are variable, and often the VLDL and LDL levels are found to be increased.[45,160]

INDICATIONS

Cholestyramine is indicated only for type II hyperlipoproteinemia, especially type IIa, in which there is elevation only of LDL (elevated plasma cholesterol, normal triglyceride).[282] Cholestyramine may cause the plasma cholesterol levels to rise in patients with hypercholesterolemia due to an increase in VLDL or IDL.

DOSAGE

The powdered resin is mixed with a liquid and taken orally. The 9 g packets contain 5 g of active drug. It is usually easiest to take when mixed with orange juice, grapefruit juice, lemonade, applesauce, puddings, gelatins, yogurt, or oatmeal. The initial dose of 16 g/day is slowly increased every 2 to 4 weeks to a maximum dose of 32 g/day. It may be taken in two, three, or four divided doses. In patients with type IIa hyperlipoproteinemia, cholestyramine usually lowers plasma cholesterol by 20 to 25 percent below the level achieved by diet.[222,283] In patients with homozygous type II hyperlipoproteinemia (homozygous familial hypercholesterolemia), the addition of nicotinic acid may at times be of benefit.[222]

SIDE EFFECTS

The major side effects of cholestyramine are gastrointestinal. Constipation is common in older patients, but can be alleviated with bran supplements or stool softeners. Nausea, vomiting, cramps, and abdominal distension may occur, but usually respond to an adjustment in dosage. Increased flatulence may be noted. Rare side effects include hyperchloremic acidosis in children, intestinal obstruction, steatorrhea, and elevation in alkaline phosphatase.

Cholestyramine may interefere with the absorption of fat-soluble vitamins and acidic compounds such as digitalis, thiazides, warfarin, thyroid preparations, tetracycline, and phenylbutazone. These medications should be taken at least 1 h before cholestyramine. Supplementary multivitamins should probably be given to all patients on cholestyramine therapy.

Nicotinic acid (niacin)[260,274,284–286]

Nicotinic acid, when given in doses much in excess of its requirements as a vitamin, inhibits fatty acid mobilization from adipose tissue, depresses plasma free fatty acid and triglyceride levels, and decreases the synthesis of VLDL. The decrease in VLDL occurs within hours, whereas plasma cholesterol and LDL levels may decrease to a lesser degree within days, presumably secondary to the decrease in VLDL.

INDICATIONS

Nicotinic acid is primarily useful in conditions with increased levels of VLDL and LDL (types II, IV, and V hyperlipoproteinemia). It is also useful as an adjunct to diet and cholestyramine in some patients with type II hyperlipoproteinemia (or familial hypercholesterolemia), especially in type IIb patients who have an increase in plasma triglyceride level on cholestyramine therapy.

DOSAGE

Nicotinic acid is available in 100 mg and 500 mg tablets. In adults the initial dose is 100 mg three times a day with meals. The daily dose is increased by 200 to 300 mg every 4 to 7 days until the maintenance dose of 3 to 9 g/day is reached. Plain nicotinic acid is preferable to buffered or prolonged-release analogues.

SIDE EFFECTS

Intense cutaneous flushing and pruritus, which occurs within 1 to 2 h and may last up to several hours, is the most common side effect. Many patients develop a tolerance to these effects, which usually become much less bothersome within a few weeks. Mild nausea, vomiting, or diarrhea can usually be alleviated by taking the drug with meals. Nicotinic acid may produce abnormal glucose tolerance, glycosuria, hyperuricemia, and abnormal liver function tests. Accordingly, it should be used only with special caution and with careful monitoring in patients with diabetes mellitus, gout, or liver disease. Nicotinic acid may potentiate the hypotensive effects of ganglioplegic antihypertensive drugs. Long-term therapy with nicotinic acid may cause hyperpigmentation and dry skin. In patients with previous myocardial infarction studied in the Coronary Drug Project, nicotinic acid was associated with an increased incidence of atrial arrhythmias but with no definite benefit upon mortality.[108]

Clofibrate (chlorophenoxyisobutyric acid, Atromid-S)

Clofibrate is a branched-chain fatty acid ester (ethyl parachlorophenoxyisobutyrate). It enhances the catabolism and decreases the synthesis of VLDL and thus decreases plasma VLDL, intermediate low-density lipoprotein (ILDL), and triglyceride levels. Its effects upon LDL and HDL are variable.[287] It also has definite effects on blood coagulation and fibrinolysis.

INDICATIONS

Clofibrate is most useful in the treatment of hyperlipoproteinemias associated with elevated levels of VLDL, ILDL, or elevated triglyceride (types III, IV, and V). It is most useful in combination with diet and the achievement of ideal body weight in the management of patients with type III hyperlipoproteinemia. Its effectiveness in types IV and V is less clear. It has limited value in controlling elevations of LDL, as in patients with type II (see above).

DOSAGE

It is prepared in 500 mg capsules and is administered orally at a total dose of 1.5 to 2.0 g/day, divided into two to four doses.

SIDE EFFECTS

Side effects are usually very mild. Occasionally, this drug may cause nausea, diarrhea, or weight gain. Rarely, it may cause myositis, skin rash, or abnormal liver function tests. In male patients with previous myocardial infarction who were given clofibrate in the Coronary Drug Project (CDP), there was an increased incidence of cholelithiasis,[108a] arrhythmias, new angina pectoris, thromboembolism, and intermittent claudication. In the CDP study of men who had already sustained a myocardial infarction, clofibrate had no beneficial effect on recurrent infarction or mortality.[108]

Clofibrate potentiates the effects of warfarin sodium (Coumadin) and may have similar effects upon other protein-bound drugs such as diphenylhydantoin (Dilantin).

d-Thyroxine (Choloxin)

The dextrorotatory isomer of thyroxine has been reported to lower plasma cholesterol levels without undue hypermetabolism by enhancing the catabolism of LDL.[288–290] Its effects on VLDL are variable.

INDICATIONS

Indications for d-thyroxine are limited to conditions associated with elevated LDL. In patients with previous myocardial infarction in the CDP, there was an excess of cardiovascular morbidity and mortality, and the drug was withdrawn from the study. Currently, it has only limited use as a primary hypolipidemic agent, and it should not be used in patients with angina pectoris or myocardial infarction.

DOSAGE

d-Thyroxine is available in 2- and 4-mg tablets. The initial dose is 2 mg daily, with the daily dose slowly increased by 1 to 2 mg/month, up to a maintenance dose of 4 to 8 mg/day.

SIDE EFFECTS

As noted in the CDP,[108] d-thyroxine was associated with an excess mortality in patients with previous myocardial infarction, particularly those with ventricular premature complexes. Additional side effects are abnormal glucose tolerance, glycosuria, liver dysfunction, and neutropenia. It also increases the hypoprothrombinemic effects of warfarin sodium.

β-Sitosterol (Cytellin)

Sitosterols are plant sterols with structures similar to that of cholesterol. They usually are not well absorbed, and they lower plasma cholesterol by interfering with the absorption of cholesterol. The usual dosage is 3 to 6 g (15 to 30 ml of suspension) $^{1}/_{2}$ h prior to meals and at bedtime; it is often mixed in fruit juice or tea. Side effects include diarrhea, nausea, or bloating.

Rarely, significant amounts of β-sitosterol can be absorbed and produce a type of xanthomatosis. In general, sitosterol should be considered a second line medication in the treatement of hypercholesterolemia.

Colestipol

This investigational anion exchange resin sequesters bile acids and increases the catabolism of LDL in a manner similar to the action of cholestyramine. The recommended dosage is 15 to 25 g, given in individual doses of 5 g. Indications and side effects are similar to those for cholestyramine.[227,291]

Para-aminosalicylic acid–ascorbic acid (PAS-C)

This combination of a known antitubercular drug and ascorbic acid decreases levels of both cholesterol and triglyceride. The mechanism of action is unknown, but it may be a selective interference with cholesterol absorption.[228,292] The drug is supplied as 500 mg tablets and the usual daily dosage is 6 to 8 g, divided in two doses. The most frequent side effects are nausea, vomiting, and diarrhea. Rarely, it may induce a hypersensitivity reaction or a goiter. It is contraindicated in the presence of liver disease, renal disease, or gastric ulcer.

Neomycin sulfate

This antibiotic is produced from *Streptomyces fradiar;* the mechanism of its cholesterol-lowering effect is unknown. Its main use is as an adjunct to clofibrate in the treatment of type II hyperlipidemia. Neomycin sulfate is given orally as 350-mg tablets, three or four times a day with meals. It may produce mild abdominal distress or diarrhea. It has the potential to produce ototoxicity or nephrotoxicity and should not be used in patients with otologic or renal insufficiency.

Probucol (Lorelco)

This new compound is used to treat hypercholesterolemia. It is a bisphenol which is only about 2 to 8 percent absorbed. The mechanism by which it lowers plasma cholesterol is unknown. It has variable effects upon triglyceride levels and it is not recommended for the treatment of hypertriglyceridemia. Side effects include diarrhea, flatulence, nausea, vomiting, and abdominal pain. It is supplied in 250-mg tablets; the recommended dosage is 500 mg twice daily with the morning and evening meals. It may be useful to treat some patients with hypercholesterolemia or type IIa hyperlipoproteinemia,[292a] but its usefulness and long-term effects are not well established.

Norethindone acetate (Norlutate)

This progestational agent enhances the activity of postheparin lipolytic activity, promoting the plasma clearance of chylomicra and VLDL.[293] It is most useful in women with type V hyperlipidemia who cannot tolerate nicotinic acid or clofibrate. The dosage is 5 mg/day. It may produce fluid retention, breast enlargement, nausea, anorexia, decreased glucose tolerance, cholestatic jaundice.

Oxandralone (Anavar)

This anabolic steroid produces a decrease in the plasma triglyceride level of patients with types IV and V hyperlipoproteinemia.[294] It appears to enhance the peripheral hydrolysis of triglycerides via postheparin lipolytic activity. Since it may produce virilism in females, its use is restricted to males. It is most useful in patients with type V who cannot take nicotinic acid. The usual dosage is 2.5 mg three times a day. Abnormal liver function, salt and water retention, leukopenia, and aggravation of prostatic carcinoma may occur. It is contraindicated in growing children.

CLINICAL EXAMPLES OF THE SPECTRUM OF THERAPEUTIC INTERVENTION

It is now clear that significant inroads in the control of the atherosclerotic process can be best achieved when significant preventive measures are instituted early. It ought to be added that, until further evidence is accumulated, the *preventive* measures employed should *not* add significant risks of their own. When evidence of coronary atherosclerotic heart disease (CAHD) becomes evident on the clinical horizon, the potential for deceleration or reversal of the atherosclerotic process is somewhat diminished, but reasonable goals can be set and achieved if the physician and the patient are willing to collaborate. The degree of therapeutic intervention should be a decision, taken by physician and patient together, based on considerations such as specific risk factors, attainable goals, desires of the patient, and available therapeutic measures (see Table 62H-6 and Tables 62H-9 through 13). The patient's need for understanding and support, and a degree of flexibility in the implementation of the therapeutic recommendations, should always be kept in mind by the physician to avoid undue concern and possible emotional harm deriving from the therapeutic measures.

In order to illustrate how the acquired knowledge can be channeled into therapeutic recommendations, five clinical examples are shown below.

Case 1 Asymptomatic, very high risk: Maximal intervention The patient is a 6-year-old son of a widowed schoolteacher, brought in by the mother for a preschool examination. The father died at age 28 after 2 years of angina pectoris; he had a disorder of lipid metabolism, characterized by type IIa of Fredrickson, recognized for 10 years prior to his sudden death. The boy's body weight is at the 50th percentile for his age and height. He has a blood pressure of 110/70, tendinous xanthomata, and small bilateral xanthelasmas. Chest x-rays and an electrocardiogram are within normal limits. Cholesterol level is 520 mg/dl, triglycerides 80 mg/dl. When repeated 2 weeks later, cholesterol and triglycerides are 510 mg and 85 mg, respectively. The mother is informed of the high risk related to the son's lipid disorder and the genetics of the condition; she is then asked to cooperate on a series of the therapeutic measures. A screening for other disorders, extending to the thyroid and renal functions, does not reveal any abnormality. Since there is no excess body weight, the immediate recommendation is a change in diet. The NIH-NHLI low-cholesterol (less than 300 mg/day), polyunsaturate-rich diet, is recommended to be followed strictly for 2 to 3 months. At the end of that time the cholesterol level is measured again. If the diet is effective in producing a marked decrease in the cholesterol level (reasonable goal 15 to 20 percent reduction), continuation of the diet is recommended. Should the cholesterol level not be normalized by diet alone in the subsequent 6 to 12 months, a pharmacologic addition, such as cholestyramine, will be introduced. Alternative pharmacologic agents for this condition are clofibrate (Atromid-S) and nicotinic acid. Cardiological consultations at least once a year are indicated.

Comment Maximal intervention with diet and drugs is indicated to prevent the severe cardiovascular consequences of untreated type IIa hyperlipoproteinemia.

Case 2 Asymptomatic with moderate risk: Medium to maximal intervention A 45-year-old police officer, former high school football player, is seen for routine checkup. Father died suddenly at age 55; mother, 72 years of age, is living and well. Patient smokes $1^1/_2$ packs of cigarettes per day and drinks two beers per day and occasional social drinks. He is relatively sedentary, participates in no physical activities besides requirements of his job, and is asymptomatic for heart disease or angina. Habitual diet is rich in calories, saturated fats, and carbohydrates. On physical examination, blood pressure is 150/95, weight 212 pounds (125 percent of desirable body weight). Cardiovascular examination is not remarkable. Electrocardiogram and chest x-rays are within normal limits. Cholesterol level is 290 mg/dl, triglycerides 210 mg/dl. Possible secondary causes of his hyperlipidemia are ruled out.

It is obvious that several risk factors are operating in this middle-aged man. Although no cardiovascular abnormalities have emerged as yet on the clinical horizon, the cluster of risk factors (obesity, smoking, hyperlipidemia, sedentary life, borderline hypertension, rich diet) makes this patient a high risk for development of coronary atherosclerotic heart disease.

Suggested measures The patient is given information regarding the risk of CAHD. Cessation of smoking and a hypocaloric diet with limitation in refined carbohydrates are recommended, together with reduction of the alcohol consumption. At a visit two months later, there is moderate reduction in triglyceride level to 160 mg/dl; cholesterol level is 270 mg/dl. Patient has lost 10 pounds of body weight and is willing to continue in the prescribed program. Measures of diet are reinforced and, at this point, a program of gradual and moderate exercise is progressively introduced. Three months later, the cholesterol and triglycerides have progressively declined to near normal levels. The patient has lost 20 pounds of body weight, the blood pressure is now 130/85. Patient is encouraged to continue losing weight until ideal weight of 180 pounds is reached and to enforce correction of the other risk factors.

Comment Although it may appear at first sight that the measures recommended are excessive for the clinical manifestations in this patient, we feel that the combination of the risk factors in this individual requires medium to maximal intervention to decelerate or even reverse the underlying atherosclerotic process.

Case 3 Asymptomatic, low risk: Medium intervention An 18-year-old male college freshman, seen in the pre-college examination gave a family history of diabetes mellitus (mother and one aunt) and overweight in the entire family. The patient has poor dietary habits, eating all kinds of snacks at odd times. Participates in sports occasionally and without regular training. Drinks approximately 20 beers per week; smokes two packs of cigarettes per day, occasionally a marihuana cigarette. Physical examination: body weight is 35 pounds above his ideal weight, blood pressure is 130/76. The cardiovascular examination is within normal limits, the chest x-ray is unremarkable. Random blood sugar is 145 mg/dl, a 2 h postprandial blood sugar is 150 mg/dl. After suitable preparation, a glucose tolerance curve reveals borderline values for diabetes. Cholesterol is 280 mg/dl, triglycerides 250 mg/dl. When seen 2 weeks later, the lipid levels are still abnormal. The patient is informed of the mild carbohydrate abnormality and of the several risk factors in part related to his life-style. He appears cooperative and wants to be educated about proper health practices. A therapeutic program is presented, consisting of hypocaloric diet, cessation of smoking, reduction in alcohol consumption, with a positive note for early and possible effective correction of the lipid abnormality and of the carbohydrate abnormality. The diet is reduced in total calories, saturated fats, and refined carbohydrates. The patient is offered a number of pamphlets containing information prepared by the American Heart Association for his continuing education. He is to be seen at regular intervals for follow-up of deranged parameters and continuing encouragement.

Comment Although the family tendency for diabetes may be in part responsible for the carbohydrate intolerance in this patient, it is obvious that a number of risk factors are present and related to his life-style (obesity, excessive alcohol consumption, smoking, hyperlipidemia). It follows from the previous discussion that, unless major efforts at controlling risk factors are made, this subject is a prime candidate for accelerated atherosclerosis and premature CAHD. This may represent an instance of preventive medicine at the time when no cardiovascular abnormalities are noted, but the preventive effort has to start early in life (possibly even in childhood and adolescent years) to be most effective.

Case 4 Symptomatic, moderate risk: Minimal intervention A 55-year-old stockbroker, former polo player, socially prominent, married three times, drinks two to three highballs per day, smokes an occasional cigar. No regular exercise. Notable in the diet is the consumption of two eggs and large amounts of bacon each morning. He also shows preference for marbled steaks and rich desserts. Of note in the medical history, he has experienced angina pectoris only upon marked exertion or emotional upset for the past year and a half. He has also developed impotence of psychological nature because of anginal pain during intercourse. On physical examination, blood pressure is 150/85, weight is within normal limits. Cardiovascular examination reveals normal auscultatory findings. The electrocardiograms show nonspecific ST-T changes, the patient had a 2 mm ST-segment depression of his ECG at a heart rate of 140 at stage 5 during treadmill test-

ing. Cholesterol level is 350 mg/dl, triglycerides 210 mg/dl.

It is fairly evident that this patient has advanced atherosclerosis. It is also recognized that, unless major and drastic changes in the risk factors—particularly the lipid levels—are introduced, there is minimal chance for reversal or deceleration of the atherosclerotic process. Patient is informed of the level of risk present and of the measures intended for secondary prevention. He declines coronary angiography at this time. The evidence is offered to the patient and the decision is made jointly by the patient and the physician and is based on the anticipated cooperation of the patient.

Recommendations The following recommendations are offered: reduction in the amount of alcohol intake; major modifications in the diet with cholesterol restrictions to less than 300 mg/day and reduction of cholesterol level with the diet. The patient can be placed on a very mild exercise program supervised by a physician. Subsequent follow-ups will indicate whether diet alone is sufficient to promote cholesterol reduction, or whether, additionally, hypolipidemic drugs have to be introduced. The patient is advised to seek relief of work tension, to delegate responsibilities, and to avoid deadlines. Furthermore, he is advised to enlarge his areas of interest and recreation. Coronary angiography may be indicated to determine the extent of the lesions and to seek other modes of therapy (see Chap. 62E).

Comment Chances of a major improvement in the atherosclerotic process of this patient are small, judging from present knowledge. If a therapeutic attempt is made at all, however, it should be maximal intervention. Lack of cooperation from the patient should lead to a common decision not to rely on expected benefits of poorly applied therapeutic measures.

Case 5 CAHD, symptomatic, advanced: Minimal or no intervention An 82-year-old lady who has had two myocardial infarctions in the last 15 years. She is otherwise active and tends a garden. She is very particular about her diet, loves eggs and buttered toast and enjoys a sherry drink after dinner. Smokes five to ten cigarettes per day. She takes care, alone, of a four-room house. Of note is the presence of morning cough. Additional history findings: occasional short-lived episodes of ankle swelling, mild dyspnea on exertion, and, at times, angina pectoris brought about by irritation with neighbors.

On physical examination, the cardiovascular exam reveals a displaced apex, a sustained palpable S_4, ectopic precordial impulse, grade 2/6 apical holosystolic murmur; the lungs are clear. X-rays of the chest show a tortuous aorta and a modestly enlarged heart. The electrocardiogram is compatible with an old anterior myocardial infarction and occasional PVCs (premature ventricular complexes) are seen. Blood pressure is 160/85, weight is 89 pounds (90 percent of desirable body weight). Cholesterol level is 320 mg/dl, triglycerides 110 mg/dl.

Comment In spite of obviously recognizable risk factors (age, cigarette smoking, diet, and cholesterol elevation), it is important to consider in this patient that the chances of affecting the atherosclerotic process are minimal and that upsetting the lifelong habits by drastic recommendations will have the effect of producing a change in the quality of life for the patient without necessarily affecting its length.

Recommendations No intervention. Patient may be told that reduction in cigarette smoking may contribute to improvement of "chronic bronchitic" process. Although reduction of eggs in the diet is left to the decision of the patient, it is important under these circumstances *not* to convey the impression to the patient that "nothing" can be done for her "cardiovascular health" in view of age and advanced stage of the disease.

TREATMENT RESPONSIBILITY

The patient

Ultimately each patient is responsible for his own health, including the maintenance of cardiovascular health. Each patient has a responsibility to become familiar with materials appropriate for his other educational experiences that deal with both the prevention of disease and the recognition of early symptoms of disease. Although changing personal habits and behavior modification are very difficult, each patient has to assume some responsibility for certain areas such as the elimination of smoking, correction of obesity if present, selection of a healthy prudent diet, and measurement of one's blood pressure at appropriate intervals. Such preventive measures can be justified on many grounds in addition to the possible benefit on atherosclerosis.

The physician

The physician has a major responsibility for giving the patient access to information regarding health and disease while in the office or clinic. Ideally, each waiting room should be a health education room with appropriate reading materials and audio-visual materials to supplement the physician, assistants, and perhaps dietitian. In addition, based upon the patient's history, physical examination, and routine laboratory tests, the physician makes recommendations and sets goals regarding health maintenance, including a defined plan for follow-up visits and laboratory examinations. Because of his knowledge of the patient's total problems and personality, including the factors listed in Table 62H-7 the physician should be able to select goals that are both reasonable and not harmful. The physician might find the use of an algorithm, such as the one depicted in Fig. 62H-1, both practical and informative.

Health organizations

The American Heart Association (AHA) has as its major goal the prevention of heart disease. In order to accomplish this, the AHA has an active program of providing educational materials for both the public and the physician. In addition, the AHA very

actively supports basic cardiovascular research and teaching.

Government[295]

The federal government actively influences medical care through the Food and Drug Administration, for which it establishes guidelines for labeling of food products and for the use of pharmaceutical agents, and the National Heart and Lung Institute, which supports basic cardiovascular research and a number of special projects dealing with lipids and atherosclerosis.

A continuous national program of public education regarding health affairs would be advisable and highly beneficial. Ideally, this program should include health education in the public schools from kindergarten through high school, unless there were objections on appropriate grounds from individual parents. Television could provide an excellent means of continuing adult education both for health maintenance and for the recognition of early symptoms of possible dysfunction.

Food industry

The food industries have a responsibility to maintain a close liaison with nutritionists, basic scientists, and physicians regarding the large area of interrelations between nutrition and health. At present in the United States, food products are required to be labeled with a description of basic contents. The industry should make changes in food processing when these are feasible and are reasonably established as being in the best interests of the public.

IS "FINAL PROOF" NECESSARY?

Extensive evidence, reviewed in this chapter, in Chap. 62B, and elsewhere,[1-38,44] supports the following conclusions: (1) the incidence of premature atherosclerotic heart disease is strongly associated with the concentration of plasma cholesterol; (2) a diet rich in cholesterol and saturated fatty acids produces hypercholesterolemia and atherosclerosis in most species; (3) the plasma cholesterol concentration can be safely and at times remarkably lowered by modification of the usual diet by ways that are acceptable to a large number of people; (4) the long-term use of natural vegetable oils in the recommended amounts has not produced any known long-term toxic effects in human beings, and experiments in animals have not revealed any toxic effects of a diet rich in vegetable oil and linoleic acid provided that the diet contains an adequate amount of alpha tocopherol; and (5) experimental atherosclerotic plaques may show considerable regression if existing risk factors are removed or corrected and if the atherogenic diet is replaced by a low cholesterol diet rich in linoleic acid. Epidemiologic evidence indicates that perhaps over 30 percent of adult males in the United States have serum cholesterol values above 260 mg/dl, that the majority have values above the desirable levels of 140 to 200 mg/dl, and that the etiology of this type of hypercholesterolemia is presumably due to diet alone. Many epidemiologic animal and clinical investigations support the current opinion that atherosclerosis is a multifactorial disease syndrome that may be produced by different pathogenic mechanisms in different individuals and different species. These studies also support the conclusion that the lifelong diet is the single most important key factor in human atherosclerosis. On the other hand, we do not yet have final absolute, unequivocal proof that a cholesterol-reducing diet will prevent or lessen the incidence of atherosclerotic coronary heart disease. We believe that the evidence relating diet to coronary heart disease is very strong, however, and that therefore it is appropriate to make dietary recommendations to the general public and not only to individuals identified as having increased risk. Even though one may want to modify the dietary habits of the general public as little as possible, some of the dietary ingredients can and should be replaced, particularly the replacement of saturated fats by polyunsaturated fats. The food industry and government can be of great help in supporting the recommendations of the AHA and other health agencies and in providing suitable food products.

The argument is frequently heard that physicians should refrain from recommending modification of the CAHD risk factors, in particular the high lipid levels, until uncontroversial evidence is provided for a beneficial effect of the proposed modification on the atherosclerotic process. We disagree with that argument and would like to answer it as follows: (1) removal or correction of one or more risk factors can be beneficial to the patient in ways other than reducing or decelerating the atherosclerotic process (e.g., cessation of cigarette smoking will reduce the incidence of lung cancer, correction of hypertension will reduce complications such as strokes, etc.); (2) for the beneficial effect of cessation of cigarette smoking on the incidence of lung cancer and the correction of hypertension on incidence of stroke, sufficient indirect evidence was present in the literature to justify removal of these factors for several years *prior* to "final proof"; (3) time is of the essence. We do not think that it is necessary to wait for absolute final proof to initiate measures as early as possible in the life of an individual to affect and prevent the changes of atherosclerosis that are known to be associated, by epidemiologic studies, with the presence of one or more risk factors. Thus, in our opinion, it would be unwise to wait for final proof that a small reduction in plasma lipids reduces significantly the atherosclerotic process to initiate measures that should begin early in the life of an individual. In other words, evidence sufficient to recommend "primary prevention" is more than adequate in the epidemiologic and clinical

studies, and we should not be idly waiting for additional (and certainly controversial) evidence to convince the public of the importance of the preventive measures. A lifelong habit of moderate caloric intake, the reduction of ingestion of animal fats and excessive refined carbohydrates, coupled with physical activity, the avoidance of cigarette smoking, and the maintenance of blood pressure within limits are all measures already suggested by population and clinical studies that are essential to the control and deceleration of the atherosclerotic process. Thus, in our opinion final proof is not necessary. The removal or correction of the risk factors early in life, including correction of the "abnormal" lipid levels, is the only hope of a successful attack on the major pathologic process (atherosclerosis) which affects the life of so many people in Western, industrialized countries. A sample of the concerned statements by health agencies and ad hoc study groups follows.

The American Heart Association statement[189] concluded that the data from population studies and from clinical trials "provide sufficient evidence to warrant taking *prudent* action at this time, in the population at large." THe AHA general dietary recommendations include the following: (1) caloric intake adjusted to achieve and maintain ideal body weight; (2) reduction in calories from total fat to no more than 35 percent of total calories, with no more than 10 percent from saturated fatty acids, no more than 10 percent from polyunsaturated fatty acids, and the remainder monounsaturated; (3) average daily cholesterol intake no greater than 300 mg (less in persons with severe hypercholesterolemia); (4) intake of carbohydrates in complex natural forms, such as vegetables, fruits, grains, or cereals, rather than refined sugar; (5) avoidance of excess salt (<5 to 6 g/day). A similar dietary recommendation for the general public was made the the Intersociety Commission for Heart Disease Resources.[16]

In 1972, a joint statement on diet and coronary heart disease was made by the Food and Nutrition Board,[298] noting that the risk of developing CHD is positively correlated with the level of cholesterol in the plasma, especially at levels greater than 220 mg/dl. The statement also noted that no more than approximately one-third of American men and a less definitely known proportion of women have plasma cholesterol levels at or below 200 mg/dl while consuming their usual diets. They recommended that measurement of the plasma lipid profile, particularly plasma cholesterol, become a part of all health maintenance physical examinations and that all persons who fall into "risk categories" on the basis of their plasma lipids be given appropriate dietary advice to lower cholesterol consumption and to decrease substantially the intake of saturated fats by substituting polyunsaturated vegetable oils for part of the saturated fat in the diet. This statement emphasized that "the evidence now available is sufficient to discourage further temporizing with this major national health problem."

The American Health Foundation[299] recommended the following guidelines for general use: (1) adjustment of total calories to avoid obesity; (2) decreasing the total dietary fat to approximately 35 percent of total daily calories with approximately isocaloric amounts of saturated, monosaturated, and polyunsaturated fatty acids; (3) limiting the average daily cholesterol intake to less than 300 mg daily; (4) adjusting carbohydrate intake so complex types will predominate; and (5) reducing salt intake to about 5 g/day (adjusted to climatic and working conditions).

The Joint Working Party of the Royal College of Physicians of London and the British Cardiac Society made the following recommendations for the whole community: reducing the amount of saturated fats in the diet and substituting partially polyunsaturated fats, maintaining a desirable body weight, discouraging smoking, controlling blood pressure, and encouraging physical activity in all ages.[46] They noted that the recommendation applied to children as much as to adults. They also noted that a comprehensive public and professional education program was needed with the cooperation of the food manufacturers, educational authorities, and the mass media.

The Medical Boards of Finland and Sweden[300,301] jointly presented dietary recommendations for the entire population that should be started early in life. These recommendations were to decrease the total fat consumption, particularly of saturated fats, and to use relatively more polyunsaturated fats. They stressed that the serum cholesterol is generally increased by the consumption of foods high in cholesterol content and also recommended a reduction in the consumption of sugar. Similar recommendations have been made by the Netherlands Nutritional Council.[302,303]

At present, we would emphasize the necessity of individualizing all therapeutic measures whenever possible. Coronary atherosclerosis is a multifactorial condition, and all therapeutic measures are more likely to have significant benefit when started early. Finally, we would emphasize the importance of putting recommendations regarding diet and change in life habits into perspective for each patient (see Table 62H-6). This is particularly true in patients who already have angina pectoris or a myocardial infarction. In such patients, it is obviously more appropriate to direct one's major efforts toward the recognition and relief of pain rather than an excessive concern regarding dietary minutiae.

Our enthusiasm for making positive therapeutic recommendations must always be tempered by the realization of how little we know.

REFERENCES

1 Kannel, W. B., Dawber, T. R., Friedman, G. D., Glennon, W. E., and McNamara, P. M.: Risk Factors in Coronary Heart Disease: An Evaluation of Several Serum Lipids as Predictors of Coronary Heart Disease, *Ann. Intern. Med.*, 61:88, 1964.

2 Stamler, J., Berkson, D. M., Lindberg, H. A., Hall, Y., Miller, W., Mojonnier, L., Levinson, M., Cohen, D. B., and Young, Q. D.: Coronary Risk Factors: Their Impact, and Their Therapy in the Prevention of Coronary Heart Disease, *Med. Clin. North Am.*, 50:229, 1966.

3 Stamler, J.: Atherosclerotic Coronary Heart Disease—Etiology and Pathogenesis: The Coronary Risk Factors, in J.

Stamler, "Lectures on Preventive Cardiology," Grune & Stratton, Inc., New York, 1967, p. 107.

4 Blumenthal, H. T. (ed.): "Cowdry's Arteriosclerosis: A Survey of the Problem," 2d ed., Charles C Thomas, Publisher, Springfield, Ill., 1967.

5 Slack, J.: Risks of Ischaemic Heart-disease in Familial Hyperlipoproteinaemic States, *Lancet*, 2:1380, 1969.

6 Keys, A. (ed.): Coronary Heart Disease in Seven Countries, *Circulation*, 41(suppl. 1):1, 1970.

7 Jones, R. J. (ed.): "Atherosclerosis" (proceedings, second international symposium, Chicago), Springer-Verlag, Heidelberg, 1970.

8 Kannel, W. B., Castelli, W. P., Gordon, T., and McNamara, P. M.: Serum Cholesterol, Lipoproteins, and the Risk of Coronary Heart Disease: The Framingham Study, *Ann. Intern. Med.*, 74:1, 1971.

9 Epstein, F. H.: International Trends in Coronary Heart Disease Epidemiology, *Ann. Clin. Res.*, 3:293, 1971.

10 Epstein, F. H., and Ostrander, L. D., Jr.: Detection of Individual Susceptibility toward Coronary Disease, *Prog. Cardiovasc. Dis.*, 13:324, 1971.

11 Dawber, T. R., and Thomas, H. E., Jr.: Prevention of Myocardial Infarction, *Prog. Cardiovasc. Dis.*, 13:343, 1971.

12 McNamara, J. J., Molot, M. A., Stremple, J. F., and Cutting, R. T.: Coronary Artery Disease in Combat Casualities in Vietnam, *J.A.M.A.*, 216:1185, 1971.

13 Castelli, W. P., and Moran, R. F.: Lipid Studies for Assessing the Risk of Cardiovascular Disease and Hyperlipidemia, *Hum. Pathol.*, 2:153, 1971.

14 Arteriosclerosis: A Report by the National Heart and Lung Institute Task Force on Arteriosclerosis, vol. 1, DHEW Publication no. (NIH) 72-137, National Institutes of Health, Bethesda, 1971.

15 Arteriosclerosis: A Report by the National Heart and Lung Institute Task Force on Arteriosclerosis, vol. 2, DHEW Publication no. (NIH) 72-219, National Institutes of Health, Bethesda, Md., 1972.

16 Report of Inter-society Commission for Heart Disease Resources: Primary Prevention of the Atherosclerotic Diseases. *Circulation*, 42:A-55, 1970. (Revised April, 1972.)

17 Keys, A., Aravanis, C., Blackburn, H., Van Buchem, F. S., Buzina, R., Djordjevic, B. S., Fidanza, F., Karvonen, M. J., Menotti, A., Puddu, V., and Taylor, H. L.: Probability of Middle-aged Men Developing Coronary Heart Disease in Five Years, *Circulation*, 45:815, 1972.

18 Stone, N. J., and Levy, R. I.: Hyperlipoproteinemia and Coronary Heart Disease, *Prog. Cardiovasc. Dis.*, 14:341, 1972.

19 Wissler, R. W., and Geer, J. C. (eds.): "The Pathogenesis of Atherosclerosis," The Williams & Wilkins Company, Baltimore, 1972.

20 Stamler, J.: Epidemiology of Coronary Heart Disease, *Med. Clin. North Am.*, 57:5, 1973.

21 Kato, H., Tillotson, J., Nichaman, M. Z., Rhoads, G. G., and Hamilton, H. B.: Epidemiologic Studies of Coronary Heart Disease and Stroke in Japanese Men Living in Japan, Hawaii and California: Serum Lipids and Diet, *Am. J. Epidem.*, 97:372, 1973.

22 Wilhelmsen, L., Wedel, H., and Tibblin, G.: Multivariate Analysis of Risk Factors for Coronary Heart Disease, *Circulation*, 48:950, 1973.

23 Waldenström, J., Larsson, T., Ljungstedt, N. (eds.): "Early Phases of Coronary Heart Disease: The Possibility of Prediction," Nordiska Bokhandelns Forlag, Stockholm, 1973.

24 Porter, R., and Knight, J. (eds.): "Atherogenesis: Initiating Factors," Ciba Foundation Symposium 12, Associated Scientific Publishers, Amsterdam, 1973, p. 288.

25 Hagerup, L. M.: Coronary Heart Disease Risk Factors in Men and Women: From the Population Study in Glostrup, Denmark, *Acta Med. Scand.,* suppl. no. 557, 1974.

26 Rissanen, V., and Pyorala, K.: Aortic and Coronary Atherosclerosis in the Finnish Population: A Study of a Series of Violent Deaths, *Atherosclerosis,* 19:221, 1974.

27 Dock, W.: Atherosclerosis: Why Do We Pretend the Pathogenesis is Mysterious? *Circulation,* 50:647, 1974.

28 Blackburn, H.: Progress in the Epidemiology and Prevention of Coronary Heart Disease, *Prog. Cardiol.,* 3:1, 1974.

29 Bierman, E. L., and Glomset, J. A.: Disorders of Lipid Metabolism, in R. H. Williams (ed.), "The Textbook of Endocrinology," 5th ed., W. B. Saunders Company, Philadelphia, 1974, p. 890.

30 Schettler, G., and Weizel, A.: Atherosclerosis III: Proceedings of the Third International Symposium, Springer-Verlag, New York, Heidelberg, 1974, p. 1034.

31 Keys, A.: Coronary Heart Disease: The Global Picture, *Atherosclerosis,* 22:149, 1975.

32 Dolder, M. A., and Oliver, M. F.: Myocardial infarction in Young Men: Study of Risk Factors in Nine Countries, *Br. Heart J.,* 37:493, 1975.

33 Kannel, W. B., Doyle, J. T., McNamara, P. M., Quickenton, P., and Gordon, T.: Precursors of Sudden Coronary Death, *Circulation,* 51:606, 1975.

34 Heyden, S.: Epidemiological Data on Dietary Fat Intake and Atherosclerosis with an Appendix on Possible Side Effects, in A. J. Vergroesen (ed.), "The Role of Fats in Human Nutrition," Academic Press, London, 1975, p. 43.

35 Stemmermann, G. N., Steer, A., Rhoads, G. G., Lee, K., Hayashi, T., Nakashima, T., and Neehn, R.: A Comparative Pathology Study of Myocardial Lesions and Atherosclerosis in Japanese Men Living in Hiroshima, Japan, and Honolulu, Hawaii, *Lab. Invest.,* 34:592, 1976.

36 Elmfeldt, D., Wilhelmsen, L., Wedel, H., Vedin, A., Wilhelmsson, C., and Tibblin, G.: Primary Risk Factors in Patients with Myocardial Infarction, *Am. Heart J.,* 91:412, 1976.

37 Ostrander, L. D., and Lamphiear, D. E.: Coronary Risk Factors in a Community: Findings in Tecumseh, Michigan, *Circulation,* 53:152, 1976.

38 Brand, R. J., Rosenman, R. H., Sholtz, R. I., and Friedman, M.: Multivariate Prediction of Coronary Heart Disease in the Western Collaborative Group Study Compared to the Findings of the Framingham Study, *Circulation,* 53:348, 1976.

39 Kannel, W. B.: Some Lessons in Cardiovascular Epidemiology from Framingham, *Am. J. Cardiol.,* 37:269, 1976.

40 Kannel, W. B., McGee, D., and Gordon, T.: A General Cardiovascular Risk Profile: The Framingham Study, *Am. J. Cardiol.,* 38:46, 1976.

41 Kannel, W. B.: Prevention of Cardiovascular Disease, *Curr. Probl. Cardiol.,* 1:1, 1968.

42 Backburn, H.: Concepts and Controversies about the Prevention of Coronary Heart Disease, in H. I. Russek (ed.), "Cardiovascular Problems," University Park Press, Baltimore, 1976, p. 123.

43 Wissler, R. W., Vesselinovitch, D., and Getz, G. S.: Abnormalities of the Arterial Wall and Its Metabolism in Atherogenesis, *Prog. Cardiovasc. Dis.,* 18:341, 1976.

44 Paoletti, R., and Gotto, A. M., Jr. (eds.): "Atherosclerosis Reviews," vol. 1, Raven Press, New York, 1976, p. 265.

45 Levy, R. I., and Rifkind, B. M. (eds.): "Hyperlipidemia: Diagnosis and Therapy," Grune & Stratton, Inc., New York, 1977.

46 Joint Working Party of the Royal College of Physicians of London and the British Cardiology Society: Prevention of Coronary Heart Disease, *Br. Med. J.,* 1:881, 1976.

47 Levy, R. I., and Glueck, C. J.: Hypertriglyceridemia, Diabetes Mellitus, and Coronary Vessel Disease, *Arch. Intern. Med.,* 123:220, 1969.

48 Gertler, M. M., and White, P. D.: "Coronary Heart Disease: A 25 Year Study in Retrospect," Medical Economics Company, Oradell, N.J., 1976, p. 208.

49 Cornfield, J.: Joint Dependence of Risk of Coronary Heart Disease on Serum Cholesterol and Systolic Blood Pressure: A Discriminant Function Analysis, *Fed. Proc.,* 21(suppl. 2):58, 1962.

50 Golubjatnikov, R., Paskey, T., and Inhorn, S. L.: Serum Cholesterol Levels of Mexican and Wisconsin School Children, *Am. J. Epidemiol.,* 96:36, 1972.

51 Thomas, C. B., Ross, D. C., and Duszynski, K. R.: Youthful Hypercholesteremia: Its Associated Characteristics and Role in Premature Myocardial Infarction, *Johns Hopkins Med. J.,* 136:193, 1975.

52 Keys, A.: Serum Cholesterol and the Question of "Normal," in E. S. Benson and P. E. Strandjord (eds.), "Multiple Laboratory Screening," Academic Press, Inc., New York, 1969, p. 147.

53 Wynder, A. E. L., and Hill, P.: Blood Lipids: How Normal is Normal? *Prev. Med.,* 1:161, 1972.

54 Wright, I. S.: Correct Levels of Serum Cholesterol: Average vs. Normal vs. Optimal, *J.A.M.A.,* 236:261, 1976.

55 McGrandy, R. B., and Hegsted, D. M.: Quantitative Effects of Dietary Fat and Cholesterol on Serum Cholesterol in Man, in A. J. Vergroesen (ed.), "The Role of Fats in Human Nutrition," Academic Press, London, 1975, p. 211.

56 Castelli, W. P.: CHD Risk Factors in the Elderly, *Hosp. Pract.,* 11:113, 1976.

57 Coronary Drug Project Research Group: The Natural History of Patients After Recovery From Myocardial Infarction, in press.

58 Anderson, J. T., Keys, A., and Grande, F.: The Effects of Different Food Fats on Serum Cholesterol Concentration in Man, *J. Nutr.,* 62:421, 1957.

59 Ahrens, E. H., Jr., Hirsch, J., Insull, W., Jr., Tsaltas, T. T., Blomstrand, R., and Peterson, M. L.: The Influence of Dietary Fats on Serum-lipid Levels in Man, *Lancet,* 1:943, 1957.

60 Moore, R. B., Anderson, J. T., Taylor, H. L., Keys, A., and Frantz, I. D., Jr.: Effect of Dietary Fat on the Fecal Excretion of Cholesterol and its Degradation Products in Man, *J. Clin. Invest.,* 47:1517, 1968.

61 Grundy, S. M., and Ahrens, E. H., Jr.: The Effects of Unsaturated Dietary Fats on Absorption, Excretion, Synthesis, and Distribution of Cholesterol in Man, *J. Clin. Invest.,* 49:1135, 1970.

62 Quintao, E., Grundy, S. M., and Ahrens, E. H., Jr.: Effects of Dietary Cholesterol on the Regulation of Total Body Cholesterol in Man, *J. Lipid Res.,* 12:233, 1971.

62a Wilson, W. S., Hulley, S. B., Burrows, M. I., and Nichaman, M. Z.: Serial Lipid and Lipoprotein Responses to the American Heart Association Fat-controlled Diet, *Am. J. Med.,* 51:491, 1971.

63 Wissler, R., Vesselinovitch, D., Hughes, R., Turner, D., and Frazier, L. E.: Atherosclerosis and Blood Lipids in Rhesus Monkeys Fed Human Table Prepared Diets, *Circulation,* 43 and 44(suppl. 2):11, 1971. (Abstract.)

64 Mattson, F. H., Erickson, B. A., and Kligman, A. M.: Effect of Dietary Cholesterol on Serum Cholesterol in Man, *Am. J. Clin. Nutr.,* 25:589, 1972.

65 Havel, R. J.: Mechanisms of Hyperlipoproteinemia, *Adv. Exp. Med. Biol.,* 26:57, 1972.

66 Connor, W. E., and Lin, D. S.: The Intestinal Absorption of Dietary Cholesterol by Hypercholesterolemic (type II) and Normocholesterolemic Humans, *J. Clin. Invest.,* 53:1062, 1974.

67 Nestel, P. J., Havenstein, N., Homma, Y., and Cook, L. J.: Increased Sterol Excretion with Polyunsaturated-fat-High-cholesterol Diets, *Metabolism*, 24:189, 1975.

67a Hodges, R. E., Salel, A. F., Dunkley, W. L., Zelis, R., McDonough, P. F., Clifford, C., Hobbs, R. K., Smith, L. M., Fan, A., Mason, D. T., and Lykke, C.: Plasma Lipid Changes in Young Adult Couples Consuming Polyunsaturated Meats and Dairy Products, *Am. J. Clin. Nutr.*, 28:1126, 1975.

68 Mustard, J. F., Pacham, M. A.: Factors Influencing Platelet Function: Adhesion, Release, and Aggregation, *Pharmacol. Rev.*, 22:97, 1970.

69 Schnetzer, G. W., III: Platelets and Thrombogenesis: Current Concepts, *Am. Heart J.*, 83:552, 1972.

70 Hornstra, G.: Specific Effects of Types of Dietary Fat on Arterial Thrombosis, in A. J. Vergroesen (ed.), "The Role of Fats in Human Nutrition," Academic Press, London, 1975, p. 303.

71 O'Brien, J. R., Etherington, M. D., and Jamieson, S.: Acute Platelet Changes After Large Meals of Saturated and Unsaturated Fats, *Lancet*, 1:878, 1976.

72 Chapman, J. M., Massey, F. J., Jr.: The Interrelationship of Serum Cholesterol, Hypertension, Body Weight, and Risk of Coronary Disease: Results of the First Ten Years Follow-up in the Los Angeles Heart Study, *J. Chronic Dis.*, 17:933, 1964.

73 Freis, E. D.: Hypertension and Atherosclerosis, *Am. J. Med.*, 46:735, 1969.

74 Pick, R., Johnson, P. J., and Glick, G.: Deleterious Effects of Hypertension on the Development of Aortic and Coronary Atherosclerosis in Stumptail Macaques (Macaca Speciosa) on an Atherogenic Diet, *Circ. Res.*, 35:472, 1974.

75 Roberts, J. C., Jr., Moses, C., and Wilkins, R. H.: Autopsy Studies in Atherosclerosis, *Circulation*, 20:511, 1959.

76 Epstein, F. H.: Hyperglycemia: A Risk Factor in Coronary Heart Disease, *Circulation*, 36:609, 1967.

77 Robertson, W. B., and Strong, J. P.: Atherosclerosis in Persons with Hypertension and Diabetes Mellitus, *Lab. Invest.*, 18:538, 1968.

78 Kannel, W. B.: Diabetes and Cardiovascular Disease—The Framingham Study: 18-year Followup, *Cardiol. Digest*, 11:11, 1976.

79 Keys, A., Aravanis, C., Blackburn, H., Van Buchem, F. S. P., Buzina, R., Djordjevic, B. S., Fidanza, F., Karvonen, M. J., Menotti, A., Puddu, V., and Taylor, H. L.: Coronary Heart Disease: Overweight and Obesity as Risk Factors, *Ann. Intern. Med.*, 77:15, 1972.

80 Ashley, F. W., Jr., and Kannel, W. B.: Relation of Weight Change to Changes in Atherogenic Traits: The Framingham Study, *J. Chronic Dis.*, 27:103, 1974.

81 Ostrander, L. D., Lamphiear, D. E., Block, W. D., Johnson, B. C., and Epstein, F. H.: Biochemical Precursors to Atherosclerosis: Studies in Apparently Healthy Men in a General Population, Tecumseh, Michigan, *Arch. Intern. Med.*, 134:224, 1974.

82 Mann, G. V.: The Influence of Obesity on Health, *N. Engl. J. Med.*, 291:178 and 226, 1974.

83 National Diet-Heart Study: Final Report, *Circulation*, 37(suppl. 1), 1968.

84 Paul, O., Lepper, M. H., Phelan, W. H., Dupertuis, G. W., MacMillan, A., McKean, H., and Park, H.: A Longitudinal Study of Coronary Heart Disease, *Circulation*, 28:20, 1963.

85 Wilhelmsen, L., Tibblin, G., and Werko, L.: A Primary Prevention Study of Gothenburg, Sweden, *Prev. Med.*, 1:153, 1972.

86 Halperin, M., Cornfield, J., and Mitchell, S. C.: Effect of Diet on Coronary Heart Disease Mortality, *Lancet*, 2:438, 1973.

87 Sacks, F. M., Castelli, W. P., Donner, A., and Kass, E. H.: Plasma Lipids and Lipoproteins in Vegetarians and Controls, *N. Engl. J. Med.*, 292:1148, 1975.

88 Christakis, G., Rinzler, S. H., Archer, M., Winslow, G.,

Jampel, S., Stephenson, J., Friedman, G., Fein, H., Kraus, A., and James, G.: The Anti-Coronary Club: A Dietary Approach to the Prevention of Coronary Heart Disease—A Seven-Year Report, *Am. J. Public Health*, 56:299, 1966.

89 Christakis, G., Rinzler, S. H., Archer, M., and Kraus, A.: Effect of the Anti-Coronary Club Program on Coronary Heart Disease Risk-Factor Status, *J.A.M.A.*, 198:597, 1966.

90 Rinzler, S. H.: Primary Prevention of Coronary Heart Disease by Diet, *Bull. N.Y. Acad. Med.*, 44:936, 1968.

91 Turpeinen, O., Miettinen, M., Karvonen, M. J., Roine, P., Pekkarinen, M., Lehtosuo, E. J., and Ahvirta, P.: Dietary Prevention of Coronary Heart Disease: I. Observations on Male Subjects, *Am. J. Clin. Nutr.*, 21:255, 1968.

92 Turpeinen, O.: Primary Prevention of Coronary Heart Disease by Diet, *Ann. Clin. Res.*, 3:433, 1971.

93 Miettinen, M., Turpeinen, O., Karvonen, M. J., Elosuo, R., and Paavilainen, E.: Effect of Cholesterol-lowering Diet on Mortality from Coronary Heart Disease and Other Causes: A Twelve-year Clinical Trial in Men and Women, *Lancet*, 2:835, 1972.

94 Dayton, S., and Pearce, M. L.: Prevention of Coronary Heart Disease and Other Complications of Arteriosclerosis by Modified Diet, *Am. J. Med.*, 46:751, 1969.

95 Dayton, S., Pearce, M. L., Hashimoto, S., Dixon, W. J., and Tomiyasu, U.: A Controlled Clinical Trial of a Diet High in Unsaturated Fat in Preventing Complications of Atherosclerosis, *Circulation*, 40(suppl. 2):1, 1969.

96 Stamler, J.: Acute Myocardial Infarction: Progress in Primary Prevention, *Br. Heart J.*, 33(suppl.):145, 1971.

97 Stamler, J.: Primary Prevention of Sudden Coronary Death, *Circulation*, 51 and 52(suppl. 3):258, 1975.

98 Stamler, J.: The Current Status of the Chicago Coronary Prevention Evaluation Program: A 10-year Follow-up, in press.

98a Styblo, K., Meijer, J., Arntzenius, A. C., Deltaas, J. H., van Geuns, H. A., Mellema, T. L., and Sluyter, D. P.: CB Heart Project in the Netherlands: Results of Intervention in High Risk Individuals, *Heart Bull.*, 8:47, 1977.

99 Heady, J. A.: A Cooperative Trial on the Primary Prevention of Ischaemic Heart Disease Using Clofibrate: Design, Methods, and Progress, *Bull. WHO*, 48:243, 1973.

100 Oliver, M. F.: Ischaemic Heart Disease: A Primary Prevention Trial Using Clofibrate, Personal communication (quoted by Blackburn[28]).

101 Krasno, L. R., and Kidera, G. J.: Clofibrate in Coronary Heart Disease. Effect on Morbidity and Mortality, *J.A.M.A.*, 219:845, 1972.

102 Feinstein, A. R.: The Clofibrate Trials: Another Dispute about Contratrophic Therapy, *Clin. Pharmacol. Ther.*, 13:953, 1972.

103 Ahrens, E. H., Jr.: The Management of Hyperlipidemia: Whether, Rather than How, *Ann. Intern. Med.*, 85:87, 1976.

103a Epstein, F. H.: Preventive Trials and the "Diet-Heart" Question: Wait for Results or Act Now? *Atherosclerosis*, 26:515, 1977.

104 Gordon, T., and Thom, T.: The Recent Decrease in CHD Mortality, *Prev. Med.*, 4:115, 1975.

105 Hegyeli, R. J.: Personal communication to RCS, November, 1976.

106 Leren, P.: The Oslo Diet Heart Study: Eleven-Year Report, *Circulation*, 42:935, 1970.

107 Leren, P.: The Effect of Plasma Cholesterol Lowering Diet in Male Survivors of Myocardial Infarction, *Acta Med. Scand. Suppl.* 466:1, 1966.

108 Coronary Drug Project Research Group: Clofibrate and Niacin in Coronary Heart Disease, *J.A.M.A.*, 231:360, 1975.

108a Coronary Drug Project Research Group: Gallbladder Disease as a Side Effect of Drugs Influencing Lipid Metabolism, *N. Engl. J. Med.,* 296:1185, 1977.

109 Nash, D. T., Gensini, G., Simon, H., Arno, T., and Nash, S. D.: The Erysichthon Syndrome. Progression of Coronary Atherosclerosis and Dietary Hyperlipidemia, *Circulation,* 56:363, 1977.

110 Trial of Clofibrate in the Treatment of Ischaemic Heart Disease: Five-year Study by a Group of Physicians of the Newcastle upon Tyne Region, *Br. Med. J.,* 4:767, 1971.

111 Report by a Research Committee of the Scottish Society of Physicians: Ischaemic Heart Disease: A Secondary Prevention Trial Using Clofibrate, *Br. Med. J.,* 4:775, 1971.

112 The Coronary Drug Project Research Group: Aspirin in Coronary Heart Disease, *J. Chornic Dis.,* 29:625, 1976.

113 Buchwald, H., Moore, R. B., and Varco, R. L.: Surgical Treatment of Hyperlipidemia, *Circulation,* 49(suppl. 1):11, 1974.

114 Buchwald, H.: Partial Ileal Bypass Operation in the Management of the Hyperlipidemias, in R. Vareo and J. P. Delaney (eds.), "Controversy in Surgery," W. B. Saunders Company, Philadelphia, 1976, p. 625.

115 Strong, J. P. (ed.): Atherosclerosis in Primates, in "Primates in Medicine," vol. 9, S. Karger, New York, 1976, p. 401.

116 Wilens, S. L.: The Resorption of Arterial Atheromatous Deposits in Wasting Disease, *Am. J. Pathol.,* 23:793, 1947.

117 Constantinides, P.: "Experimental Atherosclerosis," Elsevier Publishing Company, New York, 1965.

118 Armstrong, M. L., Warner, E. D., and Connor, W. E.: Regression of Coronary Atheromatosis in Rhesus Monkeys, *Circ. Res.,* 27:59, 1970.

119 DePalma, R. G., Hubay, C. A., Insull, W., Jr., Robinson, A. V., and Hartman, P. H.: Progression and Regression of Experimental Atherosclerosis, *Surg. Gynecol. Obst.,* 131:663, 1970.

120 Tucker, C. F., Catsulis, C., Strong, J. P., and Eggen, D. A.: Regression of Early Cholesterol-induced Aortic Lesions in Rhesus Monkeys, *Am. J. Pathol.,* 65:493, 1971.

121 Armstrong, M. L., and Megan, M. B.: Lipid Depletion in Atheromatous Coronary Arteries in Rhesus Monkeys after Regression Diets, *Circ. Res.,* 30:675, 1972.

122 Vesselinovitch, D., Wissler, R. W., Fisher-Dzoga, K., Hughes, R., and Dubien, L.: Regression of Atherosclerosis in Rabbits: Part I. Treatment with Low-fat Diet, Hyperoxia and Hypolipidemic Agents, *Atherosclerosis,* 19:259, 1974.

123 Kritchevsky, D., Davidson, L. M., Shapiro, I. L., Kim, H. K., Kitagawa, M., Malhotra, S., Nair, P. P., Clarkson, T. B., Bersohn, I., and Winter, P. A. D.: Lipid Metabolism and Experimental Atherosclerosis in Baboons: Influence of Cholesterol-free, Semi-synthetic Diets, *Am. J. Clin. Nutr.,* 27:29, 1974.

123a Wissler, R. W., Vesselinovitch, D., Borensztajn, J., and Hughes, R.: Regression of Severe Atherosclerosis in Cholestyramine-treated Rhesus Monkeys with or without a Low-fat, Low-cholesterol diet, *Circulation,* 52(suppl. II):II-16, 1975.

124 Vesselinovitch, D., Wissler, R. W., Hughes, R., and Borensztjn, J.: Reversal of Advanced Atherosclerosis in Rhesus Monkeys: Part I. Light-microscopic Studies, *Atherosclerosis,* 23:155, 1976.

124a Weber, G., Fabbrini, P., Resi, L., Jones, R., Vesselinovitch, D., and Wissler, R. W.: Regression of Arteriosclerotic Lesions in Rhesus Monkey Aortas after Regression Diet—Scanning and Transmission Electron Microscope Observations of the Endothelium, *Atherosclerosis,* 26:535, 1977.

125 Gresham, G. A.: Is Atheroma a Reversible Lesion? *Atherosclerosis,* 23:379, 1976.

125a Barndt, R., Blankenhorn, D. H., Crawford, D. W., and Brooks, S. H.: Regression and Progression of Early Femoral Atherosclerosis in Treated Hyperlipoproteinemic Patients, *Ann. Int. Med.,* 86:139, 1977.

126 The Health Consequences of Smoking: A Public Health Service Review, 1967, Public Health Service Publication no. 1696; and suppl., Public Health Service Publication no. 1696-2.

127 Doyle, J. T.: Cigarette-smoking and Coronary Atherosclerosis, in W. Likoff, B. L. Segal, and W. Insull, Jr. (eds.): "Atherosclerosis and Coronary Heart Disease," The Twenty-fourth Hahnemann Symposium, Grune & Stratton, Inc., New York, 1972, p. 35.

128 Aronow, W. S.: Smoking, Carbon Monoxide, and Coronary Heart Disease, *Circualtion,* 48:1169, 1973. (Editorial.)

129 Astrup, P.: Carbon Monoxide, Smoking, and Cardiovascular Disease, *Circulation,* 48:1167, 1973.

130 Wald, N., Howard, S., Smith, P. G., and Kjeldsen, K.: Association between Atherosclerotic Diseases and Carboxyhaemoglobin Levels in Tobacco Smokers, *Br. Med. J.,* 1:761, 1973.

131 Strong, J. P., and Richards, M. L.: Cigarette Smoking and Atherosclerosis in Autopsied Men, *Atherosclerosis,* 23:451, 1976.

132 Gordon, T., Kannel, W. B., McGee, D., and Dawber, T. R.: Death and Coronary Attacks in Men after Giving up Cigarette Smoking: A Report from the Framingham Study, *Lancet,* 2:1345, 1974.

133 Remein, Q. R., and Wilkerson, H. L. C.: The Efficiency of Screening Tests for Diabetes, *J. Chronic Dis.,* 13:6, 1961.

134 Build and Blood Pressure Study, 1959, Society of Actuaries, Metropolitan Life Insurance Company, Statistical Bulletin 40:3, 1959.

135 Durnin, J. V. G. A., and Womersley, J.: Body Fat Assessed from Total Body Density and Its Estimation from Skinfold Thickness: Measurements in 481 Men and Women Aged from 16 to 72 Years, *Br. J. Nutr.,* 32:77, 1974.

136 Standard for Definitions of Overweight and Obesity, in G. A. Blay (ed.), "Obesity in Perspective," DHEW Publication no. (NIH) 75-708, 1973, p. 7.

137 Seltzer, C. C., and Mayer, J.: A Simple Criterion of Obesity, *Postgrad. Med.,* 38:A101, 1965.

138 Page, I. H.: A Personal View on Diet and Atherogenesis, *Mod. Med.,* 39:49, 1971.

139 Mann, J. I., Vessey, M. P., Thorogood, M., and Doll, R.: Myocardial Infarction in Young Women with Special Reference to Oral Contraceptive Practice, *Br. Med. J.,* 2:241, 1975.

139a Mann, J. I., and Inman, W. H. W.: Oral Contraceptives and Death from Myocardial Infarction, *Brit. Med. J.,* 2:245, 1975.

139b Beral, V.: Cardiovascular Disease Mortality Trends and Oral Contraceptive Use in Young Women, *Lancet,* 2:1047, 1976.

140 Glueck, C. J., Heckman, F., Schoenfeld, M., Steiner, P., and Pearce, W.: Neonatal Familial Type II Hyperlipoproteinemia: Cord Blood Cholesterol in 1,800 Births, *Metabolism,* 20:597, 1971.

141 Kwiterovich, P. O., Jr., Levy, R. I., and Fredrickson, D. S.: Neonatal Diagnosis of Familial Type II Hyperlipoproteinaemia, *Lancet,* 1:118, 1973.

142 Chase, H. P., O'Quin, R. J., and O'Brien, D.: Screening for Hyperlipidemia in Childhood, *J.A.M.A.,* 230:1535, 1974.

143 Tan, M. H., Wilmshurst, E. G., Gleason, R. E., and Soeldner, J. S.: Effect of Posture on Serum Lipids, *N. Engl. J. Med.,* 289:416, 1973.

144 Byers, S. O., Friedman, M., Elek, S. R., Diamant, J., and Neuman, R.: Neurogenic Hypercholesterolemia: Influence of Autonomic Drugs, *Atherosclerosis,* 24:189, 1976.

145 Fredrickson, D. S.: It's Time to be Practical, *Circulation,* 51:209, 1975. (Editorial.)

146 Miller, G. J., and Miller, N. E.: Plasma-High-Density-Lipoprotein Concentration and Development of Ischaemic Heart-Disease, *Lancet,* 1:16, 1975.

146a Rhoads, G. G., Gulbrandsen, C. L., and Kagan, A.: Serum Lipoproteins and Coronary Heart Disease in a Population Study of Hawaii Japanese Men, *N. Engl. J. Med.,* 294:293, 1976.

146b Gordon, T., Castelli, W. P., Hames, C. G., Hjortland, M. C., Kannel, W. B., and Dawber, T. R.: High Density Lipoproteins as Protective Factor against Coronary Heart Disease: The Framingham Study, *Am. J. Med.,* 62:707, 1977.

146c Miller, N. E., Forde, O. H., Thelle, D. S., and Mjos, O. D.: The Tromso Heart-study, *Lancet,* 1:965, 1977.

146d Castelli, W. P., Doyle, J. T., Hjortland, M. C., Hulley, S. B., Kagan, A., and Zukel, W. J.: HDL Cholesterol and Other Lipids in Coronary Heart Disease: The Cooperative Phenotyping Study, *Circulation,* 55:767, 1977.

147 Fredrickson, D. S., and Lees, R. S.: A System for Phenotyping Hyperlipoproteinemia, *Circulation,* 31:321, 1965. (Editorial.)

148 Fredrickson, D. S., Levy, R. I., and Lees, R. S.: Fat Transport in Lipoproteins: An Integrated Approach to Mechanisms and Disorders, *N. Engl. J. Med.,* 276:34, 94, 148, 215, and 2773, 1967.

149 Levy, R. I., Fredrickson, D S.: Diagnosis and Management of Hyperlipoproteinemia, *Am. J. Cardiol.,* 22:576, 1968.

150 Fredrickson, D. S., Levy, R. I., Kwiterovich, P. O., and Jover, A.: The Typing of Hyperlipoproteinemia: A Progress Report (1968), in W. L. Holmes, L. A. Carlson, and R. Paoletti, "Drugs Affecting Lipid Metabolism," Plenum Press, New York, 1969, p. 307.

151 Beaumont, J. L., Carlson, L. A., Cooper, G. R., Feifer, Z., Fredrickson, D. S., and Strasser, T.: Classification of Hyperlipidemias and Hyperlipoproteinemias, *Bull. WHO,* 43:891, 1970.

152 Levy, R. I.: Classification and Etiology of Hyperlipoproteinemias, *Fed. Proc.,* 30:829, 1971.

153 Fredrickson, D. S.: An International Classification of Hyperlipidemias and Hyperlipoproteinemias, *Ann. Intern. Med.,* 75:471, 1971.

154 Beaumont, J. L., Carlson, L. A., Cooper, G. R., Fejfar, Z., Fredrickson, D. S., and Strasser, T.: WHO Memorandum: Classification of Hyperlipidaemias and Hyperlipoproteinaemias, *Circulation,* 45:501, 1972.

155 Fredrickson, D. S.: A Physician's Guide to Hyperlipidemia, *Mod. Concepts Cardiovasc. Dis.,* 41 (no. 7):31, 1972.

156 Fredrickson, D. S., and Levy, R. I.: Familial Hyperlipoproteinemia, in J. B. Stanbury, J. B. Wyngaarden, and D. S. Fredrickson (eds.), "The Metabolic Basis of Inherited Disease," 3d ed., McGraw-Hill Book Company, New York, 1972, p. 545.

157 Morganroth, J., and Levy, R. I.: The Diagnosis and Management of the Hyperlipoproteinemias, in E. Donoso (ed.), "Drugs in Cardiology," Stratton Intercontinental, New York, 1975, p. 127.

158 Fisher, W. R., and Truitt, D. H.: The Common Hyperlipoproteinemias: An Understanding of Disease Mechanisms and Their Control, *Ann. Intern. Med.,* 85:497, 1976.

159 Glueck, C. J., Fallat, R. W., and Moulton, R.: Hyperlipidemic States: Diagnosis and Treatment in N. O. Fowler (ed.): "Cardiac Diagnosis and Treatment," 2d ed., Harper and Row, Publishers, Incorporated, New York, 1976, p. 614.

160 Levy, R. I.: Hyperlipoproteinemia: Concepts of Diagnosis and Management, *Curr. Probl. Cardiol.,* 1(3):1, 1976.

160a Havel, R. J.: Classification of Hyperlipidemias, *Ann. Rev. Med.,* 28:195, 1977.

161 Glueck, C. J., and Tsang, R. C.: Pediatric Familial Type II Hyperlipoproteinemia: Effects of Diet on Plasma Cholesterol in the First Year of Life, *Am. J. Clin. Nutr.,* 25:224, 1972.

162 Goldstein, J. L., Albers, J. J., Hazzard, W. R., Schrott, H. R.,

Bierman, E. L., and Motulsky, A. G.: Genetic and Medical Significance of Neonatal Hyperlipidemia, *J. Clin. Invest.,* 52:35A, 1973.

163 Kwiterovich, P. O., Levy, R. I., and Fredrickson, D. S.: Familial Hyperbetalipoproteinemia (Type II Hyperlipoproteinemia) in Children, *J. Clin. Invest.,* 52:49A, 1973.

164 Fredrickson, D. S., and Breslow, J. L.: Primary Hyperlipoproteinemia in Infants, *Annu. Rev. Med.,* 24:315, 1973.

165 Stone, N. J., Levy, R. I., Fredrickson, D. S., and Verter, J.: Coronary Artery Disease in 116 Kindred with Familial Type II Hyperlipoproteinemia, *Circulation,* 49:476, 1974.

166 Tsang, R. C., Fallat, R. W., and Glueck, C. J.: Cholesterol at Birth and Age 1: Comparison of Normal and Hypercholesterolemic Neonates, *Pediatrics,* 53:458, 1974.

167 Tsang, R. C., and Glueck, C. J.: Perinatal Cholesterol Metabolism, *Clin. Perinat.,* 2:275, 1975.

168 Quarfordt, S., Levy, R. I., and Fredrickson, D. S.: On the Lipoprotein Abnormality in Type III Hyperlipoproteinemia, *J. Clin. Invest.,* 50:754, 1971.

169 Hazzard, W. R., O'Donnell, T. F., and Lee, Y. L.: Broad-β Disease (Type III Hyperlipoproteinemia) in a Large Kindred, *Ann. Intern. Med.,* 82:141, 1975.

170 Morganroth, J., Levy, R. I., and Fredrickson, D. S.: The Biochemical, Clinical and Genetic Features of Type III Hyperlipoproteinemia, *Ann. Intern. Med.,* 82:158, 1975.

171 Blankenhorn, D. H., Chin, H. P., and Lau, F. Y. K.: Ischemic Heart Disease in Young Adults: Metabolic and Angiographic Diagnosis and the Prevalence of Type IV Hyperlipoproteinemia, *Ann. Intern. Med.,* 69:21, 1968.

172 Stone, M. C., and Dick, T. B. S.: Prevalence of Hyperlipoproteinaemias in a Random Sample of Men and in Patients with Ischaemic Heart Disease, *Br. Heart J.,* 35:954, 1973.

173 Brown, D. F., and Daudiss, K.: Hyperlipoproteinemia: Prevalence in a Free-living Population in Albany, N.Y., *Circulation,* 47:558, 1973.

174 Wood, P. D., Stern, M. P., Silvers, A., Reaven, G. M., and Von der Groeben, J.: Prevalence of Plasma Lipoprotein Abnormalities in a Free-living Population of the Central Valley, California, *Circulation,* 45:114, 1972.

175 Salel, A. F., Riggs, K., Mason, D. T., Amsterdam, E. A., and Zelis, R.: The Importance of Type IV Hyperlipoproteinemia as a Predisposing Factor in Coronary Artery Disease, *Am. J. Med.,* 57:897, 1974.

176 Ahrens, E. H., Jr., Hirsch, J., Oette, K., and Farquhar, J. W.: Carbohydrate-induced and Fat-induced Lipemia, *Trans. Assoc. Am. Physicians,* 74:134, 1961.

177 Malmros, H.: Dietary Prevention of Atherosclerosis, *Lancet,* 2:479, 1969.

178 Stone, N. J.: When to Worry About Plasma Lipids, *Cardiovasc. Med.,* 1:143, 1976.

179 Goldstein, J. L., Schrott, H. G., Hazzard, W. R., Bierman, E. L., and Motulsky, A. G.: Hyperlipidemia in Coronary Heart Disease: II. Genetic Analysis of Lipid Levels in 176 Families and Delineation of a New Inherited Disorder, Combined Hyperlipidemia, *J. Clin. Invest.,* 52:1544, 1973.

180 Rose, H. G., Kranz, P., Weinstock, M., Juliano, J., and Haft, J. I.: Inheritance of Combined Hyperlipoproteinemia: Evidence for a New Lipoprotein Phenotype, *Am. J. Med.,* 54:148, 1973.

181 Glueck, C. J., Fallat, R., Buncher, C. R., Tsang, R., and Steiner, P.: Familial Combined Hyperlipoproteinemia: Studies in 91 Adults and 95 Children from 33 Kindreds, *Metabolism,* 22:1403, 1973.

182 Goldstein, J. L., and Brown, M. S.: Familial Hypercholesterolemia: A Genetic Regulatory Defect in Cholesterol Metabolism, *Am. J. Med.,* 58:147, 1975.

183 Goldstein, J. L., and Brown, M. S.: Hyperlipidemia in Coronary Heart Disease: A Biochemical Genetic Approach, *J. Lab. Clin. Med.,* 85:15, 1975.

184 Brown, M. S., and Goldstein, J. L.: Familial Hypercholesterolemia: Genetic, Biochemical and Pathophysiologic Considerations, *Adv. Intern. Med.,* 20:273, 1975.

185 Goldstein, J. L., and Brown, M. S.: Lipoprotein Receptors, Cholesterol Metabolism and Atherosclerosis, *Arch. Pathol.,* 99:181, 1975.

186 Motulsky, A. G.: Current Concepts in Genetics: The Genetic Hyperlipidemias, *N. Engl. J. Med.,* 294:823, 1976.

187 Levy, R. I., Bonnell, M., and Ernst, N. D.: Dietary Management of Hyperlipoproteinemia, *J. Am. Diet. Assoc.,* 58:406, 1971.

188 Fredrickson, D. S., Levy, R. I., Bonnell, M., and Ernst, N.: Dietary Management of Hyperlipoproteinemia, DHEW Publication no. (NIH) 75-110. Washington, D.C., 1974.

189 Committee on Nutrition, American Heart Association: Diet and Coronary Heart Disease, American Heart Association (EM 379), 1973.

190 Williams, C. L., and Wynder, E. L.: A Blind Spot in Preventive Medicine, *J.A.M.A.,* 236:2196, 1976.

191 Stead, E. S., and Warren, G. K.: "Low-fat Cookery," rev. ed., McGraw-Hill Company, New York, 1959.

192 Keys, A., and Keys, M.: "Eat Well and Stay Well," rev. ed., Doubleday & Company, Inc., Garden City, N.Y., 1963.

193 Havenstein, N., and Richardson, E.: "The Anti-Coronary Cookbook," rev. ed., Grosset & Dunlap, Inc., New York, 1971.

194 Bond, C-B. Y., Dobbin, E. V., Gofman, H. F., Jones, H. C., and Lyon, L.: "The Low Fat, Low Cholesterol Diet," Doubleday & Company, Inc., Garden City, N.Y., 1971.

195 The American Heart Association Cookbook, rev. ed., David McKay Company, New York, 1975, p. 454.

196 Smith, L. K., Luepker, R. V., Rothchild, S. S., Gillis, A., Kochman, L., and Warbasse, J. R.: Management of Type IV Hyperlipoproteinemia: Evaluation of Practical Clinical Approaches, *Ann. Intern. Med.,* 84:22, 1976.

197 Albrink, M. J.: Triglycerides, Lipoproteins, and Coronary Artery Disease, *Arch. Intern. Med.,* 109:345, 1962.

198 Carlson, L. A., and Bottiger, L. E.: Ischaemic Heart Disease in Relation to Fasting Values of Plasma Triglycerides and Cholesterol: Stockholm Prospective Study, *Lancet,* 1:865, 1972.

199 Brown, M. S., and Goldstein, J. L.: Receptor-mediated Control of Cholesterol Metabolism, *Science,* 191:150, 1976.

200 Fredrickson, D. S., Levy, R. I., and Lindgren, F. T.: A Comparison of Heritable Abnormal Lipoprotein Patterns as Defined by Two Different Techniques, *J. Clin. Invest.,* 47:2446, 1968.

201 Strong, J. P., and McGill, H. C., Jr.: The Pediatric Aspects of Atherosclerosis, *J. Atheroscler. Res.,* 9:251, 1969.

202 Glueck, C. J., Fallat, R. W., and Tsang, R.: Hypercholesterolemia and Hypertriglyceridemia in Children, *Am. J. Dis. Child.,* 128:569, 1974.

203 Lauer, R. M., Conner, W. E., Leaverton, P. E., Reiter, M. A., and Clarke, W. R.: Coronary Heart Disease Risk Factors in School CHildren: The Muscatine Study, *J. Pediatr.,* 86:697, 1975.

203a Frerichs, R. R., Srinivasan, S. R., Webber, L. S., and Berenson, G. S.: Serum Cholesterol and Triglyceride Levels in 3,446 Children from a Biracial Community—Bogalusa Heart Study, *Circulation,* 54:302, 1976.

203b Srinivasan, S. R., Frerichs, R. R., Webber, L. S., and Berenson, G. S.: Serum Lipoprotein Profile in Children from a Biracial Community—Bogalusa Heart Study, *Circulation,* 54:309, 1976.

204 Dyerberg, J., Bang, H. O., and Nielsen, J. A.: Plasma Lipids and Lipoproteins in Patients with Myocardial Infarction and in a Control Material, *Acta Med. Scand.,* 187:353, 1970.

205 Werkö, L.: Can We Prevent Heart Disease? *Ann. Intern. Med.,* 74:278, 1971.

206 Heinle, R. A., Levy, R. I., Fredrickson, D. S., and Gorlin, R.: Lipid and Carbohydrate Abnormalities in Patients with Angiographically Documented Coronary Artery Disease, *Am. J. Cardiol.,* 24:178, 1969.

207 Enger, S. C., and Ritland, S.: Serum Lipoprotein Pattern in Myocardial Infarction, *Acta Med. Scand.,* 187:365, 1970.

208 Falsetti, H. L., Schnatz, J. D., Greene, D. G., and Bunnell, I. L.: Serum Lipids and Glucose Tolerance in Angiographically Proved Coronary Artery Disease, *Chest,* 58:111, 1970.

209 Patterson, D., and Slack, J.: Lipid Abnormalities in Male and Female Survivors of Myocardial Infarction and their First-degree Relatives, *Lancet,* 1:393, 1972.

210 Aro, A.: Serum Lipids and Lipoproteins in First Degree Relatives of Young Survivors of Myocardial Infarction, *Acta Med. Scand.,* (suppl. 553), 1973.

211 Nikkila, E. A., and Aro, A.: Family Study of Serum Lipids and Lipoproteins in Coronary Heart Disease, *Lancet,* 1:954, 1973.

212 Gustafson, A.: Serum Lipoproteins in Coronary Heart Disease, in J. Waldenstrom, T. Larsson, and N. Ljungstedt (eds.), "Early Phases of Coronary Heart Disease: The Possibility of Prediction," Nordiska Bokhandelns Vorlag, Stockholm, 1973, p. 201.

213 Goldstein, J. L., Hazzard, W. R., Schrott, H. G., Bierman, E. L., and Motulsky, A. G.: Hyperlipidemia in Coronary Heart Disease: I. Lipid Levels in 500 Survivors of Myocardial Infarction, *J. Clin. Invest.,* 52:1533, 1973.

214 Hazzard, W. R., Goldstein, J. L., Schrott, H. G., Motulsky, A. G., and Bierman, E. L.: Hyperlipidemia in Coronary Heart Disease: III. Evaluation of Lipoprotein Phenotypes of 156 Genetically Defined Survivors of Myocardial Infarction, *J. Clin. Invest.,* 52:1569, 1973.

215 Glueck. C. J., Fallat, R. W., Tsang, R., and Buncher, C. R.: Hyperlipemia in Progeny of Parents with Myocardial Infarction before Age 50, *Am. J. Dis. Child.,* 127:70, 1974.

216 Cohn, P. F., Gabbay, S. I., and Weglicki, W. B.: Serum Lipid Levels in Angiographically Defined Coronary Artery Disease, *Ann. Intern. Med.,* 84:241, 1976.

217 Rifkind, B. M. (ed.): Clinics in Endocrinology and Metabolism, "Disorders of Lipid Metabolism," vol. 2, no. 1, W. B. Saunders Company, Philadelphia, 1973, p. 151.

218 Friedewald, W. T., Levy, R. I., and Fredrickson, D. S.: Estimation of the Concentration of Low-Density Lipoprotein Cholesterol in Plasma, Without Use of the Preparative Ultracentrifuge, *Clin. Chem.,* 18:499, 1972.

219 Brown, M. S., and Goldstein, J. L.: Expression of the Familial Hypercholesterolemia Gene in Heterozygotes: Mechanism for a Dominant Disorder in Man, *Science,* 185:61, 1974.

220 Levy, R. I., Fredrickson, D. S., and Stone, N. J.: Cholestyramine in Type II Hyperlipoproteinemia: A Double-blind Trial, *Ann. Intern. Med.,* 79:51, 1973.

221 Moutafis, C. D., Myant, N. B., Mancini, M., and Oriente, P.: Cholestyramine and Nicotinic Acid in the Treatment of Familial Hyperbetalipoproteinaemia in the Homozygous Form, *Atherosclerosis,* 14:247, 1971.

222 Levy, R. I., Fredrickson, D. S., Shulman, R., Bilheimer, D. W., Breslow, J. L., Stone, N. J., Lux, S. E., Sloan, H. R., Krauss, R. M., and Herbert, P. N.: Dietary and Drug Treatment of Primary Hyperlipoproteinemia, *Ann. Intern. Med.,* 77:267, 1972.

223 Levy, R. I., and Rifkind, B. M.: Lipid Lowering Drugs and Hyperlipidaemia, *Drugs,* 6:12, 1973.

224 Levy, R. I., Morganroth, J., and Rifkind, B. M.: Drug Therapy: Treatment of Hyperlipidemia, *N. Engl. J. Med.,* 290:1295, 1974.

225 Buxtorf, J. C., Beaumont, V., Jacotot, B., and Beaumont,

J.-L.: Regression de xanthomes et medicaments hypolipide-miants, *Atherosclerosis*, 19:1, 1974.

226 Faergeman, O.: Effects and Side-effects of Treatment of Hypercholesterolemia with Cholestyramine and Neomycin, *Acta Med. Scand.*, 194:165, 1973.

227 Lees, A. M., McCluskey, M. A., and Lees, R. S.: Results of Colestipol Therapy in Type II Hyperlipoproteinemia, *Atherosclerosis*, 24:129, 1976.

228 Kuo, P. T., Fan, W. C., Kostis, J. B., and Hayase, K.: Combined Para-aminosalicylic Acid and Dietary Therapy in Long-term Control of Hypercholesterolemia and Hypertriglyceridemia (Types IIa and IIb Hyperlipoproteinemia), *Circulation*, 53:338, 1976.

229 Lansen, R., Glueck, C. J., and Tsang, R.: Special Diet for Familial Type II Hyperlipoproteinemia, *Am. J. Dis. Child.*, 128:67, 1974.

230 Tsang, R. C., and Glueck, C. J.: Hyperlipidemia and the Heart: Part IV. Treatment of Pediatric Hyperlipidemia, *Pract. Cardiol.*, 2:37, 1976.

231 Buchwald, H., and Varco, R. L.: Partial Ileal Bypass for Hypercholesterolemia and Atherosclerosis, *Surg., Gynecol., and Obstet.*, 124:1231, 1967.

232 Buchwald, H., Moore, R. B., Frantz, I. D., Jr., and Varco, R. L.: Cholesterol Reduction by Partial Ileal Bypass in a Pediatric Population, *Surgery*, 68:1101, 1970.

233 Gomes, M. M. R., Bernatz, P. E., Kottke, B. A., Juergens, J. L., and Titus, J. L.: Ileal Bypass in Treatment of Hyperlipidemia: Rationale and Present Status, *Mayo Clin. Proc.*, 45:229, 1970.

234 Thompson, G. R., and Gotto, A. M., Jr.: Ileal Bypass in the Treatment of Hyperlipoproteinaemia, *Lancet*, 2:35, 1973.

235 Schwartz, M. Z., Varco, R. L., and Buchwald, H.: Treatment of Heterozygous Type II Hyperlipidemia by Partial Ileal Bypass in a Pediatric Population, *J. Pediatr. Surg.*, 11:411, 1976.

236 Moore, R. B., Varco, R. L., and Buchwald, H.: Metabolic Surgery in the Hyperlipoproteinemias, *Am. J. Cardiol.*, 31:148, 1973.

237 Balfour, J. F., and Kim, R.: Homozygous Type II Hyperlipoproteinemia Treatment: Partial Ileal Bypass in Two Children, *J.A.M.A.*, 227:1145, 1974.

238 Starzl, T. E., Chase, H. P., Putnam, C. W., Porter, K. A.: Portacaval Shunt in Hyperlipoproteinaemia, *Lancet*, 2:940, 1973.

239 Starzl, T. E., Chase, H. P., Putnam, C. W., and Nora, J. J.: Follow-up of Patient with Portacaval Shunt for the Treatment of Hyperlipidaemia, *Lancet*, 2:714, 1974.

240 Stein, E. A., Pettifor, J., Mieny, C., Heimann, K. W., Spitz, L., Bersohn, I., Saaron, I., and Dinner, M.: Portacaval Shunt in Four Patients with Homozygous Hypercholesterolaemia, *Lancet*, 1:832, 1975.

241 Starzl, T. E., and Putnam, C. W.: Portal Diversion: Treatment for Glycogen Storage Disease and Hyperlipidemia, *J.A.M.A.*, 233:955, 1975.

242 Chase, H. P., and Morris, T.: Cholesterol Metabolism following Portacaval Shunt in the Pig, *Atherosclerosis*, 24:141, 1976.

243 Apstein, C. S., George, P. K., Zilversmit, D. B., Feldman, H. A., and Lees, R. S.: Cholesterol Reduction with Intensive Plasmapheresis, *Clin. Res.*, 22:459A, 1974.

244 Thompson, G. R., Lowenthal, R., and Myant, N. B.: Plasma Exchange in the Management of Homozygous Familial Hypercholesterolaemia, *Lancet*, 1:1208, 1975.

245 Thompson, G. R., and Myant, N. B.: Low Density Lipoprotein Turnover in Familial Hypercholesterolaemia after Plasma Exchange, *Atherosclerosis*, 23:371, 1976.

246 Lupien, P.-J., Moorjani, S., and Awad, J.: A New Approach to the Management of Familial Hypercholesterolaemia: Removal of Plasma-cholesterol Based on the Principle of Affinity Chromatography, *Lancet*, 1:1261, 1976.

247 Roberts, W. C., Levy, R. I., and Fredrickson, D. S.: Hyper-lipoproteinemia: A Review of the Five Types with First Report of Necropsy Findings in Type III, *Arch. Pathol.*, 90:45, 1970.

248 Fredrickson, D. S., Morganroth, J., and Levy, R. I.: Type III Hyperlipoproteinemia: An Analysis of Two Contemporary Definitions, *Ann. Intern. Med.*, 82:150, 1975.

249 Havel, R. J.: Hyperlipoproteinemia: Problems in Diagnosis and Challenges Posed by the "Type III" Disorder, *Ann. Intern. Med.*, 82:273, 1975.

250 Zelis, R., Mason, D. T., Braunwald, E. B., and Levy, R. I.: Effects of Hyperlipoproteinemias and Their Treatment on Peripheral Circulation, *J. Clin. Invest.*, 49:1007, 1970.

251 Deegan, T., and Hayward, P. J.: Serum Lipid Changes Following Myocardial Infarction, *J. Atheroscler. Res.*, 5:267, 1965.

252 Brown, D. F., Kinch, S. H., and Doyle, J. T.: Serum Triglycerides in Health and in Ischemic Heart Disease, *N. Engl. J. Med.*, 273:947, 1965.

253 Brunzell, J. D., Schrott, H. G., Motulsky, A. G., and Bierman, E. L.: Myocardial Infarction in the Familial Forms of Hypertriglyceridemia, *Metabolism*, 25:313, 1976.

254 Lieber, C. S.: Effects of Ethanol upon Lipid Metabolism, *Lipids*, 9:103, 1974.

255 Ginsberg, H., Olefsky, J., Farquhar, J. W., and Reaven, G. M.: Moderate Ethanol Ingestion and Plasma Triglyceride Levels: A Study in Normal and Hypertriglyceridemic Persons, *Ann. Intern. Med.*, 80:143, 1974.

256 Barboriak, J. J., and Hogan, W. J.: Preprandial Drinking and Plasma Lipids in Man, *Atherosclerosis*, 24:323, 1976.

257 Zelis, R., Amsterdam, E. A., Spann, J. E., Jr., and Mason, D. T.: Type IV Hyperlipoproteinemia: Clofibrate without Dietary Therapy, *J.A.M.A.*, 222:326, 1972.

258 Schonfeld, G., and Kudzma, D. J.: Type IV Hyperlipoproteinemia: A Critical Appraisal, *Arch. Intern. Med.*, 132:55, 1973.

259 Gotto, A. M., Jr.: Type V Hyperlipoproteinaemia, *J. Clin. Endocrinol. Metab.*, 2:11, 1973.

260 Yeshurun, D., and Gotto, A. M., Jr.: Drug Treatment of Hyperlipidemia, *Am. J. Med.*, 60:379, 1976.

261 Slack, J., and Nevin, N. C.: Hyperlipidaemic Xanthomatosis: I. Increased Risk of Death from Ischaemic Heart Disease in First Degree Relatives of 53 Patients with Essential Hyperlipidaemia and Xanthomatosis, *J. Med. Genet.*, 5:4, 1968.

262 Carter, C. O., Slack, J., and Myant, N. B.: Genetics of Hyperlipoproteinaemias, *Lancet*, 1:400, 1971.

263 Stanley, P., Chartrand, C., and Davignon, A.: Acquired Aortic Stenosis in a Twelve-year-old Girl with Xanthomatosis: Successful Surgical Correction, *N. Engl. J. Med.*, 273:1378, 1965.

264 Wennevold, A., and Jacobsen, J. G.: Acquired Supravalvular Aortic Stenosis in Familial Hypercholesterolemia: A Hemodynamic and Angiocardiographic Study, *Am. J. Med.*, 50:823, 1971.

265 Darmady, J. M., Fosbrooke, A. S., and Lloyd, J. K.: Prospective Study of Serum Cholesterol Levels during First Year of Life, *Br. Med. J.*, 2:685, 1972.

266 Tsang, R., Glueck, C. J., Evans, G., and Steiner, P. M.: Cord Blood Hypertriglyceridemia, *Am. J. Dis. Child.*, 127:78, 1974.

267 Brown, M. S., and Goldstein, J. L.: Familial Hypercholesterolemia: Defective Binding of Lipoproteins to Cultured Fibroblasts Associated with Impaired Regulation of 3-Hydroxy-3-Methylglutaryl Coenzyme: A Reductase Activity, *Proc. Natl. Acad. Sci. U.S.A.*, 71:788, 1974.

268 Moutafis, C. D., Simons, L. A., Myant, N. B., Adams, P. W., and Wynn, V.: The Effect of Cholestyramine on the Faecal Excretion of Bile Acids and Neutral Steroids in Familial Hypercholesterolemia, *Atherosclerosis*, 26:329, 1977.

269 Matthews, R. J.: Type III and IV Familial Hyperlipoproteinemia: Evidence that These Two Syndromes are Different Phenotypic Expressions of the Same Mutant Gene(s), *Am. J. Med.,* 44:188, 1968.

270 Schreibman, P. H., Wilson, D. E., and Arky, R. A.: Familial Type IV Hyperlipoproteinemia, *N. Engl. J. Med.,* 281:981, 1969.

271 Glueck, C. J., Tsang, R., Fallat, R., Buncher, C. R., Evans, G., and Steiner, P.: Familial Hypertriglyceridemia: Studies in 130 Children and 45 Siblings of 36 Index Cases, *Metabolism,* 22:1287, 1973.

272 Levy, R. I., Fredrickson, D. S.: The Current Status of Hypolipidemic Drugs, *Postgrad. Med.,* 47:130, 1970.

273 Lees, R. S., and Wilson, D. E.: The Treatment of Hyperlipidemia, *N. Engl. J. Med.,* 284:186, 1971.

274 Parsons, W. B., Jr.: Use of Nicotinic Acid Compounds in Treatment of Hyperlipidemia, in H. R. Casdorph (ed.), "Treatment of the Hyperlipidemic States," Charles C Thomas, Publisher, Springfield, Ill., 1971, p. 335.

275 Levy, R. I., and Langer, T.: Hypolipidemic Drugs and Lipoprotein Metabolism, *Adv. Exp. Med. Biol.,* 26:155, 1972.

276 Havel, R. J., and Kane, J. P.: Drugs and Lipid Metabolism, *Annu. Rev. Pharmacol.,* 13:287, 1973.

277 Azarnoff, D. L.: Individualization of Treatment of Hyperlipoproteinemic Disorders, *Med. Clin. North Am.,* 58:1129, 1974.

278 Kritchevsky, D. (ed.): "Hypolipidemic Agents," Springer-Verlag Inc., New York, 1975, p. 488.

279 Kritchevsky, D., Paoletti, R., and Holmes, W. L. (eds.): "Lipids, Lipoproteins and Drugs," Plenum Press, New York, 1975, p. 515.

280 Levy, R. I.: Drug Therapy of Hyperlipoproteinemia, *J.A.M.A.,* 235:2334, 1976.

281 Rifkind, B. M., and Levy, R. I.: Hyperlipidemia and Vascular Disease, in E. K. Chung (ed.) "Controversy in Cardiology: The Practical Clinical Approach," Springer-Verlag New York Inc., New York, 1976, p. 99.

282 Levy, R. I., Fredrickson, D. S., Stone, N. J., Bilheimer, D. W., Brown, W. V., Glueck, C. J., Gotto, A. M., Herbert, P. N., Kwiterovich, P. O., Langer, T., LaRosa, J., Lux, S. E., Rider, A. K., Shulman, R. S., and Sloan, H. R.: Cholestyramine in Type II Hyperlipoproteinemia: A Double-blind Trial, *Ann. Intern. Med.,* 79:51, 1973.

283 Blum, C. B., Havlik, R. J., and Morganroth, J.: Cholestyramine: An Effective, Twice-daily Dosage Regimen, *Ann. Intern. Med.,* 85:287, 1976.

284 Miettinen, T. A.: Influence of Nicotinic Acid in Cholesterol Synthesis in Man, in "Metabolic Effects of Nicotinic Acid and Its Derivatives," K. F. Gey and L. A. Carlson (eds.), Hans Huber Medical Publisher, Berne, Switzerland, 1971, p. 649.

285 Nikkila, E. A.: Effect of Drugs on Plasma Triglyceride Metabolism, *Adv. Exp. Med. Biol.,* 26:113, 1972.

286 Magide, A. A., Myant, N. B., and Reichl, D.: The Effect of Nicotinic Acid on the Metabolism of the Plasma Lipoproteins of Rhesus Monkeys, *Atherosclerosis,* 21:205, 1975.

287 Rose, H. G., Haft, G. K., and Juliano, J.: Clofibrate-induced Low Density Lipoprotein Elevation: Therapeutic Implications and Treatment by Colestipol Resin, *Atherosclerosis,* 23:413, 1976.

288 Rakow, A. D., Klör, H. U., Küter, E., Ditschuneit, H. H., and Ditschuneit, H.: Treatment of Type II Hyperlipoproteinemia with D-thyroxine, *Atherosclerosis,* 24:369, 1976.

289 Bechtol, L. D., and Warner, W. L.: Dextrothyroxine for Lowering Serum Cholesterol: Analysis of Data on 6066 Patients, *Angiology,* 20:565, 1969.

290 Krikler, D. M., Lefevre, D., and Lewis, B.: Dextrothyroxine with Propranolol in Treatment of Hypercholesterolaemia, *Lancet,* 1:934, 1971.

291 Cooper, E. E., and Michel, A. M.: Colestipol Hydrochloride, A New Hypolipidemic Drug: A Two-year Study, *South. Med. J.,* 68:303, 1975.

292 Barter, P. J., Connor, W. E., Spector, A. A., Armstrong, M., Connor, S. L., and Newman, M. A.: Lowering of Serum Cholesterol and Triglyceride by Para-aminosalicylic Acid in Hyperlipoproteinemia, *Ann. Intern. Med.,* 81:619, 1974.

292a Salel, A. F., Zelis, R., Sodhi, H. S., Price, J., and Mason, D. T.: Probucol: A New Cholesterol-lowering Drug Effective in Patients with Type II Hyperlipoproteinemia, *Clin. Pharm. Therap.,* 20:690, 1976.

293 Glueck, C. J., Levy, R. I., and Fredrickson, D. S.: Norethindrone Acetate, Post-heparin Lipolytic Activity, and Plasma Triglycerides in Familial Types I, III, IV and V Hyperlipoproteinemia, *Ann. Intern. Med.,* 75:345, 1971.

294 Glueck, C. J.: Effects of Oxandrolone on Plasma Triglycerides and Postheparin Lipolytic Activity in Patients with Types III, IV, and V Familial Hyperlipoproteinemia, *Metabolism,* 20:691, 1971.

295 Lowe, C. U.: The Role of Government in Implementing Good Nutritional Practice, *Bull. N.Y. Acad. Med.,* 47:647, 1971.

296 McGandy, R. B., Hall, B., Ford, C., and Stare, F. J.: Dietary Regulation of Blood Cholesterol in Adolescent Males: A Pilot Study, *Am. J. Clin. Nutr.,* 25:61, 1972.

297 Ford, C. H., McGandy, R. B., and Stare, F. J.: An Institutional Approach to the Dietary Regulation of Blood Cholesterol in Adolescent Males, *Prev. Med.,* 1:426, 1972.

298 Food and Nutrition Board, National Academy of Sciences—National Research Council and Council on Foods and Nutrition, American Medical Association: Diet and Coronary Heart Disease: A Joint Statement, *Prev. Med.,* 1:559, 1972.

299 American Health Foundation: Position Statement on Diet and Coronary Heart Disease, *Prev. Med.,* 1:255, 1972.

300 Keys, A.: Prevention of Coronary Heart Disease: Official Recommendations from Scandinavia, *Circulation,* 28: 227, 1968.

301 Keys, A.: Official Collective Recommendations on Diet in the Scandinavian Countries, *Nutr. Rev.,* 26:259, 1968.

302 den Hartogs, C.: Report of the Netherlands Nutritional Council: Recommendations on Amount and Nature of Dietary Fat, *Voeding,* 34:552, 1973.

303 Vergroesen, A. J., and Gottenbos, J. J.: The Role of Fats in Human Nutrition: An Introduction, in A. J. Vergroesen (ed.): "The Role of Fats in Human Nutrition," app. 2, Academic Press, Inc., New York, 1975.

Nonatherosclerotic Causes of Myocardial Ischemia and Necrosis

A
Rare Causes of Coronary Artery Disease

NANETTE KASS WENGER, M.D.

Atherosclerosis is the most common cause of coronary artery disease. Since many other processes may involve the coronary arteries, however, it is not accurate to use the term coronary artery disease as synonymous with coronary atherosclerosis. This chapter will review briefly some of the relatively rare, nonatherosclerotic causes of coronary artery disease.[1,2] Additional causes, such as coronary artery spasm, are discussed in Chap. 63B.

CONGENITAL ANOMALIES OF THE ORIGIN OF CORONARY ARTERIES[1-4]

The increasing use of coronary angiography has resulted in the more frequent detection of anomalies in the origin, number, size, distribution, and anatomic course of the coronary arteries. Most of these variations are not important clinically although they may be of great importance at the time of surgery for congenital heart disease, valve disease, or coronary artery disease, when it is critical to avoid inadvertent transsection of an aberrant coronary artery at ventriculotomy. Recognition at angiography of anomalous origin of a coronary artery or branch is important in avoiding misdiagnosing coronary occlusion.

Anomalous origin of the left coronary artery from the pulmonary artery (Bland-White-Garland syndrome)[5]

This rare condition is the most important significant congenital anomaly of the coronary arteries. It occurs in approximately 1 in 300,000 children,[10] and its incidence among all types of congenital heart disease is between 1 in 200 to 400, with a 2:1 ratio of females to males.[6-9] It is usually fatal in the first year, although about 15 percent of patients have coronary collateral circulation adequate for survival to adult life, and one lived to 64 years.[11] In utero and for a short period immediately after birth, blood flow in the anomalous coronary artery occurs, with good perfusion pressure, from the pulmonary artery to the myocardium. Because of the rapid decrease in pulmonary artery pressure after birth (see Chap. 7), however, blood flow in the anomalous vessel rapidly decreases and eventually reverses. In some infants, the rate of decrease of the pulmonary artery pressure is hindered by left ventricular failure due to ischemia. Subsequently, the anomalous vessel receives blood from the normal right coronary artery via collaterals and empties into the pulmonary artery, thereby producing a type of "coronary steal."[7] This may produce ischemia and/or infarction of the myocardium normally supplied by the left coronary artery unless the intercoronary collaterals are unusually adequate. Mitral regurgitation may be produced by ischemia or infarction of the left ventricular wall at the base of the papillary muscles or of the papillary muscles themselves, as well as by left ventricular dilatation.[12] The areas of infarction may have focal calcification, and the left ventricle may have marked endocardial fibroelastosis.

Wesselhoeft et al.[12] reviewed 140 reported cases in addition to 7 cases of their own and classified the clinical spectrum and mode of presentation in the following four groups:

THE INFANTILE SYNDROME

This is the largest group (82 percent) of patients with this condition. The diagnosis should be considered in infants who appear normal at birth but who, at about 10 weeks of life, develop acute episodes of respiratory distress, cyanosis, irritability, and profuse cold sweating. The episodes typically occur during or after feedings. There may or may not be other evidence of congestive heart failure. Repeated respiratory infections and failure to thrive are characteristic. The heart is enlarged, the left ventricular apical impulse is prominent, and there may be a short systolic murmur. Occasionally, a faint continuous murmur is heard along the lower left sternal border when there is a good coronary collateral circulation. The electrocardiogram (Fig. 63A-1) classically shows evidence of anterolateral myocardial infarction and frequently suggests left ventricular hypertrophy. Supraventricular tachyarrhythmias may be seen. The horizontal vectorcardiogram characteristically shows

FIGURE 63A-1 Anomalous origin of the left coronary artery from the pulmonary artery. Electrocardiogram of a 4-month-old infant showing evidence of anterolateral myocardial infarction.

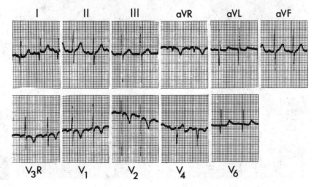

a clockwise loop, oriented posteriorly and to the left. The chest roentgenogram usually shows cardiomegaly, often with an aneurysmal left ventricular bulge due to myocardial thinning, and may show left atrial enlargement and pulmonary vascular congestion. These children may appear well between attacks, but usually die suddenly before 2 years of age.

MITRAL REGURGITATION

This presentation can be seen in infants, adolescents or adults who present with the murmur of mitral regurgitation, congestive heart failure, cardiomegaly and atrial arrhythmias.[12] The electrocardiogram may give a clue to the etiology.

CONTINUOUS MURMUR SYNDROME

This small subgroup of patients who reach adult life may be asymptomatic, although a few have angina pectoris. The predominant feature is a continuous precordial murmur, presumably due to good coronary collateral flow between the right and left coronary arteries, which may be mistaken for a patent ductus arteriosus. The electrocardiographic abnormalities of left axis deviation and/or anterolateral myocardial infarction may suggest the diagnosis.

SUDDEN DEATH IN ADOLESCENTS OR ADULTS

The majority of patients in this group are asymptomatic, although a few may have angina pectoris or palpitations. The age at which sudden death has occurred may range from 16 to 60 years. Arrhythmias, particularly ventricular, have a poor prognosis.

TREATMENT

The initial goal of therapy is to control the congestive heart failure and tachyarrhythmias. As soon as is feasible, diagnostic studies, including catheterization of the right side of the heart and selective arteriography of the right coronary artery, should be performed to determine the coronary anatomy and the extent of intercoronary collateral flow from angiography and to estimate the volume of the left-to-right shunt (Fig. 63A-2). In patients with at least a detecta-

FIGURE 63A-2 Anomalous origin of the left coronary artery from the pulmonary artery. *A* and *B*. Roentgenograms of the chest of a 10-month-old child showing massive cardiomegaly and congestive heart failure. *C* and *D*. Aortograms of a 2½-year-old child with this syndrome. In *C*, the large right coronary artery, RCA, is seen to fill from the base of the aorta. The left coronary artery, LCA, does not fill from the aorta. The contrast material passes from the right coronary artery, RCA, with retrograde flow into the left coronary artery, LCA, and subsequent filling of the main pulmonary artery. In *D*, extensive collateral communications (see arrows) at the cardiac apex between the right coronary artery and the anomalous left coronary artery are seen.

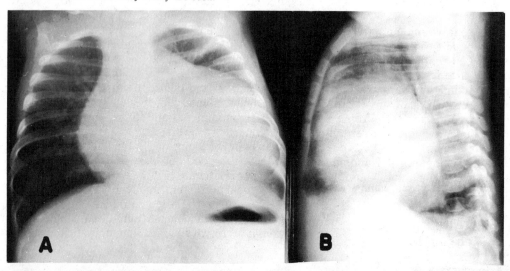

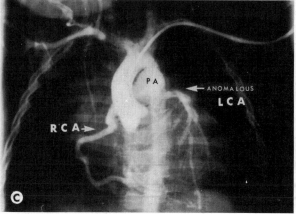

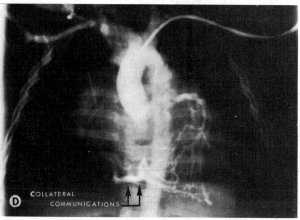

ble left-to-right shunt (from the right coronary artery to the left coronary artery to the pulmonary artery) and with an anomalous left coronary artery of reasonable size, surgery should be attempted to improve myocardial blood flow and to prevent myocardial infarction or sudden death. Medical management is the preferred treatment in infancy, with surgery reserved for the symptomatic infant who does not respond to medical management because of the high mortality of surgery in infancy and the increased incidence of graft stenosis and occlusion. Surgery consists of obliteration of the anomalous orifice of the left coronary artery and, whenever technically feasible, revascularization of the left coronary artery.[13-16] In infants, revascularization is usually attempted utilizing the left subclavian artery.[15] In older individuals, saphenous vein aortocoronary bypass grafting is utilized. Recently, the Texas Heart Institute group has recommended that direct implantation of the aberrant left coronary artery into the aorta be performed both in infants and in adults, citing its safety and efficacy.[16a]

In general, the operative mortality is less for adults than for children; abnormal exercise stress tests may even revert to normal postoperatively.[13] Improvement of the vectorcardiogram postoperatively is a favorable prognostic sign. However, even after successful bypass grafting, the collateral vessels do not regress. However, regression of the mitral regurgitation is not uncommon. An increased incidence of sudden death, presumably due to arrhythmia, is encountered even after successful surgical repair. Adult patients with this syndrome who develop coronary atherosclerosis have less atherosclerosis in the low-pressure left coronary artery than in the right coronary artery.

Anomalous origin of the right coronary artery from the pulmonary artery appears to be associated with a good prognosis and surgical intervention is not required, however, sudden death has been described.[1] Anomalous origin of both coronary arteries from the pulmonary trunk is almost always fatal.[17,18]

Anomalous origin of a coronary artery from the aorta

An anomalous origin of the coronary artery or coronary artery branch from the aorta is found in approximately 1 out of 200 patients undergoing coronary arteriography.[19] Although few of these ectopic origins are of hemodynamic significance, their recognition is important especially in the evaluation of patients with coronary artery disease or patients undergoing surgery for congenital heart disease (see below). The most common significant anomaly in this group is an ectopic circumflex coronary artery, arising from the right coronary sinus of Valsalva or from the main trunk of the right coronary artery. When the entire left coronary artery arises from the right coronary (anterior) sinus of Valsalva, this condition is associated with a high incidence of exercise-related sudden death. Coronary revascularization is indicated in the presence of ischemic pain or heart failure.[9] Lactate production during pacing, a decrease in coronary sinus blood flow with exercise,

and/or an abnormal exercise stress test may help detect patients predisposed to ischemia.

The left coronary artery may also arise from the proximal portion of the right coronary artery; the right coronary artery may arise from the left coronary artery sinus of Valsalva; and the left anterior descending branch of the left coronary artery may arise from the proximal right coronary artery or from the right coronary (anterior) sinus of Valsalva.

Single coronary artery or congenital absence of the right or left coronary artery

In this rare condition a proximal coronary artery fails to form normally. If there are no associated defects, however, adequate coronary collaterals may develop, there may be no symptoms, and the condition may only be discovered at autopsy. Atherosclerosis does not appear to occur prematurely; but if coronary atherosclerosis develops in the single coronary artery, the patient has no other adequate source of collateral blood flow and is in increased jeopardy.[20,21] Patients with tetralogy of Fallot may have a single coronary artery (see below).

Hypoplasia of one coronary artery

This condition may occur in either the left or the right coronary artery, and it may occur alone or in association with other cardiac anomalies. It also is usually compatible with longevity, although sudden death may occur.

Short left coronary artery

In most adults the main left coronary artery is 9 to 12 mm in length. At the time of cardiac surgery it is important to know if this artery is shorter when cannulating the left coronary artery in order to perfuse both branches.

Atresia of the left coronary artery ostium

Mullins et al.[22] reported a 14-year-old boy with syncope, shortness of breath, and premature ventricular beats who had a successful repair of this condition by a saphenous vein graft to the anterior descending division of the left coronary artery.

Congenital absence of the left circumflex coronary artery

This anomaly has occurred in association with the systolic click syndrome. There is an associated segmental myocardial dysfunction; the question is raised as to whether this segmental contraction disorder may cause the functional abnormality of the mitral valve apparatus.[22a]

ABNORMAL CORONARY ARTERY PATTERNS IN CONGENITAL HEART DISEASE

Abnormal distribution of the coronary arteries in association with congenital heart disease usually does not lead to cardiac dysfunction, although the pattern of distribution may be of great importance at the time of surgery. Coronary artery anomalies may present problems both with coronary artery cannulation and with inadvertent coronary artery transsection at ventriculotomy. This is particularly important with tetralogy of Fallot, corrected transposition of the great vessels, or complete transposition of the great vessels.

Tetralogy of Fallot

Patients with this anomaly have an abnormal coronary arterial pattern in 4 to 9 percent of cases.[1] The most frequent abnormal pattern is an anomalous origin of the left anterior descending branch from the right coronary artery or from a separate ostium in the right sinus of Valsalva.[23] From this origin, the left anterior descending artery courses over the anterior surface of the right ventricular outflow tract to its normal location in the anterior interventricular sulcus. This abnormal origin of the left anterior descending branch may be difficult to distinguish from the conal branch of the right coronary artery, which normally crosses the right ventricular outflow tract or pulmonary artery and which is regularly enlarged in tetralogy of Fallot due to the right ventricular hypertrophy.

A single coronary artery may also be seen in patients with tetralogy of Fallot. It originates with equal frequency from the right and left sinus of Valsalva. When the single artery originates from the right sinus, the left anterior descending and left circumflex artery may both pass behind the right ventricular outflow tract, or the left anterior descending artery may pass over the anterior surface of the right ventricle, producing the same potential hazard at surgery as an anomalous origin of the left anterior descending artery. An additional variation is an independent origin of the left circumflex artery from the posterior aortic sinus. Inadvertent injury to an anomalous coronary artery at the time of surgery for repair of tetralogy may produce myocardial infarction and death.[24]

Corrected transposition of the great vessels

An "abnormal" coronary artery pattern is typically present in this anomaly. The right coronary artery usually arises above the right coronary sinus and then branches into an anterior descending branch, which crosses the "right" ventricular outflow tract to the anterior interventricular sulcus, and a branch which courses in the atrioventricular sulcus to the posterior aspect of the heart.

Complete transposition of the great vessels

The two most common coronary arterial patterns in this anomaly are (1) normal origin of the left coronary artery from the left aortic sinus and anomalous origin of the right coronary artery from the posterior sinus, and (2) origin of the anterior descending artery from the left sinus and of both the right coronary artery and the circumflex artery from the posterior sinus. The major concern is the presence of an anomalous vessel at the site of incision into either ventricle at the time of surgical repair.

CORONARY ARTERY FISTULA OR ANOMALOUS COMMUNICATION OF A CORONARY ARTERY WITH A CARDIAC CHAMBER OR MAJOR VESSEL (SO-CALLED "CORONARY ARTERIOVENOUS FISTULA")

Congenital coronary artery fistula

Coronary arteriovenous fistula is the most common hemodynamically significant coronary artery anomaly. It is thought to be due to embryonic arrest of obliteration of the intertrabecular sinusoids, resulting in persistence of the coronary artery–cardiac chamber communication. This condition, in which a normally arising coronary artery communicates directly with a cardiac chamber or a major vessel, without an interposed capillary bed, is found in about 1 of 500 patients undergoing coronary angiography;[19] the incidence in general cases of congenital heart disease appears to be only 1 in 50,000 with no sex predilection. Although coronary artery fistula is usually an isolated anomaly, it may occur in association with severe stenosis or atresia of the semilunar valves.[25] Fistulas from the right coronary artery are more common than from the left coronary artery.

Clinically, the hallmark of a coronary artery fistula is a murmur which characteristically is continuous and which often is in an unusual location, loud and superficial, and associated with a thrill. Most patients have no symptoms. Some patients with a large left-to-right shunt may have symptoms of congestive heart failure. There is a tendency for heart failure to occur either in early infancy or beyond 40 years of age.[26] Angina pectoris may be present in adult patients, but almost always in association with significant coronary atherosclerosis.[1,19] The diagnosis should be suspected in a patient with a precordial continuous murmur or with symptoms and signs of a left-to-right shunt with or without congestive heart failure (see Chap. 55). The murmur tends to be loudest over the fistula, and this may assist in determining the chamber with which it communicates. In addition to symptoms and signs of congestive heart failure, supraventricular tachycardia may occur, particularly in patients with large left-to-right shunts. If the volume of left-to-right shunt flow is unusually large, the pulse pressure may be increased, the apex impulse may be hyperdynamic, and the pulmonic component of the second heart sound may be accentuated. The chest film may show cardiomegaly and increased pulmonary blood flow. Occasionally, the cardiac silhouette has an unusual pseudoaneurysmal appearance in association with evidence of a left-to-right shunt; this combination may suggest aneurysmal dilatation of a coronary artery in communication with a cardiac chamber. At cardiac catheterization of the right side of the heart, it may be possible to detect the vessel or chamber with which the fistula communicates by detecting an increase in oxygen content. In most patients pressures in the pulmonary artery and right intracardiac chambers are within normal limits.[27] Aortography or, preferably, coronary arteriography is definitive and typically demonstrates the involved coronary arteries to be markedly dilated, tortuous, and elongated (Fig. 63A-3). The vessels sometimes have aneurysmal dilatations.

Congenital coronary artery fistulas most frequently communicate with the right atrium or right ventricle. In one review[28] the fistula terminated in the right atrium, coronary sinus, or superior vena cava in 66 cases of 200 cases. The coronary sinus or superior vena cava were much less frequent sites of communication. In this series, the fistula entered the right ventricle in 78 cases. A possible clue to this location is a diastolic accentuation of the continuous murmur, presumably due to systolic constriction of the fistula. Communication of the fistula with the pulmonary trunk is rare[29,30] and may be suspected if the area of maximal murmur and thrill is somewhat higher along the left sternal border. Coronary artery fistula to the

left atrium is very rare and usually communicates with the left coronary artery system. Of six reported instances of coronary artery fistula to the left ventricle, five have involved the right coronary artery.

Bacterial infection ("endocarditis" or "endarteritis") of the fistula has been reported in up to 10 percent of patients with coronary fistula and may be the first clue to the diagnosis. Prophylactic antibiotic treatment should be given for dental care, etc. (see Chap. 60).

Surgical closure of a coronary artery fistula has a low operative mortality and should be considered in all patients with this condition.[31–33] Fistula closure does not effect a decrease in the size of the dilated proximal coronary artery. The major indications for surgery are to prevent bacterial infection, congestive heart failure,[35] thrombosis, myocardial ischemia, and rupture of an aneurysm of the involved artery. It is not known whether fistulas induce premature atherosclerosis. Ideally, surgical correction obliterates the fistula at the point of entry into the vessel or cardiac chamber without interfering with flow in the parent vessel or its branches. Electrocardiographic monitoring is recommended during occlusion of the fistula; ligation may be performed safely if there is no evidence of myocardial ischemia. If surgery is not elected, the patient should be carefully educated regarding antibiotic prophylaxis against bacteremia and potential infection of the fistula during dental procedures, etc.

Acquired coronary artery fistula

Coronary artery fistula may occur after either penetrating or nonpenetrating chest injury as well as following cardiac surgery. The continuous murmur may not appear until several weeks to months after the injury as the fistula increases in size with time. Clinically, acquired fistulas are very similar to congenital fistulas. The right coronary artery is most frequently involved because of its location and, perhaps, because trauma to the left coronary artery often produces death prior to hospitalization.[36] The electrocardiogram may show evidence of myocardial infarction. Surgical closure of an acquired coronary artery fistula is usually easier than that of a congenital fistula, which may have multiple communications or tracts.[37] See Chap. 87.

CORONARY ARTERY ANEURYSM

Congenital coronary artery aneurysm

The most common site of single or localized congenital coronary artery aneurysm is the right coronary artery. They are encountered primarily in male patients. Prior to 1960, the diagnosis was made at

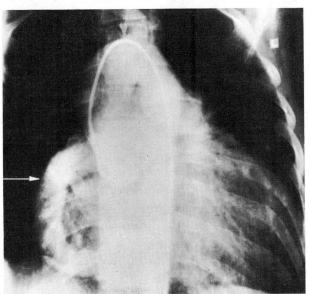

FIGURE 63A-3 Coronary artery fistula. Ascending aortogram of a 20-year-old male demonstrating a dilated, tortuous right coronary artery that communicates with the right ventricle. *(Source: P. N. Symbas et al., Congenital Fistula of Right Coronary Artery to Right Ventricle Complicated by Actinobacillus actinomycemcomtians Endarteritis, J. Thorac. Cardiovasc. Surg., 53:379, 1967.)*

autopsy examination as an incidental finding or in patients who had rupture of the aneurysm or myocardial infarction from peripheral coronary embolization of thrombus material from the aneurysm. Currently, the condition is most frequently diagnosed during life by coronary arteriography in patients with angina pectoris or myocardial infarction. Unfortunately, the diagnosis is still only rarely made during life, despite the fact that congenital aneurysms comprise about 20 percent of coronary aneurysms.

In general, whenever angina pectoris or myocardial infarction occurs in a young person, one should suspect either congenital aneurysm or anomalous origin of a coronary artery. Congenital aneurysm may be associated with a systolic murmur or a continuous murmur similar to that of a coronary artery fistula. The chest roentgenogram may reveal cardiomegaly with an unusual round shadow along the cardiac border, occasionally with dense, ringlike calcification in the wall of the aneurysm.[38] The diagnosis of coronary artery aneurysm was suspected in an asymptomatic infant because of the fluoroscopic finding of an asynchronously pulsating mass in the atrioventricular groove. Ischemic electrocardiographic changes may become evident on exercise stress testing in patients with a normal resting electrocardiogram. Myocardial infarction is usually caused by embolization from a thrombus in the aneurysm to a distal coronary artery. Rarely, the aneurysm may rupture.

Therapy consists of aorto–coronary artery bypass grafting and, whenever feasible, resection of the aneurysm.[39] However, additional aneurysmal dilatation may occur even after successful graft surgery; careful patient follow-up is recommended.[39]

Bjork and Bjork[40] described a 55-year-old man with systolic and diastolic heart murmurs known since the age of 20 who developed angina pectoris and was found to have a huge (10-mm diameter) left artery descending coronary artery leading to a 30-mm diameter coronary aneurysm at the apex of the heart. During diastole the aneurysm filled rapidly and protruded into the left ventricular cavity. During systole, it emptied most of its contents retrogradely into the dilated left anterior descending artery, producing a type of coronary steal. Operation was successful.

Acquired coronary artery aneurysm

Acquired coronary artery aneurysms, which also occur more frequently in males, are usually atherosclerotic, traumatic, or inflammatory. The most frequent cause is atherosclerosis, there are usually multiple aneurysms, and the most frequent location is the right coronary artery. Middle-aged patients with cyanotic heart disease also sometimes have aneurysmal dilatation and tortuosity of the coronary arteries of uncertain cause.[41]

Localized atherosclerotic aneurysm of the coronary arteries

This condition tends to occur in older individuals and is frequently associated with abdominal aortic aneurysm.[42] In most patients the diagnosis is made by coronary arteriography (Fig. 63A-4) or at autopsy; rarely, a round calcified shadow within the cardiac silhouette on the chest roentgenogram may suggest the diagnosis. There is no sharp dividing line between the mild to moderate areas of ectasia due to atherosclerosis—which are relatively frequently encountered at coronary arteriography—and the more

FIGURE 63A-4 Atherosclerotic coronary artery aneurysms. A. Selective arteriography of the left anterior descending (LAD) coronary artery in the right anterior oblique (RAO) position. A large, saccular atherosclerotic aneurysm in the proximal LAD is indicated by the arrows. B. Selective arteriography of the right coronary artery in the RAO position in a different patient. There are large areas of atherosclerotic aneurysmal dilatation both above and below an area of moderate obstruction. SANA = Sinoatrial node artery. *(Courtesy Drs. Spencer King and John Douglas.)*

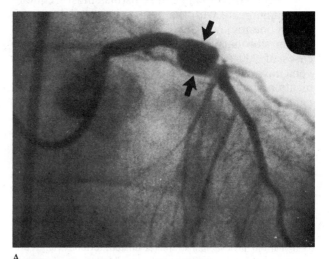

A

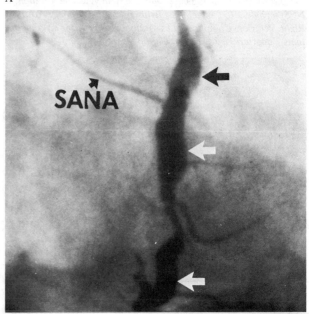

B

pronounced areas of ectasia sufficiently dilated to be called aneurysm. Diffuse coronary artery ectasia is discussed below.

Clinically, atherosclerotic coronary artery aneurysms can seldom be diagnosed prior to coronary arteriography. There may be a slight tendency for the patients to have more atypical angina pectoris and more pain at rest,[43] but this is seldom of diagnostic value. Both systolic and, more rarely, diastolic murmurs have been noted occasionally. In a few instances calcification within the aneurysm can be seen on the chest roentgenogram.

Patients with coronary artery aneurysms, especially atherosclerotic, tend to have thrombi within the aneurysm, particles of which may break off and produce embolism of distal coronary arteries with myocardial infarction.[43,44] Accordingly, chronic anticoagulant and/or antiplatelet therapy should be considered, especially if the aneurysms are large or multiple. Surgical treatment of atherosclerotic coronary aneurysms is controversial and is generally reserved for patients with evidence of distal coronary arterial emboli.[33,43] In general, coronary artery surgery is somewhat less successful than it is for other conditions in which the remainder of the vessels are often less diseased. The purpose of surgery in these patients is to prevent myocardial infarction, rupture or infection of the aneurysm, or a type of coronary steal syndrome.

Traumatic coronary artery aneurysm

This may occur after either penetrating or nonpenetrating chest trauma. The latter may be related to cardiac contusion and coronary artery dissection or the development of a false aneurysm (pulsating hematoma). Traumatic aneurysm of the coronary arteries is often associated with extensive myocardial damage, coronary artery fistula, or aneurysm of the ventricular myocardium (see Chap. 87).[43,45]

Inflammatory coronary artery aneurysm

The most common inflammatory cause of coronary artery aneurysms is *periarteritis nodosa. Systemic lupus erythematosus* and *progressive systemic sclerosis*[46] are rare causes. These are discussed under "Coronary Arteritis" below and in detail in Chap. 88. Additional causes include *necrotizing arteritis* and the *Ehler-Danlos syndrome.*[47] *Mycotic aneurysms of*

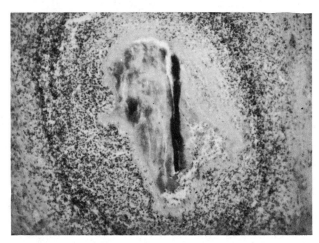

FIGURE 63A-5 Mycotic aneurysm of the coronary artery due to an infective embolus. The patient had bacterial endocarditis of the mitral valve.

the coronary arteries occasionally occur in patients with bacterial endocarditis (Fig. 63A-5). One patient with rheumatic carditis developed myocardial infarction due to thrombosis of a coronary artery aneurysm.[48] *Syphilitic coronary artery aneurysm* of the main left coronary artery may rarely occur (Fig. 63A-6), with or without severe narrowing of the ostium of the left coronary artery (see Chap. 85).[2,49]

Mucocutaneous lymph node syndrome (MLNS or Kawasaki syndrome)

This is an unusual acute illness[50,51] of infants and young children of unknown etiology. The children have fever, mucocutaneous involvement, and swelling of the cervical lymph nodes; 1 to 2 percent of patients die suddenly. Most patients develop acute cardiomegaly and electrocardiographic abnormalities of myocardial ischemia or infarction, and many have evidence of mitral regurgitation. Coronary arteriography may demonstrate diffuse, irregular aneurysms of the main coronary arteries which have a severe arteritis. Death may occur due to thrombosis within an aneurysm; rupture of an aneurysm; from heart failure resulting from thrombosis within an aneurysm; rupture of an aneurysm; or mitral regurgitation

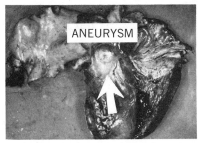

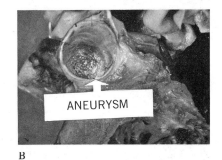

FIGURE 63A-6 Syphilitic aneurysm of the coronary artery. *A.* Marked saccular aneurysmal dilatation of the coronary artery due to syphilitic arteritis. *B.* Cross section of the coronary artery aneurysm.

secondary to papillary muscle ischemia or infarction. Glucocorticosteroid therapy has sometimes been thought to be effective and aortocoronary bypass surgery may improve ventricular function. The long-term prognosis is unknown. Interestingly, some lesions apparently regress spontaneously.[51]

Idiopathic diffuse coronary artery aneurysmal dilatation

Hallman et al.[3] described in four children an unusual syndrome of idiopathic coronary artery thickening and sclerosis with areas of aneurysmal dilatation. The intima was noted to have marked acid mucopolysaccharide deposits, and there were areas of myocardial scarring.

CORONARY ARTERY ECTASIA (DIFFUSE ANEURYSM)

There is a definite, but somewhat poorly defined, group of patients who have a primary, generalized irregular aneurysmal dilatation of the main coronary arteries with or without obstructive lesions (Fig. 63A-7).[52] The cause is thought to be coronary atherosclerosis with degenerative changes in the musculoelastic fibers of the media and marked thinning of the vessel wall. A genetic predisposition or weakness of the arterial walls is suggested by the apparent increased incidence of abdominal and lower extremity arterial aneurysms.

FIGURE 63A-7 Coronary artery ectasia (diffuse aneurysms). Right coronary artery arteriogram in the RAO position. Extensive ectasia of the right coronary artery is demonstrated. The patient also had moderate ectasia in the left coronary system without marked obstruction. *(Courtesy of Drs. Spencer King and John Douglas.)*

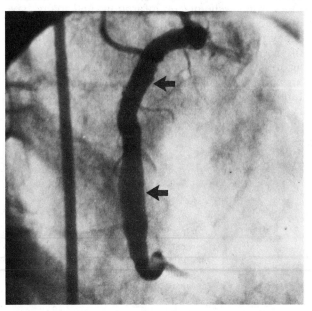

Clinically, there is a slightly greater incidence of atypical angina pectoris at rest and of recurrent episodes of prolonged pain or recurrent myocardial infarction. The latter are probably caused by downstream embolization of thrombus material formed within the areas of estasia.[2] There is an increased incidence of hypertension, family history of myocardial infarction and electrocardiographic abnormalities.[52] Coronary bypass surgery may be indicated for obstructive atherosclerotic disease (see Chaps. 62E and 62F). Most patients with this syndrome should be maintained indefinitely on anticoagulation therapy.[2] If this is not feasible, long-term antiplatelet therapy with aspirin (1 g/day) may be considered, although there are no data yet available regarding this therapy. The overall prognosis is probably less favorable than with other types of coronary atherosclerotic heart disease.

CORONARY ARTERY DISSECTION (DISSECTING ANEURYSM OR DISSECTING HEMATOMA)

Primary coronary artery dissection

Spontaneous primary dissection of a coronary artery is very rare. Of the reported cases, a substantial number have occurred in young women in the postpartum state.[2,53,54] Interestingly, histopathologic alterations in human aortic media have been reported during apparently normal pregnancy.[58] The anterior descending branch of the left coronary artery is most frequently involved usually within 2 cm of the aortic ostium.[53] Hypertension and atherosclerosis do not appear to be significant factors, although cystic medionecrosis and arteritis may be present. Characteristically, there is extensive medial destruction and hematoma producing coronary occlusion; an intimal tear is not often identified. The dissection may be demonstrated by coronary arteriography and coronary bypass surgery performed.[55] Aneurysmectomy may also be necessary.

Primary coronary artery dissection may also occur following cannulation of the coronary arteries during open heart surgery, especially if there is severe local coronary atherosclerosis or coronary artery anomalies.[56,57] It can also occur after coronary bypass graft surgery. It is also recognized as a complication of selective coronary arteriography[55] and of malfunction of an aortic valve ball-valve prosthesis.[57]

Secondary coronary artery dissection

Secondary dissection, which is much more common than primary dissection, is an extension of the process involving the ascending aorta to the main branches of the coronary arteries. Characteristically it produces symptoms and signs of myocardial ischemia and infarction in addition to those from the aortic dissection. The retrograde dissection may also produce aortic regurgitation or leakage into the pericardial space with hemopericardium or cardiac tamponade. The relative rarity of secondary coronary artery dissection is attributed to the early fatal extension of the aortic dissection into the pericardium, before the dissection extends into the coronary arteries. See also Chap. 103.

CORONARY EMBOLISM

Coronary embolism should be suspected with the acute onset of severe pain thought to be due to myocardial ischemia (see Chap. 62E) particularly in patients with any of the following characteristics or circumstances: prosthetic mitral or aortic valve,[59] bacterial or fungal endocarditis (Fig. 63A-5),[60] mitral stenosis, calcific mitral or aortic valvular disease, atrial fibrillation, congestive cardiomyopathy, ventricular aneurysm, fibroelastosis with mural thrombi, marantic endocarditis, left atrial myxoma,[61] or during catheterization of the left side of the heart, coronary arteriography,[62] or cardiac surgery. Coronary embolism should be suspected as a cause of both myocardial infarction and of sudden death in young adults. Paradoxical coronary embolism may also occur[63-65] in patients with congenital heart disease. Coronary emboli due to fat, air, parasites, or tumor occur rarely.[61] Calcific coronary embolization is commonly seen with replacement of a calcified aortic or mitral valve.[65a] Embolization of a necrotic fragment of myocardium to a coronary artery occurred in a patient with acute myocardial infarction and papillary muscle rupture.[65b]

Coronary embolism most often involves the left anterior descending coronary artery and may produce sudden death or serious dysrhythmias and extensive myocardial infarction, perhaps because of the lack of time to develop an effective collateral circulation. Diagnosis can be made only by coronary arteriography. Embolic lesions can eventually completely resolve, even after producing complete obstruction.[66] Many instances of documented myocardial infarction without obstructive coronary artery disease at the time of coronary arteriography or autopsy are probably due to coronary embolism, as well as to intravascular thrombosis, coronary artery dissection, or subintimal hemorrhage with resolution. Coronary spasm may also produce myocardial infarction (see Chaps. 62D and 62E). As noted in Chap. 62C, coronary atherosclerotic plaques may rupture their contents into the lumen of the vessel and produce downstream coronary embolization.

When coronary embolism is diagnosed early, urgent coronary embolectomy and/or saphenous vein aortocoronary bypass grafting may prevent further loss of myocardium.

CORONARY OSTIAL DISEASE

Narrowing of the coronary ostia is one of the classic types of cardiovascular disease produced by syphilis[67] (see Chap. 85). Coronary ostial stenosis may also occur in patients with pulseless (Takayasu's) disease

or in patients with coronary fibrosis (fibrous hyperplasia), with or without fibromuscular disease of the renal arteries. As noted below, the latter syndrome is sometimes associated with methysergide (Sansert) therapy. Atherosclerosis may produce isolated ostial stenosis although it is usually associated with significant atherosclerosis elsewhere in the coronary arteries.[68] Atherosclerotic ostial stenosis tends to occur more frequently in the right coronary ostium.

The development of angina pectoris or myocardial infarction several months to a few years after open heart surgery with cannulation of the coronary arteries may be related to ostial stenosis with intimal thickening and a disrupted elastic membrane.[69] The clinical presentation is of disabling angina pectoris, beginning several months postoperatively, and progressing to fatal myocardial infarction. In patients who have had an aortic ball-valve prosthesis implanted, the high-speed, lateral systolic jets of blood striking the ostia may also produce ostial stenosis; this rarely occurs with a central-flow tilting disc valve.[70,71] Aortocoronary anastomosis may be required to bypass the stenosed ostium. Left coronary ostial involvement carries the same ominous prognosis as does left main coronary artery critical obstruction.

CORONARY FIBROSIS (FIBROMUSCULAR HYPERPLASIA)

Severe fibromuscular hyperplasia and intimal proliferation, without lipid or calcium deposition, may occur in the coronary arteries and produce angina pectoris, myocardial infarction and mitral regurgitation. It may occur as an isolated lesion or in association with fibromuscular disease of the renal arteries.[2,72] The condition should be suspected in young women with evidence of coronary artery disease in association with evidence of renal artery disease. There is a strong tendency for involvement of the coronary ostia, the main left coronary artery, or the proximal portion of the left anterior descending coronary artery. There is strong suggestive evidence that methysergide (Sansert) therapy may produce the arterial lesions as well as retroperitoneal fibrosis and cardiac valve fibrosis.[2,73]

ABNORMAL CORONARY ARTERY HISTOLOGY IN CONGENITAL HEART DISEASE

Primary changes may occur in the coronary arteries proximal to a coronary artery fistula or in the right coronary artery when the left coronary artery originates from the pulmonary artery. The changes are focal fibrous intimal thickening and marked medial thickening.[74] *Secondary changes* in the coronary arteries occur in the presence of systemic hypertension. These changes are intimal and medial thickening with accelerated atherosclerosis.[75]

Pulmonary or aortic atresia and intact ventricular septum

In pulmonary atresia with an intact interventricular septum, there may be extensive myocardial sinusoids with enlarged ostia in the right ventricle. These thin-walled sinusoids carry blood from the right ventricular cavity to anomalous epicardial vessels with thick walls of collagenous and elastic fibers, but no smooth-muscle cells. These vessels may develop severe intimal changes and endarteritis due to the high systolic pressure they sustain.[1,76,77] In patients with aortic atresia and an intact ventricular septum, the enlarged ostia of sinusoids communicate with the left ventricular cavity and there may be similar enlarged, tortuous, epicardial arterial trunks. Myocardial infarction may occur in the hypoplastic ventricles of patients with either pulmonary or aortic atresia due to a combination of poor perfusion, decreased oxygenation, and severe coronary arterial lesions.[1]

Coarctation of the aorta

The coronary arteries in this anomaly, which are subjected to the high pressure in the proximal aorta, have an increase in lumen area and have medial thickening and elastosis with accelerated atherosclerosis.[78,79]

Supravalvular aortic stenosis

The coronary arteries in this anomaly are subjected to the high left ventricular systolic pressure; as a consequence, they are large and dilated and often show medial hypertrophy with splitting of the internal elastic membrane.[80]

CORONARY ARTERITIS

The most common conditions associated with coronary arteritis are syphilis, infective endocarditis, polyarteritis nodosa, systemic lupus erythematosus, rheumatoid arthritis, and pulseless (Takayasu's) disease. Extremely rare causes are salmonellosis, tuberculosis, and typhus.

Infectious diseases

SYPHILITIC CORONARY ARTERITIS

Syphilis may produce coronary ostial stenosis from an obliterative arteritis of the proximal 3 to 4 mm of the coronary arteries, usually in association with syphilitic aortitis and often in association with luetic aortic regurgitation. Coronary ostial stenosis occurs in about 20 percent of patients with syphilitic aortitis. Clinically, this ostial stenosis is difficult to suspect prior to coronary arteriography or aortography unless there is angina pectoris out of proportion to the severity of the aortic regurgitation. The infrequency of myocardial infarction is attributed to the gradual progression of the occlusive process allowing formation of of a collateral circulation. Less commonly a syphilitic gumma may occlude a coronary artery. Saphenous vein aortocoronary bypass grafting is the procedure of choice. Syphilitic heart disease is discussed in detail in Chap. 85.

ENDOCARDITIS

Coronary arterial lesions in infective endocarditis are usually thought to be secondary to embolization (Fig. 63A-5). In addition, Saphir et al.[81] described obliterative vascular changes, occasionally with resultant myocardial infarction, in coronary vessels that traverse areas of inflammation or micro-abscess. As noted previously, infective endocarditis is also a major cause of coronary embolism. Infective endocarditis is discussed in detail in Chap. 77.

SALMONELLOSIS

Patients with disseminated salmonellosis may develop a purulent thromboarteritis and thrombosis of a coronary artery with fatal myocardial infarction.[82] See also Chaps. 79A and 80.

TUBERCULOSIS

In patients with miliary tuberculosis, tubercles may occur in the intima of the coronary arteries. In patients with myocardial tuberculosis, there may be occlusion of the smaller coronary arteries due to diffuse tuberculous infiltration and noncellular intimal proliferative lesions.[83] Serial electrocardiographic changes in a young patient with active advanced tuberculosis should suggest coronary artery or myocardial tuberculosis. Tuberculosis is discussed in greater detail in Chaps. 79A and 80.

TYPHUS

Patients with epidemic typhus (*Rickettsia prowazekki*) may develop arteritis and thrombosis of the smaller coronary arteries.[84] Only rarely are these of clinical significance. Coronary arteritis is not a feature of scrub typhus (*R. orientalis*) or of Rocky Mountain spotted fever, in which myocarditis occurs (see Chaps. 79A, 80, and 82).

Collagen diseases

The cardiovascular manifestations of the collagen diseases are discussed in detail in Chap. 88, and only aspects of involvement of the coronary arteries will be summarized here.

POLYARTERITIS NODOSA

Lesions of the coronary arteries may produce angina pectoris or myocardial infarction in children or adults with polyarteritis (periarteritis) nodosa. The inflammatory, necrotizing, obliterative arteritis of both the large and small coronary arteries occurred in 60 to 70 percent of cases in one series.[85] Aneurysmal dilata-

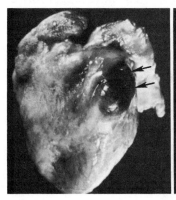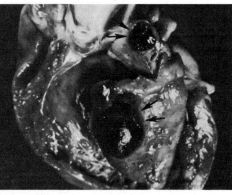

FIGURE 63A-8 Coronary artery aneurysmal dilatation due to polyarteritis of infancy. *(Courtesy of Dr. Dorothy Brinsfield.)*

tion and nodule formation in the coronary arteries may produce a characteristic "peas in the pod" appearance (Fig. 63A-8).[86] Intimal thrombosis or thrombosis of an aneurysm may produce coronary occlusion and myocardial infarction, although the relatively slow rate of occlusion may allow an adequate collateral circulation to develop. Rupture of an aneurysm may cause sudden death.

Polyarteritis of infancy (or *necrotizing arteritis of infancy*) is a fulminating disease predominantly, and occasionally selectively, involving the coronary arteries. It is the most frequent cause of coronary thrombosis in infancy and may cause sudden, unexpected death. The classic syndrome in infancy includes fever, rash, conjunctivitis, hypertension, angina pectoris or its equivalent, congestive heart failure, central nervous system abnormalities, ischemic gangrene of an extremity, leukocytosis with eosinophilia, and an abnormal urinary sediment. The electrocardiogram may show large Q waves in all the precordial leads, and the chest roentgenogram may show generalized cardiomegaly, at times with a localized bulge from a ventricular aneurysm. Glucocorticosteroid therapy may be of benefit;[86] aneurysm regression has been described with corticosteroid and azathioprine therapy.[86a] See Chap. 88.

SYSTEMIC (DISSEMINATED) LUPUS ERYTHEMATOSUS (SLE)

Most of the cardiovascular symptoms and signs in patients with SLE are due to pericarditis, myocarditis, and hypertension. The smaller coronary arteries, however, are often involved in the diffuse vasculitis of SLE with fibrinoid degeneration and fibrosis. These processes are rarely recognized clinically; they may cause focal myocardial necrosis.[87,88] However, severe arteritis of a main coronary artery with angina pectoris and myocardial infarction has been described.[87,88] See Chap. 88.

RHEUMATIC FEVER

The smaller coronary arteries are conspicuously involved in rheumatic fever with inflammation, fibrinoid degeneration, and intimal fibrotic proliferation. Young patients with rheumatic fever may develop myocardial infarction secondary to obliterative coro-

nary arteritis[89] or to coronary embolism of a rheumatic valvular vegetation. It is possible that the chronic rheumatic vasculitis contributes to the left ventricular dysfunction occasionally encountered in patients with mitral stenosis.[90] See Chaps. 58 to 60.

RHEUMATOID ARTHRITIS (BOUILLAUD'S DISEASE)

In most patients with long-standing rheumatoid arthritis who develop angina pectoris or myocardial infarction, it is due to coronary atherosclerosis.[91] In some patients, however, it is due to severe coronary arteritis and intimal thickening. This appears to be more common in patients with diffuse necrotizing arteritis or in patients receiving glucocorticosteroid therapy. See also Chap. 82.

ANKYLOSING SPONDYLITIS

The development of major extracardiac and intercoronary anastomoses was described in an elderly patient with rheumatoid spondylitic aortitis who had occlusion of the left coronary artery ostium.[92]

Disease of the small and medium coronary arteries

James and others[93-98] have described medial degeneration and necrosis and intimal hyperplasia of the small and medium coronary arteries in a variety of conditions, including the following: obscure cardiomyopathy, primary pulmonary hypertension, scleroderma, Marfan's syndrome, the congenital cardioauditory syndrome with prolonged Q-T interval, and congenital deafness (surdocardiac or Jervell-Lange-Nielson syndrome), congenital prolongation of the Q-T interval with normal hearing (Romano-Ward syndrome), progressive muscular dystrophy, and Friedreich's ataxia.[99] The sinoatrial and atrioventricular node arteries may also be prominently involved. These changes in the small coronary vessels may contribute to the arrhythmias, syncope, chest pain, conduction defects, nonspecific electrocardiographic changes, and sudden death occasionally encountered in these syndromes. See also Chaps. 79A, 79B, and 82.

NONATHEROSCLEROTIC CORONARY THROMBOSIS

Parasitic coronary thrombosis

Malarial parasites and parasitized red blood cells usually plug small coronary vessels but can occasionally occlude larger coronary arteries.[100] An adult *Schistosoma haematobium* was found in the left circumflex coronary artery without resultant myocardial infarction at the postmortem examination of a patient with schistosomiasis.[101]

Hematologic coronary thrombosis

Thrombotic occlusion in the coronary arterial system has been reported to produce myocardial infarction in association with a number of hematologic diseases, including thrombotic thrombocytopenic purpura,[94] sickle-cell anemia,[102] leukemia,[103] polycythemia vera,[104] and primary thrombocytosis.[105] On occasion, acute myocardial infarction may be the initial manifestation of polycythemia vera. Fatal complete heart block in a patient with thrombotic thrombocytopenic purpura resulted from occlusion of a small coronary artery and ischemic necrosis of the bundle of His.[95]

INHERITED DISORDERS OF METABOLISM

Mucopolysaccharidoses

This group of inherited diseases is characterized by the abnormal tissue deposition and/or urinary excretion of mucopolysaccharides. At least six syndromes of mucopolysaccharidoses involve the heart (see Chap. 52), and two syndromes, Hurler's and Hunter's syndromes, involve the coronary arteries. Hurler's syndrome, which is transmitted as an autosomal recessive trait, has a more severe course than Hunter's syndrome, which is an X-linked recessive trait. In both syndromes there is an intracellular accumulation of chondroitin sulfate B and heparitin sulfate.

Both Hurler's syndrome and Hunter's syndrome are characterized by gargoylism and dwarfism, coarse facial features, mental deficiency, hepatosplenomegaly, and stiff joints. Both are associated with premature death from cardiac involvement; there is accumulation of fibroelastic connective tissue cells filled with storage material in the cardiac valves, great vessels, coronary arteries, endocardium, myocardium, and epicardium (see Chap. 52). The extramural coronary arteries have severe intimal thickening produced by increased amounts of collagen and by the presence of large numbers of clear cells and smooth-muscle cells, both of which are distended by acid mucopolysaccharide deposits. Medial smooth-muscle cells are less involved and contain mostly lamellar bodies.[106] The involvement of

the coronary arteries may be severe enough to produce occlusion of the vessel lumen and myocardial ischemia or infarction.[106–108] The clinical syndromes are obvious when full-blown; mild instances of *forme fruste* should be considered in infants or children with valvular heart disease or symptoms of coronary artery disease. (See also Chaps. 52 and 82.)

Disorders of protein metabolism

Primary oxalosis refers to two rare disorders of oxalic acid metabolism. They have an autosomal recessive inheritance and are characterized by the excessive synthesis of oxalic acid which accumulates in major tissues, including the heart. The coronary arteries may show calcium oxalate deposits.[109] Death usually occurs about age 14 from nephrolithiasis.[108] See also Chap. 82.

Disorders of amino acid metabolism

Alkaptonuria is due to the absence of homogentisic oxidase. This causes an increased accumulation and excretion of homogentisic acid with arthritis, dark urine, and pigmentation of cartilage and other tissues. Death is frequently caused by myocardial infarction due to atheromatous plaques with a characteristic blue-black pigmentation.[1] See also Chap. 82.

Disorders of lipid metabolism

HYPERLIPOPROTEINEMIA
The genetics of the varieties of hyperlipoproteinemia are discussed in Chap. 52, and the recognition, management, and prevention are discussed in Chaps. 62E, 62F, and 62H.

FABRY'S DISEASE
This condition is characterized by the accumulation of ceramide trihexoside in the small blood vessels of most organs. It is caused by a deficiency of ceramide trihexosidase, which is inherited as a sex-linked recessive trait. Clinically, the cardiovascular features are systemic hypertension due to involvement of the renal vessels, cardiomegaly, congestive heart failure, angina pectoris, and myocardial infarction. This syndrome is discussed further in Chap. 82.

SANDHOFF'S DISEASE
This condition results from deficient activity of total hexosaminidase (A and B). It is characterized by the neural and visceral accumulation of glycosphingolipid G_{M2} ganglioside, its asialo derivative, and globoside. Clinically, there is retardation of development and cardiomegaly with or without mitral regurgitation within the first few months of life. Sandhoff's disease is distinguished from other causes of cardiomyopathy in infancy by central nervous system symptoms and the presence of cherry red maculae, as in Tay-Sachs disease.[1,110] The major symptom of both diseases is the deterioration of the central nervous system; patients usually die in the first years of life from complications brought on by the neuro-

logic involvement. The gross and light microscopic findings in the heart are very similar to those of Hurler's syndrome.[110] The coronary arteries in Sandhoff's disease may be narrowed by intimal proliferation of fibroblasts. The diagnosis can be established by the finding of globoside in the urinary sediment or by the measurement of globoside or hexosaminidase activity in plasma or other tissues.[110] See also Chap. 82.

G$_{M1}$ GANGLIOSIDOSIS

This is a rare condition in which G$_{M1}$ ganglioside accumulates in the central nervous system and, to a lesser degree, in the viscera. Cardiac involvement is present in about one-third of the cases but is usually not of clinical significance.[111] Rarely, atheromatous plaques with balloon cells of foamy PAS-negative cytoplasm may occur in the coronary arteries or aorta. See also Chap. 82.

FAMILIAL HIGH-DENSITY LIPOPROTEIN DEFICIENCY (TANGIER DISEASE)

This rare familial disorder is characterized by severe deficiency or absence of normal high-density lipoprotein in plasma and by storage of cholesterol esters throughout the body. The combination of enlarged, orange-yellow tonsils and low plasma cholesterol levels (30 to 125 mg/dl) with normal or elevated triglyceride levels (150 to 330 mg/dl) is pathognomonic. Corneal deposits, peripheral neuropathy, and hepatosplenomegaly are common. Cholesterol esters may also accumulate in the coronary arteries although it is not yet proven that Tangier disease is associated with accelerated atheromatosis or other occlusive vascular disease.[112,113] See Chap. 52.

Homocystinuria

This anomaly is associated with extensive changes in the media of the coronary arteries, with thinning and an increase in ground substance between the muscle fibers. Intimal proliferation is also seen. These changes may lead to coronary dilatation and thrombosis with myocardial infarction.[111,114,114a] See also Chaps. 52 and 103.

Gout

In addition to the epidemiologic association between gout or hyperuricemia and coronary atherosclerotic heart disease (Chap. 62B), gout can be associated with the accumulation of urate crystals in the walls of the coronary arteries as well as in the heart valves and myocardium.[115.]

MISCELLANEOUS CAUSES OF CORONARY ARTERY DISEASE

Hypertension

Hypertension in children due to chronic renal disease, polycystic kidneys, pheochromocytoma, Cush-

ing's syndrome, or the adrenogenital syndrome may be associated with accelerated coronary atherosclerosis and even myocardial infarction.[89] See Chaps. 62B and 62H.

Amyloidosis

Patients with primary cardiac amyloidosis frequently have amyloid infiltration of the intima and media of the coronary arteries[116] (Fig. 63A-9), which can produce coronary occlusion. Occasionally, there is extensive amyloid deposition in the smaller coronary arteries, although this small-vessel involvement is rarely associated with angina pectoris or myocardial infarction unless there is associated coronary atherosclerosis.[117] Amyloid infiltration of the sinoatrial and atrioventricular nodes may explain the frequent arrhythmias in amyloidosis.[117] Amyloid heart disease is discussed in greater detail in Chap. 88.

Pulseless (Takayasu's) disease

The fibrous intimal and subendothelial proliferation with arteritis may produce angina pectoris from involvement of the coronary ostia, as noted above, or of the coronary arteries.[118] Myocardial infarction and death have been described due to ostial disease. Exercise testing to detect occult coronary arterial involvement should be performed in all patients with Takayasu's disease; angina pectoris or a positive exercise test is an indication for arteriography. Coronary artery aortocoronary bypass surgery may be indicated for such patients with severe, localized coronary disease.[119] See also Chaps. 103 and 104.

Thromboangiitis obliterans (Buerger's disease)

Most of the coronary artery disease in patients with this disease is atherosclerotic, but on occasion the coronary arteries may be sclerosed or narrowed by

FIGURE 63A-9 Amyloid heart disease. Photomicrograph demonstrating amyloid deposition in a coronary arteriole (X 250).

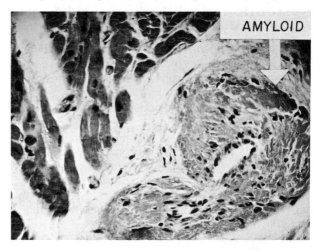

hyalinized, calcific plaques. These may cause sudden death in young males with the syndrome.[120] See Chap. 104.

Fibroelastosis

Congenital occlusive fibroelastosis may involve both coronary arteries and produce myocardial infarction and death in the newborn.[77]

Medial calcification of the coronary arteries in infancy (infantile coronary sclerosis)

Idiopathic medial necrosis with subsequent calcification is a rare manifestation of a generalized vascular disease of infancy that also involves the pulmonary and renal arteries and the large arteries of the extremities and may be associated with other congenital anomalies.[121-123] The sex distribution is equal.

The coronary arteries are grossly white, opaque, and cordlike, with narrowed lumens. Microscopically, there is degeneration and calcification of the media and the tunica elastica with fibroelastic intimal proliferation.[121-123] The etiology is unknown, but among the suggested factors are abnormalities of calcium metabolism, hypoxia, infection, allergy, or a congenital defect in elastic tissue formation. It is frequently associated with endocardial fibroelastosis, and occasionally occurs in families, suggesting that it may be genetically determined.[122]

Clinically, symptoms usually begin in the first few weeks of life and mimic those of anomalous origin of the left coronary artery from the pulmonary artery. There are episodes of acute respiratory distress with dyspnea, cyanosis, tachypnea associated with feeding difficulty and vomiting. Congestive heart failure is notably absent. Sudden death before the age of 2 is common. The electrocardiogram is compatible with myocardial ischemia or infarction. Calcification of the coronary arteries can often be detected on chest roentgenograms or by cardiac fluoroscopy. There is no satisfactory therapy.

Systemic arterial disease with myocardial infarction

A generalized occlusive disease of the small and medium-sized arteries with marked fibrous intimal thickening and myocardial infarction has been reported in two infants.[124]

Neuromuscular diseases

Involvement of the small coronary arteries with medial degeneration and intimal proliferation is particularly likely to occur in *Friedreich's ataxia* and *progressive muscular dystrophy*.[93-99] SA and AV node artery involvement explains the frequent intractable arrhythmias. These are discussed in greater detail in Chap. 88.

Tumor

Several varieties of primary and secondary tumors may obstruct the coronary ostia or a coronary artery. These include fibroma, rhabdomyoma, rhabdomyosarcoma, metastatic carcinoma,[125] and metastatic Hodgkin's disease nodules.[126]

Trauma

Both penetrating[126a] and nonpenetrating trauma to the heart may produce several types of coronary artery injury, including thrombosis with myocardial infarction in an apparently normal coronary artery; the left anterior descending artery is most frequently involved. Bypass graft surgery may be lifesaving.[127,128] Coronary artery fistula (see above) and coronary artery rupture also occur.[129] Cardiac trauma is discussed in detail in Chap. 87.

Radiation fibrosis

As noted in Chap. 101, radiation can produce a type of cardiomyopathy. In addition, it has been suggested that therapeutic radiation may produce intimal thickening and medial fibromuscular proliferation and fibrosis sufficient to cause myocardial infarction.[130] Radiation may also predispose to coronary atherosclerosis,[131] particularly in patients with coronary risk factors.[131a] See also Chap. 82.

Nontraumatic rupture of a coronary artery

Nontraumatic rupture of a coronary artery at the site of an atheromatous plaque may produce fatal cardiac tamponade.[132]

Progeria

This rare type of premature senility and dwarfism produces the appearance of old age in childhood. Atherosclerosis and angina pectoris may occur before the age of 10, and coronary atherosclerotic heart disease is the most common cause of death.

Rejection cardiomyopathy

The coronary vessels of the transplanted human heart are unusually susceptible to the development of atherosclerosis, particularly in the presence of marked hypercholesterolemia. In addition, the rejection phenomena may result in extensive intimal proliferation, necrotizing arteritis, and fibrinoid necrosis of the coronary vessels. Therapy with immunosuppressive agents and corticosteroid hormones may reverse the rejection process.

REFERENCES

1 Neufeld, H. N., and Blieden, L. C.: Coronary Artery Disease in Children, *Prog. Cardiol.*, 4:119, 1975.

2 Razavi, M.: Unusual Forms of Coronary Artery Disease, in D. G. Vidt (ed.), "Cleveland Clinic Cardiovascular Consultations," F. A. Davis Company, Philadelphia, 1975, p. 25.

3 Hallman, G. L., Cooley, D. A., and Singer, D. B.: Congenital Anomalies of the Coronary Arteries: Anatomy, Pathology, and Surgical Treatment, *Surgery*, 59:133, 1966.

4 Blake, H. A., Manion, W. C., Mattingly, T. W., and Baroldi, G.: Coronary Artery Anomalies, *Circulation*, 30:927, 1964.

5 Bland, E. F., White, P. D., and Garland, J.: Congenital Anomalies of the Coronary Arteries: Report of an Unusual Case Associated with Cardiac Hypertrophy, *Am. Heart J.*, 8:787, 1933.

6 George, J. M., and Knowlan, D. M.: Anomalous Origin of the Left Coronary Artery from the Pulmonary Artery in the Adult, *N. Engl. J. Med.*, 261:993, 1959.

7 Baue, A. E., Baum, S., Blakemore, W. S., and Zinsser, H. F.: A Later State of Anomalous Coronary Circulation with Origin of the Left Coronary Artery from the Pulmonary Artery: Coronary Artery Steal, *Circulation*, 36:878, 1967.

8 Askenazi, J., and Nadas, A. S.: Anomalous Left Coronary Artery Originating from the Pulmonary Artery. Report on 15 Cases, *Circulation*, 51:976, 1975.

9 Chaitman, B. R., Lespérance, J., Saltiel, J., and Bourassa, M. G.: Clinical, Angiographic, and Hemodynamic Findings in Patients with Anomalous Origin of the Coronary Arteries, *Circulation*, 53:122, 1976.

10 Keith, J. D.: Anomalous Origin of the Left Coronary Artery from the Pulmonary Artery, *Br. Heart J.*, 21:149, 1959.

11 Abbott, M. E.: Congenital Cardiac Disease: Anomalies of the Coronary Arteries, in Osler, W., and McCrae (eds.), *Mod. Medicine*, 4:612, Lea and Febiger, Philadelphia, 1927.

12 Wesselhoeft, H., Fawcett, J. S., and Johnson, A. L.: Anomalous Origin of the Left Coronary Artery from the Pulmonary Trunk. Its Clinical Spectrum, Pathology, and Pathophysiology Based on a Review of 140 Cases with Seven Further Cases, *Circulation*, 38:403, 1968.

13 Thomas, C. S., Jr., Campbell, W. B., Alford, W. C., Jr., Burrus, G. R., and Stoney, W. S.: Complete Repair of Anomalous Origin of the Left Coronary Artery in the Adult, *J. Thorac. Cardiovasc. Surg.*, 66:439, 1973.

14 Chiariello, L., Meyer, J., Reul, G. J., Jr., Hallman, G. L., and Cooley, D. A.: Surgical Treatment for Anomalous Origin of Left Coronary Artery from Pulmonary Artery, *Ann. Thorac. Surg.*, 19:443, 1975.

15 Pinsky, W. W., Fagan, L. R., Mudd, J. F. G., and Willman, V. L.: Subclavian-Coronary Artery Anastomosis in Infancy for the Bland-White-Garland Syndrome. A Three-Year and Five-Year Follow-up, *J. Thorac. Cardiovasc. Surg.*, 72:15, 1976.

16 Matsumoto, A., Sato, S., Kondo, J., Kumada, J., Goto, H., Kohno, M., Matsumura, H., and Niimura, I.: Definitive Surgical Treatment of Anomalous Origin of Left Coronary Artery. A New Technique Approach Used Successfully in a Seven-Month-Old Male Infant, *J. Thorac. Cardiovasc. Surg.*, 72:249, 1976.

16a Grace, R. R., Angeline, P., and Cooley, D. A.: Aortic Implantation of Anomalous Left Coronary Artery Arising from Pulmonary Artery, *Am. J. Cardiol.*, 39:608, 1977.

17 Colmers, R. A., and Siderides, C. I.: Anomalous Origin of Both Coronary Arteries from Pulmonary Trunk. Myocardial Infarction in Otherwise Normal Heart, *Am. J. Cardiol.*, 12:263, 1963.

18 Feldt, R. H., Ongley, P. A., and Titus, J. L.: Total Coronary Arterial Circulation from Pulmonary Artery with Survival to Age Seven. Report of Case, *Proc. Staff Meet. Mayo Clin.*, 40:539, 1965.

19 Leguizamon, E. E., Sheldon, W. C., and Jones, F. M., Jr.: Unpublished study, quoted by M. Razani in reference no. 2.

20 Sharbaugh, A. H., and White, R. S.: Single Coronary Artery. Analysis of the Anatomic Variation, Clinical Importance, and Report of Five Cases, *JAMA*, 230:243, 1974.

21 Spring, D. A., and Thomsen, J. H.: Severe Atherosclerosis in the "Single Coronary Artery." Report of a Previously Undescribed Pattern, *Am. J. Cardiol.*, 31:662, 1973.

22 Mullins, C. E., El-Said, G., McNamara, D. G., Cooley, D. A., Treistman, B., and Garcia, E.: Atresia of the Left Coronary Artery Ostium. Repair by Saphenous Vein Graft, *Circulation*, 46:989, 1972.

22a Gentzler, R. D., II, Gault, J. H., Liedtke, A. J., McCann, W. D., Mann, R. H., and Hunter, A. S.: Congenital Absence of the Left Circumflex Coronary Artery in the Systolic Click Syndrome, *Circulation*, 52.

23 Meyer, J., Chiariello, L., Hallman, G. L., and Cooley, D. A.: Coronary Artery Anomalies in Patients with Tetralogy of Fallot, *J. Thorac. Cardiovasc. Surg.*, 69:373, 1975.

24 Berry, B. E., and McGoon, D. C.: Total Correction for Tetralogy of Fallot with Anomalous Coronary Artery, *Surgery*, 74:894, 1973.

25 Krongrad, E., Ritter, D. G., Hawe, A., Kincaid, O. W., and McGoon, D. C.: Pulmonary Atresia or Severe Stenosis and Coronary Artery-to-Pulmonary Artery Fistula, *Circulation*, 46:1005, 1972.

26 Wedell, H. G., and Teloh, H. A.: Congenital Communication between the Right Coronary Artery and Right Atrium, *Q. Bull. Northwestern Univ. Med. School*, 33:285, 1959.

27 Nadas, A. S., and Fyler, D. C.: "Pediatric Cardiology," 3d ed., W. B. Saunders Company, Philadelphia, 1972.

28 Oldham, H. N., Jr., Ebert, P. A., Young, W. G., and Sabiston, D. C. Jr.: Surgical Management of Congenital Coronary Artery Fistula, *Ann. Thorac. Surg.*, 12:503, 1971.

29 Gobel, F. L., Anderson, C. F., Baltaxe, H. A., Amplatz, K., and Wang, Y.: Shunts between the Coronary and Pulmonary Arteries with Normal Origin of the Coronary Arteries, *Am. J. Cardiol.*, 25:655, 1970.

30 Amplatz, K., Aguirre, J., and Lillehei, C. W.: Coronary Arteriovenous Fistula into Main Pulmonary Artery. Preoperative Diagnosis by Selective Aortography, *JAMA*, 172:1384, 1960.

31 Sakakibara, S., Yokoyama, M., Takao, A., Nogi, M., and Gomi, H.: Coronary Arteriovenous Fistula. Nine Operated Cases, *Am. Heart J.*, 72:307, 1966.

32 Jaffe, R. B., Glancy, D. L., Epstein, S. E., Brown, B. G., and Morrow, A. G.: Coronary Arterial-Right Heart Fistulae. Long-Term Observations in Seven Patients, *Circulation*, 47:133, 1973.

33 Rittenhouse, E. A., Doty, D. B., and Ehrenhaft, J. L.: Congenital Coronary Artery-Cardiac Chamber Fistula. Review of Operative Management, *Ann. Thorac. Surg.*, 20:468, 1975.

34 Edwards, J. E., Gladding, T. C., and Weir, A. B., Jr.: Congenital Communication between the Right Coronary Artery and Right Atrium, *J. Thorac. Cardiovasc. Surg.*, 35:662, 1958.

35 Neufeld, H. N., Lucas, R. V., Jr., Lester, R. G., Adams, P., Jr., Anderson, R. C., and Edwards, J. E.: Origin of Both Great Vessels from the Right Ventricle without Pulmonary Stenosis, *Br. Heart J.*, 24:393, 1962.

36 Reyes, L. H., Mattox, K. L., Gaasch, W. H., Espada, R., and Beall, A. C., Jr.: Traumatic Coronary Artery-Right Heart Fistula. Report of a Case and Review of the Literature, *J. Thorac. Cardiovasc. Surg.*, 70:52, 1975.

37 Anderson, G. P., Adicoff, A., Motsay, G. J., Sako, Y., and Gobel, F. L.: Traumatic Right Coronary Arterial-Right Atrial Fistula, *Am. J. Cardiol.*, 35:439, 1975.

38 Wilson, C. S., Weaver, W. F., Zeman, E. D., and Forker, A. D.: Bilateral Nonfistulous Congenital Coronary Arterial Aneurysms, *Am. J. Cardiol.*, 35:319, 1975.

39 Mattern, A. L., Baker, W. P., McHale, J. J., and Lee, D. E.: Congenital Coronary Aneurysms with Angina Pectoris and Myocardial Infarction Treated with Saphenous Vein Bypass Graft, *Am. J. Cardiol.*, 30:906, 1972.

40 Bjork, V. O., and Bjork, L.: Intramural Coronary Artery Aneurysm: A Coronary Artery Steal Syndrome, *J. Thorac. Cardiovasc. Surg.*, 54:50, 1967.

41 Perloff, J. K., Urschell, C. W., Roberts, W. C., and Caulfield, W. H., Jr.: Aneurysmal Dilation of the Coronary Arteries in Cyanotic Congenital Cardiac Disease. Report of a Forty-Year-Old Patient with the Taussig-Bing Complex, *Am. J. Med.*, 45:802, 1968.

42 Daoud, A. S., Pankin, D., Tulgan, H., and Florentin, R. A.: Aneurysms of the Coronary Artery. Report of Ten Cases and Review of Literature, *Am. J. Cardiol.*, 11:228, 1963.

43 Berkoff, H. A., and Rowe, G. G.: Atherosclerotic Ulcerative Disease and Associated Aneurysms of the Coronary Arteries, *Am. Heart J.*, 90:153, 1975.

44 Wilson, C. S., Weaver, W. F., and Forker, A. D.: Bilateral Arteriosclerotic Coronary Arterial Aneurysms Successfully Treated with Saphenous Vein Bypass Grafting, *Am. J. Cardiol.*, 35:315, 1975.

45 Cheng, T. O., and Adkins, P. C.: Traumatic Aneurysm of Left Anterior Descending Coronary Artery with Fistulous Opening into Left Ventricle and Left Ventricular Aneurysm after Stab Wound of Chest. Report of Case with Successful Surgical Repair, *Am. J. Cardiol.*, 31:384, 1973.

46 Chaithiraphan, S., Goldberg, E., O'Reilly, M., and Jootar, P.: Multiple Aneurysms of Coronary Artery in Sclerodermal Heart Disease, *Angiology*, 24:86, 1973.

47 Imahori, S., Bannerman, R. M., Graf, C. J., and Brennan, J. C.: Ehlers-Danlos Syndrome with Multiple Arterial Lesions, *Am. J. Med.*, 47:967, 1969.

48 Rae, M. V.: Coronary Aneurysms with Thrombosis in Rheumatic Carditis. Unusual Occurrence Accompanied by Hyperleukocytosis in a Child, *Arch. Pathol.*, 24:369, 1937.

49 Denham, S. W.: Syphilitic Aneurysm of the Left Coronary Artery, *Arch. Pathol.*, 51:661, 1951.

50 Kitamura, S., Kawashima, Y., Fujita, T., Mori, T., Oyama, C., Fujino, M., Kozuka, T., Nishizaki, K., and Manabe, H.: Aorto-coronary Bypass Grafting in a Child with Coronary Artery Obstruction due to Mucocutaneous Lymphnode Syndrome. Report of a Case, *Circulation*, 53:1035, 1976.

51 Kato, H., Koike, S., Yamamoto, M., Ito, Y., and Yano, E.: Coronary Aneurysms in Infants and Young Children with Acute Febrile Mucocutaneous Lymph Node Syndrome, *J. Pediatr.*, 86:892, 1975.

52 Markis, J. E., Joffe, C. D., Cohn, P. F., Feen, D. J., Herman, M. V., and Gorlin, R.: Clinical Significance of Coronary Arterial Ectasia, *Am. J. Cardiol.*, 37:217, 1976.

53 Smith, J. C.: Dissecting Aneurysms of Coronary Arteries, *Arch. Pathol.*, 99:117, 1975.

54 Claudon, D. G., Claudon, D. B., and Edwards, J. E.: Primary Dissecting Aneurysm of Coronary Artery. A Cause of Acute Myocardial Ischemia, *Circulation*, 45:259, 1972.

55 Harrison, L. H., Jr., Gregg, D. L., Itscoitz, S. B., Redwood, D. R., and Michaelis, L. L.: Delayed Coronary Artery Dissection after Angiography. A Case Description with Successful Operative Treatment, *J. Thorac. Cardiovasc. Surg.*, 69:880, 1975.

56 Fishman, N. H., Youker, J. E., and Roe, B. B: Mechanical Injury to the Coronary Arteries During Operative Cannulation, *Am. Heart J.*, 75:26, 1968.

57 Bulkley, B. H., and Roberts, W. C.: Isolated Coronary Arterial Dissection. A Complication of Cardiac Operations, *J. Thorac. Cardiovasc. Surg.*, 67:148, 1974.

58 Manalo-Estrella, P., and Barker, A. B.: Histopathologic Findings in Human Aortic Media Associated with Pregnancy, *Arch. Pathol.*, 83:336, 1967.

59 Gonzalez-Crussi, F., Mandy, S., Johnson, J. E., III, and

Green, J. R., Jr.: Teflon Embolism of Coronary Arteries, *J. Thorac. Cardiovasc. Surg.*, 54:53, 1967.

60 Wenger, N. K., and Bauer, S.: Coronary Embolism. Review of the Literature and Presentation of Fifteen Cases, *Am. J. Med.*, 25:549, 1958.

61 Sybers, H. D., and Boake, W. C.: Coronary and Retinal Embolism from Left Atrial Myxoma, *Arch. Pathol.*, 91:179, 1971.

62 Torre, A. de la, Jacobs, D., Aleman, J., and Anderson, G. A.: Embolic Coronary Artery Occlusion in Percutaneous Transfemoral Coronary Arteriography, *Am. Heart J.*, 86:467, 1973.

63 From, A. H. L., Wang, Y., Eliot, R. S., and Edwards, J. E.: Coronary Arterial Embolism in Persistent Truncus Arteriosus: Report of a Case Following Cardiac Catheterization, *N. Engl. J. Med.*, 272:1204, 1965.

64 Watt, D. A. L.: Paradoxical Coronary Embolism, *Br. Heart J.*, 28:570, 1966.

65 Schatz, J. W., and Fischer, J. A.: Paradoxic Coronary Embolism in a Patient with Mid-systolic Click Syndrome, *Chest*, 66:587, 1974.

65a Steiner, I., Hlava, A., and Procházka, J.: Calcific Coronary Embolization Associated with Cardiac Valve Replacement. Necropsy X-ray Study, *Br. Heart J.*, 38:816, 1976.

65b Hammer, W. J., Ferrans, V. J., and Roberts, W. C.: Myocardial Embolus to Coronary Artery. Result of Rupture of Papillary Muscle during Acute Myocardial Infarction, *Chest*, 68:843, 1975.

66 Henderson, R. R., Hansing, C. E., Razavi, M., and Rowe, G. G.: Resolution of an Obstructive Coronary Lesion as Demonstrated by Selective Angiography in a Patient with Transmural Myocardial Infarction, *Am. J. Cardiol.*, 31:785, 1973.

67 Schrire, V., Barnard, C. N., and Beck, W.: Syphilitic Coronary Ostial Occlusion, *S. Afr. Med. J.*, 40:553, 1966.

68 Rissanen, V.: Occurrence of Coronary Ostial Stenosis in a Necropsy Series of Myocardial Infarction, Sudden Death, and Violent Death, *Br. Heart J.*, 37:182, 1975.

69 Trimble, A. S., Bigelow, W. G., Wigle, E. D., and Silver, M. D.: Coronary Ostial Stenosis: A Late Complication of Coronary Perfusion in Open-Heart Surgery, *J. Thorac. Cardiovasc. Surg.*, 57:792, 1969.

70 Roberts, W. C., and Morrow, A. G.: Late Postoperative Pathological Findings after Cardiac Valve Replacement, *Circulation*, 35 & 36(suppl. 1):48, 1967.

71 Yates, J. D., Kirsh, M. M., Sodeman, T. M., Walton, J. A., Jr., and Brymer, J. F.: Coronary Ostial Stenosis. A Complication of Aortic Valve Replacement, *Circulation*, 49:530, 1974.

72 Brill, I. C., Brodeur, M. T. H., and Oyama, A. A.: Myocardial Infarction in Two Sisters Less Than 20 Years Old, *JAMA*, 217:1345, 1971.

73 Hudgson, P., Foster, J. B., and Walton, J. N.: Methysergide and Coronary Artery Disease, *Am. Heart J.*, 74:854, 1967.

74 Neufeld, H. N., Lester, R. G., Adams, P., Jr., Anderson, R. C., Lillehei, C. W., and Edwards, J. E.: Congenital Communication of a Coronary Artery with a Cardiac Chamber or the Pulmonary Trunk ("Coronary Artery Fistula"), *Circulation*, 24:171, 1961.

75 Neufeld, H. N., Wagenvoort, C. A., Ongley, P. A., and Edwards, J. E.: Hypoplasia of Ascending Aorta. An Unusual Form of Supravalvular Aortic Stenosis with Special Reference to Localized Coronary Arterial Hypertension, *Am. J. Cardiol.*, 10:746, 1962.

76 Oppenheimer, E. H., and Esterly, J. R.: Some Aspects of Cardiac Pathology in Infancy and Childhood: II. Unusual Coronary Endarteritis with Congenital Cardiac Malformations, *Bull. Johns Hopkins Hosp.*, 119:343, 1966.

77 MacMahon, H. E., and Dickinson, P. C. T.: Occlusive Fibroelastosis of Coronary Arteries in the Newborn, *Circulation*, 35:3, 1967.

78 Vlodaver, Z., and Neufeld, H. N.: The Coronary Arteries in Coarctation of the Aorta, *Circulation*, 37:449, 1968.

79 Neufeld, H. N.: Studies of the Coronary Arteries in Children and their Relevance to Coronary Heart Disease, *Eur. J. Cardiol.*, 1:479, 1974.

80 Ogden, J. A.: Congenital Anomalies of the Coronary Arteries, *Am. J. Cardiol.*, 25:474, 1970.

81 Saphir, O., Katz, L. N., and Gore, I: The Myocardium in Subacute Bacterial Endocarditis, *Circulation*, 1:1155, 1950.

82 Hennigar, G. R., Thabet, R., Bundy, W. E., and Sutton, L. E., Jr.: Salmonellosis Complicated by Pancarditis. Report of a Case with Autopsy Findings, *J. Pediatr.*, 43:524, 1953.

83 Gouley, B. A., Bellet, S., and McMillan, T. M: Tuberculosis of the Myocardium: Report of Six Cases, with Observations on Involvement of Coronary Arteries, *AMA Arch. Intern. Med.*, 51:244, 1933.

84 Allen, A. C., and Spitz, S.: A Comparative Study of the Pathology of Scrub Typhus (Tsutsugamushi Disease) and Other Rickettsial Diseases, *Am. J. Pathol.*, 21:603, 1945.

85 Holsinger, D. R., Osmundson, P. J., and Edwards, J. E.: The Heart in Periarteritis Nodosa, *Circulation*, 25:610, 1962.

86 Chamberlain, J. L., III, and Perry, L. W.: Infantile Periarteritis Nodosa with Coronary and Brachial Aneurysms: A Case Diagnosed during Life, *J. Pediatr.*, 78:1039, 1971.

86a Glanz, S., Bittner, S. J., Berman, M. A., Dolan, T. F., Jr., and Talner, N. S.: Regression of Coronary-Artery Aneurysms in Infantile Polyarteritis Nodosa, *N. Engl. J. Med.*, 294:939, 1976.

87 Bonfiglio, T. A., Botti, R. E., and Hagstrom, J. W. C.: Coronary Arteritis, Occlusion, and Myocardial Infarction due to Lupus Erythematosus, *Am. Heart J.*, 83:153, 1972.

88 Benisch, B. M., and Pervez, N.: Coronary Artery Vasculitis and Myocardial Infarction with Systemic Lupus Erythematosus, *N.Y. State J. Med.*, 74:873, 1974.

89 Bor, I.: Myocardial Infarction and Ischaemic Heart Disease in Infants and Children: Analysis of 29 Cases and Review of the Literature, *Arch. Dis. Child.*, 44:268, 1969.

90 Grismer, J. T., Anderson, W. R., and Weiss, L.: Chronic Occlusive Rheumatic Coronary Vasculitis and Myocardial Dysfunction, *Am. J. Cardiol.*, 20:739, 1967.

91 Coronary Occlusion in Rheumatoid Arthritis, *Br. Med. J.*, 1:707, 1970.

92 Sanerkin, N. G.: Extracardiac Anastomosis in Coronary Ostial Occlusion, *Br. Heart J.*, 30:440, 1968.

93 James, T. N.: An Etiologic Concept Concerning the Obscure Myocardiopathies, *Prog. Cardiovasc. Dis.*, 7:43, 1964.

94 Fraser, G. R., Froggatt, P., and James, T. N.: Congenital Deafness Associated with Electrocardiographic Abnormalities, Fainting Attacks, and Sudden Death. A Recessive Syndrome, *Q. J. Med.*, 33:361, 1964.

95 James, T. N.: Pathology of Small Coronary Arteries, *Am. J. Cardiol.*, 20:679, 1967.

95a James. T. N.: De Subitaneis Mortibus. VIII. Coronary Arteries and Conduction System in Scleroderma Heart Disease, *Circulation*, 50:844, 1974.

96 James, T. N.: Congenital Deafness and Cardiac Arrhythmias, *Am. J. Cardiol.*, 19:627, 1967.

97 Varnauskas, E., Ivemark, B., Paulin, S., and Ryden, B.: Obscure Cardiomyopathies with Coronary Artery Changes, *Am. J. Cardiol.*, 19:531, 1967.

98 Phillips, J., and Ichinose, H.: Clinical and Pathologic Studies in the Hereditary Syndrome of a Long QT Interval, Syncopal Spells, and Sudden Death, *Chest*, 58:236, 1970.

99 James. T. N., and Fisch, C.: Observations on the Cardiovascular Involvement in Friedreich's Ataxia, *Am. Heart J.*, 66:164, 1963.

100 Merkel, W. C.: *Plasmodium falciparum* Malaria: The Coronary and Myocardial Lesions Observed in Autopsy in Two Cases of Acute Fulminating *P. falciparum* Infection, *AMA Arch. Pathol.*, 41:290, 1946.

101 Gazayerli, M.: Unusual Site of a Schistosome Worm in the Circumflex Branch of the Left Coronary Artery, *J. Egypt Med. Assoc.*, 22:34, 1939.

102 Oliveira E., and Gomez-Patino, N.: Falcemic Cardiopathy: Report of a Case, *Am. J. Cardiol.*, 11:686, 1963.

103 Fomina, L. G.: A Case of Myocardial Infarct in Acute Leukemia, *Sov. Med.*, 24:141, 1960.

104 Wirth, L.: Myocardial Infarction as the Initial Manifestation of Polycythemia Vera, *Milit. Med.*, 125:544, 1960.

105 Spach, M. S., Howell, D. A., and Harris, J. S.: Myocardial Infarction and Multiple Thrombosis in a Child with Primary Thrombocytosis, *Pediatrics*, 31:268, 1963.

106 Renteria, V. G., Ferrans, V. J., and Roberts, W. C.: The Heart in the Hurler Syndrome. Gross Histologic and Ultrastructural Observations in Five Necropsy Cases, *Am. J. Cardiol.*, 38:487, 1976.

107 Lindsay, S.: The Cardiovascular System in Gargoylism, *Br. Heart J.*, 12:17, 1950.

108 Hudson, R. E. B.: "Cardiovascular Pathology," vols. 1–3, Edward Arnold Publishers (Ltd.), London, 1965, 1965, and 1970.

109 Stauffer, M.: Oxalosis. Report of a Case with a Review of the Literature and Discussion on Pathogenesis, *N. Engl. J. Med.*, 263:386, 1960.

110 Blieden, L. C., Desnick, R. J., Carter, J. B., Krivit, W., Moller, J. H., and Sharp, H. L.: Cardiac Involvement in Sandhoff's Disease. An Inborn Error of Glycosphingolipid Metabolism, *Am. J. Cardiol.*, 34:83, 1974.

111 Blieden, L. C., and Moller, J. H.: Cardiac Involvement in Inherited Disorders of Metabolism, *Prog. Cardiovasc. Dis.*, 16:615, 1974.

112 Fredrickson, D. S.: Inheritance of High Density Lipoprotein Deficiency (Tangier Disease), *J. Clin. Invest.*, 43:228, 1964.

113 Fredrickson, D. S., Gotto, A. M., and Levy, R. I.: Familial Lipoprotein Deficiency (Abeta Lipoproteinemia, Hypobeta Lipoproteinemia and Tangier Disease), in J. B. Stanbury, J. B. Wyngaarden, and D. S. Fredrickson (eds.): "The Metabolic Basis of Inherited Disease," 3d ed., McGraw-Hill Book Company, New York, 1972, p. 493.

114 Schimke, R. N., McKusick, V. A., Huang, T., and Pollack, A. D.: Homocystinuria. Studies of 20 Families with 38 Affected Members, *JAMA*, 193:87, 1965.

114a James, T. N., Carson, N. A. J., and Froggatt, P.: De Subitaneis. Mortibus IV. Coronary Vessels and Conduction System in Homocystinuria, *Circulation*, 49:367, 1974.

115 Pund, E. E., Jr., Hawley, R. L., McGee, H. J., and Blount, S. G., Jr.: Gouty Heart, *N. Engl. J. Med.*, 263:835, 1960.

116 Brandt, K., Cathcart, E. S., and Cohen, A. S.: A Clinical Analysis of the Course and Prognosis of Forty-two Patients with Amyloidosis, *Am. J. Med.*, 44:955, 1968.

117 Barth, R. F., Willerson, J. T., Buja, L. M., Decker, J. L., and Roberts, W. C.: Amyloid Coronary Artery Disease, Primary Systemic Amyloidosis and Paraproteinemia, *Arch. Intern. Med.*, 126:627, 1970.

118 DeSanctis, R. W.: Case Records of the Massachusetts General Hospital, Case 46-1967, *N. Engl. J. Med.*, 277:1025, 1967.

119 Young, J. A., Sengupta, A., and Khaja, F.-U.: Coronary Arterial Stenosis, Angina Pectoris, and Atypical Coarctation of the Aorta due to Nonspecific Arteritis. Treatment with Aortocoronary Bypass Graft, *Am. J. Cardiol.*, 32:356, 1973.

120 Saphir, O.: Thromboangitis Obliterans of the Coronary Arteries and Its Relation to Arteriosclerosis, *Am. Heart J.*, 12:521, 1936.

121 Stryker, W. A.: Coronary Occlusive Disease in Infants and in Children, *Am. J. Dis. Child.*, 71:280, 1946.

122 Chipman, C. D.: Calcific Sclerosis of Coronary Arteries in an Infant, *Can. Med. Assoc. J.,* 83:955, 1960.

123 Lev, M., Craenen, J., and Lambert, E. C.: Infantile Coronary Sclerosis with Atrioventricular Block, *J. Pediatr.,* 70:87, 1967.

124 Rosenberg, H. G.: Systemic Arterial Disease with Myocardial Infarction. Report on Two Infants, *Circulation,* 47:270, 1973.

125 Calvelo, M. G., and Korns, M. E.: Left Ventricular Obstruction Caused by Metastatic Sarcoma, *Arch. Pathol.,* 21:222, 1971.

126 Javier, B. V., Yount, W. J., Crosby, D. J., and Hall, T. C.: Cardiac Metastasis in Lymphoma and Leukemia, *Dis. Chest.,* 52:481, 1967.

126a Espada, R., Whisennand, H. H., Mattox, K. L., and Beall, A. C., Jr.: Surgical Management of Penetrating Injuries to the Coronary Arteries, *Surgery,* 78:755, 1975.

127 Jokl, E., and Greenstein, J.: Fatal Coronary Sclerosis in a Boy of Ten Years, *Lancet,* 2:659, 1944.

128 Stern, T., Wolf, R. Y., Reichart, B., Harrington, O. B., and Crosby, G.: Coronary Artery Occlusion Resulting from Blunt Trauma, *JAMA,* 230:1308, 1974.

129 Heyndrickx, G., Vermeire, P., Goffin, Y., and Bogaert, P. V.: Rupture of the Right Coronary Artery due to Nonpenetrating Chest Trauma, *Chest,* 65:577, 1974.

130 Dollinger, M. R., Lavine, D. M., and Foye, L. V., Jr.: Myocardial Infarction due to Postirradiation Fibrosis of the Coronary Arteries: Case of Successfully Treated Hodgkin's Disease with Lower Esophageal Involvement, *JAMA,* 195:316, 1966.

131 Tracy, G. P., Brown, D. E., Johnson, L. W., and Gottlieb, A. J.: Radiation-Induced Coronary Artery Disease, *JAMA,* 228:1660, 1974.

131a McReynolds, R. A., Gold, G. L., and Roberts, W. C.: Coronary Heart Disease after Mediastinal Irradiation for Hodgkin's Disease, *Am. J. Med.,* 60:39, 1976.

132 Hallén, A., Nyström, S. O., Sanner, E., and Willén, R.: Non-traumatic Rupture of a Coronary Artery. Report of a Case, *Scand. J. Thorac. Cardiovasc. Surg.,* 4:215, 1970.

B
The Clinical Recognition and Management of Nonatherosclerotic Causes of Myocardial Ischemia and Necrosis

MICHAEL V. HERMAN, M.D., and
RICHARD GORLIN, M.D.

Angina pectoris is ordinarily associated in the mind of the clinician with coronary atherosclerosis.[1] It is obvious that while atherosclerosis constitutes its greatest cause, angina pectoris can arise in any clinical condition in which there is augmented cardiac workload or cardiac muscle mass or reduced perfusion (Table 63B-1). Thus, it is readily accepted

TABLE 63B-1
Causes of myocardial ischemia and necrosis

1. Coronary atherosclerosis
2. Myocardial hypertrophy
   a Valvular heart disease
   b Idiopathic hypertrophy with and without obstruction
   c Hypertension
3. Rare causes of coronary artery involvement (see Chap. 63A)
4. Anginal syndrome without identifiable cause

that aortic stenosis and/or insufficiency, occasionally mitral insufficiency, hypertension, and diseases affecting the right side of the heart in similar fashion can bring about a situation in which myocardial ischemia with or without angina pectoris can occur. Similarly, idiopathic ventricular hypertrophy may set the stage for myocardial ischemia. Rare causes of nonatherosclerotic coronary artery involvement and myocardial ischemia are discussed in Chap. 63A.

Interest in recent years, however, has centered on a group of patients with angina in whom no obvious or identifiable cause (such as valvular or hypertensive heart disease) could be determined, and in whom coronary arteriography revealed normal, large vessels. The first of these reports appeared in 1967.[2,3] Since this time, there have been numerous reports from various clinical centers around the country documenting the fact that angina pectoris, myocardial ischemia, and even frank necrosis can occur when their etiology remains obscure but is clearly not atherosclerotic.[4-6] This is called the syndrome of *angina-like chest pain without identifiable cause.*

CLINICAL CHARACTERISTICS (Table 63B-2)

The group of patients with this syndrome shows an equal distribution of sex and is in no way different from groups of patients with coronary atherosclerosis with respect to the prevalence of hypertension or smoking, while the incidence of diabetes mellitus and hyperlipidemia is clearly less. As with coronary atherosclerotic angina, not all patients have effort-induced pain, the pain of many of them occurring under unpredictable conditions and often (more frequently than during exercise) at rest.

The electrocardiogram tends to be abnormal in approximately half the subjects,[2,5] with the most common alteration being nonspecific ST-T change.

TABLE 63B-2
Clinical features of angina-like chest pain without identifiable cause

Pain	Atypical or classic angina pectoris
Physical findings	Normal, little evidence for noncardiac sources of pain
ECG	Often abnormal (ST-T changes) at rest and/or with exercise
Incidence	Equal frequency in men and women
Metabolic disorders	Less prevalent than in coronary atherosclerosis patients
Physiologic function	Normal O_2 extraction and coronary blood flow
Myocardial ischemia	May be elicited under stress

Patterns of myocardial infarction, bundle branch block, left axis deviation, and left ventricular hypertrophy have all been reported in various series. The response to exercise is abnormal in up to 20 percent to 25 percent of cases reported; females have an abnormal response more frequently than males. Only one group has reported abnormal physical findings in a significant number of cases.[5]

PATHOPHYSIOLOGY

The physiology of the coronary circulation as studied by blood flow and oxygen extraction are within normal limits.[2] Bemiller has recorded abnormal left ventricular function, however.[5] Several groups have described lactate production by the heart in patients with this syndrome.[2,4,5] The correlation between evidence of ischemia and other aspects of the syndrome was not definite. In this regard, Maseri et al. have demonstrated transient asymptomatic ischemic episodes (ST-segment changes) during prolonged electrocardiographic monitoring of patients with this syndrome.[7]

ETIOLOGIC POSSIBILITIES (Table 63B-3)

When the syndrome was first described, it was evident that multiple etiologies might be involved. It has been shown that this condition is not due to the misinterpretation of the arteriogram through serial arteriography in the same subject. There is no evidence that the syndrome is related to gallbladder disease, hiatus hernia, or cervical disc disease with any more likelihood than in any other group of patients with chest pain.[8] Oxyhemoglobin dissociation defects have been suggested, but this would seem unlikely from the work of Vokonas et al.[9] Among the etiologies which may be contributing to this group of patients are cardiomyopathy, small-vessel disease, and coronary artery spasm.

Cardiomyopathy

The various forms of cardiomyopathy can be associated with chest pain, and, of course, the angiograms of the coronary arteries are normal. Such myopathy may or may not be associated with hypertrophy, but

TABLE 63B-3
Possible etiologic factors of anginal syndrome without identifiable cause

1. Cardiomyopathy
    a Idiopathic
    b Hypertrophic
        (1) Without obstruction
        (2) Idiopathic hypertrophic subaortic stenosis
    c Mitral valve prolapse
2. Small-vessel disease (unsettled)
3. Coronary artery spasm (unsettled)
4. Angiographic misinterpretation (rare)
5. Oxyhemoglobin dissociation defect (unlikely)
6. Psychosomatic factors (common)

there are subtle forms, as described by Kreulen et al.,[10] in which only changes in end-diastolic pressure with stress or subtle changes in ventricular mass can give a clue concerning cardiomyopathy. This may well be the reason for some of the abnormal findings reported by Bemiller.[5] Cardiomyopathy in its earlier stages may indeed manifest itself as a chest pain syndrome. This is particularly true for *idiopathic hypertrophic subaortic stenosis.*

Idiopathic hypertrophic subaortic stenosis (IHSS) (see Chap. 81B) may present in a rather cryptic fashion, with patients exhibiting angina pectoris and/or the intermediate coronary syndrome. In such patients, the resting and/or postexercise electrocardiogram may show characteristic changes of subendocardial ischemia. The echocardiogram in these patients often provides the first important objective findings to establish the correct diagnosis: systolic anterior motion of the mitral valve and an increase in the ratio of septal to free-wall thickness of the left ventricle. Cardiac catheterization, with the appropriate left ventricular–aortic pressure gradients (rest, postextrasystole, nitroglycerin, isoproterenol) and the angiographic picture, finalizes the diagnosis.

Barlow's syndrome

A certain number of patients with unusual forms of chest pain may have Barlow's syndrome or prolapse of the mitral valve (see Chap. 60B).[11] This syndrome, originally characterized by a late systolic click and murmur, usually presents with either chest pain or arrhythmias, and inferolateral ST-T changes are the rule. The exercise electrocardiogram is often abnormal as well. As with the above-described disorder (IHSS), echocardiography has shown that the clinical features of mitral valve prolapse may appear in only partial expression. There may be a click, a murmur, or electrocardiographic abnormalities, which can occur separately or together or may be absent or evanescent. Both chest pain and an abnormal exercise electrocardiogram may be present in this syndrome. The diagnosis can be difficult and may require echocardiography and cineventriculography.

Our awareness of the two syndromes just discussed, and in particular of how to diagnose them, will help in separating the causes for chest pain with normal coronary arteries into distinct entities. In this regard, the coronary arteriogram should not be the sole arbiter of whether or not the patient has heart disease underlying a chest pain syndrome. Only a complete echocardiographic, ventriculographic, and hemodynamic study can serve to recognize other subtler and new forms of heart disease.

Small-vessel disease of the myocardium

Small-vessel disease of the heart without involvement elsewhere is very rare. Those patients who exhibit small-vessel cardiac disease usually have conduction disturbances and/or arrhythmias. Shirey did not find small-vessel disease by transthoracic needle biopsy of such patients,[12] although Rider et al., utilizing a right ventricular biopsy, did describe, in preliminary fashion, an abnormally thickened subendothelial lamina in 20- to 50-μm vessels in a few patients.[13] The significance of this latter observation remains to be determined.

Spasm of the coronary arteries

Recent studies provide strong evidence that the large coronary arteries in human beings can undergo varying degrees of spasm.[14–20] On occasion, this spasm can be sufficient to severely impede or totally obstruct coronary blood flow. Maseri et al.[7] have suggested that this may be termed *primary angina pectoris,* that is, an acute reduction in coronary blood supply which is responsible for the transient myocardial ischemia. Such spastic changes can take place in the complete absence of any evidence of coronary atherosclerosis. The vascular alterations bring about a major perfusion deficit evidenced by thallium 201 scintographic scanning, electrocardiographic change, and generalized alteration in left ventricular function.

The electrocardiographic changes that may occur seem to depend on the degree of occlusion. If there is only partial occlusion there will be subendocardial ischemia with ST-segmental depression, whereas if there is complete or nearly complete occlusion, there will be transmural ischemia with ST-segmental elevation. The clinical findings associated with this condition are discussed in detail in Chap. 62E (Prinzmetal's variant angina).

Psychosomatic factors

It is obvious that many patients with chest pain do not have heart disease and that a large percentage of the patients have emotional problems (see Chaps. 62E and 96).

MANAGEMENT

The response to therapy is clearly mixed and not as clear-cut as in patients with atherosclerotic angina. From a consideration of the multiple etiologic possibilities, this is not surprising. For example, if this syndrome is due to a forme fruste of hypertrophic cardiomyopathy, then obviously propranolol may be the therapy of choice. The same may be true with a prolapsed mitral valve. On the other hand, if there is evidence that this is primary angina pectoris and has a vasospastic component, then appropriate therapy may be the elimination of beta-adrenergic blockade and substitution of intensive nitrate therapy. Thus, the clinician should not be content with simply reaching a diagnosis of angina pectoris and normal coronary arteries, but should make an attempt to achieve a diagnostic differentiation so that therapy can be implemented.

PROGNOSIS

From all reports in the literature, the outlook for patients with this syndrome, irrespective of specific etiology, is generally good.[4–6] For example, in Kemp's follow-up of 200 patients over a 6-year period, there were a total of six deaths.[4] Bemiller[5] and Dreifus[6] have reached similar conclusions.

The majority of patients experience improvement in pain with time. Only 15 of the original 200 subjects reported by Kemp experienced aggravation of pain.[4] Only one new myocardial infarction occurred although 18 individuals had to be hospitalized repeatedly for recurring chest pain.[4]

SUMMARY

Myocardial ischemia and necrosis can occur in the absence of coronary atherosclerosis. Various cardiac disease states, such as valvular disease, hypertension, vasculitis, and cardiomyopathy, particularly of the hypertrophic variety, can result in an imbalance between oxygen demands and supply. Other more occult disorders such as the syndrome of angina (and occasional objective evidence of ischemia) in patients without obvious heart disease and coronary artery spasm are now being appreciated. Thus, a flexible view must be taken by the physician in the approach to the patient with angina and ischemia or myocardial necrosis.

REFERENCES

1 Zoll, P. H., Wessler, S., and Blumgart, H. L.: Angina Pectoris—A Clinical and Pathologic Correlation, *Am. J. Med.,* 11:331, 1951.

2 Kemp, H. G., Elliott, W. C., and Gorlin, R.: The Anginal Syndrome with Normal Coronary Arteriography, *Trans. Assoc. Am. Physicians,* 80:59, 1967.

3 Likoff, W., Segal, B. L., and Kasparian, H.: Paradox of Normal Selective Coronary Arteriograms in Patients Considered to Have Unmistakable Coronary Heart Disease, *N. Engl. J. Med.,* 276:1063, 1967.

4 Kemp, H. G., Vokonas, P. S., Cohn, P. F., and Gorlin, R.: The Anginal Syndrome Associated with Normal Coronary Arteriograms: Report of a Six-Year Experience, *Am. J. Med.,* 54:735, 1973.

5 Bemiller, C. R., Pepine, C. J., and Rogers, A. K.: Long-Term Observation in Patients with Angina and Normal Coronary Arteriograms, *Circulation,* 47:36, 1973.

6 Waxler, E. B., Kimbiris, D., and Dreifus, L. S.: The Fate of Women with Normal Coronary Arteriograms and Chest Pain Resembling Angina Pectoris, *Am. J. Cardiol.,* 28:25, 1971.

7 Maseri, A., Mimmo, R., Chierchia, S., Marchesi, C., Pesola, A., and L'Abbate, A.: Coronary Artery Spasm as a Cause of Acute Myocardial Ischemia in Man, *Chest,* 68:625, 1975.

8 Forrester, J. S., Herman, M. V., and Gorlin, R.: Non-coronary Factors in the Anginal Syndrome, *N. Engl. J. Med.,* 283:786, 1970.

9 Vokonas, P. S., Cohn, P. F., Klein, M. D., Laver, M. B., and

Gorlin, R.: Hemoglobin Affinity for Oxygen in the Anginal Syndrome with Normal Coronary Arteriograms, *J. Clin. Invest.*, 54:409, 1974.

10 Kreulen, T. H., Gorlin, R., and Herman, M. V.: Ventriculographic Patterns and Hemodynamics in Primary Myocardial Disease, *Circulation*, 47:299, 1973.

11 Jeresaty, R.: Mitral Valve Prolapse-Click Syndrome, *Prog. Cardiovasc. Dis.*, 15:623, 1973.

12 Shirey, E. K., Hawk, W. A., Mukerji, D., and Effler, D. B.: Percutaneous Myocardial Biopsy of the Left Ventricle: Experience in 198 Patients, *Circulation*, 46:112, 1972.

13 Rider, A. K., Billingham, M. E., and Harrison, D. C.: Small Vessel Coronary Disease: Biopsy Evidence of Intramyocardial Arteriopathy, *Circulation*, 50(suppl. 3):109, 1974.

14 Cheng, T. O., Bashour, T., Kelser, G. A., Jr., Weiss, L., and Bacos, J.: Variant Angina of Prinzmetal with Normal Coronary Arteriograms: A Variant of the Variant, *Circulation*, 47:476, 1973.

15 Gianelly, R., Mugler, F., and Harrison, D. C.: Prinzmetal's Variant of Angina Pectoris with Only Slight Coronary Atherosclerosis, *California Med.*, 108:129, 1968.

RECOGNITION AND MANAGEMENT OF NONATHEROSCLEROTIC MYOCARDIAL ISCHEMIA AND NECROSIS

16 Whiting, R. B., Klein, M. D., Vander Veer, J., and Lown, B.: Variant Angina Pectoris, *N. Engl. J. Med.*, 282:709, 1970.

17 Christian, N., and Botti, R. E.: Prinzmetal's Variant Angina Pectoris with Prolonged Electrocardiographic Changes in the Absence of Obstructive Coronary Disease, *Am. J. Med. Sci.*, 263:225, 1972.

18 Oliva, P. B., Potts, D. E., and Pluss, R. G.: Coronary Arterial Spasm in Prinzmetal Angina: Documentation by Coronary Arteriography, *N. Engl. J. Med.*, 288:745, 1973.

19 Dhurandhar, R. W., Watt, D. L., Silver, M. D., Trimble, A. S., and Adelman, A. G.: Prinzmetal's Variant Form of Angina with Arteriographic Evidence of Coronary Arterial Spasm, *Am. J. Cardiol.*, 30:902, 1972.

20 Hart, N. J., Silverman, M. E., and King, S. B.: Variant Angina Pectoris Caused by Coronary Artery Spasm, *Am. J. Med.*, 56:269, 1974.

Systemic Arterial Hypertension

64
Introduction and Classification

ELBERT P. TUTTLE, JR., M.D., and
W. DALLAS HALL, M.D.

The interrelationship of categories of disease entities is constantly modified by changing definitions. The evolution of taxonomy of disease is in a continuous state of flux as a result of medical progress. It has been emphasized by Feinstein[1] that proper nomenclature and categorization are basic to research and understanding in clinical medicine. This is particularly true in the field of hypertension.

When we consider systemic hypertension as a whole, the need for redefinition of the problem becomes obvious. General usage of the term can best be illustrated by the Venn diagram of Fig. 64-1. Hypertensive disease includes six categories. Some patients have high blood pressure without known cause, referred to as *essential hypertension* (category 1). Some have high blood pressure with a disease known to be its cause, referred to as *secondary hypertension* (category 2). Either of these essential

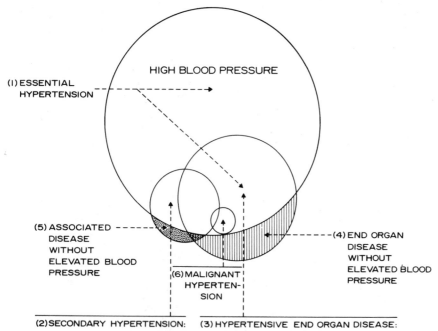

HIGH BLOOD PRESSURE

(I) ESSENTIAL HYPERTENSION

(5) ASSOCIATED DISEASE WITHOUT ELEVATED BLOOD PRESSURE

(6) MALIGNANT HYPERTENSION

(4) END ORGAN DISEASE WITHOUT ELEVATED BLOOD PRESSURE

(2) SECONDARY HYPERTENSION:

Renal parenchymal disease
Renal artery stenosis
Coarctation of the aorta
Pheochromocytoma
Glucocorticoid excess
Mineralocorticoid excess
Hypercalcemia
Drug-induced
Atherosclerosis
Diabetes mellitus
Myxedema
Disseminated lupus
Scleroderma
Dermatomyositis
Pseudoxanthoma elasticum
Periarteritis nodosa
Excess salt loading
Toxemia of pregnancy
Hyperdynamic circulation

(3) HYPERTENSIVE END ORGAN DISEASE:

Anatomic
 Arteriolar hypertrophy
 Left ventricular hypertrophy
 Nephrosclerosis
 Retinopathy
 Cerebral thrombosis and hemorrhage
Functional
 Congestive heart failure
 Uremia
 Visual dysfunction
 Encephalopathy
Malignant
 Multiple end organ decompensation
 Accelerated cerebro-nephro-adrenal
  pathophysiology

FIGURE 64-1 Venn diagram illustrating general usage of the terms hypertension and high blood pressure. Hypertensive disease includes at least six categories (see text).

or secondary groups may have consequences of their high blood pressure manifested in anatomic changes of parenchymal organs (category 3). Thus hypertensive patients may evidence cardiomegaly and left ventricular hypertrophy (i.e., hypertensive cardiovascular disease), involvement of the retinal vessels (i.e., hypertensive retinopathy), or sclerosis of the renal arterioles with impaired kidney function (i.e., nephrosclerosis). Patients with end-organ change from either type of hypertension may subsequently become normotensive with therapy or with counterbalancing comorbid disease states (category 4). They may still be considered to suffer from hypertensive disease of the end organ. Those patients with diseases known to be able to cause hypertension but who never develop high blood pressure are excluded from the hypertensive population and are indicated in Fig. 64-1 by the dark area (category 5).

A need for clearer taxonomic discrimination is also illustrated by the condition called *malignant hypertension* (category 6). Debate has continued over the question of whether papilledema and retinal hemorrhages or impaired renal function is required for the diagnosis. One solution is offered in Fig. 64-2, an expansion of a segment of Fig. 64-1.

Many authorities recognize malignant hypertension primarily by its circulatory and end-organ manifestations: marked elevation of blood pressure, encephalopathy, retinopathy, heart failure, and uremia. This picture can occur as a consequence of necrotizing arteriolonephrosclerosis, acute glomerulonephritis, pseudoxanthoma elasticum, or bilateral renal artery stenosis. Differentiation among these etiologies may be difficult. Moreover, each of these diseases may be present without causing the malignant circulatory syndrome.

Others diagnose malignant hypertension on the basis of pathophysiologic criteria: arteriolar necrosis in the kidney, elevated secretion of renin, and secondary hyperaldosteronism. Patients with these findings often do not present a classic circulatory picture. In fact, these conditions may exist with only a modest elevation in blood pressure if the hypertensive patient is sodium-depleted, is hypoalbuminemic, or has impaired myocardial contractility such as from past myocardial infarction. In addition, glomerular filtration rate may be within the normal range in the early stages. Studies or statements concerning malignant hypertension should thus specify as many as

possible of the aforementioned circulatory, anatomic, and metabolic parameters. It is worthwhile to recall the overlap and disparity of these circulatory and pathophysiologic features, illustrated in Fig. 64-2.

Variations of hypertension in different population groups have been the subject of widespread study. The effects of age, sex, race, diet, and psychosocial stress on the prevalence of high blood pressure have been assessed through numerous community studies.[2-5] In light of the large number of diseases which can lead to elevated blood pressure, as well as a modest number which can reduce it, such studies are very difficult to interpret. Comorbidity must be considered and a general medical profile of the population is desirable prior to drawing inferences concerning the prevalence or consequences of hypertension. For instance, the frequency of diabetes mellitus, urinary tract infection, and toxemia of pregnancy should be defined as well as factors such as diet, oral contraceptive intake, or the distribution of race.

Racial differences in the incidence and prevalence of hypertension have been noted. Studies of Comstock,[6] McDonough et al,[7] and Wilber[8] show that the Negro develops hypertension more frequently than the white. A study of the Jamaican Negro by Miall[9] showed pressures lower than others reported, but racial comparison in the same community was not carried out. There is little doubt that hypertension is more frequent in the adult Negro in biracial communities of the United States. The age at which blood pressure segregation first appears is a subject of current investigation.

If racial differences in the prevalence of "essential hypertension" exist, then it is obvious that the fraction of all hypertensive patients who have renal artery stenosis, primary aldosteronism, or low renin hypertension will differ among population groups. For example, the frequency of hypertension from unilateral renal artery stenosis is both absolutely and fractionally lower in the southern American Negro than in the white. The same considerations apply to studies of genetic factors in essential hypertension.

Until the causes of essential hypertension are further elucidated, the medical problems of estimating prognosis and evaluating therapeutics must be faced. A major step forward has been made with the recognition that high blood pressure can be controlled and overall morbidity reduced thereby. Yet to be analyzed are the effects of blood pressure reduction on the prognosis of conditions such as established nephrosclerosis, chronic glomerulonephritis, and diabetic nephrosclerosis.

A number of subsets of essential hypertension are now beginning to be recognized with the aid of new analytic techniques. Specifically, the various combinations of renin level, aldosterone secretion, and α- and β-adrenergic activity lead to the definition of sets with potentially different causes, natural histories, and responses to drugs.[10,11] For example, Laragh's

FIGURE 64-2 Expansion from section 6 of Fig. 64-1 called *malignant hypertension*. Usually the syndrome of malignant hypertension combines both elements of end-organ decompensation and malignant cerebro-nephro-adrenal physiology, but they do not always coexist.

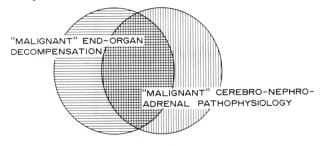

group[12,13] has identified low, normal, and high renin subsets of essential hypertension based on the value of plasma renin activity related to the 24-h excretion of sodium. Others[14,15] have defined the low renin group by finding suppressed renin activity despite efforts to stimulate renin release with agents such as diuretics. Patients with essential hypertension have been further characterized according to low, normal, or elevated extracellular fluid content or plasma volume;[16] low, normal, or elevated enzymatic indicators of sympathetic nervous system activity such as catecholamines[17] or dopamine beta hydroxylase;[18] low or normal chemical indicators of vasodepressor activity such as plasma prostaglandins (PGA)[19] or urinary kallikrein;[20] low, normal, or elevated physiologic indicators of cardiac performance such as cardiac output;[21] and low, normal, or elevated vascular or adrenal responsiveness to adrenergic or metabolic modulation.[22,23]

These metabolic and physiologic profiles should be considered in context of the dynamic feedback control of blood pressure, described in the next chapter. Patient subsets will exist in relatively stable categories because of paralysis of their normal metabolic and physiologic compensatory mechanisms. This may occur when one system component becomes overriding, such as with primary aldosteronism (persistent aldosterone excess, expanded plasma volume, and suppressed plasma renin activity) or pheochromocytoma (catecholamine excess, constricted plasma volume, and cardiac stimulation). Other patient subsets will manifest dynamically changing profiles according to constantly active feedback stimulation or suppression of the metabolic, physiologic, and vascular controls of blood pressure.

The assignment of hypertensive patients to one or another discrete category frequently reflects the classification scheme based upon the technical expertise and area of interest of the particular group of investigators. Further study will undoubtedly refine these profiles and locate them in their respective positions in the composite view of the circulation.

REFERENCES

1 Feinstein, A. R.: "Clinical Judgment," The Williams & Wilkins Company, Baltimore, 1967.

2 Stamler, J., Stamler, R., and Pullman, T. N. (eds.): "The Epidemiology of Hypertension," Grune & Stratton, Inc., New York, 1967.

3 Paul, O.: "Epidemiology and Control of Hypertension," Stratton Intercontinental Medical Book Corp., New York, 1975.

4 Kannel, W. B., and Sorlie, P.: Hypertension in Framingham, in O. Paul (ed.), "Epidemiology and Control of Hypertension," Stratton Intercontinental Medical Book Corp., New York, 1975, p. 553.

5 Johnson, B. C., Epstein, F. H., and Kyelsberg, M. O.: Distributions and Familial Studies of Blood Pressure and Serum Cholesterol Levels in a Total Community—Tecumseh, Michigan, *J. Chronic Dis.,* 18:147, 1965.

6 Comstock, G. W.: An Epidemiologic Study of Blood Pressure Levels in a Bi-racial Community in the Southern United States, *Am. J. Hyg.,* 65:27, 1957.

7 McDonough, J. R., Garrison, G. E., and Hames, C. G.: Blood Pressure and Hypertensive Disease among Negroes and Whites, *Ann. Intern. Med.,* 61:208, 1964.

8 Wilber, J. A.: Detection and Control of Hypertensive Disease in Georgia, U.S.A., in J. Stamler, R. Stamler, and T. N. Pullman (eds.), "The Epidemiology of Hypertension," Grune & Stratton, Inc., New York, 1967, p. 439.

9 Miall, W. E., Kass, E. H., Ling, J., and Stuart, K. L.: Factors Influencing Arterial Pressure in the General Population in Jamaica, *Br. Med. J.,* 2:497, 1962.

10 Laragh, J. H., Baer, L., Brunner, H. R., Buhler, F. R., Sealey, J. E., and Vaughan, E. D.: Renin, Angiotensin, and Aldosterone System in Pathogenesis and Management of Hypertensive Vascular Disease, *Am. J. Med.,* 52:633, 1972.

11 Dustan, H. P., Tarazi, R. C., and Bravo, E. L.: Physiologic Characteristics of Hypertension, *Am. J. Med.,* 52:610, 1972.

12 Sealey, J. E., and Laragh, J. H.: Searching Out Low Renin Patients: Limitations of Some Commonly Used Methods, *Am. J. Med.,* 53:303, 1973.

13 Brunner, H. R., Sealey, J. E., and Laragh, J. H.: Renin Subgroups in Essential Hypertension: Further Analysis of their Pathophysiologic and Epidemiologic Characteristics, *Circ. Res.,* 32–33(suppl. 1):99, 1973.

14 Crane, M. G., Harris, J. J., and Johns, V. J.: Hyporeninemic Hypertension, *Am. J. Med.,* 52:457, 1972.

15 Jose, A., Crout, J. R., and Kaplan, N. M.: Suppressed Plasma Renin Activity in Essential Hypertension: Roles of Plasma Volume, Blood Pressure, and Sympathetic Nervous System, *Ann. Intern. Med.,* 72:9, 1970.

16 Dustan, H. P., Tarazi, R. C., Bravo, E. L., and Dart, R. A.: Plasma and Extracellular Fluid Volumes in Hypertension, *Circ. Res.,* 32–33(suppl. 1):73, 1973.

17 Engelman, K., Portnoy, B., and Sjoerdsma, A.: Plasma Catecholamine Concentrations in Patients with Hypertension, *Circ. Res.,* 27(suppl. 1):141, 1970.

18 Shanberg, S. M., Stone, R. A., Kirshner, N., Gunnells, J. C., and Robinson, R. R.: Plasma Dopamine-β-hydroxylase: A Possible Aid in the Study and Evaluation of Hypertension, *Science,* 183:523, 1974.

19 Lee, J. B.: Cardiovascular-Renal Effects of Prostaglandins: The Antihypertensive, Natriuretic Renal "Endocrine" Function, *Arch. Intern. Med.,* 133:56, 1974.

20 Margolius, H. S., Geller, R., Pisano, J. J., and Sjoerdsma, A.: Altered Urinary Kallikrein Excretion in Human Hypertension, *Lancet,* 2:1063, 1971.

21 Julius, S., Pascual, A. B., Sannerstedt, R., and Mitchell, C.: Relationship between Cardiac Output and Peripheral Resistance in Borderline Hypertension, *Circulation,* 43:382, 1971.

22 Grim, C. E., Peters, T. J., and Maher, J. F.: Low Renin Hypertension: A State of Inappropriate Secretion of Aldosterone, *J. Lab. Clin. Med.,* 78:816, 1971.

23 Julius, S., Esler, M. D., and Randall, O. S.: Role of the Autonomic Nervous System in Mild Human Hypertension, *Clin. Sci. Molec. Med.,* 48:2435, 1975.

65
Etiology and Pathogenesis of Systemic Arterial Hypertension

ELBERT P. TUTTLE, JR., M.D., and
W. DALLAS HALL, M.D.

The explosion of knowledge arising from both basic biological research and targeted efforts to control a major public health problem has generated a massive growth of literature on hypertension in the past 15 years. The problems posed by the study of hypertension extend across the entire range of circulatory investigation. The mechanisms of regulation of the blood pressure are the subject of so vast a literature that only a selective and interpretive summary can serve the purpose of the present discussion. No effort has been made to be exhaustive in the review of reports. The authors have attempted to provide a schematic formulation to include the observations of a considerable number of active investigators. It will serve its purpose if an adequate mnemonic for the supporting observations is provided or if it is challenging enough to provoke discussion.

Blood pressure is a force which is mathematically the product of cardiac output and peripheral resistance. Elevation of blood pressure may result from any disturbance of the circulation which leads to an increase in cardiac output, peripheral resistance, or both. Since pressure varies directly with flow, any increase in blood flow or cardiac output will be initially associated with an increase in blood pressure. This initial elevation of blood pressure may be either inhibited or enhanced by various acute or chronic compensatory readjustments, ultimately acting through either cardiac output or peripheral resistance. The normal regulation of blood pressure is evidenced by its stability within a range of 50 percent above or below its basal value in healthy persons, despite variations in cardiac output ranging from one-third to five times basal output. If blood pressure elevation is frequent, prolonged, and great enough, it will induce hypertrophy of heart and blood vessels, so that the greater pressure can be generated with no increase in the stimulus. Progressive hypertrophy leads to progressive elevation in the blood pressure until vascular damage occurs and the course of the disease is secondarily accelerated. The morbidity of hypertension derives from the workload imposed on the heart and the injury to blood vessels at their points of least resistance. A number of recent international symposiums or monographs[1-9] provide extensive compendiums of current thought regarding the causes and pathogenesis of hypertension. To make available continuing group discussion of new developments, the reports[10] of the Council for High Blood Pressure Research of the American Heart Association have brought selected topics to print each year. Additional symposiums and reviews on special topics pertaining to hypertension have been published dealing with angiotensin, catecholamines, adrenal hormones, central nervous system, hemody-namics, vascular reactivity, vasodilator substances, and the kidney as they relate to hypertension.

Hypertension in its manifold forms can be understood only if all types are examined to ascertain where and how the normal regulatory mechanisms are circumvented. Special efforts must be made to distinguish the differences in physiology among the hypertensions of known cause so as to throw light on those of unknown cause.

BLOOD PRESSURE CONTROL AS A REGULATED SYSTEM

The concept of a regulated system in its simpler forms has been outlined by Peterson[11] in a discussion of the feedback regulation of the mechanical properties of blood vessels. In a regulated system of this type a negative feedback consists of the use of a portion of the energy associated with a physical force as a signal to a control mechanism to minimize the "error signal," or the deviation of the force from some basal value. An example is the use of a portion of the energy associated with a rise in blood pressure to stimulate neural receptors which induce reflexes to return the pressure toward normal. Negative feedback tends to stabilize a system, provided it is appropriately sensitive. Positive feedback, on the contrary, utilizes a portion of the energy associated with a force to increase any deviation from some initial value. This occurs, for instance, if a rise in blood pressure causes hypertrophy of blood vessels, which causes a further rise in blood pressure.

The complexity of blood pressure regulation can only be hinted at, as the regulatory mechanisms are multiple, are hierarchically arranged, regulate each other, are distributed in space at different points in the circulation, and change in time. Figure 65-1 is a schematic representation of some of the circuits and components which regulate blood pressure.

The basic effector organs determining the blood pressure are the heart, both ventricles and atria, the blood vessels (including arteries, capillaries, and veins), and the blood. Their functional characteristics arise from their mechanical properties of elasticity, viscosity, their dimensions (area of lumen, thickness of wall, and length of the blood vessels and heart chambers), and volume of the blood. There are also basic time-related biologic characteristics of the heart, including rate, rhythm, contractility, and synchronization, which are regulated. Each of these components may be varied to produce a resultant blood pressure. Complex feedback loops regulate each organ, and whether any functional characteristic of any one of the organs acts to stabilize or disturb the system depends on the properties of the whole regulatory system as well as on the characteristics of the effector organ.

As illustrated in Fig. 65-1, neural and humoral

NEURAL CONTROL LOOPS ———— EFFECTOR ORGANS ———— HUMORAL CONTROL LOOPS
VIA BRAIN   VIA KIDNEY

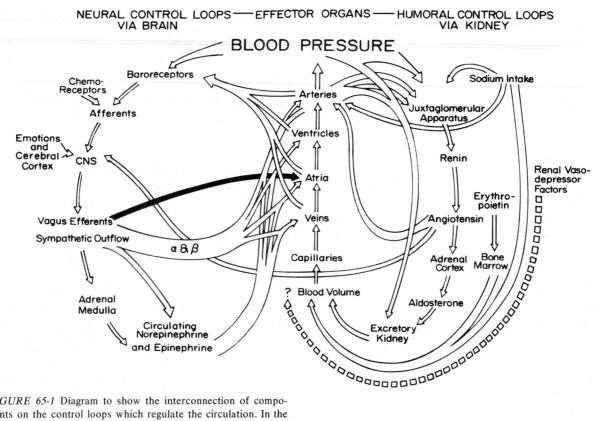

FIGURE 65-1 Diagram to show the interconnection of components on the control loops which regulate the circulation. In the central column are the effector units which impart or receive the energy carried by the blood flowing under pressure. At each side are the circuits which receive information on the state of the circulation based on the transmural pressure differential and the elastic and viscous properties of the vessel walls. This information is transformed and transmitted back to the effector units to regulate the blood pressure.

control loops regulate cardiovascular function in human beings. The neural loop comprises signals traversing the central and peripheral nervous systems. The humoral loop operates through the kidney, which acts as both an endocrine and excretory organ. Each loop may activate effector organs in series. The two loops are semi-independent, but may occasionally operate synergistically as manifest by the control of renal artery tone and innervation of the juxtaglomerular apparatus by sympathetic nerves or the effects of angiotensin on elements of the neural loop.

In the diagram no effort has been made to indicate the direction of blood pressure influence of each component. It is apparent that disturbance at some points will produce a widespread integrated response; at others, an isolated change. In either case these may be modulated by negative feedback or exacerbated by positive feedback. The major process of cardiac and vasomuscular *hypertrophy* is a positive feedback of major importance which could not be included in the diagram. It potentiates cardiovascular response to stimulus by strengthening the effector organ. Another change operating as a positive

feedback is the resetting of the sensitivity of the pressoreceptors after a new level of pressure has been established even over a period of days. When an elevated pressure has been maintained for a few days, the pressoreceptors adapt to preserve it there.

Insufficient information is available to state with certainty the role of each component in each clinical and experimental form of hypertension. A definite state of operation must be assignable to each component, however, and only when these are known will hypertension be comprehensible. A highly plausible analog model of the circulation using specific transfer functions to represent each component of the circulatory loop has been proposed by Guyton and coworkers.[12] An important component in this system is the concept of long-term autoregulation of tissue blood flow, which may in part manifest itself anatomically as the vascular hypertrophy referred to above. Thus, hypertension initially resulting from increased cardiac output and/or blood volume can become converted to hypertension associated with high peripheral resistance and normal cardiac output.

Sophisticated systems analysis of the circulation supported by extensive theoretic and empiric investigation led Guyton to propose that the single function in the entire circulation which *has* to be disturbed in order for hypertension to exist is the volume-regulating performance of the kidney as a function of the systemic arterial pressure. Because this variable operates and is integrated continuously over time, it has infinite feedback gain. This means that regardless of the cause of elevated pressure extended beyond the duration of a few minutes, the kidney will react to modulate the blood pressure rise unless its blood supply or excretory function is compromised. This hypothesis implies then that the cardiac output and peripheral resistance can assume any combination of values that may be calculated to produce a normal blood pressure provided the urinary output of sodium bears a normal relationship to systemic pressure. If the peripheral resistance is raised for the body as a whole but not for the kidney, the kidney will reduce cardiac output proportionately by excreting sodium and reducing blood volume. The lack of overt natriuresis in most patients with clinical hypertension implies a defect in this regulatory feedback. Conversely, if the blood pressure is reduced by a fall of peripheral resistance while the kidney maintains normal function (as with the creation of an arteriovenous fistula), the blood volume and cardiac output will increase to restore pressure toward normal.

The significance of this concept for the pathogenesis and etiology of hypertension cannot be overemphasized. In all forms of hypertension it becomes appropriate to examine the function of the kidney, and in therapy it supports the often-stated concept that the control of sodium balance by diet and diuretic therapy is the cornerstone of the initial management of hypertension. Whether by intrinsic renal disease or from metabolic, hormonal, or neural influences originating elsewhere in the body, the kidney must operate on an abnormal pressure-excretion function curve for hypertension to persist.[13]

A number of corollaries derive from the recognition of blood pressure as a complexly regulated variable: (1) Abnormal function of a portion of the circulatory system need not manifest itself in an abnormal blood pressure. For example, elevation of catecholamines, aldosterone, or renin need not necessarily change cardiac output, peripheral resistance, or blood pressure. (2) Elevation of the blood pressure always means that some regulatory or effector mechanisms have been driven to function outside their physiologic range. Physiologic indicators, such as the cardiac output, the peripheral resistance, or the blood volume, must be abnormal. (3) Simultaneous abnormalities may compensate for or reinforce each other. Slow progression of high blood pressure may result from gradual loss of negative feedback or from gradual progression of an initial abnormality. (4) If any of the feedback mechanisms become positive, i.e., tend to increase rather than minimize a change of pressure, then an unstable system results, with progressively rising blood pressure. This occurs in accelerated and malignant hypertension.

We will now examine individual components of the control loops. The major areas to be considered are (1) neural, (2) renal, (3) endocrine and metabolic, and (4) cardiovascular.

NEURAL FACTORS

Neural causes of hypertension may be conceived of at every point in the reflex arcs which regulate the blood vessels.[14,15] Decreased sensitivity of stretch receptors, interruption of the parasympathetic out-

flow, or stimulation of sympathetic outflow can all theoretically and experimentally lead to an integrated response, increasing cardiac output and vasomotor tone. The effect of chronic carotid sinus nerve stimulation in reducing the blood pressure of hypertensive human beings demonstrates in reverse the potential of inactivation of sinus impulses either peripherally or centrally in producing hypertension.[16]

Neurologic influences on blood pressure such as those arising from the carotid sinus may recruit hormonal and excretory mechanisms and modify renal handling of water and sodium as is evident from the vagus nerve afferent pathways which modulate antidiuretic hormone output and the stimulus to renin secretion via the β-adrenergic innervation of the kidney. Direct intracranial stimuli in focal areas, from generalized increase of intracranial pressure, or from intrathecal injection of vasodilators have also been found to produce a rise in blood pressure. Blood pressure regulation is frequently disrupted during acute cerebrovascular events, leading to either hypertensive crisis or shock. There is no evidence that pathologic central nervous system lesions cause essential hypertension or any large number of cases of hypertension. Sandok and Whisnant have provided a review of the brain and hypertension.[17]

A large body of data indicates that psychologic and emotional stimuli of various sorts can produce elevation in blood pressure.[18–20] The pattern of hypertension thus induced has not been fully described. Recent experiments in operant conditioning of primates[21] and in biofeedback[22,23] in human beings have suggested that psychologic factors can indeed chronically alter blood pressure.

Brod et al. have studied carefully a group of hypertensive human beings and a group of normal individuals under experimental emotional stress.[24] He found in both a pattern of hypertension with either increased total peripheral resistance or increased cardiac output or both. Both groups showed increased vascular resistance in kidney and skin but vasodilatation and increased flow in muscular vascular beds. The similarity of this pattern of flow to that seen in muscular exercise (or the emotional preparation for it) has led to consideration of essential hypertension as a psychogenically induced response to stress. Neurologically this can be imagined as introduced by cortical or reflex inhibition of the depressor relay stations in the brain or by direct stimulation of the sympathetic centers, including the vasodilator centers described by Uvnäs.[25]

The power of isometric muscle contraction to raise the arterial pressure has recently received attention.[26] The graded rise of pressure with graded contractile effort on the part of isolated muscles might well reflect central nervous system (CNS) stimulation of the blood pressure. The mechanism of this phenomenon remains obscure. It is brought about by increased cardiac output of undiscovered destination in normotensive individuals or by increased peripheral resistance in some who are hypertensive.[27] Of note is that the pressor response to handgrip persists despite control of blood pressure with thiazide, hydralazine, reserpine, or guanethidine.[28]

In some cases of labile hypertension[29] and in the syndrome of the hyperdynamic circulation,[30] elevated cardiac output attributable to β-adrenergic overactivity has been shown to account for all or a portion of the hypertension, but in some, excess α-adrenergic activity and depressed parasympathetic tone contribute.[31] The pattern of autonomic activity in mild human hypertension has been carefully studied and suggests augmented integrated CNS activation of vasopressor mechanisms. These CNS-mediated mechanisms include α- and β-adrenergic stimulation, renin release, and parasympathetic vasodepressor inhibition.[32]

Of great interest in support of the presence of a neurogenic component in renovascular hypertension are the effectiveness of sympathetic blocking agents in reducing renin secretion and in lowering blood pressure, the drop to control-animal pressures after pithing in renal-hypertensive rats and dogs,[33] and the resetting of the carotid sinus to regulate pressure at the new high level in chronic hypertension of both renal and unknown origin.[34] Destruction or severe depression of the nervous system will usually reduce elevated blood pressure of whatever origin, and this is accomplished without the peripheral ischemia which would be anticipated if the total effect were from depression of cardiac output. This does not necessarily imply that the neural pressor outflow to the circulation is greater than normal in hypertension. It may well mean only that the circulatory effector organs are responding more vigorously to a normal level of stimulation.[35] Under these conditions, reduction of nervous outflow below normal would still have the effect of depressing blood pressure.

A generalized participation of the sympathetic nervous system in the generation and maintenance of hypertension could result from increased effectiveness of a normal or even reduced sympathetic outflow by several mechanisms. The recently analyzed complex physiology of the sympathetic nerve endings and vascular receptors has been summarized by Carlsson.[36] Sympathetic tone may be influenced by rate of catecholamine synthesis, the activity of dopamine-β-hydroxylase in converting dopamine to norepinephrine,[37] the capacity of storage sites, the avidity of neuron membrane uptake systems, and the relative rates of catabolism by monamine oxidase and phenylethanolamine-N-methyltransferase. It has also recently been shown that norepinephrine released from peripheral neurons has almost exclusively a vasoconstrictor effect through the alpha receptors, but that circulating norepinephrine has some vasodilator component through beta receptors.[38] Dopamine, the precursor of norepinephrine, also appears to have both vasoconstrictor and vasodilator effects on blood vessels.[39]

Recent research on the vascular effects of the ubiquitous prostaglandins demonstrates that wherever sympathetic discharge occurs there is a variable counterbalancing action of vasodilator lipids. This modulates the intensity of sympathetic response according to the needs of the tissues. Both a direct vasodilator action and an inhibition of catecholamine release give these substances the power to suppress locally the response to sympathetic stimulation. The cumulative effect of these local vasodilator or anti-vasoconstrictor forces is to reduce what it would be without them when there is a state of augmented sympathetic tone. Blockade of prostaglandin synthesis by drugs such as indomethacin, aspirin, or meclofenamate may cause variable elevation of the blood pressure, depending on the level of adrenergic outflow.[40]

Two mechanisms have been demonstrated to relate sympathetic activity to metabolic and humoral variables. In experimental DOCA–salt-load hypertension in rats there is evidence that storage capacity for exogenous and endogenous catecholamines is reduced.[41] A similar change, but to a lesser degree, was seen with DOCA and salt loading separately. The effect of this change would be delivery of a greater fraction of endogenous norepinephrine to vascular and cardiac receptor sites. If confirmed, this would provide a powerful link between the humoral and neural control loops.

Another link between the two control loops has been demonstrated in the potentiation of vasoconstrictor response to the catecholamine-releasing substances like tyramine in animals treated with sub-pressor doses of angiotensin.[42] With the chronic administration of doses of angiotensin which were originally subpressor, labile and then fixed hypertension of severe degree developed. It is possible that these two new phenomena are related, since angiotensin leads to aldosterone secretion and sodium retention.

RENAL FACTORS

A second major integrative system regulating the blood pressure arises in the kidney. Goldblatt et al.[43] in 1934 demonstrated that constriction of the renal arteries would consistently produce hypertension. Later work by Kohlstaedt, Helmer, and Page[44] and by Braun-Menendez and his colleagues[45] demonstrated that there is a protein called *renin* released from the kidney and a protein substrate which together produce a nonprotein pressor substance in plasma which causes the hypertension.[46] The name *angiotensin* was agreed upon for the peptide, and it was subsequently characterized and synthesized. The exact mechanism and conditions of renin release and the loci of action of angiotensin are still under investigation. Some of the conditions of release are noted in the discussion of the juxtaglomerular apparatus. The renin-angiotensin system is thought to act by three routes: by direct vasoconstriction, by sodium retention and expansion of plasma volume via stimulation of aldosterone secretion,[47] and by increasing the effect of sympathetic stimulation[48] or by direct stimulation of the sympathetic nervous system.[49]

The demonstration by Edelman and Hartroft with fluorescent antibodies[50] and by Bing and Kazimierczak with microseparation techniques[51] that renin is found in or near the juxtaglomerular apparatus and that hypergranulation of these cells generally correlates with chronic conditions releasing angiotensin[52] provides a histologic technique for estimating renin secretion. These and other techniques indicate that renin release and local angiotensin formation occur predominantly in the renal cortex. Conditions causing high kidney perfusion pressure or increased body sodium stores suppress juxtaglomerular apparatus hypergranularity. Conversely, low kidney perfusion pressures, contracted blood volume, and decreased body sodium stores stimulate renin secretion.

In chronic experimental renovascular hypertension, after the initial rise of circulating renin the peripheral blood level gradually falls and may fall to the normal range.[53] The hypertension persists. It may at this point be cured by relief of vascular stenosis or in dogs by the administration of antirenin.[54] This course of events is quite compatible with the operation of a feedback, negative with respect to renin release, positive with respect to hypertension. Possible mechanisms are through stimulation of aldosterone and sodium retention, or the sympathetic nervous system. This would explain why a fall in cardiac output is the first hemodynamic event when renal ischemia is relieved.[55] The model of Guyton predicts this on the basis of long-term autoregulation.[12]

In humans the continued excessive release of renin can be demonstrated in renal vein blood from the ischemic kidney in unilateral renal artery stenosis,[56] and, in 50 to 75 percent of cases, in the peripheral vein blood.[57] A good kidney on the opposite side will reduce the tendency to hypertension by inhibition of its own renin release and accelerated excretion of sodium. However, renin release continues from the ischemic kidney. On the other hand, with bilateral involvement of the kidneys, the hypertension may be more severe and renin release may ultimately be suppressed, as when an experimental rat with one ischemic kidney is nephrectomized on the opposite side. The dynamic interplay of such feedback loops has not been experimentally clarified in disease states in human beings. It should be apparent, however, that failure to show markedly elevated blood renin levels does not rule out excessive renin release as a possible initial and continuing cause of hypertension. When malignant arteriolonecrosis develops, even the retention of salt and water and the extremely high pressures may be insufficient to suppress renin levels in certain patients.

The mechanism of the link between renin and stimulation of the sympathetic nervous system appears to be a complex one. Perfusion of the caudal half of the medulla of the brain with low concentrations of angiotensin II leads to suppression of the cardioinhibitory outflow along the vagus.[49] McCubbin and Page have shown a peripheral potentiation of sympathetic activity.[48] Although infusion of angiotensin does not increase the pressor response to infusion of norepinephrine, it does increase the response to maneuvers that stimulate the release of endogenous norepinephrine. The responses to injected tyramine and a sympathetic ganglion-stimulating agent (dimethylphenyl-piperazinium iodide, DMPP) are enhanced. This may account for evidence of increased sympathetic activity in high renin hypertension and prevent a fully effective negative-feedback response on the part of the nervous system.

The sometime therapeutic practices of bilateral nephrectomy and transplantation of kidneys, made possible by the recent development of maintenance hemodialysis, have thrown additional light on the role of the kidney in hypertension. It has been shown that in the majority of renal failure patients with hypertension, bilateral nephrectomy results in a fall in blood pressure at comparable levels of hematocrit and volume load even when the preoperative circulating renin levels are not elevated. There is good evidence that, in the patient with end-stage renal disease, renin levels are higher than would be predicted from the exchangeable sodium and intravascular volume[58] and also that, in those patients with hypertension, the blood pressure and total peripheral resistance are proportional to the exchangeable sodium and intravascular volume. There is a possibility, then, that even low levels of renin from scarred and shrunken end-stage kidneys can have a multiplier effect via expanded volume and volume-sensitive vessels or via the autonomic nervous system to produce severe hypertension in patients with renal failure.[59]

In addition to the well-documented and well-characterized mechanism of the renal pressor system, renal depressor systems have been discovered. Renoprival hypertension was demonstrated in the nephrectomized dog by Grollman and his colleagues.[60] He found it to be aggravated by salt and protein in the diet of the totally nephrectomized dog sustained by chronic dialysis. Ureterocaval anastomosis, producing an "endocrine kidney," showed that protection against hypertension was not related to external excretion of urine. The fall in pressure in the experimental renal hypertensive rats of Wilson when their clipped kidneys were repaired occurred only when a functioning, though not necessarily an excreting, kidney was preserved.[61] This suggests that renal inactivation of some extrarenal hypertensive factor or the release of a substance acting to reduce vasomotor tone may well play a role in keeping blood pressure down. Muirhead and his colleagues showed that the major antihypertensive action was derived from the medulla rather than from the cortex of the dog kidney.[62]

Three antihypertensive substances have recently been extracted from the kidney. The vasodilator prostaglandins,[63] a small neutral antihypertensive lipid,[64] and a phospholipid renin inhibitor[65] are all of possible significance in blood pressure control.

Prostaglandin E, which is found in high concentration in the renal medulla, not only is a powerful local vasodilator, reducing intrarenal resistance, but it is a powerful stimulant of renal sodium excretion. Thus by its vasomotor as well as its volume effect this lipid hormone may be a significant determinant of blood pressure.[66] Primary excess of assayed prostaglandin A, probably reflecting prostaglandin E, leads to interesting metabolic consequences; hypotension, sodium and potassium wasting, secondary hyperreninemia, and secondary hyperaldosteronism known as *Bartter's syndrome*.[67] Whether the opposite of this picture which would represent low renin hypertension ever results from insufficient prostaglandin E remains to be seen. Lee[68] has demonstrated reduced plasma levels of prostaglandin A_2 in patients with essential hypertension as contrasted with normotensive controls.

As has been pointed out by Guyton, the capacity of the kidney to excrete sodium and water at any given pressure is a critical determinant of the blood pressure because its rate is integrated continuously. There is increasing evidence that in many, if not all, forms of hypertension an excretory defect is involved. In renal disease it may be an anatomic defect from nephron destruction; in essential hypertension it may be physiologic from vascular constriction[69] or from biochemically augmented sodium reabsorption or, as a genetic factor, in the inheritance of small kidneys.

ENDOCRINE AND METABOLIC FACTORS

The relationship of endocrine and metabolic factors to hypertension is complex. Humoral agents from the kidney fall in this category and have been considered. Specific agents from the adrenal glands will now be discussed.

Adrenal hormones

The adrenal medullary hormones, norepinephrine and epinephrine, are causes of hypertension in pheochromocytoma. Interesting aspects of this type of hypertension are the apparent compensations made by the body which give certain unique characteristics to the physiology of pheochromocytoma. In contrast to patients with essential hypertension, patients with pheochromocytoma often have a fall in blood pressure in changing from a lying to a standing position. This may indicate suppression of the carotid and similar regulatory reflexes, or the usually associated reduction of blood volume and extracellular fluid volume. Volume depletion is further evidenced by urgent necessity of expanding blood volume to prevent shock after removal of a pheochromocytoma.[70]

Experimental data from the authors' laboratory indicate that prolonged infusion of norepinephrine induces, after transient sodium retention, a negative sodium balance and positive potassium balance compatible with suppression of aldosterone secretion.[71] These evidences of compensation suggest that negative-feedback loops are at work protecting the body from the malfunction of a single mechanism.

Oversecretion of aldosterone is a second adrenal cause of hypertension. Hypertension is a frequent concomitant of primary hyperaldosteronism.[72] The mechanism of the effect of this hormone on the blood pressure is not clearly understood. It most resembles the effect of massive sodium loading, producing an increase in extracellular volume, blood volume, and intracellular and vascular sodium content. It may have a positive inotropic action on the heart. Reduction of storage sites for norepinephrine, as described earlier in discussing DOCA hypertension, would predispose to hypertension.[41] A pressor response to ganglionic blockade in patients with primary aldosteronism is evidence that neural mechanisms above the terminal neuron are acting in a protective manner. The observation of Conn that peripheral blood renin activity is suppressed and nonstimulable in patients with aldosterone-secreting tumors is another example of the functioning of the negative feedback to minimize the rise of blood pressure.[72]

Analysis in depth of the syndrome of "primary aldosteronism" over the years reveals a family of disturbances related in ways not yet elucidated.[73] In addition to the single autonomous secreting adenoma surrounded by atrophied gland, macro- or micronodular hyperplasia of both glands or normal-appearing glands may produce the syndrome. Some glands autonomously secrete excessive amounts of mineralocorticoid. In others hypersecretion is suppressible by the administration of deoxycorticosterone and in still others by glucocorticoids. Investigations to date make it clear that ACTH provides the major stimulus for steroidal precursor production. Moreover, overstimulation of specific aldosterone production may result from either angiotensin or chronic elevations of serum potassium. Enzymatic deficiencies such as 11-β-hydroxylation or 17-α-hydroxylation also result in oversecretion of hypertensogenic corticosteroids. In addition to all of these mechanisms, we are forced to the conclusion that adrenal zona glomerulosa hypersecretion with secondary renin suppression can result from the trophic effect of additional stimuli as yet unidentified.

Recent investigation of factors modulating secretion of aldosterone has thrown some additional light on its control by factors other than ACTH and renin-generated angiotensin. Sodium depletion in nephrectomized animals and human beings,[74,75] elevation of serum potassium concentration,[76,77] the angiotensin heptapeptide,[78] and possibly a non-ACTH pituitary factor[79] have been reported or implied to stimulate aldosterone secretion. Serum potassium concentration, at least, appears to be a factor operating in the physiologic range.

The associated clinical features of Cushing's syndrome, of the adrenogenital syndrome, or of hypogonadism in conjunction with hypertension lead to the detailed analysis of adrenal function necessary to establish the respective diagnoses.

Critical to the understanding of the mechanism of hypertension is information on the levels of aldosterone and renin activity in the various types of the disease. There is little doubt that in malignant hypertension they are elevated, providing a positive feedback.[80] This may constitute the critical difference between benign and malignant hypertension. There has been long debate as to whether aldosterone secretion is elevated or not in benign essential hypertension. The difficulty is due in part to the many factors of diet that affect aldosterone secretion and in part to the difficulty of the measurement. The problem is made worse by the lack of definite criteria for differentiation between renal and essential hypertension and for diagnosis of the malignant phase of the disease.

The gradual accumulation of data, gathered under meticulously controlled circumstances, has begun to throw new light upon the interplay of renin and aldosterone in the catchall category of benign essential hypertension. From the work of Laragh and his colleagues over the years, we now have the patterns and confidence limits of aldosterone secretion as a function of sodium intake for normal individuals and for a considerable number of individuals with various types of hypertension.[80] It is clear that a number of patients with essential hypertension secrete less than normal amounts of aldosterone and/or renin, but there are others who secrete more. In addition to this, these groups may have different natural histories of their disease and different responses to drugs. All this provides strong support to the concept stated earlier that important new major subsets of essential hypertension are on the verge of being discovered and that their discrimination etiologically and physiologically will add much to the precision of pharmacologic management.

In the search for an explanation of "low renin" hypertension in which aldosterone secretion is not elevated but which responds well to spironolactone therapy, an intense investigation has been undertaken of hormonal analogues which might act physiologically like aldosterone. Melby et al. have identified one subset of patients with excessive production of 18-hydroxydeoxycorticosterone (18-OHDOC).[81] Another compound with mineralocorticoid activity, found in the urine of hypertensive, low renin patients, has been identified as 16-β-hydroxyde-hydroepiandrosterone.[82] Efforts are currently under way to ascertain whether this hormone plays a role in low renin hypertension.

The preponderance of evidence at present would suggest that the acceleration of the course of hypertensive disease in "malignant hypertension" is most readily accounted for by the breakdown of protective negative-feedback loops that delay the progression and reduce the severity of benign hypertension. Indeed, the recruitment of positive feedback seems to intervene so that the course is accelerated. The most common pattern seen is the development of renal microvascular disease, elevated renin secretion, stimulated aldosterone secretion, renal conservation of sodium and water from both vascular disease and hormonal influences, and thence dramatic exacerbation of the hypertension and secondary end-organ damage. Not every step in this sequence occurs simultaneously, and cases are reported in which one or another system component may be either normal or seemingly inappropriate. The essential characteristic of malignant hypertension, however, is the conversion of negative to positive feedback in the circulation as a whole.

Sodium

The role of the external balance of sodium in hypertension has received much consideration. Dahl and Love[83] have emphasized the hypertensinogenic potentialities of sodium in rats and man. Dahl[84] selected and bred two strains of rats, one of which develops hypertension on high sodium intake and one of which does not. Widespread clinical and experimental experience from the work of Kempner[85] and Grollman and Harrison[86] documents that in the hypertensive patient sodium intake is a major determinant of blood pressure. In a person predisposed to hypertension, a high sodium intake will induce clinical manifestations earlier and in more severe degrees. Conversely, systemic hypertension is extremely rare in patients with Addison's disease. This rarity is believed to be in part due to the reduced body stores of sodium.

A number of epidemiologic studies of populations have endeavored to detect a correlation between blood pressure and sodium intake.[87] In general, a positive correlation has been found, but the difficulties in estimating sodium intake for large groups are formidable, and many discrepancies in the correlation have been disclosed. These may well be due to other environmental or psychosocial circumstances or to group differences in the excretion of sodium loads.

Little evidence is available on differences in a person's ability to handle a sodium load. There is little question that if disease states are included, the sodium titration curve, i.e., the total body sodium content required to excrete a given daily intake of sodium, varies widely in individuals. Preliminary studies in the author's laboratory indicate that the weight which must be reached at steady state to excrete increasing sodium intake follows a sigmoid curve (Fig. 65-2). Variations in the slope and intercept of this curve in a large number of individuals have not been evaluated, and genetic and racial differences of this sort have not been explored in human beings. Variations in the excretion of sodium, as well as variations in intake, may well be a significant determinant of hypertension in individuals and in groups. A report by Helmer and Judson[88] suggests a marked tendency toward sodium retention in a small group of Negroes compared with whites with hypertension and low peripheral renin activity. It has also been shown that the genetic predisposition to sodium-induced hypertension in inbred strains of rats is due to the presence or absence of several renal factors which are not operative in hypertension-resistant animals.[89]

The mechanism of the effect of sodium on blood pressure is obscure. In hypertension, restriction of sodium intake and diuretics which induce negative sodium balance cause contraction of plasma volume

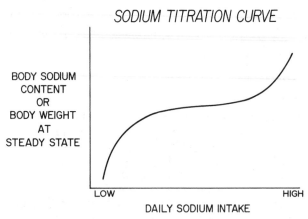

FIGURE 65-2 A curve representing the concept of a sodium titration curve in the intact organism, derived from preliminary studies in man. The slope and level of this curve vary markedly among individuals and between health and disease. The characteristics of the curve depend on the integrated function of heart, vessels, kidneys, endocrine glands, and metabolic factors such as carbohydrate intake. It has not been studied in the various types of hypertension.

transiently, but even after restoration of plasma volume[90] the pressure remains down. An effect of sodium depletion in increasing storage of norepinephrine has been reported in rats.[91] This could account for part of the blood pressure-reducing effect of sodium depletion. The mean plasma volume of groups of untreated patients with essential hypertension is reduced, particularly with diastolic blood pressure above 105 mm Hg.[92] This finding argues against primary salt loading as a cause of hypertension and, again, may represent a protective feedback. It must be emphasized, however, that studies of racial and genetic differences in this regard are generally lacking in human beings. When sodium balance does become positive, as in the malignant phase, the hypertension becomes more severe. Note has been taken of the fact that in hypertension, blood vessels have increased sodium and water content.[93] An increase in vascular stiffness is also found.[94] It is not clear whether the increased content of sodium and water is a cause or an effect of the increased stiffness of the vessel walls. The hypothesis that body sodium content influences the reactivity of cardiovascular muscle to neural or humoral stimuli on the basis of a dimensional or a biochemical change has been frequently advanced. This has been difficult to support with quantitative data which cannot be otherwise explained, but there appears to be an effect of sodium on blood pressure greater than can be exclusively attributed to changes in blood volume already present.

The role of sodium in hypertension is that in any condition in which circulatory regulation is impaired, whether from hypertension or from autonomic insufficiency, blood pressure is inordinately sensitive to changes in blood volume, varies directly with body sodium content, and varies more widely than in a person with normal feedback. Overload of sodium may cause hypertension in persons with very heavy intake, with impaired sodium-handling mechanisms, or with impaired circulatory regulation.

Ions other than sodium also participate in blood pressure regulation.[95] As examples, Overbeck et al.[96] have demonstrated a blunted vasodilator effect of potassium in hypertensive men, and Haddy et al.[97] have shown a direct vasoconstrictive effect of calcium on arteriolar tone.

Catabolism of pressor substances

Derangement of the metabolism of catecholamines has been considered possibly to account for essential hypertension.[98] Evidence suggesting the delayed breakdown of norepinephrine has not been widely accepted.[99] From the control mechanism standpoint, one would postulate that failure to destroy norepinephrine, for instance, would suppress its secretion, but much depends on the site of catabolism.

Angiotensin is rapidly destroyed in normal plasma. Evidence for delay in its destruction or sensitivity to lower levels in some people has been presented by Wood.[100] Individuals showing this trait in a nonhypertensive state have relatives with significantly more hypertension than controls.

Other studies on the inactivation of angiotensin by human hypertensive plasma in bioassay in the rat show differences in the rate of inactivation in various types of hypertension.[101] Marked differences in the blood pressure response to injected angiotensin have also been found in various types of hypertension.[102] Studies of this type are still in too early a phase to fit any clear-cut pattern, but certainly from data currently available it is clear that there are marked differences in the reactivity to and degradation of angiotensin in various forms of hypertension. In general, when blood levels are high, so are the levels of catabolic enzymes or angiotensinases.

CARDIOVASCULAR FACTORS

Characteristics of the cardiovascular system itself, rather than disturbances originating in external control organs, may cause hypertension. The cardiovascular system is the effector organ and the source of information which provides the basis of blood pressure regulation. Strain or stretch of the blood vessel wall is detected by neural stretch receptors. This is the major type of information on which short-term regulation of the blood pressure is based.

The stretch or strain of the arterial wall has been studied in detail by Peterson.[103] It is the result of the transmural pressure differential, roughly equaling the blood pressure at that point, and of the dimensions and viscoelastic properties of the vessel wall. Thus if a vessel becomes hypertrophied and resistant to stretch or if it actively participates in contraction as blood pressure rises, there may be little added stretch to signal that rise in blood pressure has taken place. It has been shown that application of norepinephrine to the wall of the carotid sinus will cause it to constrict in a manner which will cause reflex changes in blood pressure.[104] It has been stated by Peterson that in normal anesthetized dogs the carotid sinus is the most distensible portion of the arterial tree. Whether this is true in hypertensive individuals has not been clearly ascertained. If in vasoconstriction many receptor sites constrict as effectors in a manner to prevent stretch under the higher pressure, then the negative-feedback loop will not be adequately activated. It has indeed been shown that by some mechanism the carotid sinus mechanism does become adapted in hypertensive persons so that it begins to regulate blood pressure about a new higher level.

The cardiovascular system is also the *effector* which generates the blood pressure via anatomic and metabolic properties of the heart and blood vessels. The force and rate of myocardial contraction and the mechanical properties of the vessel walls are final determinants of the blood pressure. If the effector organs hypertrophy, they may execute more work with the same neural or hormonal stimulus. Like the muscles of the athlete in training, the myocardium and peripheral vascular muscles undergoing progressive hypertrophy are capable of doing more work, raising the blood pressure even higher, though the stimulus remains the same.

A combination of increased resistance of receptor sites to stretch and increased strength of effector organ contraction in response to a given stimulus would provide the positive feedback to make hypertension a progressive disease. This combination is provided by the muscular hypertrophy of heart and blood vessels. This does not account for the original elevation of blood pressure but may well explain the observation that in the population as a whole, it is those whose blood pressure is originally high in whom progressively rising pressure develops with age.[105]

Many observations support the concept that in spite of the hypertrophy of blood vessels in hypertension, the lumen is not irrevocably diminished but that continued stimulation is required to sustain the increased peripheral resistance. A modest reduction of lumen/wall thickness ratio even under conditions of maximal reflex (thermal) dilatation has been demonstrated by Folkow[35] and Sivertsson.[106] Of greater importance is their demonstration of the augmented responsiveness of these hypertrophied resistance vessels to many different neural and humoral stimuli. The rapid relief of correctable forms of hypertension frequently seen, even after long duration, when the cause (pheochromocytoma, coarctation of the aorta, or renal artery stenosis) is relieved; the response of the experimental animal to pithing; and the marked drop in pressure to hypotensive levels occasionally seen with parenteral sympathetic blocking agents all support the concept that in benign essential hypertension the vascular caliber is not irreversibly reduced. It can be postulated that in benign hypertension the increased peripheral resistance is attributable to hypertrophied vessels responding to stimulation and not to simple encroachment on the lumen by the thickened wall.

Increasing evidence is accumulating to support the concept that long-term autoregulation of tissue blood flow is a significant factor in converting high output hypertension to high resistance hypertension. In dogs and in anephric man studied on hemodialysis, sodium overload initially induces hypertension with high cardiac output, but as the load is maintained, peripheral resistance increases, and either pressure rises higher or the cardiac output is suppressed toward normal or subnormal levels. The long-term effects of diuretics as antihypertensives may produce an initial fall in cardiac output followed by a reduction of resistance to reduce blood pressure chronically. Thus, there is not only the process of arteriolar wall hypertrophy and arteriolar elongation but the reduction of cross-sectional area of the peripheral vascular bed to contribute to the elevated resistance seen in most forms of hypertension.

In summary, the blood pressure is a regulated complex variable with at least two identifiable control systems which are partially interlocked. Depending upon the point of pathologic disturbance, certain negative-feedback loops can counteract a force tending to elevate blood pressure. In most situations when elevation of blood pressure reaches a certain point, slow-moving positive feedback loops make it progressive. Ultimately, more powerful positive feedback may lead to an accelerated or malignant state.

The stimulus to hypertension may come from outside the control loops as from the cerebral cortex, chemoreceptors, or excessive sodium intake, or from within the control loops by change in activity of one or more components damaged by disease. The initial pathologic change of function need be only minimal and may be unmeasurable, but over a long period of time hypertrophy of heart and vessels allows greater responses to the same stimulus, so that the disease progresses. At a point, damage to renal vessels triggers the release of renal substances which rapidly lead to accelerated rise of pressure and decompensation of brain, heart, and kidneys.

Normalizing the blood pressure should halt the progression of the disease by interrupting positive feedback. The apparent cure of a few patients after long-term control of their blood pressure may be an illustration of the reversal of the changes which lead to the progression of hypertension.

REFERENCES

1 Laragh, J. H. (guest ed.): Symposium on Hypertension, *Am. J. Med.*, 60:733, 1976.

2 Cohn, J. N. (guest ed.): "Hypertension–1974, *Arch. Intern. Med.*, 133:911, 1974.

3 Sonnenblick, E. H. (ed.): Hypertension, Pressor Agents, and Cardiovascular Injury, I & II, *Prog. Cardiovasc. Dis.*, 17:1, 1974.

4 Onesti, G., Kim, K. E., and Moyer, J. H. (eds.): "Hypertension: Mechanisms and Management," Grune & Stratton, Inc., New York, 1973.

5 Pickering, G. W.: "Hypertension," 2d ed, Longman, Inc., New York, 1974.

6 Laragh, J. H. (ed.): "Hypertension Manual," Yorke Medical Books, New York, 1973.

7 Genest, J., and Koiw, E. (eds.): "Hypertension, 1972," Springer-Verlag OHG, Heidelberg, 1972.

8 Reader, R. (ed.): Hypertensive Mechanisms, *Circ. Res.,* vol. 27 (suppl. 2), 1970.

9 Cort, J. H., Fencl, V., Hejl, L., and Jirka, J. (eds.): "The Pathogenesis of Essential Hypertension," Proceedings of the Prague Symposium, 1960, The Macmillan Company, New York, 1962.

10 "Hypertension," Proceedings of the Council for High Blood Pressure Research, vols. I to XXIV, American Heart Association, New York, 1953–1976 [*Circ. Res.,* 11–40(suppl.), 1962–1977].

11 Peterson, L. H.: Systems Behavior, Feedback Loops, and High Blood Pressure Research, *Circ. Res.,* 12(pt. 2):585, 1963.

12 Guyton, A. C., Coleman, T. G., and Granger, H. J.: Circulation: Overall Regulation, *Ann. Rev. Physiol.,* 34:13, 1972.

13 Guyton, A. C., Coleman, T. G., Cowley, A. W., Jr., Scheel, K. W., Manning, R. D., Jr., and Norman, R. A., Jr.: Arterial Pressure Regulation: Overriding Dominance of the Kidneys in Long-term Regulation and in Hypertension, *Am J. Med.,* 52:584, 1972.

14 Kezdi, P. (ed.): "Baroreceptors and Hypertension," Pergamon Press, New York, 1967.

15 Julius, S., and Esler, M. D. (eds.): "The Nervous System in Hypertension," Charles C Thomas, Publisher, Springfield, Ill., 1976.

16 Brest, A. N., Wiener, L., and Bacharach, B.: Carotid Sinus Nerve Stimulation in the Treatment of Hypertension, in G. Onesti, K. E. Kim, and J. H. Moyer (eds.), "Hypertension: Mechanisms and Management," Grune & Stratton, Inc., New York, 1973.

17 Sandok, B. A., and Whisnant, J. P.: Hypertension and the Brain, *Arch. Intern. Med.,* 133:947, 1974.

18 Hall, W. D., and Gunnells, C.: National Conference on Emotional Stress and Heart Disease: Emotional Stress and Hypertension, *J.S.C. Med. Assoc. (suppl.)* 72:82, 1976.

19 Henry, J. P., and Cassel, J. C.: Psychosocial Factors in Essential Hypertension: Recent Epidemiologic and Animal Experimentation Evidence, *Am. J. Epidemiol.,* 90:171, 1969.

20 Simonson, E., and Brozek, J.: Russian Research on Arterial Hypertension, *Ann. Intern. Med.,* 50:129, 19.

21 Benson, H., Herd, J. A., Morse, W. H., and Kelleher, R. T.: Behavioral Induction of Arterial Hypertension and its Reversal, *Am. J. Physiol.,* 217:30, 1969.

22 Benson, H., Rosner, B. A., Marzetta, B. R., and Klemchuk, H. M.: Decreased Blood Pressure in Pharmacologically Treated Hypertensive Patients Who Regularly Elicited the Relaxation Response, *Lancet,* 1:289, 1974.

23 Kristt, D. A., and Engel, B. T.: Learned Control of Blood Pressure in Patients with High Blood Pressure, *Circulation,* 51:370, 1975.

24 Brod, J., Fencl, V., Hejl, Z., and Jirka, J.: Circulatory Changes Underlying Blood Pressure Elevation during Acute Emotional Stress (Mental Arithmetic) in Normotensive and Hypertensive Subjects, *Clin. Sci.,* 18:269, 1959.

25 Uvnäs, B.: Sympathetic Vasodilator Outflow, *Physiol. Rev.,* 34:608, 1954.

26 Donald, K. W., Lind, A. R., McNicol, G. W., Humphreys, P. W., Taylor, S. H., and Staunton, H. P.: Cardiovascular Responses to Sustained (Static) Contractions, *Circ. Res.,* 20 and 21(suppl. 1):15, 1967.

27 Tarazi, R. C., and Dustan, H. P.: Beta Adrenergic Blockade and Response to Static Exercise, *Clin Pharmacol. Ther.,* 12:303, 1971.

28 Lamid, S., and Wolff, F. W.: Drug Failure in Reducing Pressor Effects of Isometric Handgrip Stress Test in Hypertension, *Am. Heart J.,* 86:211, 1973.

29 Frohlich, E. D., Tarazi, R. C., and Dustan, H. P.: Re-examination of the Hemodynamics of Hypertension, *Am. J. Med. Sci.,* 257:9, 1969.

30 Frohlich, E. D., Tarazi, R. C., and Dustan, H. P.: Hyperdynamic Beta-adrenergic Circulatory State: Increased Beta Receptor Responsiveness, *Arch. Intern. Med.,* 123:1, 1969.

31 Julius, S., Pascual, A. V., Sannerstedt, R., and Mitchell, C.: Relationship Between Cardiac Output and Peripheral Resistance in Borderline Hypertension, *Circulation,* 43:382, 1971.

32 Julius, S., Esler, M. D., and Randall, O. S.: Role of the Autonomic Nervous System in Mild Human Hypertension, *Clin. Sci. Mol. Med.,* 48:243 s, 1975.

33 Taquini, A. C., Jr.: Neurogenic Control of Peripheral Resistance in Renal Hypertension, *Circ. Res.,* 12(pt. 2):562, 1963.

34 McCubbin, J. W., Green, J. H., and Page, I. H.: Baroreceptor Function in Chronic Renal Hypertension, *Circ. Res.,* 4:205, 1956.

35 Folkow, B.: The Hemodynamic Consequences of Adaptive Structural Changes of the Resistance Vessels in Hypertension, *Clin. Sci.,* 41:1, 1971.

36 Carlsson, A.: Pharmacology of the Sympathetic Nervous System, in F. Gross (ed.), "Antihypertensive Therapy," Springer-Verlag OHG, Berlin, 1966, p. 5.

37 Shanberg, S., Stone, R., Kirshner, N., Gunnels, J., and Robinson, R.: Plasma Dopamine-β-Hydroxylase: A Possible Aid in the Study and Evaluation of Hypertension, *Science,* 183:523, 1974.

38 Glick, G., Epstein, S. E., Wechsler, A. S., and Braunwald, E.: Physiological Differences between the Effects of Neuronally Released and Bloodborne Norepinephrine on Beta Adrenergic Receptors in the Arterial Bed of the Dog, *Circ. Res.,* 21:217, 1967.

39 Goldberg, L. I.: The Dopamine Vascular Receptor, *Biochem. Pharmacol.,* 24:651, 1975.

40 Vane, J. R., and McGiff, J. C.: Possible Contributions of Endogenous Prostaglandins in the Control of Blood Pressure, *Circ. Res.,* 36(suppl. 1):68, 1975.

41 Champlain, J. de, Krakoff, L. R., and Axelrod, J.: Catecholamine Metabolism in Experimental Hypertension in the Rat, *Circ. Res.,* 20:136, 1967.

42 McCubbin, J. W., Demoura, R. S., and Page, I. H.: Arterial Hypertension Elicited by Subpressor Amounts of Angiotensin, *Science,* 149:1394, 1965.

43 Goldblatt, H., Lynch, J., Nanzal, R. F., and Summerville, W. W.: Studies on Experimental Hypertension: I. Production of Persistent Elevation of Systolic Blood Pressure by Means of Renal Ischemia, *J. Exper. Med.,* 59:347, 1934.

44 Kohlstaedt, K. G., Helmer, O. M., and Page, I. H.: Activation of Renin by Blood Colloids, *Proc. Soc. Exp. Biol. Med.,* 39:214, 1938.

45 Braun-Menendez, E., Fasciolo, J. C., Leloir, L. F., and Munoz, J. M.: The Substance Causing Renal Hypertension, *J. Physiol.,* 98:283, 1940.

46 Braun-Menendez, E.: Pharmacology of Renin and Hypertension, *Pharmacol. Rev.,* 8:25, 1956.

47 Biron, P., Koiw, E., Nowaczynski, W., Brouillet, J., and Genest, J.: Effect of Intravenous Infusions of Valine-5-angiotensin II and Other Pressor Agents on Urinary Electrolytes and Corticosteroids, Including Aldosterone, *J. Clin. Invest.,* 40:338, 1961.

48 McCubbin, J. W., and Page, I. H.: Renal Pressor System and Neurogenic Control of Arterial Pressure, *Circ. Res.,* 12(pt. 2):553, 1963.

49 Joy, M. D., and Lowe, R. D.: The Site of Cardiovascular Action of Angiotensin II in the Brain, *Clin. Sci.,* 39:327, 1970.

50 Edelman, R., and Hartroft, P. M.: Localization of Renin in Juxtaglomerular Cells of Rabbit and Dog through the Use of Fluorescent-antibody Technique, *Circ. Res.*, 9:1069, 1961.

51 Bing, J., and Kazimierczak, J.: Renin Content of Different Parts of the Juxtagomerular Apparatus, *Acta Pathol. Microbiol. Scand.*, 54:80, 1962.

52 Hartroft, P. M.: Juxtaglomerular Cells, *Circ. Res.*, 12(pt. 2):525, 1963.

53 Miksche, L. W., Miksche, U., and Gross, F.: Effect of Sodium Restriction on Renal Hypertension and on Renin Activity in the Rat, *Circ. Res.*, 27:973, 1970.

54 Wakerlin, G. E.: Antibodies to Renin as Proof of the Pathogenesis of Sustained Renal Hypertension, *Circulation,* 17:653, 1958.

55 Ledingham, J. M., and Cohen, R. D.: Circulatory Changes during Reversal of Experimental Hypertension, *Clin. Sci.*, 22:69, 1962.

56 Judson, W. E., and Halmer, O. M.: Diagnostic and Prognostic Value of Renin Activity in Renal Venous Plasma in Renovascular Hypertension, *Hypertension,* 13:79, 1965.

57 Cohen, E. L., Rovner, D. R., and Conn, J. W.: Postural Augmentation of Plasma Renin Activity, *J.A.M.A.*, 197:973, 1966.

58 Weidman, P., Beretta-Piccoli, C., Steffen, F., Blumberg, A., and Reubi, F. C.: Hypertension in Terminal Renal Failure, *Kidney Int.*, 9:294, 1976.

59 Onesti, G., Kim, K. E., Greco, J. A., del Guercio, E. T., Fernandes, M., and Swartz, C.: Blood Pressure Regulation in End-Stage Renal Disease and Anephric Man, *Circ. Res.*, 36(suppl. 1):148, 1975.

60 Grollman, A., Muirhead, E. E., and Vanatta, J.: Role of the Kidney in Pathogenesis of Hypertension as Determined by a Study of the Effects of Bilateral Nephrectomy and Other Experimental Procedures on the Blood Pressure of the Dog, *Am. J. Physiol.*, 157:21, 1959.

61 Wilson, C.: The Kidney and Essential Hypertension, in K. D. Bock and P. T. Cottier (eds.), "Essential Hypertension," Springer-Verlag OHG, Berlin, 1960, p. 405.

62 Muirhead, E. E., Brown, G. B., Germain, G. S., and Leach, B. E.: The Renal Medulla as an Antihypertensive Organ, *J. Lab. Clin. Med.*, 76:641, 1970.

63 Bergstrom, S., Carlson, L. A., and Weeks, J. R.: The Prostaglandins: A Family of Biologically Active Lipids, *Pharmacol. Rev.*, 20:1, 1968.

64 Muirhead, E. E., Brooks, B., Kosinski, M., Daniels, E. G., and Hinman, J. W.: Renomedullary Antihypertensive Principle in Renal Hypertension, *J. Lab. Clin. Med.*, 67:778, 1967.

65 Smeby, R. R., Sen, S., and Bumpus, F. M.: A Naturally Occurring Renin Inhibitor, *Circ. Res.*, 21(suppl. 2):129, 1967.

66 McGiff, J. C., Terragno, N. A., and Itskovitz, A. D.: Role of Renal Prostaglandins as Revealed by Inhibition of Prostaglandin Synthetase, in J. H. Robinson and J. R. Vane (eds.), "Prostaglandin Synthesis Inhibitors," Raven Press, New York, 1974, p. 259.

67 Fichman, M. P., Talfer, N., Zia, P., Speckart, P., Golub, M., and Rude, R.: Role of Prostaglandins in the Pathogenesis of Bartter's Syndrome, *Am. J. Med.*, 60:785, 1976.

68 Lee, J. B.: Cardiovascular-renal Effects of Prostaglandins: The Antihypertensive, Natriuretic Renal "Endocrine" Functions, *Arch. Intern. Med.*, 133:56, 1974.

69 Hollenberg, N. K., and Adams, D. R.: The Renal Circulation in Hypertensive Disease, *Am. J. Med.*, 60:773, 1976.

70 Brunjes, S., Johns, V. J., and Crane, M. G.: Pheochromocytoma: Post Operative Shock and Blood Volume, *N. Engl. J. Med.*, 262:393, 1960.

71 Tuttle, E. P., Jr.: Saluresis and Potassium Retention Induced by Pressor Amines, *Clin. Res.*, 8:89, 1960 (abstract).

72 Conn, J. W.: Aldosteronism and Hypertension: Primary Aldosteronism versus Hypertensive Disease with Secondary Aldosteronism, *Arch. Intern. Med.*, 107:813, 1961.

73 Biglieri, E. G., Stockight, J. R., and Schambelan, M.: Adrenal Mineralocorticoids Causing Hypertension, *Am. J. Med.*, 52:623, 1972.

74 Read, V. H., McCaa, C. S., Bower, J. D., and McCaa, R. E.: Effect of Hemodialysis on the Metabolic Clearance Rate of Aldosterone in Anephric Man, *J. Clin. Endocrinol. Metab.*, 36:773, 1973.

75 McCaa, R. E., Bower, J. D., and McCaa, C. S.: Relative Influence of Acute Sodium and Volume Depletion on Aldosterone Secretion in Nephrectomized Man, *Circ. Res.*, 33:555, 1973.

76 Laragh, J. H., and Stoerk, A. C.: A Study of the Mechanism of Secretion of the Sodium-Retaining Hormone (Aldosterone), *J. Clin. Invest.*, 36:383, 1957.

77 McCaa, R. E., Ott, C. E., and McCaa, C. S.: Relation between Plasma Potassium Concentration and Aldosterone Secretion in Nephrectomized Dogs, *Int. Res. Comm. Syst.*, 2:1263, 1974.

78 Peach, M. J., and Chiu, A. T.: Stimulation and Inhibition of Aldosterone Biosynthesis in Vitro by Angiotensin II and Analogs, *Circ. Res.*, 35(suppl. 2):7, 1974.

79 Williams, G. H., Rose, L. I., Dluhy, R. G., Dingman, J. R., and Lavler, D. P.: Aldosterone Response to Sodium Restriction and ACTH Stimulation in Panhypopituitarism, *J. Clin. Endocrinol.*, 32:27, 1971.

80 Laragh, J. H., Baer, L., Brunner, H. R., Buhler, F. R., Sealey, J. E., and Vaughan, E. D.: Renin, Angiotensin and Aldosterone System in Pathogenesis and Management of Hypertensive Vascular Disease, *Am. J. Med.*, 52:633, 1972.

81 Melby, J. C., Dale, S. L., and Wilson, T. E.: 18-Hydroxydeoxycorticosterone in Human Hypertension, *Circ. Res.*, 28(suppl. 2):143, 1971.

82 Sennett, J. A., Brown, R. D., Island, D. P., Yarbro, L. R., Watson, J. T., Slaton, P. E., Hollifield, J. W., and Liddle, G. W.: Evidence for a New Mineralocorticoid in Patients with Low-Renin Essential Hypertension, *Circ. Res.*, 36(suppl. 1):2, 1975.

83 Dahl, L. K., and Love, R. A.: Etiological Role of Sodium Chloride Intake in Essential Hypertension in Humans, *J.A.M.A.*, 164:397, 1957.

84 Dahl, L. K., Heine, M., and Tassinari, L.: The Effects of Chronic Excess Salt Ingestion: Vascular Reactivity in Rats, *Circulation,* 30(suppl. 2):11, 1964.

85 Kempner, W.: Treatment of Hypertensive Vascular Disease with Rice Diet, *Am. J. Med.*, 4:545, 1948.

86 Grollman, A., and Harrison, T. R.: Effect of Rigid Sodium Restriction on Blood Pressure and Survival of Hypertensive Rats, *Proc. Soc. Exp. Med.*, 60:52, 1945.

87 Dahl, L. K.: Possible Role of Salt Intake in the Development of Essential Hypertension, in A. N. Brest and J. H. Moyer (eds.), "Hypertension—Recent Advances: The Second Hanemann Symposium on Hypertensive Disease," Lea & Febiger, Philadelphia, 1961, p. 53.

88 Helmer, O. M., and Judson, W. E.: Metabolic Studies on Hypertensive Patients with Low Plasma Renin Activity not due to Hyperaldosteronism, *Circulation,* 36(suppl. 2):140, 1967.

89 Dahl, L. K., Knudsen, K. D., and Iwai, J.: Genetic Influence of the Kidney in Hypertension-prone Rats, *Circ. Res.*, 27-(suppl. 2):277, 1970.

90 Wilson, I. M., and Freis, E. D.: The Relationship between Plasma and Extracellular Fluid Volume Depletion and the Anti-hypertensive Effect of Chlorothiazide, *Circulation,* 20:1028, 1959.

91 Champlain, J. de, Krakoff, L., and Axelrod, J.: Relationship between Sodium Balance, Blood Pressure, and Norepinephrine Storage, *Clin. Res.*, 15:197, 1967 (abstract).

92 Dustan, H. P., Tarazi, R. C., and Bravo, E. L.: Physiologic

Characteristics of Hypertension, *Am. J. Med.*, 52:610, 1972.

93 Tobian, L.: A Viewpoint Concerning the Enigma of Hypertension, *Am. J. Med.*, 52:595, 1972.

94 Feigl, E. O., Peterson, L. H., and Jones, A. W.: Mechanical and Chemical Properties of Arteries in Experimental Hypertension, *J. Clin. Invest.*, 42:1640, 1963.

95 Bohr, D. F.: Reactivity of Vascular Smooth Muscle from Normal and Hypertensive Rats: Effects of Several Cations, *Fed. Proc.*, 33:127, 1974.

96 Overbeck, H. W., Derifield, R. S., Pamnani, M. B., and Sozen, T.: Attenuated Vasodilator Responses to K^+ in Essential Hypertensive Man, *J. Clin. Invest.*, 53:678, 1974.

97 Haddy, F., Scott, J. B., Florio, M., Daugherty, R. M., Jr., and Huizerga, J. N.: Local Vascular Effects of Hypokalemia, Alkalosis, Hypercalcemia and Hypomagnesemia, *Am. J. Physiol.*, 204:202, 1963.

98 Mendlowitz, M., Gitlow, S., and Nafachi, N.: Cause of Essential Hypertension, *Perspect. Biol. Med.*, 2:354, 1959.

99 Sjoerdsma, A.: Relationships between Alterations in Amine Metabolism and Blood Pressure, *Circ. Res.*, 9:734, 1961.

100 Wood, J. E.: Genetic Control of Neutralization of Angiotensin and Its Relationship to Essential Hypertension, *Circulation*, 25:225, 1962.

101 Hickler, R. B., Lauler, D. P., and Thorn, G. W.: Plasma Angiotensinase Activity in Patients with Hypertension and Edema, *J. Clin. Invest.*, 42:635, 1963.

102 Kaplan, N. M., and Silah, J.: Effects of Angiostensin II on the Blood Pressure in Humans with Hypertensive Disease, *J. Clin. Invest.*, 43:635, 1963.

103 Peterson, L. H.: Properties and Behavior of Living Vascular Wall, *Physiol. Rev.*, 42(suppl. 5):309, 1962.

104 Peterson, L. H., Feigl, E., and Gouras, P.: Properties of the Carotid Sinus Mechanism, *Fed. Proc.*, 19:40, 1960 (abstract).

105 Stamler, J., Lindberg, H. A., Berkson, D. M., Shaffer, A., Miller, W., and Poindexter, A.: Epidemiologic Analysis of Hypertension and Hypertensive Disease in the Labor Force of a Chicago Utility Company, in "Hypertension," vol. VII, Proceedings of the Council for High Blood Pressure Research, American Heart Association, New York, 1958, p. 23.

106 Sivertsson, R.: The Hemodynamic Importance of Structural Vascular Changes in Essential Hypertension, *Acta Physiol. Scand.*, vol. 79(suppl. 343), 1970.

66
Pathology of Systemic Hypertension Including Background and Complications

RICHARD P. LYNCH, M.D., and
JESSE E. EDWARDS, M.D.

The lesions seen in the patient with hypertension can be separated into two categories. The first of these concerns background diseases that may result in a state of hypertension. The second category concerns the pathologic features of the established state of hypertension.

BACKGROUND DISEASES

The great majority of the cases of hypertension are of the so-called essential, or idiopathic, type, with no known cause for the state of hypertension. Those cases for which a background disease may be present can be divided into hormonal, renal, and obstructive varieties.

Hormonal

A wide variety of hormonal disturbances are found to be associated with hypertension.[1] In some instances, the endocrine disturbance is the direct cause of the hypertension; in other instances the relationship is less direct or remains at the level of empirical association only.

ADRENAL

Disorders of the adrenal glands are responsible for about 1 percent or less of cases of hypertension.[2]

The tumor of the adrenal medulla which is responsible for hypertension is the well-known pheochromocytoma. This tumor is usually solid and causes varying degrees of enlargement of the gland. In some instances, the tumor may be of large proportions and bilateral. Cystic changes and hemorrhage are commonly found in the large tumors. An occasional concomitant of bilateral pheochromocytomas is medullary carcinoma of the thyroid gland.[3] This association appears to have a familial basis.[4] Another frequently associated finding is necrosis of myocardial fibers which may lead to electrocardiographic changes similar to those seen with myocardial infarction.[5]

Lesions of the adrenal cortex are responsible for hypertension as part of two well-recognized syndromes, namely, primary aldosteronism and Cushing's disease. Primary aldosteronism is usually the result of an adenoma of the adrenal cortex,[6] but some cases appear to be related to bilateral adrenal cortical hyperplasia.[7] The adenomas may be quite small. The well-developed syndrome is easily recognizable, but in the early stages normokalemia may be present, making the diagnosis difficult.[8] Primary aldosteronism is, however, a relatively rare cause of hypertension among patients with so-called essential hypertension and normal serum potassium concentration.[9]

The other adrenal cortical lesion resulting in hypertension is Cushing's disease. Well-known manifestations include obesity of the trunk, hirsutism, and amenorrhea in the female. In about 80 percent of the cases in adults, the lesion causing this syndrome is bilateral adrenal cortical hyperplasia. This appears to be secondary to excessive ACTH stimulation by the pituitary gland. In most of the remaining cases, the cause is an adenoma of one of the adrenal glands; there are occasional cases caused by unilateral carcinoma of the adrenal gland.

An uncommon cause of hypertension in children is the hypertensive type of the adrenogenital syndrome.[10] In this syndrome there is an enzymatic block which limits cortisol synthesis. There is resultant progressive adrenal cortical hyperplasia involving the zona reticularis.

THYROID

Hypertension may develop as a result of severe and prolonged hyperthyroidism. This hypertension is usually systolic only.[11] Occasional patients with myxedema show mild diastolic hypertension.

PITUITARY

As just mentioned, many cases of Cushing's disease are secondary to hypersecretion of ACTH by the pituitary gland. In most instances, no specific lesion is found in the gland, but some patients will have a basophil adenoma with resultant hypersecretion of ACTH and hypertension consequent to the adrenal cortical hyperfunction.

PARATHYROID

In hyperparathyroidism resulting either from hyperplasia of the glands or an adenoma, hypertension occurs in about one-third of the cases.[12] This is generally believed to be related to the secondary renal involvement of the disease. It has recently been suggested that hypercalcemia may have a direct effect on blood pressure independent of renal damage.[13]

ESTROGEN-RELATED

In some series,[14,15] a small percentage of women taking combination estrogen-progesterone medication develop hypertension while on medication. This is more likely related to the estrogen portion of the medication. While the hypertension in most cases is mild or moderate in degree, a wide range of severity may be represented.[16]

Renal

Renal disease as a cause of hypertension may take the form of (1) hormonal-secreting tumors, (2) parenchymal disease, such as glomerulonephritis or pyelonephritis, or (3) vascular disease.

HORMONAL-SECRETING TUMORS

It has been apparent for some time that most cases of hypertension are associated with disorders of the renin-angiotensin-aldosterone mechanism. The hormone renin is secreted by the juxtaglomerular cells in the kidneys. There have been described at least eight cases of tumors of the juxtaglomerular apparatus with resultant severe hypertension.[17-20] These cases have occurred in a young age group, from 8 to 38 years, and most have been cured by nephrectomy. A case of Wilm's tumor with renin secretion and consequent hypertension has also been described.[21]

PARENCHYMAL DISEASE

In some patients with hypertension, renal disease appears to be fundamental in initiating the hypertensive state.

Glomerulonephritis is commonly associated with hypertension especially in the chronic state. In such patients the kidney shows a great reduction in size, especially in the chronic protracted form of glomerulonephritis. The changes in each organ are rather uniform, the reduction involving all portions of the

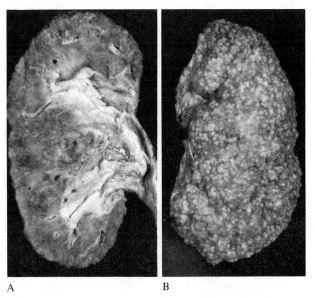

A   B

FIGURE 66-1 Kidney in chronic glomerulonephritis. *A.* Cut surface. Uniformly thin cortex. *B.* External surface. Uniform granularity and reduction in size.

renal cortex (Fig. 66-1). The kidney may be finely or coarsely granular. The coarse granularity may be a manifestation of foci of tubular dilatation protruding above the surface.

Pyelonephritis may present a remarkably variable pathologic picture. It is most characteristically a bilateral disease but with considerable variation from one area to another, resulting in gross irregularity of the kidneys. In instances of unilateral disease the uninvolved kidney may be enlarged, representing compensatory hypertrophy. The hypertension seen in a small percentage of cases of pyelonephritis is probably secondary to the vascular lesions which occur in the areas of inflammation. These are characterized by intimal fibrous thickening with considerable reduction in the lumina of the involved arteries. These changes have been compared by Weiss and Parker[22] with the changes occurring in the senile ovary representing disuse and atrophy of the vessels. There may be vascular narrowing in the areas uninvolved by the pyelonephritis. These changes are considered secondary to the hypertension generated by the pyelonephritis. In some patients with pyelonephritis, lesions may be seen which appear to have been formed as underlying causes of the inflammatory process. Most commonly, these lesions are obstructive in nature. They include obstructive disease in the prostate, neoplasms, ureteropelvic stricture, and calculi (Fig. 66-2).

In diabetic patients with the Kimmelstiel-Wilson syndrome, the kidney may not be greatly reduced in size but often has a pale, glossy appearance. The specific histologic lesion is nodular thickening of the glomerular basement membrane (Fig. 66-3). The thickening may be diffuse, in which case it is not specific for the syndrome. There are also extensive

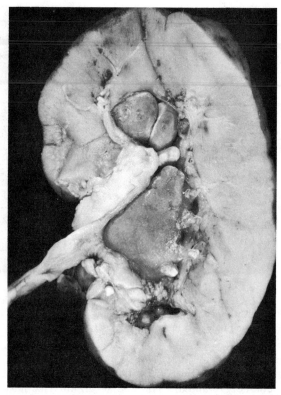

FIGURE 66-2 Cut surface of kidney with staghorn calculi in calyces.

FIGURE 66-3 Kidney in Kimmelstiel-Wilson disease. *A*. External surface. Kidney has a pale, translucent appearance. *B*. Photomicrograph. Nodular glomerulosclerosis (H&E; ×325).

occlusive vascular changes which probably play an important role in creating the hypertensive state seen so frequently in diabetic patients.

The amyloid kidney shows considerable variation in its gross appearance. It is often a large, pale kidney as classically described, but even more often it is reduced in size. Only a small proportion of patients with amyloidosis involving the kidneys is hypertensive.

The typical congenital polycystic kidney is greatly enlarged and characterized by bilateral involvement (Fig. 66-4). There may be associated cystic disease of the liver, and there is a tendency for patients with his condition to have congenital aneurysms of the circle of Willis. Hypertension is associated quite frequently with bilateral polycystic disease. The major cause of death is renal failure. About 10 percent of the patients die from subarachnoid hemorrhage resulting from rupture of an aneurysm of the circle of Willis.

Virtually every collagen disease is associated, at least in some instances, with hypertension. About one-fourth of the patients having systemic lupus erythematosus will manifest hypertension.[23] Polyarteritis is also frequently associated with hypertension. Progressive systemic sclerosis (scleroderma) is frequently associated with renal disease. In one series, half of the patients who died had renal involvement.[24] This assumed a form of malignant hypertension which, pathologically, was virtually indistinguishable from malignant nephrosclerosis.

Most other renal diseases are associated in some instances with hypertension. These include gout,[25] congenital hypoplasia,[26] irradiation,[27] trauma,[26] and toxemia of pregnancy. Toxemia of pregnancy is essentially a glomerular disease, and the mechanism of hypertension is similar to that in glomerulonephritis.

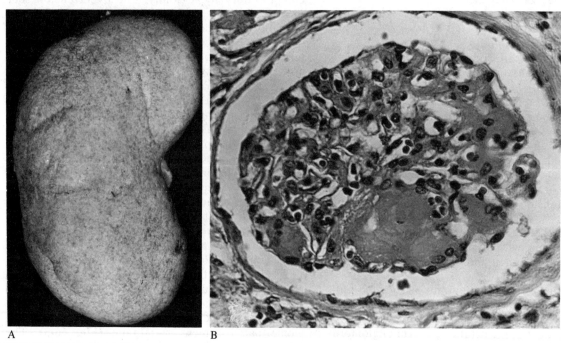

A

B

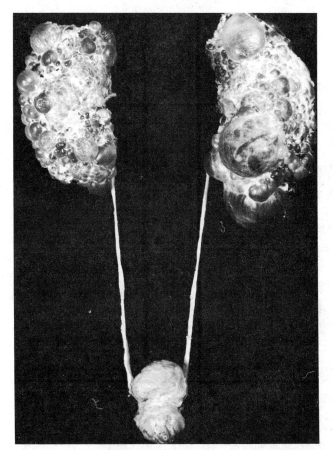

FIGURE 66-4 Kidneys and bladder in case of congenital polycystic kidneys.

unilateral renal disease and resultant hypertension. An uncommon cause of embolism is that seen as a result of dislodgement of atherosclerotic material from the aorta. This will most commonly be bilateral with involvement of intrarenal vessels and associated scarring of the kidneys, representing areas of infarction or atrophy (Fig. 66-6). The occlusive lesions may be the ultimate cause of elaboration of pressor substance leading to hypertension.[33] Atheromatous embolization may rarely be unilateral and result in so-called malignant hypertension.[34]

Rare cases of hypertension resulting from syphilitic renal arteritis have been claimed.[35]

Obstructive

The classic example of an obstructive lesion causing hypertension is coarctation of the aorta. This condition is now commonly diagnosed correctly. The basis for the hypertension has been a subject of debate as to whether it is primarily an obstructive phenomenon caused by the stenosis of the aorta or is the result of nonpulsatile flow of blood to the kidneys. Support of the latter explanation is supplied by the fact that although the systolic pressure is below normal in the compartment below the coarctation, diastolic hypertension exists both proximal and distal to the coarctation.

COMPLICATIONS

In the proper sense of the term, all the lesions seen as the result of a sustained state of hypertension are probably best considered as complications. Initial sites of complications are the myocardium and the systemic arterioles and small arteries. As a result of changes in the arterial vessels, ultimate complications may occur in various organs, particularly the kidneys and the brain. The lungs become affected as a result of changes in the heart, brain, or kidneys. In the following discussion, complications will be considered according to the anatomic sites at which they occur.

Systemic arterioles

As systemic hypertension is primarily a vasospastic disease, the arterioles, initially, are histologically normal.[36] The earliest structural change is medial hypertrophy (Fig. 66-7A). There is well-documented experimental evidence that arterioles undergo alternating patterns of constriction and dilatation, with leakage of plasma constituents into the vascular media.[37–39] It is unknown as to whether such changes apply to human arterioles.

Later changes include focal hyalinization of the medial layer and intimal fibrous thickening and medial atrophy beyond internal lesions.[40] The latter

VASCULAR
Most commonly, unilateral renal arterial disease is derived from atherosclerosis, a process primarily one of aortic atherosclerosis with renal arterial ostial narrowing (Fig. 66-5A). The process may reside in the renal artery, of which the ostium is normal (Fig. 66-5B and C). Involvement of intrarenal branches with only segmental effect upon the kidney may also result in hypertension (Fig. 66-5D). In rare instances, a renal artery aneurysm may have thrombosis with resultant renal arterial narrowing. A renal artery aneurysm in the absence of arterial stenosis rarely causes hypertension.[28]

A relatively recently described entity is *fibromuscular hyperplasia* of one or both renal arteries.[29] It has also been called *fibromuscular dysplasia* or *arterial fibrodysplasia*. In large series of cases of renovascular hypertension, this condition is responsible for about half as many cases of renal artery stenosis as atherosclerosis.[30,31] This is seen in a relatively young age group and is much more common in females. It demonstrates pathologic alternating areas of atrophy and hyperplasia of the media of the renal artery with associated fibrosis.[32]

A renal arteriovenous fistula serves as a basis for hypertension because of ischemia of the kidney beyond the fistula, resulting from diversion of arterial blood into the venous blood system.

Embolism to a major renal artery can result in

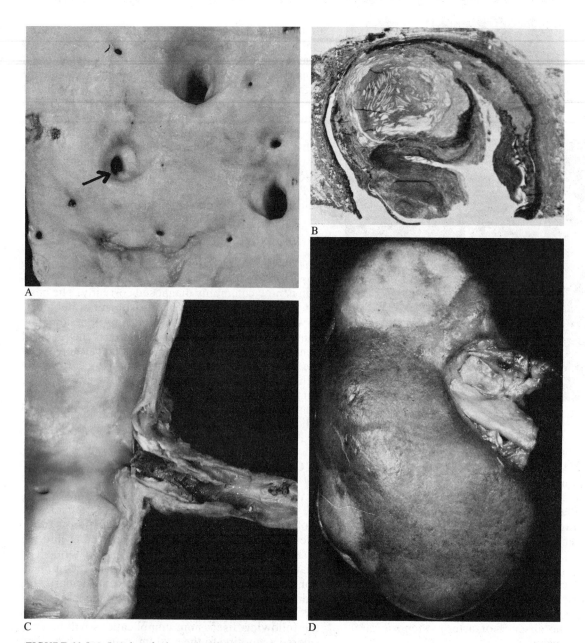

FIGURE 66-5 A. Interior of atherosclerotic abdominal aorta from behind. Narrowing of left renal artery ostium (arrow). Orifice of superior mesenteric artery above. *B.* Photomicrograph. Atherosclerosis of renal artery with greatly reduced lumen (elastic tissue stain; ×10). *C.* Stenosis with secondary thrombosis of left renal artery near origin from aorta. *D.* External surface of kidney. Segmental infarcts (pale areas) secondary to thrombosis of intrarenal arteries.

causes luminal narrowing. In general, there is a relationship between the type of intimal disease and the severity of hypertension. In milder forms of hypertension, the intimal disease is characterized by deposit of relatively acellular connective tissue. In the severe forms of hypertension, especially the rapidly progressive types (malignant hypertension), the intimal thickening is characterized by concentric cellular proliferation[41] (so-called onion-peel thickening) (Fig. 66-7*B*). Focal necrosis of all layers of the arterial walls occurs in severe hypertension.

Arteriolar changes may occur in all parts of the systemic circulation, including such organs as the myocardium, retina, kidney, pancreas, and brain.[42] The secondary effects of luminal narrowing (and possibly associated vasospasm) may take the form of microinfarcts.

Hypertension may affect the major arteries through its tendency to stimulate atherogenesis. In this way, and as a primary effect on specific organs, it may also affect the heart, the kidney, and the brain.[43]

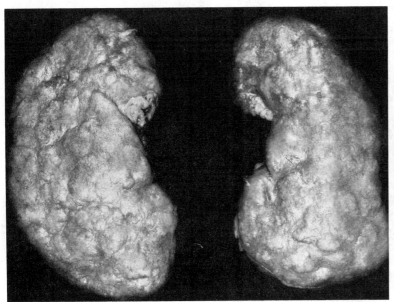
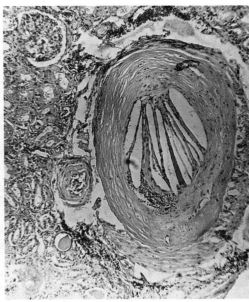

A

B

FIGURE 66-6 Kidneys in atheromatous embolism. *A.* External surface. Irregular scarring and atrophy. *B.* Photomicrograph. Atheromatous embolus in intrarenal artery (H&E; ×80).

Heart

The primary effect of hypertension on the heart is concentric hypertrophy of the left ventricle. Also, as hypertension is a factor favoring atherogenesis, coronary atherosclerosis with its own peculiar complications may be observed in the hypertensive subject.[44] Another complication of hypertension is cardiac failure. This is attended by left ventricular dilatation. The concomitant elevation of left ventricular diastolic pressure is associated with elevation of pressure in the left atrium (which becomes hypertrophied and dilated) and with pulmonary hypertension. The latter effect of the failing left ventricle is manifested by right ventricular hypertrophy and by structural changes in the pulmonary vascular bed which qualitatively are like those observed in mitral stenosis.

An additional effect of left ventricular failure is the tendency toward the development of mural thrombi, particularly in the left atrial appendage and at the apex of the left ventricle (Fig. 66-8). A potential consequence of such thrombi is systemic embolism.

In hypertension, the peripheral manifestations of cardiac failure are like those of right ventricular failure, from any cause. These include hepatic congestion, edema, accumulation of fluid in the serous cavities, iliofemoral venous thrombosis, and pulmonary embolism.

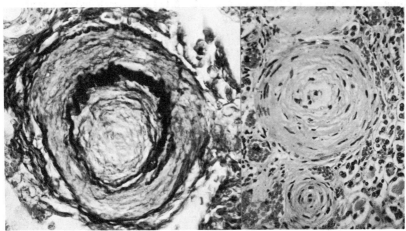

A

B

FIGURE 66-7 Photomicrographs of a small renal arterial vessel in primary (essential) systemic hypertension. *A.* Medial hypertrophy. Extreme degree of nonspecific intimal thickening, causing obliteration of lumen (elastic tissue stain; ×450). *B.* A small artery and an arteriole, each showing concentric intimal fibrous thickening (H&E; ×250).

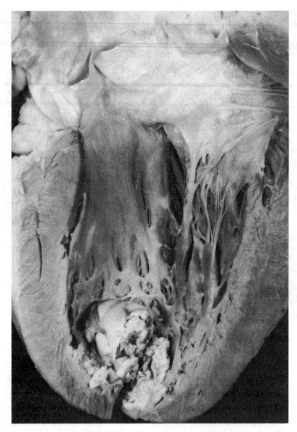

FIGURE 66-8 Left ventricle in hypertensive subject. In addition to hypertrophy of the wall, there is a mural thrombus at the apex.

Fibrinous pericarditis occurs uncommonly in those cases of essential hypertension which become complicated by uremia.

Aorta

In hypertensive subjects, cystic medial necrosis of the aorta occurs to a greater degree than in normotensive subjects of comparable age. A consequence of the combined effects of cystic medial necrosis and of hypertension is dissecting aneurysm of the aorta. This lesion may take one of two forms: (1) the classic type, in which extensive intramural dissection of blood occurs within the aortic wall[45] (Fig. 66-9); (2) the so-called incomplete dissecting aneurysm, which has received less attention than the first type. This lesion is characterized by a tear of the aortic wall like that of the primary tear of classic dissecting aneurysm. The difference between the two conditions is that in the incomplete variety no intramural dissection of blood takes place. At the site of the tear, where the aortic wall is consequently weak, a saccular aneurysm may occur. A particular site of predilection for this lesion is the junction of the aortic arch and the descending aorta (Fig. 66-10).

As hypertension stimulates the development of

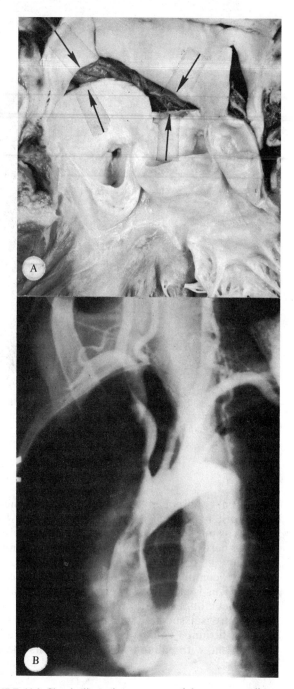

FIGURE 66-9 Classic dissecting aneurysm of the aorta complicating hypertension. *A.* In the ascending aorta a horizontal tear (between arrows) represents the primary laceration of dissecting aneurysm of the aorta. A typical intramural hematoma extended from this site. *B.* Aortogram in the case shown in *A.* There is distortion of the ascending and descending aorta, together with evidence of a false channel in the wall of the vessel. Narrowing of the brachiocephalic artery is also demonstrated.

atherosclerosis in the coronary and cerebral arteries, so may it affect the aorta. Aortic atherosclerosis may lead to aneurysm formation, particularly of the abdominal portion. Examples of occlusive thrombosis may occur. Ulceration of aortic atheromata (Fig. 66-11) may lead to widespread embolism of atheromatous material. The latter phenomenon tends to involve small arteries, and because of the disseminat-

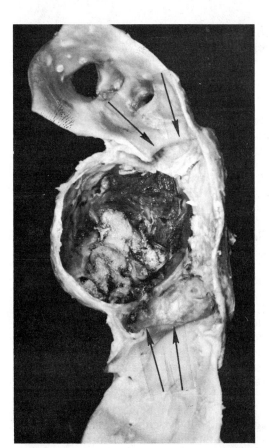

FIGURE 66-10 A saccular aneurysm at the junction of the aortic arch and descending aorta. This type of aneurysm may follow incomplete dissecting aneurysm of the aorta. Sudden interruption in the continuity of the aortic wall is apparent at the arrows.

FIGURE 66-11 Extensive ulcerative atherosclerosis which occurs in hypertensive patients is demonstrated in this thoracic aorta.

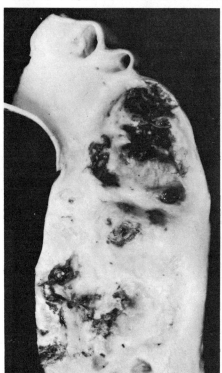

ed distribution a clinical picture simulating periarteritis nodosa may be obtained.[46,47]

It is to be emphasized that the atherosclerotic complications in the aorta are not to be confused with the unrelated problem of dissecting aneurysm.

Kidney

The renal complications of hypertension are primarily related to the small arterial and arteriolar lesions described. These lead to the changes known collectively as nephrosclerosis (Fig. 66-12). As a consequence of chronic focal arterial insufficiency, focal segments of the cortex show structural changes. These are characterized by glomerular hyalinization, by atrophy of associated tubules, and by an increase in surrounding stroma. At the sites of such changes here are depressions of the cortical surface. As the loss of renal substance is of a relatively slight order, the kidney of the hypertensive subject is only a little reduced in size. If chronic renal failure is present, dilatation of those cortical tubules in zones between atrophic foci occurs. Collections of such tubules bulge above the surface of the kidney and, together with the depressions of atrophy, are responsible for a uniformly granular character of the outer surface of the organ.

Infarction of the kidney may occur either as a

FIGURE 66-12 Nephrosclerosis. *A.* Gross specimen of kidney. External view shows fine granularity. Characteristically, the kidney is not greatly reduced in size. *B.* Lower-power photomicrograph showing areas of atrophy of the cortex alternating with zones of relatively intact cortex with dilated tubules.

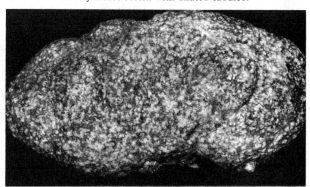

A

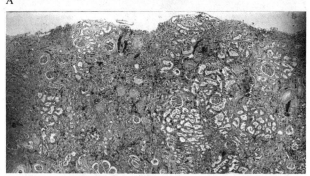

B

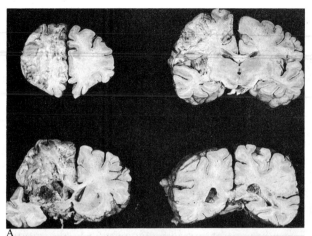

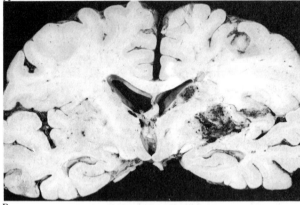

FIGURE 66-13 Cerebral infarction. *A.* Cross sections of the brain showing extensive recent infarction of the left hemisphere. *B.* Cross section of a brain showing two areas of discoloration representing infarction with secondary hemorrhage.

chance complication of embolism from intracardiac thrombi or as a manifestation of arterial occlusion from a complicating dissecting aneurysm.

Brain

The cerebral complications of hypertension are numerous and assume a wide variety of appearances.

The simplest changes are of microscopic size and are characterized by perivascular atrophy and/or microinfarction. Gross infarction of the brain occurs commonly in hypertensive subjects (Fig. 66-13*A*). In some instances of cerebral infarction there is clear evidence for the embolism from intracardiac thrombosis or, less commonly, from occlusion of a carotid artery by a dissecting aneurysm. In some cases, in which embolism may be excluded, occlusion of a regional artery by a thrombus developing in an atherosclerotic segment of an artery may be demonstrated. Most often, however, in cerebral infarction no occluded artery is identifiable. It remains to be determined whether, in such circumstances, an organic occlusion or a vasospastic episode is responsible for the ischemia that leads to infarction.

Cerebral hemorrhage may complicate hypertension. This process may assume one of several forms. In some instances (perhaps most commonly) the hemorrhage is secondary within areas of infarction (Fig. 66-13*B*). In other instances, hemorrhage into the substance of the brain appears to be a primary complication. Small but significant hemorrhages involve the substance of the brainstem or cerebellum. Most commonly the primary cerebral hemorrhages are located within the cerebrum, cause extensive destruction of the hemisphere of origin, and frequently rupture into the ventricular septum.

Hypertension is commonly associated with those

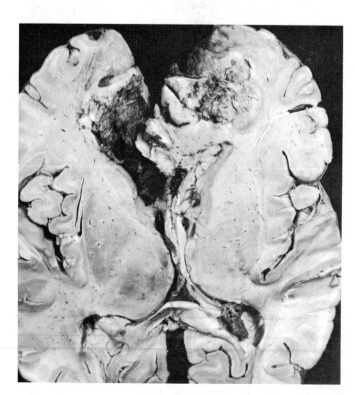

FIGURE 66-14 Frontal section of the brain in a patient with a recurrent rupture of an aneurysm of the anterior communicating cerebral artery. As a complication of the second episode of rupture, hemorrhage has extended into each frontal lobe.

cases of subarachnoid hemorrhage which result from rupture of a so-called congenital aneurysm of the circle of Willis. In these, the hypertension may have played a role, not only in rupture of the aneurysm, but also in its very development. Classically, rupture of an aneurysm of the circle of Willis is responsible for subarachnoid hemorrhage. If a patient recovers from such an episode, a subsequent rupture tends to cause hemorrhage into the cerebral substance (Fig. 66-14).

Lung

Pulmonary manifestations are common as late complications in systemic hypertension. Acute pulmonary edema may occur as a manifestation of left ventricular failure, or it may stem from the increased intracranial pressure of a cerebral complication.

Pulmonary vascular disease of the type seen in chronic pulmonary venous obstruction may be observed in cases of long-standing left ventricular failure. The various manifestations of pulmonary embolism may be observed as complications of congestive cardiac failure.

If uremia develops, the lungs show signs of this process. These include deposit of hyaline membranes along the surfaces of the alveoli and respiratory bronchioles. Congestion, edema, and bronchopneumonia are common pulmonary findings in uremia.

REFERENCES

1 Kornel, L., Riddle, M., and Schwartz, T. B.: The Management of Hypertension Associated with Disorders of Function of the Endocrine Glands ("Endocrine Hypertension?"), *Med. Clin. North Am.,* 55(1):23, 1971.

2 Kaplan, N. N.: Adrenal Causes of Hypertension, *Arch. Intern. Med.,* 133:1001, 1974.

3 Schimke, R. N., Hartmann, W. H., Prout, T. E., and Rimoin, D. L.: Syndrome of Bilateral Pheochromocytoma, Medullary Thyroid Carcinoma and Multiple Neuromas: A Possible Regulatory Defect in the Differentiation of Chromaffin Tissue, *N. Engl. J. Med.,* 279:1, 1968.

4 Schimke, R. N., and Hartmann, W. H.: Familial Amyloid-producing Medullary Thyroid Carcinoma and Pheochromocytoma: Distinct Genetic Entity, *Ann. Intern. Med.,* 63:1027, 1965.

5 Van Vliet, P. K., Burchell, H. B., and Titus, J. L.: Focal Myocarditis Associated with Pheochromocytoma, *N. Engl. J. Med.,* 274:1102, 1966.

6 Conn, J. W., Cohen, E. L., Rovner, D. R., and Nesbit, R. M.: Normokalemic Primary Aldosteronism: A Detectable Cause of Curable "Essential" Hypertension, *J.A.M.A.,* 193:200, 1965.

7 Van Buchem, F. S. P., Doorenbos, H., and Elings, H. S.: Primary Aldosteronism Due to Adrenocortical Hyperplasia, *Lancet,* 2:335, 1956.

8 Conn, J. W., Rovner, D. R., Cohen, E. L., and Nesbit, R. M.: Normokalemic Primary Aldosteronism: Its Masquerade as "Essential" Hypertension, *J.A.M.A.,* 195:21, 1966.

9 Fishman, L. M., Küchel, O., Liddle, G. W., Michelakis, A. N., Gordon, R. D., and Chick, W. T.: Incidence of Primary Aldosteronism: Uncomplicated "Essential" Hypertension: A Prospective Study with Elevated Aldosterone Secretion and Suppressed Plasma Renin Activity Used as Diagnostic Criteria, *J.A.M.A.,* 205:497, 1968.

10 Bongiovanni, A. M., and Root, A. W.: The Adrenogenital Syndrome, *N. Engl. J. Med.,* 268:1283, 1963.

11 Danowski, T. S., Sarver, M. E., D'Ambrosia, R. D., and Moses, C.: Hydrocortisone and/or Desiccated Thyroid in Physiologic Dosage: X. Effects of Thyroid Hormone Excesses on Clinical Status and Thyroid Indices, *Metabolism,* 13:702, 1964.

12 Rosenthal, F. D., and Roy, S.: Hypertension and Hyperparathyroidism, *Br. Med. J.,* 4:396, 1972.

13 Earll, J. M., Kurtzman, N. A., and Moser, R. H.: Hypercalcemia and Hypertension, *Ann. Intern. Med.,* 64:378, 1966.

14 Briggs, E., Browning, J., Mack, A., Naismith, L., Taylor, L., and Wilson, E.: Blood-Pressure in Women after One Year of Oral Contraception, *Lancet,* 1:467, 1971.

15 Laragh, J. H.: Oral Contraceptive-induced Hypertension—Nine Years Later, *Am. J. Obstet. Gynecol.,* 126(1):141, 1976.

16 Weinberger, M. H.: Oral Contraceptives and Hypertension, *Hosp. Practice,* 10(5):65, 1975.

17 Brown, J. J., Lever, A. F., Robertson, J. I. S., Fraser, R., Morton, J. J., and Tree, M.: Hypertension and Secondary Hyperaldosteronism Associated with a Renin-secreting Renal Juxtaglomerular-Cell Tumour, *Lancet,* 2:1228, 1973.

18 Schambelan, M., Howes, E. L., Jr., Stockigt, J. R., Noakes, C. A., and Biglieri, E. G.: Role of Renin and Aldosterone in Hypertension Due to a Renin-Secreting Tumor, *Am. J. Med.,* 55:86, 1973.

19 Gherardi, G. J., Arya, S., and Hickler, R. B.: Juxtaglomerular Body Tumor: A Rare Occult but Curable Cause of Lethal Hypertension, *Hum. Pathol.,* 5:236, 1974.

20 Conn, J. W., Cohen, E. L., Lucas, C. P., McDonald, W. J., Mayor, G. H., Blough, W. M., Jr., Eveland, W. C., Bookstein, J. J., and Lapides, J.: Primary Reninism, Hypertension, Hyperreninemia, and Secondary Aldosteronism Due to Renin-Producing Juxtaglomerular Cell Tumors, *Arch. Intern. Med.,* 130:682, 1972.

21 Ganguly, A., Gribble, J., Tune, B., Kempson, R. L., and Luetscher, J. A.: Renin-secreting Wilms' Tumor with Severe Hypertension: Report of a Case and Brief Review of Renin-secreting Tumors, *Ann. Intern. Med.,* 79:835, 1973.

22 Weiss, S., and Parker, F., Jr.: Pyelonephritis: Its Relations to Vascular Lesions and to Arterial Hypertension, *Medicine (Baltimore),* 18:221, 1939.

23 DuBois, E. L., and Tuffanelli, D. L.: Clinical Manifestations of Systemic Lupus Erythematosus: Computer Analysis of 520 Cases, *J.A.M.A.,* 190:104, 1964.

24 Rodman, G. P.: The Natural History of Progressive Systemic Sclerosis (Diffuse Scleroderma), *Bull. Rheum. Dis.,* 8:301, 1963.

25 Rakic, M. T., Valkenburg, H. A., Davidson, R. T., Engels, J. P., Mikkelsen, W. M., Neel, J. V., and Duff, I. F.: Observations on the Natural History of Hyperuricemia and Gout, *Am. J. Med.,* 37:862, 1964.

26 Dunn, J., and Brown, H.: Unilateral Renal Disease and Hypertension, *J.A.M.A.,* 166:18, 1958.

27 Dean, A. L., and Abels, J. C.: Study by the Newer Renal Function Tests of an Unusual Case of Hypertension following Irradiation of One Kidney and the Relief of the Patient by Nephrectomy, *J. Urol.,* 52:497, 1944.

28 Cummings, K. B., Lecky, J. W., and Kaufman, J. J.: Renal Artery Aneurysms and Hypertension, *J. Urol.,* 109:144, 1973.

29 Wylie, E. J., and Wellington, J. S.: Hypertension Caused by Fibromuscular Hyperplasia of the Renal Arteries, *Am. J. Surg.,* 100:183, 1960.

30 Foster, J. H., and Oates, J. A.: Recognition and Management of Renovascular Hypertension, *Hosp. Practice,* 10(10):61, 1975.

31 Stanley, J. C., and Fry, W. J.: Renovascular Hypertension Secondary to Arterial Fibrodysplasia in Adults: Criteria for Operation and Results of Surgical Therapy, *Arch. Surg.,* 110: 922, 1975.

32 Stanley, J. C., Gewertz, B. L., Bove, E. L., Sottiurai, V., and

Fry, W. J.: Arterial Fibrodysplasia: Histopathologic Character and Current Etiologic Concepts. *Arch. Surg.,* 110:561, 1975.

33 Retan, J. W., and Miller, R. E.: Microembolic Complications of Atherosclerosis: Literature Review and Report of a Patient, *Arch. Intern. Med.,* 118:534, 1966.

34 Dalakos, T. G., Streeten, D. H. P., Jones, D., and Obeid, A.: "Malignant" Hypertension Resulting from Atheromatous Embolization Predominantly of One Kidney, *Am. J. Med.,* 57:135, 1974.

35 Price, R. K., and Skelton, R.: Hypertension Due to Syphilitic Occlusion of the Main Renal Arteries, *Br. Heart J.,* 10:29, 1948.

36 Castleman, B., and Smithwick, R. H.: The Relation of Vascular Disease to the Hypertensive State: II. The Adequacy of the Renal Biopsy as Determined from a Study of 500 Patients, *N. Engl. J. Med.,* 239:729, 1948.

37 Brunner, H. R., and Gavras, H.: Vascular Damage in Hypertension, *Hosp. Practice,* 10(3):97, 1975.

38 Giese, J.: Renin, Angiotensin and Hypertensive Vascular Damage: A Review, *Am. J. Med.,* 55:315, 1973.

39 Byrom, F. B.: The Evolution of Acute Hypertensive Arterial Disease, *Prog. Cardiov. Dis.,* 17:31, 1974.

40 Naeye, R. L.: Arteriolar Abnormalities with Chronic Systemic Hypertension: A Quantitative Study, *Circulation,* 35:662, 1967.

41 MacMahon, H. E.: Malignant Nephrosclerosis: 50 Years Later, *J. Hist. Med.,* 21:125, 1966.

42 Heptinstall, R. H.: Relation of Hypertension to Changes in the Arteries, *Prog. Cardiov. Dis.,* 17:25, 1974.

43 Kinsey, D., and Whitelaw, G. P.: The Hypertensive Patient: Method of Study, *Am. J. Surg.,* 107:5, 1964.

44 Mulcahy, R., Hickey, N., and Maurer, B.: Coronary Heart Disease in Women: Study of Risk Factors in 100 Patients Less han 60 Years of Age, *Circulation,* 36:577, 1967.

45 Lindsay, J., Jr., and Hurst, J. W.: Clinical Features and Prognosis in Dissecting Aneurysm of the Aorta: A Reappraisal, *Circulation,* 35:880, 1967.

46 Richards, A. M., Eliot, R. S., Kanjuh, V. I., Bloemendaal, R. D., and Edwards, J. E.: Cholesterol Embolism: A Multiple-System Disease Masquerading as Polyarteritis Nodosa, *Am. J. Cardiol.,* 15:696, 1965.

47 Case Records of the Massachusetts General Hospital (Case 8-1972), *N. Engl. J. Med.,* 286:422, 1972.

67
The Detection of Hypertension

J. EDWIN WOOD, III, M.D.

Systemic arterial diastolic hypertension is among the three most important public health problems facing us today.[1] Hypertension affects 23 million American adults, coronary artery disease and cigarette smoking being the only important rivals for this dubious honor. Hypertension has achieved this role of central importance for several reasons. First, hypertension is extremely common with as much as 20 percent of the adult population destined to suffer from this disorder of the circulation. Second, the disease is characterized by serious consequences of morbidity and mortality due especially to its ability to accelerate the development of atherosclerosis, which in turn results in strokes, coronary artery disease, and other vascular problems. Additionally, renal failure and heart failure are important serious complications of all forms of hypertension. Finally, hypertension may suddenly move into an accelerated phase called *malignant hypertension,* which is often fatal. The third reason for the central importance of hypertension as a public health problem is the utter simplicity of making a diagnosis. While extraordinarily complex and sophisticated techniques have been developed for categorizing and subcategorizing patients with elevated blood pressure, none has superseded the simple measurement of blood pressure in the arm with a pneumatic cuff. The fourth point of great importance is that it has been established beyond doubt for many patients with hypertension, and convincingly for the remaining patients, that treatment is very effective in prolonging life and reducing morbidity. The treatment is easy to administer and requires only a modest amount of attention by the patient.

It is important to recognize that 80 percent or more of the patients with abnormal blood pressure fall into the category of essential hypertension. Without question, these patients are best treated with oral medications. A large number of those remaining patients whose hypertension is due to renal disease, or even those older patients with renal vascular hypertension, are also best treated with oral medications. Therefore, it is a specious argument to suggest that populations should not be surveyed for hypertension because it is economically impractical to determine which of those patients found to have elevated blood pressure have surgically correctable lesions such as hyperaldosteronism, pheochromocytoma, or other unusual causes for hypertension.

It is established that large numbers of people are unaware of the fact that they have elevated blood pressure or, if aware of it, have not taken it seriously.[1a] Recent data imply that this problem is improving due to the public programs for hypertension detection.[2] Contrary to previous teaching it is well accepted that a case may be considered adequately worked up when a carefully administered history and physical examination along with minimum laboratory data have been obtained.[3] Required laboratory studies are determinations of serum creatinine or BUN, potassium, cholesterol, uric acid, hematocrit, and random blood sugar levels. Urinalysis includes tests for protein, sugar, and blood. A microscopic examination of the urine sediment is important if a history of urinary tract disease is present, if the diastolic blood pressure exceeds 115 mm Hg, or if proteinuria or hematuria are present. Also, an electrocardiogram must be made and a chest x-ray taken.

Health planning groups preparing a hypertension detection program should recognize that identifying the individual who has hypertension represents only half the job. Lines of access to the diagnostic studies described above and of access to adequate treatment must be identified for the patient. It is frustrating and counterproductive for the individual to be told that his blood pressure is high only to find that there is no resource for diagnosis and treatment or, worse yet, to have those resources available but indifferent to the patient's need for treatment. Detection programs are most successful when coupled with public education programs and professional education programs that emphasize the four points reviewed at the outset of this chapter.

EARLY DETECTION

A hypertensive patient is best served if the hypertension is detected early in the natural history of the disorder, so that the damaging effects of elevated blood pressure that gradually occur over the years can be interrupted. Since hypertension either is asymptomatic or produces symptoms that are not specific such as headache, measurement of blood pressure is the only reasonable approach to finding of cases. Heretofore, we have relied on the chance detection of hypertension through health examination that the patient sought out for himself, life insurance examination, military service examination, employment physicals, and so on. This traditional approach has been supplemented in more recent years by positive public health efforts applied to the general population. This is often done by voluntary agencies such as the American Heart Association, but, as is always true, the knowledgeable and interested physician is the key to the success of such programs. As noted above, the greatest potential problem associated with population surveys is the lack of diagnostic and therapeutic follow-up. Public education programs help with the problem in that the patient will then take responsiblity for the follow-through himself.

TARGET POPULATIONS

Those patients who are at greatest risk from hypertension and for whom proper therapy has the greatest value are the young people in the 15- to 30-year-old group. Black people have a particularly high prevalence of hypertension. Thus, these groups deserve special attention in the design of a community screening program. All people in an age range of 15 to 65 years and regardless of race should be screened, however, in that large numbers will have undetected elevations of blood pressure (Table 67-1).

The importance of detection and treatment of patients in the older age groups who have systolic hypertension remains to be established. It cannot be recommended at this time that these patients be singled out for detection by public health survey.

BLOOD PRESSURE CRITERIA FOR DIAGNOSIS OF HYPERTENSION

The distribution of blood pressure levels in a population takes the form of a bell-shaped curve skewed

TABLE 67-1

Estimated reservoir of undetected and untreated individuals with elevated blood pressure

	Baldwin Co., Ga., 1962	National health survey, 1960-1962	Alameda Co., Calif., 1966
Populations surveyed	n = 3,084	n = 6,672	n = 2,495
% with elev. B.P. ≥ 160 sys. ≥ 95 dia.	17.5%	15.2%	13.0%
% pop. on med. for hypertension	6.0%	6.5%	5.9%
% with elev. B.P. on med. for hypertension	18.3%	23.2%	16.9%†
Total hypertensive pop.*	630	1,214	420†
(% unknown)	(41.0%)	(42.8%)	
% of total hypertensive pop. on med.	29.7%	35.7%	35.7%†
% of total hypertension "under control"	14.0%	16.3%	22.6%†
% of those on med. "under control"	47.0%	45.6%	63.3%†

*Total hypertensive pop. = those with B.P. ≥ 160 systolic, and/or 95 diastolic at time of survey plus those on medication for hypertension with survey pressures below those levels.
†In determining proportion on medication, etc., systolic level of 165 instead of 160 was used.
SOURCE: J.E. Wood, et al., Guidelines for the Detection, Diagnosis, and Management of Hypertensive Populations, *Circulation*, 44:A-263, 1971.

toward the higher blood pressure levels. Those patients with the highest pressures are at the greatest risk for complications for hypertension; those at the lowest levels, least so. The inevitable question occurs as to what point on the curve represents abnormality. Again, it is specious to argue that since no single level can be agreed upon by investigators and physicians as separating normality from abnormality, we should, therefore, not embark on any major population surveys.

Clinical experience, survey data, and treatment data lead to the general conclusion that a systolic blood pressure greater than 140 or a diastolic blood pressure greater than 90 is potentially abnormal for poeple over 40 and that a systolic blood pressure greater than 130 and a diastolic blood pressure greater than 80 is potentially abnormal for those under the age of 40. A further point of importance is that most authorities agree that a systolic blood pressure greater than 160 and a diastolic blood pressure greater than 95 is definitely abnormal. This information can be converted to a chart depicting the criteria for rescreening and referral of individuals as shown in Fig. 67-1.

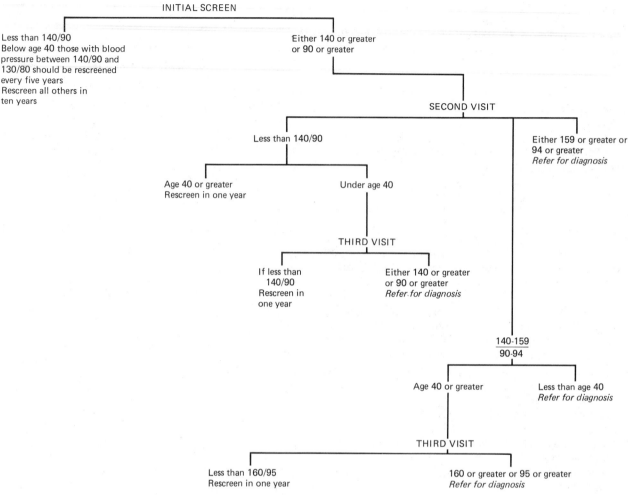

FIGURE 67-1 Blood pressure criteria for rescreening and referral. (*From J. E. Wood et al., Guidelines for the Detection, Diagnosis, and Management of Hypertensive Populations, Circulation, 44:A-263, 1971.*)

METHODS AND EQUIPMENT

Numerous studies have been carried out showing that various problems can be encountered through use of presently available standard equipment for the measurement of blood pressure. The psychologic state of the patient clearly affects blood pressure level. Size of the upper arm affects the accuracy of measurement of blood pressure. Prior use of cigarettes and possibly coffee may have an effect on blood pressure. Additionally, there is the problem of biases that the person measuring blood pressure may have. Finally, inattention to the results may be due to fatigue during the course of measuring large numbers of blood pressures. It is obvious that a simple device which could be applied on a large scale and which would result in an accurate written record of each blood pressure would be extremely useful. Various devices have been designed which reduce the effects of bias and meet some of the other problems noted, but these have the disadvantages of being difficult to apply, expensive, and not rugged enough for use in surveys.[4] Therefore, until a practical recording device can be developed, it would seem best to accept the potential for inaccuracy of our present methods with the expectation that errors introduced into blood pressure measurement by the problems of bias, rushed circumstance of mass survey, the nervous patient, or the inexperienced person measuring the blood pressure can be compensated for by the more careful review of the situation of those individuals identified as having elevated blood pressure. Most importantly, the various problems that creep into mass screening tend to result in falsely high blood pressure, so that more careful subsequent study may alert the individual to the possibility that his blood pressure may be found to be high in the future but assure him that his blood pressure is normal at the present time.

RESCREENING

Individuals may reject the results of population surveys or even individual examinations and may fail to heed the advice that they have further studies. It is important to recognize, however, that such patients have been alerted to their hypertension and that future blood pressure measurements which again result in high readings will eventually impress upon these persons that they have a problem requiring care. Therefore, the low rate of compliance with advice following initial screening should not be viewed as a program that has failed to do its job. A most important concept is that of combining a hypertension screening program with a general risk factor program for coronary disease. Thus, measuring blood pressure, taking a smoking history, and measuring serum cholesterol can be combined to produce a "risk factor profile" that has great potential for allowing such patients to reduce their risk of morbidity or mortality.

CONCLUSION

Elevated systemic arterial diastolic blood pressure is a common disorder which carries great risk to the individual but happily is easily detected and easily treated. The health care professions are as much challenged by this set of circumstances as were the health care professionals in the days of rampant infectious diseases.

REFERENCES

1 Moser, M.: Report of the Joint National Committee on Detection, Evaluation, and Treatment of High Blood Pressure, U. S. Government Printing Office, Washington, D.C., September 1976.
1a Wilber, J. A., and Barrow, J. G.: Hypertension: A Community Problem, *Am. J. Med.,* 52:653, 1972.
2 "Hypertension Detection and Following Study," Report of National Heart and Lung Institute, 1973–74.
3 Guidelines for the Detection, Diagnosis, and Management of Hypertensive Populations, Report of Inter-Society Commission for Heart Disease Resources, *Circulation,* 64:A263, 1971.
4 Labarthe, D. R., Hawkins, C. M., and Remington, R. D.: Evaluations of Performance of Selected Devices for Measuring Blood Pressure, *Am. J. Cardiol.,* 32:546, 1974.

68
Differential Diagnosis of Systemic Hypertension

ALBERT N. BREST, M.D., and
JOHN H. MOYER, M.D.

It has long been traditional to undertake a full diagnostic work-up in every patient with diastolic blood pressure elevation. During recent years, however, this approach has become increasingly controversial. Whereas some hypertension experts continue to insist that the genesis of hypertension should be characterized as accurately as possible in every patient (so as to allow the most reasoned therapeutic

approach), others argue for a less extensive work-up (so as to reduce the financial burden to the patient).[1,2] Although the specific approach remains unsettled, all parties agree it is important to identify secondary hypertension—especially the potentially curable forms of blood pressure elevation. Certainly, particular attention should be given to the patient with accelerated or malignant hypertension, the young hypertensive patient, and the hypertensive patient who is unable to tolerate or fails to respond to ordinary therapeutic regimens. There is, in addition, no disagreement that every hypertensive patient should have a complete history and physical examination. Only the extent of the laboratory work-up remains controversial.

BLOOD PRESSURE MEASUREMENT

The diagnosis of hypertension per se is made on the basis of the blood pressure reading. Blood pressures lower than 140/90 mm Hg have traditionally been regarded as normal when found in adult patients. Slightly higher systolic and diastolic blood pressures are accepted in older persons. However, there is less agreement as to the acceptable normal values for elderly subjects. An extensive study of 5,757 apparently healthy individuals between 65 and 106 years of age revealed that after age 65 blood pressure does not show a consistent rise with advancing years as it does below that age.[3] From the findings in this study, it was concluded that blood pressures higher than 160/100 mm Hg should be considered abnormal in elderly men, and that levels higher than 170/90 mm Hg are abnormal in elderly women. The World Health Organization has recommended that the values of 140 to 160/90 to 95 mm Hg be considered borderline hypertension in adults and any values above 160/95 mm Hg be considered hypertension. The definition of pediatric hypertension is less clear. However, it appears that arbitrary values of 130/85 to 140/85 to 90 should be considered hypertensive for children of all ages.[4]

In addition to the usual extremity differences, the examiner must be cognizant of the expected differences between pressure readings in the supine position and those in the erect position.[5] Normally, the systolic blood pressure falls and the diastolic pressure tends to rise as the erect position is assumed. However, regardless of position—supine or erect—the blood pressure in the lower extremities is normally higher than that in the upper extremities. The finding of lower blood pressure in the lower extremities than in the upper suggests aortic coarctation.

Having established that blood pressure elevation exists, one should next determine whether the hypertension is labile or fixed. This determination is important both from the diagnostic and the prognostic standpoints. Labile blood pressure readings may in some cases reflect a prehypertensive state, whereas in other cases they may represent episodic hypertension such as that associated with pheochromocytoma.

Another form of blood pressure elevation closely related to labile hypertension is the hyperdynamic β-adrenergic circulatory state. Typically, patients with this disorder complain of palpitation, rapid heart action, and/or excessive sweating. Like patients with labile hypertension, those with the hyperdynamic β-adrenergic circulatory state demonstrate hemodynamic evidence of a hyperkinetic circulation (increased heart rate, cardiac output, and left ventricular ejection rate); in contrast, however, they also demonstrate exaggerated responsiveness of β-adrenergic receptor sites to the specific β-adrenergic stimulant isoproterenol.[6]

SYSTOLIC HYPERTENSION

Systolic hypertension is a clinical entity distinct from diastolic blood pressure elevation. It should not be taken for granted that systolic hypertension in an older individual is due necessarily to aortic arteriosclerosis, even though this cause is the most frequent. Instead, all other diagnostic considerations should be ruled out by appropriate means.

Various high output syndromes may be associated with systolic hypertension (see Table 68-1), including anemia, thyrotoxicosis, nutritional deficiency, and arteriovenous fistula. Masked thyrotoxicosis, in particular, may be overlooked in the older patient; hyperkinetic heart syndrome should be remembered in the young subject with systolic blood pressure elevation.[7] Clinical situations characterized by increased cardiac stroke volume and accompanying systolic hypertension include complete heart block and aortic regurgitation. Also to be considered in the differential diagnosis, regardless of the age of the patient, is coarctation of the aorta, a mechanical cause for systolic blood pressure elevation.

The diagnosis of systolic hypertension due to aortic arteriosclerosis should be made only after all other potential causes for systolic blood pressure elevation have been excluded.

TABLE 68-1
Etiology of systolic hypertension

1 High output situations
  a Anemia
  b Thyrotoxicosis
  c Beriberi
  d Arteriovenous fistula
  e Hyperkinetic heart syndrome
2 Increased cardiac stroke volume
  a Third-degree AV heart block
  b Aortic insufficiency
3 Mechanical: coarctation of aorta
4 Diminished arterial elasticity: atherosclerosis

DIASTOLIC HYPERTENSION

As with systolic hypertension, there are numerous known causes for diastolic blood pressure elevation (Table 68-2). It is estimated that responsible lesions can be identified in approximately 10 percent of the hypertensive population. The most common known causes include renal parenchymal and renal arterial diseases. Less frequent is hypertension which is adrenal in origin, and the neurogenic types of diastolic hypertension are least common. Oral contraceptive hypertension is an additional category of potentially curable secondary hypertension, the incidence of which is unknown.[8] Differentiation of these various disorders is dependent on the history and physical findings plus appropriate laboratory studies.

Aside from the traditional differential diagnostic approach (renal, endocrine, and neurogenic causes versus essential hypertension), some hypertension experts now advocate a new taxonomy of hypertension based on the behavior of plasma renin activity[9] (Table 68-3). This newer diagnostic classification places enormous, and conceivably undue, importance on a single laboratory parameter. As yet, the precise clinical usefulness of this newer diagnostic approach is not fully determined.

CLUES TO THE CAUSES OF SYSTEMIC HYPERTENSION

History and physical findings

The age of the patient at the onset of hypertension may provide an important clue to the diagnosis of secondary hypertension. Essential hypertension usually becomes manifest between the ages of 20 and 50 years, although it is by no means rare for the disease to be initiated earlier.[4] On the other hand, the finding of diastolic blood pressure elevation in younger individuals should heighten the clinical suspicion of secondary hypertension, especially if the hypertension is of moderate or greater severity. Presence of diastolic hypertension in individuals under 20 years

TABLE 68-2
Etiology of diastolic hypertension (traditional differential diagnosis)

1 Primary essential hypertension
2 Secondary hypertension
  a Renal hypertension
    (1) Renal arterial disease
    (2) Renal parenchymal disease
  b Endocrine hypertension
    (1) Pheochromocytoma
    (2) Primary aldosteronism
    (3) Cushing's syndrome
    (4) Hypertensive form of adrenogenital syndrome
    (5) Hyperparathyroidism (with renal impairment)
    (6) Acromegaly
  c Neurogenic hypertension
    (1) Brain tumors
    (2) Cerebrovascular accidents
    (3) Diencephalic syndrome
  d Oral contraceptive hypertension

Etiology of diastolic hypertension (differential diagnosis based on plasma renin activity)

1 Normoreninemic hypertension
   a Normal-renin essential hypertension
   b Renal parenchymal hypertension
   c Pheochromocytoma
   d Cushing's syndrome
2 Hyperreninemic hypertension
   a High-renin essential hypertension
   b Accelerated or malignant hypertension
   c Renal arterial hypertension
   d Renin-secreting kidney tumors
   e Oral contraceptive hypertension
3 Hyporeninemic hypertension
   a Low-renin essential hypertension
   b Primary aldosteronism
   c Iatrogenic: mineralocorticoid or licorice ingestion
   d 11-β-Hydroxylase deficiency
   e 17-α-Hydroxylase deficiency
   f Adrenal carcinoma
   g Ectopic ACTH-secreting tumors
   h Idiopathic deoxycorticosterone and
      18-hydroxycorticosterone excess

of age suggests a high probability of renal parenchymal or renal arterial disease. The adrenogenital syndrome (tumor or congenital enzyme deficiency) should always be considered in hypertensive patients under 5 years of age. In contrast, onset in middle-aged or older subjects is suggestive of atherosclerotic renal arterial hypertension. Pheochromocytoma and hyperaldosteronism may be encountered in any age group.

Although essential hypertension is commonly associated with a strong family history of elevated diastolic blood pressure, the absence of a familial background does not negate the diagnosis. Contrariwise, the finding of a positive family history does not exclude secondary blood pressure elevation. Pheochromocytoma, hereditary nephritis, polycystic kidney disease, and diabetes with renal involvement are among the several disorders in which there may be coexisting hypertension and positive family history.[10,11]

The finding of labile blood pressure elevation in patients with a strong familial incidence of essential hypertension suggests a so-called prehypertensive state. On the other hand, the occurrence of intermittent hypertension associated with signs and symptoms of catecholamine excess suggests pheochromocytoma. It is noteworthy that symptomatic paroxysms of headache, excessive perspiration, palpitation, nervousness, and/or tremor usually accompany blood pressure elevation in patients with pheochromocytoma, regardless of whether the blood pressure elevation is paroxysmal or sustained.[12]

Hypokalemia-induced muscle weakness may be associated with a host of conditions characterized by coexisting hypertension and hypokalemia.[13] Muscle weakness is particularly prominent in primary aldosteronism. In the latter disorder, the muscle weakness is accompanied typically by nocturnal polyuria and polydipsia, both of which reflect hypokalemia-induced nephrogenic diabetes insipidus.

Oral contraceptive agents can cause hypertension in susceptible women, and the diagnosis should be suspected from the history of drug intake. The presence of oral contraceptive hypertension may be proved by remission following discontinuation of the contraceptive agent, although it often takes 3 or 4 months for blood pressure to return to normal after stopping the drug.[8]

Clues to underlying renal parenchymal disease also may be provided by the clinical history. A past history of kidney infections, voiding difficulties, urinary tract instrumentation, or calculus disease may point to underlying pyelonephritis, whereas a past history of proteinuria or hematuria may relate to undiagnosed glomerulonephritis.

Pertinent physical findings which have prognostic significance include hypertensive alterations in the retina and the findings of cardiomegaly. The fundi usually mirror the degree of accompanying angiospasm and/or arteriolar sclerosis, whereas left ventricular enlargement suggests that the hypertension has been severe and/or long-standing. On the other hand, certain physical findings have diagnostic value. A bruit heard in the flanks or anteriorly over the renal vasculature suggests the presence of renal arterial occlusive disease. Postural hypotension may be an additional physical finding in patients with adrenal hypertension, particularly pheochromocytoma or primary aldosteronism.[14] Palpation of bilateral flank masses in patients with diastolic hypertension suggests polycystic kidney disease, and delayed or absent femoral pulses imply aortic occlusive disease and possible aortic coarctation. Finally, certain disorders responsible for secondary hypertension (e.g., Cushing's syndrome or acromegaly) may be accompanied by physical findings which are sufficiently characteristic per se to permit diagnosis or at least to suggest strongly the underlying disturbance.

Laboratory studies

The laboratory investigation of diastolic hypertension may be divided into three categories: routine diagnostic, prognostic, and special diagnostic studies (see Table 68-4). The authors believe that the routine diagnostic tests should be performed in all hypertensive patients. Prognostic studies are employed primarily to provide a measure of the severity and significance of the hypertensive state rather than a diagnostic appraisal. *Special diagnostic tests are performed when the history and physical findings and/or routine diagnostic studies suggest the need for further diagnostic evaluation.*

Routine diagnostic tests

Included in this category are the urinalysis, intravenous pyelogram, and determination of serum potassium level. Each may provide an important diagnostic clue to the underlying hypertensive disorder.

TABLE 68-4
Diagnostic work-up for patients with diastolic hypertension

1 Routine diagnostic studies
   a Urinalysis
   b Intravenous pyelogram
   c Serum potassium
2 Prognostic tests
   a Electrocardiogram
   b Chest roentgenogram
   c BUN (blood urea nitrogen), creatinine
   d Blood glucose
   e Serum cholesterol
3 Special diagnostic studies
   a PAH (para-aminohippuric acid) and insulin clearance
   b Percutaneous renal biopsy
   c Renal scan
   d Isotope renography
   e Renal and adrenal arteriography
   f Differential renal function studies
   g Pharmacologic (histamine, phentolamine, tyramine, or glucagon) tests
   h Catecholamine excretion
   i Glucocorticoid excretion
   j Aldosterone secretion or excretion
   k Plasma renin activity
   l Adrenal venography
   m Skull roentgenograms, EEG (electroencephalogram), other cerebral studies

TABLE 68-5
Syndromes characterized by low serum potassium levels and hypertension

1 Primary aldosteronism
2 Congenital aldosteronism
3 Cushing's syndrome
4 Accelerated hypertension with secondary aldosteronism
   a Renal arterial hypertension
   b Malignant hypertension
   c Renin-secreting renal tumor
5 Potassium-wasting renal parenchymal disease
6 Diuretic-induced hypokalemia in hypertensive patients
7 Pseudo primary aldosteronism: chronic licorice ingestion

Specific urinary findings may identify or at least suggest the fundamental disorder. For example, red blood cell and white blood cell casts are generally considered pathognomonic of glomerulonephritis and pyelonephritis, respectively. An alkaline urine implies the presence of alkalosis, a characteristic finding in primary aldosteronism. The presence of bacteriuria suggests possible pyelonephritis. On the other hand, proteinuria may occur with either renal hypertension or essential hypertension with accompanying renal functional impairment.

The intravenous pyelogram not infrequently provides an important clue to clinically unsuspected renal disorders.[15] From the hypertensive standpoint, not only is the pelvocalyceal structure important, but also of significance are the comparative lengths of the kidneys as well as the appearance time, concentration, and excretion of contrast medium in the renal pelves. Difference in the renal lengths of 1.5 cm or more suggests unilateral renal dysfunction. In studying the appearance time and differential concentration and excretion of opaque medium by the kidneys during intravenous pyelography, it is important that serial studies be made at 1-min intervals for the first 5 min following rapid injection of contrast medium, rather than at the usual 5-min intervals.[16] By this method, minor initial delayed appearance of contrast medium may be detected in an ischemic kidney, whereas this same disparity in renal function may go undetected in the standard 5-, 10-, and 20-min films. Delay in appearance of contrast medium in early minute-sequence films, with increased concentration and delayed excretion in later films, and evidence of ureteral collateral circulation on the involved side, singly or in combination, strongly suggest a renal arterial lesion. On the other hand, even using rapid-sequence pyelography, occasional patients with unilateral or bilateral renal arterial lesions may have normal pyelograms. Furthermore, minor differences in renal mass and in the appearance time, concentration, and excretion of contrast medium may occur at times in normal individuals.

The finding of hypokalemia suggests possible adrenal hypertension, e.g., primary or congenital aldosteronism or Cushing's syndrome. On the other hand, as already mentioned, low serum potassium levels may be seen with other disorders, as well (see Table 68-5). It is noteworthy, in this regard, that a single normal value for serum potassium does not necessarily exclude any of these hypertensive situations.

Prognostic tests

The electrocardiogram, chest roentgenogram, and routine renal function studies do not, in general, provide any specific diagnostic clues to the type of diastolic hypertension. On the other hand, they may provide important prognostic information. Thus the electrocardiogram can indicate whether left ventricular hypertrophy and ischemia are present. Likewise the chest roentgenogram can confirm the presence of cardiomegaly; however, with the exception of aortic coarctation, in which characteristic aortic and/or rib changes may be found, chest roentgenogram examination is not helpful in establishing a causal diagnosis. Similarly, renal function studies can provide information concerning accompanying renal functional impairment, but they are not diagnostic per se. Measurement of blood glucose and serum cholesterol is also useful, because they are often elevated in hypertension and represent additional risk factors for subsequent development of atherosclerosis.

Special diagnostic tests

Additional tests of renal, endocrine, or neurogenic status are indicated when the history and physical findings or the routine diagnostic studies suggest the need for further diagnostic work-up. Also, severe unexplained hypertension in the young, malignant hypertension in any age group, and failure to respond to ordinary therapeutic regimens should be considered further indications for special diagnostic survey studies.

Percutaneous renal biopsy and the renal scan may, in some cases, provide definitive clues to hypertensive disorders which are renal parenchymal in origin. The renal scintiscanner[17] utilizes mercurial diuretics tagged with ^{203}Hg. With the renal scan, the viable renal parenchyma is outlined, and nonviable tissue composed of tumor, cyst, infarction, or atrophied structures stands out by contrast. Overall, this test appears to have limited application in the diagnosis of hypertension. However, in an occasional instance, a specific diagnostic problem; e.g., polycystic kidney disease or renal infarction may be clarified with the use of this test. Furthermore, the renal scan is sometimes valuable in the renal evaluation of patients who are hypersensitive to contrast medium. Definitive histologic diagnosis of renal parenchymal disease can be established by percutaneous renal biopsy; e.g., the diagnosis of acute proliferative glomerulonephritis or lupus erythematosus may be so established when other diagnostic studies are indefinite.

Random sampling of plasma renin activity has proved to be confusing and generally inaccurate in the differentiation of hyper-, hypo-, and normoreninemic hypertension (Table 68-3). However, stimulated renin measurements appear to be much more reliable.[18] The patient is given 60 mg furosemide by mouth, and 5 h later plasma renin activity is measured. This test may be used to identify those patients requiring further evaluation for remediable secondary hypertension.

Renal artery stenosis is being recognized as an increasingly frequent cause of blood pressure elevation; renal arterial hypertension is, in fact, the most common known potentially curable form of diastolic hypertension. In addition to the intravenous pyelogram, studies which may be helpful in the diagnosis of renovascular hypertension include isotope renography, renal arteriography, differential renal function studies, and measurement of plasma renin activity.

The isotope renogram, utilizing ^{131}I-labeled Hippuran, is not a specific diagnostic study, but it does provide a qualitative indication of individual renal functional capacity. Perhaps the chief value of the renogram is the availability of a simultaneous cross comparison of renal vascular flow. The advantages of this study are as follows: (1) the test is easy to perform, (2) reactions to the test are rare, (3) the study may be completed in 30 min, (4) the test may be repeated several times in a given day, and (5) the cost is reasonable. Some investigators believe that the renogram is superior to the excretory pyelogram for screening hypertensive patients. Morris and De-Bakey report that 90 percent of their patients with proved renal arterial hypertension had abnormal renograms,[19] and Hunt found the renogram to be distinctly abnormal in 36 of 37 patients with renal arterial hypertension.[20] Stewart and Haynie found the renogram to be highly reliable in diagnosing unilateral main artery occlusion but less accurate in the diagnosis of bilateral renal artery occlusion.[21] Although positive renograms and excretory pyelograms do not always coincide in the same patient, a combination of the two may identify a renal artery

lesion in a larger number of cases than either study used alone.[22]

The definitive diagnosis of unilateral or bilateral renal arterial disease ultimately depends on renal arteriography. Since renal arterial insufficiency may be present despite normal pyelography, differential renal function studies, or isotope renography, renal angiography is recommended whenever the clinical picture suggests the possible occurrence of this lesion. Either translumbar or percutaneous (transfemoral or transbrachial) arteriography is satisfactory. However, most radiologists appear to prefer the transfemoral retrograde aortic technique. In addition to studies made with the tip of the catheter placed just below the origin of the renal arteries, it is extremely valuable to selectively catheterize the renal arteries for direct injection of contrast medium to delineate the distal part of the main renal artery and the primary and intrarenal branches.[23] It must be recognized that renal arteriography serves only to identify an anatomic lesion in the renal arteries. Whether or not an occlusive lesion is responsible for the hypertension depends on a correlation of the arteriographic findings with the clinical situation and the data obtained from other diagnostic procedures. In fact, Eyler et al. found that a large number of patients with stenotic lesions of the renal arteries were normotensive.[24] When it is uncertain whether a lesion is responsible for the patient's hypertension, measurement of renin activity and/or differential renal function studies should be performed.

The application of differential renal function tests in the diagnosis of renal ischemia is based on the experimental work of White.[25] He found that constriction of a renal artery in the dog led to marked reduction in the volume of sodium concentration of urine obtained from the involved kidney as compared with urine collected simultaneously from the contralateral kidney. On the basis of these findings, Connor et al. proposed that a 50 percent or greater decrease in volume excreted and a 15 percent or greater decrease in sodium concentration indicated renal artery obstruction and reversible renovascular hypertension.[26] These criteria have proved reliable but too restrictive. Subsequently, Howard and Connor and their coworkers modified their indications of a "positive" test by the addition of creatinine clearance to the study.[27] An increase in the urine creatinine concentration is felt to be confirmatory evidence of greater water reabsorption as a cause of the decreased volume from the suspected kidney. Modifications of the differential renal function study have been described by Stamey,[28] Birchall et al.,[29] and Rapaport.[30] The practical differences in the results obtained with these methods have been small. Although still clinically useful, the magnitude of the procedure and the asociated morbidity and occasional mortality have made many clinicians reluctant to use differential renal function studies.

Mounting evidence indicates that the renin-angiotensin system plays a substantive role in the pathogenesis of renal arterial hypertension. Accordingly, the measurement of plasma renin activity has been used increasingly in selecting for operation those patients who are likely to benefit from renal revascularization or nephrectomy. The measurement of renin activity in the renal venous blood and in the inferior vena cava has become a valued clinical procedure. Preparation of such patients by sodium depletion and by keeping them upright for 3 to 4 h prior to renal venous sampling increases the sensitivity of the test by increasing the ratio of, and differences between, the renin activity in the two renal veins.[31] The measurement of renin activity in peripheral blood is generally considered a less sensitive indicator of renal ischemia. More recently, pharmacologic blockade with angiotensin antagonists has been advocated as a means of identifying angiotensinogenic hypertension and also of estimating surgical curability.[32] However, the ultimate usefulness of this testing procedure is still uncertain.

The clinical suspicion of pheochromocytoma should be tested by specific pharmacologic and chemical studies (see Chap. 71).

Adrenal lesions other than pheochromocytoma which may be responsible for diastolic hypertension include Cushing's syndrome, primary aldosteronism, and the hypertensive form of adrenogenital syndrome.

Cushing's syndrome can be diagnosed by demonstrating an excessive secretion of glucocorticoid hormone.[33] Elevated plasma and/or urine levels of 17-hydroxycorticoid at a time when the patient is not under acute exogenous stress strongly favor the diagnosis. Sometimes, patients with Cushing's syndrome have 17-hydroxycorticoid excretions in the high-normal range, and the diagnosis must be established with other tests. Screening procedures suggesting the diagnosis include a 24-h urine collection containing more than 10 mg of 17-hydroxycorticoids, a diabetic glucose tolerance curve, eosinophil count of less than 100 per cubic millimeter, and loss of the normal diurnal steroid excretion pattern. In patients with Cushing's syndrome, an equal or greater 17-hydroxycorticoid and 17-ketosteroid excretion occurs during the night, as compared with the day.

Hypokalemic alkalosis in a hypertensive patient, particularly when associated with an elevated serum sodium concentration and neutral or alkaline urine, is strongly suggestive of primary aldosteronism. An important diagnostic point is the demonstration of a liberal potassium level in a patient on a normal dietary intake of sodium and potassium. However, the crucial diagnostic findings involve an evaluation of the renin-angiotensin system under specific test conditions.[34] Specifically, the diagnosis depends on the demonstration of (1) elevated aldosterone secretion despite sodium loading and (2) low plasma renin activity despite sodium restriction and upright posture. These two fundamental phenomena depend on the relatively autonomous nature of aldosterone secretion in primary aldosteronism. Adrenal tumors causing primary aldosteronism can be accurately diagnosed and lateralized preoperatively in almost all cases by appropriate clinical tests, adrenal vein sampling for aldosterone,[35] and adrenal venography.[36] More recently, adrenal imaging with ^{131}I-19-iodocholesterol has been used to locate the adrenal tumor.[37]

Congenital adrenal hyperplasia may be accompanied by hypertension.[38,39] The 11-β-hydroxylase deficiency is characterized by virilization of the infant, hypertension, hypokalemia, and high levels of deoxycorticosterone and 11-deoxycortisol. The 17-α-hydroxylase deficiency causes hypogonadism, hypertension, hypokalemia, high levels of deoxycorticosterone and low urinary 17-ketosteroids.

In hyperparathyroidism resulting from either an adenoma or hyperplasia of the glands, hypertension occurs in about 50 percent of the cases.[40] The blood pressure elevation is generally felt to be related to the secondary renal involvement of the disease. About 30 percent of patients with acromegaly have significant diastolic hypertension.[41] Conceivably, increased adrenocortical steroid production could cause elevation of blood pressure, but evidence of adrenocortical overactivity is lacking. Appropriate diagnostic studies are indicated if the clinical signs and symptoms suggest either of these disorders.

Finally, neurogenic lesions including brain tumor, cerebrovascular accident, and diencephalic syndrome may, at times, be responsible for diastolic hypertension. Their presence is generally suspected from the history and/or physical findings. Skull roentgenograms, electroencephalogram, brain scan, pneumoencephalogram, and/or cerebral angiography may be employed to confirm or deny the presence of these lesions.

In summary, all patients with hypertension (systolic or diastolic) should be evaluated in an effort to establish the cause of the abnormality. Only in this way will all potentially correctable hypertensive lesions be detected, and only in this manner can an intelligent therapeutic approach be followed.

REFERENCES

1 Melby, J. C.: Extensive Hypertensive Work-up: Pro, *J.A.M.A.*, 231:399, 1975.

2 Finnerty, F. A., Jr.: Extensive Hypertensive Work-up: Con, *J.A.M.A.*, 231:402, 1975.

3 Master, A. M., and Lasser, R. P.: Blood Pressure Elevation in the Elderly Patient, in A. N. Brest and J. H. Moyer (eds.), "Hypertension: Recent Advances: Second Hahnemann Symposium on Hypertensive Disease," Lea & Febiger, Philadelphia, 1961, p. 24.

4 Londe, S., and Goldring, D.: High Blood Pressure in Children: Problems and Guidelines for Evaluation and Treatment, *Am. J. Cardiol.*, 37:650, 1976.

5 Burch, G. E., and DePasquale, N. P.: "Primer of Clinical Measurement of Blood Pressure," The C. V. Mosby Company, St. Louis, 1962.

6 Frohlich, E. D., Tarazi, R. C., and Dustan, H. P.: Hyperdynamic Beta-Adrenergic Circulatory State: Increased Beta-Receptor Responsiveness, *Arch. Intern. Med.,* 123:1, 1969.

7 Gorlin, R.: The Hyperkinetic Heart Syndrome, *J.A.M.A.,* 182:823, 1962.

8 Laragh, J. H.: Oral Contraceptive Hypertension, *Postgrad. Med.,* 53:98, 1972.

9 Laragh, J. H.: Renin, Angiotensin and Aldosterone System in Pathogenesis and Management of Hypertensive Vascular Disease, *Am. J. Med.,* 52:633, 1972.

10 Carman, C. T., and Brashear, R. E.: Pheochromocytoma as an Inherited Abnormality, *N. Engl. J. Med.,* 263:419, 1960.

11 Whalen, R. E., and McIntosh, H. D.: Spectrum of Hereditary Renal Disease, *Am. J. Med.,* 33:282, 1966.

12 Gifford, R. W., Jr., Kvale, W. F., Maher, F. T., Roth, G. M., and Priestley, J. T.: Clinical Features, Diagnosis and Treatment of Pheochromocytoma: A Review of 76 Cases, *Mayo Clin. Proc.,* 39:281, 1964.

13 Conn, J. W.: Aldosteronism in Man, *J.A.M.A.,* 183:169, 1963.

14 Kinsey, D., Whitelaw, G. P., and Smithwick, R. H.: A Screening Test for Adrenal or Unilateral Renal Forms of Hypertension Based upon Postural Change in Blood Pressure, *Angiology,* 11:336, 1960.

15 Brest, A. N., Heider, C., and Moyer, J. H.: Diagnosis of Renal Hypertension: Medical Aspects, *J.A.M.A.,* 178:718, 1961.

16 Martin, J. F.: Urographic Diagnosis of Renovascular Disease, *Postgrad. Med.,* 40:289, 1966.

17 Sodee, D. B.: The Screening of Renal Hypertension Utilizing the Mercury-197 Chlormerodrin Uptake Study and Scan, *J. Urol.,* 94:313, 1965.

18 Wallach, L., Nyarai, I., and Dawson, K. G.: Stimulated Renin: A Screening Test for Hypertension, *Ann. Intern. Med.,* 82:27, 1975.

19 Morris, G. C., and DeBakey, M. E.: Diagnosis of Renal Vascular Disease, *Am. J. Cardiol.,* 9:756, 1962.

20 Hunt, J. C.: Clinical Aspects: Symposium on Hypertension Associated with Renal Disease, *Mayo Clin. Proc.,* 36:707, 1961.

21 Stewart, B. H., and Haynie, T. P.: Critical Appraisal of the Renogram in Renal Vascular Disease, *J.A.M.A.,* 180:454, 1962.

22 Dennis, J. M., Wolfel, D. A., and Young, J. D.: Diagnosis of Renovascular Hypertension: Role of the Radiologist, *Radiol. Clin. North Am.,* 1:61, 1963.

23 Kaufman, J. J., Lupu, A. N., and Maxwell, M. H.: Renovascular Hypertension: Clinical Characteristics, Diagnosis, and Treatment, *Cardiovasc. Clin.,* 1(1):79, 1969.

24 Eyler, W. R., Clark, M. D., Garman, J. E., Rian, R. L., and Meininger, D. E.: Angiography of the Renal Areas Including a Comparative Study of Renal Arterial Stenosis in Patients with and without Hypertension, *Radiology,* 78:879, 1962.

25 White, H. L.: "Excretion of Sodium in Relation to Glomerular Filtration," (transactions, second conference on renal function), Josiah Macy, Jr., Foundation, New York, 1950, p. 127.

26 Connor, T. B., Berthrong, M., Thomas, W. C., and Howard, J. E.: Hypertension Due to Unilateral Renal Disease: With a Report on a Functional Test Helpful in Diagnosis, *Johns Hopkins Med. J.,* 100:241, 1957.

27 Howard, J. E., and Connor, T. B.: Hypertension Produced by Unilateral Renal Disease, *Arch. Intern. Med.,* 100:62, 1962.

28 Stamey, T. A.: The Diagnosis of Curable Unilateral Renal Hypertension by Ureteral Catheterization, *Postgrad. Med.,* 29:496, 1961.

29 Birchall, R., Batson, H. M., Jr., and Brannan, W.: Contribution of Differential Renal Studies to the Diagnosis of Renal Arterial Hypertension with Emphasis on the Valve of U sodium/U creatine, *Am. J. Med.,* 32:164, 1962.

30 Rapaport, A.: Modification of the "Howard Test" for the Detection of Renal Artery Obstruction, *N. Engl. J. Med.,* 263:1159, 1960.

31 Vermillion, S. E., Sheps, S. G., Strong, C. G., Harrison, E. G., Jr., and Hunt, J. C.: Effect of Sodium Depletion of Renin Activity of Renal Venous Plasma in Renovascular Hypertension, *J.A.M.A.,* 208, 2302, 1969.

32 Streeten, D. H. P., Anderson, G. H., Freiberg, J. M., and Dalakos, T. G.: Use of an Angiotensin II Antagonist (Saralasin) in the Recognition of "Angiotensinogenic" Hypertension, *N. Engl. J. Med.,* 76:899, 1972.

33 Herrera, M. G., Cahill, G. F., Jr., and Thorn, G. W.: Cushing's Syndrome, Diagnosis and Treatment, *Am. J. Surg.,* 107:144, 1964.

34 Hickler, R. B.: Clinical Experiences with Primary Aldosteronism, *Cardiovasc. Clin.,* 1(1):177, 1969.

35 Melby, J. C., Spark, R. F., Dale, S. L., Egdahl, R. H., and Kahn, P. C.: Diagnosis and Localization of Aldosterone-producing Adenomas by Adrenal-Vein Catheterization, *N. Engl. J. Med.,* 277:1050, 1967.

36 Starer, F.: Percutaneous Suprarenal Venography, *Br. J. Radiol.,* 38:675, 1965.

37 Hogan, M. J., McRae, J., Schambelan, M., and Biglieri, E. G.: Location of Aldosterone-producing Adenomas with ^{131}I-19-Iodocholesterol, *N. Engl. J. Med.,* 294:410, 1976.

38 Bongiovanni, A. M., and Root, A. W.: The Adrenogenital Syndrome, *N. Engl. J. Med.,* 268:1283, 1342, 1391, 1963.

39 Biglieri, E. G., Herron, M. A., and Brust, N.: 17-Hydroxylation Deficiency in Man, *J. Clin. Invest.,* 45:1946, 1966.

40 Hellstrom, J., Birke, G., and Edvall, C. A.: Hypertension in Hyperparathyroidism, *Br. J. Urol.,* 30:13, 1958.

41 Gordon, D. A., Hill, F. M., and Ezrin, C.: Acromegaly: A Review of 100 Cases, *Can. Med. Assoc. J.,* 87:1106, 1962.

69
Parenchymal Renal Disease

A
The Major Disease Categories

ELBERT P. TUTTLE, JR., M.D.

The multiple types of function performed by the kidney are critical to the circulation. They may be summarized as (1) the regulation of body content of inorganic metabolites by selective excretion, (2) endocrine secretion of trophic and direct-acting hormones, and (3) specific functions in intermediate metabolism of organic substances which influence remote processes in the body. All three types of function may be compromised to varying degrees by parenchymal diseases of the kidney.

The body content of water, sodium, potassium,

chloride, calcium, and hydrogen ion is critically dependent on renal regulation and has marked significance for the circulation. Positive or negative balances of each and several may result from disease of the kidney. In addition to altered physiologic regulation, change in responsiveness to drugs is commonly seen with primary renal disease.

The endocrine secretions of the kidney which affect the circulation are renin-angiotensin,[1] erythropoietin,[2] and probably one or more blood pressure–reducing agents.[3] Renin and erythropoietin may be released by the kidney in excessive or insufficient amounts in various diseases of the kidney. The prostaglandins,[4] a small neutral antihypertensive lipid,[5] and a phospholipid renin inhibitor,[6] each acting as a vasodilator or blood pressure depressant, have all been extracted from animal kidneys. Moreover, considerable evidence has recently pointed toward local hormonal actions, particularly of prostaglandin E in modifying intrarenal blood flow and the renal excretion of sodium.[6a] Deficiency of one or more of these factors in advanced disease has been postulated as the cause of "renoprival hypertension." The relationships of excretory and secretory functions of the kidneys to the regulation of the blood pressure are indicated in Fig. 65-1.

The disturbances in intermediate metabolism which occur in renal disease are best typified by the processes of protein catabolism and reabsorption. One example of protein filtration and catabolic reabsorption is seen in the renal clearance of immunoreactive insulin. By arteriovenous differences it is cleared at a rate of 190 ml/min, while the clearance measured by excretion techniques is less than 1 ml/min. Thus, with blood levels at 14 microunits/ml, approximately 3 to 5 units per day are destroyed in the normal kidney.[7] Loss of this action may account in part for the reduced insulin requirement in diabetics with advanced renal destruction. This process is also important as a prototype for the destruction of large amounts of serum proteins in nephritis and nephrosis. External losses in the urine and internal catabolic reabsorption of filtered proteins by the tubules at rates exceeding the 12 g/day or more which can be synthesized and resynthesized diminish the mass of oncotically active material in the plasma and alter the distribution of water and salt between intravascular and interstitial compartments. This leads to the edema of nephrosis.

The various types and stages of parenchymal renal disease lead to alterations in the types of function outlined above, so that the circulation is often disturbed. The combinations of influences are numerous, and a specific diagnosis of circulatory physiology is a mandatory part of every diagnosis of renal disease. What will be found will depend not only on the pathologic process in the kidney, but on diet, drugs, and other circulatory, cardiac, or metabolic disease.

PYELONEPHRITIS

Although there is considerable agreement that hypertension and pyelonephritis have a high coincidence in human beings,[8] it is not clear whether pyelonephritis causes hypertension or hypertension predisposes to pyelonephritis. The situation is clouded by the fact that diagnostic criteria for pyelonephritis are poorly defined. Sterile vascular[9] and obstructive lesions[10] can produce in the kidney anatomic evidence of scarring, tubular dilatation, and inflammation, which are taken by many to be diagnostic of pyelonephritis. Until the definite diagnosis of pyelonephritis is restricted to cases in which bacteria can be proved to be present in the kidney or to have been present in the past, the specificity of the diagnosis will be low, and misinterpretation of clinicopathologic correlations will occur.

Several important phenomena occur in pyelonephritis which may exert strong influence on the circulation: (1) Focal scarring of the kidney leads to perivascular fibrosis and distortion of blood vessels; (2) the mass of renal tissue is reduced in chronic pyelonephritis; (3) the kidney of pyelonephritis becomes incapable of maximum sodium conservation or excretion.

The vascular lesion in pyelonephritis is illustrated in studies from the author's laboratory. Figure 69A-1 illustrates the proliferation of bacteria, highlighted by staining with specific fluorescent antibodies, in the immediate perivascular area of the kidney. Figure 69A-2 shows the edge of a focal pyelonephritic scar in the upper pole of a nephrectomy specimen. The tortuosity of blood vessels in this scarred area is illustrated by the repeated appearance of the medium-sized artery in the plane of the section. Figure 69A-3*B* shows a selective renal arteriogram of the same kidney. The tortuous, angulated vessels may be compared with a normal vascular pattern shown in Fig. 69A-3*A*.

The possibility that renal ischemia due to renal

FIGURE 69A-1 Light spots in the vicinity of the blood vessel are *Escherichia coli* stained by specific antibody labeled with fluorescein.

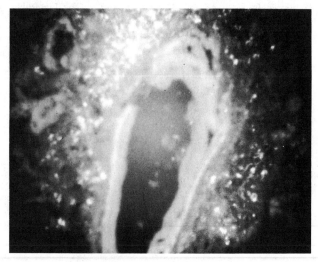

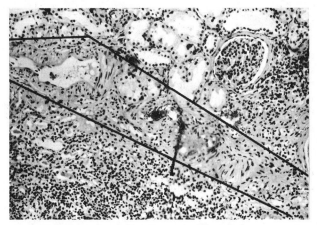

FIGURE 69A-2 Pyelonephritic scar; near the edge of the scar can be seen a tortuous arteriole twisting in and out of the plane of section.

vascular damage in pyelonephritis may produce hypertension is supported by the reports of relief of hypertension following nephrectomy in cases in which unilateral disease was present.[11] The extension of this concept to account for the relationship of pyelonephritis to hypertension has been postulated by Kincaid-Smith.[12]

In end-stage pyelonephritis the situation is somewhat different. Excessive release of renin cannot be demonstrated by bioassay of renal vein or peripheral blood. Indeed, in the 40- to 60-g kidneys of this stage, so few nephrons survive that little renin-forming tissue remains.

The demonstration of a potent blood pressure–depressing substance from the kidney by several groups[13,14] raises the possibility that loss of renal mass, enough, for instance, to produce the anemia of erythropoietin deficiency, would suffice to reduce significantly a blood pressure–lowering action of the kidney. Experimental support for the hypothesis of renoprival hypertension in animals has been referred to in Chap. 65. Hypertension may thus ensue from lack of antagonist. The blood pressure–lowering effect of renal transplantation in nephrectomized patients maintained by chronic dialysis supports the hypothesis that this mechanism is physiologically significant in human beings.[15] Prevention of experimental renoprival hypertension in the dog by implantation of nonexcretory renal tissue in the peritoneum has been demonstrated,[16] but this has not been demonstrated in hypertension with pyelonephritis in human beings. The vascular pattern in advanced chronic pyelonephritis, with great loss of tissue relative to blood vessel volume, is shown in Fig. 69A-3C, a selective renal arteriogram in a patient with long-standing disease, hypertension, and azotemia.

One reason for the variability of hypertension in pyelonephritis is the varying state of sodium balance in the disease. In some instances pyelonephritis is a salt-wasting disease and creates a degree of sodium depletion which can mask a marked tendency to hypertension. In many patients with severe chronic pyelonephritis this condition is achieved deliberately or inadvertently with rigorous restriction of dietary sodium. Conversely many patients with severe pyelonephritis cannot readily excrete large loads of salt. They can be made hypertensive on high sodium intakes. A single patient may be manipulated from one extreme to the other. This unusual sensitivity of the blood pressure to sodium intake in pyelonephritis undoubtedly obscures the relationship of pyelonephritis and hypertension. It is the author's impression that the underlying tendency toward hypertension is present in severe chronic pyelonephritis, in part from vascular disease, in part from loss of protective renal excretory and secretory mass.

A corollary of these considerations is the action of the pyelonephritic kidney in congestive heart failure. Impairment of maximum sodium conservation in the pyelonephritic kidney constitutes a built-in diuretic which can deplete the patient of salt as required, with careful control of sodium intake. The same may be said of the inability to conserve water in the isosthenuric stage. The impaired ability to manufacture ammonia makes acidifying agents more potent diuretics in many pyelonephritic patients, but the risk of inducing severe metabolic acidosis is correspondingly increased.

In cardiac patients it is mandatory to endeavor to differentiate between the azotemia resulting from the impaired renal perfusion of severe heart failure or vascular disease and the azotemia from destruction

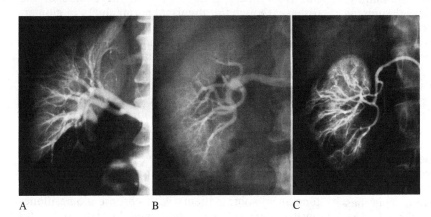

A   B   C

FIGURE 69A-3 A. Normal renal arteriogram. B. Arteriogram (from the patient in Fig. 69A-2) in acute and chronic pyelonephritis. Note the tortuosity of vessels compared with normal vessels. C. Late chronic pyelonephritis. Note the shrunken kidney, atrophy of tissue, and dense crowding of atrophic vessels. (Photographs courtesy of Dr. Richard S. Foster.)

of functioning nephrons by intrinsic renal disease. Toxic effects of overdosage of pharmacologic agents are much more likely in the presence of intrinsic renal disease. Renal concentrating ability, kidney size, excretion of radiographic contrast materials, the power to acidify the urine, sodium excretion on minimum intake, and abnormalities of the urine sediment are the clinical tools which aid in this differentiation.

NEPHROTIC SYNDROME

Recent research into the nature of nephrosis has thrown new light on some intermediate aspects of pathogenesis of the disturbance. It has been shown to occur when antibody combines with antigen of glomerular basement membrane or with the focal deposition in the basement membrane of antigen-antibody complexes formed elsewhere in the circulation.[17,18] Yet some cases of nephrosis in human beings show deposits in basement membrane which are not immunologic in origin. The extent of involvement of capillaries other than in the glomerulus is variable. It is clearly present in diabetes[19] and may be a component of some types of idiopathic nephrosis. The pathogenesis of the nephrotic syndrome is therefore quite diverse.[20]

A relationship of blood coagulation and the nephrotic syndrome has been pointed out.[21] Levels of plasma clotting factors, especially fibrinogen, have been found elevated in many nephrotic patients and have returned to normal when remission was induced by adrenal corticosteroids.[22] Thrombotic and embolic disease, originating in the renal vein, as well as in both upper and lower extremities, has been seen. Whether the clotting disturbance is a cause or an effect of the nephrotic syndrome is uncertain.

Under conditions of the classic syndrome of idiopathic nephrosis, the depletion of circulating albumin is partially or virtually compensated by the retention of salt and water. Arterial and venous pressures are low to normal, in spite of the presence of pitting edema. If either pressure is elevated, an additional diagnosis must be sought to account for the finding. An additional glomerulovascular disease such as glomerulonephritis, diabetes mellitus, or disseminated lupus may be present in patients with arterial hypertension, and should be sought by biopsy. Congestive heart failure, pericarditis, or pulmonary embolization is suggested by a high venous pressure and heavy albuminuria. A relatively rare contributing cause of anasarca and congestive heart failure in the diabetic with nephropathy is diffuse atherosclerotic narrowing of the multiple small branches of the renal artery just prior to their entry into the renal parenchyma. On the author's service a nephrotic syndrome in a patient with a pheochromocytoma disappeared when the adrenal tumor was removed. This has been previously but rarely seen by others.[23] The presence of albuminuria and glomerular pathology does not exclude etiologic diagnosis of pheochromocytoma.

Acute glomerulonephritis imposes special burdens on the heart and blood vessels. In combination, the water and sodium retention, the attendant increase of circulating blood volume,[24] the dilutional anemia, the increased peripheral resistance, and frequently a high cardiac output[25] increase both pressure work and flow work of the heart to produce a total load which leads to congestive heart failure. With a state of ventricular overload in the absence of hypertrophy and under the biochemical handicap of anemic blood, the heart is unable to maintain its compensation.

The cause of the circulatory disturbance in acute glomerulonephritis is quite obscure. The circulatory hallmarks of the disease, edema and hypertension, have been thought to arise from primary pathologic change limited to the renal glomerulus but causing remote effects through a humoral mechanism. Reports are in conflict,[26,27] but it is unlikely that renin is released in increased amounts in acute glomerulonephritis.[28] Diminution of glomerular filtration is not the cause, for glomerular filtration may remain normal.

The autonomic nervous system may contribute to the circulatory disturbance. If a purely humoral hypertension were involved, the negative feedback loops of the pressoreceptor system should lead to bradycardia and increased parasympathetic stimulus to the myocardium, as is seen with infusions of norepinephrine or angiotensin. On the contrary, in acute glomerulonephritis a tachycardia and hyperdynamic circulation are often seen, and the blood pressure is exquisitely sensitive to sympathetic blockade. Thus, if the hypertension is essentially a humoral one, the humor has the capacity to recruit the autonomic system. Fortunately a combined attack upon the sodium retention with sympatholytic drugs and diuretics brings a prompt response. It is not clear that the cardiac glycosides are clinically beneficial in the congestive-overload type of heart failure that occurs in acute glomerulonephritis, but there seems to be no contraindication to their use.

The circulatory effects of chronic glomerulonephritis depend on the stage of the disease. In the early or "latent" stage of the chronic glomerulonephritis, often the blood pressure is still normal, and the edema and abnormalities of electrolyte metabolism result from the abnormal handling of protein, not from heart failure. Late in the course of the disease, though the abnormal permeability of glomerular capillaries to protein often persists, severe reduction of glomerular filtration minimizes albumin loss, and the nephrotic syndrome disappears. Either because of vascular disease or loss of renal mass, or in part because of reconstitution of the intravascular oncotic material, at this stage of the disease hypertension appears or becomes more severe. In the late stages of glomerulonephritis severe hypertension is a major problem. The relative contributions of renal ischemia and of loss of renal vasodepressor function are obscure. Bilateral nephrectomy, followed by chronic dialysis, has resulted in reduction in hypertension in some patients with chronic glomerulonephritis, but they have remained hypertensive until successful transplantation was accomplished.[15]

A number of less common types of renal disease affect the circulation in a manner similar to that of renal diseases already mentioned. Disseminated lupus erythematosus, diabetic nephropathy, and pseudoxanthoma elasticum behave in a physiologic manner similar to acute, subacute, or chronic glomerulonephritis. Polycystic renal disease, renal tubular acidosis, and renal injury from analgesic abuse behave like chronic pyelonephritis.

REFERENCES

1 Peart, W. S.: The Renin-Angiotensin System, *Pharmacol. Rev.*, 17:143, 1965.

2 Weyer, E. M., and Fisher, J. W. (eds.): Erythropoietin, *Ann. N.Y. Acad. Sci.*, 149:1, 1968.

3 Masson, G. M. C. (ed.): Antihypertensive Function of Kidneys, in I. H. Page and J. W. McCubbin (eds.), "Renal Hypertension," The Year Book Medical Publishers, Inc., Chicago, 1968, p. 296.

4 Bergstrom, S., Carlson, L. A., and Weeks, J. R.: The Prostaglandins: A Family of Biologically Active Lipids, *Pharmacol. Rev.*, 20:1, 1968.

5 Muirhead, E. E., Brooks, B., Kosinski, M., Daniels, E. G., and Hinman, J. W.: Renomedullary Antihypertensive Principle in Renal Hypertension, *J. Lab. Clin. Med.*, 67:778, 1967.

6 Sen, S., Smeby, R. R., and Bumpus, F. M.: Isolation of a Phospholipid Renin Inhibitor from Kidney, *Biochemistry*, 6:1572, 1967.

6a Lee, J. B.: Cardiovascular-Renal Effects of Prostaglandins. The Antihypertensive, Natriuretic Renal "Endocrine" Functions, *Arch. Intern. Med.*, 133:56, 1974.

7 Chamberlain, M. J., and Stimmler, L.: The Renal Handling of Insulin, *J. Clin. Invest.*, 46:911, 1967.

8 Brod, J.: Chronic Pyelonephritis, in D. A. K. Black, "Renal Disease," F. A. Davis Company, Philadelphia, 1962, p. 293.

9 Allen, A. C.: "The Kidney," 2d ed., Grune & Stratton, Inc., New York, 1962, p. 627.

10 Freedman, L. R., Warner, A. S. Beck, D., and Paplanus, S.: Experimental Pyelonephritis: IX. The Bacteriological Course and Morphological Consequences of Staphylococcal Pyelonephritis in the Rat, with Consideration of the Specificity of the Pathological Changes Observed, *Yale J. Biol. Med.*, 34:40, 1962.

11 Butler, A. M.: Chronic Pyelonephritis and Arterial Hypertension, *J. Clin. Invest.*, 16:889, 1937.

12 Kincaid-Smith, P.: Vascular Obstruction in Chronic Pyelonephritic Kidneys and Its Relation to Hypertension, *Lancet*, 2:1263, 1955.

13 Booth, E., Hinman, J. W., Daniels, E. G., Kosinski, M., and Muirhead, E. E.: Antihypertensive Renal Factor, *J. Clin. Invest.*, 42:918, 1963. (Abstract.)

14 Hickler, R. B., Saravis, C. A., Mowbray, J. F., Lauler, D. P., Vagnucci, A. I., and Thorn, G. W.: Renomedullary Vasopressor Factor, *J. Clin. Invest.*, 42:942, 1963. (Abstract).

15 Kolff, W. J., Nakamoto, S., Poutasse, E. F., Straffon, R. A., and Figueroa, J. E.: The Effect of Bilateral Nephrectomy and Transplantation on Hypertension in Man, *Circulation*, 30(suppl. 2):23, 1964.

16 Muirhead, E. E., Stirman, J. A., and Jones, F.: Renal Autoexplantation and Protection against Renoprival Hypertensive Cardiovascular Disease and Hemolysis, *J. Clin. Invest.*, 29:266, 1960.

17 Drummond, K. N., Michael, A. F., Good, R. F., and Venier, R. L.: The Nephrotic Syndrome of Childhood: Immunologic, Clinical and Pathologic Correlations, *J. Clin. Invest.*, 45:620, 1966.

18 Dixon, F. J.: The Pathogenesis of Glomerulonephritis, *Am. J. Med.*, 44:493, 1968.

19 Siperstein, M. D., Norton, W., Unger, R. H., and Madison, L. L.: Muscle Capillary Basement Membrane Width in Normal, Diabetic, and Pre-Diabetic Patients, *Trans. Assoc. Am. Physicians*, 79:330, 1966.

20 Smith, F. G., Gonick, H., Stanley, T. M., and McIntosh, R. M.: The Nephrotic Syndrome: Current Concepts, *Ann. Intern. Med.*, 76:463, 1972.

21 Kendall, A. G., Lohmann, R. C., and Dossetor, J. B.: Nephrotic Syndrome: A Hypercoagulable State, *Arch. Intern. Med.*, 127:1021, 1971.

22 Lieberman, E., Heuser, E., Gilchrist, G. S., and Landing, B. H.: Thrombosis, Nephrosis and Corticosteroid Therapy, *J. Pediatr.*, 73:320, 1968.

23 Rizzuto, V. J., Mazzara, J. J., and Grace, W. J.: Pheochromocytoma with Nephrotic Syndrome, *Am. J. Cardiol.*, 16:432, 1965.

24 Eisenberg, S.: Blood Volume in Patients with Acute Glomerulonephritis, *Am. J. Med.*, 27:241, 1959.

25 De Fazio, V., Christensen, R. C., Regan, T. J., Baer, L. J., Morita, Y., and Hellems, H. K.: Circulatory Changes in Acute Glomerulonephritis, *Circulation*, 20:190, 1959.

26 Massani, Z. M., Finkielman, S., Worcel, M., Agrest, A., and Paladini, A. C.: Angiotensin Blood Levels in Hypertensive and Non-hypertensive Diseases, *Clin. Sci.*, 30:473, 1966.

27 Gunnells, J. C.: Circulating Vasoconstrictor Materials in Hypertension, *Circulation*, 30(suppl. 3):90, 1964.

28 Fukuda, M., Greene, J. A., and Vander, A. J.: Plasma Renin Activity during Development of Experimental Antiserum Glomerulonephritis, *J. Lab. Clin. Med.*, 71:148, 1968.

B
Chronic Renal Failure and Dialysis

SUSAN K. FELLNER, M.D.

Nephrologists sometimes joke that the heart is a simple pump designed to deliver 20 percent of its output to the kidney—that elegant regulator of the body's volume and chemical composition. Regardless of one's point of view, it is clear that the kidney has a multiplicity of functions which, when deranged, have profound effects upon cardiovascular function. In recent years, clearer understanding of the pathophysiology of renal failure coupled with new techniques of therapy have greatly prolonged the survival of patients with advanced renal disease managed either conservatively or with chronic hemodialysis. Circulatory disturbances in these patients are prevalent and threatening problems, requiring recognition of a number of interrelated physiologic factors followed by meticulous medical management. The consequences of certain aspects of impaired renal function will be examined in relationship to their effects on the circulation in chronic renal disease.

SODIUM

Patients with severe impairment of renal function are able to preserve sodium balance to a remarkable degree by varying the fractional reabsorption of filtered sodium. Whereas normal individuals excrete less than 1 percent of filtered sodium on a 4-g sodium diet, those with severe renal insufficiency can excrete 10 percent of filtered sodium. The mechanism by which increased sodium excretion is achieved appears to be related to the inhibition of tubular reabsorption of sodium in response to expansion of the extracellular fluid volume and is not related to variations in aldosterone secretion.[1]

Despite preservation of sodium regulation within limits, patients with chronic renal failure are prone to develop sodium overload and either severe hypertension or vascular congestion or both. Possibly the effects of chronic acidosis upon cardiovascular dynamics are an important added variable. When such patients develop congestive heart failure clearly related to volume overload, therapy consists of one or more of the following: (1) regulation of sodium intake, (2) diuresis with large doses of potent diuretics (ethacrynic acid or furosemide), (3) correction of acidosis, (4) plasmaphoresis, or (5) dialysis.

Conversely, patients with chronic renal disease may become sodium depleted as a consequence of rigid dietary restriction, renal disease in which derangement of medullary and interstitial architecture results in "sodium wasting," or overly enthusiastic treatment with diuretics of congestive heart failure. Diuresis sufficient to relieve pulmonary edema in severe heart failure may reduce cardiac output to the extent that glomerular filtration is further impaired. Likewise, overly vigorous therapy with antihypertensive drugs can reduce renal plasma flow, thereby worsening existing renal insufficiency.

It must be emphasized that in the course of chronic renal failure, a single patient may have problems with sodium overload or sodium depletion. Careful attention to the state of sodium and volume balance is imperative in each patient's management.

POTASSIUM

The effects of hyperkalemia upon the heart and the acute treatment of hyperkalemia with bicarbonate, insulin and glucose, calcium, and ion-exchange resins are well known and will not be dealt with here.

The chronically diseased kidney is able to increase secretion of potassium sufficiently to keep the level of serum potassium below 6 mEq/liter until the terminal stages of renal failure with oliguria are reached, or unless other circumstances modify excretion or load. If sodium intake is rigidly restricted, insufficient sodium is delivered to the distal tubule for active reabsorption and creation of luminal electronegativity necessary for potassium secretion. Severe heart failure will also limit distal exchange because of avid proximal sodium reabsorption. In this setting, diuretics are helpful in preventing hyperkalemia by increasing distal delivery of sodium. Worsening of acidosis will increase extracellular potassium levels when cellular potassium is released from cells as hydrogen ions enter. Potassium is also released into the plasma in those circumstances associated with cellular destruction such as pneumonia, gastrointestinal bleeding, transfusion of old blood, or shock.

Despite the fact that chronic renal failure is often associated with reduced total body stores of potassium,[2] hypokalemia is rarely seen, even in those conditions in which secondary aldosteronism or distal tubular potassium wasting is a prominent feature of the earlier stage of the disease. Patients undergoing chronic hemodialysis provide an important exception. Dialysate potassium in most centers is about 2.0 mEq/liter. These patients are therefore subject to wide shifts of serum potassium during dialysis, at which time problems with spontaneous arrhythmias or digitalis intoxication may occur. Consequently, some patients may require adjustment of dietary potassium intake or administration of potassium on dialysis.

CALCIUM

Total serum calcium is usually reduced in chronic renal failure, primarily as a result of diminished synthesis of active metabolites of vitamin D by the diseased kidney, particularly in the setting of high levels of intracellular phosphate. Furthermore, when hyperphosphatemia is present, complexing of calcium with phosphate reduces the amount of ionized calcium available for electrochemical activity. Serum phosphate is maintained at nearly normal values through stimulation of parathyroid hormone secretion until the glomerular filtration rate falls to about 25 ml/min, at which point the increased secretion of parathormone is no longer able to prevent phosphate retention by further inhibition of tubular reabsorption.[3]

Disorders of calcium and phosphorus metabolism in chronic renal disease have a variety of effects upon the cardiovascular system, including vascular calcifications, myocardial calcification, and hypotension. When the product of serum calcium and phosphorus concentration expressed in milligram per hundred milliliter exceeds levels of 70 to 80, metastatic calcifications are likely to occur in the cornea of the eye, the interstitial tissues, the lung, the renal tubules, and the media of small and medium-sized arteries. Such arterial calcifications can result in coronary occlusion or peripheral vascular ischemia to the point of gangrene.[4]

An unusual and potentially fatal variety of metastatic calcification involves the atrioventricular node and conducting system of the heart, resulting in atrioventricular block.[5] In addition, some patients with persistently elevated calcium-phosphorus product may develop a calcific cardiomyopathy characterized clinically by intractable heart failure and atrioventricular block, and pathologically by meta-

Restriction of dietary phosphate and treatment with oral phosphate binding gels is helpful in reducing serum phosphorus both for patients on conservative management and those undergoing chronic dialysis.

Occasionally, patients with chronic renal failure and hypocalcemia demonstrate relative hypotension and evidence of low cardiac output, which are reversible with the infusion of calcium. Shackney and Hasson[7] have reviewed the cardiovascular effects of hypocalcemia, suggesting several possible causes of hypocalcemic hypotension: (1) myocardial contractility is reduced in the presence of low concentrations of ionized calcium; (2) the magnitude of the contractile response of vascular smooth muscle varies directly, within limits, with calcium concentration; (3) release of norepinephrine from adrenal medulla and from sympathetic postganglionic fibers varies directly with the concentration of calcium. When faced with the clinical problem of hypotension and/or low cardiac output, one should consider the possibility of low levels of ionized, uncomplexed calcium as an etiologic factor. Care must be taken not to precipitate digitalis intoxication with rapid infusion of calcium. In the chronic situation, measures aimed at raising serum calcium include treatment with oral calcium preparations or vitamin D analogues or dialysis against a bath with a high calcium concentration. It is imperative that serum phosphorus be reduced toward normal levels first, in order to prevent the creation of a dangerously high calcium-phosphorus product.

ACIDOSIS

Metabolic acidosis resulting from the titration of total-body buffer stores by hydrogen ions is an invariable concomitant of chronic renal failure. Patients with renal insufficiency develop heart failure from a variety of causes, e.g., volume overload, hypertension, and anemia, to name but a few. Severe metabolic acidosis may convert a state of marginal myocardial compensation to one of failure with pulmonary edema. Two explanations for the circulatory effects of acidosis can be offered. One is a reduction in left ventricular contractility.[8] The other is constriction of the venous system.[9]

In patients already overloaded with salt and water and who are severely oliguric, dialysis may offer the only solution to relieving congestive overload and acidosis. In nonoliguric patients, rigid salt restriction and administration of sodium bicarbonate or other alkaline salts is a satisfactory mode of therapy.

ANEMIA

The pathogenesis of the anemia of renal insufficiency is complex, resulting from the failure of renal endocrine function (erythropoietin), the failure of renal excretory function, and the etiology of the renal disease itself.[10]

When it is felt that anemia per se is contributing to disturbed cardiovascular function, restoration of the hematocrit to the range of 20 to 25 percent with cautious transfusion of packed red blood cells may be helpful in patients not undergoing chronic hemodialysis. Currently, most dialysis centers have abandoned the practice of repeated blood transfusions to achieve some arbitrary level of hematocrit. Not only has the high cost of blood and the risk of hepatitis been circumvented, but it has been found that most patients respond to the stimulus of severe anemia with erythropoiesis sufficient to achieve hematocrits equal to or better than those previously produced with transfusion.[11]

Further stimulation of erythropoiesis in dialyzed patients has been shown to occur with the use of androgenic steroids.[12]

AZOTEMIA

When glomerular filtration falls, urea accumulates in the blood because of failure of excretion. Accumulation of urea and other specific products of nitrogen metabolism produce many of the symptoms and abnormal physiology of the uremic syndrome. These can be minimized by institution of an appropriate renal failure diet[13] containing regulated amounts of sodium, potassium, and high biologic-value protein, along with full vitamin supplements. Such therapy generally is begun when renal function falls below 25 percent of normal.

Azotemia in the absence of severe renal insufficiency can occur from overproduction of urea and from excessive tubular reabsorption. Excessive tubular reabsorption of urea occurs in those clinical situations in which there is reduction of renal perfusion, *independent* of the volume of the extracellular fluid compartment. For example, congestive heart failure, severe nephrotic syndrome, constrictive pericarditis, and hepatic cirrhosis with ascites have in common the delivery of an inadequate arterial volume to the kidney despite the fact that these conditions are typically associated with an expansion of the total extracellular fluid compartment. Enhanced proximal tubular reabsorption of sodium (and water) ultimately favors the reabsorption of urea as well. Because proximal sodium reabsorption results in diminished urine volume, urine flow is slowed and passive reabsorption of urea is enhanced in the distal tubule and collecting ducts. In this setting, azotemia is worsened by such catabolic states as infection, surgery, and treatment with corticosteroids.

Patients with severe congestive heart failure may demonstrate excessive production as well as reabsorption of urea resulting in serum levels of over 100 mg/100 ml. This increased urea production may derive from skeletal muscle breakdown as a consequence of circulatory hypoxemia.[14]

The diagnosis of *prerenal azotemia* is aided by the findings of serum urea/creatinine ratio of 20:1 or greater; urine of high osmolality with very low concentrations of sodium (unless diuretics have been given); and a urine sediment which contains only occasional granular casts.

EXCRETION OF DRUGS

Modification of the dosage of drugs which depend wholly or in part upon renal excretion has been conveniently tabulated by Bennett et al.[15] A guide to the use of cardiovascular and antihypertensive drugs and diuretics is shown in Table 69B-1.

SPECIFIC COMPLICATIONS

In addition to the effects of disturbed renal physiology upon the cardiovascular system, there are several specific complications which affect patients with chronic renal failure or those undergoing chronic dialysis.

Bacterial endocarditis in dialysis patients

Bacterial endocarditis has been considered a rare complication of acquired arteriovenous fistulas in man.[16] Lillehei and associates[17] were able to produce bacterial endocarditis without deliberate introduction of bacteria in normal dogs in whom they created very large arteriovenous fistulas. These animals had greatly increased cardiac outputs and plasma volumes. They concluded that severe increases in cardiac workload were sufficient to predispose to the development of bacterial endocarditis.

Since the introduction of chronic dialysis for the treatment of end-stage renal disease, a whole new population of patients with acquired arteriovenous fistulas has emerged. These fistulas are of several types: the external silastic shunt (Quinton-Scribner), the subcutaneous arteriovenous fistula (Brescia), generally created between the radial artery and a nearby vein, and the bovine heterograft subcutaneous fistula. Although subcutaneous fistulas must be punctured with large bore needles for each dialysis, they have the advantage of being freer of the complications of clotting and infection.

Reports of bacterial endocarditis in hemodialysis patients began to appear in the medical literature in 1966. Among these are two large series, that from the Atlanta Regional Nephrology Center of Emory University,[18] and a report from the Regional Kidney Disease Center in Minnesota.[19] Table 69B-2 compares the findings from these two centers. A variety of gram-positive and gram-negative organisms infected the valves of the left side of the heart in 14 of 17 patients. Three patients had right-sided lesions. Except for one patient with acute renal failure undergoing peritoneal dialysis, all patients in both series had external silastic arteriovenous shunts.

In the Atlanta series, one patient had rheumatic heart disease and one had calcification of the aortic valve. However, a case can be made for the existence of heart disease in all of these patients as a consequence of very longstanding volume overload and hypertension prior to the institution of dialysis. Seven of the eight patients had renal diseases characterized by a prolonged time course, significant renal insufficiency having been present for more than 10 years before chronic dialysis was begun.

While drug addicts have taught us that valvular heart disease is not a prerequisite for the development of bacterial endocarditis, the presence of heart disease certainly favors its occurrence. Patients with chronic volume overload, hypertension, and anemia may be analogous to Lillehei's dogs[17] in whom the stress of greatly increased workload was sufficient to predispose to bacterial endocarditis.

The Atlanta group has not had a patient with bacterial endocarditis since 1970. It is felt that aggressive management of all infections, prompt removal of infected shunts, and the change to subcutaneous fistulas as the vascular access for hemodialysis in most patients have helped to prevent this complication. Leonard et al.[19] feel that antibiotic therapy alone does not alter the outcome of bacterial endocarditis in dialysis patients and that only surgical intervention with valve replacement offers a chance for survival. Of their two dialysis patients who survived, one had undergone valve replacement. In contrast, 50 percent of the Atlanta patients survived with antibiotic therapy alone.

The following factors may predispose chronic dialysis patients to the development of bacterial endocarditis: (1) circulatory stress from the arteriovenous shunt or fistula; (2) increased cardiac workload from chronic hypervolemia, hypertension, and anemia; (3) the shunt itself becoming a nidus for infection; (4) impaired resistance to infection characteristic of end-stage renal disease.

Pericarditis

Pericarditis is a common complication of acute and chronic renal failure and usually resolves following dialysis. Paradoxically, pericarditis occurs in approximately 15 percent of patients undergoing chronic hemodialysis. Several groups have recently reviewed the clinical features and management of uremic pericarditis.[20,21,22]

CLINICAL FEATURES
Fever frequently associated with chills, leukocytosis, chest pain, pericardial friction rub at some time during the illness, and gallop rhythm are commonly present. Pulmonary vascular congestion is nearly always seen on chest x-ray; documentation of the presence of effusion can be made reliably and noninvasively with echocardiography (see Chap. 32A). While supraventricular arrhythmias are frequently seen on the electrocardiogram, other classic changes associated with pericarditis are observed in a minority of patients. Likewise, few patients demonstrate Kussmaul's sign or paradoxical pulse (pulsus para-

TABLE 69B-1
Use of cardiovascular, antihypertensive, and diuretic agents in renal failure

Drug	Route of excretion	Normal half-life, h	Maintenance dose intervals				Significant dialysis of drug†	Toxic effects *remarks
			Normal	Renal failure				
				Mild	Moderate	Severe		
Antiarrhythmic agents*								*All agents in this subgroup: excretion enhanced in acid urine; blood levels best guide to therapy
Lidocaine*	Hepatic* (Renal:<20%)	.1-.2(part)** 1.2-2.2 (part)	IV drip or boluses	Unchanged	Unchanged	Unchanged	?	*Subgroup remarks **Biexponential pharmacokinetics: clearance depends on hepatic blood flow; specific nomograms available[350]‡
Procainamide* (Pronestyl)	Renal (60%)* (Nonrenal)	2.5-4.5	Q3h	Q3h	Q4.5-6h** (×1.5-2)	Q6-9h** (×2-3)	Yes (H)	*Subgroup remarks **Usual clinical practice to decrease size and frequency of dose
Propranolol (Inderal)	Hepatic*	3.2(PO)* .1(part IV)** 2.8(part IV)	Q6h	Unchanged	Unchanged	Unchanged	No (H)	*Clearance depends on hepatic blood flow; threshold exists: PO dose <30 mg completely extracted by normal liver **Biexponential pharmacokinetics (complex in uremia); blood levels best guide
Quinidine*	Renal	3-16	Q6h	Unchanged	Unchanged	Unchanged	Yes (HP)	*Subgroup remarks
Antihypertensive agents*								*Blood pressure response best guide
Diazoxide*	Renal (Nonrenal: 20%)	22-31	IV bolus	Unchanged	Unchanged	Unchanged**	Yes (HP)	*Subgroup remarks **Decrease dose size if given very frequently; very rapid injection needed for therapeutic response
Guanethidine*	Nonrenal Renal (25-40%)	48-72(part)** 216-240(part)	Q24h	Q24h	Q24-36h (×1.5)	Q36-48h (×1.5-2)		*Subgroup remarks **Biexponential pharmacokinetics; tricyclic antidepressants decrease therapeutic effectiveness; may decrease renal blood flow
Hydralazine* (Apresoline)	Hepatic** Gastrointestinal (? Renal)	2-7.8	Q8h	Q8h	Q8h	Q8-16h (×2)	No (HP)	*Subgroup remarks **Genetic variation in metabolism exists
Methyldopa* (Aldomet)	Renal* Hepatic	1.4-2 (part,95%)** 5.2-8.1 (part,5%)	Q6h	Q6h	Q9-12h (×1.5-2)	Q12-18h** (×2-3)	Yes (HP)	*Subgroup remarks **Biexponential pharmacokinetics; 5% part may increase to 50% in severe renal failure with retention of active metabolites Prolonged hypotension; hepatitis (HAA negative)
Minoxidil*	Nonrenal	4.2**	Q24h	Unchanged	Unchanged	Unchanged	?	Prolonged hypotension (may be due to tissue binding) *Subgroup remarks **Plasma half-life (does not reflect extensive tissue binding)
Reserpine*	Nonrenal	4.5(part)** 48-168(part)	Q24h	Unchanged	Unchanged	Unchanged	No (HP)	Excessive sedation; gastrointestinal bleeding *Subgroup remarks **Biexponential pharmacokinetics for drug and metabolites

(Table continues on p. 1408.)

TABLE 69B-1   (continued)

Drug	Route of excretion	Normal half-life, h	Maintenance dose intervals Normal	Renal failure Mild	Renal failure Moderate	Renal failure Severe	Significant dialysis of drug†	Toxic effects *remarks
Cardiac glycosides*								*Add to uremic gastrointestinal symptoms; blood levels best guide to therapy (about 12h after dose)[387]; computer dosage programs available[386,395]; usual clinical practice to decrease size and frequency of dose. Toxicity may be enhanced by dialysis K^+ removal
Digitoxin	Hepatic** Renal: metabolites	72-144***	Q24h	Q24h	Q24h	Q24-36h** (×1.5)	No (HP)	*Subgroup remarks **Converted to digoxin (8%); conversion increased in uremia ***Blood level depends on plasma protein concentration and drug binding
Digoxin*	Renal (Nonrenal: 15%)	36	Q24h	Q24h	Q36h (×1.5)	Q36-72h** (×1.5-3)	No (HP)	*Subgroup remarks **Decrease loading dose to ⅔ normal[394] if using for inotropic purposes
Ouabain*	Renal (50%) Fecal (30%)	22	Q12-24h	Q24h (×2)	Q24-36h (×2-3)	Q36-48h (×3-4)	No (HP)**	*No change in dosage size needed **15% of dosage given during dialysis removed in 4h
Diuretics								
Acetazolamide	Renal	8	Q6h	Q6h	Q12h (×2)	Avoid*	?	*Ineffective
Ethacrynic acid	Hepatic Renal	? 2-4	Q6h as needed for diuresis	Q6h	Q6h	Avoid*	?	Ototoxic; volume depletion *Use alternate if possible
Furosemide	Renal (Nonrenal)	Biphasic 0.4 & 2	Q6h as needed for diuresis	Unchanged	Unchanged	Unchanged*	?	Rare ototoxicity; volume depletion; may augment antibiotic nephrotoxicity *Has been used in large doses in renal failure
Mercurials	Renal	Biphasic 36 & 288	Q24h	Q24h	Avoid	Avoid	?	Systemic mercury accumulation; nephrotoxic
Metolazone	Renal	8	Q24h	Unchanged	Unchanged	Unchanged*	No (H)	Volume depletion *Has been used in large doses in renal failure
Spironolactone	Hepatic	10 min but active metabolite to 20h	Q6h	Q6h	Q6H*	Avoid*	?	*Hyperkalemia
Thiazides*	Renal	3	Q12h	Q12h	Q12h	Avoid**	?	Hyperuricemia; volume depletion *Prototype: chlorothiazide **Ineffective
Triamterene	Hepatic	2	Q12h	Q12h	Q12h	Avoid*	?	*Hyperkalemia Folic acid antagonist

†H indicates hemodialysis; P, peritoneal dialysis.
‡Numbers refer to bibliography available from the National Auxiliary Publications Service.
SOURCE: Permission from Bennett et al., and *J.A.M.A.*[15]

TABLE 69B-2
Bacterial endocarditis in dialysis patients

	Atlanta	Minnesota
No. dialysis patients	8	9
Valve		
Aortic	2	3
Mitral	4	1
Aortic and mitral	1	3
Tricuspid	1	1*
"Right ventricular"		1
Organism		
S. aureus	3	4
S. epidermis		1
P. aeruginosa	3	
Klebsiella	1	
L. monocytogenes		2
C. pseudodiphthericum		1
Enterococcus	1	1
Antecedent infection	7	7
Mortality	50%	78%

*Tricuspid *and* aortic.

doxicus) early in their illness. The presence of uremic pericarditis may be heralded by recurrent episodes of shunt clotting or by the appearance of refractory hypotension during dialysis.

COMPLICATIONS
Cardiac tamponade often appears suddenly and dramatically during hemodialysis. Hypotension, unresponsive to saline infusion, associated with neck vein distension is characteristic. In this situation, reversal of heparin anticoagulation with protamine sulfate followed by emergency pericardiocentesis of the invariably bloody effusion is indicated.[23] Hypotension in the absence of significant pericardial effusion and ventricular arrhythmias suggest coexistent myocarditis, a potentially fatal complication.[20]

Chronic and subacute constrictive pericarditis are relatively uncommon sequelae of uremic pericarditis in dialysis patients. In the Newark group,[22] 40 of 231 dialysis patients had pericarditis. Among these, only one patient with constrictive pericarditis was identified. Subacute constrictive pericarditis is distinguished from the chronic form by its evolution over a period of weeks. Blood pressure and pulse pressure are not invariably low, but ascites, pleural effusions, elevated venous pressure, peripheral edema, pericardial rub, and low voltage on the electrocardiogram are generally present.[24]

Adhesive pericarditis, characterized by pericardial fibrosis with tight adhesion to the epicardium, was an unexpected autopsy finding in eight of Comty's dialysis patients who died of other causes.[20] Of these, two had not demonstrated clinical evidence of pericarditis.

POSSIBLE ETIOLOGIC FACTORS
Bacterial infection (in shunt, surgical wounds, respiratory tract, or blood) preceded pericarditis in 14 of Comty's 25 patients.[20] Viral studies in 5 patients failed to implicate viral infections as a cause of pericarditis. Increased tissue catabolism resulting in greater abnormalities of body chemistries may be a mechanism whereby infection predisposes to uremic pericarditis. Poor biochemical control was noted in another 8 patients immediately prior to the onset of pericarditis. However, the association of pericarditis with infection, inadequate dialysis, or gross derangements in biochemical control of uremia has not been a consistent finding in other studies. Likewise, there is disagreement as to whether major surgical procedures in the absence of infection favor the development of pericarditis.

TREATMENT OF UREMIC PERICARDITIS
For patients with uncomplicated pericarditis, a period of augmented hemodialysis (with regional heparinization or with an artificial kidney in which low clotting times can be maintained) is begun. Indomethacin, 25 mg, three or four times daily is effective in controlling pain and fever. While corticosteroids also result in rapid improvement in pain, fever, and size of effusion, side effects are more common. In particular, their catabolic effect worsens azotemia. An interesting alternative to systemic steroids is the instillation of "nonabsorbable" steroids into the pericardial sac, as reported by Buselmier et al.,[25] for patients who do not respond to more conservative management. If, as the Minnesota group suggests, such therapy can circumvent a major surgical procedure, it is certainly worth a trial. To date, too few patients have been treated in this fashion to draw any conclusions regarding the efficacy of this therapy.

Percutaneous drainage of uremic pericardial effusion with or without a catheter left in place should be limited to the patient with tamponade. Because of the presence of fibrinous adhesions between the parietal and visceral layers of the pericardium, pericardiocentesis may be difficult and potentially dangerous.

Those patients who are unresponsive to conservative management or who have had recurrent tamponade require surgery. Ribot and colleagues[22] recommend subxiphoid pericardiostomy with creation of a 7-cm window (with drain) as a safe and effective procedure. However, because a pericardial window has been associated with closure requiring reexploration or the development of late constriction, other groups recommend wide pericardiectomy.[21,26]

A pericardial window was associated with a 33 percent recurrence rate of tamponade in the experience of Dean et al.,[26] who reserve creation of a window for emergencies. They performed wide anterior pericardiectomy in 22 uremic patients of whom 20 survived; the result was felt to be excellent in 19.

Functional aortic insufficiency

Patients with chronic renal failure frequently have some combination of fluid overload, hypertension, and anemia which favors the development of functional aortic insufficiency.[27] Not only may the classic diastolic murmur be present, but peripheral signs as well. Treatment with diuretics, antihypertensive agents, or dialysis usually results in disappearance of the murmur. Two patients whose murmurs did not entirely disappear after therapy had normal aortic valves at autopsy. Another two patients whose signs of aortic insufficiency cleared after therapy also had normal aortic valves at death.[27]

It is important to recognize functional aortic insufficiency in patients with chronic renal failure so as not to deny them chronic hemodialysis or transplantation on the basis of valvular heart disease.

"Uremic heart and lung"

Whether or not uremia in and of itself results in myocardial failure and "pneumonitis" has been a subject of long debate. Clearly, circulatory congestion is a frequent concomitant of chronic renal failure for several reasons: (1) classic myocardial failure from hypertensive heart disease, (2) severe venous congestion (with elevated venous pressure, cardiac dilatation, pulmonary congestion, and generally normal circulation time) from sodium retention, and (3) severe anemia which likewise can result in venous congestion. Gueron et al.[28] emphasize the necessity of excluding such known causes of heart failure before considering a diagnosis of uremic cardiomyopathy for which there is no pathologic proof. In the original description of uremic cardiomyopathy by Bailey, Hampers, and Merrill,[29] the diagnosis was made on the basis of the clinical findings of global cardiomegaly, atrial and ventricular arrhythmias, typical electrocardiographic changes, sensitivity to digitalis, and the reversal of syndrome following dialysis. Whether dialysis simply improved volume overload, hypertension, anemia, or calcium-phosphorus abnormalities—or removed a cardiotoxic factor—cannot be determined.

Prosser and Parsons[30] agree that anemia, hypertension, hypervolemia, ionic changes of uremia, and coincident pericardial and coronary artery disease are etiologic factors in the heart failure of patients with chronic renal failure. Nevertheless, they believe that there still is an intrinsic cardiomyopathic element to uremic heart failure. They cite the following data in support of their contention: (1) In isolated rat heart preparations, perfusates containing combinations of urea, creatinine, guanadinosuccinic acid and methyl guanidine had a cardiac depressant effect. (2) It is known that intracellular sodium concentration is abnormally high in uremia, and this might result in impaired myocardial function. (3) Vitamin D is necessary for the proper functioning and structure of sarcoplasmic endoreticulum in muscle cells. Possibly, the vitamin D deficiency of chronic renal failure leads to functional impairment of myocardial cells.

Pulmonary edema in patients with chronic renal failure is usually the result of cardiac failure or congestive overload, or both. However, a pattern of pulmonary edema extending from the hilum in a sharply defined butterfly configuration can be seen in uremia in the absence of obvious pulmonary vascular congestion. Whether or not this pattern is specific for uremia has been a subject of debate. The peripheral clear areas seen on chest x-ray may be the consequence of hyperventilation in response to uremic acidosis. Alveolar fluid, which is rich in protein and fibrin, might result from increased capillary permeability, possibly caused by "uremic toxins."[31,32] Seldin, Carter, and Rector do not favor the existence of a specific uremic pneumonitis. The pulmonary picture does not occur in all uremic patients nor can it be correlated with the level of azotemia. Left ventricular failure or noncardiac venous congestion is present in patients who do exhibit the typical x-ray findings.[32]

Uremic pleuritis can develop in the absence of primary pulmonary disease and appears to be secondary to uremia per se. Dialysis generally is effective in resolving pleuritic pain, but effusions take weeks to improve. Furthermore, some patients on maintenance hemodialysis may develop hemorrhagic pleural effusions.[33]

Effects of arteriovenous fistula

Arteriovenous shunts or fistulas pose a potential hemodynamic burden to patients undergoing chronic hemodialysis. Payne et al.[34] have studied exercise-induced hemodynamic effects of arteriovenous fistulas in 8 stable dialysis patients. These patients showed no significant change in resting cardiac output, heart rate, stroke volume, arterial pressure, or systemic vascular resistance when their shunts or fistulas were occluded. However, a small but significant increase in cardiac output occurred during exercise with the fistula open. The increased cardiac output was due to the combined small increases in stroke volume and heart rate.

Despite the findings of Payne et al.[34] and despite the fact that there are many factors predisposing to heart failure in dialysis patients, the arteriovenous fistula itself has been implicated as a cause of heart failure in some patients. Ahearn and Maher[35] have described 2 dialysis patients in whom this was felt to be the case. A positive Branham's sign in one, increased fistula flow measured by ultrasonic flowmeter, and prompt resolution of heart failure following surgical revision of the fistula occurred. Thus increased flow through the arteriovenous fistula should be considered in the differential diagnosis of heart failure in dialysis patients.

Autonomic insufficiency

During the course of hemodialysis, it is not unusual for patients to develop hypotension related to excessive ultrafiltration with consequent contraction of plasma volume. Infusion of saline ordinarily returns blood pressure to prehypotensive levels. However, some patients do not respond to volume repletion with restoration of normotension, and in addition, they do not have appropriate increases in pulse rate during hypotension. Kersh and coworkers[36] postulate that autonomic dysfunction may contribute to hemodialysis-induced hypotension in such patients.

They describe 6 patients who showed evidence of autonomic insufficiency and depressed peroneal nerve conduction as well. During hemodialysis-induced hypotension, they had a fall in total systemic resistance, a fixed heart rate, a lack of responsiveness to volume expansion, but a response to norepinephrine. Furthermore, these patients had markedly subnormal responses of heart rate to the Valsalva maneuver and inhalation of amyl nitrate. Autonomic nervous system dysfunction is likely another manifestation of the generalized neuropathy seen in chronic renal failure.

Accelerated cardiovascular disease

An increased prevalence of death from cardiovascular disease has been clearly shown in two large studies of dialysis patients. The National Dialysis Registry of the United States[37] and the European combined report of regular dialysis and transplantation[38] show that approximately 50 percent of chronic dialysis patients die of cardiovascular causes. The United States group comprised 11,000 patients of whom about two-thirds were men. Their mean age was 43.8 years. The European population was likewise relatively young, with a mean age of about 40 years. Of the 1,146 cardiovascular deaths recorded in the National Dialysis Registry, 35 percent were from heart disease, 7 percent from cerebrovascular disease, and 5 percent from other vascular disease.[37] However, it is not known what percentage of the cardiac deaths were due to pericarditis, hypertensive heart disease, endocarditis, arrhythmia or other non-atherosclerotic causes. Lindner et al. from Seattle[39] have reported the survival experience of 39 dialysis patients, followed for 1 to 13 years. Their mean age at the beginning of dialysis therapy was 37 years. There were 23 deaths, with 8 from myocardial infarction, 3 from stroke and 3 from refractory congestive heart failure. Thus it has become clear that patients undergoing maintenance hemodialysis are dying at a younger age and from a greater percentage of cardiovascular causes than the population without chronic renal failure.

A variety of physiologic and biochemical abnormalities characteristic of uremia have been implicated in the development of accelerated cardiovascular disease in patients with chronic renal failure. These are shown in Fig. 69B-1. Two recent papers have extensively reviewed many of these pathophysiologic factors.[40,41]

CARBOHYDRATE ABNORMALITIES

It is generally accepted that carbohydrate intolerance in uremia is largely a consequence of resistance to peripheral insulin utilization. Additionally, uremic patients have a delayed and increased release of immunoreactive insulin. When regular hemodialysis is begun, there is improvement in hyperglycemia and an increase in glucose clearance, associated with further elevation of immunoreactive insulin levels.

HYPERLIPIDEMIA

Increased levels of plasma triglycerides are present in most patients with chronic renal failure whether or not they are dialyzed. Because hypertriglyceridemia is directly related to increases in immunoreactive insulin, and because postheparin lipolytic activity is reduced in uremia, it is postulated that a defect in both synthesis and catabolism of very low-density lipoprotein is present. Hypertriglyceridemia has been reported by various investigators to improve or to worsen after institution of regular hemodialysis. Worsening of hyperlipidemia might be secondary to continued increases in immunoreactive insulin and to the high carbohydrate renal failure diet. In addition to insulin, growth hormone, parathyroid hormone, and glucagon are potentially lipogenic. Each of these polypeptide hormones is increased in chronic renal failure.

Most studies show only a modest increase in cholesterol. Thus, the typical electrophoretic pattern

FIGURE 69B-1 Possible etiologic factors in the development of cardiovascular disease in dialysis patients.

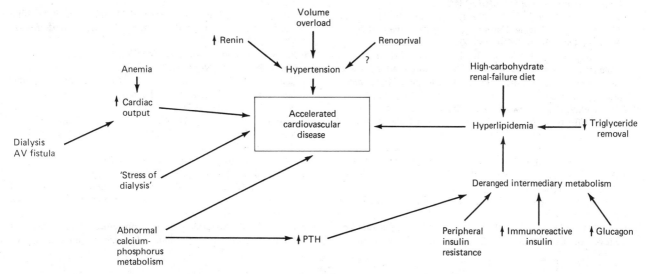

of the hyperlipidemia of patients with renal failure is Type IV.

HYPERTENSION

The pathophysiology of hypertension in patients with chronic renal failure is discussed in Chap. 65 of this book. To summarize, the hypertension of the majority of patients with chronic renal failure, whether or not they are undergoing dialysis, is related to expansion of the plasma volume with excessive amounts of salt and water. A minority of patients is hypertensive on the basis of hyperreninemia, usually from malignant hypertension. Prolonged and sustained hypertension prior to the institution of dialysis and poor control of hypertension despite dialysis in some patients are the most important risk factors for the development of cardiovascular disease in the chronic dialysis population. The need for early and aggressive control in patients with renal insufficiency cannot be overemphasized.

OTHER RISK FACTORS

Calcific cardiomyopathy, peripheral vascular calcifications, and changes in cardiac output related to arteriovenous fistulas and anemia have been discussed earlier in this chapter.

REFERENCES

1 Slatapolsky, E., Elka, I. O., Weerts, C., and Bricker, N. S.: Studies on the Characteristics of the Control System Governing Sodium Excretion in Uremic Man, *J. Clin. Invest.*, 47:521, 1968.

2 Bilbrey, G. L., Carter, N. W., White, M. G., Schilling, J. F., and Knochel, J. D.: Potassium Deficiency in Chronic Renal Failure, *Kidney. Int.*, 4:423, 1973.

3 Massry, S. G., Guest, E.: Divalent Ions in Renal Failure, *Kidney Int.*, 4(2), 1973.

4 Friedman, S. A., Novack, S., and Thomason, G. E.: Arterial Calcifications and Gangrene in Uremia, *N. Engl. J. Med.*, 280:1392, 1969.

5 Henderson, R. R., Santiago, L. M., Spring, D. A., and Harrington, A. R.: Metastatic Myocardial Calcification in Chronic Renal Failure, *N. Engl. J. Med.*, 284:1252, 1971.

6 Arora, K. K., Lacy, J. P., Schact, R. A., Martin, D. G., and Gutch, L. F.: Calcific Cardiomyopathy in Advanced Renal Failure, *Arch. Intern. Med.*, 135:603, 1975.

7 Shackney, S., and Hasson, J.: Precipitous Fall in Serum Calcium, Hypotension and Acute Renal Failure after Intravenous Phosphate Therapy for Hypercalcemia, *Ann. Intern. Med.*, 66:906, 1967.

8 Wildenthal, K., Mierzwiak, D. S., Myers, R. M., and Mitchell, J. H.: Effects of Acute Lactic Acidosis on Left Ventricular Performance, *Am. J. Physiol.*, 214:1352, 1968.

9 Harvey, R. M., Enson, Y., Lewis, M. L., Greenough, W. B., Ally, K. M., and Panno, R. A.: Hemodynamic Effects of Dehydration and Metabolic Acidosis in Asiatic Cholera, *Trans. Assoc. Am. Physicians*, 79:177, 1966.

10 Erslev, A. J.: Anemia of Chronic Renal Disease, *Arch. Intern. Med.*, 126:774, 1970.

11 Crockett, R. E., Baillod, R. A., Lee, B. W., Moorhead, J. F., Stevenson, C. M., Varghese, Z., and Sheldon, S.: Maintenance of Fifty Patients on Intermittent Hemodialysis without Blood Transfusion, *Proc. Eur. Dial. Transplant. Assoc.*, 4:17, 1967.

12 Eschbach, J. W., and Adamson, J. W.: Improvement in the Anemia of Chronic Renal Failure with Fluoxymesterone, *Ann. Intern. Med.*, 78:527, 1973.

13 Giovanetti, S., Balestri, P. O., Biagini, M., Menechini, G., and Rindi, P.: Implications of Dietary Therapy, *Arch. Intern. Med.*, 126:900, 1970.

14 Domenet, J. G., and Evans, D. W.: Uraemia in Congestive Heart Failure, *Q. J. Med.*, 38:117, 1969.

15 Bennett, W. M., Singer, I., and Coggins, C. J.: A Guide to Drug Therapy in Renal Failure, *J.A.M.A.*, 214:1468, 1970.

16 Hook, E., Wainer, H., McGee, T., and Sellers, T., Jr.: Acquired Arteriovenous Fistula with Bacterial Endarteritis and Endocarditis, *J.A.M.A.*, 164:1450, 1957.

17 Lillehei, C. W., Bobb, J. R. R., and Visscher, M. P.: Occurrence of Endocarditis with Valvular Deformities in Dogs with Arteriovenous Fistulas, *Ann. Surg.*, 132:577, 1950.

18 Fellner, S. K.: Cardiovascular Complications of Chronic Renal Failure and Dialysis, in Hurst et al. (eds.), "The Heart," 3d ed., McGraw-Hill Book Company, New York, 1974, p. 1202.

19 Leonard, A., Raij, L., Comty, C. M., Wathen, R., Rattazzi, T., and Shapiro, F. L.: Experience with Endocarditis in a Large Kidney Disease Program, *Trans. Am. Soc. Artif. Intern. Organs*, 19:298, 1973.

20 Comty, C. M., Cohen, S. L., and Shapiro, F. L.: Pericarditis in Uremia and its Sequels, *Ann. Intern. Med.*, 75:173, 1971.

21 Marini, P. V., and Hull, A. R.: Uremic Pericarditis: A Review of Incidence and Management, *Kidney Int.*, 7(suppl. 2):S163, 1975.

22 Ribot, S., Frankel, H. J., Gielchinsky, I., and Gilbert, L.: Treatment of Uremic Pericarditis, *Clin. Nephrology*, 2:127, 1974.

23 Beaudry, C., Nakamoto, S., and Kolff, W. J.: Uremic Pericarditis and Cardiac Tamponade in Chronic Renal Failure, *Ann. Intern. Med.*, 64:990, 1966.

24 Reyman, T. A.: Subacute Constrictive Uremic Pericarditis, *Am. J. Med.*, 46:972, 1969.

25 Buselmier, T. J., Simmons, R. L., von Hartitzsch, B., Najarian, J. S., and Kjellstrand, C. M.: Persistent Uremic Pericardial Effusion: Pericardial Drainage and Localized Steroid Instillation as Definitive Therapy, *Abstr. Am. Soc. Nephr.*, 6th Ann. Meeting, Washington, D.C., November, 1973, p. 18.

26 Dean, R. H., Killen, D. A., Daniel, R. A., and Collins, H. A.: Experience with Pericardiectomy, *Ann. Thorac. Surg.*, 15:378, 1973.

27 Matalon, R., Mousalli, A. R. J., Nidus, B. D., Katz, L. A., and Eisinger, R. P.: Functional Aortic Insufficiency: A Feature of Renal Failure, *N. Engl. J. Med.*, 285:1522, 1971.

28 Gueron, M., Berlyne, G. M., Nord, E., and Ben Ari, J.: The Case Against a Specific Uraemic Cardiomyopathy, *Nephron*, 15:2, 1975.

29 Bailey, G. L., Hampers, C. L., and Merrill, J. P.: Reversible Cardiomyopathy in Uremia, *Trans. Am. Soc. Artif. Intern. Organs*, 13:263, 1967.

30 Prosser, D., and Parsons, V.: The Case for a Specific Uraemic Cardiomyopathy, *Nephron*, 15:4, 1975.

31 Schwartz, E. E., and Onesti, G.: The Cardiopulmonary Manifestations of Uremia and Renal Transplantation, *Radiol. Clin. North Am.*, 10:569, 1972.

32 Seldin, D. W., Carter, N. W., and Rector, F. C., Jr.: Consequences of Renal Failure and Their Managements, in M. B. Strauss and L. G. Welt (eds.), "Diseases of the Kidney," Little, Brown and Company, Boston, 1971, p. 240.

33 Galen, M. A., Steinberg, S. M., Lowrie, E. F., Lazarus, J. M., Hampers, C. L., and Merrill, J. P.: Hemorrhagic Pleural Effusions in Patients Undergoing Chronic Hemodialysis, *Ann. Intern. Med.*, 82:359, 1975.

34 Payne, R. M., Soderblom, R. E., Lobstein, P., Hull, A. R., and Mullins, C. B.: Exercise-induced Hemodynamic Effects of

Arteriovenous Fistulas Used for Hemodialysis, *Kidney Int.,* 2:344, 1972.

35 Ahearn, D. J., and Maher, J. F.: Heart Failure as a Complication of Hemodialysis Arteriovenous Fistula, *Ann. Intern. Med.,* 77:20, 1972.

36 Kersh, E. S., Kronfield, S. J., Unger, A., Popper, R. W., Cantor, S., and Cohn, K.: Autonomic Insufficiency in Uremia as a Cause of Hemodialysis-Induced Hypotension, *N. Engl. J. Med.,* 649:650, 1974.

37 Bryan, F.: National Dialysis Registry, Proceedings of the 6th Annual Contractors' Conference of the Artificial Kidney Program of the National Institute of Arthritis, Metabolism and Digestive Diseases, 1973, p. 201.

38 Parsons, F. M., Brunner, F. P., Gurland, H. J., and Harlen, H.: Combined Report of Regular Dialysis and Transplantation in Europe, *Proc. Eur. Dial. Transplant Assoc.,* 8:3, 1971.

39 Lindner, A., Charra, B., Sherrard, D. J., and Scribner, B. H.: Accelerated Atherosclerosis in Prolonged Maintenance Hemodialysis, *N. Engl. J. Med.,* 290:697, 1974.

40 Lazarus, J. M., Lowrie, E. G., Hampers, C. L., and Merrill, J. P.: Cardiovascular Disease in Uremic Patients on Hemodialysis, *Kidney Internat.,* 7(suppl. 2):S167, 1975.

41 Bagdade, J. D.: Atherosclerosis in Patients Undergoing Maintenance Hemodialysis, *Kidney Int.,* 7(suppl. 3):S370, 1975.

70
Unilateral Renal Disease

WILLIAM C. WATERS, III, M.D.

INTRODUCTION

The existence of a causal link between kidney disease and high blood pressure was recognized clearly as early as the era of Richard Bright, but practical therapeutic applications of this clinical insight have only been made in recent years. Efforts to document and explain this connection were largely in vain until 1934, when Goldblatt demonstrated a mechanism for the production of hypertension by interference with the arterial supply to one or both kidneys.[1] This innovation has provided a new stimulus for the clinical investigator and an entirely new therapeutic avenue for the practical clinician.

Goldblatt's silver clamp, applied to one of the renal arteries of a dog, resulted in blood pressure elevation which appeared within a few days, reached its peak in a week, but usually did not persist indefinitely unless the opposite kidney was removed or its arterial supply was compromised; in the rat, the unilateral constriction was sufficient to cause permanent hypertension.[2] In most species, including human beings, relief of the one-sided obstruction is often followed by a dramatic disappearance of the hypertension. Although the normal contralateral kidney is subject to the same changes of arteriolar nephrosclerosis seen in spontaneously occurring hypertension, the ischemic kidney may at times be protected from the effects of the elevated blood pressure. On the other hand, renal biopsy material in human subjects indicates that the ischemic kidney may suffer arteriosclerotic damage as well, and even this finding does not necessarily preclude successful therapy of the hypertension by surgical repair of the vascular lesion.

The precise sequence whereby interference with renal arterial supply leads to systemic hypertension has not been adequately defined. Reduction in blood flow alone seems an insufficient explanation, since the initial fall in perfusion of the affected kidney is soon followed by a return to normal of renal blood flow after hypertension becomes established. Likewise, anoxia in the renal circulation does not lead to hypertension. It has been proposed that a fall in the blood pressure distal to the point of obstruction may constitute the stimulus, since wide gradients have been observed in patients at the time of surgical treatment, but a number of experimental studies suggest that hypertension may be produced and sustained even while the tension in the distal renal artery is at control levels. More attention has been focused in recent years on the drop in pulse pressure produced by narrowing of the arterial lumen, and on the elaboration of pressor substances by the kidney under such conditions. Certainly hemodynamic changes, however difficult to measure, must eventually be found to constitute the prime stimulus, and it seems likely that mean flow is the central determinant of pressor activity by the kidney.

In any event, after interference with the renal vascular supply, physiologic changes take place in the kidney which lead to systemic arterial hypertension, and much evidence indicates that this mechanism is humoral. Denervation or removal of the kidney to a remote site in the circulation does not interfere with production of renovascular hypertension—on the other hand, interruption of renal venous drainage prevents it. Similarly, as early as 1898, it was demonstrated that when renal cortical extracts with the physical characteristics of protein were injected, they were capable of inducing systemic hypertension.[3] Later work has indicated that extracts of the venous blood from kidneys with arterial constriction have a greater hypertensive effect than blood draining normal kidneys. It has been further demonstrated that certain renal extracts (renin) exhibit the biochemical properties of a catalyst,[4] with the capacity to accelerate the conversion of a plasma factor to the potent physiologic pressor amine angiotensin. Refinements of investigative approach have now rather clearly elucidated the production of the pressor agent:

Plasma α_2-globulin $\xrightarrow{\text{renin}}$

Angiotensin I (a decapeptide, inactive) $\xrightarrow[\text{enzyme}]{\text{converting}}$

Angiotensin II (an octapeptide, highly active vasopressor)

The structure of angiotensin II is known, it has been synthesized,[5] and this mechanism thus constitutes an attractive hypothesis to explain human renal hypertension and its relief by removal of the offending kidney or repair of the defective arterial supply.

The role of this sequence in clinical hypertension is supported by the finding of pressor activity in blood from the systemic circulation or renal vein of animals with experimental renal vascular lesions and in renal venous blood from the affected kidney (but not the normal kidney) of patients with renovascular hypertension.[6] Further, administration of hog renin in serial doses to dogs with renovascular hypertension results in a rising titer of antirenin and a progressive decline of the blood pressure toward normal.[7] Most impressive of all have been the increasingly consistent reports of elevated plasma renin level (expressed as angiotensin activity determined by bioassay or radioimmunoassay) in patients with renovascular hypertension, but not in patients with essential hypertension.[8] In addition, selective renal venous and inferior caval blood samples show augmented renin activity from the ischemic side and low values from the intact side, with intermediate values in mixed central venous blood below the point of the renal veins.[9]

It should be pointed out, however, that a body of evidence remains to suggest that the renin-angiotensin mechanism is not alone responsible for chronic renal hypertension. Dogs with renovascular hypertension often do not maintain their hypertensive levels; experimental animals with chronic renal arterial hypertension exhibit no increase in renin-angiotensin activity. Doubt is cast upon the evidence accumulated through the use of hog renin by the argument that the substance is impure and that rabbits do not exhibit the antihypertensive response to serial renin injections. Furthermore, tachyphylaxis to renin occurs in many species: rabbits with renovascular hypertension respond initially to renin, and after developing tachyphylaxis, they return to the previous elevated pressure rather than to normotensive levels. When renin tachyphylaxis has occurred, angiotensin II is no longer effective. Though it appears certain, then, that the renin-angiotensin system participates in the production of experimental and human renovascular hypertension, there is still reason to question that this mechanism is solely responsible for the sustained blood pressure elevation that ensues. Indeed, the variable clinical results obtained after nephrectomy or vascular repair are consistent with this observation, as is the frequent finding of gradual return of the blood pressure to normal after successful surgery.

An important additional humoral mechanism in the sustained hypertension of renal vascular disease is the renin-angiotensin-aldosterone axis. A role of renal humoral influences in the regulation of aldosterone production had been suspected since the observation was made that renin administered to rats resulted in hypertrophy of the zona glomerulosa of the adrenal cortex. Subsequently, it has been shown that the customary stimuli for aldosterone secretion (such as inferior vena cava ligation or phlebotomy) are ineffective in the nephrectomized animal. Most convincing of all is the observation that administration of renin, renal extract, or angiotensin II causes an increased aldosterone excretion in animals which have previously been hypophysectomized and nephrectomized; human subjects respond to angiotensin injection with a striking increase in aldosterone production. On the other hand, patients with renal hypertension may or may not show increased aldosterone secretion rate; experimental animals tend to exhibit accelerated aldosterone production only when their hypertensive disease is in a malignant phase.

Of great academic as well as clinical interest has been the finding by many observers of the antihypertensive action of the kidney.[10] Renoprival hypertension develops when bilateral nephrectomy is performed in experimental animals and is corrected by retransplantation; transplantation of a normal kidney to an animal with renovascular hypertension results in improvement of the blood pressure level. The apparently highly important effect of the normal kidney in regulation of blood pressure has been most dramatically demonstrated by the variable antihypertensive effect obtained from renal venous blood draining a kidney which is perfused with blood passing through a cannula at different pressures.[11] In this series of experiments, the blood pressure–lowering effect of the kidney was more or less quantitatively related to the height of the perfusing arterial pressure. The possible role of prostaglandins in the antihypertensive process is currently being explored, but it appears that prostaglandin inhibition does not dramatically affect the course of experimental renovascular hypertension.[12]

HUMAN HYPERTENSION AND UNILATERAL RENAL DISEASE

If obstruction of the renal artery or of the kidney itself produces hypertension in experimental animals, it is to be expected that a variety of spontaneously occurring diseases of the kidney will cause blood pressure elevation in human beings. When the disease is unilateral, the possibility of surgical cure is present, as shown by an impressive number of clinical examples. Table 70-1 presents those lesions correction of which at times has produced favorable results.

INCIDENCE AND CLINICAL FEATURES

As with any entity under active investigation, the real incidence of curable hypertension due to unilateral renal disease is unknown. Present evidence would suggest that perhaps 2 to 3 percent of all individuals

TABLE 70-1
Causes of reversible hypertension due to unilateral renal disease

I Intrinsic unilateral renal disease
  A Congenital hypoplastic kidney
  B Pyelonephritis
    1 Pyogenic
    2 Tuberculous
  C Irradiation
  D Trauma
  E Renal neoplasm
  F Unilateral renal vein thrombosis
  G Obstruction uropathy
II Renal artery lesions
  A Intrinsic
    1 Atherosclerotic plaque
    2 Thrombosis or embolism
    3 Fibromuscular hyperplasia
    4 Renal artery aneurysm
    5 Other: thromboangiitis obliterans, periarteritis, syphilitic arteritis
  B Extrinsic compression
    1 Tumor involving renal pedicle
    2 Retroperitoneal fibrosis

in the hypertensive population, after thorough diagnostic study, have sufficient findings to warrant nephrectomy or vascular repair. Of this group, only 50 percent have an unequivocal cure (blood pressure lower than 140/90 mm Hg for longer than 1 year), and an additional 25 to 35 percent show definite improvement.

Clinical suspicion of unilateral renal origin for hypertension may be aroused by a history or findings of the underlying process, such as pyelonephritis or ureteral obstruction (see Table 70-1), but very often such patients are asymptomatic. In the group with renal vascular hypertension, cases reported to date may or may not fit into a pattern.[13] Most of these patients have been male (possibly 3:1), and a surprising proportion of them have reported a recent episode of trauma to the renal area or a spontaneously occurring bout of flank pain. Albuminuria is frequent, though not invariable, and bruits are frequently found. Although many such bruits are innocent, several characteristics suggest significant renal vascular stenosis: loudness, tendency to carry over into diastole, high-pitched character, and radiation into the back or flank. It is the opinion of some observers that renovascular hypertension, like that with pheochromocytoma, often exhibits orthostatic variation, although such was not the case in a large recent study.[13] Unlike essential hypertension, in which the blood pressure elevation is *usually* benign, and unlike primary aldosteronism, in which it is *almost invariably* benign,[14] renal hypertension may produce malignant grades of hypertensive vascular disease. Indeed, those patients who have exhibited a good response to surgical treatment have in general had, before surgery, quite high blood pressure of recent onset, frequently with retinopathy.[13] Whether the selection of such patients has been partially artificial and stimulated by the urgency of their condition or whether malignant progression is in fact characteristic of renovascular hypertension remains to be determined by further experience. Certainly benign hypertension has also responded to surgical intervention, even after intervals of many years since appearance of the elevated blood pressure.

DIAGNOSIS

Clinical criteria

Because of the relative rarity of unilateral renal disease as a cause of hypertension and because of the expense of morbidity associated with definitive investigation, attempts have been made to establish criteria for the selection of hypertensive patients for further study.[13] Most authorities agree that one or more of the following findings warrants a search for curable causation: absence of family history of hypertension; onset before age 30 or after age 50, particularly if the patient is under 60; abrupt appearance of hypertension or acceleration of previously benign hypertension; failure of adequate response to medical therapy of significant hypertension; abdominal bruit; unexplained flank pain; trauma to a kidney; and radiographic evidence of asymmetry of renal outlines, particularly if progressive decrease in renal size has been demonstrated on serial roentgenograms. It is likely that accelerated or malignant hypertension should be added to this list, since prognosis without drastic therapy is grave and since very severe hypertension is rather characteristic of a renal vascular insult.

Ancillary studies

The advisability of prior selection is made more evident when one considers the fact that no one diagnostic procedure is final in predicting surgical cure; this fact is indicated further by the multiplicity of methods which have been employed. Among the means which have gained clinical acceptance are the plain abdominal film, intravenous urography, radioactive scanning procedures, aortography, direct differential studies of ureteral urine, and, importantly, the plasma renin determination on peripheral and renal venous blood.

Intravenous urography[15]

This conventional procedure may reveal, in the hypertensive patient, such obvious lesions as a hypoplastic kidney on one side, a renal tumor, unilateral hydronephrosis, or evidence of preponderantly unilateral pyelonephritis. In renal vascular disease, one or more of the following more subtle findings may be apparent: unilateral reduction in renal mass (greater than 2 cm); delayed appearance of dye on the affected side; greater relative concentration of dye in the collecting system of the diseased side when contrast material does appear ("paradoxical hyperconcentration"); and at times notching of the pelvis and upper ureter of the affected side by collateral arterial channels. These findings are much more regularly demonstrated when the rapid-sequence technique (1-, 2-, 3-, and 5-min films) and either urea-washout or hydrated pyelogram are used. A review of the massive literature on this subject indicates that approximately 85 percent of cases of eventually cured renovascular hypertension show some abnormality of the intravenous urogram when these techniques are employed, making it the most valuable single screening procedure. False negative results have been widely reported, but most recent studies suggest this is true only 2 percent of the time; obviously, this procedure will be useless in instances of bilateral renal artery stenosis and in segmental arterial disease. On the other hand, and more rarely, apparent false positive results may occur. Delineation of the anatomy of the urinary tract is nevertheless important in assisting interpretation of subsequent studies.

Radioactive "renogram"

After injection of radioactive Diodrast or Hippuran, a time curve of appearance and disappearance of radioactivity over each kidney is inscribed and compared. Characteristically, the kidney affected by renovascular hypertension exhibits a delayed appearance and delayed disappearance of dye, with impairment of the "vascular spike." Because of artifacts and false positive results this procedure has come to be regarded as of doubtful routine clinical value. However, more sophisticated instrumentation, using multiple crystals, computer analysis, and better probe placement, promises to give this technique a higher position among diagnostic maneuvers.

Radioactive scan

Renal tubular mass can be assessed by recording the bilateral accumulation of injected radiomercury or technitium. Though results to date suggest this to be a useful and accurate means for estimating comparative renal size, it does not permit measurement of those physiologic disturbances most characteristic of renovascular disease (see next paragraph), nor does it aid in distinguishing renal vascular disease from other unilateral disease.

Differential excretion studies

The kidney affected by renal vascular disease exhibits abnormalities of excretory function such that a reduction in water excretion and an even greater reduction in sodium excretion occur on the side of the vascular abnormality. There is thus in highly controlled circumstances an almost invariable finding of decreased water excretion (50 percent or greater) and decreased sodium concentration (15 percent or greater) on the side of the lesion in

patients who are later shown to have curable renal vascular hypertension.[16] However, false negative tests and technical problems have stood in the way of this technique as a routinely valuable means of distinguishing renal vascular disease from other unilateral disease of the kidney. In the hands of certain experienced workers, particularly when urea infusion, vasopressin administration, and other techniques are used, the procedure can be of considerable value.[17]

Aortography

Visualization of the aorta and renal arteries by means of translumbar puncture or retrograde catheterization of the aorta has made an enormous contribution to the study and management of suspected cases of renal vascular disease.[18] The chief virtues of this method are direct demonstration of the vascular obstruction, provision of a preoperative "map" of the surgical territory, and demonstration of segmental arterial or bilateral main arterial disease. However, although reports of false positive findings are only occasional, it is to be expected that functionally unimportant vascular lesions will be demonstrated, especially since such lesions may be present even in the nonhypertensive population. Furthermore, false negative results have been obtained in patients who subsequently made a favorable response to surgery. Nonetheless, growing experience with the technique, refinements such as selective renal angiography, and the low mortality-morbidity rates in experienced hands appear to establish the technique as the most valuable and crucial study now available for patients with suspected reversible hypertension. Selective renal angiography in particular appears to offer great assistance in delineation of segmental renal arterial disease; it also offers an opportunity to evaluate the distal renal arterial tree preoperatively.

Renin in peripheral and renal venous plasma

Development of methods for determination of plasma renin activity (by means of bioassay) and of angiotension action and circulating angiotension (radioimmunoassay method) have added greatly to the evaluation of patients with a suspected renal origin for their hypertension.[19] In patients with primary parenchymal renal disease, several groups of workers have identified at least three groups of hypertensives: those with low, with high, and with intermediate levels of plasma renin activity. Presumably the low-renin group involves patients with inappropriate sodium retention and increased plasma volume while the high-renin group represents those with pathologic elevations of renin due to elaboration by the diseased kidney or kidneys. In unilateral disease, particularily renal artery disease, a high rate of prediction of surgical cure has been found when the venous effluent from the affected kidney is greater than one and one-half times the value for the opposite, normal, side. Utilizing multiple correlations Maxwell and others have indicated that an abnormal intravenous pyelogram, renal artery lesion, recent onset of hypertension, and greater than 1.5:1 renal renin difference correlates with surgical cure in greater than 95 percent of patients.[18] Preoperative preparation of the patient with a diuretic (e.g., 80 mg furosemide the afternoon before study) taken together with salt and fluid restriction overnight greatly enhances the likelihood of unmasking the offending renal vascular lesion. Because of the high correlation rate, some authorities recommend bilateral renal venous renin studies prior to considering proceeding with aortography. Laragh and his coworkers suggest that the "renin profile," or plasma renin value adjusted for sodium excretion, will alone be adequate to identify patients with renal vascular disease.[19]

On the other hand, some patients who experience cure of hypertension by renal vascular surgery have shown bilaterally normal renal venous renins, and some observers report that as high as 15 percent have curable renal vascular hypertension which cannot be predicted by the most careful renin studies. Certainly a combined approach, utilizing renin studies together with the aortographic map, renal size, and clinical picture is the preferred approach at the present time. Use of renin antagonists, such as Saralasin, are promising for the future.

Surgical approach

Some observers hold to the principle that even in documented unilateral renal vascular hypertension a trial of drug therapy is warranted before patients are subjected to surgical intervention. It has been particularly advocated in patients over 55 years of age. Furthermore, increasing experience has indicated that the older idea that renal vascular hypertensives will not respond to drug therapy is by no means always true. For example, propranolol therapy of the patient with high renin activity may be dramatically effective in cases of small vessel disease of the kidney and in large vessel disease as well. In general, however, authorities agree that the risk of surgical intervention is fully warranted by the prospect of cure when the patient has adequate renal function, when the hypertension is producing "target organ" changes, when cerebral and coronary disease are not far advanced, when the patient is less than 60 years of age, and when the surgeon's experience with this type of renal vascular surgery is adequate. The surgical (operative and postoperative) mortality rates have ranged from 3 to 10 percent in various centers, but over half these deaths have derived from nonsurgical causes such as coronary and cerebral vascular disease. Thus the patient whose only serious affliction is hypertension may be expected to have a far more favorable outlook.

The surgical approach has included simple nephrectomy, subtotal nephrectomy, and endarterectomy with or without patch graft, splenorenal anastomosis, bypass grafts, and even dilatation of renal arteries in the case of fibromuscular dysplasia. The choice of procedure will, of course, be dictated by the lesion, together with the patient's condition. While in complicated medical problems a nephrectomy is the simplest operation, the potentiality for preservation of renal tissue will more often dictate the advisability of the more complicated procedure.

In summary, unilateral renal disease, particularly that due to renal vascular abnormalities, is an uncommon but frequently reversible cause for systemic hypertension which deserves clinical consideration in every hypertensive patient. When the patient has no family history of hypertension, is outside the age group for essential hypertension, reports a recent onset or acceleration of the condition, or presents suggestive physical or radiographic evidence of unilateral renal disease, he or she should be considered for definitive study, the most prominent aspects of which are likely to be aortography and renal vein catheterization for renin. With adequate confirmation of evidence for a unilateral renal origin for the hypertension, with indications that the hypertension is significant, with assurances of adequate renal function, and with expectations for reasonable surgical risk, the patient should be offered the opportunity to receive the benefit which experienced surgical hands can provide.

REFERENCES

1 Goldblatt, H., Lynch, J., Hanzal, R. B., and Summerville, W. W.: Studies in Experimental Hypertension: I. The Production of Persistent Elevations of Systolic Blood Pressure by Means of Renal Ischemia, *J. Exp. Med.,* 59:347, 1934.

2 Wilson, C., and Byrom, F. B.: The Vicious Circle in Chronic Bright's Disease: Experimental Evidence from the Hypertensive Rat, *Q. J. Med.,* 10:65, 1941.

3 Tigerstedt, R., and Bergman, P. G.: Niere und Kreislauf, *Scand. Arch. Physiol.,* 8:223, 1898.

4 Braun-Menendez, E., Fasciolo, J. D., Lelior, L. F., and Munoz, J. M.: The Substance Causing Renal Hypertension, *J. Physiol.,* 98:283, 1940.

5 Page, I. H., and Bumpus, F. M.: Angiotensin, *Physiol. Rev.,* 41:331, 1961.

6 Morris, R. E., Jr., Ranson, P. A., and Howard, J. E.: Studies in the Relationship of Angiotensin to Hypertension or Renal Origin, *J. Clin. Invest.,* 41:1386, 1962. (Abstract.)

7 Wakerlin, G. E., Bird, R. B., Brennan, B. B., Frank, M. H., Kremen, S., Kuperman, I., and Skorn, J. H.: Treatment and Prophylaxis of Experimental Renal Hypertension with "Renin," *J. Lab. Clin. Med.,* 41:708, 1953.

8 Veyrat, R., deChamplain, J., Boucher, R., and Genest, J.: Measurement of Human Arterial Renin Activity in Some Physiological and Pathological States, *Can. Med. Assoc. J.,* 90:215, 1964.

9 Fitz, A. E.: Renal Venous Renin (RVR) in Evaluation of Renovascular Hypertension, *Clin. Res.,* 14:376, 1966.

10 Muirhead, E. E., Hinman, J. W., Daniels, E. G., Kosinski, M., and Brooks, B.: Refined Antihypertensive Medullorenal Extract and the Protective Action of the Kidney against Hypertension, *J. Clin. Invest.,* 40:1065, 1961.

11 Tobian, L., Winn, B., and Janecek, J.: The Influence of Arterial Pressure on the Antihypertensive Action of a Normal Kidney, a Biological Servomechanism, *J. Clin. Invest.,* 40:1085, 1961.

12 Romero, J. C., Ott, C. E., Aguilo, J. J., Torres, V. E., and Strong, C. G.: Role of Prostaglandins in the Reversal of One-Kidney Hypertension in the Rabbit, *Circ. Res.,* 37:683, 1975.

13 Simon, M. D., Franklin, S. S., Bleifer, K. H., and Maxwell, M. H.: Clinical Characteristics of Renovascular Hypertension, *JAMA*, 220:1209, 1972.

14 Conn, J. W.: Aldosteronism and Hypertension, *Arch. Intern. Med.*, 107:813, 1961.

15 Bookstein, J. J., Abrams, H. L., Buenger, R. E., Lecky, J., Franklin, S. S., Reiss, M. D., Bleifer, K. H., Klatte, E. C., Var Varady, P. D., and Maxwell, M. M.: Radiologic Aspects of Renovascular Hypertension, *JAMA*, 220:1225, 1972.

16 Connor, T. B., Thomas, W. C., Jr., Haddock, L., and Howard, J. E.: Unilateral Renal Disease as a Cause of Hypertension: Its Detection by Ureteral Catheterization Studies, *Ann. Intern. Med.*, 52:544, 1960.

17 Stamey, T. A., Nudelman, I. J., Good, P. H., Schwentker, F. N., and Hendricks, F.: Functional Characteristics of Renovascular Hypertension, *Medicine*, 40:347, 1961.

18 Bookstein, J. J., Abrams, H. L., Buenger, R. E., Lecky, J., Franklin, S. S., Reiss, M. D., Bleifer, K. H., Klatte, E. C., and Maxwell, M. M.: Radiologic Aspects of Renovascular Hypertension: Part I. Aims and Methods, *JAMA*, 220:1218, 1972.

19 Laragh, J.: New Treatment Strategy Based on Renin-Sodium Index, *Hypertension*, 2:6, 1976.

71
Pheochromocytoma

AARON H. ANTON, PH.D.

PHEOCHROMOCYTOMA AND HYPERTENSION

Labbé, Tinel, and Doumer described the association of hypertension with adrenal tumors in 1922. In 1926 C. H. Mayo successfully removed adrenal tumors associated with hypertension. Pincoffs in 1929 made the first correct preoperative diagnosis of pheochromocytoma, with successful removal of the tumor. In the same year Rabin demonstrated large quantities of a pressor agent, presumed to be epinephrine, in a pheochromocytoma. Since that time rapid progress has been made in the chemistry, pathology, and diagnosis of this important tumor.[1]

Pheochromocytoma is considered to be a relatively rare cause of hypertension, but its true frequency is unknown. Although variable, statistics from several studies suggest the following approximate incidence of this tumor in the United States: 0.05 percent at autopsy, 0.5 percent among hypertensive individuals, 1 per 50,000 hospital admissions, 1 per 500,000 annual population with about 600 new cases per year. Pheochromocytomas have been found in all age groups, with the peak incidence in the fourth to fifth decades of life, but there does not seem to be a sex difference. A high incidence of the tumor occurs in patients with neurofibromatosis (von Recklinghausen's disease). A number of familial cases have been reported and as part of the Sipple syndrome (multiple endocrine adenomatosis type 2A) in which there is a positive family history, hyperparathyroidism, medullary carcinoma of the thyroid gland, and bilateral pheochromocytoma.[1-4]

Anatomy and pathology[1-4]

Pheochromocytomas arise from chromaffin elements either in the adrenal gland or in the extramedullary chromaffin tissue. As outlined in Fig. 71-1, neural crest tumors, which include the pheochromocytoma and neuroblastoma, originate from the same germ layer as do the other elements of the central and peripheral nervous systems. The sympathogonia, which are the parent cells of the peripheral nervous system, can develop along two main lines. The normal pathway of one line of development results in the formation of the sympathetic ganglions, whereas abnormally, several neoplasms may develop, of which the neuroblastoma is the most malignant and mainly occurs in children. Along the other line of development, the sympathogonia normally give rise to the adrenal medulla, and abnormally to the pheochromocytoma. In addition to their common embryologic origin, these cells, both normal and abnormal, have been found to be biochemically similar in that they produce catechols, e.g., norepinephrine, the type and amount depending on the particular tissue. Pheochromocytomas may be found in the celiac, renal, adrenal, aortic, and hypogastric plexuses, and elsewhere in the retroperitoneal and paraaortic regions, including the organs of Zuckerkandl. In addition, tumors have been found in the thorax, urinary bladder, testes, ovaries, and elsewhere. Approximately 90 percent of pheochromocytomas occur in the adrenal gland, and about 10 percent of these are bilateral. The majority of tumors occur in the right adrenal. Approximately 2 percent of extramedullary tumors are multiple.

Pheochromocytomas may or may not be encapsulated and vary greatly in size. They may weigh less than 3 g or more than 3,000 g. "Nonchromaffin" tumors, such as ganglioneuromas and neuroblastomas, have been found to secrete catecholamines and in some cases to elevate blood pressure.[5,6] Accordingly, a more appropriate classification of pheochromocytomas and similar tumors would be on the basis of chemical content rather than on staining characteristics.

Malignancy, which occurs in less than 10 percent of the cases, cannot be distinguished histopathologically, and can be diagnosed clinically only by the appearance of metastases at sites where normally there is no neural crest tissue. However, the observation by Anton et al.[7] of an increased secretion of dihydroxyphenylalanine (dopa), the first catechol on the biosynthetic pathway to norepinephrine (see Fig. 71-2), in association with a malignant pheochromocytoma suggests a biochemical identification of malignancy.

In Table 71-1 are compared the urinary catecholamines in normal persons with those in patients who have neural crest tumors. Note that in the patient with the malignant tumor (Case 2) the DA, DM, HVA and the NE, NM, VMA pathways are both exaggerated, whereas only the latter is increased in the

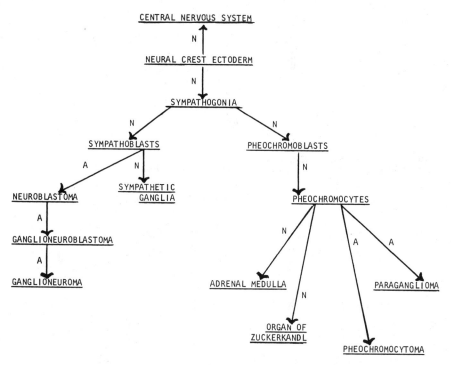

FIGURE 71-1 Embryologic origin of neural chest tumors. N, normal pathway; A, abnormal pathway.

patient with benign tumor. In this respect the malignant pheochromocytoma biochemically resembles the neuroblastoma (Case 3), an embryologically more primitive neural crest tumor. The postoperative return toward normal urinary catecholamine levels in the patient with benign tumor confirmed the clinical diagnosis of a benign pheochromocytoma, which was completely and successfully resected. A similar decrease was not seen in the patient with the malignant

tumor, and widespread metastases were found at the operation.

The plasma catecholamines from these subjects are shown in Table 71-2. Exaggeration of the DA, DM pathway in the patient with malignant tumor may be compared with the elevated NE and E in the patient with the benign tumor. Analysis of blood samples obtained during inferior vena cava catheterization revealed that the highest amount of dopa was

TABLE 71-1
Catecholamines and their metabolites in urine

Subject	Diagnosis	NE	E	DM	DA	NM	M	VMA	HVA
Control subjects (5)		0.55 (0.22– 1.14)	0.26 (0.22– 0.69)	2.96 (2.30– 3.93)	<0.1	4.82 (2.39– 10.4)	4.43 (2.09– 6.82)	122.0 (70.3– 210)	67.5 (5.0– 230)
Case 1	Benign pheochromocytoma (preoperative)	13.90	1.80	1.40	<0.1	714.0	38.0	2,192.0	100.0
	Benign pheochromocytoma (postoperative, 2 days)	0.96	0.52	4.20	<0.1	19.2	11.7	353.0	87.5
Case 2	Malignant pheochromocytoma (preoperative)	90.9	5.09	169.0	32.2	557.0	4.23	2,710.0	575.0
	Malignant pheochromocytoma (postoperative, 1 day)	61.4	4.36	82.0	24.3	492.0	2.19	1,640.0	
	Malignant pheochromocytoma (postoperative, 2 weeks)	119.0	5.81	353.0	99.5	890.0	1.72	3,270.0	550.0
Case 3	Neuroblastoma	23.9	<2.0	951.0	320.0	1,118.0	39.8	5,663.0	9,750.0

NOTE: Expressed in micrograms per 25 mg creatinine. Figures in parentheses represent the range. < = based on fluorimetry and paper chromatography. NE, norepinephrine; E, epinephrine; DM, dopamine; DA, dopa; NM, normetanephrine; M, metanephrine; VMA, vanillylmandelic acid; HVA, homovanillic acid. Multiply these figures by 50 to obtain the approximate amounts excreted over 24 h.
SOURCE: Anton et al.,[7] courtesy of *American Journal of Medicine*.

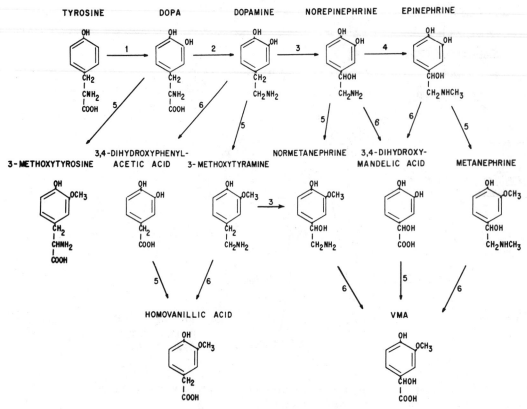

FIGURE 71-2 Biosynthesis and inactivation of the catechol-amines. The "activating" enzymes are (1) tyrosine hydroxylase; (2) aromatic L-amino acid decarboxylase; (3) dopamine-β-hydroxylase; (4) phenylethanolamine-N-methyl transferase. The "inactivating" enzymes are (5) catechol-O-methyl transferase; (6) monoamine oxidase.

at the level of the twelfth thoracic vertebra; this was the site of the metastatic nodules that subsequently were observed at surgery. Analysis of one of these nodules revealed catecholamine levels higher than those found in human adrenal glands. The appearance during surgery of large amounts of NE and E in the plasma of the patient with malignant tumor probably was a consequence of the homeostatic response to the stress of surgery, in which it was necessary to overcome the tolerance to the endogenous catecholamines as well as to counteract the adrenergic blockade of the phenoxybenzamine (Dibenzyline) which the patient had been receiving. Note the striking decrease in plasma catecholamines postoperatively in the patient with the benign tumor; a similar decrease was not observed in the patient with the malignant tumor.

Chemical content[1,5,7–9]

The steps in the biosynthesis and metabolism of the catecholamines are shown in Fig. 71-2. The precursors of catecholamines are found in pheochromocytomas and may be excreted along with catecholamine metabolities in the urine. The biosynthetic pathway

has been demonstrated in tissue culture, in which, starting with tyrosine, the pheochromocytoma cells produced dopa, dopamine, norepinephrine, and epinephrine.[9] The tumor also contains the catechol-O-methyl transferase and monoamine oxidase enzymes which render the catecholamines biologically inactive. Other tissues, particularly liver and kidney, can also carry out these metabolic steps before the metabolites are excreted into the urine. Therefore, an examination only of urinary catechols conceivably could lead to a biased viewpoint as to the functional activity of the tumor itself. Because of differing rates of catecholamine production and metabolism by different tumors, the excretion of precursors, catecholamines, and metabolites may vary considerably in patients with pheochromocytoma.[10] Norepinephrine is usually the only catecholamine found in extraadrenal tumors, whereas varying amounts of norepinephrine and epinephrine are found in adrenal tumors. Pheochromocytomas containing predominantly epinephrine are extremely rare.[11]

The cardiovascular and metabolic changes produced by pheochromocytoma are considered to be primarily due to the release of norepinephrine and epinephrine. The precursor, dopamine, also has pharmacologic actions,[12] but because of its low potency it is difficult to assess its effects in the syndrome. The cardiovascular actions of norepinephrine and epinephrine are described in Chap. 109. Recently, we carried out hemodynamic and catecholamine studies during resection of a pheochromocytoma in a patient

TABLE 71-2
Plasma catecholamines, μg/liter

Sample	NE	E	DM	DA
	Control Subjects (6)			
	0.55 (0.35–0.97)	0.30 (0.15–0.48)	<0.05	<0.10
	Benign pheochromocytoma			
Preoperative	974.	95.6	<15.0	<15.0
Postoperative, 2 days	0.96	0.42	<0.05	<0.10
	Malignant pheochromocytoma			
Preoperative	<7.0	<2.0	3.84	135.
Inferior vena cava catheterization: Tenth thoracic vertebra	<7.0	<2.0	33.9	108.
Twelfth thoracic vertebra	<11.0	<2.0	21.9	194.
First lumbar vertebra	<6.5	<2.0	21.1	107.
Third lumbar vertebra	<4.5	<2.0	27.9	62.7
During surgery, after anesthesia	60.6	2.8	17.8	74.7
Midpoint of operation	95.6	8.8	18.8	93.3
After closure of incision	65.8	7.6	22.4	74.4
Postoperative, 2 weeks	<4.5	<2.0	10.3	74.4
Postoperative, 5 weeks	<8.0	<2.0	22.6	138.

NOTE: Figures in parentheses represent the range. < = based on fluorimetry and paper chromatography. NE, norepinephrine; E, epinephrine; DM, dopamine; DA, dopa.
SOURCE: Anton et al.,[7] courtesy of *American Journal of Medicine*.

anesthetized with enflurane.[13] For the first time, cardiac performance was evaluated noninvasively by systolic time interval measurements before, during, and after removal of the tumor. The plasma norepinephrine and epinephrine changes that occurred during the operation are shown in Table 71-3A. (The urine and tumor tissue data, which are not shown, confirmed that the patient had a norepinephrine-secreting pheochromocytoma.) The corresponding hemodynamic results are tabulated in Table 71-3B and show that cardiac performance improved immediately after the tumor was excised. Thus, as peripheral resistance and blood pressure decreased after removal of the excess vasoconstricting norepinephrine, the cardiac index increased, the pre-ejection period shortened, the left ventricular ejection time lengthened, and the ratio PEP/LVET decreased. These systolic time interval data, reflecting a predominant peripheral vasoconstriction, are consistent with our finding that the patient's tumor secreted mainly norepinephrine. No arrhythmias were encountered during the operation even though the patient's systolic blood pressure reached 205 mm Hg. This suggests that enflurane, unlike cyclopropane and halothane, does not significantly sensitize the heart to catecholamine-induced arrhythmias.

The catecholamines produce hyperglycemia and an increase in plasma free fatty acids, apparently through the activation of adenyl cyclase, an enzyme which converts ATP to cyclic 3',5'-AMP. Cyclic AMP in turn activates phosphorylase and lipase,

TABLE 71-3A
Plasma catecholamines, μg/liter

	Norepinephrine	Epinephrine
Control (upper normal values)*	0.97	0.48
Patient:		
Preoperative	6.4	0.8
After induction	6.5	1.3
Exploration	9.1	1.8
After resection	1.1	0.6
Postoperative, 1 week	0.2	0.2

SOURCE: Kreul et al.;[13] courtesy of *Anesthesiology*.
*Data from several hundred analyses.

TABLE 71-3B
Hemodynamic characteristics of pheochromocytoma

	Cardiac index (L/min/m²)	Stroke index (ml/beat/m²)	Heart rate (beats/min)	Mean BP (mm Hg)	TPR* (mm Hg/L/min)	PEP (ms)	LVET (ms)	$\frac{PEP}{LVET}$
Normal values†	3.17 ± 0.2	40.6 ± 2	78 ± 2	95.4 ± 3	17 ± 1.4	86 ± 3	287 ± 5	0.30 ± .01
Patient:‡								
Before anesthesia	3.42	45.0	76	159	24	100	276	0.36
After induction	3.73	37.3	100	127	18	102	231	0.44
After resection	4.64	50.4	92	87	10	82	290	0.28

*Calculated from mean blood pressure (mm Hg) and cardiac output (L/min).
†Normal values are the means ± 1 standard error of data from 12 patients without heart disease coming for elective operations; mean age 49 ± 3, range 31–70 years. Data were collected before induction.
‡The patient's cardiac index, stroke index, and total peripheral resistance were calculated from the results of duplicate cardiac outputs at each event. PEP, LVET, heart rate, and mean blood pressure are the averages of continuous on-line measurements during each 5-min period necessary to perform each duplicate cardiac output measurement.
SOURCE: Kreul et al.;[13] courtesy of *Anesthesiology*.

which liberate glucose and free fatty acids from glycogen and triglycerides, respectively.[14] Epinephrine is more potent in this respect than norepinephrine, but there is little diagnostic significance in this difference because of the massive amounts of norepinephrine produced by the tumor. Also, the abnormal carbohydrate and fat metabolism in patients with pheochromocytoma may be partly due to an altered response to insulin.[15]

Clinical aspects[1-4,16,17]

Pheochromocytomas may be divided into two main types, depending on whether the hypertension is paroxysmal or persistent. In addition, cases of pheochromocytoma have been discovered without elevation of blood pressure. Patients with paroxysmal hypertension may experience attacks at intervals varying from more than one every hour to one in several months. The duration of the attacks also varies from a few seconds to several days. Factors which may precipitate a paroxysm are listed in Table 71-4, and the symptoms associated with the attack are indicated in Table 71-5. Blood pressure recorded during the attack in these patients almost invariably reaches levels greater than 200 mm Hg systolic and 100 mm Hg diastolic. After an attack the patient may be extremely fatigued and prostrate.

Patients with persistent hypertension usually have fewer symptoms than those with paroxysmal hypertension. In patients without characteristic symptoms, elevated urinary and/or plasma catechols allow the clinician to differentiate the pheochromocytoma from essential or malignant hypertension. Since the clinical syndrome is related to the hypersecretion of norepinephrine and epinephrine by the tumor, knowledge of their pharmacology provides the basis for a rational approach to medical management of the patient during the interim between diagnosis of the disease and surgery. For example, peripheral vasoconstriction from activation of α-adrenergic receptors by the catecholamines explains the hypertension, pallor, hemoconcentration, and decreased vascular space; administration of the α-adrenergic

TABLE 71-5
Symptoms in 100 patients with pheochromocytoma

Symptom	Patients (no. or %)
Headache	80
Perspiration	71
Palpitation (with or without tachycardia)	64
Pallor	42
Nausea (with or without vomiting)	42
Tremor or trembling	31
Weakness or exhaustion	28
Nervousness or anxiety	22
Epigastric pain	22
Chest pain	19
Dyspnea	19
Flushing or warmth	18
Numbness or paresthesia	11
Blurring of vision	11
Tightness in throat	8
Dizziness or faintness	8
Convulsions	5
Neck-shoulder pain	5
Extremity pain	4
Flank pain	4
Tinnitus	3
Dysarthria	3
Gagging	3
Bradycardia (noted by patient)	3
Back pain	3
Coughing	1
Yawning	1
Syncope	1
Unsteadiness	1
Hunger	1

SOURCE: Thomas et al;[16] courtesy of *Journal of the American Medical Association.*

blocker, phenoxybenzamine, will tend to correct these abnormalities. Again, the positive inotropic and chronotropic effects on the heart from activation of cardiac β-adrenergic receptors can account for tachycardia, palpitations, and occasional arrhythmias; these can be resolved with the β-adrenergic blocker propranolol. Such observations have established the close biochemical and physiologic relationship that is characteristic of the pheochromocytoma. However, we recently studied a patient in whom we documented increased plasma and urinary catecholamines while she remained asymptomatic except for a headache that was not characteristic of this tumor.[18]

The presence of a pheochromocytoma in a patient is an extremely treacherous and life-threatening situation. Although a few cases of pheochromocytoma have been symptomatic for longer than 25 years,[19] there is no way of telling when the release of catecholamines will produce a fatal attack. Patients with pheochromocytoma may die from cerebral vascular accidents, myocardial infarction, cardiac arrhythmias, acute pulmonary edema, intestinal lesions, or shock.[1,20,21] This was the tragic outcome 24 h after a patient was recently admitted to our institution, vomiting and complaining of severe upper right quadrant pain and headache.[22] The tentative diagnosis was acute cholecystitis (cholelithiasis has been reported in 10 to 30 percent of patients with pheo-

TABLE 71-4
Factors precipitating paroxysms in pheochromocytoma

Change of posture (bending, stooping, lateral flexion)	Hyperventilation
	Emotional stress
Exertion	Postural hypotension
Trauma to side of abdomen	Carotid sinus pressure
Local heat	Change in temperature
Perirenal air insufflation	Sleep
General anesthesia	Laughing
Parturition	Sexual intercourse
Meals	Shaving
Alcohol	Gargling
Histamine (as in gastric analysis)	Straining at stool
Amobarbital sodium sedation	Sneezing
Tetraethylammonium (TEA) chloride	Having blood pressure taken
Pain	Urination (pheochromocytoma of bladder)

SOURCE: Green;[17] courtesy of *Henry Ford Hospital Medical Bulletin.*

chromocytoma), and she was treated, in part, with propantheline. In retrospect, the anticholinergic activity of this medication in the presence of high levels of circulating catecholamines may have contributed to the patient's cardiovascular instability. Over the next 24 h her blood pressure fluctuated from 240/150 to 130/110 mm Hg. An electrocardiogram showed supraventricular tachycardia which did not respond to propranolol. In 24 h after admission, the patient suddenly developed intractable shock and cardiac arrest. At autopsy, a 50-g extraadrenal pheochromocytoma was found. Based on the analysis of plasma and tumor tissue, it was an epinephrine-secreting neoplasm; an extraadrenal epinephrine-producing pheochromocytoma occurs infrequently. It is imperative, therefore, once a pheochromocytoma is diagnosed, that precautions be taken to prevent occurrence of a fatal attack. It is advisable to have the patient's condition watched carefully, with frequent recordings of blood pressure. Intravenous phentolamine (Regitine) should be administered immediately in the event of an attack.

Oral administration of the α-adrenergic blocking agent phenoxybenzamine (Dibenzyline) has been recommended as soon as the condition is diagnosed.[23] The usual dose range is from 40 to 80 mg/day in divided doses, but both smaller and larger doses have been required. Administration of phenoxybenzamine may result in orthostatic hypotension and sedation.

The β-adrenergic blocking agent, propranolol, may also be required to selectively block excessive tachycardia or arrhythmias. Recommended dosage of propranolol for this indication is 60 mg/day in divided doses, but again the dose must be individualized. Propranolol should not be used in the absence of an α-adrenergic blocking agent because of the possibility of marked increase in peripheral resistance with precipitation of acute cardiac failure.

Pheochromocytoma has also been treated experimentally with α-methyltyrosine,[24] a drug which blocks the formation of catecholamines by inhibiting tyrosine hydroxylase, the rate-limiting step in the biosynthetic pathway (see Fig. 71-2). The toxicity of this drug precludes it from being released for general use, but it should form the basis for development of better medical management of patients with neural crest tumors.

Pheochromocytoma in pregnancy

Pheochromocytoma is a rare complication of pregnancy and poses a serious threat to the well-being of the mother and fetus. Approximately 94 cases have been reported up to 1972, with about a 45 percent maternal and a 35 percent fetal mortality rate.[25–27] The mortality was significantly less if the tumor was detected prior to term. Vigilant medical care of these patients is necessary along with an understanding of the interaction between adrenergic mechanisms, cardiovascular function, and fluid balance in order to prevent and treat the sudden catastrophic complications that may occur.

Clinical evidence indicates that pregnancy exacerbates the symptoms of a coexisting but relatively quiescent pheochromocytoma. It is not known how this comes about, but endocrine changes and pressure by the fetus on the tumor may increase its production of catecholamines. In the absence of pregnancy, the patient may experience a remission of her altered cardiovascular status. We diagnosed a pheochromocytoma in a multipara at 24 weeks of gestation.[26] Urinary analysis revealed markedly elevated catecholamine levels. Phenoxybenzamine and propranolol were instituted to control the hypertension and tachycardia, respectively. Intravenous phentolamine was also required before adequate control of blood pressure was obtained. At exploratory laparotomy the morning following her hospitalization a large unresectable retroperitoneal tumor was found. The patient underwent Cesarean section at 31 weeks of gestation and delivered a 2,085-g living male infant. The mother has continued taking the phenoxybenzamine and propranolol for more than 3 years on an outpatient basis and has remained asymptomatic. The child is normal in every respect.

In another case,[27] we diagnosed a pheochromocytoma at 21½ weeks' gestation in a 15-year-old primigravida. (To our knowledge this is the youngest person whose pregnancy was complicated by a pheochromocytoma.) At 25½ weeks' gestation, phenoxybenzamine, 20 to 60 mg/day, was started to control her hypertension. In spite of this medication, a hypertensive crisis occurred at the time her membranes ruptured spontaneously at 26 weeks' gestation, and an infusion of phentolamine was required to reduce her blood pressure from 240/130 to 160/80 mm Hg. About 24 h later she was delivered of a severely growth-retarded female infant who died shortly after birth. On the tenth postpartum day a norepinephrine-secreting extraadrenal pheochromocytoma was successfully excised. In addition to the delivery of an abnormal fetoplacental unit, the patient suffered a weight loss during the second trimester and her intravascular volume failed to expand, resulting in episodes of orthostatic hypotension. This pathophysiology can be attributed to the chronic vasoconstriction caused by the elevated levels of circulating norepinephrine, which among other things, compromised uteroplacental perfusion. The outcome of this case supports the recommendation that, if at all possible, a pheochromocytoma in pregnancy should be resected as soon as the diagnosis is established. If the patient is near term, both Cesarean section and tumor excision can be done at the same time. Earlier in the pregnancy, removal of the tumor alone should be done.

Physical examination and nondiagnostic laboratory tests[1]

The physical examination may be entirely negative. Patients with pheochromocytoma are usually thin, but cases have been described in obese patients.[18] The skin is frequently moist and may be flushed, particularly during an attack. All degrees of hypertensive retinal changes have been observed, including hemorrhages, exudates, and papilledema. The hands may be red or cyanotic. In approximately 10 to 15 percent of cases the tumor is large enough to be palpated; the attack may be precipitated by deep palpation. The cardiac examination may be negative or reveal the presence of arrhythmias[28] or cardiomegaly. Orthostatic hypotension is seen in some but not all patients.[4,27]

Fasting blood sugar level is elevated in about half the patients, usually only slightly above normal values. Glycosuria, if present, is usually intermittent. The basal metabolic rate is also elevated in about half the patients, but there are no characteristic changes in level of cholesterol or protein-bound iodine.

Differential diagnosis[1]

Because of the variety of symptoms and metabolic changes produced by pheochromocytoma, a long list of diseases must be considered.[4,17] Among the more commonly confused diagnoses are essential and malignant hypertension, thyrotoxicosis, diabetes with hypertension, congestive heart failure, neuroses with anxiety attacks, and acute abdominal emergencies. Pheochromocytoma must be considered in all hypertensive or hypotensive reactions during anesthesia or pregnancy, unexpected hypertensive or hypotensive reactions to antihypertensive agents, and hypotension after administration of phenothiazine tranquilizers.[29]

In the light of two reports of patients simulating the pheochromocytoma syndrome by self-administration of sympathomimetic amines, this possibility, although rare, should not be ruled out. In the case reported by Aguilar-Parada et al.,[30] the patient went so far as to allow one of her adrenal glands to be removed and still did not reveal the pharmacologic basis for her symptoms even when faced with the possibility of losing her remaining adrenal gland.

Diagnostic tests[1]

CHEMICAL METHODS
A number of highly sensitive and specific physicochemical methods are now available for estimating the parent catecholamines and most of their metabolites in urine and tissue.[31,34] Although the upper limits of normal urinary levels will be noted in this section, it should be emphasized that these figures will vary with the laboratory, according to the analytic procedure used. Laboratories either report their data as the total amount of substance excreted per 24 h or relate their results to a constant amount of urinary creatinine. We prefer the latter method since it will account, in part, for changes in renal function; also, it is difficult to collect all specimens voided during a 24-h period.

The upper limit of normal for the urinary excretion of free norepinephrine and epinephrine is approximately 100 μg/24 h[32] or less than 0.1 μg/mg creatinine[8] (see Table 71-1). Of this amount, more

than 60 percent is norepinephrine. Most pheochromocytomas excrete more than 300 μg catecholamines per 24 h (0.3 μg/mg creatinine) and several have been reported with catecholamine excretion rates greater than ten times this amount. In general, the measurement of total concentration of catecholamines is adequate for diagnostic purposes. Analyses of the main catecholamine metabolites, metanephrine, normetanephrine, and vanillylmandelic acid (VMA) (see Fig. 71-2), also are used for diagnostic purposes. These metabolites are excreted in far greater quantities than the parent amines and can be measured more easily.

A word of caution, however, is in order about the so-called simple colorimetric screening techniques, particularly for VMA, that are used in some laboratories. These crude tests are significantly influenced by phenolic acids of dietary origin, e.g., coffee and certain vegetables and fruits, so that they yield many false positive tests.[33] Since this may result in needless anxiety, expense, and surgery to a patient, it is advisable to use the highly specific procedures that are now available. This precaution also applies to the parent amines and their methoxy derivatives.[31,34]

The upper limit of normal for metanephrine plus normetanephrine is about 1 mg/24 h[32] or 1 μg/mg creatinine[8] (see Table 71-1). The normal value for urinary VMA is in the range of 7 mg/24 h[32] or 10 μg/mg creatinine[8] (see Table 71-1), and values much above these figures are highly suggestive of a pheochromocytoma.

There has been considerable debate as to whether it is better to measure the parent amines in the urine or one of the metabolites. The present consensus is that because of convenience and diagnostic accuracy, the analysis for urinary metanephrine and normetanephrine appears to be the most useful biochemical screening test for pheochromocytoma. The procedure for norepinephrine and epinephrine is technically more difficult, and that for VMA is less accurate diagnostically. However, in order to detect the few (less than 10 percent) cases in which only one of the catechols is elevated, a battery of analyses is necessary. The results of such analyses not only will indicate the presence of a neural crest tumor, but may provide an idea of its size,[10] whether it is a pheochromocytoma or neuroblastoma,[7,8] if it is malignant,[7] and the effect on it of therapy, e.g., drugs, surgery, radiation.[3,5] An example of this last technique is demonstrated in Fig. 71-3, in which the urinary levels of VMA and HVA (homovanillic acid) were used not only to establish the diagnosis of neuroblastoma but also as a guide in the successful treatment of this patient. Since not many laboratories are able to carry out a battery of analyses, most clinicians must still resort to a pharmacologic test together with the determination of one or two of the catechols.

The need to determine more than one metabolite in order to establish the diagnosis of a tumor does not necessarily mean that a particular test is inadequate; such a need may be the result of variations in metabolism of catecholamines by the tumor.[10] It is important in carrying out the chemical tests that directions for the collection of specimens be fol-

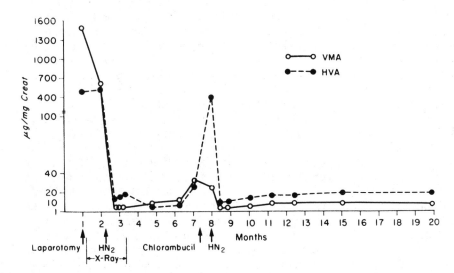

FIGURE 71-3 Urinary excretion values of VMA (vanillylmandelic acid) and HVA (homovanillic acid) in a child with neuro-blastoma before, during, and after thera-py. *(After Greer et al., Arch. Neurol., 13:139, 1965;* [5] *courtesy of Archives of Neurology and Psychiatry.)*

lowed exactly, particularly with respect to the parent amines which are unstable at pH near or above neutrality. It is advisable to analyze for free rather than total catecholamines in order to avoid interference by certain catecholamine-containing foods[35] which are excreted in the conjugated form. During the analysis for total amines these conjugates are hydrolyzed and would give rise to an artifactual elevation of urinary amines. Catecholamine-depleting agents such as reserpine and guanethidine, broad-spectrum antibiotics, methyldopa,[36] and the phenothiazines are some of the drugs which may produce spurious urinary values. The VMA test may be altered by monoamine oxidase inhibitors and disulfiram (Antabuse) and by ingestion of food items containing vanillin. False positive reactions may be obtained in conditions other than pheochromocytoma which increase secretion of catecholamines and their metabolites. A partial listing includes hypoglycemia, thyrotoxicosis, angina pectoris, myocardial infarction, renal disease, jaundice, lymphoma, and brain tumors. Fortunately many of these conditions do not enter into the differential diagnosis or can be ruled out by clinical means or other laboratory tests.

PLASMA CATECHOLAMINES

The measurement of plasma catecholamines is considered to be a less satisfactory method for the detection of pheochromocytoma than the determination of the amines in urine. This may be true insofar as screening is concerned, but more precise information about the tumor can be obtained from plasma. The objection to the use of plasma probably is due to the facts that it is more difficult to obtain, that a limited amount is available in comparison with urine, and that the analytical procedures are somewhat more involved and must be used at their ultimate sensitivity in order to detect the small amounts of catecholamines normally present. This last factor is actually an advantage in that even a slight elevation in plasma levels is readily detected and assumes

significance, since the wide fluctuations of urinary catecholamines within and among individuals are not seen in plasma. Also, as pointed out earlier, a more realistic evaluation of the type (benign or malignant) and functional capacity of the tumor can be obtained from plasma, since other tissues, e.g., liver and kidney, confuse the picture by also contributing catecholamine metabolites to the urine. In addition, the measurement of plasma catecholamines can be extremely helpful in localizing a tumor by differential venous catheterization. In fact some surgeons will not schedule surgery for a patient with a positively diagnosed pheochromocytoma until it has been localized using this technique. In the case shown in Fig. 71-4, we localized the tumor at the bifurcation of the aorta, and on the basis of the catecholamines found in the plasma,[7] diagnosed it as a benign pheochromocytoma; both predictions were confirmed at surgery.

FIGURE 71-4 Location of a pheochromocytoma by sampling at various levels from the inferior vena cava. The highest amounts of catecholamines appeared at the site (arrow) where the tumor was found at surgery.

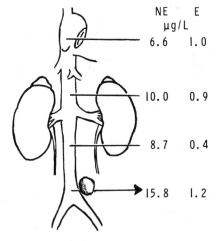

PHARMACOLOGIC TESTS[1,37–40]

Two pharmacologic tests have been commonly used in the diagnosis of pheochromocytoma: the phentolamine test for patients with blood pressure elevations above 170/110 mm Hg, and the provocative histamine test for patients with lower blood pressure levels. The phentolamine test is based on the principle that this α-adrenergic blocking agent will lower the elevated blood pressure by blocking the alpha (vasoconstrictor) effects of the catecholamines. Since the proper execution of this test is imperative for correct interpretation, a detailed summary follows:

An intravenous infusion of 5 percent glucose in water is started, and the patient is allowed to rest in bed, preferably in a quiet, darkened room, until blood pressure is stabilized at the basal level. Blood pressure recordings should then be obtained at least every 10 min for 30 min. After this period, 5 mg phentolamine is injected rapidly into the rubber tubing of the intravenous set and flushed into the vein. Blood pressure should be recorded immediately after the injection, at 30-sec intervals for the first 3 min, and at 60-sec intervals for the following 7 min. An immediate drop in blood pressure of more than 35 mm Hg systolic and 25 mm Hg diastolic is considered a positive response. Usually a maximal depressor effect is evident within 2 min after the injection, and pressure usually returns to the base line within 15 to 30 min, but a more rapid return is also possible. False positive tests occur in uremia and in patients taking sedatives, narcotics, anesthetics, antihypertensive agents, sympathomimetic amine nose drops, and a number of other drugs. It is advisable to discontinue use of sedatives and narcotics at least 48 h before the test and of catecholamine-depleting agents such as reserpine at least 2 weeks prior to the test. False positive test results may also occur because of release of catecholamines in an anxious patient.

The histamine test was introduced by Roth and Kvale in 1945. The basis of this test is the provocation of catecholamine release from the tumor by histamine. This release probably is due to the direct stimulation of the tumor, which does not appear to be innervated.[37] However, the initial histamine-induced decrease in blood pressure would reflexly activate the sympathetic nervous system. An exaggerated response occurs, probably because of an excessive release of norepinephrine from the adrenergic nerve endings, the granules of which are saturated with the amine from the elevated levels in the circulation. A cold pressor test is first performed, and after the blood pressure has returned to basal levels, a rapid intravenous injection of 0.025 or 0.05 mg histamine base in 0.25 or 0.5 ml isotonic saline solution is administered. The test is considered positive if the systolic pressure rises 20 mm Hg or more above the highest reading obtained with the cold pressor test. The rise in blood pressure usually becomes evident within 2 min following the injection of histamine and is accompanied by the characteristic symptoms of attack. The hypertensive response may be immedi-

ately terminated by administration of phentolamine; when the blood pressure is lowered, additional diagnostic significance is provided.

In recent years three additional provocative tests have been introduced, each supposedly safer and more specific than the phentolamine and histamine tests. These are the tyramine,[38] the glucagon,[39] and the tilt[37] tests. The first two, like the histamine test, are based on a drug-induced increase in blood pressure. The tilt test, unlike the others, is based on an exaggerated urinary norepinephrine response to tilting. An objection to this procedure is that it requires the patient to remain in essentially two positions of 3 h each for a total of 6 h. With respect to the tyramine test, several investigators have reported it to be inadequate in their hands.[40] The glucagon test, the usefulness of which also has been questioned,[4] appears to avoid the side effects of the histamine challenge. In 1970 Lawrence, who had introduced the glucagon test 5 years earlier, pointed out that a false positive response to this hormone had not been encountered.[41] In 1973, however, we reported positive blood pressure responses to the glucagon test in two patients with paroxysmal hypertension.[42] In Fig. 71-5, we show their blood pressures as a composite since the responses to the challenge with glucagon were essentially the same; above the figure are tabulated the plasma catecholamines, expressing

FIGURE 71-5 Plasma catecholamines and blood pressure responses to intravenous glucagon in two patients, only one of whom (case #1) had a pheochromocytoma. *(After White, Levy, and Anton, Res. Comm. Chem. Path. Pharmacol., 5:252, 1973;[42] courtesy of PJD Publications Ltd.).*

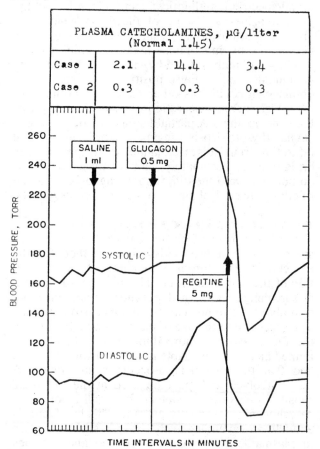

norepinephrine and epinephrine as a unit in micrograms per liter. In Case 1 the hypertension induced by the glucagon was correlated with a marked increase in plasma catecholamines (also in urine) and was followed by the successful resection of a pheochromocytoma. In contrast to this, plasma and urine catecholamines were normal in patient 2 and did not change with the glucagon-induced increase in blood pressure. A diagnosis of labile essential hypertension was made and treatment with hydrochlorothiazide was instituted. Since discharge from the hospital, this patient's blood pressure has remained below 140/90 mm Hg and she has been asymptomatic. Therefore, we conclude that this represents a false positive response to the glucagon test.

HAZARDS OF THE PROVOCATIVE TESTS

Since most of the pharmacologic tests are based on the activation of the sympathetic nervous system in one way or another, they share the hazards of precipitating a disastrous hypertensive crisis and inducing serious cardiac arrhythmias. Even with phentolamine, an agent which blocks α-adrenergic responses (but not the cardiac β-adrenergic effects of the catecholamines), tachycardia commonly occurs. This agent as well as the others must be administered very cautiously to patients with myocardial insufficiency. Severe hypotensive reactions and death[43] as well as hypertensive crisis[44] have been reported during the phentolamine test. Therefore, sympathomimetic agents, such as norepinephrine and metaraminol, and a rapid-acting hypotensive drug such as the ganglionic blocker trimethaphan (Arfonad) or the direct-acting vascular smooth muscle dilator sodium nitroprusside should be immediately available.

In the face of hypotension induced by an α-adrenergic blocking agent such as phentolamine, a pressor drug which acts by other than an adrenergic mechanism may have to be used; angiotensin is such an agent and should be available. It also is possible that the hypotensive crisis induced by an alpha blocker in the patient with pheochromocytoma may be due to the sudden expansion of the vascular space as the vasoconstriction is counteracted.[45] In this situation intravenous fluid therapy is indicated.

A major objection to the histamine test is the frequent occurrence of side effects such as nausea, vomiting, headache, and flushing. More serious and even fatal reactions also have occurred, since there may be a precipitous fall in blood pressure in the absence of a tumor or a hypertensive crisis in the presence of one.

The serious cardiac arrhythmias that may occur with these agents are less of a threat to the patient since the introduction of the β-adrenergic blocking agents. Propranolol (Inderal), for example, is given intravenously in doses of 2 to 5 mg (0.05 to 0.1 mg/kg). It has been suggested that propranolol not be used in the absence of alpha blockade; otherwise, the vasoconstrictor alpha effects of the catecholamines would be unopposed and a dangerous rise in blood pressure might occur.[45] β-adrenergic blocking agents are also contraindicated in asthmatics and in patients with incipient or frank heart failure (see also Chap.

109). In these circumstances intravenous lidocaine (Xylocaine), in doses of 50 to 100 mg, is preferred.

ROENTGEN TECHNIQUES[46]

Radiologic studies have frequently yielded information leading to the diagnosis and localization of pheochromocytomas. Tumors have been observed in chest roentgenograms and plain abdominal films. Intravenous urography has resulted in the localization of a number of tumors because of evidence of distortion of the ureters of calyxes and displacement of the kidney. Whether to proceed to more elaborate studies such as retroperitoneal pneumography or aortography is debatable because of the hazards involved.

Figure 71-6A shows a large calcified tumor which on intravenous urography was found to be distorting the right ureter. Figure 71-6B shows the same tumor with retroperitoneal carbon dioxide insufflation. The patient was a 27-year-old woman with typical attacks of paroxysmal hypertension. The mass was found on surgical intervention to be a 7- by 5- by 5-cm tumor of the organ of Zuckerkandl, with invasion of the aorta. In removing the tumor, it was necessary to remove a section of the aorta. The patient was normotensive and well 10 years after surgical treatment.[47]

Summary of diagnostic techniques

It is now possible to detect pheochromocytoma by a number of adequate methods. Ideally every hypertensive patient and every patient with unexplained "attacks" suggestive of pheochromocytoma should undergo at least one of the screening procedures. The chemical procedures are superior to the pharmacologic methods because of greater safety and diagnostic accuracy. Moreover, in contrast to the controversy, uncertainty, and potential hazards associated with the pharmacologic tests, there is unanimity of opinion that the determination of the urinary catecholamines and their metabolites is by far the ideal diagnostic test for pheochromocytoma. It should be remembered that pheochromocytomas can be missed even by the best screening methods because of low rates of catecholamine secretion and because of errors in collection or technique. Therefore the most important factors in the diagnosis of this disease are the clinical judgment and persistence of the physician. Indeed, many pheochromocytomas have been successfully removed only after repeated diagnostic tests and in some cases after repeated surgical explorations.[48]

Surgical procedures

Several excellent papers are available which discuss in detail the surgical aspects of pheochromocytoma.[2,49]

Surgeons should be prepared to explore both adrenals and the entire abdominal cavity to search

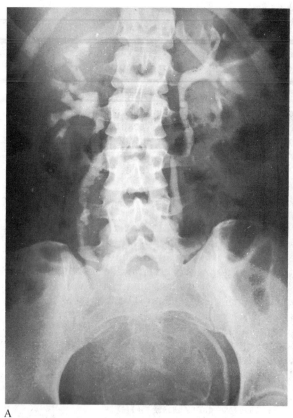

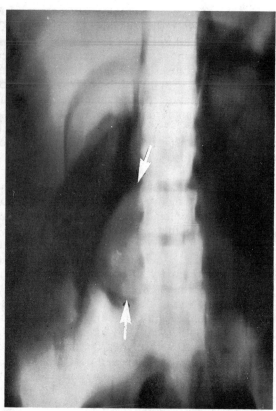

A   B

FIGURE 71-6 A. Intravenous pyelogram demonstrating dislocation of the right ureter by a paraaortic mass. *B.* The same lesion after retroperitoneal carbon dioxide insufflation. Note the calcification of the lesion. *(After Amerson and Goldberg, Postgrad. Med., 34:25, 1963;*[47] *courtesy of Postgraduate Medicine.)*

for multiple and extraadrenal tumors. Hume[2] recommends a transverse incision in the upper part of the abdomen, which provides exposure of both adrenal areas, both sympathetic chains, and the abdominal aorta. In addition, the surgeon should be capable of carrying out extensive vascular surgical procedures, since large vessels are sometimes involved.

Preoperative, operative, and postoperative periods are all particularly hazardous in these patients, and special precautions are required. It is now well recognized that these hazards can be reduced to a minimum by the proper pharmacologic preparation of the patient preoperatively.[32,45,50–52] Essentially this is accomplished by blocking the α-adrenergic receptors with phenoxybenzamine (40 to 100 mg/day for several days before and including the morning of surgery) in order to bring the hypertension under control. This will nullify the vasoconstrictor effect of the catecholamines and allow the dilatation of the vascular bed prior to surgery rather than precipitating this event acutely when the tumor is removed. Some physicians prefer to use phentolamine when required, rather than the long-lasting phenoxybenzamine, because of possible problems with persistence of α-adrenergic blockade after surgery. If phentolamine is used, the patient must be watched continuously and a constant intravenous infusion of saline solution or 5 percent dextrose in water must be maintained in the event a rapid injection of phentolamine is needed. Blockade of the β-adrenergic receptors with propranolol in addition to phenoxybenzamine may also be necessary as described earlier.[45]

Although there is some difference of opinion among anesthesiologists as to which anesthetic to use for the operation,[13,50–52] it is recognized that certain of the inhalational agents, e.g., cyclopropane and halogenated hydrocarbons such as halothane, lower the threshold to the arrhythmogenic activity of the catecholamines, large amounts of which may be released from the tumor when it is manipulated by the surgeon. For this reason, and because of the flammability of ether and fluroxene and the potential nephrotoxicity of methoxyflurane, we recently elected to use enflurane for resection of a pheochromocytoma in one of our patients.[13] In agreement with others, we found this anesthetic to be relatively safe in that no arrhythmias occurred during the operation, and as used by us, there was no significant depression of the heart (see Tables 71-3*A* and 71-3*B*).

It is advisable that the internist or cardiologist be present during the operation. Blood pressure should be recorded frequently, preferably continuously by an intraarterial technique. The electrocardiogram should be monitored because of the dangers of arrhythmias and sudden cardiac arrest. Phentolamine should be administered intravenously whenever the blood pressure rises, including during the period of induction with the anesthetic. A direct-acting vasodilator such as sodium nitroprusside or the ganglionic blocker trimethaphan should be available in case the pressure-lowering effect of the α-adrenergic blocking agent is inadequate.[53] Since the blood volume may be decreased in patients with pheochromocytoma, plasma volume expanders are useful in prevention and management of postoperative hypotension. Blood lost during the operation should be adequately replaced. If the patient has been properly prepared for surgery and his vascular volume maintained, pressor agents such as norepinephrine may not be required even after the tumor has been removed. However, it is advisable not to let the systolic pressure fall below 100 mm Hg in order to assure adequate perfusion of the vital organs. Particular caution is needed in the case of the atherosclerotic elderly individual who requires a higher than normal blood pressure to maintain good perfusion of his central nervous system. Finally, in the event of bilateral adrenalectomy, administration of hydrocortisone will be required.

REFERENCES

1 Herman, H., and Mornex, R.: "Human Tumours Secreting Catecholamines," The Macmillan Company, New York, 1964.

2 Hume, D. M.: Pheochromocytoma in the Adult and in the Child, *Am. J. Surg.*, 99:458, 1960.

3 Remine, W. H., Chong, G. C., Van Heerden, J. A., Sheps, S. G., and Harrison, E. G., Jr.: Current Management of Pheochromocytoma, *Ann. Surg.*, 179:740, 1974.

3a Tisherman, S. E., Gregg, F. J., and Danowski, T. S.: Familial Pheochromocytoma, *J.A.M.A.*, 182:152, 1962.

4 Poutasse, E. F., and Gifford, R. W., Jr.: Pheochromocytoma Diagnosis and Treatment, *Prog. Cardiovasc. Dis.*, 8:235, 1965.

5 Greer, M., Anton, A. H., Williams, C. M., and Echevarria, R. A.: Tumors of Neural Crest Origin, *Arch. Neurol.*, 13:139, 1965.

6 Voorhess, M. L., and Gardner, L. I.: Studies of Catecholamine Excretion by Children with Neural Tumors, *J. Clin. Endocrinol.*, 22:126, 1962.

7 Anton, A. H., Greer, M., Sayre, D. F., and Williams, C. M.: Dihydroxyphenylalanine Secretion in a Malignant Pheochromocytoma, *Am. J. Med.*, 42:469, 1967.

8 von Studnitz, W., Kaser, H., and Sjoerdsma, A.: Spectrum of Catechol Amine Biochemistry in Patients with Neuroblastoma, *N. Engl. J. Med.*, 269:232, 1963.

9 Cabana, B. E., Prokesch, J. C., and Christiansen, G. S.: Study of the Biogenesis of Catecholamines in Pheochromocytoma Tissue Culture, *Arch. Biochem.*, 106:123, 1964.

10 Crout, R. J., and Sjoerdsma, A.: Turnover and Metabolism of Catecholamines in Patients with Pheochromocytoma, *J. Clin. Invest.*, 43:94, 1964.

11 Engelman, K., and Hammond, W. G.: Adrenaline Production by an Intrathoracic Phaeochromocytoma, *Lancet*, 1:609, 1968.

12 Goldberg, L. I.: Cardiovascular and Renal Actions of Dopamine, *Pharmacol. Rev.*, 24:1, 1972.

13 Kreul, J. F., Dauchot, P. J., and Anton, A. H.: Hemodynamic and Catecholamine Studies during Pheochromocytoma Resection under Enflurane Anesthesia, *Anesthesiology*, 44:265, 1976.

14 Sutherland, E. W., Robison, G. A., and Butcher, R. W.: Some Aspects of the Biological Role of Adenosine 3',5'-Monophosphate (Cyclic AMP), *Circulation*, 37:279, 1968.

15 Spergel, G., Bleicher, S. J., and Ertel, N. H.: Carbohydrate and Fat Metabolism in Patients with Pheochromocytoma, *N. Engl. J. Med.*, 278:803, 1968.

16 Thomas, J. E., Rooke, E. D., and Kvale, W. F.: The Neurologist's Experience with Pheochromocytoma, *J.A.M.A.*, 197:754, 1966.

17 Green, H. L.: Pheochromocytoma: A Survey of Current Concepts, *Henry Ford Hosp. Med. Bull.*, 8:103, 1960.

18 Taubman, I., Pearson, O. H., and Anton, A. H.: An Asymptomatic Catecholamine-Secreting Pheochromocytoma, *Am. J. Med.*, 57:953, 1974.

19 Bell, M. A., Blakemore, W. S., and Rose, E.: Some Vagaries of Pheochromocytoma: Four Illustrative Cases, *Ann. Intern. Med.*, 57:406, 1962.

20 Van Vliet, P. D., Burchell, H. B., and Titus, J. C.: Local Myocarditis Associated with Pheochromocytoma, *N. Engl. J. Med.*, 274:1102, 1966.

21 Brown, R. B., and Borowsky, M.: Further Observation on Intestinal Lesion Associated with Pheochromocytoma, *Ann. Surg.*, 151:683, 1960.

22 Sobonya, R. E., Weaver, J. P., and Anton, A. H.: Extra-Adrenal Epinephrine-Producing Pheochromocytoma with Fatal Shock, *Res. Comm. Chem. Pathol. Pharmacol.*, 5:241, 1973.

23 Engelman, K., and Sjoerdsma, A.: Chronic Medical Therapy for Pheochromocytoma, *Ann. Intern. Med.*, 61:229, 1964.

24 Sjoerdsma, A., Engelman, K., and Spector, S.: Inhibition of Catecholamine Synthesis in Man with Alpha-Methyl-Tyrosine, an Inhibitor of Tyrosine Hydroxlase, *Lancet*, 2:1092, 1965.

25 Schenker, J. G., and Chowers, I.: Pheochromocytoma and Pregnancy, *Obstet. Gynecol. Surv.*, 26:739, 1971.

26 Simanis, J., Amerson, J. R., Hendee, A. F., and Anton, A. H.: Unresectable Pheochromocytoma in Pregnancy: Pharmacology and Biochemistry, *Am. J. Med.*, 53:381, 1972.

27 Brenner, W. E., Yen, S. S. C., Dingfelder, J. R., and Anton, A. H.: Pheochromocytoma: Serial Studies during Pregnancy, *Am. J. Obstet. Gynecol.*, 113:779, 1972.

28 Durant, J., and Soloff, L. A.: Arrhythmic Crisis of Phaeochromocytoma, *Lancet*, 2:124, 1962.

29 Lund-Johansen, P.: Shock after Administration of Phenothiazines in Patients with Pheochromocytoma, *Acta Med. Scand.*, 172:525, 1962.

30 Aguilar-Parada, E., Rivadeneyra, J., Torres-Leon, A. G., and Serrano, P. A.: Pseudophenochromocytoma, *J.A.M.A.*, 218:884, 1971.

31 Anton, A. H., and Sayre, D. F.: Fluorometric Assay of Catecholamines, Serotonin and Their Metabolites, in S. A. Berson (ed.), "Methods in Investigative and Diagnostic Endocrinology," vol. 1 (part 2), The Biogenic Amines, I. J. Kopin, (ed.), North-Holland Publishing Co., Amsterdam-London, 1972, p. 398.

32 Sjoerdsma, A., Engelman, K., Waldmann, T. A., Cooperman, L. H., and Hammond, W. G.: Pheochromocytoma: Current Concepts of Diagnosis and Treatment, *Ann. Intern. Med.*, 65:1302, 1966.

33 von Studnitz, W., Engelman, K., and Sjoerdsma, A.: Urinary Excretion of Phenolic Acids in Human Subjects on a Glucose Diet, *Clin. Chim. Acta*, 9:224, 1964.

34 Nagatsu, T.: Biochemistry of Catecholamines, University Park Press, Baltimore, Md., 1973.

35 Crout, J. R., and Sjoerdsma, A.: The Clinical and Laboratory Significance of Serotonin and Catechol Amines in Bananas, *N. Engl. J. Med.*, 261:23, 1959.

36 Gifford, R. W., and Tweed, D. C.: Spurious Elevation of Urinary Catecholamines during Therapy with Alpha-methyldopa, *J.A.M.A.*, 182:493, 1962.

37 Harrison, T. S., Bartlett, J. D., Jr., and Seaton, J. F.: Exag-

gerated Urinary Norepinephrine Response to Tilt in Pheochromocytoma, *N. Engl. J. Med.*, 277:725, 1967.

38 Engelman, K., aand Sjoerdsma, A.: New Test for Pheochromocytoma: Pressor Responsiveness to Tyramine, *J.A.M.A.*, 189:81, 1964.

39 Lawrence, A. M.: Glucagon Provocative Test for Pheochromocytoma, *Ann. Intern. Med.*, 66:1091, 1967.

40 Sheps, S. G., and Maher, F. T.: Comparison of the Histamine and Tyramine Hydrochloride Tests in the Diagnosis of Pheochromocytoma, *J.A.M.A.*, 195:265, 1966.

41 Lawrence, A. M.: Glucagon and Pheochromocytoma, *Ann. Intern. Med.*, 73:852, 1970.

42 White, L. W., Levy, R. P., and Anton, A. H.: Comparison of Biochemical and Pharmacological Testing for Pheochromocytoma, *Res. Comm. Chem. Pathol. Pharmacol.*, 5:252, 1973.

43 Roland, C. R.: Pheochromocytoma in Pregnancy: Report of a Fatal Reaction to Phentolamine (Regitine) Methanesulfonate, *J.A.M.A.*, 171:1806, 1959.

44 Marriott, H. J. L.: An Alarming Pressor Reaction to Regitine, *Ann. Intern. Med.*, 46:1001, 1957.

45 Prichard, B. N. C., and Ross, E. J.: Use of Propranolol in Conjunction with Alpha Receptor Blocking Drugs in Pheochromocytoma, *Am. J. Cardiol.*, 18:394, 1966.

46 Pendergrass, H. P., Tristan, T. A., Blakemore, W. S., Sellers, A. M., Jannetta, P. J., and Murphy, J. J.: Roentgen Technics in the Diagnosis and Localization of Pheochromocytoma, *Radiology*, 78:725, 1962.

47 Amerson, J. R., and Goldberg, L. I.: Pheochromocytoma: Diagnosis and Treatment, *Postgrad. Med.*, 34:25, 1963.

48 Effersoe, P., Gertz, T. C., and Lund, A.: Pheochromocytoma: A Case Report of Successful Thoraco-abdominal Operation after Nine Negative Surgical Explorations, *Acta Chir. Scand.*, 103:43, 1952.

49 Scott, H. W., Jr., Riddell, D. H., and Brockman, S. K.: Surgical Management of Pheochromocytoma, *Surg. Gynecol. Obstet.*, 120:707, 1965.

50 Fabian, W.: The Experts Opine, *Surv. Anesthesiol.*, 19:567, 1975.

51 Crout, J. R., and Brown, B. R.: Anesthetic Management of Pheochromocytoma: The Value of Phenoxybenzamine and Methoxyflurane. *Anesthesiology*, 30:29, 1969.

52 Perry, L. B., and Gould, A. B., Jr.: The Anesthetic Management of Pheochromocytoma: Effect of Preoperative Adrenergic Blocking Drugs, *Anesth. Analg.*, 51:36, 1972.

53 Nourok, D. S., Gwinup, G., and Hamwi, G. J.: Phentolamine-Resistant Pheochromocytoma Treated with Sodium Nitroprusside, *J.A.M.A.*, 183:841, 1963.

72
Primary Aldosteronism

WILLIAM C. WATERS, III, M.D.

Interest in the relatively small group of patients with curable hypertension received an enormous impetus with the discovery in 1955 of the syndrome of primary aldosteronism. Applying basic physiologic information already obtained by earlier investigators to a patient with hypertension, hypokalemia, and alkalosis, Conn and his associates demonstrated in-creased urinary excretion of the potent mineralocorticoid aldosterone and subsequently established the cause to be an adrenal cortical adenoma.[1] Although expectations of a high incidence of this syndrome were not originally fulfilled, an enthusiastic search has nonetheless been pursued, with increasing reports of atypical cases accumulating.

From a historical point of view, identification of the syndrome has had the effect of stimulating new interest in the concept of reversible hypertension, of bringing into focus the dynamic influence of aldosterone in a variety of clinical states, and perhaps most of all, in helping to define the role of renin and in identifying the "low renin" hypertensive.

PHYSIOLOGY AND PATHOPHYSIOLOGY

Aldosterone, the 17-aldehyde of corticosterone, is the most physiologically potent mineralocorticoid known. An effect of minute amounts can be demonstrated in the intestine, in sweat glands, in salivary secretions, and possibly even upon transmembrane sodium potassium transport of muscle cells. By far its most striking effect, however, is in facilitating sodium reabsorption and potassium excretion by the distal renal tubular epithelial cell;[2] indeed, the entire spectrum of abnormalities found in the clinical syndrome of primary aldosteronism can be traced to its action at this locus.

In the distal renal tubule, the electrochemical gradient established by the active transport of sodium from tubular urine to peritubular blood must be matched by an equivalent migration of anion (from urine to blood) or by an equivalent exchange of cation (from blood to urine).[3] Thus, under the accelerating effect of increased aldosterone activity, chloride may accompany the reabsorbed sodium (with resultant salt and water retention), or potassium and hydrogen may be exchanged for sodium (with resultant potassium depletion and alkalosis). Once potassium depletion has occurred, hydrogen ion loss is further encouraged, although recent work indicates that chloride depletion may be more important than potassium deficit in sustaining the elevated plasma bicarbonate concentration.[4] The clinical and biochemical disturbances of the full syndrome—hypertension, hypokalemia, and alkalosis—ensue.

A substantial body of data indicates that aldosterone in the human being is normally secreted by the zona glomerulosa of the adrenal cortex at a rate of 180 to 330 μg/day and is excreted in the urine both as free aldosterone and as the metabolically inactive degradation product tetrahydroaldosterone.[5] Unlike the secretion of other adrenal hormones, including cortisol, aldosterone is elaborated relatively independently of the influence of adrenocorticotropic hormone. On the other hand, its release is exquisitely sensitive to a variety of other stimuli, particularly those involving changes in circulatory dynamics. Constriction of the inferior vena cava, acute hemorrhage, and salt depletion are known to be regularly associated with increased secretion rates of aldosterone; similarly, saline loading or albumin infusion causes a reduction in aldosterone activity. Carpenter, Davis, and associates[6] have clearly demonstrated the role of angiotensin in stimulating aldosterone release. Thus, reduction in the flow rate to the renal juxtaglomerular apparatus results in increased renin activity, leading to angiotensin activation; angiotensin in turn stimulates adrenal cortical aldosterone production or release. Hence, the renin-angiotensin-aldosterone axis must be recognized as an important homeostatic system in the regulation of extracellular and intravascular volumes.

Considerable information concerning the pathogenesis of primary aldosteronism is contributed by a study of normal subjects given pharmacologic doses of the hormone. Nelson and others[7] found that normal adults receiving large doses of aldosterone daily developed positive salt and water balance, hypokalemia, alkalosis, and hypertension. It is significant that after a 3-kg weight gain, a new steady state was attained, and thereafter the patients "escaped" from the effects of the drug. At this level, like patients with the clinical syndrome, these subjects exhibited no edema. Suggested explanations for the "escape phenomenon" have included absence of an adrenal salt-losing factor and hypervolemia with increased renal plasma flow and overload of the distal tubular sodium-reabsorptive mechanism. Recent investigation regarding "third factor,"[8] a natriuretic agent, would suggest a role of this presumed hormone in inhibiting proximal-tubular sodium reabsorption under conditions of volume expansion, At any rate, it appears clear that both experimentally and clinically the syndrome of uncomplicated aldosterone excess only very rarely includes edema formation, and the presence of edema in a given case would suggest either complicating heart failure or that the aldosteronism is due to the cause of the edema formation ("secondary aldosteronism"—see "Differential Diagnosis").

Patients with primary hyperaldosteronism classically exhibit depressed plasma renin activity (usually determined as angiotensin II by radioimmunoassay), presumably because of the hypervolemia which necessarily accompanies the syndrome. Whether this mechanistic sequence is indeed correct is somewhat challenged by a recent study indicating that renin activity can be suppressed by doses of DOCA so small that weight gain, hypertension, and edema do not occur.[9] In any event, the low plasma renin value is essential for the diagnosis of primary aldosteronism, as it is now understood.

The converse however is not true, since a sizable number of essential hypertensive patients have low plasma renin values. The mechanism and significance of the latter finding has been much debated and is discussed below.

INCIDENCE

As of March, 1963, Conn[10] tabulated 145 reported cases of primary aldosteronism and indicated knowledge of about 50 more. Subsequently he proposed that perhaps many cases of "innocent" adrenal cortical tumors found at autopsy may in fact represent forms of the syndrome masked by the normal electrolyte findings but demonstrable by other methods,[11] and suggested that as many as 20 percent of hypertensive patients may have this curable form of hypertension. Others have failed to find such cases of inapparent aldosteronism, even on intensive study; still further reports have dealt with instances of diffuse hyperplasia and adenomatous hyperplasia associated with normal serum electrolyte patterns but with increased secretion rates of aldosterone, suppressed renin, and a variable response to surgery.[12,13]

Increasing recognition of the entity of low-renin hypertension with normal or low plasma aldosterone, and with responsiveness to spironolactone, has focused attention on the presence of other probably hypermineralocorticoid states. The frequency of such entities has been variously estimated between 5 and 30 percent of "essential hypertensive" persons.[14]

Final definition of the incidence of primary aldosteronism per se must await further study. At present, considering the size of the hypertensive population and the intensive search being undertaken in many centers, it must still be regarded as a rather uncommon disorder.

Females have predominated over males in the ratio of 2.7:1, and by far the greatest age incidence falls in the 30- to 40-year age group (approximately 70 percent of total cases). Primary aldosteronism is therefore predominantly a disease of young and middle-aged females.

SYMPTOMATOLOGY

The presenting symptoms of patients with primary aldosteronism can be traced to the underlying disturbance of fluid volume, potassium metabolism, and acid-base equilibrium. By far the most common complaints are muscle weakness and polyuria, both being present in approximately three-fourths of patients. The muscle weakness may be chronic or episodic and may be responsive in at least some cases to the administration of adequate quantities of potassium salts even prior to surgical intervention. In some cases[10] the weakness has appeared only after administration of thiazide diuretics. The polyuria is related to a concentration defect produced in the kidney by potassium depletion. This "potassium-depletion nephropathy" is characterized pathologically by vacuolar degeneration of renal tubular epithelial cells and clinically by a vasopressin-resistant isosthenuria.[15] The nephropathy is not specific for primary aldosteronism but may occur in any disease state attended by significant total body potassium depletion. Other symptoms have included headache, paresthesias, intermittent paralysis, tetanic manifestations, including dysesthesias, and a sensation of fatigue. In a small percentage of cases no symptoms at all have been present, and the diagnosis has been made after the discovery of abnormal serum electrolyte concentrations in patients being evaluated for hypertension. Considerable attention has been directed in recent years to a group of patients with hypertension, no typical symptoms, and normal serum electrolyte concentrations, in whom laboratory and pathologic data suggest an incomplete form of the syndrome (see "Incidence" and "Laboratory Findings").

PHYSICAL FINDINGS

Hypertension has been a regular finding in all typical cases. The elevation of blood pressure has been mild to moderate (160/100 to 200/120 mm Hg) with rare exceptions, and it has been repeatedly emphasized that malignant progression is not a characteristic of primary aldosteronism, although a few well-documented cases have been reported.[16] A syndrome resembling primary aldosteronism, but without hypertension, has been described by Bartter et al.,[17] in which aldosterone secretion and excretion are increased, hypokalemic alkalosis is present, and renin activity is elevated. This high renin level, together with the apparent activation of the cells of the juxtaglomerular apparatus, suggests that the hyperaldosteronism in this syndrome should be classified as secondary.

Retinopathy, usually confined to vascular attenuation and arteriovenous crossing changes, has been seen in approximately one-half of patients. Though papilledema, as noted above, is almost universally absent, hemorrhages and exudates are occasionally noted. Cardiomegaly has been reported in some 40 percent of cases, although findings of congestive heart failure such as neck vein distension, pulmonary congestion, hepatomegaly, and peripheral edema have been exceptional. Signs of neuromuscular irritability, including positive Chvostek's and Trousseau's signs, or frank tetany, have been demonstrable in approximately 10 to 15 percent of patients but only very exceptionally in males. Overt paralysis, reported in a few instances, has been confined to females.

LABORATORY FINDINGS

The diagnostic cluster of laboratory findings in primary aldosteronism includes hypertension, hypokalemic alkalosis, high urine potassium, low plasma renin, and elevated plasma aldosterone level—though all may not be present simultaneously.

Hypokalemia was present at some time in the majority of patients thus far demonstrated to have a functioning aldosteronoma. The average serum potassium level is below 3.0 mEq/liter and is usually persistently in this range. However, some patients reach these low levels only episodically. Occasional individuals may show normal serum potassium concentrations, with paroxysmal drops to hypokalemic levels. A few cases[10] have had their metabolic disturbance unmasked only after therapy with thiazide diuretics, and it has been suggested that suspicion of an aldosteronoma should be aroused by the development of symptoms of muscular weakness occurring within a few days of institution of diuretic therapy. However, mild degrees of hypokalemia are common with thiazide administration in any group, and such slight reductions should of course not be considered diagnostic.[18] As noted, reports indicate a group of patients who never manifest electrolyte abnormalities in the course of their primary aldosteronism; however, the preliminary nature of these reports make an assessment of the incidence of this incomplete syndrome very difficult at the present time. *Metabolic alkalosis,* as manifested by an elevated bicarbonate concentration of plasma and normal or elevated blood pH, is present in the majority of cases but is not invariable. Most such patients exhibit a CO_2 content of blood plasma in the range of 32 to 38 mEq/liter. *Hypernatremia* is frequent, although not constant, but hyponatremia is virtually never present and, as noted below, militates against the diagnosis of primary aldosteronism. Serum chloride concentration is depressed reciprocally with the bicarbonate elevation. In many cases low serum magnesium levels have been demonstrated.

Patients with primary aldosteronism can be shown at some time to have increased urinary *excretion of aldosterone* and/or tetrahydroaldosterone. Double-dilution isotope studies reveal increased endogenous secretion rates of aldosterone; Porter-Silber chromogens (17-hydroxysteroids and 17-ketosteroids), on the other hand, are within normal limits. *Plasma aldosterone* measurements, made through the technique of radioimmunoassay, are regularly elevated, and the aldosteronoma may be lateralized by determination of aldosterone levels in the blood obtained by bilateral adrenal venous catheterization.

Such elevations are made significant if simultaneous *plasma renin* values are suppressed and do not rise with sodium restriction or diuretics. Plasma renin activity values are reliably obtained currently by means of radioimmunoassay for angiotensin II. Plasma renin values (as expressed in units of angiotensin activity determined by bioassay) are regularly lower than normal, and they fail to rise significantly on ambulation, salt restriction, or even when natriuretic agents are given.[19]

Potassium excretion is usually within normal limits (40 to 80 mEq/liter) in spite of hypokalemia and tissue potassium depletion. Potassium-depletion nephropathy is frequently present and is manifested by decreased concentrating ability which is resistant to vasopressin. Exaggerated ammonia production results in a tendency to a persistently *alkaline urine.*

Other studies have demonstrated low sweat and salivary sodium concentrations, while total body exchangeable sodium is high and body exchangeable potassium is low as determined by radioisotopic measurement methods. An increased plasma volume, with slight decrease of the hematocrit value, is usual. The electrocardiogram may show changes of decreased T vector and prominent U waves consistent with hypokalemia, but diagnostic changes may be absent.

DIAGNOSIS

The diagnosis of typical primary aldosteronism will thus not be difficult in the young to middle-aged female with mild to moderate hypertension, hypokalemic alkalosis, increased urinary potassium concentration, alkaline urine, increased plasma aldosterone level, low plasma renin, and normal urinary 17-hydroxysteroids and 17-ketosteroids. Such is not the case, however, when the serum potassium level is normal, plasma CO_2 is within normal limits, or aldosterone assays are in an equivocal range. It is in such instances that plasma renin determinations, especially after sodium depletion, are of crucial value. Indeed, the presently controversial nature of the syndrome of primary aldosteronism with normal serum electrolytes suggests that such patients should receive the intensive study which can be afforded in a medical center before exploration is considered. Furthermore, it seems desirable to demonstrate low plasma renin values before and after sodium restriction, even in the typical case. The increasing availability of such determinations has made the plasma renin assay a routine clinical study. Even with the aid of such determinations, it appears that a heterogeneous group of hypertensive patients is appearing. As many as one-third of certain groups of hypertensive patients may have suppressed plasma renin concentrations without demonstrable aldosterone excess; other unidentified mineralocorticoids have been suggested.[20] Biglieri has proposed four types of primary aldosteronism: (1) classic adenoma, (2) classic syndrome with hyperplasia (responding poorly to surgery), (3) "indeterminate aldosteronism" in which administration of DOCA suppresses aldosterone secretion (no surgery indicated), and (4) glucocorticoid-responsive aldosteronism, in which dexamethasone is effective.[21] To this group certainly must be added the enlarging group of patients with low renin hypertension, low plasma aldosterone, and usually normal electrolytes who respond to spironolactone. These findings have been ascribed to excessive production of mineralocorticoids other than aldosterone, including 16β-hydroxydehydroepiandrosterone.[22] In any event correction of hypertension and of metabolic abnormalities with spironolactone has been shown to have diagnostic value as well as therapeutic merit in the patient whose surgical candidacy is marginal.[20]

Further attempts to demonstrate the lesion preoperatively, as by retroperitoneal air or carbon dioxide insufflation, have proved discouraging, since the great majority of tumors weigh less than 6 g and generally are less than 3 cm in diameter. On the other hand, differential adrenal venous catheterization for aldosterone has proved a promising means of lateral-izing the tumor, and may become standard procedure when facilities and local expertise permit. The final proof of diagnosis is exploration. In the slightly atypical case, however, careful evaluation to exclude other possibilities is essential. Other entities which may produce confusion are discussed in the following section, "Differential Diagnosis."

DIFFERENTIAL DIAGNOSIS

By far the most common cause of hypokalemic alkalosis in any given hypertensive patient is prior therapy with *thiazide diuretics*. Thus, in the evaluation of any hypertensive patient for possible reversible causes, detailed history regarding the many forms of diuretics must be pursued; such agents as furosemide and ethacrynic acid may also produce a "contraction alkalosis" associated with hypokalemia. Even after discontinuation of therapy for a week or more, persistent potassium depletion and/or chloride deficit may perpetuate the hypokalemic alkalosis. Further confusion may result from an increased urinary aldosterone secretion rate caused by the extracellular fluid volume depletion which diuretics may produce.[23] It is thus suggested that such patients be given a period of 3 to 4 weeks without diuretics and that during the first week without therapy adequate provision of potassium chloride, 15 mEq three times daily, be given. On the other hand, *sodium depletion*, resulting from either diruetic therapy or dietary salt restriction, may mask the electrolyte abnormalities of primary aldosteronism, and an adequate or—as some authors have recommended—increased sodium allowance should be given.

Considerable conceptual as well as diagnostic difficulties may be encountered in the infrequent patient with *malignant hypertension* and "secondary aldosteronism." A sizable proportion of patients with fulminating hypertensive disease may exhibit hypokalemia, alkalosis, and aldosterone secretion rates even higher than that seen in primary aldosteronism.[5] Such patients, when explored, have been found to have not adenomas but either bilateral adrenal hyperplasia or normal adrenal glands and have shown either an unfavorable or a poor response to subtotal adrenalectomy; thus the preoperative recognition of this group is of obvious clinical importance. It has been suggested that the presence of malignant hypertension is itself adequate evidence for the absence of an aldosteronoma, but the recent well-documented reports of accelerated hypertension cured by removal of a tumor[16] indicates that caution should be used before applying this dictum too rigidly. Other features may serve to distinguish the two groups: the patient with malignant hypertension generally has a less pronounced hypokalemia (3.2 to 3.8 mEq/liter), and alkalosis is less regularly present and less severe; the patient with accelerated hypertension often has hyponatremia, a rare finding indeed in the patient with adenoma. Similarly, reports of clinical symptoms of muscle weakness and polyuria in the secondary group are scanty. In malignant hypertension of other etiologies, the plasma renin value is very high; thus, a low renin value in this setting would point to aldosteronism. It should be noted, however, that malignant hypertension is not at all uncommon in the juvenile form of primary aldosteronism. This syndrome includes hypokalemia, alkalosis, and greatly increased aldosterone production; is more common in young males; may occur with hyponatremia; is associated with normal or hyperplastic adrenals; and is usually cured by total adrenalectomy.

Patients with hypertension and *incidental potassium depletion* (e.g., individuals with chronic diarrhea) can generally be screened out by an adequate history and by the demonstration of low levels of urinary potassium. Certain patients with unilateral *renal arterial disease* have had hypokalemic alkalosis and elevated aldosterone excretion rates, abnormalities which have responded to unilateral nephrectomy or vascular repair.[24] Although studies suggest that this combination is rare, preoperative exclusion of renovascular hypertension seems desirable before adrenal exploration is carried out. *Potassium-wasting renal disease* in patients with hypertension rarely may serve as a source of confusion, but since most such cases represent aberrant forms of Fanconi's syndrome or instances of primary renal tubular acidosis, evidence for other tubular defects (hyperchloremic acidosis, hypophosphatemia, hypouricemia, renal glycosuria, etc.) will be demonstrable. Patients with other forms of *hyperadrenalism* (Cushing's disease, neoplasms with ACTH production) will exhibit increased urinary 17-hydroxysteroid and 17-ketosteroid excretion rates.

A small group of interesting patients with benign hypertension, the full biochemical spectrum of primary aldosteronism, but with normal adrenal glands has been reported. The hypertension has usually not responded to surgical intervention, but Conn has nonetheless recommended that subtotal adrenalectomy be performed at the time of diagnostic surgical procedure, since a small percentage may be cured but more importantly because the biochemical picture suggests in this group that the renin-angiotensin-aldosterone axis has been activated and malignant progression may be in the offing.[10] Further experience will be necessary to define the status of this group. Possibly some of these patients may represent variants of the syndrome of presumed occult hypermineralocorticoidism alluded to by Liddle[22] and Melby.[20] Chronic ingestion of large amounts of *licorice* has been incriminated in the production of a syndrome of hypokalemic alkalosis and hypertension (but with low aldosterone secretion); it appears that glycyrrhizinic acid is the active ingredient responsible for the metabolic abnormalities.[25]

In the assessment of a patient for adrenal exploration for aldosteronoma, then, the following findings should probably be demonstrated: hypertension, hypokalemic alkalosis, renal potassium wasting, increased secretion and/or excretion of aldosterone or elevated plasma aldosterone, normal 17-hydroxysteroids and 17-ketosteroids, normal or elevated serum sodium concentration, and low plasma renin before and after ambulation and sodium deprivation. Papilledema will almost always be absent, and reasonable suspicion of surgically reversible renal vascular disease should be investigated. Ideally, the suspect should be removed from exposure to thiazide diuretics for several weeks and have normal or high potassium and sodium intake prior to study. Application of such rigid criteria will, however, fail to identify a number of atypical groups, including the juvenile with aldosteronism, the rare aldosteronoma which is producing malignant hypertension, and the as yet uncertain number of normokalemic patients with the disorder.

THERAPY

Emphasis has been placed on precise diagnosis of the aldosterone-producing tumor, because surgical results have been so encouraging. Previous reports indicated that 70 percent of patients are cured of their hypertension, 25 percent exhibit improvement, and only a few succumb or are not benefited by extirpation of the adenoma.

A more recent study, however, indicates only about half such patients are cured, with improvement in another 2 percent. This report, like others, confirms the strong correlation between response to spironolactone and subsequent response to surgery, and it is likely that all such patients should exhibit biochemical and blood pressure correction with 300 to 400 mg spironolactone per day prior to surgical exploration.[26]

In the vast majority of instances the tumor has been single, and in nearly all cases the pathologic changes have been confined to a single adrenal gland. Since the adenoma appears twice as frequently on the left, it should be explored first; if an adenoma is encountered, unilateral adrenalectomy should be performed and exploration of the contralateral adrenal deferred. Reexploration should be considered only if the metabolic abnormalities and hypertension persist; in this regard it should be noted that hypokalemic alkalosis generally disappears within 1 to 2 weeks, while the hypertension may require months to subside. Criteria for subtotal adrenalectomy in patients with bilateral hyperplasia are still uncertain; this procedure is probably indicated when the full biochemical spectrum is present. However, the normokalemic group with suppressed renin concentrations continues to remain an enigma.[21]

Medical considerations in the preoperative preparation of the patient are worthy of note. Attempts to replenish potassium in the patient should be made, employing oral potassium supplements, until the serum potassium level is within a normal range. Furthermore, since the status of the remaining adrenal gland is unknown, stress doses of glucocorticoids should be employed when removal of the adrenal is accomplished. Similarly, since atrophy of mineralocorticoid-producing adrenal tissue occurs with aldosteronoma, postoperative hypoaldosteronism is to be anticipated, and adequate sodium provision together with potassium restriction should be aimed at. Long-acting vasodepressor agents such as reserpine and guanethidine should probably be avoided for a minimum of 3 weeks prior to operation.

REFERENCES

1 Conn, J. W.: Primary Aldosteronism, *J. Lab. Clin. Med.,* 45:661, 1955.
2 Bartter, F. C.: The Role of Aldosterone in Normal Homeostasis and in Certain Disease States, *Metabolism,* 4:369, 1956.
3 Berliner, R. W., Kennedy, T. J., Jr., and Orloff, J.: Relationship between Acidification of Urine and Potassium Metabolism: Effect of Carbonic Anhydrase Inhibition on Potassium Excretion, *Am. J. Med.,* 11:274, 1951.
4 Kassirer, J. P., Appleton, F. M., Chazan, J. A., and Schwartz, W. B.: Aldosterone in Metabolic Alkalosis, *J. Clin. Invest.,* 46:1558, 1967.
5 Laragh, J. H., Ulick, S., Januszewicz, V., Deming, O. B., Kelly, W. C., and Lieberman, S.: Aldosterone Secretion and Primary and Malignant Hypertension, *J. Clin. Invest.,* 39:1091, 1960.
6 Carpenter, C. C. J., Davis, J. O., and Ayers, C. R.: Relation of Renin, Angiotensin II, and Experimental Renal Hypertension to Aldosterone Secretion, *J. Clin. Invest.,* 40:2026, 1961.
7 August, J. T., Nelson, D. H., and Thorn, G. W.: Response of Normal Subjects to Large Amounts of Aldosterone, *J. Clin. Invest.,* 37:1549, 1958.
8 Bricker, N. S.: The Control of Sodium Excretion with Normal and Reduced Nephron Populations, *Am. J. Med.,* 43:313, 1967.
9 Shade, R. E., and Grim, C. E.: Suppression of Renin and Aldosterone by Small Amounts of DOCA in Normal Man, *J. Clin. Endocrinol. Metab.,* 40:652, 1975.
10 Conn, J. W.: Aldosteronism in Man, part II, *J.A.M.A.,* 183:169, 1963.
11 Conn, J. W., Rovner, D. R., Cohen, E. L., and Nesbit, R. M.: Normakalemic Primary Aldosteronism, *J.A.M.A.,* 195:111, 1967.
12 Davis, W. W., Newsome, H. H., Jr., Wright, L. D., Jr., Hammond, W. G., Easton, J., and Bartter, F. C.: Bilateral Adrenal Hyperplasia as a Cause of Primary Aldosteronism with Hypertension and Suppressed Renin Activity, *Am. J. Med.,* 42:642, 1967.
13 Gunnells, J. C., Grim, C. E., and Bath, N. M.: The Clinical Spectrum of Primary Aldosteronism, *Clin. Res.,* 16:61, 1968 (abstract).
14 Genest, J., Nowaczynski, W., Kuchel, O., Boucher, R., Rojo-Ortega, J. M., Costantopoulos, G., Ganten, D., and Messerli, F.: The Adrenal Cortex and Essential Hypertension, *Recent Prog. Horm. Res.,* 32:377, 1976.
15 Relman, A. S., and Schwartz, W. B.: The Kidney in Potassium Depletion, *Am. J. Med.,* 24:764, 1958.
16 Kaplan, N. M.: Primary Aldosteronism with Malignant Hypertension, *N. Engl. J. Med.,* 269:1281, 1963.
17 Bartter, F. C., Pronove, P., Gill, J., and MacCardle, R. C.: Hyperplasia of Juxtaglomerular Complex with Hyperaldosteronism and Hypokalemic Alkalosis, *Am. J. Med.,* 33:811, 1962.
18 Kaplan, N. M.: Hypokalemia in the Hypertensive Patient, *Ann. Intern. Med.,* 66:1079, 1967.
19 Lauler, D. P.: Preoperative Diagnosis of Primary Aldosteronism, *Am. J. Med.,* 41:855, 1966.
20 Spark, R. F., and Melby, J. C.: Hypertension and Low Plasma Renin Activity: Presumptive Evidence for Mineralocorticoid Excess, *Ann. Intern. Med.,* 75:831, 1971.
21 Biglieri, E. G., Stockigt, J. R., and Schambelan, M.: Adrenal Mineralocorticoids Causing Hypertension, *Am. J. Med.,* 52:623, 1972.
22 Lowder, S. C., and Liddle, G. W.: Effects of Guanethidine and Methyldopa on a Standardized Test for Renin Responsiveness, *Ann. Intern. Med.,* 82:757, 1975.
23 Venning, E. H., Dyrenfurth, I., Dossetor, J. B., and Beck, J. C.: Effect of Chlorothiazide upon Aldosterone Excretion and Sodium and Potassium Balance in Essential Hypertension, *J. Lab. Clin. Med.,* 60:79, 1962.
24 Laidlaw, J. C., Yendt, E. R., and Gornall, A. G.: Hypertension Caused by Renal Artery Occlusion Simulating Primary Aldosteronism, *Metabolism,* 9:612, 1960.
25 Lois, L. H., and Conn, J. W.: Preparation of Glycyrrhizinic Acid, Electrolyte-active Principle of Licorice: Its Effect upon Metabolism and upon Pituitary-Adrenal Function in Man, *J. Lab. Clin. Med.,* 47:20, 1956.
26 Ferriss, J. B., Brown, J. J., Fraser, R., Haywood, E., Davies, D. L., Kay, A. W., Lever, A. F., Robertson, J. I. S., Owen, K., and Peart, W. S.: Results of Adrenal Surgery in Patients with Hypertension, Aldosterone Excess, and Low Plasma Renin, *Br. Med. J.,* 1:135, 1975.

73
Treatment of Systemic Hypertension

J. CAULIE GUNNELLS, JR., M.D.,
EDWARD S. ORGAIN, M.D., and
WILLIAM L. MCGUFFIN, JR., M.D.

PRIMARY ARTERIAL (ESSENTIAL) HYPERTENSION

Primary arterial (essential) hypertension remains a vascular disorder of complex and as yet undefined etiology.[1-3] Unquestionably, neurogenic, endocrine, renal, vascular, hormonal, and probably other as yet undisclosed mechanisms contribute components of variable magnitude in individual patients. However, knowledge of the complex mechanisms underlying hypertension is slowly evolving,[3,3a,4] and the therapeutic horizon is brightening with the steady acquisition of new and effective drugs for treatment.[5-8] Since the precise etiology of primary arterial hypertension is still unknown, current therapy is both empiric and, to a large degree, nonspecific. More specific and even curative therapy will become available when the causes of hypertension are discovered or the importance of each contributing factor is clearly defined. Our hopes have never been higher than at present because of important contributions made in the last 10 years concerning the underlying pathophysiology and the treatment of hypertension.

Physicians are not in complete accord as to what

constitutes normal in contrast to elevated blood pressure. Borderline blood pressures probably range from 140/90 to 159/94 mm Hg. When three consecutive readings on separate occasions disclose levels of 160/95 and above, sustained hypertension very probably exists.[9]

Evidence is now available to indicate that hypertension must be controlled, whether it is labile or fixed, systolic or diastolic, at any age or in either sex, in the prevention of atherothrombotic disease. Insurance and other statistics have clearly demonstrated that morbidity rates rise and that life-span shortens with even minimal increases in either systolic or diastolic blood pressure.[10] Morbidity and mortality rates in both mild and severe hypertensive states have been reduced by medical measures. Mortality in hypertension has resulted primarily from both mechanical factors and vascular complications affecting such vital organs as the brain, heart, and kidneys. Congestive heart failure, formerly a frequent complication of hypertension can be successfully treated and even prevented by good blood pressure control. Atherogenesis, although a separate entity, is closely associated with and accelerated by the appearance of hypertension.[11] It is well established that there is an unquestioned association between hypertension and coronary disease[12-15] and between hypertension and the development of cerebrovascular disease, particularly atherothrombotic brain infarction (stroke).[16] Hypertension appears to be an important factor in the genesis of microaneurysms and of cerebral hemorrhages which are less common in the controlled as compared to the uncontrolled hypertensive patient. Unfortunately, the recurrence rate for stroke survivors is not reduced significantly by antihypertensive therapy.[17] Prolonged medical control of recumbent diastolic pressure levels in a few hypertensive patients may possibly reverse the hypertensive process and reset the barostatic mechanisms. Very rarely, however, can all medication be discontinued without the return of hypertension.

The idealistic aims of therapy, therefore, are to control the blood pressure, both systolic and diastolic, at strictly normal levels, 24 h each day in both recumbent and erect positions and to prevent the onset and progression of vascular damage. Recent evidence indicates that even partial control of blood pressure exerts a salutary effect on morbidity and mortality.[18] Some clinicians will not treat mere figures during the long asymptomatic phase of benign hypertension, since they regard the value of such therapy as unproved, annoying because of side effects, injurious because of toxic drug reactions, and expensive because of necessary repetitive clinical and laboratory observations. The number of such physicians is dwindling because of repeated statistical demonstrations of lowered morbidity and mortality when blood pressures are well controlled by therapy. This fact has become irrefutable, and the failure to treat sustained hypertension is certainly untenable. There is still little general agreement as to when treatment for hypertension first should be instituted. Statistics now clearly indicate an unfavorable implication in terms of total death rate, death from coronary disease, major cardiovascular events, and cerebrovascular episodes for those patients whose diastolic pressures fall in the range of 85 to 104 mm Hg[19] or 90 through 114 mm Hg.[20] Because of these facts, opinion as to the importance of the initiation of antihypertensive therapy at earlier periods in the hypertensive process and at lower levels of both systolic and diastolic pressure certainly is undergoing radical change. Therefore, it would seem prudent to watch those patients whose resting recumbent pressures repeatedly reach borderline levels and to begin active treatment when resting pressures consistently rise above these levels. The efficacy of antihypertensive therapy in the more severe grades of hypertension (diastolic pressures of 115 through 129 mm Hg) has been established satisfactorily.[21] Young patients, particularly males and blacks, certainly deserve treatment for their hypertensive disease at lower levels of both systolic and diastolic pressures than do older patients.

It must be emphasized that the patient should be treated as a whole individual and not merely his blood pressure. Inquiry must be made with regard to the ingestion of estrogens,[22] licorice,[23] and sodium bicarbonate compounds[24] which have been shown to be associated with the development of hypertension. It is the duty of the physician to provide for the patient a regimen of treatment especially tailored not only to his needs but also to his ability to follow it. Although many patients suffering from hypertension have personality problems, psychiatric therapy is rarely needed. The primary physician can, by common sense measures, allay fears, tensions, and anxieties and can help the patient replete his mental and physical reserves. A long-term program must be arranged in which rest, recreation, vacation periods, and workloads are properly balanced. Blood pressure has been lowered in some patients, generally with mild hypertension, by psychophysiologic interventions such as biofeedback, yoga, relaxation, and meditation.[25-27] The levels of blood pressure reduction usually have been small. However, the hypertensive process with its concomitant vascular and tissue changes often demands vigorous attack with every means at one's disposal, including rest, diet, drugs, and occasionally surgery.

DIETARY THERAPY

Insurance statistics have emphasized for years the very poor prognostic label carried by obesity. Data exist which link adiposity to an increased risk for the development of hypertension. Obese hypertensive patients experience a greater risk of coronary heart disease than the nonobese, and mortality rates for obese hypertensive individuals are higher than rates for those with obesity alone or hypertension alone.[28] Weight reduction, therefore, by simple caloric restriction is universally desirable for the obese patient.

There is little question that the sodium ion plays

an important role in the development and maintenance of hypertension,[29–31] and that sodium restriction from 9 to 22 mEq/day may aid very materially in reducing blood pressure. The mechanisms by which lowering the blood pressure is achieved by sodium restrictions are not as yet clarified; however, reductions in extracellular fluid volume and circulating plasma volume, as well as alterations of blood vessel reactivity, have been suggested. Low sodium diets favor the development of both orthostatic hypotension and postural syncope; therefore, particular caution is suggested when drugs attenuating sympathetic activity are administered concurrently with significant sodium restriction. The introduction of diuretic agents has decreased the necessity for rigid sodium restriction below approximately 44 mEq/day except in the most severe hypertensive states. In view of the probable relationship of hypertension and of hyperlipidemia to atherogenesis, it is not only desirable but important to determine the serum cholesterol and triglyceride levels, as well as the lipoprotein pattern according to Fredrickson's classification[32] by the lipid electrophoretic method, in order that an appropriate dietary program involving restriction of saturated fats, cholesterol, and carbohydrate, if necessary, may be prescribed.[33]

Since obesity contributes greatly to the expression of hyperlipidemia, weight reduction must be an integral part of therapy, particularly for those at higher risk and for the young. Fat intake generally is limited to 40 to 50 g/day, the restriction pertaining primarily to saturated fats so that the ratio of unsaturated fats becomes 2:1 or even 3:1; cholesterol is limited to not more than 300 mg/day or below. When renal disease, accompanied by albuminuria, impaired renal function, and azotemia, complicates hypertension, protein should be restricted to levels compatible with the creatinine clearance. The rigid or modified rice-fruit diet regimen of Kempner,[34] although most difficult for the patient to follow for extended periods, is useful in the initial several weeks of therapy for those who exhibit extensive retinopathy (hemorrhages, exudates, papilledema) and varying degrees of renal failure. It must be remembered that patients who suffer from renal insufficiency are often salt losers and therefore detailed monitoring of the blood electrolyte pattern must be performed. As the patient's condition improves, with his hypertension controlled, a rapid adjustment to a more normal and tolerable diet then may be made.

DRUG THERAPY

The ideal drug for widespread application to large groups of hypertensive patients must provide effective control of both systolic and diastolic blood pressure (recumbent and standing) when administered orally and yet must be free of serious toxic or undesirable effects. No drug is available at present that clinically or experimentally fulfills these requirements. The sedative and tranquilizing drugs remain useful for the tense, anxious patient who exhibits fluctuating blood pressure levels. During the past two decades, the continuous production of new and effective compounds possessing different pharmacologic actions has revolutionized the treatment of hypertension. With the development of these many new compounds, two general approaches to the therapy of hypertension have evolved over the past several years. One approach has been characterized by sequential or step-care therapy, in which the hypertensive problem is approached by the stepwise addition of differing antihypertensive compounds to achieve blood pressure control. In this system, the therapy is usually initiated with a diuretic, and thereafter, drugs are added in a manner outlined in Tables 73-1, 73-6, and 73-7. An alternative approach to therapy has been antihypertensive therapy based on the defined physiologic characteristics of the hypertensive process and is based on the specific pharmacologic action of the drug directed toward the major patholophysiologic alteration that has been defined or outlined as producing the high blood pressure.[35,36] Clinicians utilizing this approach to therapy usually separate their patients into one group characterized by volume-excess, or so-called volume-dependent, hypertension in contrast to the second major physiologic group which is defined as vasoconstrictor hypertension. The former group of patients has been felt to respond most efficiently to the diuretic compounds with the latter group being most responsive to the vasodilator or renin-lowering drugs characterized primarily by hydralazine and propranolol. The volume hypertensive diseases have also been subgrouped as low renin essential hypertension whereas the vasoconstrictor group of hypertensive diseases have been subgrouped as high renin essential hypertension. The subgrouping of essential hypertension into low renin, normal renin, and high renin categories by Laragh and his coworkers has received great attention not only in designing what some feel as a specific pharmacotherapeutic approach to hypertension but also in assigning prognosis to the hypertensive process as to the risk of developing cardiovascular morbidity and mortality.[37] Based on Laragh's observations, the patients with low renin essential hypertension appear to be at lower risk for cardiovascular morbidity and mortality as a result of their hypertension than patients with normal and high renin essential hypertension. The conclusions as to prognosis of the hypertensive process and the rationale of therapy based on renin subgroups have been the subject of great controversy. A recent report by Woods et al.,[38] utilizing renin subgrouping in the choice of antihypertensive therapy, failed to demonstrate the previously outlined or suggested specificity of renin subgrouping in the choice of two antihypertensive drugs (propranolol and chlorthalidone) having widely differing mechanisms of antihypertensive action.

The most commonly used classes of compounds in the treatment of hypertension today are as follows: diuretics, vasodilators, adrenergic inhibitors or sympatholytic agents, and adrenergic receptor blockers (alpha and beta receptors) (Table 73-1).

TABLE 73-1
Antihypertensive Drugs

Diuretics

Benzothiadiazine and other related compounds
  All thiazides
  Chlorthalidone
  Metolazone
Loop diuretics
  Furosemide
  Ethacrynic acid
Potassium-sparing agents
  Spironolactone
  Triamterene
  Amiloride*

Vasodilators

Hydralazine
Minoxidil*
Prazosin
Guancydine*
Diazoxide†
Sodium nitroprusside†

Adrenergic inhibitors or sympatholytic agents

Central and peripheral inhibitors
  Reserpine compounds
  Guanethidine
  Guanadrel*
  Bethanidine*
  Debrisoquin*
  Methyldopa
  Clonidine
Monamine oxidase inhibiting agents
  Pargyline
Ganglionic blocking agents
  Pentolinium
  Mecamylamine
  Trimethaphan†
Adrenergic receptor blockers
  Alpha receptor
  Phentolamine
  Phenoxybenzamine
Beta receptor
  Propranolol
  Practolol*
  Alprenolol*
  Prindolol*

Selective antagonists

Angiotensin II
Saralasin (P-113) (L-sarcosine-8-alanine angiotensin II)*,†
Converting enzyme
CEI (SQ20881)*, †

Miscellaneous

Prostaglandins*
Magnesium sulfate
Yoga, biofeedback, meditation techniques
Sedatives and tranquilizers

*Drugs not currently available for general or uncontrolled use in U.S.A.
†Available for intravenous use only.

Diuretic compounds

The introduction of benzothiadiazine (thiazide) diuretic drugs in 1957 created an important and welcome addition to the therapeutic armamentarium for hypertension. These diuretic drugs are generally useful and effective when employed alone; however, their most valuable characteristic is the potentiation of the action of other antihypertensive drugs, thereby permitting dosage reduction or even discontinuance of one drug when several hypotensive compounds must be administered simultaneously.[39] Commonly available and frequently used, diuretic compounds in the treatment of hypertension may be categorized chemically as follows: benzothiadiazine (thiazides), phthalimidine (chlorthalidone), quinethazone-quinazolinone (metolazone), aryloxyacetic acid (ethacrynic acid), anthranilic acid (furosemide), aldosterone antagonist (spironolactone), and phenylpteridine (triamterene) (Table 73-2). From the standpoint of site or mechanism of action, these drugs can be placed into three major groups: (1) the benzothiadiazine or thiazide drugs (including chlorthalidone and metolazone) with the predominant site of action(s) in the late portion of the ascending limb and early distal tubule; (2) the "loop diuretics"—furosemide and ethacrynic acid—having the major site of action in the loop of Henle and ascending limb; and (3) the potassium-sparing or distal tubule diuretics—spironolactone and triamterene.[40,41]

The precise mechanism by which all diuretics act to lower blood pressure has not been clarified completely. An action common to all the above diuretics is the ability to produce, under appropriate circumstances, negative sodium balance. Most investigators would agree that this function probably constitutes the major if not the most important role of this group of compounds in the management of hypertension.

TABLE 73-2
Diuretic compounds

Generic name	Proprietary name	Equivalent mg. dose
Benzothiadiazine (thiazides):		
Benzthiazide	Exna	50
Benzydroflumethiazide	Naturetin	5.0
Chlorothiazide	Diuril	500
Cyclothiazide	Anhydron	2.5
Hydrochlorothiazide	Esidrix	50
	Hydrodiuril	50
	Oretic	50
Hydroflumethiazide	Saluron	50
Methyclothiazide	Enduron	2.5
Polythiazide	Renese	2.0
Trichlormethiazide	Metahydrin	2.0
	Naqua	2.0
Phthalimidine: chlorthalidone	Hygroton	50–100
Quinethazone: metolazone	Zaroxolyn	2.5–5.0
Aryloxyacetic acid: ethacrynic acid	Edecrin	50
Anthranilic acid: furosemide	Lasix	20–40
Aldosterone inhibitor: spironolactone	Aldactone A	25
Phenylpteridine: triamterene	Dyrenium	100

For further information on diuretic compounds, see Chap. 109.

BENZOTHIADIAZINES (THIAZIDES)

The thiazide compounds possess powerful diuretic and saluretic activity through their ability to inhibit renal tubular reabsorption of sodium at distal sites in the nephron. Initial and long-term hypotensive effects, thought to correlate with diminished blood volume,[42] also appear to relate to negative sodium balance, since neither the prevention of a reduction in plasma volume nor its restoration to normal by volume expanders completely reverses the arterial pressure changes. Late effects evident without disturbance in fluid volume or serum electrolyte patterns have been ascribed to decreased blood vessel reactivity and altered vascular sodium ion gradients.

A large number of benzothiadiazine drugs are currently available with wide variations in dosage and duration of action. Structural alterations of the basic formula have varied potency on an individual basis, but there is no outstanding superiority of one drug over another in terms of potency, natriuretic effectiveness, side effects, or more favorable sodium-potassium excretion ratios when appropriate doses of each drug are prescribed. It should be noted that these drugs have a rather flat dose-response curve and their potency or effectiveness cannot be augmented by increasing the dose;[43] this is in contrast to such agents as furosemide which possess a linear dose-response curve and can be used to augment or enhance the diuretic effectiveness of the benzothiadiazines when needed. The thiazide diuretic drugs are simple to use and are generally well tolerated but may cause dizziness, nausea, weakness, paresthesias, fatigue, gastric irritation, and muscle cramps. Hypersensitivity reactions, including skin rashes, purpura, thrombocytopenia, leukopenia, agranulocytosis, jaundice, and pancreatitis, have been observed. When a sensitivity reaction occurs—e.g., purpura from benzothiadiazine—a compound of different chemical structure should be substituted in order to avoid interruption of the antihypertensive program. The serum electrolyte pattern must be watched carefully in patients on prolonged thiazide therapy. A pattern of hypokalemic alkalosis is the most commonly detected abnormality, but one must be aware of the possibility of hyponatremia.[44] Hyponatremia usually does not occur unless there is associated severe dietary sodium restriction or coexistent renal insufficiency. In general, when diuretics are chronically administered, it is not necessary to restrict dietary sodium below levels of 1,000 to 1,500 mg/day. Hypokalemia is a more common complication of diuretic therapy and may occur suddenly and without associated clinical symptoms.[45] The utmost care must be taken to avoid digitalis intoxication secondary to excessive potassium loss. The majority of patients do not require supplementary potassium replacement therapy provided that adequate dietary intake of foods high in potassium can be maintained in conjunction with appropriate reduction in dietary sodium intake. Should supplemental potassium be necessary, it may be provided by the administration of liquid potassium chloride, 40 to 80 mEq/day, since other potassium salts may not restore or maintain the serum potassium adequately. Moreover, if there is the usual associated metabolic alkalosis, the chloride ion is helpful to fully correct both the hypokalemia as well as the alkalosis. A large number of liquid potassium preparations are available commercially; among the more commonly used ones are: K-Lor, Kay Ciel, Kaochlor, and K-Lyte. Equally effective and probably less expensive and as well tolerated in most patients is a 10 percent solution of potassium chloride. All liquid potassium preparations are associated with some incidence of unpleasant side effects such as unpalatability, nausea, vomiting, abdominal cramps, and occasionally diarrhea.

Earlier experiences with small bowel ulceration and/or obstruction following the ingestion of enteric-coated potassium chloride tablets led to the withdrawal of these preparations from the market. However, the recent availability in this country of Slow-K, a slow-release tablet preparation in which the potassium chloride is incorporated into a wax matrix, has led to a return of the use of potassium chloride replacement therapy in tablet form. This compound is effective, convenient, well tolerated and has not been associated with other enteric-coated tablets and also appears to have greater patient acceptability than comparable doses of liquid potassium chloride compounds.

The adjunctive use of the potassium-sparing diuretic agents such as triamterene or spironolactone may be useful in those patients in whom it is difficult to maintain a normal serum potassium concentration; however, one must be careful to avoid the potential serious side effects of hyperkalemia when utilizing these drugs alone or in combination with other diuretic drugs. In patients with renal insufficiency, the use of spironolactone and triamterene is generally considered to be contraindicated. Potassium supplements must be administered with caution, and the thiazide diuretic agents must also be used with caution, in view of their potential to induce the above described serious electrolyte abnormalities as well as to produce an associated decrease in renal blood flow and glomerular filtration rate which may ensue with the administration of these agents. The elevation of blood glucose level or the production of overt diabetes in patients predisposed to abnormal carbohydrate tolerance (diabetic and prediabetic persons) has been reported with the use of thiazide diuretics and therefore a careful inquiry for a history of diabetes mellitus is mandatory.[46] Induction of abnormal carbohydrate metabolism in nondiabetic patients has not been observed. Similarly the production of hyperuricemia with attacks of acute gout in susceptible individuals has been produced by thiazide agents. This hyperuricemia, when present, can be reversed by either the use of a uricosuric agent such as probenecid or the administration of the zanthine oxidase inhibitor, allopurinol.[47]

CHLORTHALIDONE (PHTHALIMIDINE)

Chlorthalidone possesses a similar mechanism of action, degree of induced hypotension, and frequency in type of side effects as previously described for thiazide diuretic drugs.[48] The primary difference between chlorthalidone and the thiazide agents is the duration of action; chlorthalidone exhibits pharmacologic activity up to 48 h as compared to 12 to 24 h for the various thiazide compounds. Except for this duration of action, the compound, when used in appropriate dosage schedules, possesses no specific advantage or disadvantage over the benzothiadiazine drugs listed in Table 73-2.

METOLAZONE (QUINETHAZONE-QUINAZOLINONE)

The quinethazone-quinazolinone drugs have a site and mechanism of action similar to the benzothiadiazines.[49] Metolazone (Zaroxolyn) differs structurally from quinethazone (Hydromox), a change which results in a greater diuretic potency on a weight basis. Despite a rapid onset of action (maximum natriuresis usually in 3 h), metolazone has also been shown to have a long duration (27 to 72 h) of action. In this respect, the drug is in many ways comparable to chlorthalidone. Metolazone lacks no specific advantage relative to a lower incidence of hypokalemia, hyperuricemia, carbohydrate intolerance, etc. Similarly, its antihypertensive potency is equivalent to the benzothiadiazines and chlorthalidone (phthalimidine) compounds. These longer active diuretic compounds are more useful and effective in treating hypertension than the shorter acting diuretic compounds.

FUROSEMIDE AND ETHACRYNIC ACID

Furosemide and ethacrynic acid are two of the most potent diuretics available.[13,50,51] Although the two agents are different in chemical structure (furosemide is a sulfonamide compound, and ethacrynic acid is a derivative of phenoxyacetic acid), they will be considered together because of their similar pharmacologic effects. The two drugs have their primary or main site of action in the inhibition of active chloride transport in and along the ascending limb of the loop of Henle rather than an inhibitory action on sodium transport as previously reported.[52] Considerable controversy remains as to the presence or action of these drugs on the proximal tubule in standard pharmacologic doses. Both drugs are most effective by oral and intravenous routes. When given orally, the diuretic effectiveness exists for 6 to 8 h in contrast to only 2 to 4 h by the intravenous route. An additional feature of these two compounds, in contrast to the thiazide drugs, is the presence of a rather wide and steep dose-response curve and the observation that these drugs retain their effectiveness in the presence of serum electrolyte imbalance, acid-base disturbances, and impaired renal function. In the presence of a normal to slightly expanded intravascular volume, the administration of either agent may produce a slight transient increase in both glomerular filtration rate and renal plasma flow which will be followed by a decrease in these parameters with the subsequent diuresis and volume contraction associated with the pharmacologic action of the drug. The antihypertensive action or potential of both drugs is similar to that of the thiazide drugs. In general, the diuretic effect of furosemide and ethacrynic acid should be considered greater than the antihypertensive effects; consequently, these agents may be more likely to produce adverse alterations in serum electrolytes and subsequent renal function. Therefore, caution should be exercised in the use of high or excessive doses in acute clinical situations or the prolonged administration of standard doses. These drugs may have their widest and most useful application in patients with severe hypertension and associated renal insufficiency and congestive heart failure. Their value in potentiating the antihypertensive effects of other pharmacologic drugs (e.g., vasodilators) in the so-called refractory patient has been demonstrated and emphasized. In general, the usual or common side effects are those observed with the use of thiazide compounds. Ethacrynic acid has been said to be associated with a higher incidence of gastrointestinal side effects than furosemide. In addition, transient and occasionally permanent hearing loss has been reported after the administration of ethacrynic acid either alone or in combination with the ototoxic aminoglycoside antibiotics.[53] Gastrointestinal bleeding and acute pancreatitis along with leukopenia, thrombocytopenia, and fatal agranulocytosis have also been reported as possible side effects of both agents. In contrast to the thiazide compounds, the incidence of alterations in carbohydrate intolerance appears to be much lower with these compounds; however, the frequency of hyperuricemia is similar.

SPIRONOLACTONE AND TRIAMTERENE

Spironolactone and triamterene have similar effects on patterns of electrolyte excretion, but they operate through different mechanisms.[54] Both compounds increase the urinary excretion of sodium chloride and decrease the excretion of potassium, ammonium, and titratable acid. Spironolactone acts as a specific antagonist or competitive inhibitor of aldosterone and other mineralocorticoids, whereas the exact mechanism by which triamterene produces its diuretic action is unknown. The site of action of both agents is in the distal convoluted tubule. An understanding of the mechanism of action of these two compounds can be most helpful in therapeutic applications: spironolactone will be most useful or effective in those patients exhibiting evidence of normal or increased aldosterone or other mineralocorticoid activity, whereas triamterene is effective in the absence of these hormones. As diuretics, both compounds are less effective than the benzothiadiazines or the phthalimidines, but they are able to potentiate the diuretic action of these structurally unrelated compounds. When spironolactone is administered in doses of 25 mg four times daily, side effects are minimal. However, occasional drowsiness and/or mental confusion, malaise and easy fatigability, nausea and anorexia, skin eruptions, and gynecomastia have been observed. Hyperkalemia is rarely encountered except in the presence of renal insufficiency or when potassium supplements are given concomitantly. In contrast, hyperkalemia and death have been reported from triamterene when used both alone and in conjunction with thiazide diuretic. Both the antihypertensive and diuretic effects of spironolactone and triamterene must be considered modest; their major efficacy is in combined therapy with other antihypertensive agents. In view of the mechanism of action of spironolactone, this drug has been proposed as a rather specific treatment for the initial and long-term medical management of patients with hypertension in association with mineralocorticoid excess, as seen in patients with Conn's syndrome, idiopathic hyperaldosteronism, and other variants of these disorders as well as in low renin essential hypertension;[55] these clinical hypertensive subgroups constitute a portion of the volume-excess hypertensive diseases (see above).[3a]

The vasodilator drugs

The vasodilator compounds which have been used as antihypertensive agents include hydralazine, minoxidil, guancydine, prazosin, nitroprusside, and diazoxide. The vasodilator drugs relax arteriolar smooth muscle and thus decrease peripheral vascular resistance. These compounds vary in potency; e.g., minoxidil is more effective than either hydralazine or guancydine. As a group, the vasodilators (1) produce retention of sodium and water with expansion of the extracellular fluid and plasma volumes; (2) increase sympathetic activity reflexly, increase heart rate and cardiac output; and (3) in hypotensive doses cause a rise in plasma renin activity probably due to an increased sympathetic discharge to the kidney.[56,57]

HYDRALAZINE HYDROCHLORIDE (APRESOLINE)

Hydralazine primarily induces peripheral vasodilatation; decreases peripheral vascular resistance; elevates the heart rate, stroke volume, and cardiac output; and increases the renal, coronary, and hepatic circulations. Hydralazine is best administered in a gradual fashion, beginning with an oral dose of 10 mg four times daily, increasing by 10 to 25 mg/dose but not exceeding a total of 200 mg/day except for brief periods. It may be administered parenterally, intramuscularly, or intravenously every 2 to 4 h in doses of 5 to 25 mg with increments depending on the blood pressure response. Small doses often produce mild headache, nasal congestion, tachycardia, nausea, vomiting, numbness and tingling; these side effects tend to diminish as the drug is continued. When larger oral doses (300 to 400 mg) of the drug are administered daily for prolonged periods, various toxic reactions have been observed including fever, pancytopenia, pyridoxine deficiency, neuropathy, gastrointestinal bleeding, acute psychoses, and a

collagen-like illness. In its milder form, this illness resembles acute rheumatoid arthritis which subsides spontaneously on withdrawal of the drug. In more severe form, the illness may simulate acute systemic lupus erythematosus in whole or in part causing fever, arthralgia, pleurisy, pericarditis with or without effusion, and lupus erythematosus (LE) cells in the peripheral blood. This full-blown reaction may require steroid therapy for its resolution or it may result in long-term disability and even death. In the sensitive patient, small doses of hydralazine (e.g., 10 mg, four times daily) will induce recurrence of arthritis or reappearance of LE cells. Serious toxicity has resulted predominantly when drug doses have exceeded 200 mg/day over a period of several months. Recent observations concerning hydralazine toxicity have been made: (1) that only one-half of the population with a low level of hepatic acetyl transferase activity is susceptible to clinical hydralazine toxicity; (2) both antihydralazine antibodies, suggesting hypersensitivity, and anti-DNA antibodies, suggesting lupus erythematosus, are demonstrable in toxic patients; (3) significant remissions of serious hypertension, although rare, seem to occur more frequently in once toxic patients; and (4) survival time from the onset of therapy is suggestively better in toxic patients than in similarly treated matched patients with no history of toxicity.[58]

Because hydralazine produces cardiac stimulation, its administration should proceed with appropriate caution in patients who exhibit evidence of coronary atherosclerosis or congestive heart failure, either overt or impending. When used alone, its antihypertensive potency is weak and certainly limited. Its principal value lies in its ability to help potentiate the effects of other drugs, notably in combination with a diuretic and propranolol.

MINOXIDIL*

Minoxidil is a piperidino-pyrimidine derivative that directly relaxes arteriolar smooth muscle, thereby producing its hypotensive action by a reduction in peripheral vascular resistance.[56,59] As with other vasodilators, minoxidil administration is associated with a reflex tachycardia and increased cardiac output. This drug in hypertensive patients also results in salt and water retention with resultant edema and weight gain that may gradually counteract the hypotensive action of the drug. An associated rise in plasma renin activity accompanies the use of minoxidil. Relative to hydralazine, minoxidil is a more potent vasodilator and reductions of mean arterial pressure up to 35 mm Hg have been achieved in some hypertensive patients.[56]

The drug is rapidly absorbed on oral administration with peak plasma levels being achieved in 1 h and the onset of hypotensive action within 2 h. The serum half-life is approximately $4^{1}/_{2}$ h; however, the

*Hereafter drugs marked with an asterisk (*) remain under study and are not currently available for general or uncontrolled use in the United States.

duration of action may be up to 24 h.[60] The prolonged duration of action may be due to high affinity binding of the drug in the wall of arteriolar smooth muscle which has been demonstrated in animal studies. The drug produces no depression of the glomerular filtration rate or renal plasma flow and has been found to be highly effective and most useful in patients with severe hypertension and associated renal functional impairment who have been unresponsive to combination therapy involving the majority of currently available hypertensive drugs. It has been reported to be especially effective in the high renin hypertension of chronic renal failure; such patients were previously considered to require bilateral nephrectomy for blood pressure control.[61]

The oral dose of minoxidil for blood pressure control in severe hypertension ranges from 2 to 4 mg/day. Because of the concomitant fluid retention, tachycardia, and increase in plasma renin activity associated with this drug, it is not used as a single agent but in combination with a potent diuretic as well as with a drug such as propranolol to control or reduce the well-recognized consequences of vasodilator therapy.

Side effects are related primarily to the results of its vasodilator action. However, impressive hypertrichosis and an associated coarsening of facial features have been a disturbing side effect in some patients, especially young females. A careful assessment for the presence of coronary insufficiency should be pursued because of the possible development of angina pectoris as a result of the cardiostimulatory effects of this drug. Two additional disturbing features include the documentation of unexplained pulmonary hypertension[60] in several patients receiving the drug and the development of a right atrial degenerative myocardial lesion in dogs after prolonged oral administration; the latter lesion has not been reported in other species.[56]

Because of this excellent proved hypotensive effect in patients known to be "refractory" to multiple drug regimens, it is hoped that minoxidil will exhibit a significant advance in the management of severe or accelerated hypertensive cardiovascular disease when it is made commercially available.

PRAZOSIN

Prazosin hydrochloride, a new antihypertensive agent, is a quinazoline derivative which is orally active and has been shown to exert its antihypertensive action in animals and man primarily as a result of peripheral arteriolar vasodilatation via two mechanisms:[62-64] (1) a direct relaxation of vascular smooth muscle, (2) a peripheral adrenergic sympatholytic effect having a unique site of action that may be distal to the α-adrenergic receptor. Its antihypertensive effect is produced with no apparent venous pooling or significant changes in cardiac output, heart rate, renal blood flow, or glomerular filtration rate.

Sodium retention and weight gain have not followed brief or long-term administration of the drug in hypotensive doses.

The drug is well tolerated orally with minimal side effects.[62] The antihypertensive effect is gradual in onset with optimal effect in mild hypertension in approximately 4 weeks; requiring, however, up to approximately 8 weeks in more severe hypertensive disease. The usual maximal dose is 15 to 20 mg/day given in 2 to 4 divided doses. The antihypertensive effect is potentiated when used in combination with a thiazide diuretic. The drug may be used in combination with beta blockers and clonidine and possibly with other antihypertensive agents. Prazosin is effective alone and in combination with a diuretic in patients with mild to moderately severe hypertension with and without evidence of target organ damage. The drug is estimated to have a clinical potency equal to that of methyldopa and other comparable hypotensive agents.[63] Prazosin has demonstrated a comparable effect on supine and standing blood pressure. The development of tolerance to its hypotensive action has not been observed. Prazosin has been relatively free of subjective side effects, the majority of which have included lethargy, lightheadedness, headache, and mild nausea, and with only 9 percent of patients in a large study exhibiting side effects of sufficient magnitude to require discontinuance of the drug. Hematologic and biochemical abnormalities have been virtually absent. One unique feature of the drug has been the presence of postural symptoms following the initial dose of the drug which subsequently cleared.[62]

GUANCYDINE*

Guancydine is a new antihypertensive agent which acts primarily by decreasing peripheral resistance through its action on vascular smooth muscle. The antihypertensive action of this vasodilator shares the problem of fluid retention, increased cardiac output, tachycardia, and increased plasma renin activity that is seen with this category of hypotensive agents. The simultaneous administration of a diuretic plus propranolol (or alternatively guanethidine or reserpine) negates these unpleasant and undesirable features and enhances the antihypertensive effectiveness of the drug. Renal hemodynamics are not adversely affected by guancydine and postural hypotension has not been observed.

Guancydine produces a prompt reduction in blood pressure after oral administration. Doses in the range of 1,000 mg/day (four equally divided doses) are associated with optimum balance between hypotensive action and tolerable side effects. Blood levels of the drug do not necessarily correspond to effective hypotensive therapy. When administered in conjunction with a diuretic plus propranolol or guanethidine, guancydine is effective in patients with severe hypertension; however, serious side effects consisting of anxiety, paresthesias, electrocardiographic changes of ischemia, gynecomastia, and headache may seriously limit widespread use of this drug when made commercially available.[65]

Postganglionic adrenergic blocking agents

This group of drugs selectively inhibits adrenergic (sympathetic) neuron function[66] by mechanisms involving (1) biosynthesis, storage, release, and depletion of adrenergic effector substances (principally norepinephrine); (2) interference with impulse transmission along sympathetic neuron pathways, or (3) blockade at adrenergic receptor sites. These compounds tend to produce an incomplete "chemical sympathectomy" which avoids the very annoying symptoms that result from parasympathetic blockade.

RAUWOLFIA SERPENTINA (RESERPINE) COMPOUNDS

The *Rauwolfia* alkaloids (prototype reserpine) cross the blood-brain barrier, deplete the cerebral stores of serotonin, and produce both the central sedative action of the drug and its psychic effects (anxiety, depression, etc.). The released serotonin may activate the parasympathetic nervous system, cause gastric stimulation, and induce peptic ulcer. *Rauwolfia* compounds deplete the heart and blood vessels of their superficial and deep stores of norepinephrine and thus effectively reduce sympathetic nervous system activity, both centrally and peripherally.[67] Re-uptake and rebinding of the released norepinephrine appear to be prevented. There is little difference in the antihypertensive effects of the powdered whole root or its derivatives when equivalent doses are given (Table 73-3).

The principal action of reserpine is one of decreasing peripheral vascular resistance. Reserpine can decrease heart rate, myocardial contraction, and cardiac output by decreasing sympathetic nervous system stimulation of the blood vessels and the heart secondary to depletion of norepinephrine stores in the sympathetic nerve endings and to an action on the hypothalamus and vasomotor center. It also decreases plasma renin activity.

Although tranquilizing and mildly sedative in action, the *Rauwolfia* compounds produce unpleasant symptoms of fatigue, loss of energy, nasal congestion, drowsiness, dreams, nightmares, and weight gain. Bradycardia is a useful parasympathomimetic expression of the drug, whereas stimulation of peptic ulcer, colitis, and diarrhea is not. The physician must be alerted to detect early signs of parkinsonism and

TABLE 73-3
Rauwolfia serpentina compounds

1 Powdered whole root: Raudixin, 50–100 mg, once or twice daily
2 Alseroxylon fraction: Rauwiloid, 2.0–4.0 mg, once or twice daily
3 Alkaloids: 0.25–0.75 mg, once or twice daily
   a Reserpine (Serpasil, etc.)
   b Rescinnamine (Moderil)
   c Deserpidine (Harmonyl)
4 Synthetic analogue: syrosingopine (Singoserp) 0.25–1.0 mg, three to four times daily

symptoms of mild anxiety and depression because continued *Rauwolfia* administration after symptoms of depression develop may result in prolonged severe depression which fails to improve when the drug is discontinued and may require electroshock therapy. When reserpine is given alone in oral form, 0.1 to 0.25 mg once or twice daily, its action is mild, requiring several weeks to develop. Occasionally, striking effects are noted from extremely small oral doses. Larger doses may increase side effects without contributing additional hypotensive action. Parenteral intramuscular injection of 1 to 3 mg generally creates a good hypotensive response in 1 to 3 h, an effect which may last 6 to 24 h. *Rauwolfia* compounds should not be administered to patients who already exhibit fatigue states, anxiety, agitation, depression, or an active peptic ulcer. Reactivation of a previous peptic ulcer may be avoided by the use of a strict program involving bland diet with six meals a day, antispasmodics, and the liberal ingestion of antacids.

The *Rauwolfia* compounds seem most suitable for the mildly hypertensive patient who suffers from tension, tachycardia, and angina pectoris. They are quite effective when used in combination with other drugs, particularly diuretics and vasodilators. Unpleasant symptoms produced by other hypotensive agents may be ameliorated and drug dosage may be concurrently reduced.

Retrospective studies recently have indicated an association between the use of *Rauwolfia* derivatives and breast cancer in the United States,[68] England,[69] and Finland.[70] The risk seems statistically significant at the 5 percent level. It has been thought that perhaps enhancement of the pituitary release of prolactin might be the mechanism involved, but with other drugs which enhance prolactin release such as methyldopa, phenothiazines, and tricyclic antidepressants there has been no cancer association; thus, this attractive hypothesis is less likely to be true.

GUANETHIDINE

Guanethidine sulfate (Ismelin) inhibits sympathetic activity at the peripheral nerve terminals, presumably by at least two mechanisms: (1) interruption of the neuron terminal which triggers release of norepinephrine; and (2) depletion of the adrenergic effector substance, norepinephrine.[66] It also decreases plasma renin activity. Guanethidine decreases both cardiac output, heart rate, and peripheral resistance. Unlike reserpine, it does not cross the blood-brain barrier and therefore does not deplete serotonin or norepinephrine in the central nervous system, nor does it cause central nervous system depression. Following an intravenous injection, blood pressure rises temporarily, suggesting an initial release of norepinephrine stores. Unlike reserpine, guanethidine may produce a significant or very little reduction in the pressor action of indirectly acting amines, such as tyramine. By displacing guanethidine from the neuron terminal, amphetamine rapidly will restore transmitter function of the neuron and reverse the hypotensive effect of guanethidine. Tricyclic antidepressant drugs, imipramine (Tofranil) and desipramine (Pertofrane or Norpramin), prevent concentration of guanethidine at its site of action and antagonize its antihypertensive effects.[71,72] Guanethidine is a potent antihypertensive compound. For ambulatory patients,[73] guanethidine is administered orally, beginning with 10 mg once or twice daily and increasing to a total of 200 mg/day, if necessary. Extremely gradual titration to therapeutic levels is mandatory because significant orthostatic hypotension, particularly when the patient first arises in the morning or during exercise, often results even though there is little effect on recumbent blood pressure. Blood pressure responses are noted at variable dosage levels, independent of the severity of the hypertension. Tolerance requiring progressively increased drug dosage may appear in one-third of the patients under prolonged administration. Unpleasant symptoms such as dizziness, fainting, weakness, fatigue, abdominal discomfort, nausea, and loss of ejaculation are not strictly dose-related. Fluid retention occurs in approximately one-third of treated patients, more frequently in women.

Because postural hypotension is created regularly, caution is observed when cerebral or coronary arteriosclerosis or renal disease is present. In view of its marked orthostatic effects on blood pressure and the incidence of its disagreeable side effects, guanethidine alone would appear to have definite but limited utility in the treatment of severely hypertensive patients. The advantages of combined therapy with a diuretic and/or hydralazine and/or methyldopa to avoid intolerable side effects and obtain maximal drug effectiveness should be stressed.

BETHANIDINE SULFATE*

This compound inhibits the release of norepinephrine at the postganglionic neuroeffector junction without blocking the effect of circulating norepinephrine. Like guanethidine, bethanidine is effective in moderate and severe hypertension but is characterized by faster onset and shorter duration of action. After a single oral dose, 10 to 30 mg,[74] the hypotensive effect of bethanidine usually appears within 1 to 2 h, reaches a maximum in about 4 h, and is present for not more than 8 to 12 h. Side effects are similar to guanethidine. The drug may be given alone (average daily dose 120 mg) but it is most effective in combination with other compounds.

GUANADREL*

Guanadrel sulfate is an adrenergic blocking agent with hypotensive action similar to guanethidine. Its clinical effect is considerably shorter than guanethidine, lasting 6 to 8 h. With guanadrel it may be possible to achieve significantly better control of blood pressure through the day with fewer morning complaints and less diarrhea.[75]

DEBRISOQUIN SULFATE* (DECLINAX)

Debrisoquin sulfate (Declinax) is a postganglionic adrenergic blocking agent whose mode of action presumably is the prevention of the release of norepinephrine from its peripherally located stores at the neuroeffector junction. It has limited utility as an antihypertensive compound when used alone because it primarily affects orthostatic rather than recumbent blood pressure.[76] Debrisoquin is not available for prescription in the United States and along with most of the other postganglionic adrenergic blocking agents, probably will find its ultimate usefulness in combination with other drugs.

METHYLDOPA (ALDOMET)

This compound blocks the decarboxylase enzyme system which converts dopa (3,4-dihydroxyphenylalanine) to dopamine (3,4-dihydroxyphenylethylamine), the immediate precursor of norepinephrine, and to 5-hydroxytryptophan, the precursor of serotonin (Fig. 73-1). The action of methyldopa is not yet clarified. Its activity lies in the levorotatory isomer and is not correlated with the degree of decarboxylase inhibition. The terory of the formulation of a weak or false transmitter from the decarboxylation of methyldopamine and its subsequent metabolism to methylnorepinephrine, which in turn displaces norepinephrine from the nerve terminals, is not its major action. There is evidence that methyldopa decreases the release of renin from the kidney and that its primary effect may be centrally mediated by mechanisms which decrease sympathetic vasomotor outflow.[77,78] Methyldopa decreases peripheral arteriolar resistance with little or no effect on heart rate or cardiac output.

Methyldopa may be prescribed orally in conventional fashion 250 mg three or four times a day, increasing to 500 mg four times a day after several weeks. If satisfactory lowering of blood pressure is not achieved, an oral diuretic is added to the regimen, because methyldopa may cause expansion of plasma and extracellular fluid volume. The duiretic greatly enhances the hypotensive effects of methyldopa and avoids increasing the unpleasant symptoms which will appear when larger doses, i.e., 3 to 4 g of the drug per day, are given. The average dose required falls between 1 and 2 g/day. The intravenous administration of 250 mg to 1 g has a pronounced hypotensive effect after a delay of 1 to 3 h, but the effect may last 12 to 18 h.

Hypotensive effects of the drug are mild in the

FIGURE 73-1 Biosynthesis of norepinephrine and serotonin.

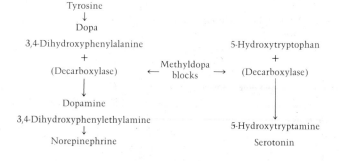

average patient and somewhat greater in the upright than in the recumbent position. Orthostatic hypotension is less with methyldopa than with guanethidine. Enthusiasm has been expressed for its use in patients who exhibit mild to malignant hypertension and even renal insufficiency. Side effects commonly encountered in ambulatory patients include dry mouth and sedation, but rarely parkinsonism, a syndrome more often associated with reserpine. With less frequency, symptoms of gastrointestinal irritation, weakness, impotence, depression, headache, arthralgia, weight gain, lactation, and acute febrile episodes with chills and aching may be observed. Alterations in liver function and liver damage[79,80] have been observed but the exact incidence of these changes is still unknown. The appearance of a febrile episode demands an immediate check of hepatic function, since alterations in liver function appear most frequently during such events. Methyldopa-induced granulomatous hepatitis[81] and methyldopa-induced submassive hepatic necrosis[82] have recently been reported. Some patients who take methyldopa exhibit a positive direct Coombs' test; however, the incidence of actual hemolysis is quite low.[83] The laboratory abnormality alone is considered benign but in combination with anemia is considered an indication for discontinuing the drug. Positive LE cell tests, rheumatoid factor, and red blood cell antibodies have also been reported. Methyldopa is contraindicated in depressive states as well as in liver disease, and caution has been suggested in the presence of either angina pectoris or congestive heart failure.

Guanethidine and methyldopa have equal effects upon standing diastolic pressure but reduction of mean blood pressure may be more rapidly achieved with guanethidine.[84]

Monoamine oxidase inhibitors: pargyline hydrochloride (Eutonyl)

Monoamine oxidase (MAO) inhibitors when used for hypertension present very serious hazards; for example, severe hypertensive crises may develop from foods which contain tyramine (cheddar cheese, pickled herring, chopped liver, certain wines, and beer) due to the tyramine-activated release of norepinephrine. Similar crises have been observed from meperidine hydrochloride (Demerol), and hyperthermic crises have resulted from imipramine hydrochloride (Tofranil). Monoamine oxidase inhibitors would appear to offer more risks than advantages as antihypertensive agents, and thus are now very rarely used.

α-ADRENERGIC RECEPTOR BLOCKING AGENTS

These compounds act principally at the peripheral receptor areas to block the action of circulating adrenergic hormones (epinephrine and norepinephrine) and sympathetic nervous stimulation.[66] The major hemodynamic action is the lowering of peripheral resistance. The two currently available drugs in this category are phentolamine and phenoxybenzamine. These agents have been used primarily in the diagnostic evaluation of patients suspected of having pheochromocytoma or paraganglioma, and in such patients these compounds may be used in preoperative preparation and management. When these drugs have been administered alone for the treatment of hypertension, their use has been impractical and for the most part ineffective. Their short- and long-term administration is associated with side effects such as headache, nausea and vomiting, excessive orthostatic tachycardia, and fatigue without satisfactory reduction in blood pressure. However, the use of α-adrenergic receptor blocking drugs in combination with other antihypertensive drugs deserves further exploration.

β-ADRENERGIC RECEPTOR BLOCKING AGENTS

The group of drugs comprising the β-adrenergic blocking agents are propranolol, practolol, alprenolol, and prindolol. Of these, only propranolol is available for prescription in the United States. The antihypertensive effect of this drug seems to be mediated by decrease in cardiac output, an attenuation of reactive changes in plasma volume during therapy, and a complex effect on vasoconstrictor mechanisms mediated by the renin-angiotensin system and by the central nervous system.[85-87] Cardiac output decreases by about 18 percent, reflecting depression of myocardial contractility and decreased venous return. Peripheral resistance tends to rise initially but falls under continued administration. Pharmacologically, beta blockade allows α-adrenergic action to be unopposed and thus vasoconstriction would be expected. Propranolol seems to be most effective in the high and normal renin groups of hypertension at dosage levels of 40 mg every 6 h (160 mg/day) up to 120 mg four times daily (480 mg/day); plasma levels adequate to suppress rises in plasma renin require much larger doses; e.g., 2,000 mg/day may be needed for maximal antihypertensive action.

Regardless of how propranolol acts, it is considered to be an effective antihypertensive agent. Propranolol may be accompanied by multiple and varied side effects which include central nervous system effects (insomnia, bad dreams, hallucinations, fatigue, depression, paresthesias, ataxia, dizziness). Rarely does it produce significant drowsiness, depression, gastrointestinal side effects or impotence. Hypoglycemia may occur in diabetic patients receiving insulin. The major contraindication is congestive heart failure, impending or overt, because propranolol produces a negative inotropic effect upon heart muscle.

It seems to be useful for mild to moderate hypertension, particularly along with salt restriction and a diuretic. It has been combined with diuretics and vasodilators with good results even in severe hypertensive states. It would seem far more useful in combination with other drugs than as a single drug for hypertension.

Propranolol is particularly useful in the hypertensive individual who suffers from angina pectoris and/or ventricular irritability. Care should be taken not to produce excessive bradycardia. Drug dosage should begin with 10 to 20 mg four times daily; increments of 20 mg every week or two up to 120 mg or more four times daily must be made gradually and cautiously.

It has been suggested that propranolol administered in divided doses twice a day instead of four times daily may be effective in the treatment of hypertension.

It is regrettable that the following drugs are not yet available for prescription in the United States: bethanidine, guanadrel, debrisoquin, minoxidil, guancydine, alprenolol, practolol, and prindolol.[88]

Adrenergic inhibitors or sympatholytic agents

CLONIDINE (CATAPRES)

Clonidine, a relatively new antihypertensive agent, is an imidazoline derivative whose hypotensive effect is produced or has been attributed to an inhibition of efferent outflow from sympathetic centers of the central nervous system resulting in a decreased sympathetic activity to the heart, kidney, and peripheral vessels.[89–91]

Clonidine is effective both orally and parenterally; however, intravenous administration is associated with a brief pressor response which may be exaggerated in patients with severe or accelerated hypertension. Therefore the use of this drug by this route needs further investigation prior to being recommended for use in acute hypertensive crises, particularly with the availability of equally or more potent agents not possessing this undesirable feature. Effective hypotensive action is demonstrable usually within 1 h after oral administration with maximal response in 2 to 4 h. Antihypertensive effectiveness is usually lost after 24 h in most patients. In patients with renal insufficiency the effective pharmacologic half-life appears to be increased. After oral clonidine administration, cardiac output, heart rate, peripheral resistance, and plasma renin activity all decrease. Blood pressure is lower both in the lying and the standing position.[91] The drug is effective in mild as well as in the more severe forms of hypertensive disease.[92] Clonidine's antihypertensive action is potentiated by concomitant diuretic therapy and is additive to the combined effects of vasodilators and beta-blockade therapy.[89]

The oral dosage schedule is usually instituted with 0.1 mg/day, increasing at 1- to 2-week intervals by 0.1 to 0.2 mg/day. Prominent side effects have included sedation, dryness of the mouth, headache, and constipation. This sedative effect tends to be more severe with increased dose levels, but this side effect as well as others may diminish with continued therapy. Some report that the sedative effect may be minimized by giving the larger or major portion of the dose at bedtime. Clonidine's antihypertensive

action has also been reported to be interfered with by the tricyclic antidepressants, as is true also of guanethidine. In addition, the drug may potentiate insulin-induced hypoglycemia.[89]

A unique withdrawal syndrome has been reported with this drug when long-term administration is abruptly discontinued. Blood pressure may revert to pretreatment levels and acute hypertensive crises have been reported. The withdrawal syndrome is associated with sympathetic nervous system overactivity and is treated by the administration of an alpha or beta blocker or reinstitution of clonidine therapy.[89] The existence of this syndrome may pose a potential hazard with this drug in unreliable patients and in patients using this drug and undergoing nonelective surgical procedures.

Clonidine alone or in combination with a diuretic is an effective antihypertensive agent and useful substitute in patients who have experienced intolerable side effects to previously available antihypertensive agents; moreover, the addition of low-dose clonidine to the drug regimens of patients lacking ideal blood pressure control may establish normotension.[89]

Diazoxide

Diazoxide is a nondiuretic compound related to the benzothiadiazine group that decreases systolic and diastolic arterial pressure in all types of hypertension by direct relaxant action on the smooth muscle of the arterioles. The decrease in peripheral resistance is accompanied by a reflex increase in heart rate and cardiac output. Effects on renal plasma flow and glomerular filtration rate are variable.[93]

Oral administration of diazoxide is occasionally utilized for severe drug-resistant hypertension. During continued oral use, this drug induces diabetes mellitus, significant salt and water retention, hirsutism, and parkinsonism.[94] Primarily it has been utilized intravenously for severe malignant hypertension and for hypertensive emergencies. Because of sodium retention and expanded extracellular fluid volume when diazoxide is administered on a daily basis, a diuretic compound should be added to the antihypertensive program. Its adverse major reactions (sodium and water retention and hyperglycemia) may be controlled by appropriate measures.[93]

Selective antagonists

ANGIOTENSIN II (SARALASIN: 1-SARCOSINE-8-ALANINE AII, P-113)*

Recent interest has been directed to specific therapeutic maneuvers by blocking receptor sites. With the understanding of the renin-angiotensin-aldosterone feedback loop and the known activity of angiotensin II on vascular receptors along with the development of the angiotensin II analogue known as saralasin (P-113), it has been shown that the rapid intravenous administration of this compound to sodium- or volume-depleted patients with hypertension produces a rapid and effective reduction in blood pressure when the hypertension is associated with a high renin state, as is seen in functionally significant unilateral renal artery stenosis. Whereas the drug is not effective in lowering blood pressure in patients with hypertension of the low or normal renin variety, great interest has been attached to this drug as a possible rapid-screening test for the identification of patients for further study in the detection of surgically curable renal artery stenosis.[95] This drug has also been recently demonstrated to possess an agonist action, especially in patients with low-renin hypertension.

CONVERTING ENZYME (CEI, SQ20881)

A chloride-dependent converting enzyme is essential for the metabolic degradation of the decapeptide (angiotensin I) to the active octapeptide (angiotensin II) in the renin-angiotensin cascade. Inhibition of this enzyme limits the production of A II, the potent vasoconstrictor. The development of a specific inhibition of this enzyme has lead to its effective intravenous use in the identification of certain hypertensive diseases associated with or produced by excessive A II production. The lack of an available oral preparation limits the therapeutic application of this compound at this time; however, its demonstrated hypotensive action in limited clinical trials has been of great interest and provides great possibilities for further clinical and laboratory application.[96]

GANGLIONIC BLOCKING AGENTS

These anticholinergic (ganglionic blocking) compounds produce blockade of both sympathetic and parasympathetic ganglia.[66] Pharmacodynamically they lower peripheral vascular resistance, cardiac output, and venous pressure; renal blood flow is diminished as blood pressure falls. Although ganglionic blockade is always incomplete, these compounds remain among the most potent but the most difficult of all the antihypertensive agents to employ in clinical practice. Wide fluctuations between recumbent hypertension and postural hypotension are common, and unpleasant reactions related primarily to parasympathetic blockade are very frequent.

Ganglionic blocking agents are not satisfactory drugs when prescribed alone for the therapy of hypertension. However, the physician should gain familiarity with at least a single compound, e.g., pentolinium, which he can use both orally and parenterally with confidence should the need arise.

PROSTAGLANDINS*

A group of unsaturated fatty acid compounds recognized collectively as prostaglandins (prostaglandins E, F, and A) have been isolated from a number of body fluids and tissues. Special cardiovascular interest has been attached to the prostaglandins of the E and A categories because of their ability (1) to lower blood pressure and (2) to induce natriuresis, whereas compounds in the F class have demonstrated predominant nonvascular smooth muscle-stimulating activity. Recent investigation has demonstrated the existence of prostaglandins A_2 and E_2 in the renal medulla, and both compounds have lowered blood pressure in experimental animals. These observations lend support to the presence of a renal medullary antihypertensive function in addition to the previously demonstrated cortical hypertensive function of the kidney mediated through the renin-angiotensin system.

In patients with essential hypertension, the intravenous infusion of prostaglandin A_1 at high infusion rates (2.1 to 11.2 µg/kg/min) has been associated with a significant fall in blood pressure after an apparent initial intrarenal vasodilatation producing natriuresis and kaliuresis, followed by a return of these renal changes to normal or control levels at the time of subsequent arterial pressure reduction. Side effects of bradycardia and hypokalemia were observed in patients receiving higher doses; other significant untoward effects have not been recorded.[97]

The possible role of the prostaglandins in the treatment of essential hypertension and their regulatory role in the depressor and natriuretic functions of the kidney await further study.

For the reader's convenience the most common toxic reactions produced by the various drugs are listed in Table 73-4.

Surgical therapy

Approximately four decades ago, sympathectomy was introduced as a surgical procedure for hypertension. Successive alterations in surgical approach, involving more extensive procedures, were then followed by an effort to denervate larger areas of the vascular bed, reduce vasoconstrictor reflexes and vascular resistance, and thus lower blood pressure (Table 73-5). Blood pressure was reduced satisfactorily in about one-third to one-half of sympathectomized patients; dramatic results were obtained in a few. In general, it was felt that lowering of the blood pressure was directly proportional to the extent of the sympathectomy, and inversely proportional to the severity of the disease.

The introduction of the newer hypotensive drugs during the past three decades has swung the pendulum of therapy away from surgical treatment so that now sympathectomy is rarely performed. It has been suggested that a limited splanchnicectomy (from the eighth to the twelfth dorsal vertebrae), performed bilaterally in a one-stage operation and supplemented by drug therapy, is preferred to the previous sympathectomies of much greater extent.[98] It should be noted that blood pressure becomes more responsive to antihypertensive drugs after sympathectomy. At the present time, those patients for whom sympathectomy might be indicated would include the younger hypertensive patient below the age of 50, who possesses satisfactory renal function and who has failed to respond to a completely adequate medical program, including diet and the newer antihypertensive compounds, or the hypertensive patient who is unable to follow an effective medical program because of multiple drug sensitivities, economic or

TABLE 73-4
Drug reactions

1 Diuretics
  a Sensitivity reactions
  b Electrolyte depletion
  c Gout
  d Diabetes
2 Hydralazine
  a Collagen-like (LE) syndrome
3 Rauwolfia compounds
  a Depression, anxiety states
  b Parkinsonism
  c Peptic ulcer
4 Guanethidine
  a Postural hypotension
  b Parasympathetic stimulation
  c Impotence
5 Methyldopa
  a Febrile illness
  b Liver toxicity
  c Hemolytic anemia (Coombs' positive)
  d Positive LE cell test
  e Rheumatoid factor
  f Red blood cell antibodies
6 Pargyline
  a Hypertensive crises—tyramine-containing foods—amphetamines, vasopressor drugs, appetite depressors
  b Hypotensive crises—meperidine (Demerol)
  c Hyperthermic crises—imipramine (Tofranil)
7 Phenoxybenzamine
  a Headache
  b Nausea
  c Vomiting
  d Tachycardia
8 Propranolol
  a Bradycardia
  b Heart block
  c Heart failure
  d Shock
  e Bronchial asthma
9 Anticholinergic compounds
  a Orthostatic hypotension—syncope, arterial thrombosis
  b Parasympathetic blockade
  c Cycloplegia
  d Ileus
  e Bladder atony
  f Impotence
10 Clonidine
  a Sedation
  b Dry Mouth
  c Dizziness
  d Headache
  e Fatigue
  f Hypertensive rebound on abruptly discontinuing the drug

geographic considerations, or low level of intellectual function.

Drug combinations

In the management of mild hypertensive disease, single compounds such as a diuretic administered alone or in combination with a low dose of a vasodilator, *Rauwolfia* compounds, or other adrenergic

TABLE 73-5
Surgical therapy: sympathectomy

Adson: Subdiaphragmatic splanchnicectomy, celiac ganglionectomy, L_1 and L_2 (1932)
Peet: Supradiaphragmatic splanchnicectomy and lower dorsal ganglionectomy $T_{10}-T_{12}$ (1933)
Smithwick: Thoracolumbar sympathectomy T_6-L_2 (1938)
Poppen: Thoracolumbar sympathectomy T_4-L_2 (1947)
Grimson: Subtotal to total paravertebral sympathectomy, stellate ganglions, T_1-L_1 (1940)

inhibitors may result in normotension. For the more severe hypertensive states, it is fundamental to attack the hypertensive mechanism(s) at multiple sites using various combinations of several drugs, each possessing a different mode of pharmacologic action. Each drug should be administered as a separate tablet and titrated gradually to optimally tolerated doses before other drugs are added. When a satisfactory hypotensive response is achieved or when significant side effects occur, the dose of one or more drugs may be added, reduced, or discontinued. Smaller yet effective doses of several drugs can be used in combination, and thus unpleasant or serious reactions may be diminished or abolished. In the more severe hypertensive diseases, until the effective and tolerated dose of each drug is established, multiple drugs in a single tablet or capsule should not be prescribed, because the dose of one ingredient cannot be altered without changing the dose of others in the combination. However, in the milder forms of hypertension, appropriate uses of combination tablets may have the added advantage of single daily dose administration and possibly decreased cost, thereby increasing patient compliance. In so doing one may avoid the often common problem of cessation of therapy seen with complicated drug regimens.

The physician must avoid the much too prevalent tendency to surrender easily or switch from one drug to another before the effectiveness or tolerance of each prescribed drug is established firmly. Often the initial unpleasant side effects gradually diminish or disappear without appreciable change in drug dosage as subjective tolerance develops.

Excellent results have been achieved with various combinations of drugs, but as yet, the most useful and effective combination for most hypertensive patients has not been firmly established. Of considerable interest has been the recent use in moderate and severe essential hypertension of a combination consisting of an oral diuretic, e.g., hydrochlorothiazide 50 mg twice daily, propranolol in doses of 80 to 160 mg/day in combination with hydralazine 40 to 400 mg/day. This drug combination apparently is not associated with postural hypotension, tachycardia, other significant hemodynamic disturbances, impairment of renal function, or major adverse symptoms in patients so treated, and the combination has the additional advantage of a pharmacologic attack on the pathophysiologic alterations that produce the hypertensive process; namely, the initial treatment with a diuretic produces a natriuresis and volume contraction which in the majority of hypertensive patients is the cornerstone or basis of all subsequent pharmacotherapy. The addition of propranolol with its attendant beta blockade produces a reduction in cardiac output along with a lowering of the pulse rate together with a reduction in plasma renin activity. The overall long-term effects of oral propranolol therapy on peripheral resistance remains a subject of some controversy. If the blood pressure is not thereby brought under control, the subsequent addition of hydralazine, a vasodilator, provides yet another pharmacologic assault on one of the more common underlying factors in the hypertensive process, namely, an increase in peripheral resistance. The peripheral vasodilatation produced by hydralazine thereby adds another and differing mechanism of action to produce normotension. Moreover, the prior administration of a diuretic and propranolol prevents the well-recognized undesirable side effects of vasodilator therapy, namely, tachycardia, increased cardiac output, sodium retention, and a rise in plasma renin activity.

It is well to remember that *Rauwolfia* derivatives often ameliorate the unpleasant symptoms of other drugs and reinforce their hypotensive activity. The oral diuretics greatly enhance the hypotensive activity of other antihypertensive compounds, and if the patient is receiving digitalis, it is wise to use one of the potassium-sparing compounds, such as spironolactone or triamterene. Because of salt loss, the enhancement of other antihypertensive compounds by diuretics, particularly ganglionic blocking agents, guanethidine, methyldopa, and clonidine, may be entirely orthostatic and may result in postural syncope. This reaction must be anticipated in order to prevent potentially tragic injury. Hydralazine likewise tends to augment the effects of other compounds when given in combination.

For the mildly hypertensive patient, it is simpler to begin therapy with an oral diuretic agent (benzothiadiazine, chlorthalidone, etc.), either alone or in combination with spironolactone (or triamterene), in order to preserve serum potassium levels, particularly if large daily doses of the diuretic are contemplated and needed. To this program may be added a *Rauwolfia* compound, hydralazine, a low dose of methyldopa, or clonidine. This combination is simple, well tolerated, and usually effective, particularly for the milder grades of hypertension. Reserpine with chlorthalidone provides an effective hypotensive combination related possibly to the prolonged diuretic action of chlorthalidone; however, serum potassium levels must be watched closely and potassium supplements added to preserve normal levels. If additional drug therapy is needed, one may add to the program in a stepwise fashion as outlined in Table 73-6.

Patients presenting with sustained mild to moderate hypertension (diastolic pressure 90 to 115 mm Hg) also usually offer no therapeutic difficulties in blood pressure control unless they exhibit multiple drug sensitivities, which fortunately plague only a few individuals. An acceptable drug sequence treatment program for patients in this category is outlined in Table 73-6. The selection of the particular drug at step 2 is highly individualized in most patients and is

TABLE 73-6
Mild to moderate hypertension*
(Diastolic pressure 90–115 mm Hg)

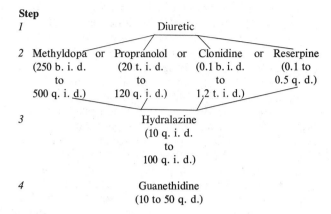

Step

1   Diuretic

2 Methyldopa or Propranolol or Clonidine or Reserpine
   (250 b. i. d.   (20 t. i. d.   (0.1 b. i. d.   (0.1 to
      to   to   to   0.5 q. d.)
   500 q. i. d.)   120 q. i. d.)   1.2 t. i. d.)

3   Hydralazine
                         (10 q. i. d.
                           to
                        100 q. i. d.)

4   Guanethidine
                      (10 to 50 q. d.)

*Dosages given in mg.

often more dependent on the physician's preference and familiarity with its side effects, dosage schedules, etc., rather than selection based on a specific pharmacologic action relative to the mechanism(s) of the hypertensive process. In patients with this level of hypertension, rarely is it necessary to add step 4; however, a reasonable alternative is the substitution of low-dose guanethidine at step 2. This drug in combination with a diuretic is a useful effective antihypertensive regimen and offers the advantage of single-dose low-cost daily therapy, a feature which should assist in improving patient compliance.

Patients suffering from moderately severe hypertension (diastolic pressure 115 to 130 mm Hg) often require a more intensive drug regimen or sequence as outlined in Table 73-7. Reserpine is rarely effective in this category of patients, and because of annoying

TABLE 73-7
Moderately severe hypertension*
(Diastolic pressure 115-130 mm Hg)

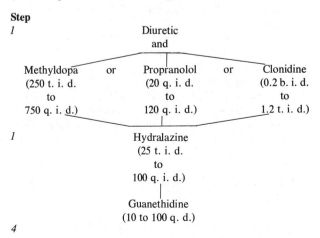

Step

1   Diuretic
                          and

 Methyldopa   or   Propranolol   or   Clonidine
 (250 t. i. d.   (20 q. i. d.   (0.2 b. i. d.
    to   to   to
 750 q. i. d.)   120 q. i. d.)   1.2 t. i. d.)

1   Hydralazine
                        (25 t. i. d.
                         to
                      100 q. i. d.)

                        Guanethidine
                    (10 to 100 q. d.)

4

*Dosages given in mg.

side effects that are often additive to other more effective drugs it has been eliminated at step 2 in the treatment regimen.

The presence of severe hypertension (diastolic pressure usually 130 mm Hg or higher) is often found in patients who are quite ill and almost always demonstrate the presence of or potential for severe target organ damage. Prognosis depends to a large extent on the integrity of renal function. When moderate to severe azotemia is present, the survival time is shortened. Lowering of blood pressure may produce further transient renal impairment. However, reduction of blood pressure in patients suffering from advanced hypertensive disease complicated by renal insufficiency does not necessarily result in deterioration of renal function and usually results in improved survival rates. Therapeutic programs for this group of patients are best initiated in a hospital setting, where careful control of diet and drugs can be monitored by appropriate laboratory procedures and blood pressure recordings at frequent intervals in both the recumbent and upright posture. When immediate action seems urgently needed or when oral medication seems momentarily contraindicated because of nausea, vomiting, renal insufficiency, or irregular drug absorption, parenteral administration of the drugs outlined in the section "Hypertensive Emergencies" may be desirable for the *initiation* of therapy in conjunction with the usual dietary program. As the patient's condition permits, drugs are administered orally and parenteral therapy is withdrawn. A useful oral drug program in this group of patients is outlined in Table 73-8. It should be emphasized that in these patients the diuretic drug of choice may be furosemide or ethacrynic acid rather than a thiazide. These potent diuretics may lead rapidly to electrolyte depletion when sodium is restricted to as low as 500 mg/day, especially when renal function is impaired. Blood pressure should be restored toward normal gradually, since abrupt falls in blood pressure may lead to vascular collapse and a precipitous decrease in renal function. Further adjustments in diet and drugs after blood pressure control has been achieved may allow even the severely hypertensive patient to delete from his program all except moderate salt restriction and a lesser number of antihypertensive compounds.

Treatment regimens should be individualized to each patient's needs and his ability to follow various physical, dietary, and drug programs coupled with the physician's understanding of the antihypertensive pharmacology of the drugs prescribed.

HYPERTENSIVE EMERGENCIES

As one of many medical emergencies, acute hypertensive crises[99] may arise and present an abrupt threat to a patient's life. Such emergencies include hypertensive encephalopathy,[100] usually associated

TABLE 73-8
Severe hypertension*
(Diastolic pressure usually 130 mm Hg or higher)

Step

1 — Diuretic and

| Propranolol (40 q. i. d. to 160 q. i. d.) + Hydralazine (25 q. i. d. to 100 q. i. d.) | or | clonidine (0.2 b. i. d. to 1.2 t. i. d.) + Hydralazine (25 q. i. d. to 100 q. i. d.) | or | Methyldopa (250 q. i. d. to 750 q. i. d.) + Hydralazine (25 q. i. d. to 100 q. i. d.) or Guanethidine (20 to 100 q. d.) |

2 — Guanethidine (20 to 100 q. d.) | Guanethidine (20 to 100 q. d.) or Hydralazine (25 q. i. d. to 100 q. i. d.)

3 — Minoxidil (2.5 b. i. d. to 15 t. i. d.)

*Dosages given in mg.

with excessive diastolic levels (above 140 mm Hg), increased cerebrovascular resistance, cerebral edema, and elevated spinal fluid pressure. They complicate the course of primary hypertension or the acute forms of hypertension secondary to renal infarction, toxemia of pregnancy, or glomerulonephritis. In these situations, it is mandatory to administer hypotensive agents in parenteral form in order to obtain the maximum effect from each milligram of drug and to achieve optimal reduction in blood pressure. For an acute emergency, the drug selected should possess a predictable therapeutic action of known intensity and duration, preferably without undesirable side effects.

The simplest and oldest compound for general use is reserpine, administered intramuscularly, 1.0 to 3.0 mg (average 2.5 mg), every 4 to 12 h. Further injections to provide maintenance therapy depend on the duration of each response, which generally ranges from 4 to 12 h. Such moderate and gradual reduction of blood pressure is of particular utility in the accelerated phase of hypertension in which headache, vomiting, confusion, papilledema, convulsions, cerebral edema, elevated spinal fluid pressure, and variable reduction in renal function are present and in which abrupt lowering of blood pressure may be disastrous, inducing irreversible shock, coma, and uremia. A prominent and limiting side effect of parenteral reserpine is the intense somnolence which interferes with the monitoring of central nervous system signs in patients with hypertensive encephalopathy.

Similarly, methyldopa, 250 mg to 1.0 g, administered intravenously, can produce satisfactory blood pressure responses in 1 to 3 h and lasting 12 to 18 h. The favorable hemodynamic action of methyldopa recommends its use in renal insufficiency. Also, hydralazine hydrochloride may be injected intramuscularly or intravenously, 5.0 to 20 mg or more, every 4 to 6 h, or by continuous intravenous drip for acute hypertensive disease associated with renal insufficiency, toxemia of pregnancy, or glomerulonephritis.

Diazoxide is an extremely potent vasodilating agent and is effective when given intravenously in 150- to 300-mg doses as a bolus in a 10- to 15-s period. If only a slight reduction in arterial pressure occurs or if the reduction is brief (i.e., 30 to 60 min instead of 3 to 15 h), additional doses of diazoxide (150 to 300 mg) should be administered every 15 to 30 min until the desired effect is achieved and maintained.[101] A 35 percent average reduction in mean arterial pressure occurs during the first 2 min, leveling off at an average 20 percent below control levels for an average duration of 3 to 15 h. Because diazoxide tends to retain sodium, it should be administered sequentially or in combination with an intravenous diuretic.

Trimethaphan camphorsulfonate (Arfonad), a tertiary amine ganglionic blocking agent, is administered in concentrations of 0.1 to 1.0 g/100 ml intravenously at a rate of 3.0 to 4.0 mg/min. Hypotension is achieved within minutes, and upon discontinuance of the drug, blood pressure rises rapidly. The rapid onset and brief duration of its action offer advantages both for immediate depression of blood pressure when needed and for continuous regulation of blood pressure at desired levels.

Sodium nitroprusside (Nipride) is probably the ideal drug for the treatment of all hypertensive emergencies.[102,103] As outlined by Palmer and Lassiter,[102] such an agent should possess rapid action, specific effect on resistance vessels, little to no effect on other smooth muscle or cardiac muscle systems, immediate reversibility, lack of effect on central or autonomic nervous systems, no tachyphylaxis, and high potency/low toxicity therapeutic ratio. The pharmacology of nitroprusside is widely applicable to these criteria. Moreover, the current commercial availability of this drug as a 50-mg lyophilized powder to be administered intravenously at a rate of 1 µg/kg/min from a light-protected bottle has led to a more widespread use and more effective physiologic treatment of the hypertensive crisis. The need for constant patient monitoring during the administration of this drug is not a contraindication to its use, since patients requiring this drug are acutely and gravely ill and are best cared for in specialized units trained in the administration of such compounds. Nitroprusside is degraded to thiocyanate and when infused for prolonged periods at high rates, particularly in the presence of renal insufficiency, thiocyanate levels in the serum may reach toxic proportions (greater than 12 mg per 100 ml); therefore, monitoring of thiocyanate levels is a useful procedure in patients receiving nitroprusside as is close observation for the clinical manifestations of thiocyanate toxicity.

In general, reserpine intramuscularly and methyldopa intravenously are simple and safe to use when the critical condition allows 1 or 2 h for therapy to become effective. However, when an immediate effect within minutes becomes mandatory—e.g., in pulmonary edema or dissecting aneurysm—diazoxide, trimethaphan, or nitroprusside are preferred. It should be remembered that an intravenous diuretic (e.g., ethacrynic acid, 50 to 100 mg, or furosemide, 80 to 160 mg) can be administered with any of the above drugs. As soon as it is feasible and the patient's clinical condition permits, a transition from the parenteral to the oral mode of therapy should be made so that the hypertensive process may be controlled over a long period of time and to allow complete regression of the acute hypertensive changes.

The treatment of hypertensive emergencies requires considerable skill, based on a background of knowledge regarding the physiologic disturbances involved, including the status of the kidneys, brain, and heart, and a practical pharmacologic familiarity with effective hypotensive drugs.

SECONDARY (NONESSENTIAL) HYPERTENSION

Acute glomerulonephritis

The pathophysiologic alterations in acute glomerulonephritis involve primarily a decrease in glomerular filtration rate with a relatively normal renal blood flow associated with the retention of salt and water, edema, generalized arteriolar spasm, hypertension, and occasionally encephalopathy. Cardiac output, circulation time, and arteriovenous oxygen differences remain essentially normal; blood volume and extracellular fluid volume are increased. Major cardiovascular manifestations of nephritis—hypertension and edema—are the consequences of the expanded vascular volume resulting from the defect in sodium and water excretion in acute nephritis.

Hypertension and edema as manifestations of acute nephritis are common, but may be absent in mild cases. Hypertension has been attributed to vasospasm from neurogenic or hormonal influences and to expansion of the extracellular and intravascular fluid volumes. Usually the blood pressure is elevated only moderately, in the range of 140 to 160 mm Hg systolic and 90 to 110 mm Hg diastolic. Few patients exhibit rises in diastolic pressure higher than 150 mm Hg; blood pressures above 200/120 mm Hg are unusual. Although acute glomerulonephritis is more common in children, hypertension is said to occur with approximately the same frequency and severity as in older groups.[104]

Mild elevations in blood pressure often do not influence the clinical course of the disease and may not require treatment. If the diastolic blood pressure is below 90 mm Hg and the urine volume is normal, rest and sedation are all that may be indicated. Although decreased urine output and edema may be present without hypertension, the clinical association of these findings is usual. In this setting, when blood pressure rises above 100 mm Hg diastolic, even without overt signs of either cardiac or cerebral involvement, more aggressive antihypertensive therapy should be instituted. Basic therapy should begin with dietary sodium and fluid restriction to limit further the expanded intravascular volume. In children, the pharmacologic control of hypertension can be obtained by the use of reserpine, 80 to 150 μg/kg given intramuscularly once every 12 to 24 h. In more resistant cases, hydralazine 100 μ/kg may be added. In adults, blood pressure elevations of mild degree can usually be controlled with standard oral doses of reserpine, hydralazine, methyldopa, or clonidine. Parenteral therapy may be instituted with doses of 1.0 to 3.0 mg reserpine and/or 5.0 to 20 mg hydralazine intramuscularly. In the milder forms of acute nephritis, antihypertensive therapy is usually needed only for a brief period, and drug toxicity does not present a problem in the absence of significant renal insufficiency.

In more severe form, when there is marked fluid retention and the diastolic pressure exceeds 120 mm Hg and cerebral symptoms of hypertensive encephalopathy appear, a life-threatening emergency exists which must be controlled by appropriate therapy. In general, antihypertensive therapy at this time is approached using as guidelines those programs outlined under the section "Hypertensive Emergencies" earlier in this chapter. In addition, a more direct approach aimed toward the resolution of the inflammatory and exudative processes within the glomeruli themselves may be taken with the use of corticosteroids as adjunctive therapy. Likewise, careful attention must be directed toward correction of the expanded intravascular volume as a result of sodium and water retention. The judicious and appropriate use of newer intravenous diuretics in the form of ethacrynic acid or furosemide are especially advantageous. An older form of therapy, parenteral magnesium sulfate, has demonstrated efficacy in selected patients with acute nephritis.

An effective treatment schedule with magnesium sulfate is as follows: Magnesium sulfate is administered intravenously as a 3 to 4 percent solution (water or D5W) at a dose calculated at 250 mg/kg. The solution is administered over a 45- to 60-min period with the initial administration being given at a rate of 4 to 6 ml/min, until the patient demonstrates skin flushing or complains of warmth. If during this initial period the respiratory rate falls to 6 to 8/min, the intravenous rate is slowed, and the remaining solution is given over the projected 45- to 60-min treatment period. This dosage schedule may achieve a serum magnesium level of 5 to 7 mg/100 ml and has not been associated with serious side effects in the presence of acute renal insufficiency associated with acute nephritis. The dosage schedule (250 mg/kg) may be repeated in 6 h if not initially effective. The antidote is calcium gluconate. In patients who are refractory to these maneuvers, the role of dialysis, either peritoneal or hemodialysis, should not be neglected to carry these patients through this particular phase of the nephritic process. The importance of treating other signs of central nervous system dysfunction by the appropriate use of sedatives (barbiturates) and anticonvulsants (Dilantin sodium) has been demonstrated.

Chronic parenchymal renal disease

Most chronic parenchymal renal diseases are conventionally associated with gradual deterioration in renal function and the development of renal insufficiency and hypertension. A majority of the patients have significant reduction in both glomerular filtration rate and renal plasma flow, although the correlation between these parameters and the level of associated blood pressure is not always predictable. The failure to demonstrate a specific or unifying mechanism for the hypertension of chronic renal disease therefore leaves the general therapeutic approach in these patients similar to that pursued in patients with primary hypertension. However, treatment maneuvers designed to lower blood pressure in the presence of renal insufficiency present special hazards which deserve emphasis. The physician must frequently reassess the overall level of renal function and the beneficial or detrimental effect of blood pressure reduction on this crucial parameter. It appears clear that blood pressure reduction must be achieved to prevent further renal functional impairment as a result of the hypertensive process, but it is likewise true that excessively rapid and inappropriate blood pressure reduction is capable of compromising renal function even further and at times at a remarkably rapid rate. Measures, most notably drug therapy with the exception of hydralazine and methyldopa, generally reduce cardiac output, renal blood flow, and glomerular filtration rate. This is particularly true of the ganglionic blocking agents which exhibit their greatest hypotensive effect in the upright posture and depend on the kidney for their excretion, thereby presenting the additional danger of cumulative toxicity.

In the patient with parenchymal renal disease whose hypertension is mild to moderate and for the most part asymptomatic, reserpine in oral doses of 0.25 to 1.0 mg daily is a safe and potentially effective hypotensive agent when used alone or in combination with hydralazine. Methyldopa probably should be reserved for the patient with moderate-to-severe hypertension. For the reasons mentioned above, we prefer to avoid the use of guanethidine when possible. Appropriate sodium restriction is most beneficial in controlling blood pressure in parenchymal renal disease. Special care must be taken to provide adequate sodium intake in order to prevent progressive sodium depletion with the disastrous results of volume contraction and acceleration of renal insufficiency, likewise, the injudicious administration of dietary sodium may well expand the intravascular volume, leading to possible left ventricular failure and also an increase in blood pressure or the observation that increasing amounts of antihypertensive agents are necessary to achieve previous blood pressure control.[105-107] In general, the majority of patients with renal disease can tolerate a level of dietary sodium intake within the range of 40 to 80 mEq/day without significant alteration in renal function if blood pressure is controlled. However, it must be emphasized that this level of sodium restriction must be reevaluated in relation to changing levels of renal function as a result of the primary disease as well as to the use of adjunctive agents such as diuretics and other antihypertensive maneuvers. Diuretic drugs may be used when renal insufficiency is complicated by hypertension and/or edema, but their use in the presence of azotemia may lead to symptomatic hyponatremia, especially when combined with rigid dietary sodium restriction. The choice of diuretics is of importance. The thiazides may alter renal function, and therefore it is suggested that they be used sparingly (every other day instead of daily) or not at all in those patients with glomerular filtration rates of 30 ml/min or below. Ethacrynic acid and furosemide have the advantage of potency even in the presence of renal insufficiency; however, their inappropriate and/or prolonged use may be associated with electrolyte disturbance and other untoward side effects (see "Diuretic Compounds"). Because of the well-known hazards and frequency of hyperkalemia in renal insufficiency, the use of the potassium-sparing diuretics (spironolactone and triamterene) is not advised in these patients.

Accelerated or malignant hypertension adds to the gravity of the prognosis in renal disease. Resting diastolic pressures of 125 mm Hg or greater, severe hypertensive retinopathy, encephalopathy, and left ventricular failure all represent unquestioned indications for aggressive treatment. The recent demonstration of the usefulness of intravenous diazoxide combined with furosemide in these patients, in particular those with associated azotemia, deserves emphasis.[107] The details of this and other therapeutic approaches in the treatment of hypertensive emergencies is outlined earlier in this chapter.

The primary aim of antihypertensive therapy in the presence of renal disease is the gradual and progressive reduction of blood pressure to normal or near-normal levels by means of rest, diet, and drugs with special attention being placed on the preservation of renal function.[105] Other general measures in the management of azotemia must also be instituted as deemed necessary. The role of a single or repetitive hemodialysis should not be overlooked in the management of these patients. Uremia as well as hypertension can often be controlled with this therapy. Patients with chronic renal failure and volume overload (low renin state) respond to hemodialysis with a lowering of blood pressure more readily than do patients with high renin (vasoconstrictor) hypertension and chronic renal failure.[108] Recent emphasis has been directed toward nephrectomy as adjunctive therapy for control of hypertension in this latter group of patients with terminal renal failure. However, more recent reports,[61] have stressed the value of minoxidil in the control of hypertension in these patients thereby negating the numerous adverse effects of the removal of native kidneys in the dialysis

population with previously severe and uncontrolled hypertension. Should renal insufficiency be progressive and irreversible, renal transplantation would be desirable—a maneuver which further substantiates the critical role of the kidney in the production of hypertension in the presence of severe renal insufficiency.

REFERENCES

1 Ledingham, J. M.: The Etiology of Hypertension, *Practitioner*, 207:5, 1971.

2 Page, I. H.: Arterial Hypertension in Retrospect, *Circ. Res.*, 34:133, 1974.

3 Guyton, A. C., Coleman, T. G., Cawley, A. W., Manning, R. D., Jr., Norman, R. A., and Ferguson, J. D.: A Systems Analysis Approach to Understanding Long Range Arterial Blood Pressure and Hypertension, *Circ. Rec.*, 35:15, 1974.

3a Laragh, J. H., (ed.): "Hypertension Manual," Yorke Medical Books, New York, 1974.

4 Sambhi, M. P., Crane, M. G., and Genest, J.: Essential Hypertension: New Concepts About Mechanisms (UCLA Conference), *Ann. Intern. Med.*, 79:411, 1973.

5 Page, L. B., and Sidd, J. J.: Medical Management of Primary Hypertension, *N. Engl. J. Med.*, 287:960, 1018, and 1974, 1972.

6 Sheps, S. G., and Kirkpatrick, R. A.: Hypertension: Subject Review, *Mayo Clin. Proc.*, 50:709, 1975.

7 Goldberg, L. I.: Current Therapy of Hypertension: A Pharmacologic Approach, *Am. J. Med.*, 58:489, 1975.

8 Koch-Weser, J.: Correlation of Pathophysiology and Pharmacotherapy in Primary Hypertension, *Am. J. Cardiol.*, 32:499, 1973.

9 The National High Blood Pressure Education Program: Guidelines for the Evaluation of and Management of the Hypertensive Patient, DHEW (NIH) 76-744, 1973.

10 Lew, E. A.: High Blood Pressure, Other Risk Factors and Longevity: The Insurance Viewpoint, *Am. J. Med.*, 55:281, 1973.

11 Hollander, W.: Hypertension: Antihypertensive Drugs in Atherosclerosis, *Circulation*, 48:1112, 1973.

12 Kannel, W. B., Schwartz, M. J., and McNamara, P. M.: The Framingham Study, *Dis. Chest*, 56:43, 1969.

13 Kannel, W. B., Gordon, T., and Schwartz, M. J.: Systolic versus Diastolic Blood Pressure and Risk of Coronary Heart Disease (the Framingham Study), *Am. J. Cardiol.*, 27:335, 1971.

14 Kannel, W. B.: Role of Blood Pressure in Cardiovascular Morbidity and Mortality, *Prog. Cardiovasc. Dis.*, 17:5, 1974.

15 Roberts, W. C.: The Hypertensive Diseases: Evidence that Systemic Hypertension Is a Greater Risk Factor to the Development of Other Cardiovascular Diseases than Previously Suspected, *Am. J. Med.*, 59:523, 1975.

16 Kannel, W. B., Wolf, P. A., Verter, J., and McNamara, P. M.: Epidemiologic Assessment of the Role of Blood Pressure in Stroke (the Framingham Study), *J.A.M.A.*, 214:301, 1970.

17 Hypertension—Drug Cooperative Study Group: Effect of Antihypertensive Treatment on Stroke Recurrence, *J.A.M.A.*, 229:409, 1974.

18 Paguchi, J., and Freis, E. D.: Partial Reduction of Blood Pressure in Prevention of Complications in Hypertension, *N. Engl. J. Med.*, 291:329, 1974.

19 Oglesby, P.: Risks of Mild Hypertension: A Ten-Year Report, *Br. Heart J.*, 33(suppl.):116, 1971.

20 Veterans Administration Cooperative Study Group on Anti-

hypertensive Agents: Effects of Treatment Morbidity in Hypertension: II. Results in Patients with Diastolic Blood Pressure Averaging 90 Through 114 mm Hg, *J.A.M.A.*, 213: 1143, 1970.

21 Veterans Administration Cooperative Study Group on Antihypertensive Agents: Effects of Treatment on Morbidity in Hypertension, *J.A.M.A.*, 202:1028, 1967.

22 Laragh, J. H.: Oral Contraceptive Hypertension, *Postgrad. Med.*, 53:98, 1972.

23 Coster, M. D., and David, G. K.: Reversible Severe Hypertension due to Licorice Ingestion, *N. Engl. J. Med.*, 278:1381, 1968.

24 Lowder, S. C., and Brown, R. D.: Hypertension Corrected by Discontinuing Chronic Sodium Bicarbonate Ingestion: Subsequent Transient Hypoaldosteronism, *Am. J. Med.*, 58:727, 1975.

25 Patel, C.: Randomised Controlled Trial of Yoga and Bio-Feedback in Management of Hypertension, *Lancet*, 2:93, 1975.

26 Kristt, D. A., and Engel, B. T.: Learned Control of Blood Pressure in Patients with High Blood Pressure, *Circulation*, 51:370, 1975.

27 Abboud, F. M.: Relaxation, Autonomic Control and Hypertension, *N. Engl. J. Med.*, 294:107, 1976.

28 Chiang, B. N., Perlman, L. V., and Epstein, F. H.: Overweight and Hypertension: A Review, *Circulation*, 39:403, 1969.

29 Fregley, M. J. (ed.): Seminar on the Role of Salt in Cardiovascular Hypertension: I, II, and III, *Am. J. Cardiol.*, 8:526, 684, and 863, 1961.

30 Freis, E. D.: Salt Volume and the Prevention of Hypertension, *Circulation*, 53:589, 1976.

31 Dustin, H. R., Tarazi, R. C., and Bravo, E. L.: Diuretic and Diet Treatment of Hypertension, *Arch. Intern. Med.*, 133: 1007, 1974.

32 Fredrickson, D. S., Levy, R. I., and Lees, R. S.: Fat Transport in Lipoproteins: An Integrated Approach to Mechanisms and Disorders, *N. Engl. J. Med.*, 276:34, 94, 148, 215, and 273, 1967.

33 Lees, R. S., and Wilson, D. E.: The Treatment of Hyperlipidemia, *N. Engl. J. Med.*, 284:186, 1971.

34 Kempner, W.: Treatment of Hypertensive Vascular Disease with Rice Diet, *Am. J. Med.*, 4:545, 1948.

35 Koch-Weser, J.: Correlation of Pathophysiology and Pharmacotherapy in Primary Hypertension, *Am. J. Cardiol.*, 32:499, 1973.

36 Koch-Weser, J.: Individualization of Antihypertensive Drug Therapy, *Med. Clin. North Am.*, 58:1027, 1974.

37 Brunner, H. R., Sealey, J. E., and Laragh, J. H.: Renin Subgroups in Essential Hypertension: Further Analysis of Their Pathophysiological and Epidemiological Characteristics, *Circ. Res.*, 32 and 33(suppl. 1):99, 1973.

38 Woods, J. W., Pittman, A. W., Pulliam, C. C., Wark, E. E., Jr., Waider, W., and Allen, C. A.: Renin Profiling in Hypertension and Its Use in Treatment with Propranolol and Chlorthalidone, *N. Engl. J. Med.*, 294:1137, 1976.

39 Finnerty, F. A.: Relationship of Extracellular Fluid Volume to the Development of Drug Resistance in the Hypertensive Patient, *Am. Heart J.*, 81:563, 1971.

40 Earley, L. E.: Diuretics, *N. Engl. J. Med.*, 276:966, 1023, 1967.

41 Laragh, J. H.: The Proper Use of Newer Diuretics, *Ann. Intern. Med.*, 67:606, 1967.

42 Tarazi, R. C., Dustan, H. P., and Edward, D.: Long-term Thiazide Therapy in Essential Hypertension, *Circulation*, 41:709, 1970.

43 McLeod, P. J., Ogilvie, R. I., and Ruedy, J.: Effects of Large and Small Doses of Hydrochlorothiazide in Hypertensive Patients, *Clin. Pharmacol. Ther.*, 11:733, 1970.

44 Fichman, M. P., Vorherr, H., Kleeman, C. R., and Telfer, N.: Diuretic-induced Hyponatremia, *Ann. Intern. Med.*, 75:853, 1971.

45 Kosman, M. E.: Management of Potassium Problems during Long-Term Diuretic Therapy, *J.A.M.A.*, 230:743, 1974.

46 Kohner, E. M., Dollery, C. T., Lowry, C., and Schumer, B.: Effect of Diuretic Therapy on Glucose Tolerance in Hypertensive Patients, *Lancet*, 1:986, 1971.

47 Nicotero, J. A., Schieb, E. T., Martinez, R., Rodnan, G. P., and Shapiro, A. P.: Prevention of Hyperuricemia by Allopurinol in Hypertensive Patients Treated with Chlorothiazide, *N. Engl. J. Med.*, 282:133, 1970.

48 Bryant, J. M., Schvartz, N., Torosdag, S., Fletcher, J., Jr., Fertig, H., Schwartz, M. S., Quan, R. B. F., McDermott, J. J., and Spencer, T. B.: The Antihypertensive Effects of Chlorthalidone: A Comparative Analysis with Benzthiazide Compounds, *Circulation*, 25:522, 1962.

49 Materson, B. J., et al.: Antihypertensive Effects of Metolazone (Zaroxolyn), *Curr. Ther. Res.*, 16:890, 1974.

50 Kirkendall, W. M., and Stein, J. H.: Clinical Pharmacology of Furosemide and Ethacrynic Acid, *Am. J. Cardiol.*, 22:162, 1968.

51 Kim, K. E., et al.: Ethacrynic Acid and Furosemide, *Am. J. Cardiol.*, 27:407, 1971.

52 Burg, M. B.: Renal Chloride Transport and Diuretics, *Circulation*, 53:587, 1976.

53 Meriwether, W. D., Mangi, R. J., and Serpich, A. A.: Deafness Following Standard IV Dose of Ethacrynic Acid, *J.A.M.A.*, 216:795, 1971.

54 Liddle, G. W.: Aldosterone Antagonists and Traimterene, *Ann. N. Y. Acad. Sci.*, 139:466, 1966.

55 Spark, R. F., and Melby, J. C.: Hypertension and Low Plasma Renin Activity: Presumptive Evidence for Mineralocorticoid Excess, *Ann. Intern. Med.*, 75:831, 1971.

56 Koch-Weser, J.: Vasodilator Drugs in the Treatment of Hypertension, *Arch. Intern. Med.*, 133:1017, 1974.

57 Chidsey, C. A., III, and Gottlieb, T. B.: The Pharmacologic Basis of Antihypertensive Therapy: The Role of Vasodilator Drugs, *Prog. Cardiovasc. Dis.*, 15:99, 1974.

58 Perry, H. M., J.: Late Toxicity to Hydralazine Resembling Systemic Lupus Erythematosus or Rheumatoid Arthritis, *Am. J. Med.*, 54:58, 1973.

59 DuCharme, D. W., Freyburger, W. A., Graham, B. E., and Carlson, R. G.: Pharmacologic Properties of Minoxidil: A New Hypotensive Agent, *J. Pharmacol. Exp. Ther.*, 184:662, 1973.

60 Wilburn, R. L., et al.: Long-Term Treatment of Severe Hypertension with Minoxidil, Propranolol and Furosemide, *Circulation*, 52:706, 1975.

61 Pettinger, W. A., and Mitchell, H. C.: Minoxidil: An Alternative to Nephrectomy for Refractory Hypertension, *N. Engl. J. Med.*, 289:167, 1973.

62 Proceeding of a Prazosin Symposium, San Francisco, California, May 1974, *Postgrad. Med.*, November 1975.

63 Bloom, D. S., Rosendorf, C., and Kramer, R.: Clinical Evaluation of Prazosin as the Sole Agent for the Treatment of Hypertension: A Double-Blind Cross-over Study with Methyldopa, *Curr. Ther. Res.*, 18:144, 1975.

64 Rougier, M., and Lahon, H. F. J.: Prazosin: A New Antihypertensive Agent, *Br. J. Clin. Pract.*, 28:280, 1974.

65 Clark, D. W., and Goldberg, L. I.: Guancydine: A New Antihypertensive Agent: Use with Quinethazone and Guanethidine or Propranolol, *Ann. Intern. Med.*, 76:579, 1972.

66 Frohlich, E. D.: Inhibition of Adrenergic Function in the Treatment of Hypertension, *Arch. Intern. Med.*, 133:1033, 1974.

67 Bein, H. J.: The Pharmacology of *Rauwolfia*, *Pharmacol. Rev.*, 8:435, 1956.

68 Report from the Boston Collaborative Drug Surveillance Program: Reserpine in Breast Cancer, *Lancet*, 2:669, 1974.

69 Armstrong, B., Stevens, N., and Doll, R.: Retrospective Study of the Association between the Use of *Rauwolfia* Derivatives and Breast Cancer in English Women, *Lancet*, 2:672, 1974.

70 Heinonen, O. P., Shapiro, S., Tuominen, L., et al.: Reserpine Use in Relationship to Breast Cancer, *Lancet*, 2:675, 1974.

71 Nies, A. S.: Adverse Reactions and Interactions Limiting the Use of Antihypertensive Drugs, *Am. J. Med.*, 58:495, 1974.

72 Ober, K. F., and Wang, R. I. H.: Drug Interactions with Guanethidine, *Clin. Pharmacol. Ther.*, 14:190, 1973.

73 Eagan, J. T., and Orgain, E. S.: A Study of 38 Patients and Their Responses to Guanethidine: A New Antihypertensive Agent, *J.A.M.A.*, 175:550, 1961.

74 Shen, D., Gibaldi, M., Throne, M., Bellward, G., Cunningham, R., Israili, Z., Dayton, P., and McNay, J.: Pharmacokinetics of Bethanidine in Hypersensitive Patients, *Clin. Pharmacol. Ther.*, 17:363, 1975.

75 Hansson, L. Pascual, A., and Julius, S.: Comparison of Guanadrel and Guanethidine, *Clin. Pharmacol. Ther.*, 14:204, 1973.

76 Orgain, E. S., and Kern, A.: Debrisoquin in the Therapy of Hypertension, *Arch. Intern. Med.*, 125:255, 1970.

77 Henning, M.: Studies on the Mode of Action of α-Methyldopa, *Acta Physiol. Scand.(Suppl.)*, 322:1, 1969.

78 Gaffney, T. E., Privitera, P. J., and Mohammed, S.: The Multiple Sites of Action in Methyldopa, in G. Onesti, K. E. Kim, and J. H. Moyer (eds.), "Hypertension: Mechanisms and Management," Grune & Stratton, Inc., New York, 1973.

79 Toghill, P. J., Smith, P. G., Benton, P., et al.: Methyldopa Liver Damage, *Br. Med. J.*, 3:545, 1974.

80 Tysell, J. E., Jr., and Knauer, M.: Hepatitis Induced by Methyldopa (Aldomet): Report of a Case and a Review of the Literature, *Digestive Dis.*, 16:849, 1971.

81 Miller, A. C., Jr., and Reid, W. M.: Methyldopa-Induced Granulomatous Hepatitis, *J.A.M.A.*, 235:2001, 1976

82 Rehman, O. U., Keith, T. A., and Gall, E. A.: Methyldopa-Induced Submassive Hepatic Necrosis, *J.A.M.A.*, 224:1390, 1973.

83 Murad, F.: Immunohemolytic Anemia during Therapy with Methyldopa, *J.A.M.A.*, 203:149, 1968.

84 Tarpley, E. L.: Controlled Trial of Guanethidine and Methyldopa in Moderate Hypertension, *Curr. Ther. Res.*, 16:1187, 1974.

85 Holland, O. B., and Kaplan, N. M.: Propranolol in the Treatment of Hypertension, *N. Engl. J. Med.*, 294:930, 1976.

86 Nies, A. S., and Shand, D. G.: Clinical Pharmacology of Propranolol, *Circulation*, 52:6, 1975.

87 Buhler, F. R., Laragh, J. H., et al.: Anti-Hypertensive Action of Propranolol: Specific Anti-Renin Responses in High and Normal Renin Forms of Essential, Renal, Renal Vascular, and Malignant Hypertension, *Am. J. Cardiol.*, 32:511, 1973.

88 Freis, E. D.: Letters to the Editor: The Drug Lag, *J.A.M.A.*, 235:473, 1976.

89 Pettinger, W. A.: Clonidine: A New Antihypertensive Drug, *N. Engl. J. Med.*, 293:1179, 1975.

90 Mroczek, W. J., Davidov, M., and Finnerty, F. A.: Prolonged Treatment with Clonidine: Comparative Hypertensive Effects Along and with a Diuretic Agent, *Am. J. Cardiol.*, 30:536, 1972.

91 Onesti, G., Schwartz, A. B., Kim, K. E., Pas-Martinez, V., and Swartz, C.: Antihypertensive Effect of Clonidine, *Circ. Res.*, 28 and 29 (suppl. 2):53 and 69, 1971.

92 Rosenman, R. H.: Combined Clonidine-Chlorthalidone Therapy in Hypertension, *Arch. Intern. Med.*, 135:1236, 1975.

93 Kosman, M. E.: Evaluation of Diazoxide (Hyperstat IV), *J.A.M.A.*, 224:1422, 1973.

94 Fang, P., MacDonald, I., et al.: Oral Diazoxide in Uncontrolled Malignant Hypertension, *Med. J. Aust.*, 2:621, 1974.

95 Streeten, D. H. P., Phil, D., Anderson, G. H., Freiberg, J. M., and Dalakos, T. B.: Use of an Angiotensin II Antagonist (Saralasin) in the Recognition of "Angiotensinogenic" Hypertension, *N. Engl. J. Med.*, 292:657, 1975.

96 Gavras, H., Brunner, H. R., Laragh, J. H., Sealey, J. E., Gavras, I., and Vukovich, R. A.: An Angiotensin Converting-Enzyme Inhibitor to Identify and Treat Vasoconstrictor and Volume Factors in Hypertensive Patients, *N. Engl. J. Med.*, 291:817, 1974.

97 Lee, J. B., McGiff, J. C., Kannegiesser, H., Aykent, Y. Y., Mudd, J. G., and Frawley, T. F.: Prostaglandin A₁: Antihypertensive and Renal Effects, *Ann. Intern. Med.*, 74:703, 1971.

98 Whitelaw, G. P., Kinsey, D., and Smithwick, R. H.: Factors Influencing the Choice of Treatment in Essential Hypertension, *Am. J. Surg.*, 107:220, 1964.

99 Sheps, S. G.: Hypertensive Crisis, *Postgrad. Med.*, 49:95, 1971.

100 Gifford, R. W., and Westbrook, E.: Hypertensive Encephalopathy: Mechanisms, Clinical Features, and Treatment, *Prog. Cardiovasc. Dis.*, 17:115, 1974.

101 Koch-Weser, J.: Drug Therapy: Diazoxide, *N. Engl. J. Med.*, 294:1271, 1976.

102 Palmer, R. F., and Lasseter, K. C.: Drug Therapy: Sodium Nitroprusside, *N. Engl. J. Med.*, 292:294, 1975.

103 Tuzel, I., Limjuco, R., and Kahn, D.: Sodium Nitroprusside in Hypertensive Emergencies, *Curr. Ther. Res.*, 17:95, 1975.

104 Schwartz, W. B., and Kassirer, J. P.: Clinical Aspects of Acute Post-Streptococcal Glomerulonephritis, in M. B. Strauss and L. G. Welt (eds.), "Diseases of Kidney," Little, Brown and Company, Boston, 1971.

105 Shapiro, A. P.: Hypertension in Renal Parenchymal Disease, *Disease-A-Month*, September 1969.

106 Hunt, J. C., Strong, C. G., Harrison, E. S., Jr., Furlow, W. L., and Leary, F. J.: Management of Hypertension of Renal Origin, *Am. J. Cardiol.*, 26:280, 1970.

107 Mroczek, W. J., Davidov, M., Gavrilovich, L., and Finnerty, F. A., Jr.: The Value of Aggressive Therapy in the Hypertensive Patient with Azotemia, *Circulation*, 40:893, 1969.

108 Wiedmann, P., Maxwell, N. H., Jupu, A. N., Lewin, A. J., and Massry, S. G.: Plasma Renin Activity and Blood Pressure in Terminal Renal Failure, *N. Engl. J. Med.*, 285:757, 1971.

Heart Disease Secondary to Diseases of the Lungs and Pulmonary Arteries

74
Pulmonary Hypertension

S. GILBERT BLOUNT, JR., M.D., and
ROBERT F. GROVER, M.D., Ph.D.

INTRODUCTION

In the unexpanded fetal lung, the pulmonary vascular resistance is high and the pulmonary blood flow is low. Dawes has shown active pulmonary vasoconstriction to be the dominant factor determining pulmonary vascular resistance in the fetal lamb.[1] He significantly increased blood flow through the unexpanded lung by increasing the oxygenation of fetal arterial blood or by infusing the vasodilator acetylcholine. Conversely, fetal hypoxemia caused an increase in pulmonary vascular resistance and decreased pulmonary blood flow. This evidence strongly suggests that the fetal pulmonary circulation is regulated by hypoxia.

The first breaths following birth transform the lung from a collapsed, fluid-filled, underperfused organ to its expanded, air-filled, fully perfused postnatal state. Pulmonary vascular resistance falls as the lung expands and the alveoli are aerated. Pulmonary blood flow increases rapidly, and the lung functions to oxygenate blood and remove carbon dioxide for the infant beginning extrauterine life. The pulmonary arterial pressure then falls to below aortic pressure; unless the ductus arteriosus closes, blood flows from systemic to pulmonary circulation, producing a left-to-right shunt. The ductus arteriosus may open and close intermittently during the first few days of life. Hemodynamic studies of normal human infants during the first hours of life frequently demonstrate a large left-to-right shunt through a patent ductus arteriosus.[2] Right-to-left shunting of blood has also been demonstrated, indicating that significant fluctuations in pulmonary vascular resistance may occur after birth.[3] However, by the end of the first week of life, the normal ductus arteriosus is functionally closed, and the postnatal pulmonary circulatory pattern becomes established.

Bradykinin, a potent vasoactive peptide, may play an important role in the circulatory adjustments to extrauterine life. Of all the substances formed in the body, kinins are the most potent vasodilators known; they are highly effective in dilating pulmonary arterioles.[4] Paradoxically, bradykinin constricts the umbilical arteries and veins and also the ductus arteriosus.[5] Bradykinin is formed from its inactive precursor, kininogen, by the action of an enzyme, kallikrein. This enzyme is activated by several factors, including a rise in blood oxygen tension and a fall in the temperature of umbilical arterial blood, which occur at the time of birth.[6] These observations have led to the hypothesis that bradykinin concentration in the circulation may rise at birth, dilate the pulmonary arterioles, constrict the ductus arteriosus (and the umbilical vessels), and thereby aid in establishing the postnatal pulmonary circulation.[7] An obvious corollary to this hypothesis is that a failure to activate bradykinin at birth could result in a persistence of a high pulmonary vascular resistance and patency of the ductus arteriosus.

The most striking histologic feature of the fetal pulmonary vascular bed is the thick muscular media of the small muscular pulmonary arteries. These vessel walls appear thinner with vascular dilatation in the postnatal period. It is widely accepted that this thinning process represents an actual decrease in muscle mass within the media of the vessels.[8] The development of increased pulmonary vascular resistance and pulmonary hypertension after birth has been largely attributed to failure of this decrease in vascular musculature; this may indeed be true. However, the authors believe that existence of a greater muscle mass in the fetal lung than in the normal infant lung has not been definitely established; the thickness of the fetal vessels may merely represent vasoconstriction. Thinning of the pulmonary vessel walls continues during the first year and a half of life, resulting in the normal adult vessel structure. This normal involution of pulmonary arterial smooth muscle occurs as long as no abnormal stimulus produces pulmonary vasoconstriction.[9,10]

Once the structural transition in the pulmonary vascular bed has been completed, the pulmonary circulation assumes its familiar hemodynamic characteristics of low pressure, low resistance, and high compliance. Normal man resting supine at sea level has a mean pulmonary arterial pressure, i.e., the average pressure throughout the cardiac cycle and during several respiratory cycles, of 12 mm Hg; there is no significant variation over the age range of 4 to 70 years.[11,12]

The change in pulmonary arterial pressure in the

normal lung due to increased pulmonary blood flow has been studied by two different methods. One method diverts the total right ventricular output through the left lung by inflating an occluding balloon within the lumen of the artery to the right lung. Blood flow is approximately doubled in the left lung, without change in cardiac output or other major circulatory adjustments. This maneuver produces a small but consistent rise in pulmonary arterial pressure of 5 mm Hg.[13,14] The second and more complex method is more physiologic. A supine subject exercises by pumping a bicycle ergometer with his legs. Moderate exercise may double the cardiac output, but very heavy exercise is required to produce a threefold increase in the cardiac output. Though this exercise serves to increase the total pulmonary blood flow, associated alterations in respiratory dynamics and cardiac function may also influence the pulmonary circulation. Under the above circumstances, mean pulmonary arterial pressure may increase as much as 15 mm Hg (Fig. 74-1). These modest elevations of pulmonary arterial pressure in response to increased blood flow through the normal lung must be borne in mind when evaluating the hemodynamics of left-to-right shunts.

CONDITIONS LEADING TO PULMONARY HYPERTENSION

The term *pulmonary hypertension* implies an elevation of the pulmonary arterial pressure to levels above the accepted limit of normal, i.e., 35/15 mm Hg. The maintenance of a normal pulmonary arterial blood pressure is dependent on a physiologic relationship between the volume of pulmonary arterial blood flow per unit of time and the resistance to that flow. The most important and best-understood factors responsible for elevation of pulmonary arterial blood pressure include (1) elevation of pulmonary capillary and/or left atrial pressure, (2) decrease in cross-sectional area of the total pulmonary vascular

bed, and (3) significant increase in pulmonary arterial blood flow. Pulmonary blood volume, blood viscosity, bronchopulmonary arterial anastomoses, intrapulmonary pressure, and intrathoracic pressure may play some part in the development of pulmonary hypertension; however, these mechanisms are probably of minor importance. Pulmonary hypertension may result when one or more of these mechanisms are involved; if it is of sufficient severity and duration, pathologic changes are produced within the pulmonary vascular bed which initiate or further the obstructive element and heighten the pulmonary vascular resistance. The following discussion emphasizes these three factors. Other factors, such as hypoxia, which influenced the pulmonary blood pressure are also discussed.

Elevation of pulmonary capillary pressure and/or left atrial pressure

The elevation of pulmonary capillary pressure usually results from obstruction to pulmonary venous blood flow. This obstruction may be as distal as the left ventricle or as proximal as the pulmonary vein, encompassing many forms of obstruction at sites in between.

Normal mean left atrial pressure ranges between 2 and 12 mm Hg. A study of the components of the normal left atrial pressure tracing revealed the *a* wave to have an average mean pressure of 10 mm Hg (range, 4 to 16 mm Hg) and the *v* wave to average 13 mm Hg (range, 6 to 21 mm Hg).[15] The normal mean pulmonary arterial pressure of about 12 to 18 mm Hg produces an average pressure gradient of about 6 to 11 mm Hg across the pulmonary vascular bed. However, at the end of diastole, the pressure in the pulmonary artery falls to a level equal to that in the left atrium, and the left atrial *a* wave is superimposed

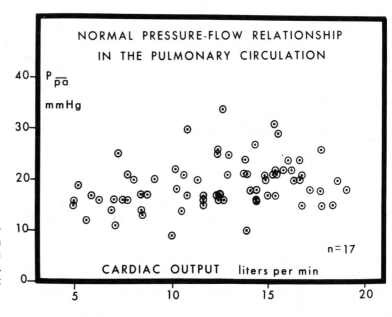

FIGURE 74-1 When pulmonary blood flow is increased through the normal lung, the rise in mean pulmonary artery pressure (P_{PA}) is minimal. Data are from 17 normal young men studied at sea level. Cardiac output was measured by Fick's method at rest and during supine leg exercise.[93]

upon the pulmonary arterial pressure wave.[16] Recently, there has been considerable interest in the clinical application of this phenomenon. Simply by monitoring the (diastolic) pulmonary arterial pressure, obtained by a flow-directed catheter, one can detect failure of the left ventricle from elevation of the left atrial pressure, reflecting the rising left ventricular end-diastolic pressure.[17] However, the limitations of this technique are being recognized. Finite time is required for pulmonary arterial diastolic pressure to equilibrate the left atrial pressure, and in tachycardia equilibration does not occur.[18] Also, the presence of pulmonary vascular disease will invalidate this indirect estimation of left atrial pressure.

The left atrial and pulmonary capillary pressures may become elevated in the normal person during severe exercise or with other conditions resulting in greatly increased pulmonary arterial blood flow. Experimental conditions producing pulmonary capillary pressure elevation include the rapid intravenous injection of saline solution and the use of methoxamine or other potent systemic vasoconstrictive substances.[19] Any other situation causing redistribution of blood into the pulmonary vascular bed could also produce elevation of the left atrial and pulmonary capillary pressures. This would suggest that the mechanism is a passive increase in volume, distending the pulmonary venous and capillary systems and increasing the transmural pressure. In human beings the pulmonary blood vessels are affected by both active and passive mechanisms, and alterations in pulmonary vascular resistance are not necessarily directly related to change in vessel size.[20]

Variations in intrapulmonary and intrathoracic pressure must also be considered as contributing to the elevation of pulmonary capillary pressure and thereby the pulmonary arterial pressure. Although this mechanism is probably of minor significance, it seems feasible that increased alveolar pressure might be transmitted to the pulmonary capillary bed; if widespread, it might affect the pulmonary arterial pressure.

Conditions associated with obstruction to pulmonary venous flow elevate the pulmonary arterial pressure in a retrograde and passive manner; they will be considered next.

INCREASE IN RESISTANCE TO LEFT VENTRICULAR FILLING

Increase in the residual diastolic blood volume in the failing left ventricle results in an increased resistance to left ventricular filling. The left ventricular failure may result from an obstructive defect, such as systemic hypertension or obstruction to left ventricular outflow, or it may be due to myocardial inadequacy secondary to coronary artery disease or primary or secondary myocardial disease. Hypertrophy of the left ventricle for whatever cause without an elevation of residual diastolic blood volume, probably most marked in some patients with cardiomyopathy, will greatly decrease the compliance of the left ventricle

and thereby increase the resistance to filling with resultant elevation of left atrial pressure and decrease in cardiac output.[21] The pulmonary hypertension secondary to such conditions is due to the retrograde transmission of the elevated pulmonary venous pressure across the capillary bed and is usually of moderate degree. The occasional further rise of pulmonary arterial pressure is suggestive of a reflex vasoconstrictive element in the pulmonary hypertension; it produces an increase in the gradient between the pulmonary arterial and left atrial pressures.[22] Constrictive pericarditis, marked myocardial fibrosis, and restrictive endocarditis may also effect this change; in these conditions, there is rarely a vasoconstrictive element, and the gradient across the capillary bed is normal or modestly increased. The pulmonary arterial systolic pressure is usually between 40 and 60 mm Hg.

MITRAL VALVULAR DISEASE

Left atrial pressure rises when the mitral valve orifice is decreased beyond a critical area. As there are no valves in the left atrial–pulmonary venous–capillary system, a rise in left atrial pressure is transmitted to and across the pulmonary capillary bed, elevating the pulmonary arterial pressure. With mild degrees of mitral valve stenosis, the pulmonary hypertension may be purely passive in nature, with preservation of a normal pressure gradient across the pulmonary vascular bed.

However, in certain individuals with mitral stenosis of such severity as to elevate the left atrial pressure to 25 mm Hg or higher, the pulmonary arterial pressure may rise out of proportion to the left atrial pressure. This varies considerably among individuals and is considered a manifestation of individual variability of pulmonary vascular reactivity. This rise in pulmonary arterial pressure is in excess of that which can be accounted for by retrograde pressure transmission. The increased pressure gradient results from the additive factor of an elevated pulmonary vascular resistance, which further raises the pulmonary arterial pressure. The mechanism of this increase in pulmonary vascular resistance remains controversial. Some investigators consider this an active form of pulmonary hypertension mediated by a reflex response to a critical level of pulmonary venous pressure.[22,23] As noted above, this mechanism may vary considerably from one individual to the next; it is rarely noted with slight or moderate left atrial pressure elevation, as is seen with left ventricular failure or myocardial disease. Supporting evidence for a reflex vasoconstrictive mechanism for pulmonary hypertension in patients with severe mitral stenosis is the sudden, dramatic fall in pulmonary arterial pressure within a few weeks after successful mitral valvotomy or mitral valve replacement.[24,25]

The studies of Wood also suggest a vasoconstrictive element; he reported a fall in pulmonary arterial pressure and resistance and a rise in cardiac output and left atrial pressure following acetylcholine injection into the pulmonary artery of patients with mitral stenosis and marked pulmonary hypertension.[26] The acetylcholine is inactivated in the lungs and produces no direct effect on the systemic circulation. In the authors' laboratory a similar response has been noted following the intrapulmonary arterial administration of tolazoline hydrochloride. The study of Silove et al.[22] adds evidence supporting the presence of a reflex vasoconstrictive mechanism; such studies, though suggestive, are not conclusive in substantiating a vasoconstrictor effect.

It is also possible that no vasoconstrictive element need be postulated; a sudden significant rise in pulmonary arterial pressure may occur when a critical area of the pressure-volume curve of the pulmonary vascular bed is reached.[27]

OBSTRUCTION PROXIMAL TO THE MITRAL VALVE

Several more unusual abnormalities may also produce an elevated pulmonary arterial pressure by a mechanism similar to that previously described. Such conditions include supramitral valvular obstruction, left atrial myxoma, cor triatriatum, congenital stenosis of pulmonary veins as they enter the left atrium, mediastinitis involving the pulmonary veins, and total anomalous pulmonary venous connections with a long and narrow common venous trunk.

Decrease in total cross-sectional area of the pulmonary vascular bed

Structural changes reducing the total cross-sectional area of the pulmonary vascular bed result in increased resistance to pulmonary arterial blood flow. However, the remarkable distensibility of the pulmonary vasculature provides a considerable compensatory reserve;[11,13] the total area of the pulmonary vascular bed must be reduced by more than 50 percent before a significant elevation of pulmonary arterial pressure results.[28-30] It is well recognized that patients do not develop pulmonary hypertension following pneumonectomy if the remaining lung is normal.[9] Studies involving selective lobectomy in animals have suggested that the distensibility of the lower lobes may not be as great as that of the upper lobes.[30] Hence, not only the volume (mass) of lung tissue removed but also its anatomic location may be an important determinant of the resultant change in pulmonary vascular resistance.

Significant compromise of the pulmonary vascular bed may result from compression of the pulmonary vessels, as is seen with extensive parenchymal fibrosis of the lung; it may be secondary to reduction of the vessel lumen produced by primary infectious or granulomatous involvement of the vessel wall, or it may stem from great hypertrophy of the musculature of the media. Obstruction may also occur from within, as is the case in widespread miliary emboli or thrombosis involving the small pulmonary arterial vessels; the total pulmonary bed is so reduced as to result in severe pulmonary hypertension.

PULMONARY EMBOLI

Pulmonary hypertension may occur when pulmonary emboli cause widespread obstruction and obliteration of the pulmonary vasculature. The clinical picture of pulmonary embolization may vary considerably; catastrophic, sudden, massive pulmonary embolization resulting in acute right ventricular failure is familiar to all. However, recurrent episodes of pulmonary embolism involving lesser areas of the pulmonary vascular bed may present entirely different and perplexing clinical syndromes.

The so-called primary, or essential, pulmonary hypertension presents a difficult problem in differential diagnosis. The pathogenesis of essential pulmonary hypertension is not clear. Some writers doubt its existence as a specific entity and consider the changes in the pulmonary vasculature to be secondary to recurrent miliary embolization;[31] some data obtained from animal experiments tend to substantiate this view. The difference between pulmonary hypertension caused by clinically evident recurrent episodes of pulmonary embolism and the more silent clinical picture of so-called primary pulmonary hypertension may be only a function of the size and localization of the emboli. In the former condition, larger emboli occlude vessels of greater size, whereas in so-called primary pulmonary hypertension the emboli are situated more peripherally in vessels of 0.1 to 1.0 mm in diameter. Wagenvoort and Wagenvoort in a publication[32] based on studies of pulmonary vessels in lung tissue from 156 patients with a clinical diagnosis of primary pulmonary hypertension concluded that the alterations in 110 patients were initiated by vasoconstriction. They stated that various stimuli which they did not identify might bring about vasoconstriction in the presence of a hyperreactive pulmonary vasculature. They therefore concluded that the pulmonary vascular lesions in the majority of patients with primary pulmonary hypertension were consistent with a vasoconstrictive pathogenesis. However, intense vasoconstriction is considered to exist in some individuals living at high altitude, and yet histologic examination of the lungs of some of these persons has been surprisingly unremarkable.[33,34] Therefore, the exact etiology of this entity remains in doubt.

There is an apparent association between primary pulmonary artery hypertension and appetite suppressants, particularly aminorex fumarate.[35] Analysis of the case records reveals that some of the patients were obese, some were on oral contraceptives, while others had varicose veins, and yet others gave a history of recent pregnancy or abortion. All these circumstances are known to predispose to venous thrombosis and, thus possibly to pulmonary emboli. However, even after exclusion of such patients there apparently remains a group with no obvious cause for the development of pulmonary artery hypertension, and it is in this group that aminorex may possibly play a role in etiology. Lung biopsies and/or necropsies have revealed recent or old pulmonary emboli in some patients. In others no such findings were apparent, and the only changes present were nonspecific intimal thickening and fibrosis and hyalinization of the media—changes compatible with pulmonary artery hypertension of a variety of causes. It is noteworthy that in geographic areas other than Central Europe, pulmonary hypertension has not been reported in clinical studies of individuals taking aminorex fumarate.[36] Furthermore, all attempts, including our own,[37] to induce pulmonary hypertension in animals with aminorex have failed. Thus, at present, the relationship between aminorex and pulmonary artery hypertension, if one does exist, is certainly not established.

Most likely it will ultimately be determined that many disease processes may result in the clinical picture of idiopathic pulmonary hypertension.[38,39] The clinical features of this entity are described later in this chapter. Experimental and clinical studies have indicated the difficulty of determining whether pulmonary vascular changes in patients with pulmonary hypertension represent thrombus formation due to primary vessel disease or whether they represent the vascular reaction to multiple pulmonary emboli. Recurrent miliary pulmonary emboli can effect changes within small pulmonary vessels which are morphologically indistinguishable from the subintimal thickening noted in patients with idiopathic pulmonary hypertension.[38] It is entirely possible that patients now considered to have primary or idiopathic pulmonary hypertension may indeed have recurrent miliary pulmonary emboli. The source of the miliary emboli is not always clear, although silent thrombi are not infrequently found at careful routine postmortem examination. The fact that young women are the most frequently afflicted might suggest a disorder of blood clotting related to the menstrual cycle. It is also now reasonably well established that there is an increased tendency to venous thrombosis and pulmonary embolism in women taking oral contraceptives.[40] In fact, the pulmonary vascular changes referred to above may result not necessarily from miliary emboli but rather from pulmonary vascular thrombosis in situ due to a coagulation defect.

PULMONARY VASCULAR OBSTRUCTION RESULTING FROM DISORDERS IN BLOOD CLOTTING

Theoretically, several phenomena associated with blood coagulation could produce pulmonary hypertension. These include fibrin deposition and fibrinolysis, platelet clumping and disaggregation, and the release of vasoactive substances, e.g., prostaglandins, serotonin. It has been postulated, but not proved, that the conversion of fibrinogen to fibrin, followed by fibrinolysis, occurs continuously in normal human beings.[41] An estimated 25 percent of the total body store of fibrinogen is replaced every 24 h.[42] Hence, there may be a dynamic equilibrium between fibrin deposition and fibrin removal. Should this equilibrium be disturbed, a net accumulation of fibrin could result. A failure to dissolve fibrin would be anticipated if plasminogen activator were deficient or if fibrinolysis were inhibited. It has been demonstrated that certain apparently normal individuals have a

defective mechanism for generating plasminogen activator, e.g., in response to exercise.[43] Also, fibrinolysis is defective in a variety of disease states.[44,45] The lung is a source of both plasminogen activator and fibrinolysin inhibitor (Trasylol), and the concentrations of both vary among individuals of the same species as well as among individuals of different species.[46] Hence, marked variations in the lung's ability to dissolve fibrin may exist. However, the potential role of deficient fibrinolysis in the pathogenesis of pulmonary hypertension is still speculative.

Numerous stimuli are capable of producing aggregation of blood platelets, one of the most potent being adenosine diphosphate (ADP). When an animal is given a single intravenous injection of ADP, transient pulmonary hypertension results. Histologic examination of the lungs reveals occlusion of small pulmonary arteries by platelet clumps. Therefore, the pulmonary hypertension is apparently caused by platelet microemboli which subsequently disperse. However, when this process occurs repeatedly for several weeks, pathologic changes develop in the intima and media of the small pulmonary arteries.[47] A normal endogenous source of ADP is red blood cells. This probably explains the pulmonary hypertension observed following the intravenous injection of small quantities of hemolyzed blood.[48] Pulmonary hypertension associated with thrombocytopenia has been reported.[49] In these cases, autopsy revealed disseminated pulmonary arterial thromboses, suggesting that abnormal platelet clumping may be one cause of primary pulmonary hypertension.

MEDIAL HYPERTROPHY

Diffuse thickening of the walls of the small muscular pulmonary arteries may be due to medial hypertrophy or to vasoconstriction. When these processes are of sufficient severity to reduce the vascular lumen to the point where vascular resistance is greatly increased, pulmonary hypertension results. The apparent thickening of the vessel wall has been designated as medial hypertrophy; however, an increased wall-to-lumen ratio can be caused by lumen reduction as well as by increased thickness of the vessel wall. Thus, medial hypertrophy may indicate hypertrophy or vasoconstriction or a combination of the two.

Increased pressure within a vessel is the stimulus for vasoconstriction, which then leads to increased work of the media and, in turn, to further hypertrophy. Although this vasoconstriction may be reversible in an early phase, at a later stage it may become fixed because of the persistent shortening of the elastic and muscular coats of the artery. This phenomenon, which has been designated as arterial contracture,[50] may be a limiting factor in the regression of the vascular changes described above. Constriction of small muscular arteries with hypertrophied media accounts, in part, for the pulmonary hypertension normally observed in the infant in the immediate postnatal period. If this medial hypertrophy does not regress in a normal manner, increased pulmonary vascular resistance persists; this occurs in certain patients with large ventricular septal defects and other comparable lesions. The resultant pulmonary hypertension apparently traumatizes the pulmonary arteries. With the passage of time, constriction and later contracture, intimal proliferation, fibrosis, thrombosis, and atherosclerosis may make their appearance, further reducing the lumen of the small pulmonary vessels.[29] Their effect is not always additive, however, for as the obstructive lesions become more extensive, there frequently is concomitant medial atrophy and thinning with dilatation. Consequently, the magnitude of the increased pulmonary vascular resistance may change little over long periods of time, despite an alteration in the nature of the vascular obstruction.[51]

The authors have been interested in the effect of the vasodilating agent tolazoline on pulmonary vascular resistance, particularly in patients with ventricular septal defects and pulmonary hypertension.[52] Tolazoline, a drug of complex action, produces vasodilatation by several mechanisms, one of which is stimulation of histamine H_2 receptors,[53] which is probably the most important factor in the vasodilatation produced in human beings. The authors' studies of children with severe pulmonary hypertension demonstrated that tolazoline reduced pulmonary arterial pressure; this was often associated with an increase, and never with a decrease, in pulmonary arterial blood flow (see also "Increase in Pulmonary Arterial Blood Flow," below). The authors believe that a vasodilator such as tolazoline is most effective when the increased pulmonary vascular resistance is primarily a consequence of generalized constriction of hypertrophied small muscular arteries; when the smooth muscle relaxes, vasodilatation can occur. This responsive situation is found most frequently in the first years of life. When pulmonary hypertension has been present for years, obliterative changes such as intimal proliferation and fibrosis, thrombosis, and atherosclerosis may be present in the smaller pulmonary arteries.[51] If these lesions are widespread and account for a large portion of the increased pulmonary vascular resistance, a vasodilator cannot be expected to lower pulmonary vascular resistance appreciably. However, both the magnitude and duration of increased pulmonary vascular resistance are probably important in determining the age at which a given patient will lose his responsiveness to tolazoline.[51] The authors have found the response to tolazoline to help in predicting preoperatively which children with high pulmonary vascular resistance would show a decrease in pulmonary arterial pressure and resistance following closure of ventricular septal defect.[51]

Pulmonary hypertension has been induced in the rat by the feeding of *Crotalaria spectabilis*,[54] an annual shrub which is found throughout tropical and subtropical areas of the world. Rats fed the seeds of this plant develop a form of pulmonary vascular disease characterized by hypertrophy of the media of small muscular pulmonary arteries and by the development of a muscular media in the pulmonary arterioles. These changes are comparable with those found in human beings with significant elevation of pulmonary artery blood pressure. However, the manner in which *Crotalaria* adversely affects human beings in the West Indies when ingested as "bush tea" is by

causing venoocclusive disease of the liver. The development of pulmonary hypertension and significant changes in the small muscular pulmonary arteries has not been reported to occur in man.[55]

Pulmonary hypertension has been documented in patients ingesting other substances such as the drugs aminorex fumarate mentioned earlier in this chapter and also more recently following biguanide (phenformin) therapy.[98] This intriguing possibility of dietary pulmonary hypertension has recently been reviewed by Fishman.[55] The manner by which pulmonary hypertension developed after ingestion of these substances is unknown. It has been postulated that the initiating mechanism may be the release of certain metabolites of ingested foods that act as vasoactive substances and initiate vasoconstriction of very small muscular pulmonary arteries. Another consideration is that the primary insult caused by these unknown metabolites involves the endothelium of the small muscular pulmonary arteries or precapillary vessels and that platelet aggregation develops following the damage to the endothelium and leads to thrombi and occlusive disease of these vessels. The association of severe liver disease and pulmonary hypertension has been observed,[100-102] and this may be more than coincidental. Metabolites of ingested substances normally altered in their passage through the liver may in the presence of severe liver disease gain access to the pulmonary circulation in a relatively unaltered state and by one or more of the mechanisms discussed above result in changes in the small pulmonary arteries that lead to the development of pulmonary hypertension. These conjectures are without foundation in fact at present but make for interesting speculation.

"FUNCTIONAL" REDUCTION OF THE PULMONARY VASCULAR BED

Constriction of the small muscular pulmonary arteries (100 to 300 μm in diameter) increases the resistance to pulmonary blood flow. Alveolar hypoxia frequently provides the stimulus for such vasoconstriction. Patients with marked alveolar hypoventilation associated with pulmonary parenchymal disease, such as chronic bronchitis and/or emphysema, often have a significant element of hypoxic vasocontriction.[29,56] Central nervous system disease, paralytic states, chronic airway obstruction,[57] obesity, or any condition leading to alveolar hypoventilation can lead to pulmonary hypertension. Normal human beings are exposed to increasing alveolar hypoxia as they ascend to high altitude and are subjected to lowered total atmospheric pressure. This hypoxia, if marked and prolonged, produces marked pulmonary hypertension, as is seen in the Indian populations living above 14,000 ft in the Andes.[58] However, no elevation of pulmonary arterial pressure is seen in the residents of Bogota, Colombia, at an elevation of 8,300 ft, or at lower altitudes.[59] Whether or not pulmonary hypertension will develop at a given altitude is therefore dependent on the degree of hypoxia. Also of importance, however, is the pulmonary vascular reactivity of the population involved. Work from the authors' laboratory revealed a remarkable degree of pulmonary hypertension in certain individuals living in Colorado at the modest altitude of 10,200 ft.[60] These pressure elevations were much greater than would have been predicted from studies of Peruvian Indians living at similar altitudes in the Andes. Further investigation of these population differences is indicated.

Pulmonary hypertension at high altitude results from increased resistance to blood flow through the lung. Since the pressure elevation is immediately lowered by oxygen administration, hypoxic vasoconstriction is implied. The pulmonary vascular resistance is so grossly elevated that one would expect obvious medial hypertrophy of the small muscular pulmonary arteries. However, histologic examination of the lungs of these adult high-altitude dwellers has been surprisingly unremarkable; only with quantitative techniques has a subtle increase in vascular smooth muscle been demonstrated.[33,34] The general normality of these pulmonary arteries suggests some other form of structural alteration, such as loss of compliance or contracture.[50] It is also noteworthy that airway hypoxia can produce medial hypertrophy and hyperplasia in small pulmonary arteries in the *absence* of pulmonary hypertension,[61] and so the muscular media is not increased as a consequence of an elevated intravascular pressure. When an individual is born in a hypoxic environment at high altitude, the muscular fetal pulmonary arteries do not undergo the usual rapid regression; the hypoxia continues to influence the pulmonary circulation significantly, just as it normally does before birth. Hypoxic pulmonary hypertension may therefore be considered a residual phenomenon from intrauterine life (Fig. 74-2). These

observations broaden our interpretation of the significance of pulmonary hypertension. In most normal persons living at high altitude, the moderate pulmonary hypertension produces no symptoms, no decrease in exercise tolerance, and no apparent adverse effects later in life.[58,60] This pulmonary hypertension may well be completely reversible (Fig. 74-3).[62]

Alveolar hypoxia produces pulmonary hypertension by increasing resistance to blood flow through the lung. The major increase in resistance occurs at the precapillary level, but some additional increase in resistance may also develop distal to the capillary bed. The hypoxic stimulus acts via the perivascular environment of the pulmonary blood vessels; in the absence of airway hypoxia, intravascular hypoxemia does not produce pulmonary vasoconstriction. The exact mechanism involved in hypoxic pulmonary vasoconstriction remains elusive. However, it is certainly a local phenomenon, since it occurs in isolated perfused lungs[63] and even in small blocks of lung tissue.

Calcium ions are required for excitation-contraction coupling within vascular smooth-muscle cells. The source of this calcium can be either extracellular or an intracellular pool. McMurtry et al.[63] have shown that verapamil will selectively inhibit pulmonary vasoconstriction induced by airway hypoxia, but not that induced by humoral agents such as angiotensin II or prostaglandin $F_{2\alpha}$. The action of verapamil is to block the transmembrane influx of extracellular calcium. These findings imply that the mode of action of hypoxia is to depolarize the cell membrane, permitting the influx of extracellular calcium which then causes contraction of the vascular smooth-muscle cell. Further, the selective action of verapamil implies that the vasoconstriction effect of hypoxia is not mediated by a humoral agent which acts on the intracellular calcium pool. In other words, the pulmonary vascular actions of hypoxia appear to be direct and not humorally mediated.

During airway hypoxia, humoral agents are released within the lung[64,65] which modulate the pulmo-

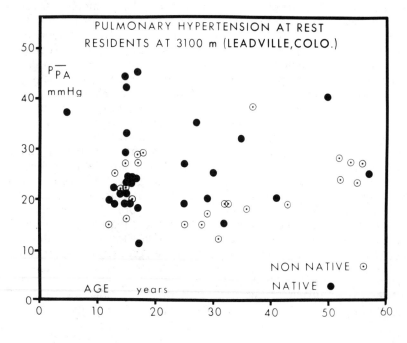

FIGURE 74-2 Residence at the moderate altitude of 10,200 ft (3,100 m) for several years to a lifetime is often associated with the development of significant pulmonary hypertension. Mean pulmonary artery pressure (P_{PA}) at rest in the supine posture is plotted in relation to age for 30 persons born in Leadville (●) and 24 persons who moved to Leadville at various ages after birth (⊙). *(Data from published and unpublished observations of Grover et al.[87,94])*

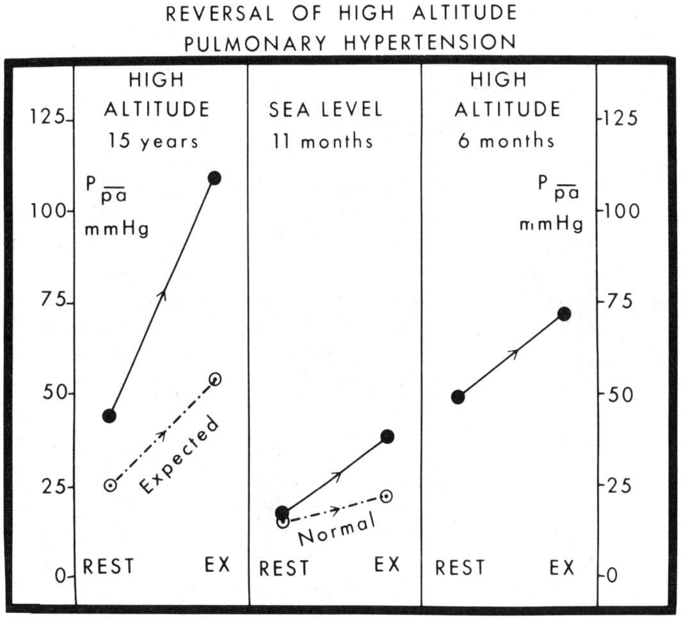

REVERSAL OF HIGH ALTITUDE
PULMONARY HYPERTENSION

FIGURE 74-3 Among adolescents living at moderate altitude (Leadville, Colo., 10,200 ft) a 15-year-old girl was found with unusually severe pulmonary hypertension. Her mean pulmonary artery pressure (P_{PA}) at rest and during exercise (solid line) were much higher than expected, on the basis of data from 28 adolescents also living in Leadville. She moved to sea level, and after 11 months, her P_{PA} was virtually normal. She then returned to Leadville; 6 months later her pulmonary hypertension had returned. This indicates that even when marked pulmonary hypertension develops from the hypoxia of moderate altitude, it may be reversible.[62]

nary vascular response and thereby attenuate the direct vasoconstriction action of hypoxia. Thus, inhibition of prostaglandin synthesis by meclofenamate augments the hypoxic pressor response,[66] presumably by blocking the formation of a dilator prostaglandin. Further, this observation reinforces the concept that the pulmonary pressor effect of hypoxia is not mediated by a constrictor prostaglandin such as $PGF_{2\alpha}$. Similarly, blockade of histamine H_2 dilator receptors with metiamide augments the hypoxic pressor response, while blockade of histamine H_1 constrictor receptors with chlorpheniramine fails to attenuate the pressor response.[67] These observations imply that during airway hypoxia, histamine is released to modulate the pulmonary vasoconstriction, but not to mediate the hypoxic pressor effect. Since the source of this histamine is probably the pulmonary perivascular mast cell, the hyperplasia of these mast cells during chronic hypoxia[68] may function to attenuate (but not mediate) the severity of chronic hypoxic pulmonary hypertension.

It is of great importance to appreciate that the elevated pulmonary vascular resistance secondary to alveolar hypoxia is a reversible form of pulmonary hypertension.[56,62] Thus, in the patient with chronic obstructive airway disease entering the hospital with acute respiratory failure, often precipitated by a respiratory infection, and with an element of heart failure, the main therapeutic effort should be directed toward elevation of the oxygen tension of the alveolar air, thereby abolishing the vasoconstriction of small pulmonary arteries and effectively lowering the pulmonary artery pressure.[69]

Although the most current evidence indicates that humoral agents do not mediate the pulmonary vasoconstrictor effects of hypoxia, it is now clear that humoral agents do account for a major portion of the pulmonary hypertensive response to pulmonary

microembolism. This is indicated by the observations that pretreatment with antihistamine or inhibitors of prostaglandin synthesis prevents over half of the increase in pulmonary vascular resistance following microembolism of the lung in the dog.[70] These humoral agents are probably released from blood platelets which aggregate on the emboli, since inhibitors of platelet function or induction of thrombocytopenia also markedly reduce the pulmonary hypertensive response to microembolism.[71] The identity of the humoral agents responsible for pulmonary vasoconstriction during platelet aggregation is uncertain. Although exogenous $PGF_{2\alpha}$ has a strong pulmonary pressor action in the dog,[72] it is probable that the more potent thromboxanes[73] which are formed concurrently with the prostaglandins in vivo actually account for the acute pulmonary hypertensive response to microembolism observed in the intact animal.

Increase in pulmonary arterial blood flow

Increased pulmonary arterial blood flow rarely causes elevated pulmonary arterial blood pressure when it occurs after the normal regression of the so-called fetal pulmonary vascular pattern.[9] The capacious normal pulmonary vascular bed has a great reserve; blood flow is rarely of such magnitude as to produce significant disproportion between the volume of flow and the overall cross-sectional area of the pulmonary vascular bed.[27] Treadmill exercise studies performed in the authors' laboratory on normal individuals revealed that increases of cardiac output to 16 to 18 liters/min produced pulmonary arterial systolic pressures of only 35 to 40 mm Hg. Furthermore, many patients with atrial septal defects catheterized in the author's laboratory had normal pulmonary arterial pressures in the presence of pulmonary artery blood flows of approximately 15 liters/min. When significant pulmonary hypertension exists in the presence of elevated pulmonary arterial blood flow, it would appear certain that there is a coexistent decrease in the cross-sectional area of the pulmonary vascular bed. Thus, increased pulmonary arterial blood flow can be significant in the presence of a decreased pulmonary vascular bed; this combination produces a significant increase of pulmonary vascular resistance, with resulting pulmonary hypertension. This is the usual situation in patients with intracardiac septal defects and large left-to-right shunts who have significantly increased pulmonary arterial blood pressure.[74]

However, quite a different situation results if pulmonary blood flow is greater than normal from the time of birth. This occurs as an "experiment of nature" in patients with congenital absence of one pulmonary artery as an isolated defect. One lung receives the entire output of the right ventricle, and from the time of birth, blood flow through this lung is twice normal. The incidence of pulmonary hypertension was 19 percent[9] in the 32 reported cases of this isolated anomaly. The mechanism of production of pulmonary hypertension in this situation has been postulated as follows:[10] a basic property of smooth muscle is that it will contract in response to the stimulus of stretch. The fetal small pulmonary arteries have a thick media of smooth muscle; these arteries increase in diameter at birth to accept the normal increase in pulmonary blood flow following expansion of the lung. If the pulmonary blood flow is excessive, these muscular arteries may be stretched to the point where they react by constriction. A cycle of stretch-constriction is established, which may lead to hypertrophy of the media, and the increased resistance presented by the constricted vessels results in the pulmonary hypertension.[75] The elevated intraluminal pressure also tends to stretch the arteries and acts as an added stimulus to augment the vasoconstriction, perpetuate the hypertension, and lead to contracture, a fixed state.[50]

An experimental model of increased pulmonary blood flow from the time of birth was developed by Vogel et al.[10] Normally, each lung receives approximately one-half of the cardiac output from the right ventricle. However, if the branch of the pulmonary artery supplying the left lung is ligated, then blood flow through the right lung must double. When ligation of the left pulmonary artery was performed on neonatal calves in the authors' laboratory, the animals invariably developed progressive pulmonary hypertension over several weeks, leading to right-sided heart failure. Following publication of these results,[10] other investigators attempted to duplicate this model, but the calves rarely developed pulmonary hypertension. These divergent results are explained by the fact that the authors' laboratory is located in Denver at an altitude of 5,300 feet, and

consequently there is a mild atmospheric hypoxia. This mild hypoxic stimulus is inadequate to produce pulmonary vasoconstriction in the normal calf. However, in the calf with ligation of the left pulmonary artery, the combined stimulus of hypoxia plus increased blood flow through the left lung is sufficient to produce pulmonary hypertension. Furthermore, it became apparent that this calf model required the presence of both stimuli, since increased pulmonary blood flow along (left pulmonary artery ligation) in the absence of atmospheric hypoxia at sea level failed to produce pulmonary hypertension. When normotensive calves with left pulmonary artery ligation at sea level were transported to Denver, they then developed pulmonary hypertension. Conversely, when pulmonary hypertensive calves with left pulmonary artery ligation in Denver were taken to sea level, they became normotensive.[76] This elegant series of experiments provides an explanation for the fact that among patients with congenital left-to-right shunts (ventricular septal defect, patent ductus, arteriosus), the reported incidence of pulmonary hypertension is greater in communities at higher altitudes, such as Denver and Mexico City. An interesting corollary is that at these higher altitudes there is a lower incidence of neonatal heart failure in infants with large ventricular septal defects, since the increased pulmonary vascular resistance tends to prevent a massive left-to-right shunt.

This implies that an initially normal hyperreactive neonatal pulmonary vascular bed responds to an abnormal stimulus by widespread pulmonary vasoconstriction. The usual medial smooth-muscle involution is prevented, and the persisting medial "hypertrophy" maintains the pulmonary vascular resistance at a high level. If the abnormal stimulus were removed, the vascular media would presumably undergo "disuse atrophy," and the pulmonary arteries would become normal. The high intraluminal pressure is traumatic to the pulmonary arteries, for with the passage of time secondary vascular changes develop: intimal proliferation and thickening, atherosclerosis, thrombosis, and extensive vascular occlusion. Heath and Edwards[77] described six grades of structural changes in the pulmonary arteries and indicated that the first three grades represented reversible changes should the basic congenital cardiovascular defect be corrected. Grades 5 and 6, however, were considered irreversible, and grade 4 was described as variable, depending on the individual's response. Once this vascular damage has occurred, pulmonary hypertension is probably irreversible.[99]

Pulmonary hypertension increases the risk involved in surgical intervention of patients with congenital heart disease. In patients with pulmonary hypertension who have had successful ventricular septal defect closure, the elevated pulmonary vascular resistance regressed toward normal when medial hypertrophy and cellular intimal proliferation were the only vascular abnormalities. This is true even with pulmonary vascular resistance equal to systemic resistance, with bidirectional shunting and cyanosis. It is not generally recognized that such cases of Eisenmenger's reaction may be operable if detected early when medial hypertrophy is the predominant pulmonary vascular abnormality.[51] Only an occasional patient surviving surgical treatment has demonstrated regression of pulmonary vascular resistance when additional vascular lesions were present.

ACUTE PULMONARY EDEMA OF HIGH ALTITUDE WITH PULMONARY HYPERTENSION

Among normal healthy men ascending to altitudes above 9,000 ft, a small number will develop acute pulmonary edema. This adverse reaction to altitude may occur on the man's first ascent to altitude, as has been the extensive experience with India's soldiers taken to the Himalayas,[59] and also among mountain climbers.[78] Somewhat paradoxically, it is not uncommon in fully acclimatized residents of high altitude upon reascent following sojourn at sea level.[59] Recovery is usual, and the individual may then remain at high altitude without further episodes of pulmonary edema. However, these susceptible individuals are likely to have a recurrence of acute pulmonary edema with subsequent ascents.[79] Apparently the *transition* from low to high altitude is important in precipitating this condition in the susceptible individual.

The etiology of high-altitude pulmonary edema (HAPE) is unknown. Originally, it was thought to result from acute left ventricular failure, but now there seems to be little evidence to support this view. Most cases have occurred in young men with no indication of impaired left ventircular function. Radiographically, the heart is characteristically not enlarged in HAPE. Hemodynamic studies during the acute phase of HAPE revealed a normal left atrial pressure in one man with a probe-patent foramen ovale.[79] Pulmonary artery "wedge" pressures have been normal in all cases, but this must be interpreted with caution, since the mechanical process of "wedging" the catheter interrupts blood flow through the vascular segment distal to the catheter. More probably, the true pulmonary capillary pressure is elevated in the edematous areas of the lung, even though left-sided heart pressures are normal. Thus, the possibility of constriction of small pulmonary veins at the postcapillary level, with resulting elevation of pulmonary capillary pressure, is not excluded.

Only a small number of patients with HAPE have been studied by cardiac catheterization during their acute illness, but pulmonary hypertension has been a consistent finding.[80] Although the high pulmonary artery pressure might be a passive reflection of an elevated pulmonary capillary pressure, it might conceivably be the initial factor causing the edema. Following this suggestion by Hultgren,[81] investigations were carried out in five men who had experienced several well-documented episodes of HAPE while mountain climbing. Clinically, all were normal and free from cardiac and pulmonary disease. At sea level, their hemodynamics, including arterial blood gases, cardiac output, and right-sided heart pressures

at rest and during exercise, were entirely normal. The pulmonary arterial pressor response to acute hypoxia was entirely normal in three men but somewhat exaggerated in the other two.

To simulate the conditions under which these men had developed HAPE in the past, they were transported rapidly to high altitude and then climbed for several hours at 12,000 ft. Following this, about 30 h after they left sea level, cardiac catheterization was performed at 10,200 ft. None of the men developed HAPE by clinical examination or chest roentgenogram. However, all had impairment of blood oxygenation, with abnormal widening of the alveolar-to-arterial oxygen difference, particularly during exercise. In spite of hyperventilation and respiratory alkalosis, significant pulmonary hypertension was present in all five men at rest and increased dramatically during exercise (Fig. 74-4), but "wedge" pressures remained normal. Thus, these men had a clearly abnormal response to exposure to altitude, and the development of pulmonary hypertension without detectable pulmonary edema suggests that the pulmonary hypertension may be at least in part important in edema production.

FIGURE 74-4 When man ascends to the moderate altitude of 10,200 ft for a few days, significant pulmonary hypertension does not usually develop. This is indicated by the solid line giving average data for eight normal young men from sea level studied after 10 days at altitude. In contrast, five men (CB, RG, RI, CH, and TW) with past histories of high-altitude pulmonary edema developed marked pulmonary hypertension after 1 day at this same altitude. Compare with Fig. 74-1.[81]

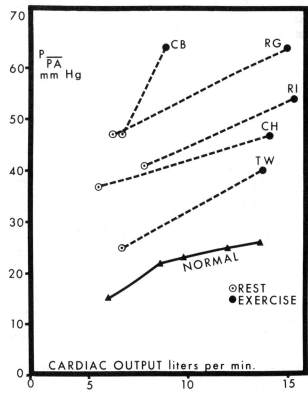

The mechanism responsible for increasing pulmonary vascular resistance in these men is not known. Hypoxic pulmonary vasoconstriction alone cannot explain these findings, since acute relief of hypoxia at high altitude did not normalize the pulmonary arterial pressures. This implies the presence of some form of vascular obstruction in addition to vasoconstriction. Postmortem examination performed in a very few fatal cases of HAPE has revealed widespread platelet and fibrin thrombi in the pulmonary capillaries.[82] Conceivably, then, a coagulopathy is the primary abnormality in individuals who develop HAPE. We postulate that this would be manifest in the lung by the temporary thrombotic occlusion of large numbers of pulmonary capillaries. Those regions of the lung where capillaries were not occluded would then carry the entire cardiac output. In addition, these dilated vessels would be exposed to an abnormally elevated perfusion pressure, resulting in "overperfusion pulmonary edema" with the patchy distribution on chest roentgenogram which is characteristic of HAPE. This postulated mechanism would then extend to include spontaneous lysis of the capillary thrombi over the succeeding 2 or 3 days, with a virtually complete return of normal pulmonary hemodynamics and gas exchange. In support of this hypothesis is the recent report by Gray et al.[83] that in normal men taken to high altitude, circulating platelet count falls and platelet aggregates are trapped in the lung. Maher et al.[84] have also detected a transient hypercoagulable state in normal men on exposure to high altitude. When these normal responses are considered in conjunction with the report of deficient fibrinolysis in subjects susceptible to HAPE,[85] extensive intravascular obstruction of pulmonary capillaries could result. However, the validity of this hypothesis has not been established and awaits the outcome of continuing investigation.

INDIVIDUAL VARIABILITY OF PULMONARY VASCULAR REACTIVITY

It is now appreciated that there exist great differences in pulmonary vascular reactivity between individuals of the same species and individuals of different species.[86] A given stimulus often provokes a spectrum of responses, varying in magnitude from one individual to the next; these inherent differences in reactivity are indeed characteristic of biologic systems.

Chronic hypoxia tends to accentuate latent differences of pulmonary vascular reactivity among normal individuals. In a study at the authors' laboratory, 28 normal high school students who lived at an altitude of 10,200 ft had catheterization of the right side of the heart; in about 25 percent, severe pulmonary hypertension developed during exercise[87] or when the students were breathing 13 percent oxygen.[87] In contrast to these hyperreactors, another

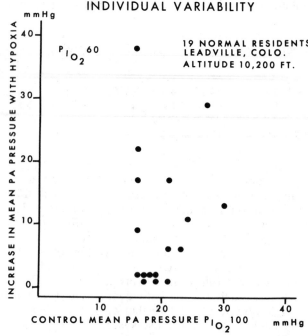

FIGURE 74-5 When normal high-altitude residents are made acutely hypoxic by lowering the inspired oxygen tension ($P_{I_{O_2}}$) from 100 to 60 mm Hg, some individuals have virtually no increase in mean pulmonary arterial pressure (hyporeactors), while other individuals have a marked pressure increase of 15 to 40 mm Hg (hyperreactors).

group demonstrated virtually no rise in pulmonary arterial pressure when breathing 13 percent oxygen and exhibited only a modest rise during exercise (Fig. 74-5).

Marked individual variability exists among cattle also. We have found that among steers exposed to the chronic hypoxia of high altitude, pulmonary arterial pressure increases to only 40 to 50 mm Hg in some individuals, whereas the same stimulus raises pressures to over 100 mm Hg in other individuals.[88] This has led to the concept that some cattle are susceptible (S) to hypoxic pulmonary hypertension while others are resistant (R) to it. Furthermore, it has now been established that the S and R traits are genetically determined;[89] the progeny of S cattle are pulmonary hyperreactors, and the progeny of R cattle are pulmonary hyporeactors.[90] These differences in reactivity appear to be inherent in the pulmonary vasculature itself, since they can be demonstrated with stimuli other than hypoxia, namely, $PGF_{2\alpha}$. Human pulmonary vascular reactivity also may well be genetically determined. In studying the human population at high altitude in Colorado, we found one family in which three of five children had excessively high pulmonary arterial pressures.[87] From our work with a variety of animal species, we believe that it is probably the thickness of the muscular media of the pulmonary arteries which is genetically determined and which in turn establishes the reactivity of the pulmonary vascular bed[91] (Fig. 74-6).

This individual variability in relation to pulmonary

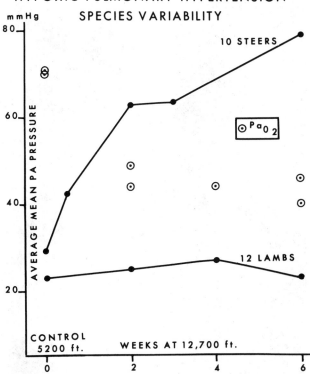

FIGURE 74-6 When normal lambs and steers were taken to high altitude, the arterial oxygen tension (P_{a,O_2}) decreased from 70 to 40 to 45 mm Hg (open circles), indicating that both species were equally hypoxic. However, only the steers developed significant pulmonary hypertension.

vascular reactivity is an important feature in understanding the problems of pulmonary hypertension.

CLINICAL RECOGNITION OF PULMONARY HYPERTENSION

The causes of pulmonary hypertension are varied, but the clinical picture in the fully developed state is essentially the same; minor variations are dependent on the specific cause of the pulmonary hypertension. The purest example is probably primary (essential) pulmonary hypertension, frequently designated as idiopathic pulmonary hypertension. Both these terms are inadequate and misleading in the opinion of the authors. McGuire and associates[31] questioned the existence of primary pulmonary hypertension. They indicated that this entity could be accepted only in the presence of isolated right ventricular hypertrophy, recorded elevated pulmonary artery pressure with a normal pulmonary artery "wedge" pressure, and (at necropsy) the absence of occlusive lesions in the pulmonary vascular tree. The authors hold that such requirements are mutually exclusive and that pulmonary hypertension, with resulting right ventricular hypertrophy sufficient to cause death, is not possible when there are normal or minimal occlusive changes in the pulmonary vasculature. Although it is probable that diffuse vasoconstriction can involve the small muscular pulmonary arteries and affect

pulmonary vascular resistance and may be the initiating process in some instances, one would expect changes in the pulmonary vasculature secondary to prolonged vasoconstriction. Thus, it is considered improbable that a normal pulmonary vasculature is compatible with the degree of pulmonary hypertension noted in patients with primary pulmonary hypertension. Therefore, within the meaning of the terminology as outlined by McGuire and associates,[31] primary pulmonary hypertension does not exist. The condition under present consideration, then, consists or isolated right ventricular hypertrophy and pulmonary hypertension *with* occlusive pulmonary vascular disease, which is always secondary to some primary disease or abnormal process, usually obscure and unknown. It is probable that patients currently diagnosed as having primary pulmonary hypertension will ultimately be proved to have disease of polyglot origin. However, the authors believe, as discussed earlier in this chapter, that the underlying cause in many of these patients may eventually be demonstrated to be either recurrent miliary embolization or intravascular thrombosis within the lung itself due to disorders of blood clotting.

The familial occurrence of primary pulmonary hypertension has been well established. A recent report by Inglesby and associates[95] documented the occurrence of primary pulmonary hypertension in a kindred with impaired fibrinolytic mechanisms. Antiplasmin levels were significantly elevated in all 7 of the 10 members of the family, in four generations, in whom coagulation studies had been done. Thus, Inglesby et al. suggested that the impaired ability to lyse recurrent miliary pulmonary emboli may have been responsible for the development of the primary pulmonary hypertension.

The diagnosis usually is made after exhaustive study has failed to reveal any primary disease that could result in the development of the pulmonary hypertension. It is a rare disorder; Paul Wood[92] observed only 17 instances in a consecutive series of 10,000 patients. Although it is found at all ages and in both sexes, it would seem predominantly to involve young women.

Exertional dyspnea and fatigue are the most common presenting complaints, but a syncopal episode is not infrequently the initial symptom. Symptoms tend to appear late in the natural history of the disease, since pulmonary hypertension, per se, does not cause distress any more than does systemic hypertension. It is only when the cardiac output becomes relatively low and fixed that symptoms appear. Thus, the findings of advanced pulmonary hypertension in a patient exhibiting mild symptoms of recent onset should suggest immediately the diagnosis of primary pulmonary hypertension. Patients with a similar degree of pulmonary hypertension secondary to some overt primary disease will usually develop symptoms earlier because of the fundamental disease process. Chest pain of anginal type, hoarseness, hemoptysis, and palpitation also may be evident. Other symtpoms may develop secondary to the low fixed cardiac output or to congestive heart failure. None of these is characteristic of the primary entity, since they occur in the face of advanced pulmonary hypertension, whatever the cause.

The findings on physical examination, in general, depend on the presence and extent of right ventricular hypertrophy, the degree of pulmonary hypertension, the level of cardiac output, and the state of cardiac compensation. The patient usually is acyanotic, although evidence of peripheral cyanosis may be present. Prominent *a* waves in the deep jugular veins should immediately suggest the diagnosis of idiopathic pulmonary hypertension, as this finding usually reflects right ventricular pressure in excess of left ventricular pressure, and there are few other entities which lead to pulmonary hypertension of this magnitude. The extremities may be cool and the peripheral pulses small, reflecting the low cardiac output. Clubbing of the fingers is rarely, if ever, present, and when present with central cyanosis it should suggest another diagnosis, such as Eisenmenger's reaction. The precordium is quiet, reflecting normal or decreased cardiac output. Palpation reveals a forceful sustained thrust along the lower left sternal border and thrust and shock over the second left intercostal space. Auscultation usually discloses no murmurs of significance, although a soft systolic ejection murmur may be audible over the pulmonary area. Rarely, a diastolic murmur of pulmonary insufficiency also may be detected. A systolic ejection click may be present in the pulmonary area, followed by a single or finely split second heart sound, with the second component greatly increased in intensity. A fourth heart sound is at times audible along the lower left sternal border and is transmitted toward the apex, reflecting the resistance to filling of the hypertrophied right ventricle. In the more advanced stage, when failure has ensued, the murmur of tricuspid insufficiency and a right ventricular gallop sound may appear, together with the findings of heart failure and fluid retention.

The electrocardiogram displays the findings of right ventricular hypertrophy of varying severity, often advanced, depending on the stage of the disease process. Abnormalities reflecting right atrial hypertrophy are common. Though there are no pathognomonic findings in the electrocardiogram, changes indicative of severe right ventricular hypertrophy suggest this entity. There is probably no other form of acquired pulmonary hypertension that results in similar degrees of right ventricular hypertrophy.

The radiologic examination (Fig. 74-7) reveals a prominent main pulmonary artery and primary pulmonary branches; the peripheral lung fields usually appear normal or show a decrease in vascular markings. There are no findings suggestive of primary pulmonary parenchymal disease. The aorta is not unusual in appearance. The overall heart size may be

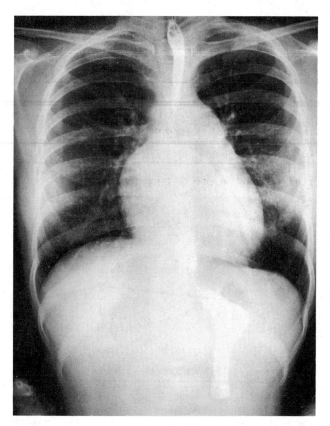

FIGURE 74-7 Posteroanterior roentgenogram of the chest of a patient with primary pulmonary hypertension. There is minimal overall cardiac enlargement, but the silhouette indicates enlargement of the right atrium and configuration compatible with right ventricular hypertrophy. The main pulmonary artery is prominent; the aorta is small and the superior vena cava rather prominent, but the periphery of the lung fields actually appears somewhat clear.

slightly enlarged, with a configuration suggesting right atrial and right ventricular hypertrophy. However, right ventricular hypertrophy is a difficult radiographic diagnosis, and more dependable information about right ventricular hypertrophy is obtained from the electrocardiogram. Late in the course of the disease, with the development of congestive heart failure, the heart dilates and may increase greatly in size. The main pulmonary artery area then actually appears less prominent because of the dilatation of the outflow tract of the right ventricle.

Recognition of secondary forms of pulmonary hypertension is most important, as mitral valve disease or another remediable lesion must always be considered as a cause of the clinical picture. Rheumatic mitral stenosis may first appear as severe pulmonary hypertension, with subtle findings to indicate the presence of mitral valve obstruction. The symptoms are those of low cardiac output, rather than the usual symptoms associated with mitral stenosis, which reflect elevated pulmonary capillary pressure: severe exertional dyspnea, orthopnea, exertional cough, acute paroxysmal pulmonary edema, and hemoptysis. On auscultation, the murmur of mitral stenosis may not readily be detected because of the low cardiac output and the rotation of the heart due to right ventricular hypertrophy. The murmur of mitral stenosis may at times not be evident even after careful evaluation with the possible diagnosis of mitral stenosis in mind. Radiologic examination may reveal only a prominent main pulmonary artery and right-sided enlargement, with little or no evidence of left atrial enlargement. Cardiac catheterization may demonstrate only a high pulmonary artery pressure and low cardiac output, with minimal elevation of pulmonary capillary pressure; in fact, the latter may, on rare occasions, be within normal limits.

Careful radiologic evaluation, including fluoroscopy, may be helpful in suggesting the underlying lesion. An even slightly enlarged left atrium should raise the suspicion of mitral stenosis; Kerley B lines, if present, are helpful, and careful search should be made for calcification in the area of the mitral valve, as its presence is tantamount to the diagnosis of mitral valve disease until proved otherwise. P waves compatible with left atrial enlargement are a helpful electrocardiographic abnormality suggesting the diagnosis of mitral valve disease. Catheterization of the left side of the heart, however, may be the only method by which mitral stenosis can be ruled out and the diagnosis of primary pulmonary hypertension established with reasonable certainty. Admittedly, there is a risk at cardiac catheterization in patients with severe pulmonary hypertension and a relatively low fixed cardiac output; nevertheless, this procedure is justified, if performed with care, to rule out a possible correctable lesion.

Echocardiographic studies should indicate the presence or absence of mitral stenosis, although the features are frequently not related to the severity of the stenosis. The echocardiographic features of patients with primary pulmonary hypertension have included a reduced diastolic descent of the anterior mitral valve leaflet similar to that observed in patients with mitral stenosis but with normal motion of the posterior leaflet.[96] The pattern of pulmonic valve motion has also been evaluated in patients with primary pulmonary hypertension, and with increasing experience the pattern may reflect the severity of the pulmonary hypertension, but, of course, would not in itself indicate the cause of the pulmonary hypertension.[97] Indeed echocardiography with increasing experience will doubtlessly greatly reduce the need for invasive studies such as cardiac catheterization.

Patients with severe pulmonary hypertension, particularly when central cyanosis is present, should be suspected of having an intracardiac or intervascular shunt. Patients with Eisenmenger's reaction may have a clinical picture indistinguishable from that of primary pulmonary hypertension, although they usually present a history of cardiovascular involvement over many years, if not for life. Cardiac catheterization is again essential in ruling out a small left-to-right shunt or in establishing the presence and level of the right-to-left shunt.

Diseases of the pulmonary parenchyma must also be ruled out by careful evaluation of the clinical picture and radiologic findings. If this evaluation is carefully performed, pulmonary function tests should but rarely have to be resorted to in establishing the presence of parenchymal disease. Pulmonary artery pressure elevation of the order observed in

patients with primary pulmonary hypertension is but rarely encountered in pulmonary parenchymal disease; even moderate pulmonary artery pressure elevation appears late in the course of the disease, well after the clinical picture has suggested primary pulmonary parenchymal disease for many years.

Finally, diseases involving the pulmonary vasculature, either primarily or as the result of widespread systemic disease with pulmonary involvement, must be considered in the differential diagnosis of primary pulmonary hypertension. Any patient presenting findings of significant pulmonary hypertension should be carefully evaluated for the presence of a systemic disease process.

REFERENCES

1. Dawes, G. S.: Vasodilation in the Unexpanded Foetal Lung, in R. F. Grover (ed.), "Progress in Research in Emphysema and Chronic Bronchitis," S. Karger A. G., Basel, 1963, p. 153.

2. Adams, F. H., and Lind, J.: Physiologic Studies on the Cardiovascular Status of Normal Newborn Infants (with Special References to the Ductus Arteriosus), *Pediatrics,* 19:431, 1957.

3. Assali, N. S., Morris, J. A., Smith, R. W., and Munson, W. A.: Studies on Ductus Arteriosus Circulation, *Circ. Res.,* 13:478, 1963.

4. Campbell, A. G. M., Dawes, G. D., Fishman, A. P., Hyman, A. I., and Perks, A. M.: The Release of a Bradykinin-like Pulmonary Vasodilator Substance in Foetal and New-born Lambs, *J. Physiol. (Lond.),* 195:83, 1968.

5. Eltherington, L. G., Stoff, J., Hughes, T., and Melmon, K. L.: Constriction of Human Umbilical Arteries: Interaction between Oxygen and Bradykinin, *Circ. Res.,* 22:747, 1968.

6. Heymann, M. A., Rudolph, A. M., Nies, A. S., and Melmon, K. L.: Bradykinin Production Associated with Oxygenation of the Fetal Lamb, *Circ. Res.,* 25:521, 1969.

7. Melmon, K. L., Cline, M. J., Hughes, T., and Nies, A. S.: Kinins: Possible Mediators of Neonatal Circulatory Changes in Man, *J. Clin. Invest.,* 47:1295, 1968.

8. Wagenvoort, C. A., Neufeld, N. N., and Edwards, J. E.: The Structure of the Pulmonary Arterial Tree in Fetal and Early Postnatal Life, *Lab. Invest.,* 10:751, 1961.

9. Pool, P. E., Vogel, J. H. K., and Blount, S. G., Jr.: Congenital Unilateral Absence of a Pulmonary Artery: The Importance of Flow in Pulmonary Hypertension, *Am. J. Cardiol.,* 10:706, 1962.

10. Vogel, J. H. K., Averill, K. H., Pool, P. E., and Blount, S. G., Jr.: Experimental Pulmonary Arterial Hypertension in the Newborn Calf, *Circ. Res.,* 13:557, 1963.

11. Bevegard, S., Holmgren, A., and Jonsson, B.: The Effect of Body Position on the Circulation at Rest and during Exercise, *Acta Physiol. Scand.,* 49:279, 1960.

12. Granath, A., Jonsson, B., and Strandell, T.: Circulation in Healthy Old Men, Studied by Right Heart Catheterization at Rest and during Exercise in Supine and Sitting Position, *Acta Med. Scand.,* 176:425, 1964.

13. Brofman, B. L., Charms, B. L., Kohn, P. M., Elder, J., Newman, R., and Rizika, M.: Unilateral Pulmonary Artery Occlusion in Man: I. Control Studies, *J. Thorac. Surg.,* 34:206, 1957.

14. Charms, B. L., Brofman, B. L., Elder, J. C., and Kohn, P. M.: Unilateral Pulmonary Artery Occlusion in Man: II. Studies in

Patients with Chronic Pulmonary Disease, *J. Thorac. Surg.,* 35:316, 1958.

15 Braunwald, E., Brockenbrough, E. D., Frahm, C. J., and Ross, J., Jr.: Left Atrial and Left Ventricular Pressures in Subjects without Cardiovascular Disease, *Circulation,* 24:267, 1961.

16 Kaltman, A. J., Herbert, W. H., Conroy, R. J., and Kossmann, C. E.: The Gradient in Pressure across the Pulmonary Vascular Bed during Diastole, *Circulation,* 34:377, 1966.

17 Bouchard, R. J., Gault, J. H., and Ross, J., Jr.: Evaluation of Pulmonary Arterial End-diastolic Pressure as an Estimate of Left Ventricular End-diastolic Pressure in Patients with Normal and Abnormal Left Ventricular Performance, *Circulation,* 44:1072, 1971.

18 Herbert, W. H.: Limitations of Pulmonary Artery End-diastolic Pressure, *N.Y. State J. Med.,* 72:229, 1972.

19 Stanfield, C. A., and Yu, T. N.: Hemodynamic Effects of Methoxamine in Mitral Valve Disease, *Circ. Res.,* 8:859, 1960.

20 Oakley, C., Glick, G., Luria, M. N., Schreiner, B. V., Jr., and Yu, P. N.: Some Reguatlory Mechanisms of the Human Pulmonary Vascular Bed, *Circulation,* 26:917, 1962.

21 Goodwin, J. F.: Congestive and Hypertrophic Cardiomyopathies, *Lancet,* 1:731, 1970.

22 Silove, E. D., Tavernor, W. D., and Berry, C. L.: Reactive Pulmonary Arterial Hypertension after Pulmonary Venous Constriction in the Calf, *Cardiovasc. Res.,* 6:36, 1972.

23 Van Bogaret, A., and Tosetti, R.: Experimental Pulmonary Hypertension, *Br. Heart J.,* 25:771, 1963.

24 Braunwald, E., Braunwald, N. S., Ross, J., Jr., and Morrow, A. G.: Effects of Mitral Valve Replacement on the Pulmonary Vascular Dynamics of Patients with Pulmonary Hypertension, *N. Engl. J. Med.,* 273:509, 1965.

25 Dalen, J. E., Matloff, J. M., Eavans, G. L., Hoppin, F. G., Jr., Bhardwaj, P., Harken, D. E., and Dexter, L.: Early Reduction of Pulmonary Vascular Resistance after Mitral Valve Replacement, *N. Engl. J. Med.,* 277:387, 1967.

26 Wood, P.: The Vasoconstrictive Factor in Pulmonary Hypertension, in W. R. Adams and I. Veith (eds.), "Pulmonary Circulation," Grune & Stratton, Inc., New York, 1959, p. 294.

27 Fowler, N. O.: The Normal Pulmonary Arterial Pressure-Flow Relationship during Exercise, *Am. J. Med.,* 47:1, 1969.

28 Downing, S. E., Pursel, S. E., Vidone, R. A., Brandt, H. M., and Liebow, A. A.: Studies on Pulmonary Hypertension with Special Reference to Pressure-Flow Relationships in Chronically Distended and Undistended Lobes, in R. F. Grover (ed.), "Progress in Research in Emphysema and Chronic Bronchitis," S. Karger A. G., Basel, 1963, p. 76.

29 Grover, R. F., and Weil, J. V.: Pulmonary Hypertension and Pulmonary Hypertensive Heart Disease, in H. F. Conn and R. V. Conn, Jr. (eds.), "Current Diagnosis," 3d ed., W. B. Saunders Company, Philadelphia, 1971, p. 291.

30 Lategola, M. T., Massion, W., and Schilling, J. A.: The Effect of Bilateral Pulmonary Resection on Total Oxygen Uptake and Total Pulmonary Hemodynamics in the Dog, *J. Thorac. Surg.,* 37:606, 1959.

31 McGuire, J., Scott, R. C., Helm, R. A., Kaplan, S., Gall, E. A., and Biehl, J. P.: Is There an Entity Primary Pulmonary Hypertension? *Arch. Intern. Med.,* 99:917, 1957.

32 Wagenvoort, C. A., and Wagenvoort, N.: Primary Pulmonary Hypertension, *Circulation,* 42:1163, 1970.

33 Arias-Stella, J., and Saldana, M.: The Muscular Pulmonary Arteries in People Native to High Altitude, in R. F. Grover (ed.), "Progress in Research in Emphysema and Chronic Bronchitis," S. Karger A. G., Basel, 1963, p. 292.

34 Naeye, R. L.: Children at High Altitude: Pulmonary and Renal Abnormalities, *Circ. Res.,* 16:33, 1965.

35 Hatano, S., and Strasser, T., (eds.): "Primary Pulmonary Hypertension," World Health Organization, Geneva, Switzerland, 1975.

36 Kew, M. C.: Aminorex Fumarate: A Double-blind Trial and Examination for Signs of Pulmonary Arterial Hypertension, *S. Afr. Med. J.,* 44:421, 1970.

37 Byrne-Quinn, E., and Grover, R. F.: Aminorex (Menocil) and Amphetamine: Acute and Chronic Effects on Pulmonary and Systemic Haemodynamics in the Calf, *Thorax,* 27:127, 1972.

38 Berthrong, M., and Cochran, T. H.: Pathological Findings in Nine Children with "Primary" Pulmonary Hypertension, *Johns Hopkins Med. J.,* 97:69, 1959.

39 Berthrong, M.: Discussion, in R. F. Grover (ed.), "Progress in Research in Emphysema and Chronic Bronchitis," S. Karger A. G., Basel, 1963, p. 239.

40 Wood, J. E.: Oral Contraceptives, Pregnancy, and the Veins, *Circulation,* 38:627, 1968.

41 Hjort, P. F., and Hasselback, R.: A Critical Review of the Evidence for a Continuous Hemostasis in Vivo, *Thromb. Diath. Haemorrh.,* 6:580, 1961.

42 Macfarlane, A. S.: Measurement of Synthesis Rates of Liver-produced Plasma Proteins, *Biochem. J.,* 89:277, 1963.

43 Cash, J. D., and Allan, A. G. E.: The Fibrinolytic Response to Moderate Exercise and Intravenous Adrenaline in the Same Subjects, *Br. J. Haematol.,* 13:376, 1967.

44 Almér, L. O., and Nilsson, I. M.: On Fibrinolysis in Diabetes Mellitus, *Acta Med. Scand.,* 198:101, 1975.

45 Isacson, S., and Nilsson, I. M.: Defective Fibrinolysis in Blood and Vein Walls in Recurrent "Idiopathic" Venous Thrombosis, *Acta Chir. Scand.,* 138:313, 1972.

46 Astrup, T., Glas, P., and Kok, P.: Lung Fibrinolytic Activity and Bovine High Mountain Disease, *Proc. Soc. Exp. Biol. Med.,* 127:373, 1968.

47 Reeves, J. T., Jokl, P., Merida, J., and Leathers, J. E.: Pulmonary Vascular Obstruction Following Administration of High-Energy Nucleotides, *J. Appl. Physiol.,* 22:475, 1967.

48 Silove, E. D.: Effects of Haemolysed Blood and Adenosine Diphosphate on the Pulmonary Vascular Resistance in Calves, *Cardiovasc. Res.,* 5:313, 1971.

49 Wang, Y., From, A. H. L., Krivit, W., Segal, M. A., and Edwards, J. E.: Disseminated Pulmonary Arterial Thrombosis Associated with Thrombocytopenia: Occurrence in Identical Twins, *Circulation,* 32(suppl. 2): 215, 1965.

50 Short, D. S.: The Problem of Medial Hypertrophy in Pulmonary Hypertension, in R. F. Grover (ed.), "Progress in Research in Emphysema and Chronic Bronchitis," S. Karger A. G., Basel, 1963, p. 219.

51 Vogel, J. H. K., Grover, R. F., Jamieson, G., and Blount, S. G., Jr.: Long-Term Physiologic Observations in Patients with Ventricular Septal Defect and Increased Pulmonary Vascular Resistance, *Adv. Cardiol.,* 11:108, 1974.

52 Grover, R. F., Reeves, J. T., and Blount, S. G., Jr.: Tolazoline Hydrochloride (Priscoline): An Effective Pulmonary Vasodilator, *Am. Heart J.,* 61:5, 1961.

53 Sanders, J., Miller, D. D., and Patil, P. N.: Alpha Adrenergic and Histaminergic Effects of Tolazoline-like Imidazolines, *J. Pharmacol. Exp. Ther.,* 195:362, 1975.

54 Kay, J. M., and Heath, D.: "*Crotalaria spectabilis:* The Pulmonary Hypertension Plant," Charles C Thomas, Publisher, Springfield, Ill., 1971.

55 Fishman, A. P.: Dietary Pulmonary Hypertension, *Circ. Res.,* 35:657, 1974.

56 Abraham, A. S., Cole, R. B., and Bishop, J. M.: Reversal of Pulmonary Hypertension by Prolonged Oxygen Administration to Patients with Chronic Bronchitis, *Circ. Res.,* 23:147, 1968.

57 Levy, A. M., Tabakin, B. S., Hanson, J. S., and Narkewicz, R. M.: Hypertrophied Adenoids Causing Pulmonary Hypertension and Severe Congestive Heart Failure, *N. Engl. J. Med.,* 277:506, 1967.

58 Peñaloza, D., Sime, F., Banchero, N., Gamboa, R., Cruz, J., and Marticorena, E.: Pulmonary Hypertension in Healthy Men Born and Living at High Altitudes, *Am. J. Cardiol.*, 11:150, 1963.

59 Reeves, J. T., and Grover, R. F.: High Altitude Pulmonary Hypertension and Pulmonary Edema, *Prog. Cardiol.*, 4:99, 1975.

60 Grover, R. F.: The High Altitude Resident of North America, *Scientia (Milan)*, 103:9, 1968.

61 Naeye, R. L.: Children at High Altitude: Pulmonary and Renal Abnormalities, *Circ. Res.*, 16:33, 1965.

62 Grover, R. F., Vogel, J. H. K., Voigt, G. C., and Blount, S. G., Jr.: Reversal of High Altitude Pulmonary Hypertension, *Am. J. Cardiol.*, 18:928, 1966.

63 McMurtry, I. F., Davidson, A. B., Reeves, J. T., and Grover, R. F.: Inhibition of Hypoxic Pulmonary Vasoconstriction by Calcium Antagonists in Isolated Rat Lungs, *Circ. Res.*, 38:99, 1976.

64 Bergofsky, E. H.: Mechanisms Underlying Regulation of Regional Pulmonary Blood Flow in Normal and Diseased States, *Am. J. Med.*, 57:378, 1974.

65 Fishman, A. P.: Hypoxia and the Pulmonary Circulation: How and Where It Acts, *Circ. Res.*, 38:221, 1976.

66 Weir, E. K., McMurtry, I. F., Tucker, A., Reeves, J. T., and Grover, R. F.: Prostaglandin Synthetase Inhibitors Do Not Decrease Hypoxic Pulmonary Vasoconstriction, *J. Appl. Physiol.*, 41:714, 1976.

67 Tucker, A., Weir, E. K., Reeves, J. T., and Grover, R. F.: Failure of Histamine Antagonists to Prevent Hypoxic Pulmonary Vasoconstriction in Dogs, *J. Appl. Physiol.*, 40:496, 1976.

68 Kay, J. M., Waymire, J. C., and Grover, R. F.: Lung Mast Cell Hyperplasia and Pulmonary Histamine Forming Capacity at High Altitude, *Am. J. Physiol.*, 226:178, 1974.

69 Grover, R. F., and Weil, J. V.: Pulmonary Hypertension and Pulmonary Hypertensive Heart Disease, in H. F. Conn and R. B. Conn, Jr. (eds.), "Current Diagnosis," 3d ed., W. B. Saunders, Company, Philadelphia, 1971, p. 291.

70 Tucker, A., Weir, E. K., Reeves, J. T., and Grover, R. F.: Pulmonary Microembolism: Attenuated Pulmonary Vasoconstriction with Prostaglandin Inhibitors and Antihistamines, *Prostaglandins*, 11:31, 1976.

71 Mlczoch, J., Tucker, A., Weir, E. K., Reeves, J. T., and Grover, R. F.: Platelet Mediated Pulmonary Hypertension and Hypoxemia during Pulmonary Microembolism, *Chest*, in press.

72 Weir, E. K., Reeves, J. T., Droegemueller, W., and Grover, R. F.: 15-Methylation Augments the Cardiovascular Effects of Prostaglandin $F_{2\alpha}$, *Prostaglandins*, 9:369, 1975.

73 Kolata, G. B.: Thromboxanes: The Power Behind the Prostaglandins? *Science*, 190:770, 1975.

74 Lucas, R. V., Jr., Adams, P., Jr., Anderson, R. C., Meyne, N. G., Lillehei, C. W., and Varco, R. C.: The Natural History of Isolated Ventricular Septal Defect, *Circulation*, 24:1372, 1961.

75 Wood, P.: Pulmonary Hypertension, with Special Reference to the Vasoconstrictive Factor, *Br. Heart J.*, 20:557, 1958.

76 Vogel, J. H. K., McNamara, P. G., Hallman, G., Rosenberg, H., Jamieson, G., and McCrady, J. D.: Effects of Mild Chronic Hypoxia on the Pulmonary Circulation in Calves with Reactive Pulmonary Hypertension, *Circ. Res.*, 21:661, 1967.

77 Heath, D., and Edwards, J. E.: The Pathology of Hypertensive Pulmonary Vascular Disease, *Circulation*, 18:533, 1958.

78 Houston, C. S.: Pulmonary Edema at High Altitude, in R. F. Grover (ed.), "Normal and Abnormal Pulmonary Circulation," S. Karger A. G., Basel, 1963, p. 313.

79 Fred, H. L., Schmidt, A. M., Bates, T., and Hecht, H. H.: Acute Pulmonary Edema of Altitude, Clinical and Physiologic Observations, *Circulation*, 25:929, 1962.

80 Hultgren, H. N., Lopez, C. E., Lundberg, E., and Miller, H.: Physiologic Studies of Pulmonary Edema at High Altitude, *Circulation*, 29:393, 1964.

81 Hultgren, H. N., Grover, R. F., and Hartley, L. H.: Abnormal Circulatory Responses to High-Altitidue Pulmonary Edema, *Circulation*, 44:759, 1971.

82 Arias-Stella, J., and Kruger, H.: Pathology of High Altitude Pulmonary Edema, *Arch. Pathol.*, 76:147, 1963.

83 Gray, G. W., Bryan, A. C., Freedman, M. H., Houston, C. S., Lewis, W. F., McFadden, D. M., and Newell, G.: Effect of Altitude Exposure on Platelets, *J. Appl. Physiol.*, 39:648, 1975.

84 Maher, J. T., Levine, P. H., and Cymerman, A.: Human Coagulation Abnormalities during Acute Exposure to Hypobaric Hypoxia, *J. Appl. Physiol.*, 41:702, 1976.

85 Singh, I., Chohan, I. S., and Mathew, N. T.: Fibrinolytic Activity in High Altitude Pulmonary Oedema, *Indian J. Med. Res.*, 57:210, 1969.

86 Grover, R. F., Vogel, J. H. K., Averill, K. H., and Blount, S. G., Jr.: Pulmonary Hypertension: Individual and Species Variability Relative to Vascular Reactivity, *Am. Heart J.*, 66:1, 1963.

87 Vogel, J. H. K., Weaver, W. F., Rose, R. L., Blount, S. G., Jr., and Grover, R. F.: Pulmonary Hypertension on Exertion in Normal Man Living at 10,150 Feet (Leadville, Colorado), *Med. Thorac.*, 19:461, 1962.

88 Grover, R. F., Reeves, J. T., Will, D. H., and Blount, S. G., Jr.: Pulmonary Vasoconstriction in Steers at High Altitude, *J. Appl. Physiol.*, 18:567, 1963.

89 Grover, R. F., Will, D. H., Reeves, J. T., Weir, E. K., McMurtry, I. F., and Alexander, A. F.: Genetic Transmission of Susceptibility to Hypoxic Pulmonary Hypertension, *Prog. Resp. Res.*, 9:112, 1975.

90 Will, D. H., Hicks, J. L., Card, C. S., and Alexander, A. F.: Inherited Susceptibility of Cattle to High Altitude Pulmonary Hypertension, *J. Appl. Physiol.*, 38:491, 1975.

91 Tucker, A., McMurtry, I. F., Reeves, J. T., Alexander, A. F., Will, D. H., and Grover, R. F.: Lung Vascular Smooth Muscle as a Determinant of Pulmonary Hypertension at High Altitude, *Am. J. Physiol.*, 228:762, 1975.

92 Wood, P.: "Diseases of the Heart and Circulation," 2d ed., Eyre & Spottiswoode (Publishers), Ltd., London, 1957.

93 Alexander, J. K., Hartley, L. H., Modelski, M., and Grover, R. F.: Reduction of Stroke Volume during Exercise in Man following Ascent to 3,100 m Altitude, *J. Appl. Physiol.*, 23:849, 1967.

94 Hartley, L. H., Alexander, J. K., Modelski, M., and Grover, R. F.: Subnormal Cardiac Output at Rest and during Exercise in Residents at 3,100 m Altitude, *J. Appl. Physiol.*, 23:839, 1967.

95 Inglesby, T. V., Singer, J. W., and Gordon, D. S.: Abnormal Fibrinolysis in Familial Pulmonary Hypertension, *Am. J. Med.*, 55:5, 1973.

96 Goodman, D. J., Harrison, D. C., and Popp, R. L.: Echocardiographic Features of Primary Pulmonary Hypertension, *Am. J. Cardiol.*, 33:438, 1974.

97 Weyman, A. E., Dillon, J. C., Feigenbaum, H., and Chang, S.: Echocardiographic Patterns of Pulmonic Valve Motion with Pulmonary Hypertension, *Circulation*, 50:905, 1974.

98 Bergman, H., Fahlen, M., Helder, G., Ryden, L., Wallentin, I., and Zettergren, L.: Phenformin and Pulmonary Hypertension, *Br. Heart J.*, 8:824, 1973.

99 Wagenvoort, C. A., and Wagenvoort, N.: "Pathology of Pulmonary Hypertension," John Wiley & Sons, New York, 1977.

100 Naeye, R. L.: "Primary" Pulmonary Hypertension with Coexisting Portal Hypertension: A Retrospective Study of Six Cases, *Circulation*, 22:376, 1960.

101 Cohen, N., and Mendlow, H.: Concurrent "Active Juvenile Cirrhosis" and "Primary Pulmonary Hypertension," *Am. J. Med.*, 39:127, 1965.

102 Levine, O. R., Harris, R. C., Blanc, W. A., and Mellins, R. B.: Progressive Pulmonary Hypertension in Children with Portal Hypertension, *J. Pediatr.*, 83:964, 1973.

75

Pulmonary Embolism and Acute Cor Pulmonale

LEWIS DEXTER, M.D., and
JAMES E. DALEN, M.D.

That, therefore, which according to the ordinary nomenclature is called suppurative phlebitis, is neither suppurative, nor yet phlebitis, but a process which begins with a coagulation, with the formation of a thrombus in the blood, and afterwards presents a stage in which the thrombi soften, so that the whole history of the process is contained in the history of the thrombus.

RUDOLF VIRCHOW, 1858[1]

Pulmonary embolism is the most common form of acute pulmonary disease in the adult hospital population. It is the most common immediate cause of death at the Peter Bent Brigham Hospital. Most lethal episodes of pulmonary embolism are preceded by less massive episodes. If pulmonary embolism can be detected when it first occurs, highly effective therapy is available to prevent further embolism. However, these therapeutic measures cannot be introduced unless a diagnosis can be made. Diagnosis is notoriously difficult.

INCIDENCE OF PULMONARY EMBOLISM

Frequency

Pulmonary emboli are found in approximately 10 percent of all autopsies in general hospitals and in about 25 percent in hospitals giving custodial care. In patients dying in congestive heart failure, postmortem data indicate an incidence of 30 to 50 percent. It has been estimated[1a] that the total incidence of pulmonary embolism in the United States is of the order of 630,000 per year, of whom 200,000 die. Thus, it ties with stroke as the third most common cause of death in the United States.

Age and sex

The incidence of pulmonary embolism increases with age, being rare under 20 and infrequent under 30. It becomes progressively more common with advancing years. There is no sex or race predilection.

ORIGIN OF THROMBI

In over 90 percent of cases, the site of formation of venous thrombi is in the calves of the legs.[2] A thrombus may propagate upward as a bland thrombus without inflammatory reaction (phlebothrombosis), or there may be an inflammatory (nonbacterial) reaction, in which case it is referred to as *thrombophlebitis*. In either event, it propagates up the vein and may break off to become an embolus at any time. The volume of embolic material liberated depends on the extent of its propagation and the point from which it breaks loose. A clot extending from calf to iliac vein has a volume of approximately 100 ml. Another site of origin of clots is the pelvis, but here the venous volume is much smaller than that of the legs except in the case of the uterine veins post partum. How often emboli originate in the right atrium of patients with atrial fibrillation and congestive heart failure is not known. The potential volume of clot that may form within the right side of the heart is much less than that formed in the leg veins. However, irrespective of precise incidence, the legs are usually the site of origin and from a therapeutic viewpoint should be considered as the source.[3]

FACTORS PREDISPOSING TO VENOUS THROMBOSIS AND EMBOLISM

In 1856 Virchow suggested three possible causes of venous thrombosis: stasis of blood, abnormality of venous wall, and abnormal state of coagulation.[4] Since that time little progress has been made in further identification of fundamental causes.

Stasis results from prolonged bed rest (e.g., following fractures, operations, debilitating diseases of all types), pregnancy, obesity, and especially congestive heart failure. The latter is by far the most important disease predisposing to thromboembolism. Prolonged chair sitting, at home or in the office, on long automobile or plane trips, and especially when the legs are crossed, is an aggravating factor because the legs remain immobile. The blood hardly moves out of the dependent legs until the foot or leg is moved at which point the muscles squeeze blood very effectively out of the legs (muscle pump) thereby overcoming stasis. Prolonged chair sitting alone is rarely a cause of venous thrombosis, but when added onto the predisposing factors mentioned above, it becomes a highly significant factor in producing venous thrombosis.[5]

Abnormality of venous wall occurs from trauma, surgical procedures, phlebosclerosis (which is common in older people), inflammatory diseases of veins (Buerger's disease, typhoid fever, arterial insufficiency, and gangrene), and degenerative lesions (atherosclerosis, diabetes mellitus).

A hypercoagulable state has been postulated to

occur during pregnancy and in those taking oral contraceptives. Whether or not this is really true remains controversial.[6] The most clear-cut example of a hypercoagulable state is antithrombin III deficiency.[7] Antithrombin III inactivates factors XII, XI, IX, and Xa of the intrinsic clotting system. The deficiency appears to be a genetic defect. When the deficiency is severe, venous thrombosis and fatal pulmonary embolism are the usual cause of death, even at a young age. Other members of the family deficient in this factor are similarly afflicted. It has been estimated that about 2 percent of venous thromboembolism is due to this deficiency.

Abnormalities of the clotting mechanism also include thrombocytosis (postoperative, postpartum, postsplenectomy, idiopathic thrombocythemia); sickle-cell anemia; and the presence of cold agglutinins, cryoglobulins, cryofibrinogens, and macroglobulins. Raised levels of circulating fibrinogens, or thromboplastin, platelet "stickiness," sludging, and the presence of certain types of carcinoma (pancreas, stomach, ovaries) have all been implicated as causes of intravascular thrombosis, but their role is neither clear nor constant.

DIAGNOSIS OF VENOUS THROMBOSIS

The clinical recognition of venous thrombosis is disappointing. In only about 30 percent of patients with pulmonary embolism is venous thrombosis detectable clinically.[3] The recognition of "silent" venous thrombosis has recently been greatly improved by four methods: phlebography, impedance plethysmography, Doppler ultrasound, and the radioactive fibrinogen test.

Phlebography was introduced by DosSantos in 1938; later by Bauer and again more recently a number of improvements have been introduced.[8] Although the technique is cumbersome, time-consuming, at times produces discomfort, and requires expertise in execution and interpretation, it is the single most accurate method for detecting venous thrombosis of the legs. It is not practical as a screening procedure but is ideal for confirming the diagnosis of venous thrombosis and provides an accurate assessment of the nature, location, and extent of thrombus. Impedance plethysmography is noninvasive and simple to perform and has had an accuracy of about 98 percent in detecting venous thrombosis.[9] Doppler ultrasound detection is a quick and simple way of detecting complete venous occlusion but has many limitations.[3] Its virtue is in the presence of a positive finding. A negative result does not rule out venous thrombosis.

The radioactive fibrinogen test depends on the preferential uptake of ^{125}I-labeled human fibrinogen by a forming thrombus. The leg is then scanned by an external scintillation counter. Over a thrombus there is a greater number of counts than elsewhere. There has been about an 85 percent correlation between this fibrinogen test and venography.[3] It misses very small clots in the calves of the leg and clots above

Poupart's ligament. The recent availability of ^{125}I human fibrinogen in the United States will make this test available on a wider scale than heretofore.

PATHOGENESIS OF EMBOLISM

When a clot breaks loose, it travels up the vein without hindrance into the right side of the heart. Most frequently the clot is broken up into multiple small particles by the churning and pumping action of the right ventricle and then passes into the pulmonary arterial system. Its distribution in the lungs follows closely the distribution of blood flow, i.e., it is found mainly in the lower lobes and to a lesser extent in the upper lobes. Emboli usually lodge in both lungs and in several lobes.[10] The rising pulmonary arterial pressure may pound the particles farther down in the vascular system. The immediate effect is usually total blockage of the circulation through the embolized vessel. As the pressure in the pulmonary artery rises, blood "worms" its way past the clot, so that partial revascularization occurs within minutes. Resolution of emboli proceeds at a slower rate, and lysis is the result of circulating plasmin (fibrinolysin). In patients without heart or pulmonary disease, resolution of clots may be complete in 2 weeks.[11] In some, it takes longer. In patients with cardiac and pulmonary disease, resolution is often incomplete, but chronic cor pulmonale from pulmonary embolism, though it occurs, is rare.[1a]

The immediate cause of embolism is usually not apparent, but sometimes it occurs on arising from bed, straining at stool, exertion, or hyperventilation, all of which maneuvers result in distension of veins of the legs, thereby promoting the breaking off of clots.

RESPONSE OF THE LUNG TO EMBOLI

Three different reactions to embolism in the lung may occur—pulmonary infarction, acute cor pulmonale, or unexplained acute dyspnea.[12]

In pulmonary infarction, the circulation is so much compromised that the pulmonary parenchyma is destroyed, but the bronchial collateral circulation is sufficient to maintain the viability of fibrous tissue. Septic embolism may give rise to a pulmonary abscess wherein both pulmonary tissue and fibrous tissue are destroyed. This is now seen almost exclusively in unclean manipulations in the evacuation of the pregnant uterus.

Acute cor pulmonale refers to pulmonary and right ventricular hypertension caused by embolic plugging of the pulmonary arterial system with resultant circulatory obstruction. This occurs only if the embolism is sufficiently massive to occlude more than 60 percent of the pulmonary circulation. Acute cor pulmonale produces a rise of pressure in right ventricle and pulmonary artery proximal to the obstruction, and a reduction of blood flow (cardiac output) through the lung.

If pulmonary infarction does not occur, and if the embolism is not sufficiently massive to cause acute cor pulmonale, the patient's primary symptom may be acute dyspnea.

PATHOLOGIC PHYSIOLOGY

Pulmonary infarction

The lung has two circulations, the pulmonary and the bronchial. The pulmonary artery subserves the purpose of gas exchange. The bronchial circulation supplies the pulmonary structures down to, but not including, the alveoli.

The pulmonary artery rises from the right ventricle and divides into two main branches, which further divide into lobar branches. These and the next division extend out almost to the pleural surface. Subsequent branches are short, resembling twigs on a tree. The number and sizes of the various divisions are shown in Table 75-1. The pulmonary capillaries are large, surround the alveoli as a mesh, and are extensively anastomotic among themselves. The capillaries empty into venules and then into larger and larger veins, finally culminating in four main venous trunks emptying into the left atrium.

The bronchial arteries arise from the aorta or one of the first two intercostal arteries. They supply the trachea, bronchi, and mediastinal structures. They also supply the vasa vasorum of the pulmonary artery. In the dog, about two-thirds of the bronchial venous blood empties into the pulmonary veins and one-third into the azygos, hemiazygos, and intercostal veins of the systemic circulation.

Pulmonary and bronchial arterial systems are anastomotic in three regions. There is a potential, if not actual, connection between bronchial artery and pulmonary artery, especially in various pulmonary disease conditions. There is normally an extensive anastomosis between bronchial capillaries and pulmonary capillaries and between bronchial veins and pulmonary veins.

Flow from bronchial vessels to pulmonary vessels is normally less than 1 percent of the cardiac output. Increase of bronchial collateral flow occurs following pulmonary arterial occlusion by ligation or embolism, in tumors, and in inflammatory lesions of all sorts, particularly bronchiectasis.

Pulmonary infarction cannot be produced experimentally in animals by ligation of the right or left main branch of the pulmonary artery or by microembolization. Ligation of a lobar branch rarely produces infarction, provided that the remainder of the circulation is normal. The collateral circulation is sufficient to maintain the viability of the pulmonary parenchyma. Pulmonary infarction regularly takes place on occlusion of pulmonary arteries ranging in size from lobar arteries down to vessels about 2 mm in diameter if the collateral flow from bronchial arteries is interfered with by ligation of the bronchial arteries, pulmonary veins, or lobar veins; by compression from pleural effusion; or by lowering the systemic (bronchial arterial) blood pressure. In other words, pulmonary infarction seems to occur when two sets of conditions coexist: (1) when middle-sized pulmonary arteries are occluded and (2) when the collateral circulation from bronchial arteries is compromised by pulmonary venous hypertension or systemic hypotension.

Pulmonary infarction in human beings appears to occur as it does in the experimental animal. It occurs as a result of embolization of middle-sized vessels when bronchial collateral circulation is interfered with by pulmonary congestion from heart failure or by systemic hypotension. A curious and unexplained finding is that only about 10 percent of occlusions of middle-sized vessels result in pulmonary infarction.[13] This is true both in the experimental animal and in human beings. Thus, pulmonary infarction radiologically and histologically represents the exception rather than the rule when middle-sized vessels are occluded with embolic material. Infarcts occur in the lower lobes rather than in the upper lobes for two reasons: (1) flow to the lower lobes is greater than that to the upper lobes, at least in the upright position, so that the lower lobes receive more emboli; (2) the lower lobes in the upright position are more congested than are the upper lobes.

Circulatory obstruction (acute cor pulmonale)

The lung is a high-flow, low-pressure organ. All the cardiac output passes through the lung. Under basal conditions this amounts to 3.1 liters/min/m² body surface. This flow may be increased about threefold without any appreciable change in pulmonary arterial pressure. Table 75-2 compares the low pressures that exist in the normal lung with the relatively high pressures that exist in the systemic circuit. The lung is a low-resistance organ. Its resistance is only about one-fifteenth that of the systemic circuit. There is an enormous pulmonary vascular reserve. The cross-

TABLE 75-1
Number of emboli required to produce pulmonary hypertension

Artery	Diameter of artery and emboli, mm	No. of arteries	No. of emboli
Lobar	5.0	8	7
First order	4.0	12	28
Second order	2.3	43	60
Third order	1.0	1,021	1,600
Lobular	0.3	16,000	20,000
Atrial	0.17	64,000	90,000

SOURCE: L. Dexter and G. T. Smith, Quantitative Studies of Pulmonary Embolism, in "Transactions of the American Clinical and Climatological Association," vol. 75, Waverly Press, Inc., Baltimore, 1964, p. 72; with permission of authors, recorder, and publisher.

TABLE 75-2
Pressures (mm Hg) and resistances (dynes-s-cm⁻⁵) in normal human beings

Pressures:			Pressures:		
Systemic vein, mean		5	Pulmonary vein, mean		7
Right atrium, mean		0	Left atrium, mean		5
Right ventricle, S/ED*		25/0	Left ventricle, S/ED		120/5
Pulmonary artery,			Aorta	120/80	(95)
S/ED		25/9 (15)	Systemic capillaries,		
Pulmonary capillaries,			mean		25
mean		9	Resistance:		
Resistance:			Systemic vascular		1,200
Pulmonary vascular		80			

*Systolic/end-diastolic

sectional area of the pulmonary vasculature both in dogs and in human beings must be reduced by over one-half before any change in pressure or flow through the organ can be detected. Pneumonectomy does not result in pulmonary hypertension provided the opposite lung is normal. The amount of embolic material required to produce a 5- to 10-mm Hg rise of pressure in the pulmonary artery in an 8-kg dog, this being the first sign of circulatory embarrassment, is shown in Table 75-1, where the size and number of embolic particles are compared with the size and number of different branches of the pulmonary artery. A small number of large particles and increasing numbers of small particles are required to produce incipient pulmonary hypertension. At the precapillary level, 22 million *Lycopodium* spores are required.[14]

There has been a controversy over the years regarding the presence or absence of reflex vasoconstriction as a result of thromboembolism. It has been postulated that the powerful pulmonary vasoconstrictor serotonin might be released from platelet thrombi and thus give rise to pulmonary hypertension on a vasoconstrictor basis, in addition to the mechanical plugging by the emboli. Such a mechanism has not as yet been proved. Bradykinin and vasoactive fibrinopeptides from the breakdown of fibrinogen and fibrin are currently under investigation for the role they play in the pulmonary circulatory disturbance. There is good experimental evidence that diffuse pulmonary vasoconstriction occurs as a result of embolization of *arterioles* in the lung but not as a result of *arterial* occlusion. Thromboemboli occlude mainly arteries, not arterioles (Table 75-3). Furthermore, the amount of thromboembolic material in the lungs of patients dying of pulmonary embolism is uniformly of such magnitude as to account for the circulatory changes on the basis of simple me-

TABLE 75-3
Location of emboli in 34 human lungs

Arteries	Size, mm	No. of cases	Frequency
Elastic	>1.0	8	Few
Muscular	0.1–1.0	34	Common
Arterioles	0.03–0.1	13	Rare

SOURCE: L. Dexter and G. T. Smith, Quantitative Studies of Pulmonary Embolism, *Am. J. Med. Sci.,* 247:37, 1964; with permission of authors, editor, and publisher.

TABLE 75-4
Arterial volume of human lungs

Lungs	No. of cases	Arterial volume, ml/m²
Normal:		
Right	12	62±3.3
Left	14	55±4.0
Embolized:		
Right	10	21±9.8
Left	26	22±11.6

SOURCE: L. Dexter and G. T. Smith, Quantitative Studies of Pulmonary Embolism, *Am. J. Med. Sci.,* 247:37, 1964; with permission of authors, editor, and publisher.

chanical obstruction[15] (Table 75-4 and Fig. 75-1). Reports of a single small embolus producing death have not been confirmed by more recent studies utilizing postmortem arteriography.[13,15] Other types of embolic material (fat, air, amniotic fluid) do occlude arterioles, and it may well be that there is an element of diffuse vasoconstriction in these unusual types of embolism.

With reduction of more than 50 to 60 percent of the cross-sectional area of the pulmonary arteries, circulatory and respiratory changes appear. Pressure

FIGURE 75-1 A postmortem pulmonary arteriogram from a patient who died of pulmonary embolism. Note the large avascular parenchymal areas due to thromboembolic occlusion of medium and small muscular arteries. The volume of injection mass required to fill the pulmonary arterial vasculature in this lung has been reduced by two-thirds. *(From G. T. Smith, G. J. Dammin, and L. Dexter, Postmortem Arteriographic Studies of the Human Lung in Pulmonary Embolization, J.A.M.A., 188:143, 1964; with permission of the authors, editor, and publisher.)*

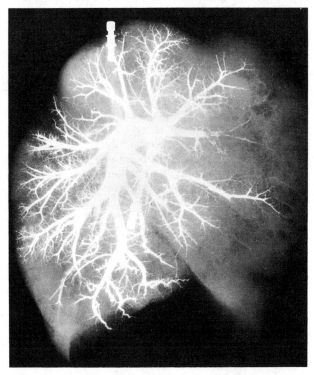

becomes elevated in the pulmonary artery proximal to the obstruction and in the right ventricle. The right ventricular systolic pressure may rise to 60 or 70 mm Hg and may return toward normal in the course of 30 to 60 min or longer. This fall of pressure may be due to several factors: (1) revascularization by blood being forced past the embolus; (2) slippage of the embolic material further down the pulmonary arterial system where the cross-sectional area is larger; (3) opening up of new vessels in unoccluded areas of the lung; and (4) eventual lysis of the clots.[10,16] An abrupt rise of systolic pressure may be so disadvantageous to the right ventricle as to result in acute dilatation, a rise in its diastolic pressure, and a corresponding rise in systemic venous pressure (right ventricular failure).[17] The cardiac output, initially high, falls; pulse rate usually rises; and peripheral circulatory failure may appear. Manifestations may be syncope, collapse, or frank shock. Coronary blood flow increases at first, largely because of hypoxemia, but if hypotension and shock transpire, it decreases.[18,19] There is no evidence to support the concept of a pulmonary-coronary reflex. Hyperventilation occurs regularly. Breathing is one of two types: it is either rapid and shallow or deep and gasping. Tachypnea, shallow breathing, elevation of the diaphragm, and abnormal blood gases are characteristic responses to acute pulmonary embolism.[20]

CLINICAL PICTURE

Minor degrees of embolism probably occur frequently, but since they produce no circulatory or respiratory disturbance, they go completely unnoticed. Virtually no information is available concerning the fate of such emboli. It is presumed that lysis of such clots can be handled effectively under normal circumstances.

Pulmonary infarction

The time elapsing between embolic occlusion and manifestations of pulmonary infarction must vary considerably. It has been reported to occur anywhere from 2½ to 79 h following wedging of a cardiac catheter into a branch of the pulmonary artery for the measurement of pulmonary capillary wedge pressure in human beings. Pulmonary infarction causes some disability, never death. Death from embolism is due to circulatory obstruction (acute cor pulmonale). Pulmonary infarction may be looked upon as a fortuitous event in that it draws the physician's attention to the fact that embolism has occurred. It is of great diagnostic importance. It must be emphasized, however, that infarction is inconstantly present even though embolism has occurred. Furthermore, the manifestations of pulmonary infarction may be mimicked by a variety of other pulmonary diseases. The symptoms are often but not always

TABLE 75-5
Symptoms and signs of pulmonary infarction (97 cases)

Symptoms	Number	Percent
Tachypnea	87	90
Tachycardia	85	88
Fever	77	79
Pleurisy	71	73
Cough	56	58
Friction rub	44	45
Hemoptysis	38	39
Icterus	22	23
Chill	3	3

abrupt in onset, vary in severity, and follow the pattern shown in Table 75-5.

SYMPTOMS AND SIGNS
The common manifestations[21,22] of pulmonary infarction are a rise of temperature, pulse, and respiration. This triad has been emphasized for many years by surgeons. It is seen just as commonly in medical patients, particularly patients with cardiac disease. It is one of the important clues to the presence of pulmonary infarction. Temperature rises characteristically to 101 or 102°F, occasionally higher. A rise to 104° accompanied by a shaking chill suggests a septic infarct, although this is not invariably the case. The pulse rate rises characteristically to about 120 but depends in part on associated pleural pain. It is sometimes accompanied by an arrhythmia, either atrial (fibrillation or flutter) or ventricular (premature beats), in which case the pulse rate may become extremely rapid. Tachypnea tends to follow the course of the fever as well as that of the pleural pain.

Pleuritic pain is the next most common manifestation of pulmonary infarction. It may be transient, or it may last for days. It is most commonly located over the lower part of the chest, but with irritation of the diaphragm there may be radiation to the shoulder regions. There may be tenderness of the overlying chest wall.

Cough is frequent; it may be dry or it may be productive of sputum.

Hemoptysis occurs in over one-third of cases. The blood may be dark or bright red, or it may be mixed with sputum. Hemoptysis should always suggest pulmonary infarction to the physician. It may, of course, occur as a result of heart disease alone or as a result of a variety of other diseases of the lung.

A friction rub may be heard transiently over the infarcted area. Both pain and friction rub may disappear with the development of an effusion.

Pleural effusions in association with infarction often are bloody but are at times serous.

LABORATORY FINDINGS
Characteristically the white blood cell count rises to 10,000 or 15,000, and occasionally higher. There is usually a modest preponderance of polymorphonuclear cells.

In the serum, there is characteristically a rise of lactic dehydrogenase (LDH) activity and in about one-half of cases no rise of activity of glutamic oxaloacetic transaminase (SGOT). Although a rise of LDH level in the face of a normal SGOT level was initially considered to be diagnostic of pulmonary embolism, this has been shown repeatedly to be not the case. Values of LDH level may be normal in the presence of embolism, and many other diseases can produce an increase in LDH level. These enzyme changes are not useful diagnostic tools.

Characteristic radiologic findings of pulmonary infarction are best seen 12 to 24 h after embolization. These findings consist of an area of consolidation somewhere in the periphery of the lung, usually the lower lobes. There is a rounded profile facing the hilus. The shadow extends out to the pleural surface. Such a picture is found in 15 to 30 percent of cases. In another 15 to 30 percent, shadows suggesting patchy pneumonitis or pulmonary edema may be present, pleural fluid may appear, and there may be elevation of the diaphragm and diminished diaphragmatic excursions on the affected side. In perhaps 30 percent of cases the roentgenogram is normal. It should be noted that a normal chest x-ray in a patient with acute dyspnea is consistent with pulmonary embolism without infarction.

Pulmonary infarction produces no significant electrocardiographic findings.

Circulatory obstruction[21,22]

Manifestations of circulatory obstruction are hyperventilation, pulmonary hypertension, right ventricular failure, and reduced cardiac output.

RESPIRATION AND ARTERIAL BLOOD GASES
Pulmonary embolism results in hyperventilation. The breathing is shallow and rapid. At the onset of embolism tachypnea is probably present in all cases. The precise respiratory rate is one of the most neglected physical signs in clinical medicine. In pulmonary embolism, it is all-important. At the onset of embolism, it is "invariably" over 20 and frequently above 30. Respiratory distress may appear in transient episodes lasting only a few minutes; more commonly it persists for about 48 h. This hyperventilation is reflected in the arterial blood gases, which demonstrate a reduction in P_{CO_2} and mild respiratory alkalosis. The arterial P_{O_2} is decreased (< 90 mm Hg) in nearly every patient with acute pulmonary embolism, even when embolism is minor.[22]

PULMONARY HYPERTENSION AND RIGHT VENTRICULAR FAILURE
The rise of pressure in the pulmonary artery is of course generated by the right ventricle and occurs with great rapidity, i.e., in the course of a few beats. If embolism is sufficiently massive to occlude more than 60 percent of the pulmonary circulation, the sudden strain put on the right ventricle results in its dilatation and in the rise of its diastolic filling pressure, right atrial pressure, and systemic venous pressures. Venous distension and hepatic enlargement

and tenderness ensue. Tachycardia is the rule. The pulmonic component of the second heart sound may become accentuated and even palpable. The venous pulse may exhibit large *a* waves if cardiac rhythm is normal sinus. There may also be large *v* waves as a result of tricuspid incompetence. Rarely atrial fibrillation or atrial flutter suddenly appears.

The sudden appearance of signs of right ventricular failure, distended neck veins, parasternal heave, and gallop rhythm in a patient without heart disease is highly suggestive of acute, massive pulmonary embolism.

REDUCTION OF CARDIAC OUTPUT

Syncope and shock: Pulmonary embolism may produce transient dizziness or actual syncope lasting for only a few minutes. With massive embolism a typical shock picture supervenes. The patient is cold, clammy, and sweaty, and the blood pressure is low or unobtainable by cuff method. The patient is weak and pale. The pulse is rapid, small, and thready. This circulatory collapse may persist for hours.

Anginal pain: Crushing substernal pain indistinguishable from that of an acute coronary occlusion with myocardial infarction may occur as a result of massive embolism and is attributable to the reduction of coronary blood flow because of low aortic pressure in the face of a high right ventricular work load because of pulmonary and right ventricular hypertension. This pain, together with heart failure and shock, and the electrocardiogram may be indistinguishable at the onset from the picture of posterior myocardial infarction. Sometimes it takes several days for the pattern of one or the other to evolve. Fortunately medical treatment of these two conditions does not differ basically.

LEFT VENTRICULAR FAILURE
It is not quite clear why the left ventricle should fail in this condition, since it is located distal to the circulatory obstruction and its work load in terms of pressure and flow is reduced. The normal heart does not fail in shock except perhaps terminally. Left ventricular failure as a result of pulmonary embolism is seen almost exclusively in patients with underlying disease of the left ventricle. Pulmonary edema may occur in these patients as a complication of pulmonary embolism. Thus, the manifestations of global heart failure with pulmonary edema and hepatomegaly and venous distension may occur as a result of embolism.

OTHER MANIFESTATIONS
Cyanosis is common and may occur as a fleeting episode or may be present for a number of days. Usually clinically detectable cyanosis is accompanied by an arterial oxygen saturation less than 85

percent. Even when cyanosis is not apparent, hypoxemia is almost always evident from analysis of arterial blood gases.

Apprehension is a common symptom and is similar to that seen in association with coronary occlusion. It is a sensation of impending disaster. The symptom is usually observed after the embolism has occurred, and in retrospect it sometimes turns out to be the initial manifestation of embolism, there being no other symptoms or signs to account for the patient's anxiety.

Radiologic findings may consist of an area of translucency essentially devoid of vascular markings in an area distal to the obstruction of a major vessel, or the vascular markings in one lobe or even in one lung may be considerably diminished as compared with those of the opposite lung. Another finding is dilatation of the main trunk of the pulmonary artery, the right ventricle, right atrium, and azygos vein and a regression toward normal in ensuing days. Heart size may change temporarily because of dilatation of the right ventricle and of the main trunk of the pulmonary artery. All these changes occur immediately following embolic occlusion. The frequency with which such findings are detected depends on the size and location of the embolus, the degree of pulmonary hypertension that ensues, the care with which the roentgenograms are interpreted, and comparison of sequential films.

Electrocardiographic changes of acute pulmonary embolism are diagnostic in only about 10 percent of cases and are best observed immediately after the embolic event. These near diagnostic changes occur only when embolism has been sufficiently massive to cause acute cor pulmonale.[21,23]

They may consist of right axis deviation, S-1, Q-3 pattern, depressed ST-1 and ST-2, flat or inverted T-2 and T-3, and P pulmonale in the standard leads. In the precordial leads, there may be clockwise rotation of the heart, upright R waves with inverted ST segments over the right precordium, or an rsR′ configuration in V_1 suggesting incomplete right bundle branch block. Inferior myocardial infarction may be confused electrocardiographically with acute pulmonary embolism because of the presence of Q waves and inverted T waves in leads II, III, and aV_F. Vectorcardiography has not increased diagnostic precision. Other changes which have no diagnostic implications consist of nonspecific T-wave changes, and these are found in about 75 percent of cases. Posterior rotation of the mean T vector with inverted T waves in the right precordial leads may be noted.

Natural course of pulmonary embolism[1a]

From the foregoing, it is seen that pulmonary embolism is abrupt in onset. Depending on the size of the embolus, the episode of disability is mild, moderate, or devastating. Of the patients who die, about one-half die within $1/2$ h of the onset, two-thirds within 1

h, and three-fourths within 1 h. Those who recover begin to improve promptly. Follow-up studies of patients with angiographically documented acute pulmonary embolism have indicated that in some patients the pulmonary angiogram and right-sided heart pressures may be completely normal 2 to 3 weeks after the acute episode. Although resolution may take longer in some patients, persistence of embolic obstruction with consequent chronic cor pulmonale is rare. Most patients surviving the acute episode do well if further embolism is prevented.

Chronic recurrent pulmonary embolism and chronic cor pulmonale

Repeated episodes of pulmonary embolism may eventually lead to sustained pulmonary hypertension, right ventricular hypertrophy, chronic right ventricular failure, and death. Shortness of breath is the presenting symptom, followed by easy fatigability and eventually by abdominal distension. There may or may not be a clear-cut history of embolic episodes or of phlebitis. Physical signs may include venous distension with prominent *a* waves and *v* waves, a sternal lift denoting right ventricular hypertrophy, an accentuated pulmonic component of the second heart sound, occasionally a pulmonic systolic murmur, a holosystolic murmur in the lower parasternal area due to tricuspid incompetence, and enlarged liver, ankle edema, but rarely ascites. The electrocardiogram characteristically is indicative of right ventricular hypertrophy. A roentgenogram of the heart shows enlargement of the right ventricle, main trunk of the pulmonary artery, and hilar vessels. The proximal branches of the pulmonary artery may be dilated, whereas the peripheral branches are constricted, giving the comma sign. Peripheral lung fields are oligemic.

Definitive treatment should be instituted, because individuals with these conditions are thrombophilic and the disorder is life-threatening. Many authorities recommend ligation of the inferior vena cava plus anticoagulants for 2 or 3 months postoperatively.

Differentiation from so-called primary pulmonary hypertension may be impossible during life, the latter being a postmortem diagnosis. Patients suspected of having primary pulmonary hypertension should be considered to have recurrent pulmonary embolism and treated accordingly.

DIAGNOSIS AND SPECIAL TESTS

Diagnosis is rarely easy or straightforward. From the foregoing description it is apparent that embolism must be large before any symptoms whatsoever appear, and even then they may not be sufficiently characteristic to be pathognomonic of the condition.

Pulmonary infarction may be easily confused with bronchitis, bronchopneumonia, neoplasm, pleurisy of other cause, atelectasis, or fever of unknown origin. Acute cor pulmonale may at first appear to be a simple syncopal attack, circulatory collapse, an accentuation of preexisting heart failure, or acute myocardial infarction.

Pulmonary embolism is especially difficult to recognize in patients with prior congestive heart failure. Heart disease is one of the most common predispositions to pulmonary embolism, and when it occurs in this setting the mortality is inordinately high. For this reason, one must maintain a constant vigilance for signs or symptoms of venous thromboembolism in patients with heart disease.

A number of clinical clues are helpful although not diagnostic. If any of the following are present, one must think in terms of pulmonary embolism but at the same time realize that other possibilities exist: (1) any pulmonary or cardiac abnormality in the presence of deep phlebitis of the legs; (2) congestive heart failure without obvious cause; (3) unexplained dyspnea and tachypnea; (4) blood-streaked or grossly bloody sputum; (5) pleurisy; (6) unexplained rise of temperature and more rapid pulse and respiration; (7) unexplained deterioration in chronic pulmonary disease; (8) "refractory" heart failure.

Special techniques (pulmonary angiography and lung scanning) have greatly enhanced the diagnosis of pulmonary embolism (see Chaps. 29B and 29C). These two procedures should be regarded as complementary, not competitive. Pulmonary angiography has been found to be safe in experienced hands even in desperately ill patients. Selective injection of radiopaque material into the pulmonary artery with sequential films is currently the most accurate method of establishing the diagnosis. It requires a well-trained team and is not simple to perform.[24–27]

Lung perfusion scanning[27a] consists of the intravenous injection of ^{131}I-tagged human serum albumin which by appropriate heating, acidification, and agitation consists of aggregates of particles of approximately 50 to 150 μm in size. Many of these particles are caught in the lung and remain there for a period of 2 h or more. External scanning of the normal lung reveals homogeneous dissemination of radioactive particles. Large embolic occlusions result in areas of absent radioactivity. Lung scans are most consistent with pulmonary embolism when they show abnormalities in the presence of a normal roentgenogram of the chest (see Chaps. 29B and 29C). When there are pulmonary abnormalities, the scan must be interpreted in relation to these abnormalities. Lung scans are simple to perform and can be performed repeatedly. A normal lung scan excludes pulmonary embolism.

Ventilation scanning[27a] of the lungs consists of inhaling radioactive xenon, holding the breath, and scanning the lung. This ventilation scan is then compared with the perfusion scan. The characteristic findings in pulmonary embolism are multiple segmental perfusion defects that ventilate normally.

Upon suspicion of embolism: (1) The patient should receive 7,500 to 10,000 units heparin intravenously immediately, followed by (2) routine chest x-ray and (3) electrocardiogram. (4) Arterial blood oxygen tension should be obtained; if the arterial P_{O_2} is above 90 mm Hg, it is unlikely that pulmonary embolism is present. (5) If the deep veins of the legs are normal by contrast phlebography or by imped-

ance phlebography, pulmonary embolism is unlikely. If at this point, pulmonary embolism *is* a likely possibility, (6) perfusion and ventilation lung scanning should be carried out. If the perfusion scan is normal, pulmonary embolism has not occurred. If positive, it is consistent with but not diagnostic of pulmonary embolism. If there is a segmental perfusion-ventilation mismatch, there is a strong but not completely diagnostic likelihood of pulmonary embolism. If clinical suspicion is still high but the above tests are nondiagnostic or equivocal, (7) pulmonary angiography should be performed. If positive, a therapeutic plan should be instituted. If negative, pulmonary embolism can be considered not to have occurred. The majority of patients should have pulmonary angiography, especially if surgical intervention is contemplated.

MORTALITY AND PROGNOSIS

The mortality rate of each episode of embolism of a size sufficient to produce symptoms lies between 20 and 38 percent. Between one-third and one-half the patients have subsequent episodes of embolism, and in 20 percent the subsequent embolus is fatal.

TREATMENT[28,29]

Treatment or prophylaxis should be instituted when there is a "generous suspicion" that embolism has occurred, because of the likelihood of further episodes, the high mortality rate of each episode, and the efficacy of prophylaxis. Therapy should not be deferred until the diagnosis is confirmed by lung scanning or pulmonary angiography.

Treatment is directed toward supportive measures during the acute episode and prevention of subsequent episodes.

Treatment of attack

For the acute attack, intravenous heparin is the treatment of choice. There is evidence that heparin in a dosage higher than that required to block thrombin-fibrinogen interaction has a specific effect in relieving bronchoconstriction and perhaps the high pulmonary vascular resistance. Several papers have shown striking success by using a high dosage of heparin intravenously in patients with massive pulmonary embolism, in whom the prognosis is usually considered to be ominous. Table 75-6 represents a recommended dosage of heparin which is tailored to the severity of the thromboembolic process.

The incidence of bleeding is determined not by the dose of heparin but by a defect in the wall of a blood vessel. Therefore, contraindications to anticoagulants must be observed; anticoagulants must not be given to potential bleeders, e.g., those with active

TABLE 75-6
Recommended dosage of heparin for types of thromboembolism

Type of thromboembolism	Heparin dosage
Venous thrombosis; no embolism	7,500 U I.V. q. 6 h. for 7 days. Clotting time at 5 h. Warfarin on day 2 with 5-day changeover from heparin.
Minor embolism without hypotension or shock	7,500–10,000 U. I.V. q. 4–6 h. for 7 days as above.
Massive embolism with hypotension and shock	12,500–15,000 U. I.V. stat; then 10,000–15,000 U. I.V. q. 4 h. until stable; then 7,500–10,000 U. (as indicated by clotting time) q. 4–6 h. for 7–10 days.

peptic ulcer, esophageal varices, any hemorrhagic diatheses, severe liver or kidney disease, severe hypertension, intracranial disease, and those who have had recent surgery on brain, spinal cord, joints, or genitourinary tract. For apprehension, pain, and respiratory distress, intravenous morphine sulfate may be required. Meperidine hydrochloride (Demerol) is less effective. Oxygen should be administered by nasal catheter or oxygen mask. Hypotension and shock may require an intravenous infusion of isoproterenol, 1 mg diluted in 500 ml of 5 percent dextrose in water, or the more potent 1-norepinephrine bitartrate (Levophed), 2 ml of 0.2 percent in 500 ml of 5 percent dextrose in water. The rate of infusion is determined by the response of the blood pressure.

For either shock or heart failure, rapid digitalization is indicated but with due caution because of hypoxia, which predisposes to myocardial irritability.

Embolectomy[30]

Embolectomy (Trendelenburg's operation) was introduced at the turn of the century but met with only occasional success. The introduction of cardiopulmonary bypass has made the performance of embolectomy more feasible. However, the surgical risk of embolectomy remains over 50 percent, partly because of misdiagnosis and partly because the operation is often performed on patients who are in profound shock. Many, or perhaps most, patients who require embolectomy die before it can be performed. Conversely, many patients who survive embolectomy might have survived with less vigorous therapy.

The primary indication for embolectomy is the presence of shock, resistant to vasopressors, in a patient with bilateral central pulmonary emboli documented by pulmonary angiography. In this set of circumstances, embolectomy may be lifesaving. In the absence of shock, pulmonary embolectomy is not indicated even if massive pulmonary embolism is documented by angiography. Such patients will survive without embolectomy if further embolism is prevented.

Fibrinolytic therapy[28]

The search for an agent that will safely dissolve thromboemboli in human beings has been long and complex. The two agents that have been most extensively studied are streptokinase and urokinase. The efficacy of urokinase in the treatment of acute pulmonary embolism in human beings has been assessed in a random, national cooperative trial sponsored by the National Heart and Lung Institute.

In this trial, conducted at 16 different hospitals, patients were treated by a common protocol. One-half the patients were treated with a 12-h infusion of urokinase, while the other group was treated with a 12-h infusion of heparin. After completion of the 12-h infusion, therapy was the same in both groups. Pulmonary angiography and catheterization of the right side of the heart were repeated after the infusion of heparin or urokinase, and multiple lung scans were obtained over a period of 2 weeks.

The repeat pulmonary angiograms demonstrated more resolution of embolism in the group treated with urokinase. It should be noted that the degree of resolution was quite modest, 1.56 on a scale of 4. Five days after treatment, the resolution as determined by lung scan was the same in both groups. The hospital mortality was the same for both groups.

Hemorrhagic complications were significant. Moderate or severe bleeding occurred in 27 percent of the heparin group and in 45 percent of the patients treated with urokinase.

Although these early results are somewhat encouraging, the modest degree of resolution and the major bleeding complication indicate that urokinase is not yet appropriate for clinical use.

A second study compared a 24-h infusion of urokinase with that of streptokinase in 167 patients with angiographically confirmed pulmonary embolism. Urokinase and streptokinase were equally effective. There was no significant increase of benefit from 24 h of infusion over 12 h. Significant bleeding occurred in more than one-third of the patients and was sufficiently severe in 14 percent as to require transfusion. It is concluded that the role of these agents in the management of thromboembolism remains to be determined.

Prevention of another attack

Prevention of another embolic episode requires recognition of the first one and then consists of general measures to prevent venous thrombosis: anticoagulants and/or venous interruption.

GENERAL MEASURES
These measures consist of early ambulation, elevation of the legs in order to prevent venous stasis, use of elastic stockings or Ace bandages in an effort to maintain superficial venous collapse and increased velocity of flow in deep veins, avoidance of pressure points that obstruct venous return, and leg exercises.

ANTICOAGULANTS[29]
Heparin, the cornerstone of therapy, is continued for 7 to 10 days as outlined in Table 75-6. Anticoagula-

tion with warfarin is usually begun on the second to fourth day of heparin therapy. It is vital that treatment be maintained at a high level as long as there is an underlying predisposition to thromboembolism. In the patient who has had a fracture, this should be 2 months after the cast is removed and the patient becomes ambulatory. In the cardiac patient or other patients with a continued predisposition to embolism, anticoagulant treatment should be permanent.

In recent years, heparin at blood concentrations too low to produce an anticoagulant effect as judged by conventional clotting tests has been used with the purpose of preventing thromboembolism. The dose of heparin usually used is 5,000 units every 8 or 12 h. Because of conflicting reports, the efficacy of low dose heparin among certain patients is unclear and its final place in prophylaxis against venous thromboembolism remains to be established.

VENOUS INTERRUPTION[31]

Ligation of the superficial femoral veins bilaterally has had a high failure rate in preventing embolism because of passage of the clot by way of the deep femoral vein. The procedure has been abandoned. Bilateral common femoral vein ligation is simple to perform and entails essentially no risk, but further embolism has occurred in 5 to 10 percent of cases, usually because the clot was above the tie at time of surgery. Interruption of the vena cava just below the renal veins has a risk of 2 to 5 percent in patients without heart disease. If the patient is in left-sided heart failure, the inhospital risk has been 20 percent; if he is in left- and right-sided heart failure, the risk is 50 percent. Essentially the same risk exists for femoral vein ligation, which indicates not the operative risk but the high mortality rate of thromboembolism in patients with prior heart failure. If a pelvic source of embolism exists, the left ovarian vein also must be ligated. This does not result in interruption of pregnancy or of future pregnancies. Interruption of the vena cava is highly (98 percent) effective in the prevention of further embolism. Although it has been said that it results in considerable leg vein disability, most authorities claim an equal degree of disability from leg vein thrombosis in controls who were not operated on. Interruption of the inferior vena cava is indicated (1) when embolism occurs in patients receiving anticoagulants, (2) when anticoagulants are contraindicated, (3) when diseases predisposing to venous thrombosis and pulmonary embolism are prominent and persistent, (4) when septic embolism occurs, and (5) in some patients with massive embolism in whom further embolism would be fatal.

To avoid general anesthesia and a major surgical operation, Mobin-Uddin devised a transvenous catheter method for interruption of the inferior vena cava with an intracaval device of an umbrella design.[32] Indications for this procedure have been recurrent embolism despite adequate anticoagulant therapy; conditions in which anticoagulants are contraindicated; massive embolism with shock; following pulmonary embolectomy; high-risk patients with deep venous thrombosis awaiting a surgical procedure; iliofemoral thrombosis not responding to anticoagulants; and patients undergoing hip nailing. In 2,215

patients in whom this filter was implanted, recurrent embolism was reported in 3 percent, fatal in 0.8 percent. Filter migration with 28-mm filters has been reduced to about 1 percent. Other complications are largely on the basis of inexperience. This appears to be another useful procedure of prophylaxis.

PREGNANCY

The treatment of pulmonary embolism during pregnancy presents a therapeutic problem. Preventive measures must continue throughout pregnancy and the puerperium. Heparin does not cross the placental barrier, presents no hazard to the fetus, but is difficult to administer for more than 2 weeks. Coumarin derivatives cross the placenta and result in an 18 percent fetal mortality. Interruption of the pregnancy to avert further embolism is not satisfactory because of the loss of the fetus. Ligation of femoral veins does not protect against emboli arising from pelvic and gluteal veins. Interruption of the inferior vena cava *and* left ovarian vein is a highly effective preventive procedure. It entails a surgical risk of about 2 percent in experienced hands. There is little risk of miscarriage after the first trimester, and there is no interference with future pregnancies. The above points indicate that interruption of the inferior vena cava is the treatment of choice to prevent further pulmonary embolism during pregnancy.[33]

SPECIAL TYPES OF EMBOLISM[*]

Fat embolism[34,35]

The entrance of free globules of fat into systemic veins most often occurs after fractures of long bones, especially of the tibia and femur after automobile accidents. It may also occur following direct injury of subcutaneous fat tissue by contusion, concussion, or burns; childbirth or poisoning; the use of a pump oxygenator; or simulated high-altitude flights. Some less common causes include alcoholism, fatty metamorphosis of the liver, decompression sickness, sickle-cell crisis, multiple blood transfusions, sternal splitting incisions for cardiac surgery, and external cardiac massage.

The exact pathophysiology of the fat embolism syndrome is unknown and probably is different in different patients. At least some of the fatty emboli are due to the release of depot fat from traumatized bone and tissues,[34,36,37] since myeloid tissues can occasionally be identified in the pulmonary vessels. There is also evidence that physicochemical alterations in the natural emulsion of circulating fats result in the production of macroglobules of fat that act as emboli. Other mechanisms that have been suggested as contributing to the syndrome include defects in the coagulation system,[38,39] traumatic shock, excess

[*]This section was written by Robert C. Schlant, M.D.

free fatty acidemia, and the liberation of toxic free fatty acids in the lungs from the embolic fat by enzymatic hydrolysis.[40] The often sudden drop in hematocrit is usually related to blood losses in fractured extremities, extensive pulmonary hemorrhages, or, rarely, an associated disseminated intravascular coagulation (DIC).

The fat droplets are of varied size and obstruct branches of the pulmonary artery of all sizes, including arterioles and capillaries. In addition, there is often extensive intrapulmonary hemorrhage and damage to the pulmonary parenchyma. The fat globules that traverse the pulmonary circulation block arterioles and capillaries of the brain, skin, kidney, heart, and other organs.

Clinically, there is usually a lucid interval of 6 h to several days following the trauma before the first symptoms or signs of fat embolism appear. Most features of the syndrome result from fat emboli either to the lungs or to the brain. The manifestations of the pulmonary fat emboli are basically those described above, although patients with fat embolism syndrome are perhaps more likely to have copious bronchial secretions, which may be hemorrhagic. The cerebral symptoms, which may occur simultaneously with or after the pulmonary symptoms, include headache, restlessness, increasing irritability, disorientation, delirium, convusions, stupor, and coma.

The signs of systemic fat embolism include petechiae, especially of the anterior chest, axillary folds, neck, fundi, and conjunctiva. Rarely, fat emboli may be seen in the retinal vessels. Biopsy of the skin petechiae may demonstrate fat globules. In other patients, the petechiae, whether spontaneous or induced, are related to the frequently associated thrombocytopenia. A frozen section of clotted blood examined for fat may be of early diagnostic value, particularly in patients with an arterial P_{O_2} less than 60 mm Hg.[41] Serum calcium may be decreased, presumably because of the interaction between the increased fatty acids and calcium, whereas serum lipase and tributyrinase concentrations are usually elevated. The findings of fat droplets in sputum or urine are suggestive but not diagnostic.[42] The chest roentgenogram may show diffuse, fluffy infiltrates or only hazy, fine stippling throughout both lungs.

There is no specific therapy for fat embolism, and the most important principle is the maintenance of pulmonary function. It is important to correct the arterial hypoxia, which is almost always present and occasionally quite marked, by whatever means are necessary: a mask, an endotracheal tube, or even a tracheostomy and assisted circulation. Although 100 percent oxygen may be initially necessary, this should later be reduced to 40 percent to avoid oxygen toxicity. Frequent determinations of arterial blood gas concentrations are necessary. Recently, massive doses of corticosteroids have been shown to be very useful and lifesaving, although there are no adequately controlled clinical trials.[43,44] The use of low doses of heparin has frequently been recommended in order to decrease platelet adhesiveness. Theoretically, however, the stimulatory effect of heparin upon lipase activity in the lung might be detrimental by increasing the amount of toxic fatty acids in the lungs. Also unproven are the alleged therapeutic benefits of low molecular weight dextran,[45] intravenous ethyl alcohol, hypothermia, or various detergents.

Air embolism[46]

Air may enter the nervous system in the course of intravenous infusions, pneumoperitoneum, knee-chest position in the puerperium, uterine douches, surgical procedures on the neck or brain, retroperitoneal air injection, irrigation of nasal sinuses, tubal or vaginal insufflation, or rapid decompression. The lethal dose varies with the age, condition, and position of the patient and the rapidity of air entry. It varies between 5 and 15 ml/kg. Death results either from an "air lock" in the right ventricle or from air embolism to the lungs with obstruction in addition to secondary reflex pulmonary vasoconstriction.[46,47] It is likely that only very minute (if any) volumes of air traverse the pulmonary capillaries. Clinically, air embolism is associated with the sudden onset of dyspnea, shock, and cyanosis in association with a loud continuous churning or "mill-house" murmur or noise over the precordium produced by the air and blood in the right ventricle.

Treatment consists of correction of the cause; turning the patient on the left side with the head in a dependent position in an effort to displace the air bolus from the right ventricular outflow tract to the right ventricular apex and to trap the air in the superior portion of the right atrium; aspiration of air through a needle or catheter inserted into the right ventricle; and the administration of artificial respiration with 100 percent oxygen. Closed-chest cardiac massage has also been used successfully, particularly when the air embolism occurs during a neurosurgical or neck operation.[48]

Amniotic fluid embolism[49-55]

Amniotic fluid embolism as a cause of maternal mortality was first described in 1926 by Meyer[49] and was more firmly established as a clinical syndrome in 1941 by Steiner and Lushbaugh.[50] The incidence has been variably stated from 1 in 8,000 to 1 in 37,323 live births. It remains one of the more common causes of maternal death during labor, delivery, and the immediate postpartum period. Predisposing factors are increased age and parity, premature placental separation, intrauterine fetal death, oversized baby, prolonged and vigorous labor with tumultuous uterine contractions, uterine rupture, large doses of oxytocin, and meconium contamination of amniotic fluid.

The amniotic fluid containing meconium, epithelial squamae, mucin, amorphous debris, lipids, bile pigments, or lanugo enters the maternal circulation either through the venous sinuses of the uteroplacental site or through the endocervical veins. The pulmonary embolic manifestations are primarily due to the solid contents of the amniotic fluid, since most experiments have indicated that filtered amniotic fluid produces minimal pulmonary vascular response. Occasionally, amniotic fluid material can be detected in the vessels of the heart, kidneys, and brain.[51]

In about half the patients who survive the initial pulmonary embolic event, diffuse intravascular coagulation (DIC) develops. This is due to the entry into the circulation of a large amount of thromboplastic substances contained in the amniotic fluid. The coagulation process is initiated, leading to the utilization of factors V and VIII, prothrombin, and fibrinogen. If utilization proceeds more rapidly than repletion, deficiencies of these factors develop. The fibrinolytic enzyme system is activated as a compensatory mechanism, resulting in the production of large amounts of fibrin degradation products, which act as inhibitors of thrombin, interfere with normal fibrin polymerization, and impair platelet function. This process results in severe vaginal hemorrhage. Fibrin deposition throughout the microvasculature aggravates the pulmonary embolic manifestations and also produces hypoperfusion and profound alteration of function of almost every organ in the body.

Clinically, most episodes occur near the end of the first stage of labor and are manifest by the abrupt onset of severe dyspnea, hypotension and shock, tachypnea, tachycardia, cyanosis, evidence of acute cor pulmonale and of pulmonary edema, and apprehension which may rapidly progress to semicoma or coma. Generalized convulsions, cardiac arrest, and death may occur suddenly. Chest pain rarely occurs. About 25 to 50 percent of patients die within the first hour, and the survivors are still at great risk of life from either irreversible shock or the subsequent development of profuse vaginal bleeding. There may be bleeding from venipuncture sites and all body orifices or into skin and mucosa.

The laboratory findings in severe instances reflect gross deficiencies of all coagulation factors, especially low fibrinogen levels in the blood and a low platelet count.

Treatment[52,53] consists of (1) the usual general supportive measures for thromboembolism; (2) immediate evacuation of the uterus to remove the basic cause of the diffuse intravascular coagulation process; (3) for hemorrhage, administration of fresh blood or plasma and platelets; and (4) if bleeding persists, the addition of low doses of heparin (5,000 units) as an antithrombin agent. Fibrinogen has been advocated, and its pros and cons have recently been discussed by Jewett.[54] Its benefit is that it promotes clotting and hemostasis. Its disadvantage is that it may produce more deposition of fibrin. The handling of such catastrophes is greatly assisted by monitoring blood pressure, central venous pressure, pulmonary artery pressure with a Swan-Ganz catheter, and urinary output.

Tumor embolism[55–59]

In addition to usual forms of pulmonary metastases resulting from the dissemination of malignant tumors, acute and subacute cor pulmonale may be produced by emboli of malignant tissue cells to the pulmonary arteries and capillaries. These emboli may originate from the primary site of the tumor or from other sites, such as the liver or inferior vena cava, to which the tumor has spread. Tumor emboli occur with virtually any type of malignancy, and their frequency is surely higher than the rarity of reported cases would indicate. Tumor emboli are relatively more common in patients with renal carcinoma, primary hepatic carcinoma, gastric carcinoma, and trophoblastic tumors (chorioepithelioma). Since trophoblastic tumors, even with extensive pulmonary metastases, may respond well to chemotherapy,[56,57] it is imperative to consider this diagnosis whenever a female patient has symptoms of acute dyspnea, pleurisy, cough, or hemoptysis or unexplained signs of pulmonary hypertension following a hydatidiform mole, an abortion, or a normal pregnancy. Occasionally, the pulmonary emboli may not occur until several years after the initiating pregnancy, and the patient may be asymptomatic in the interval, although usually there is amenorrhea, excessive bleeding or discharge, or other disturbances of menses. Since uterine curettage is often negative, diagnosis is best established by estimations of urinary gonadotropin excretion. The radiologic changes in the lungs resulting from metastasis by trophoblastic tumors may take one or more of the following forms: (1) discrete, usually well-defined, and rounded opacities; (2) snowstorm patterns with multiple, small, less-well-defined opacities; and (3) changes resulting from embolic occlusion of the pulmonary arteries without invasion of the lung parenchyma. Of great interest is the recent study of 50 asymptomatic puerperal patients, 13 of whom had pulmonary scan defects thought to be due to asymptomatic trophoblastic emboli.[58]

Cor pulmonale, i.e., right-sided heart failure, occasionally results from hematogenous or lymphogenous spread of tumor. It can be subacute, occurring over the course of a week or 10 days, or slowly growing, when the clinical picture is that of chronic right-sided heart failure.[59]

Rare causes of embolism[60–61]

Among the many very rare forms of pulmonary emboli are those due to cotton fiber; talc or other particulate matter in contaminated heroin; hair; barium sulfate crystals after barium enema; vegetable material; bullets; cardiac catheters; indwelling catheters; bone marrow; brain tissue; parasites; cardiac vegetations; "foam cells" from rupture of atheromata of the large pulmonary artery; liver cells; and bile thromboemboli.

REFERENCES

1 Virchow, R. L. K.: "Cellular Pathology as Based upon Physiological and Pathohistology," translated by Frank Chance, 7th Am. ed., Robert M. DeWitt, New York, 1860, p. 236.

1a Dalen, J. E., and Alpert, J. S.: Natural History of Pulmonary Embolism, *Prog. Cardiovasc. Dis.*, 17(4):259, 1975.

2 Couch, N.: Deep Vein Thrombosis: Causes, Diagnosis, Prevention and Treatment, in J. E. Dalen (ed.), "Pulmonary Embolism," Medcom Press, New York, 1973, p. 6.

3 Kakkar, V. V., and Corrigan, T. P.: Detection of Deep Vein Thrombosis: Survey and Current Status, *Prog. Cardiovasc. Dis.*, 17(3):207, 1974.

4 Virchow, R.: Die Propfbildungen und Verstopfungen in den Gefässen, *Handb. spec. Path. u. Ther,* Erlangen, 1854.

5 Dexter, L.: The Chair and Venous Thrombosis, *Trans. Am. Clin. Climatol. Assoc.,* 84:1, 1973.

6 Handin, R. I.: Thromboembolic Complications of Pregnancy and Oral Contraceptives, *Prog. Cardiovasc. Dis.,* 16(3):395, 1974.

7 Rosenberg, R. D.: Actions and Interactions of Antithrombin and Heparin, *N. Eng. J. Med.,* 292:146, 1975.

8 Rabinov, K., and Paulin, S.: Roentgen Diagnosis of Venous Thrombosis in the Leg, *Arch. Surg.,* 104:134, 1972.

9 Wheeler, H. B., O'Donnell, J. A., Anderson, F. A., Jr., and Benedict, K., Jr.: Occlusive Impedance Phlebography: A Diagnostic Procedure for Venous Thrombosis and Pulmonary Embolism, *Prog. Cardiovasc. Dis.,* 17(3):199, 1974.

10 Dalen, J. E., Mathur, V. S., Evans, H., Haynes, F. W., PurShahriari, A. A., Stein, P. D., and Dexter, L.: Pulmonary Angiography in Experimental Pulmonary Embolism, *Am. Heart J.,* 72:509, 1966.

11 Dalen, J. E., Banas, J., Brooks, H., Evans, G., Paraskos, J., and Dexter, L.: Resolution Rate of Acute Pulmonary Embolism in Man, *N. Engl. J. Med.,* 280:1194, 1969.

12 Dexter, L., and Dalen, J. E.: The Pathophysiology of Pulmonary Embolism, in J. E. Dalen (ed.), "Pulmonary Embolism," Medcom Press, New York, 1973, p. 22.

13 Smith, G. T., Dammin, G. J., and Dexter, L.: Postmortem Arteriographic Studies of the Human Lung in Pulmonary Embolism, *J.A.M.A.,* 188:143, 1964.

14 Hyland, J. W., Piemme, T. E., Alexander, S., Haynes, F. W., Smith, G. T., and Dexter, L.: Behavior of Pulmonary Hypertension Produced by Serotonin and Emboli, *Am. J. Physiol.,* 205:591, 1963.

15 Dexter, L., and Smith, G. T.: Quantitative Studies of Pulmonary Embolism, *Am. J. Med. Sci.,* 247:641, 1964.

16 Mathur, V. S., Dalen, J. E., Evans, H., Haynes, F. W., PurShahriari, A. A., Stein, P. D., and Dexter, L.: Pulmonary Angiography One to Seven Days after Experimental Pulmonary Embolism, *Invest. Radiol.,* 2:304, 1967.

17 McIntyre, K. M., and Sasahara, A. A.: Hemodynamic and Ventricular Responses to Pulmonary Embolism, *Prog. Cardiovasc. Dis.,* 17(3):175, 1974.

18 Stein, P. D., Alshabkhoun, S., Hatem, C., PurShahriari, A. A., Haynes, F., Harken, D. E., and Dexter, L.: Coronary Artery Blood Flow in Acute Pulmonary Embolism, *Am. J. Cardiol.,* 21:32, 1968.

19 Stein, P. D., Alshabkhoun, S., Hawkins, H. F., Hyland, J. W., and Jarrett, C. E.: Right Coronary Blood Flow in Acute Pulmonary Embolism, *Am. Heart J.,* 77:356, 1969.

20 Stein, M., and Levy, S. E.: Reflex and Humoral Responses to Pulmonary Embolism, *Prog. Cardiovasc. Dis.,* 17(3):167, 1974.

21 Szucs, M. D., Brooks, H. L., Grossman, W., Banas, J. S., Meister, S. G., Dexter, L., and Dalen, J. E.: Diagnostic Sensitivity of Laboratory Findings in Acute Pulmonary Embolism, *Ann. Intern. Med.,* 74:161, 1971.

22 Sasahara, A. A.: Current Problems in Pulmonary Embolism, *Prog. Cardiovasc. Dis.,* 17(3):161, 1974.

23 Stein, P. D., Dalen, J. E., McIntyre, K. M., Sasahara, A. A., Wenger, N. K., and Willis, P. W., III: The Electrocardiogram in Acute Pulmonary Embolism, *Prog. Cardiovasc. Dis.,* 17(4):247, 1975.

24 Stein, P. D., O'Connor, J. F., Dalen, J. E., PurShahriari, A. A., Hoppin, F. G., Hammond, D. T., Haynes, F. W., Fleischner, F. G., and Dexter, L.: The Angiographic Diagnosis of Acute Pulmonary Embolism: Evaluation of Criteria, *Am. Heart J.,* 73:730, 1967.

25 Sasahara, A. A., Stein, M., Simon, M., and Littmann, D.: Pulmonary Angiography in the Diagnosis of Thromboembolic Disease, *N. Engl. J. Med.,* 270:1075, 1964.

26 Dalen, J. E., Brooks, H. L., Johnson, L. W., Meister, S. G., Szucs, M. M., and Dexter, L.: Pulmonary Angiography in Acute Pulmonary Embolism: Indications, Techniques, and Results in 367 Patients, *Am. Heart J.,* 81:175, 1971.

27 Tow, D. E., and Simon, A. L.: Comparison of Lung Scanning and Pulmonary Angiography in the Detection and Follow-up of Pulmonary Embolism: The Urokinase-Pulmonary Embolism Trial Experience, *Prog. Cardiovasc. Dis.,* 17(4):239, 1975.

27a Wagner, H. N., and Strauss, H. W.: Radioactive Tracers in the Differential Diagnosis of Pulmonary Embolism, *Prog. Cardiovasc. Dis.,* 17(4):271, 1975.

28 Genton, E., and Hirsh, J.: Observations in Anticoagulant and Thrombolytic Therapy in Pulmonary Embolism, *Prog. Cardiovasc. Dis.,* 17(5):335, 1975.

29 Clagett, G. P., and Saltzman, E. W.: Prevention of Venous Thromboembolism, *Prog. Cardiovasc. Dis.,* 17(5):345, 1975.

30 Sautter, R. D., Myers, W. O., Ray, J. F., III, and Wenzel, F. J.: Pulmonary Embolectomy: Review and Current Status, *Prog. Cardiovasc. Dis.,* 17(5):371, 1975.

31 Crane, C.: Venous Interruption for Pulmonary Embolism: Present Status, *Prog. Cardiovasc. Dis.,* 17(5):329, 1975.

32 Mobin-Uddin, K., Utley, J. R., and Bryant, L. R.: The Inferior Vena Cava Umbrella Filter, *Prog. Cardiovasc. Dis.,* 17(5):391, 1975.

33 Evans, G., Dalen, J. E., and Dexter, L.: Pulmonary Embolism during Pregnancy, *J.A.M.A.,* 206:320, 1968.

34 Peltier, L. F.: The Diagnosis and Treatment of Fat Embolism, *J. Trauma,* 11:661, 1971.

35 Herndon, J. H., Riseborough, E. J., and Fischer, J. E.: Fat Embolism: A Review of Current Concepts, *J. Trauma,* 11:673, 1971.

36 Gauss, H.: The Pathology of Fat Embolism, *Arch. Surg.,* 9:593, 1924.

37 Kerstell, J.: Pathogenesis of Post-Traumatic Fat Embolism, *Am. J. Surg.,* 121:712, 1971.

38 Bradford, D. S., and Dick, H. M.: Fat Embolism: Report of a Case and Discussion of Current Concepts of Pathogenesis and Treatment, *Clin. Orthop.,* 65:218, 1969.

39 Bradford, D. S., Foster, R. R., and Nossel, H. L.: Coagulation Alterations, Hypoxemia, and Fat Embolism in Fracture Patients, *J. Trauma,* 10:307, 1971.

40 Fonte, D. A., and Hausberger, F. X.: Pulmonary Free Acids in Experimental Fat Embolism, *J. Trauma,* 11:668, 1971.

41 Dines, D. E., Linscheid, R. L., and Didier, E. P.: Fat Embolism Syndrome, *Mayo Clin. Proc.,* 47:237, 1972.

42 Tedeschi, C. G., Castelli, W., Kropp, G., and Tedeschi, L. G.: Fat Macroglobulinemia and Fat Embolism, *Surg. Gynecol. Obstet.,* 11:177, 1967.

43 Liljedahl, S., and Westermark, L.: Aetiology and Treatment of Fat Embolism: Report of Five Cases, *Acta Anaesthesiol. Scand.,* 11:177, 1967.

44 Fischer, J. E., Turner, R. H., Herndon, J. H., and Riseborough, E. J.: Massive Steroid Therapy in Severe Fat Embolism, *Surg. Gynecol. Obstet.,* 132:667, 1971.

45 Rokkanen, P., Lahdensuu, M., Kataja, J., and Julkunen, H.: The Syndrome of Fat Embolism: Analysis of Thirty Consecutive Cases Compared to Trauma Patients with Similar Injuries, *J. Trauma,* 10:299, 1971.

46 Berglund, E., and Josephson, S.: Pulmonary Air Embolization

in the Dog: I. Hemodynamic Changes in Repeated Emboliza-
tions, *Scand. J. Clin. Invest.*, 26:97, 1970.

47 Josephson, S.: Pulmonary Air Embolization in the Dog: II.
Evidence and Location of Pulmonary Vasoconstriction, *Scand.
J. Clin. Lab. Invest.*, 26:113, 1970.

48 Ericsson, J. A., Gottlieb, J. D., and Sweet, R. B.: Closed-Chest
Cardiac Massage in the Treatment of Venous Air Embolism,
N. Engl. J. Med., 270:1353, 1964.

49 Meyer, J. R.: Embolia Pulmonar Amino-Caseosa, *Brasil Med.*,
2:301, 1926.

50 Steiner, P. E., and Luschbaugh, C. C.: Maternal Pulmonary
Embolism by Amniotic Fluid as a Cause of Obstetric Shock
and Unexpected Deaths in Obstetrics, *J.A.M.A.*, 117:1245,
1941.

51 Liban, E., and Raz, S.: A Clinicopathologic Study of Fourteen
Cases of Amniotic Fluid Embolism, *Am. J. Clin. Pathol.*,
51:477, 1969.

52 Williams, W. J., Beutler, E., Erslev, A. J., and Rundles, R. W.:
"Hematology," McGraw-Hill Book Company, New York,
1972.

53 Wintrobe, M. D.: "Clinical Hematology," 7th ed., Lea &
Febiger, Philadelphia, 1974.

54 Jewett, J. F.: Amniotic-Fluid Infusion, *N. Engl. J. Med.*,
292:973, 1975.

55 Peterson, E. P., and Taylor, H. B.: Amniotic Fluid Embolism:
An Analysis of 40 Cases, *Obstet. Gynecol.*, 35:787, 1970.

56 Bagshawe, K. D., and Noble, M. I. M.: Cardiorespiratory
Aspects of Trophoblastic Tumors, *Q. J. Med.*, 35:39, 1966.

57 Li, M. C.: Trophoblastic Disease: Natural History, Diagnosis,
and Treatment, *Ann. Intern. Med.*, 74:102, 1971.

58 Ross, M., Nowicki, K., and Rangarajan, N. S.: Asymptomatic
Pulmonary Embolism During Pregnancy, *Obstet. Gynecol.*,
37:131, 1971.

59 Durhan, J. R., Ashley, P. F., and Dorenclamp, D.: Cor pulmonale Due to Tumor Emboli: Review of Literature and Report of
a Case, *J.A.M.A.*, 175:757, 1961.

60 Mehta, S., and Rubenstone, A. I.: Pulmonary Bile Thromboemboli: A Report of Two Cases, *Am. J. Clin. Pathol.*, 47:490,
1967.

61 Dimmick, J. E., Bove, K. E., McAdams, A. J., and Benzing, G.,
III: Fiber Embolization—Hazard of Cardiac Surgery and Catheterization, *N. Engl. J. Med.*, 292:685, 1975.

76
Chronic Cor Pulmonale

NEIL T. FELDMAN, M.D., and
ROLAND H. INGRAM, JR., M.D.

Chronic elevation of pulmonary arterial pressure due
to decrease in the effective pulmonary vascular
cross-sectional area leads to right ventricular hypertrophy. Chronic cor pulmonale has been defined as
some combination of hypertrophy and dilatation of
the right ventricle due to hypertension of the pulmonary circulation, the cause of which lies within the
pulmonary parenchyma and/or within the pulmonary
vascular system between the origin of the main
pulmonary artery and the entry of the pulmonary
veins into the left atrium.[1] This definition specifically
excludes pulmonary vascular changes resulting from

chronic increases in left atrial pressure and chronic
increases in pulmonary blood flow due to left-to-right
intracardiac shunts. Even when so strictly defined,
chronic cor pulmonale includes many disease states
with diverse etiologies, different pathophysiologic
alterations, and varying clinical characteristics.

INCIDENCE

The true incidence of chronic cor pulmonale is
difficult, if not impossible, to define. The factors
creating the difficulty are that the primary diagnosis
is often entered on the death certificate without any
mention of the complication of chronic cor pulmonale, the infrequency with which chronic cor pulmonale is diagnosed clinically, and the nonuniform
application of rigorous pathologic criteria for diagnosing cor pulmonale at the postmorten table.[2] Nonetheless, one can appreciate the potential incidence by
noting that in the United States the mortality rate
from chronic bronchitis and emphysema, the most
common cause of cor pulmonale, was 30,000 in 1970.
This death rate is expected to double every 5 years. A
significant portion of those afflicted with chronic
bronchitis and emphysema can be expected to have
episodes of acute cor pulmonale with respiratory
failure and to develop chronic cor pulmonale at some
time during their illness, which is often terminal. In
this country and in Western Europe the number of
cases of cor pulmonale secondary to other etiologies
is much less common. Despite the uncertainties in
the true incidence of chronic cor pulmonale, many
sources still quote an incidence somewhere between
7 and 10 percent of all heart disease in the United
States. Thus, the disorder is common enough to
require careful attention from cardiologists.

PULMONARY VASCULAR HYPERTENSION

Normal pulmonary circulation

In order to appreciate the interpretation of pulmonary vascular hypertension in pathophysiologic
terms, a brief review of the anatomy and physiology
of the normal pulmonary circulation is often helpful.
Normal pulmonary arteries have thinner walls and
are less muscular than systemic arteries of comparable lumen size, and innervation is relatively sparse.[3]
Less smooth muscle and fewer nerve endings set a
structural basis for more modest vasomotor responses of the pulmonary circulation as compared with the
systemic circulation. Thus, normally the pulmonary
vasculature is a low-resistance circuit which allows
the entire cardiac output to pass through at minimal
driving pressures and hence at a minimal energy
expenditure for the right ventricle. The distension of

larger vessels and recruitment of parallel vessels at the arteriolar and capillary level allow large flow increases that can be accommodated with only small increases in driving pressure. The use of the parallel vascular channels not only decreases the pulmonary vascular resistance but also increases the effective gas exchange surface area.

Reduction of the pulmonary vascular bed

Since the pulmonary circulation is a low-resistance system with large reserves which accommodate large increases of blood flow, rather severe alterations must exist before the occurrence and persistence of pulmonary hypertension. Increased pulmonary vascular resistance results from reduction of the effective vascular cross-sectional area and from an increased viscosity of the blood. An increase in blood flow will aggravate the preexisting pulmonary hypertension. The pulmonary vessels are uniquely and continuously subjected to and influenced by fluctuations in surrounding pressures of the pleural and air spaces. Some investigators have proposed that the wide swings in airway and pleural pressures in obstructive pulmonary diseases contribute to the chronic pulmonary hypertension in these diseases; however, there is not adequate proof for this mechanism. The mechanisms which appear to be established will be considered in sequence with reference to Fig. 76-1.

1 Diffuse anatomic changes in pulmonary arterioles are often secondary to chronic pulmonary hypertension. In

the context of this chapter, the most prominent cause of chronic pulmonary hypertension is some disorder of the pulmonary parenchyma, the reversibility of which will determine the improvement to be expected in the pulmonary vasculature. The onset of anatomic changes intensifies existing pulmonary hypertension and helps to make the process to a great degree irreversible.

a Intimal thickening, whether due to elastosis, fibrosis, or lipid-laden macrophages, often has a patchy distribution and is a regular postmortem finding in subjects beyond the age of 40 who did not have pulmonary hypertension during life.[4] Therefore, the extent of intimal change must be great to account for worsening or perpetuation of pulmonary hypertension. The reversibility of intimal change is unknown, but the fibrotic variety is presumably irreversible.

b Inflammatory changes most often are in association with a systemic illness such as allergic vasculitis or with diffuse inflammatory lung lesions. Inflammatory changes have also been noted secondary to pulmonary hypertension of any cause. By inference the lesions are reversible with subsidence of the inflammatory process unless fibrinoid necrosis and fibrosis result.

c Hypertrophy and hyperplasia of the medial smooth muscle in pulmonary arterioles are regular findings in long-standing pulmonary hypertension and have been shown to be reversible to some extent.[5]

2 Diffuse pulmonary arteriolar constriction is clearly the most reversible of the processes contributing to pulmonary hypertension.

a Alveolar hypoxia has been known to produce pulmonary vasoconstriction since the pioneer studies by Liljestrand and Von Euler in 1948. More recently Fishman has critically reviewed the spate of studies which followed the initial discovery.[6] The bulk of evidence favors a local regional arteriolar constriction rather than a reflex vasoconstriction. Hypoxic vasoconstriction experimentally appears below an alveolar P_{O_2} of 60 mm Hg when the pH of the blood is normal. The resulting diversion of blood flow from lung regions which are hypoventilated represents a compensatory role for hypoxic vasoconstriction which serves to equalize regional ventilation-perfusion abnormalities. However, the wide dispersal of ventilation-perfusion ratios in diffuse parenchymal diseases and the continuous alveolar hypoxia with chronic hypoventilation negate the regionally compensatory role, and pulmonary hypertension results. The arteriolar constriction is quickly reversible following correction of the alveolar hypoxia whether by improving ventilation-perfusion relationships or by giving oxygen therapeutically. The vasoconstrictive response of the pulmonary vasculature to hypoxia has been shown by Fowler and Read to occur in only two-thirds of normal subjects.[7] These authors postulated that the vascular responders to hypoxia are those who would be more prone to develop chronic cor pulmonale with diseases producing widespread alveolar hypoxia. Recently Lindsay and Read have presented evidence in support of this hypothesis.[8]

b Acidemia has been shown clinically to act synergistically with hypoxia in worsening pulmonary hyperten-

FIGURE 76-1 Factors which clinically or experimentally produce or intensify pulmonary hypertension in chronic cor pulmonale are schematically outlined. The factors in parentheses have been shown only experimentally to produce pulmonary vascular smooth muscle contraction. For discussion refer to text.

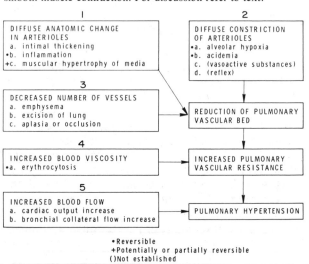

1
DIFFUSE ANATOMIC CHANGE IN ARTERIOLES
a. intimal thickening
•b. inflammation
+c. muscular hypertrophy of media

2
DIFFUSE CONSTRICTION OF ARTERIOLES
•a. alveolar hypoxia
•b. acidemia
c. (vasoactive substances)
d. (reflex)

3
DECREASED NUMBER OF VESSELS
a. emphysema
b. excision of lung
c. aplasia or occlusion

REDUCTION OF PULMONARY VASCULAR BED

4
INCREASED BLOOD VISCOSITY
•a. erythrocytosis

INCREASED PULMONARY VASCULAR RESISTANCE

5
INCREASED BLOOD FLOW
a. cardiac output increase
b. bronchial collateral flow increase

PULMONARY HYPERTENSION

•Reversible
+Potentially or partially reversible
( )Not established

sion.[9] Acidemia alone also has been shown to produce significant increases in pulmonary vascular resistance.[10]

  c Many biologically produced vasoactive substances in the form of various amines, polypeptides, and prostanoic acid relatives have been shown to produce pulmonary vasoconstriction experimentally. Although these substances are present in the body, their role in the production of pulmonary hypertension in human beings remains to be defined.

  d In keeping with the sparsity of smooth muscle and nerves in pulmonary vessels, the reflex effects are minimal. Most often changes in pulmonary arterial pressure are secondary to the more prominent effects on cardiac function in intact animals and in human beings. However, there is evidence suggesting that both arterial and venous constriction occur in response to sympathetic nerve stimulation under controlled flow conditions in dogs.[11] Even if such changes were to be found in human subjects, their physiologic importance would still be uncertain.

3 A decrease in the number of pulmonary vessels need not be associated with significant pulmonary hypertension at resting cardiac outputs. During exercise the normal fall in pulmonary vascular resistance depends in large part on parallel vascular channel recruitment.[3] In the absence of this reserve through loss of vessels, the pulmonary vascular pressure rises to hypertensive levels with an increase in cardiac output. Should a diffuse vascular narrowing process be present as well, or the loss of vessels be extensive enough, then pulmonary hypertension would be present at rest. Extensive resection of lung tissue and severe emphysema best exemplify the decrease in numbers of vessels, though aplasia of pulmonary vessels and chronic vascular occlusions must also be included.

4 Erythrocytosis increases the viscosity of blood whether it is secondary to chronic hypoxemia or an overproduction by the bone marrow from some other cause. In the face of arterial hypoxemia, an increase in oxygen-carrying capacity represents an adaptive mechanism. An increase in blood viscosity with higher hematocrits may offset the benefits of an increased oxygen-carrying capacity. The mechanism by which increased viscosity worsens pulmonary hypertension is not a simple and straightforward one. The viscosity of blood, which is a non-Newtonian fluid, is an inverse function of shear rate.[12] The effects of an increasing hematocrit and a decreasing shear rate associated with slowing of blood flow would be additive and would require a greater driving pressure for a given flow of blood. However, the translation of the basic experimental data into the clinical practice of performing phlebotomy has been made without supportive clinical hemodynamic data. Nonetheless, erythrocytosis with a hematocrit greater than 55 percent is a potential factor in increasing pulmonary hypertension.

5 An increase in pulmonary blood flow due to an increase in cardiac output or to increased bronchial arterial collateral flow accentuates pulmonary hypertension when there is a restricted pulmonary vascular bed. Cardiac output increases may be associated with exercise, infection, or some other increased metabolic state.

Bronchial arterial collateral flow is seldom quantitatively significant except in the case of bronchiectasis.

RIGHT VENTRICULAR RESPONSE TO PULMONARY HYPERTENSION

The analogy has often been made between the left ventricle in systemic arterial hypertension and the right ventricle in pulmonary hypertension. The basic observation is that right ventricular hypertrophy occurs in association with long-standing pulmonary hypertension. Since there is no fundamental difference in configuration and pumping action of the two ventricles before birth, the difference that exists in the adult has been attributed to the difference in resistance to flow.[13] The normal adult right ventricle has relatively thin walls and is crescentic in shape on coronal section of the heart; its pumping action is more akin to that of a bellows in contrast to the concentric contraction of the left ventricle. The right ventricle is better able to handle an increase in volume output than to meet an increased pressure load; whereas the left ventricle is better designed to function in the face of a pressure load.[13] An important change in both configuration and mass of the right ventricle occurs in response to a chronic pressure load. The time base and pressure load required to bring about the right ventricular changes are yet to be studied in patients, so there are no guidelines for prediction available. The increase in right ventricular mass and the alteration of myocardial contractility following pulmonary artery banding in cats is surprisingly rapid and occurs in a matter of days as shown by Spann and colleagues.[14] It is doubtful that the response is as rapid in human beings. In patients with chronic cor pulmonale an additional factor not accounted for by most animal models is the inevitable alteration in blood gases which, in addition to the pressure load, must influence the function of the myocardium. A schematic diagram containing a proposed sequence of events is shown in Fig. 76-2.

LEFT VENTRICULAR FUNCTION IN CHRONIC COR PULMONALE

For some time pathologists have known that left ventricular hypertrophy is found in some patients with chronic cor pulmonale.[15] Neither coronary atherosclerosis, systemic arterial hypertension, valvular disease, nor cardiomyopathy could be found to account for the hypertrophy of the left ventricle. Although the actual cause for left ventricular hypertrophy in association with chronic obstructive pulmonary disease remains speculative,[15a] an explanation for left ventricular dysfunction has been offered

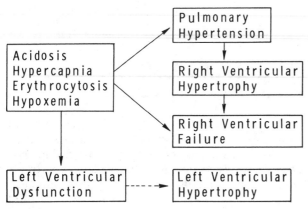

FIGURE 76-2 In the course of chronic cor pulmonale the several factors which lead to right and left ventricular dysfunction are shown schematically. For discussion refer to text.

by Fishman.[15] Combinations of hypoxemia, hypercapnia, acidosis, polycythemia, and diminution of cardiac output are apparently sufficient to depress left ventricular function. Dysfunction with elevation of left ventricular end-diastolic pressure might well be the stimulus for hypertrophy. Since the myocardium is a continuous syncytium of functioning muscle, it is quite possible that both ventricles might to some extent undergo hypertrophy despite the absence of an increased hemodynamic load on the left ventricle. On the other hand, more recent studies have indicated that left ventricular dysfunction is relatively uncommon in patients with cor pulmonale,[17] and, when present, can usually be ascribed to coexistent coronary artery disease.[18] The controversy will undoubtedly continue.

DISEASES ASSOCIATED WITH CHRONIC COR PULMONALE

One or several of the mechanisms for pulmonary hypertension may be operative in the various diseases associated with chronic cor pulmonale. The extent to which each of the mechanisms contributes depends upon the causative disease. Table 76-1 lists diagnoses according to the primary anatomic site of disease or to the primary process leading to chronic cor pulmonale. The list is not exhaustive but does serve as a framework in which to place additional causes with similar processes and anatomic derangements. Irrespective of the category, both pulmonary parenchymal and vascular changes will have occurred by the time cor pulmonale has developed. Thus, arterial hypoxemia with an abnormal alveolar-to-arterial gradient for oxygen is a feature common to all forms.

Many forms of chronic cor pulmonale are associated with alveolar hypoventilation in addition to arterial hypoxemia. Alveolar hypoventilation is defined as an elevation of the arterial P_{CO_2} above 45 mm

TABLE 76-1
Sites of disease and diagnoses associated with cor pulmonale

Pulmonary parenchyma and intrathoracic airways
  Chronic obstructive pulmonary disease*
  Bronchiectasis
  Cystic fibrosis*
  Restrictive lung diseases†
  Pneumoconioses
Chest wall and neuromuscular apparatus‡
  Kyphoscoliosis
  Amyotrophic lateral sclerosis
  Myasthenia gravis
  Myopathies
Inadequate ventilatory drive‡
  Obesity-hypoventilation syndrome
  Failure of automatic control ventilation
  Chronic mountain sickness
Upper airway obstruction‡
  Hypertrophied tonsils and adenoids (infants and children)
Pulmonary vessels
  Primary pulmonary hypertension
  Recurrent pulmonary emboli
  Pulmonary arteritis
  Primary veno-occlusive disease

*Disorders often associated with *net* alveolar hypoventilation.
†Net alveolar hypoventilation terminally.
‡Disorders associated with *general* alveolar hypoventilation.

Hg. The degree of arterial P_{CO_2} elevation is in direct proportion to the inadequacy of alveolar ventilation in relation to metabolic production of carbon dioxide. *Net* alveolar hypoventilation is associated with a normal or increased minute volume. The increased "wasted" ventilation and pulmonary blood flow to inadequately ventilated lung regions leads to hypercapnia despite the normal or increased minute volume. *General* alveolar hypoventilation is associated with an overall decrease in minute volume. The differences in the therapeutic and prognostic implications of the net and general forms of alveolar hypoventilation are significant. In the case of general alveolar hypoventilation the lung parenchyma, airways, and vessels are relatively normal anatomically, and the response of the cor pulmonale to establishing adequate ventilation can be quite dramatic.[19]

Pulmonary parenchyma and intrathoracic airways

CHRONIC OBSTRUCTIVE LUNG DISEASE

To some degree in a given patient, both chronic bronchitis and emphysema almost always are present in combination, but cor pulmonale is restricted to those with functionally significant bronchitis with or without emphysema.[20,21] The obstructive process is diffuse but regionally unequal; this results in maldistribution of inspired air. The reversible bronchial pathologic changes are due to secretions, bronchospasm, mucosal edema, and bronchial wall inflammatory changes. Irreversible fibrotic and atrophic changes may occur in some airways. The distribution of blood flow in relation to ventilation determines the extent and type of the gas exchange derangement found in a given patient. Underventilated lung regions will have hypoxia of both alveolar gas and pulmonary capillary blood. In such regions of low ventilation-perfusion ratios, hypoxic, hypercapnic, and acidotic pulmonary arterial constriction results in some diminution of perfusion to the underventilated region. However, if many such regions are present within the nonuniform lung, pulmonary hypertension supervenes. If the nonuniformity persists and hypoventilated regions with alveolar hypoxia and hypercapnia predominate (net alveolar hypoventilation) cor pulmonale develops.

The extent of the contribution of emphysematous capillary destruction to the pulmonary hypertension is difficult to assess. However, since a patient with predominant emphysema has normal or only slightly elevated pulmonary arterial pressure at rest, the contribution of capillary destruction appears to be minor. Although probably minor as a contributor to pulmonary hypertension at rest, capillary bed destruction with loss of effective alveolar gas exchange surface appears to limit exercise performance.[22]

Erythrocytosis secondary to chronic hypoxemia may be prominent, especially in bronchitic patients. An increase in blood viscosity, red blood cell mass, and blood volume is thought to further compromise the pressure-flow relationships of the constricted and restricted pulmonary vascular bed. However appealing this pathophysiologic mechanism might appear, measurable improvement in either pulmonary hemodynamics or gas exchange or exercise tolerance in patients has not been objectively demonstrated following phlebotomy for secondary erythrocytosis.[23] A double-blind study of phlebotomy in secondary polycythemia did, however, demonstrate an improvement in dyspnea and a decrease in fatigability and headache.[24]

An increase in cardiac output and hence pulmonary blood flow would indeed be an important factor in accentuating the pulmonary hypertension. Measurements of cardiac output during a clinically stable period in these persons or in patients with chronic obstructive pulmonary disease have not often demonstrated an increase in cardiac output in relation to oxygen consumption. Should an increase in cardiac output play an important role in accentuating pulmonary hypertension, no direct therapy can be recommended for the hyperkinetic circulatory state. If a hyperdynamic circulation is present, it is most often secondary to fever and infection or occurs as a result of abnormalities of gas exchange. Collateral channels between the bronchial arteries and veins and the pulmonary circulation are exaggerated in pulmonary emphysema. The collateral flow does not appear to be quantitatively significant, but it is possible that it may contribute to pulmonary hypertension in the presence of a restricted vascular bed. The summation of the various mechanisms leading to alteration of the pressure-flow relationship in the pulmonary vascular bed produces the pulmonary hypertension which in time leads to chronic cor pulmonale. Of all the mechanisms cited, alveolar hypoxia with hypoxic vasoconstriction is the dominant reversible factor.

Clinical manifestations of chronic cor pulmonale with failure are increasing dyspnea, weight gain from fluid retention, and often episodes of cough syncope.

The patient is often cyanotic at rest. The neck veins are distended and do not collapse with inspiration. Pulsations of neck veins are prominent, with giant v waves and rapid y descents indicating tricuspid valvular regurgitation. Right ventricular hypertrophy is indicated by a palpable lower left parasternal or subxiphoid heave. On auscultation, an S_3 gallop accentuated by inspiration and a loud pulmonic second sound are often heard. A lower left parasternal holosystolic murmur accentuated by inspiration usually indicates tricuspid valvular regurgitation. Examination of the lung reveals diffuse rhonchi and wheezes in both phases of respiration. Pedal edema, ascites, and tender hepatic enlargement may be present. Clubbing of the digits is not unusual. The remainder of the clinical signs and symptoms are those that may be found in chronic obstructive lung disease which is not complicated by right ventricular failure.

Reversal of the pulmonary hypertension is based on relief of bronchospasm, treatment of the infection which led to mucosal changes and hypersecretion, and the establishment of bronchial drainage. An increase in regional ventilation serves to alleviate alveolar hypoxia, which in turn relieves pulmonary arterial constriction and improves arterial oxygenation and carbon dioxide elimination. Thus, relief of the obstructive process is the keystone to the therapy and prevention of episodic respiratory insufficiency with right ventricular decompensation. The chest films in Fig. 76-3 are of a patient who had a rewarding and not unusual response to therapy. The response to infusion of aminophylline, which is used mainly as a bronchodilator, also has beneficial hemodynamic effects, as is shown in Fig. 76-4 from the studies of Parker et al.[25]

Avoiding inhalation of irritants, especially cigarette smoke, and episodes of purulent bronchitis is basic to the preventive management. Digitalis preparations and diuretics are often added to the bronchopulmonary drainage and bronchodilator and antibiotic regimens used in therapy of chronic obstructive pulmonary disease when pulmonary hypertension increases and right ventricular failure occurs. Providing adequate oxygenation is essential in the management of acute episodes. If there is increasing hypercapnia and acidosis during oxygen therapy, mechanical ventilatory assistance or control may be necessary. Return to an unassisted air-breathing status must then await successful therapy of the airway disease. The role of phlebotomy is still unclear, but most physicians recommend removal of blood when the hematocrit exceeds 55 to 60 percent.

Ambulatory oxygen therapy appears to be beneficial in the severely hypoxemic ($P_{a,O_2} < 50$ mm Hg) patient with cor pulmonale. There are data demonstrating that pulmonary artery hypertension and polycythemia are partially reversible with continuous low-flow oxygen therapy and may even be improved by nighttime oxygen alone.[26,27] Prior to initiating chronic oxygen therapy it is important to demonstrate that an improvement in hypoxemia is not

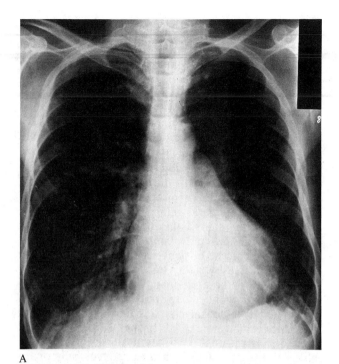

A

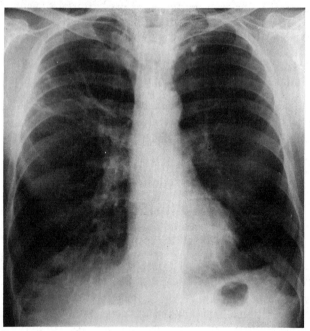

B

FIGURE 76-3 Chest roentgenograms are shown for a 67-year-old man who had chronic obstructive pulmonary disease with evidence of severe emphysema and chronic bronchitis complicated by chronic cor pulmonale and chronic respiratory insufficiency. The film at the top, A, was taken upon admission for an "acute-on-chronic" respiratory insufficiency episode in association with frank right ventricular failure. Bronchopulmonary drainage, antibiotic therapy, improved ventilation and blood oxygenation, aminophylline infusions, and diuretic therapy resulted in symptomatic improvement and a decrease in heart size as shown in B.

Infusion of Aminophylline in COPD
With Cor Pulmonale

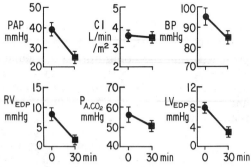

FIGURE 76-4 The mean values ($\pm$SEM) of pulmonary artery pressure (PAP), right ventricular end-diastolic pressure (RV_{EDP}), left ventricular end-diastolic pressure (LV_{EDP}), and mean systemic blood pressure (BP) along with cardiac index (CI) and arterial P_{CO_2} (P_{A,CO_2}) are shown for nine patients with chronic cor pulmonale (Parker et al.[25]). The control values are taken prior to a 1.0-g aminophylline infusion, and the 30-min values are taken at the completion of the infusion. Note that there is no decrease in cardiac output, a significant fall in pulmonary artery pressure and end-diastolic pressures of both ventricles, and a significant improvement in ventilation. *(Plotted from tabular data with the permission of Dr. J. O. Parker.)*

associated with worsening of hypercapnea to dangerous levels.

Asthma rarely, if ever, leads to chronic cor pulmonale unless it is complicated by chronic bronchitis.[21] It is clear, however, that asthma complicated by chronic bronchitis deserves a separate classification because the episodic onset merges over several years into a "wheezy" chronic obstructive pulmonary syndrome. Other than the historical background and prominence of wheezes, the clinical manifestations do not merit special emphasis. Pathophysiologic sequences and therapeutic measures are similar to those applied to chronic obstructive lung disease.

BRONCHIECTASIS

Bronchietasis is associated with dilatation and distortion of airways and with lung tissue destruction and fibrosis which may lead to pulmonary hypertension and chronic cor pulmonale. In such cases, mismatching of ventilation and blood flow, fibrosis with restriction of the pulmonary vascular bed, and extensive anastomoses of the bronchial circulation with the pulmonary circulation contribute to the pulmonary hypertension. A history of chronic cough with copious quantities of purulent secretions leads one to suspect bronchiectasis. The diagnosis is established with certainty only from typical bronchographic findings. Bronchopulmonary drainage, prevention of superimposed acute infections, and prompt antibiotic treatment of any acute infection are the primary therapeutic measures.

CYSTIC FIBROSIS

Cystic fibrosis is also complicated by bronchiectasis. The same pathophysiologic mechanisms and thera-

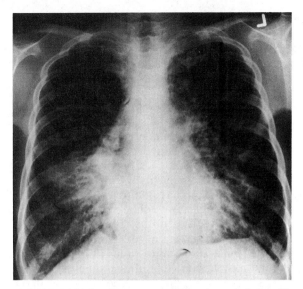

FIGURE 76-5 The chest roentgenogram shown is from a 17-year-old boy with cystic fibrosis complicated by extensive bronchiectasis, chronic respiratory insufficiency, and chronic cor pulmonale. In addition to cardiac enlargement there are extensive infiltrates throughout both lung fields with lingular and right middle lobe infiltrates being most obvious.

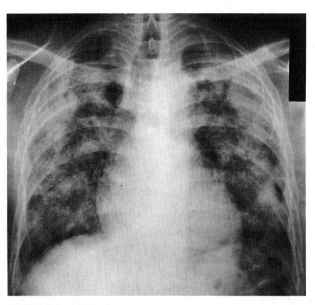

FIGURE 76-6 This chest roentgenogram was taken on a 52-year-old man with an 18-year occupational exposure to silica dust. Extensive apical pleural fibrosis and a diffuse reticulonodular parenchymal infiltrate are seen. The heart shadow is enlarged, and the patient had severe right-sided heart failure with functional tricuspid valvular regurgitation. Therapeutic measures were mainly ineffective.

peutic principles apply as in other forms of bronchiectasis.[28] In addition to the extremely viscid secretions characteristic of this disorder, the collapsibility of large bronchi renders the cough mechanism relatively ineffective for bronchopulmonary drainage.[29] Figure 76-5 illustrates a typical chest roentgenogram of a patient with cystic fibrosis complicated by chronic cor pulmonale.

RESTRICTIVE LUNG DISEASES

Chronic diffuse interstitial pulmonary diseases, especially when complicated by fibrosis of interstitial tissue and secondary vascular changes, can lead to severe pulmonary hypertension and cor pulmonale. There are many etiologies for diffuse interstitial processes. Granulomatous diseases, such as sarcoid, diffuse interstitial fibrosis in association with connective tissue disorders, radiation pneumonitis, histiocytosis X, and some pneumoconioses related to occupational exposures are a few examples. Most often the chronic interstitial process is idiopathic, and even lung biopsy specimens serve only to confirm that there is an interstitial pneumonitis of unknown cause which was suspected clinically and roentgenographically. Progression of the usual interstitial process may eventuate in a honeycomb pattern, representing extensive fibrosis with cystic areas that are lined with bronchial epithelium. Such regions do not participate in gas exchange and on occasion rupture to give a spontaneous pneumothorax.

There is usually severe dyspnea on exertion, often associated with symptoms of acute hyperventilation, such as circumoral and digital paresthesias and light-headedness. Tachypnea at rest is prominent. Fine end-inspiratory dry rales along with the above-mentioned signs of pulmonary hypertension and right ventricular hypertrophy and failure are found. The pulmonary hypertension is due mainly to anatomic changes, and if they are severe enough to produce cor pulmonale, therapy is rarely effective in reversing events. To the extent that inflammatory changes are operative, glucocorticoids or immunosuppressive therapy might be expected to aid in abating both the pulmonary hypertension and gas exchange abnormalities. However, by the time that pulmonary hypertension has become severe and cor pulmonale with failure occurs, there is usually little to offer other than digitalis, diuretics, and continuous oxygen therapy. Despite the implied irreversibility of the pulmonary hypertension, the response to therapy can be rewarding, if not lasting.

Certain etiologies for both diffuse interstitial diseases and acinar-filling processes respond well to treatment, but the decision to treat must be made well in advance of the onset of severe pulmonary hypertension. Desquamative interstitial pneumonia, hypersensitivity pneumonitis, pulmonary alveolar proteinosis, and chronic eosinophilic pneumonia are diseases that belong in this category.

PNEUMOCONIOSES

The inflammatory and fibrotic response to a large variety of silica-containing inorganic dusts produces restrictive and/or obstructive abnormalities of lung function. A typical roentgenographic picture (Fig. 76-6) along with an appropriate history of dust expo-

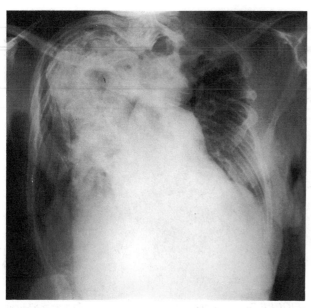

FIGURE 76-7 An example of kyphoscoliosis in association with neurofibromatosis is shown. The patient has general alveolar hypoventilation and chronic cor pulmonale. The response to therapy was rewarding. The size of the cardiac silhouette is difficult to evaluate in the presence of the thoracospinal deformity.

sure are needed to make the diagnosis. Some forms appear to be relatively benign; whereas those with massive fibrosis are apt to develop chronic cor pulmonale that is largely refractory to treatment.

Chest wall and neuromuscular apparatus

Musculoskeletal abnormalities lead to general alveolar hypoventilation through mechanical impedance of thoracic cage movement, muscle weakness and paralysis, or insufficient ventilatory drive. The lungs and airways are not primarily diseased, and mechanical support—or if possible, some measure to improve chest bellows performance—improves ventilation and thereby reverses hypoxic and hypercapnic pulmonary arterial constriction.

KYPHOSCOLIOSIS
Kyphoscoliosis must be severe to result in sufficient chest wall restriction to cause general alveolar hypoventilation. A kyphotic angle exceeding 100° or an angle of scoliosis in excess of 120° may be associated with cor pulmonale.[30] Cardiac enlargement is often difficult to detect from chest roentgenograms, as can be seen in Fig. 76-7. Unfortunately, surgical improvement of the skeletal abnormality often fails to improve the respiratory function. Therapy is designed to avoid complicating bronchopulmonary infections. Any acute respiratory insufficiency episode is treated promptly with both mechanical ventilation and antibiotics. Sedatives and narcotics are contraindicated.

NEUROMUSCULAR DISORDERS
Neuromuscular disorders such as muscular dystrophy, poliomyelitis, amyotrophic lateral sclerosis, myasthenia gravis, and cervical cord lesions at or below the level of the third cervical vertebra are associated with general alveolar hypoventilation. Should the hypoventilation leading to pulmonary hypertension be of sufficient duration and severity, right ventricular hypertrophy and, ultimately, failure may occur. Mechanical ventilatory support is the only treatment for the hypoventilation. Cuirass-type respirators work well during sleep and allow quiet waking activity. The lack of adequate respiratory muscular activity also impairs cough as a tracheobronchial clearance mechanism and predisposes these patients to develop pneumonias. Postural drainage, avoidance of aspiration and inhaled irritants, and prompt therapy of pneumonias are crucial in the management of these patients. Immobility often leads to thrombophlebitis which may result in complicating pulmonary emboli.

Inadequate ventilatory drive

EXTREME OBESITY
Extreme obesity has been associated with general alveolar hypoventilation, cor pulmonale, and right ventricular failure. The viewpoint that the hypoventilation disorder is due to mechanical impedance of chest wall motion by adipose tissue is difficult to accept as the sole basis for the syndrome, since many extremely obese patients do not have this disorder. Hyposensitivity to carbon dioxide, whether acquired or preexistent, probably serves as a background factor for the development of the alveolar hypoventilation. In some obese subjects upper airway obstruction, apparently due to the relaxation of pharyngeal and cervical muscles, develops during sleep.[31] These periods of obstructive apnea cause repeated arousals and chronic sleep deprivation which leads to hypersomnolence during the day.

The afflicted obese patient is usually cyanotic, drowses easily (sometimes while speaking), and snores loudly. Facial twitches and spasmodic jerks of the limbs punctuate the impromptu slumber. The description is similar to the one Charles Dickens gave for his fat boy in *The Posthumous Papers of the Pickwick Club.* Burwell et al. were struck by the similarity between Dickens' description and the findings in their patients.[32] Hence, the name *Pickwickian syndrome* was applied to the disease of these patients. The best therapy for the obesity-alveolar hypoventilation syndrome is weight loss, which usually leads to recovery. Congestive heart failure and respiratory insufficiency are often precipitated by intrabronchial infections; and such infections should be assiduously avoided or promptly treated. Mechanical ventilator therapy is required for increasing hypoventilation and heart failure. Therapeutic measures and precautions that apply to the therapy of respiratory insufficiency in chronic obstructive lung disease also apply to the obesity-hypoventilation syndrome. Progesterone is a respiratory stimulant known to increase the minute ventilation and carbon dioxide responsiveness of obese hypoventilators.[33] Recently, sublingual medroxyprogesterone was shown to produce a substantial improvement in hypoxemia, hypercapnea, and cor pulmonale in a group of Pickwickian patients.[34] It is well to remember that these obese, immobile, polycythemic patients are prone to have pulmonary embolic episodes which, unless constantly suspected, are difficult to detect in this clinical setting.

FAILURE OF AUTOMATIC CONTROL OF VENTILATION

General alveolar hypoventilation in the absence of extreme obesity, chest wall restriction, cervicothoracic spinal cord diseases, or muscular abnormalities has been attributed to an abnormality in the central nervous system control of ventilation. The name *Ondine's curse* was first applied to the syndrome of failure of automatic control of ventilation by Severinghaus and Mitchell.[35] The reference is to a play entitled *Ondine* by Jean Giraudoux.[36] In it, Hans, after being forsaken by Ondine, ceases to have automatic body functions and must consciously will himself to breathe if he is to live. More recently Mellins et al.[37] have reviewed the literature on Ondine's curse. Most cases have been seen following encephalitis, meningitis, or brainstem surgery. The pathogenesis and treatment are similar to that outlined for other forms of general alveolar hypoventilation. Electrical stimulation of the phrenic nerve as a respiratory pacemaker appears to be a promising and rational therapeutic approach to this disorder.

CHRONIC MOUNTAIN SICKNESS

A loss of tolerance to hypoxia may occur in some previously acclimatized high-altitude residents usually residing at altitudes above 14,000 ft. Although the cause for the loss of acclimatization is unknown, increasing erythrocytosis, general alveolar hypoventilation with insensitivity to hypoxic and hypercapnic stimuli to breathing, and chronic cor pulmonale develop. The only therapeutic approach available is to transport the patient to a lower altitude.

Upper airway obstruction

In recent years a clinical syndrome in infants and children has been described in which chronic upper airway obstruction due to hypertrophied tonsils and adenoids is characterized by general alveolar hypoventilation, pulmonary hypertension, and congestive heart failure. The importance of the syndrome lies in the dramatic response to tonsillectomy and adenoidectomy.[38] The pathogenesis of the disorder, which is more common in Negroes, is not clear. It is possible that extreme reactivity of the pulmonary vascular bed to hypoxia and hypercapnia is a significant factor. However, an inadequate ventilatory response to altered blood gases must be present to allow the development of hypoxia and hypercapnia. Following surgical removal of tonsils and adenoids and after clinical recovery, the patients are hyporesponsive to inhaled carbon dioxide in comparison with the response of normal children.[39]

Primary pulmonary vascular diseases

Diseases which primarily affect the pulmonary vasculature always produce some alteration of the pulmonary parenchyma as well. In contrast to restrictive parenchymal diseases, however, the pulmonary hypertension may be severe when both the vital capacity and gas exchange ability of the lung are only minimally impaired. The diagnosis often rests on this disparity.[40] Intimal thickening, hyperplasia of medial smooth muscle, and obliteration of vessels by surrounding fibrosis are frequent pathologic findings. Therapeutic measures must be based on preventing progression of the disease process if the etiology is known and is treatable. Whatever the underlying cause, embolic episodes must be prevented.

PRIMARY PULMONARY HYPERTENSION

Primary pulmonary hypertension affects young women more often than men and older women.[41] A familial form has been described.[42] A defect in fibrinolysis which might lead to pulmonary microemboli was found in one kindred.[43] The clinical course is characterized by progression of exertional dyspnea and symptoms of acute respiratory alkalosis during exertion. Syncope with exercise is found in approximately 25 percent. Death from refractory heart failure occurs within 6 months to several years. The physical findings are related to right ventricular hypertrophy and pulmonary hypertension. There are relatively few abnormal physical findings in the lungs. Therapeutic measures are mainly supportive, i.e., digitalis, diuretics, and oxygen. Vasodilating drugs are not useful, since no drug is selective for the pulmonary vasculature and since vasoconstriction plays a minimal role in producing the pulmonary hypertension. It has been suspected that silent thromboembolic episodes either cause or frequently complicate the pulmonary vascular disease. Whatever the role of thromboembolism, it is agreed that continuous anticoagulant therapy is desirable if there is no contraindication.

RECURRENT PULMONARY EMBOLI

Recurrent silent pulmonary emboli can present as progressive pulmonary hypertension with cor pulmonale and respiratory failure.[44] The symptoms and signs are identical to those of primary pulmonary hypertension. Any age or sex can be affected. The background historical factors that lead one to suspect this disorder are chronic inflammatory and venous changes in the legs or a history of chronic inflammatory disease of the pelvic organs. The therapeutic principle is to prevent further embolic episodes and to allow regression of vascular changes secondary to previous emboli.

MISCELLANEOUS PULMONARY VASCULAR DISEASES

Sickle-cell anemia is associated with occlusive pulmonary vascular disease. Pulmonary infarctions and extensive vascular changes occur secondary to aggregation of the abnormal red blood cells.[45] Two additional factors contributing to the pulmonary hypertension are a sclerocythemic hyperviscosity syndrome and, after several infarctions, an increase in bronchial collateral circulation.[46] The best prophylaxis is to avoid sickle-cell crises, but this cannot be done with any certainty at present.

Schistosomiasis is probably the commonest cause of pulmonary hypertension worldwide, although it is rare in the United States. The pulmonary hypertension is secondary to ova emboli from adult female worms residing in the pelvic and mesenteric veins. Prevention of further embolization by eradicating the adult worms is the only therapy.

Arteritis of the small pulmonary arteries occurs in association with systemic arteritis and in connective tissue disorders, especially lupus erythematosus and rheumatoid arthritis. The major clinical manifestations are most often related to involvement of other organ systems and pulmonary parenchyma. Therapy, whether immunosuppressive or glucocorticoid, is usually given because of other organ system involvement.

Most patients with scleroderma who develop cor pulmonale do so because of the development of interstitial fibrosis. In a few patients with this disease cor pulmonale develops in the absence of fibrosis.[47] Lesions in the pulmonary artery and arterioles are seen which are nonspecific and resemble those seen in pulmonary hypertension from a variety of causes.

Pulmonary veno-occlusive disease is a rare cause of pulmonary hypertension in children and young adults.[48] Widespread occlusion of the pulmonary veins by thrombi leads to localized pulmonary edema and Kerley B lines on the chest roentgenogram. The disease is of unknown etiology and therapy with anticoagulants does not appear to be effective.

A twentyfold increase in the number of cases of pulmonary hypertension occurred in Switzerland apparently in relation to ingestion of an anorexigenic drug, aminorex.[49] The mechanism is unknown and the association with the drug is not fully proven. Attempts at experimental induction in animals have to date been unsuccessful.[50]

An East African plant used in herbal remedies and belonging to the genus *Crotalaria* has been suggested as a cause of pulmonary hypertension.[51] When fed to rats, right ventricular hypertrophy and hypertensive pulmonary vascular disease are produced. Although not known to produce pulmonary hypertension in human beings, a history of ingesting herbal remedies should be sought in pulmonary hypertension of obscure origin.

ELECTROCARDIOGRAPHIC FINDINGS

There are many electrocardiographic findings that may be associated with chronic cor pulmonale. The P wave axis is often greater than +60°, with peaked waves in the inferior leads (II, III, aV_F) and V_1, often with prominent Ta waves producing depression of the PR segment. Whether P wave changes truly reflect right atrial hypertrophy is debatable. The peak QRS voltage is often low. Mean QRS frontal axis is often vertical or directed to the right ($\geq +90°$), and posterior rotation is often indicated by rS or QS patterns in the precordial leads. The latter finding may be confused with the pattern of a previous anteroseptal infarction. The mean QRS axis may be directed posteriorly, superiorly, and to the right so that there is an apparent left axis deviation in the standard and augmented limb leads.[52] This pattern of apparent left axis deviation along with low voltage is most often associated with emphysema in which there is minimal air flow obstruction.[53]

Less commonly in chronic obstructive pulmonary disease and more commonly in other etiologies, one finds tall R waves in the right precordial leads or varying degrees of right bundle branch block. It is well to remember that a normal electrocardiogram does not exclude the diagnosis of chronic cor pulmonale.

Both atrial and ventricular arrhythmias may occur with episodes of increasing hypoxemia with or without hypercapnia. Rapid decreases in arterial P_{CO_2} during ventilatory therapy are frequently associated with an array of alarming arrhythmias, especially if the patient has had renal compensation for a chronically elevated $PA_{,CO_2}$.[54] Although the arrhythmias have been attributed to alterations in blood gases, one study has described microscopic abnormalities in the sinus node tissue in 25 of 30 patients who died with chronic cor pulmonale.[55]

ROENTGENOGRAPHIC ABNORMALITIES

The diverse etiologies for chronic cor pulmonale create many patterns of parenchymal, pleural, and skeletal abnormalities which often give the diagnostic clue to the type of disease present.[56] Review of the divergent patterns in Figs. 76-3 and 76-5 to 76-7 will amplify this point. The roentgenographic findings of pulmonary hypertension, irrespective of the underlying disease, are dilatation of the main pulmonary artery and its major branches with prompt tapering to narrow branches. Often in chronic obstructive pulmonary disease complicated by right ventricular failure and respiratory insufficiency, the vascular shadows at the apex and superior hilar regions are distended with relative narrowing of vascular shadows at the lung base which angiographically can be shown to represent a reversal of the normal pulmonary blood flow distribution found in the upright human being. Right ventricular hypertrophy is indicated by enlargement of the heart shadow anteriorly, an upward tilt or lateral displacement of the left border of the heart, and enlargement of the right border of the heart. However, a rather significant change in heart size can be present and remain undetected unless previous films are available for comparison. When right ventricular failure occurs, the superior vena caval and azygos venous shadows are prominent. Pleural effusions and Kerley B lines are rarely found in right ventricular failure alone and suggest a complicating pneumonia in the case of pleural effusion or left ventricular failure when both effusions and Kerley B lines are present.

REFERENCES

1 Chronic Cor Pulmonale: Report of an Expert Committee of the World Health Organization, *Circulation,* 27:594, 1963.

2 Mitchell, R. S., Maisel, J. C., Dart, G. A., and Silvers, G. W.: The Accuracy of the Death Certificate in Reporting Cause of Death in Adults: With Special Reference to Chronic Bronchitis and Emphysema, *Am. Rev. Resp. Dis.,* 104:844, 1971.

3 Fishman, A. P.: Dynamics of the Pulmonary Circulation, in W. F. Hamilton (ed.), "Handbook of Physiology," sect. 2, "Circulation," vol. II, American Physiological Society, Washington, D.C., 1963, p. 1667.

4 Wagenvoort, C. A., Heath, D., and Edwards, J. E.: "The Pathology of the Pulmonary Vasculature," Charles C Thomas, Publisher, Springfield, Ill., 1964.

5 Hasleton, P. S., Heath, D., and Brewer, D. B.: Hypertensive Pulmonary Vascular Disease in States of Chronic Hypoxia, *J. Pathol. Bacteriol.,* 95:431, 1968.

6 Fishman, A. P.: Respiratory Gases in the Regulation of the Pulmonary Circulation, *Physiol. Rev.,* 41:214, 1961.

7 Fowler, K. T., and Read, J.: Effect of Alveolar Hypoxia on Zonal Distribution of Pulmonary Blood Flow, *J. Appl. Physiol.,* 18:244, 1963.

8 Lindsay, D. A., and Read, J.: Pulmonary Vascular Responsiveness in the Prognosis of Chronic Obstructive Lung Disease, *Am. Rev. Resp. Dis.,* 105:242, 1972.

9 Enson, Y., Guitini, C., Lewis, M. L., Morris, T. Q., Ferrer, M. I., and Harvey, R. M.: The Influence of Hydrogen Ion Concentration and Hypoxia on the Pulmonary Circulation, *J. Clin. Invest.,* 43:1146, 1964.

10 Fishman, A. P., Fritts, H. W., Jr., and Cournand, A.: Effects of Breathing Carbon Dioxide upon the Pulmonary Circulation, *Circulation,* 22:220, 1960.

11 Kadowitz, P. J., Joiner, P. D., and Hyman, A. L: Influence of Sympathetic Stimulation and Vasoactive Substances on the Canine Pulmonary Veins, *J. Clin. Invest.,* 56:354, 1975.

12 Wells, R. E., Jr., and Merrill, E. W.: Influence of Flow Properties of Blood upon Viscosity-Hematocrit Relationships, *J. Clin. Invest.,* 41:1591, 1962.

13 Brecher, G. A., and Galletti, P. M.: Functional Anatomy of Cardiac Pumping, in W. F. Hamilton (ed.), "Handbook of Physiology," sect. 2, "Circulation," vol. II, American Physiological Society, Washington, D.C., 1963, p. 759.

14 Spann, J. F., Jr., Mason, D. T., and Zelis, R. F.: The Altered Performance of the Hypertrophied and Failing Heart, *Am. J. Med. Sci.,* 258:291, 1969.

15 Fishman, A. P.: The Left Ventricle in "Chronic Bronchitis and Emphysema," *N. Engl. J. Med.,* 285:402, 1971.

15a Rao, B. S., Cohn, K. E., Eldridge, F. L., and Hancock, E. W.: Left Ventricular Failure Secondary to Chronic Pulmonary Disease, *Am. J. Med.,* 45:229, 1968.

16 Baum, G. L., Schwartz, A., Llamas, R., and Castillo, C.: Left Ventricular Function in Chronic Obstructive Lung Disease, *N. Engl. J. Med.,* 285:361, 1971.

17 Burrows, B., Kettel, L. J., Niden, A. H., Rabinowitz, M., and Diener, C. F.: Patterns of Cardiovascular Dysfunction in Chronic Obstructive Lung Disease, *N. Engl. J. Med.,* 286:912, 1972.

18 Steele, P., Ellis, J. H., VanDyke, D., Sutton, F., Creagh, E., and Davies, H.: Left Ventricular Ejection Fraction in Severe Chronic Obstructive Airways Disease, *Am. J. Med.,* 59:21, 1975.

19 Fishman, A. P., Goldring, R. M., and Turino, G. M.: General Alveolar Hypoventilation: A Syndrome of Respiratory and Cardiac Failure in Patients with Normal Lungs, *Q. J. Med.,* 35:261, 1966.

20 Duffell, G. M., Marcus, J. H., and Ingram, R. H., Jr.: Limitation of Expiratory Flow in Chronic Obstructive Pulmonary Disease: Relation of Clinical Characteristics, Pathophysiological Type and Mechanisms, *Am. Intern. Med.,* 72:365, 1970.

21 Thurlbeck, W. M., Henderson, J. A., Fraser, R. G., and Bates, D. V.: Chronic Obstructive Lung Disease: A Comparison between Clinical, Roentgenologic, Functional and Morphologic Criteria in Chronic Bronchitis, Emphysema, Asthma and Bronchietasis, *Medicine,* 49:81, 1970.

22 Marcus, J. H., McLean, R. L., Duffell, G. M., and Ingram, R. H., Jr.: Exercise Performance in Relation to the Pathophysiologic Type of Chronic Obstructive Pulmonary Disease, *Am. Heart J.,* 70:466, 1965.

23 Rakita, L., Gillespie, D. G., and Sancetta, S. M.: The Acute and Chronic Effects of Phlebotomy on General Hemodynamics and Pulmonary Functions of Patients with Secondary Polycythemia Associated with Pulmonary Emphysema, *Am. Heart J.,* 70:466, 1965.

24 Dayton, L. M., McCullough, R. E., Scheinhorn, D. J., and Weil, J. V.: Symptomatic and Pulmonary Response to Acute Phlebotomy in Secondary Polycythemia, *Chest,* 68:785, 1975.

25 Parker, J. O., Kelkar, K., and West, R. O.: Hemodynamic Effects of Aminophylline in Cor Pulmonale, *Circulation,* 33:17, 1966.

26 Abraham, A. S., Cole, R. B., and Bishop, J. M: Reversal of Pulmonary Hypertension by Prolonged Oxygen Administration to Patients with Chronic Bronchitis, *Circ. Res.,* 23:147, 1968.

27 Petty, T. L.: Outpatient Oxygen for Chronic Airway Obstruction, *J. A. M. A.,* 228:1541, 1974.

28 Goldring, R. M., Fishman, A. P., Turino, G. M., Cohen, H. I., Denning, C. R., and Andersen, D. H.: Pulmonary Hypertension and Cor Pulmonale in Cystic Fibrosis of the Pancreas, *J. Pediatr.,* 65:501, 1964.

29 Mellins, R. B., Levine, O. R., Ingram, R. H., Jr., and Fishman, A. P.: Obstructive Disease of the Airways in Cystic Fibrosis, *Pediatrics,* 41:560, 1968.

30 Bergofsky, E. H., Turino, G. M., and Fishman, A. P.: Cardiorespiratory Failure in Kyphoscoliosis, *Medicine,* 38:263, 1959.

31 Kryger, M., Quesney, L. F., Holder, D., Gloor, P., and MacLeod, P.: The Sleep Deprivation Syndrome of the Obese Patient: A Problem of Periodic Nocturnal Upper Airway Obstruction, *Am. J. Med.,* 56:531, 1974.

32 Burwell, C. S., Robin, E. D., Whaley, R. D., and Bickelmann, A. G.: Extreme Obesity Associated with Alveolar Hypoventilation: A Pickwickian Syndrome, *Am. J. Med.,* 21:811, 1956.

33 Lyons, H. A., and Huang, C. T.: Therapeutic Use of Progeste-

rone in Alveolar Hypoventilation Associated with Obesity, *Am. J. Med.,* 44:881, 1968.

34 Sutton, F. D., Zwillich, C. W., Creagh, C. E., Pierson, D. J., and Weil, J. V.: Progesterone for Outpatient Treatment of Pickwickian Syndrome, *Am. Intern. Med.,* 83:476, 1975.

35 Severinghaus, J. W., and Mitchell, R. A.: Ondine's Curse—Failure of Respiratory Center Automaticity While Awake, *Clin. Res.,* 10:122, 1962.

36 Giraudoux, J.: "Ondine, a Romantic Fantasy in Three Acts," English version by M. Valency, Samuel French, Inc., New York, 1956.

37 Mellins, R. B., Balfour, H. H., Jr., Turino, G. M., and Winters, R. W.: Failure of Automatic Control of Ventilation (Ondine's Curse): Report of an Infant Born with This Syndrome and Review of the Literature, *Medicine,* 49:487, 1970.

38 Bland, J. W., Jr., Edwards, F. K., and Brinsfield, D.: Pulmonary Hypertension and Congestive Heart Failure in Children with Chronic Upper Airway Obstruction: New Concepts of Etiologic Factors, *Am. J. Cardiol.,* 23:830, 1969.

39 Ingram, R. H., and Bishop, J. B.: Ventilatory Response to Carbon Dioxide after Removal of Chronic Upper Airway Obstruction, *Am. Rev. Resp. Dis.,* 102:645, 1970.

40 Williams, M. H., Jr., Adler, J. J., and Colp, C.: Pulmonary Function Studies as an Aid in the Differential Diagnosis of Pulmonary Hypertension, *Am. J. Med.,* 47:378, 1969.

41 Walcott, G., Burchell, H. B., and Brown, A. L., Jr.: Primary Pulmonary Hypertension, *Am. J. Med.,* 49:70, 1970.

42 Hood, W. B., Spencer, H., Lass, R. W., and Daley, R.: Primary Pulmonary Hypertension: Familial Occurrence, *Br. Heart J.,* 30:336, 1968.

43 Inglesby, T. V., Singer, J. W., and Gordon, D. S.: Abnormal Fibrinolysis in Familial Pulmonary Hypertension, *Am. J. Med.,* 55:5, 1973.

44 Wilhelmsen, L., Selander, S., Soderholm, B., Paulin, S., Varnauskas, E., and Werko, L.: Recurrent Pulmonary Embolism, *Medicine,* 42:335, 1963.

45 Moser, K. M., and Shea, J. G.: The Relationship between Pulmonary Infarction, Cor Pulmonale, and the Sickle States, *Am. J. Med.,* 22:561, 1957.

46 Heath, D., and Thompson, I. M.: Bronchopulmonary Anastomoses in Sickle-Cell Anaemia, *Thorax,* 24:232, 1969.

47 Case Records of the Massachusetts General Hospital (Case 2-1972), *N. Engl. J. Med.,* 286:91, 1972.

48 Rosenthal, A., Vawter, G., and Wagenvoort, C. A.: Intrapulmonary Veno-occlusive Disease, *Am. J. Cardiol.,* 31:78, 1973.

49 Gertsch, M., Salzmann, C., Scherrer, M., Stucki, P., and Wyss, F.: Haufen sich die Primar Vascularen Formen des Chonischen Cor Pulmonale? *Schweiz. Med. Wochenschr.,* 98:1579 and 1695, 1968.

50 Kay, J. M., Smith, P., and Heath, D.: Aminorex and the Pulmonary Circulation, *Thorax,* 26:262, 1971.

51 Heath, D., Shaba, J., Williams, A., Smith, P., and Kombe, A.: A Pulmonary Hypertension-producing Plant from Tanzania, *Thorax,* 30:399, 1975.

52 Oram, S., and Davies, P.: The Electrocardiogram in Cor Pulmonale, *Prog. Cardiovasc. Dis.,* 9:341, 1967.

53 Shmock, C. L., Pomerantz, B., Mitchell, R. S., Pryor, R., and Maisel, J. C.: The Electrocardiogram in Emphysema with and without Chronic Airways Obstruction, *Chest,* 60:328, 1971.

54 Ayers, S. M., and Grace, W. J.: Inappropriate Ventilation and Hypoxemia as Causes of Cardiac Arrhythmias, *Am. J. Med.,* 46:495, 1969.

55 Thomas, M. A., and Wee, A. S. T.: The Sinus Node in Cor Pulmonale, *Isr. J. Med. Sci.,* 5:831, 1969.

56 Fraser, R. G., and Paré, J. A. P.: "Diagnosis of Diseases of the Chest," vols. I and II, W. B. Saunders Company, Philadelphia, 1970.

Diseases of the Endocardium

77
Endocarditis

EDWARD R. DORNEY, M.D.

The endocardium and heart valves may be affected by a variety of diseases—congenital, infectious, immunologic, and endocrine. The pathologic spectrum includes ulceration, overgrowth of tissue, shortening or rupture of chordae tendineae and valves, and verrucous formation. Two entities, bacterial endocarditis and nonbacterial endocarditis, are discussed in this chapter. A third, Libman-Sacks endocarditis, is discussed in Chap. 88.

BACTERIAL ENDOCARDITIS

In the preantibiotic era, the course of bacterial endocarditis was one of unswerving progression to an inevitable conclusion. The natural history of the disease, which presented a predictable sequence of signs and symptoms, was exhaustively studied and accurately cataloged.[1-4] With the introduction of effective antibiotic therapy by Loewe et al. in 1944,[5] however, this pattern was interrupted, and early recognition, before the classic picture developed, became necessary. In addition to adequate therapy, the innovation of intracardiac surgical procedures in the past decade has further altered the picture of the disease, so that the classic clinical descriptions, classifications, and prognoses of the preantibiotic era no longer pertain.

Before treatment was available, the clinical distinction between acute and subacute bacterial endocarditis was primarily made on the basis of the survival time of the patient. Those surviving after 8 weeks were said to have subacute cases, while those succumbing in less than 8 weeks were said to have had acute cases. Today, with adequate treatment, a survival of 65 to 80 percent of all patients with endocarditis is expected in modern hospitals.[6,7] It is still possible to classify certain cases as acute because of fulminating onset or rapid progression, but it is not possible to predict which of the seemingly indolent cases will suddenly result in valve ulceration or crippling cerebral embolization.[8] One cannot consistently predict the severity of the disease from the type of bacteria involved.[7] In view of these facts, the distinction between acute and subacute bacterial endocarditis loses its clinical significance, since all cases should be considered imminently lethal and full therapy should be instituted as soon as the diagnosis is made.

Pathology

The basic lesion of bacterial endocarditis is a friable, verrucous vegetation which is engrafted on the surface of a heart valve, the endocardial lining of a heart chamber, or the endothelium of a blood vessel.[9] These vegetations usually are located in areas altered by rheumatic, congenital, or syphilitic heart disease but may also be found on apparently normal surfaces.[10]

The active vegetations are composed of three layers: The first or innermost layer is usually the thickest and accounts for three-fourths to seven-eighths of the entire vegetation. This layer is made up of platelets, fibrin, white blood cells, red blood cells, some bacteria, strands of collagen, and varying amounts of necrosis. The middle layer is composed primarily of bacteria and the outer layer mostly of fibrin with varying amounts of bacteria present.[9] As healing progresses, the exposed areas of the vegetation become covered with fibrous tissue, and there are invasion and phagocytosis of the bacterial layer by leukocytes, calcification of some of the bacterial areas, and hyalinization and calcification of the necrotic innermost core of the vegetation.

In the preantibiotic era the pathologic distinction between acute and subacute bacterial endocarditis was sometimes made on the basis of the size of the vegetation, the amount of necrosis present, and the presence or absence of prior endocardial disease, but the distinction was not always certain.[11] The use of potent antibiotics has made the differentiation even more tenuous because of the changes introduced by healing.[11]

Previous rheumatic endocarditis is the most common substrate for bacterial endocarditis. The mitral valve is the site most frequently involved, followed by the aortic, tricuspid, and pulmonic valves, in that order. Involvement of these valves may result in perforation of the leaflets or in secondary spread of the infection to the chordae tendineae or papillary muscles, with consequent necrosis and rupture. Vegetations large enough to cause obstruction to a valve orifice have been noted.[12] Extension into the aortic valve ring with abscess formation may result in fistulas between the aorta and the right ventricle or between the aorta and either of the atria. It also can result in complete heart block from destruction of the conduction system or in purulent pericarditis from rupture into the pericardial sac.

In congenital heart disease, the ventricular septal defect is the single lesion most often involved and accounts for approximately 50 percent of the cases. It is followed in frequency by the patent ductus arteriosus, pulmonic stenosis, and aortic stenosis.[5,6] Fallot's tetralogy, before or after shunting procedures, is the most commonly involved of the cyanotic lesions and in some series ranks second only to the ventricular septal defect.[13,14] Atrial septal defects are seldom involved, and when endocarditis has been reported with this lesion, the vegetations are seen on the pulmonic and tricuspid valves.

Postoperative endocarditis following finger fracture of a valve, insertion of a plastic patch or valve leaflet, a stich in the endocardium, or a Starr valve or other prosthesis has been reported.[15-17] Elek has shown that the presence of silk suture material reduced by 10,000 times the size of a bacterial inoculum needed to produce infection.[18]

Endocarditis has also been reported in association with coarctation of the aorta,[13] peripheral arteriovenous fistula, aneurysm of the aorta, idiopathic hypertrophic aortic stenosis (asymmetric septal hypertrophy), postinfarction mural thrombosis, and "click-murmur" syndrome. Cardiac lesions other than valvular or endocardial vegetations, such as valve ring abscess, myocarditis, or mural abscess, are less commonly seen. Myocarditis has taken the form of perivascular collections of lymphocytes,[19] miliary infarctions, or focal inflammatory reaction in the interstitial tissue and is second in frequency only to the endocardial lesion. Valve ring abscess is easily overlooked at postmortem examination, as stressed by Sheldon and Golden, and therefore may be more common than is actually reported.[20] It should be suspected in any case of continuing sepsis or recurrent disease despite adequate treatment. Pericardial involvement is rare and when present is usually the result of external rupture of a mural or valve ring abscess or is secondary to uremia. Gross myocardial infarction due to embolization of a major coronary artery has been reported.

The Bracht-Wächter body has been interpreted as being pathognomonic of bacterial endocarditis. This is a collection of lymphocytes in the myocardium and is not specific for the disease.[11]

Osler's node, a painful, red, indurated area appearing usually in the pads of the fingers or toes and lasting for several hours to several days, is made up of an endothelial swelling and perivasculitis of the small vessels just below the malpighian layer of the skin. These lesions are of uncertain origin, do not ulcerate, and are considered to be nonbacterial.[21] Janeway's lesion is a painless, hemorrhagic nodular lesion found in the palms of the hands and on the soles of the feet. These lesions show a definite tendency to ulceration, and biopsy material has demonstrated polymorphonuclear infiltration of the capillaries surrounding tissues with marked necrosis. Bacteria have been cultured from the area of these lesions which were identical to those found in the blood.[21]

Because of the central location in the circulation of the primary lesion and the friable structural characteristics of the endocardial vegetations, peripheral arterial embolism is a comon finding in bacterial endocarditis. Embolization may continue for several months after bacteriologic cure.[6] Bland and septic infarction and abscess formation have been reported in all the organs of the body and are most commonly recognized in the kidney, brain, and spleen.

Bacterial embolization to the walls of small arteries may result in mycotic aneurysms ranging in size from 1 to 2 mm to several centimeters.[21] These lesions may destroy a vital organ such as the brain by hemorrhage or may cause death by exsanguination.[7]

In addition to gross renal infarction secondary to embolization of a major branch of a renal artery, glomerulitis, most likely due to microembolization of bacteria, and also glomerulonephritis, indistinguishable from acute glomerulonephritis, were common findings in the preantibiotic era.[22] They are seen today in long-standing untreated cases of endocarditis and in those which have been inadequately treated. More recently the demonstration of low serum β/C globulin levels and immunoglobulin deposits along the glomerular basement membrane of the kidneys supports the concept of immune-mediated renal disease in bacterial endocarditis. Levy[23] has recently discussed the possibility that the rheumatoid factor, found in over 50 percent of patients with bacterial endocarditis, might serve as a protection against the development of this type of nephritis.

Pathogenesis

The question of why endocarditis develops in certain patients with rheumatic valvular or congenital cardiovascular disease and not in others with similar lesions is largely unanswered. From the experimental work of Highman and Altland, which demonstrated increased susceptibility to endocarditis in rats subjected to high altitudes in a pressure chamber, the similar experiences of Nedzel with the use of Pitressin, and the observations of Allen and Sirota and of Angrist and Marquiss, it seems that many factors in addition to bacteremia and cardiac deformities are involved. Lillehei has shown that the creation of a large peripheral arteriovenous fistula will lead to valvular endocarditis in 75 percent of dogs surviving for 4 weeks. Chronic impairment of cardiac lymphatic flow has been demonstrated to make the dog particularly susceptible to the development of endocarditis after injection of staphylococci. Garrison and Freedman[24] have developed a technique for the production of "marantic" vegetations in rabbits by the insertion of a polyethylene catheter in the atria or the ventricular chambers. These vegetations can be reproducibly infected with various bacteria and provide an excellent model for study of the disease and response to treatment and prophylaxis.

There is good evidence to show that transient bacteremia is a common day-to-day occurrence. Various writers have attempted to establish a possible source of bacteremia in bacterial endocarditis, with about a 40 percent positive result in the series studied. Bacteremia secondary to tooth extration, cleaning, and filling has been frequently noted.[25] Bactermia has been reported with genitourinary manipulations[26] such as prostatic massage, catheterization, or cystoscopy or after normal obstetric deliveries, with infections of the upper part of the respiratory tract, and with pyoderma. In recent years bacteremia following cardiac surgical procedure or cardiac catheterization has also become important. The self-administration of narcotics by the intravenous route is a common precipitating cause in endocarditis, particularly that of the variety restricted to the right side of the heart.[27,28] The size of the inoculum of bacteria must be of importance in the establishment of infection since relatively few people with valvular disease develop endocarditis despite frequent exposure to bacteremia during everyday life as well as with medical procedures.

Areas of localization of vegetations within the heart are remarkably constant and have been the basis for the main theories concerning the pathogenesis of the disease itself. The lesions are found on the ventricular surface of the aortic valve in aortic insufficiency, with satellite lesions in the anteromedial leaflet of the mitral valve, the chordae tendineae, and papillary muscles. They are found on the coapting surfaces of the mitral valve on the atrial side in mitral insufficiency, with some extension to the atrial wall where the regurgitant jet impinges. In ventricular septal defects, they may be on the defect itself but frequently involve the area of the jet lesion on the right ventricular wall or the septal leaflet of the tricuspid valve (Fig. 77-1).

Many theories have been advanced to explain this localization of lesions. It has been suggested that trauma in the area of impingement of the valves, with the increased pressure applied to the surfaces, forces bacteria into the endothelium, or that exposure to a greater volume impact of the bloodstream against the damaged valve may be responsible. Other suggestions, well described elsewhere, have merit in individual cases but do not explain the majority of instances.[11]

Rodbard proposed that a high-velocity flow from an area of increased pressure through a narrowed orifice into a low-pressure area results in the destruction of laminar flow just distal to the orifice.[29] This results in disruption of the endothelial nutrition in the area and at the same time increases the local bacterial count, thereby setting the stage for infection. He has devised an ingenious set of experiments which lends considerable credence to his theory. His model would also explain the endocarditis on the aortic valve in syphilitic disease, when the pathologic lesion is in the valve ring, and localization of the bacterial implants in congenital heart disease, e.g., bicuspid

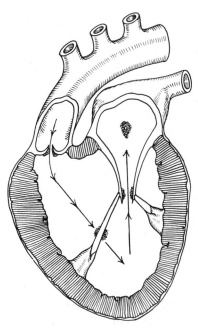

FIGURE 77-1 The high-velocity streams in mitral and aortic insufficiency and sites of endocarditic lesions. The arrow at the left indicates a high arterial pressure that generates regurgitant flow from aorta to ventricle. The vena contracta and the endocarditis lesions appear at the ventricular surface of the aortic valves. The stream through the incompetent aortic valve may produce lesions on the chordae tendineae of the aortic leaf of the mitral valve. If the mitral valves cannot seat properly during ventricular systole, the regurgitant stream (arrow at right) will pass to the sink of the left atrium, and endocarditis will tend to become engrafted on the atrial surface of the mitral valve. The atrial endocardium in line with the regurgitant jet stream may show a fibrous reaction. *(Reproduced by permission of the author and the American Heart Association, Inc., from S. Rodbard, Blood Velocity and Endocarditis, Circulation, 27:18, 1963.)*

aortic valve, when the valve surfaces remain intact (Fig. 77-2).

Organisms involved

Bacterial endocarditis is not a reportable disease, and the overall incidence cannot be accurately estimated. Reports from several large institutions, as tabulated by Kerr and others, show a variation of from 1 in 1,000 admissions to 1 in 6,000 admissions.[8,30]

Actually this disease should no longer be termed bacterial endocarditis, since it has now been proved due to various forms of fungi and to *Rickettsia*[31,32] and viruses as well as bacteria. It would be more descriptive to use the term endocarditis preceded by the name of the appropriate microorganism.

Thayer[33] in 1931 reported a representative series of 536 cases of proved bacterial endocarditis. His statistics showed a 62.5 percent incidence of streptococci (all types), 14.7 percent due to pneumococci, 12.5 percent due to staphylococci, and 6.9 percent

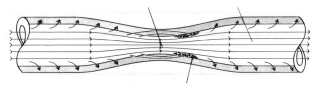

FIGURE 77-2 Flow through a permeable tube. A high-pressure source (at left) drives fluid through an orifice into a low-pressure sink. The curved arrows leaving the stream and entering the wall in the upstream segment represent the normal perfusion of the lining layer. Velocity is maximal, and perfusing pressure is low immediately beyond the orifice where the momentum of the stream converges the streamlines to form a vena contracta. The low pressure in this segment results in reduced perfusion and may cause a retrograde flow from the deeper layers of the vessel into the flowing stream. (Reproduced by permission of the author and the American Heart Association, Inc., from S. Rodbard, Blood Velocity and Endocarditis, Circulation, 27:18, 1963.)

due to gonococci. With the advent of antibiotics and the reduction of the mortality rate from above 98 percent to 30 percent, the comparative incidence of bacteria has been difficult to tabulate, since postmortem studies are no longer representative of the disease as a clinical entity. In addition, during this period most writers have reported under the heading of *subacute* bacterial endocarditis, thereby weighting the frequency of organism occurrence toward the less-virulent *Streptococcus viridans*.[8] Several reports tabulating both clinical and pathologic material and including all infectious endocarditis seen at various teaching hospitals are now available.[7,34–38] All these series obtained during the antibiotic era have shown a marked reduction in the occurrence of the pneumococci and gonococci as compared with that of Thayer,[33] with a concomitant increase in the frequency of staphylococcal infection. Several of these writers[6,7] have also shown that the *Streptococcus faecalis* has become the third most common organism, exceeded only by *S. viridans* and staphylococci. This increase in frequency of *S. faecalis* has also been noted by others.[26,30,39] Although *S. faecalis* has a tendency to produce green hemolysis on blood agar, it can be differentiated from other group D streptococci and from *S. viridans* by its ability to grow in 6.5 percent saline agar. Despite this fact, *S. faecalis* has been included in the *S. viridans* group by many writers, among them Thayer[33] and Wilson.[35] It should, however, be considered as a separate entity because of its growth characteristics in culture, its resistance to antibiotics, and the clinical picture that it produces.

The increasing importance of the group with consistently negative blood cultures but with clinical and pathologic evidence of bacterial endocarditis has been recently emphasized.[6,7,36,40] This group accounted for 13 percent of the series of Vogler, Dorney, and Bridges[7] and for 16 percent of that of Morgan and Bland.[6]

Wilson,[35] Kerr,[30] and Afremow[8] have noted the overall decrease in the frequency of bacterial endo-

carditis since the introduction of antibiotics. The reasons for this decrease in occurrence and the change in bacteria involved are multiple. Adequate antibiotic prophylaxis following genitourinary, obstetric, and gynecologic procedures and during dental manipulations has undoubtedly cut down on bacteremia and implantation of the more sensitive streptococci.[25] It may be that the decrease in rheumatic endocarditis noted during the same period is responsible for the reduction of *S. viridans* endocarditis, since it represents the common substrate for this particular organism. Penicillin therapy of pneumonia has reduced the frequency and severity of pneumococcal infections and has also afforded control of the gonococcus. At the same time the indiscriminate and prolonged use of antibiotics has encouraged the emergence of antibiotic-resistant strains, and overgrowth of gram-negative bacteria,[16] and the development of fungi. The aging population with the increasing frequency of long hospitalizations and genitourinary manipulations has favored the development of endocarditis on normal heart valves by the more invasive organisms such as staphylococci and *Streptococcus faecalis*.[26,30]

The introduction of cardiac surgical procedures has undoubtedly affected the prevalence of some organisms. Hoffman has estimated that the occurrence of endocarditis after finger fracture of the mitral or aortic valve would average about 1 percent and the organism involved is most often *Staphylococcus*. Open heart surgical procedure with placement of prosthetic valves, suture material, or endocardial patches results in a still higher percentage of infection than the closed techniques. Geraci et al. have estimated that the incidence of infection is about 10 percent of the patients having had partial or total prosthetic valve replacement.[15] *Pseudomonas aeruginosa*,[15,16] *Staphylococcus aureus*,[15] and *S. epidermidis* and a variety of fungi[15] are prevalent on the postoperative pump group. Bacteria usually considered to be nonpathogenic (*Achromobacter*, *Sarratia marcescens*, *Corynebacterium*, and *S. epidermidis*) have also been reported in this circumstance. *Streptococcus viridans* is rarely encountered in postoperative material. Recent studies have shown, however, that prevention of endocarditis in the postoperative state may be possible with proper use of antibiotics.[17]

Clinical manifestations

The similarity of bacterial endocarditis to other diseases, severe and insignificant, together with the lack of definitive signs and symptoms early in the disease, makes the diagnosis difficult. Friedberg has found that the diagnosis of virus infection or influenza is made commonly in the first few weeks of illness. To this should be added the group of bacterial endocarditis presenting with signs of other catastrophic illnesses such as stroke, peripheral vascular occlusion, hemorrhage, congestive heart failure, or uremia in which the attention is directed away from the true cause of the disease and toward one of its manifestations.

Classically, bacterial endocarditis has been described as a disease in which a patient comes to the physician with an orgainc heart murmur, fever, splenomegaly, petechiae, and peripheral embolic manifestations. In a series of 148 cases collected by the author from the teaching hospitals of Emory University, 74 percent had no evidence of embolization on admission, 60 percent had no petechiae, 61 percent had no splenomegaly, and 88 percent had no clubbing of the fingers. Four percent had no heart murmur.[7]

It would be better to think of bacterial endocarditis as a group of syndromes rather than as a single stereotyped entity. The disease is caused by a variety of microorganisms, so that fever will be present to a greater or lesser degree depending on the virulence of the particular organism and the quantity present in the blood at any given time. In some patients there will be afebrile periods. Shaking chills and profuse sweats may be present, or there may be a feeling of lassitude and anorexia with no awareness of fever. A murmur is not always present early in the disease, and there are no infallible criteria which will distinguish the "functional," or "innocent," murmur from the sound caused by an organic deformity.[10,41-43] Arthralgias are common, and septic arthritis has been seen. Clubbing of the fingers is rare in cases which are treated early, but it may be found in as many as 25 percent of patients later in the course of the disease.[37] In recent years Osler's nodes and Janeway's lesions have become relatively rare. Osler's nodes were seen only once in the author's series of cases, and Janeway's lesions were never seen.[7] Petechiae are found more frequently and tend to be located in the mucous membranes of the mouth, in the conjunctiva, and the necklace area, or about the wrists and ankles.[7,37] Splinter hemorrhages and small red to black streaks under the fingernails may be seen but are not diagnostic of the disease.[44] For example, they may be secondary to trauma, trichinosis, rheumatic fever, infectious mononucleosis, or cryoglobulinemia or may be without obvious cause. Roth's spots are hemorrhagic areas with a white center which are seen in the retina and the conjunctiva. At any state of the disease, they may appear suddenly, remain for several days, and gradually fade, leaving no residual mark. These spots are not diagnostic of bacterial endocarditis; they may also be seen with various forms of anemia, leukemia, and scurvy. Abscess formation may also be seen in the retina.

Since the bacterial vegetations are located in the center of the circulation in left-sided endocarditis, embolic episodes may occur to any systemic artery. Abscess formation, hemorrhage, or infarction of various organs will again alter the clinical picture according to the organ involved and the type of involvement.

NEUROLOGIC SYNDROMES
Bacterial endocarditis may at first resemble meningitis, subarachnoid hemorrhage, hemiplegia, coma, convulsions, or toxic psychosis, particularly in the older age groups.[10] Particularly suspicious is sudden hemiplegia in young adults, brain abscesses in the presence of cyanotic congenital heart disease, or subarachnoid hemorrhage in a patient with a heart

murmur. In pneumococcal pneumonia with meningitis, endocarditis of the aortic valve should be sought. It may occur in 25 to 30 percent of cases.[45] Chorea has been reported.

HEMATOLOGIC SYNDROMES
A normochromic, normocytic anemia occurs in 60 to 70 percent of cases of bacterial endocarditis. Fever, anemia, and murmur should always suggest bacterial endocarditis. Murmur may be absent or "due to anemia." Blood cultures may be sterile or fever may be absent as a result of the indiscriminate use of antibiotics. The combination of fever, anemia, petechiae, and splenomegaly does not always mean primary hematologic disease, and when these signs are present, blood cultures should be taken. Phagocytic monocytes may appear in the peripheral blood in great numbers in bacterial endocarditis. Anemia, fever, and monocytes in the peripheral blood may suggest bacterial endocarditis rather than leukemia. Cultures are frequently negative when these cells are present.[46] Bacterial endocarditis may present as generalized or local purpura or simulate multiple myeloma with an increase of plasma cells in the blood and elevated globulin levels.

PERIPHERAL VASCULAR DISEASE
The sudden onset of peripheral gangrene in a patient with fever and/or murmur may be due to bacterial endocarditis. Small emboli may lodge in terminal arterioles and produce gangrenous infarctions of various acral portions of the body (i.e., tip of the nose, pinna of the ear, fingers, and toes). Larger emboli may present as peripheral vascular occlusions and simulate atherosclerotic occlusive disease. When large emboli occur, it is wise to consider the possibility of endocarditis due to fungi.

RENAL INVOLVEMENT
The kidney is second only to the spleen in frequency of embolic involvement in bacterial endocarditis.[21,39] When renal infarction occurs in the presence of a heart murmur or fever, bacterial endocarditis should be suspected. Persistent hematuria is a helpful diagnostic point in the evaluation of fever and murmur. In the aged, the appearance of a syndrome simulating acute glomerulonephritis should start the search for a heart murmur or bacteremia.[41] Embolic glomerulonephritis may appear with pyuria and hematuria and may be mistaken for pyelonephritis.

SPLENIC INFARCTION
The spleen is the most common site of embolic infarction in bacterial endocarditis.[39] Pain in the left upper quadrant with radiation to the left shoulder is the usual complaint. There may be local tenderness, abdominal rigidity, and friction rub. Rupture of the spleen may also occur.[7] Differential diagnosis from pulmonary embolism at times may be difficult.

CARDIOVASCULAR SYNDROMES

The literature on bacterial endocarditis has referred to "changing murmurs" as a part of the diagnosis of this disease. It does not mean a change in the intensity of an already present murmur but the appearance of a new organic murmur such as that due to aortic insufficiency or mitral regurgitation. This is virtually diagnostic of bacterial endocarditis if it occurs with evidence of acute sepsis.[41] In the presence of fever, rupture of a chorda tendinea, or papillary muscle with the characteristic associated murmur or the appearance of a continuous murmur of aortic–right ventricular fistula has the same significance. Acute myocardial infarction occurring during a prolonged fever is strongly suggestive of bacterial endocarditis. The sudden appearance of congestive heart failure in a patient with previously well-compensated rheumatic or congenital disease should suggest the need for blood cultures.

PERICARDITIS

Pericarditis is said to be rare in bacterial endocarditis. It may occur, however, with staphylococcal infection, embolism to a coronary artery with myocardial infarction, uremic pericarditis, rupture of a mycotic aneurysm into the pericardial sac, and coexistent rheumatic carditis. Echocardiography and selective culturing can be helpful in identifying involved valves when multiple murmurs are present, and replacement of a valve is felt to be necessary for treatment.

RIGHT-SIDED BACTERIAL ENDOCARDITIS

When bacterial endocarditis is localized to the right side of the heart, murmurs are less common and are seen in only 35 percent of cases. Pulmonary symptoms such as cough and pleuritic pain are common, as are findings of consolidation, pleural friction rub, or pleural fluid. Peripheral embolization is rare. Blood cultures will be positive, as in left sided endocarditis.[28] Right-sided bacterial endocarditis should be suspected in narcotic addicts with septicemia and fever,[28] in infants with fever following septic skin lesions, and in fever following cardiac surgical treatment. A triad of heroin addiction, bacteremia, and pulmonary infarction in the absence of obvious cause is strongly suggestive of staphylococcal tricuspid endocarditis, although other organisms such as *Candida albicans* and gram-negative bacteria are also frequently seen.

BACTERIAL ENDOCARDITIS FOLLOWING CARDIAC SURGICAL PROCEDURE

Bacterial endocarditis following cardiac surgical treatment does not resemble the usual disease. Petechiae, peripheral emboli, and splenomegaly are rare. Anemia may be difficult to evaluate in the postsurgical state, and murmurs seldom change. Infective endocarditis should be suspected if fever persists, unexplained, after 5 to 7 days in the postoperative period or if it recurs 4 to 6 weeks after discharge from the hospital.[15] A syndrome of fever, lymphocytosis, and splenomegaly of unknown cause may rarely occur following open heart surgical procedures using bypass techniques, and this may cause confusion with endocarditis. Fever and anemia, with or without a murmur, occurring after insertion of a valvular prosthesis may simulate bacterial endocarditis; this condition is probably a traumatic hemolytic anemia secondary to a disrupted valve. Fungal endocarditis should be suspected with persistent fever and negative blood cultures in the postoperative period, particularly if large emboli are present. Fungemia may be absent in as many as 50 percent of the cases. Diagnosis can sometimes be made from culture of emboli. Precipitant tests for *Candida* may be useful in this situation.[47]

BACTERIAL ENDOCARDITIS FOLLOWING GYNECOLOGIC AND GENITOURINARY PROCEDURES

Bacterial endocarditis should be suspected in any patient who sustains a persistent fever following a genitourinary or gynecologic procedure. The bacteria involved in these areas frequently attack normal valves, and a murmur may not be present initially.[10,26] The responsible organism is frequently the enterococcus. The occurrence of peripheral arterial occlusion in a postoperative patient with fever should direct attention to the possibility of bacterial endocarditis.[10] Unexplained persistent fever in the postpartum patient with a murmur suggests the need for blood cultures.

CHRONIC DISEASE

Fever occurring during the course of lymphoma, metastatic malignant disease, or myelofibrosis may be due to endocarditis.[10] The appearance of a new murmur, particularly of aortic insufficiency, together with fever is doubly significant.

Diagnosis

The single most important factor in the diagnosis of bacterial endocarditis is a high index of suspicion. Once suspicion has been aroused, the next step in diagnosis is the procuring of blood cultures. When clinical findings suggest the disease, blood cultures should be incubated in both aerobic and anaerobic media.[48] Blood is best obtained from the antecubital vein, since it is easily available and since it has been shown that the bacterial yield of the venous blood from this source closely approximates that of arterial blood.[49,50] An occasional case will show a positive marrow culture when both venous and arterial blood are sterile.[49] If routine aerobic and anaerobic blood cultures are not productive, special techniques designed to bring out "L" forms or fungi should be instituted. Cultures should not be discarded before 3 weeks to allow for growth of some of the slower organisms such as the *Bacteroides* group, which might otherwise be overlooked. Cultures are positive in bacterial endocarditis in 60 to 90 percent of cases reported, depending on the adequacy of the laboratory and the prior use of antibiotics. It has been demonstrated that the first four blood cultures will provide over 90 percent of the positive returns and that usually all cultures or no cultures will be positive.[42,51] If antibiotics have been given prior to obtaining blood cultures, then more cultures will be required over a period of 2 to 3 days.[50] Penicillinase incorporated in the culture media will sometimes increase the yield of positive cultures. Bacteremia in this disease is relatively constant, so that the time of the future is not significant unless chills are occurring regularly.[50] In this case the bacteremia is usually heaviest approximately 1 h prior to the chill.[50]

With the exception of the positive blood culture, the laboratory is of little aid in the diagnosis of bacterial endocarditis. Anemia may be found in up to 70 percent of cases. The white blood cell count may be normal, low, or elevated. Normal counts are just as prevalent as elevated counts.[42] Sedimentation rate is elevated in 90 percent of cases but is of no differential aid in the work-up of fever of unknown origin except as an important negative finding when bacterial endocarditis is being considered. Considerable attention has been given to the presence of phagocytic monocytes in the peripheral blood. These cells were first described by Van Nuys and associated with bacterial endocarditis by Leede and Suntheim. The cells are about 20 to 30 μ in diameter and have an abundant, finely reticulated cytoplasm and one or two large, oval nuclei. The cytoplasm may contain bacteria or red blood corpuscles in various stages of degeneration. They may be seen in the fingertip blood but are best obtained by earlobe punctures. According to Hill and Bayrd, these cells are most commonly seen in cases of endocarditis with negative blood cultures.[46] They are not diagnostic, however, and have been reported in septicemia without endocarditis, tuberculosis, rheumatic fever, and many other conditions.

Since bacterial endocarditis may appear in so many disguises and since blood cultures are not always positive, criteria must be set up for treatment without bacterial proof. In cases with negative bacterial cultures, particularly with a prolonged intermittent course and raised gamma globulin level, serologic tests for *Rickettsia burnetii* should be carried out[32] in addition to blood cultures. Friedberg has said that "unexplained fever for more than a week or ten days in a patient with significant cardiac murmur should form the basis of a presumptive diagnosis of bacterial endocarditis." He cautions against the overenthusiastic application of this principle, particularly in children, adolescents, and young adults. Such a decision to treat the patient for bacterial endocarditis should not be made lightly, nor should the hunt for another cause of symptoms be abandoned because treatment for endocarditis has been decided upon. Once therapy is instituted, however, it should be carried out for its full duration unless it becomes obvious that the diagnosis of endocarditis is in error. Echocardiography may be of some help in identifying valvular lesions when cultures are negative or if valve excision is considered and murmurs are identified at more than one valve area.

Treatment[36]

The treatment of bacterial endocarditis should be directed toward the immediate and total eradication of the infecting organism. To this end, killing doses of specific antibiotics should be given promptly and continued sufficiently long to ensure complete elimination of the bacteria without dependence on host factors.[52] Several principles should be kept in mind when approaching the problem:

1 Bactericidal agents should be used.[39] In this disease the morphologic structure of the vegetation is such that the bacteria are inaccessible to the leukocytes which would ordinarily be expected to destroy them once growth had been inhibited by bacteriostatic agents.[53] When bacteriostatic wide-spectrum antibiotics are used, the colonies of bacteria remain deep within the vegetations and begin to multiply shortly after the treatment is discontinued. There is no place for the exclusive use of bacteriostatic agents in the treatment of bacterial endocarditis regardless of the in vitro sensitivity tests.[41,52] The only exceptions to this statement at the present time are the presence of "L" forms or when *Rickettsia* or *Bacteroides* is the infecting agent.

2 The dose of antibiotics should be sufficiently high to effect a serum concentration at least four times greater than the concentration needed to kill the causative bacteria in vitro.[54] This may be tested by making serial dilutions of the patient's serum inoculated with approximately 50,000 organisms of a fresh young culture of his own bacteria. After 24 h of incubation in a 5 percent carbon dioxide atmosphere, the clear tubes are subcultured for 48 h on semisolid thioglycolate medium.[54] This type of test is particularly helpful, since it has been demonstrated that there may be a total lack of correlation between the usual in vitro antibiotic-sensitivity tests and the results of therapy.[35,52,53,55] Sensitivity tests provide an optimal condition for the interaction of the drug and organism which does not always exist in the patient. The end point of these tests may indicate bacterial activity or merely inhibition of growth. These may be differentiated by subculturing the apparently clear tubes. This method may be used as a general index of the sensitivity of a particular organism. In most cases it is possible to predict by experience the dosage of penicillin or other antibiotic needed in the treatment of a specific organism once its sensitivity is known. The adequacy of the dosage may then be evaluated by the clinical response and the serum inhibition tests.[55]

Recent experimental endocarditis studies have demonstrated synergism between penicillin and vancomycin with aminoglycoside antibiotics such as gentamicin and streptomycin, which greatly enhances the rapidity and efficiency of sterilization of the verrucae by these agents.[56,57]

3 The drug used should be able to penetrate fibrin.[52,53] In this disease the bacteria are deep within the vegetation and must be reached by the antibiotics if cure is to take place. The excellent results seen with penicillin therapy may be in part related to its ability to penetrate fibrin, in contrast to a drug such as polymyxin which is potent in the test tube but disappointing in vivo and has only limited fibrin-penetrating ability.

4 Treatment should be continued long enough to effect a cure. The trend today seems to be toward shorter courses of treatment. Though this has been successful with the *Streptococcus viridans* group,[54] it has not been so for the *S. faecalis* (the enterococci) or the staphylococci.

5 Once adequate serum levels have been demonstrated and clinical response in the form of a feeling of well-being is experienced by the patient, treatment should not be abandoned if fever or petechiae reappear or embolization should occur. Fever is not uncommonly caused by the penicillin itself during treatment, and this may respond to the use of Benadryl hydrochloride (diphenhydramine hydrochloride).[7] Fever may also be due to phlebitis at the site of intravenous infusion or sterile abscess formation if the intramuscular route is used. Petechiae and peripheral emboli may occur for many weeks after the disease is totally eradicated.[21] If the dosage of penicillin is found to be inadequate as indicated by serum dilution tests, it is better to double the dose than to increase in small increments. This is a potentially lethal disease which demands early aggressive treatment if disability and/or death are to be prevented. It is far better to overtreat than to undertreat.

Penicillin G or one of the semi-synthetic penicillinase-resistant varieties, alone or in combination with aminoglycoside antibiotics, remains the backbone of therapy in bacterial endocarditis.[58]

Various methods of administration of penicillin have been suggested.[52] Initially, intermittent intramuscular dosage was employed with injections given at 2-, 3-, or 4-h intervals. More recently, a continuous intravenous drip through a No. 25 pediatric scalp vein needle inserted in a small vein of the hand or arm has been employed.[7] Heparin, 25 mg/1,000 ml 5 percent dextrose and water, is added to minimize the tendency of local phlebitis formation which occurs with high dosages of penicillin. A polyethylene catheter may be inserted into the vena cava in selected cases where peripheral veins are not adequate. The experimental work of Eagle, which demonstrated the superiority of intermittent over continuous doses of penicillin in controlling infection in animals,[53] has not proved to be a significant factor in the treatment of bacterial endocarditis.

Oral penicillin treatment of endocarditis has been advocated from time to time, but the variability of the absorption of penicillin from the gastrointestinal tract of the same patient and from patient to patient makes this an unsatisfactory method of treatment for this disease.[39,52,59] This unreliability of absorption also holds true for the newer penicillinase-resistant penicillins,[60] and these drugs are not recommended at this time.

In addition to antibiotics, other medications, such as the anticoagulants and fibrinolytic enzymes, have been employed as adjuvants in the treatment of bacterial endocarditis. These agents have been used for either preventing formation of the vegetations or breaking down the already formed verrucae to allow better penetration of the antimicrobial drugs. Anticoagulants have been abandoned in the treatment of bacterial endocarditis because they have shown no therapeutic benefit and because of the increased danger from bleeding if embolization should occur. They are now used only in the treatment of thrombophlebitis and pulmonary emboli occurring during the course of left-sided bacterial endocarditis. Fibrinolytic enzymes have been used in experimental animals with no clear-cut indication of therapeutic value, and in addition they may produce toxic reactions.

Probenecid (Benemid) has been recommended by many writers.[52,59,60] This drug, given in doses of 0.5 g every 6 h by mouth, will increase the penicillin level of the blood about four times and will prolong the duration of effect of an individual injection to about 12 h. This drug may not be necessary, since any desired level of penicillin may be maintained by intravenous administration as described previously. Nausea and vomiting are seen in 7 percent of cases.

When penicillin is used in high concentrations, it must be remembered that the sodium salt contains 40 mg sodium per million units and the potassium salt contains 65 mg potassium. This could be a significant factor in patients with congestive heart failure or renal insufficiency.

Myoclonic jerks, hyperreflexia, seizures, and coma have been reported in patients in whom inordinately high concentrations of penicillin have accumulated in the cerebrospinal fluid because of either excessive dosage or failure of renal excretion.

In the author's experience, penicillin reactions have not constituted a great problem. If a history of previous penicillin sensitivity in the form of rash or itching is obtained, the usual dose is started intravenously with 50 mg Benadryl hydrochloride added to the infusion. Epinephrine, Solu-Cortef, and equipment for providing an airway are held immediately available when the infusion is started. Other writers have recommended penicillin desensitization,[55] concomitant use of adrenal steroids, or the use of antibiotics other than penicillin.[61] Penicillin desensitization in itself is hazardous and may provide no protection[61] against subsequent anaphylactic reactions. In those cases where itching and rash become a problem despite Benadryl hydrochloride, prednisone has been used orally to control this reaction. The author has found it necessary to discontinue treatment in only one case because of uncontrolled reaction to the penicillin. Previous anaphylactic-type reaction would constitute an indication for the use of another antibiotic.

If repeated attempts at therapy with appropriate antibiotics in sufficient dosage are unsuccessful, or more important, if *intractable* heart failure should occur secondary to valvular insufficiency during therapy, then replacement of the damaged valve should be undertaken while therapy is continued.[62,63] When murmurs exist in two or more valve areas, the decision for surgery has to be made, multiple quantitative blood cultures taken proximal and distal to each valve can be helpful in localizing the site of infection.[64] Echocardiography may also be useful in this situation since verrucae on the valves can at times be identified.

After treatment is completed, blood cultures should be drawn at 2, 4, and 6 weeks and a close check kept on temperature during this period. Physical activity during treatment is limited according to the individual situation. Bed rest is employed with heart failure or other evidence of myocarditis during treatment, whereas in uncomplicated cases the patient is allowed such freedom as can be permitted by a mobile infusion stand. The duration of disability following treatment is also dictated by the stage of compensation of the individual patient. Strenuous exercise should be restricted for several weeks following treatment.

STREPTOCOCCUS VIRIDANS

In most cases of *Streptococcus viridans* endocarditis, the minimum inhibiting dose of penicillin as measured by tube dilution is less than 0.1 unit/ml.[39,59,65] It has been demonstrated by Tompsett et al.[65] and by Geraci[54,59] that this group of bacteria may be treated with a combination of 1 million units of aqueous procaine penicillin G intramuscularly every 12 h, 1 g streptomycin and 1 g dihydrostreptomycin given alternately every 12 h, and 0.5 g Benemid given orally every 6 h. The treatment is continued for 14 days. It should be noted that this short-term therapy is recommended only for the most sensitive of the *S. viridans* group, those inhibited by 0.1 unit of penicillin per milliliter or less. Tompsett et al., using a schedule of 500,000 units of penicillin G intramuscularly every 2 h plus 0.5 g dihydrostreptomycin every 6 h or 1 g every 12 h intramuscularly, obtained a 91 percent cure rate with 33 cases of *S. viridans* endocarditis which had sensitivities of 0.4 unit/ml or less.[65] It is interesting that 7 of his 33 cases had a resistance greater than 0.1 unit/ml, but in each of these there was also a bacteriologic cure on this regimen. Tan[66] reported on 49 patients with *S. viridans* with a minimal inhibitory concentration of 0.2 μ or less who were treated for 2 weeks. Of these, 13 were treated with parenteral penicillin G alone, 9 with parenteral penicillin G plus streptomycin, and 27 with oral penicillin V plus streptomycin. The patients in the group treated with penicillin alone relapsed but were cured by a repeat of lesser therapy with parenteral penicillin. Wolfe[67] treated 100 cases with parenteral penicillin G in the mean dose of 11.4 million units per day for 30.4 days and streptomycin 1.2 g per day for 13.4 days with no bacteriologic failures and only two episodes of ataxia attributable to the streptomycin. These subsided spontaneously. Since there is a small percentage of cases with *S. viridans* which are not controlled by the 2-week regimen, it would seem logical to extend the duration of the treatment in an attempt to include these cases.[65]

The suggested treatment for *S. viridans* endocarditis is 10 million units of aqueous crystalline penicillin G given as a continuous intravenous infusion in 5 percent dextrose and water with 25 mg heparin added to each 1,000 ml. In addition 1 g streptomycin should be given each day intramuscularly. This dosage should be continued for 3 weeks. The penicillinase-resistant penicillins, oxacillin and methicillin, should not be used in the treatment of *S. viridans*.[60,68] Vancomycin has been utilized for treatment of *S. viridans* when serious penicillin sensitivity was present.[69] This should be combined with streptomycin 0.5 g given intramuscularly twice a day. More recently clindamycin (Cleocin) has been used in penicillin-sensitive individuals in a dose of 450 mg given intramuscularly every 8 h.[70]

STREPTOCOCCUS GROUP D (FECALIS, BOVIS, EQUINUS)

The best therapy at the present time for enterococcus infection is a combination of penicillin G and streptomycin given in high dosage for a prolonged period of time.[54,71] Although the need for streptomycin has been questioned by some, when large doses of penicillin are used, the suggested method of treatment is to give 20 million units of penicillin each day as a continuous intravenous drip supplemented with 1 g streptomycin intramuscularly. Treatment should be continued for 4 weeks. Once therapy is established, the efficacy of the dosage should be tested by serum inhibition studies done 2 h after a dose of streptomycin. If the serum is not lethal for the pateint's bacteria at greater than 1:4 dilution, then the penicillin should be increased to 40 million units and inhibition studies repeated. Weinstein[72] has demonstrated in four patients that a combination of 1 million units of intravenous penicillin and 60 to 100 mg of gentamicin intramuscularly every 8 h is equally effective in treatment of enterococcal endocarditis. He has also demonstrated that in vitro this combination is effective against a greater percentage of enterococcus isolates than the penicillin-streptomycin combination. Vancomycin 500 mg intravenously every 6 h in combination with streptomycin 1 g intramuscularly each day provides an acceptable alternative to penicillin-sensitive patients or in those in whom the penicillin-streptomycin treatment was ineffective.[73] On the basis of in vitro bactericidal activity, intravenous ampicillin 12 g a day with 1 g streptomycin has been suggested as an alternative for the penicillin-streptomycin therapy of enterococcal endocarditis, but sufficient clinical trials of the drug used in this manner are not available at the present time for evaluation.[74] Cephalosporin and clindamycin, used either alone or in combination with aminoglycoside, such as gentamicin or streptomycin, have not proved adequate in enterococcal infections. In penicillin-sensitive patients erythromycin 1 g intravenously every 6 h may be effective.

Streptococcus bovis and *equinus* contain the group D antigen but are much more sensitive to penicillin in vitro and in vivo than the enterococcus varieties, and probably could be treated with penicillin alone. Until more information is available, infection by these agents should be treated the same as enterococcus infection, with penicillin or vancomycin plus and aminoglycoside as described above for enterococcus.[75]

STAPHYLOCOCCUS

The treatment of *Staphylococcus* endocarditis depends on the resistance of the organism and its ability to produce penicillinase. Sensitivity of the organism should be established by the tube-dilution method and the absence of penicillinase production demonstrated by the techniques of Haight. Penicillin G–sensitive *Staphylococcus aureus* or *Staphylococcus epidermidis* should be treated with 50 million units of aqueous, crystalline penicillin G in a 24-h intravenous drip in addition to 0.5 g streptomycin intramuscularly every 12 h. If this combination fails to provide a clinical response within 2 to 3 days, or if the serum bactericidal level is less than 1:4 dilution of the patient's serum, then the penicillin dose should be doubled, or gentamicin 5 mg/kg substituted for streptomycin. Vancomycin 500 mg every 6 h intravenously and gentamicin 5 mg/kg given in divided dose every 8 h may be substituted for penicillin in the allergic patient, or keflin 12 g intravenously with streptomycin or gentamicin may be used. There is some crossover sensitivity with penicillin, but this is not usually a problem. Treatment should be carried out for at least 4 weeks. Recurrence of fever during treatment may mean the emergence of a penicillinase-producing resistant staphylococcus, and cultures should be repeated.[65] The duration of the treatment has not been established with certainty for vancomycin or cephalothin, but 4 weeks is probably necessary with this particular type of bacteria. Staphylococci which are more resistant than usual to penicillin but which do not produce penicillinase should also be treated with penicillin G and streptomycin, vancomycin, or cephalothin. Methicillin (Staphcillin) and non-penicillinase-producing staphylococci as in penicillin G and should not be used with these bacteria.[68]

For resistant penicillinase-producing staphylococci, one of the penicillinase-resistant varieties of penicillin is the treatment of choice.[54,55,60,68] For practical purposes, resistance in a clinically identified staphylococcus is synonymous with penicillinase production.[60,68] Treatment for resistant penicillinase-producing staphylococci consists of nafcillin (Unipen) 12 g a day given either intramuscularly or intravenously in combination with 1 g streptomycin each day or gentamicin 5 mg/kg in divided doses every 8 h, oxacillin 12 g intravenously along with streptomycin or gentamicin, vancomycin 500 mg intravenously every 6 h in combination with intramuscular streptomycin or intravenous gentamicin, or methicillin 18 to 24 g intravenously and gentamicin. Treatment should be continued for a period of 4 weeks, and serum inhibition tests should be repeated during therapy to ensure a continuing adequacy of the levels.

ENDOCARDITIS WITH NEGATIVE BLOOD CULTURES[34]

For those cases of bacterial endocarditis in which the diagnosis is clinically certain but bacteriologically unproven, the usual starting therapy is 25 million units of aqueous, crystalline penicillin G given as a 24-h intravenous drip with 1 g streptomycin intramuscularly. If there is no response in 2 to 3 days, and the cultures remain negative, the penicillin dose is doubled, and if this is unsuccessful, gentamicin 5 mg/kg may be substituted for the streptomycin. If, at the outset, disease seems rapidly progressive or the possibility of staphylococcal infection exists, nafcillin 3 g every 4 h intravenously should be added to the regimen.

Since there is no combination of drugs which will cover all possible bacteria, therapy should be begun with an agent or agents which will cover the bacteria most commonly involved in that particular type of clinical presentation. If routine cultures continue to remain negative, a further search for fungi and other more fastidious organisms should be carried out along with antibody titers for *Rickettsia*. Percipitin tests for *Candida* may be helpful.

POSTOPERATIVE ENDOCARDITIS

The therapy for bacterial endocarditis following cardiac surgical treatment presents a different problem from that of the usual case. In this situation there is a nidus of infection, often at the site of a suture or prosthesis, which cannot always be reached or eradicated by the usual antibiotic regimens. Two groups of patients have been identified.[77,78] The first occurring in the immediate postoperative period up to 60 days, and those occurring at any time thereafter. The first group will many times contain particularly resistant bacteria or fungi which respond poorly to antibacterial therapy. Treatment with the appropriate antibiotic should be instituted, but because of resistance to antibiotics and for other reasons such as overwhelming sepsis or production of large emboli, surgery may be required early in the course of treatment. Endocarditis occurring later in the postoperative state should be treated with the usual antibacterial regimen for the organism involved, and surgery carried out only if the prosthesis has become dislodged or otherwise compromised, or if heart failure or other indications for surgery in endocarditis are present.

GRAM-NEGATIVE ENDOCARDITIS

Treatment of endocarditis caused by the gram-negative bacteria has not been satisfactorily delineated. These bacteria are still a rare cause of disease in the absence of suture material or prosthetic valves, and no large body of experience in their treatment is available. For this reason, one must rely on the in vitro sensitivity studies to indicate the proper choice of therapeutic agent. There have been several reports of successful treatment of *Pseudomonas aeruginosa* endocarditis with an aminoglycoside-carbenicillin combination (carbenicillin 30 to 40 g, gentamicin 100 mg), sometimes together with polymyxin or tobramycin and combined with excision of infected valves.[79] The cure rate seems to be definitely related to excision of infected valves or prostheses. *Pseudomonas cepacia* has been treated successfully with trimethoprim sulfamethoxazole and polymyxin accompanied by surgical removal of the infected valve.[80] *Serratia marcescens* has been successfully treated with the combination of carbenicillin-gentamicin along with valvular excision.[81] Ampicillin 12 g a day intravenously has been successful with various strains of *Hemophilus, E. Coli, Proteus mirabilis,* and *Salmonella.* As with the other gram-negative bacteria, excision of the infected valve may be necessary if response to antibiotic treatment is not adequate. Cephalothin is effective against certain gram-negative bacteria; it has been particularly effective against the motile *Aerobacter* forms and may be potentiated with streptomycin or kanamycin in this setting. Gentamicin has been used, and massive doses of penicillin G have also been successfully employed in the treatment of *Salmonella typhimurium* endocarditis.[82]

FUNGAL ENDOCARDITIS

Amphotericin B, alone or in combination with 5-fluorocytosine, is the drug of choice for endocarditis caused by *Histoplasma, Candida, Rhodotorula, Aspergillis,* and blastomycosis. The optimal dosage of amphotericin has not been decided at present, but cures have been elicited by starting with a dose of 0.25 mg/kg body weight and gradually increasing to a maximally tolerated daily dose, usually 75 to 80 mg/day, which is then continued for a period of 6 months.[54,83] It appears, however, that fungal[84] endocarditis is rarely curable with the drug therapy alone. Excellent results with treatment of *Candida* endocarditis have been reported by Utley,[85] who recommends surgical removal of the infected valve and irrigation of the heart at surgery with amphotericin B solution followed by intravenous amphotericin therapy for a minimum of 10 to 12 weeks.

MISCELLANEOUS ORGANISMS

Endocarditis due to *Rickettsia burnetii* has been successfully treated with intermittent dosage of tetracycline or, if this fails, by surgical removal of the infected valve, followed by administration of tetracycline for a period of several months.[32] Gonococci, β-hemolytic streptocci, and pneumococci should be treated with 20 million units of penicillin G by continuous intravenous drip for a period of 4 weeks. *Bacteroides* presents a difficult problem because of resistance of certain strains to presently available antibiotics. Individual sensitivity tests should be done with this organism. Good results with some strains have been reported with the use of large doses of penicillin and more recently with clindamycin given in a dose of 340 mg intramuscularly every 8 h.[70,86]

Prognosis

The prognosis of the patient who has undergone successful antibacterial treatment depends on several factors, the most important of which is the residual valvular damage. Studies have shown that valvular damage in the form of valve perforations or increased insufficiency, particularly of the aortic valve, is responsible for the greatest morbidity and mortality in the posttreatment period.[6,7,87] Such patients are

frequently candidates for corrective valve surgical procedures. Robinson and Ruedy,[87] in studying autopsy material of bacterial endocarditis, have also noted this increased tendency to valvular perforations and congestive heart failure in their fatal cases. Uremia secondary to acquired nephritis of bacterial endocarditis is no longer a common cause of death during or after treatment.[6,7] Cerebral vascular accidents[6] and coronary embolization[6] in the posttreatment period have been recorded as occasional causes of death. It is difficult to assess the functional importance of the myocarditis which occurs with bacterial endocarditis, since patients demonstrating severe congestive heart failure have also invariably had severe valvular lesions. Some writers have felt that the myocarditis produced during bacterial endocarditis was the primary factor in congestive heart failure.[52] Robinson and Ruedy[87] have noticed the coincidence of valvular perforations and congestive heart failure in their autopsy series and, in reviewing charts, were able to correlate the onset of failure with the appearance of clinical signs of perforation. They also felt that the morphologic changes in the myocardium could not explain the frequency of heart failure, since they were present with equal frequency in patients with and without congestive heart failure.[87]

In general the fate of survivors has been good.[6,7] In the author's series from Emory University, 82 percent survived for 5 years.[7] All but 1 of the 10 deaths which occurred after treatment came within the first 5 years after discharge from the hospital. Four occurred within the first year. Morgan and Bland reported 10-year survival in their patients.[6] Of their 17 deaths, 11 occurred within 25 months after discharge from the hospital.

Relapse following treatment is less common today than when smaller doses of antibiotics were used and now occurs in about 5 to 10 percent of cases. Relapse almost invariably occurs within 6 to 8 weeks after therapy. Reinfection is estimated by several writers to occur in about 2 to 4 percent of patients.[7]

Prophylaxis

It has been demonstrated that significant bacteremia may occur in patients with oral sepsis with or without dental manipulations, following tooth extraction, transurethral prostatic resection, urethral catheterization, and in many other clinical situations. Since bacteremia plus valvular damage or congenital cardiac deformity may result in bacterial endocarditis, an attempt should be made either to control bacteremia or to prevent implantation and multiplication of the bacteria in the epithelium of the heart.

Studies of bacteremia before and after the use of antibiotics in the procedures mentioned show that bacteremia cannot be eliminated but can be substantially reduced.[88] This effect, plus the inhibiting action of the drug before the bacteria can be established in the heart valves, may logically be assumed to prevent bacterial endocarditis, although statistical proof of this fact is not available.[52] Experimental work in the rabbit model has given some insight into the activity of antibiotics against bacteria which settle on marantic vegetations.[89,90] Many questions still exist, however, as to the comparability of this and other animal-model experiments with natually occurring infections.

All patients with rheumatic or syphilitic valvular disease or congenital cardiac abnormalities should be given antibiotic prophylaxis in the situations which will be discussed in the following sections.

DENTAL

Instruction of the patient with valvular or congenital heart disease in meticulous oral hygiene and care of the teeth and gums is the first step in prophylaxis against bacterial endocarditis.

Any dental procedure—filling, cleaning,[25] extractions, root canal work, or installation of a bridge—may result in bacteremia. Multiple extractions particularly should be avoided in the presence of dental sepsis because of the increase in intensity of the bacteremia in this situation. Bacteremia usually persists for less than 30 min following extractions. *Streptococcus viridans* is the organism present in the bacteremia in over 90 percent of the cases. Preliminary use of penicillin for several days before extraction may result in the emergence of resistant strains of streptococci.

Several suggestions for prophylaxis have been made on the basis of recent animal work. Durack[91] suggested benzyl penicillin 2 million units plus procaine penicillin 600,000 units plus streptomycin 1 g intramuscularly 30 min before the procedure. An alternative for individuals who are penicillin-sensitive would be vancomycin 1 g intravenously before the procedure. Kaye[92] used the same penicillin-streptomycin approach, but would give an additional 600,000 units of procaine penicillin intramuscularly on each of the 2 days following the procedure. For patients who are hypersensitive to penicillin, cefazolin 1 g plus streptomycin 0.5 g by intramuscular injection 30 min before the procedure, with additional doses every 8 h for 72 h is recommended. Erythromycin 500 mg four times a day for 72 h starting 1 h before the procedure has been suggested for individuals who are hypersensitive to penicillin but must take oral prophylaxis.

Until more information is available concerning human prophylaxis in this relatively uncommon disease, 1.2 million units of procaine penicillin given 2 h before the dental procedure, and repeated once in 8 to 12 h if bleeding is still apparent, could be used for all routine dental work. Obviously infected areas would require continuation of medication at 8-h intervals. Cefazolin 1 g 2 h before the procedure, repeated as with the penicillin-streptomycin, could be used in penicillin-sensitive individuals. Vancomycin 500 mg intravenously could also be used. If intravenous or intramuscular medication cannot be used and the individual is penicillin-sensitive, eryth-romycin 500 mg four times a day beginning 1 h before the procedure and continuing for 2 days is an alternative. If, for any reason, intramuscular or intravenous antibiotic cannot be used in the non-penicillin-sensitive patient, then penicillin V 2 million units taken 1 h before the procedure and continued at 6-h intervals for 48 h is suggested.

Necessary dental work in the patient with endocarditis should be accomplished during the course of therapy.

GENITOURINARY

Streptococcus faecalis (enterococcus) is the chief group of bacteria found after genitourinary manipulation or surgical treatment.[26] The present procedure is to give procaine penicillin 2 million units intramuscularly or 500 mg of ampicillin plus 1 g streptomycin 30 min before the procedure and repeated every 12 h thereafter for 3 days. Kaye[92] has suggested using aqueous penicillin G 20 million units intravenously daily with streptomycin 1 g intramuscularly every 12 h or with gentamicin 1.7 mg/kg intramuscularly every 8 h starting 1 h before the procedure and continuing for 72 h.

PREGNANCY

Treatment should start with the onset of labor with 1.2 million units of procaine penicillin plus 1 g streptomycin intramuscularly and should be continued for 3 days in the postpartum period.

GASTROINTESTINAL TRACT

Procedures likely to cause trauma to soft tissues, particularly if infection is present, should be treated with prophylactic antibiotics as outlined for genitourinary disease. If staphylococcal infection is suspected, oxacillin, 1 g intramuscularly plus 0.5 g streptomycin should be given about 2 h before the procedure and continued for 2 days at 4-h intervals.

TONSILLECTOMY

Patients undergoing tonsillectomy should be given prophylaxis in the same manner as those undergoing dental procedures.

CARDIAC SURGERY

Prevention of infective endocarditis in the immediate postoperative period in bypass surgical procedures is a difficult problem. A multitude of bacteria, including *Staphylococcus aureus, S. epidermatis, pseudomonas sepacia, Corynebacterium, Pseudomonas aerogenosa,* and many other forms including fungi have been reported as infecting agents. There is no single antibiotic or antibiotic combination which could cover all of these possibilities adequately, so attention should be directed to prevention of the most common immediate postoperative infecting agent, which is *S. aureus* or *epidermatis.* One suggestion is 12 g/day of methicillin starting the night before operation and continuing into the third postoperative day or until all intracardiac monitoring lines have been removed. Some physicians have suggested that gentamicin be started immediately after surgery and be continued as long as the methicillin but we have not subscribed to this practice. The danger of such broad spectrum coverage of antibiotics is that it may predispose to superinfection with fungi. Our own recommendation is 1 g of oxacillin intravenously beginning 1 h preoperatively and repeated every 6 h for 4 days in the postoperative state. Meticulous care of equipment, a reduction of operative technique, and rigid attention to antiseptic technique in the interoperative and postoperative periods are still the mainstay of prophylaxis in this situation. In the studies by Kluge,[93] the chief source of contamination in the operating room is the air directly in the area of the operative site and the blood used for transfusion. Attempts at prophylaxis definitely include efforts directed toward correction of these problems.

INTRACARDIAC PROSTHESES

The author has seen bacterial endocarditis due to hemolytic *Staphylococcus aureus*, *Streptococcus viridans*, and nonhemolytic *Staphylococcus epidermidis* following dental procedures in patients with prosthetic mitral and aortic valves which have been in place from 1 to 4 years. For this reason it is recommended that all patients with prosthetic valves be given 1 g of nafcillin plus 0.5 g streptomycin intramuscularly 1 h prior to dental manipulation and on the mornings of the 2 subsequent days in the case of extractions. In the presence of penicillin sensitivity, vancomycin or erythromycin, as previously described, could be substituted.

NONBACTERIAL THROMBOTIC ENDOCARDITIS

Nonbacterial thrombotic endocarditis (NBTE)—terminal endocarditis, marantic endocarditis, cachexic endocarditis, endocarditis simplex, degenerative verrucous endocarditis—was first described by Ziegler[94] in 1888 and was distinguished from other forms of endocarditis by Libman[95] in 1923. The present nomenclature was applied by Gross and Friedburg in 1936.[94] Except for a prediction by Libman concerning the role of NBTE,[96] this disease was considered by most writers to be a terminal occurrence[94,95] with no clinical significance until Allen and Sirota suggested that it might actually be the first step in the formation of bacterial endocarditis. Angrist and Marquiss agreed with this idea and suggested that in addition the nonbacterial lesions might also represent a healed form of bacterial endocarditis and could be the cause of postcure embolization. There is little evidence to show that NBTE is a residual of infectious endocarditis, but more recent clinical and laboratory studies seem to indicate that histologically similar lesions induced by indwelling catheters in the right side of the heart do serve as a nidus for infective endocarditis in both animals and human beings.[89,97] Several reports are now available which show that the spontaneously occurring nonbacterial vegetations are, indeed, responsible for peripheral arterial embolization and may be the cause of death.[96,98–103]

Horowitz and Ward[101] have attempted to relate disseminated intravascular coagulation, pulmonary hyaline membrane disease, and NBTE through the mediation of tissue thromboplastin, which is presumably released from an infected bowel tissue. A somewhat similar suggestion was previously made by McKay[102] in a case of disseminated intravascular coagulation in nonbacterial endocarditis associated with metastatic colon carcinoma.

The lesions appear in five types: (1) small univerrucous lesions, barely visible, consisting of a single nodule up to 3 mm high seen along the line of closure of the valves; (2) a large univerrucous nodule which is more firmly adherent to the valve proper and which may be smooth or shaggy in appearance and up to 7 mm in size; (3) a small multiverrucous lesion composed of as many as three nodules firmly attached to the valve and spread along the line of closure like a beaded ridge, grossly resembling the verrucae of acute rheumatic fever;[44] (4) a large multiverrucous lesion consisting of a friable, granulomatous mass up to 7 mm high, spread for several centimeters across the area of closure to the valve (this may be loosely attached to the valve and would be likely to produce emboli); (5) healed lesions, which take the form of a fibrous tab or nodule resembling valve tissue at the valve margin, particularly at the corpora Arantii (Lambl's excrescences), and may occur in normal or diseased valves and appear to be the result of a collagen degeneration within the valve leaflet which has provided a nidus for thrombosis.[98,99]

This disease is not restricted to individuals with prolonged illness or cachexia, and has been reported in illness of 1 day to several years' duration.[98,99] Various malignancies, usually with metastasis, are the most common accompanying illness, but the verrucae have been found with acute pneumonia, pulmonary emboli, peritonitis secondary to perforated viscus, ruptured abdominal aneurysm, and many other acute diseases. Also, two cases have been reported in patients with organic psychosis.[98,99,104,105] Males and females are about equally affected. The ages reported have ranged from 18 to 90 years. Murmurs are present in about one-third of the cases and are usually systolic and are related to previous rheumatic or atherosclerotic disease. The valves on the left side of the heart are the most commonly affected, with only occasional reports of tricuspid or pulmonic involvement.[97,99] Significant aortic regurgitation has resulted from interference with coaptation of the aortic valve leaflets by large "marantic" vegetation.[106] The vegetations should be demonstrable by echocardiography, which provides an easily available noninvasive method of identification.

The importance of these lesions lies in their ability to cause peripheral arterial embolization and to mimic the clinical findings of bacterial endocarditis, particularly if fever is present from some other cause. It may be, as suggested by some writers, that these lesions do form a site for implantation of bacteria and may account for some of the bacterial endocarditis seen on previously normal valves.

At the present time, there is no definite therapy for

NBTE, although anticoagulation may have some place in prevention of repeated embolic episodes.

LIBMAN-SACKS ENDOCARDITIS

See discussion of lupus erythematosus in Chap. 88.

REFERENCES

1 Horder, T.: Infective Endocarditis, with an Analysis of 150 Cases and with Special References to the Chronic Form of the Disease, *Q. J. Med.,* 2:290, 1909.

2 Libman, E., and Celler, H.: The Etiology of Subacute Infective Endocarditis, *Am. J. Med. Sci.,* 140:516, 1910.

3 Osler, W.: Chronic Infective Endocarditis, *Q. J. Med.,* 2:219, 1909.

4 Osler, W.: Gulstonian Lectures on Malignant Endocarditis, *Lancet,* 1:415–418, 459–464, 505–508, 1885.

5 Loewe, L., Rosenblatt, P., Greene, H., and Russell, M.: Combined Penicillin and Heparin Therapy of Subacute Bacterial Endocarditis: Report of Seven Consecutive Successfully Treated Patients, *JAMA,* 124:144, 1944.

6 Morgan, W., and Bland, E.: Bacterial Endocarditis in the Antibiotic Era, *Circulation,* 19:753, 1959.

7 Vogler, R., Dorney, E., and Bridges, H.: Bacterial Endocarditis, *Am. J. Med.,* 32:910, 1962.

8 Afremow, M.: A Review of 202 Cases of Bacterial Endocarditis, 1948–1952, *Ill. Med. J.,* 107:67, 1955.

9 Allen, A.: Nature of Vegetations of Bacterial Endocarditis, *AMA Arch. Pathol.,* 27:661, 1939.

10 Vogler, R., and Dorney, E.: Bacterial Endocarditis in the Normal Heart, *Bull. Emory Univ. Clin.,* 1:21, 1961.

11 Gould, S.: "Pathology of the Heart," 2d ed., Charles C Thomas, Publisher, Springfield, Ill., 1960.

12 Libman, E.: A Study of the Endocardial Lesions of Subacute Bacterial Endocarditis, *Am. J. Med.,* 13:544, 1952.

13 Vogler, R., and Dorney, E.: Bacterial Endocarditis in Congenital Heart Disease, *Am. Heart J.,* 64:198, 1962.

14 Nadas, A.: "Pediatric Cardiology," 2d ed., W. B. Saunders Company, Philadelphia, 1963.

15 Geraci, J., Dale, A., and McGoon, D. P.: Bacterial Endocarditis and Endarteritis Following Cardiac Operations: Addendum, *Wis. Med. J.,* 62:302, 1963.

16 Sykes, C., Beckwith, J., Muller, W., and Wood, J.: Postoperative Endoauriculitis Due to *Pseudomonas aeruginosa* Cured by a Second Operation, *Arch. Intern. Med.,* 110:113, 1962.

17 Stein, P., Harken, D., and Dexter, L.: The Nature and Prevention of Prosthetic Valve Endocarditis, *Am. Heart J.,* 71:393, 1967.

18 Elek, S.: Experimental Staphylococcal Infections in the Skin of Man, *Ann. N.Y. Acad. Sci.,* 65:85, 1956.

19 Thayer, W.: Studies on Bacterial (Infective) Endocarditis, *Johns Hopkins Hosp. Rep.,* 22:1, 1926.

20 Sheldon, W., and Golden, A.: Valve Ring Abscess of the Heart, a Frequent but Not Well Recognized Complication of Acute Bacterial Endocarditis, *Circulation,* 4:1, 1951.

21 Kerr, A.: "Subacute Bacterial Endocarditis," Charles C Thomas, Publisher, Springfield, Ill., 1955.

22 Bell, E.: Glomerular Lesions Associated with Endocarditis, *Am. J. Pathol.,* 8:639, 1932.

23 Levy, R., and Hong, R.: The Immune Nature of Sub Acute Bacterial Endocarditis (S.B.E. Nephritis), *Am. J. Med.,* 54:645, 1973.

24 Garrison, P., and Freedman, L.: Experimental Endocarditis. 1. Staphylococcal Endocarditis in Rabbits Resulting from Placement of a Polyethylene Catheter in the Right Side of the Heart, *Yale J. Biol. Med.,* 42:394, 1970.

25 Harvey, W., and Capone, M.: Bacterial Endocarditis Related to Cleaning and Filling Teeth, *Am. J. Cardiol.,* 7:793, 1961.

26 Koenig, M., and Kaye, D.: Enterococcal Endocarditis, *N. Engl. J. Med.,* 264:257, 1961.

27 Hussey, H., and Katz, S.: Infections Resulting from Narcotic Addiction: Report of 102 Cases, *Am. J. Med.,* 9:186, 1950.

28 Bain, R., Edwards, J., Scheifley, C., and Geraci, J.: Right-sided Endocarditis and Endarteritis: A Clinical and Pathological Study, *Am. J. Med.,* 24:98, 1958.

29 Rodbard, S.: Blood Velocity and Endocarditis, *Circulation,* 27:18, 1963.

30 Kerr, A.: Bacterial Endocarditis—Revisited, *Mod. Concepts Cardiovasc. Dis.,* 33:831, 1963.

31 Evans, A.: Rickettsia Endocarditis, *Br. Med. J.,* 1:1613, 1963.

32 Kristinsson, A., and Bentall, H.: Medical and Surgical Treatment of Q Fever Endocarditis, *Lancet,* 2:693, 1967.

33 Thayer, W.: Bacterial or Infective Endocarditis, *Edinburgh Med. J.,* 38:237, 1931.

34 Cherubin, C. E., and Neu, H. C.: Infective Endocarditis at the Presbyterian Hospital at New York City 1938–1962, *Am. J. Med.,* 51:83, 1971.

35 Wilson, L.: Etiology of Bacterial Endocarditis, *Ann. Intern. Med.,* 58:946, 1963.

36 Blount, J.: Bacterial Endocarditis, *Am. J. Med.,* 38:909, 1965.

37 Pankey, G.: Subacute Bacterial Endocarditis at the University of Minnesota Hospital, 1939 through 1959, *Ann. Intern. Med.,* 55:550, 1961.

38 Pankey, G.: Acute Bacterial Endocarditis at the University of Minnesota Hospital, 1939 through 1959, *Am. Heart J.,* 64:583, 1962.

39 Hunter, T., and Patterson, P.: Bacterial Endocarditis, *Disease-A-Month,* November 1956, p. 1.

40 Williams, T., Viroslav, J., and Knight, V.: Management of Endocarditis—1970, *Am. J. Cardiol.,* 26:186, 1970.

41 Segal, B., Likoff, W., and Moyer, J.: "The Theory and Practice of Auscultation," F. A. Davis Company, Philadelphia, 1964, p. 313.

42 Dormer, A.: Bacterial Endocarditis: Survey of Patients Treated between 1945 and 1956, *Br. Med. J.,* 1:63, 1958.

43 MacGregor, G.: Murmurless Bacterial Endocarditis, *Br. Med., J.,* 1:1011, 1956.

44 Gross, N., and Tall, R.: Clinical Significance of Splinter Hemorrhages, *Br. Med. J.,* 2:1496, 1963.

45 Austrian, R.: The Syndrome of Pneumococcal Endocarditis, Meningitis, and Rupture of the Aortic Valve, *Trans. Am. Clin. Climatol. Assoc.,* 68:40, 1956.

46 Hill, R., and Bayrd, E.: Phagocytic RE Cells in Subacute Bacterial Endocarditis with Negative Cultures, *Am. Intern. Med.,* 52:310, 1960.

47 Gaines, D. J., and Remington, J. S.: Diagnosis of Deep Infection with *Candida, Arch. Intern. Med.,* 132:699, 1973.

48 Washington, J.: Blood Cultures. Principles and Techniques, *Mayo Clin. Proc.,* 50:91, 1975.

49 Bennett, I.: Bacteremia, *Veterans Admin. Tech. Bull.,* 2, 1954.

50 Bennett, I., and Beeson, P.: Bacteremia: A Consideration of Some Experimental and Clinical Aspects, *Yale J. Biol. Med.,* 26:241, 1953–1954.

51 Belli, J., and Waisbren, B.: The Number of Blood Cultures Necessary to Diagnose More Cases of Bacterial Endocarditis, *Am. J. Med. Sci.,* 232:284, 1956.

52 Finland, M.: Treatment of Bacterial Endocarditis, *N. Engl. J. Med.,* 250:372, 419, 1954.

53 Eagle, H.: Experimental Approach to the Problem of Treatment Failure with Penicillin, *Am. J. Med.,* 13:389, 1952.

54 Geraci, J.: Antibiotic Therapy of Bacterial Endocarditis, *Heart Bull.,* 12:90, 1963.

55 Glaser, R., and Ripkind, D.: The Diagnosis and Treatment of Bacterial Endocarditis, *Med. Clin. North Am.,* 47:1285, 1963.

56 Watanakunakorn, C., and Glotzbecker, C.: Enhancement of the Effects of Anti-staphyloccal Antibiotics by Aminoglycosides, *Antimicrob. Agents Chemother.,* 6:802, 1974.

57 Durack, D., Pelletier, L., and Petersdorf, R.: Chemotherapy of Experimental Streptococcal Endocarditis, *J. Clin. Invest.,* 53:829, 1974.

58 Romansky, M., Foulke, C., Olson, R., and Holmes, J.: Ristocetin in Bacterial Endocarditis, *Arch. Intern. Med.,* 107:480, 1961.

59 Geraci, J.: The Antibiotic Therapy of Bacterial Endocarditis, *Med. Clin. North Am.,* 42:1107, 1958.

60 Klein, J., and Finland, M.: The New Penicillins, *N. Engl. J. Med.,* 269:1074, 1963.

61 Grieco, M., Dubin, M., Robinson, J., and Schwartz, M.: Penicillin Hypersensitivity in Patients with Bacterial Endocarditis, *Ann. Intern. Med.,* 60:204, 1964.

62 Wilcox, B., Proctor, H., Rackney, C., and Peters, R.: Early Surgical Treatment of Valvular Endocarditis, *JAMA,* 200:820, 1967.

63 Braniff, B., Shumway, N., and Harrison, D.: Valve Replacement in Active Bacterial Endocarditis, *N. Engl. J. Med.,* 276:1464, 1967.

64 Pazin, G., Peterson, K., Griff, F., Shaver, J., and Ho, M.: Determination of the Site of Infective Endocarditis, *Ann. Intern Med.,* 82:748, 1975.

65 Tompsett, R., Robbins, W., and Bernsten, C.: Short-term Penicillin and Dihydrostreptomycin Therapy of Streptococcal Endocarditis, *Am. J. Med.,* 24:57, 1958.

66 Tan, J., Kaplan, S., Terhune, C., and Hamburger, M.: Success for Two Week Treatment Schedule for Penicillin Sensitive *Streptococcus viridans* Endocarditis, *Lancet,* 2:1340, 1971.

67 Wolfe, J., and Johnson, W.: Penicillin-sensitive Streptococcal Endocarditis: In Vitro and Clinical Observations on Penicillin-Streptomycin Therapy, *Ann. Intern. Med.,* 81:178, 1974.

68 Hewitt, W.: The Penicillins: A Review of Strategy and Tactics, *JAMA,* 185:264, 1963.

69 Friedberg, C., Rosen, K., and Bienstock, P.: Vancomycin Therapy for Bacterial Endocarditis Due to *S. viridans* or Enterococcus in Patients Intolerant of Penicillin or Streptomycin (presented at the 49th Annual Session, American College of Physicians), Boston, Apr. 5, 1968.

70 Romig, D., Cox, F., Poblod, D., and Quinn, E.: Clindamycin, A New Alternate Antibiotic for Bacterial Endocarditis (program and abstracts of Eleventh Interscience Conference on Antimicrobial Agents), October 1971, p. 50.

71 Tompsett, R., and Pizette, M.: Enterococcal Endocarditis, *Arch. Intern. Med.,* 109:146, 1962.

72 Weinstein, A., and Moellering, R.: Penicillin and Gentamicin Therapy for Enterococcal Infection, *JAMA,* 223:1030, 1973.

73 Westenfelder, G., Paterson, P., Reisberg, B., and Carlson, G.: Vancomycin-Streptomycin Synergism in Enterococcal Endocarditis, *JAMA,* 223:37, 1973.

74 Beaty, H., Turck, M., and Petersdorf, R.: Ampicillin in the Treatment of Enterococcal Endocarditis, *Ann. Intern. Med.,* 65:701, 1966.

75 Watanakunakorn, C.: *Streptococcus bovis* Endocarditis, *Am. J. Med.,* 56:256, 1974.

76 Murray, H., Weakley, F., Mann, J., and Arthur, R.: Combination Antibiotic Therapy in Staphylococcal Endocarditis, *Arch. Intern. Med.,* 136:480, 1976.

77 Dorney, E., and King, S.: Bacterial Endocarditis Following Prosthetic Cardiac Valve Surgery in Early and Late Occurrence, *Circulation,* 41(suppl 3):150, 1970.

78 Wilson, W., Jaumin, P., Danielson, G., Guiliani, E., Washington, J., and Geraci, J.: Prosthetic Valve Endocarditis, *Ann. Intern. Med.,* 83:751, 1975.

79 Archer, G., Fekety, F., and Supena, R.: *Pseudomas aeruginosa* Endocarditis in Drug Addicts, *Am. Heart J.,* 88:570, 1974.

80 Noriega, E., Rubinstein, E., Simberkoff, M., and Rahal, J.: Subacute and Acute Endocarditis Due to *Pseudomonas cepacia* in Heroin Addicts, *Am. J. Med.,* 59:29, 1975.

81 Mills, J., and Drew, D.: *Serratia marcescens* Endocarditis: A Regional Illness Associated with Intravenous Drug Abuse, *Ann. Intern. Med.,* 84:29, 1976.

82 Weinstein, L., Lerner, P., and Chew, W.: Clinical and Bacteriologic Studies of the Effect of "Massive" Doses of Penicillin G on Infections Caused by Gram-negative Bacilli, *N. Engl. J. Med.,* 271:525, 1964.

83 Weinstein, L., and Schlesinger, J.: Treatment of Infective Endocarditis 1973, *Prog. Cardiovasc. Dis.,* 16:275, 1973.

84 Kaye, J., Bernstein, S., Tsuji, H., Redington, H., Milgram, M., and Bern, J.: Surgical Treatment of *Candida* Endocarditis, *JAMA,* 203:621, 1968.

85 Utley, J., Mills, J., and Rowe, B.: Role of Valve Replacement in the Treatment of Fungal Endocarditis, *J. Thorac. Cardiovasc. Surg.,* 69:255, 1975.

86 Felner, J., and Dowell, V.: Bacteroides Bacteremia, *Am. J. Med.,* 50:787, 1971.

87 Robinson, M., and Ruedy, J.: Sequelae of Bacterial Endocarditis, *Am. J. Med.,* 32:922, 1962.

88 Hook, E., and Kaye, D.: Prophylaxis of Bacterial Endocarditis, *J. Chronic Dis.,* 15:635, 1962.

89 Durack, D., and Beeson, P.: Experimental Endocarditis. 1. Colonization of a Sterile Vegetation, *Br. J. Exp. Pathol.,* 53:44, 1972.

90 Durack, D., and Beeson, P.: Experimental Bacterial Endocarditis. 2. Survival of Bacteria in Endocardial Vegetation, *Br. J. Exp. Pathol.,* 53:50, 1972.

91 Durack, D.: Current Practice in Prevention of Bacterial Endocarditis, *Br. Heart J.,* 37:478, 1975.

92 Kaye, D.: "Infective Endocarditis," University Park Press, Baltimore, 1976, p. 260.

93 Kluge, R., Calia, F., McLaughlin, J., and Hornick, R.: Sources of Contamination in Open Heart Surgery, *JAMA,* 230:1415, 1974.

94 Gross, L., and Friedberg, C.: Non-bacterial Thrombotic Endocarditis, *AMA Arch. Intern Med.,* 58:620, 1936.

95 Libman, E.: Characterization of Various Forms of Endocarditis, *JAMA,* 80:813, 1923.

96 Libman, E.: The Varieties of Endocarditis and Their Clinical Significance, *Trans. Assoc. Am. Physicians,* 53:345, 1938.

97 Green, J., and Cummings, K.: Aseptic Thrombotic Endocardial Vegetations, *JAMA,* 225:1525, 1973.

98 Barry, W., and Scarpelli, D.: Non-bacterial Thrombotic Endocarditis, *Arch. Intern. Med.,* 109:79, 1962.

99 MacDonald, R., and Robbins, S.: The Significance of Nonbacterial Thrombotic Endocarditis: An Autopsy and Clinical Study of 78 Cases, *Ann. Intern. Med.,* 46:255, 1957.

100 Boas, N., and Barnett, R.: Coronary Embolism with Myocardial Infarction: Complication of Verrucous Endocarditis, *JAMA,* 170:1804, 1959.

101 Horowitz, C., and Ward, P.: Disseminated Intravascular Coagulation, Non-bacterial Thrombotic Endocarditis and Occult Pulmonary Hyaline Membrane Disease: An Interrelated Triad? *Am. J. Med.,* 51:272, 1971.

102 McKay, D., and Wable, G.: Disseminated Thrombosis in Colon Cancer, *Cancer,* 8:970, 1955.

103 McDonald, R., and Robbins, S.: The Significane of Non-bacterial Thrombotic Endocarditis: An Autopsy and Clinical Study of 78 Cases, *Ann. Intern. Med.,* 46:255, 1957.

104 Rosen, P., and Armstrong, B.: Nonbacterial Thrombotic Endocarditis in Patients with Malignant Neoplastic Disease, *Am. J. Med.,* 54:23, 1973.

105 Chino, F., Kodama, A., Otake, M., and Dock, Donald: Nonbacterial Thrombotic Endocarditis in a Japanese Autopsy Sample. A Review of 80 Cases, *Am. Heart J.,* 90:190, 1975.

106 Walter, Paul: personal communication.

78
Rare Causes of Endocardial Disease

NANETTE KASS WENGER, M.D.

Certain diseases seem to involve the pericardium and the epicardial portion of the myocardium, others involve the entire myocardium, and still others involve the endocardial portion of the myocardium. Actually, such diseases are rarely isolated to one of these anatomic areas of the heart but often involve at least two areas. For example, the epicardium is almost always involved to some degree when pericarditis is present. The myocardium is often involved to some degree when the disease process is located mainly in the endocardium. Therefore it is quite appropriate for some of the "endocardial" diseases to be discussed in Chap. 81B. The purpose of the present chapter is to further highlight those diseases that may predominantly affect the endocardium although the remainder of the myocardium may also be involved.

CARCINOID SYNDROME

In 1952, Biörck et al.[1] described the relation between heart disease and malignant carcinoid tumors with metastases. Valvular lesions on the right side of the heart occur in more than half of the patients with the carcinoid syndrome.[2] Heart failure is the leading cause of death in metastatic carcinoid disease, although cardiac involvement does not appear to alter the prognosis in patients with the carcinoid syndrome.

Pathophysiology

Cardiac involvement occurs late in the course of carcinoid disease, almost invariably associated with hepatic metastases. An exception occurs with ovarian primary carcinoid tumors, which discharge their endocrine products directly into the systemic venous circulation.[3] The fibrotic endocardial lesions were formerly attributed to the potent concentration of serotonin (5-hydroxytryptamine) reaching the right side of the heart, altering endocardial permeability, and allowing deposition of platelets and subsequent fibrosis of the endocardium. Serotonin, normally inactivated by the liver, is, in effect, secreted by the hepatic carcinoid metastases. However, serotonin administration has not produced comparable lesions in experimental animals; the kinin peptides, possibly bradykinin, may play a part in the pathogenesis of the cardiac disease. The concentration of bradykinin in the right side of the heart is ten times that in the brachial and femoral arterial blood; bradykinin also increases cardiac output and alters endothelial permeability. Lung monoamine oxidase inactivates serotonin and had been invoked to explain the rarity of carcinoid lesions on the left side of the heart. However, left-sided carcinoid lesions are not as rare as originally indicated, even in the absence[2,4] of a right-to-left intracardiac shunt or pulmonary carcinoid metastases.

Pathology

At postmortem examination,[2] there is pearly white thickening of the pulmonic and tricuspid valve cusps and of the ventricular endocardium, with retraction, thickening, and fusion of the chordae tendineae (Fig. 78-1). Microscopic examination shows an unusual acellular hyalinized collagenous material, rich in acid mucopolysaccharide, completely devoid of elastic fibers, deposited on an intact endocardial surface. Ultrastructural studies suggest that these plaques result from healing of a superficial endocardial lesion, possibly initiated by bradykinin.[4a] Metastatic carcinoid lesions may be found in the myocardium (Fig. 78-2).

Clinical manifestations

HISTORY
Patients describe paroxysmal flushing and diarrhea, at times associated with edema and with wheezing. There may be abdominal pain and weight loss. Cardiovascular symptoms, when present, are those of

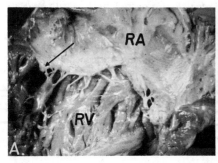

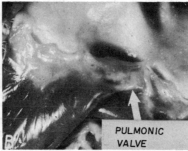

FIGURE 78-1 Valvular changes in carcinoid heart disease. *A.* The tricuspid valve shows nodular thickening along the valve margin (arrow), with scarring and retraction of the valve and the chordae tendineae. *B.* The pulmonic valve shows thickening and retraction of all leaflets.

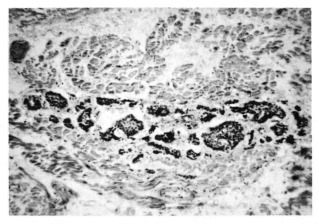

FIGURE 78-2 Carcinoid, metastatic to the myocardium. Nests of small, regular cells are arranged in an organoid pattern (×150).

right ventricular failure; fatigue and progressive exertional dyspnea occur, with edema as a late finding.

PHYSICAL EXAMINATION

The major cardiac manifestations of the carcinoid syndrome are pulmonic stenosis (Fig. 78-3), tricuspid insufficiency and stenosis, and right-sided heart failure. Tricuspid insufficiency occurs more commonly than pulmonic stenosis. Rarely, the murmur is audible only during a cutaneous flush, although the cardiac murmur often increases in intensity during a flushing episode.

The clinical presentation[2] includes cutaneous flushes, telangiectasia, intestinal hypermotility, and bronchoconstriction. Hypotensive crises may occur with the episodic flushing, diarrhea, and wheezing. Hepatomegaly, ascites, peripheral edema, dyspnea, "cyanosis," and distended neck veins do not necessarily connote carcinoid valvular heart disease with heart failure, as they may result solely from hepatic enlargement secondary to metastatic carcinoid.[3]

Left-sided cardiac lesions are unusual, but may produce the murmurs of mitral stenosis or regurgitation and even more rarely of aortic valve disease.

LABORATORY EXAMINATION

The *electrocardiogram* is not diagnostic. Low voltage is the most common electrocardiographic abnormality, but its mechanism is not clear. Right ventricular hypertrophy, right bundle branch block, and prominent P waves are seen.

Chest x-ray is rarely of value in diagnosing carcinoid heart disease; there may be minimal right-sided dilatation, but hypertrophy is unusual.

The elevated *urinary excretion of 5-HIAA* is diagnostic of a carcinoid tumor. Hypoproteinemia is common and may add to the peripheral manifestations of cardiac failure.

The valvular lesions can be confirmed at *cardiac catheterization*. The right atrial pressure may be disproportionately elevated for the degree of tricuspid insufficiency; right atrial endocardial thickening prevents the atrium from expanding during ventricular systole.[5] However, there is often no correlation between the severity of the valvular lesions and the severity of the heart failure. Cardiac catheterization findings of hyperkinemia without pulmonic or tricuspid valvular disease have been described;[6] it is suggested that hyperserotoninemia produces hyperkinemia; this, coupled with the episodic increased cardiac output associated with flushing, might result in congestive heart failure. However, increased cardiac output has also been noted in patients with the carcinoid syndrome without apparent cardiac involvement,[4] although most patients with carcinoid heart disease have a normal or low cardiac output.

Therapy

Digitalis and diuretic therapy may help control the edema and ascites. Therapy[2] with serotonin antagonists has been useful in controlling symptoms. The tumor chemotherapy most effective to date is with cyclophosphamide. Surgical correction of symptomatic valvular lesions is advocated,[7] and a tricuspid valve prosthesis may, at times, be needed.

ENDOMYOCARDIAL DISEASES

See Chaps. 55 and 81B.

FIGURE 78-3 Carcinoid heart disease. Right ventricular angiocardiogram demonstrates moderate pulmonic stenosis. At cardiac catheterization there was a 39 mm Hg systolic gradient across the pulmonic valve. *A.* One second after injection of contrast material. *B.* One and one-half seconds after injection of contrast material.

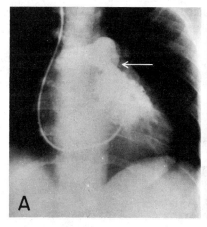
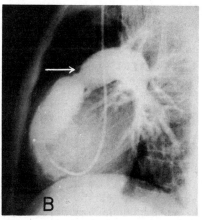

Endomyocardial fibrosis (EMF; Davies' disease)

See Chap. 81B.

Idiopathic mural endomyocardial disease (Becker's disease)

See Chap. 81B.

Fibroplastic parietal endocarditis with eosinophilia (Loeffler's disease, Loeffler's endocarditis)

See Chap. 81B.

VIRAL ENDOCARDITIS

Viruses have produced endocardial and valvular lesions in experimental animals,[8] and the endocardium is also involved in cases of viral myocarditis. There may be a viral cause of some of the poorly understood forms of endocardial and valvular disease.[9]

MURAL INFECTIVE ENDOCARDITIS

Infective endocarditis, discussed in Chap. 77, characteristically involves the heart valves, but may also affect the endocardial lining of the cardiac chambers. Infective endocarditis confined to the mural endocardium is rare[10] and results from extension of the infective process from another site, generally myocardium or lung.

TAKAYASU'S ARTERIOPATHY

Endocardial thickening and valvular involvement, histologically identical with the intimal arterial changes of Takayasu's arteriopathy, are encountered at necropsy. Extension of this process to the cardiac valves probably explains the cardiac murmurs reported in this disease.[11]

CARDIOMYOPATHY

See Chap. 81B.

ENDOCARDIAL FIBROSIS ASSOCIATED WITH METHYSERGIDE THERAPY[12]

Methysergide therapy for migraine has been known to cause inflammatory fibrosis of the retroperitoneal space. Recently, this has also been described in the pleuropulmonary space, great vessels, coronary ostia, heart valves, and endocardium. (See Chaps. 63A and 82.)

Pathology

Fibrous sheets of dense collagenous material cover normal underlying endocardium, heart valves, and chordae tendineae. The lesions mimic those of the carcinoid syndrome, except that carcinoid is predominantly right-sided whereas methysergide lesions are left-sided for the most part. Methysergide is chemically similar to serotonin.

Clinical manifestations

Symptoms of congestive heart failure may appear. Mitral and aortic valve murmurs, often with progressive increase in intensity, and evidence of congestive heart failure are noted. There are no specific electrocardiographic or roentgenologic features.

Treatment

Methysergide therapy should be discontinued. This often results in complete or partial regression of the murmurs and heart failure. Indeed, cessation of therapy for 2 or 3 months is recommended before cardiac catheterization or consideration of valve replacement is entertained. On occasion, however, valve replacement may be necessary.

Prevention

Methysergide should be avoided in patients with known valvular disease, cardiac decompensation, and collagen or fibrotic disorders.

Dosage should be kept below 8 mg daily, and intermittent methysergide therapy is recommended. This appears to decrease the fibrotic complications.

REFERENCES

1 Biörck, G., Axén, O., and Thorson, A.: Unusual Cyanosis in a Boy with Congenital Pulmonary Stenosis and Tricuspid Insufficiency: Fatal Outcome after Angiocardiography, *Am. Heart J.*, 44:143, 1952.

2 Grahame-Smith, D. G.: The Carcinoid Syndrome, *Am. J. Cardiol.*, 21:376, 1968.

3 Stephan, E., and DeWit, J.: Carcinoid Heart Disease from Primary Carcinoid Tumour of the Ovary: Haemodynamic and Cine Coronary Angiocardiographic Study after Operation, *Br. Heart J.*, 36:613, 1974.

4 Roberts, W. C., and Sjoerdsma, A.: The Cardiac Disease Associated with the Carcinoid Syndrome (Carcinoid Heart Disease), *Am. J. Med.*, 36:5, 1964.

4a Ferrans, V. J., and Roberts, W. C.: The Carcinoid Endocardial Plaque. An Ultrastructural Study, *Hum. Pathol.*, 7:387, 1976.

5 Roberts, W. C., Mason, D. T., and Wright, L. D., Jr.: The Nondistensible Right Atrium of Carcinoid Disease of the Heart, *Am. J. Clin. Pathol.*, 44:627, 1965.

6 Schwaber, J. R., and Lukas, D. S.: Hyperkinemia and Cardiac Failure in the Carcinoid Syndrome, *Am. J. Med.*, 32:846, 1962.

7 Carpena, C., Kay, J. H., Mendez, A. M., Redington, J. V., Zubiate, P., and Zucker, R.: Carcinoid Heart Disease: Surgery for Tricuspid and Pulmonary Valve Lesions, *Am. J. Cardiol.,* 32:229, 1973.

8 Burch, G. E., DePasquale, N. P., Sun, S. C., Hale, A. R., and Mogabgab, W. J.: Experimental Coxsackie Virus Endocarditis, *JAMA,* 196:349, 1966.

9 Carstens, H. B.: Postnatal Mumps Virus Infection Associated with Endocardial Fibroelastosis, *Arch. Pathol.,* 88:399, 1969.

10 Buchbinder, N. A., and Roberts, W. C.: Active Infective Endocarditis Confined to Mural Endocardium: A Study of Six Necropsy Patients, *Arch. Pathol.,* 93:435, 1972.

11 Chhetri, M. K., Pal, N. C., Neelakantan, C., Chowdhury, N. D., and Basu Mullick, K. C.: Endocardial Lesion in a Case of Takayasu's Arteriopathy, *Br. Heart J.,* 32:859, 1970.

12 Bana, D. S., MacNeal, P. S., LeCompte, P. M., Shah, Y., and Graham, J. R.: Cardiac Murmurs and Endocardial Fibrosis Associated with Methysergide Therapy, *Am. Heart J.,* 88:640, 1974.

Diseases of the Myocardium

79
Pathology of Myocardial Diseases

WILLIAM C. ROBERTS, M.D., and
VICTOR J. FERRANS, PH.D., M.D.

The purpose of this chapter is to describe the morphologic changes that are observed at necropsy in patients with inflammatory heart muscle disease (myocarditis) and noninflammatory heart muscle disease (cardiomyopathy). The taxonomy offered here has been created from the pathologist's viewpoint. A clinical taxonomy for cardiomyopathies is offered by Dr. John Goodwin in Chap. 81A. The disorders discussed here will be presented in the order shown in Table 79-1 (see also Fig. 79-1).

TABLE 79-1
Heart muscle diseases

Inflammatory cardiomyopathy (myocarditis)

I Known infectious agent (bacteria, viruses, parasites, rickettsias, spirochetes and treponemas, fungi)
  A Primary
  B Secondary
II Unknown agent (idiopathic)
III Associated with another known condition
  A Collagen disease
    1 Acute rheumatic fever
    2 Rheumatoid arthritis
    3 Systemic lupus erythematosus
    4 Other
  B Sarcoidosis

Noninflammatory cardiomyopathy

I Idiopathic
  A Dilated type
  B Hypertrophic type
    1 With subaortic stenosis
    2 Without subaortic stenosis
II Endomyocardial disease
  A With eosinophilia (Löffler's fibroplastic parietal endocarditis)
  B Without eosinophilia (endomyocardial fibrosis of Davies)
III Infiltrative
  A Amyloid
  B Iron (hemosiderosis)
  C Glycogen
  D Lipids and mucopolysaccharides
  E Calcium

INFLAMMATORY HEART MUSCLE DISEASES

Known infectious agent

In contrast to noninflammatory ones, inflammatory cardiomyopathies are infrequently observed today at necropsy. Acute myocarditis is now commonly seen at necropsy only in patients with "overwhelming" systemic acute infections, in those receiving immunosuppressive therapy, and in those with infective endocarditis[1,2] (see Fig. 79-2).

Virtually every known bacterium, virus, parasite, rickettsia, spirochete and treponema, and fungus has been shown to produce myocarditis. The myocardial involvement is rarely primary but is associated with involvement of other body organs and tissues. The specific types of organisms and their effect on the heart are discussed elsewhere (see Chap. 80).

Unknown agent

An occasional patient at necropsy is observed to have foci of polymorphonuclear- or mononuclear-cell myocardial inflammation unassociated with stainable organisms or positive cultures. Most of these patients have received antibiotic therapy so that possibly the organisms, although not the inflammatory response, were eradicated.

Associated with another known condition

COLLAGEN DISEASE

Focal specific inflammatory infiltrates, namely Aschoff bodies and rheumatoid nodules, are recognized lesions in the heart in acute rheumatic fever and rheumatoid arthritis, respectively.[3] Fortunately, fatal acute rheumatic fever is infrequent today; when it does occur, the cardiac inflammatory response often has been altered by corticosteroid therapy. Rheumatoid nodules in the myocardium may be less affected by corticosteroid therapy than are Aschoff bodies. The latter occur in about 3 percent of patients with fatal rheumatoid arthritis. Aschoff bodies are found in most patients dying during the acute episode of rheumatic fever and in about 5 percent of patients with chronic mitral stenosis.[3a]

At one time, focal myocarditis was believed to be fairly common in systemic lupus erythematosus (SLE). In the corticosteroid era, however, myocarditis is extremely rare.[4]

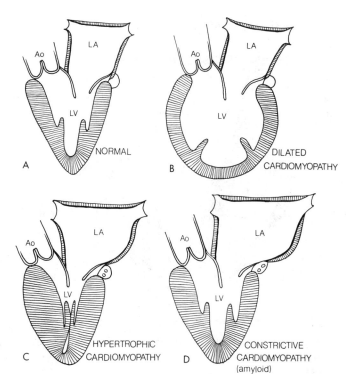

FIGURE 79-1 Diagram illustrating the various types of cardio-myopathies compared to the normal. In hypertrophic cardio-myopathy, the left ventricular cavity is small, and in the restrictive variety, as illustrated by amyloidosis, the left ventricular cavity is of normal size. In the dilated type, the largest circumference of left ventricle is not at its base but about midway between apex and base.

SARCOIDOSIS

A neglected cause of cardiac dysfunction is cardiac sarcoidosis, i.e., the replacement of portions of myocardial wall by sarcoid granulomas.[5] Hard granulo-

FIGURE 79-2 Cardiac candidiasis. This 14-year-old boy (A68-309) had lymphosarcoma for 17 months with terminal acute leukemic phase. He received a variety of chemotherapeutic agents including prednisone, and terminally he developed *Candida albicans* septicemia. At necropsy, he had *Candida* abscesses in most body organs including heart. Shown in *A* is a low-power (X 3) photomicrograph of left ventricular wall showing multiple *Candida* abscesses. *B.* Close-up of one of the myocardial abscesses, X 182. Periodic acid–Schiff stains on each. The patient never had evidence of cardiac dysfunction.

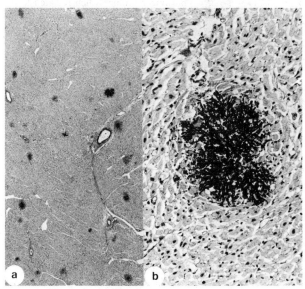

mas are found in the heart in about 20 percent of patients with sarcoidosis studied at necropsy. Although sarcoid lesions are never limited to the heart, most patients with cardiac sarcoidosis have symptoms resulting primarily from cardiac dysfunction. In other words, a patient with sarcoidosis either has dominant cardiac involvement or the heart is spared.[5] The cardiac deposits preferentially involve (1) the cephalad portion of the ventricular septum, producing severe conduction disturbances, particularly complete heart block; (2) the left ventricular papillary muscles and the adjacent free walls, producing papillary muscle dysfunction; or (3) right or left ventricular free walls, which, after corticosteroid therapy, may scar and lead to the development of ventricular aneurysms (Figs. 79-3 and 79-4). Ventricular arrhythmias, particularly tachycardia, are frequent consequences. Sudden death is common and may be the initial manifestation of sarcoidosis.

NONINFLAMMATORY HEART MUSCLE DISEASES

Idiopathic dilated cardiomyopathy

An idiopathic cardiomyopathy may be defined as a disease of the myocardium not resulting from coronary, valvular, congenital, hypertensive, or pulmonary heart disease.[6] Idiopathic cardiomyopathy is of two types: the ventricular dilated type and the hypertrophic (nonventricular dilated) type. Morphologic differences between these two types are summarized in Table 79-2.

CARDIAC SARCOIDOSIS

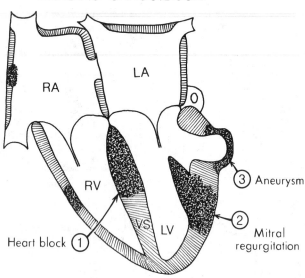

SARCOID GRANULOMA OR SCAR

FIGURE 79-3 Diagram showing the more frequent locations of sarcoid granulomas in the heart and their more frequent functional consequences.

Idiopathic cardiac enlargement, heart disease of unknown origin, primary myocardial disease, and *congestive cardiomyopathy* are other terms which have been used to describe what we prefer to call idiopathic dilated cardiomyopathy (DC). The reason we prefer the latter term is that the major morphologic feature of this condition is dilatation of both

TABLE 79-2
Morphologic differences between idiopathic dilated and hypertrophic cardiomyopathies

		Dilated type	Hypertrophic type
1	Dilated ventricular cavities	+	0
2	Intracardiac thrombi	+	0
3	Asymmetric septal hypertrophy	0	+
4	Myocardial fiber disorientation	0	+
5	Endocardial plaque, LVOT*	0	+
6	Thickened mitral valve	0	+
7	Abnormal intramural coronary arteries	0	+
8	Ventricular scarring	0-+	+
9	Thickened ventricular walls	0-+	+
10	Increased cardiac weight	+	+
11	Dilated atrial cavities	+	+

*LVOT = left ventricular outflow tract.

ventricular cavities (Fig. 79-5). Although the degree of dilatation of both ventricular cavities is usually similar, occasionally one ventricle is more dilated than the other one. The ventricular dilatation is associated with poor ventricular contractions, which in turn produce low ejection fractions and high end-systolic volumes. The latter appear to limit atrial emptying, which in turn leads to high atrial end-diastolic volumes with resulting atrial dilatation.

The large end-systolic ventricular volumes lead to relative stasis of blood and frequent thrombus formation. The most frequent locations of thrombi in

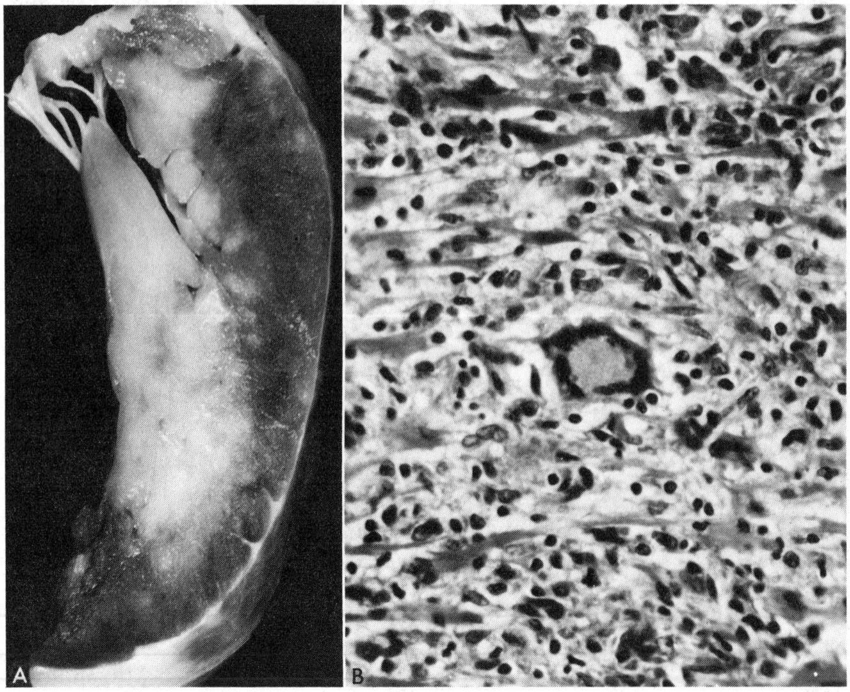

FIGURE 79-4 Cardiac sarcoidosis. Shown here is a longitudinal section through anterolateral *(A)* papillary muscle in a 26-year-old woman (PGGH #A-70-541) who had been asymptomatic until 10 days before her death, when dyspnea appeared. The dyspnea rapidly worsened, and when hospitalized on the day of death, she was in acute pulmonary edema. The blood pressure was 80/70 mm Hg, heart rate 160 beats per minute, and a grade 3 to 4/6 pansystolic blowing murmur, which radiated to the axilla, was audible. Chest roentgenogram showed congested lungs, cardiomegaly, and prominent hilar adenopathy. Electrocardiogram showed nonspecific ST-T wave changes and atrial hypertrophy. She developed complete heart block and died shortly thereafter.

At necropsy, large firm white deposits were present in the walls of all four cardiac chambers and completely replaced both left ventricular papillary muscles *(A)*. On histologic section, the firm white areas represented hard granulomas typical of sarcoidosis *(B)*. (Hematoxylin and eosin stain; X 400.) Similar hard granulomas were present in lymph nodes, liver, spleen, and lung. Stains for acid-fast organisms, other bacteria, and fungi were negative.

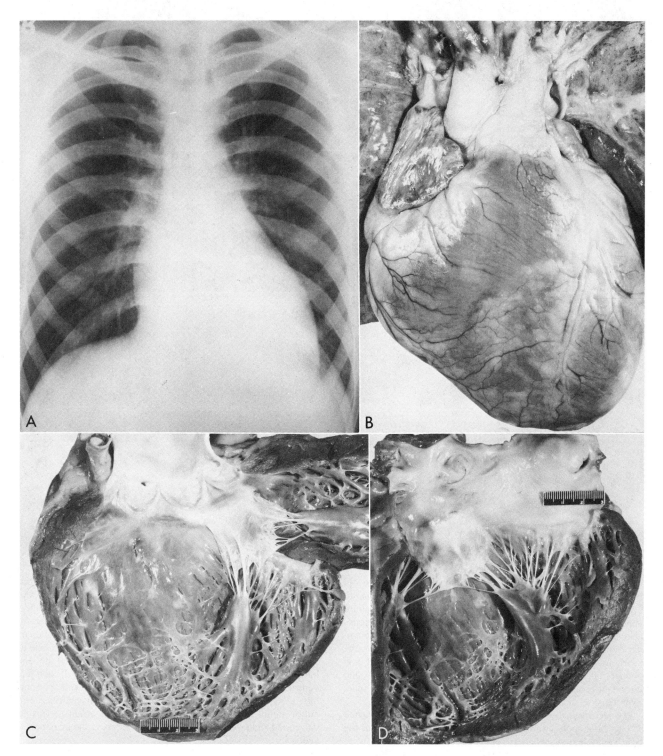

FIGURE 79-5 Idiopathic dilated cardiomegaly in a 22-year-old white man (A61-56) who had been well until 5 years before death when he had the onset of pleuritic-type pain followed by congestive cardiac failure. Electrocardiogram showed nonspecific T-wave changes. After a 4-month hospitalization, he was entirely well until 2 months before death when an upper respiratory infection prompted overt congestive heart failure. Thereafter, the heart failure progressively worsened and the heart enlarged. A grade 2/6 apical systolic murmur appeared.

At necropsy, the heart weighed 570 g, and both ventricles were very dilated (*A* to *D*). The valves and coronary arteries were normal. Histologic sections of left ventricular wall showed only mild interstitial fibrosis. *A.* Chest roentgenogram during last week of life. *B.* Anterior aspect of heart. The pericardial sac contained 50 ml of serous fluid. *C.* Opened left ventricle, aortic valve, and aorta. Small, focal endocardial thickenings are present. *D.* Opened left atrium, mitral valve, and left ventricle. The mitral anulus is not dilated.

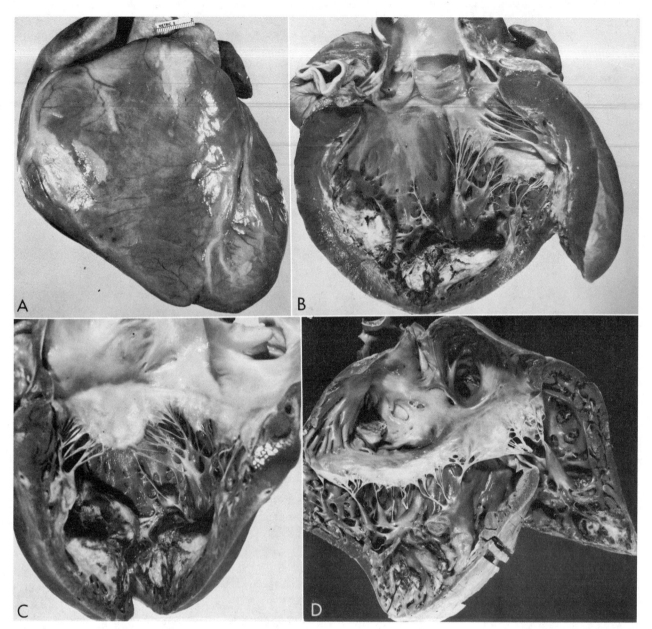

FIGURE 79-6 Idiopathic dilated cardiomegaly in a 36-year-old black man (A69-199), a habitual alcoholic, who had been well until 2 years before death when evidence of congestive cardiac failure appeared. The latter gradually worsened, and various arrhythmias also appeared. Finally, pulmonary infiltrates, proved to be secondary to pulmonary emboli, precipitated death. By radiograph the heart was markedly enlarged. Electrocardiogram showed low voltage, Q- and T-wave changes suggesting old infarction, and intraventricular conduction defect. He never had chest pain, hypertension, or a precordial murmur.

At necropsy, the heart plus the intracardiac thrombi weighed 750 g. "Milk spots" were present over the anterior surface of the right ventricle and at the left ventricular apex (A). Thrombi were present in the apex of both ventricles (B to D) and in the right atrial appendage (D). Histologically, large foci of replacement and interstitial fibrosis were seen in the left ventricular wall. Both left ventricular papillary muscles were atrophied and severely scarred. A. Heart as viewed anteriorly. The notch present at the junction of the right and left ventricular apices was considered at one time to be diagnostic of the African condition, endomyocardial fibrosis, but this is not the case, as shown by this patient. B. Opened left ventricle, aortic valve, and aorta showing the large apical thrombus. C. Opened left atrium, mitral valve, and left ventricle. The mitral anulus is not dilated. D. Opened right atrium, tricuspid valve, and right ventricle showing a thrombus at the apex of the ventricle.

patients with DC are in order of frequency left ventricle, right ventricle, right atrial appendage, and left atrial appendage (Fig. 79-6). About 75 percent of these patients have left ventricular thrombi at necropsy. We have never observed thrombus in the atria or right ventricle without thrombi being present also in the left ventricle. In addition to fibrin thrombi, focal endocardial thickenings often are present near the apices of the ventricles and probably represent "healed" or organized thrombi. The intracardiac thrombi obviously may give rise to pulmonary and systemic emboli.

The hearts are always increased in weight; the average in 100 necropsy patients we have studied is just under 600 g. Despite the increased weight, the maximal thickness of left ventricular free wall and ventricular septum is often less than 1.5 cm.

Although interstitial myocardial fibrosis of varying

degree usually is present by histologic examination, left ventricular wall scarring is observed by gross inspection in only about 25 percent of the patients. Even when scarring is observed grossly, it is usually limited to papillary muscle and subendocardium (inner one-half of wall). Thus, the poor myocardial contractility cannot be explained by ventricular scarring.

The leaflets of the four cardiac valves are usually normal, but occasionally the margins of the mitral and tricuspid valve leaflets are focally thickened by fibrous tissue. The latter is most frequent in patients with atrioventricular valvular regurgitation for long periods. These valvular thickenings appear to be secondary to the regurgitation, and do not themselves cause valvular incompetence. The cause of valvular regurgitation in these patients appears to be papillary muscle dysfunction, because the tricuspid and mitral valvular annuli are usually only mildly dilated (less than 25 percent above normal).[7]

Histologic study of the myocardial walls in these patients discloses nonspecific changes. Many myocardial cells appear hypertrophied; others, atrophied. The amount of fibrous tissue between myocardial cells usually is increased. Inflammatory cells are absent. The intramural coronary arteries are normal. Electron microscopy has confirmed these histologic observations and demonstrated other nonspecific changes, including cellular edema; increased numbers of lipid droplets, lysosomes, and lipofuscin granules; dilatation of the tubules of the sarcoplasmic reticulum and the T system; mild myofibrillar damage, and various mitochondrial alterations.[8] The mitochondria vary in size; many are smaller than normal. No virus particles have been observed in the myocardium of patients with fatal cardiomyopathy. The changes in myocardium in patients with histories of habitual alcoholism are indistinguishable from those in patients without positive histories. In general, the extent of the degenerative changes in the myocardial cells correlates with the duration and severity of cardiac dysfunction.

Although it is well recognized that dilated cardiomyopathy may be confused clinically with coronary heart disease, separation of the two at necropsy may present problems if one adheres rigidly to a definition which includes "absence of coronary arterial disease." How much coronary arterial narrowing, in other words, is permissible to still allow the diagnosis of DC? We initially included in our definition[6] of this entity less than 50 percent cross-sectional luminal narrowing, but this cut-off point prevented inclusion of patients who had typical clinical features of DC, including absence of chest pain, and in whom necropsy confirmed absence of myocardial scarring but showed up to 75 percent cross-sectional luminal narrowing of a major coronary artery. Because fatal coronary (atherosclerotic) heart disease is always associated with cross-sectional luminal narrowing of greater than 75 percent,[9] a 75 percent cut-off point appears more reasonable. Furthermore, there is apparently no reduction in flow through a tube (coronary artery) until more than 75 percent of the cross-sectional area of its lumen is obliterated. Obviously, the associated coronary atherosclerosis presents no

problem in the younger patients, but it might in the older ones.

Idiopathic hypertrophic cardiomyopathy

Hypertrophic cardiomyopathy (HC) is strikingly different both functionally and morphologically from dilated cardiomyopathy (DC) (Table 79-2). The major problem is a *hyper*contracting left ventricle rather than the *hypo*contracting ventricle of DC. The morphologic counterpart of this hypercontracting ventricle is a massive ventricular muscle mass and small ventricular cavities. HC is the classic example of the "muscle-bound heart"; DC, in contrast, is the classic example of the flabby heart, mostly cavity with comparatively little myocardial mass.

In his original description, Teare applied the term *asymmetrical hypertrophy of the heart* to this condition. Subsequently, other terms including functional subaortic stenosis, diffuse muscular subaortic stenosis, idiopathic hypertrophic subaortic stenosis, hypertrophic obstructive cardiomyopathy, and asymmetric septal hypertrophy (ASH) have been applied. The terms which include the word stenosis or obstruction appear inappropriate, because obstruction is more often absent than present.[10] The terms which emphasize asymmetry of the walls bordering the left ventricular cavity have served a useful purpose in emphasizing the characteristic morphologic feature of this condition, but it is now apparent that the ventricular septum may be thicker than the left ventricular free wall in an occasional patient with a condition other than HC (Table 79-3). In addition, a few patients with HC do not have ASH (i.e., septum thicker than free wall), and on rare occasion the left ventricular free wall may not be hypertrophied in HC.

Study at necropsy of nearly 70 patients with HC has demonstrated the following characteristic features of this condition (Figs. 79-7 to 79-11): (1) disproportional hypertrophy of the ventricular septum (95 percent); (2) disorientation of myocardial fibers in the ventricular septum (100 percent); (3) small or normal-sized left and right ventricular cavi-

TABLE 79-3
Causes of ASH

1 Hypertrophic cardiomyopathy
  a With obstruction (IHSS)
  b Without obstruction
2 Aortic stenosis
  a Valvular
  b Discrete subvalvular
  c Supravalvular
  d Tunnel
3 Systemic hypertension
4 Pulmonary hypertension (RVFW > LVFW)*
5 Posterobasal myocardial infarct
6 Parachute mitral valve syndrome

*RVFW = right ventricular free wall, LVFW = left ventricular free wall.

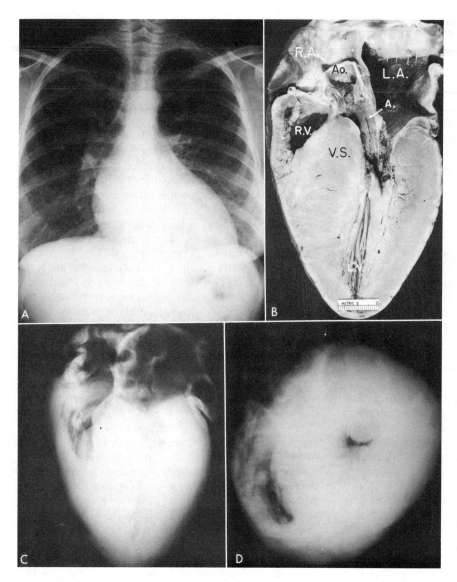

FIGURE 79-7 Hypertrophic cardiomyopathy of the obstructive type. This 36-year-old woman (A67-121) developed congestive cardiac failure during her second pregnancy at age 32. When studied at age 34, she had a grade 3/6 precordial systolic murmur, loudest over the apex, and audible third and fourth heart sounds. Electrocardiogram showed bilateral bundle branch block with left axis deviation and prolongation (0.23 s) of the P-R interval. Catheterization disclosed a 75 mm Hg peak systolic pressure gradient at rest between left ventricle (160/18) and femoral artery (85/50), and a 125 mm Hg gradient with provocation (Valsalva). The premature ventricular response was positive for HC. She died during an episode of rapid heart action. She was known to have multiple premature ventricular contractions on occasions.

At necropsy, the heart was enlarged (*A*), weighing 450 g; the left ventricular cavity was small (*B* to *D*), and the ventricular septum (V.S.) was much thicker than the left ventricular (L.V.) free wall. There was little room in the left ventricular cavity for the mitral leaflets, and contact lesions (fibromas) were present on the ventricular aspect of the anterior (*A*) mitral leaflet and on the adjacent left ventricular mural endocardium (*B*). Ao. = aorta, R.V. = right ventricle. This is the typical "muscle-bound" heart in which the ventricular cavities are minute in comparison to the mass of ventricular muscle. Both right (R.A.) and left (L.A.) atria are dilated.

ties (95 percent); (4) mural endocardial plaque in the left ventricular outflow tract (75 percent); (5) thickened mitral valve (75 percent); (6) dilated left atrium (100 percent); and (7) abnormal intramural coronary arteries (50 percent).

Disproportional septal hypertrophy was observed by Teare in his initial description of HC.[11] The thickest portion of the septum is not that portion immediately beneath the aortic valve, however, but that part located about midway between aortic valve and left ventricular apex. This level corresponds approximately to the apex of right ventricle. The *maximal thickness of ventricular septum* in our adult patients averaged 3.0 cm, and the *maximal thickness of left ventricular free wall*, 1.8 cm.

When the echocardiogram measures what is believed to be the thickest portion of ventricular septum, the echo beam simultaneously delineates only that portion of left ventricular free wall which is located behind posterior mitral leaflet. In normal subjects and in patients with left ventricular hypertrophy from such causes as aortic valve stenosis and systemic hypertension, the thickest portion of left ventricular free wall is located about 2 cm caudal to the base of left ventricle, i.e., the area measured by echocardiography. In patients with the *obstructive type* of HC, this posterobasal portion of left ventricular free wall represents the thickest portion of free wall. In the patients with the *nonobstructive type* of HC, however, the portion of left ventricular free wall directly behind the posterior mitral leaflet is not thickened and the thickest portion of free wall is located more caudally, i.e., not measurable by echocardiogram. Differences in the configuration of the posterobasal left ventricular free wall between the obstructive and nonobstructive types are diagrammed in Fig. 79-10. Thus, by examination of the posterobasal portion of left ventricular free wall, an

FIGURE 79-8 Hypertrophic cardiomyopathy. This 33-year-old man (A68-185) had no systolic pressure gradient at rest between left ventricle and brachial artery, but a 33 mm Hg gradient was provoked by isoproterenol. He died of sudden unilateral hemiparesis which appeared 6 days after the catheterization. He had been asymptomatic when examined at age 26 when a grade 2 to 3/6 precordial systolic murmur, loudest at the apex, was heard. Catheterization at that time showed a 30 mm Hg peak systolic gradient at rest between left ventricle and brachial artery, and it rose to 85 mm Hg with ouabain provocation. He became symptomatic (exertional and nocturnal dyspnea) 6 months before death, when atrial fibrillation appeared. The precordial murmur then was only intermittently audible.

At necropsy, the heart weighed 450 g; both atria were dilated, but neither ventricle was dilated (A). The ventricular septum was thicker than the left ventricular free wall (B). A mural endocardial plaque was present in the left ventricular outflow tract, and the corresponding anterior mitral leaflet was thickened (C and D). The longitudinal cut of heart in D clearly shows that the ventricular septum is thicker than the left ventricular free wall.

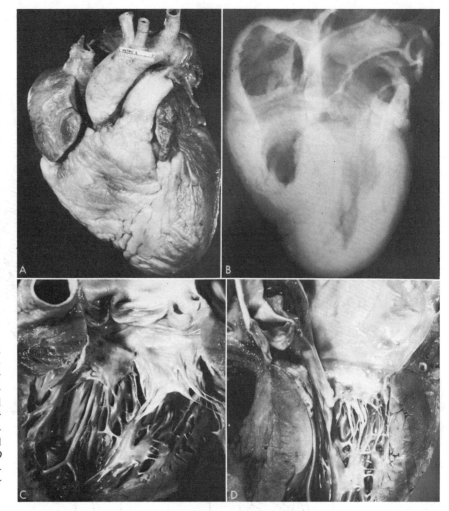

FIGURE 79-9 Hypertrophic cardiomyopathy of the nonobstructive type. This 33-year-old woman (A67-70) became mildly symptomatic when 15 years of age. She had three pregnancies without difficulty, but during the fourth she had overt congestive cardiac failure. When evaluated at age 28, she had exertional dyspnea, chest pain, and occasional episodes of dizziness. Several other family members also had HC. A grade 2/6 precordial systolic murmur, loudest at the apex, and a fourth heart sound were audible. Electrocardiogram showed left bundle branch block and premature ventricular contractions. The cardiac silhouette was enlarged by radiograph. No systolic gradient was present between left ventricle (108/34 mm Hg) and brachial artery (114/64 mm Hg) at rest. By age 30, the angina, dyspnea, and dizziness were worse and more frequent; syncope had occurred once. On repeat catheterization, still no systolic gradient was present between left ventricle (97/30 mm Hg) and femoral artery (102/58) at rest, but a 9 mm Hg gradient was provoked by isoproterenol. The premature ventricular contraction response was normal. Repeat catheterization 2 years later showed virtually identical findings. The left ventricular angiocardiogram was interpreted as showing "cavity obliteration." She was found dead in bed at home 4 months later.

At necropsy, the heart weighed 430 g. The ventricular septum was much thicker than the left ventricular free wall, which was of normal thickness. The mitral leaflets were only slightly thickened, and no endocardial mural plaque was present in the left ventricular outflow tract. Both atria were dilated.

This case is typical of the nonobstructive variety of hypertrophic cardiomyopathy and is characterized by normal thickness of at least the basal portion of the left ventricular free wall.

accurate determination can be made as to whether the patient had the obstructive or the nonobstructive form of HC.

A second major anatomic feature of HC is focal disorganization of myocardial fibers in the ventricu-

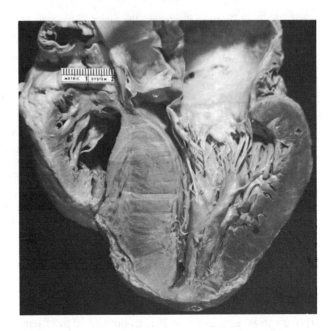

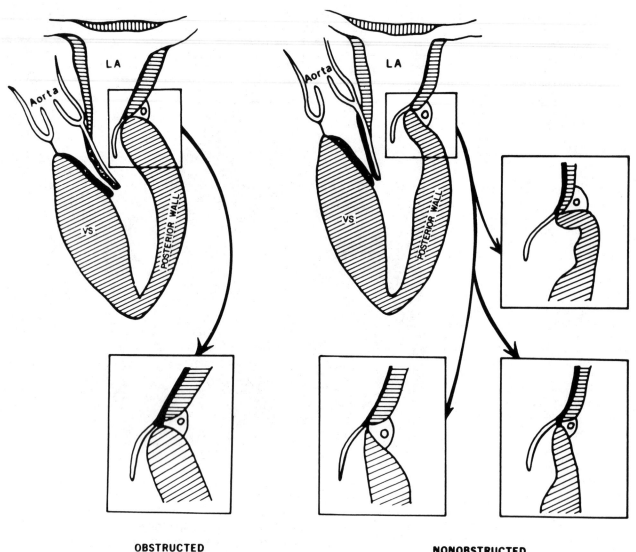

OBSTRUCTED

NONOBSTRUCTED

FIGURE 79-10 Diagram illustrating the major differences between the obstructive and nonobstructive types of hypertrophic cardiomyopathy. In the obstructive type, the most basal portion of posterior and lateral left ventricular free walls is rounded and thick. In the nonobstructive type, the left ventricular free wall beneath the posterior mitral leaflet is thinned and pointed.

lar septum (Fig. 79-11). In Teare's original description he observed by histologic examination a "bizarre arrangement of muscle bundles" and "considerable variation in size" of the myocardial fibers in the ventricular septum.[11] This myocardial fiber disarray in the septum occurs in patients of all ages (including infants) with HC of either the obstructive or nonobstructive variety.[10] The size and extent of the foci vary, and between them are large areas of myocardium in which the muscle cells are hypertrophied but normally arranged (in parallel). The areas of disarray are composed of cells that are arranged in whorls or at random, the cells being wider (transverse diameters up to 80 µm, average 28 µm; normal 10 to 15 µm) and often shorter than normal. The abnormalities in

cellular architecture are not absolutely unique to HC, but they are clearly more severe and widespread in this condition than in any other.

Not only does disorganization between *myocardial fibers* occur, but in addition, ultrastructural studies[12] have shown disarray of *myofibrils* and *myofilaments* within individual cells (Fig. 79-11). Again, the abnormalities of myofibrils and myofilaments are not absolutely specific for HC, but when disorganization of these subcellular components is found in other cardiac conditions, the abnormal cells are in small numbers. The individual septal myocardial cells in HC also frequently show increased amounts of Z-band material and nonspecific changes of cellular hypertrophy and degeneration.

Myofiber disarray in the left and right ventricular free walls is more difficult to determine by light microscopy than that in the ventricular septum. Ultrastructural examination of the left and right ventricular free walls, however, discloses many bizarrely shaped, disorganized, cells in the ventricular

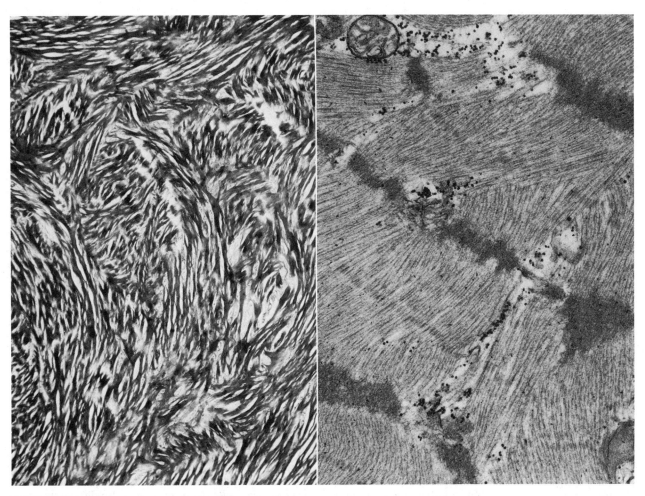

FIGURE 79-11 Histologic (left) and ultrastructural (right) features of ventricular septum of hypertrophic cardiomyopathy. *Left:* From a 19-year-old man with the obstructive type. There is marked disorganization of muscle bundles and bizarre arrangement of muscle cells. Masson's trichrome stain, X 60. *Right:* From a 39-year-old woman with the obstructive type. There is marked abnormal orientation of the myofibrils and widening of the Z bands, X 47,000.

free walls of patients *without obstruction* whereas the bizarrely shaped and disorganized myocardial fibers are virtually entirely absent from the ventricular free walls in the patients *with obstruction.*[10] Thus, the disorientation of groups of myocardial cells and the disarray of myofibrils and myofilaments within individual myocardial cells is not the result of left ventricular outflow obstruction or high intraventricular systolic pressures.

Another major anatomic characteristic of hypertrophic cardiomyopathy is lack of ventricular cavity dilatation. The left ventricular cavity usually has a flattened S shape. The development of ventricular dilatation is an extremely rare occurrence in HC. In contrast to the ventricular cavities, both atrial cavities at necropsy virtually always are dilated.

In adults, the mural endocardium of the left ventricular outflow tract is usually thickened by fibrous tissue. This thickening is in direct apposition to the anterior mitral leaflet, which also is thickened by fibrous tissue. The caudal margin of the mural endocardial outflow plaque corresponds to the distal margin of the anterior mitral leaflet. This caudal margin probably represents the site of obstruction. If that is the case, then the fibrous thickening of the left ventricular outflow tract (including both mural endocardium and anterior mitral leaflet) should be restricted to the patients with obstruction. We found this outflow thickening in 95 percent of our necropsy patients with hemodynamically confirmed left ventricular outflow obstruction at rest and in only 45 percent of the patients without obstruction. Furthermore, the thickening was distinctly more severe in the patients with obstruction.

Not only is the anterior mitral leaflet thickened, but often, more frequently in the patients with obstruction, the posterior mitral leaflet is as well. The thickening of both leaflets is probably the consequence of the small left ventricular cavity in this condition. It is important to recall that the mitral valve resides in the left ventricle, which, being small, causes abnormal contact of the leaflets with themselves and also causes the anterior one to contact the septum. In the patients without obstruction, the basal portion of the left ventricular cavity is larger than in the patients with obstruction because of the thinning of the basal portion of free wall posteriorly and laterally. The focal fibrous thickening of the posterior mitral leaflet probably results from abnormal contact during ventricular systole because there is not enough room in the ventricular cavity to easily accommodate the leaflets and chordae. The ventricle and mitral leaflets in this respect may be regarded as being similar to an accordion. The mitral leaflet thickening in HC is somewhat analogous to that which occurs normally as a consequence of aging. With aging, the left ventricular cavity becomes smaller, presumably in response to the lowered cardiac output; the mitral leaflets, thicker; the left ventricular muscle, less compliant; and the left atrium dilates in response to increased work required to fill the small left ventricle. Similar mechanisms appear to be accelerated in hypertrophic cardiomyopathy.

Most patients with HC have some degree of mitral regurgitation. It is not related to anular dilation, since the mitral anulus in this condition is smaller than normal. Furthermore, the leaflet thickening, in and of itself, is not extensive enough to cause valvular regurgitation. The most likely explanation appears to be abnormal bending of the papillary muscles, particularly the anterolateral one. These structures may be bent abnormally by the bulging ventricular septum with resulting excessive tension on the chordae tendineae preventing closure of the mitral orifice. Although they are usually present in the papillary muscles in HC, focal scars cannot account for the regurgitation. Although it is usually mild in HC, mitral regurgitation may be the predominant clinical feature of this condition. Mitral valve replacement in HC is hazardous since the small left ventricular cavity is rarely capable of freely accommodating a prosthesis.[13]

Endomyocardial disease with and without eosinophilia

Löffler in 1936 described two patients with "fibroplastic parietal endocarditis with blood eosinophilia."[6] In 1957 Bousser summarized reports of 13 patients with "eosinophilic leukemia," and a number of reports have appeared describing each of these two conditions.[6] In each, there is endocardial fibrosis of one or both ventricles and severe eosinophilia. Death is usually the result of congestive cardiac failure. From examination of previous reports and of our eight necropsy patients,[6] it appears that the clinical and morphologic features of eosinophilic leukemia and Löffler's endocarditis are similar and that these two conditions are indeed the same disease. Certain similarities also exist between endomyocardial fibrosis of the African (EMF) and endomyocardial fibrosis with eosinophilia, described by others as Löffler's endocarditis or eosinophilic leukemia. The mural endocardial thickening in the ventricles is seen in both conditions, and blood eosinophilia may occur in EMF.

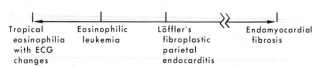

FIGURE 79-12 Diagram illustrating spectrum of endomyocardial disease with and without eosinophilia.

The possibility that Löffler's fibroplastic parietal endocarditis, eosinophilic leukemia (without abnormal myelopoiesis), and EMF are the same disease at different stages of development is an attractive hypothesis (Fig. 79-12). Patients with eosinophilia associated with a transient, benign, febrile illness, such as tropical eosinophilia or Löffler's pneumonia, may represent one end of the spectrum. Patients with severe EMF and no blood eosinophilia may represent the other end. Between these two extremes there may be patients who still have eosinophilia but have less extensive endocardial scarring. The latter process is still active, and thus eosinophilia is still present, but as the inflammatory process dies down, cardiac scar tissue remains and eosinophilia disappears.

Infiltrative cardiomyopathies

These include various infiltrates into the walls of the cardiac chambers. The infiltrates may be localized to *myocardial interstitium* (amyloid) or to the interior of *myocardial cells* (iron, glycogen, lipids, calcium).

AMYLOID

Amyloid may be deposited in any portion of the heart, and the deposits may be large (grossly visible) or small (microscopic-sized).[14] When cardiac dysfunction results from cardiac amyloidosis, the amyloid deposits are grossly visible and diffusely distributed throughout the ventricular walls, which have firm, rubbery consistencies (Fig. 79-13). Histologically, most ventricular myocardial cells are surrounded by amyloid fibrils. Thus, not only is ventricular motion restricted but most myofibers are constricted by the amyloid deposits. In addition to its being in the myocardial interstitium, amyloid is deposited in the walls and in the lumens of the intramural coronary arteries, in mural endocardium (particularly in the atria), in valvular endocardium, in epicardium, and in both conduction tissue and cardiac nerves. The endocardial deposits do not produce valvular dysfunction. The deposits in the lumens of the small coronary arteries, however, may lead to focal myocardial ischemia with resulting necrosis and fibrosis. The amount of amyloid deposition in the conducting myocardium is minimal in comparison to that present in contracting myocardium. Nevertheless, conduction and rhythm disturbances are more common in these patients than in those of similar age and sex

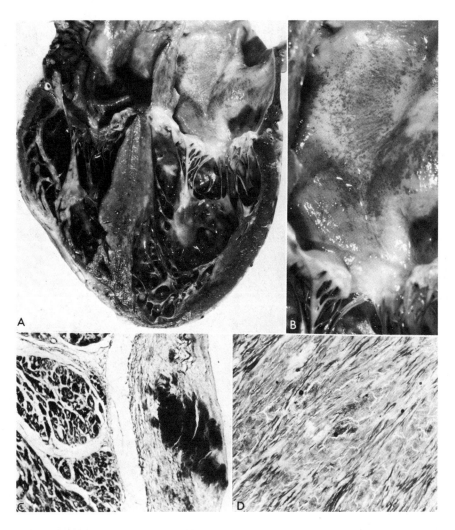

FIGURE 79-13 Cardiac amyloidosis. Shown in *A* is the posterior half of the heart in an 86-year-old man (A68-18) who had angina pectoris and healed myocardial infarction as well as large amyloid deposits. A close-up of left atrial endocardium is shown in *B*. The waxy lesions on this endocardium represent amyloid deposits and are indicative of extensive ventricular amyloid deposits. *C*. Photomicrograph of left atrial endocardial amyloid deposit, X 107. *D*. Amyloid has infiltrated extensively a left ventricular papillary muscle, X 32. Crystal violet stain, (*C* and *D*).

without cardiac amyloidosis. Amyloid may be viewed as an "acellular cancer" in that the deposits infiltrate within and between normal tissues, but no cells are present in the proliferating material.

Although the ventricular walls are made rigid by heavy amyloid deposits, the ventricular cavities are not dilated unless another cardiac condition also is present. Thus, cardiac amyloidosis joins hypertrophic cardiomyopathy and constrictive pericarditis as causes of congestive cardiac failure in the absence of ventricular cavity dilatation. The atria, in contrast, usually are dilated. The enlargement of the cardiac silhouette on roentgenogram in this condition may well be related to the atrial dilatation. Most patients with symptomatic cardiac amyloidosis have electrocardiographic low voltage, conduction or rhythm disturbances, and congestive cardiac failure unresponsive to digitalis therapy. Diagnosis of clinically significant cardiac amyloidosis should be questioned in the absence of congestive cardiac failure and electrocardiographic low voltage.[14]

IRON

For years it was debated whether or not iron deposition in the heart could cause cardiac dysfunction. It is now clear, just as with amyloid, that cardiac dysfunction will occur if the cardiac iron deposits are large enough;[15] cardiac dysfunction does not occur in patients with only microscopically visible iron deposits, and cardiac dysfunction usually does occur when the deposits are grossly visible. In contrast to amyloid deposits which are between myocardial cells, the iron deposits are within myofibers (Fig. 79-14). The iron deposits are most extensive in ventricular myocardium, less in atrial myocardium, and least in conducting as contrasted to working myocardium. Most patients with large cardiac iron deposits have abnormal electrocardiograms, mainly arrhythmias and conduction disturbances, and congestive cardiac failure. In contrast to amyloid, the ventricular cavities typically are dilated. Thus, the iron heart is a weak heart, not a strong one.

GLYCOGEN

A deficiency of one or more of the enzymes involved in the biosynthesis and degradation of glycogen produces glycogen storage disease, of which at least eight types have been described.[6] Cardiac involvement occurs in types II, III, and IV. Most patients with glycogen storage causing cardiomegaly belong

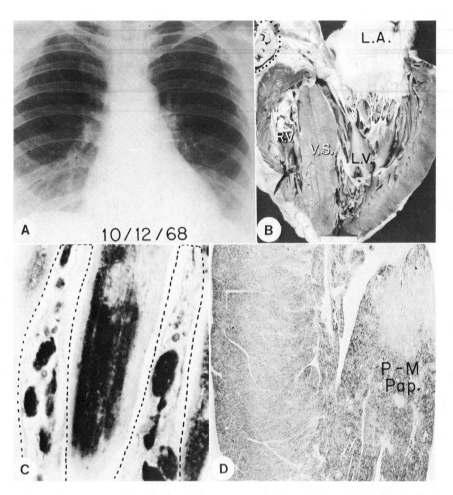

FIGURE 79-14 Cardiac hemosiderosis in a 42-year-old woman (68-327) with sickle-cell anemia. She had received 260 units of blood when congestive cardiac failure developed 6 years before death. Chest roentgenogram *(A)* showed cardiomegaly. By the time of death she had received 359 units of blood (90 g iron). At necropsy, the walls of the right and left ventricles and left atrium were rusty brown due to extensive iron deposits *(B).* The right atrial wall in contrast was tan *(B)* and only minute particles of iron were present in it by histologic examination. *C.* Photomicrograph of several myocardial cells showing huge deposits of iron in them. Despite large deposits of iron in working myocardium, no iron deposits were observed in conducting myocardium. Longitudinal section of left ventricular wall including posteromedial (P-M) papillary muscle is shown in *D.* Foci of necrosis and fibrosis are present. The necrotic and fibrotic areas probably are anatomic indicators of chronic myocardial hypoxia, a result of the chronic anemia. Prussian blue iron stains; X 628 *(C),* X 3 *(D).*

to type II (Pompe's disease), defined as a deficiency of α-1,4-glucosidase, a lysosomal enzyme that hydrolyzes glycogen to glucose. As a result the heart enlarges, sometimes to a marked degree, and congestive cardiac failure supervenes. Survival rarely extends beyond infancy or early childhood. Microscopically, the muscle cells show a characteristic lacework pattern, with large, clear central spaces (which represent the sites of glycogen deposition) and a peripheral rim of compressed cytoplasm. Endocardial fibroelastosis of at least the left ventricle usually is present also. Although the deposits of glycogen usually involve all myocardial cells relatively uniformly, on occasion the fibers in the ventricular septum may contain disproportionately excessive quantities of glycogen and lead to subaortic stenosis. Myocardial involvement occurs to a variable extent in type III glycogenosis (glycogen-debranching enzyme deficiency). In type IV glycogenosis (branching enzyme deficiency) deposits of abnormal glycogen are found free in the cytoplasm of cardiac muscle cells, hepatocytes, and a variety of other cell types. These glycogen deposits are basophilic and are composed of nonbranching fibrils that measure 40 to 80 Å in diameter and resemble those in basophilic degeneration of the heart.

LIPIDS

Infiltration of cytoplasm of cardiac muscle cells by lipid droplets (fatty degeneration) is a nonspecific finding in many disorders, including hypoxia. *Fabry's disease* (angiokeratoma corporis diffusum universale) may be singled out among the lipid storage diseases as one in which extensive and clinically significant (producing cardiomegaly and congestive cardiac failure) accumulations of glycolipid also are present in endothelium and vascular smooth muscle and in most other body tissues. The disease results from a deficiency of ceramide trihexosidase, an enzyme which hydrolyzes ceramide trihexoside. This glycolipid accumulates in the form of birefringent granules composed of concentric or parallel lamellae spaced 40 to 65 Å apart. In ordinary histologic preparations, the deposits are dissolved, and the cardiac muscle cells resemble those in type II glycogenosis.

CALCIUM

Calcium is most commonly observed in the heart in the coronary arteries, mitral anulus, aortic and scarred mitral valve cusps, in large myocardial scars, and in pericardium. In these circumstances the calcific deposits are extracellular. Calcific deposits, however, also may occur within individual myocardial cells. This occurrence most commonly is observed in patients with fatal prolonged shock or renal failure. Its cause is uncertain, although severe hypoxia is the most likely explanation because the lesion may be produced experimentally by this means.[6] High serum levels of calcium also may be a factor. The myofibers infiltrated by calcium are always necrotic. Massive myocardial calcification may occur and produce cardiac dysfunction.

REFERENCES

1 Roberts, W. C., Bodey, G. P., and Wertlake, P. T.: The Heart in Acute Leukemia. A Study of 420 Autopsy Cases, *Am. J. Cardiol.*, 21:388, 1968.

2 Arnett, E. N., and Roberts, W. C.: Active Infective Endocarditis: A Clinicopathologic Analysis of 137 Necropsy Patients, *Curr. Probl. Cardiol.*, 1(7):1–76, 1976.

3 Roberts, W. C., Kohoe, J. A., Carpenter, D. F., and Golden, A.: Cardiac Valvular Lesions in Rheumatoid Arthritis, *Arch. Intern. Med.*, 122:141, 1968.

3a Virmani, R., and Roberts, W. C.: Aschoff Bodies in Operatively Excised Atrial Appendages and in Papillary Muscles: Frequency and Clinical Significance, *Circulation*, 55:559, 1977.

4 Bulkley, B. H., and Roberts, W. C.: The Heart in Systemic Lupus Erythematosus and the Changes Induced in it by Corticosteroid Therapy. A Study of 36 Necropsy Patients, *Am. J. Med.*, 58:243, 1975.

5 Roberts, W. C., McAllister, H. A., Jr., and Ferrans, V. J.: Sarcoidosis of the Heart: A Clinicopathologic Study of 35 Necropsy Patients and Review of 78 Previously Reported Necropsy Patients, *Am. J. Med.*, (in press).

6 Roberts, W. C., and Ferrans, V. J.: Pathologic Anatomy of the Cardiomyopathies. Idiopathic Dilated and Hypertrophic Types, Infiltrative Types, and Endomyocardial Disease with and without Eosinophilia, *Hum. Pathol.*, 6:287, 1975.

7 Bulkley, B. H., and Roberts, W. C.: Dilatation of the Mitral Anulus. A Rare Cause of Mitral Regurgitation, *Am. Heart J.*, 59:457, 1975.

8 Ferrans, V. J., Massumi, R. A., Shugoll, G. I., Ali, N., and Roberts, W. C.: Ultrastructural Studies of Myocardial Biopsies in 45 Patients with Obstructive or Congestive Cardiomyopathy, in "Recent Advances in Studies on Cardiac Structure and Metabolism," E. Bajusz and G. Rona (eds.) with A. J. Brink and A. Lochner, vol. 2, "Cardiomyopathies," University Park Press, Baltimore, 1973, p. 231.

9 Roberts, W. C., and Buja, L. M.: The Frequency and Significance of Coronary Arterial Thrombi and Other Observations in Fatal Acute Myocardial Infarction. A Study of 107 Necropsy Patients, *Am. J. Med.*, 52:425, 1972.

10 Epstein, S. E., Clark, C. E., Maron, B. J., Redwood, D. R., Henry, W. L., Roberts, W. C., Ferrans, V. J., and Morrow, A. G.: Asymmetric Septal Hypertrophy, *Ann. Intern. Med.*, 81:650, 1974.

11 Teare, D.: Asymmetrical Hypertrophy of the Heart in Young Adults, *Br. Heart J.*, 20:1, 1958.

12 Ferrans, V. J., Morrow, A. G., and Roberts, W. C.: Myocardial Ultrastructure in Idiopathic Hypertrophic Subaortic Stenosis. A Study of Operatively Excised Left Ventricular Outflow Tract Muscle in 14 Patients, *Circulation*, 45:769, 1972.

13 Roberts, W. C.: Operative Treatment of Hypertrophic Obstructive Cardiomyopathy. The Case against Mitral Valve Replacement, *Am. J. Cardiol.*, 32:377, 1973.

14 Buja, L. M., Khoi, N. B., and Roberts, W. C.: Clinically Significant Cardiac Amyloidosis. Clinicopathologic Findings in 15 Patients, *Am. J. Cardiol.*, 26:394, 1970.

15 Buja, L. M., and Roberts, W. C.: Iron in the Heart. Etiology and Clinical Significance, *Am. J. Med.*, 51:209, 1971.

80
Myocarditis

NANETTE KASS WENGER, M.D.

Hence this inflammation almost always terminates fatally; but the death which it usually occasions may happen instantly or somewhat slowly. Thus *carditis* has been known to become fatal in a very few days; while in other instances, when the disease has attained to its highest degree, the most alarming symptoms partially disappear, and a sort of convalescence is established; sometimes even the patient is restored to apparent health; he then flatters himself with a near and perfect cure; but the most intelligent physician perceives only a transformation, or degeneration of the disease into another affection slower, but not less severe, as *a chronic organic* disease is then established, mortal in all cases.

JEAN NICOLAS CORVISART 1806[1]

INTRODUCTION

Epidemiology and incidence

Myocarditis, an inflammatory process involving the heart, has been described with almost every known bacterial, viral, rickettsial, mycotic, and parasitic disease. It occurs in patients of all ages and in a variety of populations. The incidence of specific etiologic agents for infectious myocarditis varies with the age of the patients surveyed; with the geographic location; with the endemic or epidemic occurrence of infectious diseases; with the sophistication of public health measures, especially immunization and sanitation programs; with the availability of effective medication; and with a specific patient's associated disease and/or therapy.

Prior acute myocarditis or chronic recurrent infectious myocarditis is a possible cause of diffuse myocardial disease and has been implicated as a cause of postinfectious asthenia. The specific etiologic diagnosis of infectious myocarditis must often be based on the extracardiac manifestations of the disease, as the clinical cardiovascular syndromes and the pathologic myocardial alterations are strikingly similar for many different etiologic agents. Most commonly, the cardiovascular manifestations are but a minor presentation of a systemic infection in which the noncardiac symptoms predominate.

It is not possible to ascertain the true incidence of myocarditis, as the vast majority of patients recover spontaneously; indeed diphtheritic and Chagas' myocarditis are the major exceptions to the generally favorable prognosis. Myocarditis is difficult to diagnose clinically, particularly in a mild case without impairment of cardiovascular function; electrocardiographic abnormalities are usually nonspecific, and the bacteriologic, biochemical, and immunologic tests used to identify the causative organisms are of value only when positive. However, myocarditis, as diagnosed by areas of focal or diffuse inflammation, is encountered in 4 to 10 percent of routine postmortem examinations. Electrocardiographic abnormalities suggestive of myocarditis, in the absence of other clinical evidence of myocarditis, occur in 10 to 33 percent of patients with the common infectious diseases. The diagnosis of myocarditis by this method appears completely dependent on the frequency of electrocardiographic recordings, particularly during convalescence.

Clinical manifestations

The typical clinical picture of myocarditis consists of fatigue, dyspnea, palpitations, and occasionally precordial discomfort. These early nonspecific symptoms occur during the first few weeks of a systemic infection and are followed by cardiac enlargement, a cardiac murmur or a pericardial friction rub, a faint first heart sound, distension of the neck veins, gallop sounds, and pulsus alternans.[1a] Particularly in a patient with viral infection, there is risk of early left ventricular failure being misinterpreted as viral pneumonia.

There is persistent fever, but the tachycardia is disproportionate to the degree of fever. This excessive tachycardia, both at rest and with effort, should alert the clinician to the diagnosis of myocarditis. Supraventricular or ventricular arrhythmias are common. Pulmonary or systemic embolization may be evident. This symptom complex is associated with frequent but nonspecific electrocardiographic alterations: rhythm disturbances, conduction defects, low voltage, and ST-T abnormalities. The combination of precordial discomfort and electrocardiographic abnormalities may be misinterpreted as myocardial infarction.

These more diagnostic clinical manifestations of myocarditis rarely occur at the height of the infectious illness but rather become evident during convalescence as the systemic infection is subsiding. In many instances, the cardiovascular and electrocardiographic abnormalities should determine the duration of convalescence recommended after an acute infectious illness in an attempt to minimize myocardial damage.

Although most patients recover rapidly, a significant number have recurrent or chronic myocarditis, and some patients succumb to a fulminant acute illness. Indeed, acute myocarditis is not an unusual cause of sudden death in young adults.

Pathology (see Chap. 79)

Pathologic examination of the hearts of the patients who die of apparent acute myocarditis reveals a spectrum of abnormalities including cardiac dilatation and hypertrophy, mural thrombi, interstitial cellular infiltrates, and myofiber degeneration. Routine histologic examination of the heart rarely affords an etiologic diagnosis; the availability of electron microscopy and newer immunofluorescent techniques may permit more frequent and accurate identification of specific forms of infectious myocarditis. Even when a causative organism is isolated, it is often not known whether direct invasion and tissue damage by the infectious agent or a toxic, allergic, or hypersensitivity response to this agent is responsible for the clinical, electrocardiographic, and pathologic manifestations. Furthermore, histologic myocardial abnormalities in patients dying of presumed myocarditis may also be attributed to the corticosteroid hormones, pressor amines, digitalis, and other drugs administered during the illness or to the nonspecific stress effect described by Selye.

Infectious myocarditis, as diagnosed by electrocardiographic or histologic abnormalities,[2] is encountered during a systemic infection in many patients who present trivial or no clinical evidence of cardiovascular involvement.

BACTERIAL MYOCARDITIS

Diphtheria

Myocarditis occurs in 10 to 25 percent of patients with clinical diphtheria and is responsible for the majority of diphtheria fatalities.

PATHOPHYSIOLOGY

The diphtheria circulating endotoxin produces a disturbance of cellular respiration, apparently acting as a competitive analogue once the host's cytochrome b is depleted; thus, organs with high energy requirements (heart, nerves, etc.) are first affected.[3] These alterations of cellular metabolism may result in electrocardiographic depolarization abnormalities even without irreversible necrosis of the myocardial cell. Diphtheria toxin appears to have a special affinity for the conduction system, and damage to this is a prominent feature of diphtheritic myocarditis.

PATHOLOGY

Pathologic examination of the heart reveals a flaccid, dilated, pale myocardium. Microscopic myocardial abnormalities include hyaline necrosis and myocytolysis, with extensive intracellular fat accumulation and glycogen depletion; diphtheria toxin interferes with fatty acid oxidation and inhibits protein synthesis. Unlike most other forms of myocarditis, the parenchymatous changes are extensive and appear disproportionate to the interstitial infiltrate. The SA and AV nodes are notably free of fatty infiltration, but extensive necrosis may occur throughout the conduction system.[4] Extensive mitochondrial damage is evident at electron microscopy. Diphtheritic valvular endocarditis has also been described.

History The earliest cardiovascular symptoms are not related to myocarditis but to toxemia and respiratory obstruction; hypoxia is due to membrane formation and edema.

Physical examination The early clinical findings of myocarditis include tachycardia, soft heart sounds, and gallop rhythm which progress to overt heart failure and circulatory collapse. The peripheral circulatory collapse, due primarily to vasomotor paralysis, is associated with a marked sinus tachycardia; both vasomotor paralysis and myocarditis, with decreased cardiac output and shock, may be responsible for the tachycardia.

Laboratory examination Electrocardiographic abnormalities and elevated serum levels of cardiac enzymes may be the earliest evidence of myocarditis. ST-T electrocardiographic changes (Fig. 80-1), the first evidence of acute myocarditis, usually appear in the second week of illness; conduction abnormalities, especially bundle branch block, follow. The development of bundle branch block is associated with a 50 percent mortality.[5] An atrioventricular conduction disturbance, characteristically complete heart block, is an ominous sign which warns of incipient congestive heart failure and peripheral circulatory failure; an 80 to 100 percent mortality rate is reported among patients who develop complete heart block. Marked elevation of the serum transaminase levels likewise signals a poor prognosis. Most electrocardiographic abnormalities regress, in survivors, within several months.

TREATMENT
Intubation should be accomplished with positive-pressure ventilation, if necessary; and penicillin G or erythromycin and diphtheria antitoxin should be administered. Digitalis must be administered cautiously because of the high incidence of complete heart block. Electrocardiographic monitoring is requisite for all patients with abnormal electrocardiograms. Temporary[6] or permanent implanted cardiac pacemakers[7] and mechanically assisted circulation may markedly reduce the fatalities from diphtheritic myocarditis. Nevertheless, primary prevention by immunization against diphtheria is the approach of choice.

CLINICAL COURSE
In general, the early onset of myocarditis and the presence of severe electrocardiographic abnormalities indicate a grave prognosis. The patient should be kept at bed rest as long as electrocardiographic abnormalities or undue tachycardia on exertion are present; these may persist for 6 to 8 weeks after the onset of diphtheria. Regression of electrocardiographic abnormalities parallels the recovery from myocarditis.[3] The patient who recovers from diphtheritic myocarditis may have persistent atrioventricular conduction abnormalities for months or years, but this is generally the sole evidence of residual heart disease.

Tuberculosis

Myocardial tuberculosis occurs more frequently in children, probably because they have an increased incidence of miliary tuberculosis.

PATHOLOGY
The pathologic myocardial manifestations of tuberculosis include large caseous nodules, miliary lesions, diffuse myocarditis, and pericarditis. Tubercle bacilli may reach the heart by direct extension or by lymphatic or hematogenous spread.

Single or multiple yellow-white tuberculous nodules are most common in the right atrium and usually occur by direct extension from the hilar lymph nodes. These classic tubercles (Fig. 80-2) have central caseation and surrounding granulation tissue with mononuclear and giant cells. The miliary lesions often follow the course of the coronary blood vessels. Diffuse tuberculous myocarditis is a curiosity rarely diagnosed ante mortem. The perivascular and interstitial infiltrate is nonspecific, and diagnosis depends on the identification of tubercle bacilli.

CLINICAL MANIFESTATIONS
As with the syphilitic gumma, the tuberculous myocardial nodule[8] may be completely asymptomatic or may produce symptoms by interfering with cardiac rhythm, cardiac conduction, or intracardiac blood flow; it may mimic myocardial infarction. The sudden onset of arrhythmia in a young patient with tuberculosis may signal myocardial or coronary artery tuberculous involvement. The author observed a patient in whom a large tuberculoma of the right ventricular outflow tract interfered with intracardiac blood flow, simulating valvular obstruction[9] (Fig. 80-3). Rupture of a myocardial tubercle into a cardiac chamber may cause disseminated tuberculosis; fatal rupture of a tuberculous myocardial abscess and of a tuberculous myocardial aneurysm have been described. A tuberculous granuloma should be considered in evaluating a calcified mass in the myocardium.[10]

TREATMENT
A three-drug regimen of isoniazid, rifampin, and ethambutol or streptomycin is recommended. Rarely, incision and drainage of a tuberculoma may be required to restore adequate cardiac pumping function.[9]

Typhoid fever (*Salmonella*)

The clinical manifestations of typhoid fever are due to an endotoxin. The most common cardiovascular complication at the height of the typhoid fever

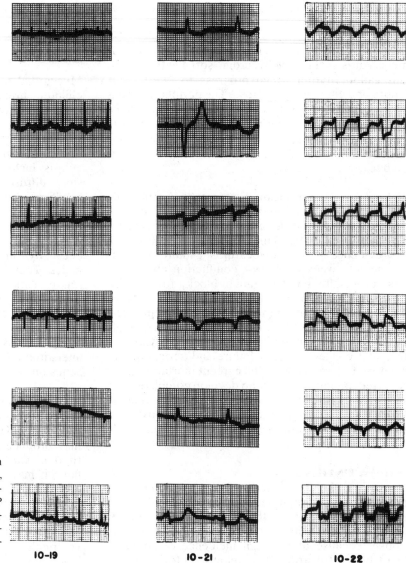

FIGURE 80-1 Fatal diphtheritic myocarditis in an 8-year-old girl. 10/19, sinus tachycardia; 10/21, complete heart block, multiple ectopic ventricular beats, marked ST-T changes; 10/22, no P waves seen, rapid tachycardia with marked alteration in QRS contour, and profound ST-T changes. A. Extremity leads. B. Precordial leads (facing page).

10-19   10-21   10-22

A

infection is peripheral circulatory failure. Typhoid myocarditis is more commonly encountered in patients severely ill with typhoid fever and in children. It seems more common with chloramphenicol-resistant typhoid.

PATHOLOGY
Pathologic changes include myofiber cloudy swelling, fragmentation, hyaline degeneration, and a mononuclear cell interstitial infiltrate. Occasionally, there is evidence of coronary endarteritis, endocarditis, or pericarditis;[11] ventricular rupture has been reported. We have encountered a subendocardial Salmonella typhimurium abscess, 2 in. in diameter, mimicking a cardiac tumor (see Fig. 86-19). A Salmonella abscess in the atrial septum caused complete AV dissocia-

tion;[12] asymptomatic Salmonella abscesses have also been reported.

CLINICAL MANIFESTATIONS
Evidence of myocarditis generally appears in the second or third week of illness and includes bradycardia, tachycardia, gallop rhythm, hypotension, cardiac enlargement, and congestive heart failure. Electrocardiographic abnormalities[13] have been described in 40 to 60 percent of patients during convalescence from typhoid fever; these include conduction disturbances, abnormal Q waves, and ST-T changes; the electrocardiogram may simulate myocardial infarction. Electrocardiographic changes may, at times, antedate clinical evidence of myocarditis or x-ray evidence of cardiac enlargement.[14]

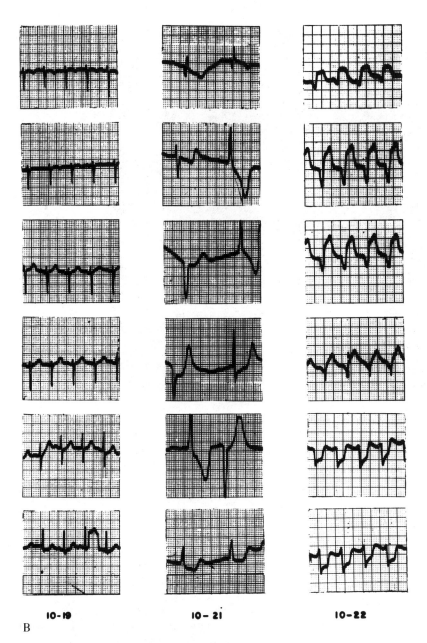

10-19   10-21   10-22

B

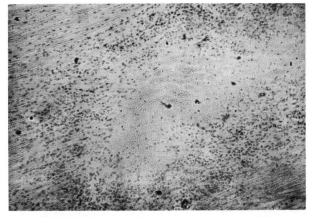

FIGURE 80-2 Myocardial granuloma in miliary tuberculosis. Caseating granuloma replacing myocardial fibers.

Tachycardia and circulatory instability after exercise often persist for 1 to 3 months after disappearance of the electrocardiographic abnormalities; they represent residual myocarditis, and the patient must be treated appropriately.

TREATMENT

Chloramphenicol is the drug of choice for serious *Salmonella* infections, with ampicillin or trimethoprim-Gantanol serving as alternatives, especially for chloramphenicol-resistant infections.

Vasopressor drugs may be needed to treat circulatory collapse. Digitalis and diuretic therapy should be continued for longer than the clinical picture sug-

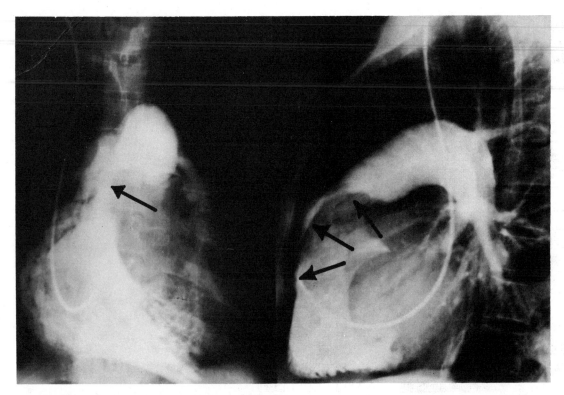

FIGURE 80-3 Right ventricular angiocardiogram demonstrating a mass obstructing (arrow) the right ventricular outflow tract. Upon surgical intervention, a lemon-sized mass was found, arising from the right ventricle and containing thick, caseous material. The mass was presumed to be a tuberculoma.

gests, as their premature discontinuation may cause recurrence of evidence of heart failure. Sensitivity to digitalis has been described, requiring that it be administered cautiously.[15]

SCARLET FEVER, ACUTE RHEUMATIC FEVER (β-HEMOLYTIC STREPTOCOCCUS)

Scarlet fever

PATHOLOGY
Most patients with fatal scarlet fever have pathologic evidence of myocarditis. These changes include subendothelial and perivascular round-cell infiltrates and hyaline or granular muscle necrosis.[16] Valve vegetations may be present.

CLINICAL MANIFESTATIONS
Conduction disturbances and arrhythmias may be encountered in scarlet fever, often after defervescence; however, derangement of cardiac function of the severity of the cardiac enlargement, congestive heart failure, and cardiac murmurs associated with acute rheumatic fever is most unusual. Nevertheless,

sudden death has been reported in scarlet fever myocarditis; and electrocardiographic changes of P-Q and Q-T interval prolongation and ST-T alterations occur.

Rheumatic fever

PATHOLOGY
The myocarditis of acute rheumatic fever is part of a pancarditis, and Aschoff's bodies are the diagnostic myocardial lesion. (See Chap. 58.)

CLINICAL MANIFESTATIONS
Valvulitis characteristically produces the hemodynamic impairment in rheumatic fever. However, on occasion, the dominant abnormality may be myocarditis with resultant heart failure.

TREATMENT
Penicillin G is the recommended treatment for both scarlet fever myocarditis and acute rheumatic fever myocarditis; in addition salicylates and corticosteroid hormones are used to suppress the inflammatory response in rheumatic myocarditis.

Meningococcemia

Acute interstitial myocarditis is present in over three-fourths of fatal meningococcal infections; it occurs more frequently with meningococcemia than with meningitis alone and more often when *Neisseria meningitidis* groups B and C are implicated than with group A.

PATHOLOGY

Pathologic abnormalities include epicardial and endocardial petechiae, myocardial hemorrhages, focal necrosis, polymorphonuclear cell infiltrates, myofiber degeneration, and capillary thrombosis; associated endocarditis and pericarditis are rare. AV node inflammation was recently shown to be the cause of sudden cardiac death in protracted meningococcemia.[17]

CLINICAL MANIFESTATIONS

The circulatory collapse, congestive heart failure, disseminated intravascular coagulation, and ST-T electrocardiographic changes encountered in the Waterhouse-Friderichsen syndrome reflect both the peripheral circulatory effect of meningococcal endotoxin and the myocarditis of the disease.

TREATMENT

Penicillin G is recommended, since many group B and C strains are resistant to sulfa drugs. Corticosteroid hormones are indicated only when there is evidence of adrenal insufficiency. Disseminated intravascular coagulation is best treated with heparin. Fluid restriction and digitalis administration are indicated for congestive heart failure. Hypotension should be treated with isoproterenol, as levarterenol may potentiate the endotoxic vascular endothelial damage.[18] A temporary cardiac pacemaker may avert sudden death in patients with conduction defects.[17]

Bacterial endocarditis

The clinical cardiovascular manifestations and electrocardiographic abnormalities of bacterial endocarditis generally reflect the severity of the valvulitis, rather than the myocarditis.

PATHOLOGY

Myocardial histologic abnormalities in bacterial endocarditis include minute infarcts, cloudy myofiber swelling, fatty degeneration, petechial hemorrhages, microabscesses, and perivascular inflammation.[19] Valve vegetations are frequent.

CLINICAL MANIFESTATIONS

Conduction abnormalities are not uncommon in patients with aortic valve endocarditis; the infection extends from the aortic valve to the conduction system. Myocarditis may augment the severity of the heart failure due to infective valvulitis.

TREATMENT (see Chap. 77)

Recommended therapy depends on the causative organism and its sensitivity. Electrical pacing of the heart may be lifesaving in patients who develop complete heart block.[20]

Staphylococcal, pneumococcal, gonococcal infection

PATHOLOGY

Myocardial abscesses and valve vegetations occur with staphylococcal, pneumococcal, and gonococcal infection but are usually associated with sepsis or acute endocarditis.

CLINICAL MANIFESTATIONS

Congestive heart failure and shock may be present, and there are often ST-T electrocardiographic changes. However, myocardial abscesses are classically silent.

TREATMENT

Penicillin G is recommended for pneumococcal and gonococcal infections, and penicillinase-resistant penicillin for staphylococcal infections.

Clostridial infection (gas gangrene)[20a]

Clostridium perfringens requires devitalized, hypoxic tissue for the development of infection. This occurs in myocardial infarction.

PATHOLOGY

Multiple abcess formation; with cystic spaces of gas production, occurred in a patient with myocardial infarction and gangrene of the foot.

CLINICAL MANIFESTATIONS

The above-described patient died of abcess rupture with purulent pericarditis.

Brucellosis

PATHOLOGY

Myofiber degeneration and granulomatous lesions constitute the histologic alterations.

CLINICAL MANIFESTATIONS

Bacterial endocarditis, pericarditis, and electrocardiographic ST-T changes have been reported in brucellosis.[21]

TREATMENT

There is clinical response to tetracycline and to streptomycin therapy; the value of corticosteroid hormones is uncertain.

Tetanus (*Clostridium tetani*)

PATHOLOGY

Pathologic alterations include myofiber necrosis, edema, a mononuclear cell infiltrate, and nerve cell degeneration. A cardiotoxic lysin is implicated.[22]

CLINICAL MANIFESTATIONS

Frequent, life-threatening cardiac arrhythmias and cardiac arrest have been reported in patients with tetanus; these complications are probably related to hypoxia and electrolyte derangements.

TREATMENT

Continuous cardiac monitoring and maintenance of ventilation are most important. Tetanus antitoxin and penicillin should be administered. Since the cardiovascular complications reflect sympathetic overactivity, propranolol is recommended for control of arrhythmias, and bethanidine for the hypertension. Tetanus immunization is preventive.

Tularemia

PATHOLOGY
Perivascular mononuclear cell myocardial infiltrates and myofiber cloudy swelling have been reported in tularemia.

CLINICAL MANIFESTATIONS
There are no associated clinical or electrocardiographic abnormalities. Pericarditis with effusion may result in constrictive pericarditis.

TREATMENT
Streptomycin therapy is recommended.

Melioidosis

Systemic melioidosis, due to the bacillus *Pseudomonas Pseudomallei,* is endemic in Southeast Asia.

PATHOLOGY
At postmortem examination of the patient described below, a 4-cm left ventricular abscess was found, with surrounding necrotic myocardium; the abscess cavity was filled with purulent debris. Numerous smaller myocardial abscesses were also present.

CLINICAL MANIFESTATIONS
A recent case in a 58-year-old soldier in Vietnam had the clinical and electrocardiographic features of acute myocardial infarction.[23]

TREATMENT
A combination of tetracycline and a sulfonamide is recommended for melioidosis.

Acute nasopharyngitis, tonsillitis, bronchopneumonia, pertussis

PATHOLOGY
Pathologic evidence of the acute myocarditis includes mononuclear cell interstitial infiltrates and muscle necrosis.

CLINICAL MANIFESTATIONS
Hypotension, cyanosis, arrhythmias, ST-T electrocardiographic changes, congestive heart failure, and even sudden death have been described in isolated cases of acute nasopharyngitis, tonsillitis, bronchopneumonia, and pertussis; cardiac symtpoms become evident at the time of subsidence of the acute infection.[24]

TREATMENT
Therapy depends on the specific organism and its sensitivity.

SPIROCHETAL MYOCARDITIS

Syphilis

PATHOLOGY
The myocardial manifestations of syphilis include diffuse miliary interstitial gummatous myocarditis and localized gumma of the myocardium.

Diffuse gummatous myocarditis is characterized by an interstitial infiltrate of fibroblastic or myxomatous tissue and mononuclear cells, associated with muscle fragmentation and vasculoation. As is usual in tertiary syphilis, spirochetes cannot be demonstrated in the myocardium; however, spirochetes can be frequently identified in similar lesions in congenital syphilis. Boss et al.[25] suggested that the diffuse myocarditis represented a hypersensitivity response to the syphilitic infection. Saphir attributed the myocardial changes to syphilitic or atherosclerotic vascular disease; he required a true gumma to diagnose syphilitic myocardial disease.

Localized myocardial gummas, solitary or multiple, are encountered more frequently, often as unexpected findings at postmortem examination (Fig. 80-4). The gray-white nodule has a central necrotic area surrounded by granulation tissue, mononuclear cells, fibroblasts, and giant cells (Fig. 80-5). Associated syphilitic aortitis is frequent.

CLINICAL MANIFESTATIONS
The major clinical abnormalities are arrhythmias; conduction abnormalities; and valvular pseudostenosis, which generally occurs when a gumma impinges on the ventricular outflow tract. The characteristic location of a gumma in the left ventricular myocardium at the base of the interventricular septum accounts for the clinical manifestations: conduction system abnormalities of heart block and bundle branch block,[26] or symptomatic pseudostenosis of

FIGURE 80-4 Syphilitic gumma of the myocardium. Cross section through gumma of right ventricular wall.

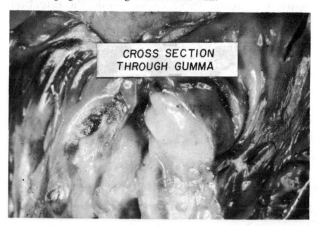

CROSS SECTION THROUGH GUMMA

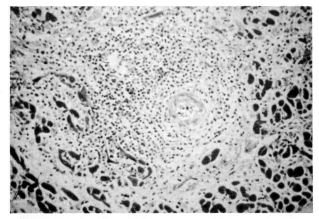

FIGURE 80-5 Syphilitic gumma of the myocardium. Perivascular and interstitial inflammatory infiltrate and interstitial fibrosis (×150).

the aortic or pulmonic valves. Fatal rupture of a gummatous aneurysm of the left ventricle has been reported. Diffuse syphilitic myocarditis may mimic the clinical and electrocardiographic picture usually associated with myocardial infarction.

TREATMENT
Penicillin G therapy is recommended.

Leptospirosis (Weil's disease)

Cardiovascular manifestations occur in about 10 percent of patients with leptospirosis, predominantly in the second week of illness as the fever and systemic toxicity subside.

Myocarditis occurs more commonly with *Leptospira icterohaemorrhagiae* but has also been reported with *Leptospira pomona* infection.[27]

PATHOLOGY
The pathologic myocardial lesion[28] is characterized by focal hemorrhage, pronounced interstitial edema, areas of myocardial degeneration and necrosis, and an inflammatory cell infiltrate (Fig. 80-6). This occurs primarily in the subendocardial region and papillary muscles, and frequently involves the conduction system. Rare leptospirae have been demonstrated in the interstitial lesions. Metabolic, allergic, and toxic causes have been suggested for the myocarditis.

CLINICAL MANIFESTATIONS
Cardiovascular manifestations of leptospirosis include arrhythmias, cardiac enlargement, gallop rhythm, and congestive heart failure. Leptospiral endocarditis and pericarditis have also been described, the latter probably secondary to uremia.[29]

Nonspecific transient electrocardiographic abnormalities occur in over one-half of patients with leptospirosis. T-wave changes are most common; sinus bradycardia, ventricular premature beats, paroxysmal atrial flutter and fibrillation, atrioventricular conduction defects, and prolonged P-Q and Q-T intervals are also described. Metabolic disturbances—uremia, hyperbilirubinemia, and elec-

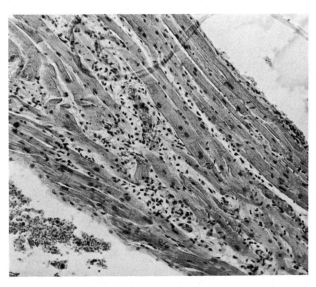

FIGURE 80-6 Leptospirosis involving the myocardium. There is focal interstitial infiltration of mononuclear cells and lymphocytes with fragmentation of muscle substance (×150).

trolyte abnormalities—may in part explain the electrocardiographic abnormalities, which characteristically disappear during convalescence.

TREATMENT
Penicillin G or tetracycline should be administered; however, evidence is lacking for antibiotic effectiveness except in the earliest stage of leptospiral infection.

CLINICAL COURSE
There is an ominous prognosis when severe bradycardia, complete heart block, and hypotension occur. Death from parenchymatous and interstitial myocarditis has been reported in patients with Weil's disease whose hepatic and renal status was improving. The author has seen a 38-year-old man with fatal leptospirosis who, at the end of the first week of illness, developed sinus bradycardia, arrhythmia, terminal congestive heart failure, and shock.

Relapsing fever, louse-borne

Myocarditis is the commonest cause of death in fatal cases of relapsing fever, due to the spirochete *Borrelia recurrentis*. Death is often sudden and unexpected, occurring shortly after the initiation of therapy. The physiologic abnormalities of endotoxic shock are thought to overwhelm a damaged myocardium.[30]

PATHOLOGY
The diffuse myocarditis, particularly near the small arteries, is characterized by a lymphocytic and plasmacytic infiltrate with interstitial edema. There are petechial hemorrhages but no myocardial necrosis.

CLINICAL MANIFESTATIONS

The illness is characterized by fever, chills, vomiting, abdominal pain, delirium, and often coma. The disease resolves by crisis, either spontaneous or shortly after antibiotic administration. The crisis includes chills; vasoconstriction; increased fever, tachycardia, tachypnea, and hypertension; and lasts for 10 to 30 min. A hypotensive phase follows with vasodilation and flushing, but continued fever and tachycardia. Recovery and defervescence begin after about 2 h, although hypotension, evidence of venous pressure elevation, and gallop rhythm may persist for 8 to 12 h. Arrhythmia in the hypotensive phase is thought to cause the sudden death.[30]

LABORATORY EXAMINATION

Diagnosis is made by demonstrating spirochetes in the peripheral blood smear.

The crisis is characterized by acute neutropenia and respiratory alkalosis. Neutropenia progresses in the hypotensive phase; spirochetes disappear from the blood, and a metabolic acidosis develops.

Chest x-ray is usually normal, but electrocardiographic conduction abnormalities are typical, as is Q-T interval prolongation.

TREATMENT

Tetracycline is recommended; penicillin is also used.

RICKETTSIAL MYOCARDITIS

Myocarditis is common in rickettsial diseases, particularly scrub typhus (tsutsugamushi disease).

Typhus

PATHOLOGY

Classifications of myocarditis frequently state that myocardial involvement is invariably seen in rickett-

FIGURE 80-7 Myocardial involvement in typhus. *A*. Perivascular inflammatory infiltrate (×150). *B*. Perivascular nodule, with partial obliteration of the vessel lumen. Infiltrate consists of mononuclear cells with occasional polymorphonuclear leukocytes (×350).

sial infections and that vasculitis is the characteristic pathologic lesion. There is a focal acute interstitial mononuclear cell infiltrate but no myofiber damage. The disparity between the pathologic severity of scrub typhus myocarditis and the minimal degree of clinical cardiovascular impairment appears related to the preservation of myocardial fibers. Endothelial proliferation and perivascular infiltrates involve the small blood vessels (Fig. 80-7).

Minor focal myocardial lesions in epidemic typhus *(Rickettsia prowazekii)* are in part attributable to a coronary arteritis. There is an acute subendocardial and perivascular interstitial infiltrate, without significant myocardial degenerative changes. The few post-mortem studies after subsidence of the acute illness show no evidence of permanent myocardial damage.

CLINICAL MANIFESTATIONS

Transient congestive heart failure, arrhythmias, and nonspecific electrocardiographic changes[31] occur frequently in the acute phase of scrub typhus, usually during the second week of illness.[32] The circulatory failure may be peripheral in origin.[32] There are no residual cardiac symptoms.

TREATMENT (see end of section)

Rocky Mountain spotted fever

PATHOLOGY

Similar myocardial lesions to those of typhus occur in Rocky Mountain spotted fever but are even less prominent in this disease (Fig. 80-8).

CLINICAL MANIFESTATIONS

The cardiovascular complications of Rocky Mountain spotted fever reflect the widespread vasculitis: hypovolemia, hypotension, increased interstitial fluid with pulmonary and peripheral edema, thrombocytopenia, (?) disseminated intravascular coagulation, etc.

TREATMENT (see also end of section)

Therapy includes colloid-containing fluids to correct the hypovolemia, oxygen and assisted ventilation if needed, and heparin for coagulation abnormalities, in addition to antimicrobial therapy.[33]

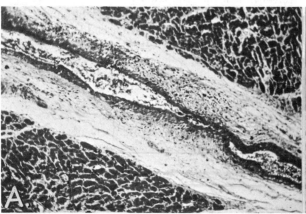
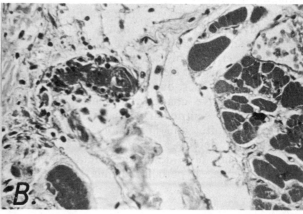

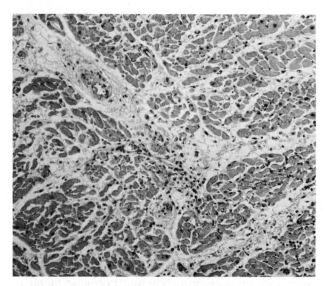

FIGURE 80-8 Rocky Mountain spotted fever. Focal interstitial infiltration of the myocardium with lymphocytes and mononuclear leukocytes (×150).

Q fever

PATHOLOGY
Because patients with Q fever usually recover, minimal postmortem evidence is available.

CLINICAL MANIFESTATIONS
Q fever (Rickettsia burnetii) is rarely associated with cardiac symptoms in the absence of underlying heart disease; fatal Q fever endocarditis has occurred in patients with diseased heart valves or recent cardiac surgery.[34] Pericarditis, however, is common.

The myocarditis is of variable severity.[35] Transient cardiomegaly and electrocardiographic changes of "myopericardial disease" and arrhythmia[36] have been described, with occasional residual electrocardiographic abnormalities and congestive heart failure after Q fever myocarditis.

TREATMENT
Tetracycline and chloramphenicol are currently considered to be the drugs of choice for these rickettsial infections. There is little data available regarding the long-term follow-up of patients with rickettsial myocarditis.

VIRAL MYOCARDITIS

Virus replication in the heart results in a temporary or permanent change in myocardial structure and function.[37]

Recently, considerable emphasis has been placed on myalgia as presaging cardiac involvement in viral infections.[37a]

Viral myocarditis may cause congestive heart failure, life-threatening arrhythmias, and conduction disturbances; it may also cause sudden death. Prior viral myocarditis has been implicated as a cause of chronic cardiomyopathy.[2] Myocardial histopathologic changes have been described with almost all known viral infections, but Coxsackie, echo, and poliomyelitis viruses are most commonly isolated from human hearts.

In viral myocarditis, there is a characteristic latent period between the acute systemic infection and the onset of clinical myocarditis. This strongly implicates activation of an autoimmune mechanism, possibly related to alteration of the myocardial cell by virus replication.[38] However, the rarity of clinically apparent viral myocarditis relative to the total number of viral infections makes it impractical and unrealistic to institute therapy designed to suppress autoimmune responses.

Alternative explanations for viral myocarditis include direct cellular destruction by the virus or viral alteration of cellular energy systems. "Conditioning factors" such as malnutrition, pregnancy, bacterial infection, ethanol intake, corticosteroid hormone therapy, ionizing radiation, heat/cold stress, etc., may be important in the production of the initial viral infection and in the activation of latent or dormant viruses.[39]

Viral infections may produce congenital cardiac malformations, with resultant impairment of cardiac function. Additionally, alteration of pulmonary or systemic vascular resistance during viral infections may compromise cardiac function. Viral infections commonly cause pericarditis, and less often, valvulitis.

The routine availability of diagnostic viral laboratory tests will enable identification of specific forms of viral myocarditis. This is a prerequisite for the development of special viral vaccines (as for rubella), of viricidal drugs, of interferon-inducers, etc.[39]

Coxsackie B

Coxsackie virus infections commonly occur in epidemics and are more prevalent in summer and early fall. The Coxsackie B virus seems especially cardiotropic in human beings; this enterovirus is the most common cause of viral heart disease, although Coxsackie pericarditis occurs more commonly than myocarditis.[40]

Recent evidence suggests that occult Coxsackie B myocarditis, demonstrable only at pathologic examination, may be extremely common in infants and children. Coxsackie myocarditis in the neonate may be acquired either transplacentally or from nursery contacts.

Coxsackie virus infection in the mother may also be responsible for congenital heart disease in the fetus.[41] Coxsackie myocarditis may be particularly virulent during pregnancy.

Coxsackie B 1-5 and A 4,16 are most commonly implicated.

PATHOLOGY
On histologic examination of the myocardium, focal inflammatory cells, usually mononuclear, are seen, with myofiber necrosis, particularly involving the inner third of the myocardium.

Electron microscopic studies localize Coxsackie virus particles along the tubules of the sarcoplasmic reticulum of cardiac muscle. Coxsackie virus antigens have been demonstrated in both the myocardium and the mitral valve by immunofluorescent antibody studies on routine autopsy specimens, suggesting a hypersensitivity or autoimmune mechanism.

Coxsackie virus is rarely isolated from the heart later than 9 days after the onset of infection,[37] further suggesting an immunologic process.

CLINICAL MANIFESTATIONS

Coxsackie B myocarditis, often fatal in nursery epidemics, is an acute fulminating illness with fever, respiratory distress, cyanosis, extreme tachycardia or arrhythmia, cardiac dilatation, congestive heart failure, and circulatory collapse. Gallop rhythm is common, and murmurs are rare.

Typically, acute Coxsackie myopericarditis is a benign disease in the adult. However, severe Coxsackie B myopericarditis, often with pleurodynia, is reported with increasing frequency; fever, arrhythmias, severe congestive heart failure, and pericarditis with effusion are common. The disease occurs more commonly in men. The pain and electrocardiographic abnormalities may mimic myocardial infarction.

Complete recovery is characteristic, but residual electrocardiographic abnormalities, cardiac enlargement, and constrictive pericarditis have been reported,[42] as has recurrence of illness. Persistent, symptomatic complete heart block has necessitated pacemaker implantation.[42a]

LABORATORY EXAMINATION

Viral involvement of the AV node has been implicated as the cause of the arrhythmias and electrocardiographic abnormalities (Fig. 80-9). ST-segment displacement occurs frequently and T-wave abnormalities and low voltage may also be present.

Cardiac enzyme levels may be elevated, and there is often cardiac enlargement on the chest x-ray. Echocardiography best demonstrates the contribution of a pericardial effusion to the cardiac enlargement.

Viral confirmation is best done by isolation from blood or from throat or rectal swabs; antibody titer determinations require acute and convalescent serums.[40]

TREATMENT

There is no specific therapy, other than supportive measures and control of heart failure, but rest is indicated. Specifically, jogging, alcohol, reserpine, and undernutrition should be avoided. As with other viral diseases, occasional reports stress a possible contraindication to corticosteroid hormone therapy. Corticosteroid hormones inhibit interferon synthesis, appear to increase virus multiplication and virulence, and are best withheld for the first week or two of illness.[37]

The adult with Coxsackie myopericarditis, misdiagnosed as myocardial or pulmonary infarction and treated with anticoagulation, may develop the complication of hemopericardium.[42]

Echovirus

Echoviruses have been recovered from the hearts of patients dying of clinical myocarditis.[43] Types 9, 11, 19, and 22 appear especially cardiotropic. Nursery infections are not uncommon.

PATHOLOGY

Histologic abnormalities include focal myocardial necrosis and a predominantly lymphocytic inflammatory cell infiltrate.

CLINICAL MANIFESTATIONS

This is a febrile illness with rash and respiratory and gastrointestinal symptoms. Symptomless myocarditis is characteristically associated with myalgia, and an electrocardiogram is recommended for patients with this symptom.[44]

FIGURE 80-9 Coxsackie virus B myopericarditis in a 4-year-old child, confirmed by culture and rising viral antibody titer. A wandering supraventricular pacemaker was present in addition to the ST-T changes.

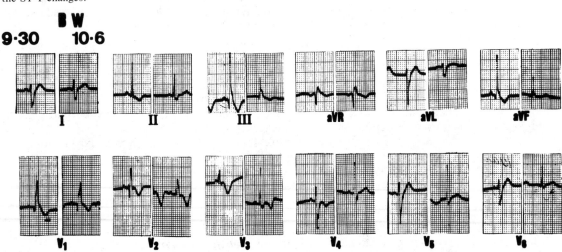

Congestive heart failure, arrhythmias, and pericarditis have been reported. Occasional acute cardiovascular collapse is described.[45] Typically, however, there is mainly tachycardia and tachypnea, and the clinical course is benign.

LABORATORY EXAMINATION
There are variable electrocardiographic conduction and rhythm abnormalities; cardiac enlargement may be seen on x-ray. There is elevation of the serum antibody neutralizing titer.

TREATMENT
Management is as recommended for Coxsackie myocarditis.

Poliomyelitis

Poliomyelitis virus, similar to the Coxsackie virus, is cardiotropic in human beings. Poliomyelitis myocarditis occurs in the majority of fatal cases of poliomyelitis.

PATHOLOGY
Pathologic evidence of poliomyelitis myocarditis occurs in 40 to 90 percent of fatal cases of poliomyelitis. Histologically, there is a focal interstitial and perivascular lymphocytic infiltrate; polymorphonuclear leukocytes are present in areas of muscle cell necrosis, but myofibers are generally intact. However, poliomyelitis virus has been recovered from heart muscle in fatal cases of poliomyelitis without pathologic evidence of myocarditis. Inflammatory and degenerative changes are also present in the superior cervical vagus ganglion and the cardiac plexus; disturbances of cardiac innervation may underlie the electrocardiographic and clinical abnormalities.

CLINICAL MANIFESTATIONS
Cyanosis, dyspnea, and tachycardia are the early manifestations. They may be followed by vascular collapse, pulmonary edema, and hypertension, the latter usually related to hypoventilation and hypoxia.

LABORATORY EXAMINATION
Electrocardiographic abnormalities are frequent but nonspecific and are partly attributable to brainstem disease, metabolic alterations, etc.[46] There may be P-Q, Q-T, and QRS prolongation and ST-T changes; the electrocardiogram may mimic that of myocardial infarction, and arrhythmias may occur.

TREATMENT
Tracheostomy is indicated, as is the use of oxygen, a respirator, and vasopressor drugs to combat vascular collapse. Immunization against poliomyelitis is the indicated preventive measure.

Influenza

Influenza, even in the absence of myocarditis, is poorly tolerated by patients with pulmonary disease or heart disease (particularly rheumatic mitral stenosis) and by pregnant women. These groups of patients, at a minimum, should receive influenza vaccine. Myocarditis occurs commonly in patients with influenza of sufficient severity to require hospitalization.

PATHOLOGY
Myofiber necrosis may be seen as early as 24 h after the onset of illness. Gross changes are evident at pathologic examination by day 5; the myocardium is pale and flabby; there is myofiber necrosis with lymphocytic, plasma cell, and monocytic infiltrates; and interstitial hemorrhage may be seen. Changes usually resolve by day 18.[47]

CLINICAL MANIFESTATIONS
The illness is characterized by fever, myalgia, headache, and cough. Since symptomless myocarditis is almost invariably associated with myalgia, this finding warrants an electrocardiographic recording.[44]

Dyspnea, palpitations, angina pectoris, and heart failure are reported in influenzal myocarditis; there is often associated pericarditis. Peripheral circulatory failure and arrhythmias are common, and sudden death during convalescence may be due to complete heart block with Stokes-Adams syncope. Cardiovascular symptoms appear as the acute influenzal illness subsides.[48]

Sudden death recently occurred in a young child hospitalized for minimal heart failure following a respiratory infection; there was no premonitory arrhythmia or hypotension. Postmortem myocardial viral cultures confirmed a Hong Kong A$_2$ influenzal myocarditis.

LABORATORY EXAMINATION
Diagnosis is by hemagglutinin-inhibition and complement-fixation titers.

The electrocardiographic abnormalities include sinus bradycardia, sinoatrial block, ectopic ventricular beats, T-wave changes, and partial and complete atrioventricular block. Electrocardiographic abnormalities appear unrelated to the severity of the illness.[47]

Cardiac enlargement and evidence of pulmonary vascular congestion are seen on chest x-ray.

TREATMENT
The therapeutic value of corticosteroid hormones is uncertain, despite occasional reports of dramatic response to therapy. Amantidine has been suggested for influenza A infections. Symptomatic complete heart block has necessitated pacemaker implantation.

Mumps

Although mumps myocarditis is diagnosed most frequently during the first week of the clinical illness, the cardiovascular disease may occasionally precede the parotitis. Myocarditis occurs more commonly in adults and when meningoencephalitis is present, but is described in 4 to 15 percent of patients with mumps.[49]

PATHOLOGY

The rare postmortem examinations show the heart to be soft and dilated. Histologic myocardial alterations include polymorphonuclear and lymphocytic infiltrates, cloudy swelling of the myofibers, and focal myocardial necrosis.[50]

CLINICAL MANIFESTATIONS

Precordial pain, dyspnea, tachycardia, and palpitations, followed by congestive heart failure, may be occasionally encountered in the patient with clinical evidence of mumps. These may be associated with pericarditis and arrhythmias. Rare deaths are reported.[49] Residual heart disease is unusual.

LABORATORY EXAMINATION

Electrocardiographic abnormalities include ST-T changes, atrioventricular block, and arrhythmias. They usually return to normal with recovery. Nonspecific, transient electrocardiographic abnormalities, without impairment of cardiac function are common and probably represent an asymptomatic mumps myocarditis.

TREATMENT

Corticosteroid hormone therapy may be of value in the rare severe cases.

Infectious mononucleosis

Cardiovascular symptoms occur in 0.7 percent of patients with infectious mononucleosis, but 6 percent have electrocardiographic abnormalities.[51] These appear 7 to 20 days after the onset of symptoms of infectious mononucleosis.

PATHOLOGY

Abnormal lymphocytes, often perivascular in location, are seen in the myocardium; focal myofiber necrosis has been described.

CLINICAL MANIFESTATIONS

Clinical evidence of myocarditis or pericarditis is unusual; occasional reports describe chest pain, cardiac dilatation, cardiac murmurs, friction rubs, gallop rhythm, and congestive heart failure, particularly in patients with severe infectious mononucleosis.[52] The combination of chest discomfort, cardiac serum enzyme level elevation, and electrocardiographic abnormalities may mimic myocardial infarction.[51,52a]

LABORATORY EXAMINATION

The occasional electrocardiographic abnormalities in infectious mononucleosis include premature ventricular beats, T-wave changes, P-Q and Q-T interval prolongation, rare Q waves, conduction disturbances, and changes compatible with pericarditis.

TREATMENT

Corticosteroid hormone therapy is of questionable value. The prognosis is excellent.

Viral hepatitis

PATHOLOGY

Histologic changes include petechial hemorrhages, lymphocytic and phagocytic infiltrates, and focal myofiber and conduction system necrosis.

CLINICAL MANIFESTATIONS

Hypotension, cardiac enlargement, pulmonary edema, and sudden death have been described,[53] as has pericardial effusion.

LABORATORY EXAMINATION

Electrocardiographic abnormalities, particularly T-wave changes, bradycardia, and arrhythmias, may be evident during the early weeks of illness in viral (infectious) hepatitis. Transient ST-T changes occurred in a patient with serum (HB Ag) hepatitis.[54]

TREATMENT

Corticosteroid hormones were reported effective in controlling Stokes-Adams attacks in a young woman with infectious hepatitis and myocarditis.

Rubella

Myocarditis is common in the infant with the congenital rubella syndrome, but may also occur in older patients with rubella. With congenital rubella there is an active myocarditis in utero which (1) may heal in utero leaving a damaged myocardium; (2) may progress after birth with variable myocardial damage; or (3) may simulate myocardial ischemia, infarction, or conduction abnormality secondary to the myocardial damage. Ventricular aneurysm may result.[5]

PATHOLOGY

Examination of the heart with rubella myocarditis shows extensive myocardial vacuolation necrosis, without interstitial inflammatory response or cellular infiltrate; only rarely is rubella virus recoverable from the myocardium,[55] and the pathologic diagnosis is often dependent on fluorescent antibody studies.

CLINICAL MANIFESTATIONS

Congenital rubella syndrome Myocarditis in the infant with congenital rubella is characterized by severe heart failure, cardiac enlargement, and electrocardiographic changes mimicking those of myocardial infarction; this myocarditis results in a high neonatal mortality rate, and infants who survive have significant morbidity.[55] The babies who survive show concomitant subsidence of the cardiac enlargement, congestive heart failure, and electrocardiographic abnormalities.

Acquired rubella Pericarditis, ST-T electrocardiographic changes, and heart block have been described as evidence of cardiac involvement in patients with rubella.

TREATMENT
Supportive treatment and standard management of heart failure are recommended.

Rubeola

PATHOLOGY
Nonspecific myocardial histologic abnormalities have been attributed to the commonly associated streptococcal bronchopneumonia.

CLINICAL MANIFESTATIONS
Pericarditis, occasionally with effusion, and transient electrocardiographic ST-T changes, atrioventricular conduction abnormalities, and arrhythmias occur in about 20 percent of patients with rubeola. These are rarely of clinical significance. Occasional reports describe persistent cardiac enlargement, heart failure, and recurrent arrhythmias.[56]

TREATMENT
The bacterial superinfection should be treated with antibiotics; the value of corticosteroid hormones is questionable.

Rabies

PATHOLOGY
Postmortem cardiac abnormalities include focal myofiber degeneration and an acute diffuse mononuclear and polymorphonuclear cell reaction, edema, and capillary dilatation. Rabies virus has been demonstrated in the myocardium.[56a]

CLINICAL MANIFESTATIONS
Tachycardia, arrhythmias, heart failure, and vascular collapse have been described with rabies. Previously unrecognized myocarditis may play an important role in the terminal stages of rabies.[56a,57]

LABORATORY EXAMINATION
ST-T electrocardiographic changes, Q waves, and electrical alternans have been described.[58]

TREATMENT
Management is for control of heart failure and circulatory collapse. Rabies vaccine and corticosteroid hormone therapy are indicated.[58] However, the prognosis is grave.

Varicella

PATHOLOGY
There is histologic evidence of focal interstitial and perivascular myocardial inflammation; myofiber necrosis may occur; eosinophilic intranuclear inclusion bodies are diagnostic. Sudden death occurred in a child with disseminated varicella; the extensive conduction system inflammation contrasted with the minor myocardial abnormalities, suggesting that the varicella virus may show a tropism for cardiac conduction tissues.

CLINICAL MANIFESTATIONS
The typical chicken pox rash is present. Severe vomiting, abdominal pain, and tachycardia occur; there may be marked facial edema. Heart failure and pericarditis in the patient with a varicella infection are usually concomitant with varicella pneumonia.

LABORATORY EXAMINATION
Bundle branch block and electrocardiographic conduction abnormalities may be present. Varicella virus may be isolated; and complement-fixation tests are positive.

TREATMENT
The therapeutic value of corticosteroid hormones is uncertain, as severe and even fatal varicella infection may occur in patients receiving corticosteroid hormone therapy.[59] Digitalis should be administered with caution, as toxicity occurs frequently.

Primary atypical pneumonia

CLINICAL MANIFESTATIONS
Evidence of myocarditis is almost invariably associated with myalgia in *Mycoplasma pneumoniae* infections, and myalgia is an indication for an electrocardiogram. Although the myocarditis is characteristically asymptomatic, gallop rhythm, a pericardial friction rub, and Stokes-Adams syncope[60] have been described.

LABORATORY EXAMINATION
Diagnosis is made by elevation of the cold agglutinin titer, *Streptococcus MG* titer, and complement-fixation antibody titer to *M. pneumoniae*. Nonspecific electrocardiographic abnormalities are evidence of an asymptomatic myocarditis in mycoplasma pneumonia.

ST-T electrocardiographic abnormalities, prolongation of AV conduction, arrhythmias, and electrocardiographic changes of pericarditis occur, although rarely, in patients with primary atypical pneumonia, with and without clinical evidence of myocarditis. It is important that these electrocardiographic changes, which may mimic those of myocardial infarction or pulmonary embolism, be correctly interpreted.

TREATMENT
Erythromycin should be administered, but does not appear to influence the course of the myocarditis. The prognosis is good, and physical activity during convalescence does not appear harmful, although bed rest for at least a week is recommended.[44]

Lymphocytic choriomeningitis

PATHOLOGY
There is no known histologic abnormality.

CLINICAL MANIFESTATIONS
Pericarditis with effusion, electrocardiographic ST-T changes, palpitations, and tachycardia have been described in patients with lymphocytic choriomeningitis.[61]

TREATMENT
The value of corticosteroid hormones is uncertain.

Psittacosis

PATHOLOGY
Histologic changes include subendocardial hemorrhages, interstitial edema, and cellular infiltrates. Occasionally, plasma cells contain the characteristic psittacosis inclusion bodies. Chlamydial (psittacosis lymphogranuloma venereum agent) infection may be an antecedent of chronic diffuse myocardial disease and may also be responsible for acquired valvular heart disease.

CLINICAL MANIFESTATIONS
Congestive heart failure, cardiac enlargement, hypotension, pericarditis with effusion, and ST-T electrocardiographic changes[62] have been reported with systemic psittacosis; mural thrombi may result in pulmonary or systemic emboli.[63]

TREATMENT
Tetracycline therapy is recommended.

Viral encephalitis

PATHOLOGY
An interstitial myocarditis with focal aggregates of lymphocytes was described at postmortem examination.[64]

CLINICAL MANIFESTATIONS
Pericarditis and electrocardiographic ST-T changes occur, although rarely, in viral encephalitis.

Herpes simplex

PATHOLOGY
Chronic inflammatory cells and histiocytes have been described in the myocardium.[65]

CLINICAL MANIFESTATIONS
Herpes simplex myocarditis has been described in adults; a recent presumptive case was characterized clinically by intractable shock.

TREATMENT
Although experimental, adenine arabinoside is recommended by some for treatment.

Cytomegalovirus

PATHOLOGY
Intranuclear cytomegalic inclusion bodies in the myocardial fibers were described in an infant with generalized cytomegalic inclusion disease.[66]

CLINICAL MANIFESTATIONS
In an infant with cytomegalic inclusion disease, the myocarditis was clinically evident as congestive heart failure.

Cytomegalovirus myocarditis in adults may be evident only as electrocardiographic ST-T changes; heart failure has been described, as has associated pericarditis.

TREATMENT
Adenine arabinoside therapy is experimental but may be beneficial.[67]

Variola

PATHOLOGY
A basophilic cell infiltrate has been noted on microscopic examination of the myocardium.

CLINICAL MANIFESTATIONS
Clinical myocarditis has not been described in variola. Postvaccinial myocarditis is discussed in Chap. 82.

Herpes zoster

CLINICAL MANIFESTATIONS
Angina pectoris and arrhythmias have occurred during herpes zoster infections.

TREATMENT
Adenine arabinoside therapy may be effective, but this is an experimental drug.

Adenovirus infection

PATHOLOGY
Type 21 adenovirus, usually associated with mild respiratory illness, has also caused fatal, diffuse, nonsuppurative myocarditis.[68]

CLINICAL MANIFESTATIONS
A respiratory infection is followed by collapse, cyanosis, and often cardiac arrest.[5]

LABORATORY EXAMINATION
The virus can be isolated, and neutralizing antibody titers support the diagnosis.

Arbovirus infection

CLINICAL MANIFESTATIONS
Patients describe a febrile respiratory illness followed by pleural or pericardial pain, breathlessness, and palpitations.[69]

Acute arbovirus (dengue and chikungunya fever) myocarditis is characterized by atrial and ventricular arrhythmias, atrioventricular block, pericarditis, and heart failure. Arrhythmia and/or embolism may result in sudden death.

Although some patients recover completely, a considerable number have residual electrocardiographic abnormalities, heart failure, and/or constrictive pericarditis.[70]

LABORATORY EXAMINATION

ST-T electrocardiographic abnormalities are often the earliest evidence of myocarditis.

Respiratory syncytial virus (RSV)[70a]

CLINICAL MANIFESTATIONS

Complete atrioventricular block and syncope, requiring a temporary transvenous pacemaker, occurred 2 weeks after a febrile respiratory infection.

LABORATORY EXAMINATION

At least a fourfold increase in RSV complement-fixation antibody titer is required to diagnose the illness.

MYCOTIC MYOCARDITIS

Actinomycosis

Actinomycotic infection may reach the myocardium either by hematogenous spread via the coronary arteries or by direct extension from the lungs or pericardium; the latter is more likely to produce clinical evidence of cardiac involvement.

PATHOLOGY

Edwards[71] described the classic lesion as a necrotizing, suppurative, fibrocaseous myocardial abscess; actinomycotic granules, composed of dense aggregates of branched filamentous organisms, are in the center of the lesion.

CLINICAL MANIFESTATIONS

Symptoms vary depending on the extent and distribution of the actinomycotic abscesses; actinomycotic myocarditis may present as valvular obstruction with a cardiac murmur, arrhythmia, congestive heart failure, endocarditis, or pericarditis.

TREATMENT

Penicillin G or tetracycline is the drug of choice.

Blastomycosis

Myocardial involvement may be produced by miliary hematogenous spread, by extension from pericardial disease, or by retrograde lymphatic spread from mediastinal lymph nodes.

PATHOLOGY

The cardiac lesion of blastomycosis is a tubercle; the central caseous area and giant cells in the surrounding granulation tissue contain *Blastomyces dermatitidis*.

CLINICAL MANIFESTATIONS

Congestive heart failure or pericarditis may occur in myocardial blastomycosis.[72]

TREATMENT

Amphotericin B therapy is recommended.

Moniliasis (candidiasis)

Systemic moniliasis occurs most frequently in infants and in debilitated adults receiving prolonged antibiotic, or immunosuppressive, therapy. These patients often have indwelling intravenous catheters.[72a]

PATHOLOGY

Cardiac involvement is described in 10 to 63 percent of cases of systemic candidosis.[72a]

There are minute multiple myocardial abscesses with necrotic myocardial cells centrally and monilial pseudohyphae, yeast forms, and inflammatory cells peripherally. Lesions are consistent with hematogenous spread, occurring predominantly in the left ventricle, with occasional His bundle involvement. The pericardium may also be involved. Systemic abcesses and positive blood cultures are usual.

CLINICAL MANIFESTATIONS

The *Candida albicans* organisms have a predilection for the brain, heart, and kidney; cardiac symptoms, however, may be minimal or absent unless endocarditis with vegetations is present.[73] Nevertheless, in patients without valvulitis, myocarditis has caused complete heart block, power failure, and sudden death; and it increases the morbidity and mortality of systemic moniliasis.

LABORATORY EXAMINATION

Left bundle branch block and first-degree and complete atrioventricular block have been reported to occur acutely. The electrocardiographic changes may mimic myocardial infarction.

TREATMENT

Amphotericin B systemically and Mycostatin orally should be given. All other antibiotics should be discontinued, and immunosuppressive drugs discontinued or decreased in dosage. The prognosis is grave.

Aspergillosis

Pulmonary symptoms predominate in aspergillosis, although cardiac involvement occurs in the generalized disease. Predisposing factors for systemic spread with cardiac involvement appear to be debilitating diseases, cytotoxic drugs, corticosteroid hormone therapy, radiation, and antibiotic therapy.[74] It is most common in patients with malignant disease and in renal and cardiac transplant recipients.

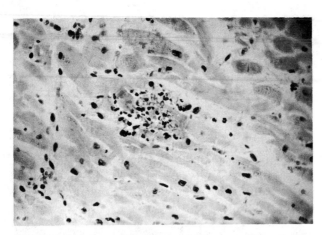

FIGURE 80-10 Aspergillus abscess of the myocardium, showing fragmented septated hyphae surrounded by polymorphonuclear leukocytes (×120).

PATHOLOGY

Focal myocardial granulomas or microabscesses contain mycelial and filamentous forms of *Aspergillus* (Fig. 80-10). These lesions produce conspicuous thrombosis of small coronary vessels and may cause myocardial necrosis and infarction.[74]

CLINICAL MANIFESTATIONS

Tachycardia, associated with electrocardiographic T-wave changes persisting for several weeks, was considered evidence of myocarditis in a patient with pulmonary aspergillosis.[75] However, there are often few electrocardiographic changes, and blood cultures are generally negative.

Rupture of a granulomatous aspergillous abscess into a cardiac chamber has been reported. Pericarditis may occur, with subsequent constrictive disease; endocarditis with *Aspergillus* vegetations has been described.[66]

TREATMENT

Therapy includes use of amphotericin B, but the prognosis once myocarditis is evident is uniformly poor.

Histoplasmosis

PATHOLOGY

The microscopic myocardial abnormalities are predominantly perivascular and consist of focal minute granulomas, myofiber destruction, and phagocytic cells glutted with *Histoplasma capsulatum*.

CLINICAL MANIFESTATIONS

Disseminated histoplasmosis may, on occasion, involve the myocardium but usually produces no impairment of function. *H. capsulatum* endocarditis and pericarditis, often with effusion, occur more frequently. Arrhythmias have been documented, and obstruction of the superior vena cava has been described.[76]

TREATMENT

The therapy is administration of amphotericin B.

Sporotrichosis

PATHOLOGY

Sporotrichum schenkii produces submiliary necrotic foci with an inflammatory cellular reaction in the myocardium; the organisms are both free and in macrophages.[77]

CLINICAL MANIFESTATIONS

Cardiac symptoms have not been described in disseminated ulcerating sporotrichosis.

TREATMENT

The disease is treated with amphotericin B and potassium iodide.

Coccidioidomycosis

PATHOLOGY

Gross and microscopic myocardial lesions have been described in cases of disseminated coccidioidomycosis. *Coccidioides immitis* spherules are in the necrotic center of miliary granulomatous myocardial lesions; there are surrounding mononuclear and giant cells. A nonspecific myocarditis with myofiber degeneration and an inflammatory cell interstitial infiltrate has also been reported.[78]

CLINICAL MANIFESTATIONS

The occasional cardiac symptoms are usually attributed to associated pericarditis; constrictive pericarditis may be a late complication.

TREATMENT

The drug of choice is amphotericin B.

Cryptococcosis

PATHOLOGY

Cryptococcus neoformans is identified in multiple myocardial granulomas (Fig. 80-11).

FIGURE 80-11 Cryptococcus neoformans myocarditis. There is a clump of *C. neoformans* between the muscle fibers, some of which show atrophy or complete replacement (×320).

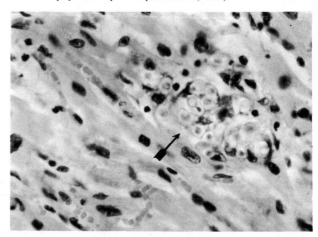

CLINICAL MANIFESTATIONS

Ventricular tachycardia, congestive heart failure, and sudden death were described in a 31-year-old man with cryptococcosis of the heart.[79] Electrocardiographic changes included P-Q and QRS prolongation.

TREATMENT

Administration of amphotericin B with 5-fluorocytosine is the treatment of choice.

PROTOZOAL MYOCARDITIS

Trypanosomiasis (Chagas' disease)

In an endemic area for *Trypanosoma cruzi,* the young patient with acquired myocardiopathy, arrhythmia, and a right bundle branch block electrocardiographic pattern probably has chronic Chagas' disease.[80] Indeed, chronic Chagas' disease is the most common form of heart disease in some areas of South America, affecting an estimated 7 million persons.[81]

The highest incidence of chronic Chagas' disease is in the third and fourth decades of life; there is a preponderance of cases in males from rural areas.[81]

ETIOLOGY AND EPIDEMIOLOGY

The reservoirs and transmitting vectors for Chagas' disease are triatomes infected with *T. cruzi,* found mainly in the tropical and subtropical Americas, but also encountered in the southwestern United States. Chagas' disease has also been transmitted by blood transfusion.[81a] The trypanosomes assume a leishmanial form in the myocardial fiber, where they multiply by binary fission; no myocardial inflammatory response occurs until the myofiber ruptures.

ACUTE CHAGAS' DISEASE

Pathology Postmortem examination during the acute illness in the rare patient who dies shows diffuse myocardial degeneration, *T. cruzi* in the myofibers, interstitial mononuclear cell and connective tissue proliferation, and endocardial mural thrombus formation.

Clinical manifestations Acute Chagas' disease, most common in early childhood, is characteristically asymptomatic and unrecognized. Patients with chronic Chagas' disease often deny a prior acute illness. Fever, sweating, muscular pain, diarrhea, and vomiting occur. Some patients also develop tachycardia, cardiomegaly, congestive heart failure, or nonspecific electrocardiographic changes, but arrhythmias are notably absent. Recovery from the acute myocarditis, with subsidence of cardiac manifestations, usually occurs within a few months, and the patient appears well for the ensuing 10 to 20 years. However, some fatalities occur with acute Chagas' disease from heart failure and/or meningoencephalitis.

Laboratory examination Diagnosis can be confirmed by a positive xenodiagnostic study, and complement-fixation tests are usually positive after 6 weeks.

Treatment We have observed a patient with laboratory-acquired acute Chagas' disease. Although she had recovered from the acute illness before diagnosis and without therapy, a course of treatment with the investigational drug Bayer 2502 was given; it is hoped that this drug can prevent the chronic manifestations of Chagas' disease by destroying intracellular trypanosomes.* An 8-aminoquinoline derivative (349 C59) may also be effective.[5]

CHRONIC CHAGAS' DISEASE

Myocardial involvement is the hallmark of chronic Chagas' disease. The clinical diagnosis of chronic *T. cruzi* disease depends on recognition of the chronic heart disease which occurs in about 50 percent of patients. The predominant cardiac manifestations of chronic Chagas' disease, particularly the arrhythmias, were emphasized by Chagas in his original description of the illness in 1910.

Pathology Pathologic descriptions[82] of chronic Chagas' myocarditis emphasize the mild cardiac muscle destruction as compared with the severe autonomic ganglion, cardiac nerve, and conduction system inflammation and degeneration; this reflects the neurotoxic properties of *T. cruzi.* The cardiac chambers are hypertrophied; diffuse interstitial myocardial fibrosis and mononuclear cell infiltrates are most prominent in the region of the sinoatrial node, the AV node, the bundle of His, and the subepicardial ganglions. Leishmanial forms of *T. cruzi* are found in degenerated myocardial fibers, especially in the right atrial wall (Fig. 80-12). Endocardial mural thrombosis often results in pulmonary embolization. Ventricular aneurysm has been described.[81a]

A circulating antibody (EVI), which appears to have high clinical specificity, can be demonstrated by immunofluorescent techniques to react with endocardium, vascular structures, and interstitium of striated muscle in 95 percent of patients with Chagas' heart disease and in 45 percent of asymptomatic individuals with *T. cruzi* infection.[83]

Clinical manifestations The clinical picture of chronic Chagas' myocarditis is one of insidious, progressive, prolonged congestive heart failure and cardiac enlargement. Mitral and tricuspid insufficiency usually become evident and pulmonary embolization is common. Precordial pain may be present. Fixed splitting of the second heart sound due to right bundle branch block is frequent. The almost invariable arrhythmias make syncope and sudden death common, in patients both with and without conges-

*Drug supplied by Dr. Myron G. Schultz, Center for Disease Control, Altanta, Ga.

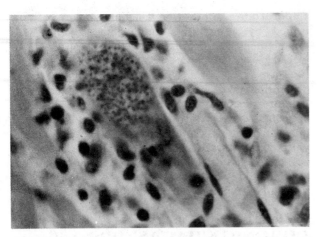

FIGURE 80-12 Note the *Trypanosoma cruzi* in its leishmanial state parasitizing the sarcoplasm of the myocardial cell. The surrounding fiber edema and acute inflammatory reaction are indicative of rupture of the myocardial cell (×125 Hematoxylin and eosin). *(Courtesy of Dr. M. Gravanis.)*

tive heart failure. Complete heart block, premature ventricular beats, and atrial fibrillation have a grave prognostic significance.

Laboratory examination Confirmatory laboratory evidence includes a positive Machado-Guerreiro complement-fixation reaction and a positive xenodiagnostic study.

Electrocardiographic abnormalities occur in 87 percent of patients with chronic Chagas' disease and are often the initial manifestation of illness. Right bundle branch block, with a superiorly oriented ÂQRS, is the most common electrocardiographic abnormality and occurs in over 50 percent of patients. Arrhythmias, atrioventricular block, conduction defects, and abnormalities of the P and T waves are common.

Arrhythmias, especially ventricular extrasystoles, may be provoked by effort; the appearance of ventricular premature beats on the exercise electrocardiogram in Chagas' myocarditis has a diagnostic value similar to ST-segment displacement in coronary atherosclerotic heart disease.

Treatment The use of propranolol or other antiarrhythmic agents in combination with ventricular demand pacing appears beneficial for the many patients who have both life-threatening ventricular tachyarrhythmias and episodes of high-degree atrioventricular block. Preliminary reports suggest that Cd-412 (Peruvoside) may be preferable to digitalis in treating the heart failure of Chagas' myocarditis; this cardiac glycoside appears to increase inotropism with little increase in myocardial excitability or atrioventricular conduction prolongation. There is no known specific therapy; preventative measures involve vector control.

Sleeping sickness (trypanosomiasis)

Severe central nervous system disease and relatively asymptomatic cardiac lesions characterize *Trypanosoma rhodesiese* and *T. Gambiense* infections, the former being more severe.

PATHOLOGY

The myocardial lesion in sleeping sickness is an interstitial and perivascular mononuclear cell infiltrate with interstitial hemorrhage, myocardial edema, and myofiber degeneration. The acute inflammatory myocarditis may be a predecessor of chronic myocardial fibrosis.

In addition to the myocarditis, there may be involvement of the endocardium, epicardium, heart valves, conducting system, and sympathetic cardiac ganglia; possible relationship to endomyocardial fibrosis is suggested.[84]

CLINICAL MANIFESTATIONS

The disease is more common in the male. Occasional patients with *T. rhodesiense* infection may have pulmonary edema or severe congestive heart failure, cardiac enlargement, and pericardial effusion. The anemia may contribute to the severity of the heart failure.

LABORATORY EXAMINATION

Electrocardiographic abnormalities occur in one-third to one-half of cases; these are most pronounced early in the disease, before therapy is instituted, and in the sicker patients. Electrocardiographic abnormalities include bradycardia, atrioventricular and bundle branch block, decreased QRS voltage, Q-T interval prolongation, premature ventricular beats, and T-wave changes.[85] Diagnosis can be made by trypanosome isolation from spinal fluid.

TREATMENT

Dramatic response to tryparsamide and Mel B has been reported, although occasional Herxheimer-like reactions may be fatal. The value of corticosteroid hormones remains questionable.[86] Both pentamidine and suramin sodium provide effective chemoprophylaxis.

Toxoplasmosis

PATHOLOGY

In both congenital and acquired toxoplasmosis, hematogenously disseminated *Toxoplasma gondii* invade the myocardial cell without causing myofiber destruction or an inflammatory reaction. The protozoa divide by binary fission and fill the myofiber with a basophilic mass of organisms. When the parasitized cell ruptures, a focal mononuclear cell inflammatory reaction to the liberated organisms occurs, associated with myofiber necrosis.

Almost constant microscopic myocardial involvement is described in toxoplasmosis; this is often without clinical evidence of cardiac disease.

CLINICAL MANIFESTATIONS

Major manifestations include fever, weakness, and evidence of cerebral involvement. The patient with toxoplasmosis myocarditis may have cardiac enlargement, heart failure, pericarditis with effusion, hypotension, arrhythmias, and Stokes-Adams syncope;[87] complete recovery from toxoplasma myocarditis is unusual.[88] The pericarditis may progress to constriction.

The almost invariable tachycardia in adults with acute toxoplasmosis may represent an otherwise inapparent myocarditis.

LABORATORY EXAMINATION

Frequent nonspecific electrocardiographic abnormalities, usually ST-T changes and conduction disturbances, have been noted in toxoplasma infections,[88] often in the absence of other clinical evidence of myocarditis. Diagnosis is by a dye test or complement-fixation test for toxoplasmosis.

TREATMENT

Recommended therapy includes use of pyrimethamine and sulfonamides. Corticosteroid hormones do not appear helpful.

Malaria

PATHOLOGY

Myocardial vessel distension and occlusion with malarial parasites and parasitized red blood cells are very frequent in falciparum malaria; there is pronounced interstitial edema and a moderate mononuclear cell infiltrate, without associated muscle necrosis or fibrosis.

Herrera[89] reported a case of *Plasmodium vivax* malaria in an 8-year-old boy who died of congestive heart failure; he described coronary vascular occlusions with numerous myocardial microinfarctions and suggested that combined vascular and parenchymal lesions may result in permanent cardiac damage from malaria.

Fatty myocardial degeneration and the deposition and phagocytosis of pigment are common in malaria, the latter presumably secondary to the hemolytic anemia.

CLINICAL MANIFESTATIONS

Cardiovascular complications, other than peripheral circulatory collapse, are rare in the patient with acute malignant tertian malaria *(Plasmodium falciparum)*, despite the extensive pathologic changes observed at postmortem examination. There is little evidence that malaria results in chronic heart disease.

Angina pectoris may occur from coronary arteriolar and capillary occlusion by malarial parasites and parasitized red blood cells. This may explain the ST-T electrocardiographic changes during the acute illness.

TREATMENT

Chloroquine and primaquine should be administered for the treatment of vivax and chloroquine-sensitive falciparum malaria. Choroquine-resistant falciparum malaria should be treated with quinine, pyrimethamine, and sulfadiazine.

Leishmaniasis

PATHOLOGY

Clasmatocytes in the myocardium are heavily laden with Leishman-Donovan bodies; muscle cell fragmentation and mononuclear cell infiltrates are the pathologic lesions presumed responsible for the occasional symptoms. These occur only in the visceral form of the kala-azar.

CLINICAL MANIFESTATIONS

Minor cardiac symptoms and signs due to *Leishmania donovani* occur only in the visceral form of kala-azar. They include occasional congestive heart failure and electrocardiographic abnormalities.[90]

TREATMENT

The treatment is administration of stibogluconate sodium.

Balantidiasis

PATHOLOGY

A granulomatous myocarditis with muscle atrophy has been described; degenerated forms of *Balantidium coli* were found in the small myocardial arteries, and an intact protozoan was identified in the myocardium.

CLINICAL MANIFESTATIONS

Balantidiasis is generally an intestinal infestation, but a case of *B. coli* myocarditis, with death from cardiac failure, was reported.[91]

TREATMENT

Oxytetracycline is the drug of choice; Diodoquin is also effective therapy.

Sarcosporidiosis

PATHOLOGY

Sarcosporidia characteristically invade cardiac and peripheral muscles; the infestations are incidental findings at microscopic tissue examination.[92] Sarcocysts have also been described in Purkinje tissue. Each sarcocyst within a muscle fiber contains several hundred basophilic bodies; the involved myocardial fiber is larger than adjacent fibers.

Sarcosporidiosis is differentiated from toxoplasmosis by the large number of parasites within each cyst, by the lack of myocardial degenerative or inflammatory reaction to the protozoan, and by the exclusive localization of Sarcosporidia in muscle.

CLINICAL MANIFESTATIONS

There is no clinical evidence of cardiac disease.

Amebiasis

PATHOLOGY

Amebic microabscesses may occur in the myocardium, or there may be a diffuse or focal myocarditis. Amebic abscesses have also involved the pericardium.

CLINICAL MANIFESTATIONS

Angina pectoris, Stokes-Adams syncope, pericarditis, and pericardial effusion have been described as evidence of amebic myocarditis. Electrocardiographic abnormalities include complete heart block and ST-T changes.[93]

TREATMENT

Therapy consists of metronidazole or emetine.

HELMINTHIC MYOCARDITIS

Trichinosis

Trichinosis is the most prevalent helminthic infestation of human beings; the most frequent and serious complication is myocarditis, which accounts for the preponderance of trichinosis fatalities.

PATHOLOGY

Circulating *Trichinella spiralis* larvae invade the heart in the acute phase of trichinosis, but never encyst in the myocardium; parasites are not present in the myocardium after the second week of illness and are presumed to have been destroyed or returned to the circulation. A focal acute myocarditis, involving both the parenchyma and interstitial tissue, begins after the second week of illness and attains its maximum severity in the fourth to eighth week. The myocarditis has been postulated to be a nonspecific inflammatory manifestation of larval invasion of the myocardium, a reaction to the death of the parasite, or a hypersensitivity or toxic response to *T. spiralis*. Focal areas of muscle necrosis occasionally contain parasites; the interstitial connective tissue is diffusely infiltrated with eosinophils and inflammatory cells.[94]

CLINICAL MANIFESTATIONS

The diagnosis of trichinosis should be considered in any patient with periorbital edema, eosinophilia, and marked muscle tenderness, even without a history of pork ingestion. Cardiac complications of trichinosis appear in the second or third week of illness, when systemic symptoms are abating.[95] Then, concomitant with cerebral involvement, the cardiac manifestations become maximal in the fourth to eighth week and subsequently subside. There may be dyspnea,

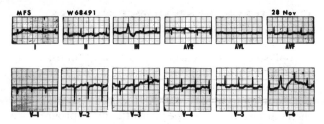

FIGURE 80-13 Trichinosis myocarditis. The electrocardiographic abnormalities include sinus tachycardia, premature ventricular beats, Q-T interval prolongation, and nonspecific ST-T alteration.

cardiac enlargement, substernal pain, arrhythmia, tachycardia, and congestive heart failure, at times mimicking the presentation of myocardial infarction.

Recovery is the rule in trichinosis myocarditis, and residual chronic heart disease is unusual.

LABORATORY EXAMINATION

Eosinophilia is characteristic. Skeletal muscle biopsy may be diagnostic.

Transient electrocardiographic abnormalities occur in about one-third of patients with trichinosis, often without cardiac symptoms; they are presumed due to the toxic, metabolic, or hypersensitivity response to *T. spiralis*, as the larvae do not encyst in the heart.[95] The electrocardiographic changes parallel the other evidence of myocarditis; they appear in the second or third week of illness, are most pronounced at about the sixth week, and then gradually disappear. Nonspecific T-wave changes are the most common electrocardiographic abnormality, with decreased QRS voltage, premature ventricular beats, and altered conduction also observed (Fig. 80-13). The electrocardiogram may mimic that of myocardial infarction.[96]

TREATMENT

Corticosteroid hormone therapy diminishes the inflammatory response in trichinosis myocarditis and produces striking clinical improvement. Thiabendazole is effective therapy.[97] Proper cooking of pork and pork products can virtually eliminate human trichinosis.

Echinococcosis (hydatidosis)

Cardiovascular manifestations constitute an important, though rare, complication of echinococcosis. Cardiac echinococcosis, first described by Dévé, is most frequently encountered in sheep-raising areas: Uruguay, Australia, New Zealand, and the Mediterranean countries. Hydatidosis is predominantly a hepatic-pulmonary disease, with 0.5 to 2 percent cardiac involvment. Most cases occur in the second to fifth decade of life, and men are more commonly affected.[98]

PATHOLOGY

Taenia echinococcus hexacanth embryos are generally believed to invade the myocardium via the coronary circulation, although lymphatic spread has recently been proposed. Left ventricular involvement has been described as most common and is attributed to the richer left ventricular coronary artery supply. Another series reported slightly more frequent right ventricular echinococcal involvement; this was explained as the result of a more direct entrance of blood into the right coronary artery. Di Bello[99] categorizes 50 percent of cysts as localized in the free wall of the left ventricle and 20 percent in the interventricular septum. The echinococcus hexacanth forms a pseudocyst in the myocardium which may produce surrounding muscle ischemia from compression, may interfere with heart valve function, or may interfere with conduction. Primary echinococcus cysts are always solitary and vary from pea size to grapefruit size. Myocardial density, particularly in the ventricles, limits cyst growth and favors the formation of daughter cysts. The cyst may rupture into a cardiac chamber or into the pericardium, depending on its location and the direction of least resistance.

CLINICAL MANIFESTATIONS

Although uncomplicated cardiac hydatid disease is characteristically silent and latent, the patient may have chest pain, palpitations, tachycardia, murmurs, congestive heart failure, Stokes-Adams syncope, or sudden death. In an endemic area, the diagnosis of cardiac echinococcosis should be suggested by the presence of echinococcus cysts elsewhere in the body, a positive intradermal reaction, history of an anaphylactic shock syndrome, and a peculiar cardiac murmur which may be due to obstruction of blood flow by a large cyst.[100]

Cardiac findings prior to cyst rupture may be related to pericarditis, valve obstruction, atrioventricular conduction abnormalities, or coronary insufficiency, depending on the size and location of the cyst.

Echinococcal cyst rupture is often evident as anaphylaxis due to sensitization to hydatid protein. The first symptoms of intracardiac rupture of the cyst may be due to pulmonary or cerebral embolization of daughter cysts. There may be acute pericarditis with tamponade.[101]

Sudden death has been reported from both pulmonary and cerebral embolism. Late complications occur from secondary pericardial echinococcosis (which may produce constrictive disease) or from metastatic echinococcosis.

LABORATORY EXAMINATION

Eosinophilia is common. The Casoni test is positive, as is the complement-fixation titer. A bizarre and often calcified cardiac shadow is seen on the chest roentgenogram.

A large myocardial echinococcus cyst may compress the surrounding heart muscle and cause ischemia; indeed, electrocardiographic ST-T ischemic changes, particularly in the precordial leads, may localize an echinococcal cyst prior to surgery. Occasional P-wave changes have been reported with atrial cysts, and atrioventricular block has been documented with septal cysts. Arrhythmias and conduction abnormalities are not unusual. The electrocardiogra-

phic abnormalities may be reversible following excision of a cardiac echinococcal cyst.

Angiocardiographic examination delineates the cyst and confirms the diagnosis;[98] coronary arteriography may aid in localization of the cyst. Recently, a hydatid cyst in the interventricular septum has been diagnosed echocardiographically.[101a]

TREATMENT

The diagnosis of cardiac hydatid disease should be made in the uncomplicated stage of the illness, prior to cyst rupture. Surgical excision of the echinococcal cyst is indicated in the asymptomatic patient, before rupture[98] into the pericardial cavity or into a cardiac chamber; this permits curative surgery.

The first successful surgical excision of a cardiac echinococcus cyst was in 1932; successful surgical treatment by both the closed and the open techniques is reported with increasing frequency.

Schistosomiasis

PATHOLOGY

Schistosoma japonicum ova and, less commonly, ova of *S. haematobium* and *S. mansoni* may localize in the myocardium. The pathologic lesion, usually an incidental finding at postmortem examination, is a microscopic pseudotubercle or granuloma[102] with an individual ovum at the center. In one report of a fatal case of *S. haematobium* myocarditis, the myocardial lesion was thought to represent an allergic response to the parasite.

CLINICAL MANIFESTATIONS

Cardiac manifestations of schistosomiasis are most commonly those of cor pulmonale, secondary to pulmonary schistosomiasis; primary symptomatic myocardial schistosomiasis is rare.[103]

LABORATORY EXAMINATION

Electrocardiographic abnormalities are common but may be due to an actual schistosomal myocarditis, to the drug therapy, to the anemia, to the frequently associated chronic renal disease and hypertension, or they may represent a hypersensitivity response.[104]

TREATMENT

Treatment includes use of potassium antimony tartrate for *S. japonicum,* and miridazole for *S. mansoni* and *S. haematobium.*

Ascariasis

PATHOLOGY

The larvae of *Ascaris lumbricoides* invade the myocardium via a coronary artery. A verminous myocardial abscess has been described in a 27-month-old child; an ascaris larva, coiled in the left ventricular muscle, was surrounded by an extensive, necrotizing inflammatory process. Ferreira's[105] description of a fertilized ascaris ovum in the left ventricular myocardium suggested an embolic origin.

CLINICAL MANIFESTATIONS
Rare instances of sudden death have occurred.

TREATMENT
Mebendazole or pyrantel pamoate is the treatment of choice. The therapeutic efficacy of corticosteroid hormones is uncertain.

Heterophyidiasis

PATHOLOGY
In patients with intestinal heterophyidiasis, the ova of various trematodes enter the general circulation and may lodge in the heart. There may be myocardial infiltrates and occlusion of small capillaries by heterophyid ova. The right ventricle was prominently involved with interstitial edema and muscle fiber fragmentation in one reported case. Heterophyid ova were found between the myofibers. Thickening and calcification of the mitral valve have also been described.[106]

CLINICAL MANIFESTATIONS
Cardiac enlargement, arrhythmia, and congestive heart failure have been reported.

TREATMENT
The therapy is use of tetrachlorethylene.

Filariasis

PATHOLOGY
Pericardial effusion, myocardial sclerosis with interstitial fibrosis and cellular infiltrates, restrictive endocardial fibrosis, and mural thrombi may be seen at postmortem examination. Filarial larvae may be identified on histopathologic examination.

CLINICAL MANIFESTATIONS
In an endemic area for filariasis, unexplained congestive heart failure in a patient with eosinophilia should suggest filarial myocarditis.[107] Cardiomegaly and predominant right-sided cardiac failure have resulted from *Loa loa* infestation.

LABORATORY EXAMINATION
The electrocardiographic abnormalities include conduction defects, arrhythmias, and low QRS voltage.

Severe restrictive filarial endocarditis has been demonstrated at cardiac catheterization; this persisted after the congestive heart failure, conduction abnormalities, and systemic allergic manifestations were controlled by corticosteroid therapy.

TREATMENT
Tatibouet[108] described a patient with *Loa loa* cardiomyopathy in whom severe congestive heart failure was not improved by digitalis and diuretic therapy;

treatment with corticosteroid hormones, presumably by suppressing the inflammatory response, effected a complete clinical remission. He suggested that the restrictive endocardial fibrosis, which mimics Loeffler's endocarditis, is an allergic reaction to the filarial parasite.

Diethylcarbamazine appears to be effective against filariasis.

Paragonimiasis

PATHOLOGY
Cardiac infestation, without cardiac symptoms, has been described in disseminated visceral infection with *Paragonimus westermani;* adult trematodes were noted at microscopic examination of the myocardium.[109]

TREATMENT
Bithionol therapy has been suggested.

Strongyloidiasis

PATHOLOGY
On microscopic examination of the myocardium, in a case of cardiac *Strongyloides* infestation, scattered filariform larvae were surrounded by lymphocytes in the interstitial tissues; cardiac muscle fibers were not involved.

LABORATORY EXAMINATION
Strongyloides stercoralis infestation of the heart, without cardiac symptoms, has been manifest[110] by nonspecific T-wave electrocardiographic abnormalities.

TREATMENT
Thiabendazole has been reported effective against human strongyloidiasis.

Cysticercosis

PATHOLOGY
Generalized infection with *Taenia solium* may involve the heart. The exudative tissue reaction to *Cysticercus cellulosae* results in fibrous encapsulation of the cyst; the parasite may eventually be resorbed, or the cyst may calcify.

CLINICAL MANIFESTATIONS
Multiple scolex-containing cysts produce no myocardial damage, and there are usually no cardiac symptoms;[111] however, congestive heart failure has been described and nonspecific P- and T-wave changes recorded.

Visceral larva migrans

PATHOLOGY
In a rare fatal case, there was generalized allergic granulomatosis; the scattered myocardial nodules had central fibrinous necrosis and surrounding epithelioid cells, giant cells, and eosinophils; the myocardial fibers were intact. A similar pathologic picture was encountered in another autopsy study which

also demonstrated fragments of the larval parasite in the granulomatous lesion. Extensive interstitial mononuclear cell infiltrates have been reported.[112]

CLINICAL MANIFESTATIONS

Patients almost invariably recover from *Toxocara canis* infestation, and there is rarely clinical evidence of cardiac disease. Congestive heart failure has been described.

TREATMENT

A case of severe recurrent myocarditis with recovery was described in a child with visceral larva migrans; cortisone therapy resulted in clinical improvement. Thiabendazole may be of value.

GENERAL COMMENTS REGARDING THE TREATMENT OF MYOCARDITIS*

The medical management of the patient with infectious myocarditis includes (1) specific therapy for the underlying infection, (2) general measures, designed primarily to decrease cardiac work, and (3) control of the complications of myocarditis: congestive heart failure, arrhythmias, and thromboembolism.

Restriction of physical activity reduces the work of the heart and is designed to decrease residual myocardial damage and promote healing. This is the only measure directed specifically at the myocarditis, as the value of drugs which suppress inflammation and/or autoimmune response remains controversial. Corticosteroid hormones appear relatively contraindicated in infectious myocarditis, particularly myocarditis of viral etiology, as suppression of systemic defense mechanisms may permit dissemination of the infection. In general the use of corticosteroid hormones appears justified only in patients with intractable heart failure, severe life-threatening arrhythmias, or severe systemic toxicity.

A regimen of modified bed rest is of the utmost importance, with the caloric requirements of a particular physical activity guiding its permission or restriction. For example, the use of a bedside commode requires less work than the use of a bedpan; and sitting in a chair may require less cardiac work than being recumbent in bed. Furthermore, the patient with considerable dyspnea may be more comfortable sitting in a chair than recumbent in bed. A passive or mild active supervised physical activity program of low-level caloric expenditure will help prevent atrophy of the muscle mass and will help decrease venous stasis and the propensity to thromboembolism.

The use of hyperbaric oxygen acutely or on a long-term basis remains experimental. Similarly, the rationale for, and the results of, the administration of polarizing solutions (glucose, insulin, and potassium) are debatable.

Control of congestive heart failure involves the reduction of systemic tissue oxygen requirements by restriction of activity, the augmentation of myocardial contractility by the administration of digitalis, and the diminution of fluid retention by sodium restriction and the use of diuretic agents. The role of preload and afterload reducing agents is under active investigation. Administration of oxygen has been described as of value in patients with congestive heart failure from acute myocarditis, but adequate data are lacking. Digitalis in doses somewhat greater than the average recommended amount may be necessary to control the congestive heart failure; patients receiving such dosages should be carefully observed for digitalis toxicity. Paradoxically, some patients with acute myocarditis seem unusually sensitive to the usual doses of digitalis. Variables determining digitalis dosage include electrolyte levels, cardiac rhythm, the severity of any associated hepatic and/or renal disease, and possibly the adequacy of myocardial oxygenation. At times, digitalis cannot completely reverse the myocardial failure in patients with acute myocarditis, particularly in the presence of very severe disease, associated anemia, arrhythmias, or pulmonary embolization. Specific therapy to combat the infection may be required before the congestive heart failure can be controlled.

In those varieties of acute myocarditis characterized by frequent arrhythmias, continuous monitoring for disturbances of cardiac rhythm is recommended. An intensive care unit, where personnel and equipment for cardiac resuscitation, cardiac defibrillation, and cardiac pacing are readily available, provides optimal care. Arrhythmias should be detected and treated early, before cardiac disturbances become life-threatening. The antiarrhythmic drugs—quinidine, procainamide, propranolol—concomitantly depress myocardial contractility and must be used with caution in the patient with myocarditis.

Anticoagulant therapy is indicated in patients with systemic or pulmonary embolization.

Intractable cardiac failure in a patient with acute myocarditis may, in time, prove an indication for temporary partial or total cardiopulmonary bypass; an external or implanted mechanical device may assist the circulation until the myocardium has recovered from the acute insult.

The early diagnosis of infectious disease and institution of appropriate chemotherapy may decrease the incidence of infectious myocarditis; the major preventive role of vaccination and immunization against infectious diseases deserves emphasis.

REFERENCES

1 Corvisart, J. N.: Essai sur les Maladies et les Lésions Organiques du Coeur, Paris, 1806, English translation by Jacob Gates, MMSS, 1812, pp. 182–189 and 299–303.

1a Woodward, T. E., Togo, Y., Lee, Y.-C, and Hornick, R. B.: Specific Microbial Infections of the Myocardium and Pericardium. A Study of 82 Patients, *Arch. Intern. Med.*, 120:270, 1967.

*With appreciation to Dr. Jonas A. Shulman, Professor of Medicine (Infectious Diseases), Emory University School of Medicine, for reviewing drug therapy.

2 Pankey, G. A.: Effect of Viruses on the Cardiovascular System, *Am. J. Med. Sci.*, 250:103, 1965.

3 Ledbetter, M. K., Cannon, A. B., II, and Costa, A. F.: The Electrocardiogram in Diphtheritic Myocarditis, *Am. Heart J.*, 68:599, 1964.

4 Morales, A. R., Vichitbhandha, P., Chandruang, P., Evans, H., and Bourgeois, C. H.: Pathologic Features of Cardiac Conduction Disturbances in Diphtheritic Myocarditis, *Arch. Pathol.*, 91:1, 1971.

5 Harris, L. C., and Nghiem, Q. X.: Cardiomyopathies in Infants and Children, *Prog. Cardiovasc. Dis.*, 15:255, 1972.

6 Matisonn, R. E., Mitha, A. S., and Chesler, E.: Successful Electrical Pacing for Complete Heart Block Complicating Diphtheritic Myocarditis, *Br. Heart J.*, 38:423, 1976.

7 Gallez, A., and Bernard, R.: La Myocardite Diphtérique: Utilisation de L'entrainement Électrosystolique Témporaire dans un Cas Compliqué de Bloc Auriculo-ventriculaire Complet, *Acta Cardiol.*, 26:88, 1971.

8 Kinare, S. G., and Deshmukh, M. M.: Complete Atrioventricular Block Due to Myocardial Tuberculosis, *Arch. Pathol.*, 88:684, 1969.

9 Rawls, W. J., Shuford, W. H., Logan, W. D., Hurst, J. W., and Schlant, R. C.: Right Ventricular Outflow Tract Obstruction Produced by a Myocardial Abscess in a Patient with Tuberculosis, *Am. J. Cardiol.*, 21:738, 1968.

10 Claiborne, T. S.: Caseating Granulomas of the Heart, *Am. J. Cardiol.*, 33:920, 1974.

11 Shilkin, K. B.: *Salmonella typhimurium* Pancarditis, *Postgrad. Med. J.*, 45:40, 1969.

12 Langaker, O. M., and Svanes, K.: Myocardial Abscess Due to *Salmonella typhimurium*, *Br. Heart J.*, 35:871, 1973.

13 Bertrand, E., Barabe, P., and Assamoi, M. O.: La Myocardite Typhoïdique, *Coeur Med. Intern.*, 10:213, 1971.

14 Laha, P. N.: Typhoid Myocarditis, *J. Assoc. Physicians India*, (editorial), 22:279, 1974.

15 Diem, L. V., and Arnold, K.: Typhoid Fever with Myocarditis, *Am. J. Trop. Med. Hyg.*, 23:218, 1974.

16 Brody, H., and Smith, L. W.: The Visceral Pathology in Scarlet Fever and Related Streptococcus Infections, *Am. J. Pathol.*, 12:373, 1936.

17 Robboy, S. J.: Atrioventricular-Node Inflammation: Mechanism of Sudden Death in Protracted Meningicoccemia, *N. Engl. J. Med.*, 286:1091, 1972.

18 Denmark, T. C., and Knight, E. L.: Cardiovascular and Coagulation Complications of Group C Meningococcal Disease, *Arch. Intern. Med.*, 127:238, 1971.

19 Saphir, O.: Myocardial Lesions in Subacute Bacterial Endocarditis, *Am. J. Pathol.*, 11:143, 1935.

20 Wang, K., Gobel, F., Gleason, D. F., and Edwards, J. E.: Complete Heart Block Complicating Baterial Endocarditis, *Circulation*, 46:939, 1972.

20a Guneratne, F.: Gas Gangrene (Abcess) of Heart, *N.Y. State J. Med.*, 75:1766, 1975.

21 Buczyńska-Hencner, S.: Three Cases of Myocarditis in the Course of Brucellosis, *Pol. Tyg. Lek.*, 20:761, 1966.

22 Murphy, K. J.: Fatal Tetanus with Brain-Stem Involvement and Myocarditis in an Ex-Serviceman, *Med. J. Aust.*, 2:542, 1970.

23 Baumann, B. B., and Morita, E. T.: Systemic Meliodosis Presenting as Myocardial Infarct, *Ann. Intern. Med.*, 67:836, 1967.

24 Gore, I., and Saphir, O.: Myocarditis Associated with Acute Nasopharyngitis and Acute Tonsillitis, *Am. Heart J.*, 34:831, 1947.

25 Boss, J. H., Leffkowitz, M., and Freud, M.: Unusual Manifestations of Syphilitic Cardiovascular Disease, *Ann. Intern. Med.*, 55:824, 1961.

26 Soscia, J. L., Fusco, J. M., and Grace, W. J.: Complete Heart Block Due to a Solitary Gumma, *Am. J. Cardiol.*, 13:553, 1964.

27 Nusynowitz, M. L.: Myocarditis and Heart Failure Due to *Leptospira pomona*, *Hawaii Med. J.*, 23:41, 1963.

28 Ch'i, L., Ts'ai-li, M., Yun-chen, C., and Wei-ju, C.: Anicteric Leptospirosis. II. Observations on Electrocardiograms, *Chinese Med. J.*, 84:291, 1965.

29 Edwards, G. A., and Domm, B. M.: Human Leptospirosis, *Medicine*, 39:117, 1960.

30 Judge, D. M., Samuel, I., Perine, P. L., and Vukotic, D.: Louse-borne Relapsing Fever in Man., *Arch. Pathol.*, 97:136, 1974.

31 Martin, M., and Bezon, A.: Curable Acute Primary Carditis Due to *Rickettsia prowazeki*, *Presse Med.*, 68:1253, 1960.

32 Woodward, T. E., McCrumb, F. R., Jr., Carey, T. N., and Togo, Y.: Viral and Rickettsial Causes of Cardiac Disease, Including the Coxsackie Virus Etiology of Pericarditis and Myocarditis, *Ann. Intern. Med.*, 53:1130, 1960.

33 Hand, W. L., Miller, J. B., Reinarz, J. A., and Sanford, J. P.: Rocky Mountain Spotted Fever: A Vascular Disease, *Arch. Intern. Med.*, 125:879, 1970.

34 Mitchell, R., Grist, N. R., Bazaz, G., and Kenmuir, A. C. F.: Pathological, Rickettsiological and Immunofluorescence Studies of a Case of Q Fever Endocarditis, *J. Pathol. Bacteriol.*, 91:317, 1966.

35 Sheridan, P., MacCaig, J. N., and Hart, R. J. C.: Myocarditis Complicating Q Fever, *Br. Med. J.*, 2:155, 1974.

36 Barraclough, D., and Popert, A. J.: Q Fever Presenting with Paroxysmal Ventricular Tachycardia, *Br. Med. J.*, 2:423, 1975.

37 Lerner, A. M., Wilson, F. M., and Reyes, M. P.: Enteroviruses and the Heart (With Special Emphasis on the Probable Role of Coxsackie Viruses, Group B, Types 1–5), 1. Epidemiological and Experimental Studies, 2. Observations in Humans, *Mod. Concepts Cardiovasc. Dis.*, 44:7, 11, 1975.

37a Lewes, D.: Viral Myocarditis, *Practitioner*, 216:281, 1976.

38 Sanders, V.: Viral Myocarditis, *Am. Heart J.*, 66:707, 1963.

39 Burch, G. E., and Giles, T. D.: The Role of Viruses in the Production of Heart Disease, *Am. J. Cardiol.*, 29:231, 1972.

40 Hirschman, S. Z., and Hammer, G. S.: Coxsackie Virus Myopericarditis. A Microbiological and Clinical Review, *Am. J. Cardiol.*, 34:224, 1974.

41 Grist, N. R., and Bell, E. J.: Coxsackie Viruses and the Heart, *Am. Heart J.*, 77:295, 1969.

42 Smith, W. G.: Coxsackie B Myopericarditis in Adults, *Am. Heart J.*, 80:34, 1970.

42a Schilken, R. M., and Myers, M. G.: Complete Heart Block in Viral Myocarditis, *J. Pediatr.*, 87:831, 1975.

43 Bell, E. J., and Grist, N. R.: Echo Viruses, Carditis, and Acute Pleurodynia, *Am. Heart J.*, 82:133, 1971.

44 Lewes, D., Rainford, D. J., and Lane, W. F.: Symptomless Myocarditis and Myalgia in Viral and *Mycoplasma pneumoniae* Infections, *Br. Heart J.*, 36:924, 1974.

45 Drew, J. H.: Echo 11 Virus Outbreak in a Nursery Associated with Myocarditis, *Aust. Paediatr. J.*, 9:90, 1973.

46 Trimbos, J. B. M. J.: Electrocardiogram and Myocardium in Poliomyelitis, *Folia Med. Neerl.*, 1963, p. 49.

47 Verel, D., Warrack, A. J. N., Potter, C. W., Ward, C., and Rickards, D. F.: Observations on the A₂ England Influenza Epidemic: A Clinicopathological Study, *Am. Heart J.*, 92:290, 1976.

48 Coltman, C. A., Jr.: Influenza Myocarditis. Report of a Case with Observations on Serum Glutamic Oxaloacetic Transaminase, *JAMA*, 180:204, 1962.

49 Kussy, J. C.: Fatal Mumps Myocarditis, *Minn. Med.*, 57:285, 1974.

50 Roberts, W. C., and Fox, S. M., III: Mumps of the Heart, Clinical and Pathologic Features, *Circulation*, 32:342, 1965.

51 Miller, R., Ward, C., Amsterdam, E., Mason, D. T., and Zelis,

R.: Focal Mononucleosis Myocarditis Simulating Myocardial Infarction, *Chest,* 63:102, 1973.

52 Nikiforov, V. N., Malkova, T. N., and Barashkova, M. N.: Changes of the Cardiovascular System in Infectious Mononucleosis, *Klin. Med.,* 44:68, 1966.

52a Hudgins, J. M.: Infectious Mononucleosis Complicated by Myocarditis and Pericarditis, *JAMA,* 235:2626, 1976.

53 Bell, H.: Cardiac Manifestations of Viral Hepatitis, *JAMA,* 218:387, 1971.

54 Miller, A. B., and Waggoner, D. M.: Cardiac Disease, Hepatic Disease and Hepatitis B Antigen, *Ann. Intern. Med.,* 79:276, 1973.

55 Ainger, L. E.: Heart Disease in Congenital Rubella Syndrome, *Cardiol. Dig.,* 2:21, 1967.

56 Giustra, F. X., and Nilsson, D. C.: Myocarditis Following Measles: Report of a Case, *AMA J. Dis. Child.,* 79:487, 1950.

56a Roux, F., Bourgeade, A., Salaiin, J. J., Bondurand, A., Ette, M., and Bertrand, E.: L'Atteinte Cardiaque dans la Rage Humaine, *Coeur Med. Intern.,* 15:37, 1976.

57 Cheetham, H. D., Hart, J., Coghill, N. F., and Fox, B.: Rabies with Myocarditis. Two Cases in England, *Lancet,* 1:921, 1970.

58 Vassa, N. T., Yajnik, V. H., Shah, S. S., Doshi, H. V., Kothari, U. R., and Joshi, K. R.: Myocarditis in Rabies—Clinical and Electrocardiographic Study of 16 Cases, *J. Assoc. Physicians India,* 22:7, 1974.

59 Moore, L. M., Henry, J., Benzing, G., III, and Kaplan, S.: Varicella Myocarditis, *Am. J. Dis. Child.,* 118:899, 1969.

60 Rosner, P., Eichenberger, G., Ferrero, C., and Koralnik, O.: Bloc Auriculo-ventriculaire Complet par Myocardite a *Mycoplasma pneumoniae, Schweiz. Med. Wochenschr.,* 96:1343, 1966.

61 Thiede, W. H.: Cardiac Involvement in Lymphocytic Choriomeningitis, *Arch. Intern. Med.,* 109:104, 1962.

62 Sutton, G. C., Morrissey, R. A., Tobin, J. R., Jr., and Anderson, T. O.: Pericardial and Myocardial Disease Associated with Serological Evidence of Infection by Agents of the Psittacosis—Lymphogranuloma Venereum Group (Chlamydiaceae), *Circulation,* 36:830, 1967.

63 Dymock, I. W., Lawson, J. M., MacLennan, W. J., and Ross, C. A. C.: Myocarditis Associated with Psittacosis, *Br. J. Clin. Pract.,* 25:240, 1971.

64 Ungar, H.: Diffuse Interstitial Myocarditis in a Case of Epidemic Encephalitis, *Am. J. Clin. Pathol.,* 18:48, 1948.

65 Bell, R. W., and Murphy, W. M.: Myocarditis in Young Military Personnel: Herpes Simplex, Trichinosis, Meningococcemia, Carbon Tetrachloride, and Idiopathic Fibrous and Giant Cell Types, *Am. Heart J.,* 74:309, 1967.

66 Buttrick, D. D., and Roberts, L.: Generalized Cytomegalic Inclusion Disease: Report of Two Cases with Associated Fungal Infection, One Involving Aspergillosis, the Second with Candidiasis, *Am. J. Dis. Child.,* 110:319, 1965.

67 Wilson, R. S. E., Morris, T. H., and Rees, J. R.: Cytomegalovirus Myocarditis, *Br. Heart J.,* 34:865, 1972.

68 Henson, D., and Mufson, M. A.: Myocarditis and Pneumonitis with Type 21 Advenovirus Infection, *Am. J. Dis. Child.,* 121:334, 1971.

69 Nagaratnam, N., Siripala, K., and deSilva, N.: Arbovirus (Dengue Type) as a Cause of Acute Myocarditis and Pericarditis, *Br. Heart J.,* 35:204, 1973.

70 Obeyesekere, I., and Hermon, Y.: Arbovirus Heart Disease: Myocarditis and Cardiomyopathy Following Dengue and Chikungunya Fever—A Follow-up Study, *Am. Heart J.,* 85:186, 1973.

70a Gills, T. D., and Gohd, R. S.: Respiratory Syncthial Virus and Heart Disease. A Report of Two Cases, *JAMA,* 236:1128, 1976.

71 Edwards, A. C.: Actinomycosis in Children. A Review of the Literature and Report of Cases, *Am. J. Dis. Child.,* 41:1419, 1931.

72 Baker, R. D., and Brian, E. W.: Blastomycosis of the Heart: Report of Two Cases, *Am. J. Pathol.,* 13:139, 1937.

72a Franklin, W. G., Simon, A. B., and Sodeman, T. M.: Candida Myocarditis without Valvulitis, *Am. J. Cardiol.,* 38:924, 1976.

73 Brooks, S. E. H., and Young, E. G.: Clinicopathologic Observations on Systemic Moniliasis. A Case Report and Review of the Literature, *Arch. Pathol.,* 73:383, 1962.

74 Williams, A. H.: *Aspergillus* Myocarditis, *Am. J. Clin. Pathol.,* 61:247, 1974.

75 Cade, J. F.: Pulmonary Aspergillosis with Myocarditis, *Med. J. Aust.,* 1:581, 1966.

76 Owen, G. E., Scherr, S. N., and Segre, E. J.: Histoplasmosis Involving the Heart and Great Vessels, *Am. J. Med.,* 32:552, 1962.

77 Collins, W. T.: Disseminated Ulcerating Sporotrichosis with Widespread Visceral Involvement: Report of a Case, *Arch. Dermatol.,* 56:523, 1947.

78 Reingold, I. M.: Myocardial Lesions in Disseminated Coccidioidomycosis, *Am. J. Clin. Pathol.,* 20:1044, 1950.

79 Jones, I., Nassau, E., and Smith, P.: Cryptococcosis of the Heart, *Br. Heart J.,* 27:462, 1965.

80 Rosenbaum, M. B.: Chagasic Myocardiopathy, *Prog. Cardiovasc. Dis.,* 7:199, 1964.

81 Puigbó, J. J., Rhode, J. R. N., Barrios, H. G., Suárez, J. A., and Yépez, C. G.: Clinical and Epidemiological Study of Chronic Heart Involvement in Chagas' Disease, *Bull. WHO,* 34:655, 1966.

81a Aldama-Luebbert, A., Nasrallah, A. T., Garcia, E., and Hall, R. J.: Ventricular Aneurysm in Chagas' Myocardiopathy: Clinical, Epidemiologic, Angiographic Features, *Texas Med.,* 72:55, 1976.

82 Mott, K. E., and Hagstrom, J. W. C.: The Pathologic Lesions of the Cardiac Autonomic Nervous System in Chronic Chagas' Myocarditis, *Circulation,* 31:273, 1965.

83 Cossio, P. M., Laguens, R. P., Diez, C., Szarfman, A., Segal, A., and Arana, R. M.: Chagasic Cardiopathy. Antibodies Reacting with Plasma Membrane of Striated Muscle and Endothelial Cells, *Circulation,* 50:1252, 1974.

84 Poltera, A. A., Cox, J. N., and Owor, R.: Pancarditis Affecting the Conducting System and All Valves in Human African Trypanosomiasis, *Br. Heart J.,* 38:827, 1976.

85 Bertrand, E., Baudin, L., Vacher, P., Seutilhes, L., Ducasse, B., and Veyret, V.: L'Atteinte du Coeur dans 100 Cas de Trypanosomiase Africaine à Trypanosoma Gambiense, *Arch. Mal. Coeur,* 60:1520, 1967.

86 de Raadt, P., and Koten, J. W.: Myocarditis in *Rhodesiense* Trypanosomiasis, *East Afr. Med. J.,* 45:128, 1968.

87 Mary, A. S., and Hamilton, M.: Ventricular Tachycardia in a Patient with Toxoplasmosis, *Br. Heart J.,* 35:349, 1973.

88 Theologides, A., and Kennedy, B. J.: Toxoplasmic Myocarditis and Pericarditis, *Am. J. Med.,* 47:169, 1969.

89 Herrera, J. M.: Lesiones cardiacas en la Malaria Vivax: Estudio de un Caso con Daños Coronario y Miocárdico (Cardiac Lesions in Vivax Malaria: Study of a Case with Coronary and Myocardial Damage), *Arch. Inst. Cardiol. Méx.,* 30:26, 1960.

90 Benhamou, E., and Foures, R.: Le Coeur dans un Cas de Kala-azar Infantile, *Arch. Mal. Coeur,* 31:81, 1938.

91 Sidorov, P.: Un Cas de Balantidose chez l'Homme Suivi d'une Myocardite Granulomateuse, *Ann. Anat. Pathol.,* 12:711, 1935.

92 Arai, H. S.: Sarcosporidiosis in Two Cases with Trichinosis, *J. Mt. Sinai Hosp.,* 15:367, 1949.

93 Lyons, E.: Amoebiasis und das Kardiovaskularsystem, *Z. Kreislaufforsch.,* 50:698, 1961.

94 Barr, R.: Human Trichinosis: Report of Four Cases, with

Emphasis on Central Nervous System Involvement, and a Survey of 500 Consecutive Autopsies at the Ottawa Civic Hospital, *Can. Med. Assoc. J.,* 95:912, 1966.

95 Gray, D. F., Morse, B. S., and Phillips, W. F.: Trichinosis with Neurologic and Cardiac Involvement: Review of the Literature and Report of Three Cases, *Ann. Intern. Med.,* 57:230, 1962.

96 Kirschberg, G. J.: Trichinosis Presenting as Acute Myocardial Infarction, *Can. Med. Assoc. J.,* 106:898, 1972.

97 Stone, O. J., Stone, C. T., Jr., and Mullins, J. F.: Thiabendazole—Probable Cure for Trichinosis, *JAMA,* 187: 536, 1964.

98 Murphy, T. E., Kean, B. H., Venturini, A., and Lillehei, C. W.: Echinococcus Cyst of the Left Ventricle: Report of a Case with Review of the Pertinent Literature, *J. Thorac. Cardiovasc. Surg.,* 61:443, 1971.

99 Di Bello, R., Urioste, H. A., and Rubio, R.: Hydatid Cysts of the Ventricular Septum of the Heart: A Study Based on Two Personal Cases and Forty-one Observations in the Literature, *Am. J. Cardiol.,* 14:237, 1964.

100 de los Arcos, E., Madurga, M. P., Leon, J. P., Martinez, J. L., and Urquia, M.: Hydatid Cyst of Interventricular Septum Causing Left Anterior Hemiblock, *Br. Heart J.,* 33:623, 1971.

101 Perez-Gomez, F., Duran, H., Tamames, S., Perrote, J. L., and Blanes, A.: Cardiac Echinococcosis: Clinical Picture and Complications, *Br. Heart J.,* 35:1326, 1973.

101a Farooki, Z. Q., Adelman, S., and Green, E. W.: Echocardiographic Differentiation of a Cystic and a Solid Tumor of the Heart, *Am. J. Cardiol.,* 39:107, 1977.

102 Lima, J. P. R.: Study of the So-called "Ectopical Lesions" in Manson's Schistosomiasis, II. Myocardial Schistosomiasis, *Rev. Inst. Med. Trop. São Paulo,* 11:290, 1969.

103 Wessel, H. U., Sommers, H. M., Cugell, D. W., and Paul, M. H.: Variants of Cardiopulmonary Manifestations of Manson's Schistosomiasis: Report of Two Cases, *Ann. Intern. Med.,* 62:757, 1965.

104 Bertrand, E., and Barabe, P.: Les Cardiopathies des Bilharzioses. Incidence Réelle à Abidjan, *Presse Med.,* 78:2426, 1970.

105 Ferreira, A.: Altercões Hepáticas por Ascaris Lumbricoides em um Caso de Infestacao Macica dos Intestinos: Localizacao de Ova de *A. lumbricoides* no Miocárdio, *Rev. Méd. Aeroáut,* 15:35, 1963.

106 Africa, C. M., de Leon, W., and Garcia, E. Y.: Visceral Complications in Intestinal Heterophyidiasis of Man, *Acta Med. Philippina,* Monograph Series, no. 1, 118, 1940.

107 Fournier, P., Pauchant, M., Voisin, C., and Leduc, M.: Contribution á l'Étude Anatomo-clinique de l'Endocardite Pariétale fibroplastique: Ses Rapports avec la Filariose, *Arch. Mal. Coeur,* 54:869, 1961.

108 Tatibouet, L., and Eusen, Y: Insuffisance Cardiaque d'Origine Filarienne (Cardiac Insufficiency of Filarial Origin), *Semaine Hôp. Paris,* 37:3418, 1961.

109 Kean, B. H., and Breslau, R. C.: Cardiac Paragonimiasis, in "Parasites of the Human Heart," Grune & Stratton, Inc., New York, 1964, pp. 104–106.

110 Kyle, L. H., McKay, D. G., and Sparling, H. J., Jr.: Strongyloidiasis, *Ann. Intern. Med.,* 29:1014, 1948.

111 Goldsmid, J. M.: Two Unusual Cases of Cysticercosis in Man in Rhodesia, *J. Helminthol.,* 40:331, 1966.

112 Becroft, D. M. O.: Infection by the Dog Roundworm *Toxocara canis* and Fatal Myocarditis, *N.Z. Med. J.,* 63:729, 1964.

81
Cardiomyopathy

A
Classification

JOHN F. GOODWIN, M.D.

Before classifying the cardiomyopathies it is necessary to define them. Cardiomyopathy is "heart muscle disease of unknown cause."[1] Confusion has been caused in the past, first, by including within the definition of cardiomyopathy the many diseases in which the heart has been involved as part of a generalized disorder affecting other systems of the body, and, second, by including conditions in which the heart is involved secondarily to the target organ. The new definition of cardiomyopathy specifies lack of knowledge of the cause. It has been proposed that diseases of the heart which result from diseases elsewhere in the body should be designated as "rare specific heart muscle disease."[1] These conditions are dealt with in Chaps. 80 and 82.

Cardiomyopathies may be classified into four main types based on disordered physiology and pathology[2,3] (see Fig. 81A-1 and Tables 81A-1 and 81A-2).

HYPERTROPHIC CARDIOMYOPATHY WITH OR WITHOUT OBSTRUCTION (HYPERTROPHIC OBSTRUCTIVE CARDIOMYOPATHY); IDIOPATHIC SUBAORTIC STENOSIS

The main feature of hypertrophic cardiomyopathy is the massive ventricular hypertrophy which affects principally the septum but may extend to involve all parts of the left ventricle and sometimes also the right ventricle. There is a genetic basis to the disease, which can occur in many members of the same family. Overt evidence of familial involvement is not usually obtained with certainty in more than approximately 30 percent of the patients, but a suggestive history can be obtained from an additional 30 percent. In the remainder there is no evidence available, probably because the severity of the disease varies widely, and patients with minor degrees of involvement may have a good prognosis and may not come to medical attention.

Gross pathology indicates the marked degree of hypertrophy and in many cases a considerable amount of myocardial fibrosis also. The papillary muscles of the mitral valve are hypertrophied, and there may be endocardial thickening, particularly in

CARDIOMYOPATHIES

With obstruction (asymmetrical septum)　　Without obstruction.

HYPERTROPHIC

Massive hypertrophy.
Reduced systolic volume.
Increased ventricular stiffness.
Difficulties in filling.
Good pump function.

Mainly left ventricle and septum.
Patchy distribution of disease.
Genetic basis.

CONGESTIVE

Moderate hypertrophy.
Massive dilatation.
Increased systolic and diastolic volumes.
Poor pump function.

Multifactorial syndrome.
Uniform distribution of disease.
Right and left ventricles.
Usually acquired basis.

OBLITERATIVE

Obliteration of ventricular cavities:
gross distortion of atrio-ventricular valves.
Compromised pump function.

Endomyocardial fibrosis (E.M.F.).
Right and left ventricles.
Hypereosinophilic syndromes.
Damage to endocardium by unknown
causes, or by eosinophilia, induces
reaction with fibrous tissue and thrombus.
Can resemble constrictive pericarditis.

RESTRICTIVE

Restriction to ventricular filling.
by rigid unyielding endocardial, subendocardial or myocardial disease which
impairs ventricular distension.
Good pump function.

Left ventricle.
Resembles constrictive pericarditis.
Cryptogenic.
Can be due to amyloid or hypereosinophilia.

FIGURE 81A-1 Diagrammatic representation of the structural and functional pathology in the four main groups of cardiomyopathy, with brief notes for amplification. *[Reproduced (slightly modified) from Goodwin[1a] with the permission of the author and publisher and the American Heart Association.]*

the region of the inflow tract of the left ventricle. The mitral valve is structurally normal but may develop changes of "wear and tear" so that secondary mitral valve abnormality may develop, and indeed calcification has been reported. The major coronary arteries are widely patent and smooth-bore, but the intramural coronary arteries may show occlusive changes. Ventricular dilatation is not usually seen in postmortem specimens, though it has been reported in patients who have died in congestive heart failure. Electron microscopy shows characteristic abnormal orientation of myofibrils, while light microscopy shows short, thick, greatly abnormal muscle fibers arranged in circular collections. These lesions are essentially patchy and may be found alongside areas of normal muscle or simple hypertrophy.

The effect of the pathologic changes is to produce a stiff, inelastic myocardium with resistance to ventricular filling. The systolic function of the heart remains good until the late stages of the disease, when the abnormal process has become generalized. The asymmetric hypertrophy of the septum is associated with gradients in systole across the outflow tract of the left ventricle in the majority of patients, though these are sometimes absent. In the natural history of the disease, gradients may develop or disappear, may never be present, or may remain established. Disappearance of the gradient suggests progression of the disease. There is some evidence that the outflow tract gradients and the disorder of filling are increased by beta-adrenergic stimulation and diminished by beta-adrenergic blockade.[3,4]

TABLE 81A-1
Characteristics of the left ventricle in the four main types of cardiomyopathy*

LV characteristics	Hypertrophic obstructive	Congestive	Obliterative	Restrictive — Cryptogenic	Restrictive — Amyloid
Hypertrophy	+++	+	±	0	+
Inflow resistance	++	0	0	0	0
Inflow restriction	0	0	+	++	++
Inflow obliteration	0	0	++	0+	0
Outflow obstruction	+	0	0	0	0
Pump function	++	Poor	±	++	Poor
Endocardium	Slight thickening	Slight thickening	Marked thickening (EMF); (eosinophils)	Fibrosis or eosinophils	Normal
Myocardium	Massive Hy; no infiltration	No infiltration	Fibrosis	Normal	Amyloid infiltration

*LV = left ventricle, Hy = hypertrophy, EMF = endomyocardial fibrosis.

TABLE 81A-2
Definitions of the ventricular diastolic faults in cardiomyopathy*

Fault	Definition	Associated features
Resistance	Decreased distensibility due to stiff muscle	Hypertrophy Fibrosis Dyskinesia (i.e., HOCM, AS, coronary artery disease)*
Restriction	Impaired diastolic volume and stretch due to organic subendocardial or myocardial lesion	Fibrosis Eosinophils Amyloid
Obliteration	Impaired filling due to intracavitary space-occupying masses which also *restrict* filling	Fibrosis EMF Thrombus Eosinophils (Loeffler's cardiomyopathy)

*HOCM = hypertrophic obstructive cardiomyopathy, AS = aortic stenosis.
EMF = endomyocardial fibrosis.

CONGESTIVE CARDIOMYOPATHY

The term congestive cardiomyopathy denotes a syndrome characterized by congestive heart failure of unknown cause. It represents a collection of disorders rather than a single disease, and there is little evidence that it occurs on genetic basis. Unlike hypertrophic cardiomyopathy, ventricular hypertrophy is moderate rather than extreme, and the left ventricle is dilated. Gross examination of the heart reveals a soft, flabby myocardium. There may be antemortem endocardial thrombus in either or both ventricles. The valves are normal, though there may be some evidence of mitral and tricuspid insufficiency due to stretching of the valve and the papillary muscles in connection with the dilatation. In contrast to hypertrophic cardiomyopathy there is no increased resistance to ventricular filling, but systolic function is extremely poor, as is shown by reduced minute and stroke volumes and increased systolic and diastolic volumes with low ejection fraction. The coronary arteries are smooth and widely patent, and evidence of significant coronary artery disease has not been found in this syndrome. The ventricles are usually uniformly, rather than patchily, involved, and both ventricles are committed to the disease.

The onset of the disease is usually insidious, with a history of progressive heart failure over a period of several months, sometimes preceded by an apparent upper respiratory tract infection. In some patients, however, the disease may be present for much longer periods, and this can be demonstrated by the presence of cardiac enlargement in chest radiographs taken many years before the onset of symptoms. It is possible that many cases do not come to attention for long periods because of milder forms of the disease. The clinicopathologic and hemodynamic descriptions are therefore based essentially on patients with severe forms of the disease who have come to medical attention because of symptoms.

By definition the causes of congestive cardiomyopathy are unknown, but certain associated risk factors can be identified, though it is not certain how important these are. These risk factors are: (1) alcohol; (2) pregnancy and the puerperium; (3) systemic hypertension; (4) previous infection, possibly viral; (5) autoimmune disorders; (6) noxious physical and chemical agents. It seems possible that one or more factors may act together in producing the disease in many instances. The associated risk factors will be dealt with in Chap. 81C.

The rare specific heart muscle diseases usually produce a congestive type of cardiomyopathy.

OBLITERATIVE CARDIOMYOPATHY

This term has been introduced to describe conditions in which the cavity of the ventricle is obliterated by abnormal tissue. This abnormal tissue may consist of fibrosis with superadded thrombus (as in endomyocardial fibrosis) or dense masses of eosinophils (as in Loeffler's eosinophilic cardiomyopathy). The effect of the obliterative process is to produce a restriction of ventricular filling due to reduction in size of the cavity.

Endomyocardial fibrosis

This is a common (though not the commonest) form of heart disease in tropical Africa and also occurs in other humid tropical zones. It is most unusual in temperate climates. The disease may involve the right or the left ventricle or both. The onset is insidious with episodes of heart failure or atrial fibrillation, apparent improvement, and then deterioration into progressive heart failure. Early in the disease febrile episodes are common but may be due to associated infections, which are extremely frequent in tropical areas. In the right-sided form of the disease obliteration of the right ventricular apex occurs progressively. The blood flow to the lungs is maintained by the enlarged hypertrophied right atrium.

The disease affects the pericardium, myocardium, and endocardium. In acute stages the endocardium is hyperemic and infiltrated by inflammatory cells. The myocardium shows septums of fibrous tissue penetrating from the thick endocardium, and when the disease is active, there are star-shaped areas where fibers are being destroyed, often near the small blood vessels. Involvement of the endocardium is not uniform. The lesions occur in the inflow tracts, most commonly in the apices of both ventricles and under the septal cusp of the tricuspid valve and the posterior cusp of the mitral valve.

The right ventricular form of the disease resembles severe constrictive pericarditis with high central venous pressure, impressive cardiac enlargement, absence of significant murmurs, and often hepatic enlargement and ascites. There may be edema of the face and proptosis. The left ventricular form of the

CHAPTER 81A **1559**
CLASSIFICATION

disease affects the entire function of the left ventricle. Left ventricular failure often occurs and severe mitral regurgitation as a result of mitral valve involvement results. Right-sided heart failure may result from the left-sided heart failure. Involvement of both ventricles may occur in the same patient.[5]

Loeffler's eosinophilic cardiomyopathy

In this condition the endocardium of the left ventricle is infiltrated with dense masses of eosinophils, progressively obliterating the left ventricular cavity and thus producing a functional disturbance similar to that found in left ventircular endomyocardial fibrosis. It is not clear whether Loeffler's disease is a single entity or the result of a number of syndromes associated with hypereosinophilia. Eosinophils can damage the endocardium and affect myocardial function.[6a] Loeffler's disease has been found in patients with eosinophilic leukemia or the hypereosinophilic syndrome.[6] This last name has been coined to describe a group of conditions in which there is marked eosinophilia of the blood associated with diffuse organ infiltration by eosinophils. There are prominent cardiac and blood abnormalities, and morbidity and mortality is significant. The syndrome should not be confused with other eosinophilic conditions associated with parasitic infections, asthma, autoimmune diseases, infections, and or collagen disease.

In Loeffler's disease the dense masses of the eosinophils in the left ventricular cavity produce both restriction to inflow and obliteration. Thrombosis may be added to the eosinophilic lesions, so that systemic embolism is not uncommon in the active phase of the disease. The eosinophils may disappear and be replaced by masses of fibrous tissue. It has been suggested[7,7a] that eosinophilic cardiomyopathy is the temperate-zone equivalent of endomyocardial fibrosis in the tropics. Certainly the pathologic lesions can bear considerable similarity, but the intense eosinophilia found in Loeffler's and allied syndromes is never present in endomyocardial fibrosis, in which there is usually only a mild eosinophilia in the early stages of the disease.

RESTRICTIVE CARDIOMYOPATHY

This term replaced the original designation of constrictive cardiomyopathy which was introduced to describe patients in whom the hemodynamic and clinical features resembled constrictive pericarditis. The term "restrictive" was substituted for "constrictive" to emphasize that the abnormality restricts ventricular filling from within rather than from without, as in constrictive pericarditis.[2] Restrictive cardiomyopathy is extremely rare and the cause usually unknown. Left ventricular hypertrophy and fibrosis with thickening of the endocardium have been described.[8] Early descriptions of constrictive or restrictive cardiomyopathy were largely based on the results of hemodynamic studies of the right side of the heart. Certain differences from constrictive pericarditis were outlined and are still of value in differential diagnosis. In restrictive cardiomyopathy the early diastolic pressure in the right ventricle is usually above zero while in constrictive pericarditis is usually at or below zero. In restrictive cardiomyopathy the end-diastolic pressures in the ventricles usually differ, whereas in constrictive pericarditis they are usually the same. There may be pulmonary hypertension in restrictive cardiomyopathy, but not in constrictive pericarditis. It must be emphasized, however, that differentiation on occasions may be impossible without exploratory thoracotomy. In some cases of restrictive cardiomyopathy described recently[8] left ventricular studies showed a steep early diastolic rise in the left ventricular pressure pulse to a plateau without a prominent a wave. In the majority of the patients systolic function of the left ventricle was normal, as is usual in constrictive pericarditis. Apparently patients with primary restrictive cardiomyopathy have a unique fault in left ventricular diastolic function manifested by restriction of left ventricular volume without reduction in the rate of ventricular filling.[8]

Amyloid heart disease

Amyloid heart disease may exist without evidence of involvement of other organs. It has been described as producing a restrictive syndrome and may also closely resemble constrictive pericarditis. The glassy amyloid deposits in the heart make the organ stiff and rigid and thus restrict the filling in this way. Cardiac pain is common, probably because deposits of amyloid occur around the small blood vessels, tending to strangle them. In some cases of amyloid heart disease left ventricular function may be preserved, and the condition then closely resembles primary restrictive cardiomyopathy. But in severe cases, when amyloid deposits are widespread, left ventricular function may be markedly disturbed. A recent study has defined the characteristics of primary amyloid disease of the heart.[9] In severe amyloid disease left ventricular contraction is impaired, and there is reduced distensibility of the left ventricle. Both early and end-diastolic pressures are elevated, and the ratio of change in pressure to volume increased. Unlike primary restrictive cardiomyopathy, both ventricles tend to fill slowly. The relationships between primary restrictive cardiomyopathy and amyloid restrictive cardiomyopathy are not yet fully defined.

The definitions of resistance to ventricular filling, obliteration of ventricular filling, and restriction to ventricular filling are set out in Table 81A-2. It will be obvious that there is some overlap, in that in conditions which involve the endocardium there may be evidence of all three abnormalities of function. For example, any obliterative lesion inevitably produces some restriction to filling. The terms should therefore be interpreted with flexibility and recognized as a useful means of documentation rather than as a fixed classification.

OTHER FORMS OF CARDIOMYOPATHY NOT YET FULLY DEFINED

Ischemic cardiomyopathy

This term has been used to describe patients with occlusive coronary artery disease who develop progressive heart failure without previous evidence of angina or myocardial infarction. The term tends to be misleading, but it is sometimes useful in distinguishing these patients from those with congestive cardiomyopathy, who have normal coronary arteries. The differential diagnosis depends upon coronary arteriography or autopsy examination, but angiographic evidence of marked ventricular dyskinesia suggests underlying occlusive coronary artery disease whereas smooth uniform hypokinesia of the left ventricle suggests congestive cardiomyopathy.

Arrhythmic cardiomyopathy

This term has been used to describe patients who develop cardiac insufficiency on the basis of multiple arrhythmias. It is doubtful whether this is a single entity as the arrhythmias are likely to be due to some underlying disease, and the term should probably be abandoned.

Familial cardiomyopathy

This term is used loosely to denote heart muscle disease occurring in families. The commonest cause is hypertrophic cardiomyopathy, though a familial tendency has occasionally been noted in congestive cardiomyopathy, and some patients are seen who do not fit exactly into any of the accepted groups of cardiomyopathy.

Cardiomyopathy and associated cardiac syndromes

There is increasing awareness that patients with the so-called floppy mitral valve, or with the long QT, syndromes may have associated myocardial disease, while personal experience suggests that the floppy mitral valve syndrome does on occasions occur in association with hypertrophic cardiomyopathy. It is possible that some patients with the syndrome of "angina with normal coronary arteries" have primary myocardial disease of as yet undetermined type. The hypothesis that cardiac pain may arise primarily from muscle disease rather than from impairment of blood supply deserves consideration. Further investigation of the characteristics of ventricular function in this group of patients is needed.

REFERENCES

1 Goodwin, J. F., and Oakley, C. M.: The Cardiomyopathies, *Br. Heart J.,* 34:545, 1972.

1a Goodwin, J. F.: Prospects and Predictions for the Cardiomyopathies, *Circulation,* 50:210, 1974.

2 Goodwin, J. F.: The Congestive and Hypertrophic Cardiomyopathies: A Decade of Study, *Lancet,* 1:731, 1970.

3 Goodwin, J. F.: Prospects and Predictions for the Cardiomyopathies, *Circulation,* 50:210, 1974.

4 Braunwald, E., Lambrew, C. T., Morrow, A. G., Pierce, G. E., Rockoff, S. D., and Ross, J. Jr.: Idiopathic Hypertrophic Subaortic Stenosis, *Circulation,* 29/30 (suppl. 4): 1, 1964.

5 Parry, E. H. O., and Ikeme, A. C.: "Cardiovascular Disease in Nigeria," Ibadan University Press, Nigeria, 1966, p. 24.

6 Chusid, M. J., Dale, D. C., West, B. C., and Wolff, S. M.: The Hypereosinophilic Syndrome: Analysis of 14 Cases with Review of Literature, *Medicine,* 54:1, 1975.

6a Chew, C. Y. C., Ziady, G. M., Rapheal, M. J., Nellen, M., and Oakley, C. M.: Primary Restrictive Cardiomyopathy: Nontropical Endocardial Fibrosis and Hypereosinophilia Heart Disease, *Br. Heart J.,* 39:399, 1977.

7 Brockington, E. F., and Olsen, E. G. J.: Loeffler's Endocardial and Davies' Endomyocardial Fibrosis, *Am. Heart J.,* 85:308, 1973.

7a Oakley, C. M., and Olsen, E. G. J.: Eosinophilia and Heart Disease, *Br. Heart J.,* 39:233, 1977.

8 Ziady, G. M., Oakley, C. M., Raphael, M. J., and Goodwin, J. F.: Primary Restrictive Cardiomyopathy, *Br. Heart J.,* 35:556, 1975.

9 Chew, C., Ziady, G. M., Raphael, M. J., and Oakley, C. M.: The Functional Defect in Amyloid Heart Disease. The "Stiff" Heart Syndrome, *Am. J. Cardiol.,* 36:438, 1975.

B

Idiopathic Hypertrophic Subaortic Stenosis (Obstructive Cardiomyopathy, Asymmetric Septal Hypertrophy)

EUGENE BRAUNWALD, M.D.

Idiopathic hypertrophic subaortic stenosis (IHSS) is a cardiomyopathy characterized by marked hypertrophy of the left ventricle, involving in particular the interventricular septum and the outflow tract.[1] During systole, the anterior leaflet of the mitral valve abuts the hypertrophied septum and may narrow this region sufficiently to produce obstruction to left ventricular ejection.

ANATOMIC CHANGES

Figure 81B-1 shows the heart of a patient with IHSS which exhibits tremendous hypertrophy of the left ventricle, with bulging of the upper portion of the ventricular septum into both ventricular cavities; on coronal section, the latter appear as mere slits. In

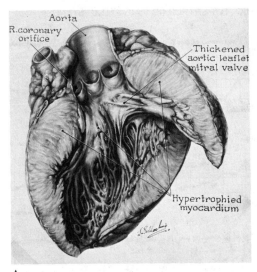

A

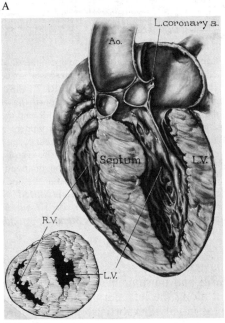

B

FIGURE 81B-1 A. Drawing of left ventricular wall and cavity of a patient with idiopathic hypertrophic subaortic stenosis. *B.* Sagittal and coronal sections showing disproportionate thickening of the ventricular septum encroaching on the two ventricular cavities. *(Reproduced by permission of the American Heart Association, Inc.; from E. Braunwald, "Idiopathic Hypertrophic Subaortic Stenosis," Monograph no. 10, 1964.)*

most instances the left ventricular hypertrophy in patients with IHSS is asymmetric; indeed, patients with classic IHSS appear to represent only one part of a spectrum of disease that has asymmetric septal hypertrophy (ASH) as its characteristic feature.[2,3] Regardless of whether obstruction to left ventricular outflow is present or absent, the septum is at least 1.3 times thicker than that portion of the left ventricular free wall directly behind the posterior mitral valve leaflet.

Microscopic examination of the left ventricle shows variable degrees of interstitial fibrosis, a disorderly arrangement of the muscle in which the cells are arranged in whorls or at random, and a bizarre type of cellular hypertrophy in which the cells are wider and shorter than normal and are stellate-shaped with disarray of myofibrils.[4] These abnormalities are localized to the upper portion of the ventricular septum in patients with obstruction to left ventricular outflow, but are more diffuse, involving both the septum and left ventricular free wall in those with minimal or no obstruction. In patients who have died suddenly the small coronary arteries, including the atrioventricular node artery, are frequently abnormally narrowed; the sinus node is frequently sclerotic; and a variety of histologic abnormalities may be present in the atrioventricular node and the bundle of His.[5]

ETIOLOGY

The anatomic, hemodynamic, and clinical features of this condition vary considerably among different patients, among different affected individuals in the same family, and even in the same patient at different stages of the disease. However, the feature which most patients have in common, i.e., ASH, appears to be genetically transmitted as a non-sex-linked autosomal dominant.[3]

The discovery of a heart murmur, an abnormal electrocardiogram or, in surveys of families of patients with documented IHSS, an abnormal echocardiogram (see below), are often presenting features of the disease.[1] Clinical findings are occasionally present in early childhood. The finding of the characteristic gross and microscopic findings in infants and stillborn children supports the concept that the disease is congenital in some instances.[6] However, in about one-third of patients at least one detailed examination revealed no evidence of a heart murmur prior to the eventual discovery of the murmur, and in them it appears likely that many of the manifestations of the disease are acquired.

As a consequence of the distortion of the left ventricle caused by massive septal hypertrophy and/or the tethering of the mitral valve by abnormally positioned papillary muscles, the mitral valve is positioned abnormally anteriorly, i.e., close to the ventricular septum, at the end of diastole. The obstruction to left ventricular outflow is caused by the abnormal forward motion of the mitral valve and the apposition of its anterior leaflet with the greatly hypertrophied ventricular septum. Thus, the mitral valve participates in the formation of the obstructive orifice, and moderately severe mitral regurgitation is often present. The severity of left ventricular hypertrophy in patients with obstruction to left ventricular outflow is not a simple function of the severity of the obstruction, and in some patients the left ventricle is hypertrophied without obstruction. In a large number of patients there is no obstruction in the basal state, but over the course of time obstruction can be provoked by various physiologic or pharmacologic stimuli, and it then becomes established, even in the basal state.[1] It has been suggested that the hyperkinetic heart syndrome may eventually develop into IHSS, but this transition has not been documented.

CLINICAL MANIFESTATIONS
Age: symptoms

The ages of patients range from birth to 85 years, but most commonly IHSS is a disease of young adults, with the majority of the patients in the third and fourth decades. The most frequent symptoms are exertional dyspnea and angina pectoris. Dizziness and "graying out" spells are also very common, especially on assuming the erect posture. Frank syncope appears less common, and when it does occur, it does not carry with it as ominous a prognosis as in patients with valvular aortic stenosis. Congestive heart failure with salt and water retention and palpitations due to arrhythmias are observed less commonly.[1]

Physical examination

A number of the male patients with IHSS have a history of unusual athletic achievement and evince considerable muscular development on physical examination. The heart is usually enlarged, with a left ventricular lift. A double apical impulse with an abnormally tall presystolic expansion wave (*a* wave) is usually present (Fig. 81B-2); in some instances there are two outward movements of the precordium during systole, resulting in a triple impulse. On superficial examination of the patient with IHSS, obstruction to left ventricular outflow may not be readily evident, and the findings, in general, suggest ventricular septal defect or mitral regurgitation. Many patients have a thrill along the lower precordium and/or at the apex; it is palpable only rarely in the jugular notch or along the carotid vessels. The peripheral pulses are brisk, and an atrial sound is usually audible (Fig. 81B-2). A protodiastolic gallop is present in more than one-half of the patients. A systolic murmur, usually grade 3/6 or louder, commences after the brief pause following the first heart sound. It is heard in almost every patient, is most prominent at the apex and along the left sternal border, and is usually not well transmitted to the neck. An additional pansystolic murmur characteristic of mitral regurgitation is often present; in patients with no or mild obstruction the murmur may be soft (grade 1 to 2/6) or even absent. The second heart sound is often single or exhibits paradoxic splitting, i.e., the aortic follows the pulmonary component. All of the physical signs may be accentuated or ameliorated by the physiologic or pharmacologic maneuvers which modify the severity of obstruction and which are reviewed below.[1]

It is important to consider some of the features that differentiate IHSS from valvular aortic stenosis.

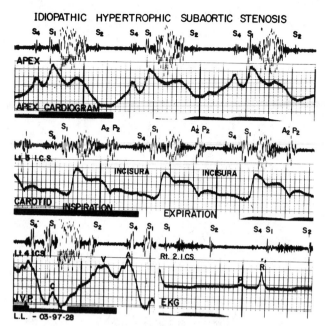

FIGURE 81B-2 Phonocardiogram recorded at the apex, the third left intercostal space (Lt. 3 I.C.S.), the fourth left intercostal space (Lt. 4 I.C.S.), and the second right intercostal space (Rt. 2 I.C.S.). S_1, first heart sound; S_2, second heart sound; S_4, fourth heart sound; J.V.P., jugular venous pulse. Note the prominent S_4 and the presystolic expansion of the apex cardiogram, the prominent *a* wave of the J.V.P., and the rapid upstroke of the indirect carotid arterial pulse. The apex cardiogram exhibits an early systolic collapse followed by a late systolic expansion. The diamond-shaped midsystolic ejection murmur is recorded best at the apex and is less prominent along the Rt. 2 I.C.S. (*Reproduced by permission of the American Heart Association, Inc.; from E. Braunwald, "Idiopathic Hypertrophic Subaortic Stenosis," Monograph no. 10, 1964.*)

The systolic thrill and murmur in IHSS are usually most prominent along the left sternal border and at the apex, whereas in valvular aortic stenosis they are most obvious at the base of the heart, with radiation to the jugular notch and along the carotid vessels. In IHSS, the characteristic systolic murmur is usually ejection in type (Fig. 81B-2), is sometimes holosystolic, and is usually medium-pitched. In valvular aortic stenosis it is always an ejection murmur and is generally low-pitched and rasping. A systolic ejection sound is unusual in IHSS; it is common in valvular aortic stenosis in the absence of valvular calcification. The diastolic blowing murmur of semilunar valve incompetence, heard along the sternal edge, is rare in IHSS but relatively common in patients with valvular aortic stenosis. In IHSS, the arterial pulse rises rapidly and is bifid (bisferiens). In valvular aortic stenosis, it is anacrotic and tends to rise slowly. In both IHSS and severe valvular stenosis (Fig. 81B-2), a prominent fourth heart sound is frequently evident, and the apex cardiogram shows a presystolic impulse, the first component of which is synchronous with the fourth heart sound (Fig. 81B-2).

Many of the above-mentioned physical findings suggest increased activity of the atrium in IHSS and may be correlated with an interesting clinical and hemodynamic feature. The stiffness (reduced disten-

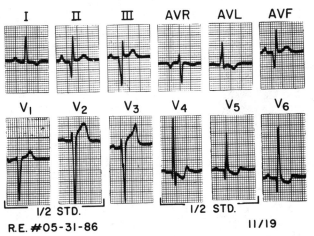

I   II   III   AVR   AVL   AVF

V₁   V₂   V₃   V₄   V₅   V₆

1/2 STD.   1/2 STD.

R.E. #05-31-86   11/19

FIGURE 81B-3 Electrocardiogram showing abnormal Q waves in leads II, III, aV$_g$, V$_5$, and V$_6$. The precordial leads exhibit the voltage criteria for left ventricular hypertrophy. *(Reproduced by permission of the American Heart Association, Inc.; from E. Braunwald, "Idiopathic Hypertrophic Subaortic Stenosis," Monograph no. 10, 1964.)*

sibility) of the greatly thickened left ventricle impedes passive ventricular filling, and a vigorous, poorly timed atrial contraction is required for proper ventricular filling. When patients with IHSS lose this important atrial contribution to ventricular filling, i.e., when they develop nodal rhythm, atrial fibrillation, or atrial flutter, their circulatory state deteriorates quite rapidly. Fortunately, these arrhythmias are not very common, but when they occur they may cause sudden collapse. The development of atrial fibrillation is a poor prognostic sign.

Electrocardiogram

The electrocardiogram is helpful in the diagnosis of IHSS; a normal tracing is extremely rare in patients with obstruction. In most instances there is evidence of left ventricular hypertrophy, but there are two other important findings. One of these is the presence of abnormal Q waves.[1,2] Most commonly, very deep, broad Q waves are found in leads II, III, and aV$_F$, and over the left precordium (Fig. 81B-3). Indeed, a significant number of patients with IHSS are referred because of these electrocardiographic findings, which may be falsely attributed to coronary artery disease. However, the abnormal Q waves are not produced by myocardial infarction but are probably related to the marked hypertrophy of the ventricular septum. The coronary arteries are usually widely patent. The second interesting electrocardiographic feature is the Wolff-Parkinson-White (W-P-W) syndrome. In approximately one-fourth of patients with IHSS the electrocardiogram shows two of the components of the triad, a short P-Q (P-R) interval and slurring of the R wave, i.e., a delta wave. QRS prolongation is seen less commonly.

Pulse tracings

The indirectly recorded carotid arterial pulse rises sharply and then falls during midsystole. There is a

secondary elevation or plateau during late systole, and the incisura is often delayed (Fig. 81B-2). The jugular venous pulse shows a prominent *a* (atrial contraction) wave.

Echocardiogram

Echocardiography has emerged as the most useful, noninvasive technique for the diagnosis and characterization of IHSS,[3] for following the progression in individual patients, and for screening relatives of affected members (Fig. 81B-4). There are two principal abnormalities: (1) an increase in the thickness of the interventricular septum (recorded immediately inferior to the level of the mitral leaflets) relative to that of the posterobasal region of the free wall (recorded at the level of the posterior mitral leaflet) from a normal value of approximately 1.0/1.0 to more than 1.3/1.0; the hypertrophied septum is relatively immobile and contracts poorly; (2) abnormal forward motion of the anterior mitral leaflets during systole in patients with obstruction; the mitral valve is also in an abnormally anterior position at end-diastole.

Roentgenogram

The conventional chest roentgenogram reveals an abnormally large cardiothoracic ratio in approximately one-half of the patients, and the left ventricle is considered to be enlarged in almost all, but the degree of enlargement correlates poorly with the systolic pressure gradient or the degree of disability. Aortic dilatation is an uncommon finding in IHSS, and the presence of marked aortic dilatation in a patient with obstruction to left ventricular outflow suggests that valvular or discrete subvalvular stenosis rather than IHSS is present. Intracardiac calcification is absent in IHSS.

Hemodynamics

The directly recorded peripheral arterial pressure rises very rapidly, falls in midsystole, and often shows a second elevation before the dicrotic notch. The withdrawal pressure tracing at the time of left-sided heart catheterization, demonstrating a subaortic gradient, is helpful in localizing the obstruction to the subvalvular region (Fig. 81B-5). In patients with IHSS and obstruction to left ventricular outflow, the systemic arterial pressure is usually within normal limits; the pulmonary artery pressure exceeds the upper limits of normal in about one-fourth of patients. A systolic pressure gradient within the right ventricular outflow tract may be recorded in about one-sixth, and the right ventricular end-diastolic pressure is often abnormally elevated. The *a* wave is the most prominent wave in the right and left atrial pressure pulses in almost every patient.[1] The resting cardiac index varies widely; though generally normal, it often exceeds the upper limits in asymptomatic patients and is depressed late in the course of the

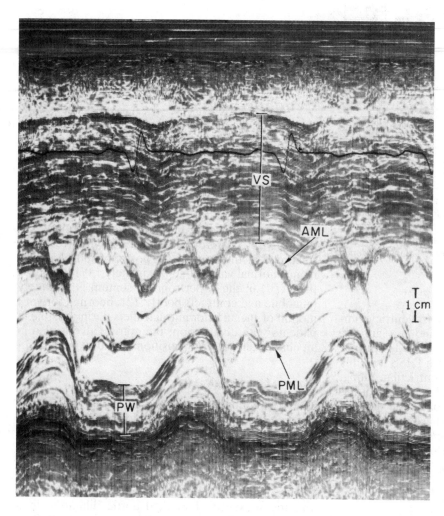

FIGURE 81B-4 Echocardiogram of a patient with IHSS. The ventricular septum (VS) is massively hypertrophied, disproportionately so when compared to the posterior wall (PW) of the left ventricle. The anterior mitral leaflet (AML) is displaced anteriorly in the ventricular cavity at the onset of systole and moves forward, coming into apposition with the septum, during systole. PML—posterior mitral leaflet. (Through the courtesy of Dr. S. E. Epstein.)

disease. The mean left atrial pressure is abnormally elevated in half the patients, while the left ventricular end-diastolic pressure exceeds the upper limit of normal in almost all of them. There is little correlation between the most common symptoms in IHSS and the severity of obstruction. In addition to obstruction to ventricular outflow, IHSS is characterized by an abnormally low ventricular compliance, an important consequence of which is impedance to ventricular filling and atrial hypertrophy.

One of the most important features of IHSS is the variability of the severity of obstruction and therefore the hemodynamic findings.[1] Large variations in the systolic pressure gradient occur in the course of a single study. In some cases a significant systolic pressure gradient may be recorded at the beginning of the catheterization, but all hemodynamic evidence of obstructions disappears after an hour or two; less frequently the opposite occurs. Forced slow respiration, discomfort or anxiety, elevation of the legs, and general anesthesia all have striking effects on the severity of obstruction. These variations in the severity of obstruction constitute one of the most important characteristics of IHSS, distinguishing it

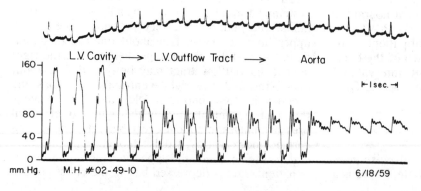

FIGURE 81B-5 Pressure tracing recorded continuously as the catheter was withdrawn from the left ventricular cavity, through the left ventricular outflow tract, and into the ascending aorta. There is a striking "atrial kick" as well as a notch on the upstroke of the left ventricular pressure pulse proximal to the obstruction. (Reproduced by permission of the American Heart Association, Inc.; from E. Braunwald, "Idiopathic Hypertrophic Subaortic Stenosis," Monograph no. 10, 1964.)

from other forms of heart disease with intracardiac or extracardiac obstruction to blood flow. Since the obstruction in IHSS results from the systolic apposition of the hypertrophied muscle constituting the walls of the left ventricular outflow tract to the anterior leaflet of the mitral valve, the principal determinants of the severity of obstruction are (1) the systolic volume of the left ventricular cavity, (2) the force of left ventricular contraction, and (3) the transmural pressure which distends the outflow tract during systole.

Analysis of the postextrasystolic arterial pulse pressure response is a useful diagnostic test for IHSS.[1] In normal individuals, and in patients with conditions other than IHSS, the cardiac cycle following a premature contraction is characterized by a ventricular contraction more forceful than normal, and consequently the arterial pulse pressure is greater than normal. Patients with IHSS share with normal subjects, and with patients with discrete obstruction to left ventricular outflow, this postextrasystolic augmentation of the force of left ventricular contraction. However, patients with IHSS and obstruction to left ventricular outflow exhibit an abnormal postpremature beat with a pulse pressure which does not exceed that of the control beat.

Patients with IHSS also exhibit characteristic responses to a variety of vasoactive drugs.[1] The intravenous administration of rapidly acting cardiac glycosides results in large and consistent increases in the pressure gradient and diminutions in the size of the stenotic orifice. Similarly, isoproterenol, amyl nitrite, and nitroglycerin intensify the obstruction in patients in whom a gradient is present in the basal state, and provoke the development of obstruction in those without obstruction in the basal state. Methoxamine and phenylephrine abolish the obstruction in patients with IHSS. During exercise, the calculated effective orifice size of the left ventricular outflow tract diminishes in most patients, and often the obstruction becomes even more severe shortly after discontinuation of exercise. The Valsalva maneuver or assumption of the erect posture also augments the systolic pressure gradient or provokes the development of obstruction in patients in whom no gradient is present in the basal state. In contrast, in patients with discrete obstruction to left ventricular outflow, the Valsalva maneuver tends to reduce the magnitude of the gradient. Changes in body position also vary the severity of obstruction. Assuming the supine position with leg elevation may abolish the gradient, while a decided intensification of the obstruction results from standing up or from being tilted into the erect position.

Angiocardiogram

The left ventricular angiocardiogram is of considerable diagnostic value in IHSS (Fig. 81B-6). It characteristically reveals marked thickening of the left ventricular wall. The left ventricular cavity tends to be unusually small and irregular and may be almost totally obliterated at the end of ejection. The left ventricular cavity is also abnormal in shape in the majority of patients, an inward concavity at the

midportion of the right inferior margin which results from the bulging of the greatly hypertrophied interventricular septum into the left ventricular cavity being the most common finding. The anterior leaflet of the mitral valve is frequently seen to be pulled forward into the left ventricular outflow tract during systole on the lateral projection, and the enormously hypertrophied papillary muscles are often visible. Mitral regurgitation is present in more than one-half of the patients.

TREATMENT

Because of the risk of sudden death, even in asymptomatic patients in whom the disease has not been recognized, strenuous physical activity is inadvisable. Digitalis should not be administered to patients with IHSS, with the exception of those with atrial fibrillation and a rapid ventricular response and in those with little or no obstruction but symptoms of reduced cardiac reserve. Use of nitroglycerin, isoproterenol, and vigorous diuresis should also usually be avoided. In the event of a syncopal episode or cardiovascular collapse, assumption of the "shock" position (with the head lowered and the legs elevated) and the infusion of phenylephrine or methoxamine are helpful in relieving the obstruction.

Since tachycardia and sympathetic stimulation of the myocardium tend to intensify obstruction and augment myocardial oxygen needs, propranolol, a beta-adrenergic receptor blocking drug, has been utilized for the treatment of symptomatic patients with IHSS. Oral doses of 20 to 60 mg four times a day diminish the frequency and intensity of attacks of angina pectoris and may reduce the frequency of syncopal attacks and of arrhythmic episodes.[7] However, symptoms secondary to cardiac decompensation are not relieved and may even be intensified by propranolol.

Patients with heart failure or those with disabling angina and syncope which is unresponsive or poorly responsive to medical therapy should be considered for surgical treatment if there is marked obstruction in the basal state (i.e., a systolic pressure gradient exceeding 60 mm Hg with a normal cardiac output). The operation consists of incising and/or partially excising the muscular ridge obstructing the left ventricular outflow tract, which is usually approached through the ascending aorta.[8] In experienced hands the mortality rate is in the neighborhood of 5 percent, and major complications such as complete heart block, mitral regurgitation, or a ventricular septal defect are incurred in another 5 percent. The remaining patients have, in general, exhibited substantial clinical improvement, and the hemodynamic effectiveness of the procedure has been documented by postoperative cardiac catheterizations and echocardiograms. In the large majority of patients these beneficial clinical and hemodynamic changes have been sustained.[8,9] However, the effects of proprano-

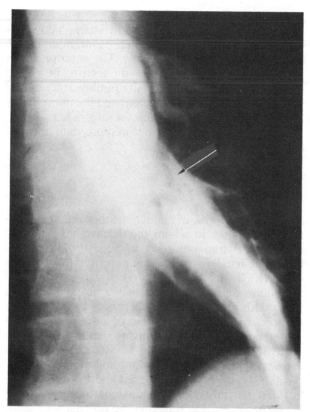 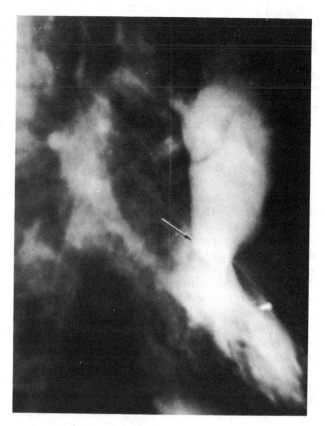

FIGURE 81B-6 Systolic angiograms in a patient with idiopathic hypertrophic subaortic stenosis. In the anteroposterior projection (left) the radiolucent band in the outflow tract (arrow) has a *W* configuration, suggesting visibility of both mitral leaflets. In the lateral projection (right) the abnormal systolic position of the mitral leaflet is shown (arrow). The leaflet is concave, with the leading edge projecting into the outflow tract opposite the hypertrophied septum and participating with the septum in the formation of the obstructing orifice. Minimal mitral regurgitation is present.

lol and of operation on the natural history of the disease remain to be elucidated.

PROGNOSIS

In a study in which 98 patients with IHSS were followed for 1 to 12 years,[10] 10 deaths due to IHSS occurred; 6 were sudden, while in 4 death followed increasing disability. The obstruction tended to be less severe in patients who succumbed, suggesting that death may not be related to progressive narrowing of the left ventricular outflow tract. Among the survivors it was observed that the older patients tended to be more severely symptomatic; although the course was extremely variable, the patients who were asymptomatic initially tended to remain so, while those who were more disabled generally deteriorated or died.[10,11]

REFERENCES

1 Braunwald, E., Lambrew, C. T., Rockoff, S. D., Ross, J., Jr., and Morrow, A. G.: Idiopathic Hypertrophic Subaortic Stenosis. Description of the Disease Based upon an Analysis of 64 Patients, *Circulation,* 29(suppl. 4):1, 1964.

2 Wolstenholme, G. E. W., and O'Connor, M.: "Hypertrophic Obstructive Cardiomyopathy," Ciba Foundation Study Group, no. 37, J. & A. Churchill, London, 1971.

3 Epstein, S. E., Henry, W. L., Clark, C. E., Roberts, W. C., Maron, B. J., Ferrans, V. J., Redwood, D. R., and Morrow, A. G.: Asymmetric Septal Hypertrophy, *Ann. Intern. Med.,* 81: 650, 1974.

4 Maron, B. J., Ferrans, V. J., Henry, W. L., Clark, C. E., Redwood, D. R., Roberts, W. C., Morrow, A. G., and Epstein, S. E.: Differences in Distribution of Myocardial Abnormalities in Patients with Obstructive and Nonobstructive Asymmetric Septal Hypertrophy (ASH). Light and Electron Microscopic Findings, *Circulation,* 50:436, 1974.

5 James, T. N., and Marshall, T. K.: DeSubitaneis Mortibus. XII. Asymmetrical Hypertrophy of the Heart, *Circulation,* 51:1149, 1975.

6 Maron, B. J., Edwards, J. E., Henry, W. L., Clark, C. E., Bingle, G. J., and Epstein, S. E.: Asymmetric Septal Hypertrophy (ASH) in Infancy, *Circulation,* 50:809, 1974.

7 Cohen, L. S., and Braunwald, E.: Amelioration of Angina Pectoris in Idiopathic Hypertrophic Subaortic Stenosis with Beta-adrenergic Blockade, *Circulation,* 35:847, 1967.

8 Morrow, A. G., Reitz, B. A., Epstein, S. E., Henry, W. L., Conkle, D. M., Itscoitz, S. B., and Redwood, D. R.: Operative Treatment in Hypertrophic Subaortic Stenosis. Techniques, and the Results of Pre- and Postoperative Assessments in 83 Patients, *Circulation*, 52:88, 1975.

9 Tajik, A. J., Giuliani, E. R., Weidman, W. H., Brandenburg, R. O., and McGoon, D. C.: Idiopathic Hypertrophic Subaortic Stenosis. Long-Term Surgical Follow-up, *Am. J. Cardiol.*, 34:815, 1974.

10 Frank, S., and Braunwald, E.: Idiopathic Hypertrophic Subaortic Stenosis. Clinical Analysis of 126 Patients with Emphasis on Natural History, *Circulation*, 37:759, 1968.

11 Shah, P. M., Adelman, A. G., Wigle, E. D., Gobel, F. L., Burchell, H. B., Hardarson, T., Curiel, R., de la Calzada, C., Oakley, C. M., and Goodwin, J. F.: The Natural (and Unnatural) History of Hypertrophic Obstructive Cardiomyopathy. A Multicenter Study, *Circ. Res.*, 34, 35(suppl. 11):179, 1974.

C
Congestive Cardiomyopathy

JOHN F. GOODWIN, M.D.

Congestive cardiomyopathy may be considered as a syndrome of isolated cardiomegaly, with dilated ventricles, inappropriate hypertrophy, and heart failure. The striking feature is the dilatation of the ventricles, and an equally appropriate term would be "dilated" cardiomyopathy. The causes of congestive cardiomyopathy are essentially unknown, diverse, and probably multiple.

PATHOLOGY (see Chap. 79)

The gross pathology of the heart reveals a flabby ventricular musculature. The heart is overweight, although the thickness of the ventricular walls may not be increased because of thinning due to dilatation. The increase in weight indicates that hypertrophy has undoubtedly occurred. The disease is diffuse and involves both ventricles. The ventricular muscle is pale and soft, and the trabeculae and papillary muscles are flattened. Antemortem thrombus may be found in either ventricle. The valves are anatomically normal, but the mitral and tricuspid valves may show dilatation of the rings and stretching of papillary muscles. The coronary arteries are of large caliber, unobstructed, and smooth. The naked-eye appearance of the necropsy specimen gives no clue as to etiology (Fig. 81C-1).

Light microscopy is usually equally disappointing. At times the myocardium may appear virtually normal though in some cases there is fibrosis, necrosis of muscle fibers, and infiltration with round cells. Fibrosis is usually most frequent in the inner third of the myocardium. Endocardial fibrosis may be found if there has been prolonged congestive heart failure. Occasionally some intimal thickening may be found in vessels in the fibrotic areas, probably secondary to the fibrosis. It has been suggested that the changes in the myocardium are secondary to inadequate perfu-

sion resulting from poor cardiac function, rather than the result of vascular disease.

Electron microscopy shows many abnormalities, particularly an excess of glycogen and an increase in mitochondria are qualitatively abnormal, often with extensive disruption of cristae. These changes, however, do not indicate any particular disease process and are probably the result of prolonged heart failure. No causal infecting or toxic agent has been discovered in the myocardium. Positive fluorescence of adenovirus antigen has been found in the necleus of some myocardial cells and interstitial cells in cardiac biopsies of the right ventricular myocardium in congestive cardiomyopathy, suggesting the possibility of virus infection.[1]

Failure to demonstrate the causal agent in the myocardium is the striking feature of congestive cardiomyopathy. Some hypertrophy of muscle fibers is always seen, but these do not appear qualitatively abnormal. The electron microscopic appearance of the myofibrils is usually normal. Unusual granules, possibly lysosome-like precursors of lipofuscin may be seen. Lysosomes are increased.

The pathology elsewhere in the body merely reflects the effects of prolonged congestive heart failure, and in some patients those of systemic and pulmonary embolism. By definition, any disease of another system excludes the diagnosis of "congestive cardiomyopathy."

EPIDEMIOLOGY

Comprehensive epidemiologic studies of congestive cardiomyopathy are lacking, probably because of difficulties in definition of the syndrome and lack of investigative facilities in many places. It appears likely, however, that congestive cardiomyopathy has

FIGURE 81C-1 Necropsy specimen of heart in congestive cardiomyopathy showing dilatation and moderate hypertrophy of the right ventricle. *(Courtesy of Dr. E. G. J. Olsen.)*

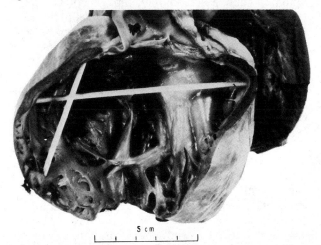

5 cm

a worldwide distribution, but its incidence is virtually unknown. It seems possible that the condition is commoner in underdeveloped tropical countries than it is in the West, but there is no certainty of this. Undoubtedly the disease is much commoner than was previously realised. It seems likely that the apparent increase in frequency is due to improved diagnosis and increased awareness of the condition. Few causal factors have been incriminated with certainty, but many have been suspected. These include malnutrition, alcohol, infections (possibly virus), immunologic disorders, pregnancy, and the puerperium, and hypertension. Certain toxic agents, notably cobalt, emetine, irradiation, and daunorubicin have been shown to damage the myocardium and can produce a syndrome indistinguishable from congestive cardiomyopathy. These conditions, however, appear to be examples of quite specific direct cardiac damage which leads to heart failure and are not within the strict definition of congestive cardiomyopathy.

CLINICAL MANIFESTATIONS

The initial symptoms are usually those of breathlessness on exertion, but episodes of nocturnal dyspnea due to left ventricular failure may occur. Nocturnal dyspnea may be preceded by irritating nocturnal dry cough. Fatigue is usually due to a low cardiac output and stroke volume. The symptoms of left-sided heart failure may be rapidly followed by those of right-sided heart failure, with swelling of the ankles, distension and discomfort in the abdomen due to a congested liver, and sometimes pulsation in the neck due to tricuspid regurgitation.

The physical signs are those of congestive heart failure without obvious cause. When the disease is fully established, the patient is breathless on slight exertion or sometimes even at rest. The skin is cool, pale, and often slightly cyanosed. The peripheral veins are constricted, and the arterial pulse is small in volume. There is commonly, though not always, a tachycardia at rest. The jugular venous pressure is elevated, sometimes substantially, but unless it is grossly raised, the external jugular veins are not distended and venous hypertension must be recognized by pulsation of the deep neck veins. When the patient is in sinus rhythm, there is usually a prominent *a* wave followed by a poor *x* descent (often due to tricuspid incompetence) and a prominent *v* wave. When there is atrial fibrillation, the *a* wave disappears, and there is a single wave due to a combination of right atrial filling and tricuspid regurgitation. The heart is enlarged. Usually the left ventricular impulse can be felt outside the midclavicular line and is commonly of poor quality, suggesting dilatation of the left ventricle. Pulsation to the left of the sternum may be due to right ventricular dilatation. In patients with a long history, the left ventricular impulse may

be more forceful. On auscultatation systolic murmurs of mitral and tricuspid reflux are often heard, but are rarely loud and often diminish with treatment. Persistent, very loud systolic murmurs suggest organic valvular disease. Gallop rhythm is the rule; a third heart sound due to rapid filling is commonly heard, indicating a dilated poorly functioning left ventricle. Frequently a fourth heart sound indicating stiffness of the abnormal ventricle is heard also but it may be of such low frequency as to be inaudible. When the heart rate exceeds 100 beats per minute, the third and fourth heart sounds may summate, producing a single sound in the middle of diastole—a summation gallop. The second heart sound will show reversed splitting if there is left bundle branch block. Pulmonary valve closure is accentuated when there is pulmonary hypertension. The blood pressure is usually normal or low, the pulse pressure often being reduced owing to the poor cardiac output. In some patients an associated pericardial effusion may be present. This can be difficult to detect in the presence of severe myocardial failure, but increase in the central venous pressure and reduction in the arterial pressure on inspiration may indicate a degree of tamponade. The heart sounds may be soft and the cardiac impulse impalpable when a large effusion is present. Examination of the lungs may reveal basal râles, though these are a poor sign of left ventricular failure. Pleural effusion may be present and may be detectable clinically. When right-sided heart failure is severe, there may be considerable enlargement of the liver which may pulsate in presystole, when there is sinus rhythm, and in systole when there is atrial fibrillation and severe tricuspid regurgitation. Ankle edema is common, and there may be sacral edema if the patient has been in bed for a long period. Ascites may be present.

Examination of other systems is essentially negative. There is no abnormal skin color or pigmentation other than that due to heart failure. There are no lymph gland enlargements; the spleen is rarely enlarged except occasionally when heart failure has been prolonged. The central and peripheral nervous systems are normal.

SPECIAL INVESTIGATIONS

Examination of the blood is usually unrewarding. The hemoglobin is commonly normal or slightly reduced though slightly elevated values may be found. A reduction in hemoglobin levels is usually due to slight bone marrow depression, and an increase to chronic hypoxia or possibly the effect of diuretics. The white blood cell count is usually normal. The erythrocyte sedimentation rate (ESR) is often elevated, for reasons that have not been explained. Serum proteins are usually normal, but abnormal globulins may be found and are probably the result of hepatic insufficiency due to heart failure. Occasionally abnormal enzyme activity, possibly from the same cause, may be found. Serum iron level is normal or occasionally low. Where they have been measured, levels of vanillylmandelic acid in urine have been normal.[2] Attempts to isolate virus from the blood of patients with chronic congestive cardiomyopathy have not been successful.

Phonocardiography

Phonocardiography confirms the clinical findings and shows the third and fourth heart sounds and usually the systolic murmurs of mitral and tricuspid insufficiency when these are present. Accentuation of pulmonary valve closure may be shown but is not often striking.

Electrocardiography

Electrocardiography usually shows nonspecific changes (Fig. 81C-2). The T waves are flat or gently inverted. There is often some atrial enlargement and a modest degree of left ventricular hypertrophy, which in some cases, however, may be marked if disease is of long standing. Commonly the QRS complex is of low voltage. The frontal plane axis is abnormal in 40 percent. The commonest arrhythmia is atrial fibrillation, which occurs in 25 percent, but atrial flutter, junctional rhythms, supraventricular tachycardia, first-degree or complete heart block, and ventricular tachycardia have all been noted.[2] Left bundle branch block is present in 10 percent of patients. In a small number of patients q waves may be seen in the precordial leads, which may suggest myocardial infarction (Fig. 81C-2). They are due to multiple areas of necrosis or fibrosis scattered through the left ventricle and septum.[3]

Echocardiography

There is dilatation of both ventricles, with poor movement of the posterior wall of the left ventricle, and paradoxic movement of the septum. There is usually a pronounced atrial wave ("kick") of the anterior mitral cusp due to the high left ventricular end-diastolic pressure. The amplitude of the movement of the cusp may be increased, but it is not

thickened, and the diastolic closure rate is either normal or increased. Both systolic and diastolic volumes of the left ventricle are increased and the ejection fraction reduced. The rate of circumferential shortening of the myocardial fibers is reduced. There may be evidence of associated pericardial effusion.

Chest radiography

There is considerable cardiomegaly due mainly to enlargement and dilatation of both ventricles. The left and right atria may be enlarged, the right atrium often more than the left, as the result of tricuspid regurgitation. The pulmonary vasculature shows evidence of a high left atrial pressure with increase in size of the upper lobe vessels and reduction in size of the lower lobe vessels, but this feature is not usually marked. The main pulmonary arteries are slightly enlarged (Fig. 81C-3). Pleural effusions may be present, and in some patients there may be evidence of pulmonary infarction. When a pericardial effusion is present, the heart may show considerable enlargement with the usual flask-shaped pattern. But this characteristic appearance is not invariable, and a pericardial effusion of some size may be present without any definite radiologic features.

Hemodynamics

The hemodynamics are essentially those of failure of the heart as a pump. In the early stages of the disease

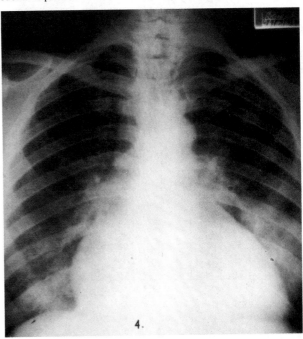

FIGURE 81C-3 Six-foot posteroanterior chest radiograph in congestive cardiomyopathy. The heart is greatly enlarged, including the pulmonary arteries and right atrium. The superior vena cava is prominent due to right-sided heart failure. Incipient pulmonary edema is present due to left-sided heart failure.

FIGURE 81C-2 Electrocardiographic abnormalities in a series of 74 patients with congestive cardiomyopathy. *(From A. Kristinsson, "Diagnosis, Natural History and Treatment of Congestive Cardiomyopathy," Ph.D. Thesis, University of London, 1969.)*

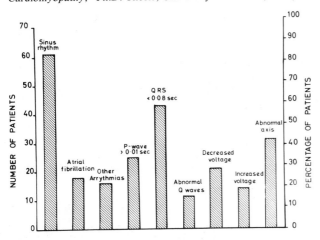

the reduced stroke volume may be compensated for by tachycardia which maintains the cardiac output. The minute volume, however, does not rise normally on exercise, which produces an increase in end-diastolic pressure in the left ventricle and thus dyspnea. In the late stages of the disease both minute volume and stroke volume are seriously compromised. It is possible however that for quite a long periods the advantage of dilatation may allow the patient a reasonable effort tolerance without symptoms. This advantage is the stimulation of an increased force of contraction by the increased end-diastolic fiber length, achieving the same stroke with less myocardial fiber shortening. Eventually, however, the disadvantages of dilatation greatly outweigh the advantages. According to Laplace's law dilatation is accompanied by greater mural tension and pressure, and these invoke a greater metabolic need and oxygen demand. There is in addition a decreased rate of fiber shortening, diminished maximal rate of increase in pressure (max dp/dt), and diminished velocity of ejection. Dilatation, therefore, is essentially a disadvantageous feature. The disadvantages of dilatation are to some extent overcome by compensatory hypertrophy, which tends to maintain overall cardiac function although the function of individual myocardial units is depressed. It might be expected, therefore, that the greater the hypertrophy, the better the compensation and the better the prognosis, and as will be seen later there is some evidence to suggest that this may be the case in some patients. The reduced cardiac output and stroke volume are accompanied by an increase in left ventricular end-diastolic pressure (Fig. 81C-4). The ejection fraction, which is reduced, is inversely related to left ventricular end-diastolic pressure.[2] Systolic and diastolic ventricular volumes, measured both by echocardiography and angiocardiography, are increased.

Reduced oxygen saturation of mixed venous blood is found in most patients and results in a high arteriovenous difference. Pulmonary artery pressure and pulmonary vascular resistance are often modestly raised as a result of the left ventricular failure, but severe degrees of pulmonary hypertension are unusual.

Angiocardiography

Angiocardiography reveals a diffusely enlarged left ventricle with generalized hypokinesis and very poor overall contraction. The normal pear-shaped contour of the left ventricle is replaced by diffuse globular enlargement. Areas of dyskinesia are not usually seen, but may be occasionally evident, and these make distinction from ischemic heart disease with myocardial infarction difficult. Filling defects in the left ventricle due to intramural thrombus may be seen. The left atrium is usually slightly, but never grossly, enlarged, and mitral regurgitation is slight, or at the most moderate, but practically never extreme.

Systolic time intervals

The ratio of pre-ejection period (PEP) to left ventricular ejection time (LVET) is abnormal in congestive cardiomyopathy. The PEP/LVET ratio varies inversely with the ejection fraction.[4] Ratios greatly above normal have been found in our laboratory.

COMPLICATIONS

The complications of congestive cardiomyopathy are mainly those of severe heart failure. Atrial fibrillation, which occurs in around 20 percent of patients, increases the risks of embolism. Embolism from the left ventricle may occur in the absence of atrial fibrillation and is presumably related to the formation of friable thrombus in the poorly contracting cavity. The symptoms that are produced will depend on the site of the embolism. Pulmonary embolism is not uncommon, particularly when congestive heart failure is severe, and patients with a low cardiac output and extensive peripheral edema are immobilized. It is

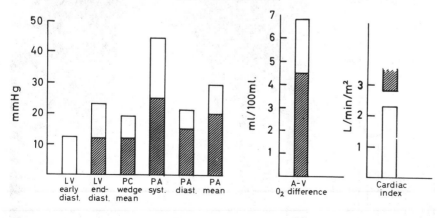

THE HAEMODYNAMIC FINDINGS IN 30 CATHETERISATIONS OF THE RIGHT HEART AND 14 CATHETERISATIONS OF THE LEFT HEART (AVERAGE VALUES)

NORMAL VALUES

FIGURE 81C-4 Results of hemodynamic study in congestive cardiomyopathy. (From A. Kristinsson, "Diagnosis, Natural History and Treatment of Congestive Cardiomyopathy," Ph.D. Thesis, University of London, 1969.)

usually secondary to deep venous thrombosis in the lower extremities but occasionally may result from the formation of thrombus in the right atrium, particularly if there is atrial fibrillation. Repeated small pulmonary emboli may progressively obliterate the pulmonary vascular bed and aggravate right-sided heart failure. Sudden death is usually due to ventricular fibrillation as a result of the cardiomyopathy but may occasionally be a result of obstruction to the pulmonary circulation by a series of emboli. Repeated pulmonary embolism may be suspected if there is progression of right-sided heart failure, attacks of unexplained tachycardia, disturbances of consciousness, or fever. Clinical examination will reveal signs of increasing pulmonary hypertension and central venous pressure with sometimes evidence of pleural reaction when the infarct is peripheral. Hemoptysis and icterus may occur when pulmonary infarction develops, but it must be emphasized that repeated and widespread pulmonary embolism can occur without any symptoms of infarction of the lungs.

NATURAL HISTORY

The course of the disease is usually steadily downhill, and death commonly ensues within 6 months to 5 years after the onset of symptoms. The first symptoms are usually those of heart failure, not infrequently preceded by an apparent upper respiratory infection. With energetic treatment the heart failure usually remits, and the patient improves but relapses after a period of months, or very occasionally, years. Recurring episodes of heart failure become increasingly difficult to control until finally the patient is in a state of severe congestive heart failure from which recovery is most unlikely. Death may occur suddenly, at any time, from ventricular fibrillation or occasionally pulmonary embolism, though sudden death is not particularly common and serious arrhythmias are not usually a problem. The development of atrial fibrillation is nearly always accompanied by deterioration and marks a further stage in the progress of the disease. Morbidity may be greatly increased at any time by the effects of systemic embolism, particularly when the embolism produces cerebral damage such as hemiplegia.

So far no particular form of treatment has been shown conclusively to influence the natural history. Early control of heart failure, prolonged bed rest, and prevention of pulmonary and systemic embolism all have a part to play.

POTENTIATING CONDITIONS; POSSIBLE CAUSAL RELATIONSHIPS; RISK FACTORS

A number of conditions have been related to, speculated upon, or identified with the syndrome of congestive cardiomyopathy. These are *systemic hypertension, pregnancy and the puerperium, immunologic disorders, virus infections,* and *chemical and physical agents which produce toxic effects on the myocardium.* Occlusive disease of the small coronary vessels, as in diabetes, and marked thyrotoxicosis have also been suggested as causes. These factors will be considered individually.

Alcohol

It has long been known that consumption of large quantities of alcohol over long periods may be followed by congestive heart failure with gross cardiomegaly. The hemodynamic clinical, radiologic, and electrocardiographic features of alcoholic cardiomyopathy are indistinguishable from those of congestive cardiomyopathy except that usually the heart failure remits if alcohol is abandoned and recurs when consumption is resumed. Eventually permanent cardiac damage occurs, and progressive deterioration sets in despite abstinence. Alcoholic cardiomyopathy is common in the United States, in parts of South Africa and Australia, and in Western Europe. The consumption of large quantities of beer has resulted in the so-called beer drinkers' heart, but factors such as fluid overload and excessive salt consumption may be involved in addition to alcohol. In many instances alcoholic cardiomyopathy is associated with heavy consumption of both spirits and wine.

The incidence of alcoholic cardiomyopathy is difficult to determine. It is said to be common in alcoholic persons, who have been shown to have diminished cardiac performance as compared with normal subjects when stressed by angiotensin.[5] Alcohol in large doses causes acute depression in myocardial function which is enhanced by barbiturates.[5] The quantity of alcohol consumed by individual patients is often hard to assess, but it is clear that most patients with congestive cardiomyopathy do not have an excessive alcoholic intake and that this is not the cause of the disease, although alcohol in small amounts may be injurious to a heart already damaged by other causes.

Alcoholic cardiomyopathy is not usually associated with marked nutritional deficiencies, and these are not considered to be important factors.[5]

Beriberi heart disease due to deficiency of vitamin B_1 produces a different clinical picture; that of high-output cardiac failure with warm extremities, bounding pulses, and edema. However a "dry" form without signs of high cardiac output has been described (Sho-shin beriberi).

Heart disease due to *cobalt,* which has been used as a frothing agent in beer, produces a congestive type of cardiomyopathy perhaps unrelated to alcohol.

The pathology of alcoholic cardiomyopathy is not specific and resembles that of congestive cardiomyopathy except that fibrosis is perhaps more common. Electron microscopic appearances are nonspecific also, although recently generalized swelling of the sarcoplasmic reticulum without disorganization has been suggestive as a characteristic feature.[5a] Vascular inflammation in the small coronary arteries has been described.[5b] An interesting and unexplained feature of alcoholic disorder is the dissociation between alcoholic liver disease and heart disease, the two organs rarely being involved in the same patients, as if the toxic effect of alcohol selects one or other organ, but not both, in the same individual. It is probable that individual susceptibility or an underlying abnormality of the heart potentiates the toxic effects of alcohol upon the myocardium.

The way in which alcohol affects the heart is uncertain. During acute administration a significant rise in osmolality occurs which is associated with an increase in plasma volume, presumably indicating a transfer fluid from the extravascular space.[4] A direct action of alcohol on the cardiac cell, possibly by affecting intracellular transfer of calcium or myosin ATP-ase activity might contribute to the late stage of myocardial depression. It has also been suggested that acetaldehyde, the first metabolite of alcohol, can significantly depress ventricular function, and this may have a role in the pathogenesis of alcoholic cardiomyopathy. Altered lipid metabolism produced by alcohol and changes in lipid composition may be responsible for the early changes in the mitochondria which occur in the cardiomyopathy. Possibly magnesium deficiency may play a part. It has been shown that feeding alcohol daily to mice can produce ultrastructural abnormalities of the myocardium despite adequate nutrition. Individual variability in response and the concentration of the alcohol in the blood in unit time may be of significance.

There is little evidence to suggest that alcohol is an important cause of congestive cardiomyopathy, but it is perfectly possible that it is an additive or conditioning factor in patients who already have cardiac damage from some other cause and that its possible importance should not be underestimated.

Systemic hypertension

High blood pressure may be associated with congestive cardiomyopathy. In a series of 74 of our patients 19 had blood pressures in excess of 140/90 mm Hg. Hypertension was present only during congestive heart failure in 7, was initially absent and later present in 3, occasionally present in 4, and consistently present in 5.[2]

Hypertension during heart failure is well known and is due either to increased catecholamine secretion, reduced renal blood flow, or both. When hypertension is present before the onset of heart failure, the syndrome of congestive cardiomyopathy could be ascribed to abnormal response of the afterload imposed on the left ventricle by the hypertension, producing dilatation and modest hypertrophy rather than progressive compensatory hypertrophy without dilatation. The low blood pressure sometimes found during severe congestive heart failure could be ascribed to a fall in cardiac output.

Hypertension and congestive cardiomyopathy are often common diseases in the same geographic populations, and it has been suggested that congestive cardiomyopathy may be "masked" hypertensive heart disease in West Africans.[6]

Hypertension has been shown to develop after heart failure has been controlled in congestive cardiomyopathy, again suggesting that the heart failure might have been of hypertensive origin rather than due to initial heart muscle disease. If so, the response of the myocardium to hypertension has been unusual, perhaps because of an underlying myocardial disorder. While hypertension may be the cause in some patients with congestive cardiomyopathy, it is apparently not an important factor in the majority of patients.

Pregnancy and the puerperium

The term peripartal cardiomyopathy has been given to a syndrome of cardiac failure occurring during the later part of pregnancy, or in the puerperium, without obvious cause and without evidence of prior heart disease. Heart failure in association with pregnancy has been recognized for over 100 years, but recently attention has been drawn to the condition again. The etiology remains obscure. The clinical, hemodynamic, and pathologic features are those of congestive cardiomyopathy, and it has been suggested that the occurrence of pregnancy is no more than fortuitous. However, the absence of heart disease before the pregnancy and a tendency to recurrence with subsequent pregnancies suggests that it is a specific condition. It appears to be more common in black than in white patients, in multiparous older women, and in the presence of twin pregnancy and toxemia. Malnutrition has been blamed as a cause but never proved. Possible adverse effects of lactation have been blamed.[7] Toxemia of pregnancy in association with peripartal cardiomyopathy is not common, but toxemia can cause a rapidly reversible form of heart failure in the postnatal period. It has been suggested that postpartum cardiomyopathy may exist in different forms. Three main groups have been postulated: those due to toxemia, those due to preexisting hypertensive heart disease, and those due to myocarditis of specific or nonspecific type. Recently it has been suggested that transient hypertension developing rapidly in the postpartum period might be responsible for heart failure that recurred with subsequent pregnancies.[8]

Peripartal cardiac failure is particularly common among the agricultural population of northern Nigeria in the region of Zaria, where ancient customs surrounding childbirth still survive and multiple pregnancies are the rule. Following delivery the women subject themselves to a constant heat load for many days. At this time the consumption of salt is particularly high. It has been suggested that perhaps the combination of excessive heat load and excessive salt consumption may be the cause of the heart failure. As in other parts of Nigeria, hypertension is particularly common, and this may be a factor also.[9]

Although commoner in black than white peoples, peripartal cardiomyopathy can occur in the absence of obvious risk factors such as alcoholism, malnutrition, toxemia, or hypertension. The possibility of viral infection has been considered when Coxsackie B infection has occurred in the puerperium.

The pathology is nonspecific and similar to that of congestive cardiomyopathy. Fibrosis may be extensive, and inflammatory changes with necrosis may be found. The coronary arteries are normal. Possibly the incidence of mural thrombi and embolism may be greater than in other forms of congestive cardiomyopathy.

The time of onset is usually in the latter months of pregnancy or within the first 10 weeks of the puerperium.

There is a marked tendency to recurrence, mortality being greater in patients with persistent cardiac enlargement than in those in whom the heart size returns to normal after the first attack. Subsequent pregnancy in a patient who retains cardiac enlargement carries a poor prognosis for the mother.

In view of the risk of recurrence in subsequent pregnancies it is likely that the disorder is a specific entity, the cause of which remains unknown. However, conditioning factors may well be necessary for its development, as in other forms of congestive cardiomyopathy, and these could be metabolic, immunologic, infective, or hypertensive.

Immunologic disorders

Although immunoglobulin binding in heart muscle cells in patients with congestive cardiomyopathy has been described, immunologic factors do not appear to play a primary role in etiology or pathogenesis of congestive cardiomyopathy. Reactive antibody responses are more likely to represent a secondary immunologic phenomenon, perhaps as a result of previous infection.[10]

The relation of virus infection to congestive cardiomyopathy

Using immunofluorescent techniques evidence of Coxsackie B antigen in the myocardium has been found in a third of routine postmortem specimens, and it has been claimed that immunofluorescent Coxsackie B viral antigen has even been found on cardiac valves. Coxsackie B antigen has also been found in the heart of a patient with evidence of pancarditis in life. Animal studies have shown clearly that acute infection of the myocardium can be produced by the Coxsackie viruses. A number of mechanisms may be important in the production of myocardial injury by viruses. These are: direct invasion of the myocardial cell; involvement of the central nervous system and a direct effect on the myocardium; myocardial metabolic disturbances; myocardial vascular disturbances; combination of myocardial toxins; and antigen-antibody reactions.[11] So-called conditioning factors such as trauma may influence the virulence of the virus.

The onset of congestive cardiomyopathy may be associated with symptoms suggesting an infection, sometimes of the upper respiratory tract, which could possibly be of viral origin, and it has been suggested that congestive cardiomyopathy could be

the result of previous viral myocarditis. There is, however, very little information regarding the transition from acute myocarditis to chronic congestive cardiomyopathy, and little evidence to implicate virus infection in patients with established congestive cardiomyopathy. The transition from acute pyrexial illness with involvement of the myocardium to a chronic state of cardiomyopathy has been described in individual cases, and persistent cardiac abnormalities have been recognized in a third of a group of patients 5 years after acute myocarditis. The development of congestive cardiomyopathy has been described after arbovirus infections in Ceylon. An increased incidence has been found of complement-fixing antibodies to various viruses, including poliomyelitis, Coxsackie B, and influenza in the blood of patients with idiopathic cardiomyopathy as compared to controls. In one patient, positive fluorescence for adenovirus antigen in the nuclei of the myocardial cells from a biopsy of the right ventricular myocardium has been demonstrated.[1] Our own preliminary studies have demonstrated an increase in titer in the blood of antibodies to Coxsackie B_4 virus in patients with congestive cardiomyopathy and in those with acute myopericarditis, as compared to controls. Possibly, when the heart is damaged by acute virus infection, further damage results from autoimmune processes.

Further investigation of virus infections of the myocardium as cause of congestive cardiomyopathy may be the most fruitful line of enquiry to pursue. Failure to demonstrate evidence of a previous infective process in the myocardium does not exclude a previous virus infection.

Allied conditions and experimental studies

It is possible that clues to the causation of congestive cardiomyopathy might be obtained from similar cardiac disorders due to a known toxic cause, or from experimental studies in animals.

Daunorubicin cardiomyopathy

The cardiomyopathy produced by daunorubicin provides an example of a direct myocardial toxic action with specific effects on enzyme function leading often to progressive pump failure and death. Daunorubicin is an antibiotic which is particularly effective in acute myeloblastic leukemia but has also been used in other leukemias. The mechanism of cardiac toxicity is incompletely understood, but it is likely that it is connected with binding of the drug to DNA in nuclei and mitochondria. Once bound, the drug is only very slowly liberated from the cell. Cardiac muscle cells cannot reproduce themselves, and hence any inhibition of protein synthesis resulting from alteration in the DNA end plates could persist. Cumulative interference with the processes of normal protein regeneration, replenishment and growth might explain the delayed onset of signs of toxicity and also the fact that adults appear to be more vulnerable than children, and the elderly most vulnerable of all. It has been shown that cardiac toxicity is dependent upon the dose in children but not always in adults. Cardiac symptoms do not usually occur for between 3 to 6 months after starting treatment but can be delayed for weeks or months after treatment has been completed. Symptoms due to heart failure may develop with remarkable rapidity, sinus tachycardia with gallop rhythm, hypotension, dyspnea, tachypnea, and signs of left ventricular insufficiency predominate at this stage. Because of the rapidity of the onset of heart failure the heart may not be greatly enlarged, although signs of increased left atrial pressure may appear in the lung fields. Early electrocardiographic changes are slight and consist of reduction in voltage of the QRS and ST-segment and repolarization abnormalities. There are few detailed studies of cardiac function but noninvasive tests have shown progressively diminishing stroke volume and diminished velocity of contraction.

At necropsy there is generalized ventricular dilatation unless death occurs very rapidly after the onset of cardiac failure. As in congestive cardiomyopathy, mural thrombosis in the ventricles is not infrequently seen. Endocardial fibrosis may occur, causing restrictive features. Ultrastructural examination shows degenerating atrophic myocardial cells, alteration of nuclear chromatin, and changes in the mitochondria.

Cardiac damage as a result of daunorubicin results from a direct toxic effect of the drug on the cardiac muscle cell, producing progressive cardiac insufficiency.[12] Daunorubicin cardiomyopathy, when produced in animals, could prove a useful model on which the effect of additional conditioning agents such as hypertension, alcohol, infections, etc., might be studied. The need for a search for a toxic agent in congestive cardiomyopathy that might act in the same or a similar way as daunorubicin is evident.

Cobalt cardiomyopathy

In 1965 investigators in Quebec and in Omaha observed an endemic cardiomyopathy with the characteristics of congestive cardiomyopathy, some cases terminating fatally with predominantly right-sided congestive failure. The cause of the cardiac damage was finally traced to small amounts of cobalt introduced into the beer as a frothing agent. At autopsy the hearts were enlarged and overweight, the chambers being dilated and often containing mural thrombi. Histopathologic changes consisted of hyaline necrosis and dystrophic vacuolar degeneration of cardiac muscle cells. There was swelling of muscle fibers, uneven staining of the sarcoplasm, and disorganization of contractile elements. Fatty tissue replacement of the myofibrils was noted. Fibrosis was variable. Extracardiac lesions consisted of pleural effusions and thromboembolism involving many arteries. Additional features were pericardial effusion, polycythemia, and a tendency for involvement of the thyroid gland.

Experimental studies in which rats were given cobalt produced similar results, but it was found that conditioning factors, particularly protein deficiency, were necessary for reproduction of the human type of the disease. In the experimental model the primary abnormality appeared to be mitochondrial damage due to an enzymatic block of oxidative decarboxylation of pyruvate and alpha-ketoglutarate levels.[13] Ultrastructural studies demonstrated depression of the activity of the mitochondrial oxidative enzyme succinate dehydrogenase. A feature which differed from the human form was a tendency to polypoid vegetative endocarditis.

Cobalt cardiomyopathy seems now to have disappeared as a result of removal of traces of cobalt from beer. From the experimental studies it seems possible that in human beings conditioning factors, particularly low protein intake, may have facilitated the toxicity of cobalt. An anomaly that has never been satisfactorily explained is the observation that the quantities of cobalt in beer were exceedingly small and less than those given for the treatment of pernicious anemia. It seems likely that the full story of cobalt cardiomyopathy has not yet been told. In general the changes in the myocardium appear to have been more severe than in congestive cardiomyopathy on histopathologic studies. It seems unlikely that ingestion of minute quantities of cobalt is a factor in the causation of congestive cardiomyopathy.

Parasitic cardiomyopathy
(see Chap. 80)

The most important form is that due to South American trypanosomiasis or Chagas' disease. The infecting parasite, *Trypanosoma cruzei,* is transmitted to human beings by a bedbug vector which drops from the ceiling at night and enters the body by biting the eye or other parts of the face. Acute, followed by chronic, heart disease follows. In the acute form there are two local manifestations: first, an elastic, hard, but not painful edema around the eye, often unilateral and accompanied by conjunctival infection and discoloration of the skin, and second, lymphadenopathy involving the preauricular and cervical lymph nodes. There may be fever, sweating, anorexia, vomiting, and diarrhea. Hepatosplenomegaly and edema are common. The acute cardiomyopathy is due to multiplication of the parasite in the cardiac muscle fibers with a severe interstitial cellular reaction with polymorphonuclear neutrophils. Parasites can be identified within the cardiac muscle fibers. The cardiovascular signs consist of tachycardia and arterial hypotension and gallop rhythm and cardiac enlargement. The electrocardiogram shows prolonged P-R and Q-T intervals, flattening or inversion of T waves and depression of the ST segment with low-voltage QRS complexes. The cardiovascular signs may disappear completely, and the patient then enters the latent phase of the disease which may last for up to 20 years. The chronic phase is often ushered in by symptoms of arrhythmias such as palpitations or syncope, and the electrocardiogram may show right bundle branch block and multiple ectopic beats. The disease then progresses to heart failure. At any stage complete atrial or ventricular block with Adams-Stokes attacks or sudden death may occur. A small apical aneurysm of the left ventricle is common. Thrombosis may develop in the aneurysm and embolism follow.

The features of Chagasic cardiomyopathy have little or nothing in common with those of congestive cardiomyopathy, and the infective agent can be readily demonstrated in the myocardium. It is useful to consider it as a contrast to congestive cardiomyopathy, where no evidence of an infective agent is usually found.

Catecholamines and congestive cardiomyopathy

It has been known for some time that administration of large quantities of catecholamines to human beings may produce subendocardial necrosis. Animal experiments have shown that administration of catecholamines will increase the rate of protein synthesis and induce hypertrophy without preceding decompensation. The natural course of the hereditary cardiomyopathy of syrian hampsters can be accelerated by digitalis and catecholamines if given in a vulnerable phase of the disease, while beta blocking agents can inhibit the effect of catecholamines. It has been suggested that high sympathetic tone in humans with cardiomyopathy will induce an increased rate of protein synthesis, hypertrophy, necrosis, and deterioration in heart function.[14] It remains to be seen whether excessive catecholamine discharge or secretion is a factor in the etiology of congestive cardiomyopathy in human beings.

Ventricular hypertrophy in congestive cardiomyopathy

Some degree of hypertrophy is almost invariable in congestive cardiomyopathy. Many hearts are substantially overweight, and although the thickness of the ventricular muscle may not be greatly increased, the excessive weight must denote considerable hypertrophy, for dilatation stretches and reduces the thickness of the ventricular wall. Whatever the underlying disorder, the exact stimuli to myocardial hypertrophy are not yet fully understood. One stimulus might be an increase in tension of the myocardial fibers resulting from dilatation. An increase in oxygen consumption and energy production as a result of myocardial damage might act as a signal to the genetic apparatus activating RNA through chromosomal DNA. In some conditions, such as aortic regurgitation, ventricular dilatation is the result of an obligatory increase in ventricular volume as a result of the regurgitation. It seems likely that the dilatation thus acts as a stimulus to the hypertrophy which is necessary to achieve the extra power of contraction required. It is notable that the massively dilated and hypertrophied left ventricle of chronic aortic regurgitation may retain adequate cardiac function for many years, although the function of individual units of hypertrophied myocardium is reduced, and thus extreme cardiomegaly militates against successful aortic valve replacement. However, hypertrophy in these circumstances is clearly compensatory, at least up to a point. Three stages of compensatory hypertrophy have been defined: first, the stage of damage; second, the stage of stable hyperfunction; and third, the stage of exhaustion. In the first stage energy production, oxygen consumption, and oxidative phosphorylation increase, as does the synthesis of protein and DNA and RNA. In the second stage there is decrease in myocardial catecholamine stores and an increase in lactic acid synthesis. Reduction of contractility begins at this stage. In the third stage there is a fall in ATP-ase activity and decrease in the activity of mitrochondrial enzymes as a prelude to established heart failure.[15]

When the dilatation is the result of direct myocardial damage, the situation may be different, though little experimental data is available, for most of the experimental work on hypertrophy has been related to that which has been produced by increased ventricular afterload. In such circumstances adaptive hypertrophy can develop in a matter of days. In rats, both altitude hypoxia and physical training produce an increased capacity for energy transport, but not hypertrophy. Previous exercise training to hypoxia at altitude prevents disturbances of metabolic function in the stages of hypofunction. When experimental coarctation of the aorta has been produced in rats, myocardial hypertrophy develops within a few days, and only a minority of the animals die in heart failure during the first week. If hypertrophy is prevented by the administration of actinomycin D, the majority die within the first week. Actinomycin D has no direct effect on myocardial function.[16] Similar results have been obtained when protein synthesis is inhibited by a protein-free diet.

Although hypertrophy occurs in congestive cardiomyopathy, ventricular dilatation is much more impressive, and it has been suggested[17,18] that agents that damage the myocardium may interfere with contractile function by preventing calcium binding by troponin and that the deficient contractile function that follows results in ventricular dilatation, increased wall tension, and failure of the RNA/DNA response needed to produce hypertrophy. This speculation is based on personal experience which suggests that the prognosis is directly related to the degree of hypertrophy and that patients live longest who have the greatest degree of hypertrophy. There are of course notable exceptions to this generalization, but the theory deserves further study.

Failure to discover any characteristic feature in the myocardium in congestive cardiomyopathy suggests that the appearances may represent merely a graveyard of dead tissue without indicating the cause of the damage. Examination of the finer processes of myocardial chemistry and cellular biology beyond the boundaries of structure and ultrastructure are required. Studies of enzyme function carried out on biopsy specimens have yielded interesting information which will be dealt with later in this chapter.

The coronary arteries in congestive cardiomyopathy

General experience is uniform that the major coronary arteries are normal. They are widely patent with smooth lumens and show only occasional minimal narrowing, presumably due to small incidental plaques of atheroma. Occlusive changes have been described in small intramural coronary arteries of sizes between 80 to 500 pm, but it is not known whether these changes are the result of the myocardial disorder or the cause. Endomyocardial biopsy studies in patients with congestive cardiomyopathy have not revealed occlusive changes or other abnormalities in arterioles included in the biopsy specimens.

The distinction from ischemic heart disease due to atherosclerosis of the major coronary arteries can be difficult, for chest pain is present in a small number of patients with congestive cardiomyopathy, and the electrocardiogram may suggest anterior infarction. These appearances are probably due to multiple areas of damaged myocardium which interfere with interventricular conduction with loss of positive forces.[3]

The contractile pattern of the left ventricle is different in ischemic heart disease due to coronary occlusion and in congestive cardiomyopathy. In the former there are usually one or more areas of dyskinesia due to old infarction, whereas in the latter the left ventricle is diffusely hypokinetic without regional abnormalities of wall movement. Occasionally, however, regional dyskinesia may be seen in congestive cardiomyopathy, presumably reflecting larger areas of scarring and fibrosis than is usual.

Diabetes and congestive cardiomyopathy

When heart disease occurs in diabetic subjects, it is almost invariably due to organic occlusive disease of the major coronary arteries or hypertension or both. Congestive cardiomyopathy in diabetic subjects has been ascribed to occlusive disease in the small coronary arteries akin to that which may be found in other arteries of similar size elsewhere in the body in diabetic patients.

Thyroid heart disease and congestive cardiomyopathy

The relationship of disturbed thyroid function to congestive cardiomyopathy is not known. Classically thyrotoxicosis produces a high-output type of heart failure in young persons in sinus rhythm, or a low-output type of heart failure in older subjects with toxic nodular goiter and atrial fibrillation. It is

thought that excessive thyroid hormone damages the myocardium in some way. Occult thyrotoxicosis, in which clinical evidence of thyroid dysfunction is absent, may present with severe right-sided heart failure which may persist for many years. Although thyroid function tests are usually normal in congestive cardiomyopathy, it is wise to look for any evidence of disturbed thyroid function, as it is a treatable condition. Similarly, congestive heart failure in myxedema, with pericardial effusion is well recognized, but a relationship to congestive cardiomyopathy has not been established.

"Ischemic" cardiomyopathy

The term ischemic cardiomyopathy has been applied to patients who develop severe cardiac insufficiency and pump failure on a basis of occlusive coronary artery disease, and in whom the emphasis of the disease is on progressive heart failure rather than on episodes of infarction and angina. Although in 90 to 95 percent of patients with appreciable coronary artery disease ischemic pain or infarction is common, in the remaining small proportion a syndrome of progressive heart failure may dominate the picture, and the patient may present with the syndrome of congestive cardiomyopathy. It seems confusing, however, to refer to this condition as "ischemic" cardiomyopathy since it is clearly the result of coronary artery disease and should be described as such.

An alternative view may be taken in patients with apparent ischemic cardiac pain which occurs in the absence of demonstrable coronary artery disease. In such patients it is customary to consider conditions such as coronary artery spasm, coronary embolism, or primary thrombosis, while the association of cardiac pain with "normal" coronary arteries is well recognized in such conditions as prolapse of the mitral valve and hypertrophic cardiomyopathy. It is possible that in certain circumstances primary disease of the myocardial elements may be the cause of ischemic pain in the absence of vascular abnormality. This thesis has yet to be explored.

DIFFERENTIAL DIAGNOSIS OF CONGESTIVE CARDIOMYOPATHY

The differential diagnosis is that of the causes of congestive heart failure. Organic valvular or congenital heart disease can usually be readily differentiated, and the principal differential diagnoses are from ischemic heart disease, hypertensive heart disease, and specific heart muscle disease.

Ischemic heart disease

In ischemic heart disease, there is almost invariably a history of cardiac pain, angina of effort, unstable angina, or cardiac infarction. There may be a family history of heart disease, and clinical examination may reveal the stigmata of metabolic arterial disease such as arcus cornealis, plaques of cholesterol on the skin or tendons, and evidence of poor carbohydrate tolerance. It must be admitted that many patients with ischemic heart disease do not show any of these abnormalities. Examination of the heart may be clinically quite normal although third or fourth heart sounds are quite common in chronic coronary artery disease. Abnormal, diffuse, or paradoxic pulsation of the left ventricle, superior and internal to the impulse, and suggesting a cardiac aneurysm is a strong pointer towards ischemic heart disease. The electrocardiogram can be most helpful by showing clear evidence of previous infarction in ischemic heart disease. Occasionally the appearances can be misleading, as has already been mentioned. Conduction defects may occur both in ischemic heart disease and congestive cardiomyopathy, but left bundle branch block is slightly more common in cardiomyopathy. Absolute proof is dependent upon the demonstration of coronary artery disease by selective coronary arteriography and of regional dyskinesia by left ventricular angiography. But in 90 percent of patients the diagnosis of congestive cardiomyopathy can be made with accuracy by clinical methods and bedside diagnosis.

Hypertensive heart disease

The relation of hypertension to congestive cardiomyopathy has already been discussed. Patients with established hypertensive heart disease usually have marked left ventricular hypertrophy and evidence of long-standing hypertensive vascular disease elsewhere in the body, particularly in the optic fundi, before heart failure develops. Moreover, episodes of left ventricular failure are usually related to substantial increases in systemic blood pressure, often on an acute basis. Difficulty may arise in the differential diagnosis when heart failure persists despite only moderate hypertension. Diagnosis then is likely to lie between hypertensive heart disease, coronary artery disease, and congestive cardiomyopathy, the presence of definite cardiac pain favoring the diagnosis of ischemic heart disease.

Rare specific heart muscle disease (see Chaps. 80 and 82)

It is of vital importance, faced with a patient with apparent congestive cardiomyopathy, to exclude specific heart muscle diseases for which there may be specific treatment. This can usually be done by bedside diagnosis. Full clinical examination should usually suffice to exclude conditions such as diffuse systemic sclerosis, systemic lupus erythematosus, polyarteritis, hemochromatosis, peripheral myopathy, or Friedreich's ataxia. Sarcoidosis of the myocardium may be more difficult to distinguish and should be suspected when there are multiple arrhythmias or heart block, both of which are uncommon in congestive cardiomyopathy. Examples of some useful clinical clues are

1 Diffuse systemic sclerosis: Raynaud's phenomenon, telagiectasia, calcinosis around the terminal phalanges, hypertension, dysphagia, renal impairment
2 Systemic lupus erythematosus: hypertension, joint involvement, renal lesions, hemolytic anemia, pericarditis, possibly liver involvement
3 Polyarteritis nodosa: peripheral neuropathy, hypertension, pericarditis, renal disease, abdominal pain, pulmonary involvement
4 Sarcoidosis: arrhythmias and heart block, lung changes, positive liver biopsy, positive lymph gland biopsy, salivary gland enlargement, ocular involvement, negative tuberculin reaction, erythema nodosum
5 Hemochromatosis: pigmentation, diabetes mellitus, cirrhosis of the liver, high serum iron level, family history
6 Peripheral skeletal myopathy: limb-girdle weakness
7 Friedreich's ataxia: cerebellar signs

Cardiac features which may be useful in the differential diagnosis are a tendency for arrhythmias and heart block in sarcoidosis and the peripheral myopathies, and the presence of pericardial friction in polyarteritis, systemic lupus erythematosus, or virus infection.

Hypertrophic cardiomyopathy
(see Chap. 81A)

Occasionally when obstruction to left ventricular outflow is absent hypertrophic cardiomyopathy may be difficult to distinguish from congestive cardiomyopathy, particularly when atrial fibrillation or heart failure has developed. A past history of angina is commoner in hypertrophic cardiomyopathy than in congestive cardiomyopathy, as is a history of syncope. The jerky, ill-sustained arterial pulse, while not as striking as in patients with obstruction, may still be retained in those without obstruction and contrasts with the small-volume pulse of congestive cardiomyopathy. If sinus rhythm has persisted in hypertrophic cardiomyopathy, the presence of a left atrial beat is strong evidence. The powerful left ventricular thrust of hypertrophic cardiomyopathy, with its ill-sustained character, is not usually seen in congestive cardiomyopathy. However, in some patients with congestive cardiomyopathy of long standing who have considerable left ventricular hypertrophy the differential diagnosis may be difficult. It is exceptional to find an atrial beat in congestive cardiomyopathy, and its presence virtually denies the diagnosis. The electrocardiogram in hypertrophic cardiomyopathy is likely to show considerably greater voltage in leads reflecting left ventricular action potentials than in congestive cardiomyopathy. The echocardiogram is of value in differential diagnosis, for the septum will be disproportionately thick in hypertrophic cardiomyopathy, and the left ventricular cavity will be small, whereas in congestive cardiomyopathy the septum will be of normal thickness and the ventricular cavity dilated. Diastolic closure rate of the mitral valve is likely to be slow in hypertrophic cardiomyopathy but rapid in congestive cardiomyopathy. Final differentiation in difficult patients may depend upon left ventricular angiography, which shows the characteristic abnormally shaped cavity with massive hypertrophy in hypertrophic cardiomyopathy as compared with the diffusely dilated, poorly contractile left ventricle with moderate hypertrophy in congestive cardiomyopathy.

Constrictive pericarditis and restrictive cardiomyopathy
(see Chap. 84)

Lesions producing cardiac constriction or restriction may sometimes be confused with congestive cardiomyopathy. The major differential diagnostic point is usually the character of the jugular venous pulse, which shows the typical M-shaped pattern with prominent *a* and *v* waves and sharp *x*, and particularly *y* descents. Unlike congestive cardiomyopathy the cardiac impulse may be impalpable, and the heart appears to be of normal size. A third heart sound is invariable in constrictive pericarditis except in a few exceptionally severe cases. It tends to occur earlier than in congestive cardiomyopathy. Hemodynamic studies reveal equal pressures in end-diastole in both ventricles and equal left and right atrial pressures in constrictive pericarditis, whereas in congestive cardiomyopathy the corresponding pressures are usually higher in the left side of the heart. Left ventricular angiography in constrictive pericarditis usually reveals normal contraction as opposed to grossly impaired contraction in congestive cardiomyopathy. A paradoxic arterial pulse is common in constrictive pericarditis, as is increase in the venous pressure on inspiration. These features are both uncommon in congestive cardiomyopathy. Thus the differential diagnosis from constrictive pericarditis should not be difficult, but differentiation between congestive cardiomyopathy and restrictive cardiomyopathy can cause problems, for the heart in restrictive cardiomyopathy is not infrequently enlarged, and the differential diagnosis clinically may depend mainly upon the character of the venous pulse and the paradox in the arterial pulse. The final proof depends upon angiography and cardiac catheterization.

Other causes of congestive cardiac failure

The onset of congestive cardiac failure is not in itself a diagnosis and the question "What is the cause of the heart failure?" must always be asked. Common causes of heart failure that are not always appreciated are recurrent pulmonary embolism; infective endocarditis; severe anemia; thyrotoxicosis; and pericardial effusion with tamponade. Rarer causes are atrial myxoma; tricuspid stenosis; and obliterative pulmonary hypertension. Occasionally in extremely severe aortic stenosis with heart failure and a low cardiac output, murmurs may be trivial and the anacrotic nature of the pulse obscured by the extremely low cardiac output. Demonstration of calcification in the aortic valve may provide crucial evidence. Finally, the presence of signs of unexpectedly high cardiac output such as peripheral vasodilatation and warm extremities should suggest a cause such as thyrotoxicosis, severe anemia, arteriovenous fistula, chronic liver disease, cor pulmonale, extensive Paget's disease, or beriberi.

Not infrequently patients with a chronic pericardial effusion are misdiagnosed as having congestive cardiomyopathy because of the apparent cardiomegaly on chest radiography. The differential diagnosis can be made quite readily, for the patient with a large chronic pericardial effusion has no signs of heart muscle disease and notably no gallop rhythm, although the signs of tamponade may not be present if effusion is chronic. The electrocardiogram tends to be normal or to show only slight reduction of voltage of the QRS-ST complex, the T waves remaining normal. The echocardiogram should provide certain differentiation by showing the presence of the effusion and usually normal ventricular function. A third heart sound in the presence of a pericardial effusion suggests either that there is associated heart muscle disease or that constrictive pericarditis is developing.

TREATMENT OF CONGESTIVE CARDIOMYOPATHY

The treatment of congestive cardiomyopathy remains unsatisfactory and is likely to do so until the causes are identified. Control of heart failure with digitalis and diuretics is essential. It is important to advise complete withdrawal of alcohol. There is no evidence that smoking is deleterious to patients with congestive cardiomyopathy, but its adverse effects on the heart and circulation make it sensible to advise against it.

Prolonged bed rest may have a part to play in certain patients and, in distinction to ischemic heart disease, physical activity should be restricted and only reduced activity allowed for the 12 months following the first episode of heart failure.

The use of steroids is sometimes advocated for congestive cardiomyopathy. No definite evidence of their value has been shown, though symptomatic improvement may be produced. Steroids do not appear to cause any deterioration in congestive cardiomyopathy, but experimental work has shown that myocardial lesions in mice produced by Coxsackie B virus can be increased by the administration of steroids. In view of the possibility of virus infection being implicated in some patients with congestive cardiomyopathy the routine use of steroids is not advised. They may, however, have an important part to play in certain specific heart muscle diseases, particularly sarcoidosis and the connective tissue disorders.

Recently the effect of some new inotropic agents and agents which reduce the afterload on the left ventricle have been studied. An example of the former is glucagon, which stimulates adenyl cyclase systems to produce cyclic AMP without stimulating ectopic activity and can produce improvement in myocardial function in patients who are acutely ill. The improvement, however, is not sustained after 48 to 72 h, possibly because of the exhaustion of severely damaged muscle cells or the occupation of glucagon receptors in the myocardium.[19] Personal experience confirms that intravenous glucagon can improve myocardial function temporarily and may be useful in a crisis. A bolus of 3 mg or 1 to 2 mg/h may be used in an infusion. Bolus injection is followed by a transient rise and then a fall in pre-ejection period with an initial increase in heart rate and an initial increase and then reduction in left ventricular ejection time. The PEP/LVET ratio tends to fall and then to rise. Phentolamine, which blocks alpha receptors, and unloads the left ventricle by producing peripheral vasodilatation may have a direct inotropic effect in heart failure. Experience has shown (T. Hardason, personal communication) an increase in left ventricular ejection time, a fall in pre-ejection period, and a fall in the PEP/LVET ratio, suggesting a true increase in inotropic activity. As with glucagon the effects were transient.[20]

Salbutamol, a beta-adrenergic stimulant widely used for the treatment of bronchial asthma, can produce striking improvement in cardiac function when given intravenously. Our acute studies in congestive cardiomyopathy (B. Sharma, personal communication) showed an increase in cardiac output and stroke volume and a fall in left ventricular end-diastolic pressure with only a slight increase in heart rate and fall in systemic blood pressure. The improvement may be considered essentially to be due to reduction in afterload of the left ventricle with a secondary inotropic effect, but a primary inotropic effect has also been postulated.

Of the three drugs the most effective is probably salbutamol, which can be given by continuous intravenous infusion at a rate of 2 to 8 μg/min. Recently the use of beta-adrenergic blockade in certain patients with congestive cardiomyopathy has been suggested.[14] In the only report so far available 7 patients with congestive cardiomyopathy were selected on the basis of an increased heart rate at rest. All patients were on oral treatment with digitalis and diuretics and were treated with either alprenolol or practolol for an average of 5.4 months. They were in a steady state or were progressively deteriorating when the treatment was started. Virus infection of the heart was thought to have occurred previously in 6 of the 7 patients. All patients improved clinically, and noninvasive studies showed improvement in left ventricular function. It was considered that excessive catecholamine activity might have been an important factor in the development of the cardiomyopathy, but it is possible that these patients were suffering from the effects of acute infection of the heart and might have improved spontaneously.

Without further data it would be unwise to treat patients with congestive cardiomyopathy with beta-adrenergic blocking agents in view of their myocardial depressant action, which is likely to be unfavorable in patients with severely depressed contractile function. Further studies of catecholamine secretion

and output in congestive cardiomyopathy are clearly needed in order to define those patients who may benefit from this apparently paradoxic form of treatment.

The long-term treatment of congestive cardiomyopathy with newer drugs remains difficult. Salbutamol has been shown to be ineffective when given orally, and phentolamine is not available in an oral form, though phenoxybenzamine could presumably be used as an alternative. Nitrites have been shown to improve left ventricular failure in ischemic heart disease and might possibly have a place.

Anticoagulants should be advised when a patient is immobilized for long periods, particularly in the presence of a low cardiac output and peripheral edema as is common in congestive cardiomyopathy. If there is severe hepatic congestion, depression of factor VII may occur, and the prothrombin time may be prolonged, so that the dose of anticoagulants required to prevent venous thrombosis and embolism may be quite small. When either systemic or pulmonary embolism has occurred, heparin should be given initially followed by oral anticoagulants. The possibility of low-dose intramuscular heparin (50 mg every 12 h) as a prophylaxis for venous thrombosis should be considered. It is very unlikely that heparin in this dosage will have any effect on established thrombosis, however.

Surgical treatment of congestive cardiomyopathy

As it would be expected, there is really no possibility of surgical treatment. Pericardiotomy has been suggested and carried out in the past, but the rationale is not clear and convincing evidence of lasting improvement has not been published. In severe and intractable cases in young persons the possibility of cardiac transplantation may have to be considered.

Endomyocardial biopsy in congestive cardiomyopathy

The place of biopsy has not yet been fully defined. There are four main objectives however: first, to obtain a definitive diagnosis; second, to follow the progress of treatment by serial biopsies, as in cardiac transplantation; third, to determine prognosis; and fourth, to investigate and correlate histochemical and biochemical function of the deranged myocardial cell.[21]

With regard to diagnosis, endomyocardial biopsy has so far proved disappointing. This is not surprising in congestive cardiomyopathy since even extensive ultrastructural study after death has failed to elucidate the causes. Biopsy may be valuable in the rare specific heart muscle diseases where lesions such as sarcoidosis may be discovered or important abnormalities in arterioles might be detected.

As a tool for investigating further the abnormal

processes involved in congestive cardiomyopathy biopsy is of great importance, and already enzyme abnormalities have been detected. Enzymes on the various subcellular organelles have been assayed in both control and diseased cardiac muscle. Reduced levels of mitochondrial dehydrogenases and of myofibrillar ATP-ase with threefold increase in lactic dehydrogenases were found in patients with depressed myocardial function. It has been suggested that diminished myocardial contractility in congestive cardiomyopathy is associated with impairment of mitochondrial energy production and thus with anaerobic glycolysis.[22] It remains to be seen whether these changes will be consistent in a larger series and whether they will lead to the detection of a specific fault or toxic agent.

In the present state of knowledge endomyocardial biopsy should not be used as a routine investigation in all patients with heart muscle disease or as an occasional diagnostic exercise, but should be performed as part of an intensive research protocol into the causes and management of congestive cardiomyopathy.

REFERENCES

1 Kawai, C.: Idiopathic Cardiomyopathy, A Study on the Infectious-Immune Theory as a Cause of the Disease, *Jpn. Circ. J.*, 35:765, 1971.

2 Kristinsson, A.: "Diagnosis, Natural History and Treatment of Congestive Cardiomyopathy," Ph.D. thesis, University of London, 1969, p. 35.

3 Gau, G. T., Goodwin, J. F., Oakley, C. M, Olsen, E. G. J., Rahimtoola, S. H., Raphael, M. J., and Steiner, R. E.: Q Waves and Coronary Arteriography in Cardiomyopathies, *Br. Heart J.*, 34:1034, 1972.

4 Weissler, A. M., Lewis, R. P., and Leighton, R. F.: The Systolic Time Intervals as a Measurement of Left Ventricular Performance in Man, in "Progress in Cardiology," vol. 1, P. N. Yu and J. F. Goodwin (eds.), Lea & Febiger, Philadelphia, 1972, p. 155.

5 Regan, T. J.: Alcoholic Cardiomyopathy, in N. O. Fowler (ed.), "Myocardial Disease," Grune & Stratton, Inc., New York, 1973, p. 233.

5a Bulloch, R. T., Pearce, M. B., Murphy, M. D., Jenkins, B. J., and Davis, J. L.: Myocardial Lesions in Idiopathic and Alcoholic Cardiomyopathy, *Am. J. Cardiol.*, 29:15, 1972.

5b Factor, S. M.: Intramyocardial Small-vessel Disease in Chronic Alcoholism, *Am. Heart J.*, 92:561, 1976.

6 Brockington, I. F., and Edington, G. M.: Adult Heart Disease in Western Nigeria. A Clinico-pathological Synopsis, *Am. Heart J.*, 83:27, 1972.

7 Seftel, H., and Susser, M.: Maternity and Myocardial Failure in African Women, *Br. Heart J.*, 23:43, 1961.

8 Brockington, I. F.: Postpartum Hypertensive Heart Failure, *Am. J. Cardiol.*, 27:650, 1971.

9 Davidson, N. McD., and Parry, E. H. O.: Peripartum Cardiac Failure. An Explanation for the Observed Geographic Distribution in Nigeria, *Bull. WHO*, 51:203, 1975.

10 Hess, E. V., and Karsner, A.: Immunological Studies in Myocardial Diseases, in N. O. Fowler, (ed.), "Myocardial Diseases," Grune & Stratton, Inc., New York, 1973, p. 281.

11 Burch, G. E., and Giles, T. D.: Viral Cardiomyopathy, in "Recent Advances in Studies on Cardiac Structure and Metabolism," E. Bajusz and G. Rona (eds.), vol. 2, "Cardiomyopathies," University Park Press, Baltimore, 1973, p. 121.

12 Editorial: Daunorubicin and the Heart, *Br. Med. J.*, 2:431, 1974.

13 Rona, G., and Chapel, C. I.: Pathogenesis and Pathology of Cobalt Cardiomyopathy, in "Recent Advances in Studies on Cardiac Structure and Metabolism," E. Bajusz and G. Rona (eds.), vol. 2, "Cardiomyopathies," University Park Press, Baltimore, 1973, p. 407.

14 Waagstein, F., Hjalmarson, A., Varnauskas, E., and Wallentin, I.: Effect of Chronic Beta Adrenergic Receptor Blockade in Congestive Cardiomyopathy, *Br. Heart J.*, 37:1022, 1975.

15 Meerson, F. Z.: The Myocardium in Hyperfunction, Hypertrophy and Heart Failure, *Circ. Res.*, 25(suppl. 2):35, 1969.

16 Meerson, F. Z.: Mechanisms of Hypertrophy of the Heart and Experimental Prevention of Acute Cardiac Insufficiency, *Br. Heart J.*, 33(suppl.):100, 1971.

17 Goodwin, J. F.: The Congestive and Hypertrophic Cardiomyopathies: A Decade of Study, *Lancet*, 1:733, 1970.

18 Goodwin, J. F.: Prospects and Predictions for the Cardiomyopathies, *Circulation*, 50:210, 1974.

19 Glick, G.: Glucagon, A Perspective, *Circulation*, 45:513, 1972, (editorial).

20 Goodwin, J. F.: Relationships among Hypertrophy, Hypertension and Coronary Arterial Patterns and Pharmacological Responses in Cardiomyopathies, in "Recent Advances in Studies on Cardiac Structure and Metabolism," N. S. Dhalla and G. Rona (eds.), vol. 3, "Myocardial Metabolism," University Park Press, Baltimore, p. 431.

21 Brooksby, I. A. B., Coltart, D. J., and Webb-Peploe, M. M.: Progress in Endomyocardial Biopsy, *Mod. Concepts Cardiovasc. Dis.*, 44:65, 1975.

22 Peters, T. J., Wells, C., Oakley, C. M., Brooksby, I. A. B., Webb-Peploe, M. M., and Coltart, D. J.: Enzyme Studies in Myocardial Biopsies in Congestive Cardiomyopathy, *Br. Heart J.*, 37:380, 1975.

D
Obliterative and Restrictive Cardiomyopathies

JOHN F. GOODWIN, M.D.

OBLITERATIVE CARDIOMYOPATHY

Obliterative cardiomyopathy has been defined in Chap. 81A. The essence of the condition is obliteration of the ventricular cavities, impairment of myocardial function, and distortion of the atrioventricular valves. The prototype is *endomyocardial fibrosis (EMF)* found in tropical, humid zones of the world in a wide belt running through the equatorial regions.[1,2]

Endomyocardial fibrosis

PATHOLOGY

The disease affects mainly the endocardium but also involves the myocardium and the pericardium. In the acute initial illness the pericardium is infiltrated by inflammatory cells and is hyperemic. The myocardium is affected both by septal fibrous tissue, which penetrates from the endocardium, and by destruction of muscle fibers in star-shaped areas, often around small blood vessels, where the fibers are replaced by fibroblasts. The endocardium is patchily involved, and lesions occur essentially in the inflow tract of the ventricles, at the apices, and under the septal cusp of the tricuspid valve and the posterior cusp of the mitral valve. The atrial endocardium is not usually affected. Early lesions show scattered hyperemia with lymphocytes and proliferating fibroblasts. Small thrombi may be adherent to the endocardial surface. In late cases a wedge of thrombus may obliterate the apex of the ventricle, and the endocardium is a mass of thick collagenous fibrous tissues with sparse chronic inflammatory cells. Calcification may occur in places. The disease may involve either or both ventricles. When the left ventricle is involved, it forms a rigid cavity lined with fibrous tissue at the apex, which may eventually become completely obliterated. The papillary muscles are bound down by fibrous tissue into a firm bed so that they become rigid and short, and the septal muscles and their chordae become stuck against the septum. As a consequence the mitral valve becomes grossly regurgitant. In the right ventricle the slow obliteration of the cavity draws in the endocardium, which can be seen as notch on the surface of the ventricle in severe cases.

As a result of the inflammation of the pericardium there is commonly an effusion which may be massive and is particularly associated with the right-sided form of the disease.

Microscopic examination reveals disorganization of the endocardium, accumulation of acid mucopolysaccharides, and proliferation of fibroplastic tissue. Thrombus may overlie a dense layer of collagen which is separated from the myocardium by loose connective tissue, small blood vessels, and occasionally inflammatory cells.

INCIDENCE
Endomyocardial fibrosis is not the commonest form of heart disease seen in tropical countries, but in tropical Africa it accounts for approximately 10 percent of all cardiac diseases. It is mainly a disease of older children and young adults, but can occur in later adult life, and involves both sexes.

EPIDEMIOLOGY AND SYMPTOMS
The disease is commonest by far in the rain forest regions of Equatorial Africa and has only very recently been described in people who have not resided in these areas for some time. There have been very few cases in Europeans, and such sufferers have always spent several years in equatorial zones.

The disease usually begins with an acute initial illness consisting of edema and breathlessness associated with fever. The symptoms commonly remit, and the individual may remain well until the established disease declares itself. Following the initial illness, there may be progressive tiredness and general ill health with prolonged fever. Swelling of the abdomen is due to ascites and may be associated with dyspnea and cough due to left ventricular failure.

There is usually tachycardia. Episodes of atrial fibrillation may occur. In the established disease the clinical picture is usually one of severe right-sided heart failure and in many respects may resemble constrictive pericarditis. If the left ventricle is also involved, there will be dyspnea, rales in the chest, and often evidence of mitral regurgitation. Episodes in the acute illness may be related to seasonal events and tend to appear in the rainy season.

ETIOLOGY
The cause of endomyocardial fibrosis is unknown, but it seems certain that it is related in some way to the tropical environment. The presence of fever, and the irregular exacerbation of the disease suggest an infective origin, and it has been noted in Uganda that the disorder affects predominantly people of immigrant origin who come from areas where endemic malaria is low to live in an area with a high rate of malarial transmission. EMF tends to involve predominantly people in the lower socioeconomic groups, but it is not found in many areas where malnutrition is common, so it cannot be ascribed to this cause. Filariasis has been suggested as a possible cause, but proof is lacking.

The plantain, which forms the staple diet of East and West African groups, contains large quantities of 5-hydroxytryptamine, and the possibility of EMF being a form of carcinoid heart disease has been considered. Immunologic studies suggest that the groups most prone to develop EMF tend to be different in their immunologic background from those less susceptible. The immunologic pattern is represented by high levels of malarial antibody immunoglobulin and IgM circulating autoantibodies to thyroid and gastric parietal cell mucosa. These immunologic patterns may merely be the result of infection.

The most appealing theory is that of an infective agent, possibly a virus, which is insect-borne by some vector which is particularly active in the rainy season.

CLINICAL MANIFESTATIONS: RIGHT VENTRICULAR EMF
In the *right ventricular* form the clinical picture is closely similar to that of severe constrictive pericarditis. There is substantial ascites, but without peripheral edema. The liver is enlarged. The face may be puffy, and there is occasionally exophthalmus. The jugular venous pressure is greatly elevated, with a large systolic wave and sharp *y* descent. The pressure rises on inspiration. Ventricular pulsation is not impressive, and the right atrium occupies most of the area usually taken up by the ventricles. There may be a pansystolic murmur of the tricuspid regurgitation at the left sternal edge, and a third heart sound is frequent. The heart sounds may be soft owing to the accompanying pericardial effusion. The arterial pulse is small and wanes with inspiration. There is tachycardia. Central cyanosis may be seen, probably due

to areas of the lungs which are perfused but not ventilated owing to occupation by the enormous right atrium of areas where the lungs should be. Those areas of lung which are perfused but not ventilated serve as intrapulmonary shunts, allowing systemic venous blood to reach the pulmonary veins and thence the systemic arteries. Angiocardiographic studies have shown that the azygos vein fills from the right atrium, suggesting that blood might flow through the azygos system to the pulmonary veins, bypassing the right side of the heart.[2,3]

Radiography The cardiac silhouette is massive due mainly to the enormous right atrium, and the lung fields may appear underfilled. The appearances are similar to those of a very large pericardial effusion. Occasionally calcification can be seen in the right region of the fibrosed right ventricular apex. Small pleural effusions are not infrequently found.

Electrocardiography The electrocardiogram is diffusely abnormal but not diagnostic. Low-voltage QRS complexes and flat T waves or T-wave inversion may be found. The P waves are tall, indicating right atrial enlargement.

CLINICAL MANIFESTATIONS: LEFT VENTRICULAR EMF

In *left ventricular* endomyocardial fibrosis the chief complaints are dyspnea and cough, but there may also be symptoms of right-sided heart failure. Cardiovascular signs are those of a low cardiac output, mitral regurgitation, and pulmonary hypertension. The jugular venous pulse shows a sharp *a* wave, and the arterial pulse is of small volume. Sinus rhythm is usually present, but atrial fibrillation may occur. The pulse pressure is small. Both ventricles may be enlarged, but the left ventricular impulse is often unremarkable. Vigorous pulmonary arterial pulsation may be felt, and the pulmonary closure sound may be loud and the split narrow. There is usually a pansystolic murmur in the mitral area, followed by an early third heart sound. The murmur of mitral regurgitation tends to be diminuendo and to disappear before the second heart sound, due to the meeting by the normal anterior cusp of the mitral valve with the disordered posterior cusp and subsequent restriction of regurgitation at the end of systole. In some patients mitral regurgitation may be slight or absent, and then the signs may not suggest the true cause of the left ventricular failure.

Radiography The chest radiograph shows moderate cardiac enlargement with signs of raised left atrial pressure and some enlargement of the left atrium. When mitral regurgitation is severe, the left atrium tends to be substantially increased in size. The left atrium seldom if ever reaches the aneurysmal size of the right atrium. A linear streak of calcification may be seen in the region of the obliterated apex of the left ventricle.

Electrocardiography The electrocardiogram shows left ventricular hypertrophy and left atrial enlargement. There may be evidence of right ventricular hypertrophy as a result of the pulmonary hypertension. Left ventricular endomyocardial fibrosis of slight or moderate degree may coexist with severe right ventricular disease, in which case the signs of the right ventricular disease predominate and may conceal those of the left. *Disease of both ventricles* is much commoner than lone disease of either. Severe pulmonary hypertension in substantial left ventricular disease cannot occur if the right ventricle is also appreciably involved. In general, therefore, the majority of patients with endomyocardial fibrosis present with signs of right-sided disease.

Hemodynamics The peculiar nature of the disease, with its reduction in ventricular volume, restriction of filling, and impairment of myocardial function, embodies many of the hemodynamic abnormalities that may be found in the other types of cardiomyopathy. The most important of these abnormalities are the restriction of ventricular filling produced by reduction in ventricular cavity size by the obliterative process, and the atrioventricular valvular regurgitation which results from involvement of the papillary muscles. When the right ventricle is involved, the incompetent tricuspid valve impairs the forward output, and the right atrial pressure pulse shows a high right atrial pressure dominated by a systolic wave due to the regurgitation. The restrictive element is shown by the presence of steep *x* and *y* descents and high mean pressure in the right atrium. The obliterative-restrictive process in the ventricle produces a pattern similar to constrictive pericarditis, with a dip-and-plateau contour. There is a sharp early diastolic dip with a high end-diastolic plateau and poor systolic wave. Pressures in the right atrium and right ventricle in systole may be similar. Inspiration may increase the central venous pressure and diminish the arterial pressure, but less commonly than in constrictive pericarditis. Obliteration of the ventricular cavity reduces the stroke volume, so that a compensatory tachycardia is needed to maintain an adequate minute volume. The involvement of the myocardium secondary to the endocardial process produces impairment of systolic function also. In severe right ventricular disease the right atrium may assume an enormous size and may be responsible for maintaining the circulation, and blood flow occurs into the pulmonary artery at the end of ventricular diastole.

Left ventricular endomyocardial fibrosis produces generalized impairment of left ventricular function by the processes just described in the right ventricle. Mitral regurgitation may be striking, left ventricular end-diastolic pressure is elevated, and the ejection fraction and stroke volume are reduced. Some degree of pulmonary hypertension commonly results from the left ventricular failure and mitral regurgitation.

Angiocardiography The right ventricular type shows the enormously dilated right atrium and obliteration of the right ventricle except for a small area in the region of the outflow tract. The lung fields appear underfilled. The presence of a pericardial effusion is denoted by a gap between the contrast medium and the right atrium in the outer border of the right cardiac silhouette. In the left-sided type the apex of the left ventricle may be completely obliterated, and severe mitral regurgitation into the large left atrium is seen. There may be a linear strip of calcium in the obliterated body of the left ventricle.

COMPLICATIONS

Embolic phenomena occur in about 15 percent of patients with EMF. Bacterial endocarditis is uncommon, occurring in only about 2 percent. Additional rheumatic heart disease may occur.

OTHER INVESTIGATIONS

There are no consistent biochemical abnormalities in the blood except for disordered liver function in advanced cases when impairment of Bromsulphalein excretion may occur. Needle biopsy of the liver reveals centrilobular fibrosis. Ascitic and pericardial fluids are usually blood-stained or serous and contain leukocytes and 4 to 5 g of protein per 100 ml. The blood count shows a slight degree of anemia and a mild to moderate eosinophilia.[2,3]

DIFFERENTIAL DIAGNOSIS

In right-sided EMF when the heart is of moderate size, the differential diagnosis is from constrictive pericarditis, an important distinction being the absence of pericardial calcification in EMF. However, calcification does not always occur in constrictive pericarditis, particularly in the early stages, so the sign is not a reliable one in individual cases. Angiocardiography may demonstrate the thickened pericardium in constrictive pericarditis and the distortion of the right ventricle in endomyocardial fibrosis, respectively. The hemodynamics are very similar. When the heart is not greatly enlarged in EMF, differentiation may also be required from restrictive cardiomyopathy. When the heart is substantially enlarged, the diagnosis must also be made from pericardial effusion of tuberculous or pyogenic origin. It must be remembered that in areas where endomyocardial fibrosis is common, tuberculous pericarditis and pyogenic pericarditis are also common, much more than in temperate zones at the present time. When the heart is enormous, the distinction must be made not only from a pericardial effusion but also from other conditions such as severe Ebstein's syndrome. The characteristic auscultatory features and the right bundle branch block in Ebstein's syndrome are absent in EMF. Angiocardiography should clarify the diagnosis. Right atrial myxoma can mimic constrictive pericarditis closely and should be considered if the heart is not grossly enlarged. Echocardiography can be very helpful, but angiography is usually needed to establish this diagnosis.

TREATMENT

The treatment of EMF is unrewarding, because the cause is unknown. It is directed toward the control of heart failure with diuretics. As in constrictive pericarditis digitalis is of little value because the lesion is essentially a mechanical one and the tachycardia is necessary to maintain an adequate cardiac output. However, when rapid atrial fibrillation is present, digitalis is essential to slow the ventricular rate. It should be used with care, however. Ascites may be tapped when abdominal distension is extreme, but tapping should be avoided except when essential because of the added protein loss entailed. Instead fluid should be rigidly restricted and diuretics used carefully.

Surgical treatment has been considered. The possibility of constructing a conduit between the right atrium and the pulmonary artery or of replacing the tricuspid valve has been envisaged in the right ventricular type, but virtually no practical experience has been gained, since cardiac surgery is usually not available in the areas where endomyocardial fibrosis is most prevalent. Excision at the obliterating mass in the left ventricle may be possible. Replacement of the mitral valve in the left-sided lesion has been undertaken.[3a] It seems doubtful whether surgical procedures involving valve replacement alone would be successful in view of the disorganization of the ventricles.

Becker's disease

This condition of idiopathic mural endomyocardial disease was described by Becker in 1963.[4] It occurs in southern Africa, where the tropical climate apparently necessary for the development of endomyocardial fibrosis does not occur.

The pathologic lesion is one of endocardial fibrosis with hypoplastic elastic tissue and with narrowing and occlusion of endocardial vessels. The cause is unknown, and the clinical and hemodynamic features are apparently those of congestive cardiomyopathy without features of restriction or obliteration. The edema in the endocardium results in subendocardial necrosis, and the blood supply from the cavity of the heart to the inner one-third of the myocardium is diminished by thrombus formation.

The relationship between Becker's disease, endomyocardial fibrosis, primary cryptogenic cardiomyopathy, endocardial fibroelastosis, and Loeffler's cardiomyopathy is uncertain. Possibly the five conditions represent different responses of the endocardium to different types of damage.

Loeffler's eosinophilic cardiomyopathy

Association of eosinophilia with deposits in the ventricular cavities has been long known since the original description at the end of the last century. There have been many subsequent descriptions of heart disease associated with severe eosinophilia. Endomyocardial disease appears to be the usual cardiac lesion, and in the early stages masses of eosinophils may partially obliterate the ventricular cavities and restrict filling. In the later stages chronic fibroplastic parietal endocardial changes occur with grey-white, fibrous endocardial scarring. The lesions often predominate in the left ventricle, producing a rigid, immobile cavity. The elastic and collagen proliferation and the inflammatory infiltrates may extend into the underlying myocardium.

THE EOSINOPHILIAS

The causes of eosinophilia in Loeffler's disease have been divided into three types: first, *leukemic*, usually eosinophilic, sometimes myeloid; second, *reactive*, the underlying disease being polyarteritis, Hodgkin's disease, reticular endothelial tumors, carcinomas, sensitivity to drugs, parasitic infections, and asthma; third, *unknown*.[5]

The term "hypereosinophilic syndrome" has been coined to describe a condition characterised by persitent marked eosinophilia of the blood combined with diffuse infiltration of organs with eosinophils, and associated with significant cardiac and immunologic abnormalities.[6]

In a recent review of the hypereosinophilic syndrome[7] 84 percent of the patients were noted to have some evidence of cardiac disease, the most frequent finding being congestive heart failure of both right and left ventricles. One-fifth of the patients with clinical evidence of disease had cardiomegaly with congestive heart failure. Cardiac murmurs were common, frequently arising in the mitral valve. A majority of patients had a greatly increased total white blood cell count up to or above 100,000 cells/mm. Eosinophilia was usually profuse, being from 30 to 75 percent in the majority and only under 10 percent in 2 of 57 patients. The eosinophils frequently appeared morphologically abnormal, often being described as larger than usual or having unusual staining characteristics. Eosinophilic metamyelocytes and primitive blast cells were not infrequently found in peripheral blood. The chromosomal analysis was sometimes abnormal, and the erythrocyte sedimentation rate was elevated in 70 percent of patients, although the platelet count was usually normal; cryoglobulinemia could occur. Coombs' tests were occasionally positive, but the lupus erythomatosus test was negative.

The prognosis is poor. Within 3 years, 80 percent of patients die; 20 percent within the first month after the onset of the disease.

CARDIAC LESIONS

The extensive literature on eosinophilic heart disease has recently been reviewed.[4a] Endocardial disease has been described in both ventricles but appears to be more common in the left. Three stages have been distinguished: first, fibrosis; second, thrombosis, an accumulation of mural thrombus being firmly attached to the wall, sometimes producing partial cavity obliteration; third, an acute, extensive area of inner ventricular myocardial damage in patients with a short illness. Approximately 20 percent of patients have valvular lesions with particular involvement of the posterior mitral cusp in the fibrosis. Sometimes warty deposits and friable vegetations have been found on valves. Bacterial infection of mural thrombus has occurred. Pericardial effusion has been described.

Four histologic patterns have been noted: first, an acute myocardial inflammation, in which there is patchy necrosis and myocardial infiltration with lymphocytes, plasma cells, and eosinophils; second, a thick layer of thrombus with infiltration of the underlying endocardium; third, organization of the endocardial thickening consisting mainly of dilated blood vessels, chronic inflammatory cells, and collagen, sometimes with superimposed thrombus; finally, a prominent layer of hyaline fibrous tissue in the thickened endocardium.[5]

CLINICAL MANIFESTATIONS

There may be hepatosplenomegaly and lymph gland enlargement. The cardiac signs will depend upon the stage of the disease, the organs involved, and the degree of obliteration of the ventricles. The features most commonly seen are those of restrictive cardiomyopathy with the characteristic venous pulse and raised central venous pressure. Gallop rhythm is common. The heart is not always obviously enlarged (Fig. 81D-1), and the cardiac output may be maintained by good pump function, so that the clinical signs of low cardiac output are absent and the blood

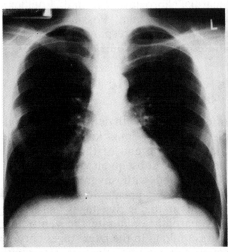
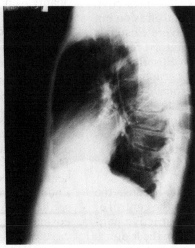

A   B

FIGURE 81D-1 Chest radiographs of a patient with restrictive cardiomyopathy due to eosinophilic heart disease. *A.* Six-foot posteroanterior film showing minimal cardiac enlargement and normal pulmonary vasculature and lung fields. *B.* Lateral film showing minimal enlargement of the right ventricle only.

pressure is normal. In severe cases there may be gross right-sided and left-sided heart failure and signs of systemic embolism. Pericardial effusion may aggravate the signs of tamponade produced by the syndrome, the heart sounds may be soft, and the heart silhouette grossly enlarged on radiography.

Hemodynamics In distinction to endomyocardial fibrosis few detailed hemodynamic studies have been reported in eosinophilic cardiomyopathy because of its rarity. But like EMF the character of the lesions and their distribution produces a combination of reduction in cavity volume and restriction to filling. In two personal cases the pattern was that of restrictive cardiomyopathy, which will be discussed in the next section, "Restrictive Cardiomyopathy." Cardiac output is maintained by tachycardia which compensates for the reduced stroke volume, and in mild cases there is good pump function.

Angiocardiography Through angiocardiography one can see the deformity of both ventricles by dense masses of fibrous tissues, with variable obliteration of the cavity. If there is merely endocardial thickening, the chambers may appear normal. In the early stages of the disease pump function remains good, and contraction may appear normal with normal volumes and ejection fractions.

COMPLICATIONS

Systemic embolism is common. It may precede the onset of cardiac symptoms. The other complications include those of severe heart failure in late cases.

TREATMENT

The treatment of eosinophilic cardiomyopathy is unsatisfactory but should be directed both at the underlying eosinophilic disease and at the cardiac complications. When clear evidence of eosinophilic leukemia is present, the use of appropriate antimetabolic treatment may be helpful. In other cases steroid and immunosuppressive drugs have been used with varying success. Antiparasitic therapy has been tried but without success. Cyclophosphamide, methotrexate, and busulphan have all been shown to decrease the leukocytosis, but neither the eosinophilia nor the symptoms have improved significantly. Vincristine has been shown to reduce eosinophilia as well as the total white cell blood count. Prednisone can produce partial or complete remission.[7]

If progressive cardiac damage is to be avoided, it seems essential to reduce the total eosinophil count. Plasmaphoresis has been considered, but there are no reports on its use.

Cardiac therapy is as for congestive heart failure, with the use of anticoagulants if embolism has occurred. However, in view of the high incidence of embolism, anticoagulants may be considered on a prophylactic basis once the diagnosis has been made.

Eosinophils and the endocardium

It seems likely that eosinophils in the blood in large quantities actively damage the endocardium, producing an exuberant inflammatory reaction. The reasons for this and the way in which it occurs are not clear, but the eosinophils in such patients have abnormal characteristics suggesting an autoimmune disorder.[7a]

Relationship of endomyocardial fibrosis to eosinophilic cardiomyopathy

Any connection between the two diseases has been denied in the past, but the many similarities must give rise to speculation that they might in fact represent different parts of the spectrum of one disease. The similarity of the histologic changes is striking, eosinophilic cardiomyopathy showing no differences from endomyocardial fibrosis.[5] The two major differences are the geographic localization of endomyocardial fibrosis to the tropics and of eosinophilic cardiomyopathy to the temperate zones, on the one hand, and the marked eosinophilia in eosinophilic cardiomyopathy compared with EMF, on the other. Profuse eosinophilia has never been described in endomyocardial fibrosis. A less striking difference is the greater incidence of embolism in eosinophilic cardiomyopathy. It has been suggested, therefore, that endomyocardial fibrosis is a late form of eosinophilic cardiomyopathy due to a parasitic infection via eosinophilia.[5] The information available at this time does not permit a satisfactory answer to this problem. It would be wise to regard both endomyocardial fibrosis and eosinophilic cardiomyopathy as diseases characterised by an endomyocardial reaction to some toxic agent, probably blood-borne. It seems unlikely that the same agent is at work in both diseases in view of the difference in eosinophilia and the accumulating data suggesting that eosinophils themselves in large amounts directly damage the endocardium. Since profuse eosinophilia has not been demonstrated even in acute cases of EMF, it is difficult to incriminate the eosinophil in the etiology of this disease.

RESTRICTIVE CARDIOMYOPATHY

Restrictive cardiomyopathy has been defined in Chap. 81A. It is said to be present when diastolic ventricular volume and stretch are impaired by organic subendocardial or myocardial lesions. Good contractile function is usually, though not always, maintained.

Restrictive cardiomyopathy is a very rare condition, and its exact characteristics have not yet been fully defined. As has been pointed out, there is a relationship between obliterative and restrictive cardiomyopathy, since patients with obliterative lesions of necessity have a restrictive element to their ventricular function because of the reduction in ventricular cavity size and the rigidity imposed by the endomyocardial lesions producing the obliteration.

Pathology of restrictive cardiomyopathy

Whatever the underlying disease, the heart muscle tends to be rigid and inelastic, and there is frequently endocardial thickening. Except in very severe cases of widespread myocardial disease, the ventricular cavities are not dilated. Obliterative lesions are not present, and endocardial thrombosis is uncommon. The atrioventricular and semilunar valves are normal.

Hemodynamics of restrictive cardiomyopathy

The hemodynamic picture is similar to that of constrictive pericarditis but with certain differences. The abnormal process in the myocardium and endocardium tends to restrict filling of the ventricles in the same way. Thus, there is an early diastolic dip in the right and left ventricular pressure pulses followed by a high end-diastolic pressure which is preceded by a plateau. The atrial pressure pulses show large *a* and *v* waves, and sharp *x* and *y* descents. The central venous pressure may rise on inspiration and the arterial pressure may fall, as in tamponade, though less frequently than in constrictive pericarditis. Stroke volume is reduced, but minute volume is maintained by a tachycardia. When the left ventricle only is involved, there is rapid early filling, but little increase in volume in mid and late diastole.[7b] The heart shows variable enlargement depending upon the severity and extent of the disease, and may be normal in size.

Angiocardiography tends to show a smooth symmetric thick-walled left ventricle. Systolic contraction is normal in the early stages, but becomes impaired with increasing severity. Valvular regurgitation is not usually seen.

The differences from constrictive pericarditis are, first, that the end-diastolic pressures in the two ventricles tend to be different in restrictive cardiomyopathy whereas they are identical in constrictive pericarditis: in restrictive cardiomyopathy the pressure in the left ventricle often exceeds the right in end-diastole, and the early diastolic dip in the right ventricular pressure pulse frequently does not approach zero, whereas in constrictive pericarditis it is often at or below zero. Second, there is often pulmonary hypertension in restrictive cardiomyopathy but rarely in constrictive pericarditis. These differences reflect the generalized constriction in constrictive pericarditis, which involves both ventricles equally, rather than the unequal involvement of the two ventricles in restrictive cardiomyopathy. The low early diastolic dip and normal pulmonary arterial pressure are probably due to the good systolic function of the ventricles in constrictive pericarditis (except in very severe cases) as compared with the impaired left ventricular function in many cases of restrictive cardiomyopathy. These differences are not absolute, and considerable overlap can occur. They are useful clues, however, to differentiating between the two conditions; yet sometimes exploratory thoracotomy is essential to reveal the true diagnosis.

Clinical manifestations

The clinical picture, as is to be expected, often resembles constrictive pericarditis.[8] The arterial pulse tends to be small in volume, regular in rhythm, and rapid in rate. Atrial fibrillation occasionally occurs but is uncommon. The jugular venous pressure is elevated, sometimes extremely so, and shows large *a* and *v* waves with sharp *x* and *y* descents, especially the *y*. The venous pressure may rise further on inspiration. When atrial fibrillation is present, there may be an element of tricuspid regurgitation so that the *x* descent is partially or completely obliterated. The cardiac impulse is usually not striking, though in advanced cases there may be evidence of both left and right ventricular enlargement. Diastolic pulsation, as seen in constrictive pericarditis, does not occur. Pulmonary valve closure may be accentuated due to pulmonary hypertension, and the split may be narrow. Significant murmurs are usually absent. There is a constant early third heart sound arising from the left ventricle. In severe cases there may be evidence of congestive heart failure. In many cases pump function is well maintained and symptoms tend to be those of tiredness and fatigue due to inability to elevate the cardiac output adequately on effort, or palpitations due to compensatory tachycardia. Cardiac pain may occur, particularly when amyloid disease is the cause.

Within the general framework of the term restrictive cardiomyopathy three different groups may be identified: *primary cryptogenic, amyloid,* and *eosinophilic.* Their characteristics will now be mentioned.

Primary cryptogenic restrictive cardiomyopathy

Until recently it was thought that amyloid disease was the commonest cause of restrictive cardiomyopathy, and indeed it still remains a common cause. The term *primary* or *cryptogenic cardiomyopathy* has been given to patients with a distinctive hemodynamic picture of unknown cause. As with other types of restrictive cardiomyopathy the clinical picture resembles that of constrictive pericarditis, particularly when the right ventricle is involved in addition to the left. Usually, however, the disease is confined to the left ventricle. Signs of left ventricular enlargement with a loud third heart sound, raised central venous pressure, and the characteristics of restriction are the major physical signs.

The hemodynamics of the left ventricle have been studied in detail.[9] The left ventricular diastolic pressure shows a steep early diastolic rise to a plateau usually above zero. The end-diastolic pressure has ranged between 18 and 40 mm Hg. Instantaneous pressure-volume relationships have shown a normal pattern at the beginning of diastole, but toward the end of diastole the pressure tends to climb steeply to high levels, while the left ventricular volume fails to increase correspondingly. Angiocardiography shows a small, thick-walled left ventricle with a smooth, symmetric outline and normal systolic contraction.

Little is known about the pathologic appearances, but where autopsy studies have been carried out, there was moderate left ventricular hypertrophy and fibrosis with thickening of the endocardium but no cellular infiltration. The prognosis in the small number of patients studied appears to be poor. Nothing is known of the relationship of the pathologic changes in these patients to endomyocardial fibrosis or to endocardial fibroelastosis. As with endomyocardial fibrosis and eosinophilic cardiomyopathy, these patients may have a reaction of the left ventricle to some toxic stimulus. The possibility that they represent the end stage of eosinophilic cardiomyopathy when the eosinophils have disappeared from the endocardium cannot be ruled out, but the absence of thrombosis in primary restrictive cardiomyopathy and of the other characteristic changes found in eosinophilic cardiomyopathy suggest that this probably is not the case.

Amyloidosis

Amyloidosis is a rare disease. It is characterised by the accumulation of a protein polysaccharide complex which contains specific binding sites for anti–gamma globulin antiserum as well as other serum proteins such as fibrinogen, albumen, and complement.

Amyloidosis is frequently classified as *primary* or *secondary* according to its distribution. It is doubtful however whether there is any fundamental difference in the two types, but the differentiation has some clinical usefulness. In *primary amyloidosis* deposits of amyloid material are found mainly in the tongue, gastrointestinal tract, heart, blood vessels, peripheral nerves, skin, periarticular structures, and mucous membranes. The *secondary* type develops in patients with long-standing wasting or suppurative disorders, such as tuberculosis or rheumatoid arthritis, and occurs mainly in the liver, spleen, and lymph nodes, in addition to the kidneys and adrenal glands. There is considerable overlap in distribution between the primary and secondary types.[10]

Amyloidosis, usually in distribution of the so-called primary type, occurs in around 10 percent of patients with multiple myeloma and occasionally in patients with lymphoma. In primary amyloidosis a monoclonal immunoglobulin and a bone marrow plasmacytosis is found in a high proportion of cases. Free light chains may be found in the urine in patients with amyloidosis with or without associated myeloma. Possibly these light polypeptide chains form insoluble complexes with amyloid and are distributed according to the location of the complementary carbohydrate. It has been suggested that the spectrum of the amyloidoses reflects the underlying plasma cell dyscrasias.[10]

Amyloidosis may also occur on a familial basis. In one type patients are usually in the third or fourth decade of life and suffer cardiovascular insufficiency, peripheral neuropathy, hepatosplenomegaly, and

occular and gastrointestinal abnormalities. Elevation of serum lipoprotein and an abnormal protein found between the alpha and beta globulins may be present. In another type amyloidosis involves primarily the kidneys, liver, spleen, and adrenals and develops late in the course of familial Mediterranean fever.

A nephrotic syndrome is a common sequel to either primary or secondary amyloidosis.

CARDIAC AMYLOIDOSIS
Involvement of the heart occurs mainly in the primary form but may also be found in the familial type and in old age. In the primary type of amyloid disease the heart may be the only organ affected in a clinically detectable way, and patients present with the syndrome of restrictive cardiomyopathy. When the disease is evident elsewhere, there may be macroglossia and thickening of the conjunctiva (Fig. 81D-2). A carpal tunnel syndrome may be caused by compression due to amyloid deposits. Deposits may also be found in the rectus sheath. There may be mild lymphadenopathy or hepatic and splenic enlargement.

Cardiac involvement is unusual in the secondary form of amyloidosis. Senile cardiac amyloidosis occurs twice as commonly in the male as in the female. It may present as heart failure and intolerance to digitalis, while heart block has been described. However, senile cardiac amyloidosis is often an incidental finding during a postmortem examination, and its clinical significance is uncertain.[11]

THE PATHOLOGY OF CARDIAC AMYLOIDOSIS
The waxy amyloid material is deposited in the intercellular spaces between the myofibrils, often in rela-

FIGURE 81D-2 Macroglossia in primary amyloid disease. The tongue is large, glassy, and stiff.

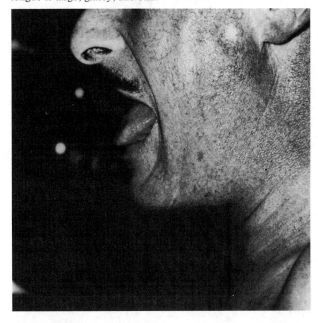

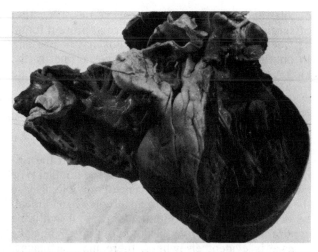

FIGURE 81D-3 Necropsy specimen of the heart in amyloid disease. The left ventricle is not dilated, and there is moderate hypertrophy.

tion to blood vessels. Capillaries are reduced in number, and myocardial cellular atrophy may result from interference with blood supply. Compression of myofibrils may also cause necrosis and atrophy. The disease may be diffuse or localized in distribution, and the amyloid tissue may be recognised by specific staining properties with Congo red. Electronmicroscopy reveals a fine fibrillary structure.

The myocardium is firm and waxy, and the heart has a stiff, rigid consistency (Fig. 81D-3). Amyloid may be found widely distributed in the atria and ventricles and papillary muscles. It is also found in the media of small coronary arteries, in the pericardium, and in the conduction system. It often appears selectively to involve the sinoatrial node. The involvement of the endocardium may produce rigidity of the valves.

CLINICAL PICTURE OF CARDIAC AMYLOIDOSIS

In addition to the lesions of tongue and mucous membranes there may be purpura or peripheral neuropathy, but the abnormal signs may be confined to the heart. In many cases the appearances are those of restrictive cardiomyopathy already described. When amyloid disease is extensive, left ventricular systolic function is impaired, and a different syndrome emerges. This has recently been described in detail in a small series of patients.[12] Patients tend to be severely ill with marked cardiac failure and low cardiac output. A history of cardiac pain is common, and there is cardiomegaly on the chest radiograph. A pericardial effusion may be present. The hemodynamics reveal elevation of both right ventricular and left ventricular systolic pressures. Both early and late (end-) diastolic pressures in the left ventricle are also substantially elevated. The cardiac index is low, and the ejection fraction substantially reduced.

Electrocardiography shows low-voltage complexes but no specific repolarization changes, although sometimes evidence of atrioventricular block. Q waves may be found in chest leads, perhaps referable to interference with myocardial blood supply by the amyloid deposits.

Echocardiography demonstrates normal left ventricular dimensions in diastole but reduced amplitude of pulsation of the septum and posterior wall and an increased systolic dimension. A pericardial effusion may also be detected.

Angiocardiography reveals marked trabeculation of the left ventricle with impressive papillary muscle indentations without distortion of the shape of the cavity. Systolic emptying is impaired, and poor contractile function is demonstrated by the grossly reduced ejection fraction.

Simultaneous measurements of volume and pressure in diastole[12] have demonstrated poor compliance of the left ventricle. The ratio between change in pressure and change in volume was greater than normal, which led to slow filling throughout diastole.

The main differentiation from restrictive cardiomyopathy due to less severe and disseminated amyloid disease or to other causes is the impaired systolic function and the slow filling of the left ventricle throughout diastole. In constrictive pericarditis and milder forms of restrictive cardiomyopathy rapid filling occurs early in diastole with little further filling in late diastole.

TREATMENT

The therapy of amyloid is highly unsatisfactory and most patients die within a few years of the disease becoming fully developed. Standard treatment for heart failure should be employed and may improve the prognosis somewhat.

Restrictive cardiomyopathy due to eosinophilic disease

Eosinophilic cardiomyopathy has been fully described under the section "Obliterative Cardiomyopathy." When the ventricular lesion in eosinophilic cardiomyopathy is confined to endocardial thickening without obliterative masses, the hemodynamic picture is one of restrictive cardiomyopathy with good pump function: severe congestive heart failure does not usually occur. If the disease can be arrested at this stage, the prognosis may be reasonably favorable.

Echocardiography demonstrates good posterior ventricular wall and septal movement with normal end-systolic cavity dimensions (Fig. 81D-4). *Left ventricular angiography* shows good contraction with a normal ejection fraction. The pressure-volume characteristics are those of primary restrictive cardiomyopathy.

It must be emphasised that the restrictive cardiomyopathies are still an ill-understood and poorly defined group. Much has still to be learned about the underlying causes and effects on ventricular function.

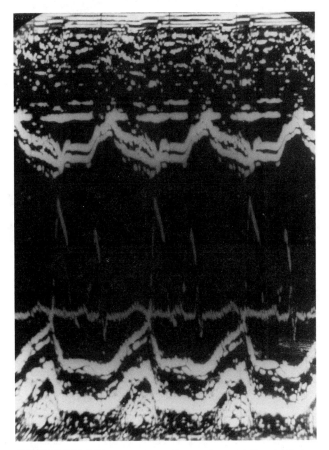

FIGURE 81D-4 M-scan echocardiogram in restrictive cardiomyopathy due to eosinophilic heart disease. There is good movement of the posterior wall of the left ventricle and of the ventricular septum. The left ventricle is not dilated, and the mitral valve is normal.

Endocardial fibroelastosis

Although endocardial fibroelastosis (EFE) does not fit neatly into the classification of cardiomyopathies, it cannot be ignored in any consideration of diseases involving the myocardium and the endocardium. Endocardial fibroelastosis is a condition which essentially involves the left ventricle of infants and children, often on a familial basis. The endocardium is grossly thickened in consistency and white in color. The myocardium is relatively unaffected. The endocardial thickening may extend to involve the mitral valve apparatus, which may be plastered down as if coated with wax. Some degree of endocardial fibroelastosis results from long-standing heart failure.

Severe endocardial fibroelastosis is commonly described in two forms: the *primary*, or idiopathic, form in which other heart disease is absent; and the *secondary* form in which there is left-sided congenital heart disease such as coarctation of the aorta, aortic stenosis, mitral stenosis, or atresia. The disease is noted for the early development of severe heart failure which is often unresponsive to medical treatment. Occasionally symptoms may be delayed until the age of 5 years.[13] The clinical picture is one of congestive cardiomyopathy, but the left ventricle

appears peculiarly spherical and immobile, the cavity being smooth and not indented. Severe mitral regurgitation is common though not the rule. Many infants succumb to the disease, but some recover and are left with varying degrees of left ventricular insufficiency and mitral regurgitation.

The cause is unknown. Mumps virus infection has been suggested, as has disease of the cardiac lymphatics, but neither theory has been confirmed.

The existence of endocardial fibroelastosis as a specific entity has indeed been questioned, and it has been affirmed that the process is merely secondary to severe heart failure resulting from congenital lesions. This problem still remains unresolved, and the difficulty is aggravated by the fact that in life the diagnosis of endocardial fibroelastosis is usually one of exclusion, and often the disease cannot be distinguished from viral myocarditis, though the presence of severe mitral regurgitation would suggest EFE.

The pathology of EFE is entirely different from endomyocardial fibrosis and the obliterative cardiomyopathies. Obliteration of the ventricular cavity does not occur, secondary thrombosis is extremely uncommon, and the process does not tend to extend into the myocardium. The relation to primary restrictive cardiomyopathy is unknown, but this condition may possibby represent an adult form of endocardial fibroelastosis.

REFERENCES

1 Davies, J. N. P.: Endomyocardial Fibrosis in Africans, *East Afr. Med. J.,* 25:10, 105, 1968.

2 Parry, E. H. O.: Endomyocardial Fibrosis, in G. Wolstenholme and M. O'Connor (eds.), "Cardiomyopathies," Ciba Foundation Symposium, Churchill, London, 1964, p. 322.

3 Somers, K., and Fowler, J. N.: Endomyocardial Fibrosis. Clinical Diagnosis, in G. A. Shaper (ed.), "Introduction to the Cardiomyopathies," *Cardiologia,* 52:25, 1968.

3a Lepley, D., Aris, A., Korns, M. E., Walker, J. A., and D'Cunha, R. M.: Endomyocardial Fibrosis: A Surgical Approach, *Ann. Thorac. Surg.,* 18:626, 1974.

4 Becker, B. J. P., Chatgadakis, C. B., and Verne-Lennon, B.: Cardiovascular Collagenosis with Parietal Endocardial Thrombosis, *Circulation,* 7:345, 1953.

4a Oakley, C. M., and Olsen, E. G. J.: Eosinophilia and Heart Disease (Editorial), *Br. Heart J.,* 39:233, 1977.

5 Brockington, I., and Olsen, E. J. G.: Loeffler's Endocarditis and Davies' Endomyocardial Fibrosis, *Am. Heart J.,* 85:308, 1973.

6 Hardy, W. R., and Anderson, R. E.: The Hypereosinophilic Syndrome, *Ann. Intern. Med.,* 68:1220, 1968.

7 Chusid, M. A., Dale, D. C., West, P. C., and Wolff, S. M.: The Hypereosinophilic Syndrome, *Medicine,* 54:1, 1975.

7a Spry, C. J. F., and Tai, P. C.: Studies on Blood Eosinophils. II. Patients with Löffler's Cardiomyopathy, *Clin. Exper. Immunol.,* 24:423, 1976.

7b Chew, C. Y. C., Ziady, G. M., Raphael, M. J., Nellen, M., and Oakley, C. M.: Primary Restrictive Cardiomyopathy. Nontropical Endomyocardial Fibrosis and Hypereosinophilic Heart Disease, *Br. Heart J.,* 39:399, 1977.

8 Hetzel, P. S., Wood, E. H., and Burchell, H. P.: Pressure Pulses in the Right Side of the Heart in a Case of Amyloid Disease and in a Case of Idiopathic Heart Failure Simulating Constrictive Pericarditis, *Proc. Mayo Clin.*, 28:107, 1953.

9 Ziady, G. M., Oakley, C. M., Raphael, M. J., and Goodwin, J. F.: Primary Restrictive Cardiomyopathy, *Br. Heart J.*, 37:556, 1975.

10 Humphrey, I. C., and Owens, A. H.: Immunoglobulins of Plasma Cell Dyscrasias, in A. M. Harvey, R. J. Jones, A. H. Owens, Jr., and R. H. Ross (eds.), "The Principles and Practice of Medicine," Appleton-Century-Crofts, New York, 1972, p. 1220.

11 Pomerance, A.: The Pathology of Senile Cardiac Amyloidosis, *J. Pathol. Bacteriol.*, 91:357, 1966.

12 Chew, C., Ziady, G. M., Raphael, M. J., and Oakley, C. M.: The Functional Defect in Amyloid Heart Disease: "The Stiff Heart Syndrome," *Am. J. Cardiol.*, 36:438, 1975.

13 Nadas, A.: "Paediatric Cardiology," 2d ed., W. B. Saunders Company, Philadelphia, 1963, p. 269.

82
Myocardial Involvement in Systemic Disease

NANETTE KASS WENGER, M.D.

INTRODUCTION[1-6]

Myocardial structural and functional abnormalities may be encountered in a wide variety of systemic diseases.[1] As a rule, the systemic manifestations of the disease overshadow the myocardial abnormalities, but the latter occasionally dominate the clinical presentation.

The myocardial lesions associated with systemic disease may be diffuse or localized. When the myocardium is *diffusely* involved, the clinical picture may resemble that of myocarditis or cardiomyopathy (see Chaps. 80 and 81). Under such circumstances, there may be cardiac enlargement and progressive congestive heart failure; arrhythmias, embolic phenomena, and sudden death are not uncommon. On the other hand, a myocardial abnormality may be recognized only by an abnormal electrocardiogram, or it may be identified as an incidental finding at postmortem examination. When the myocardial involvement is *localized,* it may produce cardiac arrhythmias, obstruction to blood flow, or electrocardiographic abnormalities, or it may be an incidental finding at autopsy. Both the diffuse and localized myocardial lesions may be associated with valvular (endocardial) and/or pericardial disease.[2]

The diagnostic problem in myocardial disease is complex because similar clinical syndromes may result from widely differing histologic abnormalities; in addition, related etiologic factors may produce different histologic patterns. The specific etiologic diagnosis of the myocardial disease often depends on the extracardiac manifestations of the disease, which may remove it from the designation of idiopathic myocardial disease.[3]

The systemic diseases with myocardial involvement will be considered in the following groups:

Infectious diseases
Sarcoidosis
Nutritional disorders
Metabolic disorders
Hematologic diseases
Neurologic and neuromuscular diseases
Collagen vascular diseases
Neoplastic diseases
Chemical and drug effects (toxicity and hypersensitivity)
Physical causes
Miscellaneous systemic syndromes

Cardiovascular complications of oral contraceptive use and of drug abuse will also be considered in this chapter.

INFECTIOUS DISEASES

See Chap. 80.

SARCOIDOSIS

Sarcoidosis is a multisystem granulomatous disorder which cannot yet be classified etiologically. It will be discussed as a separate entity because of the frequency of cardiac manifestations. Myocardial sarcoid occurs equally among whites and Negroes, despite the marked predominance of systemic sarcoidosis in the Negro.[7] The incidence of systemic sarcoidosis in females is usually twice that in males. The disease is characterized by relapses and spontaneous remissions.

Pathology

The autopsy incidence of myocardial sarcoidosis is about 20 percent; cor pulmonale secondary to diffuse pulmonary sarcoidosis occurs even more frequently.[8,9]

Sarcoid granulomas, often gross and extensive, infiltrate the ventricular myocardium, the ventricular septum (often damaging the conduction system),[10,11] and the heart valves. Sarcoid granulomas may occur in the atria, in the pericardium, and in the media and adventitia of the aorta.[12] The granulomas are characteristically described as being near blood vessels, often involving the vessel wall.[8] The microscopic appearance is of a noncaseating granuloma, with central multinucleate giant cells and epithelioid cells, surrounded by a cuff of lymphocytes. These granulomas may coalesce, with eventual myofiber replacement by a dense fibrotic scar. This is the anatomic basis for the electrocardiographic pattern of "myocardial infarction" which has been described. Papillary muscle infiltration may result in mitral regurgitation. Ventricular aneurysms also occur in areas of transmural myocardial destruction.[13] Histochemical and electron microscopic studies in cardiac sarcoidosis demonstrate extensive myocardial damage that accounts for the generally poor response to conventional therapy for congestive heart failure.[14]

Clinical manifestations

HISTORY

Myocardial involvement is a serious complication of sarcoidosis[13] that occurs late in the course of the disease and is evident particularly in the second and third decades of life. There is no sex predilection.[7,15] Dyspnea and palpitations are frequent. Occasionally, atypical chest pain or Stokes-Adams syncope occur. Although about 20 percent of patients with sarcoid have autopsy evidence of cardiac involvement, only about 5 percent of these individuals have cardiovascular symptoms.[16–18a]

PHYSICAL EXAMINATION

Sarcoid heart disease should be suspected in a patient with systemic sarcoidosis who develops unexplained tachycardia, cardiac arrhythmias, conduction abnormalities, cardiac murmurs, cardiac enlargement, or congestive heart failure. Complete heart block without apparent cause in a young adult should also suggest the possibility of myocardial sarcoidosis.[19,20]

Atrioventricular conduction disturbances, particularly complete heart block with Stokes-Adams syncope, are the most common clinical manifestations.[13] Ventricular arrhythmias, often difficult to control, occur next most commonly and may result in sudden death.[8] Sinus tachycardia and supraventricular arrhythmias are also described.

Congestive heart failure is common when cor pulmonale is secondary to systemic sarcoidosis but is less frequently seen in myocardial sarcoidosis. Clinical evidence of pericardial involvement is rare in myocardial sarcoid; constrictive pericarditis[9] has not been described, but pericardial effusion,[21] including hemorrhagic effusion,[22] has been reported.[23] Valve involvement is uncommon.

LABORATORY EXAMINATION

Electrocardiogram As many as 50 percent of patients with sarcoid may demonstrate an electrocardiographic abnormality. Abnormalities of rhythm, of conduction, and of repolarization occur commonly in the absence of cardiovascular symptoms.[17] Arrhythmias, ventricular and supraventricular, are often paroxysmal, and serial electrocardiograms often show varying atrioventricular and intraventricular conduction abnormalities. As in any disease with focal or localized replacement or displacement of the myocardium, the electrocardiogram may resemble that of myocardial infarction.[24] Abnormal P waves and ST-T changes are common, but nonspecific, findings.

Both exercise stress testing and ambulatory monitoring are recommended to search for ventricular dysrhythmias.[24a]

Chest x-ray The diagnosis of sarcoid is usually suspected because of hilar lymphadenopathy. The radiologic cardiac findings are variable, related to the extent of myocardial involvement, the degree of cor pulmonale, and the occurrence of pericardial effusion.

Other diagnostic tests A positive Kveim test supports the diagnosis of sarcoidosis, although its specificity has been questioned, as does a positive lymph node biopsy. Scalene node biopsy appears valuable in diagnosing sarcoid as the cause of a cardiac conduction abnormality in patients without overt signs of the disease.[24b]

Clinical course

Two-thirds of patients with myocardial sarcoid die suddenly; almost one-third of patients dying of sarcoid heart disease have had complete heart block at one time.[9] Ventricular arrhythmias are also associated with a grave prognosis. Indeed, the clinical course of symptomatic cardiac sarcoidosis tends to be short, with three-fourths of patients dying within 2 years of the onset of cardiac symptoms in one series.[18a]

Treatment

Myocardial involvement seems to be an indication for corticosteroid hormone therapy in sarcoidosis, regardless of the severity of the systemic sarcoidosis.[25] Abnormal Q waves and other electrocardiographic abnormalities, including life-threatening ventricular arrhythmias and atrioventricular and intraventricular block, have resolved both with[22,25a] and without steroid therapy. The arrhythmias are often refractory to both digitalis and many antiarrhythmic agents; in addition, these drugs may potentiate atrioventricular block.[16] β-Adrenergic blocking agents appear to decrease the severity of arrhythmias and may reduce the incidence of sudden death.[19] Quinidine, with and without propranolol, has also been described as effective.[24a]

Implantation of a permanent demand pacemaker may be useful in patients with high-degree atrioventricular block in an effort to prevent sudden death.[13]

In one young patient with a ventricular aneurysm due to cardiac sarcoidosis, multifocal premature ventricular beats and refractory ventricular tachycardia responded dramatically to aneurysm resection.[26] Rarely, mitral valve replacement has been necessary.

NUTRITIONAL DISORDERS[*27]

Beriberi (see Chap. 81C)

Oriental (Shoshin) beriberi, usually caused by malnutrition, is characterized by high output cardiac failure

---

*With appreciation to Dr. Daniel Rudman, Professor of Medicine, Emory University School of Medicine, for review of this section.

and is often associated with syncope, shock, and rapid death. In the Western Hemisphere, it has occasionally been associated with excessive beer drinking at the expense of other sources of calories.[27a] Occidental beriberi, most commonly seen in alcoholic men, presents both right and left ventricular failure, often without evidence of a hyperkinetic circulation; it is not infrequently misdiagnosed as coronary atherosclerotic heart disease, alcoholic cardiomyopathy, or diffuse myocardial disease of unknown cause.

PATHOLOGY

The myocardial anatomic lesions in beriberi[28] include biventricular dilatation and hypertrophy, hydropic degeneration of myofibers and of the conduction system, interstitial and intracellular edema, and collagen swelling. Inflammation and necrosis are notably absent. Myocardial fibrosis occurs after prolonged illness.

PATHOPHYSIOLOGY

The cardiac manifestations of beriberi are probably due not to an anatomic myocardial alteration but to a potentially reversible derangement of carbohydrate metabolism with effects similar to those of hypoxia. Inability of the myocardium to utilize oxygen and the resultant decreased metabolic demand for oxygen may decrease coronary blood flow.[29] Myocardial energy production is impaired by lack of cocarboxylase; thus, fats rather than carbohydrates must provide the major source of energy.[29] High output cardiac failure, with decreased myocardial oxygen extraction and consumption, imposes an additional workload on a heart already handicapped by this metabolic defect.[30]

In patients with oriental beriberi, severe metabolic acidosis may play an important role in the pathogenesis of the heart failure and reversal of the acidosis may be crucial in enabling survival from Shoshin beriberi.[31] High output biventricular failure, hypotension, and markedly diminished peripheral resistance were documented in a recent case at cardiac catheterization; there was a striking metabolic acidosis, with a pH of 7.09, P_{CO_2} of 10 mm Hg, and accumulation of lactic and pyruvic acids. Sodium bicarbonate therapy reversed the acidosis, and after thiamine hydrochloride administration, the hemodynamic derangements rapidly returned to normal.

In occidental beriberi, severe heart failure with a low cardiac output, depressed left ventricular work and efficiency, and a normal peripheral resistance may occur; in these cases, the myocardial rather than the peripheral vascular abnormality of beriberi appears to predominate.[29,32] Beriberi heart disease due to thiamine deficiency, therefore, must also be considered as a cause of heart failure with a low cardiac output.[33]

Excessive drinking of beer or other alcoholic beverages may predispose to beriberi, not only by providing insufficient dietary thiamine but by increasing the systemic metabolic requirement for thiamine because of its high carbohydrate content.[27a,34]

CLINICAL MANIFESTATIONS

History The presenting symptoms of beriberi heart disease include fatigue, dyspnea, orthopnea, edema, and palpitations. A history of malnutrition and/or excessive alcohol intake is usual.

Physical examination In addition to the neurologic abnormalities, the classic physical findings in the high output stage include sinus tachycardia; tachypnea; a full, bounding arterial pulse with an increased pulse pressure; elevated venous pressure with neck vein engorgement; peripheral vasodilatation; cardiomegaly; a faint S_1 and an accentuated pulmonary component of S_2; gallop rhythm; systolic murmurs; pulmonary congestion; hepatomegaly; and serous effusions and edema.

Congestive heart failure is most pronounced in patients with minimal neurologic involvement, i.e., in those best able to continue at work. Physical exertion characteristically precipitated cardiac failure in prisoners of war with beriberi.

Laboratory examination Electrocardiogram There is no characteristic electrocardiographic pattern for beriberi, but a sinus tachycardia and the absence of arrhythmias are worthy of note. Nonspecific T-wave changes and diminished QRS voltage are observed; Q-T interval prolongation is attributable to hypokalemia. The electrocardiographic abnormalities often disappear after thiamine therapy.

Chest x-ray There is generalized cardiomegaly on roentgenographic examination. Hilar vessels are prominent, often without pulmonary congestion.

Other findings Anemia and hypoproteinemia are characteristic. The thiamine pyrophosphate (TPP) level is elevated prior to thiamine administration but falls rapidly after therapy. Thiamine acts as a cofactor for transketolase, and the transketolase activity is decreased with thiamine deficiency; determination of red blood cell transketolase levels may prove the most specific laboratory test for the diagnosis of beriberi heart disease.[35] The circulation time may be rapid or normal. The arteriovenous oxygen difference is diminished, reflecting the shunting of blood.

Cardiac catheterization High output cardiac failure and increased oxygen consumption have been demonstrated at cardiac catheterization. The cardiac output is increased out of proportion to the oxygen consumption, producing a decrease in the systemic arteriovenous oxygen difference. The decreased peripheral vascular resistance, which returns to normal after thiamine therapy, may contribute to the increased cardiac output.[36]

Systolic time intervals A low PEP/ET ratio is compatible with a high cardiac output–low peripheral vascular resistance syndrome.[27a]

Diagnostic criteria: summary The diagnosis of beriberi should be considered in patients with unexplained heart failure, particularly when there is associated alcoholism or malnutrition.

Blankenhorn's criteria for beriberi heart disease include (1) absence of other etiologic factors for heart disease; (2) history of at least 3 months of gross dietary thiamine deficiency; (3) simultaneous peripheral neuritis or pellagra; (4) cardiomegaly and regular sinus rhythm; (5) edema, increased venous pressure, anemia, and hypoproteinemia; (6) minor, nonspecific electrocardiographic changes which usually disappear after therapy; and (7) response to thiamine therapy by recovery with diminution of heart size or, alternatively, autopsy proof of the diagnosis.

TREATMENT

Untreated beriberi heart disease is characterized by a high mortality rate, and the clinical response of severe heart failure to the administration of thiamine typically is dramatic. Therapy consists of thiamine, prolonged rest, adequate diet, vitamins, sodium restriction, and diuretics; digitalis alone has little effect, as it cannot correct the abnormality in myocardial energy production. Classically, therapy reverses all the symptoms and abnormal clinical and laboratory findings in beriberi. However, the development of both systemic hypertension and pulmonary edema have been described after thiamine administration and have been attributed to the rapid return of edema to the intravascular space and the sudden increase in peripheral vascular resistance.[37] The acute left ventricular failure may relate to the increase in systemic vascular resistance prior to the return to normal of myocardial function.[27a] There appears to be both a peripheral vascular and a myocardial component in beriberi heart disease, with a more rapid response of the peripheral abnormality to thiamine. Low output cardiac failure may occur, and digitalis is indicated until the myocardial defect is reversed.[32]

At times, there may be only partial regression of cardiomegaly after thiamine therapy, presumably when there is irreversible myocardial fibrosis in the later stages of the disease.

Pellagra

The cardiovascular disturbances and the electrocardiographic abnormalities in pellagra have been attributed both to the nicotinic acid deficiency and to the frequently associated beriberi.

Several studies report no evidence for heart disease due solely to pellagra. Cardiac symptoms and electrocardiographic and radiologic abnormalities were described only in patients with underlying heart disease, and no cardiac lesions attributable to pellagra were demonstrated at postmortem examination.

CLINICAL MANIFESTATIONS

Exertional dyspnea, tachycardia, palpitations, and edema are described, but all of these may not be due to heart disease. The diagnosis is usually suggested by the finding of the typical erythematous skin lesion, glossitis, diarrhea, and dementia in a patient with a diet deficient in tryptophaneniacin.

LABORATORY EXAMINATION

Electrocardiographic abnormalities are usually encountered with the visceral, rather than the dermatologic, manifestations of pellagra. Sinus tachycardia and ST-T changes are most common, with diminished QRS voltage also described. The regression of nonspecific electrocardiographic changes described in 40 percent of patients with pellagra paralleled the clinical improvement.

TREATMENT

Niacin therapy is specific, but multivitamin therapy is generally recommended. Rachmilewitz[38] demonstrated electrocardiographic improvement with niacin therapy alone, rather than with treatment of the associated beriberi; electrocardiographic abnormalities subsided after niacin was administered to patients on thiamine-deficient diets.

Scurvy

Sudden death may occur in patients with severe scurvy and is probably due to myocardial involvement.[39] At postmortem examination, the myocardium may show fatty degeneration.[40]

Right ventricular hypertrophy has been reported in babies with scurvy who die suddenly. The mechanism of the clinical abnormalities and the mechanism of sudden death are unknown. Chest pain, dyspnea, ST-segment abnormalities, and P-Q (P-R) interval prolongation have been observed in human volunteers on a vitamin C–deficient diet.[39]

The diagnosis of severe scurvy should be considered as a medical emergency, requiring immediate intravenous ascorbic acid therapy; this frequently reverses the abnormal electrocardiographic changes.[41]

Hypervitaminosis D

Gross and microscopic deposits of calcium in the heart, associated with myocardial necrosis and fatty degeneration, occur in patients with hypervitaminosis D.[42] The electrocardiographic abnormalities of hypercalcemia—shortened Q-T interval and ST-T changes—may be present. The ST-T alterations may reflect myocardial damage as well (see "Supravalvular Aortic Stenosis," in Chap. 55).

Kwashiorkor

This disease occurs in urbanized South Africa, in Bantus on a high carbohydrate, low protein diet. There is striking atrophy and disintegration of the conduction system; this may be the basis for the atrioventricular conduction disturbances encountered in these children and for the unexplained cases of sudden death.[43] Other cardiac lesions include biventricular dilatation and hypertrophy, interfibrillary edema, myofiber atrophy, minimal interstitial fibrosis, and ventricular endocardial mural thrombosis. There is no significant endocardial fibroelastosis or valvular involvement. Atrophic hearts have been described in children with kwashiorkor.[44] Hepatic fibrosis and hemosiderosis may be present.

The patients characteristically demonstrate tachycardia, cardiomegaly, low output cardiac failure, and extreme edema. Skeletal muscle wasting is particularly prominent in children. Pulmonary and peripheral emboli are common, as is sudden death, the latter often in the first week of recovery.

Nonspecific ST-T abnormalities are the most frequent electrocardiographic alterations, with sinus bradycardia, low QRS voltage, and U waves also seen.[45] Potassium therapy typically reverts the electrocardiographic abnormalities.[30] Arrhythmias are rare. The electrocardiogram becomes normal with clinical improvement. The heart is small on roentgenologic examination.

The patients respond to bed rest and adequate diet in all but the later stages of the disease, but tend to relapse with return to physical activity and an inadequate diet. Transient congestive heart failure is also observed during the recovery phase of kwashiorkor, possibly because of fluid and electrolyte shifts.[46]

Obesity (see also Chap. 89)

There is typically left ventricular or biventricular hypertrophy; isolated cor pulmonale is not seen in the absence of pulmonary embolization.[47,48] Increased cardiac output and an increased circulating blood volume are chronically present in excessively obese patients. Systemic hypertension is common.

The increase in cardiac work appears responsible for the cardiac hypertrophy and eventual myocardial failure. The heart failure initially responds well to digitalis, diuretics, sodium restriction, and limitation of activity. Weight reduction is obviously indicated, but the continuous maintenance of lean body weight seems to be very difficult for such patients.

METABOLIC DISORDERS

Amyloidosis[49–59]

See Chap. 81D.

Pheochromocytoma (see also Chap. 71)

Predominantly epinephrine-secreting pheochromocytomas may mimic a cardiomyopathy.[60] Pathologically, there may be interstitial inflammation, myofiber degeneration, and focal necrosis, with subsequent fibrosis. The catecholamine-induced myocardial damage is due to inability of the coronary circulation to meet the increased metabolic demands of the myocardium; catecholamines probably also cause constriction of the small coronary arteries.

The clinical findings are those of congestive heart failure, tachycardia, and arrhythmias. Sweating, weakness, abdominal pain, and hypotensive episodes are frequently associated manifestations. The diagnosis is often missed when hypertension is absent.[61] Associated hypertrophic obstructive cardiomyopathy has been reported. Cardiac enlargement is evident on chest x-ray, and there are nonspecific ST-T electrocardiographic abnormalities.

Adrenergic blocking agents commonly reverse the ST-T electrocardiographic abnormalities, and preoperative therapy with phenoxybenzamine and propranolol may reduce the surgical risk in patients with pheochromocytoma with cardiomyopathy.[62]

Tumor removal is associated with hemodynamic, electrocardiographic, and clinical improvement of the cardiomyopathy.

Cardiac glycogenosis (glycogen storage disease of the heart, Pompe's disease, glycogenosis type II)

Cardiac glycogenosis is an autosomal recessive disorder of carbohydrate metabolism and occurs equally in both sexes. It is characterized by the accumulation of excessive quantities of normal glycogen in cardiac muscle, skeletal muscle, and other tissues.[63] The specific metabolic defect is absence of the enzyme α-glucosidase.[64] McPhie[65] delineated five categories of glycogenosis, but cardiac involvement is prominent only in type II. Nevertheless, electrocardiographic abnormalities have been described in patients with glycogenosis other than type II;[66,67] and gross myocardial involvement, presumably the cause of death, was recorded in an infant with type III glycogenosis (Cori's disease).[68]

PATHOLOGY

At pathologic examination, the ventricles are massive with thick walls and normal chambers (Fig. 82-1), and the atria are normal. The myocardial fibers are enlarged, with diffuse and extensive vacuolation, producing a lacework pattern; the glycogen-filled

FIGURE 82-1 Glycogen storage disease of the heart. Massive thickening of the left ventricular wall and thickening of the left ventricular endocardium.

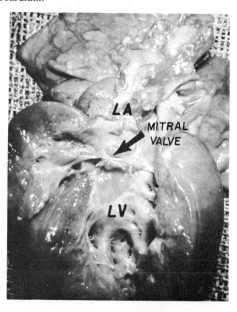

vacuoles compress the nuclei, displacing them to the periphery of the cell.[63]

CLINICAL MANIFESTATIONS

The age at onset of symptoms of glycogen storage disease is a diagnostic clue, as heart failure usually occurs between ages 2 and 6 months, and always before 18 months. The characteristic clinical presentation includes feeding difficulty, cyanosis, dyspnea, tachycardia, massive cardiac enlargement, susceptibility to respiratory infection, and terminal congestive heart failure. Generalized muscle weakness and hypotonia, large tongue, hyporeflexia, and other neurologic deficits are also present, and a similar disorder is often described in a sibling.

Glycogen storage disease with massive left ventricular hypertrophy may also present the clinical and hemodynamic picture of hypertrophic subaortic stenosis.[69] A massively hypertrophied interventricular septum, encroaching upon both the right and left ventricular outflow tracts, has also been described.[66] Digitalis therapy may be harmful in these patients with muscular outflow tract obstruction. Sudden death is common in the first year of life and is presumably due to arrhythmia. Death otherwise occurs in infancy or early childhood, usually related to heart failure or respiratory infection.

LABORATORY EXAMINATION

Demonstration of increased glycogen in a skeletal muscle biopsy confirms the diagnosis, as does the absence of α-glucosidase activity in skeletal muscle or liver biopsy tissue or in the blood leukocytes.[70] Diagnostic confirmation is also afforded by periodic acid Schiff staining of the peripheral blood lymphocytes, demonstrating glycogen granules, and by demonstration of decreased lymphocyte acid maltase activity.[71] The blood sugar level, glucose tolerance, and galactose tolerance are normal, as is the response to injected glucagon and epinephrine; these test results distinguish between Pompe's disease and other types of glycogen storage disease.

Electrocardiogram The electrocardiographic pattern is that of left ventricular hypertrophy, with strikingly increased QRS voltage and a shortened P-Q interval[72] (Fig. 82-2). Ehlers[63] believes that these electrocardiographic findings are pathognomonic and that they distinguish this abnormality from other causes of left ventricular hypertrophy in infancy. T-wave abnormalities and left axis deviation are also seen.

FIGURE 82-2 Glycogen storage disease of the heart in a 3-month-old infant. There is biventricular hypertrophy with massively increased QRS voltage and Wolff-Parkinson-White conduction.

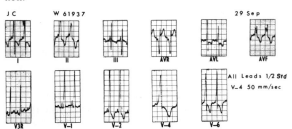

Chest x-ray Massive generalized cardiac enlargement and pulmonary congestion are characteristic (Fig. 82-3).

Echocardiography Echocardiography can delineate the enormously thickened interventricular septum and ventricular walls. Systolic anterior motion of the anterior mitral valve leaflet has also been described,[73] as has outflow tract obstruction.

Cardiac catheterization Angiocardiography usually demonstrates a massive, thick-walled left ventricle, which appears rigid, particularly when there is associated endocardial sclerosis. We have seen a patient with massive cardiomegaly and right ventricular preponderance; the angiocardiographic findings were suggestive of a tumor within the right ventricle (Fig. 82-3).

DIAGNOSTIC CRITERIA AND DIFFERENTIAL DIAGNOSIS

Di Sant'Agnese lists four criteria for the diagnosis of cardiac glycogen storage disease: (1) marked cardiomegaly, (2) lacework appearance of the myocardium, (3) clinical or histologic confirmation of the presence of normal glycogen, and (4) death within the first year of life. However, survival has been reported to the age of 34 months.[74] This condition must be differentiated from endocardial fibroelastosis, anomalous left coronary artery, coronary artery sclerosis of infancy, and acute myocarditis, all of which may produce severe heart failure in the infant.

TREATMENT

There is, at present, no specific therapy. Attempts at surgical resection of the hypertrophied interventricular septum have been unrewarding, as has been the administration of acid maltase.[71] Digitalis must be administered with caution.

Other glycogen abnormalities of the myocardium

CONGENITAL NODULAR GLYCOGENIC INFILTRATION

Congenital nodular glycogenic infiltration of the myocardium, previously designated as rhabdomyoma, is the most common cardiac "tumor" in the pediatric age group and is associated with tuberous sclerosis in approximately 50 percent of cases.[75,76] These solitary or multiple "tumors," first described by von Recklinghausen in 1862, are not encapsulated but merge with the surrounding myocardium; the cause is obscure but seems related to a disturbance of glycogen metabolism. The gray-purple nodules in the ventricle are usually incidental findings at postmortem examination, but large glycogenic masses in the interventricular septum may cause arrhythmias and AV block. Arrhythmias and sudden death in infancy are not uncommon; 52 percent fatality was reported in the first year of life, and 86 percent fatality before

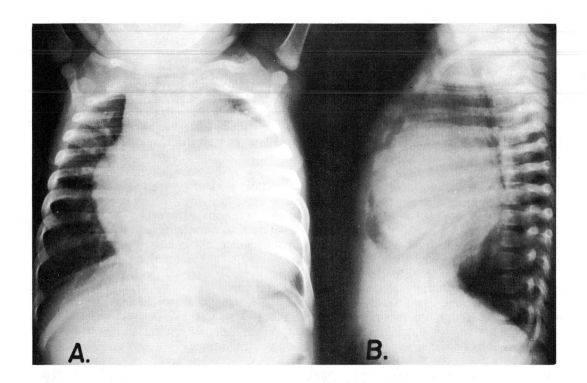

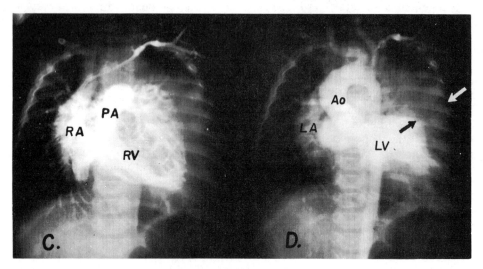

FIGURE 82-3 Glycogen storage disease of the heart. *A,B.* Massive generalized cardiomegaly with pulmonary congestion. Cardiac pulsations were normal at fluoroscopy. *C,D.* Venous angiocardiogram demonstrating distortion of the right ventricular outflow tract secondary to hypertrophy of the interventricular septum and left ventricle (between arrows).

puberty occurred in one series of patients with rhabdomyoma. Subaortic and subpulmonic stenoses have been due to rhabdomyoma.[77] Symptomatic "tumors" are potentially amenable to surgery.[77a]

GLYCOGEN IN FAMILIAL CARDIOMYOPATHY

Increased myocardial glycogen has also been reported in patients with familial cardiomyopathy; they were demonstrated to have normal function of all the enzymes characteristically absent in known forms of glycogenosis.[78]

McArdle's syndrome

McArdle's syndrome is a metabolic myopathy in which deficient glycogen breakdown in muscle is due to lack of muscle phosphorylase. There is an autosomal recessive pattern of inheritance. Clinically, there is profound skeletal muscle weakness, with pain and stiffness on exercise. Clinical cardiovascular disease is unusual.

Ratinov et al.[79] reported a patient with P-R interval prolongation, an interventricular conduction delay, increased QRS voltage, and T-wave abnormalities; these electrocardiographic changes are similar to those of other forms of cardiac glycogenosis. Myoglobinuria may be present.

Polysaccharide storage disease

The precise metabolic abnormality is not defined. Some patients have associated hepatic cirrhosis. Nonmetachromatic neutral polysaccharide is deposited in the myocardium in discrete granules or in plaques. Cellular vacuolation and abnormal glycogen deposition have been described.[67]

Dyspnea, palpitations, giddiness, and syncope may occur. Cardiac enlargement and systolic murmurs are described. Electrocardiographic abnormalities include biventricular and left ventricular hypertrophy, conduction abnormalities, Q waves, and P- and T-wave abnormalities.

Hemochromatosis

The diagnosis of hemochromatosis must be considered, especially in males, with cardiomyopathy without apparent cause, since this is a potentially remediable disease.

Hemochromatosis is a metabolic disorder characterized by excessive tissue iron deposition. It occurs predominantly in the male and in the older age group. Since the advent of insulin therapy of diabetes, cardiac failure has been the leading cause of death in hemochromatosis,[80] accounting for one-third to one-half of the fatalities. Fifteen percent of patients with hemochromatosis present with cardiac symptoms, and cardiac disease occurs even in the absence of skin pigmentation and diabetes. Cardiac involvement is characteristic in patients with hemochromatosis presenting in childhood or early adult life.[81]

PATHOLOGY

At postmortem examination,[80] the myocardium may be rusty brown; biventricular dilatation and hypertrophy are seen. The myocardial fibers are infiltrated with iron-pigment granules (Fig. 82-4); iron is not deposited in interstitial connective tissue, hence no fibrosis occurs. Myofiber fragmentation and atrophy are present. Subepicardial iron deposition is most

FIGURE 82-4 Hemochromatosis of the myocardium. Deposition of hemosiderin granules (arrow) in myocardial fibers (×430).

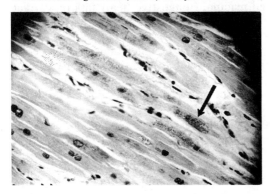

extensive; the right atrium is the least commonly involved chamber. Extensive deposition of iron pigment in the conduction system is unusual.[82]

PATHOPHYSIOLOGY

Hemochromatosis is a disease of iron storage with resultant tissue damage, but the genesis of the cardiac insufficiency is unknown. Indeed, the mechanism of iron entry into myocardial cells is unknown. There is no correlation between the degree of myocardial iron deposition, the extent of the resultant interstitial fibrosis, and the cardiac functional impairment. However, patients with grossly visible cardiac iron deposition all have heart failure.[83] The rate of iron deposition may be more important than the absolute quantity of iron; interference with an enzyme system or another metabolic abnormality has also been postulated. Cardiac iron deposition occurs only after the liver and other organs are saturated with iron; iron deposition is greater in cardiac than in skeletal or smooth muscle.[13]

The hemodynamic pattern resembling constrictive pericarditis or restrictive cardiomyopathy demonstrated at cardiac catheterization[80,84] suggests a mechanical cause of the cardiac failure, such as myocardial fibrosis; however, this is not always present.[85] Electron microscopic evidence of intracellular disruption by iron deposition—decreased mitochondria and myofibrils—suggests that iron deposition per se can cause myocardial dysfunction.[86]

CLINICAL MANIFESTATIONS

Hemochromatosis is clinically recognizable by the tetrad of liver disease, diabetes mellitus, heart disease, and skin pigmentation. Classically, the patient is dyspneic, with generalized cardiomegaly, stasis cyanosis, edema, and ascites. The presentation[80,84] includes arrhythmias, AV block, and rapidly progressive congestive heart failure which responds poorly to digitalis and diuretic therapy. Unexplained precordial pain is occasionally described. Paroxysmal atrial tachycardia and paroxysmal atrial fibrillation are the most frequent arrhythmias. The supraventricular arrhythmias relate to atrial rather than to conduction system iron deposition; iron is rarely deposited in conduction tissue. Ventricular arrhythmias are less common, despite ventricular iron deposition.

Electrocardiographic abnormalities,[87] in addition to the arrhythmias, include diminished QRS voltage, conduction disturbances, and nonspecific T-wave changes. Electrocardiographic abnormalities may be the earliest evidence of cardiac involvement.

A large globular heart with feeble pulsations and biventricular hypertrophy is seen at *radiologic* examination; it may mimic pericardial effusion, constrictive pericarditis, beriberi, or myxedema heart disease. *Echocardiography* in the early stages of the disease has been reported to show a nondilated, concentrically thickened left ventricle with diminished compliance; late in the illness, the picture is indistinguishable from a congestive cardiomyopathy.[86] Echocardiographic abnormalities may antedate clinically evident myocardial disease.

Confirmatory diagnostic evidence includes demonstration of excessive iron deposits in a sternal marrow aspirate and/or liver biopsy specimen, and the finding of an elevated serum iron level.

TREATMENT
Removal of iron by repeated venesection, except in patients with chronic refractory anemia, is the accepted therapy. Permanent pacemaker insertion successfully controlled syncopal episodes in a patient with complete heart block.[88] Death in untreated patients usually occurs within a year after the onset of cardiac symptoms. One patient[89] survived more than 3 years after the onset of cardiac disease; regression of cardiomegaly occurred after repeated phlebotomy, in which about 31 g of iron was removed. Other patients have had regression of symptoms and hemodynamic abnormalities with repeated venesection.[81,83]

Acquired hemochromatosis

Acquired hemochromatosis is seen in patients with refractory anemias requiring multiple transfusions and has similar cardiac complications.[90] These include pericarditis with and without effusion, cardiac enlargement, heart failure, atrial and ventricular arrhythmias, and atrioventricular block. The anatomic abnormalities are indistinguishable from idiopathic hemochromatosis. Chelating agents, designed to remove excess iron, may be of value.[86]

Fabry's disease (angiokeratoma corporis diffusum universale)

Cardiac failure is a common cause of death in this inherited abnormality of glycolipid metabolism, which occurs predominantly in the male. This sex-linked disorder is variably and incompletely recessive, with severest manifestations in the homozygous male and mild disease in the heterozygous female.[91] Abnormal glycolipid deposition in the blood vessel walls and in the myocardium is due to a deficiency of the enzyme ceramide trihexosidase.[92]

PATHOLOGY
At autopsy, the myofibers are fragmented, with striking vacuolation, due to glycolipid deposition; ceramide trihexoside may also be deposited in the coronary arteries (contributing to myocardial infarction), the conduction system, and the heart valves.[92a] Mitral and aortic valve abnormalities are common.[67,93] The glycolipid deposits in the lysosomes have a lamellar ultrastructure, similar to that of other lipidoses; however, the pattern of organ involvement in Fabry's disease resembles the glycogenoses more than other lipidoses. Cardiac and smooth-muscle

involvement in Fabry's disease is far more severe and extensive than in other biochemically related lipid metabolism disorders.[91]

CLINICAL MANIFESTATIONS
Angiokeratosis and corneal opacities are common. There are crises characterized by fever and burning pain in the extremities. Clinical cardiovascular manifestations occur in most patients and include left ventricular hypertrophy and ultimate cardiac failure.[94] Hypertension is common and is generally due to renal failure; angina pectoris and myocardial infarction may occur.[95] Cardiac murmurs may be heard. Evidence of renal dysfunction is characteristic.

The *electrocardiogram* may show changes of left ventricular hypertrophy or myocardial infarction.[93] Sinoatrial block, a short P-Q interval, atrial fibrillation, right bundle branch block, and nonspecific ST-T changes have been recorded. Cardiac enlargement is evident on chest x-ray and changes of pulmonary vascular congestion may appear.

There is no effective therapy.

Tay-Sachs disease

This neurodegenerative disorder, inherited as an autosomal recessive trait, especially in Jewish families, is due to hexosaminidase A deficiency. Gangliosides are important constituents of cell membranes; the deposition of abnormal gangliosides in the myocardium may explain the electrocardiographic repolarization derangements.[67]

Cardiovascular symptoms are unusual in these children with mental retardation, decerebrate rigidity, and a cherry red macula. Those affected with the disease die in early childhood. Electrocardiographic abnormalities include a wide QRS-T angle, Q-T interval prolongation, and abnormal T waves.

Sandhoff's disease

This autosomal recessive disorder of glycosphingolipid metabolism, due to hexosaminidase A and B deficiency, resembles Tay-Sachs disease. Anatomic abnormalities include endocardial fibroelastosis; redundancy and hooding of the mitral valve, with abnormal myxoid valve tissue; and coronary artery luminal narrowing due to fibroblastic proliferation[67] in a foamy, fibrocollagenous background. There is early central nervous system degeneration and a cherry red macula. Congestive heart failure, cardiac enlargement, and mitral regurgitant murmurs are present.

Electrocardiographic changes include T-wave abnormalities and those of left ventricular hypertrophy. The diagnosis is made by finding globoside in the urinary sediment or by measuring plasma activity of globoside or hexosamine.

G_{M1} gangliosidosis

Galactosidase deficiency is characteristic of this autosomal recessive trait. Foamy histiocytes with vacuolation are seen, with thickening of the mitral and tricuspid valves.[67] One-third of patients have cardiovascular involvement.

Progressive psychomotor retardation, hepatosplenomegaly, and skeletal abnormalities are present. Cardiovascular symptoms are unusual, and electrocardiographic abnormalities are nonspecific.

Niemann-Pick disease

This autosomal recessive disorder is characterized by excessive tissue sphingomyelin with foam cells in the myocardium. Clinical evidence of cardiac dysfunction is rare.

Isolated cardiac lipidosis

Isolated myofiber lipid accumulation has been reported in a few infants. The pathogenesis is unknown. Lipid accumulates in the sarcoplasm of myocardial cells, producing myofibril degeneration. The lipid is primarily triglyceride, with some free fatty acids. On electron microscopy, there are increased numbers and swelling of the mitochondria, with abnormal intramitochondrial membranes. Lipoprotein infiltration confined to the base of the heart and the conduction system produced fatal atrial tachyarrhythmias in a young infant. No other organ system was involved.[96]

The infants, who often have central nervous system symptoms, develop cardiac enlargement and heart failure. Arrhythmias are common, and they and/or the heart failure are the cause of death.[97] Conduction disturbances and biventricular hypertrophy are seen on the electrocardiogram.

Porphyria

Despite an absence of cardiac symptoms and clinical cardiovascular abnormalities in porphyria, pigment deposition and myocardial fiber disintegration with loss of nuclei and striations are frequently seen at postmortem examination.

Eliaser described electrocardiographic abnormalities, diminished QRS voltage, left axis deviation, and ST-segment displacement during an attack of acute porphyria in a patient with a normal electrocardiogram between attacks. T-wave abnormalities have also been reported with acute porphyria.[98] However, completely normal electrocardiograms have also been reported in 10 patients with porphyria, 8 recorded during an acute attack.

Mucopolysaccharidoses[99]

The genetically determined disturbances of mucopolysaccharide metabolism are distinguished biochemically by the mucopolysaccharides deposited in tissues and/or excreted in the urine (see Chaps. 62B and 55). Abnormal cytoplasmic granulations (Alder's anomaly, Reilly bodies) are present in the peripheral blood leukocytes in several types of mucopolysaccharidoses and may furnish a clue to the etiology of the cardiac disease.[100] Precise enzymatic defects have not been identified.

HURLER'S SYNDROME (GARGOYLISM, MUCOPOLYSACCHARIDOSIS I)

Clinical cardiovascular disease is present in more than 70 percent of patients with Hurler's syndrome (gargoylism). This inborn error of metabolism is characterized by the deposition of a complex macromolecular glycoprotein in the parenchymal cells and supporting connective tissue of most organ systems.[101] It is inherited both as an autosomal and as a sex-linked recessive trait.

Pathology At postmortem examination[102] the myocardial and connective tissue cells are swollen, hypertrophied, and vacuolated. Myocardial involvement is most prominent adjacent to blood vessels; large cells filled with storage material interfere with myocardial contractility. There is biventricular cardiac hypertrophy; nodulation and thickening of the heart valves, preferentially involving the mitral valve; endocardial sclerosis; and intimal proliferation of the coronary and pulmonary arteries.[102a]

Clinical manifestations Clinical signs and symptoms usually appear between the ages of 1 and 2 years, when sufficient glycoprotein has accumulated to interfere with tissue growth, structure, and function. Mental retardation, skeletal deformities, corneal opacities, and hepatosplenomegaly are characteristic.

Cardiomegaly and murmurs of valve deformity, particularly mitral regurgitation,[103] with resultant congestive heart failure, comprise the major cardiac abnormalities. Calcific mitral stenosis has been described. Clinical or electrocardiographic evidence of coronary insufficiency is rare, despite the frequent and significant coronary artery narrowing. The associated thoracic deformities, pulmonary disease, hypertension, hypoproteinemia, and anemia contribute to the cardiovascular symptoms. Cardiac failure is the cause of death in two-thirds of patients with Hurler's syndrome, with death occurring at an average age of 11 years.

There is no specific therapy.

Laboratory examination At *radiologic* examination, there is generalized cardiomegaly (Fig. 82-5) and calcification of the mitral valve ring; this is the most common cause of mitral annulus calcification in childhood. No specific *electrocardiographic* pattern is present, although Q-T prolongation and left ventricular hypertrophy are noted. *Echocardiography* may help identify valvular abnormalities and calcification, as well as muscle function abnormalities[104] (Fig. 82-6).

Excessive amounts of dermitan sulfate and heparitin sulfate are excreted in the urine.

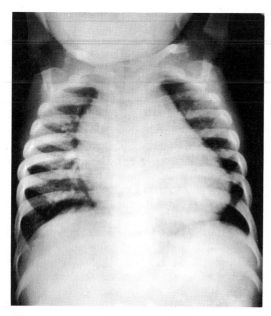

FIGURE 82-5 Generalized cardiac enlargement and prominent bronchovascular markings in a child with Hurler's syndrome.

HUNTER'S SYNDROME (MUCOPOLYSACCHARIDOSIS II)

Hunter's syndrome, inherited as an X-linked recessive trait, has the same biochemical defect as Hurler's syndrome. The clinical manifestations are milder, and corneal clouding is not grossly evident.

SANFILLIPO'S SYNDROME (MUCOPOLYSACCHARIDOSIS III)

This abnormality of heparitin sulfate metabolism is inherited as an autosomal recessive trait. Patients have severe mental retardation, hepatosplenomegaly, stiffened joints, and coarse facial features; mitral insufficiency with anterior leaflet prolapse has been described.[67]

MORQUIO SYNDROME (MUCOPOLYSACCHARIDOSIS IV)

Morquio syndrome is an abnormality of keratosulfate metabolism inherited as an autosomal recessive trait. The characteristic cardiac lesion is aortic regurgitation (Fig. 82-7) which characteristically appears after adolescence. There are skeletal deformities and corneal opacities, but no mental retardation.

SCHEIE'S SYNDROME (MUCOPOLYSACCHARIDOSIS V)

Aortic regurgitation is also the cardiac lesion in Scheie's syndrome, an abnormality of chondroitin sulfate B metabolism which is inherited as an autosomal recessive trait.

MAROTEAUX-LAMY SYNDROME (MUCOPOLYSACCHARIDOSIS VI)

No cardiac manifestations have been noted in this abnormality of chondroitin sulfate B metabolism, which is inherited as an autosomal recessive trait.

FUCOSIDOSIS

This disorder is due to fucose accumulation in tissues, with predominant progressive cerebral degeneration which produces dementia, loss of muscle strength, spasticity, and decerebrate rigidity. Cardiac enlargement and arrhythmias occur.[67] Electrocardiographic abnormalities are nonspecific, but premature ventricular beats are common.

Refsum's syndrome

This inherited disorder of lipid metabolism, with an autosomal recessive mode of transmission, is characterized by phytanic acid accumulation due to impaired oxidative degeneration.[105] Cardiovascular involvement occurs in the majority of patients.

PATHOLOGY

Microscopic examination of the myocardium shows atrophic cells and fibrosis; there is no evidence of inflammation, but the autonomic nerves, sinus node, and His bundle are abnormally prominent. This ap-

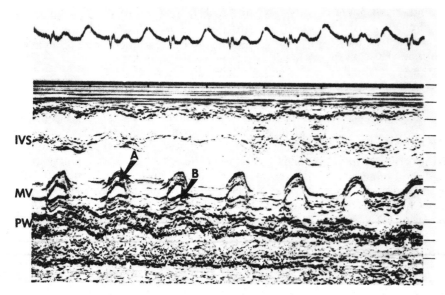

FIGURE 82-6 Hurler's syndrome. Thickening of the anterior (A) and posterior (B) leaflets of the mitral valve on an echocardiogram.

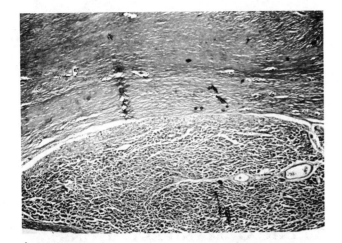

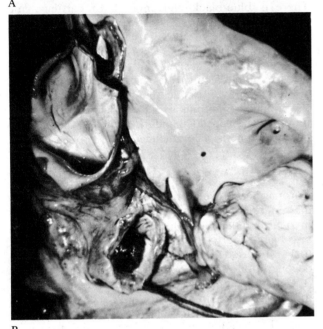

FIGURE 82-7 Morquio-Ulrich syndrome. *A.* Marked thickening of the endocardium is mainly fibrous, with sparse elastic fibers (×20). *B.* Gross specimen with thickened endocardium.

pears to be due to phytanic acid accumulation in the heart, mainly localized peripherally in the myelin sheath.

CLINICAL MANIFESTATIONS

Chronic polyneuropathy, cerebellar ataxia, and atypical retinitis pigmentosa are seen. More severe cardiac involvement is associated with ophthalmoplegia, ptosis, and facial weakness. Palpitations, Stokes-Adams syncope, and sudden death are described.

Electrocardiographic conduction and ST-T abnormalities; arrhythmias, especially complete heart block; and at times Q-T prolongation have been described as cardiovascular complications of heredopathia atactica polyneuritiformis, or Refsum's syndrome.[106] Cerebrospinal fluid protein level is elevated.

A diet low in phytanic acid and standard antiarrhythmic therapy are recommended.

Primary xanthomatosis
(see also Chaps. 62B and 62H)

Patients with familial hypercholesterolemic xanthomatosis have an increased incidence of premature atherosclerotic coronary artery disease.[107] Cardiovascular symptoms are due to a combination of coronary atherosclerotic heart disease with myocardial infarction and xanthomatous infiltration of the myocardium.

PATHOLOGY

In one patient with xanthomatosis, the coronary arteries were normal but the ventricles were hypertrophic, with focal yellow-gray patches. Focal lipid deposits and fibrosis extensively involved the interventricular septum, probably causing the arrhythmias and conduction abnormalities.[108] Acquired aortic stenosis, with foamy macrophages and cholesterol clefts in the aortic valve, has been described in hypercholesterolemic xanthomatosis.[109]

CLINICAL MANIFESTATIONS
(see Chaps. 62B and 62H)

In addition to the usual presentation of the hypercholesterolemic type of xanthomatosis as coronary artery disease or, rarely, aortic stenosis, hereditary normocholesterolemic xanthomatosis may present as congestive cardiomyopathy with congestive heart failure, arrhythmias, and conduction abnormalities.[108]

TREATMENT
See Chaps. 62B and 62H.

Hand-Schüller-Christian disease

In Hand-Schüller-Christian disease, lipid accumulation may be secondary to reticuloendothelial cell abnormality, as no disturbance of lipid metabolism has been demonstrated.[110] Xanthomatous deposits, consisting mainly of cholesterol and neutral fat, occur in many organ systems, including the myocardium, in generalized Hand-Schüller-Christian disease. The classic clinical triad includes exophthalmos, diabetes insipidus, and bony defects of the calvarium.

There is little correlation between cardiovascular infiltrates and cardiovascular symptoms. The clinical course of Hand-Schüller-Christian disease is slowly progressive.

There is no specific therapy.

Gout

Urate deposits in the heart may involve the intima of the coronary arteries; the valvular endocardium, usually of the mitral valve; the pericardium; and the myocardium. In one patient with gout,[111] a mitral valve tophus extended through the myocardium into the epicardium, compressing the left circumflex coronary artery, causing myocardial infarction. The microscopic appearance was that of a classic tophus–central amorphous material, demonstrated to be uric acid and urates, with a rim of fibrous connective tissue containing giant cells and macrophages.

Arrhythmias, including variable degrees of atrioventricular block, constitute the major clinical manifestations. Hypertension is secondary to renal disease. Pericarditis has been described.

Bigeminal rhythm in a patient with gout was unresponsive to quinidine and procainamide (Pronestyl) but subsided, on several occasions, after probenecid therapy; the arrhythmia was presumed due to a gouty deposit. Complete heart block, which appeared during an attack of gout, resolved to a Wenckebach phenomenon and then to first-degree atrioventricular block, concomitant with uricosuric therapy, a decrease in serum uric acid concentration, and disappearance of the clinical symptoms of gout; urate deposition in the conduction system was implicated.[112] Probable acute gouty pericarditis has been successfully treated with colchicine.[113]

Oxalosis

Primary oxalosis, a rare hereditary defect (autosomal recessive) in intermediary metabolism, and secondary hyperoxaluria are both characterized by calcium oxalate deposition in body tissues. At postmortem examination, refractile, yellow, rosette-like calcium oxalate crystals are seen in the myocardial fibers and interstitial tissue of the heart, in the coronary arteries, and in the cardiac conduction system.[114] Mononuclear cell infiltrates and myofiber degeneration and fibrosis occur in areas of dense crystal deposition.[115]

Patients with primary oxalosis have nephrolithiasis, nephrocalcinosis, and renal failure. Congestive heart failure may occur. Cardiac arrhythmias and conduction abnormalities have been described in patients with oxalosis, with complete heart block sometimes presenting as a medical emergency.[116,117] Hemorrhagic pericardial effusion has also been described.[67] In patients with renal insufficiency, secondary oxalosis may also cause heart failure and conduction abnormalities, including complete heart block.[118]

There is no known therapy. Pacemaker implantation may be indicated. In patients with uremia and secondary oxalosis, hemodialysis may decrease calcium oxalate deposition.[118]

Aspartyl glucosaminuria

This hereditary disease, reported primarily from Finland, is due to a lysozomal enzyme deficiency in glycolipid metabolism. Patients have a coarse facies, bony and connective tissue abnormalities, and progressive mental retardation. Systolic murmurs and

T-wave abnormalities on the electrocardiogram are described, and one patient had moderate mitral regurgitation at cardiac catheterization.[67]

Ochronosis (alkaptonuria)

This disorder is due to a deficiency of homogentisic oxidase. Areas of gray-blue to purple-black pigmentation occur in the myocardium and coronary arteries; ochronotic pigment granules are deposited preferentially in collagen and fibrous tissue but do not evoke an inflammatory cell response.[118a] Atheromata in the coronary arteries have a characteristic blue-black pigmentation.

CLINICAL MANIFESTATIONS

There is blue-black pigmentation of cartilage and other tissue; arthritis is prominent. There is only modest evidence of cardiovascular disease with hereditary or exogenous ochronosis compared with the striking anatomic lesions. Aortic and mitral valve disease with calcification may produce murmurs; aortic and left ventricular aneurysms usually produce few clinical symptoms. Homogentisic acid is present in the urine, producing dark urine. A diet low in phenylalanine is recommended.

Primary myocardial calcification

Coronary atherosclerotic heart disease with myocardial infarction is the most common cause of massive myocardial calcification. Cardiac calcification has also been reported secondary to vascular, inflammatory, and toxic causes of myofiber necrosis and degeneration.

Generalized myocardial calcification was reported in a premature infant with myofiber degnerative changes. Right ventricular calcification was described[119] in adults with endomyocardial fibrosis in Uganda. There is no apparent abnormality of calcium metabolism in these cases.

Paget's disease of bone

In addition to the high output cardiac failure encounter in patients with generalized Paget's disease, calcification of the heart valves may extend into the interventricular system and has produced complete heart block.[120]

Fibrocystic disease of the pancreas (mucoviscidosis)

Cor pulmonale, secondary to chronic pulmonary disease, is the most common form of heart disease in patients with fibrocystic disease of the pancreas.

Myocardial fibrosis has also been reported with fibrocystic disease of the pancreas in infants and young children. At postmortem examination, there is biventricular dilatation and hypertrophy, with scar tissue replacement of degenerating muscle fibers; endocardial fibroelastosis of the atria is prominent.[121] Focal necrosis is described.

The suggested causes include nutritional or metabolic deficiencies, probably related to the steatorrhea and to prolonged antibiotic therapy which alters the intestinal flora.[122,123] Viral or other infectious myocarditis, associated with pulmonary infections, is also implicated. It appears unlikely that the myocardial lesions are a primary manifestation of the cystic fibrosis.[124]

The clinical presentation includes cardiac enlargement, arrhythmias, and electrocardiographic abnormalities; the patients usually succumb to congestive heart failure.

Hypokalemia

Hypokalemia is encountered in the clinical setting of prolonged diarrhea or vomiting, familial periodic paralysis, primary aldosteronism, potassium-losing nephritis, sprue, gastrointestinal fistula, diabetic acidosis, severe alkalosis, or corticosteroid hormone and diuretic therapy, etc.; cardiovascular abnormalities are usual when the serum potassium level is less than 3 mEq/liter.

PATHOLOGY

The myocardial lesions due to hypokalemia in human beings are similar to those produced in rats by a potassium-deficient diet. Loss of muscle striation, myofiber vacuolation and fragmentation, interstitial cellular infiltrate, and varying myocardial necrosis and fibroblastic proliferation (Fig. 82-8) are most pronounced in the subendocardial layer of the ventricles and in the papillary muscles.

CLINICAL MANIFESTATIONS

Significant abnormalities of cardiovascular function are uncommon, although hypotension, tachycardia, and congestive heart failure have been reported.

The characteristic electrocardiographic pattern is of Q-U interval prolongation, widening and flattening of the T wave, ST-segment displacement, prominent U waves, diminished QRS voltage, and increased AV conduction time. These abnormalities are probably

FIGURE 82-8 Hypokalemic myocarditis. There is an interstitial inflammatory infiltrate, with myofiber fragmentation (×150).

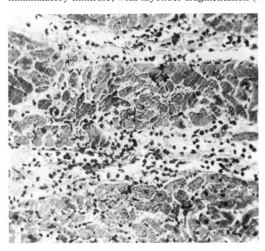

due to electrophysiologic disturbances rather than anatomic myocardial lesions. There is little relation between the serum potassium level and the extent of electrocardiographic changes, suggesting that the electrocardiographic alterations reflect myocardial potassium concentration;[125] in one patient with hypokalemic myocarditis secondary to steatorrhea, the myocardial potassium concentration was 15 mg/100 g of wet tissue, compared with a normal value of greater than 300 mg. Weaver and Burchell,[126] however, believe a specific hypokalemic electrocardiographic pattern correlates well with the serum potassium level in stable patients.

Digitalis intoxication may become manifest in patients who are receiving digitalis and become hypokalemic as a result of diuretics that produce a kaluresis. (See Chaps. 44 and 46D.)

TREATMENT

Potassium replacement is requisite and total body potassium stores must be repleted. Oral replacement therapy is often preferrable to parenteral treatment, but the latter is often required in hypokalemic patients who are receiving digitalis and have a cardiac arrhythmia.

Uremia (see Chap. 69B)

The frequent cardiovascular manifestations of uremia include left ventricular hypertrophy, congestive heart failure, arrhythmias, and pericarditis and may be due to hypertensive cardiovascular disease, electrolyte imbalance, fluid overload, anemia, coronary artery disease, the arteriovenous fistula used for hemodialysis, and/or metastatic myocardial calcification.[127] Whether a true uremic cardiomyopathy exists remains controversial.[128,129] Calcium deposition in the small myocardial arteries evokes intimal proliferation and fibrosis with resultant luminal narrowing and ischemic myocardial damage.[130] A myocardial depressant substance in uremia has been postulated; uremic compounds have been shown to depress pumping function in experimental animal hearts.[131]

CLINICAL MANIFESTATIONS

A specific clinical syndrome of uremic cardiomyopathy has been described[132] in patients treated for chronic renal failure by a low protein diet; it is characterized by massive cardiomegaly, gallop sounds, decreased mean blood pressure, pericarditis, arrhythmias, and marked sensitivity to cardiac glycosides.

The pericarditis appears related to the degree of renal failure. Uremic pericarditis is characteristically serosanguineous to hemorrhagic, hence there is danger of fatal cardiac tamponade when heparin is administered for hemodialysis. Occasionally cardiac tamponade or constrictive pericarditis occurs;[133,134]

constriction appears to be more frequent in dialyzed patients, in part due to heparin-related bleeding.

Nonspecific electrocardiographic abnormalities in patients with uremia may be attributed to the associated hypertension, anemia, electrolyte abnormalities, and pericarditis. In patients receiving chronic renal dialysis, conduction defects, complete heart block, and even sudden death appear related to metastatic calcification of the conduction system.[127,135] Patients on a high fat, low protein renal failure diet for a number of years may also have an increased incidence of coronary atherosclerotic heart disease which may produce electrocardiographic abnormalities. Constrictive pericarditis should be suspected when the cardiac silhouette decreases in size in the face of persistent or increased evidence of congestive heart failure.[134]

TREATMENT

All abnormalities of uremic cardiomyopathy improve markedly or disappear after hemodialysis. The role of the protein-restricted diet in the development of the cardiomyopathy syndrome is uncertain. Pericarditis and pericardial effusion can usually be controlled by dialysis, indomethacin therapy, and/or pericardiocentesis. Constriction may require pericardiectomy.

HEMATOLOGIC DISEASES

Leukemia

Clinical cardiovascular or electrocardiographic abnormalities occur in about 25 percent of patients with leukemia. Half of the cardiac manifestations are due to leukemic infiltrates in the myocardium; the remainder are attributable to anemia, myocardial hemorrhage, hypoxia, pericarditis, etc.

PATHOLOGY

Leukemic cellular infiltrates are observed in the myocardium in about one-half of patients dying of leukemia; this occurs more commonly in acute and stem-cell leukemia, and more frequently in myelocytic than in lymphocytic leukemia. Myocardial involvement is rare in Hodgkin's disease. Cardiac leukemic infiltration is more likely with an increased peripheral leukocyte count and an increased patient survival time.[136]

The characteristic lesion is focal leukemic infiltration of the myocardial capillaries and interstitial tissues (Fig. 82-9); dense infiltration causes muscle degeneration and necrosis. Anemia is the principal factor responsible for cardiac hypertrophy; cardiac hypertrophy is encountered more frequently with prolonged survival with the disease, hence chronic anemia.[136] In acute leukemia, cellular infiltrates (Fig. 82-10) and hemorrhage occur most frequently in the pericardium and in the walls of the right atrium and

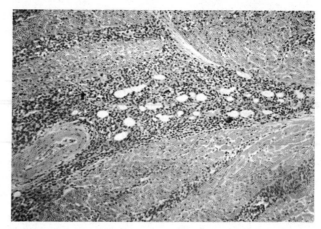

FIGURE 82-9 Acute leukemia. Focal leukemic infiltrate in the interstitium. No myocardial fiber atrophy or necrosis (×20).

left ventricle.[137] Left atrial rupture due to massive leukemic infiltration has been reported.

CLINICAL MANIFESTATIONS

Myocardial invasion and cardiovascular symptoms may occur early in the course of leukemia, particularly in acute leukemia. Occasionally, cardiac symptoms are the initial manifestations of the disease.

There is often a discrepancy between the severe cardiac involvement at autopsy and the lack of clinical disease. Cardiovascular symptoms may be overshadowed by other manifestations of acute leukemia.[137] Also, the cardiac symptoms and electrocardiographic disturbances depend on both the extent and the location of the leukemic myocardial infiltrates.

The predominant clinical manifestations are tachycardia, arrhythmias, cardiac enlargement, pericarditis, and congestive heart failure.[138] Most patients with clinical evidence of leukemic heart disease have abnormal electrocardiograms. There is no diagnostic electrocardiographic pattern, but tachycardia, premature ventricular beats, ventricular or atrial excitation abnormalities, and nonspecific ST-T changes are common. Heart block has been described. Leukemic

FIGURE 82-10 Acute myeloblastic leukemia. Cross section through the right atrial wall, at the area of the coronary sulcus, showing the right coronary artery (arrow) embedded in a massive leukemic infiltrate.

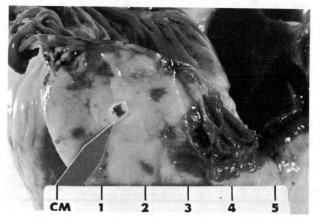

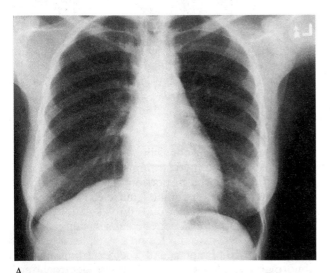

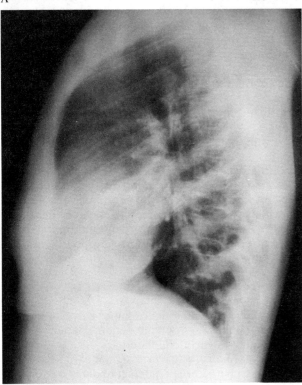

FIGURE 82-11 Sickle-cell cardiomyopathy. *A.* Minimal cardiac enlargement and straightening of the border of the left side of the heart. *B.* Diagnosis of sickle-cell problem suggested by flattened vertebrae with biconcave discs.

heart block was reported to disappear after x-ray therapy, and ST-T abnormalities reverted to normal after Myleran administration.[139]

Myeloma

Cardiac involvement with myeloma is unusual since myeloma nodules rarely involve the myocardium and pericardium. Characteristically, patients have no cardiovascular symptoms. Cardiac tamponade and digitalis-resistant atrial fibrillation, the latter due to an SA node myeloma infiltrate, have been described, however.[140]

Sickle-cell anemia

The cardiovascular manifestations of sickle-cell disease are due to the chronic anemia; to the pulmonary arterial thromboses, leading to cor pulmonale; and to the myocardial disease caused by thrombosis of small intracardiac blood vessels.[141] At postmortem examination, biventricular dilatation and hypertrophy, myofiber hypertrophy, arteritis with proliferation and thrombosis, and resultant myocardial degeneration, necrosis, and secondary fibrosis are noted.

CLINICAL MANIFESTATIONS

Cardiomegaly is present in most patients with sickle-cell anemia and is usually associated with prominent exertional dyspnea and systolic murmurs. Congestive heart failure is a late manifestation.

The frequent pulmonary systolic murmurs and mitral systolic and diastolic murmurs, coupled with the joint symptoms of sickle-cell disease, often lead to the misdiagnosis of acute rheumatic fever and chronic rheumatic heart disease.

Although dyspnea is the predominant symptom, classic symptoms and electrocardiographic changes of myocardial ischemia occurred in a 22-year-old man during a sickle-cell crisis; the electrocardiogram reverted to normal after the crisis, and myocardial infarction was not demonstrated at subsequent postmortem examination.

Anemia and sickling are readily demonstrable, and characteristic bone changes may be detected (Fig. 82-11). There is no specific electrocardiographic pattern for sickle-cell anemia, but P-Q interval prolongation and nonspecific ST-segment and T-wave changes are common.[142]

As yet, there is no satisfactory, specific therapy.

Sickle-cell trait cardiomyopathy

An obscure cardiomyopathy has been described in patients with sickle-cell trait without anemia; congestive heart failure, pulmonary thromboembolism, and sudden death were the major manifestations. Chronic alcohol ingestion seemed an important determinant, either acting directly as a myocardial toxin or facilitating sickling from resulting systemic acidosis.[143]

Polycythemia vera

The consensus in the older literature is that coronary thrombosis is a manifestation of the thrombotic tendency of polycythemia vera and is unrelated to the degree of coronary atherosclerosis. This complex problem needs additional study using more modern methods.[144]

The major cardiac manifestation of polycythemia vera is myocardial infarction, presumably secondary to intravascular thrombosis of the coronary arteries. Associated moderate systemic hypertension may also cause cardiovascular symptoms.

Essential thrombophilia

Angina pectoris and electrocardiographic changes of ischemia were associated in two patients with primary thrombocytosis and an elevated platelet count. Electrocardiographic abnormalities of myocardial infarction were also described in an 8-year-old girl with essential thrombophilia.[145]

There is characteristic elevation of the platelet count. Therapy with ^{32}P may produce a decrease in angina and concomitant electrocardiographic improvement.[146]

Thrombotic thrombocytopenic purpura

Occlusion of myocardial arterioles, particularly those supplying the conduction system, in thrombotic thrombocytopenic purpura may produce transient disturbances of cardiac rhythm and conduction; infarction of the bundle of His has been reported.[147] Arrhythmias and conduction abnormalities may occur.

Anaphylactoid purpura

Clinical and electrocardiographic evidence of myocardial damage occurs at the onset of anaphylactoid purpura.[148] The cardiac changes are similar to those of serum sickness and drug reactions, probably reflecting arteriolar and capillary periangitis. The symptoms are usually mild, and cardiac involvement may be overlooked. However, heart failure, retrosternal pain, and arrhythmias, particularly atrial fibrillation, nodal rhythm, or heart block, may develop.[149] Electrocardiographic abnormalities vary from nonspecific ST-T alterations to those of myocardial infarction.

Arrhythmias and atrioventricular conduction disturbances may occur. Corticosteroid hormone therapy is recommended.

Hereditary hemorrhagic telangiectasia

A typical telangiectatic lesion was demonstrated in the ventricle by histologic examination and postmortem coronary angiography in a patient with chest pain, syncope, left bundle branch block, and arrhythmias.[149a]

NEUROLOGIC AND NEUROMUSCULAR DISEASES

Progressive (Duchenne's) muscular dystrophy

Cardiomyopathy occurs in more than half of all patients with nonmyotonic progressive muscular dystrophy, a sex-linked, recessively inherited disorder which almost exclusively severely affects the male.[150] There is no correlation between the degree of skeletal muscle disease and the severity of cardiac symptoms or electrocardiographic abnormalities.[150] Cardiac manifestations may, indeed, antedate recognition of the neuromuscular disease; a recent report describes predominant cardiomyopathy.[151]

PATHOLOGY

The cardiac lesion consists of fatty and fibrous replacement of the myocardium, with selective scarring of the posterobasal portion of the left ventricle and posteromedial papillary muscle; this unusual focal location for myocardial fibrosis cannot yet be explained,[152] although a genetic determinant has been suggested. The anatomic lesion correlates well with the electrocardiographic and vectorcardiographic[153] abnormalities. However, comparable electrocardiographic abnormalities occur in asymptomatic female carriers without apparent anatomic lesions. There are areas of compensatory myofiber hypertrophy, but most myocardial cells are atrophic, with loss of striation, vacuolation, fragmentation, and nuclear degeneration.

James[154] noted normal main coronary arteries but described generalized noninflammatory degenerative changes in the small myocardial arteries, including those supplying the sinus and AV nodes; he suggested this as a basis for the frequent arrhythmias. Sinoatrial node artery occlusion was demonstrated cineangiographically in a patient with Duchenne's muscular dystrophy; postmortem examination showed this to be due to noninflammatory degeneration.[155] Additionally, myocardial (intramural coronary) artery abnormalities correlate poorly with the localization of myocardial vacuolation and scarring.

CLINICAL MANIFESTATIONS

The neuromuscular disease is diagnosed by the triad of peculiar waddling gait, large calves, and the "climbing up the legs" phenomenon, characteristically beginning in early childhood.

Tachycardia is the earliest sign of cardiac involvement; this characteristic clinical finding,[156] persisting during sleep,[157] is often associated with arrhythmia and cardiac enlargement (Fig. 82-12). Although an S_3 and S_4 are frequently heard, symptoms of congestive heart failure are generally absent because of the patient's prolonged inactivity or bed rest. Incipient congestive heart failure has been demonstrated by cardiac catheterization studies. Arrhythmia or infection precipitates overt cardiac failure. Mitral regurgitant murmurs may be due to papillary muscle dysfunction; faint heart sounds are described.

There may be chest pain, the latter probably musculoskeletal in origin.[158] Death is usual in the second decade, often from respiratory infection; sudden death is not uncommon.

LABORATORY EXAMINATION

The *electrocardiogram* is the earliest and most sensitive indication of cardiac involvement and is abnormal in 40 to 90 percent of patients.[158,159] The distinctive electrocardiographic changes include tall R waves in the right precordial leads and deep Q

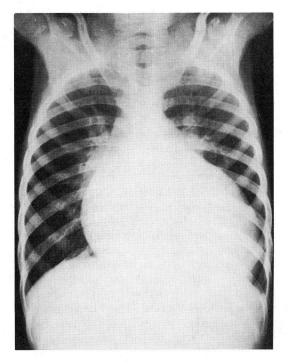

FIGURE 82-12 Generalized cardiac enlargement and pulmonary venous congestion in a 10-year-old boy with muscular dystrophy. (Courtesy of Crippled Children's Division, Georgia Department of Public Health.)

Radiologic determination of cardiac size and configuration is complicated by the thoracic deformities and elevated diaphragms, the latter due to diaphragmatic dystrophy.

Echocardiographic demonstration of a relaxation abnormality (decreased diastolic endocardial velocity) of the posterior left ventricular wall has been suggested to be more selective than the electrocardiogram in identifying early cardiac involvement.[163]

Increased cardiac output has been described in progressive muscular dystrophy. Release by the heart muscle of malic acid dehydrogenase and aldolase, suggesting increased permeability of the myocardial cell, was recently reported;[164] however, this observation is not constant,[158] and to date no distinctive enzyme profile can differentiate myocardial from skeletal muscle dystrophy.

TREATMENT

There is no specific therapy. Congestive heart failure, when present, responds to the usual management. The role of prophylactic demand pacemaker insertion in patients with conduction disturbances requires evaluation.

waves in the inferior limb leads and left precordial leads;[152] identical electrocardiographic abnormalities may be present in affected family members. This characteristic electrocardiographic pattern has also been described in asymptomatic female carriers of Duchenne's muscular dystrophy,[160] identified by elevated blood creatinine phosphokinase levels. A genetic determinant of the electrocardiographic pattern has been postulated. However, definite muscle weakness, predominantly of the pelvic girdle, has been documented in some female carriers, and the possibility of a latent cardiomyopathy deserves attention.[161]

Tachycardia is characteristic; arrhythmias and P-wave abnormalities are common; conduction defects, a short P-Q interval, and nonspecific T-wave changes are also seen (Fig. 82-13).

The *ballistocardiogram* has been reported[162] to reflect cardiac abnormality even earlier than the electrocardiogram.

Cardiomyopathy in other forms of nonmyotonic muscular dystrophy

Cardiomyopathy occurs in other forms of nonmyotonic muscular dystrophy—the limb-girdle type (Erb's), the fascioscapulohumeral type (Landouzy-Déjerine), and the limb-girdle-pseudohypertrophic type—but the manifestations are less prominent and less specific than in the Duchenne type.[165] Gallop sounds, cardiac enlargement, and minor nonspecific electrocardiographic abnormalities occur.[158] Symptoms of heart failure are unusual; cough and dyspnea are usually pulmonary in origin. Rhythm and conduction disturbances are seen. The association of fascioscapulohumeral dystrophy with persistent atrial standstill has been reported.[166]

X-Linked humeroperoneal neuromuscular disease

This X-linked recessive neuromuscular disease is associated with mild muscular disability and life-threatening cardiovascular complications. Sudden death is common in young adult life.

CLINICAL MANIFESTATIONS
The distal leg and proximal arm weakness and contractures begin in the first decade, progress slowly, and stabilize in the second decade. Palpitations, awareness of a slow pulse, and syncope are the only cardiac symptoms reported. Bradycardia is prominent, often with a diffuse and displaced apex impulse, an S_3, and nonspecific murmurs. Heart failure is notably absent.

FIGURE 82-13 Muscular dystrophy in a 10-year-old boy. The electrocardiogram mimics posterolateral wall myocardial infarction. (Courtesy of Crippled Children's Division, Georgia Department of Public Health.)

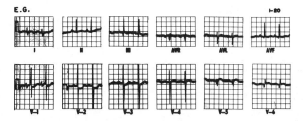

Electrocardiogram Atrial abnormalities are universal in patients with evidence of neuromuscular disease—P-wave abnormalities, atrial arrhythmias, varying degrees of atrioventricular block, and permanent atrial paralysis with a chronic junctional bradycardia.[167]

Electromyograms and muscle biopsy Both neuropathy and myopathy of the peripheral musculature are suggested by these tests.

Cardiac catheterization Ventricular function is normal.

TREATMENT

Permanent demand pacing is recommended irrespective of the atrial activity for patients with ventricular rates below 50 beats per minute, because of the high incidence of sudden cardiac death.[167]

Friedreich's ataxia

In his original description of heritable progressive spinocerebellar degeneration, Friedreich noted cardiac involvement—arrhythmia, cardiac enlargement, and congestive failure—in 5 of 6 patients. Cardiovascular disease occurs in one-third to one-half of the patients with Friedreich's ataxia, with cardiac symptoms often the initial manifestation of the disease. No relation can be documented[168] between the severity of the neurologic disease, the family history of ataxia, and the severity of the heart disease.

ETIOLOGY OF THE CARDIOMYOPATHY

The cardiac disease of Friedreich's ataxia has been attributed to scoliosis or chest deformity causing cor pulmonale, to coronary artery narrowing or occlusion, to neurogenic or toxic causes, to rheumatic or congenital factors, etc.;[168] Boyer[168] believed it to be an example of pleiotropy, i.e., a genetically determined disturbance, presumably of a metabolic pathway, having effects on several organs. The association of Friedreich's ataxia and idiopathic hypertrophic subaortic stenosis in the same patient has received recent attention; both diseases are familial, both affect the myocardium, both have similar electrocardiographic abnormalities, and both become symptomatic in the same age group; hence an etiologic link has been questioned.[169,170]

PATHOLOGY

Autopsy evidence of cardiac involvement is virtually universal in Friedreich's ataxia. Cardiac hypertrophy, fatty degeneration, diffuse reticular interstitial fibrosis, and eosinophilic and lymphocytic infiltrates are present. Collagen tissue replaces the degenerating myofibers, and compensatory hypertrophy of the remaining muscle cells occurs. Mural thrombosis is described. The coronary arteries vary from normal to diffusely involved with atheromatous lesions, with

and without obstruction. Infiltration of the Purkinje fibers of the AV node and conducting system by fibrous tissue disrupts the normal pathway of excitation; this may explain the frequent arrhythmias. The cardiomyopathy has also been attributed[171] to extensive medial degeneration and intimal hyperplasia with obliterative disease of the smaller intramural coronary arteries; arrhythmias, most commonly atrial fibrillation and paroxysmal supraventricular tachycardia, may also be due to involvement of the SA and AV node arteries.

CLINICAL MANIFESTATIONS

Friedreich's ataxia, the most common of the hereditary ataxias, is characterized by the onset in adolescence of progressive skeletal deformities, ataxia, and a scanning, dysarthric speech disturbance; death due to congestive heart failure or intercurrent infection usually occurs within 20 years after onset of symptoms. Palpitations and exertional dyspnea are common; angina pectoris is rare. The classic physical findings include inappropriate sinus tachycardia, arrhythmias, cardiac enlargement, nonspecific heart murmurs, and congestive heart failure. The congestive heart failure is rare before age 10 and is due to myocardial disease, with or without cor pulmonale. Hypertrophic obstructive cardiomyopathy may also occur. Occasional peripheral emboli may result from the endocardial mural thrombi.

Electrocardiographic abnormalities (Fig. 82-14) occur in about 90 percent of cases of Friedreich's ataxia[165] and are more frequent in patients with clinical cardiac disease; T waves suggestive of left ventricular ischemia have been described as an almost constant abnormality. ST-T changes of myocardial ischemia, AV block, and bundle branch block are the most frequent electrocardiographic disturbances. Atrial fibrillation is also seen. Both right and left ventricular hypertrophy are described. Electrocardiographic abnormalities may appear rapidly and are sometimes reversible.[165] The incidence of electrocardiographic abnormalities is unrelated to age, sex, or disease duration but is somewhat higher with severe

FIGURE 82-14 Twenty-one-year-old man with Friedreich's ataxia, congestive heart failure, and recurrent arrhythmias. There is electrocardiographic evidence of biventricular hypertrophy and nonspecific ST-T abnormalities. A wandering supraventricular pacemaker is demonstrated on the rhythm strips.

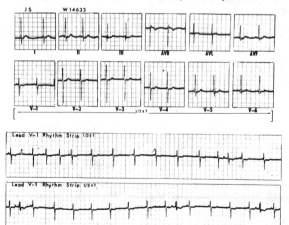

neurologic disease. There is a striking association between a family history of Friedreich's ataxia and the electrocardiographic disturbances; affected members of the same family tend to show the same electrocardiographic patterns. The electrocardiographic abnormalities and the cardiac pathologic changes correlate poorly.[172]

The *vectorcardiogram* has been suggested to show earlier evidence of cardiac involvement than the electrocardiogram and to more closely parallel the degree of neurologic involvement.[173] *Roentgenologic* examination shows generalized cardiac enlargement and pulmonary vascular congestion, in addition to the marked thoracic bony deformities.

At cardiac *catheterization* there is an increased filling pressure in both ventricles, with a small stroke volume. Serial *echocardiographic* examinations are recommended to evaluate the development of hypertrophic obstructive cardiomyopathy.[173a]

TREATMENT
There is no specific therapy. Standard management of the congestive heart failure is appropriate.

Roussy-Lévy hereditary polyneuropathy

This disorder is characterized by a combination of the clinical manifestations of peroneal muscular atrophy and Friedreich's ataxia, with the abnormalities occuring relatively independently within a family; there is an autosomal dominant pattern of inheritance. The clinical and electrocardiographic evidence of cardiomyopathy resembles that of Friedreich's ataxia.[174]

Myotonia atrophica (Steinert's disease)

Cardiac involvement usually occurs late in the course of the disease, but occasionally the cardiac abnormalities may antedate recognition of the primary disease.[175,176] Indeed, neuromuscular signs noted during an evaluation for cardiovascular disease may contribute to the earlier diagnosis of myotonia atrophica. There is no correlation between the severity of the muscular disease, the severity of the clinical cardiac disease, and the extent of the electrocardiographic abnormalities, but cardiac involvement is considered responsible for cases of sudden death.

This slowly progressive illness is inherited as an autosomal dominant, with clinical manifestations becoming evident in the third and fourth decades. The pathogenesis of the cardiac abnormalities remains obscure.

PATHOLOGY
Autopsy and endomyocardial biopsy studies usually disclose diffuse myocardial fibrosis with fatty infiltration, separation of myofibers by fibrous connective tissue, and marked variation in size and shape of the myofibers and myocardial nuclei.[175] Conduction system fibrosis is described. Electron microscopy shows vacuolation of the sarcoplasmic reticulum and mitochondrial abnormalities;[177] damage to the sarco-

plasmic reticulum has been suggested as a basis for the conduction abnormalities.[165]

Some reports describe electrocardiographic conduction and rhythm abnormalities as the only cardiovascular manifestations of myotonia atrophica; they deny anatomic alterations and suggest that the cardiac disturbances may be metabolic.[178]

CLINICAL MANIFESTATIONS
Slow muscle relaxation after contraction, muscle atrophy, increased skeletal muscle tone, expressionless face, cataracts, premature frontal baldness, and gonadal atrophy comprise the clinical manifestations of the heredofamilial muscle disorder myotonia atrophica (Steinert's disease).

Dyspnea and palpitations are common. The clinical findings[179] include a weak pulse; a split S_1 and an S_4, producing a triple rhythm; hypotension; and less commonly, cardiac enlargement and congestive heart failure. Murmurs, chest pain, or other evidence of clinical heart disease are rare. Heart failure, which occurs in only about 7 percent of patients, is a late manifestation of the illness.[165] The sinus bradycardia of myotonia contrasts sharply with the characteristic sinus tachycardia of Duchenne's muscular dystrophy and Friedreich's ataxia. Atrial flutter or fibrillation, when present, rarely require digitalis to control the ventricular response because high-degree atrioventricular block is characteristic.[165]

Murmurs, chest pain, or other evidence of clinical heart disease is rare, although recently the association of mitral valve prolapse has been described.[179a] The blood pressure is typically at the lower levels of normal. Syncope may be due to ventricular fibrillation, complete heart block, or extreme bradycardia. Sudden death has been described. Alveolar hypoventilation has resulted in hypercapnea, hypoxemia, pulmonary hypertension, and right ventricular failure.

The *electrocardiogram* is the earliest and most sensitive index of cardiac involvement and is abnormal in 60 to 85 percent of patients with myotonia atrophica.[178–180] There is a high incidence of electrocardiographic abnormalities in the absence of clinical evidence of heart disease.[181]

Atrioventricular and intraventricular conduction defects are most common and are manifest as P-Q interval prolongation, low P-wave voltage, slurred and notched QRS complexes, left axis deviation, and bundle branch block.[179] Serial studies show gradual progression of both the atrioventricular and intraventricular conduction abnormalities,[178] although intermittent bundle branch block has been described. Sinus bradycardia is the most frequent arrhythmia; with atrial flutter and fibrillation also commonly encountered.

The electrocardiographic abnormalities may mimic those of myocardial infarction (Fig. 82-15). Left axis deviation on the electrocardiogram without associated clinical heart disease in a 2-year-old child suggested the diagnosis of myotinia atrophica.[182]

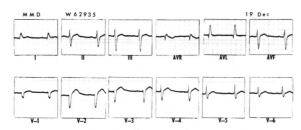

FIGURE 82-15 Electrocardiogram mimicking anterior myocardial infarction. This patient with myotonia atrophica has no symptoms referable to the cardiovascular system.

Electrocardiographic conduction defects and changes in ventricular activation on the vectorcardiogram occurred in 60 percent of patients with myotonia atrophica; their presence was consistent with the autopsy reports of myocardial involvement.[183] Electrocardiographic abnormalities are comparable in older and younger patients, suggesting that coronary atherosclerosis does not influence the electrocardiographic changes.[180] His bundle electrocardiography with atrial pacing has documented marked impairment of His-Purkinje conduction.[181]

Roentgenologic examination is typically unremarkable. Asymptomatic cardiac enlargement may be related to the bradycardia.

TREATMENT

It is possible to successfully treat Stokes-Adams syncope with a permanently implanted cardiac pacemaker.[180,184]

Myasthenia gravis

PATHOLOGY

Myofiber necrosis with acute and chronic secondary inflammatory infiltrates has been noted at postmortem examination, particularly in association with thymoma. This may represent a severe, progressive "autoimmune" myocarditis and may explain the occurrence of arrhythmias, heart failure, and electrocardiographic abnormalities.[185] Alternatively, myocardial changes may be due to hypokalemia or to the frequently associated bronchopneumonia. Minor interstitial and perivascular lymphocytic aggregations may be the only myocardial abnormalities present in other patients.

CLINICAL MANIFESTATIONS

Patients with myasthenia gravis have variable generalized weakness following use of voluntary muscles but generally present no clinical evidence of cardiac dysfunction.[186] However, tachycardia, arrhythmia, dyspnea, and precordial oppression occur in some patients. Heart failure is rare.

Nonspecific *electrocardiographic* ST-T abnormalities were reported to disappear with neostigmine therapy; transitory electrocardiographic changes of acute myocardial infarction were described during a myasthenic crisis.[187] Occasional arrhythmias are described. Terminal QRS notching, seen in 15 percent of myasthenic patients in a recent series, may be evidence of myocardial involvement; this abnormality did not regress with anticholinesterase therapy or thymectomy.[185] There is no specific vectorcardiographic or radiologic abnormality.

TREATMENT

Drugs used to treat cardiovascular problems may adversely affect the patient with myasthenia. Quinidine may aggravate the myasthenia, and procainamide and lidocaine may interfere with neuromuscular transmission; cardioversion appears preferable for arrhythmia management. Morphine may be dangerous, as vagotonic drugs have an increased effect in myasthenia patients and since morphine is potentiated by neostigmine.[188]

Tuberous sclerosis

Pale gray myocardial tumor masses, composed of mature fat tissue, have been described in patients with tuberous sclerosis;[189] further data are needed to establish the relation between these hematomatous lipomas of the heart and the cerebral tubers.

Chronic progressive external ophthalmoplegia (CPEO, Kearns' syndrome)

Patients with CPEO also manifest pigmentary degeneration of the retina, ataxia, facial and limb weakness, and cardiac abnormalities. It is not known whether this represents a primary myopathy, a denervation atrophy, or a single metabolic defect.

PATHOLOGY

Increased glycogen content and an increased number of mitochondria constitute the myocardial abnormalities.

CLINICAL MANIFESTATIONS

Dizziness and syncope may occur. Varying degrees of atrioventricular block are noted and tend to be progressive. Conduction disturbances, particularly right bundle branch block and left axis deviation, are also noted. Physical findings of complete heart block may be noted.

Abnormalities of AV conduction are demonstrated in the His bundle electrocardiogram. Ventricular function indices are normal at cardiac catheterization.

TREATMENT

Prophylactic demand pacemaker insertion is recommended because sudden death is common.[190]

Familial centronuclear myopathy

This slowly progressive wasting skeletal muscle disease begins at birth and is associated with ptosis, hyporeflexia, and cardiomyopathy. Familial occurrence is noted.

PATHOLOGY
Skeletal muscles have a nucleus centrally located in the myofiber. Fibrosis and myofiber hypertrophy occur in the myocardium.[191]

CLINICAL MANIFESTATIONS
The signs and symptoms are of congestive heart failure. Electrocardiographic and electromyographic abnormalities are nonspecific. Creatine phosphokinase levels are elevated.

TREATMENT
The standard management for congestive heart failure is recommended.

Kugelberg-Welander syndrome (juvenile progressive spinal muscular atrophy)

This syndrome is characterized by the onset in childhood or adolescence of proximal, followed by distal, limb muscle atrophy and weakness. This non-sex-linked, recessively inherited disorder has a slowly progressive course.[191a]

There is fibrosis of the atria, ventricles, and conduction system. Atrial arrhythmias and atrioventricular conduction abnormalities occur, as do cardiac enlargement and heart failure. Pacemaker therapy may be required.

COLLAGEN VASCULAR DISEASE

See Chap. 88.

NEOPLASTIC DISEASES

See Chap. 86.

CHEMICAL AND DRUG EFFECTS (TOXICITY AND HYPERSENSITIVITY)

Toxicity

ETHYL ALCOHOL[192–210]
See Chap. 81B.

FETAL ALCOHOL SYNDROMES
Some children, born of chronic alcoholic mothers, demonstrate altered growth and morphogenesis. Their typical facies includes short palpebral fissures, maxillary hypopensia, microcephaly, and ptosis. Congenital heart defects, particularly septal defects, are common.

This syndrome may reappear in later births if the alcoholism is continued.

COBALT (BEER DRINKER'S) CARDIOMYOPATHY[211–219]
See Chap. 81C.

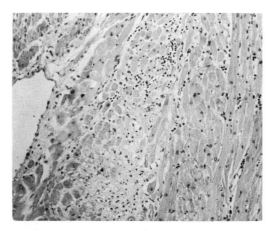

FIGURE 82-16 Emetine toxicity. Focal myocytolysis of the myocardium with interstitial and focal perivascular infiltration of lymphocytes.

EMETINE AND CHLOROQUINE
Cardiovascular toxicity is evident in the majority of patients receiving emetine. Emetine toxicity is common when treating patients who have amebiasis and schistosomiasis because of the small margin of safety between the effective and toxic drug dose. Similar, but milder, abnormalities of shorter duration occur with chloroquine, but the toxicity of combined emetine and chloroquine therapy appears additive.[220]

Pathology The pathologic changes are myocardial degeneration (Fig. 82-16) and myofiber destruction without an inflammatory response. Electron microscopic studies show selective mitochondrial damage, which appears reversible with cessation of therapy.[221]

Pathophysiology It has been suggested that the electrocardiographic abnormalities are functional, i.e., not due to structural myocardial damage, since they can be prevented or reversed by potassium administration; disturbance of potassium metabolism can be implicated as the cause of both the electrocardiographic changes and the neuromuscular toxicity observed with emetine and chloroquine therapy.[220] However, emetine inhibits mitochondrial oxidative phosphorylation; and this may account for some of the cardiotoxicity.[222]

Clinical manifestations Dyspnea and precordial pain are described with emetine and dehydroemetine toxicity. With dehydroemetine, parenteral therapy was associated with more toxicity than oral administration, and adults had more evidence of toxicity than children.[223] As with quinidine and quinine, chloroquine drug idiosyncrasy may also present as an acute cardiovascular emergency. Adrenalin appears to be an effective antidote.[224]

Arrhythmias, hypotension, tachycardia, and sudden death are encountered during emetine therapy.

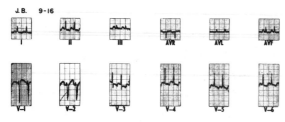

FIGURE 82-17 Emetine toxicity. Sinus tachycardia, Q-T interval prolongation, and nonspecific ST-T abnormalities are present.

Dehydroemetine toxicity has been reported to be manifest clinically by tachycardia and gallop sounds. Chloroquine toxicity is often evident as a decreased cardiac output and bradycardia.

Almost invariable *electrocardiographic* T-wave abnormalities and Q-T interval prolongation occur after the first week of emetine therapy (Fig. 82-17);[223] on occasion, electrocardiographic alterations appear only after completion of therapy. Tachycardia, P-Q interval prolongation, ST-segment displacement, and conduction disturbances have been described; terminal ventricular fibrillation was recorded. Electrocardiographic abnormalities persist or progress during continued emetine administration but characteristically regress within a month or two after cessation of therapy. The initial abnormality—precordial T-wave inversion—is usually the last to disappear.

The *electrocardiographic* abnormalities ascribed to dehydroemetine therapy are less marked and of shorter duration than those due to emetine.[223] They include sinus tachycardia, arrhythmia, decreased QRS voltage, and T-wave changes. Conduction abnormalities and arrhythmias are seen with chloroquine toxicity.

The chest *x-ray* is usually normal. SGPT (serum glutamic pyruvic transaminase) elevation and SGOT (serum glutamic oxaloacetic transaminase) elevation, which appear to be myocardial in origin, may be encountered.

Treatment Bed rest is advocated during emetine and chloroquine therapy, with frequent evaluation of the symptoms, the physical findings, and the electrocardiogram; emetine therapy appears contraindicated in patients with underlying heart disease. Most reports list the appearance of clinical cardiovascular abnormalities as an indication for immediate cessation of emetine therapy, even in the absence of the much more frequently encountered electrocardiographic alterations; this appears prudent inasmuch as the mechanism of emetine toxicity is poorly understood.

As noted, clinical and electrocardiographic abnormalities regress with cessation of drug administration, and no specific therapy is required. Occasional summaries cite electrocardiographic abnormalities as the only evidence of myocardial toxicity, with all other cardiovascular disturbances being transient and subsiding even with continuation of emetine therapy. This is not the current recommendation for care.

PHENOTHIAZINE DRUGS (CHLORPROMAZINE, THIORIDAZINE)

Arrhythmias and electrocardiographic abnormalities are common among patients receiving these psychotropic drugs; because of this toxicity, there is a relative contraindication to their use in patients with cardiovascular disease, particularly ischemic heart disease.

However, potentially hazardous cardiac arrhythmias are also encountered in patients without heart disease receiving customary therapeutic doses of these psychotropic drugs.[225]

Pathology Focal interstitial myocardial necrosis without clinical cardiac disease was reported after chlorpromazine therapy. Acid mucopolysaccharide deposition around the intramyocardial arterioles, particularly in the conduction system, subendocardium, and papillary muscles, was seen in patients receiving phenothiazine therapy who died suddenly.[226]

Pathophysiology Phenothiazine drugs alter myocardial catecholamines; increased circulating norepinephrine may predispose to cardiac arrhythmias, cardiac catecholamine depletion may depress myocardial contractility, or both mechanisms may be operative.

Hypotension, the most common cardiovascular side effect of phenothiazine drugs, may be due to inhibition of centrally mediated pressor reflexes or to α-adrenergic blockade.

These drugs have a quinidine-like effect, facilitating reentrant excitation due to decreased conduction velocity and temporal dispersion of action potential duration in different cardiac fibers.[225] The nonhomogeneous repolarization sets the stage for reentrant arrhythmias.

Clinical manifestations These patients have frequent arrhythmias,[227] supraventricular and ventricular, and syncope.

Electrocardiographic ST-T changes occur in about half of the patients receiving phenothiazine drugs and are apparently dose- and duration-related; occasional P-R and Q-T interval prolongation are also noted. T-wave amplitude decreases, and prominent U waves are seen. Intraventricular conduction disturbances are also seen, particularly with higher doses. The electrocardiogram returns to normal when phenothiazine therapy is discontinued[228] (Fig. 82-18).

Fasting and/or potassium administration "normalize" the T wave, but the clinical implications of this phenomenon remain controversial.[229]

The chest *x-ray* is usually normal.

Treatment The psychotropic drug should be discontinued. Quinidine and procainamide are not generally recommended to treat the arrhythmias, as they may

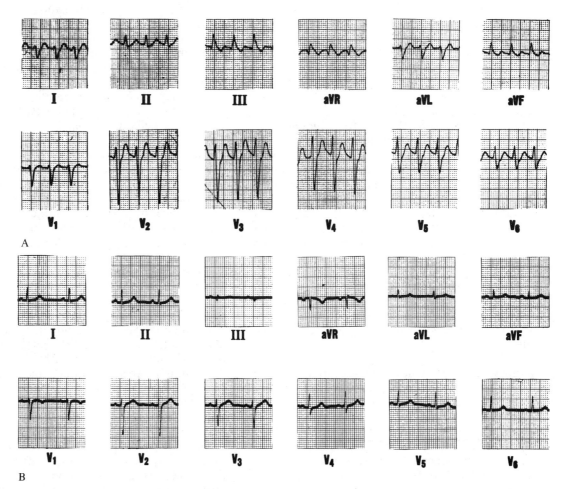

FIGURE 82-18 A. Thioridazine (Mellaril) poisoning. Normal serum electrolyte levels, *B.* Normal ECG after recovery.

further decrease conduction velocity and reinforce the arrhythmia. Lidocaine, which enhances conduction velocity, should be used.[225] Ventricular tachycardia, unresponsive to routine drug therapy, was effectively treated with an implanted pacemaker in one patient receiving thioridazine (Mellaril).[230] Pacing may be used both for overdrive suppression and to treat an underlying bradycardia after tachyarrhythmia reversion.

TRICYCLIC ANTIDEPRESSANT DRUGS

Pathophysiology These drugs block norepinephrine re-uptake at neuronal endings and antagonize the therapeutic effect of guanethidine in a similar manner. Monamine oxidase inhibitors given concomitantly with tricyclic antidepressants may result in a hypertensive crisis, as both augment the pressor effect of norepinephrine. Tricyclic antidepressant drugs in high dosage depress myocardial contractility, heart rate, and coronary blood flow; with low doses, tachycardia may occur.[231] The drugs have a quinidine-like antiarrhythmic effect.

Thus tricyclic antidepressant agents may cause cardiovascular abnormalities via their anticholinergic activity, by direct myocardial depression or by their effect on adrenergic neurons.[231a]

Clinical manifestations These drugs are associated with a variety of cardiovascular complications, including unresponsiveness to therapy for hypertension, particularly with guanethidine and clonidine, hypertensive crises, cardiac arrhythmias, heart failure, myocardial infarction, and sudden death.[231]

Electrocardiographic abnormalities may occur, particularly T-wave changes; P-R, Q-T, and QRS prolongation are described, as are conduction disturbances and supraventricular and ventricular arrhythmias.

Treatment The use of tricyclic antidepressant drugs is generally contraindicated in patients with cardiac disease. The very elderly patients also seem at increased risk of sudden death, making these drugs inadvisable for them. However, life-threatening arrhythmias also occur in patients without heart disease. In general, lidocaine should be used rather than quinidine or procainamide in managing tricyclic antidepressant drug arrhythmias (or phenothiazine arrhythmias).[225] Physostigmine has been reported to successfully control life-threatening cardiac arrhythmias in a patient with amitriptyline poisoning.[232]

With tricyclic antidepressant drug toxicity, dialysis is ineffective, and digitalis should be used with utmost caution as it may increase the arrhythmias. Beta blocking agents may increase the myocardial depression. Norepinephrine should be chosen if support of the blood pressure is indicated.[231a]

METHYSERGIDE

(see also Chaps. 63A and 78)

Methysergide (Sansert) therapy for migraine is reported to cause retroperitoneal fibrosis and pleuropulmonary fibrosis and appears to produce endocardial fibroelastosis similar to that of the carcinoid syndrome. Coronary ostial stenosis is also described.

Pathophysiology Methysergide is chemically similar to serotonin, and this may explain the similarity of these cardiac lesions to those of the carcinoid syndrome.[233]

Clinical manifestations Murmurs and hemodynamic changes of valvular stenosis and insufficiency have been described and may regress when methysergide is discontinued. Congestive heart failure may occur.[234]

Treatment Methysergide appears contraindicated in patients with coronary atherosclerotic heart disease, as it may precipitate angina pectoris or myocardial infarction.[235] It is also inadvisable in patients with valvular disease or cardiac decompensation. Drug dosage restriction and intermittent therapy may prevent fibrotic complications. Valve replacement has occasionally been necessary.

CYCLOPHOSPHAMIDE

Intermittent, massive doses of this antineoplastic agent may have some advantages in cancer chemotherapy but produce unacceptable cardiac complications. Myocardial necrosis and hemorrhagic myocarditis occur with distinctive abnormalities: capillary microthrombosis and fibrin deposition in the myocardial interstitium and in myofibers.[235a] Heart failure and/or pulmonary edema, unresponsive to therapy, result in a fatal low cardiac output state. Elevated serum enzyme levels indicate myocardial damage, and decreased voltage, T-wave changes, and Q-T interval prolongation appear on the electrocardiogram.[236]

Intensive cyclophosphamide dose regimens are not justified. Cardiac function should be monitored by clinical parameters, serum enzyme levels, and electrocardiographic changes during therapy.

DAUNORUBICIN CARDIOMYOPATHY

See Chap. 81D.

ADRIAMYCIN (DOXORUBICIN)

Adriamycin is an anthracycline antibiotic compound used as an antineoplastic agent to treat lymphoma, leukemia, and solid tumors. Cardiac toxicity is the major factor limiting its use. A single rapid infusion of 60 to 75 mg/m² is usually given at 21-day intervals.

Pathology and pathophysiology Cardiac enlargement and mural thrombi occur. There is myocardial interstitial fibrosis with cellular loss, vacuolation, and fragmentation. Electron microscopy shows loss of contractile substance with mitochondrial swelling and distortion.[237]

Adriamycin is cleared rapidly from the serum, binding to tissue (including heart) DNA and inhibiting nucleic acid synthesis.

Clinical manifestation Rapidly progressive symptoms of biventricular failure appear 1 to 6 months after completion of chemotherapy. Cardiomyopathy is unrelated to a prior history of heart disease. There is evidence of profound, intractable biventricular failure, with death commonly occurring within several weeks.[238]

Transient *electrocardiographic* abnormalities —ST-T changes, premature ventricular beats, supraventricular tachycardia—occur in 5 to 30 percent of patients during the first few days after drug administration. These changes are unrelated to subsequent cardiomyopathy and are not dose-dependent.[239] A conspicuous decrease in QRS voltage occurs with the onset of clinical cardiomyopathy, but the electrocardiogram is insensitive in detecting early myocardial dysfunction.

There is rapid cardiac dilatation and pulmonary vascular congestion on chest *x-ray*. Serial measurements of *systolic time intervals* may detect early cardiotoxicity. Depression of ventricular function [increased (preejection phase)/(left ventricular ejection time)] is more profound and recovery time longer as the cumulative dose of adriamycin increases.[240] It is uncertain whether echocardiographic or systolic time interval abnormalities can detect early cardiomyopathy in time to permit cumulative dose restriction.

Treatment Heart failure is unusual below a total dose of 550 mg/m² of adriamycin, and this is the recommendation upper limit for chemotherapy. There appears to be a synergistic effect between x-irradiation and other antitumor antibiotics and adriamycin in producing cardiotoxicity.[240a] The heart failure is relatively unresponsive to inotropic drugs and mechanical ventricular assistance.[238] Combined therapy with digitalis, diuretics, and peripheral vasodilators occasionally is of benefit.

CHRONIC ARSENIC POISONING

Acute interstitial myocarditis may occur during arsenical therapy of syphilis and is usually associated with an exfoliative arsenical dermatitis. An allergic cause is postulated for the myocarditis, although the exact allergen is not apparent.

Pathology The anatomic cardiac lesion is an interstitial myocarditis with edema, focal fibrosis, eosinophilic cell and mononuclear cell infiltrates, and endocardial thickening with mural thrombus formation.

Clinical manifestations The clinical findings include dyspnea, cardiac enlargement, and progressive congestive heart failure. Nonspecific T-wave changes and Q-T interval prolongation constitute the electrocardiographic abnormalities.[241]

There is no specific therapy.

ACUTE ARSENIC POISONING

Acute arsenic poisoning, usually due to arsenic trioxide, is the most common cause of acute heavy metal poisoning. Arsenic interferes with the function of respiratory system enzymes and may produce myocardial hypoxia. Multiple focal subepicardial hemorrhages occur within the first few hours after poisoning.

Clinical manifestations There are no cardiac symptoms, and no residual cardiovascular disease is evident in patients who recover.[242] The electrocardiographic changes are those of myocardial ischemia[242] and Q-T interval prolongation; the electrocardiographic abnormalities disappear more rapidly in patients receiving BAL (British anti-lewisite, dimercaprol) than in untreated patients.[243]

ACUTE ARSINE GAS POISONING

Arsine gas causes red blood cell hemolysis, decreasing the oxygen-carrying capacity of the blood. Both the myocardial hypoxia and the appreciable amounts of arsenic in the heart muscle at autopsy are implicated in the production of the cardiac lesions: subepicardial hemorrhage, myocardial degeneration and fragmentation, and interstitial edema.[244]

Clinical manifestations The severity of the illness relates to the extent of toxic exposure. Poisoning with arsine gas may terminate fatally as a result of acute myocardial failure. Abnormal T waves appear on the electrocardiogram. There is evidence of red blood cell hemolysis.

Therapy is supportive. BAL (British anti-lewisite) is not useful in arsine poisoning.

ANTIMONY

Fuadin, tartar emetic, Astiban, and other antimony compounds used to treat schistosomiasis frequently produce myocardial damage. Although fatal hepatic antimony toxicity usually precedes fatal cardiac toxicity, myocardial disturbances may occur early in the course of therapy and even after the completion of treatment.

Cardiovascular symptoms are uncommon, but precordial oppression has been described. Death occurs suddenly, not uncommonly from arrhythmia, with no constant or significant prior change in heart rate or blood pressure.

Almost invariable *electrocardiographic* abnormalities appear by the end of a course of antimony therapy.[245]

Nonspecific ST-T changes and a prolonged Q-T interval constitute the major electrocardiographic abnormalities;[245,246] the rare arrhythmias and conduction abnormalities have an ominous prognosis. Electrocardiographic alterations increase as the duration of a course of antimony therapy increases and usually regress after cessation of treatment.[245] Similar electrocardiographic abnormalities have been described during repeated courses of antimony compounds in the same individual. Arrhythmias and conduction abnormalities require cessation of therapy.

l-NOREPINEPHRINE, EPINEPHRINE, AND ISOPROTERENOL (see Chap. 81C)

Myocarditis, with lesions similar to those seen with pheochromocytoma,[247] may occur following therapy with *l*-norepinephrine. This is also described with epinephrine and isoproterenol therapy. Focal myocardial necrosis, an inflammatory infiltrate, edema, and epicardial hemorrhages are present.

Pathophysiology Epinephrine platelet-aggregating effects have been thought to produce myocardial necrosis; pretreatment of animals with anti-platelet aggregating agents has decreased epinephrine-induced myocardial necrosis.[248]

Ischemic electrocardiographic changes may also be due to hypertension, increased myocardial oxygen demand, coronary endothelial damage, hypokalemia, etc.

Clinical manifestations Chest pain has been reported. The electrocardiographic changes are those of myocardial injury and ischemia.

Treatment It has been suggested[249] that these changes represent a toxic myocarditis and that *l*-norepinephrine dosage should be determined on a milligram per kilogram basis, rather than by blood pressure response to therapy. The role of antiplatelet agents remains controversial.

CARBON MONOXIDE

Acute and chronic carbon monoxide poisoning may cause myocardial infarction or myocarditis. The illness is more severe with acute carbon monoxide poisoning and with higher carbon monoxide blood levels in the chronic illness. Cardiac damage is attributed both to hypoxemia, as carbon monoxide diminishes the oxygen transport capacity of the blood, and to a direct toxic effect of carbon monoxide on myocardial fiber mitochondria.[250] Carbon monoxide both replaces the oxygen in oxyhemoglobin and decreases the tissue dissociation of oxyhemoglobin.

Pathology Hemorrhagic and necrotic lesions, probably hypoxemic in origin, have a predilection for the papillary muscles and the subendocardial layer of the left ventricle. Endocardial injury may be associated with mural thrombosis.[251] Round-cell infiltration is seen in areas of muscle disruption and fragmentation. Rupture of the heart has occurred.

Clinical manifestations Clinical manifestations include chest pain,[252] palpitations, and exertional dyspnea. Sinus tachycardia and an apical systolic murmur are frequent findings. The cyanosis often seen with hypoxia is not evident; skin color is pink.

Severe carbon monoxide poisoning may produce pulmonary edema or cardiovascular collapse.[253] Carbon monoxide poisoning may produce myocardial infarction in a patient with coronary atherosclerosis, anemia, or other disease with impaired tissue oxygenation.[254]

The *electrocardiogram* is the most sensitive index of myocardial damage.[251] Electrocardiographic alterations are usually transient but may persist for weeks or months. Ischemic ST-T changes occur most frequently;[255] conduction abnormalities, bundle branch block, ventricular premature beats, and atrial fibrillation are also encountered.

In the *echocardiogram* left ventricular wall motion abnormalities and mitral valve prolapse are described; the latter may reflect the papillary muscle lesions commonly encountered with carbon monoxide poisoning.[256]

Treatment One hundred percent oxygen should be administered to relieve tissue hypoxia. Hyperbaric oxygen appears of value.[253] Bed rest is indicated when there is clinical or electrocardiographic evidence of myocardial damage.[251] Clinical recovery usually occurs within a day or two.[254] However, nonspecific chest pain and palpitations may persist for long periods of time.

COBALT (see also Chap. 81C)

Fatal cobalt cardiomyopathy occurred in a metal worker. Cobalt cardiomyopathy due to industrial exposure had not been previously described, and the case reported had no apparent sensitizing or precipitating factor.[256a]

Pathology At postmortem examination there was excessive cobalt accumulation in the myocardium, and the histologic abnormalities were like those of beer-drinker's cardiomyopathy.[256a]

Clinical manifestations This case was characterized clinically by heart failure, chest pain, cyanosis, electrocardiographic abnormalities, and shock.

HYDROCARBONS (FLUORINATED)

Aerosol inhalation toxicity appears due to fluorocarbon compounds used as aerosol propellants. Anatomic abnormalities include myofiber fragmentation and vacuolation and loss of cross-striations.[257] These potent cardiotoxins depress myocardial contractility, apparently in a dose-related fashion.[258]

Cardiac enlargement, pneumopericardium, and arrhythmias have been reported to result from hydrocarbon ingestion; the predominant pneumonitis and central nervous system toxicity may mask the car-diovascular symptoms, particularly those of left ventricular failure. Hypotension is frequent.

ST-T *electrocardiographic* changes are seen. The electrical sequelae include sinus bradycardia which progresses to AV dissociation with progressively lower escape rhythms, terminating in asystole or ventricular fibrillation; this is the probable mechanism of sudden death from "glue-sniffing."[259]

Therapy is supportive; antiarrhythmic agents may be indicated. Epinephrine should be used only with utmost caution in hydrocarbon-exposed patients, especially those exposed to halogenated hydrocarbons, because of the common arrhythmias, including ventricular fibrillation.

PHOSPHORUS

Death in the first 12 to 24 h after phosphorus poisoning is usually cardiovascular in origin. Later deaths are due to hepatic failure.

Pathophysiology Phosphorus appears to inhibit amino acid incorporation into myocardial proteins, with resultant cardiac dysfunction. A direct toxic effect of phosphorus on the myocardium and on peripheral blood vessels produces depression of myocardial contractility and lowering of systemic vascular resistance, which is unresponsive to adrenergic agents.[260] The myocardial lesion is fatty degeneration with myofiber necrosis.[261]

Clinical manifestations Ventricular fibrillation or peripheral vascular collapse is a grave prognostic sign. Other cardiovascular manifestations are rare. Electrocardiographic abnormalities occur[261] in more than 50 percent of patients with phosphorus poisoning; these changes appear related to the amount of phosphorus ingested. Nonspecific ST-T abnormalities[262] and Q-T interval prolongation are most common and regress with clinical improvement.

FLUORIDE

Excessive quantities of fluoride exert a direct toxic action on cardiac muscle. Additional cardiovascular abnormalities may result from the hypocalcemia that results from the calcium-binding effect of fluoride.[263] Treacherous cardiac arrhythmias may kill the patient.

MERCURY

ST-segment and T-wave abnormalities, Q-T interval prolongation, and occasional arrhythmias were described[264] in 42 patients with mercury poisoning; a mercury-containing fungicide had been inadvertently ingested.

LEAD

Clinical and electrocardiographic assessment of myocardial damage should be part of the management of all patients with chronic lead poisoning.

Lead poisoning from lead-contaminated stills may exacerbate the alcoholic cardiomyopathy of moonshine whiskey drinkers; cardiac function improved in one group of such patients after chelation of the lead with calcium EDTA (ethylenediaminetetraacetic acid).

Pathology and pathophysiology The myocardial dysfunction in lead poisoning may be due to the hypertensive changes of lead nephropathy and/or a direct toxic effect of lead on the myocardium.[265] Pathologic evidence of myocarditis—interstitial fibrosis, occasional inflammatory cells, and a serous exudate—has been described in patients dying of chronic lead poisoning.

Clinical manifestations Frequent cardiomyopathy and chest pain have been noted in young patients with chronic occupational lead poisoning. Heart failure also occurred. Tachycardia, gallop rhythm, and pulmonary edema were the clinical manifestations.[266]

Electrocardiographic abnormalities of sinus bradycardia, shortened P-Q interval, occasional premature ventricular beats, and nonspecific ST-T changes subsided after therapy with EDTA.

EDTA and supportive management are indicated.

SCORPION VENOM

Scorpion sting myocardial toxicity is more common than neurotoxicity, and often is the cause of death. Scorpion venom is a potent sympathetic system stimulator; the clinical cardiovascular manifestations and myocardial morphologic abnormalities after severe scorpion sting are due to the elevated level of circulating catecholamines.

Pathology The myocardial lesions in cases of fatal scorpion sting resemble those of catecholamine excess: myofiber fat droplet deposition and degenerative changes, focal necrosis, interstitial cellular infiltrates, edema, and hemorrhage. The papillary muscles and subendocardium are prominently involved; these hypoxic lesions are probably related to the myocardial inotropic effect of catecholamines.[267]

Clinical manifestations Myocarditis has been reported[268] due to the sting of a scorpion, *Tityus trinitatis* (Buthidae). Heart rate and rhythm disturbances were frequent; transient murmurs were heard. All the evidence of myocarditis was transient, returning to normal within a week. Reversible tachycardia, pulmonary edema, and peripheral circulatory failure have been described secondary to *Buthus tamulus* scorpion bites. The sting of the yellow scorpion, *Buthus quinquestriatus,* frequently results in hypertension, anxiety, profuse perspiration, and pulmonary edema.[269] Circulatory collapse may follow.

Electrocardiographic abnormalities—conduction changes, ST-T abnormalities, or Q-T interval prolongation—occurred in 76 percent of patients with *Tityus trinitatis* sting.[268] Changes mimicking myocardial infarction occurred from *Buthus tamulus* bites, and abnormal Q and T waves persisted in one case.[270] Myocardial serum enzyme levels may be elevated.

Treatment Adrenergic blocking agents appear of value in the treatment of the cardiovascular manifestations of scorpion sting and in the prevention of scorpion venom cardiomyopathy.[269]

"BLACK WIDOW" SPIDER VENOM

In addition to the common neurotoxicity accompanying "black widow" *(Lactrodectus m. tredecimguttatus)* spider bites, atrial fibrillation and marked blood pressure lability are described. Urinary catecholamine levels were elevated; beta blockade therapy was beneficial.[270a]

SNAKE VENOM

Myocardial infarction and circulatory collapse may be due to intravascular coagulation and/or direct myocardial toxicity.

Clinical manifestations Adder bites have resulted in death from circulatory collapse, and myocardial infarction secondary to severe hypotension.[271] Milder cases may have only transient angina pectoris.

Reversible T-wave electrocardiographic abnormalities were described[272] due to Malayan viper bites; intravascular coagulation was the postulated mechanism. Transient electrocardiographic changes of myocardial infarction have also occurred following adder bites and presumably were due to a direct toxic effect of the snake venom on the myocardium.

WASP VENOM

It is uncertain whether catecholamines, dopamine, norepinephrine, other substances in wasp (yellow jacket, hornet) venom, or substances produced in reaction to the venom are responsible for the cardiovascular toxicity. There is subepicardial hemorrhage; changes of myocardial infarction occur.

Clinical manifestations Chest pain is the most prominent cardiac symptom. Circulatory collapse and often reversible pulmonary edema are described.[273] The electrocardiographic changes are of myocardial ischemia or infarction.

TICK PARALYSIS

Transient evidence of toxic myocarditis—cardiac enlargement and cardiac failure—occurred after regression of the neurologic changes in a child with tick paralysis.[274] Nonspecific electrocardiographic abnormalities were also transient.

Hypersensitivity

Disease processes related to hypersensitivity are being recognized with increasing frequency. The following discussion of drug hypersensitivity considers primarily the direct damage to myocardial cells. Drug-induced cardiomyopathies[275] which result from interference with cellular metabolic activity have been discussed in the preceding section; drugs which act through an allergic mechanism, either directly on the myocardium or secondary to a coronary vasculitis, will next be considered. The drug-induced electrocardiographic abnormalities generally reflect a direct or indirect effect on the electrical activity of the heart; occasionally the drug effect is directly on the myofiber; most electrocardiographic abnormalities are reversible as the drug is metabolized or eliminated.[276]

ANAPHYLAXIS
Even in patients without apparent heart disease, sensitization by exogenous agents may result in acute anaphylaxis with primarily cardiovascular manifestations. Myocardial abnormalities occur, independent of changes in coronary blood flow.

Clinical manifestations Anaphylactic reactions to a variety of drugs are often associated with profound hypotension and have precipitated myocardial infarction in patients with underlying coronary atherosclerosis. Dyspnea, cyanosis, chest pain, syncope, and arrhythmias, often recurrent, have also been recorded; because of these manifestations, anaphylaxis has occasionally been misdiagnosed as myocardial infarction with shock.

Electrocardiographic nonspecific ST-T changes have been recorded, as have abnormalities of impulse formation and conduction. The etiology of the electrocardiographic changes in anaphylaxis is unknown; possible explanations include myocardial antigen-antibody reactions, a pharmacologic effect of the mediator substances of anaphylaxis, effects of the drugs (e.g., epinephrine) used to treat the anaphylaxis, myocardial hypoxia, etc.[277]

Treatment Histamine appears to be an important mediator of the anaphylaxis, and antihistamine therapy is generally effective.[278]

SERUM SICKNESS
Serum sickness is characterized anatomically by a generalized vasculitis and necrotizing arteritis; coronary artery and myocardial and pericardial artery involvement explain the clinical presentation.

A variety of cardiovascular abnormalities are encountered with serum sickness.[279] There may be tachycardia, arrhythmia, hypotension, the pain and friction rub of pericarditis, and the pain of myocardial infarction. Electrocardiographic changes, particularly transient ST-T and conduction abnormalities, are common. The changes may mimic myocardial infarction.

Corticosteroid hormone therapy is recommended.

SULFONAMIDE
Interstitial myocarditis, characterized by mononuclear and eosinophilic perivascular infiltrates, was described in patients who had received sulfonamide drugs.[280] In a patient with a severe sulfonamide myocarditis, granulomatous myocardial lesions, myofiber necrosis, and petechial hemorrhages were noted at autopsy examination. Similar fatal myocarditis has been due to sulfonylurea antidiabetic therapy.[281]

One group of patients with autopsy evidence of sulfonamide myocarditis[280] had no cardiac symptoms, and only about 50 percent of the patients had clinical evidence of sulfonamide hypersensitivity. However, symptomatic sulfonamide myocarditis with severe heart failure has also been described; tachycardia and cardiac enlargement were prominent. Electrocardiographic abnormalities are nonspecific. Sulfonamide cardiomyopathy has been reported to subside after digitalis and corticosteroid hormone therapy.[282]

PENICILLIN
Granulomatous and diffuse interstitial myocarditis have occurred in penicillin hypersensitivity reactions, with and without clinical cardiac symptoms and electrocardiographic abnormalities. Classic granulomatous lesions predominated in the papillary muscles; inflammatory arteritis, edema, areas of myofiber necrosis, and eosinophilic and inflammatory cellular exudates were present on microscopic examination.

Bradycardia and transient ST-T electrocardiographic changes occur in penicillin hypersensitivity and are thought to represent myocardial involvement.[283] Pericarditis with effusion has also been described.[284]

PHENYLBUTAZONE
A profound interstitial myocarditis, pathologically indistinguishable from other drug-hypersensitivity lesions, may occur with phenylbutazone therapy.

Postmortem abnormalities include focal perivascular granulomas, muscle necrosis, edema, eosinophilic and acute inflammatory cellular reaction, and fibrinoid collagen degeneration.[285,286]

Chest pain, tachycardia, hypotension, and heart failure, have been reported both during and after phenylbutazone therapy in the recommended dosage range.[285] Pericarditis has also been described. Electrocardiographic changes are compatible with myocardial ischemia.

SMALLPOX VACCINE
Myocarditis and pericarditis, both presumed due to an antigen-antibody reaction, have been described 1 to 2 weeks after smallpox vaccination. The time lag suggests that a viremia is not implicated.[287] Cardiovascular complications are less common than neurologic or dermatologic reactions. Since 1972 smallpox vaccination has not been required in the United States because the potential complications of vaccination were considered more serious than the risk of smallpox infection.

Fatal smallpox myocarditis is characterized by acute myocardial degeneration, particularly of the left ventricle, with loss of myofiber striations, myocardial necrosis, edema, and granulocytic infiltrates.[288] The illness is generally mild, with spontaneous recovery, although chest pain, dyspnea, and rapid heart rate have been described. Severe heart failure may occur.[289] Death has also occurred without premonitory cardiac symptoms.[288] The ST-T changes on the electrocardiogram and the occasional arrhythmias disappear in patients who survive.[287]

Corticosteroid hormone therapy and routine heart failure management are indicated.

CHOLERA VACCINE

Cardiovascular complications of cholera vaccine administration, as with tetanus and smallpox vaccination, suggest an allergic myocarditis. One patient had atrial fibrillation and ventricular tachycardia with syncope.[290] In this patient eosinophilia and an elevated antimyocardial antibody titer suggested an allergic myocarditis.

The *electrocardiogram* may show arrhythmias and/or changes of myocardial ischemia. Arrhythmia management is indicated.

AUREOMYCIN (CHLORTETRACYCLINE)

In allergic myocarditis due to Aureomycin hydrochloride hypersensitivity,[291] fibrinoid necrosis and a diffuse perivascular and interstitial infiltrate of eosinophils, lymphocytes, and Anitschkow myocytes were seen.

ANTITUBERCULOUS DRUGS

Streptomycin Widespread myofiber necrosis, diffuse eosinophilic and inflammatory cell infiltrates, and petechial myocardial hemorrhages were the cardiac lesions in a patient who died suddenly during a course of chemotherapy for tuberculosis; the patient had received isoniazid, para-aminosalicylic acid, and streptomycin, but since death followed an injection of streptomycin, it was presumed due to streptomycin allergy.[292] Chest discomfort was the only cardiac abnormality preceding death.

Para-aminosalicylic acid In another fatal case of myocarditis during antituberculous chemotherapy, the myofibers were fragmented, multinucleate giant cells were present, there was a generalized and perivascular inflammatory cell infiltrate, and IgG appeared localized along the myofiber sarcolemma. Heart failure, pericardial effusion, hypotension, and ventricular irritability occurred. The patient had received streptomycin, para-aminosalicylic acid, isoniazid, and ethambutol; death was attributed to aminosalicylic acid hypersensitivity, which is known to cause cardiac dilatation and transient arrhythmias.[293]

PHENINDIONE

Fatal myocarditis was described[294] due to sensitivity to phenindione (Danilone) anticoagulation.

ACETAMINOPHEN (PARACETAMOL)

Myocardial necrosis is seen with large doses of paracetamol. There are no specific clinical abnormalities. Electrocardiographic abnormalities have also occurred with large doses of paracetamol, an analgesic which is a phenacetin metabolite;[295] it is not certain whether this represents a toxic or hypersensitivity response.

RESERPINE, GUANETHIDINE

Biochemical and structural myocardial lesions occur in experimental animals after prolonged reserpine and guanethidine therapy but are apparently not related to catecholamine depletion. Focal inflammatory necrosis, change in mitochondrial architecture, deranged lipid and glycogen metabolism, and depression of mitochondrial oxidative enzymes[296] may be a toxic or hypersensitivity effect or may be related to catecholamine depletion.

LITHIUM

Lithium carbonate, used to treat manic-depressive illness, may cause electrocardiographic abnormalities and arrhythmias.[297] Lithium decreases intracellular potassium, prolonging repolarization and facilitating ectopic beats and ventricular and supraventricular arrhythmias. Palpitations may be described.

Almost invariable T-wave electrocardiographic abnormalities occur with administration of this psychotropic drug. There are no electrolyte or serum enzyme abnormalities, and the T waves return to normal when lithium is discontinued.[298] Arrhythmias may occur. Cardiovascular performance as assessed by treadmill exercise testing is unaffected.[298a]

Patients should be instructed to discontinue the drug if symptoms of arrhythmia appear. The role of supplementary potassium is unclear, as serum potassium levels are normal. Careful follow-up and electrocardiographic monitoring is recommended for patients who have ventricular arrhythmias.[298a]

PHYSICAL CAUSES

Radiation (see also Chaps. 63A and 101)

High-dose radiation therapy to the thorax may damage the heart and pericardium. With more potent sources of therapeutic radiation and with longer survival of patients with malignant disease, latent effects of cardiac radiation are likely to become more apparent. It has also been suggested that radiation may predispose to or accelerate coronary atherosclerosis, since vascular injury may accelerate lipid deposition.

PATHOLOGY

Pericardial fibrosis occurs most commonly, often with dense collagen deposition in the pericardium and epicardium; myocardium is among the most radiation-resistant tissues, but patchy fibrosis and necrosis may be seen.

The coronary arteries become thickened and hyalinized; the narrowed lumen has resulted in myocardial infarction. Endocardial fibrosis and fibroelastosis may produce cardiac murmurs by valve distortion. Fibrosis of the conduction system has produced complete heart block.

Electron microscopy shows disorganization of the mitochondria, myofibrils, nucleus, and sarcolemma, differing from abnormalities seen with ischemic myocardial disease.[299]

CLINICAL MANIFESTATIONS

The diagnosis of radiation-induced cardiac fibrosis should be considered in patients who have received extensive radiation therapy and who present unusual clinical or electrocardiographic evidence of heart disease. The cardiac disease must be correctly identified so that proper management can be instituted.

Acute pericarditis; pericardial effusion, occasionally with tamponade; and chronic pericarditis with and without constriction may occur. The occurrence of pericardial effusion is at times erroneously considered evidence of malignant involvement.[300] Cardiac murmurs may appear; and complete heart block with Stokes-Adams syncope is described.

Transient electrocardiographic abnormalities are not uncommon, and some ST-T alterations do not regress.[301] Pericardial effusion may be suggested by the chest x-ray. At times, echocardiography, pericardiocentesis, and/or cardiac catheterization are required to determine whether cardiac tamponade, constrictive pericarditis, or both are present.[300]

Electric shock

Electrocardiographic changes of myocardial ischemia and infarction have developed several weeks after severe electric shock; further study of this problem is needed.[302]

Trauma (see also Chap. 87)

Isolated focal myocardial disease has been occasionally documented among pilots killed in aircraft accidents, but not in the nonpilot air crew killed in the same accidents. Since there was no evidence that the trauma caused the myocardial damage, it seems probable that sudden cardiac death was due to the focal myocardial disease.[303]

Posttraumatic myocardial ossification has been described.[304] Ventricular aneurysm has resulted from blunt trauma.[304a]

Heatstroke

The myofiber degeneration, petechial hemorrhages, and interstitial edema may be due to direct tissue injury, to hypoxia, to metabolic abnormalities, etc.[305]

Myocardial damage due to heatstroke is evidenced by *electrocardiographic* abnormalities, including ST-T wave changes, and conduction abnormalities which appear reversible in survivors. Serum LDH isoenzyme level elevation compatible with cardiac damage is seen.

MISCELLANEOUS SYSTEMIC SYNDROMES

Rejection cardiomyopathy

Anatomic alterations include necrotizing arteritis and vascular fibrinoid necrosis, myocytolysis, edema, and a mononuclear, predominantly lymphocytic and plasma cell, reaction.

CLINICAL MANIFESTATIONS

Cardiac function deterioration may be evident as decreased exercise tolerance, increased venous pressure, and gallop rhythm. Temperature and heart rate rise. However, about three-fourths of patients remain asymptomatic.[306]

Decreased electrocardiographic voltage is the most reliable sign of late acute rejection of the transplanted heart. Arrhythmias and conduction abnormalities also occur.[306] Enlargement of the cardiac silhouette, due to cardiac dilatation and/or pericardial effusion, is encountered with rejection of the transplanted human heart. The sedimentation rate rises.

Endomyocardial (percutaneous transcatheter) biopsy, accomplished with greatest safety in the left ventricle, provides early identification of rejection cardiomyopathy.

TREATMENT

Immunosuppressive therapy and corticosteroid hormones may reverse the process[307] and permit good long-term cardiac function in most patients. Early identification of rejection cardiomyopathy by endomyocardial biopsy permits augmentation of immunosuppressive therapy and has increased recipient survival.[308]

Cardiomyopathy of aging (see also Chap. 41)

Presbycardia or senile myocardial degeneration occurs occasionally, but senile cardiac amyloidosis and degenerative calcification of the mitral and aortic valve rings and cusps[309] and fibrosis of the cardiac skeleton are probably more common in elderly patients. Myocarditis of varied cause may also occur in the elderly.[291]

A number of cardiovascular changes are observed with aging, including increased myofiber vacuolization, neutral fat deposition, and lipofuscin deposition.[310] Cardiac output decreases, presumably related to a lesser metabolic demand. There is a greater increase in heart rate and blood pressure in response to stress, and a decrease in exercise tolerance. Increased notching and slurring of the QRS complex of the electrocardiogram is seen; however, the significance of these alterations is uncertain.[311]

Rheumatoid disease (see Chap. 60B)

Rheumatoid heart disease should be suspected in patients with peripheral rheumatoid arthritis and cardiac manifestations. As the longevity of patients with rheumatoid arthritis increases, more patients may develop rheumatoid heart disease.

PATHOLOGY

Valvular, myocardial, and pericardial involvement may occur in patients with rheumatoid disease. Granulomas, histologically similar to rheumatoid nodules, occur in the epicardium and myocardium and at the bases and in the cusps of the aortic and mitral valves[312] in 3 to 20 percent of autopsied patients with rheumatoid disease.[313] This is most common with peripheral rheumatoid disease. A nonspecific interstitial myocarditis is present in 10 to 20 percent of cases. An associated diffuse arteritis involves the smaller coronary arteries in 10 to 20 percent of postmortem studies. Degeneration of the AV node and bundle of His, secondary to narrowing of their nutrient arteries, may result in heart block and associated symptoms.[313a] Pericarditis, although rarely diagnosed clinically, is evident in about 40 percent of postmortem cases. The aortic and mitral valves become fibrosed, thickened, and incompetent; calcific aortic stenosis may also develop.[312]

The high incidence of cardiac pathologic lesions contrasts sharply with the relative rarity of clinical cardiac manifestations. Cardiac amyloid may also produce clinical manifestations in the patient with rheumatoid disease.

CLINICAL MANIFESTATIONS

Congestive heart failure, disproportionate to the severity of the valvular lesions, is attributed to the associated myocardial disease. Complete heart block with Stokes-Adams syncope has been caused by rheumatoid nodular infiltrates of the interventricular septem.[314–316]

Arrhythmias and valvular insufficiency murmurs are present. Aortic regurgitation is far more common with ankylosing spondylitis than with peripheral rheumatoid disease.[317] There is no sex preponderance.

Cardiac hypertrophy due to hemodynamically significant rheumatoid valvular disease is unusual in patients without severe articular disease of long duration. Acute pericarditis, often with a rub, may be associated with effusion or tamponade; chronic constrictive rheumatoid pericarditis may develop.

The *electrocardiographic* changes are often nonspecific ST-T abnormalities. *Echocardiography* appears to be a sensitive method to detect early, asymptomatic cardiac involvement; in one series, pericardial thickening or effusion was present in almost half of the patients and mitral valve abnormalities in one-third.[318] The rheumatoid factor is often, but not invariably, positive. Other routine laboratory tests are not helpful.

TREATMENT

Standard management is recommended for heart failure. Constrictive pericarditis has, on occasion, necessitated pericardiectomy. Pacemaker therapy may be of value for the patient with complete heart block.

Ankylosing spondylitis
(see Chap. 60B)

Cardiac disease is a late complication of ankylosing spondylitis but is unrelated to the severity of the spondylitis. The progress of the disease is characteristically slow.

PATHOLOGY

Both the aortic valve and the aortic root are involved by focal medial inflammation with subsequent fibrosis. The fibrosis and endarteritis which involve the aortic root extend into the interventricular septum, replacing the atrioventricular bundle with fibrous tissue. Fibrosis may extend to the base of the anterior mitral valve leaflet, producing mitral regurgitation.

Myocardial abnormalities are nonspecific: fibrosis, perivascular lymphocytic infiltrate, increase in mucinous ground substance, etc.[319] Atrioventricular node and His bundle degeneration, secondary to nutrient artery narrowing, may explain the conduction abnormalities.[313a] Pericarditis has also been described. About 20 percent of patients have anatomic abnormalities; 12 percent have no clinical cardiac manifestations.[317]

CLINICAL MANIFESTATIONS

The disease occurs almost exclusively in men. Aortic regurgitation is the typical valvular lesion in patients with ankylosing spondylitis of long duration. Both the aortic regurgitation and the conduction abnormalities are encountered more frequently in older patients and when extensive peripheral joint involvement is present, but aortic regurgitation has preceded evidence of spondylitis.[317]

Progressive atrioventricular block has terminated fatally with either asystole or ventricular tachyarrhythmias. Cardiomyopathy, with cardiac enlargement and congestive heart failure, has been described in ankylosing spondylitis; the role of associated coronary artery disease or prior rheumatic fever requires further delineation.

Atrioventricular and intraventricular conduction defects are common electrocardiographic abnormalities, often antedating the valvular disease. First-degree atrioventricular block, with a P-Q interval commonly between 0.35 and 0.45 s may persist for many years. Conduction defects also occur in the absence of aortic regurgitation.[320] Complete heart block is common. Ankylosing spondylitis must be considered as an etiology of otherwise unexplained complete heart block. Sacroiliac and lumbar spine x-rays must be obtained to clarify the diagnosis.[321]

TREATMENT

Aortic regurgitation is typically not of sufficient severity to warrant valve replacement; complete atrioventricular block[314,320] may require pacemaker implantation.

Reiter's disease

Pericardial, myocardial, and valvular involvement are associated with the arthritis, urethritis, and conjunctivitis of Reiter's disease, particularly after recurrent attacks. The aortic valve cusps are thickened; the edges are rolled and cordlike, and the valve ring is dilated, with collagen replacement of muscle and elastica.[322]

CLINICAL MANIFESTATIONS

Acute pericarditis can be diagnosed by a pericardial friction rub, often associated with pericardial pain;

apical gallop sounds and apical systolic murmurs also occur.[323] Aortic regurgitation is a late complication in patients with severe recurrent disease. Rarely, cardiac involvement may be the sole active manifestation of Reiter's disease.[324]

The electrocardiographic abnormalities include prolongation of the P-Q interval which may progress to complete heart block,[321] widening of the QRS complex, and nonspecific ST-T changes.

TREATMENT

Pacemaker implantation may be necessitated by the complete heart block.

Cogan's syndrome

About one-third of the reported cases of Cogan's syndrome (nonsyphilitic interstitial keratitis and bilateral deafness) have cardiovascular manifestations.[325] Fibrinoid necrosis, primarily of the aortic valve, may also produce aortic regurgitation. Angiitis of the myocardial arteries may result in myocardial ischemia and necrosis.

Cardiac enlargement; heart murmurs, particularly those of aortic regurgitation; and congestive heart failure are prominent.

Behçet's disease

Recurrent oral and genital ulceration with relapsing iritis of unknown cause constitute Behçet's disease. The cardiac manifestations include cardiac enlargement, gallop sounds, pericardial friction rub, and arrhythmias.[326] Thrombophlebitis is common. Aneurysms of large arteries may occur. There are nonspecific ST-T electrocardiographic changes.

Corticosteroid therapy has been effective.

Marfan's syndrome
(see Chaps. 88 and 103)

Cardiovascular manifestations[327] in this heritable disorder of connective tissue may be due to medial cystic necrosis of the aorta, defective valve cusps, myocardial lesions, the occasionally associated congenital heart disease, and/or coronary arterial disease.

PATHOLOGY

The aortic lesion may present as diffuse or dissecting aortic aneurysm or dilatation of the aortic valve ring with aortic regurgitation. Deformed, thickened, or sacculated valve cusps and redundant chordae tendineae result in aortic and mitral regurgitation. Bacterial endocarditis may complicate the disorder. Dilatation or dissection of the pulmonary artery may occur. Cystic and noncystic medial degeneration with intimal proliferation in the myocardial, the sinus node, and AV node arteries probably are the pathologic bases for rhythm and conduction disturbances

and sudden death.[328] Myocardial abnormalities may contribute to the cardiac enlargement and failure.

CLINICAL MANIFESTATIONS

Arachnodactyly, ectopia lentis, and aortic regurgitation are the hallmarks of Marfan's syndrome. Kyphoscoliosis and pectus excavatum may contribute to the cardiovascular symptoms. Arrhythmias or conduction defects may occur. Clinical evidence of aortic dissection, the murmur of mitral regurgitation in association with the aortic regurgitation, and the appearance of heart failure are not unusual.

TREATMENT

Heart failure and arrhythmias require standard therapy; surgical correction of specific aortic or valvular abnormalities may be required.

Noonan's syndrome

Noonan's syndrome has a phenotype similar to Turner's syndrome but has no chromosome abnormalities. Congenital heart disease, particularly valvular pulmonic stenosis, is common. Left ventricular cardiomyopathy, with and without symptoms, both of the obstructive and nonobstructive variety, is also a feature.[329] Rapidly progressive obstructive cardiomyopathy, refractory to medical and surgical therapy, has also been described.[330]

Ehlers-Danlos syndrome
(see Chap. 88)

Skin fragility and hyperelasticity with joint hyperextensibility are characteristic of this inherited disorder of collagen synthesis. Inheritance patterns vary among the six types. Valvular and chordal abnormalities of the aortic and mitral valves and myocardial fibrosis, especially of the papillary muscles, are described.[331,332] Aortic dissection and spontaneous rupture of large arteries are common. Mitral valve prolapse is common and appears to progress with age. Cardiac failure, in association with mitral and/or aortic valve murmurs, occurs.

There is no specific therapy.

Pseudoxanthoma elasticum (Groenblad-Strandberg syndrome) (see Chap. 88)

Primary cardiac abnormalities are unusual in this heritable connective tissue disorder, but they may occasionally be the mode of presentation or the cause of death.[333] Cardiovascular abnormalities are present in the majority of patients.

The pathologic alteration is a pearly white endocardial thickening which may involve the heart valves; the increased collagen and elastic fibers may encase the cardiac conduction system.[333] Calcification and fragmentation of the elastica of the myocardial arteries are seen.

Characteristic crepelike cutaneous lesions and retinal angioid streaks are present. Clinical findings include cardiac enlargement, heart failure, arrhythmias, and murmurs of valve deformity which result from the endocardial thickening. Angina pectoris has been described,[334] and Stokes-Adams syncope has occurred. Premature advanced arterial disease may occur in the myocardium and peripheral vessels.

There is no specific therapy.

Weber-Christian disease (relapsing febrile nodular nonsuppurative panniculitis)

PATHOLOGY

There is usually little pathologic confirmation of cardiac involvement in Weber-Christian disease except for focal necrosis of the epicardial fat. Periarteritis and endarteritis of the myocardial and pericardial blood vessels with vascular occlusion could explain the clinical abnormalities. In a recent case, however, myocardial nodules were demonstrated, identical to those in the skin. These were granulomatous foci with central necrosis and surrounding histiocytes, lymphocytes, and eosinophils.[335]

CLINICAL MANIFESTATIONS

The disease is most common in women in the second to fourth decade and is characterized by painful subcutaneous nodules. Cardiac enlargement and heart failure may occur. There are nonspecific electrocardiographic abnormalities.[336]

There is no specific therapy.

Juvenile xanthogranuloma (nevoxanthoendothelioma)

This generally self-limiting skin disease of infants and children is amenable to radiation therapy. There is occasional visceral involvement, including cardiac, with xanthogranulomas. Xanthogranulomatous "tumors" of the epicardium were reported to produce symptomatic hemopericardium.[337]

Trisomy 17-18

Diffuse myocardial fibrosis with prominent capillary formation was described in an infant with trisomy 17-18 who died of severe cardiac failure; a viral etiology has been postulated.[338] This appears to be the first myocardial lesion described with chromosomal abnormalities.

Scleredema of Buschke

Scleredema, generally a self-limiting skin infiltration with acid mucopolysaccharides, often follows a respiratory infection and occasionally has associated systemic manifestations. There is firm, nonpitting edema of the face, neck, scalp, and thorax. Myocardial involvement has been characterized by pericardial effusion and heart failure. The cardiac problems tend to resolve as the skin infiltrate clears; hence this form of cardiomyopathy has a good prognosis.[339] ST-T electrocardiographic changes and decreased

QRS voltage are also resolved as the skin infiltrate clears.[340] Skin biopsy is diagnostic.

There is no specific therapy.

Wegener's granulomatosis

The classic triad of nonhealing midline granuloma of the nose, pulmonary infiltrate, and renal disease described by Wegener may progress to systemic involvement, presumably with an allergic panarteritis.

Myocardial abnormalities include focal necrotizing vasculitis, granulomatous lesions, fibrinoid degeneration, myofiber necrosis, and an inflammatory cell infiltrate, at times with giant cells.[341]

The clinical presentation is of cardiac enlargement, congestive heart failure, and pericarditis with effusion; the reported association with mitral stenosis appears fortuitous, related to pathologic study of the left atrial appendage removed at surgery.[342]

Cytotoxic drugs, with or without corticosteroid hormones, appear of value.

Reye's syndrome

This rapidly fatal disease of young children is characterized by encephalopathy and fatty degeneration of the viscera. The cause is unknown, but cardiac involvement may contribute to the fatal outcome.

In one study intramyocardial fat droplets were universally present in the atria and were present to a lesser extent in the ventricles. The SA and AV nodes were free of fat, but extensive fat deposition was described in the bundle of His, bundle branches, and Purkinje fibers. Electron microscopy revealed mitochondrial swelling with fragmentation of the cristae; fat droplets were present between clusters of mitochondria.[343]

Fatty accumulation in the Purkinje system suggests that bundle branch block and complete heart block may be important clinical problems. Cardiovascular symptoms or signs are unusual. No specific cardiovascular management appears warranted.

Lentiginosis

All patients with lentiginosis should be evaluated at intervals for evidence of developing cardiomyopathy. The relation to previously described familial pigmented spots with cardiac murmurs and electrocardiographic abnormalities is uncertain. An association with atrial myxoma is also suggested.[344] Skin melanin and myocardial norepinephrine are chemically related, and an enzyme defect or abnormality of precursor substances has been suggested as a cause.[345]

Clinically, there are prominent, widespread lentigenes. Cardiac enlargement and/or systolic murmurs should suggest the diagnosis of cardiomyopathy in patients with lentiginosis. There is progressive massive atrioventricular septal hypertrophy with resultant bilateral outflow tract obstruction.

The disease is often mild at onset, but increases in severity; at times progression of the cardiomyopathy is associated with increase in the number of lentiform moles. Electrocardiographic abnormalities are variable and nondiagnostic.

Surgical septectomy has had variable success, and propranolol therapy is suggested.

Q-T prolongation, ventricular arrhythmias, and sudden death
(see also Chap. 49)

Patients with Q-T interval prolongation, often with T-wave abnormalities, are prone to ventricular arrhythmias, syncope, and sudden cardiac death.[346] The Romano-Ward disease is familial with an autosomal dominant pattern of inheritance; it occurs predominantly without deafness.[347] Consanguinity is described in most families with deafness, and the inheritance pattern appears to be autosomal recessive[346] for Jervell and Lange-Nielsen's syndrome. Cardiac manifestations are identical, with and without deafness.[348] Q-T prolongation also may play a role in the sudden infant death syndrome (SIDS); this finding has been documented in parents and siblings of SIDS infants.[349] However, a series of resuscitated SIDS infants had normal Q-T intervals.[349a]

The heart is generally normal at postmortem examination, although sinus node and sinus node artery abnormalities have been reported. Occasional extensive conduction system fibrosis is reported.[350]

The mechanism of Q-T prolongation is unknown, as is the mechanism of arrhythmogenesis. Delayed ventricular repolarization increases the vulnerable period and thus the susceptibility to ventricular arrhythmias. This unequal Q-T duration in different areas of the myocardium, i.e., asynchronous, prolonged refractoriness, appears to predispose to arrhythmias.

CLINICAL MANIFESTATIONS
Palpitations and syncope are the major cardiac symptoms; the arrhythmias and syncope appear to be triggered by physical or emotional stress, and the disease is more severe in infancy and childhood. Children with congenital deafness (and their siblings) should be evaluated electrocardiographically for Q-T interval prolongation, as should children with unexplained syncope.

The cardiovascular physical examination is unremarkable, except for the arrhythmias. Neurologic evaluation is normal except for the deafness.

The Q-T interval may vary in duration even from beat to beat, and at times Q-T prolongation decreases with increasing age. In some patients, the Q-T interval is normal at rest but prolongs with exercise.[350] Despite the marked variation in electrical systole, mechanical systole as measured on the phonocardiogram remains normal in duration, and is constant.[346]

Ventricular tachycardia and fibrillation are the characteristic arrhythmias, but asystole also occurs. Atrial arrhythmias are also described, as is bradycardia. Other routine laboratory studies are normal.[351]

TREATMENT
Propranolol seems to be the therapy of choice and has been reported to decrease the frequency of arrhythmias and syncopal episodes; it appears to work via a direct "quinidine-like" antiarrhythmic effect rather than by beta blockade.[347] However, the propranolol-induced bradycardia may engender ventricular arrhythmias, and combined pacemaker-propranolol therapy may be warranted.

Digitalis and dilantin shorten the Q-T interval, and variable success has been reported with their use; the value of pacemaker therapy is equivocal. Quinidine therapy is contraindicated, as it further prolongs the Q-T interval and increases ventricular arrhythmias. Phenothiazine drugs and tricyclic antidepressant agents are contraindicated for the same reason. The effects of left stellate ganglionectomy remain unpredictable.[352]

The families of children with this disorder should be trained in cardiopulmonary resuscitation, as should personnel in schools for deaf children. These patients should be monitored electrocardiographically during dental and surgical procedures.[350] Extreme physical activity should be avoided, particularly in childhood. A suggested approach to manage asymptomatic siblings with Q-T prolongation is to do exercise stress testing; further Q-T prolongation or the appearance of T-wave abnormalities with exercise may be considered an indication for prophylactic propranolol.[348]

Mucocutaneous lymph node syndrome

See Chap. 63A.

Neurofibromatosis (von Recklinghausen's disease)

Stenotic renal arteries, with resultant hypertension, and coarctation of the abdominal aorta are the most common cardiovascular abnormalities in von Recklinghausen's disease.

The rare myocardial lesions include myocardial and epicardial neurofibromas, acquired fibromuscular stenosis of the right ventricular outflow tract,[353] and obstructive cardiomyopathy. The patient with the latter abnormality also had Ullrich-Turner syndrome.[354] Cardiac murmurs and progressive heart failure are described.

Diabetic cardiomyopathy
(see also Chap. 81C)

Heart failure in diabetic patients is almost always due to associated coronary atherosclerotic heart disease and/or hypertensive cardiovascular disease. Additionally, a specific diabetic cardiomyopathy has been claimed to occur in the absence of these disorders.[355] Epidemiologically, heart failure occurred twice as frequently in men and five times as frequently in women with diabetes in the Framingham study.[356]

PATHOLOGY

Endothelial proliferation and wall thickening with luminal narrowing due to acid mucopolysaccharide deposition are described in the small intramural coronary arteries.[355,357] Focal myocardial fibrosis results.

It is not known whether the microangiopathy or a metabolic defect in energy production underlies the cardiomyopathy. In an animal model, mucopolysaccharide infiltration of cardiac muscle produced a stiff ventricle.

CLINICAL MANIFESTATIONS

The increased incidence of heart failure, particularly involving women, seemed confined to insulin-dependent diabetics in the Framingham study.[356] Left ventricular or biventricular failure is encountered. The usual management of congestive heart failure is recommended.

Mulibrey nanism

This autosomal recessive disorder is characterized by prenatal-onset growth failure, muscular hypotonia, enlarged cerebral ventricles and cisternas, and ocular fundal changes. The major cardiac abnormality is constrictive pericarditis.[358] Patchy collagenous myocardial fibrosis occurs beneath a thickened pericardium which often has flecks of calcium.

CLINICAL MANIFESTATIONS

Symptoms and signs of cardiac failure vary in severity. Nonspecific P- and T-wave abnormalities are present on the electrocardiogram; arrhythmias may occur. Cardiac enlargement is present on x-ray examination, with diminished cardiac pulsations at fluoroscopy. Echocardiography confirms the pericardial thickening. The cardiac catheterization findings are those of constrictive pericarditis.[358]

TREATMENT

Pericardiectomy has effected marked clinical and hemodynamic improvement in the sicker patients; conservative management is recommended in milder cases of illness.

Ulcerative colitis

Recurring myopericarditis has been described during relapses of chronic ulcerative colitis.[359] Retrosternal discomfort and pleuritic chest pain are described, and a pericardial friction rub may be present. Nonspecific ST-T electrocardiographic abnormalities resolve with therapy with corticosteroid hormones.

Whipple's disease (intestinal lipodystrophy)

Clinical cardiac findings and gross cardiac lesions occur in the majority of patients with intestinal lipodystrophy; however, the extent of cardiac involvement appears unrelated to the severity and duration of Whipple's disease.

Large macrophages with PAS-positive granules, identical to those seen in the intestine, occur in the pericardium, myocardium, and heart valves. Adhesive pericarditis, focal myocardial fibrosis, and valvular fibrosis with deformity are present.[360] Rod-shaped bodies, possible bacteria, are seen in the heart valves and myocardium.[360a]

CLINICAL MANIFESTATIONS

Cardiac murmurs, particularly mitral valve murmurs; pericardial friction rubs; and congestive heart failure are encountered. Electrocardiographic abnormalities are common, but nonspecific.

TREATMENT

There is often a favorable response to antibiotic therapy.

CARDIOVASCULAR COMPLICATIONS OF ORAL CONTRACEPTIVE AGENTS

The cardiovascular complications of the use of oral contraceptive agents (estrogen and progesterone compounds) are related in great part to their effects on blood vessels, on the clotting mechanism, and on the renin-angiotensin-aldosterone system.[361]

Higher dose estrogen compounds are associated with increased cardiovascular complications, and a number of these are no longer available for use.

Pathophysiology

Estrogen causes a loss of vascular smooth-muscle tone; venous stasis, predisposing to venous thrombosis, is most prominent in the lower extremities. Vascular intimal changes are also described. Estrogen also increases platelet stickiness and affects factors which inhibit clotting and fibrinolysis; this increases the tendency to intravascular thrombosis, particularly in association with the increased venous stasis. Estrogen and progesterone increase renin and angiotensinogen production, resulting in increased angiotensin and thereby increased aldosterone concentrations. Oral contraceptives also increase serum triglyceride levels[361a] and glucose levels.

THROMBOPHLEBITIS AND PULMONARY EMBOLISM

There is an increased incidence of thrombophlebitis and thromboembolism, especially pulmonary embolism, in young women taking oral contraceptives.[362] Almost a fivefold increase in deep venous thrombosis of the legs is reported. This does not appear related to the duration of oral contraceptive use or to estrogen dosage. There is no test which can identify women prone to thromboembolic complications. It remains uncertain whether the abnormality is one of coagulation or whether it relates to intrinsic vascular wall changes. Therefore, oral contraceptive use appears contraindicated in patients with heart disease who have congestive heart failure (which increases the likelihood of peripheral venous thrombosis and pulmonary embolism), pulmonary hypertension, or cyanotic heart disease. Oral contraceptives are also inadvisable for patients with a history of heart failure, phlebitis, or thromboembolic disease. Their use by patients with severe varicose veins also appears unwise.

Excessive smoking, weight gain, and prolonged bed rest add to the risk of thromboembolism. Postoperative thrombosis is increased fourfold in patients on oral contraceptive agents; discontinuation of the agents several weeks prior to elective major surgery appears prudent.[362a] The risk is accentuated among older women who smoke cigarettes.

HYPERTENSION

Hypertension may develop in about 5 percent of patients taking oral contraceptive agents,[361a,362b] and the hypertension may appear up to 6 months after therapy is begun. The hypertension is characteristically mild.[363] After discontinuing oral contraceptives, return of the blood pressure to normal levels generally occurs within 3 to 6 months. Oral contraceptives appear contraindicated in patients with hypertension or a history of hypertension, or with renal disease or a toxemia history; all patients begun on oral contraceptives should have their blood pressure measured initially and periodically, particularly during the first 6 months of therapy.

CEREBROVASCULAR ACCIDENT

Oral contraceptives may increase the severity of migraine headaches; there is a four- to sixfold increase in the likelihood of cerebrovascular accident due to cerebral thrombosis. Their use is not recommended for patients with a history of migraine headaches, transient ischemic attacks, or other neurologic events.

MYOCARDIAL INFARCTION

Young women taking oral contraceptive agents are also predisposed to myocardial infarction; and oral contraceptive use appears to be an independent risk factor in these individuals. The increased risk appeared to diminish when oral contraceptive use was discontinued. In women with the traditional risk factors for coronary atherosclerosis (Chaps. 62B and 62H) oral contraceptive agents appear to act synergistically in increasing the risk of myocardial infarction. Oral contraceptive agents increased the risk of death from myocardial infarction 2.8 times in the 30 to 39 age group and 4.7 times in the 40 to 44 age group in one study.[364] Thus the risk of fatal myocardial infarction is greater in women using oral contraceptives, particularly in the older age groups.[364] Further investigation showed the increased risk of fatal myocardial infarction to be comparable among younger

and older women, about a threefold increase, but total complications remained greater over age 40.[364a] The coronary arterial lesions are often proximal, involving a long segment of artery, and tend to appear smooth and rounded in contrast to the usual irregular atheromatous lesions.

PULMONARY HYPERTENSION

Isolated case reports describe pulmonary hypertension apparently related to oral contraceptive usage. Pulmonary vascular intimal proliferation and/or pulmonary thromboembolism may play a role.[364b]

CARDIOVASCULAR COMPLICATIONS OF DRUG ABUSE

The increasing frequency of drug abuse and drug overdose requires its consideration in determining the etiology and the correct management of many cardiovascular emergencies.

Narcotic overdose

CLINICAL MANIFESTATIONS

The heroin (morphine and methadone) overdose patient classically presents with respiratory depression to apnea, unconsciousness, areflexia, cyanosis, and pinpoint pupils (although with profound cerebral hypoxia, the pupils may dilate). Pulmonary edema without congestive heart failure may be due to hypoxia secondary to respiratory depression, it may be an allergic response to adulterating impurities, or it may be a direct effect of opiate action. Cardiac arrhythmias are attributable both to hypoxia and to the quinine used to dilute the heroin.

TREATMENT

Nalorphine therapy is indicated.[365] Intubation may be required and positive-pressure oxygen has been of value.[366] Patients with suspected heroin overdose responding well to narcotic antagonists still require at least 24 h of observation, as pulmonary edema may be a late complication;[367] indeed pulmonary edema may recur, possibly related to development of an acute cardiomyopathy,[367a] and some patients may die of this complication.

Bacterial endocarditis
(see also Chap. 77)

Bacterial endocarditis, particularly right-sided endocarditis, is a frequent complication in patients using intravenous drugs. Tricuspid regurgitation or multiple (septic) pulmonary emboli are the frequent presenting findings. Myocardial abscesses and mycotic pulmonary arteriovenous aneurysms may also be seen.

Angiothrombotic pulmonary hypertension

Angiothrombotic pulmonary hypertension may result from repeated intravenous injection of substances intended for oral use; talc or starch particles embolize to the lung, producing small artery, arteriolar, and capillary thrombosis. The pulmonary vascular sclerosis is evident on chest x-ray as an interstitial reticulonodular infiltrate.[365]

Arterial disease

Arterial thrombosis, necrotizing arteritis, and arteriovenous fistulas occur as complications of intraarterial drug abuse.

Thrombophlebitis

Thrombophlebitis of the arms and legs, with and without bland pulmonary emboli, is commonly encountered with intravenous drug abuse. Mycotic vascular aneurysms also occur.

Cardiomyopathy

Cardiomyopathy, with severe biventricular failure, has occurred with prolonged high-dose dextroamphetamine abuse. The histologic abnormalities simulated those of pheochromocytoma myocarditis, suggesting that chronic sympathomimetic amine ingestion may lead to clinical heart disease.[368]

Arrhythmias; electrocardiographic abnormalities

AMPHETAMINES
Amphetamines and other stimulant drugs, particularly when taken parenterally, may result in serious arrhythmias and severe hypertension, the latter occasionally complicated by cerebrovascular accident.

PEHNOTHIAZINES
Phenothiazine and other psychotropic agents characteristically produce ECG abnormalities but may also be associated with hypertension, serious arrhythmias, and sudden death;[369] cardiac failure and myocardial infarction are also described.[370]

GLUE AND SOLVENT SNIFFING
Glue and solvent sniffing is associated with sudden death, presumably due to cardiac arrhythmias. Fluorinated hydrocarbons, the "inert" propellant in most aerosols, readily induce severe cardiac arrhythmias; fluorinated hydrocarbons have been detected in the blood of volunteers using nebulizers.[371]

MARIJUANA SMOKING
Marijuana potentiates atropine and epinephrine tachycardias, probably by a β-adrenergic mechanism. Therefore caution is advised in administering vasoactive drugs and anesthetics to persons smoking marijuana.[372]

COCAINE ABUSE
Cocaine and related sympathomimetic amine overdose is manifest by profound hypertension and tachycardia. This "dopaminergic crisis" responds rapidly to propranolol therapy.

MULTIPLE DRUG ABUSE
The electrocardiograms of drug-dependent patients, particularly of multiple drug users, often show conduction, depolarization, and repolarization abnormalities and bradyarrhythmias, all of which may contribute to the increased incidence of sudden death in drug-dependent individuals.[373]

The above may be further compounded by the hypotension of barbiturate abuse, the respiratory depression of narcotic abuse, and the frequent ventricular arrhythmias seen with alcohol abuse.

REFERENCES

1 Hudson, R. E. B.: The Cardiomyopathies: Order from Chaos, *Am. J. Cardiol.,* 25:70, 1970.
2 Perloff, J. K., Lindgren, K. M., and Groves, B. M.: Uncommon or Commonly Unrecognized Causes of Heart Failure, *Prog. Cardiovasc. Dis.,* 12:409, 1970.
3 Primary Myocardial Diseases and the Myocardiopathies, I and II, *Prog. Cardiovasc. Dis.,* 7:1, 1964.
4 Goodwin, J. F.: Clarification of the Cardiomyopathies, *Mod. Concepts Cardiovasc. Dis.,* 41:41, 1972.
5 Burch, G. E., and DePasquale, N. P.: Recognition and Prevention of Cardiomyopathy, *Circulation,* 42:A47, 1970.
6 Burch, G. E., Tsui, C. Y., and Harb, J. M.: Ischemic Cardiomyopathy, *Am. Heart J.,* 83:340, 1972.
7 Smith, W. P.: Primary Sarcoid Heart Disease: Report of a Case, *J. Fla. Med. Assoc.,* 51:652, 1964.
8 Chisholm, J. C., Jr.: Sarcoid Cardiomyopathy, *J. Natl. Med. Assoc.,* 58:265, 1966.
9 Porter, G. H.: Sarcoid Heart Disease, *N. Engl. J. Med.,* 263:1350, 1960.
10 Rossi, L.: Sarcoid Heart Disease, *Br. Med. J.,* 1:546, 1973.
11 Fawcett, F. J., and Goldberg, M. J.: Heart Block Resulting from Myocardial Sarcoidosis, *Br. Heart J.,* 36:220, 1974.
12 Deneberg, M.: Sarcoidosis of the Myocardium and Aorta: A Case Report, *Am. J. Clin. Pathol.,* 43:445, 1965.
13 Duvernoy, W. F. C., and Garcia, R.: Sarcoidosis of the Heart Presenting with Ventricular Tachycardia and Atrioventricular Block, *Am. J. Cardiol.,* 28:348, 1971.
14 Ferrans, V. J., Hibbs, R. G., Black, W. C., Walsh, J. J., and Burch, G. E.: Myocardial Degeneration in Cardiac Sarcoidosis: Histochemical and Electron Microscopic Studies, *Am. Heart J.,* 69:159, 1965.
15 Editorial: Sarcoid Heart Disease, *Br. Med. J.,* 4:627, 1972.
16 Wheeler, R. C., and Abelmann, W. H.: Cardiomyopathy Associated with Systemic Diseases, *Cardiovasc. Clin.,* 4:283, 1972.
17 Lie, J. T., Hunt, D., and Valentine, P. A.: Sudden Death from Cardiac Sarcoidosis with Involvement of Conduction System, *Am. J. Med. Sci.,* 267:123, 1974.
18 Stein, E., Jackler, I., Stimmel, B., Stein, W., and Siltzbach, L. E.: Asymptomatic Electrocardiographic Alterations in Sarcoidosis, *Am. Heart J.,* 86:474, 1973.
18a Matsui, Y., Iwai, K., Tachibana, T., Friue, T., Shigematsu, N., Izumi, T., Homma, A. H., Mikami, R., Hongo, O., Hiraga, Y., and Yamamoto, M.: Clinicopathological Study on Fatal Myocardial Sarcoidosis, *Ann. N.Y. Acad. Sci.,* 278:455, 1976.
19 Ghosh, P., Fleming, H. A., Gresham, G. A., and Stovin, P. G. I.: Myocardial Sarcoidosis, *Br. Heart J.,* 34:769, 1972.
20 Fleming, H. A.: Sarcoid Heart Disease, *Br. Heart J.,* 36:54, 1974.

21 Clark, E. J., and Blount, A. W.: A Fatal Case of Myocardial Sarcoidosis, *Lancet,* 2:568, 1966.

22 Gozo, E. G., Jr., Cosnow, I., Cohen, H. C., and Okun, L.: The Heart in Sarcoidosis, *Chest,* 60:379, 1971.

23 Shiff, A. D., Blatt, C. J., and Colp, C.: Recurrent Pericardial Effusion Secondary to Sarcoidosis of the Pericardium. A Biopsy-proved Case, *N. Engl. J. Med.,* 281:141, 1969.

24 Phinney, A. O., Jr.: Sarcoid of the Myocardial Septum with Complete Heart Block: Report of Two Cases, *Am. Heart J.,* 62:270, 1961.

24a Stein, E., Stimmel, B., and Siltzbach, L. E.: Clinical Course of Cardiac Sarcoidosis, *Ann. N.Y. Acad. Sci.,* 278:470, 1976.

24b Strauss, G. S., Lawton, B. R., Wenzel, F. J., and Ray, J. F., III: Detection of Covert Myocardial Sarcoidosis by Scalene Node Biopsy, *Chest,* 69:790, 1976.

25 Bashour, F. A., McConnell, T., Skinner, W., and Hanson, M.: Myocardial Sarcoidosis, *Dis. Chest.,* 53:413, 1968.

25a Friedman, H. S., Parikh, N. K., Chandler, N., and Calderon, J.: Sarcoidosis with Incomplete Bilateral Bundle Branch Block Pattern Disappearing Following Steroid Therapy: An Electrophysiological Study, *Eur. J. Cardiol.,* 4:41, 1976.

26 Lull, R. J., Dunn, B. E., Gregoratos, G., Fox, W. A., and Fisher, G. W.: Ventricular Aneurysm Due to Cardiac Sarcoidosis with Surgical Cure of Refractory Ventricular Tachycardia, *Am. J. Cardiol.,* 30:282, 1972.

27 Ziffer, H., and Baker, H.: Relationship of Some Vitamins to Cardiovascular Disease, in E. B. Feldman (ed.), "Nutrition and Cardiovascular Disease," Appleton-Century-Crofts, New York, 1976, p. 263.

27a Stefadouros, M. A., El Shahawy, M., and Witham, A. C.: Sheshin in Georgia: A Case of Acute Fulminant Cardiac Beriberi, *J. Med. Assoc. Ga.,* 65:149, 1976.

28 Rowlands, D. T., Jr., and Vilter, C. F.: A Study of the Cardiac Stigmata in Prolonged Human Thiamine Deficiency, *Circulation,* 21:4, 1960.

29 Brink, A. J., Lochner, A., and Lewis, C. M.: Thiamine Deficiency and Beriberi Heart Disease: Biochemical and Clinical Investigations, *S. Afr. Med. J.,* 40:581, 1966.

30 Alexander, C. S.: Nutritional Heart Disease, *Cardiovasc. Clin.,* 4:221, 1972.

31 Jeffrey, F. E., and Abelmann, W. H.: Recovery from Proved Shoshin Beriberi, *Am. J. Med.,* 50:123, 1971.

32 Akbarian, M., Yankopoulos, N. A., and Abelmann, W. H.: Hemodynamic Studies in Beriberi Heart Disease, *Am. J. Med.,* 41:197, 1966.

33 McIntyre, N., and Stanley, N. N.: Cardiac Beriberi: Two Modes of Presentation, *Br. Med. J.,* 3:567, 1971.

34 Campbell, G. M., and Bieder, L.: Beri-Beri Cardiomyopathy. Report of a Case, *N.Z. Med. J.,* 64:503, 1965.

35 Akbarian, M., and Dreyfus, P. M.: Blood Transketolase in Beri-Beri Heart Disease: A Useful Diagnostic Index, *JAMA,* 203:23, 1968.

36 Wagner, P. I.: Beriberi Heart Disease: Physiologic Data and Difficulties in Diagnosis, *Am. Heart J.,* 69:200, 1965.

37 Webb, D. I.: Beriberi Heart Disease with Acute Renal Failure, *Arch. Intern. Med.,* 120:494, 1967.

38 Rachmilewitz, M., and Braun, K.: Electrocardiographic Changes and the Effect of Niacin Therapy in Pellagra, *Br. Heart J.,* 7:72, 1945.

39 Sament, S.: Cardiac Disorders in Scurvy, *N. Engl. J. Med.,* 282:282, 1970.

40 Follis, R. H., Jr.: Sudden Death in Infants with Scurvy, *J. Pediatr.,* 20:347, 1942.

41 Shafar, J.: Rapid Reversion of Electrocardiographic Abnormalities after Treatment in Two Cases of Scurvy, *Lancet,* 2:176, 1967.

42 Bauer, J. M., and Freyberg, R. H.: Vitamin D Intoxication with Metastatic Calcification, *JAMA,* 130:1208, 1946.

43 Sims, B. A.: Conducting Tissue of the Heart in Kwashiorkor, *Br. Heart J.,* 34:828, 1972.

44 Smythe, P. M., Swanepoel, A., and Campbell, J. A. H.: The Heart in Kwashiorkor, *Br. Med. J.,* 1:67, 1962.

45 Swanepoel, A., Smythe, P. M., and Campbell, J. A. H.: The Heart in Kwashiorkor, *Am. Heart J.,* 67:1, 1964.

46 Shaper, A. G.: Cardiomyopathies in Children in the Tropics, *J. Trop. Pediatr.,* 11:25, 1965.

47 Amad, K. H., Brennan, J. C., and Alexander, J. K.: The Cardiac Pathology of Chronic Exogenous Obesity, *Circulation,* 32:740, 1965.

48 Alexander, J. K., and Pettigrove, J. R.: Obesity and Congestive Heart Failure, *Geriatrics,* 22:101, 1967.

49 Brigden, W.: Cardiac Amyloidosis, *Prog. Cardiovasc. Dis.,* 7:142, 1964.

50 Gafni, J., Sohar, E., and Heller, H.: The Inherited Amyloidoses: Their Clinical and Theoretical Significance, *Lancet,* 1:71, 1964.

51 Barth, W. F.: Amyloidosis: Review of Cardiac and Renal Manifestations, *Med. Ann. D.C.,* 36:228, 1967.

52 Lindberg, J.: Rupture of the Right Ventricle of the Heart in a Case of Advanced Heart Amyloidosis, *Acta Pathol. Microbiol. Scand.,* 79:53, 1971.

53 Husband, E. M., and Lannigan, R.: Electron Microscopy of the Heart in a Case of Primary Cardiac Amyloidosis, *Br. Heart J.,* 30:265, 1968.

54 James, T. N.: Pathology of the Cardiac Conduction System in Amyloidosis, *Ann. Intern. Med.,* 65:28, 1966.

55 van Buchem, F. S. P.: Cardiac Amyloidosis: Report of Six Cases, *Acta Cardiol.,* 21:367, 1966.

56 Garcia, R., and Saeed, S. M.: Amyloidosis. Cardiovascular Manifestations in Five Illustrative Cases, *Arch. Intern. Med.,* 121:259, 1968.

57 Case Records of the Massachusetts General Hospital, *N. Engl. J. Med.,* 290:1474, 1974.

58 Pomerance, A.: The Pathology of Senile Cardiac Amyloidosis, *J. Pathol. Bacteriol.,* 91:357, 1966.

59 Brownstein, M. H.: Cardiac Amyloidosis and Complete Heart Block, *N.Y. State J. Med.,* 66:397, 1966.

60 Garcia, R., and Jennings, J. M.: Pheochromocytoma Masquerading as a Cardiomyopathy, *Am. J. Cardiol.,* 27:568, 1972.

61 Baker, G., Zeller, N. H., Weitzner, S., and Leach, J. K.: Pheochromocytoma without Hypertension Presenting as Cardiomyopathy, *Am. Heart J.,* 83:688, 1972.

62 Wiswell, J. G., and Crago, R. M.: Reversible Cardiomyopathy with Pheochromocytoma, *Trans. Am. Clin. Assoc.,* 80:185, 1969.

63 Ehlers, K. H., Hagstrom, J. W. C., Lukas, D. S., Redo, S. F., and Engle, M. A.: Glycogen-Storage Disease of the Myocardium with Obstruction to Left Ventricular Outflow, *Circulation,* 25:96, 1962.

64 Hers, H. G.: α-Glucosidase Deficiency in Generalized Glycogen-Storage Disease (Pompe's Disease), *Biochem. J.,* 86:11, 1963.

65 McPhie, J. M.: Cardiac Glycogenosis, *Am. Heart J.,* 60:836, 1960.

66 Hohn, A. R., Lowe, C. U., Sokal, J. E., and Lambert, E. C.: Cardiac Problems in the Glycogenoses with Specific Reference to Pompe's Disease, *Pediatrics,* 35:313, 1965.

67 Blieden, L. C., and Moller, J. H.: Cardiac Involvement in Inherited Disorders of Metabolism, *Prog. Cardiovasc. Dis.,* 16:615, 1974.

68 Miller, C. G., Alleyne, G. A., and Brooks, S. E. H.: Gross Cardiac Involvement in Glycogen Storage Disease Type III, *Br. Heart J.,* 34:862, 1972.

69 Ehlers, K. H., and Engle, M. A.: Glycogen Storage Disease of the Myocardium, *Am. Heart J.,* 65:145, 1963.

70 Huijing, F., van Creveld, S., and Losekoot, G.: Diagnosis of

Generalized Glycogen Storage Disease (Pompe's Disease), *J. Pediatr.*, 63:984, 1963.

71 Nihill, M. R., Wilson, D. S., and Hugh-Jones, K.: Generalized Glycogenosis Type II (Pompe's Disease), *Arch. Dis. Child.*, 45:122, 1970.

72 Ruttenberg, H. D., Steidl, R. M., Carey, L. S., and Edwards, J. E.: Glycogen-Storage Disease of the Heart: Hemodynamic and Angiocardiographic Features in 2 Cases, *Am. Heart J.*, 67:469, 1964.

73 Rees, A., Elbl, F., Minhas, K., and Solinger, R.: Echocardiographic Evidence of Outflow Tract Obstruction in Pompe's Disease (Glycogen Storage Disease of the Heart), *Am. J. Cardiol.*, 37:1103, 1976.

74 Yamamoto, T., Eguchi, A., Okudaira, M., Suzuki, E., Yokoyama, T., and Tanabe, J.: Glycogen Storage Disease of the Heart: First Case in Japan, *Am. J. Cardiol.*, 5:556, 1960.

75 Goyer, R. A., and Bowden, D. H.: Endocardial Fibroelastosis Associated with Glycogen Tumors of the Heart and Tuberose Sclerosis, *Am. Heart J.*, 64:539, 1962.

76 Golding, R., and Reed, G.: Rhabdomyoma of the Heart: Two Unusual Clinical Presentations, *N. Engl. J. Med.*, 276:957, 1967.

77 Kuehl, K. S., Perry, L. W., Chandra, R., and Scott, L. P., III: Left Ventricular Rhabdomyoma: A Rare Cause of Subaortic Stenosis in the Newborn Infant, *Pediatrics*, 46:464, 1970.

77a Fenoglio, J. J., Jr., McAllister, H. A., Jr., and Ferrans, V. J.: Cardiac Rhabdomyoma: A Clinicopathologic and Electron Microscopic Study, *Am. J. Cardiol.*, 38:241, 1976.

78 Öckerman, P. A., and Berlin, S. O.: Biochemical Studies in Familial Cardiomyopathy: With Special Reference to the Differential Diagnosis from Known Types of Glycogen Storage Disease, *Acta Med. Scand.*, 176:277, 1964.

79 Ratinov, G., Baker, W. P., and Swaiman, K. F.: McArdle's Syndrome with Previously Unreported Electrocardiographic and Serum Enzyme Abnormalities, *Ann. Intern. Med.*, 62:328, 1965.

80 Wasserman, A. J., Richardson, D. W., Baird, C. L., and Wyso, E. M.: Cardiac Hemochromatosis Simulating Constrictive Pericarditis, *Am. J. Med.*, 32:316, 1962.

81 Skinner, C., and Kenmure, A. C. F.: Haemochromatosis Presenting as Congestive Cardiomyopathy and Responding to Venesection, *Br. Heart J.*, 35:466, 1973.

82 James, T. N.: Pathology of the Cardiac Conduction System in Hemochromatosis, *N. Engl. J. Med.*, 271:92, 1964.

83 Easley, R. M. Jr., Schreiner, B. F., Jr., and Yu, P. N.: Reversible Cardiomyopathy Associated with Hemochromatosis, *N. Engl. J. Med.*, 287:866, 1972.

84 Faivre, G., Gilgenkrantz, J. M., Cherrier, F., Tenette, C., and Gaucher, P.: (Hemochromatosis and Adiastole: Apropos of an Anatomical Case), *Arch. Mal Coeur*, 54:935, 1961.

85 Faivre, G., Gilgenkrantz, J. M., Cherrier, F., and Tenette, C.: Le coeur dans l'hémochromatose: Considerations hémodynamiques, *M. Monde*, 40:128, 1964.

86 Arnett, E. N., Nienhuis, A. W., Henry, W. L., Ferrans, V. J., Redwood, D. R., and Roberts, W. C.: Massive Myocardial Hemosiderosis: A Structure-Function Conference at the National Heart and Lung Institute, *Am. Heart J.*, 90:777, 1975.

87 Perrin, A.: Les complications cardiaques de l'hémochromatose: Les cardiopathies pigmentaires, *M. Monde*. 40:122, 1964.

88 Slama, R., Motte, G., Coumel, P., Passa, P., and Perrault, M.: Les blocs auriculoventriculaires de l'hémochromatose, *Presse Med.*, 79:747, 1971.

89 Grosberg, S. J.: Hemochromatosis and Heart Failure: Presentation of a Case with Survival after Three Years' Treatment by Repeated Venesection, *Ann. Intern. Med.*, 54:550, 1961.

90 Engle, M. A., Erlandson, M., and Smith, C. H.: Late Cardiac Complications of Chronic, Severe, Refractory Anemia with Hemochromatosis, *Circulation*, 30:698, 1964.

91 Ferrans, V. J., Hibbs, R. G., and Burda, C. D.: The Heart in Fabry's Disease. A Histochemical and Electron Microscopic Study, *Am. J. Cardiol.*, 24:95, 1969.

92 Duncan, C., and McLeod, G. M.: Angiokeratoma Corporis Diffusum Universale (Fabry's Disease): A Case with Gross Myocardial Involvement, *Australas. Ann. Med.*, 19:58, 1970.

92a Desnick, R. J., Blieden, L. C., Sharp, H. L., Hofschire, P. J., and Moller, J. H.: Cardiac Valvular Anomalies in Fabry Disease: Clinical, Morphologic, and Biochemical Studies, *Circulation*, 54:818, 1976.

93 Becker, A. E., Schoorl, R. Balk, A. G., and van der Heide, R. M.: Cardiac Manifestations of Fabry's Disease. Report of a Case with Mitral Insufficiency and Electrocardiographic Evidence of Myocardial Infarction, *Am. J. Cardiol.*, 36:829, 1975.

94 Burda, C. D., and Winder, P. R.: Angiokeratoma Corporis Diffusum Universale (Fabry's Disease) in Female Subjects, *Am. J. Med.*, 42:293, 1967.

95 Kemp, G. L.: Fabry's Disease Involving the Myocardium and Coronary Arteries, without Skin Manifestations, *Vasc. Dis.*, 4:100, 1967.

96 Ross, C. F., and Belton, E. M.: A Case of Isolated Cardiac Lipidosis, *Br. Heart J.*, 30:726, 1968.

97 Deacon, J. S. R., Gilbert, E. F., Viseskul, C., Herrman, J., Angevine, J. M., Opitz, J. M., and Albert, A. E.: Familial Cardiac Lipidosis, *Birth Defects*, 10:181, 1974.

98 Eilenberg, M. D., and Scobie, B. A.: Prolonged Neuropsychiatric Disability and Cardiomyopathy in Acute Intermittent Porphyria, *Br. Med. J.*, 1:858, 1960.

99 McKusick, V. A.: A Genetical View of Cardiovascular Disease, *Circulation*, 30:326, 1964.

100 Glober, G. A., Tanaka, K. R., Turner, J. A., and Lui, C. K.: Mucopolysaccharidosis, an Unusual Cause of Cardiac Valvular Disease, *Am. J. Cardiol.*, 22:133, 1968.

101 Vanace, P. W., Friedman, S., and Wagner, B. M.: Mitral Stenosis in an Atypical Case of Gargoylism: A Case Report with Pathologic and Histochemical Studies of the Cardiac Tissues, *Circulation*, 21:80, 1960.

102 Okada, R., Rosenthal, I. M., Scaravelli, G., and Lev, M.: A Histopathologic Study of the Heart in Gargoylism, *Arch. Pathol.*, 84:20, 1967.

102a Renteria, V. G., Ferrans, V. J., and Roberts, W. C.: The Heart in the Hurler Syndrome: Gross, Histologic, and Ultrastructural Observations in Five Necropsy Cases, *Am. J. Cardiol.*, 38:487, 1976.

103 Krovetz, L. J., Lorincz, A. E., and Schiebler, G. L.: Cardiovascular Manifestations of the Hurler Syndrome: Hemodynamic and Angiocardiographic Observations in 15 Patients, *Circulation*, 31:132, 1965.

104 Schieken, R. M., Kerber, R. E., Ionasescu, V. V., and Zellweger, H.: Cardiac Manifestations of the Mucopolysaccharidoses, *Circulation*, 52:700, 1975.

105 Campbell, A. M. G., and Williams, E. R.: Natural History of Refsum's Syndrome in a Gloucestershire Family, *Br. Med. J.*, 3:777, 1967.

106 Lewis, H. D., Jr., White, H. H., and Dunn, M.: Refsum's Syndrome: A Neurological Disease with Interesting Cardiovascular Manifestations, *Circulation*, 33-34(suppl. 3):157, 1966.

107 Jensen, J., Blankenhorn, D. H., and Kornerup, V.: Coronary Disease in Familial Hypercholesterolemia, *Circulation*, 36:77, 1967.

108 Lyle, W. H., Leonard, B. J., Bowden, W. E., and Miller, D. G.: Normocholesterolemic Xanthomatosis: Report of Case with Myocardial Fibrosis and Mysclerosis, *Ann. Intern. Med.*, 53:1260, 1960.

109 Rothbard, S., Hagstrom, J. W. C., and Smith, J. P.: Aortic

Stenosis and Myocardial Infarction in Hypercholesterolemic Xanthomatosis, *Am. Heart J., 73*:687, 1967.

110 Miller, A. A., and Ramaden, F.: Neural and Visceral Xanthomatosis in Adults, *J. Clin. Pathol., 18*:622, 1965.

111 Pund, E. E., Jr., Hawley, R. L., McGee, H. J., and Blount, S. G., Jr.: Gouty Heart, *N. Engl. J. Med., 263*:835, 1960.

112 Virtanen, K. S. I., and Halonen, P. I.: Total Heart Block as a Complication of Gout, *Cardiologia, 54*:359, 1969.

113 Paulley, J. W., Barlow, K. E., Cutting, P. E. J., and Stevens, J.: Acute Gouty Pericarditis, *Lancet, 1*:21, 1963.

114 Pikula, B., Plamenac, P., Ćurčić, B., and Nikulin, A.: Myocarditis Caused by Primary Oxalosis in a 4-Year-Old Child, *Virchows Arch. [Pathol. Anat.], 358*:99, 1973.

115 Hahlweg, G., and Orf, G.: Sog. Fibroplastische Myocarditis bei Oxalose, *Pathol. Microbiol.,* (Basel), 29:1, 1966.

116 Coltart, D. J., and Hudson, R. E. B.: Primary Oxalosis of the Heart: A Cause of Heart Block, *Br. Heart J., 33*:315, 1971.

117 Stauffer, M.: Oxalosis: Report of a Case, with a Review of the Literature and Discussion of the Pathogenesis, *N. Engl. J. Med., 263*:386, 1960.

118 Salyer, W. R., and Hutchins, G. M.: Cardiac Lesions in Secondary Oxalosis, *Arch. Intern. Med., 134*:250, 1974.

118a Lichtenstein, L., and Kaplan, L.: Hereditary Ochronosis: Pathologic Changes Observed in Two Necropsied Cases, *Am. J. Pathol., 30*:99, 1954.

119 Somers, K., and Williams, A. W.: Intracardiac Calcification in Endomyocardial Fibrosis, *Br. Heart J., 24*:324, 1962.

120 King, M., Huang, J.-M., and Glassman, E.: Paget's Disease with Cardiac Calcification and Complete Heart Block, *Am. J. Med., 46*:302, 1969.

121 McGiven, A. R.: Myocardial Fibrosis in Fibrocystic Disease of the Pancreas, *Arch. Dis. Child., 37*:656, 1962.

122 De Garcia-Dadoni, C. R.: Alteraciones miocárdicas en la mucoviscidosis, *Arch. Argent. Pediatr., 63*:188, 1965.

123 Mosquera, F., and Becu, L.: Necrosis miocardiaca no isquemica en el curso de la enfermedad fibroquistica del pancreas, *Arch. Argent. Pediatr., 63*:450, 1965.

124 Oppenheimer, E. H., and Esterly, J. R.: Myocardial Lesions in Patients with Cystic Fibrosis of the Pancreas, *Johns Hopkins Med. J., 133*:252, 1973.

125 Coni, N. K.: The Myocardium in Periodic Paralysis, *Postgrad. Med. J., 45*:691, 1969.

126 Weaver, W. F., and Burchell, H. B.: Serum Potassium and the Electrocardiogram in Hypokalemia, *Circulation, 21*:505, 1960.

127 Terman, D. S., Alfrey, A. C., Hammond, W. S., Donndelinger, T., Ogden, D. A., and Holmes, J. H.: Cardiac Calcification in Uremia: A Clinical, Biochemical and Pathologic Study, *Am. J. Med., 50*:744, 1971.

128 Gueron, M., Berlyne, G. M., Nord, E., and Ben Ari, J.: The Case against the Existence of a Specific Uraemic Myocardiopathy, *Nephron, 15*:2, 1975.

129 Prosser, D., and Parsons, V.: The Case for a Specific Uraemic Myocardopathy, *Nephron, 15*:4, 1975.

130 Lewin, K., and Trautman, L.: Ischaemic Myocardial Damage in Chronic Renal Failure, *Br. Med. J., 4*:151, 1971.

131 Scheuer, J., and Stezoski, S. W.: The Effects of Uremic Compounds on Cardiac Function and Metabolism, *J. Mol. Cell. Cardiol., 5*:287, 1973.

132 Bailey, G. L., Hampers, C. L., and Merrill, J. P.: Reversible Cardiomyopathy in Uremia, *Trans. Am. Soc. Artif. Intern. Organs, 13*:263, 1967.

133 Hager, E. B.: Clinical Observations on Five Patients with Uremic Pericardial Tamponade, *N. Engl. J. Med., 273*:304, 1965.

134 Moraski, R. E., and Bousvaros, G.: Constrictive Pericarditis Due to Chronic Uremia, *N. Engl. J. Med., 281*:542, 1969.

135 Arora, K. K., Lacy, J. P., Schacht, R. A., Martin, D. G., and Gutch, C. F.: Calcific Cardiomyopathy in Advanced Renal Failure, *Arch. Intern. Med., 135*:603, 1975.

136 Summers, J. E., Johnson, W. W., and Ainger, L. E.: Childhood Leukemic Heart Disease. A Study of 116 Hearts of Children Dying of Leukemia, *Circulation, 40*:575, 1969.

137 Roberts, W. C., Bodey, G. P., and Wertlake, P. T.: The Heart in Acute Leukemia: A Study of 420 Autopsy Cases, *Am. J. Cardiol., 21*:388, 1968.

138 Nogrette, P.: Le coeur dans les leucémies, les lymphorécticulosarcomes et la maladie de Hodgkin, *Coeur Méd. Intern., 5*:27, 1966.

139 Mehrotra, T. N., and McMillan, J. A.: Electrocardiographic Changes in Chronic Myeloid Leukaemia, *Br. J. Clin. Pract., 21*:366, 1967.

140 Atkinson, K., McElwain, T. J., and Mackay, A. M.: Myeloma of the Heart, *Br. Heart J., 36*:309, 1974.

141 Oliveira, E., and Gómez-Patiño, N.: Falcemic Cardiopathy: Report of a Case, *Am. J. Cardiol., 11*:686, 1963.

142 Uzsoy, N. K.: Cardiovascular Findings in Patients with Sickle Cell Anemia, *Am. J. Cardiol., 13*:320, 1964.

143 Fleischer, R. A., and Rubler, S.: Primary Cardiomyopathy in Nonanemic Patients. Association with Sickle Cell Trait, *Am. J. Cardiol., 22*:532, 1968.

144 Burch, G., and De Pasquale, N.: Erythrocytosis and Ischemic Myocardial Disease, *Am. Heart J., 62*:139, 1961.

145 Spack, M. S., Howell, D. A., and Harris, J. S.: Myocardial Infarction and Multiple Thromboses in a Child with Primary Thrombocytosis, *Pediatrics, 31*:268, 1963.

146 Bernstein, A., Simon, F., Rothfeld, E. L., and Cohen, F. B.: Primary Thrombocytosis and Anginal Syndrome, *Am. J. Cardiol., 6*:351, 1960.

147 James, T. N., and Monto, R. W.: Pathology of the Cardiac Conduction System in Thrombotic Thrombocytopenic Purpura, *Ann. Intern. Med., 65*:37, 1966.

148 MacGregor, G. A., and Vallance-Owen, J.: Cardiac Involvement in Anaphylactoid Purpura, *Lancet, 2*:572, 1957.

149 Imai, T., and Matsumoto, S.: Anaphylactoid Purpura with Cardiac Involvement, *Arch. Dis. Child., 45*:727, 1970.

149a Miller, C. L., and Murphy, M. L.: Hereditary Hemorrhagic Telangiectasia: Demonstration of a Myocardial Lesion by Postmortem Coronary Angiography, *J. Arkansas Med. Soc., 73*:64, 1976.

150 Cannon, P. J.: The Heart and Lungs in Myotonic Muscular Dystrophy, *Am. J. Med., 32*:765, 1962.

151 Norris, F. H., Jr., Moss, A. J., and Yu, P. N.: On the Possibility That a Type of Human Muscular Dystrophy Commences in Myocardium, *Ann. N. Y. Acad. Sci., 138*:342, 1966.

152 Perloff, J. K., Roberts, W. C., de Leon, A. C., Jr., and O'Doherty, D.: The Distinctive Electrocardiogram of Duchenne's Progressive Muscular Dystrophy: An Electrocardiographic-pathologic Correlative Study, *Am. J. Med., 42*:179, 1967.

153 Ronan, J. A., Jr., Perloff, J. K., Bowen, P. J., and Mann, O.: The Vectorcardiogram in Duchenne's Progressive Muscular Dystrophy, *Am. Heart J., 84*:588, 1972.

154 James, T. N.: Observations on the Cardiovascular Involvement, Including the Cardiac Conduction System, in Progressive Muscular Dystrophy, *Am. Heart J., 63*:48, 1962.

155 Demany, M. A., and Zimmerman, H. A.: Progressive Muscular Dystrophy. Hemodynamic, Angiographic, and Pathologic Study of a Patient with Myocardial Involvement, *Circulation, 40*:377, 1969.

156 Gilroy, J., Cahalan, J. L., Berman, R., and Newman, M.: Cardiac and Pulmonary Complications in Duchenne's Progressive Muscular Dystrophy, *Circulation, 27*:484, 1963.

157 Hooey, M. A., and Jerry, L. M.: The Cardiomyopathy of Muscular Dystrophy: Report of Two Cases with a Review of the Literature, *Can. Med. Assoc. J., 90*:771, 1964.

158 Perloff, J. K., de Leon, A. C., Jr., and O'Doherty, D.: The

Cardiomyopathy of Progressive Muscular Dystrophy, *Circulation,* 33:625, 1966.

159 Welsh, J. D., Lynn, T. N., Jr., and Haase, G. R.: Cardiac Findings in 73 Patients with Muscular Dystrophy, *Arch. Intern. Med.,* 112:199, 1963.

160 Mann, O., De Leon, A. C., Jr., Perloff, J. K., Simanis, J., and Horrigan, F. D.: Duchenne's Muscular Dystrophy: The Electrocardiogram in Female Relatives, *Am. J. Med. Sci.,* 255:376, 1968.

161 Emery, A. E. H.: Abnormalities of the Electrocardiogram in Female Carriers of Duchenne Muscular Dystrophy, *Br. Med. J.,* 2:418, 1969.

162 Lowenstein, A. S., Arbeit, S. R., and Rubin, I. L.: Cardiac Involvement in Progressive Muscular Dystrophy: An Electrocardiographic and Ballistocardiographic Study, *Am. J. Cardiol.,* 9:528, 1962.

163 Kovick, R. B., Fogelman, A. M., Abbasi, A. S., Peter, J. B., and Pearce, M. L.: Echocardiographic Evaluation of Posterior Left Ventricular Wall Motion in Muscular Dystrophy, *Circulation,* 52:447, 1975.

164 Wendt, V. E., Stock, T. B., Hayden, R. O., Bruce, T. A., Gudbjarnason, S., and Bing, R. J.: The Hemodynamics and Cardiac Metabolism in Cardiomyopathies, *Med. Clin. North Am.,* 46:1445, 1962.

165 Perloff, J. K.: Cardiac Involvement in Heredofamilial Neuromyopathic Diseases, *Cardiovasc. Clin.,* 4:334, 1972.

166 Baldwin, B. J., Talley, R. C., Johnson, C., and Nutter, D. O.: Permanent Paralysis of the Atrium in a Patient with Facioscapulohumeral Muscular Dystrophy, *Am. J. Cardiol.,* 31:649, 1973.

167 Waters, D. D., Nutter, D. O., Hopkins, L. C., and Dorney, E. R.: Cardiac Features of an Unusual X-Linked Humeroperoneal Neuromuscular Disease, *N. Engl. J. Med.,* 293:1017, 1975.

168 Boyer, S. H., IV, Chisholm, A. W., and McKusick, V. A.: Cardiac Aspects of Friedreich's Ataxia, *Circulation,* 25:493, 1962.

169 Gach, J. V., Andriange, M., and Franck, G.: Hypertrophic Obstructive Cardiomyopathy and Friedreich's Ataxia. Report of a Case and Review of Literature, *Am. J. Cardiol.,* 27:436, 1971.

170 Ruschhaupt, D. G., Thilenius, O. G., and Cassels, D. E.: Friedreich's Ataxia Associated with Idiopathic Hypertrophic Subaortic Stenosis, *Am. Heart J.,* 84:95, 1972.

171 James, T. N., and Fisch, C.: Observations on the Cardiovascular Involvement in Friedreich's Ataxia, *Am. Heart J.,* 66:164, 1963.

172 Ivemark, B., and Thorén, C.: The Pathology of the Heart in Friedreich's Ataxia: Changes in Coronary Arteries and Myocardium, *Acta Med. Scand.,* 175:227, 1964.

173 Gregorini, L., Valentini, R., and Libretti, A.: The Vectorcardiogram in Friedreich's Ataxia, *Am. Heart J.,* 87:158, 1974.

173a Van der Hauwaert, L. G., and Dumoulin, M.: Hypertrophic Cardiomyopathy in Friedreich's Ataxia, *Br. Heart J.,* 38:1291, 1976.

174 Lascelles, R. G., Baker, I. A., and Thomas, P. K.: Hereditary Polyneuropathy of Roussy-Lévy Type with Associated Cardiomyopathy, *Guys Hosp. Rep.,* 119:253, 1970.

175 Holt, J. M., and Lambert, E. H. N.: Heart Disease as the Presenting Feature in Myotonia Atrophica, *Br. Heart J.,* 26:433, 1964.

176 Church, S. C.: The Heart in Myotonia Atrophica, *Arch. Intern. Med.,* 119:176, 1967.

177 Bulloch, R. T., Davis, J. L., and Hara, M.: Dystrophia Myotonica with Heart Block: A Light and Electron Microscopic Study, *Arch. Pathol.,* 84:130, 1967.

178 Örndahl, G., Thulesius, O., Eneström, S., and Dehlin, O.: The Heart in Myotonic Disease, *Acta Med. Scand.,* 176:479, 1964.

179 Miller, P. B.: Myotonic Dystrophy with Electrocardiographic Abnormalities: Report of a Case, *Am. Heart J.,* 63:704, 1962.

179a Winters, S. J., Schreiner, B., Griggs, R. C., Rowley, P., and Nanda, N. C.: Familial Mitral Valve Prolapse and Myotonic Dystrophy, *Ann. Intern. Med.,* 85:19, 1976.

180 Petkovich, N. J., Dunn, M., and Reed, W.: Myotonia Dystrophica with A-V Dissociation and Stokes-Adams Attacks: A Case Report and Review of the Literature, *Am. Heart J.,* 68:391, 1964.

181 Josephson, M. E., Caracta, A. R., Gallagher, J. J., and Damato, A. N.: Site of Conduction Disturbances in a Family with Myotonic Dystrophy, *Am. J. Cardiol.,* 32:114, 1973.

182 Payne, C. A., and Greenfield, J. C., Jr.: Electrocardiographic Abnormalities Associated with Myotonic Dystrophy, *Am. Heart J.,* 65:436, 1963.

183 Fearrington, E. L., Gibson, T. C., and Churchill, R. E.: Vectorcardiographic and Electrocardiographic Findings in Myotonia Atrophica: A Study Employing the Frank Lead System, *Am. Heart J.,* 67:599, 1964.

184 Clements, S. D., Jr., Colmers, R. A., and Hurst, J. W.: Myotonia Dystrophica. Ventricular Arrhythmias, Intraventricular Conduction Abnormalities, Atrioventricular Block and Stokes-Adams Attacks Successfully Treated with Permanent Transvenous Pacemaker, *Am. J. Cardiol.,* 37:933, 1976.

185 Leomanmäki, K., Hokkanen, E., and Heikkilä, J.: Electrocardiogram in Myasthenia Gravis, Analysis of a Series of 97 Patients, *Ann. Clin. Res.,* 1:236, 1969.

186 McCrea, P. C., and Jagoe, W. S.: Myocarditis in Myasthenia Gravis with Thymoma, *Ir. J. Med. Sci.,* 454:453, 1963.

187 Kohn, P. M., Tucker, H. J., and Kozokoff, N. J.: The Cardiac Manifestations of Myasthenia Gravis with Particular Reference to Electrocardiographic Abnormalities, *Am. J. Med. Sci.,* 249:561, 1965.

188 Gibson, T. C.: The Heart in Myasthenia Gravis, *Am. Heart J.,* 90:389, 1975.

189 Pomerleau, O. F., and Schwarz, H. J.: Tuberous Sclerosis with Unusual Findings: A Case Report, *J. Maine Med. Assoc.,* 60:137, 1969.

190 McComish, M., Compston, A., and Jewitt, D.: Cardiac Abnormalities in Chronic Progressive External Ophthalmoplegia, *Br. Heart J.,* 38:526, 1976.

191 Verhiest, W., Brucher, J. M., Goddeeris, P., Lauweryns, J., and DeGeest, H.: Familial Centronuclear Myopathy Associated with "Cardiomyopathy," *Br. Heart J.,* 38:504, 1976.

191a Tanaka, H., Vemura, N., Toyama, Y., Kudo, A., Ohkatsu, Y., and Kanehisa, T.: *Am. J. Cardiol.,* 38:528, 1976.

192 Evans, W.: Alcoholic Myocardiopathy, *Prog. Cardiovasc. Dis.,* 7:151, 1964.

193 Burch, G. E., and Giles, T. D.: Alcoholic Cardiomyopathy. Concept of the Disease and Its Treatment, *Am. J. Med.,* 50:141, 1971.

194 Shanoff, H. M.: Alcoholic Cardiomyopathy: An Introductory Review, *Can. Med. Assoc. J.,* 106:55, 1972.

195 Alexander, C. S.: Alcohol and the Heart, *Ann. Intern. Med.,* 67:670, 1967.

196 Regan, T. J., Wu, C. F., Weisse, A. B., Moschos, C. B., Ahmed, S. S., and Lyons, M. M.: Acute Myocardial Infarction in Toxic Cardiomyopathy without Coronary Obstruction, *Circulation,* 51:453, 1975.

197 Brigden, W.: Alcoholic Cardiomyopathy, *Cardiovasc. Clin.,* 4:187, 1972.

198 Ferrans, V. J.: Alcoholic Cardiomyopathy, *Am. J. Med. Sci.,* 252:89, 1966.

199 Wendt, V. E., Wu, C., Balcon, R., Doty, G., and Bing, R. J.: Hemodynamic and Metabolic Effects of Chronic Alcoholism in Man, *Am. J. Cardiol.,* 15:175, 1965.

200 James, T. N., and Bear, E. S.: Effects of Ethanol and Acetaldehyde on the Heart, *Am. Heart J.,* 74:243, 1967.

201 Wendt, V. E., Ajluni, R., Bruce, T. A., Prasad, A. S., and Bing, R. J.: Acute Effects of Alcohol on the Human Myocardium, *Am. J. Cardiol.,* 17:804, 1966.

202 Whereat, A. F., and Perloff, J. K.: Ethyl Alcohol and Myocardial Metabolism, *Circulation,* 47:915, 1973.

203 Mitchell, J. H., and Cohen, L. S.: Alcohol and the Heart, *Mod. Concepts Cardiovasc. Dis.,* 39:109, 1970.

204 Delgado, C. E., Fortuin, N. J., and Ross, R. S.: Acute Effects of Low Doses of Alcohol on Left Ventricular Function by Echocardiography, *Circulation,* 51:535, 1975.

205 Gould, L.: Cardiac Effects of Alcohol, *Am. Heart J.,* 79:422, 1970.

206 Limas, C. J., Guiha, N. H., Lekagul, O., and Cohn, J. N.: Impaired Left Ventricular Function in Alcoholic Cirrhosis with Ascites. Ineffectiveness of Ouabain, *Circulation,* 49:755, 1974.

207 Spodick, D. H., Pigott, V. M., and Chirife, R.: Preclinical Cardiac Malfunction in Chronic Alcoholism. Comparison with Matched Normal Controls and with Alcoholic Cardiomyopathy, *N. Engl. J. Med.,* 287:677, 1972.

208 Ahmed, S. S., Levinson, G. E., and Regan, T. J.: Depression of Myocardial Contractility with Low Doses of Ethanol in Normal Man, *Circulation,* 48:378, 1973.

209 Gould, L., Collica, C., Zahir, M., and Gomprecht, R. F.: Ethyl Alcohol. Effects on Coronary Blood Flow in Man, *Br. Heart J.,* 34:815, 1972.

210 Regan, T. J.: Ethyl Alcohol and the Heart, *Circulation,* 44:957, 1971.

211 Sanders, M. G.: Alcoholic Cardiomyopathy: A Critical Review, *Q. J. Stud. Alcohol,* 3:324, 1970.

212 Sereny, G.: Effects of Alcohol on the Electrocardiogram, *Circulation,* 44:558, 1971.

213 Demakis, J. G., Proskey, A., Rahimtoola, S. H., Jamil, M., Sutton, G. C., Rosen, K. M., Gunnar, R. M., and Tobin, J. R., Jr.: The Natural Course of Alcoholic Cardiomyopathy, *Ann. Intern. Med.,* 80:293, 1974.

214 Rutledge, D. I., and Caputo, R.: Heart Failure in Heavy Beer Drinkers, *Lahey Clin. Bull.,* 16:177, 1967.

215 Mohiuddin, S. M., Taskar, P. K., Rheault, M., Roy, P. E., Chenard, J., and Morin, Y.: Experimental Cobalt Cardiomyopathy, *Am. Heart J.,* 80:532, 1970.

216 Alexander, C. S.: Cobalt and the Heart, *Ann. Intern. Med.,* 70:411, 1969.

217 Kesteloot, H., Roelandt, J., Williams, J., Claes, J. H., and Joossens, J. V.: An Enquiry into the Role of Cobalt in the Heart Disease of Chronic Beer Drinkers, *Circulation,* 37:854, 1968.

218 Morin, Y., Têtu, A., and Mercier, G.: Cobalt Cardiomyopathy: Clinical Aspects, *Br. Heart J.,* 33(suppl.):175, 1971.

219 Sullivan, J. F., George, R., Bluvas, R., and Egan, J. D.: Myocardiopathy of Beer Drinkers: Subsequent Course, *Ann. Intern. Med.,* 70:277, 1969.

220 Sanghvi, L. M., and Mathur, B. B.: Electrocardiogram after Chloroquine and Emetine, *Circulation,* 32:281, 1965.

221 Pearce, M. B., Bulloch, R. T., and Murphy, M. L.: Selective Damage of Myocardial Mitochondria Due to Emetine Hydrochloride, *Arch. Pathol.,* 91:8, 1971.

222 Murphy, M.L., Bulloch, R.T., and Pearce, M.B.: The Correlation of Metabolic and Ultrastructural Changes in Emetine Myocardial Toxicity, *Am. Heart J.,* 87:105, 1974.

223 Dempsey, J. J., and Salem, H. H.: An Enzymatic Electrocardiographic Study on Toxicity of Dehydroemetine, *Br. Heart J.,* 28:505, 1966.

224 Michael, T. A. D., and Aiwazzadeh, S.: The Effects of Acute Chloroquine Poisoning with Special Reference to the Heart, *Am. Heart J.,* 79:831, 1970.

225 Fowler, N. O., McCall, D., Chou, T., Holmes, J. C., and Hanenson, I. B.: Electrocardiographic Changes and Cardiac Arrhythmias in Patients Receiving Psychotropic Drugs, *Am. J. Cardiol.,* 37:223, 1976.

226 Burda, C. D.: Electrocardiographic Abnormalities Induced by Thioridazine (Mellaril), *Am. Heart J.,* 76:153, 1968.

227 Fletcher, G. F., Kazamias, T. M., and Wenger, N. K.: Cardiotoxic Effects of Mellaril: Conduction Disturbances and Supraventricular Arrhythmias, *Am. Heart J.,* 78:135, 1969.

228 Wendkos, M. H.: Cardiac Changes Related to Phenothiazine Therapy, with Special Reference to Thioridazine, *J. Am. Geriatr. Soc.,* 15:20, 1967.

229 Alvarez-Mena, S. C., and Frank, M. J.: Phenothiazine-Induced T-Wave Abnormalities. Effects of Overnight Fasting, *JAMA,* 224:1730, 1973.

230 Schoonmaker, F. W., Osteen, R. T., and Greenfield, J. C., Jr.: Thioridazine (Mellaril)-induced Ventricular Tachycardia Controlled with an Artificial Pacemaker, *Ann. Intern. Med.,* 65:1076, 1966.

231 Raisfeld, I. H.: Cardiovascular Complications of Antidepressant Therapy. Interactions at the Adrenergic Neuron, *Am. Heart J.,* 83:129, 1972.

231a Jefferson, J. W.: A Review of the Cardiovascular Effects and Toxicity of Tricyclic Antidepressants, *Psychosom. Med.,* 37:160, 1975.

232 Tobis, J., and Das, B. N.: Cardiac Complications in Amitriptyline Poisoning. Successful Treatment with Physostigmine, *JAMA,* 235:1474, 1976.

233 Graham, J. R.: Cardiac and Pulmonary Fibrosis during Methysergide Therapy for Headache, *Trans. Am. Clin. Climatol. Assoc.,* 78:79, 1967.

234 Bana, D. S., MacNeal, P. S., LeCompte, P. M., Shah, Y., and Graham, J. R.: Cardiac Murmurs and Endocardial Fibrosis Associated with Methysergide Therapy, *Am. Heart J.,* 88:640, 1974.

235 Hudgson, P., Foster, J. B., and Walton, J. N.: Methysergide and Coronary Artery Disease, *Am. Heart J.,* 74:854, 1967.

235a Appelbaum, F. R., Strauchen, J. A., Grow, R. G., Savage, D. D., Kent, K. M., Ferrans, V. J., and Herzig, G. P.: Acute Lethal Carditis Caused by High-Dose Combination Chemotherapy: A Unique Clinical and Pathological Entity, *Lancet,* 1:58, 1976.

236 O'Connell, T. X., and Berenbaum, M. C.: Cardiac and Pulmonary Effects of High Doses of Cyclophosphamide and Isophosphamide, *Cancer Res.,* 34:1586, 1974.

237 Buja, L. M., Ferrans, V. J., and Roberts, W. C.: Drug-Induced Cardiomyopathies, *Adv. Cardiol.,* 13:330, 1974.

238 Lefrak, E. A., Pitha, J., Rosenheim, S., and Gottlieb, J. A.: A Clinicopathologic Analysis of Adriamycin Cardiotoxicity, *Cancer,* 32:302, 1973.

239 Blum, R. H., and Carter, S. K.: Adriamycin. A New Anticancer Drug with Significant Clinical Activity, *Ann. Intern. Med.,* 80:249, 1974.

240 Rinehart, J. J., Lewis, R. P., and Balcerzak, S. P.: Adriamycin Cardiotoxicity in Man, *Ann. Intern. Med.,* 81:476, 1974.

240a Kushner, J. P., Hansen, V. L., and Hammer, S. P.: Cardiomyopathy after Widely Separated Courses of Adriamycin Exacerbated by Actinomycin-D and Mithramycin, *Cancer,* 36:1577, 1975.

241 Barry, K. G., and Herndon, E. G., Jr.: Electrocardiographic Changes Associated with Acute Arsenic Poisoning, *Med. Ann. D.C.,* 31:25, 1962.

242 Weinberg, S. L.: The Electrocardiogram in Acute Arsenic Poisoning, *Am. Heart J.,* 60:971, 1960.

243 Glazener, G. S., Ellis, J. G., and Johnson, P. K.: Electrocardiographic Findings with Arsenic Poisoning, *Calif. Med.,* 109:158, 1968.

244 McKinstry, W. J., and Hickes, J. M.: Emergency—Arsine Poisoning, *AMA Arch. Intern. Med.,* 100:34, 1957.

245 Honey, M.: The Effects of Sodium Antimony Tartrate on the Myocardium, *Br. Heart J.,* 22:601, 1960.

246 Somers, K., and Rosanelli, J. D.: Electrocardiographic Effects of Antimony Dimercapto-Succinate ("Astiban"), *Br. Heart J.,* 24:187, 1962.

247 Van Vliet, P. D., Burchell, H. G., and Titus, J. L.: Focal Myocarditis Associated with Pheochromocytoma, *N. Engl. J. Med.,* 274:1102, 1966.

248 Haft, J. I., Gershengorn, K., Kranz, P. D., and Oestreicher, R.: Protection against Epinephrine-Induced Myocardial Necrosis by Drugs that Inhibit Platelet Aggregation, *Am. J. Cardiol.,* 30:838, 1972.

249 Szakács, J. E., and Mehlman, B.: Pathologic Changes Induced by *l*-Norepinephrine: Quantitative Aspects, *Am. J. Cardiol.,* 5:619, 1960.

250 Hayes, J. M., and Hall, G. V.: The Myocardial Toxicity of Carbon Monoxide, *Med. J. Australia,* 1:865, 1964.

251 Anderson, R. F., Allensworth, D. C., and deGroot, W. J.: Myocardial Toxicity from Carbon Monoxide Poisoning, *Ann. Intern. Med.,* 67:1172, 1967.

252 Shafer, N., Smilay, M. G., and MacMillan, F. P.: Primary Myocardial Disease in Man Resulting from Acute Carbon Monoxide Poisoning, *Am. J. Med.,* 38:316, 1965.

253 Mosinger, M., de Bisschop, G., and Luccioni, R.: Les manifestations cardioques dans l'intoxication oxycarbonée, *Arch. Mal. Prof.,* 30:5, 1969.

254 Jaffe, N.: Cardiac Injury and Carbon Monoxide Poisoning, *S. Afr. Med. J.,* 39:611, 1965.

255 Cosby, R. S., and Bergeron, M.: Electrocardiographic Changes in Carbon Monoxide Poisoning, *Am. J. Cardiol.,* 11:93, 1963.

256 Corya, B. C., Black, M. J., and McHenry, P. L.: Echocardiographic Findings after Acute Carbon Monoxide Poisoning, *Br. Heart J.,* 38:712, 1976.

256a Barborik, M., and Dusek, J.: Cardiomyopathy Accompanying Industrial Cobalt Exposure, *Br. Heart J.,* 34:113, 1972.

257 James. F. W., Kaplan, S., and Benzing, G., III: Cardiac Complications following Hydrocarbon Ingestion, *Am. J. Dis. Child.,* 121:431, 1971.

258 Harris, W. S.: Toxic Effects of Aerosol Propellants on the Heart, *Arch. Intern. Med.,* 131:162, 1973.

259 Flowers, N. C., and Horan, L. G.: The Electrical Sequelae of Aerosol Inhalation, *Am. Heart J.,* 83:644, 1972.

260 Talley, R. C., Linhart, J. W., Trevino, A. J., Moore, L., and Beller, B. M.: Acute Elemental Phosphorus Poisoning in Man: Cardiovascular Toxicity, *Am. Heart J.,* 84:139, 1972.

261 Diaz-Rivera, R. S., Ramos-Morales, F., Garcia-Palmieri, M. R., and Ramirez, E. A.: The Electrocardiographic Changes in Acute Phosphorus Poisoning in Man, *Am. J. Med. Sci.,* 241:758, 1961.

262 Rao, S., and Brown, R. H.: Acute Yellow Phosphorus Rat Poisoning, *Ill. Med. J.,* 145:128, 1974.

263 Goodman, L. S., and Gilman, A.: "The Pharmacologic Basis of Therapeutics," 3d ed., The Macmillan Company, New York, 1965, p. 816.

264 Dahhan, S. S., and Orfaly, H.: Electrocardiographic Changes in Mercury Poisoning, *Am. J. Cardiol.,* 14:178, 1964.

265 Freeman, R.: Reversible Myocarditis Due to Chronic Lead Poisoning in Childhood, *Arch. Dis. Child.,* 40:389, 1965.

266 Kline, T. S.: Myocardial Changes in Lead Poisoning, *J. Dis. Child.,* 99:48, 1960.

267 Yarom, R., Gueron, M., and Braun, K.: Scorpion Venom Cardiomyopathy, *Pathol. Microbiol.,* 35:114, 1970.

268 Poon-King, T.: Myocarditis from Scorpion Stings, *Br. Heart J.,* 1:374, 1963.

269 Gueron, M., and Yarom, R.: Cardiovascular Manifestations of Severe Scorpion Sting: Clinicopathologic Correlations, *Chest,* 57:156, 1970.

270 Krishnankutty, P. K.: Toxic Myocarditis Due to Scorpion Bite—A Case Report, *Indian Heart J.,* 17:362, 1965.

270a Weitzman, A., Margulis, G., and Lehmann, E.: Uncommon Cardiovascular Manifestations and High Catecholamine Levels due to "Black Widow" Bite, *Am. Heart J.,* 98:89, 1977.

271 Chadha, J. S., Ashby, D. W., and Brown, J. O.: Abnormal Electrocardiogram after Adder Bite, *Br. Heart J.,* 30:138, 1968.

272 Reid, H. A., Thean, P. C. Chan, K. E. and Baharom, A. R.: Clinical Effects of Bites by Malayan Viper (*Ancistrodon rhodostoma*), *Lancet,* 1:617, 1963.

273 Levin, H. D.: Acute Myocardial Infarction following Wasp Sting. Report of Two Cases and Critical Survey of the Literature, *Am. Heart J.,* 91:365, 1976.

274 Pearn, J. H.: A Case of Tick Paralysis with Myocarditis, *Med. J. Australia,* 1:629, 1966.

275 Wenzel, D. G.: Drug-induced Cardiomyopathies, *J. Pharm. Sci.,* 56:1209, 1967.

276 Surawicz, B., and Lasseter, K. C.: Effect of Drugs on the Electrocardiogram, *Prog. Cardiovasc. Dis.,* 13:26, 1970.

277 Booth, B. H., and Patterson, R.: Electrocardiographic Changes during Human Anaphylaxis, *JAMA,* 211:627, 1970.

278 Harkavy, J.: Cardiac Manifestations Due to Hypersensitivity, *Ann. Allerg.,* 28:242, 1970.

279 Langsjoen, P. H., and Stinson, J. C.: Acute Fatal Allergic Myocarditis: Report of a Case, *Dis. Chest,* 48:440, 1965.

280 French, A. J.: Hypersensitivity in the Pathogenesis of the Histopathologic Changes Associated with Sulfonamide Chemotherapy, *Am. J. Pathol.,* 22:679, 1946.

281 Field J. B., and Federman, D. D.: Sudden Death in a Diabetic Subject during Treatment with BZ-55 (Carbutamide), *Diabetes,* 6:67, 1957.

282 MacSearraigh, E. T. M., and Patel, K. M.: Cardiomyopathy as a Complication of Sulphonamide Therapy, *Br. Med. J.,* 3:33, 1968.

283 Haden, R. F., and Langsjoen, P. H.: Manifestations of Myocardial Involvement in Acute Reactions to Penicillin, *Am. J. Cardiol.,* 8:420, 1961.

284 Schoenwetter, A. H., and Silber, E. N.: Penicillin Hypersensitivity, Acute Pericarditis, and Eosinophilia, *JAMA,* 191:672, 1965.

285 Hodge, P. R., and Lawrence, J. R.: Two Cases of Myocarditis Associated with Phenylbutazone Therapy, *Med. J. Australia,* 1:640, 1957.

286 Edelstein, J. M.: Butazolidin Angiitis and Periangiitis Simulating Aschoff Nodule, *Am. Heart J.,* 69:573, 1965.

287 MacAdam, D. B., and Whitaker, W.: Cardiac Complications after Vaccination for Smallpox, *Br. Med. J.,* 2:1099, 1962.

288 Finlay-Jones, L. R.: Fatal Myocarditis after Vaccination against Smallpox: Report of a Case, *N. Engl. J. Med.,* 270:41, 1964.

289 Matthews, A. W., and Griffiths, I. D.: Post-vaccinial Pericarditis and Myocarditis, *Br. Heart J.,* 36:1043, 1974.

290 Gavrilesco, S., Streian, C., and Constantinesco, L.: Tachycardie ventriculaire et fibríllation auriculaire, associées, après vaccination anticholérique, *Acta. Cardiol.,* 28:89, 1973.

291 Kline, I. K., Kline, T. S., and Saphir, O.: Myocarditis in Senescence, *Am. Heart J.,* 65:446, 1963.

292 Chatterjee, S. S., and Thakre, M. W.: Fiedler's Myocarditis: Report of a Fatal Case following Intramuscular Injection of Streptomycin, *Tubercle,* 39:240, 1958.

293 Barrett, D. A., II, Dalldorf, F. G., Barnwell, W. H., II, and Hudson, R. P.: Allergic Giant Cell Myocarditis Complicating Tuberculosis Chemotherapy, *Arch. Pathol.,* 21:201, 1971.

294 Kerwin, A. J.: Fatal Myocarditis Due to Sensitivity to Phenindione, *Can. Med. Assoc. J.,* 90:1418, 1964.

295 Sanerkin, N. G.: Acute Myocardial Necrosis in Paracetamol Poisoning, *Br. Med. J.,* 3:478, 1971.

296 Sun, S.-C., Sohal, R. S., Colcolough, H. L., and Burch, G. E.: Histochemical and Electron Microscopic Studies of the Ef-

fects of Reserpine on the Heart Muscle of Mice, *J. Pharmacol. Exp. Ther.,* 161:210, 1968.

297 Tangedahl, T. N., and Gau, G. T.: Myocardial Irritability Associated with Lithium Carbonate Therapy, *N. Engl. J. Med.,* 287:867, 1972.

298 Demers, R. G., and Heninger, G. R.: Electrocardiographic T-Wave Changes during Lithium Carbonate Treatment, *JAMA,* 218:381, 1971.

298a Tilkian, A., Schroeder, J. S., Kao, J., and Hultgren, H.: Effect of Lithium on Cardiovascular Performance: Report on Extended Ambulatory Monitoring and Exercise Testing before and during Lithium Therapy, *Am. J. Cardiol.,* 38:701, 1976.

299 Burch, G. E., Sohal, R. S., Sun, S.-C., Miller, G. C., and Colcolough, H. L.: Effects of Radiation on the Human Heart: An Electron Microscopic Study, *Arch. Intern. Med.,* 121:230, 1968.

300 Radiation Heart Disease, *J. Louisiana Med. Soc.,* 120:243, 1968.

301 Biran, S., Hochmann, A., and Stern, S.: Therapeutic Irradiation of the Chest and Electrocardiographic Changes, *Clin. Radiol.,* 20:433, 1969.

302 Elmino, O., and Rossi, A.: Alterazioni cardiovascolari in alcuni casi di trauma elettrico, *Folia Med.,* 48:164, 1965.

303 Stevens, P. J., and Ground, K. E. U.: Occurrence and Significance of Myocarditis in Trauma, *Aerosp. Med.,* 41:776, 1970.

304 Grossman, C. M.: Posttraumatic Ossification of the Myocardium, *J. Trauma,* 14:85, 1974.

304a Berkoff, H. A., Rowe, G. G., Crummy, A. B., and Kahn, D. R.: Asymptomatic Left Ventricular Aneurysm: A Sequela of Blunt Chest Trauma, *Circulation,* 55:545, 1977.

305 Kew, M. C., Tucker, R. B. K., Bersohn, I., and Seftel, H. C.: The Heart in Heatstroke, *Am. Heart J.,* 77:324, 1969.

306 Graham, A. F., Schroeder, J. S., Caves, P. K., Stinson, E. B., and Harrison, D. C.: Late Acute Rejection in the Human Cardiac Transplant Survivor: Clinical Diagnosis, Treatment and Significance, *Am. J. Cardiol.,* 31:136, 1973 (abstract).

307 Barnard, C. N.: Hurnan Cardiac Transplantation, *Am. J. Cardiol.,* 22:584, 1968.

308 Brooksby, I. A. B., Coltart, D. J., and Webb-Peploe, M. M.: Progress in Endomyocardial Biopsy, *Mod. Concepts Cardiovasc. Dis.,* 44:65, 1975.

309 Pomerance, A.: Pathology of the Heart with and without Cardiac Failure in the Aged, *Br. Heart J.,* 27:697, 1965.

310 Dock, W.: Cardiomyopathies of the Senescent and Senile, *Cardiovasc. Clin.,* 4:361, 1972.

311 Burch, G., and Giles, T.: Senile Cardiomyopathy, *J. Chronic Dis.,* 24:1, 1971.

312 Weintraub, A. M., and Zvaifler, N. J.: The Occurrence of Valvular and Myocardial Disease in Patients with Chronic Joint Deformity: A Spectrum, *Am. J. Med.,* 35:145, 1963.

313 Carpenter, D. F., Golden, A., and Roberts, W. C.: Quadrivalvular Rheumatoid Heart Disease Associated with Left Bundle Branch Block, *Am. J. Med.,* 43:922, 1967.

313a James, T. N.: De Subitaneis Mortibus. XXIII. Rheumatoid Arthritis and Ankylosing Spondylitis, *Circulation,* 55:669, 1977.

314 Hoffman, F. G., and Leight, L.: Complete Atrioventricular Block Associated with Rheumatoid Disease, *Am. J. Cardiol.,* 16:585, 1965.

315 Harris, M.: Rheumatoid Heart Disease with Complete Heart Block, *J. Clin. Pathol.,* 23:623, 1970.

316 Lev, M., Bharati, S., Hoffman, F. G., and Leight, L.: The Conduction System in Rheumatoid Arthritis with Complete Atrioventricular Block, *Am. Heart J.,* 90:78, 1975.

317 Bulkley, B. H., and Roberts, W. C.: Ankylosing Spondylitis

and Aortic Regurgitation. Description of the Characteristic Cardiovascular Lesion from Study of Eight Necropsy Patients, *Circulation,* 48:1014, 1973.

318 Nomeir, A. M., Turner, R., Watts, E., Smith, D., West, G., and Edmonds, J.: Cardiac Involvement in Rheumatoid Arthritis, *Ann. Intern. Med.,* 79:800, 1973.

319 Takkunen, J., Vuopala, U., and Isomäki, H.: Cardiomyopathy in Ankylosing Spondylitis. I. Medical History and Results of Clinical Examinations in a Series of 55 Patients, *Ann. Clin. Res.,* 2:106, 1970.

320 Weed, C. L., Kulander, B. G., Mazzarella, J. A., and Decker, J. L.: Heart Block in Ankylosing Spondylitis, *Arch. Intern. Med.,* 117:800, 1966.

321 Böttiger, L. E., and Edhag, O.: Heart Block in Ankylosing Spondylitis and Uropolyarthritis, *Br. Heart J.,* 34:487, 1972.

322 Cliff, J. M.: Spinal Bony Bridging and Carditis in Reiter's Disease, *Ann. Rheum. Dis.,* 30:171, 1971.

323 Neu, L. T., Jr., Reider, R. A., and Mack, R. E.: Cardiac Involvement in Reiter's Disease: Report of a Case with Review of the Literature, *Ann. Intern. Med.,* 53:215, 1960.

324 Collins, P.: Aortic Incompetence and Active Myocarditis in Reiter's Disease, *Br. J. Vener. Dis.,* 48:300, 1972.

325 Eisenstein, B., and Taubenhaus, M.: Nonsyphilitic Interstitial Keratitis and Bilateral Deafness (Cogan's Syndrome) Associated with Cardiovascular Disease, *N. Engl. J. Med.,* 258:1074, 1958.

326 Lewis, P. D.: Behçet's Disease and Carditis, *Br. Med. J.,* 1:1026, 1964.

327 Wagenvoort, C. A., Neufeld, H. N., and Edwards, J. E.: Cardiovascular System in Marfan's Syndrome and Idiopathic Dilatation of the Ascending Aorta, *Am. J. Cardiol.,* 4:496, 1962.

328 James, T. N., Frame, B., and Schatz, I. J.: Pathology of Cardiac Conduction System in Marfan's Syndrome, *Arch. Intern. Med.,* 114:339, 1964.

329 Phornphutkul, C., Rosenthal, A., and Nadas, A. S.: Cardiomyopathy in Noonan's Syndrome, Report of 3 Cases, *Br. Heart J.,* 35:99, 1973.

330 Hirsch, H. D., Gelband, H., Garcia, O., Gottlieb, S., and Tamer, D. M.: Rapidly Progressive Obstructive Cardiomyopathy in Infants with Noonan's Syndrome. Report of Two Cases, *Circulation,* 52:1161, 1975.

331 Madison, W. M., Jr., Bradley, E. J., and Castillo, A. J.: Ehlers-Danlos Syndrome with Cardiac Involvement, *Am. J. Cardiol.,* 11:689, 1963.

332 Green, G. J., Schuman, B. M., and Barron, J.: Ehlers-Danlos Syndrome Complicated by Acute Hemorrhagic Sigmoid Diverticulitis, with an Unusual Mitral Valve Abnormality, *Am. J. Med.,* 41:622, 1966.

333 Huang, S., Kumar, G., Steele, H. D., and Parker, J. O.: Cardiac Involvement in Pseudoxanthoma Elasticum: Report of a Case, *Am. Heart J.,* 74:680, 1967.

334 Gouffault, J., Lenoir, P., Pawlotsky, Y., Guillou, M., and Bourel, M.: Manifestations cardio-vasculaires de l'eastorrhexie systématisée: à propos d'un nouveau cas de syndrome de Groenblad, Strandberg et Touraine, *Sem. Hôp. Paris,* 40:2467, 1964.

335 Wilkinson, P. J., Harman, R. R. M., and Tribe, C. R.: Systemic Nodular Panniculitis with Cardiac Involvement, *J. Clin. Pathol.,* 27:808, 1974.

336 Bellonias, E., Raftopoulos, J., Costeas, F., and Bartsokas, C.: Myocardial Involvement in Weber-Christian Disease: Report of One Case and Review of Literature, *Vasc. Dis.,* 2:140, 1965.

337 Eller, J. L.: Roentgen Therapy for Visceral Juvenile Xanthogranuloma, Including a Case with Involvement of the Heart, *Am. J. Roentgenol.,* 95:52, 1965.

338 Kurien, V. A., and Duke, M.: Trisomy 17-18 Syndrome: Report of a Case with Diffuse Myocardial Fibrosis and Review of Cardiovascular Abnormalities, *Am. J. Cardiol.,* 21:431, 1968.

339 Johnson, M. L., and Ikram, H.: Scleroedema of Buschke. An Uncommon Cause of Cardiomyopathy, *Br. Heart J.,* 32:720, 1970.

340 Yogman, M., and Echeverria, P.: Scleredema and Carditis: Report of a Case and Review of the Literature, *Pediatrics,* 54:108, 1974.

341 McCrea, P. C. and Childers, R. W.: Two Unusual Cases of Giant Cell Myocarditis Associated with Mitral Stenosis and with Wegener's Syndrome, *Br. Heart J.,* 26:490, 1964.

342 Saheta, N. P.: Cardiomyopathy and Mitral Stenosis Associated with Wegener's Granulomatosis, *Indian Heart J.,* 19:144, 1967.

343 Morales, A. R., Bourgeois, C. H., and Chulacharit, E.: Pathology of the Heart in Reye's Syndrome (Encephalopathy and Fatty Degeneration of the Viscera), *Am. J. Cardiol.,* 27:314, 1971.

344 Rees, J. R., Ross, F. G. M., and Keen, G.: Lentiginosis and Left Atrial Myxoma, *Br. Heart J.,* 35:874, 1973.

345 Somerville, J., and Bonham-Carter, R. E.: The Heart in Lentiginosis, *Br. Heart J.,* 34:58, 1972.

346 Mathews, E. C., Jr., Blount, A. W., Jr., and Townsend, J. I.: Q-T Prolongation and Ventricular Arrhythmias, with and without Deafness, in the Same Family, *Am. J. Cardiol.,* 29:702, 1972.

347 Garza, L. A., Vick, R. L., Nora, J. J., and McNamara, D. G.: Heritable Q-T Prolongation without Deafness, *Circulation,* 41:39, 1970.

348 Roy, P. R., Emanuel, R., Ismail, S. A., and Tayib, M. H. E.: Hereditary Prolongation of the Q-T Interval. Genetic Observations and Management in Three Families with Twelve Affected Members, *Am. J. Cardiol.,* 37:237, 1976.

349 Maron, B. J., Clark, C. E., Goldstein, R. E., and Epstein, S. E.: Potential Role of QT Interval Prolongation in Sudden Infant Death Syndrome, *Circulation,* 54:423, 1976.

349a Kelly, D. H., Shannon, D. C., and Liberthson, R. R.: The Role of the QT Interval in the Sudden Infant Death Syndrome, *Circulation,* 55:663, 1977.

350 Phillips, J., and Ischinose, H.: Clinical and Pathologic Studies in the Hereditary Syndrome of a Long Q-T Interval, Syncopal Spells and Sudden Death, *Chest,* 58:236, 1970.

351 Chaudron, J. M., Heller, F., Van den Berghe, H. B., and Lebacq, E. G.: Attacks of Ventricular Fibrillation and Unconsciousness in a Patient with Prolonged QT Interval. A Family Study, *Am. Heart J.,* 91:783, 1976.

352 Schwartz, P. J., Periti, M., and Malliani, A.: The Long Q-T Syndrome, *Am. Heart J.,* 89:378, 1975.

353 Rosenquist, G. C., Krovetz, L. J., Haller, J. A., Jr., Simon, A. L., and Bannayan, G. A.: Acquired Right Ventricular Outflow Obstruction in a Child with Neurofibromatosis, *Am. Heart J.,* 79:103, 1970.

354 Gerbaux, A., Belfante, M., and Hiltgen, M.: Myocardiopathie obstructive, syndrome de Turner-Ullrich et maladie de von Recklinghausen, *Ann. Med. Interne. (Paris),* 125:641, 1974.

355 Rubler, S., Dlugash, J., Yuceoglu, Y. Z., Kumral, T., Branwood, D. W., and Grishman, A.: New Type of Cardiomyopathy Associated with Diabetic Glomerulosclerosis, *Am. J. Cardiol.,* 30:595, 1972.

356 Kannel, W. B., Hjortland, M., and Castelli, W. P.: The Role of Diabetes in Congestive Heart Failure: The Framingham Study, *Am. J. Cardiol.,* 34:29, 1974.

357 Hamby, R. I., Zoneraich, S., and Sherman, L.: Diabetic Cardiomyopathy, *JAMA,* 229:1749, 1974.

358 Tuuteri, L., Perheentupa, J., and Rapola, J.: The Cardiopathy of Mulibrey Nanism, a New Inherited Syndrome, *Chest,* 65:628, 1974.

359 Mowat, N. A. G., Bennett, P. N., Finlayson, J. K., Brunt, P. W., and Lancaster, W. M.: Myopericarditis Complicating Ulcerative Colitis, *Br. Heart J.,* 36:724, 1974.

360 McAllister, H. A., Jr., and Fenoglio, J. J., Jr.: Cardiac Involvement in Whipple's Disease, *Circulation,* 52:152, 1975.

360a Lie, J. T., and Davis, J. S.: Pancarditis in Whipple's Disease: Electromicroscopic Demonstration of Intracardiac Bacillary Bodies, *Am. J. Clin. Pathol.,* 66:22, 1976.

361 Wood, J. E.: The Cardiovascular Effects of Oral Contraceptives, *Mod. Concepts Cardiovasc. Dis.,* 41:37, 1972.

361a Stern, M. P., Brown, B. W., Jr., Haskell, W. L., Farquhar, J. W., Weberle, C. L., and Wood, P. S. D.: Cardiovascular Risk and Use of Estrogens or Estrogen-Progestagen Compounds. Stanford Three-Community Study, *JAMA,* 235:811, 1976.

362 Handin, R. I.: Thromboembolic Complications of Pregnancy and Oral Contraceptives, *Prog. Cardiovasc. Dis.,* 16:395, 1974.

362a Thrombosis—Perspectives on a Major Side Effect of Oral Contraceptives, *Med. J. Aust.,* 1:788, 1976.

362b Laragh, J. H.: Oral Contraceptive-Induced Hypertension—Nine Years Later, *Am. J. Obstet. Gynecol.,* 126:141, 1976.

363 Greenblatt, D. J., and Koch-Weser, J.: Oral Contraceptives and Hypertension. Report from the Boston Collaborative Drug Surveillance Program, *Obstet. Gynecol.,* 44:412, 1974.

364 Mann, J. I., and Inman, W. H. W.: Oral Contraceptives and Death from Myocardial Infarction, *Br. Med. J.,* 2:245, 1975.

364a Mann, J. I., Inman, W. H. W., and Thorogood, M.: Oral Contraceptive Use in Older Women and Fatal Myocardial Infarction, *Br. Med. J.,* 2:445, 1976.

364b Kleiger, R. E., Boxer, M., Ingham, R. E., and Harrison, D. C.: Pulmonary Hypertension in Patients Using Oral Contraceptives: A Report of Six Cases, *Chest,* 69:143, 1976.

365 Jaffe, R. B., and Koschmann, E. B.: Intravenous Drug Abuse. Pulmonary, Cardiac, and Vascular Complications, *Am. J. Roentgenol.,* 109:107, 1970.

366 Light, R. W., and Dunham, T. R.: Severe Slowly Resolving Heroin-Induced Pulmonary Edema, *Chest,* 67:61, 1975.

367 Steinberg, A. D., and Karliner, J. S.: The Clinical Spectrum of Heroin Pulmonary Edema, *Arch. Intern. Med.,* 122:122, 1968.

367a Paranthaman, S. K., and Kahn, F.: Acute Cardiomyopathy with Recurrent Pulmonary Edema and Hypotension following Heroin Overdosage, *Chest,* 69:117, 1976.

368 Smith, H. J., Roche, A. H. G., Jagusch, M. F., and Herdson, P. B.: Cardiomyopathy Associated with Amphetamine Administration, *Am. Heart J.,* 91:792, 1976.

369 Ebert, M. H., and Shader, R. I.: Cardiovascular Effects of Psychotropic Drugs, *Conn. Med.,* 33:695, 1969.

370 Alexander, C. S., and Niño, A.: Cardiovascular Complications in Young Patients Taking Psychotropic Drugs: A Preliminary Report, *Am. Heart J.,* 78:757, 1969.

371 Sniffing Syndrome, *Br. Med. J.,* 2:183, 1971.

372 Beaconsfield, P., Ginsburg, J., and Rainsbury, R.: Marijuana Smoking. Cardiovascular Effects in Man and Possible Mechanisms, *N. Engl. J. Med.,* 287:209, 1972.

373 Lipski, J., Stimmel, B., and Donoso, E.: The Effect of Heroin and Multiple Drug Abuse on the Electrocardiogram, *Am. Heart J.,* 86:663, 1973.

Diseases of the Pericardium

83
The Pathology of Pericardial Disease

REGINALD E. B. HUDSON, M.D.

ANATOMY

The pericardium is a fibroserosal double-walled sac enveloping the heart and the roots of the great vessels entering and leaving it. The inner visceral layer is adherent to the heart, but the outer parietal layer is free of it; the two layers are lined by continuous serosa and are separated by a capillary interval containing lubricating lymph, which allows the heart to move inside the sac insensibly and without friction.

The parietal layer is attached to the central tendon and adjacent muscle of the diaphragm, and by superior and inferior ligaments to the sternum. It lies in direct contact with the left half of the lower part of the sternum, and sometimes with the left fourth to sixth cartilages. Posteriorly, it is related to the descending aorta and esophagus, and laterally to the pleurae, phrenic nerves, and vessels. The fibrous layer of the sac is incomplete where penetrated by vessels; the venae cavae are covered anterolaterally and the pulmonary veins anteriorly. The aorta and pulmonary trunk, however, are completely ensheathed and one can pass a finger through the transverse sinus separating them from the atria. The spaces between vessels with partial covering form other sinuses. The oblique sinus is bounded by the left inferior pulmonary vein and the inferior vena cava, and it extends upwards behind the left atrium, separating it from the esophagus and descending aorta. A vestigial fold stretching from the left pulmonary artery to the upper left pulmonary vein, contains the remnants of the left duct of Cuvier, reduced to a small oblique vein of Marshall (or to a fibrous cord) draining into the coronary sinus.

EMBRYOLOGY OF CONGENITAL PERICARDIAL DEFECTS

The pericardial cavity arises by fusion of mesodermal spaces around the primitive heart tube in the 2-mm embryo. It communicates with the peritoneal cavity, also developing in the mesoderm, by dorsal canals in the septum transversum (the mesoderm between these cavities). The lung buds invaginate into these canals, which thus become the pleural cavities, which become sealed off from the pericardial and peritoneal cavities in the fifth week. The sealing of the foramen between the canal and the pericardial cavity is effected partly by the pleuropericardial membrane, a valvelike structure carrying the duct of Cuvier on each side from the body wall to the heart; and partly by huge enlargement of the cavities relative to the size of the communicating foramina.

Pericardial defects arise by imperfect closure of the pleuropericardial foramen; this is more likely to happen on the left side because the duct of Cuvier normally obliterates on this side; however, bilateral defects can occur. In a review, Moore[1] classified the defects into three groups:

1 (60%) Heart and left lung in a common cavity
2 (21%) Foramen between the pericardial and left pleural sacs
3 (19%) Pericardium absent or rudimentary

Defects were three times commoner in males and were commonly associated with anomalies of the heart, lungs, pleural cavities, peritoneum, or kidneys. The heart may be unduly mobile when incompletely confined by the pericardium.

The abnormality may be symptomless, but there is an ever-present risk of infection of the intercommunicating pleural and pericardial cavities, or of strangulation of a herniated part of the heart, sometimes with a portion of lung also, through a defect. The affected portion of the heart becomes intensely congested, and endocardial mural thrombus may form on an infarcted area. Sometimes an enlarged left atrial appendage protrudes through the defect; it may be mentioned here that left atriomegaly, possibly congenital, may occur without a pericardial defect. Herniation of the greater omentum through a peritoneal-pericardial defect, causing chest pain on the left side of a 28-year-old man, was cured by surgery.[2]

CYSTS AND DIVERTICULA

A true diverticulum communicates with the pericardial cavity; a cyst does not. These abnormalities form a mixed group, classified by Loehr[3] into the following three varieties:

1 Congenital true cysts, coelomic (mesodermal), lymphagiomatous, bronchial, or teratomatous
2 Acquired, secondary to hematoma, neoplasm, or parasitic disease

A cyst may be harmless, causing no symptoms, being first noted during routine radiography; it may change shape during respiration. Its precise nature, however, will usually require surgical exploration. An additional congenital type is that connected with a ventricular diverticulum.

PERICARDIAL EFFUSION

Continuous accumulation of fluid in the pericardial sac may eventually restrict venous filling of the heart (tamponade) and lower cardiac output; the obstruction to venous filling is worse during inspiration, and this is reflected in the weaker pulse (pulsus paradoxus). Eventually, fatal cardiac syncope may ensue. Other causes of venous obstruction such as aneurysm or tumor may produce similar results.

Types of effusion

HYDROPERICARDIUM
The pericardium at necropsy usually contains a few milliliters of clear transudate which is alkaline and almost devoid of albumin. When the volume exceeds, say 150 ml, the term hydropericardium is applied; the fluid is usually clear and straw-colored, but may be reddish or brownish from blood, or yellowish from jaundice. Hydropericardium occurs in heart or renal failure, in myxedema, and with pleural effusions.

HEMOPERICARDIUM
Blood in the pericardium is usually a sign of a serious illness, commonly rupture of the heart or of an aortic dissection; trauma; or, rarely, acute pericarditis, metastatic carcinoma, or hemorrhagic conditions. It soon clots and shrinks on to the serosa causing thickening.

CHYLOPERICARDIUM
Milky effusion is rare; it results from obstruction or injury to the thoracic duct, sometimes by mediastinal hygroma. The fluid is chyle or lymph and clears with ether; it contains protein, cholesterol, triglycerides, amylase, and blood cells, and it may accumulate rapidly and repeatedly until surgical remedy by ligation of the lymphatic duct and its vessels, together with pericardiectomy.

PERICARDITIS

Pericarditis may be fibrinous or serofibrinous (including "cholesterol pericarditis"), purulent, adhesive or constrictive (with or without calcification), neoplastic, or traumatic.

Fibrinous and serofibrinous pericarditis

Fibrinous or fibrous "milk patches" on the heart's surface are common at necropsy; these are unimportant. At the other extreme, visceral and parietal layers may be thickened and loosely stuck together;

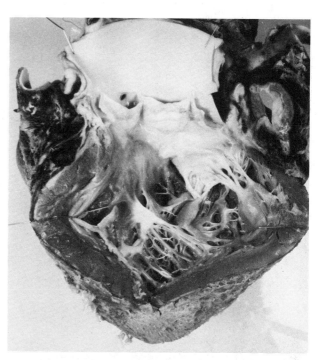

FIGURE 83-1 Shaggy fibrinohemorrhagic pericarditis in the heart of a 34-year-old woman with chronic rheumatic mitral and aortic valve disease. *(From R. E. B. Hudson, "Cardiovascular Pathology," vol. 2, Edward Arnold Publishers, Ltd., London, 1965, p. 1545, with permission of publisher.)*

on separation, each surface shows a "bread and butter" appearance of two heavily buttered slices of bread pressed together then peeled apart (Fig. 83-1). Fluid exudate may be present; it may be bloodstained and is sometimes pocketed. In Concato's polyserositis, effusions occur also in the pleurae and peritoneum, with thick, white fibrous patches ("sugar icing") on the spleen and liver surfaces; the pericarditis may become constrictive.

This form of pericarditis is commonest. It occurs in numerous diseases but may be idiopathic; electrocardiographic changes indicate surface myocardial involvement.

Purulent pericarditis (Fig. 83-2)

This is usually associated with local infection—subphrenic abscess, pacemaker leads, pneumonia, amebiasis, actinomycosis, coccidioidomycosis, osteomyelitis, or a wound. Also, it may complicate cardiac surgery, meningitis, infective endocarditis, puerperal sepsis, genitourinary infection, tularemia, or infestations such as guinea worm (dracunculosis) or hydatid disease (echinococcus). The exudate contains polymorphonuclear and red blood cells and usually also the causative agent.

Adhesive pericarditis

This is a common sequel to any acute pericarditis and is a constant sequel of cardiac surgery, often adding great difficulty to reoperation.

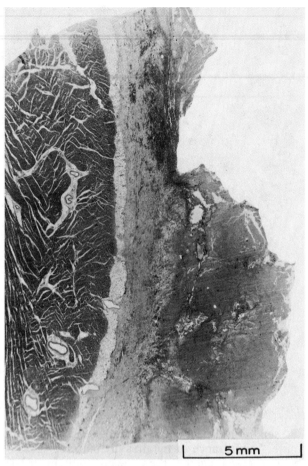

FIGURE 83-2 Suppurative pericarditis of the heart of a 30-year-old Negro; the deepest layer is fibrous. (Hematoxylin-eosin.) (From R. E. B. Hudson, "Cardiovascular Pathology," vol. 2, Edward Arnold Publishers, Ltd., London, 1965, p. 1544, with permission of publisher.)

Constrictive pericarditis

Fibrous thickening of the pericardium, often with calcification, may restrict venous return and lead to congestive heart failure.

CLINICAL TYPES OF PERICARDITIS

Rheumatic fever

Effusion is part of the carditis; the volume varies, and it may resorb completely, apart from milk patches. Sometimes adhesions result, but constriction is rare.

Acute benign pericarditis

This painful feverish condition may follow an acute upper respiratory infection or atypical pneumonia, or it may have no obvious cause. It usually resolves after 2 months or so, but may relapse; sometimes

tamponade and, rarely, constriction may follow. The fluid is lymphocytic and occasionally bloodstained. Viral etiology is often suspected and sometimes proven, e.g., with Coxsackie A or B or ECHO virus.

Chronic relapsing pericarditis

This may last up to several years; an excellent review came from Bedford[4]; most of his cases were idiopathic.

Cholesterol pericarditis

This rare effusion contains so much cholesterol that Alexander[5] likened it to gold paint; the color varies from yellow to dark green, and the cholesterol content may reach 250 mg/100 ml or more. It occurs in myxedema, hemorrhagic or constrictive pericarditis from tuberculosis, or it may have no obvious cause. The pericardium may be thickened by nonspecific inflammatory fibrosis containing cholesterol in clefts and in macrophages. Treatment is pericardiectomy.

Autoimmune pericarditis

This may follow heart operations (postcommissurotomy syndrome), cardiac infarction (Dressler's syndrome), or other cardiac trauma. It often relapses. Serum heart antibodies are usually present and provide a useful diagnostic test.[6]

Myxedema

Pericardial effusion is common as part of the hypothyroidism; it resolves with specific hormone therapy.

Uremic pericarditis

This occurs in renal failure; the fluid is clear usually but is sometimes bloodstained, and it may cause tamponade; constriction sometimes follows. The complication is now commoner because better dialysis management permits longer survival; it is less likely with peritoneal dialysis than with hemodialysis; indeed, changing to the former method may abolish the pericarditis. Nevertheless, surgical pericardiectomy may become essential in intractable cases with threatening tamponade.[7]

Tuberculous pericarditis (Fig. 83-3)

This is now much less common in the western world. It probably arises during the early dissemination to the pericardium (often the pleurae too) following primary infection, starting as a fibrinous pericarditis and going on to effusion with pericardial thickening. The effusion slowly lessens and inspissates, resulting in a fibrocaseous lesion. Bacilli may be demonstrable in the exudate directly or by animal inoculation. The final state of healing may obliterate the sac cavity, leaving a thick, adherent fibrous coating to the heart; this may undergo calcification or even bone formation and cause constriction. Sometimes, tuberculous lesions will be found in the heart itself. Tamponade

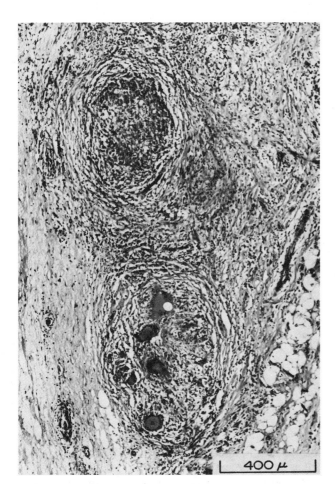

FIGURE 83-3 Tuberculous pericarditis, from the heart of a 31-year-old woman. (Hematoxylin-eosin.) *(From R. E. B. Hudson, "Cardiovascular Pathology," vol. 3, Edward Arnold Publishers, Ltd., London, 1970, p. S.865, with permission of publisher.)*

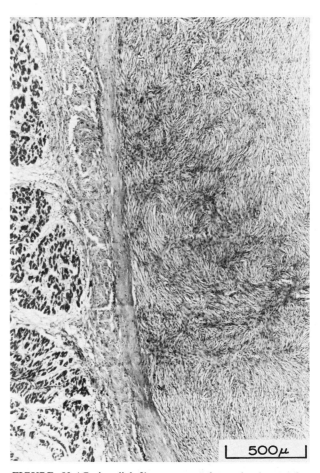

FIGURE 83-4 Pericardial fibrosarcoma; from the heart of a 74-year-old woman. The tumor arises from the clearly defined layer, and it extends from this into the dark-staining surface myocardium. (Hematoxylin-eosin.) *(From R. E. B. Hudson, "Cardiovascular Pathology," vol. 2, Edward Arnold Publishers, Ltd., London, 1965, p. 1564, with permission of publisher.)*

may occur during the effusive or late healing stage and may cause acute or chronic heart failure.

Constrictive pericarditis

It is now recognized that this serious complication may result from conditions other than tuberculosis and Pick's polyserositis. These include acute and purulent pericarditis, Coxsackie pericarditis, neoplasm, amyloidosis, trauma, presence of foreign body, systemic lupus erythematosus, and rheumatoid arthritis. Besides congestive failure, it may cause nephrotic syndrome. Localized annular constriction may cause functional valvular stenosis. Many authorities report the curative value of skilled and timely surgical pericardiectomy to relieve constriction. By contrast, pericardial calcification may be symptomless, occurring in areas of dense fibrosis; sometimes histoplasmosis has been incriminated.

Cardiac infarction

Fibrinous pericardial adhesions are almost invariably found overlying an acute infarct; they may form strong adhesions. Bloodstaining is fairly common, but frank hemorrhage indicates rupture of the heart. A chronic autoimmune pericarditis (Dressler's syndrome) has already been mentioned above.

TUMORS OF THE PERICARDIUM

Primary tumors are rare; they include benign lipoma, fibroma, hemangioma, or malignant mesotheliomas or sarcomas (Fig. 83-4 shows an example of fibrosarcoma). Rarely, a teratoma grows in the pericardium of an infant or child, usually in relation to the great vessels at the heart base; it is usually benign, but it may dwarf and compress these structures. Secondary tumors are much commoner; they include lymphomas and metastases from carcinoma of the breast, lung, thyroid, or pancreas, or from a melanoma.

A special form of "tumor" is idiopathic mediastinal fibrosis, a mysterious disease which invades the mediastinum, obstructing the superior vena cava, and compressing the pulmonary hila by dense fibrosis. It belongs to a group of similar conditions including retroperitoneal fibrosis, Riedel's struma, and sclerosing cholangitis. Methysergide (Deseril) therapy for migraine has been incriminated in a few cases. The relapsing nodular panniculitis of Weber-Christian disease may involve the pericardium.

PERICARDIAL TRAUMA

The pericardium may be damaged by all kinds of violence, but the commonest, albeit inevitable, trauma occurs in cardiac surgery. Another iatrogenic cause is therapeutic irradiation for cancer, e.g., cancer of the breast or lung, lymphoma, thymona; it may evoke effusion and lead to fibrosis of the pericardium and even of the heart itself, probably due to ischemia from capillary damage[8]; the fibrosis may become constrictive.

REFERENCES

1 Moore, R. L.: Congenital Deficiencies of the Pericardium, *Arch. Surg.,* 11:765, 1925.

2 Haider, R., Thomas, D. G. T., Ziady, G., Cleland, W. P., and Goodwin, J. F.: Congenital Pericardio-peritoneal Communication with Herniation of Omentum into the Pericardium. A Rare Cause of Cardiomegaly, *Br. Heart J.,* 35:981, 1973.

3 Loehr, W. M.: Pericardial Cysts, *Am. J. Roentgenol.,* 68:584, 1952.

4 Bedford, D. E.: Chronic Effusive Pericarditis, *Br. Heart J.,* 26:499, 1964.

5 Alexander, J. S.: A Pericardial Effusion of "Gold Paint" Appearance Due to the Presence of Cholesterin, *Br. Med. J.,* 2:463, 1919.

6 Robinson, J., and Brigden, W.: Recurrent Pericarditis, *Br. Med. J.,* 2:272, 1968.

7 Kramer, P., Wigger, W., and Scheler, F.: Management of Uraemic Pericarditis, *Br. Med. J.,* 4:564, 1975.

8 Fajardo, L. F., and Stewart, J. R.: Pathogenesis of Radiation-induced Myocardial Fibrosis, *Lab. Invest.,* 29:244, 1973.

9 Hudson, R. E. B: "Cardiovascular Pathology," Edward Arnold, London, 1965, 1970, chaps. 32, 33, S32, and S33.

84
The Recognition and Management of Pericardial Disease and its Complications

NOBLE O. FOWLER, M.D.

Acute Pericarditis. There are few diseases attended by more variable symptoms, or of more difficult diagnosis, than this. Sometimes it appears with all the symptoms of a very violent disease of the chest; at other times it proves fatal without leading us, in the least, to suspect its existence.

René Théophile Hyacinthe Laennec, 1823[1]

FUNCTIONS OF THE NORMAL PERICARDIUM

Removal of both the parietal and visceral pericardium in patients who have chronic constrictive pericarditis or acute inflammatory disease of the pericardium is followed by no recognizable disability; therefore, the pericardium is not essential for life. Yet, the pericardium has been found to have certain protective functions.[2] Since the heart dilates more readily without the pericardium, insufficiency of the tricuspid and mitral valves develops more easily when the heart is subjected to increased filling pressure after removal of the pericardium.[3] The pericardium may offer protection against pulmonary edema by limiting right ventricular filling when the left ventricle is dilated.[3] Similarly, the pericardium has been shown to limit cardiac expansion in hypervolemia. The paradoxical pulse which develops in some patients with dilated and failing hearts may be related to restriction of cardiac expansion by the normal pericardium.[4] Decline of intrapericardial pressure during ventricular systole may aid atrial filling.[5] The pericardium is believed to protect the heart from infections of the lungs and pleural space. It has been stated that the lung is protected by the pericardium from the trauma of the beating heart and that the pericardium helps to maintain the heart in an optimum functional position. Following removal of the pericardium, roentgen studies of the chest usually reveal that the heart appears somewhat larger than before such an operation.

CONGENITAL DEFICIENCY OF THE PERICARDIUM

Congenital defect of the pericardium is uncommon but has been reported in a number of articles during the last two decades. In 1959, Ellis et al.[6] described two cases which were then the ninety-eighth and ninety-ninth reported examples. In most instances the defects are partial or left-sided parietal pericardial defects; right-sided defects or total absence of the pericardium are rare.

The radiologic features suggestive of left-sided pericardial defect are:[6] a shift of the heart to the left, a long and prominent pulmonary artery segment, and apparent flattening of the left ventricular segment. Ellis et al. indicated the value of left pneumothorax in the diagnosis of left-sided pericardial defects. Nasser and associates reported six cases of pericardial defect, two with partial absence of the left pericardium and two with complete absence of the left pericardium.[7] All six patients had prominent pulmonary artery segments; with partial left defect, the left atrial appendage was prominent; with complete defects, there was levoposition of the heart and a segment of lung was interposed between aorta and pulmonary artery and another segment between the left hemidiaphragm and inferior border of the heart. Left-sided pericardial defect may simulate the following disorders: atrial septal defect, idiopathic dilatation of the pulmonary artery, pulmonic stenosis, cardiac tumor, left hilar adenopathy, corrected transposition of the great arteries, mediastinal tumor, and bronchogenic carcinoma.

Clinical findings

Five of Nasser's six patients had pectus excavatum. Pulsation of the left posterior chest wall was reported by Glancy et al.[8] as a physical sign. In four of Nasser's patients with complete left pericardial defect, the electrocardiograms showed right axis deviation in four and suggested right ventricular hypertrophy in one. Cardiovascular dynamics, in the absence of cardiac strangulation, are believed to be normal.[7]

Associated defects

Two of Nasser's six patients had atrial septal defect—one with anomalous pulmonary veins, the other with Eisenmenger's syndrome. Other associated defects reported by Hipona and associates[9] were patent ductus arteriosus in four patients; bifid heart in two; tetralogy of Fallot in two; tricuspid insufficiency in one; bicuspid aortic valve in one; bronchogenic cysts in six; and aberrant pulmonary lobe in one. Bronchial cysts and enterogenous thoracic cysts have been reported as associated defects.[6] Diaphragmatic pericardial defects may be combined into a pentalogy with abdominal wall defects, lower sternal defects, deficiency of the anterior diaphragm and congenital intracardiac defects.[10]

Echocardiographic studies of five patients with complete absence of the left pericardium showed changes mimicking right ventricular volume overload, possibly due to altered rardiac position and motion in the thorax.[11] Death, as the resalt of herniation of the heart through a partial left pericardial defect, has been reported in a 28-year-old woman, in a 2-year-old boy, and in an orangutan.[6] Strangulation of the left atrial appendage has been reported, too[12,13] (Fig. 84-1). Surgical correction is not usually recommended for total left-sided defect but has been

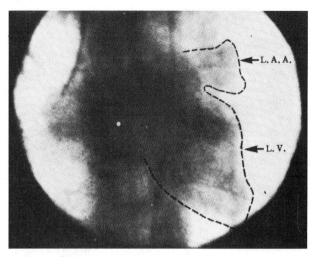

FIGURE 84-1 Angiocardiogram revealing herniated left atrial appendage (LAA) in patient with left-sided parietal pericardial defect. *(From Nasser et al., Circulation, 41:469, 1970.[7] By permission.)*

recommended for partial defects because of potential herniation and strangulation.[14]

PERICARDIAL CYSTS

Pericardial cysts and diverticula are not rare.[15] Over 80 percent of instances occur at the right anterior cardiophrenic angle (Fig. 84-2). The cysts may be congenital pericardial coelomic cysts which are usually not connected with the pericardium except by loose connective tissue. Lymphangiomatous cysts may arise from the pericardium and are usually multilocular. When the fibrous structure of the pericardium is weak, the serosa may herniate to form a diverticulum. When the diverticulum loses its con-

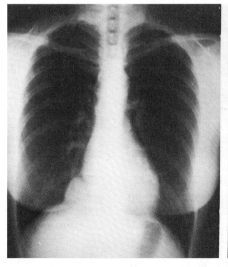
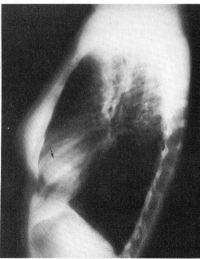

FIGURE 84-2 Pericardial cyst located in the right cardiophrenic angle. In the lateral view (right), its location is shown by an arrow. *(Courtesy of Dr. Harold Spitz, Professor of Radiology, University of Cincinnati.)*

nection with the pericardial sac, a pericardial cyst is formed.

Pericardial coelomic cysts and diverticula usually are not recognized until middle adult life. They may remain unchanged or enlarge slowly over a period of several years. Symptoms are seldom produced. Their location is usually in the right anterior cardiophrenic angle. The differential diagnosis includes foramen of Morgagni diaphragmatic hernia, large right pericardial fat pad, other mediastinal or diaphragmatic tumors, and rarely, tumors of the heart or pericardium.

PAIN OF PERICARDITIS

The pain of acute pericarditis is one of the features of major clinical interest. Nearly all patients with recognized acute nonspecific pericarditis have chest pain. In this disorder chest pain is often severe and may resemble that of myocardial infarction. Capps found that only the lower portion of the external surface of the parietal pericardium is pain-sensitive,[16] and presumably much of the pain in acute pericarditis is caused by inflammation of the adjoining diaphragmatic pleura. Hence, it is common for the pain of acute pericarditis to be referred to the left supraclavicular area. The characteristic increase of pericardial pain by deep inspiration, or by rotating the trunk, has been explained by the theory that pain fibers from the pericardium are carried in the left phrenic nerve. More recently it has been shown that the pain of acute pericarditis can be relieved by left stellate ganglion block.[17] This observation casts some doubt upon the earlier theory that the phrenic nerve carries the pain pathways from the pericardium.

PARADOXICAL PULSE IN PERICARDIAL DISEASE

A second major feature of pericardial disease is compression of the heart either by fibrosis or by pericardial fluid. When the heart is thus compressed, it is unable to fill completely. Systemic and pulmonary venous pressures rise, and systemic blood pressure falls. Eventually cardiac output declines and syncope may occur if these events transpire quickly. When the heart is compressed more gradually over a period of weeks, months, or years, peripheral edema may develop. This sequence of events is called *cardiac tamponade,* or *cardiac compression* if the cardiac restriction results from fibrosis rather than from fluid.

Many patients with cardiac tamponade or with cardiac constriction by fibrosis develop an interesting physical finding called the *pulsus paradoxus*. The paradoxical pulse is an abnormal inspiratory fall in systemic blood pressure. It is difficult to draw a sharp line between health and disease in this connection because there is normally an inspiratory decline of a few millimeters of mercury in systolic blood pres-

sure. Inspiratory decline of systolic blood pressure in excess of 8 or 10 mm Hg is probably abnormal, but the decline may be exaggerated by abnormally deep breathing. Experimental studies in our laboratory suggest that the normal decline is caused by two factors:[18] (1) there is a transmission of the increased negativity of intrathoracic pressure during inspiration to the heart and great vessels; (2) inspiration is known to increase filling of the right side of the heart and right-sided heart output. Because of the transit time in the lungs, this increase in output of the right side of the heart does not increase output of the left side until nearly the beginning of expiration. It should be pointed out that pericardial disease is not the commonest cause of a paradoxical pulse. The commonest cause is obstruction to breathing associated with bronchial asthma[19] or pulmonary emphysema. With obstruction to respiration we have been able to show experimentally that the abnormal inspiratory decline of blood pressure is caused by transmission of the unusually great fluctuations of intrathoracic pressure to the heart and great vessels.[18] There have been a number of theories concerning the paradoxical pulse of pericardial disease. Katz and Gauchat found in 1924 that with cardiac tamponade intrapericardial pressure did not fall during inspiration.[20] As a result, pulmonary venous pressure should fall more during inspiration than left atrial pressure, thus tending to decrease filling of the left side of the heart during inspiration. Later workers have confirmed this observation, but the interpretation of the data is in dispute. Dock believed that inspiratory traction by the diaphragm and mediastinum upon the taut pericardium further increased intrapericardial pressure, thus interfering with cardiac filling.[21] Dornhorst thought that the normal inspiratory increase in filling of the right side of the heart persisted during cardiac tamponade, thus raising intrapericardial pressure and interfering with left ventricular filling during inspiration.[22] We investigated this problem in experimental animals. Our studies in part confirmed the postulates of Dornhorst. We were able to show that there was indeed a persistence of the normal inspiratory increase of filling of the right side of the heart during cardiac tamponade. If this was prevented, paradoxical pulse did not develop, no matter how severe the cardiac tamponade. Furthermore, the paradoxical pulse could be simulated by increasing filling of the right side of the heart in other ways in apneic animals with cardiac tamponade.[23] In our studies, and in those of Guntheroth,[24] inspiratory decline of intrapericardial pressure was not materially reduced during tamponade. Guntheroth and associates believe that normal respiratory variations of a reduced right ventricular stroke volume are responsible for the exaggerated respiratory variations in blood pressure during cardiac tamponade. D'Cruz et al. studied three patients with cardiac tamponade by means of echocardiography. Inspiration decreased mitral valve anterior motion and decreased its EF slope, accompanied by an increase of right ventricular dimensions and decrease of left ventricular dimensions.[25] Shabetai found that both vena caval and pulmonary arterial blood flow velocity increased during inspiration in patients with cardiac tamponade but failed to increase normally during inspiration in patients with constrictive pericarditis.[24] These observations are consistent with the animal studies of the mechanism of the paradoxical pulse in cardiac tamponade and suggest that the mechanism is different in constrictive pericarditis.

Pulsus paradoxus may occur in patients with restrictive cardiomyopathy and has been described in clinical shock.[27]

ETIOLOGY OF PERICARDITIS

Predisposing factors

Pericarditis, especially constrictive pericarditis, has been reported in patients with atrial septal defect[26] and in our experience appears more common in this disorder than would be expected on the basis of chance alone. Pericarditis appears to be of increased prevalence in certain varieties of chronic anemia, e.g., in thalassemia.[28]

The clinician should remember that few diseases affect the pericardium alone. Hence, the discovery of pericarditis may be the first clue to such systemic illness as uremia, lupus erythematosus, tuberculosis, or previously unsuspected neoplastic disease. The common causes of acute pericarditis are listed in Table 84-1.[29] There seems to be little question that the commonest variety of acute pericarditis is the disease called *acute idiopathic, acute benign,* or *acute nonspecific pericarditis.* None of these names is free from objection, since the disorder is now known to be complicated occasionally by myocardiopathy with

TABLE 84-1
Etiologic classification of pericardial disease

1 Acute idiopathic or nonspecific

2 Acute myocardial infarction

3 Postmyocardial infarction syndrome (Dressler's syndrome)

4 Trauma, penetrating or nonpenetrating

5 Postthoracotomy syndrome or postcardiotomy syndrome

6 Connective tissue diseases: rheumatoid disease; rheumatic fever; disseminated lupus erythematosus; scleroderma; Takayasu's arteritis[43]

7 Specific infections
   a Bacterial infections; infective endocarditis[44]
   b Tuberculosis
   c Fungous infections: histoplasmosis, nocardiosis, blastomycosis[42]
   d Viral (Coxsackie B, influenza, ECHO)
   e Amebiasis[45]
   f Toxoplasmosis[46]
   g Meningococcal disease[47]
   h Gonococcal disease[48]

8 Primary or metastatic neoplasm, including lymphoma and leukemia

9 Radiation[49]

10 Aortic aneurysm: rupture or leakage of dissecting or nondissecting aneurysm into the pericardial sac

11 Drugs: hydralazine; psicofuranine; procainamide; anticoagulant therapy; isonicotinic acid hydrazide; penicillin

12 Chylopericardium

13 Uremia, and in association with hemodialysis[50]

14 Miscellaneous; sarcoidosis; myxedema; amyloid disease; multiple myeloma

congestive heart failure or by constrictive pericarditis.[30] Thus the term *benign* is hardly applicable in all instances. In epidemics, acute nonspecific pericarditis can be shown to be caused by Coxsackie A or B virus,[31] influenza A or B virus, or chickenpox. However, investigation of sporadic cases seldom demonstrates the cause. (Two other disorders affect principally the pericardium and have clinical features somewhat similar to those of idiopathic benign pericarditis: the postcardiotomy syndrome and the postmyocardial infarction syndrome. These diseases will be discussed later in this presentation.) Rheumatic pericarditis is not commonly found in adults but is not rare in children. The pericardium may be involved by malignant metastatic tumors, the two commonest being carcinoma of the lung in males, and carcinoma of the breast in females. Malignant melanoma is known to spread to the pericardium frequently, and lymphomas and leukemia affect the pericardium rather commonly. Primary tumors of the pericardium, such as mesothelioma, are quite rare.[32] Uremic pericarditis is common in patients with renal failure. It may be associated with cardiac tamponade. Pericarditis may occur in disseminated lupus erythematosus in as many as 48 percent of instances but is seldom the first manifestation of the disease.[33] Pericarditis may result from specific acute bacterial infections, such as pneumococcal pneumonia or septicemia of varied cause. A myocardial abscess complicating bacterial endocarditis may cause pericarditis. Amebic abscesses of the liver may burrow through the diaphragm into the pericardial space. Dissecting aneurysm involving the aortic root may produce a pericardial friction rub and the electrocardiographic changes of acute pericarditis by blood seepage even without frank rupture into the pericardial space.[34]

Traumatic pericarditis as the result of gunshot and stab wounds is familiar. More recently it has been learned that traumatic pericarditis may result from indirect trauma to the heart without penetration. It has also been learned that pericardial bleeding, caused by either direct or indirect trauma, may be followed by constrictive pericarditis.[35] At the Cincinnati General Hospital there was a recent example of this in a 20-year-old man who was stabbed in the heart. A few weeks after discharge from the hospital he was admitted again with acute pericarditis, which was followed within a matter of 6 weeks by the syndrome of cardiac compression. At thoracotomy he was found to have striking pericardial thickening. Rheumatoid arthritis has been recently emphasized as a cause of pericarditis in adults,[36,37] although it has been recognized as a cause of pericarditis in children for over 60 years. We have observed several patients with pericarditis associated with rheumatoid arthritis. In two instances, constrictive pericarditis developed and pericardial resection was necessary.[38] Irradiation of the mediastinum may be associated with pericarditis, which on occasion may lead to cardiac constriction.[39,40] Of note is the latent period following radiation therapy, which may be many months. Radiation pneumonitis may or may not occur. Histoplasmosis may affect the pericardium.[41] We reported 16 instances of acute histoplasma pericarditis from the University of Cincinnati Medical Center.[42] Actinomycosis may affect the pericardium and may closely simulate tuberculous pericarditis.[29] Cultures of the fluid and biopsy of the pericardium or lung are needed to make the distinction. Rarely drugs, such as hydralazine, which can produce a lupus-like syndrome, and psicofuranine, may be associated with pericarditis. The use of procainamide may be followed by a lupus-like syndrome, with positive lupus erythematosus cell tests and pericarditis. The use of Dilantin, isoniazid, and other drugs may be followed by pericarditis.[51]

ACUTE PERICARDITIS

History

If the patient with acute pericarditis has a complaint related specifically to the pericarditis, it is usually that of chest pain. Not infrequently, patients with acute pericarditis come to the physician complaining of other manifestations of the systemic illness which causes the pericarditis, such as fever, joint disease, skin disease, fatigue, or the symptoms of uremia. The chest pain of acute pericarditis is often quite characteristic, but at other times it is not. The pain may be of very sudden onset. It may begin over the sternum and radiate to the neck and down the left upper extremity, mimicking very closely the pain of acute myocardial infarction.[52] This syndrome seems to be more common in patients with acute nonspecific pericarditis than in those with other forms of pericarditis. Especially when it occurs in a middle-aged or older man, an erroneous diagnosis of myocardial infarction may be made. The two disorders can often be distinguished by a careful history. In acute pericarditis the pain is usually increased by deep breathing or by rotating the thorax and may be somewhat relieved when the patient sits up and leans forward. Pain along the left trapezius ridge is a common complaint. In acute myocardial infarction the pain is usually not increased by breathing or by rotation of the thorax. Pain may occur in acute pericarditis caused by tuberculosis or rheumatic fever but is usually less severe. Uremic pericarditis is usually thought to be painless. However, close questioning of the mentally obtunded uremic patient discloses that pain is not uncommon in these patients.[53] Pain usually accompanies pericarditis of the postcardiotomy syndrome and the postmyocardial infarction syndrome.

In acute pericarditis the presenting symptoms may be those of cardiac tamponade with dyspnea, orthopnea, and tachycardia in the absence of pain. Radiologic changes in the cardiopericardial silhouette or electrocardiographic changes may call attention to the disease.

Physical examination

PERICARDIAL FRICTION RUB

The characteristic pathognomonic finding of pericarditis is the pericardial friction rub, although it is not always present. The pericardial friction rub should be searched for with the patient in various positions, including sitting upright, leaning forward with the breath expelled, and on his hands and knees in bed. A pericardial rub occurs as the heart moves. The heart moves with atrial systole, ventricular systole, and ventricular diastole. Accordingly there may be three components to the pericardial rub, one during each of these phases of the cardiac cycle. Each component is a short, scratchy sound. When three components are heard, it is quite diagnostic of pericardial rub. There may be only two components to the rub, one during ventricular systole and one during ventricular diastole. In such a case the to-and-fro sound usually indicates a pericardial friction rub. A pericardial friction rub may be heard only in systole. Under such circumstances it is difficult to be certain that one is not dealing with a murmur or an extracardiac sound. The question can usually be settled by frequent observation, since a pericardial friction rub will become a to-and-fro sound or disappear within a few days. A pleuropericardial rub is usually louder at the cardiac apex or adjacent to that part of the lung where a pleural friction rub is heard, is often associated with a left pleural friction rub, and is markedly affected by breathing. A pleuropericardial rub is often diagnosed in error when a pericardial rub is, in fact, present. The reason for this error is the mistaken belief that a pericardial friction rub should not vary with respiration. In fact, the pericardial rub is often quite strikingly altered by breathing. In some instances it is audible only during moderate inspiration. Contrary to common belief, a pericardial friction rub may be heard when there is considerable pericardial effusion.

PERICARDIAL EFFUSION

The other features characteristic of acute pericarditis are the signs of pericardial effusion, which may or may not be found. The circulatory effects of acute pericardial effusion depend on its rate of accumulation. If pericardial fluid accumulates very rapidly, a few hundred milliliters can cause cardiac compression and cardiac tamponade, with elevation of the venous pressure, decrease of systemic blood pressure, and perhaps syncope or sudden death. On the other hand, a more gradual accumulation of pericardial fluid often fails to produce these symptoms and signs even when the pericardial space contains a liter or more of fluid. In patients with suspected pericardial effusion, it is important to locate the cardiac apex impulse. If the apex impulse is in normal position in the fifth left intercostal space at or inside the midclavicular line and there is percussion dullness beyond this point, pericardial effusion can be suspected. This sign is difficult to evaluate when there is left pleural effusion.

When there is rapid accumulation of pericardial fluid and rising venous pressure, a paradoxical pulse may be found. The paradoxical pulse has already been defined and its physiology has been discussed. When this finding is pronounced, the radial pulse will become attenuated or disappear during inspiration. When this sign is less pronounced, it is important to search for it with a blood pressure cuff and a stethoscope when acute or chronic pericarditis is suspected. The patient should breathe normally. The examiner should observe the level of systolic blood pressure at which arterial sounds are heard in expiration only, and then the pressure at which the sounds are heard throughout the cardiac cycle. The difference between the two indicates the magnitude of the paradoxical pulse. A value exceeding 8 to 10 mm Hg in a patient who has normal nonobstructed breathing is strongly suggestive of cardiac compression. However, an occasional patient with congestive heart failure, especially when the condition is caused by chronic myocardial disease and myocardial fibrosis, may demonstrate pulsus paradoxus.[54] Acute or chronic obstructive airway disease may be associated with a paradoxical pulse; if the systemic venous pressure is elevated because of cor pulmonale with congestive failure, then cardiac tamponade may be closely simulated. Acute cardiac infarction, when complicated by cardiogenic shock and acute pericarditis, may also be associated with a paradoxical arterial pulse and elevated systemic venous pressure in the absence of cardiac tamponade. When the venous pressure is elevated in pericarditis, the cervical veins may become more distended during inspiration, which is the reverse of the normal situation. This finding is called Kussmaul's sign. This sign is not invariably present and is not diagnostic of acute pericarditis. It may be found in vena caval obstruction and in some patients with congestive heart failure caused by myocardial or valvular disease.

OTHER PHYSICAL FINDINGS IN ACUTE PERICARDITIS

Some patients who have acute pericarditis with effusion may demonstrate Ewart's sign, an area of percussion dullness and bronchial breathing beneath the angle of the left scapula. This sign has not been helpful in our experience. It may be found in patients with dilatation of the heart and no pericardial effusion. It is frequently absent in patients with pericardial effusion. An occasional patient with pericardial effusion may demonstrate an early diastolic sound, or pericardial knock sound, between 0.06 and 0.12 s after the onset of the second heart sound. This sound may be difficult to distinguish from an early ventricular gallop rhythm at the cardiac apex. Other findings in these patients are usually those of the underlying illness. Fever is common, as is tachycardia. Cardiac murmurs are usually difficult to evaluate when there is a pericardial friction rub.

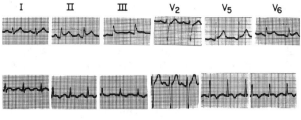

J.M. , 38 ♂ IDIOPATHIC PERICARDITIS

FIGURE 84-3 Serial electrocardiographic changes in a 38-year-old man with acute nonspecific pericarditis. The upper record demonstrates ST-segment elevation without reciprocal depression. Two days later (lower record) the elevated ST segments have returned to the isoelectric line, and the T waves are negative. There are no pathologic Q waves.

Laboratory tests

ELECTROCARDIOGRAPHY

We recently reviewed the electrocardiographic features of pericarditis.[55] The characteristic electrocardiogram of acute pericarditis is not found in all instances. Typically, in the first few days after the onset of chest pain, there is elevation of the ST segments in two or all three of the standard limb leads without reciprocal depression (Fig. 84-3). The precordial leads often show elevated ST segments in most leads. Depressed ST segments are found as a rule only in lead V_1 and in lead aV_R. There are rare exceptions to this statement. After a few days or a week, the ST segments tend to return to the base line and then the T waves become negative as the disorder enters its subacute phase (Fig. 84-3). There may be some diminution of QRS voltage, but P wave voltage tends to be maintained.[56] It is important that the electrocardiogram be distinguished from that of acute myocardial infarction (Fig. 84-4). The most distinctive feature is the development of pathologic Q waves in myocardial infarction; these do not appear in patients with acute pericarditis. In the first few days of the attack, the absence of reciprocal

FIGURE 84-4 Serial electrocardiographic changes in a 49-year-old man with acute myocardial infarction. The upper record was made the first day of chest pain, and demonstrates ST-segment elevation and tall T waves. In the lower tracing made 3 days later, there are pathologic Q waves; the T waves are now negative, while the ST segments are still elevated.

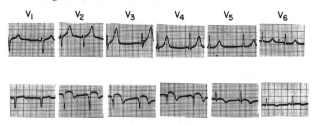

H. L. , 49 ♂ ACUTE MYOCARDIAL INFARCTION

ST-segment depression in the limb leads is usually a reliable indication of pericarditis. Characteristically, the T waves become negative in acute pericarditis only after the ST segments return to the isoelectric line. In acute myocardial infarction the T waves often become negative while the ST segments are still elevated. This differential feature is less reliable.

The cardiac rhythm is usually a normal sinus rhythm; occasionally there is paraoxysmal atrial fibrillation or flutter. Depression of the PR segment is said to occur in acute pericarditis,[56a] but it is often difficult to evaluate the PR segment because of the usual ST-segment elevation.

RADIOLOGIC STUDIES (see also Chaps. 24 and 29A,B)

In many patients with acute pericarditis, the findings on routine chest radiologic and cardiac fluoroscopy studies are normal. A few hundred milliliters of pericardial effusion do not necessarily produce a detectable radiologic change. The study of cardiac pulsations by routine fluoroscopy is an unreliable way of detecting pericardial effusion. When there are several hundred milliliters of fluid in the pericardial space then the cardiac silhouette will be increased in size. Characteristically, the lungs are less congested than in patients with congestive heart failure, and this may be a valuable sign, since at times the clinical features of cardiac dilatation may resemble those of pericardial effusion. Patients who have acute benign pericarditis often show additional pleural effusion and small areas of pneumonitis. There are similar radiologic findings in patients with postcardiotomy or postmyocardial infarction syndrome. Image-intensifier cardiac fluoroscopy may be useful in detecting pericardial effusion if the *epicardial fat line* can be shown by its decreased density inside the pericardial fluid. Radiologic demonstration of pericardial fluid or thickening is more reliable, however, if some contrast medium is employed. Cardiac scanning, following the injection of radioactive iodinated serum albumin, is free of hazard and discomfort to the patient (Fig. 84-5)[57] (see Chap. 30). This method is less sensitive than the use of an iodine-containing contrast medium or carbon dioxide. Durant showed that the injection of 50 to 100 ml carbon dioxide into the antecubital vein of a patient lying on the left side will often demonstrate pericardial thickening or effusion (Fig. 84-6).[58] Errors may result if there is right pleural effusion or disease of the adjacent right middle lobe. Angiocardiography, carried out with the patient in the sitting posture, or right lateral decubitus, is usually an effective way of detecting pericardial thickening or fluid accumulation in the pericardial space (Fig. 84-7). The distance from the lateral right border of the contrast medium to the lateral border of the cardiopericardial silhouette normally should not exceed 3 to 5 mm. It must be remembered that this space includes right atrial wall, pleura, and visceral

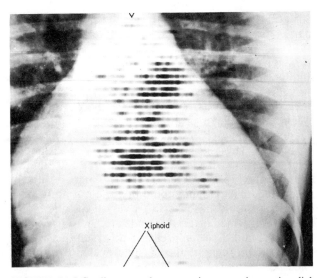

FIGURE 84-5 Cardiac scan demonstrating extensive pericardial effusion. The black dots indicate the blood within the heart chambers and great vessels; the white radiopaque area indicates the extent of the pericardial effusion.

and parietal pericardium as well as any fluid or fibrosis.

ECHOCARDIOGRAPHY (see also Chap. 32E)

Echocardiography is a rather sensitive and specific method which is useful in demonstrating pericardial effusion (Fig. 84-8).[59] At present, this test, because of

FIGURE 84-6 Identification of pericardial effusion by injection of carbon dioxide into a peripheral vein. The patient is lying on the left side. The arrow tip indicates carbon dioxide within the right atrium, and the increased pericardial thickness may be seen just above the head of the arrow.

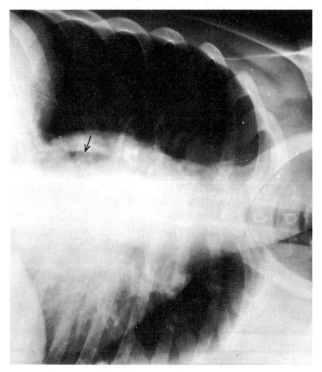

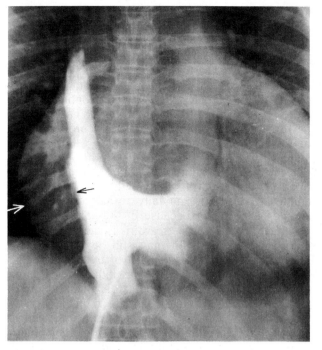

FIGURE 84-7 Angiocardiogram in pericardial effusion, showing increased distance between the right border of the cardiopericardial silhouette and the contrast medium within the right atrium. *(From N. O. Fowler, "Cardiac Diagnosis and Treatment," Harper & Row, Publishers, Inc., Hagerstown, 1976. By permission.)*

its lack of risk and its precision, has largely replaced the methods described above for demonstrating pericardial effusion. (Fig. 84-8).

OTHER TESTS

The white blood cell count is often increased in acute benign pericarditis but may be within normal limits. The serum glutamic-oxaloacetic transaminase may be slightly increased.

FIGURE 84-8 Echocardiogram showing pericardial effusion caused by a postpericardiotomy syndrome following insertion of mitral valve prosthesis. *(Courtesy of Dr. Neil Agruss.)*

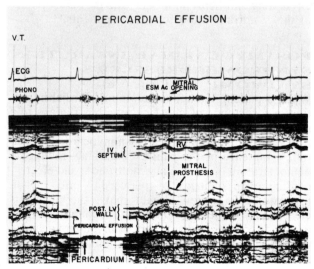

Differential diagnosis

In the patient with acute and severe chest pain, the differential diagnosis from acute myocardial infarction, pleurisy, spontaneous pneumothorax, or mediastinal emphysema must be made. Characteristically the pain of acute pericarditis is increased by deep breathing or by rotating the thorax, whereas that of acute myocardial infarction is not. If one hears a pericardial friction rub in a patient within 24 h of the onset of chest pain, acute pericarditis is more likely than acute myocardial infarction. Characteristic electrocardiographic changes are usually sufficient to make the distinction; these have already been discussed. The serum level of glutamic-oxaloacetic transaminase is nearly always increased in acute transmural myocardial infarction but is usually normal with nontransmural infarction or acute coronary insufficienty. It is increased in some patients with acute pericarditis. Therefore, a normal transaminase value is more consistent with pericarditis than with acute myocardial infarction. It is of utmost importance that acute pericarditis not be mistaken for acute myocardial infarction. The use of anticoagulants in patients with acute pericarditis may be extremely hazardous. This writer has observed three instances of severe pericardial bleeding in patients with nonspecific pericarditis who received anticoagulants. Two patients died, and one required surgical relief of cardiac tamponade. When there is doubt about the diagnosis, anticoagulants should not be used. Myocardial imaging with technetium Tc 99m pyrophosphate or thallium is of value in establishing or excluding the diagnosis of myocardial infarction.[59a]

In acute pleurisy there is only a pleural friction rub; the characteristic electrocardiographic features of acute pericarditis are missing. Since the two disorders may coexist, demonstration of fluid in the pericardial space may be necessary for the distinction. In spontaneous pneumothorax, sudden onset of chest pain and dyspnea often occur. Percussion hyperresonance and decreased or absent breath sounds confirm the diagnosis, but these signs are absent when the air collection is small, and chest roentgenograms are required. Occasional patients with left pneumothorax demonstrate a crunching or bubbling to-and-fro sound over the precordium.[60] A similar sound may be heard in acute spontaneous mediastinal emphysema, which also must be considered in the differential diagnosis of chest pain.[61] Crepitus in the soft tissues of the lower anterior neck and roentgen demonstration of mediastinal air will establish the diagnosis.

Etiologic diagnosis

As stated earlier, diagnostic studies in acute pericarditis are often required to determine the cause of the disorder. Unless the cause of the pericarditis is obvious, e.g., trauma, recent cardiac infarction, uremia, neoplasm, we generally obtain certain routine diagnostic evaluations in all patients. These include the electrocardiogram, chest radiogram, urinalysis, complete blood count, and serum urea nitrogen. We also obtain an intermediate-strength skin test with tuberculin, serial complement fixation tests for histoplasmosis, and ASO titer or streptozyme test, which bears on the possibility of rheumatic fever. Neutralyzing serum antibody studies for viral diseases are also made. It is essential to obtain a good history, with emphasis on trauma, neoplasm, radiation therapy, and drug usage, especially with regard to hydralazine, procainamide, or diphenylhydantoin.

ACUTE IDIOPATHIC PERICARDITIS

Most of the features of the commonest variety of acute pericarditis, i.e., acute idiopathic, acute benign, or acute nonspecific pericarditis, have been already discussed. There is an antecedent infection in the upper part of the respiratory tract a few weeks before the illness in approximately 28 percent of patients.[30] Acute onset of chest pain is found in about 60 percent of patients with this illness.[61] Rarely, pain is absent. Often pericardial effusion is not recognizable, but in some instances it is great enough to be detectable radiologically and may produce cardiac tamponade. The pericardial fluid is frequently bloody. Radiologic examination of the chest often demonstrates associated pleural effusion and transient areas of pulmonary infiltration.[62] The patient is usually febrile. The fever is often greatest on the first day of illness and may last for a few days to as much as 3 to 6 weeks. There are recurrences in about 23 percent of patients.[30] In the study of Johnson and associates,[63] evidence consistent with viral infection was found in 5 of 34 patients with acute benign pericarditis. The differential diagnosis from tuberculous pericarditis presents a significant problem. In endemic areas, histoplasma pericarditis may simulate idiopathic pericarditis.[42]

TUBERCULOUS PERICARDITIS

We recently reviewed the Cincinnati General Hospital experience with tuberculous pericarditis.[64] Although patients with tuberculous pericarditis may have underlying miliary tuberculosis or radiologically detectable areas of pulmonary involvement, in the majority of instances tuberculous pericarditis in adults is clinically primary and originates from tuberculosis of the mediastinal nodes. Thus, the clinical evidence of tuberculosis is not readily discernible and the etiologic diagnosis is often missed.[65] Very large amounts of pericardial effusion, a history of previous tuberculosis, a history of weight loss, or fever which persists beyond 2 to 3 weeks usually suggest that the possibility of tuberculosis should be thoroughly investigated. If both first- and second-strength purified protein derivative (PPD) skin tests are negative, tuberculosis is unlikely. Aspiration of pericardial fluid, followed by guinea pig inoculation and culture, will reveal tubercle bacilli in about 50 percent of patients who have tuberculous pericarditis with effusion. Unfortunately the 6-week waiting period for the results of this test is unacceptable to most physicians. Our policy, if the patient continues to be quite ill, with a fever after 3 weeks, has been to perform a pericardial biopsy at thoracotomy after 1 or 2 weeks of preliminary treatment with isoniazid and para-aminosalicylic acid or streptomycin. At this time, it appears that one should consider the substitution of ethambutol, 15 mg/kg/day, for para-aminosalicylic acid. The daily dosage of ethambutol should be kept low because of the danger of optic nerve toxicity. If the pericarditis is caused by tuberculosis, tubercle bacilli may still be demonstrable histologically after this amount of treatment. If the biopsy specimen shows changes indicative of some other disorder, such as rheumatoid nodules, metastatic neoplasm, or fungous disease, then the therapy would be altered accordingly. If the specimen shows caseation necrosis and no acid-fast or other organisms, long-term antituberculosis therapy must be started. (See later discussion regarding the use of triple therapy plus corticosteroids.)[65] Difficulty arises if the specimen shows only nonspecific changes of inflammation. In this event, one's decision will have to rest on judgment based on clinical evaluation of the entire picture. If tuberculosis still seems a reasonable possibility, then adequate antituberculosis therapy must be instituted.

POSTCARDIOTOMY SYNDROME

A syndrome like that of acute nonspecific pericarditis, which begins within a period of 10 days to 2 or 3 months following cardiac surgery, or direct or indirect cardiac trauma, is very likely related to the antecedent event. At the University of Cincinnati Hospitals, a postcardiotomy syndrome was found in 13.7 percent of patients subjected to mitral valvulotomy.[66] This complication is apparently even more common in some hospitals. Engle and associates found an excellent correlation between the titer of circulating anti-heart antibodies and the development of this syndrome in postoperative patients.[67]

POSTMYOCARDIAL INFARCTION SYNDROME: DRESSLER'S SYNDROME (see Chap. 62E)

When a patient has had an acute myocardial infarction, a recurrence of chest pain within 10 days to a few months may indicate the postmyocardial infarction syndrome rather than a fresh myocardial infarction.[68] Increase of the pain by breathing, radiologic demonstration of pulmonary infiltration, and electrocardiographic changes of pericarditis rather than myocardial infarction should make the diagnosis clear. This has been a relatively uncommon complication in our experience. In both postmyocardial infarction syndrome and postcardiotomy syndrome, recurrent attacks over a period of several years may take place.

OTHER VARIETIES OF PERICARDITIS

Patients who have acute pericarditis caused by rheumatic fever almost always have underlying endocarditis and myocarditis. The absence of cardiac murmurs is strong evidence against rheumatic fever as the cause of acute pericarditis. Patients who have pericarditis associated with lupus erythematosus usually have other manifestations of the illness, such as anemia, leukopenia, thrombocytopenia, skin rash, fever, arthritis, and nephritis. Uncommonly, pericarditis is the presenting feature of the illness. A positive test for lupus erythematosus cells will clarify the diagnosis. In patients with uremic pericarditis, renal failure is usually obvious. Uremic pericarditis is usually fibrinous but occasionally produces a few hundred milliliters of pericardial effusion. Occasionally, the fluid is bloody, and there may be cardiac tamponade.[69] It is important to know of a history of previous irradiation of the mediastinum so that postradiation pericarditis is not overlooked. Rheumatoid arthritis is readily apparent from the physical examination. One should not forget to inquire into the history of drug ingestion, particularly hydralazine or procainamide. In patients with persistent pericarditis of obscure etiology, one should not neglect the possibility of fungous disease, especially histoplasmosis. It may be necessary to culture a pericardial biopsy specimen to arrive at a satisfactory diagnosis.

Aspiration of the pericardial effusion may be helpful in diagnosis when the causative organism can be identified in the fluid, either directly or on culture, or by animal inoculation. The quality of the fluid is usually not too helpful, except when there is an acute pyogenic pericarditis which may complicate septicemia or result from left empyema, trauma, or mediastinitis. Sanguineous pericardial effusion may be found in a variety of disorders. It may be found in tuberculosis, carcinoma, lupus erythematosus, idiopathic benign pericarditis, rheumatoid arthritis, and even occasionally in rheumatic fever. A grossly bloody pericardial effusion, however, is very suggestive of either neoplastic invasion or of tuberculosis. In this writer's experience, a slow leak from aneurysm of the aortic root over a period of several days may also produce grossly bloody pericardial effusion. At times occult bronchogenic carcinoma may produce massive hemorrhagic pericarditis. The primary lesion may be too minute to be detected radiologically. Identification of tumor cells in pericardial fluid may confirm a neoplastic cause; however, expert cytologic examination is necessary to differentiate these cells from normal mesothelial cells. Even experts may disagree in the interpretation of cells found in the pericardial fluid. Myxedema may induce pericardial effusion (see Chap. 93). Chylopericardium may result from anomalous lymphatic drainage into the pericardium. Cholesterol pericarditis with deposits of cholesterol may occur.

Treatment

The treatment of acute pericarditis consists of relief of symptoms and the treatment of the underlying

systemic illness. In idiopathic benign pericarditis, reassurance, bed rest as long as fever and pain persist, and aspirin for relief of pain are usually all that is required. Although adrenal steroids have been shown to relieve the discomfort of this disorder,[30] the possibility of tuberculous and other varieties of infectious pericarditis can seldom be dismissed. Thus, one should use these drugs wisely and carefully in an illness which usually follows a benign course. When the diagnosis is clearly nontuberculous and pain is unrelieved by salicylates, the administration of indomethacin or corticosteroids may produce dramatic results. I usually give prednisone, 60 mg/day, in divided doses for 3 weeks (adult dosage). The dosage is reduced 5 to 10 mg/day each week to 30 mg/day and then is reduced 2.5 mg/day at weekly intervals.

The treatment of rheumatic pericarditis is that of the underlying rheumatic fever and usually requires a period of bed rest. Therapeutic doses of penicillin, for 10 days to 2 weeks, and continuous prophylactic penicillin thereafter are recommended. Since there are underlying myocarditis and endocarditis, the use of adrenal steroids for 3 to 6 weeks should be strongly considered.

When a tuberculous etiology seems possible because of the clinical setting and clinical course, the treatment should include long-term therapy for tuberculosis. The patient should be placed at bed rest as long as he or she is febrile. Isoniazid, 300 mg/day orally, is administered along with ethambutol 15 mg/kg body weight daily (adult dosage). This therapy is continued for 1 to 2 years. Streptomycin, 1 g/day intramuscularly, is given until the patient becomes afebrile. The streptomycin dosage is then reduced to 1 g twice weekly and continued for 1 year. Lyons et al. believe that the mortality and morbidity may be less when triple therapy for tuberculosis *plus* corticosteroids are used.[65] Accordingly, they would favor the use of corticosteroids in most cases. The majority of cases seen at the Cincinnati General Hospital have been diagnosed early in the course of the illness, and the patients have responded well to antituberculous chemotherapy, requiring neither adrenal steroids nor operation. If the patient is seen late in the illness or has recurrent effusion or tamponade, it is wise to add adrenal steroids to the triple therapy for tuberculosis. In our series of 20 patients, only 1 died; 7 required surgical resection.

Persistent elevation of venous pressure, unrelieved dyspnea, hepatomegaly, or ascites, despite the above drug therapy, indicate that surgical resection of the pericardium should be considered.[70]

Patients who have acute cardiac tamponade following direct trauma to the heart from stab or gunshot wounds must be treated as emergencies. The rise in intrapericardial pressure interferes with cardiac filling, and cardiac output rapidly becomes inadequate to sustain life. Intravenous infusion of saline solution or other fluid may temporarily improve blood pressure until cardiac tamponade can be relieved. It is the policy at the Cincinnati General Hospital to treat the patient by one or two needle aspirations of the pericardial space. If the symptoms of cardiac tamponade are not relieved by needle aspiration or if they return after a second aspiration, then thoracotomy is required in order to suture the lacerated myocardium or blood vessel.

Uremic pericarditis, as well as the remainder of the uremic syndrome, may be treated by peritoneal dialysis, by hemodialysis, or by renal transplant in selected instances.

When specific infectious pericarditis related to disease of the left pleural space or to septicemia is treated with the appropriate antibiotics, surgical drainage may or may not be necessary. Surgical therapy, however, must not be delayed if the response is poor.

Pericarditis in lupus erythematosus usually responds to adrenal steroid therapy, although occasionally cardiac tamponade develops and pericardial aspiration is required.

Postthoracotomy and postmyocardial infarction syndromes should be managed in the same way as acute benign pericarditis. In either of the three disorders, recurrences are common. In the event of numerous recurrences, surgical resection of the pericardium may be considered, but the results are often disappointing.

Pericardial effusion caused by certain types of neoplastic disease may be treated by instillation of thiotepa (triethylenethiophosphoramide) into the pericardial space; however, surgical resection of the pericardium may be needed.

Pericardial effusion due to myxedema rarely produces cardiac tamponade; it responds to thyroid medication. Adrenal steroid therapy may be useful in postradiation pericarditis, and in pericarditis following administration of certain drugs, such as procainamide.

NEEDLE ASPIRATION OF THE PERICARDIAL SPACE

Needle aspiration of the pericardial space may be performed in patients with acute pericarditis for one of two major purposes: (1) to confirm the diagnosis and to attempt to establish the underlying cause; (2) to relieve acute cardiac tamponade. Needle aspiration of the pericardial space is a major procedure. Laceration of a coronary artery or of the myocardium may cause death from cardiac tamponade. Either ventricular fibrillation or vagovagal arrest is another complication. Needle aspiration of the pericardium is performed with the patient's thorax at 60° from the horizontal. The needle is inserted preferably in one of two places.[71] One may employ the subxiphoid approach, with the needle inserted in the angle between the left costal margin and the xiphoid and directed toward the right shoulder. This approach is favored by this writer. A second choice is near the cardiac apex, about 2 cm inside the left border of cardiac dullness, with the needle directed toward the

fourth dorsal vertebra. The needle should have a short bevel in order to minimize the danger of laceration.

If a grossly bloody fluid is obtained, its hematocrit should be compared with the patient's blood hematocrit to be certain that the needle is not in the cardiac chambers. Failure of the bloody fluid to clot offers further assurance that it is not obtained from within the heart. The author has seen a fatality result from injection of air into a cardiac chamber when injection into the pericardial space was intended. The injection of air into the pericardial space may demonstrate the size of the heart, the thickness of the parietal pericardium, and the amount of pericardial effusion. Patients with benign pericarditis more commonly have a thin pericardium, but it may become thickened. Patients with tuberculous or neoplastic pericarditis more commonly have a thickened pericardium. In many hospitals it is a practice that aspiration of the pericardium should be performed by a thoracic surgeon in order that he may be available to deal with any emergency which may arise. During the procedure the electrocardiogram should be monitored, as well as blood pressure and venous pressure. A cardiac defibrillator and apparatus for artificial respiration should be at hand. Immediate decline of venous pressure and rise of systemic blood pressure following pericardial aspiration offer convincing proof of cardiac tamponade. If repeated aspirations are needed for the relief of cardiac tamponade, prompt surgical resection of the pericardium is indicated. In recent years we have observed three deaths caused by needle pericardiocentesis, despite the use of great care and supervision of the procedure by experienced personnel. It is our present opinion that needle aspiration of the pericardial sac should be largely limited to the emergency relief of cardiac tamponade. For the purpose of diagnosis, the procedure of open surgical drainage and biopsy of the pericardium is likely to be both safer and more informative.

CARDIAC TAMPONADE

Traditionally, cardiac tamponade has been characterized by three clinical features: a rising venous pressure, a falling arterial blood pressure, and a small quiet heart.[72] I should like to emphasize that this description applies primarily to cardiac tamponade of very rapid onset, in particular that following such cardiac trauma as gunshot or stab wounds. Strict reliance on these criteria may cause the diagnosis to be missed if one is dealing with cardiac tamponade of more gradual onset associated with neoplasm or infection. The diagnosis will not be missed if the possibility is considered in every patient who has an increased systemic venous pressure.

Cardiac tamponade may be defined as an impairment of diastolic filling of the heart caused by an unchecked rise in intrapericardial pressure. The hemodynamic manifestations of accumulation of fluid in the pericardial sac depend on the rapidity with which the fluid accumulates. If the fluid accumulates very rapidly, a few hundred milliliters of blood or other fluid can cause fatal cardiac tamponade (Fig.

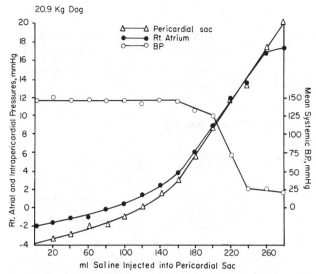

FIGURE 84-9 Graph showing the production of cardiac tamponade by serial injections of saline solution into the pericardial sac of an anesthetized dog. As more than 160 ml saline solution was injected into the pericardial sac, right atrial and intrapericardial pressures rose more steeply and blood pressure fell more abruptly. Blood pressure fell to shock levels as intrapericardial pressure exceeded 14 mm Hg. *(From N. O. Fowler, "Cardiac Diagnosis and Treatment," Harper & Row, Publishers, Inc., Hagerstown, 1976, p. 863. By permission.)*

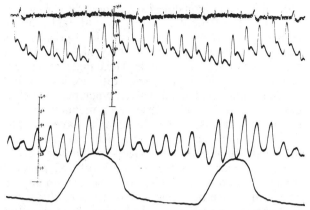

FIGURE 84-10 Pressure pulse record in patient with cardiac tamponade produced by tuberculous pericarditis. *A.* Electrocardiogram. *B.* Direct intraarterial recording of blood pressure. *C.* Right ventricular pressure pulse recording. *D.* A record of respiration; inspiration moves the trace upward. One may observe considerable paradoxical pulse in the blood pressure record; there is a very high diastolic blood pressure in the right ventricle which averages somewhat better than 20 mm Hg, the normal being 0 to 5 mm Hg. *(From N. O. Fowler, Cardiac Catheterization in Adult Heart Disease, Ann. Intern. Med., 38:387, 1953. By permission.)*

84-9). On the other hand, when fluid accumulates slowly within the pericardial sac, its fibrous wall will stretch gradually, and several liters of fluid may not produce cardiac tamponade. The diagnosis of cardiac tamponade, then, depends on the demonstration not only of pericardial fluid but also of the characteristic hemodynamic features.

Physiology

Normally, intrapericardial pressure is similar to intrapleural pressure. There is an expiratory negative pressure of a few millimeters of mercury, with a further decline of 2 to 5 mm Hg in inspiration. In tamponade the elevated intrapericardial pressure still displays an inspiratory fall.[3] Systemic venous pressure and right atrial pressure rise to maintain cardiac filling[73] (Fig. 84-9). Ventricular end-diastolic volume is reduced, ventricular end-systolic volume tends to be normal, and there is a decreased ventricular ejection fraction.[74] Although cardiac stroke volume is diminished, tachycardia at first compensates sufficiently so that a relatively normal cardiac output is maintained. However, as the pericardial pressure rises further, the heart can no longer compensate, and then cardiac output begins to decrease. At first, an increase of peripheral vascular resistance aids in maintaining blood pressure; with further tamponade, blood pressure begins to fall dramatically. With the rise of intrapericardial pressure, the left and right ventricular diastolic pressures rise, as do the right and left atrial and systemic and pulmonary venous pressures. With cardiac tamponade the systemic venous pressure is usually at least 14 cm of water and often considerably more.[75] With tamponade the pressure in the pericardial sac is at least 10 mm Hg. The

systemic arteries usually display a paradoxical pulse, which may be defined as an abnormal inspiratory decline in systolic blood pressure (greater than 10 mm Hg) (Fig. 84-10). The paradoxical pulse is almost universally present in tamponade. In my experience this finding has been a valuable clue to the recognition of this disorder when other findings are equivocal. However, with acute tamponade—for example, that caused by cardiac trauma—the arterial pulses may be impalpable.

Etiology

Cardiac tamponade is most commonly related to one of three causes: (1) trauma which may be direct or indirect, penetrating or nonpenetrating; (2) infection; (3) neoplastic disease (Table 84-2). One should be alert to the possibility of tamponade whenever pericarditis is present, especially when it is caused by one of these three conditions. One must be alert to this possibility even in the absence of known infection, trauma, or malignant disease. Often the under-

TABLE 84-2
Common causes of cardiac tamponade

1 Trauma
2 Malignant disease
3 Specific infections: bacterial, tuberculosis
4 Anticoagulants in idiopathic, uremic, or malignant pericarditis
5 Idiopathic pericarditis
6 Rupture of heart or great vessels
7 Iatrogenic (diagnostic procedures, transvenous pacing)
8 Acute rheumatic fever
9 Following cardiac operation

lying disease responsible for tamponade is inapparent when the patient is first seen with tachycardia, high venous pressure, and falling blood pressure. In many patients anticoagulants may have caused or contributed to the tamponade. The dangers of anticoagulants in patients with pericarditis are known, but at times anticoagulants are given when pericarditis is unrecognized. We have observed patients with idiopathic pericarditis, thought in error to have myocardial infarction, in whom cardiac tamponade has followed the use of anticoagulants. In one series, uremic pericarditis occurred in 25 of 152 patients treated by chronic dialysis.[76] In patients with uremic pericarditis, hemodialysis may be followed by cardiac tamponade related to the use of heparin. With myocardial infarction or malignant disease cardiac tamponade has been seen in patients receiving anticoagulants. Admittedly, we cannot be certain that the anticoagulants played a leading role in these particular patients, but heparin, given in the first few days of infarction has been associated with tamponade in a number of instances in my experience. Other causes of tamponade are neoplasm, rupture of the heart or great vessels, trauma, dissecting aneurysm, nondissecting aneurysm, and myocardial infarction. Cardiac tamponade may be iatrogenic, following diagnostic puncture of the left or right ventricle or transvenous pacing of the heart.[77] Inadvertent injection of radiopaque contrast medium into the pericardial sac may be followed by tamponade, since the contrast material is hypertonic.[78] Rarely, rheumatic fever may cause cardiac tamponade; we have observed a few examples of this.

It is important to examine the neck veins closely when patients are suspected of having cardiac tamponade. When a patient is acutely ill with high venous pressure, a paradoxical arterial pulse strongly suggests tamponade. Figure 84-10 is a recording of blood pressure, right ventricular pressure, and respiration of a patient with cardiac tamponade produced by tuberculous pericarditis. There is striking respiratory variation in blood pressure. The systolic pressure during expiration is as high as 130 mm Hg but declines to approximately 85 mm Hg during inspiration (pulsus paradoxus). The right ventricular pulse pressure is very small in expiration; the mean systolic pressure in the right ventricle is approximately normal. With inspiration the pulse pressure in the right ventricle increases. This is consonant with increased inspiratory filling of the right ventricle, which is believed to occur during cardiac tamponade as in the normal individual.[4] In cardiac tamponade the cardiac rhythm is usually that of sinus tachycardia. Occasionally one may find atrial arrhythmias, especially atrial flutter and atrial fibrillation.

Electrocardiographic findings

The electrocardiogram may show the changes typical of acute pericarditis (Fig. 84-3), but these features are often not observed and the electrocardiographic

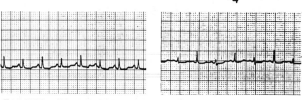

EM 38º   Cardiac Tamponade

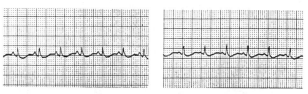

After removal   640 ml   pericardial fluid.

FIGURE 84-11 Electrical alternans of the QRS complexes of the ECG in a 38-year-old woman with cardiac tamponade. The lower record was made the day after relief of tamponade, and the alternans is no longer present. Alternans of the QRS complexes only is not diagnostic of cardiac tamponade, but total alternans involving P, QRS, and T complexes is said to be virtually limited to patients with cardiac tamponade.

changes may be relatively nonspecific. The voltage of the QRS and T complexes is often low. There may be nonspecific ST or T wave changes. Occasionally there are more specific changes. Figure 84-11 shows electrical alternans of the QRS complexes in the electrocardiogram of a 38-year-old woman with cardiac tamponade caused by metastatic malignant neoplasm. This finding is suggestive but not diagnostic of cardiac tamponade. It may occur with pericarditis without tamponade, and with emphysema, hypertensive disease, or coronary disease, among others. It has been said that if P, QRS, and T complexes all show alternans, this observation is virtually diagnostic of cardiac tamponade. However, this combination is extremely rare, in our experience.

Clinical features (Table 84-3)

One of the common antecedent conditions—infection, neoplasm, or trauma—may be recognized. Dyspnea is usually present. Typical orthopnea is often absent, but the patient may be leaning far forward in an attempt to relieve dyspnea. Sinus

TABLE 84-3
Cardiac tamponade: clinical features

1 Dyspnea
2 Orthopnea
3 Tachycardia
4 Elevated venous pressure and hepatic engorgement
5 Decreased systolic blood pressure with narrow pulse pressure
6 Pulsus paradoxus
7 Heart sounds: normal or faint
8 Chest x-ray: cardiopericardial silhouette normal or enlarged, lungs clear
9 Cardiac fluoroscopy: cardiac pulsations normal or diminished
10 ECG: ST elevation or nonspecific T wave changes; occasional electrical alternans

tachycardia is usually found. There is elevated systemic venous pressure, which can usually be appreciated by the observation of distended neck veins with the patient's trunk at 45° from the horizontal. The liver is engorged. The systolic blood pressure is usually decreased, and occasionally with severe tamponade the pulse and blood pressure are unobtainable. A paradoxical pulse is to be expected. I would emphasize that palpation of the femoral artery may be of help in finding the paradoxical pulse; the pulse may be more difficult to feel or evaluate at the wrist when the blood pressure is extremely low. Even with severe cardiac tamponade the heart sounds may be of good quality.[79] We have seen patients in whom the diagnosis of cardiac tamponade was dismissed in error because the heart sounds were well heard. However, heart sounds are often faint in tamponade of rapid onset following cardiac trauma. The cardiac apical impulse is usually not readily felt. A ventricular gallop rhythm is usually absent in cardiac tamponade, although occasionally it is found. The presence of gallop rhythm and an apical impulse displaced downward and outward are strong evidence in favor of cardiac enlargement and congestive heart failure, rather than cardiac tamponade, as the cause of elevated venous pressure and dyspnea.

Radiologic studies

Roentgenograms are often helpful. The cardiopericardial silhouette may be of normal size or only slightly increased, and the lung fields typically are clear. Pulmonary edema is uncommon in cardiac tamponade. Cardiac fluoroscopy is of limited diagnostic value in a patient suspected of having cardiac tamponade. When there is cardiac trauma with rapid onset of tamponade, the heart usually appears quiet on fluoroscopy. But in the patients with more gradual onset of tamponade the radiologist may describe pulsations of normal quality. If suggested clinically, tamponade should not be dismissed when the radiologist reports that cardiac pulsations appear normal. Occasionally, with image-intensifier fluoroscopy, one can identify an *epicardial fat line* well inside the lateral border of the cardiopericardial silhouette; this observation suggests the presence of pericardial fluid but not necessarily of tamponade. This evidence of pericardial effusion is to be expected, however, in only the minority of patients with cardiac tamponade. If cardiac tamponade is suspected and time permits, it is desirable to demonstrate that there is in fact pericardial fluid. Pericardial fluid occurs commonly in advanced biventricular congestive heart failure,[80] or in pericarditis without cardiac tamponade. The demonstration of fluid indicates that tamponade is possible, but this finding is not diagnostic of cardiac compression.

The echocardiogram is a very sensitive method of detecting pericardial effusion (Fig. 84-8),[59] and this is the method which we usually employ.

Treatment

Unless there is a desperate need for immediate pericardiocentesis because of unconsciousness or shock, we prefer to confirm the presence of pericardial fluid with echocardiography. Then if the clinical features of cardiac tamponade are also present, the usual treatment is aspiration of fluid from the pericardial sac. Dramatic improvement in blood pressure and in cardiac output may occur with removal of as little as 25 ml of fluid, although usually more is removed. If aspiration cannot be carried out promptly, blood pressure may be improved by transfusion of saline solution or plasma, or the intravenous infusion of such positive inotropic drugs as isoproterenol.[81] Blood transfusion may be desirable if the patient has suffered trauma and blood has been lost.

Once cardiac tamponade has been relieved, the therapeutic task is not finished. One must consider then the cause of the cardiac tamponade, and what should be done to prevent recurrence. The pericardial fluid should be studied to establish the cause. If the patient is receiving anticoagulants, they are discontinued promptly. Mephyton is given if the patient has been receiving warfarin. Specific therapy should be directed toward the cause. Bacterial infections require specific antibiotics; tuberculosis requires streptomycin, ethambutol, and isoniazid. Adrenal steroids may be needed in idiopathic pericarditis. Logue and associates[82] find the administration of a combination of adrenal steroids and diuretics useful in some patients in the recognition of pericardial effusion and in the prevention and management of cardiac tamponade. Such therapy reduces the size of the transverse diameter of the heart an average of 3½ cm within 1 week in patients with pericardial effusion. This reduction does not occur in patients with myocardial disease without heart failure. Surgical treatment may be indicated in any one of several possible situations. One of these exists when tamponade is a reasonably certain diagnosis and either fluid cannot be obtained or the removal of the fluid does not relieve the tamponade. Surgical treatment is essential when fluid repeatedly reaccumulates with recurrent tamponade. Surgical treatment may be the treatment of choice when tamponade is caused by trauma. In the past we have treated traumatic tamponade by aspirating the pericardial sac once or twice, and then resorting to open surgical treatment if further reaccumulation occurred. However, some authorities believe that surgical treatment should be used when there is traumatic bleeding into the pericardial sac in order to diminish the risk of later development of pericardial thickening and scarring.[83] The patient who has had cardiac tamponade should be placed in an intensive care unit, with careful monitoring of the blood pressure and the venous pressure to indicate possible recurrence.

CHRONIC PERICARDITIS

The principal symptomatic variety of chronic pericarditis is chronic constrictive pericarditis. Many patients with chronic pericarditis are asymptomatic.

Some have chronic pericardial effusion of unknown cause. If the fluid accumulates slowly, unsuspected enlargement of the cardiac silhouette may be discovered on routine radiologic examination of the chest. In such patients, tuberculosis, neoplastic disease, or scleroderma, in addition to asymptomatic idiopathic pericarditis, should be considered in the differential diagnosis. In many instances, the cause of chronic and asymptomatic pericardial effusion cannot be established. The physician should remember that myxedema may produce considerable pericardial effusion. Cholesterol pericarditis may be associated with myxedema but does not have specific etiologic implications. It may follow acute pericarditis of any cause, including tuberculosis, rheumatoid arthritis, and myocardial infarction.[85] In other patients with chronic pericarditis radiologic examination reveals calcification of the pericardium. Such patients are often asymptomatic and without significant cardiac constriction. Other patients are discovered to have pericardial adhesions or thickening at autopsy after death from an unrelated illness. External adhesions which bind the pericardium to the chest wall are no longer believed to cause cardiac enlargement or embarrassment of cardiac function. Our discussion of chronic pericarditis will deal principally with cardiac constriction. In such patients the complaints are usually similar to those of congestive heart failure except that they often begin very gradually. There is a tendency to develop ascites relatively early. Exertional dyspnea is a common complaint but may be inconspicuous in the presence of edema and ascites. Orthopnea and nocturnal dyspnea are unusual, in contrast to the course of events in ordinary forms of congestive heart failure. Fatigue with effort may be a major complaint. Chest pain is absent as a rule. There are, however, patients who pursue a course intermediate between acute pericarditis and chronic constrictive pericarditis. Such patients develop a rather acute pericarditis caused by tuberculosis, rheumatoid arthritis, acute idiopathic pericarditis, or trauma, for example, and then progress to cardiac constriction in a matter of a few weeks or months. In recent years, this form of constrictive pericarditis has been more common at the University of Cincinnati Hospitals than the classic variety of chronic constrictive pericarditis which develops slowly over several or many years. Hancock has recently described subacute effusive and constrictive pericarditis in which there are features of both tamponade and constriction of the heart.[86] Chronic constrictive pericarditis is a rare disease, and in most major hospitals only a few instances are seen in a year.[87] At the Mayo Clinic, 79 instances were observed during a 10-year period.[42]

Cause of chronic constrictive pericarditis

The cause of chronic constrictive pericarditis (Table 84-4) remains in doubt in many patients. It can be

TABLE 84-4
Etiologic classification of chronic constrictive pericarditis

1 Idiopathic
2 Specific infections
   a Bacterial infections
   b Tuberculosis
   c Fungous disease: histoplasmosis
   d Viral disease: Coxsackie B-3 virus
3 Connective tissue diseases: rheumatoid disease, lupus erythematosus
4 Neoplastic disease
   a Primary: mesothelioma or sarcoma
   b Secondary: bronchogenic carcinoma, breast cancer, lymphoma, leukemia
5 Trauma, penetrating or nonpenetrating
6 X-irradiation
7 Uremia, especially after hemodialysis[84]

shown by histologic examination of the removed pericardium that approximately 17 percent of instances are caused by tuberculosis.[87] It has been learned in recent years that idiopathic pericarditis can be followed by constrictive pericarditis.[42] A study of 72 patients with constrictive pericarditis at the Mayo Clinic revealed that in 2 the disease developed after acute idiopathic pericarditis.[88] We have observed two instances of this at the University of Cincinnati Hospitals. Acute pericarditis caused by Coxsackie B-3 virus was followed by constrictive pericarditis in one instance.[89] Cardiac trauma followed by bleeding into the pericardial space may be followed by constrictive pericarditis.[35] At the Cincinnati General Hospital one instance of constrictive pericarditis following tularemic pericarditis was observed. Constrictive pericarditis may follow irradiation pneumonitis and pericarditis,[39] it may follow rheumatoid arthritis,[38] and it may be associated with neoplastic invasion of the pericardium.[90] Histoplasmosis[91] or nocardiosis[92] may be followed by constrictive pericarditis. Rheumatic fever may be followed by adhesive pericarditis and pericardial calcification but seldom, if ever, by constrictive pericarditis. Uremic pericarditis may be followed by constrictive pericarditis.[76]

Physical examination

The physical examination of a patient with constrictive pericarditis reveals the signs of cardiac compression that were described earlier in this chapter. However, the arterial pulse pressure is often normal. An important and almost invariable sign is elevation of the venous pressure, as best judged clinically by the observation of distension of the neck veins with the patient at a 45° angle from the horizontal. The cervical venous pulse characteristically shows a deep *y* trough. In cardiac tamponade the *y* trough is not conspicuous.[24] Kussmaul's sign, viz., inspiratory swelling of the neck veins, may be present. This sign is not diagnostic of constrictive pericarditis. A paradoxical pulse is found in a minority of patients.[93] The method of examination for this sign was discussed earlier in this chapter. The heart sounds are often distant, but not invariably so. A pericardial knock sound may be heard at the cardiac apex[94] (Fig. 84-12).

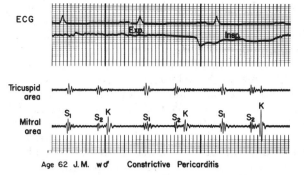

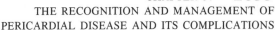

FIGURE 84-12 Phonocardiogram showing pericardial knock sound (K), following the second heart sound (S₂) by 0.09 s.

This sound follows the second heart sound by 0.06 to 0.12 s. It sounds much like a gallop at the cardiac apex but is shorter and occurs somewhat earlier in diastole. Cardiac murmurs are usually absent. The heart size is usually normal or moderately enlarged. The apex impulse is felt with difficulty, if at all. Pulmonary rales are uncommon. The liver is usually enlarged and may be firmer than normal. Cardiac cirrhosis is a common complication. Ascites is a common finding. Some dependent edema may be present but is often absent. There is usually no pericardial friction rub, but one may be heard on rare occasions. Rarely, the nephrotic syndrome may occur.

Laboratory data

ELECTROCARDIOGRAM OF CONSTRICTIVE PERICARDITIS

The electrocardiogram is often abnormal but is usually not diagnostic. Characteristic changes are low voltage of the QRS complexes, especially in the limb leads, with flattening or negativity of the T waves in most leads (Fig. 84-13). Atrial fibrillation is present in one-fourth to one-third of these patients. Atrial flutter is found in a few patients. Some patients have an electrocardiographic pattern which resembles right ventricular hypertrophy. Electrocardiographic patterns of left ventricular hypertrophy, or either right or left bundle branch block are extremely unusual.

FIGURE 84-13 Electrocardiogram of a patient with chronic constrictive pericarditis. Note the low voltage of QRS complexes and negative T waves.

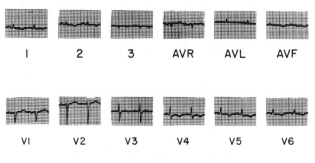

T.D. CONSTRICTIVE PERICARDITIS

RADIOLOGIC STUDIES

Radiologic studies characteristically demonstrate clear lung fields. The heart may be small but occasionally is found on radiologic study to be slightly enlarged. In more acute cardiac constriction, the cardiac silhouette may be quite large, because of a combination of pericardial thickening and pericardial fluid.[86] Calcification of the pericardium is found in 40 to 50 percent of instances, but is not diagnostic of constrictive pericarditis. Calcification of the pericardium may occur in patients who have adhesive pericarditis without cardiac constriction as a result of rheumatic fever and other illnesses. Strangely enough, cardiac fluoroscopy may reveal fairly normal cardiac pulsations in patients with constrictive pericarditis and is not invariably reliable in this respect. Angiocardiography is of much greater value and will often demonstrate thickening of the pericardium beyond the normal limit of 3 to 5 mm in patients with constrictive pericarditis. Straightening of the lateral border of the right atrium, demonstrated by angiocardiography, may suggest constrictive pericarditis (Fig. 84-14). However, this sign may be absent in constrictive pericarditis, and present with pericardial effusion.

CARDIAC CATHETERIZATION

Cardiac catheterization studies are of interest in patients with constrictive pericarditis, but the abnormalities are not specific for the disorder. Characteristic findings at cardiac catheterization are elevation of the mean right atrial pressure, an M pattern of the right atrial pressure pulse, and an early diastolic dip

FIGURE 84-14 Angiocardiogram showing straightening of the right atrial border in a patient with constrictive pericarditis confirmed at operation. This sign is not always present in constrictive pericarditis, and may be observed in patients with pericardial effusion.

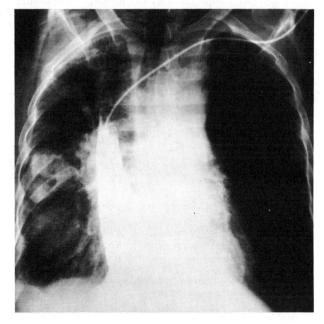

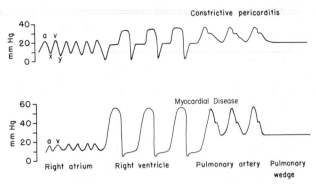

CARDIAC PRESSURES IN MYOCARDIAL AND PERICARDIAL DISEASE

FIGURE 84-15 Diagram of pressures of the right side of the heart in constrictive pericarditis as contrasted with those of myocardial disease with heart failure. Note the M pattern in the right atrial pressure pulse and the early diastolic dip in the right ventricular pressure pulse of constrictive pericarditis. The systolic right ventricular and pulmonary arterial pressures are lower in constrictive pericarditis than in myocardiopathy. In myocardiopathy, the wedge pressure exceeds the mean right atrial pressure; the two pressures are approximately equal in constrictive pericarditis. *From "Advances in Cardiopulmonary Diseases," vol. 3, edited by Banyai, Yearbook Medical Publishers, Chicago, 1966.)*

in both right and left ventricles, with an elevated end-diastolic pressure in both ventricles (Fig. 84-15). Burwell has pointed out that the characteristic finding is a pressure plateau in which the pulmonary wedge pressure, pulmonary artery diastolic pressure, right ventricular end-diastolic pressure, mean right atrial pressure, and superior vena caval pressure all tend to be identical in constrictive pericarditis.[95] However, 3 of 6 patients with myocardial fibrosis showed the same variety of pressure plateau.[96] Thus, patients with infiltrative disease of the myocardium, including amyloidosis, subendocardial fibroelastosis, and myocardial fibrosis, may demonstrate a pressure pattern similar to that of constrictive pericarditis.

Patients with biventricular heart failure also have elevated ventricular diastolic pressures, but as a rule the pulmonary wedge pressure exceeds the right atrial pressure by more than 10 mm Hg.[97] In patients with constrictive pericarditis, the pressures tend to be the same, or the pulmonary wedge pressure tends to be no more than 6 mm greater than the right atrial mean pressure. The hemodynamics of pericardial disease are contrasted with those of myocardial disease in Fig. 84-15 and Table 84-5. In constrictive pericarditis, the resting cardiac output is more likely to fall within the normal range than in myocardial disease with equivalent elevation of systemic venous pressure. Wood found relatively normal resting cardiac outputs in approximately two-thirds of 13 patients with constrictive pericarditis.[93] In cardiac tamponade the characteristic early diastolic dip in the right ventricular pressure pulse is absent.[24]

DIFFERENTIAL DIAGNOSIS

The diagnosis of constrictive pericarditis should be strongly considered in every patient who has exertional dyspnea, with or without edema, when there is persistent elevation of venous pressure after treatment for heart failure, and when there is no readily apparent variety of heart disease. The demonstration of a paradoxical pulse, clear lung fields on fluoroscopy, and a normal or moderately enlarged heart makes the diagnosis virtually certain. Echocardiography usually shows abnormal ventricular septal motion, but the findings are not usually specific.[97a] Although not diagnostic in itself, the demonstration of pericardial calcification in a patient with elevated systemic venous pressure makes constrictive pericarditis highly likely. As already pointed out, certain patients with myocardial diseases, especially those with myocardial fibrosis and amyloidosis, may present similar findings although the heart is usually larger. If the venous pressure remains elevated after maximum treatment, the use of angiocardiography to determine the thickness of the pericardium may be of critical value in making a decision as to the diagnosis. The differential diagnosis of myocardial and pericardial disease has been well presented by Burch.[98] In an occasional patient the distinction cannot be made,

TABLE 84-5
Hemodynamics of myocardial and pericardial disease

	Constrictive pericarditis	Cardiomyopathy
1 Left atrial pressure	Tends to equal RAP	10 to 20 mm Hg > RAP
2 Right atrial pressure	Usually > 15 mm Hg with prominent y trough	Usually < 15 mm Hg: normal if wedge pressure normal
3 Cardiac output	Tends to normal with normal AV difference	Usually low with increased AV difference
4 Right ventricular pressure	Consistent early diastolic dip	Early diastolic dip may disappear with therapy
5 Diastolic right ventricular pressure	Tends to equal or exceed ⅓ of systolic pressure	Usually does not equal ⅓ of systolic pressure
6 Pulmonary artery pressure	Systolic pressure usually < 40 mm Hg	Systolic pressure often 45 to 65 mm Hg
7 Respiratory variation in pressures	Tends to be absent	Usually present
8 Diastolic pressure plateau	RAP = RVDP = PADP = PWP	PWP < RAP

NOTE: RAP, right atrial pressure; AV, arteriovenous; RVDP, right ventricular diastolic pressure; PADP, pulmonary arterial diastolic pressure; PWP, pulmonary wedge pressure and it is necessary to resort to surgical exploration of the pericardium.

Treatment

The treatment of constrictive pericarditis is pericardial resection if the patient is becoming progressively disabled. Because of appreciable operative mortality, operation is not ordinarily recommended when the patient is only mildly limited in physical activity. If the patient is believed to have tuberculous pericarditis, the surgical resection should be preceded by several weeks of antituberculous therapy. Although the mortality rate for surgical resection was formerly stated to be 25 percent, it would appear that in recent years the figure has been less than this. In Wood's series, the operative mortality rate was 11 percent.[93]

REFERENCES

1 Laënnec, R. T. H.: Traité de l'auscultation médiate, William Brown, Printer, Philadelphia, 1923.

2 Holt, J. P.: The Normal Pericardium, *Am. J. Cardiol.*, 26:455, 1970.

3 Berglund, E., Sarnoff, S. J., and Isaacs, J. P.: Ventricular Function: Role of the Pericardium in Regulation of Cardiovascular Hemodynamics, *Circ. Res.*, 3:133, 1955.

4 Shabetai, R., Fowler, N. O., Fenton, J. C., and Masangkay, M.: Pulsus Paradoxus, *J. Clin. Invest.*, 44:1882, 1965.

5 Szidon, J. P., Lahiri, S., Lev, M., and Fishman, A. P.: Heart and Circulation of the African Lung Fish, *Circ. Res.*, 25:23, 1969.

6 Ellis, K., Leeds, N. E., and Himmelstein, A.: Congenital Deficiencies in the Parietal Pericardium: A Review of 2 New Cases Including Successful Diagnosis by Plane Roentgenography, *Am. J. Roentgenol. Radium Ther. Nucl. Med.*, 82:125, 1959.

7 Nasser, W. K., Helmen, C., Tavel, M. E., et al.: Congenital Absence of the Left Pericardium, *Circulation*, 41:469, 1970.

8 Glancy, D. L., Saunders, C. V., and Porta, A.: Posterior Chest Wall Pulsation in Congenital Complete Absence of the Left Pericardium, *Chest*, 65:564, 1974.

9 Hipona, F. A., Crummy, A. J., Jr.: Congenital Pericardial Defect Associated with Tetralogy of Fallot, *Circulation*, 29:132, 1964.

10 Spitz, L., Bloom, F., Milner, S., and Levin, S. E.: Combined Anterior Abdominal Wall, Sternal, Diaphragmatic, Pericardial, and Intracardiac Defects: A Report of 5 Cases and Their Management, *J. Pediatr. Surg.*, 10:491, 1975.

11 Payvandi, M. N., and Kerber, R. E.: Echocardiography in Congenital and Acquired Absence of the Pericardium, *Circulation*, 53:86, 1976.

12 Robin, E., Gangerly, S. N., and Fowler, M. S.: Strangulation of the Left Atrial Appendage Through a Congenital Partial Pericardial Defect, *Chest*, 67:354, 1975.

13 Carty, J. E., Deverall, J. B., and Losowsky, M. S.: Pericardial Defect Presenting as Acute Pericarditis, *Br. Heart J.*, 37:98, 1975.

14 Lind, T. A., Pitt, M. J., Groves, B. M., et al.: The Abnormal Left Hilum, *Circulation*, 51:183, 1975.

15 Klatte, E. C., and Yune, H. Y.: Diagnosis and Treatment of Pericardial Cysts, *Radiology*, 104:541, 1972.

16 Capps, J. A.: Pain from the Pleura and Pericardium, *Proc. Assoc. Res. Nerv. Ment. Dis.*, 23:263, 1943.

17 Weissbein, A. S., and Heller, F. N.: A Method of Treatment for Pericardial Pain, *Circulation*, 24:607, 1961.

18 Shabetai, R., Fowler, N. O., and Gueron, M.: The Effects of

Respiration on Aortic Pressure and Flow, *Am. Heart J.*, 65:525, 1963.

19 Rebuck, A. S., and Pengelly, L. D.: Pulsus Paradoxus in the Presence of Airways Obstruction, *N. Engl. J. Med.*, 288:66, 1973.

20 Gauchat, H. W., and Katz, L. N.: Observations on Pulsus Paradoxus (with Special Reference to Pericardial Effusions), *A.M.A. Arch, Intern. Med.*, 33:350, 1924.

21 Dock, W.: Inspiratory Traction on the Pericardium: The Cause of Pulsus Paradoxus in Pericardial Disease, *A.M.A. Arch. Intern. Med.*, 108:837, 1961.

22 Dornhorst, A. C., Howard, P., and Leathart, G. C.: Pulsus Paradoxus, *Lancet*, 1:746, 1952.

23 Shabetai, R., Fowler, N. O., and Fenton, J. C.: Respiratory Variation in Blood Pressure (P), *Circulation*, 28:802, 1963.

24 Shabetai, R., Fowler, N. O., and Guntheroth, W. G.: The Hemodynamics of Cardiac Tamponade and Constrictive Pericarditis, *Am. J. Cardiol.*, 26:480, 1970.

25 D'Cruz, I. A., Cohen, H. C., Prabhu, R., and Glick, G.: Diagnosis of Cardiac Tamponade by Echocardiography, *Circulation*, 52:460, 1975.

26 Yahini, J. H., Goor, D., Kraus, Y., Pauzner, Y. M., and Neufeld, H. N.: Atrial Septal Defect and Constrictive Pericarditis, *Am. J. Cardiol.*, 17:718, 1966.

27 Cohn, J. N., Pinkerson, A. L., and Tristani, F. E.: Mechanism of Pulsus Paradoxus in Clinical Shock, *J. Clin. Invest.*, 46:1744, 1967.

28 Engle, M. A.: Cardiac Involvement in Cooley's Anemia, *Ann. N. Y. Acad. Sci.*, 119:694, 1964.

29 Wolff, L., and Grunfeld, O.: Pericarditis, *N. Eng. J. Med.*, 268:419, 1963.

30 Connolly, D. C., and Burchell, N. B.: Pericarditis: A Ten Year Survey, *Am. J. Cardiol.*, 7:7, 1961.

31 Grist, N. R., and Bell, E. J.: Coxsackie Viruses and the Heart, *Am. Heart J.*, 77:295, 1969 (editorial).

32 Clinicopathologic Conference: Pericardial Disease with Effusion, Systemic Involvement and Pulmonary Edema, *Am. J. Med.*, 33:442, 1962.

33 Harvey, A. M., Shulman, L. E., Tumulty, P. A., Conley, C. L., and Schoenrich, E. H.: Systemic Lupus Erythematosus: Review of the Literature and Clinical Analysis of 138 Cases, *Medicine*, 33:291, 1954.

34 Fowler, N. O.: "Cardiac Diagnosis," Harper & Row, Publishers, Incorporated, New York, 1968.

35 Schaffer, A. I.: Case of Traumatic Pericarditis with Chronic Tamponade and Constriction, *Am. J. Cardiol.*, 7:125, 1961.

36 Kennedy, W. P. U., Partridge, E. R. H., and Matthews, M. B.: Rheumatoid Pericarditis with Cardiac Failure Treated by Pericardiectomy, *Br. Heart J.*, 28:602, 1966.

37 Franco, A. E., Levine, H. D., and Hall, A. P.: Rheumatoid Pericarditis: Report of 17 Cases Diagnosed Clinically, *Ann. Intern. Med.*, 77:837, 1972.

38 Keith, T. A., III: Chronic Constrictive Pericarditis in Association with Rheumatoid Disease, *Circulation*, 25:477, 1962.

39 Cohn, K. E., Stewart, J. R., Fujardo, L. F., and Hancock, E. W.: Heart Disease Following Radiation, *Medicine*, 46:281, 1967.

40 Bloomer, W. D., and Hellman, S.: Normal Tissue Responses to Radiation Therapy, *N. Engl. J. Med.*, 293:80, 1975.

41 Friedman, J. L., Baum, G. L., and Schwarz, J.: Primary Pulmonary Histoplasmosis, *Am. J. Dis. Child.*, 109:298, 1965.

42 Picardi, J., Kauffman, C. A., Schwarz, J., Holmes, J. C., Phair, J. P., and Fowler, N. O.: Pericarditis Caused by *Histoplasma capsulatum*: Report of 16 Cases and Review of the Literature, *Am. J. Cardiol.*, 37:82, 1976.

43 Soloway, M., Morr, T. W., and Linton, D. C., Jr.: Takayasu's

Arteritis: Report of a Case with Unusual Findings, *Am. J. Cardiol.,* 25:258, 1974.

44 Buchbinder, N. A., and Roberts, W. C.: Left-sided Valvular Active Infective Endocarditis: A Study of Forty-Five Necropsy Patients, *Am. J. Med.,* 53:20, 1972.

45 Rab, A. M., Alam, N., Hoda, A. N., and Yee, A.: Amebic Liver Abscess: Some Unique Presentations, *Am. J. Med.,* 43:811, 1967.

46 Theologides, A., and Kennedy, B. J.: Toxoplasmic Myocarditis and Pericarditis, *Am. J. Med.,* 47:169, 1969 (editorial).

47 Morse, J. R., Oretsky, M. I., and Hudson, J. A.: Pericarditis as a Complication of Meningococcal Meningitis, *Ann. Intern. Med.,* 74:212, 1971.

48 Holmes, K. K., Counts, G. W., and Beaty, H. N.: Disseminated Gonococcal Infection, *Ann. Intern. Med.,* 74:979, 1971.

49 Morton, D. L., Kagan, A. R., Roberts, W. C., et al.: Pericardiectomy for Radiation-induced Pericarditis with Effusion, *Ann. Thorac. Surg.,* 8:195, 1969.

50 Beaudry, C., Nakamoto, S., and Kolff, W. J.: Uremic Pericarditis and Cardiac Tamponade in Chronic Renal Failure, *Ann. Intern. Med.,* 64:990, 1966.

51 Alarcon-Segovia, D.: Drug-induced Lupus Syndromes, *Proc. Staff Meet. Mayo Clin.,* 44:664, 1969.

52 Barnes, A. R., and Burchell, H. B.: Acute Pericarditis Simulating Acute Coronary Occlusion: A Report of Fourteen Cases, *Am. Heart J.,* 23:247, 1942.

53 Schreiner, G. E., and Maher, J. F.: "Uremia: Biochemistry, Pathogenesis and Treatment," Charles C Thomas, Publisher, Springfield, Ill., 1961, p.301.

54 Fowler, N. O., Gueron, M., and Rowlands, D. T.: Primary Myocardial Disease, *Circulation,* 23:498, 1961.

55 Fowler, N. O.: The Electrocardiogram in Pericarditis, *Cardiovasc. Clin.,* 5:256, 1974.

56 Surawicz, B., and Lassiter, K. D.: Electrocardiogram in Pericarditis, *Am. J. Cardiol.,* 26:471, 1970.

56a Spodick, D. H.: Electrocardiographic Sequences in Acute Pericarditis: Significance of P-R Segment and P-R Vector Changes, *Circulation,* 48:575, 1973.

57 Wagner, H. N., Jr., McAfee, J. G., and Mosley, J. M.: Medical Radioisotope Scanning, *J.A.M.A.,* 174(1):162, 1960.

58 Durant, T. M.: Negative (Gas) Contrast Angiocardiography, *Am. Heart J.,* 61:1, 1961.

59 Feigenbaum, H.: Echocardiographic Diagnosis of Pericardial Effusion, *Am. J. Cardiol.,* 26:475, 1970.

59a Berman, D. S., Amsterdam, E. A., Hines, H. H., Salel, A. F., Bailey, G. J., DeNardo, G. L., and Mason, D. T.: New Approach to Interpretation of Technetium-99m Pyrophosphate Scintigraphy in Detection of Acute Myocardial Infarction, *Am. J. Cardiol.,* 39:341, 1977.

60 Semple, T., and Lancaster, W. M: Noisy Pneumothorax: Observations Based on 24 Cases, *Br. Med. J.,* 1:1342, 1961.

61 Hamman, L.: Spontaneous Mediastinal Emphysema, *Bull. Johns Hopkins Hosp.,* 64:1, 1939.

62 McGuire, J., Kotte, J. H., and Helm, R. A.: Acute Pericarditis, *Circulation,* 9:425, 1954.

63 Johnson, R. T., Portnoy, B., Rogers, N. G., and Buescher, E. L.: Acute Benign Pericarditis: Virologic Study of 34 Patients, *Arch. Intern. Med.,* 108:823, 1961.

64 Fowler, N. O., and Manitsas, G. T.: Infectious Pericarditis, *Prog. Cardiovasc. Dis.,* 16:323, 1973.

65 Lyons, H. A., Rooney, J. J., and Crocco, J. A.: Tuberculous Pericarditis, *Ann. Intern. Med.,* 68(5):1175, 1968 (abstract).

66 Keith, T. A., Fowler, N. O., Helmsworth, J. A., and Gralnick, H.: The Course of Surgically Modified Mitral Stenosis: Study of Ninety-four Patients with Emphasis on the Problem of Restenosis, *Am. J. Med.,* 34:308, 1963.

67 Engle, M. A., Zabriskie, J. S., Senterfit, L. B., et al.: Postpericardiotomy Syndrome. A New Look at an Old Condition, *Mod. Concepts Cardiovasc. Dis.,* 44:59, 1975.

68 Dressler, W.: The Post-myocardial-infarction Syndrome: A Report on Forty-four Cases, *A.M.A. Arch, Intern. Med.,* 103:28, 1959.

69 Koopot, R., Zerefos, N. S., Lavender, A. R., et al.: Cardiac Tamponade in Uremic Pericarditis, *Am. J. Cardiol.,* 32:846, 1973.

70 Rooney, J. J., Crocco, J. A., and Lyons, H. A.: Tuberculous Pericarditis, *Ann. Intern. Med.,* 72:73, 1970.

71 Kotte, J. H., and McGuire, J.: Pericardial Paracentesis, *Mod. Concepts Cardiovasc. Dis.,* 20(7):102, 1951.

72 Beck, C. A.: Two Cardiac Compression Triads, *J.A.M.A.,* 104:715, 1935.

73 Metcalfe, J., Woodbury, J. W., Richards, V., and Burwell, C. S.: Studies in Experimental Pericardial Tamponade: Effects on Intravascular Pressures and Cardiac Output, *Circulation,* 5:518, 1952.

74 O'Rourke, R. A., Fischer, D. P., Escobar, E. E., Bishop, V. S., and Rapaport, E.: Effect of Acute Pericardial Tamponade on Coronary Blood Flow, *Am. J. Physiol.,* 212:549, 1967.

75 Spodick, D. H.: Acute Cardiac Tamponade: Pathologic Physiology, Diagnosis and Management, *Prog. Cardiovasc. Dis.,* 10:64, 1967.

76 Comty, C. M., Cohen, S. L., and Shapiro, F. L.: Pericarditis in Chronic Uremia and Its Sequels, *Ann. Intern. Med.,* 75:173, 1971.

77 Morris, J. J., Jr., Whaley, R. E., McIntosh, H. D., Thompson, H. K., Brown, I. W., and Young, W. G., Jr.: Permanent Ventricular Pacemakers: Comparison of Transthoracic and Transvenous Implantation, *Circulation,* 36:587, 1967.

78 Popper, R. W., Schumacher, D., and Quinn, C. H.: Cardiac Tamponade due to Hypertonic Contrast Medium in the Pericardial Sac Following Cineangiography: Clinical Observation and Experimental Study, *Circulation,* 35:933, 1967.

79 Jones, E. W., and Helmsworth, J.: Penetrating Wounds of the Heart: Thirty Years Experience, *Arch. Surg.,* 96:671, 1968.

80 Stewart, D. J., Carson, P. H., Bahler, R. C., and Foxman, D.: Presence of Pericardial Effusions in Heart Failure, *Circulation,* 36(suppl. 2):243, 1967.

81 Fowler, N. O., and Holmes, J. C.: Hemodynamic Effects of Isoproterenol and Norepinephrine in Acute Cardiac Tamponade, *J. Clin. Invest.,* 48:502, 1969.

82 Logue, R. B., Taylor, D. R., and Carter, L. Y.: Diagnosis and Treatment of Pericardial Effusion without Pericardiocentesis: Use of Steroids and Diuretics, *Circulation,* 36(suppl. 2):174, 1967.

83 Boyd, T. F., and Strieder, J. W.: Immediate Surgery for Traumatic Heart Disease, *J. Thorac. Cardiovasc. Surg.,* 50:305, 1965.

84 Moraski, R. E., and Bousvaros, G.: Constrictive Pericarditis due to Chronic Uremia, *N. Engl. J. Med.,* 281:542, 1969.

85 Brawley, R. K., Vasko, J. S., and Morrow, A. G.: Cholesterol Pericarditis. Consideration of Its Pathogenesis and Treatment, *Am. J. Med.,* 41:235, 1966.

86 Hancock, E. W.: Subacute Effusive-Constrictive Pericarditis, *Circulation,* 43:183, 1971.

87 Paul, O., Castleman, B., and White, P. D.: Chronic Constrictive Pericarditis: A Study of 53 Cases, *Am. J. Med. Sci.,* 216:361, 1948.

88 Cooley, J. C., Clagett, O. T., and Kirklin, J. W.: Surgical Aspects of Chronic Constrictive Pericarditis, *Ann. Surg.,* 147:488, 1968.

89 Howard, E. J., and Maier, H. C.: Constrictive Pericarditis Following Acute Coxsackie Viral Pericarditis, *Am. Heart J.,* 75:247, 1968.

90 Slater, S. R., Kroop, I. G., and Zuckerman, S.: Constrictive Pericarditis Caused by Solitary Metastatic Carcinosis of the Pericardium and Complicated by Radiation Fibrosis of the Mediastinum, *Am. Heart J.,* 43:401, 1952.

91 Wooley, C. F., and Hosier, D. M.: Constrictive Pericarditis due

to *Histoplasma capsulatum, N. Engl. J. Med.,* 264:1230, 1961.

92 Susens, G. P., Al-Shamma, A., Rowe, J. C., Herbert, C. C., Bassis, M. L., and Coggs, G. C.: Purulent Constrictive Pericarditis Caused by *Nocardia asteroides, Ann. Intern. Med.,* 67: 1021, 1967.

93 Wood, P.: Chronic Constrictive Pericarditis, *Am. J. Cardiol.,* 7:48, 1961.

94 Harvey, W. P.: Auscultatory Findings in Diseases of the Pericardium, *Am. J. Cardiol.,* 7:15, 1961.

95 Burwell, C. S.: Some Effects of Pericardial Disease on the Pulmonary Circulation, *Trans. Assoc. Am. Physicians,* 64:74, 1951.

96 Burwell, C. S., and Robin, E. D.: Some Points in the Diagnosis of Myocardial Fibrosis, *Trans. Assoc. Am. Physicians,* 67:67, 1954.

97 Dye, C. L., Genovese, P. D., Daly, W. J., and Behnke, R. H.: Primary Myocardial Disease: II. Hemodynamic Alterations, *Ann. Intern. Med.,* 58:442, 1963.

97a Gibson, T. C., Grossman, W., McLaurin, L. P., Moos, S., and Craige, E.: An Echocardiographic Study of the Interventricular Septum in Constrictive Pericarditis, *Br. Heart J.,* 38:738, 1976.

98 Burch, G. E., and Phillips, J. H.: Methods in the Diagnostic Differentiation of Myocardial Dilatation from Pericardial Effusion, *Am. Heart J.,* 64:266, 1962.

Syphilis and the Cardiovascular System

85
Syphilitic Cardiovascular Disease

C. THORPE RAY, M.D.

> The organism responsible for cardiovascular syphilis, the *Treponema pallidum*, was discovered in a diseased aorta in 1906 (Reuter), but long before the discovery of the actual causative agent in syphilis the connection between that disease and aortitis was known, and for several centuries the responsibility for the production of aneurysms by syphilis was suspected (Paré, 1575, Lancisi, 1724, and Morgagni, 1761).[1-3] Gummata, long known to be of leutic origin, were early found in the heart itself.
>
> **PAUL DUDLEY WHITE, M.D., 1931**[4]

It is regrettable that modern texts do not include more than minimal historical notes about cardiovascular syphilis, one of the few truly preventable forms of heart disease. The incidence of cardiovascular syphilis decreased for several decades, so that now the disease is uncommon even in geographic areas where incidence was previously quite high. This radical change in the incidence of cardiovascular syphilis forms the basis of interesting speculation.

Certainly, penicillin is effective and has made the treatment of early syphilis much easier and cheaper than the older regimens of arsenical, bismuth, and iodide treatment. With modern penicillin treatment of early syphilis there is little likelihood of the incomplete course which was so frequent in the prolonged treatment periods prior to the advent of penicillin. However, it should be emphasized that the incidence of cardiovascular syphilis was decreasing rapidly before penicillin was available for widespread use in civilian practice. Since the stages of cardiovascular syphilis which are symptomatic and diagnosable usually occur from 10 to 30 years after the appearance of the chancre, changes in incidence of this disease attributable to the use of penicillin would have been expected only after 1956. The clearly evident decrease in incidence prior to 1955 may be attributed to natural changes in the chronic epidemic of syphilis and especially to the efforts of the public health services. The control of syphilis has been quite successful, but the increasing incidence of new infections in recent years would seem to indicate that cardiovascular syphilis will continue to occur though its incidence will be reduced.[5]

SYPHILITIC AORTITIS

The fundamental lesion of cardiovascular syphilis is aortitis, one of the most common of syphilitic lesions in the body. Localization of the spirochetes in the wall of the aorta occurs quite early after the primary infection. Initially the treponemas are in the adventitia; they then spread into the media by way of the lymphatic vessels surrounding the vasa vasorum. The vasa vasorum undergo an obliterative endarteritis, with subsequent necrosis of the elastic and connective tissue in the media and the formation of scar tissue. Active inflammation continues for many years in untreated cases, and virulent treponemas have been isolated from the wall of the aorta as long as 25 years after infection. The aortic intima becomes thickened over the areas of medial necrosis, and in the late stages the intima appears pitted and scarred, with wrinkling of the intervening tissue, an appearance which has been likened to the bark of a tree.

The incidence and severity of the syphilitic aortitis is greatest in the ascending aorta, next great in the transverse portion, and least in descending and abdominal portions of the aorta. This distribution of the lesions of syphilitic aortitis has been attributed to the rich supply of lymphatic vessels in the ascending and transverse portions of the arch. The tendency to develop more severe lesions in the first portion of the aorta leads to involvement of the coronary ostiums and the base of the aortic valve leaflets.

The incidence of aortitis in cases of untreated syphilis has been estimated to be as high as 70 to 80 percent. This is in striking contrast to the incidence of the complications of aortitis (aortic insufficiency, aneurysm, and ostial disease), which occur in about 10 percent of cases of untreated syphilis.[6] The significance of uncomplicated aortitis is that this lesion forms the basis for the symptomatic and lethal forms of cardiovascular syphilis. Furthermore, adequate treatment in the stage of uncomplicated aortitis should arrest the disease and prevent progression to the more serious complications. The longer treatment is delayed following the primary infection, the greater is the likelihood of the development of more serious lesions. It is noteworthy that an increase in the incidence of syphilitic aortic insufficiency has been reported in the aged, some of whom received treatment.[7] It is conceivable that progression to aortic insufficiency resulted from the initial damage to the media even though the treponemas were eradicated, but persistence of viable organisms following conventional treatment must be considered.

The application of the fluorescent treponemal antibody test has permitted identification of treponemas in ocular fluid, spinal fluid, liver, lymph nodes, and other tissues, even after treatment with amounts of penicillin currently considered to be adequate.[5,8–12] These organisms had the staining properties and morphologic characteristics of *Treponema pallidum.* The viability of these organisms is established by successful animal passage.[5,12] Evaluation of these findings is incomplete, particularly in regard to the pathogenicity of these organisms and the criteria for adequacy of a treatment regimen that does not eradicate the treponemas.

The diagnosis of uncomplicated syphilitic aortitis has been debated at great length. The diagnostic criteria which have been suggested consist of dilatation of the ascending aorta, a tambour aortic second sound in the absence of hypertension and atherosclerosis, a systolic aortic murmur, burning retrosternal pain, breathlessness, etc. Since the incidence of aortitis is high in untreated syphilis, these criteria might be expected to have validity when applied only to known cases of syphilis in large syphilis clinics, but attempts to employ these criteria in a general clinic have met with complete failure. A supportive

FIGURE 85-1 Linear calcification of the wall of the ascending and transverse aorta in a 63-year-old male with positive serologic tests for syphilis and mild aortic insufficiency. Areas of calcification are indicated by arrows. The ascending aorta is dilated.

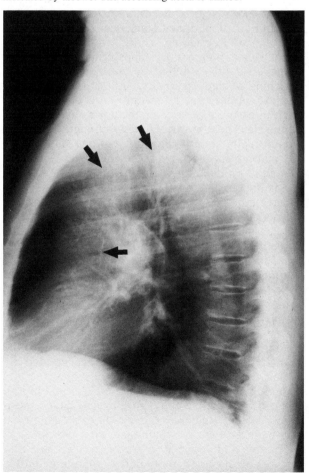

finding in the diagnosis of syphilitic aortitis is the presence of calcification of the ascending aorta, which may be present in the late stages but is of no aid in the diagnosis of early syphilitic aortitis. Calcification of the ascending aorta occurs in about 20 percent of the patients with syphilitic aortitis (Fig. 85-1). The diagnostic specificity of linear calcification of the ascending aorta is limited. In one series of consecutive cases of linear calcification of the aorta only 25 percent had positive serologic evidence of syphilis.[13] The tendency for the calcification of atherosclerosis to occur along the medial side of the ascending arch and for calcification in syphilitic aortitis to occur along the anterolateral wall offers some aid in differentiating the calcifications due to these two disorders.

The dilatation of the first 2 in. of the ascending aorta has been difficult to demonstrate without aortic root angiography. Occasionally linear calcifications permitted demonstration of a dilated root, but this segment of the aorta is centrally located and radiologically hidden by other structures of the heart and great vessels. With the use of echocardiography the dimensions of the aorta are easily assessed by a noninvasive technic (Fig. 85-2). The presence of calcification in the wall of the ascending aorta as well as movement and competency of the aortic cusps are likewise easily established by this approach. It must be recognized that dilatation of the ascending aorta with aortic valvular insufficiency may occur in diseases other than aortic insufficiency.

From the foregoing statements it is apparent that a

FIGURE 85-2 Echocardiogram in a case of syphilitic aortic insufficiency of moderate degree. The aorta is dilated, measuring 4.5 cm in this dimension. Failure of coaptation of aortic valve leaflets is apparent (see arrows marked #1) as well as vibration of the anterior leaflet in systole (see arrow marked AAVL). A systolic murmur was present as well as a typical aortic diastolic murmur.

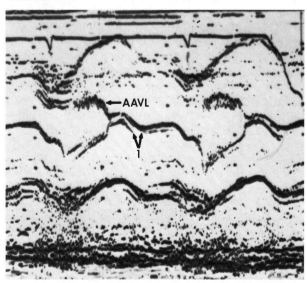

certain diagnosis of early uncomplicated syphilitic aortitis is not possible, since it produces neither signs nor symptoms. However, such a diagnosis in an established case of untreated syphilis is reasonably sound statistically, and the patient should be treated accordingly with the idea of preventing progression to the serious complications: aortic insufficiency, aortic aneurysm, and coronary ostial disease.

AORTIC INSUFFICIENCY

Aortic valvular insufficiency is the most frequent of the complications of syphilitic aortitis. The mesaortitis in the first portion of the aorta results in dilatation of the aortic valve ring so that the commissures are widened and coaptation of the valve cusps no longer occurs (Fig. 85-2). Thickening and rolling of the edge of the cusp may be present. The result of these pathologic changes is free aortic regurgitation without stenosis. Calcification in the valve cusps does not occur unless there is concomitant rheumatic or atherosclerotic disease. Depending on the degree and duration of the aortic regurgitation, variable amounts of left ventricular dilatation and hypertrophy occur. The endocardium over the septum may show a thickened plaque in the area of the regurgitant jet. The other complications of syphilitic aortitis may coexist with aortic valvular insufficiency. Disease of the coronary ostiums is present in approximately 20 percent of cases of aortic insufficiency. Aortic aneurysm may coexist with aortic valvular insufficiency but much less frequently than does ostial disease. After free aortic regurgitation is present, aneurysms do not tend to develop; however, the presence of an aneurysm does not protect against subsequent development of aortic insufficiency. Aortic insufficiency is more common among Negroes than whites (3:1) and more common in males than females (4:1). In the prepenicillin era aortic insufficiency was most commonly manifest between the ages of 35 and 55 years, or 10 to 25 years after the primary lesion, but changes in the natural history of this disease in more recent times must be considered.[7] In most cases diagnosis is made after symptoms have appeared.

The diagnosis of syphilitic aortic insufficiency is usually not difficult. Demonstration of a murmur of aortic insufficiency along with evidence of syphilis constitutes a reasonable basis for diagnosis. Evidence of syphilis consists of a history of infection, serologic evidences of syphilis, evidence of syphilis elsewhere in the body, or any combination of the three.

Using the less sensitive nontreponemal antigen tests for syphilis (VDRL, Kolmer), the serum is positive in approximately three-fourths of the cases of aortic insufficiency and the spinal fluid is positive in about one-half of the cases. The nontreponemal antigen tests are readily available, and when they are diagnostic, no further serologic testing is needed unless there is a concern about a biologic false positive result. However, when these serologic tests are not diagnostic, the more specific and more sensitive treponemal antigen tests should be employed. Reiter's protein complement fixation (RPCF) test is quite specific although not as sensitive as the *T. pallidum* immobilization (TPI) test or the fluorescent treponema antibody-absorption (FTA-ABS) test.[5,14–17] The latter is the most specific and the most sensitive of all, and its utilization may clarify the causation of aortic insufficiency when other serologic tests for syphilis are negative. Because of its high degree of specificity the FTA-ABS test is best for checking biologic false positive reactions. However, the increased sensitivity of the FTA-ABS test may not favor its use in following therapeutic response to treatment.[18]

The clinical manifestations of aortic insufficiency are discussed in detail in Chap. 60. A brief discussion is presented here for the purpose of emphasis and convenience. Slight aortic insufficiency may be present without producing any additional circulatory abnormality. At times, an abnormality of the arterial pulse contour may be detected even though the systemic diastolic blood pressure remains normal. The ascending limb of the arterial pulse is steep and the crest of the wave is brief in such cases. With more severe aortic insufficiency the diastolic blood pressure becomes low, the pulse pressure wide, and the arterial pulse contour grossly abnormal. The classic peripheral vascular signs include (1) Traube's sign, a pistol shot sound over the peripheral arteries, (2) Duroziez's sign, a diastolic murmur proximal to constriction of peripheral arteries, (3) de Musset's sign, a systolic nodding of the head, (4) Corrigan's pulse, a water hammer or collapsing arterial pulse, (5) Quincke's capillary pulse, an alternate flushing and blanching of capillary beds, and (6) Hill's sign, an increase in femoral artery pressure over brachial artery pressure of more than the normal difference of 20 mm Hg. These physical findings are interesting but are not really helpful clinically. No one should miss the murmur of aortic insufficiency that is severe enough to produce these signs, but the faint murmur that is unassociated with such signs frequently goes undetected.

The murmur of aortic insufficiency is high-pitched and heard best with the diaphragm of the stethoscope applied with firm pressure. The murmur is usually heard in the second right interspace adjacent to the sternum, along the left sternal border, and at the apex. As a rule, it is louder along the left sternal border in early diastole and decreases in intensity during diastole (decrescendo). It is useful to listen to the heart while the patient is leaning forward and holding the breath in expiration. Occasionally, the intensity of the murmur may be accentuated by having the patient lie on the stethoscope (the diaphragm being applied along the left sternal border). Occasionally, the diastolic murmur may have a musical character ascribable to eversion of a cusp which may be permanent or which may vary with time.

Harvey and associates[19] have pointed out that diseases of the aortic root such as syphilitic aortitis, dissecting aneurysm, aneurysm of a sinus of Valsalva, dilatation of the aorta due to hypertension, and rheumatoid aortitis may produce aortic regurgitation that is heard with maximum intensity along the right sternal border. The technique is to compare the intensity of the murmur as heard in the third right interspace near the sternum with the intensity of the murmur as heard in the third left interspace near the sternum. When the murmur is louder on the right, consider aortic root disease.

The murmur of mild aortic insufficiency may be similar to the murmur of pulmonary insufficiency. The ausculatory characteristics and location of the two murmurs may be identical, and when the pulse pressure is normal, these murmurs may be difficult to differentiate. When the murmur is louder along the right sternal border, it is usually due to aortic insufficiency. When there is prompt intensification of the murmur with inspiration, it is likely to be pulmonary insufficiency. When there is definite mitral stenosis due to rheumatic fever, the high-pitched murmur along the left sternal border may be due to either aortic insufficiency or pulmonary insufficiency. Statistically, while either or both can occur, most murmurs of this type are due to aortic insufficiency.[20] When aortic insufficiency is severe, it may be associated with a loud systolic murmur heard best in the second and third right interspaces adjacent to the sternum. This murmur may stimulate that of aortic stenosis and may be accompanied by a thrill. A wide pulse pressure and pulsus bisferiens indicate that aortic insufficiency is the major problem in confusing cases. The use of cineangiography with injections of contrast material in the root of the aorta will define the presence and degree of aortic insufficiency when doubt remains about the origin of a basal diastolic murmur (see Chap. 29C).

Virtually all patients with moderate aortic insufficiency associated with a wide pulse pressure will exhibit a ventricular diastolic gallop at the apex. Many patients with severe aortic regurgitation have diastolic rumbles at the apex. The Flint rumble was originally described in patients with aortic insufficiency due to syphilis but may be secondary to aortic regurgitation of any cause. The rumbling character of the murmur at the apex has been attributed to fluttering of the anterior mitral leaflet which may be easily demonstrated by echocardiography (Fig. 85-3). The differential problem becomes the following: Does the patient have aortic insufficiency as the major or only abnormality and a Flint rumble, or does he have rheumatic mitral stenosis and aortic insufficiency? The Flint rumble usually occurs in middiastole, but there may be presystolic accentuation. An opening snap and loud first sound indicate mitral stenosis. The P-Q (P-R) interval is often long in patients with aortic insufficiency, and the first heart sound may be faint. The finding of a loud first heart sound despite a long P-Q interval favors the diagnosis of mitral stenosis. Occasionally, there is a loud aortic ejection click in patients with aortic regurgitation that may be mistaken for a loud first sound. Atrial fibrillation occurs with greater frequency in patients with mitral stenosis. An abnormal systolic and diastolic thrust is palpable at the apex when aortic regurgitation is present. These pulsations do not occur when there is pure mitral stenosis. Such

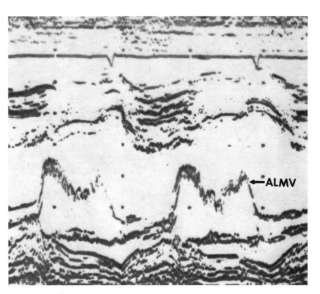

FIGURE 85-3 Echocardiogram from a case of syphilitic aortic insufficiency of moderate severity. In addition to the basal murmur of insufficiency there was a Flint rumble at the apex. Fluttering of the anterior leaflet of the mitral valve is demonstrated (see arrow marked ALMV). Normal mitral valvular motion excludes mitral stenosis as a cause of the rumble.

pulsations do not rule out mitral stenosis but suggest that aortic regurgitation is the dominant lesion. Calcification of the mitral or aortic valve cusps not only indicates mitral valve disease but signifies a rheumatic cause. Calcifications of the early portion of the aorta suggest a syphilitic cause. Such clinical findings are usually adequate to differentiate syphilitic and rheumatic valvular disease. The status of the valves, their motion, and the presence of calcification is easily determined by echocardiography, and reliable differentiation of these valvular diseases is readily available (Fig. 85-3).

When heart failure ensues, the diastolic pressure may gradually rise until a normal level is reached. The end-diastolic pressure in the left ventricle is extremely high under these circumstances, and there is often early closure of the mitral valve (Fig. 85-4). Left ventricular dilatation often results in mitral insufficiency. Tricuspid insufficiency may occur late in the course of heart failure.

The prognosis of syphilitic aortic insufficiency is generally poor. Only 30 to 40 percent of patients with this condition survive 10 years after the diagnosis is made.[22] The presence of congestive heart failure is the most important determinant of longevity in this disease. Of the patients who remained free of heart failure, 56 percent survived 15 years; but of those who had heart failure at the time of diagnosis, less than 20 percent survived 5 years and less than 6 percent survived 10 years. The average duration of life from the onset of heart failure is about 3 years. In syphilitic aortic insufficiency with heart failure, sudden death is fairly common. Exceptional patients have survived 15 to 20 years after the onset of heart

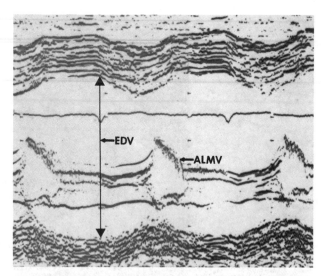

FIGURE 85-4 Echocardiogram from a case of severe syphilitic aortic insufficiency and heart failure. Fluttering of the anterior leaflet (see arrow marked ALMV) is demonstrated as well as early closure of the mitral valve. Marked dilatation of the left ventricle (see arrow marked EDV) is demonstrated, measuring 7.5 cm in this dimension. Contrast with Fig. 85-3.

failure. At the other end of the spectrum are those patients who experience a sudden onset of heart failure and who, in spite of the most rigorous treatment, progress inexorably downhill and die during the first stay in the hospital.

Several important factors influence longevity in aortic insufficiency. The degree of regurgitation and the diastolic blood pressure are important. Low diastolic pressure makes for a limited coronary blood flow. The presence and degree of ostial narrowing are equally important. It is interesting to note that those patients who survive 10 to 15 years after the onset of heart failure usually have only minimal narrowing of the coronary ostiums and those patients who survive only a short time after onset of failure usually have more severe degrees of ostial disease. The appearance of anginal pain with heart failure indicates a poorer prognosis. Under these circumstances the anginal pain is usually attributed to coronary ostial narrowing, but angina may occur in the absence of significant ostial disease when the regurgitation is severe and the diastolic pressure is low. In either event, the outlook is poorer when coronary blood flow is inadequate. The presence of other diseases, such as coronary artery atherosclerosis, hypertension, or anemia, adds a further burden to an already failing heart. Excessive physical activity may shorten life expectancy in syphilitic aortic insufficiency, and the onset of heart failure may appear quite suddenly for the first time following strenuous exertion.

The treatment of syphilitic aortic insufficiency should first be directed at heart failure if this is present. There is no particular urgency to begin administration of penicillin at this stage of the dis-

ease, since the disaster is almost complete. Once the heart failure is controlled, penicillin therapy may be started. The risk of Jarisch-Herxheimer reaction is extremely small, and no particular precautions against it are necessary. However, there are numerous case reports and many unreported individual experiences in which an unexpected increase in aortic insufficiency and heart failure or a rupture of an aneurysm followed penicillin administration. In these instances the Jarisch-Herxheimer reaction may have been important.

The following schedules of penicillin therapy are recommended:[21]

I Early syphilis (primary, secondary, latent syphilis of less than 1 year's duration)

  A Benzathine penicillin G, 2.4 million units total, administered intramuscularly by simple injection or

  B Aqueous procaine penicillin G, 4.8 million units total, administered by daily intramuscular injections of 600,000 units for 8 days or

  C Procaine penicillin G in oil with 2 percent aluminum monostearate (PAM), 4.5 million units total, by intramuscular injection of a 2.4-million-unit first dose followed by two additional doses of 1.2 million units at 3-day intervals

  D For patients who are allergic to penicillin:

    1 Tetracycline hydrochloride, 500 mg orally four times daily for 15 days or

    2 Erythromycin (stearate, ethylsucrinate as base), 500 mg orally four times daily for 15 days

II Syphilis of more than 1 year's duration (latent syphilis of indeterminate or more than 1 year's duration, cardiovascular late benign, neurosyphilis)

  A Benzathine penicillin G, 7.2 million units total, administered by intramuscular injection of 2.4 million units weekly for 3 successive weeks or

  B Aqueous procaine penicillin G, 9 million units total, given by daily intramuscular injections of 600,000 units for 15 days

  C For patients who are allergic to penicillin:

    1 Tetracycline hydrochloride 500 mg orally four times daily for 30 days or

    2 Erythomycin (stearate, ethylsucrinate, or base) 500 mg orally four times daily for 30 days

Penicillin is the treatment of choice since its effects on syphilis have been more extensively investigated, particularly in early syphilis. The dosage schedules for late syphilis have not been as extensively investigated. The persistence of viable spirochetes in various tissues following adequate treatment with penicillin raises serious questions about the drugs, dosage schedules, and the duration of treatment.

Follow-up on all cases of treated syphilis is essential. The quantitative VDRL is the best test to use in the posttreatment period. Retreatment should be considered if (1) the clinical signs or symptoms persist or recur, (2) there is a sustained fourfold increase in the titer of the quantitative VDRL test, or (3) an initially high titer of the VDRL test fails to show a fourfold decrease within a year. If treatment is indicated, the treatment schedule for late syphilis should be followed.

The medical management of severe syphilitic aortic insufficiency leaves much to be desired. The continuing physiologic burden of severe regurgitation along with poor coronary blood flow makes for a limited response to the usual measures employed in the treatment of heart failure. The only relief for the primary physiologic defects, aortic regurgitation and poor coronary flow, is by surgical correction with a Starr-Edwards or similar prosthesis (see Chap. 61). If the coronary ostiums are patent, the rise in diastolic pressure following replacement of the aortic valve will result in an increased coronary artery blood flow. If there is significant ostial narrowing, normal coronary artery blood flow may be reestablished through use of internal mammary to coronary artery anastomosis or saphenous vein aorta–coronary artery graft. The advanced age of some of these patients is a limiting factor in the surgical approach to these problems.

ANEURYSM (see Chap. 107)

Aneurysm of the aorta is a late complication of syphilitic aortitis, usually occurring from 15 to 30 years after the initial infection. Aneurysms occur about one-third as frequently as aortic insufficiency, but the same race and sex incidence is found for both lesions. As a result of damage from aortitis, the aorta may undergo generalized dilatation to form a fusiform aneurysm or a more localized dilatation to form a saccular aneurysm. In the latter, the communication with the aortic lumen may be quite large or only a centimeter in diameter. The aneurysmal sac may contain a laminated clot, with the older portion nearer the lumen of the aorta and the newer clot next to the aneurysmal wall where the additional growth occurs. The walls of large aneurysms are composed largely of fibrous tissue, and identification of remnants of the original wall of the aorta may be impossible. Approximately 50 percent of syphilitic aneurysms occur in the ascending aorta, 30 to 40 percent in the transverse arch, 15 percent in the descending aorta, and less than 5 percent in the abdominal aorta. Frequently more than one aneurysm exists in the same patient (Fig. 85-5).

Since the signs and symptoms of aneurysms result largely from compression of adjacent structures, one would expect different clinical manifestations from aneurysms in various portions of the aorta. For example, aneurysms of the ascending aorta may compress the pulmonary artery, the superior vena cava, or the right main bronchus, with predictable results from involvement of each structure. However, aneurysms in this location may enlarge in an anterolateral direction and achieve considerable size before giving rise to symptoms from impingement upon adjacent structures. The close anatomic relations of the transverse arch to the esophagus, trachea, bronchi, recurrent laryngeal nerve, and vertebrae makes for compression of vital structures with much smaller aneurysmal sacs. Dysphagia, dyspnea, stridor, cough, hemoptysis, hoarseness, and pain are frequently encountered in aneurysms of the trans-

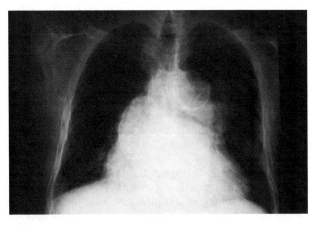

FIGURE 85-5 Radiograph demonstrating multiple aortic aneurysms (four). Calcification in the walls of the aneurysmal sacs help establish the syphilitis etiology. Severe congestive failure, and aortic, mitral, and tricuspid insufficiency were present also.

verse arch. Involvement of the orifices of the great vessels results in unequal pulses in the arms, and compression of the left stellate ganglion results in unequal pupils. Atelectasis, infection, and lung abscesses are frequent results of compression of the bronchi and lungs. The descending aorta has more space for dilatation and may undergo considerable enlargement before symptoms occur from compression of lung or erosion of vertebrae and impingement upon sensitive nerve roots. Aneurysms in this location may erode ribs and present a pulsatile mass in the left side of the chest posteriorly. Aneurysms of the abdominal aorta often present as a pulsating epigastric mass with pain in the abdomen and back.

There is always danger of rupture of syphilitic aneurysms. In the thorax, perforation is most commonly into the pericardial cavity, pleural cavities, bronchial tree, and esophagus. Aneurysms of the ascending aorta tend to perforate into the pericardial and right pleural spaces. Infrequently, there is perforation into the pulmonary artery, which causes a sudden appearance of a continuous murmur and right ventricular strain.

The diagnosis of syphilitic aortic aneurysm is made by the demonstration of the characteristic structural changes in the aorta with a history of syphilis, or evidences of syphilis elsewhere in the body. To be sure that the mass in question is an aneurysm, it must be shown to be a part of the aorta in all views. Expansile pulsation in a mass is helpful if present, but not all aneurysms demonstrate expansile pulsations, particularly very large aneurysms and those containing laminated clots. A solid tissue mass located adjacent to the aorta may reveal systolic movement which is transmitted from the aorta. Linear calcification extending along the wall of the aorta and into the wall of the mass is helpful in establishing the mass as an aneurysm (Fig. 85-5). If the aorta is displaced by extravascular solid tumor masses such as neoplasms, lymphadenopathy, dermoid cysts, substernal goiter, or enlarged thymus. Differentiation of aneurysms from such extravascular turmors is usually not too difficult, but if any doubt remains, the issue is settled by aortography (see Chaps. 29A and 107). Echocardiography is quite useful in identification of dilatation of the first part of the ascending aorta (Fig. 85-2). Differentiation of dilatation of the ascending aorta due to syphilis from that due to dissecting aneurysms may also be achieved by echocardiography.

Other diseases of the aorta which result in dilatation must be differentiated from syphilitic aneurysm. Traumatic aneurysm occurs in the region of the isthmus; the serologic tests for syphilis are negative; and there is usually a history of trauma. Coarctation of the aorta, dissecting aneurysm, Marfan's syndrome, aortic stenosis with poststenotic dilatation, and atherosclerosis may produce a dilated aorta and aortic valvular insufficiency. These various diseases have diagnostic characteristics of their own which allow differentiation from syphilis. The dilatation and elongation of the aorta with atherosclerosis forms a simple smooth arc from ascending aorta to the aortic knob. Syphilitic changes in this portion of the aorta result in more than one arc in this segment.

The prognosis of syphilitic aortic aneurysms is grave. After the onset of symptoms, the average duration of life is measured in months. In a series of 188 cases, only 18 patients were alive at the end of 2 years; of the 170 who died, the average duration of life was about 6 months. Many aneurysms are diagnosed radiologically before the onset of symptoms, and the duration of life in the asymptomatic patients might be expected to be longer than in those presenting symptoms of compression of some vital organ.

Once the aorta has dilated in either saccular or fusiform manner, the hydraulic principles are such that this weakened segment is subjected to a greater shearing force per unit length than is the adjacent aorta of normal diameter. The total force acting along the wall of the aorta is greatly increased by an increase in diameter of the aorta. The aneurysm usually continues to grow unless the lumen is filled with a large clot, which may tend to protect against further disruption of the wall.

The treatment of syphilitic aortic aneurysm is often symptomatic and directed at complications of the aneurysm such as atelectasis, infection, lung abscess, and the control of pain. Penicillin is recommended in the same dosage schedule as in aortic insufficiency. That antisyphilitic therapy will prolong life at this stage of the disease is questionable, since the aortic defect is now a mechanical one with hydraulic reasons for progression. At the present time the preferred treatment is surgical excision of the aneurysm with restoration of the continuity of the aorta (see Chap. 107).

CORONARY OSTIAL DISEASE

Involvement of the ostiums of the coronary arteries in syphilitic aortitis results in a gradual, progressive narrowing. The coronary ostiums may be so nearly occluded that one is impressed by the ability of extracoronary collateral vessels to maintain life. Because of the slowness of the occlusive process, myocardial infarction is rare; however, small areas of fibrosis throughout the myocardium are common. The incidence of ostial narrowing without other complications of aortitis is difficult to determine from published autopsy data, but the association of aortic insufficiency and coronary ostial disease is quite common.

The presence of coronary ostial narrowing is suspected when angina pectoris occurs in patients with syphilitic aortic insufficiency, but it must be remembered that angina may occur with aortic regurgitation alone. In the absence of aortic insufficiency, a diagnosis of syphilitic ostial disease as a cause of angina pectoris can be made only by coronary arteriography. Visualization of the coronary arteries is sometimes difficult under these circumstances. The coronary ostium may not admit the catheter tip and identification of a narrowed coronary ostium is dependent upon aortic root injection of the contrast material.

The outlook of coronary ostial disease is poor. It is often associated with aortic insufficiency, and the low diastolic pressure plus the narrowing of the ostiums provides an inadequate blood flow to an overloaded heart. Sudden death due to ventricular fibrillation secondary to myocardial ischemia is common in this group of patients, and they are extremely poor risks for surgical treatment or any maneuver which impairs effective coronary perfusion. Treatment of coronary ostial disease consists of the usual management of angina and heart failure, plus the same antisyphilitic regimen of penicillin as for aortic insufficiency. Occasionally, the anginal syndrome may disappear after antisyphilitic therapy. Attempts at correction of coronary ostial narrowing by ostial endarterectomy have been reported.[23-25] More extensive experience with internal mammary-coronary artery anastomoses and saphenous vein aorta–coronary artery grafts have shown this approach to reduced coronary blood flow to be successful. In syphilitic ostial disease the distal coronary arteries are usually normal, but this finding needs to be confirmed by angiography to be assured of adequate run-off following bypass surgery.

GUMMA OF THE MYOCARDIUM

Involvement of the myocardium by gumma formation is unusual. The manifestations of an isolated gumma are determined by its location. In instances of high septal involvement, bundle branch block and atrioventricular block may occur. When areas of the free wall of the ventricle are replaced by gummatous tissue, the electrocardiogram resembles that of myocardial infarction. In most instances the diagnosis of myocardial gumma is made post-mortem.

OTHER VASCULAR MANIFESTATIONS OF SYPHILIS

Syphilis is a widespread disease and commonly involves blood vessels other than the aorta. The formation of a gumma anywhere in the body depends primarily on changes in blood vessels. The changes in the central nervous system in syphilis result from an obliterative arteritis of the cerebral vessels. Syphilis primarily in the central nervous system may give rise to secondary systemic vascular disorders such as the postural hypotension seen in tabes dorsalis.

REFERENCES

1 Paré, A.: "Opera Chirurgica," Apud J. Fischerum, Francofurti and Moenum, 1612. (French translation, Paris, 1840, vol. I, p. 372, 1st French ed., 1664.

2 Lancisi: "De Novissime Observatis Abscessibus," 1724.

3 Morgangni, G. B.: "De Sedibus et Causis Morborum," Ex. typog., Remondiniana, Venice, 1761.

4 White, P. D.: Cardiovascular Syphilis, in "Heart Disease," P. D. White (ed.), The Macmillan Company, New York, 1931.

5 Sparling, P. F.: Diagnosis and Treatment of Syphilis, N. Engl. J. Med., 284:642, 1971.

6 Termini, B. A., and Music, S. I.: The Natural History of Syphilis: A Review, South. Med. J., 65:241, 1972.

7 Prewitt, T. A.: Syphilitic Aortic Insufficiency: Its Increased Incidence in the Elderly, JAMA, 211:637, 1970.

8 Nicholas, L., and Beerman, H.: Late Syphilis: A Review of Some of the Recent Literature, Am. J. Med. Sci., 254:549, 1967.

9 Smith, J. L., and Israel, C. W.: The Presence of Spirochetes in Late Seronegative Syphilis, JAMA, 199:126, 1967.

10 Yobs, A. R., Brown, L., and Hunter, E. F.: Fluorescent Antibody Technique in Early Syphilis as Applied to the Demonstration of T. pallidum in Lesions in the Rabbit and in the Human, Arch. Pathol., 77:220, 1964.

11 Cannefax, G. R., Norins, L. C., and Gillespie, E. J.: Immunology of Syphilis, Am. Rev. Med., 18:471, 1967.

12 Dunlap, E. M. C.: Persistence of Treponemes after Treatment, Br. Med. J., 2:577, 1972.

13 Higgins, C. B., and Reinke, R. T.: Nonsyphilitis Etiology of Linear Calcification of the Aorta, Radiology, 113:601, 1974.

14 Olansky, S., and Norins, L. C.: Current Serodiagnosis and Treatment of Syphilis, JAMA, 198:165, 1966.

15 Deacon, W. E., Lucas, J. B., and Price, E. V.: Fluorescent Treponemal Antibody-Absorption (FTA-ABS) Test for Syphilis, JAMA, 198:624, 1966.

16 Cohen, P., Stout, G., and Ende, N.: Serologic Reactivity in Consecutive Patients Admitted to a General Hospital: A Comparison of the FRA-ABS, VDRL, and Automated Reagin Tests, Arch. Intern. Med., 124:364, 1969.

17 Harner, R. E., Smith, J. L., and Israel, C. W.: The FTA-ABS Test in Late Syphilis: A Serological Study in 1,985 Cases, JAMA, 203:545, 1968.

18 Arwood, W. C., Miller, J. L., Stout, C. W., and Norins, L. C.: The TPI and FTA-ABS Tests in Treated Late Syphilis, JAMA, 203:549, 1968.

19 Harvey, W. P., Corrado, M. A., and Perloff, J. K.: Right-sided Murmurs of Aortic Insufficiency (Diastolic Murmurs Better Heard to the Right of the Sternum Rather than the Left), Am. J. Med. Sci., 245:533, 1963.

20 Brest, A. N., Udhoji, V., and Likoff, W. A.: A Reevaluation of the Graham Steel Murmur, N. Engl. J. Med., 263:173, 1960.

21 Syphilis: Recommended Treatment Schedules, 1976 Recommendation Established by the Veneral Disease Control Advisory Committee, Ann. Intern. Med., 85:94, 1976.

22 Webster, B., Rich, C., Jr., Dense, P. M., Moore, J. E., Nicol, C. S., and Padget, P.: Studies in Cardiovascular Syphilis: The Natural History of Syphilitic Aortic Insufficiency, Am. Heart J., 46:117, 1953.

23 Dubost, C., Blondeau, P., Piwnica, A., Weiss, M., Lenfant, C., Passelecq, J., and Guery, J.: Syphilitic Coronary Obstruction: Correction under Artificial Heart-Lung and Profound Hypothermia at 10°C, Surgery, 48:540, 1960.

24 Connolly, J. E., Eldridge, F. L., Calvin, J. W., and Stemmer, E. A.: Proximal Coronary Artery Obstruction: Its Etiology and Treatment by Transaortic Endarterectomy, N. Engl. J. Med., 271:213, 1964.

25 Beck, W., Barnard, C. N., and Schire, V.: Syphilitic Obstruction of Coronary Ostia Successfully Treated by Endarterectomy, Br. Heart J., 27:911, 1965.

Tumors of the Heart

86
Cardiac Tumors

NANETTE KASS WENGER, M.D.

INTRODUCTION

The heart reacts to injury by degenerative rather than regenerative phenomena; this paucity of mitotic activity in cardiac muscle may contribute to the rarity of primary cardiac tumors. However, cardiac tumors are not disproportionately rare when compared with the heart's percentage of total body weight, 0.4 to 0.5 percent. The low incidence of metastatic disease to the heart has been attributed to (1) the strong kneading action of the heart, (2) the metabolic peculiarities of cardiac muscle, (3) the rapid intracardiac blood flow, and (4) the restricted cardiac lymphatic connections, as cardiac metastases via lymphatic channels must spread in a retrograde manner. Cardiac tumors, though infrequent, are no longer medical curiosities, since surgical cure is often possible.

GENERAL CONSIDERATIONS

Tumors of the heart produce no characteristic symptoms unless they interfere with cardiac function; therefore, only about 5 to 10 percent of all cardiac neoplasms can be diagnosed clinically. Only minimal cardiac dysfunction may occur even with extensive myocardial invasion and destruction. The lack of symptoms may be attributable to slow tumor growth which allows for compensatory cardiac changes, and to the relative resistance of the heart valves, conduction tissue, and arteries to tumor invasion,[1] which preserves the normal cardiac hemodynamics. Myocardial metabolism is aerobic, requiring lactic acid and extracting little glucose from the blood; tumor metabolism is highly anaerobic, requiring much glucose and little oxygen, and producing lactate; these two tissues are thus almost symbiotic, which may explain the infrequent symptoms. Most often, however, symptoms of the primary neoplasm tend to overshadow the cardiac manifestations in patients with cardiac metastases.

Severe, intractable, rapidly progressive cardiac failure, sudden in onset and without apparent cause, is the hallmark of a symptomatic cardiac neoplasm. Equally suggestive[2] are (1) pericardial effusion, particularly if hemorrhagic, and unexplained pericarditis, often with a persistent pericardial friction rub; (2) unexplained, rapidly changing arrhythmias, persistent tachycardia, or complete heart block with Stokes-Adams syncope; (3) embolic phenomena with symptoms mimicking bacterial endocarditis; (4) venous thromboses; (5) pulmonary hypertension; and (6) the effects of valve blockade or the obstruction of blood flow through a cardiac chamber. Cardiac tumors often simulate valvular disease,[3] particularly mitral and tricuspid, but the murmurs and symptoms characteristically vary with position;[1] the development of pulmonic stenosis is suggestive of cardiac tumor.[4] The clinical picture of pulmonic stenosis may also result from extrinsic pressure by a mediastinal tumor. A triad of chest pain, dyspnea, and a pulmonary systolic murmur has been described, with expiratory accentuation of the murmur as the tumor compresses the pulmonary artery and diminution or disappearance of the murmur with inspiration.[5] Angina pectoris may be due to a cardiac tumor, and electrocardiographic abnormalities may simulate myocardial infarction.[6] Sudden death may occur with or without preceding symptoms. Tumor may be detected on microscopic examination of an arterial tumor embolus.

Bizarre, incongruous combinations of symptoms, physical findings, and laboratory data should suggest cardiac tumor. Metastatic tumor to the heart should be considered as the cause of otherwise unexplained cardiac symptoms in a patient with a malignant neoplasm.

Variability of findings at repeated cardiac catheterizations has been emphasized;[7] the catheterization data often correlate poorly with the clinical symptoms. Radiographic clues[8,9] include an unusual or irregular cardiac silhouette, with or without abnormal pulsations; cardiac chamber displacement or distortion; angiographic filling defects; and ectopic or peculiar cardiac calcification.

Benign and malignant primary cardiac tumors and metastatic cardiac tumors produce indistinguishable clinical manifestations. The location of the cardiac tumor generally determines the clinical manifestations, so the problem of cardiac tumors will be considered in this chapter in relation to their anatomic localization.[10]

Benign

Over three-fourths of all primary cardiac tumors are benign, and half of these are intracavitary tumors.[1] Myxomas and rhabdomyomas account for more than one-half of all primary benign cardiac tumors, with myxomas dominating the clinically manifest benign cardiac tumors. Cardiac fibromas, lipomas, angiomas, papillomas, teratomas, leiomyomas, and xanthomas are rare.[1] Although these tumors are classified as benign, many cause death by producing arrhythmias, pericardial effusion with cardiac tamponade, obliteration of cardiac chambers, valve blockade, embolic phenomena, etc. Primary cardiac tumors of infancy and childhood are almost exclusively benign; rhabdomyomas, myxomas, and fibromas are most frequent, with occasional reports of lipomas and teratomas.[12,13]

Malignant

Primary malignant tumors of the heart are almost exclusively sarcomas; they comprise over 20 percent of all primary tumors of the heart.[14,15] Sarcomas occur at all ages, equally in males and females, but are rare in infancy and childhood.

The typical clinical picture[15,16] is of relentless, unexplained cardiac failure with cardiac enlargement, hemopericardium, bizarre cardiac rhythm disturbances, chest pain, and occasionally sudden death.

METASTATIC CARDIAC TUMORS

Metastatic tumor to the heart should be suspected when a patient with malignant disease develops cardiac dysfunction without apparent cause. Acute pericarditis, often with a persistent pericardial friction rub, cardiac tamponade or constriction, rapid roentgenographic increase in heart size, onset of an ectopic tachycardia, development of second- or third-degree atrioventricular block, changing cardiac murmurs, evidence of obstruction to the great vein orifices, and progressive intractable, unexplained cardiac failure are strongly suggestive of cardiac metastases.[17,18] However, cardiac symptoms are uncommon and occur in less than 10 percent of patients with cardiac metastases; cardiac metastases do not appear to be a major factor contributing to the death of the patient. There is variable correlation between the size and extent of cardiac metastases and the clinical manifestations of heart disease; symptoms depend more on the location than on the size of the metastatic tumor.[19] For example, metastasis of a hypernephroma to the AV node produced complete heart block.[20]

There is no characteristic electrocardiographic finding in metastatic cardiac tumor, but nonspecific electrocardiographic abnormalities are common.[21] ST-T alterations are most frequent; occasionally they are pronounced and persistent, particularly when cardiac metastases produce myocardial necrosis.[22] Arrhythmias are more frequent with metastatic than with benign cardiac tumors. Atrial arrhythmias, atrioventricular block, bundle branch block, abnormal P waves, decreased QRS voltage in cases with and without[23] pericardial effusion, and changes mimicking myocardial infarction also occur.[24] The arrhythmias often do not respond to digitalis or any other standard therapy.[25] Occasionally, electrocardiographic abnormalities may provide a clue to the location of neoplasm in the heart.[26,26a]

Cardiac metastases occur with all types of primary tumors: carcinomas, sarcomas, leukemias, lymphomas, Kaposi's sarcoma, myeloma,[25] etc. No malignant tumor tends particularly to metastasize to the heart, with the possible exception of malignant melanoma, which involves the myocardium in over 50 percent of cases[17] (Fig. 86-1). Cardiac metastases occur most frequently from bronchogenic carcinoma and carcinoma of the breast, being found in one-third of cases (Fig. 86-2).

Cardiac infiltration, often macroscopic, is seen in one-half of cases of leukemia and in one-sixth of cases of lymphoma (Fig. 86-3), particularly reticulum cell sarcoma[18] (see Chap. 82) (Fig. 86-4). There is

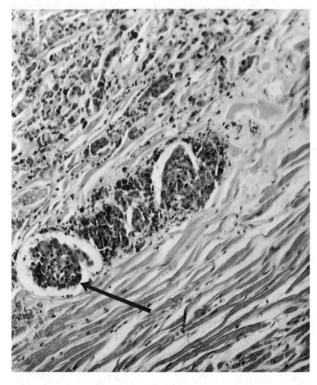

FIGURE 86-1 Malignant melanoma, metastatic to the heart. There are destruction and replacement of cardiac muscle by neoplastic tissue. A neoplastic deposit is present in a vascular channel (arrow) ($\times$150).

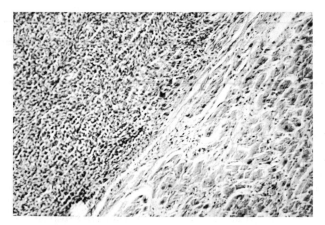

FIGURE 86-2 Cystosarcoma phylloides of the breast, metastatic to the heart. The tumor is composed of small spindled sarcoma cells (×120).

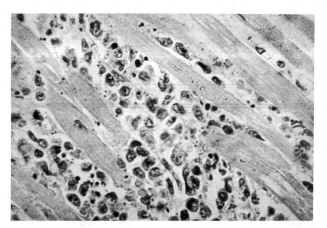

FIGURE 86-4 Myocardial invasion by reticulum cell sarcoma. There is interstitial infiltration of the myocardium by large, atypical reticulum cells (×900).

usually extensive myocardial infiltration, and occasionally, a major coronary vessel may be occluded. The incidence of cardiovascular signs and symptoms is similar with and without cardiac lymphoma; in patients with lymphoma, the cardiovascular abnormalities may be due to mediastinal or pulmonary lymphoma, anemia, hypoalbuminemia, or unrelated cardiac disease,[18] or to radiation myopericarditis and/or pneumonitis following therapy.

Metastatic cardiac tumors are sixteen[1] to forty[15] times more common than primary cardiac tumors, and carcinomatous invasion is more frequent than sarcomatous. Despite this, attention should be focused on diagnosis of the primary cardiac tumor, as resection is more likely to result in cure of the heart disease. Cardiac metastases occur most frequently over age 50, with an equal sex incidence.[19] Metastatic tumor to the heart has been described in 0.1 to 6.4 percent of unselected autopsies and in 1.5 to 20.6 percent of patients dying of malignant tumors.[19,21] The recent increased frequency of diagnosis of metastatic cardiac tumors reflects both a greater interest

FIGURE 86-3 Hodgkin's disease invasion of the myocardium. There is a polymorphic infiltrate composed of plasma cells, eosinophils, and a Reed-Sternberg cell (arrow) (×250).

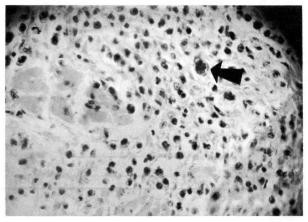

in the problem and a longer life-span of patients with malignant disease; the longer life-span, due to improved therapeutic methods, probably enables increased tumor dissemination. There does not, however, appear to be good correlation between the duration of malignant disease and cardiac metastases.

Cardiac metastases are encountered with widespread systemic tumor dissemination; only rarely is metastatic tumor limited to the heart or pericardium. Carcinomatous metastases are generally grossly visible, multiple, discrete, small, white, firm nodules; microscopically they resemble the primary tumor and the metastases in other organs. Diffuse infiltration is characteristic of sarcomatous metastases. Necrosis is uncommon.[19]

Metastatic tumors are classically thought to reach the heart by embolic hematogenous spread, by lymphatic spread, or by direct invasion, in descending order of frequency.[19] Recently, cardiac lymphatics have been reported to be the chief pathway of tumor metastases to the heart; lymphatic obstruction by tumor results in myocardial interstitial edema, and the secondary pressure on the myofibers may contribute to the eventual cardiac decompensation,[27] particularly in the patient with underlying coronary atherosclerotic heart disease.

Lymphatic spread of tumors is particularly frequent with carcinoma of the bronchus and the breast; the proximity of the heart to major mediastinal lymphatic channels explains the high incidence of cardiac metastases from mediastinal tumors.[19]

SPECIFIC CLINICAL SYNDROMES

Intracavitary tumors

GENERAL CONSIDERATIONS

Intracavitary cardiac tumors originate almost exclusively in the atria and produce symptoms by acutely or chronically interfering with cardiac filling or ejection. Left atrial tumors produce signs and symptoms of obstruction of the pulmonary circulation;[28] right atrial tumors present evidence of inflow obstruction.

Intracavitary tumors characteristically mimic valvular disease. Tumor emboli, pulmonary and systemic, constitute a serious complication. Intracavitary tumors may produce a hemolytic anemia because of mechanical trauma to red blood cells by the tumor.[2]

Structural and hemodynamic abnormalities of the atrioventricular valves have also occurred with polypoid atrial tumors, presumably in response to the friction effect of the tumor on the surfaces involved.[29]

LEFT ATRIAL MYXOMA

Background information Myxomas constitute 35 to 50 percent[30] of all primary cardiac tumors and are the most common intracavitary tumors. They occur at all ages, although they are rare in childhood, and are three times more common in women. A familial occurrence is occasionally described.[30a] Myxomas are often rapidly fatal if not recognized and surgically removed; nevertheless, one patient had a 34-year history of intermittent symptoms from an atrial myxoma, and death occurred from an unrelated cause. Many atrial myxomas have been diagnosed clinically in recent years, with the presentations of embolization, obstruction to blood flow, or constitutional manifestations.[31] Many reports of successful surgical removal of atrial myxomas appear in the literature.[32,33]

Etiology Some investigators believe cardiac myxomas develop from mural thrombi.[34] Others consider them true tumors.[34a] Local myxoma recurrences and growth of myxomatous emboli favor the neoplastic origin. Indeed, the recurrent tumor appears to grow more rapidly than did the initial myxoma.[35] A viral etiology has also been proposed as a contributing factor to the continuing growth of the myxoma.

Pathology About 75 percent of myxomas occur in the left atrium; most others are located in the right atrium. Myxomas may also occur in both atria.[35a] They are usually solitary and entirely intracavitary, arising on a pedicle from the rim of the interatrial septum near the fossa ovalis. The tumors vary in size from 0.4 to 8.0 cm and are grossly pale, glistening, gelatinous, and friable, hence their propensity to embolization (Fig. 86-5). Tumor emboli may be related to the contact between the mitral valve leaflet, the tumor, and the ventricular septum.

Calcification is not infrequent. On microscopic examination, the tumor consists of relatively loose, poorly cellular myxomatous tissue (Fig. 86-6). The histologically benign appearance contrasts with the clinically malignant behavior of the tumor.

History Left atrial myxomas produce a classic triad of obstructive, embolic, and constitutional effects.[36] Acute circulatory failure and acute paroxysmal dyspnea may result from ball-valve blockade of the mitral valve by an atrial tumor. The clinical presentation[31,37] may include syncope, epileptiform seizures, coma, shock, acute pulmonary edema, cyanosis, gangrene of the nose and toes, or episodic bizarre behavior.[7] Episodic dyspnea, unexplained syncope or seizures,

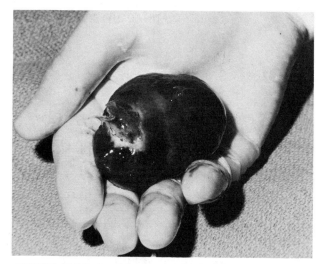

FIGURE 86-5 Left atrial myxoma with pedicle.

and paroxysmal dizziness are commonly the important clues. Symptoms often vary with positional change. Syncope seems to be a particularly ominous symptom, often warning of sudden death. Angina pectoris may result from decreased cardiac output; sudden death is not infrequent, particularly in patients with symptomatic atrial tumors.[32]

Tumor emboli may mimic bacterial endocarditis. Indeed, an unexplained peripheral embolus or an apparently embolic stroke in a young person, particularly in the presence of sinus rhythm, should suggest intracardiac myxoma.[31]

Nonspecific systemic manifestations[38] of low-grade fever, weight loss, and clubbing may occur with atrial myxomas, often causing confusion with bacterial endocarditis, lupus erythematosus, myocarditis, or even rheumatic fever.

Physical examination The size, location, and pedunculated character of the myxoma allow ball valve blockage of the mitral valve, simulating mitral stenosis. The murmur of mitral regurgitation has also been

FIGURE 86-6 Atrial myxoma composed of loose connective tissue, infiltrated by plasma cells, with prominent vascularity and stellate fibroblasts (×250).

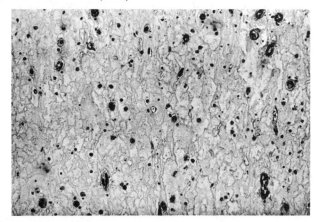

LEFT ATRIAL MYXOMA

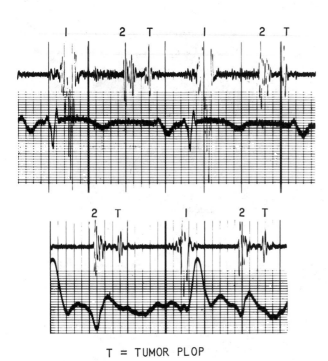

T = TUMOR PLOP

FIGURE 86-7 "Tumor plop," or opening snap, in a case of left atrial myxoma.

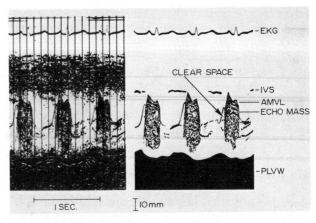

FIGURE 86-8 Echocardiogram: left atrial myxoma. Note mass of echoes behind the anterior mitral valve leaflet, preceded by the characteristic clear or echo-free space. (*Courtesy Dr. J. Felner.*)

described. The tumor mass may interfere with closure of a normal mitral valve, or alternatively "wrecking ball" trauma from the pedunculated tumor, especially when calcified, may result in valve leaflet scarring or even chordal rupture.[39]

Murmurs, blood pressure, and heart rate often vary with positional change.[10,32] The character of the murmur may change on repeated examinations, occasionally having an unusual "whoop" sound;[7] the intensity of the murmur is often disproportionate to the degree of functional impairment. Opening snaps or "tumor plops" have been recorded in atrial tumors[40] and may reflect either sudden tension of the tumor stalk at the end of its forward excursion or the impact of the tumor against the heart wall[41] (Fig. 86-7); disparity between the timing of the opening snap and the severity of clinical symptoms should suggest an atrial tumor.[7] The delay in mitral valve closure may reflect the time needed for the myxoma to move back into the left atrium.

"Endocardial" friction rubs are presumed due to physical contact of the tumor with the atrial or ventricular endocardium.[42] Clubbing may occur, mimicking congenital heart disease.[43]

Laboratory Anemia, leukocytosis, elevated sedimentation rate, and hyperglobulinemia occur with myxoma, possibly reflecting tumor emboli or tumor breakdown products. The serum globulin levels return to normal after tumor removal.

Electrocardiographic clues include unexplained arrhythmias, particularly atrial fibrillation and flutter, conduction disturbances, bundle branch block, and abnormal P waves in the absence of right ventricular hypertrophy, although right ventricular hypertrophy is not infrequent. ST-segment changes mimicking myocardial infarction have been described.[22]

Echocardiography (see also Chap. 32C) is an excellent noninvasive screening technique for patients suspected of having left atrial myxomas.[44] Mitral stenosis can be excluded by echocardiographic demonstration of normal mitral valve motion, and echoes of tumor movement can be recorded[39] (Fig. 86-8).

In patients with a prolapsing left atrial myxoma, a mass of echoes is demonstrable in the left atrium in systole, prolapses through the mitral valve in diastole, and appears as a dense mass of echoes behind the anterior mitral valve leaflet. It is characteristically preceded by an echo-free space at the mitral valve at the onset of diastole, reflecting the time required for the atrial myxoma to prolapse through the mitral orifice.

Echocardiography should be performed prior to catheterization if a left atrial myxoma is suspected, so that levophase pulmonary angiography or retrograde catheterization of the left side of the heart can be elected.[45]

Gated radionuclide cardiac imaging also appears of value in the detection of atrial myxomas and in the delineation of the pattern of tumor movement.[45a]

Apex cardiography may also help to identify a mobile left atrial tumor. A prominent notch on the upstroke of the apex cardiogram, which coincides with a notch on the upstroke of the left ventricular pressure tracing, appears related to the sudden tumor movement from the left ventricle to left atrium; this occurs simultaneously with the prolonged S_1 and prior to the c wave of the left atrial pressure tracing.[39,46]

The chest roentgenogram frequently shows pulmonary venous distension or pulmonary edema. An abnormal cardiac silhouette or unusual intracardiac calcification on x-ray examination should also suggest an intracavitary tumor (Figs. 86-9 and 86-10), but

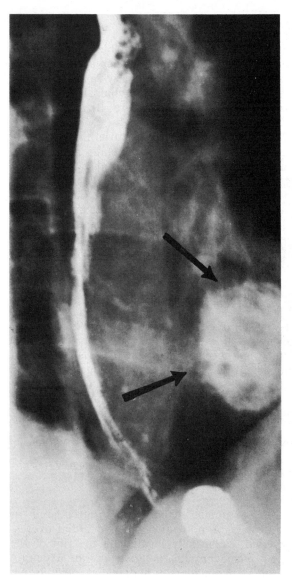

FIGURE 86-9 Calcified tumor mass (arrow) in the posterior aspect of the left atrium. At fluoroscopy this mass moved freely in a superoinferior axis within the cardiac silhouette. The tumor has been known to be present for at least 15 years and is thought to represent a calcified myxoma in a completely asymptomatic patient.

FIGURE 86-10 Mitral configuration of the heart due to a calcified left atrial myxoma. A. Left atrial enlargement, with visible right border of the left atrium (arrow). B. Roentgenogram of surgical specimen, showing calcification of the myxoma (arrow). C. Indentation of the esophagus by the enlarged left atrium (arrow).

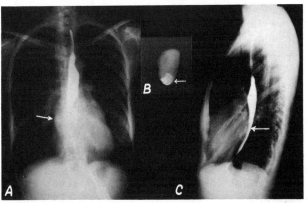

angiocardiographic demonstration of a filling defect in a cardiac chamber provides the definitive diagnosis.[8] The left atrial chamber may be visualized via a catheter passed retrograde into the aorta, left ventricle, and through the mitral valve. Transseptal puncture to enter the left atrium is unwise if a left atrial myxoma is suspected, as fragmentation of the friable tumor mass and systemic embolization may occur. At cardiac catheterization, the atrial pressure is elevated because of outflow obstruction; the pulmonary capillary pressure may also be increased.

Nonprolapsing left atrial myxomas impede flow across the mitral valve and result in a slow y descent of the left atrial pressure pulse, indistinguishable from that of mitral stenosis; there is no notch in the upstroke of the left ventricular pressure pulse. A prolapsing left atrial myxoma produces prominent c and v waves with a rapid y descent (due to sudden left atrial decompression) on the left atrial pressure tracing; as mentioned earlier, there is a notch on the upstroke of the left ventricular pressure pulse due to an abrupt decrease in left ventricular volume as the tumor returns to the atrium in early systole.[45]

On occasion, the diagnosis of cardiac myxoma may be made at histologic examination of a peripheral embolus.[47]

Differentiation from mitral stenosis Useful features which differentiate a left atrial myxoma from rheumatic mitral stenosis include[1,32] (1) absence of a history of rheumatic fever; (2) sudden onset and unusually rapid progression of symptoms; (3) intermittent signs and symptoms; (4) lack of correlation between physical findings, roentgenologic examination, and severity of symptoms; (5) positional variation of murmurs, blood pressure, heart rate, and symptoms; assuming the recumbent position may relieve valve obstruction and cause dramatic symptomatic improvement; (6) positional syncope; (7) absence of an opening snap or disparity between the timing of the opening snap and the clinical symptoms; in addition, the opening snap may be of unusually low pitch;[44] (8) normal sinus rhythm and an S_3, and (9) intracardiac calcification not characteristic of mitral valve calcification. In general, atrial fibrillation and left atrial enlargement are rare with left atrial myxomas.

Occasional reports document atrial myxomas in patients with rheumatic heart disease. Successful surgical removal was reported of a left atrial myxoma which simulated restenosis of the mitral valve in a patient who had had a prior mitral commissurotomy.

Treatment Surgical excision under direct vision using cardiopulmonary bypass[32,33] should be performed promptly, as recurrent and often fatal embolization is common prior to scheduled surgery.[47] At times valvuloplasty or even valve replacement may be necessitated by trauma to the mitral valve and/or chordae tendineae due to tumor movement.

Recurrences of resected myxomas, although unusual, have been documented with increasing frequency in recent years.[48,49] Contralateral myxoma recurrence has also been described. Therefore, wide resection of the atrial septum surrounding the tumor base is recommended, with repair of the resulting atrial defect with a Dacron patch. Careful atrial exploration for multicentric tumor foci is also warranted. Periodic follow-up of postoperative patients should include echocardiography and the determination of the hemoglobin, erythrocyte sedimentation rate, and serum protein levels. Elevation of the sedimentation rate may be of value in early identification of a recurrent tumor; this is important because systemic emboli may occur before tumor mechanical factors interfere with cardiac function.[49]

RIGHT ATRIAL MYXOMA

History The typical history is of rapidly progressive unresponsive right-sided heart failure. Dyspnea is the most common symptom; cough and cyanosis may be present. The cyanosis may vary with position, due to varying right-to-left shunting of blood. Dizziness and syncope may also be related to body position; syncope occurs in about one-third of patients. A history suggesting pulmonary embolization is occasionally obtained. Constitutional symptoms include fever, sweating, and weight loss, which occur in about one-fifth of patients..

Physical examination Classical physical findings are those of right-sided heart failure. Ninety percent of patients have either a murmur or a friction rub. Right atrial tumors may mimic constrictive pericarditis, presenting evidence of increased venous pressure: hepatomegaly, pleural effusion, ascites, and edema. They may simulate tricuspid stenosis, producing intractable right-sided heart failure by mechanical interference with right ventricular filling; indeed, right atrial myxomas may constitute the most common etiology of isolated tricuspid stenosis. They may present with right-sided heart failure and arrhythmia and mimic Ebstein's anomaly; or they may cause superior vena cava obstruction, with resultant facial edema, cyanosis, distended neck veins, edema of the upper extremities, and dilated superficial collateral veins.[37] The murmur of tricuspid regurgitation may be present even with an anatomically normal tricuspid valve, as the tumor mass may interfere with valve closure; alternatively a calcified tumor may cause actual valve destruction.

The combination of cyanosis and clubbing may mimic congenital heart disease.[43] Friction rubs, with and without murmurs, may be heard.

Laboratory Leukocytosis, elevated sedimentation rate, and hyperglobulinemia occur, as with left atrial myxomas. However, the hemoglobin level is often elevated without arterial hypoxemia.

The electrocardiographic changes include the large P waves of right atrial enlargement, low volt-

age, and evidence of right bundle branch block or right ventricular hypertrophy.

Right atrial enlargement may be evident on the chest roentgenogram; right ventricular enlargement may also be present, but pulmonary vascular congestion is notably absent, despite clinical evidence of advanced right-sided heart failure. Bizarre intracardiac calcification is not unusual.

The echocardiogram of right atrial tumor demonstrates a dense mass of echoes behind the tricuspid valve in diastole, which, because of the angulation of the transducer beam, may or may not show an early echo-free space as seen with left atrial myxoma. There has been echocardiographic documentation of one large right atrial myxoma which in late diastole moved through the tricuspid valve into the right ventricle, remaining there until the first third of ventricular systole, when it was ejected back into the right atrium. Bilateral atrial myxoma has also been diagnosed echocardiographically.[35a]

A venous angiocardiogram adequately delineates right-sided intracavitary myxomas. When a right atrial myxoma is suspected, superior vena caval injection is suggested to avoid the risk of tumor dislodgement. Selective coronary angiography has delineated the blood supply to a right atrial myxoma.[49a] Both right and left atrial myxomas commonly produce pulmonary hypertension.

Treatment See discussion of left atrial myxoma.

OTHER PRIMARY ATRIAL TUMORS

Angioma Angiomas occur as clustered, red or white, sessile or polypoid, subendocardial excrescences and are usually located on the rim of the foramen ovale; they characteristically are asymptomatic and are incidental findings at postmortem examination. Microscopically, they are endothelial-lined spaces filled with blood, lymph, and occasional thrombi with varying degrees or organization.

Lipoma Lipomas (Fig. 86-11) may be variants of myxomas or of hamartomas. They are sessile or pedunculated, usually solitary, fatty masses which may calcify and which may be found in any part of the heart, but often occur in the atria. Lipomas have, on occasion, produced valvular insufficiency,[50] arrhythmias, and electrocardiographic abnormalities, but are characteristically asymptomatic.

Osteoclastoma An extraskeletal osteoclastoma of the interatrial septum produced obstruction to pulmonary venous return and to superior and inferior vena caval flow.[51]

Sarcoma Rapidly progressive superior vena cava or tricuspid valve obstruction suggests sarcoma, because of its frequent right atrial localization,[52] rather than benign myxoma, which occurs more often on the left. The ball-valve blockade phenomenon is less common with sarcoma than with myxoma. Obstruction of the inferior vena cava occasionally occurs.

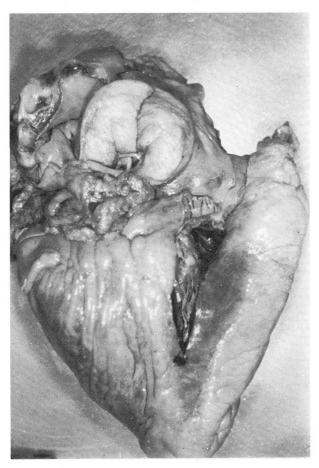

FIGURE 86-11 Gross lipoma arising from the interatrial septum. The lipoma was located over the fossa ovalis and measured approximately 4 × 3 × 2.8 cm. (*Courtesy Dr. M. Gravanis.*)

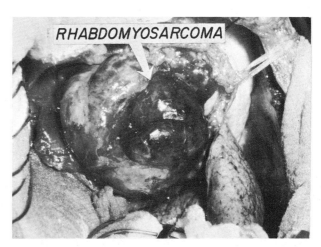

FIGURE 86-12 Rhabdomyosarcoma of the left atrium (arrow). There are enlargement of the atrial appendage and distension of the atrium, due to the tumor.

There is predominant right-sided occurrence of sarcomas, with some predilection for the atrium. Endocardial sarcomas tend to be infiltrative or sessile, firm, yellow-gray mural tumors with intracavitary extension (Fig. 86-12); they vary considerably in size and appearance. Sarcomas grow rapidly, producing a rapid change in roentgenographic contour (Fig. 86-13).

Angiocardiography is the diagnostic procedure and may reveal a filling defect due to an intracavitary sarcoma. Temporary symptomatic remission occurred after surgical removal of a primary sarcoma of the mitral valve; the patient had had the recent onset of the murmurs of mitral stenosis and mitral insufficiency, associated with hemoptysis and a hemorrhagic pleural effusion.[53] A patient with a mitral valve fibrosarcoma also had murmurs of mitral stenosis and mitral insufficiency, which gradually increased in intensity and were associated with progressive cardiac enlargement, congestive heart failure, cyanosis, and clubbing. Survival for 34 months was described in a patient with a left atrial rhabdomyosarcoma treated with tumor excision, chemotherapy, and radiation.[54]

Teratoma A malignant teratoma with widespread systemic metastases was described in a 2-year-old girl. The tumor originated in the interatrial septum and projected into the right atrial cavity.

RIGHT VENTRICULAR TUMORS

Syncope and unexplained fever are the most common presentations of right ventricular tumors. Physical findings have included the murmurs of pulmonary and tricuspid valve obstruction, diminishing on expiration; and a variety of clicks and rubs, often varying with position. Right ventricular conduction delay or right ventricular hypertrophy may be present on the electrocardiogram, and ectopic intracardiac calcification on chest roentgenogram may suggest the diagnosis.

Echocardiography often reveals an intracavitary mass of echoes, and systolic movement of the echo mass through the pulmonic valve has been described.[54a] The diagnosis is confirmed by angiography. Surgery is recommended where possible.

A pulmonic ejection systolic murmur, a delayed and accentuated pulmonic component of the second heart sound, and calcification in the area of the right ventricular outflow tract have suggested the diagnosis of a right ventricular myxoma.[55] Myxoma of the

FIGURE 86-13 Rhabdomyosarcoma of the left atrium. *A.* Mitral configuration of the heart with pulmonary congestion. *B.* Marked left atrial enlargement (arrow) with elevation of the left main bronchus.

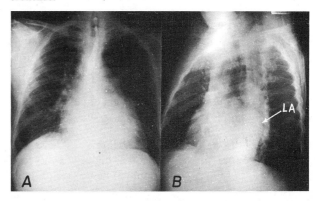

pulmonary valve has also been reported masquerading as severe pulmonic stenosis.

Rhabdomyoma, the most common cardiac tumor in infancy, usually arises from the interventricular septum. Intracavitary extension may result in outflow tract obstruction, simulating pulmonic stenosis.[56] It has been associated with both cardiac lipoma and tuberous sclerosis.

A right ventricular fibrosarcoma which clinically simulated pulmonic stenosis was successfully removed at surgery.[16] The development of a pulmonic stenosis murmur and the appearance of right ventricular hypertrophy on the electrocardiogram, associated with pericardial effusion, syncope, and chest pain, were described in a patient with a primary rhabdomyosarcoma. Some fibromas have mimicked congenital tricuspid stenosis.[60]

LEFT VENTRICULAR TUMORS

Chest pain, syncope, and/or heart failure may herald a left ventricular tumor. A fragment from an aortic valve myxoma produced fatal coronary embolism.[57]

Intracavitary left ventricular tumors often mimic aortic stenosis; narrowing of the left ventricular outflow tract by tumor may mimic hypertrophic subaortic stenosis; at times, though, the murmur and other evidence of left ventricular outflow obstruction due to tumor will vary with change in position.[58] The blood pressure may also show positional variation. Left ventricular hypertrophy is often evident on the electrocardiogram and chest roentgenogram.

Echocardiography may be of value, and precordial radioisotopic heart scans have suggested the diagnosis.[30,44] Angiography is confirmatory.

Fibromas generally arise from the subendothelium of the heart valves, particularly the aortic valve. They are characteristically solitary, small, villous, pedunculated masses of acellular, hyaline tissue covered with endothelium. Papillary heart valve tumors (fibromas) have also been thought to represent giant Lambl's excrescences and thus to be thrombotic rather than neoplastic in nature.[59] Fibromas are usually incidental findings at postmortem examination. However, some fibromas have mimicked congenital subaortic stenosis while others have caused sudden death.[61]

FIXED (NONPROLAPSING) INTRACAVITARY TUMORS

A tumor in a fixed position in relation to the semilunar valves or pulmonary veins chronically obstructs blood flow through the heart but does not produce positional changes in murmurs and symptoms. Instead, the clinical picture is of congestive heart failure: fatigue, exertional dyspnea, paroxysmal nocturnal dyspnea, and orthopnea; and palpitations from atrial fibrillation or other arrhythmias. There are elevated venous pressure, edema, hepatomegaly, ascites, and evidence of pulmonary and systemic embolization.

Echocardiography, using a suprasternal approach, has proved valuable in exploring the left atrium for nonprolapsing atrial myxomas.[61a]

INTRACAVITARY METASTATIC TUMORS

Endocardial or valvular metastatic tumor is unusual, since these areas are relatively avascular. Tumor metastases to the endocardium and heart valves probably occur by direct implantation, usually on an abnormal endothelium.[19] Endocardial and valvular metastases may be polypoid and simulate a benign myxoma;[62] they may embolize and mimic bacterial endocarditis.[19] Supraventricular arrhythmias, particularly atrial fibrillation or flutter, occur with tumor involvement of the atria; they are often resistant to digitalis and other antiarrhythmic therapy. Intracavitary metastatic tumors[19] are probably disseminated via the great veins. Metastases from carcinoma of the kidney, testis, bronchus, and thyroid invade the right atrium via the venae cavae; metastases to the left atrium, via the pulmonary veins, are usually from bronchogenic carcinoma.[63] In a patient who has an inferior vena cava tumor extended into the right atrium, mimicking a right atrial myxoma, nonvisualization of the inferior vena cava is a diagnostic clue.[63a]

Intracavitary metastatic tumors produce symptoms indistinguishable from those due to primary tumors, but the progression and severity of symptoms is more relentless. Nevertheless, the clinical presentation relates primarily to the location of the tumor. Echocardiography and angiography aid in the diagnosis.

Myocardial mural tumors

BACKGROUND INFORMATION

Primary myocardial tumors may involve the heart wall, heart valves, or the cardiac conduction system. They occur at all ages and with an equal sex incidence. Mural tumors are usually incidental autopsy findings; arrhythmias provided the clinical clue in the few tumors diagnosed antemortem. Metastatic myocardial tumors are encountered more frequently than primary myocardial tumors. Rarely, spontaneous myocardial rupture results from tumor infiltration.

As regards myocardial metastatic disease, some studies show that all areas of the myocardium are equally liable to tumor metastases and are invaded by tumor in proportion to their bulk; this would explain the preponderance of left ventricular metastases.[1,21] Other series[64] report a greater incidence of right-sided metastases, presumably because 75 percent of coronary blood flow returns to the right side of the heart and allows more embolic tumor cells to lodge there. Still other studies report an equal number of right and left ventricular metastases. Metastatic tumor encircling or compressing the epicardial coronary arteries has resulted in myocardial infarction.[65]

PATHOLOGY

Rhabdomyoma See "Glycogen Storage Disease," Chap. 82.

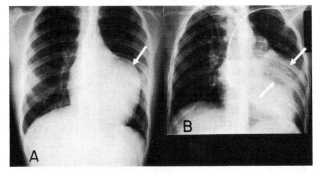

FIGURE 86-14 Hamartoma of the myocardium. *A*. Alteration of the cardiac configuration by a tumor projecting from the border of the left side of the heart (arrow). *B*. Left-sided opacification following injection of contrast material into the superior vena cava. A filling defect of the left atrium and left ventricle is produced by encroachment of the tumor mass (arrow).

Fibroma Intramural ventricular fibromas producing cardiovascular abnormalities have been surgically removed successfully.[66]

Angioma The interventricular septum is a common site for the few symptomatic angiomas; these produce complete heart block, Stokes-Adams syncope, and sudden death.[13]

Hamartoma Hamartomas are firm, white, unencapsulated nodules which usually arise in the ventricle (Fig. 86-14). They are composed of fibrous tissue with varying amounts of fat, elastic tissue, and blood vessels (Fig. 86-15). The term *mesenchymoma* is generally used synonymously with hamartoma.[67] Hamartomas generally are asymptomatic but occasionally cause arrhythmias and sudden death.

Mesothelioma Primary mesotheliomas of the AV node may produce complete heart block, Stokes-Adams syncope, and sudden death. These tiny, slow-growing cystic tumors, generally thought to be derived from epicardial rests, invade the AV node and its approaches, but characteristically spare the AV bundle and its branches. This tumor has not, to date, been diagnosed antemortem. It occurs almost exclusively in adults and predominantly in women;

FIGURE 86-15 Hamartoma of the heart. There is a haphazard arrangement of fat cells, cardiac muscle cells, and small blood vessels (×120).

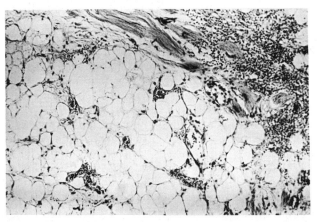

the diagnosis should be considered if otherwise unexplained complete heart block develops in a young patient.[68] Pacemaker implantation may avert sudden death.[69] Recent evidence favors an endodermal rather than mesothelial origin, and the designation "endodermal inclusion cyst" is suggested.[70] Primary malignant mesotheliomas (lymphangioendotheliomas) also selectively involve the conduction system.

Sarcoma Sarcomas are less common in the myocardium than in the endocardium or pericardium. Sarcomatous invasion and destruction of the conduction system has resulted in complete AV block with Stokes-Adams syncope.[71]

Burkitt's lymphoma Myocardial, as well as epicardial and endocardial, involvement is not infrequent in Burkitt's lymphoma, a multifocal, rapidly fatal disorder. Complete AV block has been described, and conduction abnormalities have regressed after radiation therapy.[72]

HISTORY
Myocardial mural tumors are characteristically asymptomatic. Symptoms of arrhythmias—palpitations and Stokes-Adams syncope—have suggested the diagnosis. Myocardial infarction is rare, as is congestive heart failure, but sudden death occurs with disturbing frequency in patients with myocardial (mural) tumors.

PHYSICAL EXAMINATION
Atrial fibrillation and flutter, at first transient and later permanent, are common with right atrial tumors. Tumor invasion of the AV node or of the interventricular septum may result in heart block with Stokes-Adams syncope;[20] this may be the mechanism of sudden death. Mural tumors may also present as myocardial dysfunction with cardiac enlargement, congestive heart failure with gallop rhythm and pulsus alternans, unexplained tachycardia, or occasionally angina pectoris. Pericarditis with hemorrhagic effusion may develop, as may superior vena cava obstruction.

LABORATORY
The frequent electrocardiographic abnormalities include arrhythmias, heart block, bundle branch block, abnormal P waves with atrial tumors, nonspecific ST-T alterations, and changes mimicking myocardial infarction.[22] Impaired conduction is the most frequent manifestation of myocardial tumors.

The chest roentgenogram may show an abnormal but nondiagnostic cardiac silhouette, although the cardiac contour is often normal. Echocardiography does not appear to be of diagnostic value except, perhaps, when tumor of the interventricular septum results in septal thickening.

Radioisotope scanning may help to identify myocardial tumors.[73] Angiography, including coronary angiography, aids in tumor delineation.

TREATMENT

Mural tumors are rarely amenable to surgical removal because of their extent and location. Antitumor therapy appears to increase the survival of patients developing complete heart block due to cardiac metastases.[74]

Pericardial tumors

BACKGROUND INFORMATION

Pericardial tumors are less common than those of the heart. However, pericardial metastases occur more frequently than myocardial metastases.[24] Pericardial metastases are common in intrathoracic neoplasms,[19] often occurring by direct extension.

PATHOLOGY

Malignant pericardial tumors predominate, with sarcomas being most frequent. Benign pericardial tumors include mesotheliomas, teratomas, lipomas, fibromas, neurofibromas, leiomyomas, and hemangiomas.

Teratoma Teratomas arise near the roots of the great vessels, especially the aorta. They are usually intrapericardial and produce symptoms by cardiac compression. Successful surgical removal of an intrapericardial teratoma was first reported in 1942. The typical adult teratoma contains elements from all three germinal layers[75] and is a firm, multicystic, well-encapsulated tumor.

Leiomyoma A pericardial leiomyoma has caused death by compression of the atrium.[75a]

Lymphoma Pericardial involvement is prominent in lymphoma, presumably by direct extension from mediastinal tumors; the heart, however, has been reported to be involved more frequently than the pericardium in patients with malignant lymphoma, suggesting that hematogenous dissemination is common. Pericardial effusion is encountered with myocardial and epicardial infiltration.

Sarcoma Pericardial sarcomas are diffuse and tend to deform or obliterate the cardiac contour. Many pathologic varieties occur, with a preponderance of angiosarcomas and round-cell and spindle-cell sarcomas (Fig. 86-16). Osteosarcomas have also been described.[76] Over 30 percent have distant metastases, most commonly to the lung and pleura but also to the mediastinal, tracheobronchial, and retroperitoneal lymph nodes, the pancreas, the adrenals, and the liver and kidneys.

Malignant mesothelioma Malignant pericardial mesotheliomas or coelotheliomas produce pericarditis, often with hemopericardium and tamponade, and have simulated constriction by obliteration of the pericardial cavity.[11] They frequently invade the myocardium and the conduction system and encircle and

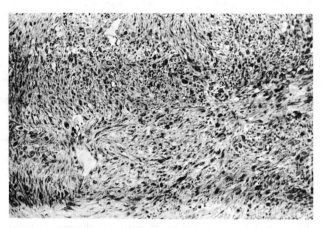

FIGURE 86-16 Pleiomorphic rhabdomyosarcoma of the heart. Spindle-cell sarcoma with large pleiomorphic rhabdomyoblasts (×120).

compress the vena cava. Tumor erosion of a coronary artery may result in myocardial infarction or acute cardiac tamponade. Tumor extension into the thorax and mediastinum is characteristic.[77] Mesotheliomas have few distinctive histologic criteria and are difficult to classify; pathologic diagnosis depends on exclusion of all other epithelial body structures as a possible source of the tumor.

HISTORY

The clinical presentation of symptomatic tumors is of acute pericarditis, with precordial pain; dyspnea and cough are more common when significant pericardial effusion occurs.

PHYSICAL EXAMINATION

The common clinical picture, particularly of malignant pericardial tumors, is of acute pericarditis, with a pericardial friction rub, and electrocardiographic ST-T changes of pericarditis. Pericardial effusion, often with tamponade, presents as cardiac enlargement, decreased cardiac pulsations, pulsus paradoxus, neck vein distension, and, at times, a superior vena caval syndrome. Atrial arrhythmias[74] and refractory heart failure may occur.

Pericardial effusion, often hemorrhagic, occurs in over one-third of metastatic cardiac tumors. Pericardial metastases are even more silent than myocardial, usually presenting only as pericardial effusion, with infrequent constrictive pericarditis.[78] Constrictive pericarditis due to metastases is especially common with bronchogenic carcinoma and carcinoma of the breast.

LABORATORY

Decreased voltage may be evident on the electrocardiogram, and atrial arrhythmias may be present. Malignant pericardial effusions may be associated with electrical alternans.

The tumor is often initially suspected because of a bizarre cardiac contour on roentgenographic examination. Frequent epicardial involvement produces irregularity of the external surface of the heart, demonstrable by roentgenographic examination or pneumopericardiography. Atypical cardiac calcification may be seen.

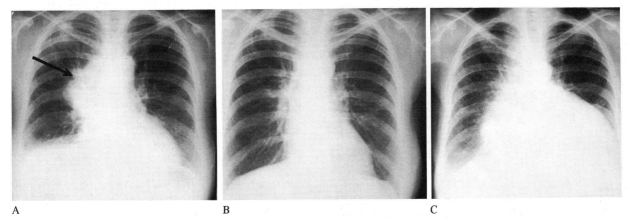

A   B   C

FIGURE 86-17 A. Bronchogenic carcinoma with mediastinal extension (arrow). *B.* Regression of the bronchogenic carcinoma after 4 months of x-ray therapy. *C.* Massive pericardial effusion, 1 year later, due to pericardial metastases from the bronchogenic carcinoma.

Hemorrhagic pericardial effusion is typical of both benign and malignant pericardial tumors (Fig. 86-17). Pericardiocentesis provides both symptomatic relief and a cytologic diagnosis, by examination of the pericardial fluid[23] (Fig. 86-18). Further diagnostic aids include pericardial biopsy and delineation of the tumor mass by echocardiography, by angiocardiography, and/or by CO_2 injection into the pericardium.

TREATMENT
Neoplastic pericardial effusion reaccumulates rapidly after therapeutic pericardiocentesis.[79] Radioisotope treatment and chemotherapy are of variable benefit. Successful obliteration of the pericardial space and control of malignant pericardial effusion have been accomplished by talc poudrage.[80] Pericar-

dial resection, however, is often the treatment of choice.

In patients with pericardial sarcomas, wide excision of the pericardium is recommended to prevent subsequent constriction secondary to recurrent, often hemorrhagic, pericardial effusion.

Pseudotumors of the heart

Any pericardial, myocardial, or intracavitary mass may simulate a cardiac tumor; hence the term *pseudotumor.*[9] Pedunculated or endothelialized thrombi, abscesses, or foreign bodies may mimic intracavitary tumors; cysts, abscesses, or hematomas may mimic intramural myocardial tumors;[81] congenital diverticuli, ventricular aneurysms, coronary artery aneurysms, or intrapericardial lesions may mimic epicardial tumors[7] (Fig. 86-19).

Therapy of cardiac tumors; general principles

Surgical excision, if feasible, is the treatment of choice for all benign cardiac tumors.[7] Occasionally malignant or metastatic cardiac tumors may also be

FIGURE 86-18 Pericardial fluid containing sheets of malignant cells forming papillary projections. The patient had adenocarcinoma of the breast, metastatic to the heart.

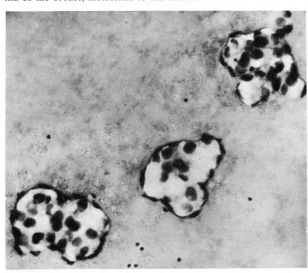

FIGURE 86-19 Pseudotumor of the heart. *Salmonella typhimurium* subendocardial abscess (arrow), 2 in. in diameter, at the apex of the left ventricle.

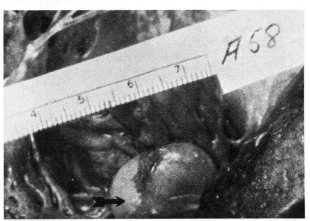

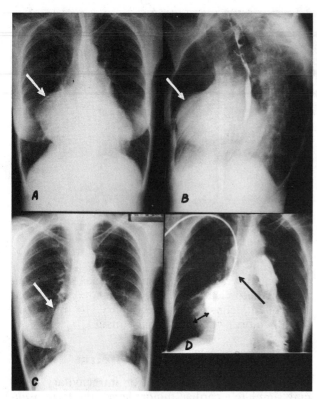

FIGURE 86-20 Myocardial metastases from carcinoma of the uterus. *A* and *B*. Large tumor mass projecting from the border of the right side of the heart (arrow). *C*. Regression of the size of the tumor mass following 2 months of radiation therapy (arrow). *D*. Right atrial angiocardiogram, prior to radiation therapy, showing projection of the tumor mass beyond the opacified right atrium and compression of the right ventricular outflow tract by the tumor mass (arrow).

amenable to surgery; often postoperative chemotherapy and radiation therapy are advisable.[54] In general, however, surgical therapy for primary malignant tumors or for metastases to the heart is usually neither possible nor desirable. Palliative radiation with roentgen therapy[82] (Fig. 86-20) or various radioisotopic substances, and systemic chemotherapy with compounds such as nitrogen mustards, folic acid antagonists, and other antimetabolites, may afford symptomatic relief. There has been angiographic documentation of regression of intracavitary metastases following chemotherapy. Symptomatic remission for months to years has been described after treatment with vincristine and cyclophosphamide and after surgery.[83] Significant palliation of cardiac symptoms with chemotherapy and radiation therapy can be expected in leukemia and lymphoma.[18,24,84,85] However, radiation to the chest may produce myocardial fibrosis and damage to the conduction system (see Chap. 101). Intrapericardial instillation of chemotherapeutic and radioisotopic substances produces no predictable results. Disappearance of heart block, presumably caused by cardiac metastases, has occurred following x-ray therapy. Radiation has also caused regression of pericardial effusion.[19,84] However, pericardiectomy may be required to prevent cardiac tamponade and appears to be the optimal management for malignant pericardial effusion.[86] Malignant disease of the heart is treated at the Emory University School of Medicine teaching hospitals by a combination of high-energy radiation and chemotherapy.

REFERENCES

1 Griffiths, G. C.: A Review of Primary Tumors of the Heart, *Prog. Cardiovasc. Dis.,* 7:465, 1965.

2 Goodwin, J. F.: Symposium on Cardiac Tumors. Introduction: The Spectrum of Cardiac Tumors, *Am. J. Cardiol.,* 21:307, 1968.

3 Besterman, E., Bromley, L. L., and Peart, W. S.: An Intrapericardial Phaeochromocytoma, *Br. Heart J.,* 36:318, 1974.

4 Babcock, K. B., Judge, R. D., and Bookstein, J. J.: Acquired Pulmonic Stenosis. Report of a Case Caused by Mediastinal Neoplasm, *Circulation,* 26:931, 1962.

5 Littler, W. A., Meade, J. B., and Hamilton, D. I.: Acquired Pulmonary Stenosis, *Thorax,* 25:465, 1970.

6 Bagby, G. C., Jr., Goldman, R. D., Newman, H. C., and Means, J. F.: Acute Myocardial Infarction Due to Childhood Lymphoma, *N. Engl. J. Med.,* 287:338, 1972.

7 Abbott, O. A., Warshawski, F. E., and Cobbs, B. W., Jr.: Primary Tumors and Pseudotumors of the Heart, *Ann. Surg.,* 155:855, 1962.

8 Steiner, R. E.: Radiologic Aspects of Cardiac Tumors, *Am. J. Cardiol.,* 21:344, 1968.

9 Abrams, H. L., Adams, D. F., and Grant, H. A.: The Radiology of Tumors of the Heart, *Radiol. Clin. North Am.,* 9:299, 1971.

10 Harvey, W. P.: Clinical Aspects of Cardiac Tumors, *Am. J. Cardiol.,* 21:328, 1968.

11 Fine, G.: Primary Tumors of the Pericardium and Heart, *Cardiovasc. Clin.,* 5:207, 1973.

12 Nadas, A. S., and Ellison, R. C.: Cardiac Tumors in Infancy, *Am. J. Cardiol.,* 21:363, 1968.

13 Van der Hauwaert, L. G.: Cardiac Tumours in Infancy and Childhood, *Br. Heart J.,* 33:125, 1971.

14 Somers, K., and Lothe, F.: Primary Lymphosarcoma of the Heart: Review of the Literature and Report of 3 Cases, *Cancer,* 13:449, 1960.

15 Bearman, R. M.: Primary Leiomyosarcoma of the Heart: Report of a Case and Review of the Literature, *Arch. Pathol.,* 98:62, 1974.

16 Goldstein, S., and Mahoney, E. B.: Right Ventricular Fibrosarcoma Causing Pulmonic Stenosis, *Am. J. Cardiol.,* 17:570, 1966.

17 Glancy, D. L., and Roberts, W. C.: The Heart in Malignant Melanoma: A Study of 70 Autopsy Cases, *Am. J. Cardiol.,* 21:555, 1968.

18 Roberts, W. C., Glancy, D. L., and De Vita, V. T., Jr.: Heart in Malignant Lymphoma (Hodgkin's Disease, Lymphosarcoma, Reticulum Cell Sarcoma and Mycosis Fungoides): A Study of 196 Autopsy Cases, *Am. J. Cardiol.,* 22:85, 1968.

19 Hanfling, S. M.: Metastatic Cancer to the Heart: Review of the Literature and Report of 127 Cases, *Circulation,* 22:474, 1960.

20 James, T. N.: Metastasis of Hypernephroma to Atrioventricular Node: Report of a Case, *N. Engl. J. Med.,* 266:705, 1962.

21 Berge, T., and Sievers, J.: Myocardial Metastases. A Pathological and Electrocardiographic Study, *Br. Heart J.,* 30:383, 1968.

22 Harris, T. R., Copeland, G. D., and Brody, D. A.: Progressive Injury Current with Metastatic Tumor of the Heart: Case Report and Review of the Literature, *Am. Heart J.,* 69:392, 1965.

23 Biran, S., Hochman, A., Levij, I. S., and Stern, S.: Clinical Diagnosis of Secondary Tumors of the Heart and Pericardium, *Dis. Chest,* 55:202, 1969.

24 Freiman, A. H.: Cardiovascular Disturbances Associated with Cancer, *Med. Clin. North Am.,* 50:733, 1966.

25 Atkinson, K., McElwain, T. J., and Mackay, A. M.: Myeloma of the Heart, *Br. Heart J.,* 36:309, 1974.

26 Rothfeld, E. L., and Zirkin, R. M.: Unusual Electrocardiographic Evidence of Metastatic Cardiac Tumor Resembling Atrial Infarction, *Am. J. Cardiol.,* 10:882, 1962.

26a Swirsky, M. H., Roth, O., and Celentano, L.: Electrocardiographic Diagnosis of a Metastatic Heart Tumor, *Conn. Med.,* 40:375, 1976.

27 Kline, I. K.: Cardiac Lymphatic Involvement by Metastatic Tumor, *Cancer,* 29:799, 1972.

28 Thomas, K. E., Winchell, C. P., and Varco, R. L.: Diagnostic and Surgical Aspects of Left Atrial Tumors, *J. Thorac. Cardiovasc. Surg.,* 53:535, 1967.

29 Carter, J. B., Cramer, R., Jr., and Edwards, J. E.: Mitral and Tricuspid Lesions Associated with Polypoid Atrial Tumors, Including Myxoma, *Am. J. Cardiol.,* 33:914, 1974.

30 Bonte, F. J., and Curry, T. S., III: Technetium-99m HSA Blood Pool Scan in Diagnosis of an Intracardiac Myxoma, *J. Nucl. Med.,* 8:35, 1967.

30a Stiltanen, P., Tuuteri, L., Norio, R., Tala, P., Ahrenberg, P., and Halonen, P. I.: Atrial Myxoma in a Family, *Am. J. Cardiol.,* 38:252, 1976.

31 Greenwood, W. F.: Profile of Atrial Myxoma, *Am. J. Cardiol.,* 21:367, 1968.

32 Wight, R. P., Jr., McCall, M. M., and Wenger, N. K.: Primary Atrial Tumor: Evaluation of Clinical Findings in Ten Cases and Review of the Literature, *Am. J. Cardiol.,* 11:790, 1963.

33 Castaneda, A. R., and Varco, R. L.: Tumors of the Heart: Surgical Considerations, *Am. J. Cardiol.,* 21:357, 1968.

34 Salyer, W. R., Page, D. L., and Hutchins, G. M.: The Development of Cardiac Myxomas and Papillary Endocardial Lesions from Mural Thrombus, *Am. Heart J.,* 89:4, 1975.

34a Symbas, P. N., Hatcher, C. R., Jr., and Gravanis, M. B.: Myxoma of the Heart: Clinical and Experimental Observations, *Ann. Surg.,* 183:470, 1976.

35 Read, R. C., White, H. J., Murphy, M. L., Williams, D., Sun, C. N., and Flanagan, W. H.: The Malignant Potentiality of Left Atrial Myxoma, *J. Thorac. Cardiovasc. Surg.,* 68:857, 1974.

35a Fitterer, J. D., Spicer, M. J., and Nelson, W. P.: Echocardiographic Demonstration of Bilateral Atrial Myxomas, *Chest,* 70:282, 1976.

36 Peters, M. N., Hall, R. J., Cooley, D. A., Leachman, R. D., and Garcia, E.: The Clinical Syndrome of Atrial Myxoma, *JAMA,* 230:695, 1974.

37 Adams, C. W., Collins, H. A., Dummit, E. S., and Allen, J. H.: Intracardiac Myxomas and Thrombi: Clinical Manifestations, Pathology and Treatment, *Am. J. Cardiol.,* 7:176, 1961.

38 Goodwin, J. F.: Diagnosis of Left Atrial Myxoma, *Lancet,* 1:464, 1963.

39 Nasser, W. K., Davis, R. H., Dillon, J. C., Travel, M. E., Helmen, C. H., Feigenbaum, H., and Fisch, C.: Atrial Myxoma: I. Clinical and Pathologic Features in Nine Cases; II. Phonocardiographic, Echocardiographic, Hemodynamic, and Angiographic Features in Nine Cases, *Am. Heart J.,* 83:694, 810, 1972.

40 Pitt, A., Pitt, B., Schaefer, J., and Criley, J. M.: Myxoma of the Left Atrium: Hemodynamic and Phonocardiographic Consequences of Sudden Tumor Movement, *Circulation,* 36:408, 1967.

41 Bass, N. M., and Sharratt, G. J. P.: Left Atrial Myxoma Diagnosed by Echocardiography, with Observations on Tumour Movement, *Br. Heart J.,* 35:1332, 1973.

42 Hubbard, T. F., and Neil, R. N.: Myxoma of the Right Ventricle: Report of a Case with Unusual Findings, *Am. Heart J.,* 81:548, 1971.

43 Talley, R. C., Baldwin, B. J., Symbas, P. N., and Nutter, D. O.: Right Atrial Myxoma. Unusual Presentation with Cyanosis and Clubbing, *Am. J. Med.,* 48:256, 1970.

44 MacVaugh, H., III, and Joyner, C. R.: Mitral Insufficiency Due to Calcified Myxoma, Treatment of Resection and Mitral Annuloplasty, *J. Thorac. Cardiovasc. Surg.,* 61:287, 1971.

45 Sung, R. J., Ghahramani, A. R., Mallon, S. M., Richter, S. E., Sommer, L. S., Gottlieb, S., and Myerburg, R. J.: Hemodynamic Features of Prolapsing and Nonprolapsing Left Atrial Myxoma, *Circulation,* 51:342, 1975.

45a Pohost, G. M., Pastore, J. O., McKusick, K. A., Chiotellis, P. N., Kapellakis, G. Z., Myers, G. S., Dinsmore, R. E., and Block, P. C.: Detection of Left Atrial Myxoma by Gated Radionuclide Cardiac Imaging, *Circulation,* 55:88, 1977.

46 Becker, L. C., and Conti, C. R.: Left Atrial Myxoma: Evidence of Tumor Movement by Apexcardiogram, *Chest,* 60:280, 1971.

47 Newman, H. A., Cordell, A. R., and Prichard, R. W.: Intracardiac Myxomas: Literature Review and Report of Six Cases, One Successfully Treated, *Am. Surg.,* 32:219, 1966.

48 Walton, J. A., Jr., Kahn, D. R., and Willis, P. W., III: Recurrence of a Left Atrial Myxoma, *Am. J. Cardiol.,* 29:872, 1972.

49 Jugdutt, B. I. Rossall, R. E. and Sterns L. P.: An Unusual Case of Recurrent Left Atrial Myxoma, *Can. Med. Assoc. J.,* 112:1099, 1975.

49a Berman, N. D., McLaughlin, P. R., Bigelow, W. G., and Morch, J. E.: Angiographic Demonstration of Blood Supply of Right Atrial Myxoma, *Br. Heart J.,* 38:764, 1976.

50 Estevez, J. M., Thompson, D. S., and Levinson, J. P.: Lipoma of the Heart: Review of the Literature and Report of Two Autopsied Cases, *Arch. Pathol.,* 77:638, 1962.

51 Dorney, P.: Osteoclastoma of the Heart, *Br. Heart J.,* 29:276, 1967.

52 Glancy, D. L., Morales, J. B., Jr., and Roberts, W. C.: Angiosarcoma of the Heart, *Am. J. Cardiol.,* 21:413, 1968.

53 Forker, E. L., January, L. E., and Lawrence, M. S.: Primary Sarcoma of the Mitral Valve, *Am. Heart J.,* 66:243, 1963.

54 Matloff, J. M., Bass, H., and Dalen, J. E.: Rhabdomyosarcoma of the Left Atrium: Physiologic Responses to Surgical Therapy, *J. Thorac. Cardiovasc. Surg.,* 61:451, 1971.

54a Chandraratna, P. A. N., Pedro, S. S., Elkins, R. C., and Grantham, N.: Echocardiographic, Angiocardiographic, and Surgical Correlations in Right Ventricular Myxoma Simulating Pulmonic Stenosis, *Circulation,* 55:619, 1977.

55 Snyder, S. N., Smith, D. C., Lau, F. Y. K., and Turner, A. F.: Diagnostic Features of Right Ventricular Myxoma, *Am. Heart J.,* 91:240, 1976.

56 Farooki, Z. Q., Henry, J. G., Arciniegas, E., and Green, E. W.: Ultrasonic Pattern of Ventricular Rhabdomyoma in Two Infants, *Am. J. Cardiol.,* 34:842, 1974.

57 Harris, L. S., and Adelson, L.: Fatal Coronary Embolism from a Myxomatous Polyp of the Aortic Valve: An Unusual Cause of Sudden Death, *Am. J. Clin. Pathol.,* 43:61, 1965.

58 de Paiva, E. C., Macieira-Coelho, E., Amram, S. S., Duarte, C. da S., and Coelho, E.: Intracavitary Left Ventricular Myxoma, *Am. J. Cardiol.,* 20:260, 1967.

59 Heath, D.: Pathology of Cardiac Tumors, *Am. J. Cardiol.,* 21:315, 1968.

60 Van der Hauwaert, L. G., Corbeel, L., and Maldague, P.: Fibroma of the Right Ventricle Producing Severe Tricuspid Stenosis, *Circulation,* 32:451, 1965.

61 Butterworth, J. S., and Poindexter, C. A.: Papilloma of Cusp of the Aortic Valve: Report of a Patient with Sudden Death, *Circulation,* 48:213, 1973.

61a Petsas, A. A., Gottlieb, S., Kingsley, B., Begal, B. L., and Myerburg, R. J.: Echocardiographic Diagnosis of Left Atrial

Myxoma: Usefulness of Suprasternal Approach, *Br. Heart J.,* 38:627, 1976.

62 Olsen, S., Bach-Nielsen, P., and Piper, J.: Polypoid Tumours of the Cardiac Auricles: Report of 3 Cases, *Acta Med. Scand.,* 171:637, 1962.

63 Rogen, A. S., and Moffat, A. D.: Unusual Secondary Tumour of Heart, *Br. Heart J.,* 29:638, 1967.

63a Kerber, R. E., Fieselmann, J., and Mischler, N.: Inferior Vena Cava Tumor Thrombus Extending into the Right Atrium and Mimicking Right Atrial Myxoma: Angiographic Differentiation, *Am. Heart J.,* 93:506, 1977.

64 Hanbury, W. J.: Secondary Tumours of the Heart, *Br. J. Cancer,* 14:23, 1960.

65 Franciosa, J. A., and Lawrinson, W.: Coronary Artery Occlusion Due to Neoplasm: A Rare Cause of Acute Myocardial Infarction, *Arch. Intern. Med.,* 128:797, 1971.

66 Geha, A. S., Weidman, W. H., Soule, E. H., and McGoon, D. C.: Intramural Ventricular Cardiac Fibroma: Successful Removal in Two Cases and Review of the Literature, *Circulation,* 36:427, 1967.

67 Childress, R. H., King, R. D., Aldrich, D. D., Buehl, I. A., King, H., and Genovese, P. D.: Successful Resection of a Benign Right Ventricular Mesenchymoma, *Am. J. Cardiol.,* 20:255, 1967.

68 Lafargue, R. T., Hand, A. M., and Lev. M.: Mesothelioma (Coelothelioma) of the Atrioventricular Node, *Chest,* 59:571, 1971.

69 Manion, W. C., Nelson, W. P., Hall, R. J., and Brierty, R. E.: Benign Tumor of the Heart Causing Complete Heart Block, *Am. Heart J.,* 83:535, 1972.

70 Sopher, I. M., and Spitz, W. U.: Endodermal Inclusions of the Heart: So-called Mesotheliomas of the Atrioventricular Node, *Arch. Pathol.,* 92:180, 1971.

71 Lenègre, J., Moreau, Ph., and Iris, L: Deux cas de bloc auriculoventriculaire complet par sarcome primitif du coeur (Two Cases of Complete Auriculoventricular Block Due to Primary Sarcoma of the Heart), *Arch. Mal. Coeur,* 56:361, 1963.

72 Cole, T. O., Attah, E. B., and Onyemelukwe, G. C.: Burkitt's Lymphoma Presenting with Heart Block, *Br. Heart J.,* 37:94, 1975.

73 Folger, G. M., Jr., and Peters, H. J.: Nodular Fibroelastosis (Fibroelastic Hamartoma): A Tumorous Malformation of the Heart, *Am. J. Cardiol.,* 21:420, 1968.

74 Redwine, D. B.: Complete Heart Block Caused by Secondary Tumors of the Heart: Case Report and Review of Literature, *Tex. Med.,* 70:59, 1974.

75 Legnami, F. A., and Corwin, R. D.: Intrapericardial Teratoma: Report of a Case, *Am. Heart J.,* 65:674, 1963.

75a Brandes, W. W., Gray, J. A. C., and MacLeod, N. W.: Leiomyoma of the Pericardium, *Am. Heart J.,* 23:426, 1942.

76 Lowry, W. B., and McKee, E. E.: Primary Osteosarcoma of the Heart, *Cancer,* 30:1068, 1972.

77 Sytman, A. L., and MacAlpin, R. N.: Primary Pericardial Mesothelioma: Report of Two Cases and Review of the Literature, *Am. Heart J.,* 81:760, 1971.

78 Deparis, M., Manigand, G., Sors, Ch., Auzepy, Ph., and Gubler, M.: Les péricardites constrictives d'origine néoplastique. A propos d'une observation anatomo-clinique, *Presse Méd.,* 75:1008, 1967.

79 McNalley, M. C., Kelble, D., Pryor, R., and Blount, S. G., Jr.: Angiosarcoma of the Heart: Report of a Case and Review of the Literature, *Am. Heart J.,* 65:244, 1963.

80 Goldman, B. S., and Pearson, F. G.: Malignant Pericardial Effusion: Review of Hospital Experience and Report of a Case Successfully Treated by Talc Poudrage, *Can. J. Surg.,* 8:157, 1965.

81 Wollenweber, J., Giuliani, E. R., Harrison, C. E., Jr., and Kincaid, O. W.: Pseudotumors of the Right Heart, *Arch. Intern. Med.,* 121:169, 1968.

82 Cham, W. C., Freiman, A. H., Carstens, P. H. B., and Chu, F. C. H.: Radiation Therapy of Cardiac and Pericardial Metastases, *Radiology,* 114:701, 1975.

83 Freeland, J. P., Sy, B. G., Ahluwalia, M. S., and Dunea, G.: Hemangiosarcoma of the Heart, *Chest,* 60:222, 1971.

84 Terry, L. N., Jr., and Kligermen, M. M.: Pericardial and Myocardial Involvement by Lymphomas and Leukemias. The Role of Radiotherapy, *Cancer,* 25:1003, 1970.

85 Garfein, O. B.: Lymphosarcoma of the Right Atrium: Angiographic and Hemodynamic Documentation of Response to Chemotherapy, *Arch. Intern. Med.,* 135:325, 1975.

86 Lokich, J. J.: The Management of Malignant Pericardial Effusions, *JAMA,* 224:1401, 1973.

87
Traumatic Heart Disease

LOREN F. PARMLEY, JR., M.D., and
PANAGIOTIS N. SYMBAS, M.D.

Traumatic injuries continue to constitute one of the major causes of mortality and morbidity in our present society. Cardiac injury, particularly from blunt injury, is often overshadowed by the more overt manifestations of cerebral, abdominal, or musculoskeletal trauma. Under these circumstances the more subtle aspects of injury to the cardiovascular system remain unnoticed, occasionally becoming manifest in a catastrophic manner either in the immediate postinjury period or hours, days, or even months after the injury. Consequently only the more serious injuries of the heart and great vessels may be clearly evident initially, and unless sought out by appropriate clinical evaluation of the injured patient, the diagnosis may be frequently overlooked. Obviously, then, an awareness of possible cardiac injury in every traumatized individual is a prerequisite to early diagnosis and treatment.

The most common cause of traumatic heart disease is mechanical injury produced by physical force. These injuries may be classified as penetrating or nonpenetrating. A penetrating injury requires a vector for the physical force—i.e., an object such as a knife or particularly a missile that penetrates the heart or great vessels by traversing the body surface, or rarely a needle that migrates through the wall of an adjacent organ such as the esophagus, or a missile fragment that is embolic to the heart from a distant intravascular location (Fig. 87-1). Nonpenetrating injuries, on the other hand, are cardiovascular lesions resulting from physical forces acting externally upon the body. These forces act through any one or a combination of several of the following six mechanisms:[1,2] (1) unidirectional force against the chest; (2) bidirectional or compressive force against the thorax; (3) indirect forces, i.e., compression of the abdomen and lower extremities, resulting in marked increase in intravascular pressure; (4) decelerative forces, particularly when imparting differential deceleration to the heart and great vessels; (5) blast forces of great magnitude; and finally, (6) concussive force, which is an empirical category indicating a jarring force that interferes with cardiac rhythm but is not of sufficient magnitude to produce a significant anatomic lesion. However, even these definitions are

not exact, for a high-velocity missile that passes adjacent to the heart may result in a contusive injury to the myocardium because of the shock wave in the tissues, and contrariwise, nonpenetrating trauma may cause a penetrating injury to the heart because of puncture by a fractured rib.

There is a subgroup of these mechanical injuries that is becoming increasingly important as the diagnostic and therapeutic techniques in the management of heart disease become more complex and refined. This is the iatrogenic trauma group comprising the complications of vigorous cardiopulmonary resuscitative procedures[3] resulting in nonpenetrating contusive injuries of the pericardium and myocardium and the diagnostic procedures of cardiac catheterization[4] and regional angiocardiography that may produce penetrating cardiac injuries. The increasing use of

FIGURE 87-1 This 22-year-old man sustained a gunshot wound of the abdomen requiring surgical repair of abdominal organs. The bullet was not evident at the time of surgery, and no attempt was made to recover it. Roentgen studies (A) obtained postoperatively revealed that the bullet was in the pelvis, and a chest film was normal. A routine chest roentgenogram 4 years later (B) revealed that the bullet was now in the heart, presumably embolic via the right iliac vein from the pelvis, where the bullet was no longer visualized on roentgen study.

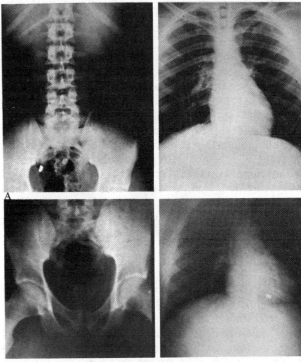

B

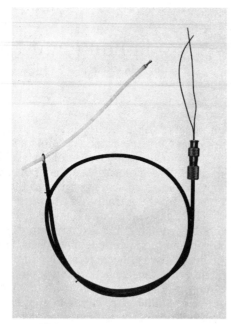

FIGURE 87-2 Photograph of a No. 6F single-opening Lehman catheter with a folded radio wire which was passed through the saphenous vein into the right ventricle in a 6-year-old hydrocephalic boy who had a ventricular-jugular shunt with a Holter catheter. As demonstrated, the migratory Holter catheter was looped with the wire, and while maintaining gentle traction on the wire, the entire combination was removed from the right ventricle via the saphenous vein. *(Reproduced with permission of Dr. Dorothy Brinsfield.)*

venous catheters for cardiovascular monitoring and electrode pacemakers has led to a corresponding increase of penetrating lesions,[5,6] thrombotic endocardial vegetations,[6a] and septic endocarditis,[6b] as well as the rarely occurring migration of therapeutic intravenous catheters to the heart or pulmonary vascular bed[7] (Fig. 87-2).

Two additional categories of heart trauma *not* due to mechanical injury are sufficiently distinctive to warrant separate classification. The first category encompasses cardiac injuries due to ionizing radiation which predominantly causes pericarditis, but may also result in myocardial injury.[8,9] The second includes the group of cardiac injuries due to electric current which most often produces either atrial or ventricular arrhythmias, but may also cause burns of the heart and great vessels. Other types of cardiac trauma are bizarre and almost defy classification; e.g., a calcified right atrial myxoma may erode a tricuspid valve because of the mechanical effect of constant beating against this structure—a form of "internal" nonpenetrating trauma.

The true incidence of traumatic heart disease is difficult to establish. Some penetrating injuries and the majority of nonpenetrating injuries of the heart are well tolerated, as clinical and experimental studies[1,10] have indicated. Consequently the majority of these lesions are infrequently diagnosed, since their initial clinical manifestations may be relatively mini-mal and the lesion may be overlooked unless specific studies are undertaken.[2,11] For this reason and because only the more severe injuries are reflected in autopsy studies,[1] the actual, relatively high incidence of traumatic heart disease is not appreciated.

PENETRATING WOUNDS

Two to four percent of penetrating wounds of the thoracoabdominal region involve the heart.[11-14] Even though the site of the penetrating wound may not involve the precordium, the possibility of cardiac injury must always receive serious consideration, particularly with missile wounds, especially those which may have traversed the mediastinum.[1] To deny the possibility of heart and great-vessel injury because of a presumed remote location of the wound may result in a false sense of security. The delayed appearance of serious clinical manifestations of penetrating heart wounds is well known.[15,16] The rapidity of death from the onset of symptoms, particularly those of cardiac tamponade, is often swift.[17] Therefore, all patients who might have incurred a penetrating heart wound should be kept under close medical and surgical observation for several days.

Almost half the individuals who have incurred stab wounds of the heart may be expected to survive for a sufficient time to reach medical treatment.[15] Gunshot or other missile injury carries with it a much more serious outlook, and perhaps only 10 to 15 percent of these injured individuals would fall in the salvageable category.

The variety of objects[18,19] that may produce penetrating heart wounds is legion, including such diverse objects as pieces of glass, needles, toothpicks, parts of dental plates, coins, and even the spine of a stingray. Obviously penetration of the heart may occur as a result of erosion by a foreign body from an adjacent organ or cavity as well as through migration of a foreign body from a more distant site.[19]

The multiplicity of heart and great-vessel lesions that may be produced by penetrating wounds is indicated in Table 87-1. Lacerating or penetrating wounds frequently result in immediate hemorrhage of varying magnitude. The severity of the hemorrhage and whether it is intra- or extrapericardial determine the clinical picture and dictate the requirements of treatment.[17] When there is intrapericardial hemorrhage with a sealed pericardial wound, cardiac tamponade is the major threat. Paradoxically this may be the mechanism that permits temporary survival, but death follows quickly unless relief is afforded. The management of penetrating wounds should be based primarily on prompt diagnosis with appropriate emergency resuscitative procedures and surgical treatment as indicated. The immediate treatment of these lesions when they manifest with massive and/or continuous intrapleural hemorrhage is surgical repair. However, when cardiac tamponade is the presenting clinical picture, the treatment has been a matter of controversy between proponents of immediate surgical treatment[1,20,21] and a group who prefer a more conservative approach[22,23] utilizing repeated pericardiocentesis when needed and relying on surgi-

TABLE 87-1
Cardiac lesions produced by penetrating wounds

> *I* Pericardial injury
> > *A* Laceration
> > *B* Hemopericardium
> > > *1* Cardiac tamponade
> > *C* Effusion, fibrinous pericarditis
> > > *1* Recurrent effusion
> > *D* Pneumopericardium
> > *E* Suppurative pericarditis
> > *F* Constrictive pericarditis
> *II* Myocardial injury
> > *A* Laceration
> > *B* Penetration or perforation
> > *C* Rupture
> > *D* Retained foreign body
> > > *1* Abscess
> > *E* Structural defects
> > > *1* Aneurysm formation
> > > *2* Septal defects
> > > *3* Aortocardiac fistula
> *III* Valvular injury
> > *A* Leaflet injury
> > *B* Papillary muscle or chordae tendineae laceration or rupture
> *IV* Coronary artery injury
> > *A* Thrombosis or laceration, with or without myocardial infarction
> > *B* Arteriovenous fistula
> > *C* Aneurysm
> *V* Embolism
> > *A* Foreign body
> > *B* Thrombus
> > > *1* Septic
> > > *2* Sterile
> *VI* Bacterial endocarditis
> *VII* Rhythm or conduction disturbances

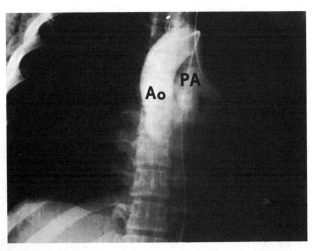

FIGURE 87-3 Aortogram demonstrating concomitant opacification of both the aorta (Ao) and the pulmonary artery (PA) through a fistula. *(Reproduced by permission of the author and publisher; from P. N. Symbas, "Traumatic Injuries of the Heart and Great Vessels," Charles C Thomas, Publisher, Springfield, Ill., 1971, p. 126.)*

cal treatment only if clots or other factors prevent adequate relief of the tamponade or if there is rapidly recurring tamponade. Although both schools of therapeutic approach have reported a low mortality rate, in the range of 2.7 to 15 percent, immediate surgical repair appears now to be the treatment of choice for all penetrating cardiac wounds, and pericardiocentesis should be used only to provide time for a safe operation. The unpredictable course of the patients with favorable response to pericardiocentesis, the propensity of these lesions to rebleed, the possibility of coronary artery injury, and the rare late development of posttraumatic constrictive pericarditis,[17] coupled with the remarkable advancement in the fields of anesthesia and cardiac surgery, greatly favor the immediate surgical treatment of the penetrating cardiac wounds.[1,24]

There are many delayed sequelae of penetrating wounds of the heart encompassing primarily the complications of infection, embolism, arrhythmias, and the creation of structural defects such as ventricular septal defect, aortocardiac or aortopulmonary communication (Fig. 87-3), and ventricular aneurysm[16] (Table 87-1). These sequelae should always be suspected in patients who have sustained penetrating wounds of the heart, or even of the chest; they dictate the necessity of frequent and careful examinations during the postinjury period. When symptoms and signs of a structural defect are detected,

cardiac catheterization and angiocardiography should be performed to define the lesion and its hemodynamic significance. Once evaluated, the proper mode of therapy, i.e., emergency or elective surgery or close observation, should be determined by a collaborative medical and surgical team approach. Appropriate medical and surgical treatment has been developed for all of the complications of penetrating cardiac wounds. Special techniques and extracorporeal circulation are now utilized for the correction of hemodynamically significant structural lesions such as interventricular septal defects, aortocardiac or aortopulmonary fistula, and traumatic ventricular aneurysm.[1]

Recurrent posttraumatic pericarditis, a phenomenon complicating approximately a fifth of all cases of penetrating heart wounds, has been compared to the postcardiotomy syndrome (Fig. 87-4). Conservative management of symptoms is the treatment of choice for this posttraumatic complication unless unrelenting cardiac tamponade or other sequelae, such as purulent or constrictive pericarditis occur which dictate surgical intervention.

Although coronary artery laceration usually results in cardiac tamponade, myocardial infarction is rarely the major complication in the absence of surgical ligation of the injured vessel.[25] In these patients, survival is dependent upon the proper reconstruction of major branches of the coronary artery system or the ligation of smaller terminal vessels. Coronary artery aneurysm[26] and arteriovenous fistula[15] are rare sequelae of injury, and treatment should be individualized.

Projectiles retained in the heart are often tolerated well.[15] However, embolization of the foreign body or associated thrombus has occurred, and the possibility of bacterial endocarditis is ever present if the

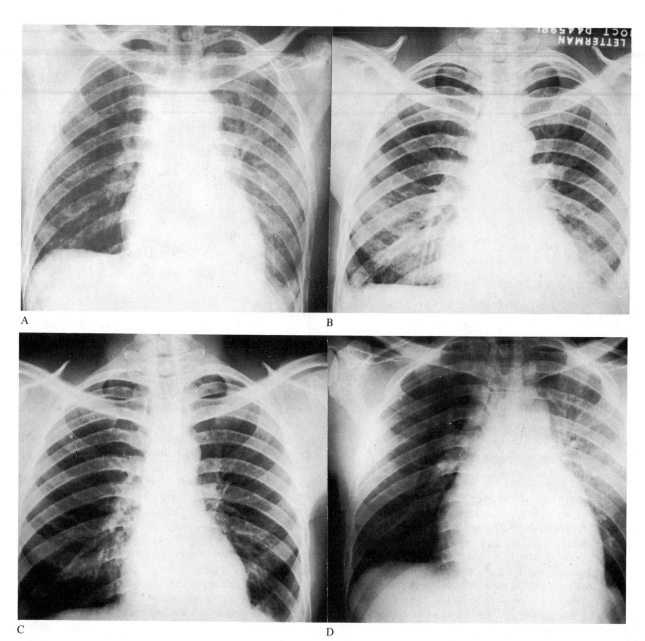

FIGURE 87-4 Series of chest roentgenograms of a 39-year-old man who incurred a penetrating stab wound of the heart. Initial films (A) (October 21, 1961) and another 2 days later (B) (October 23, 1961) reveal hemopericardium and the development of bilateral hemothorax, both clearing on conservative treatment within a week (C) (October 30, 1961) after repeated left thoracenteses. Increasing symptoms of pericarditis, spiking temperatures to 104°F, and increasing size of the cardiac silhouette, with hazy infiltration of left midlung (D) (November 3, 1961) appeared 3 days later, requiring pericardiocentesis with removal of 300 ml of sterile serosanguineous fluid. Subsequently, there was prompt clinical improvement with no recurrence of pericardial effusion.

projectile is not imbedded completely in the myocardial wall. In addition, several patients have developed a "cardiac neurosis"[27] with an almost maniacal desire for removal of the foreign body in spite of the physician's explanation and assurance. When the foreign body is located in the epicardial surface, it will frequently produce chronic pericardial effusion until removed. These possible complications and the patient's demands, as well as the relative simplicity and safety of the surgical procedure, suggest that after precise angiographic location, elective extraction may be the preferable management of projectiles in the heart.

The embolism of a foreign body caught within the heart or intravascular structures is a fascinating study in variability of action.[28] If the foreign body is found in the large venous channels, embolization may occur to the heart (Fig. 87-1) or pulmonary arteries (Fig. 87-5), and in fact, the embolus may pass back and forth within these structures. Similarly a foreign body may become embolic in a retrograde fashion, passing from an initial site in the right side of the heart to the peripheral veins or from the pulmonary artery or vein to either the right or left side of

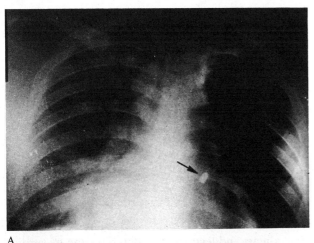

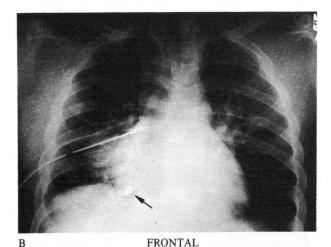

A

B   FRONTAL

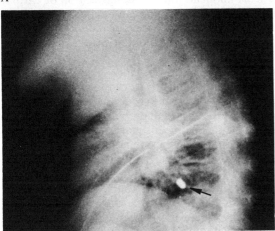

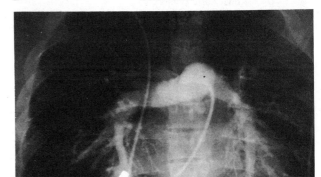

B   LATERAL

C

FIGURE 87-5 A. Chest roentgenogram of a young male who shortly before admission sustained a bullet wound in the right side of the chest, demonstrating the missile in the left hilum. *B.* Frontal and lateral views of the same patient 1 h later show that the bullet had moved to the right lower lobe. *C.* Pulmonary angiogram demonstrating the bullet embolized into the right lower lobe artery. *(Reproduced by permission of the author and publisher; from P. N. Symbas, "Traumatic Injuries of the Heart and Great Vessels," Charles C Thomas, Publisher, Springfield, Ill., 1971, pp. 94–96.)*

the heart, respectively.[15] Embolism of a foreign body from the left side of the heart to the systemic arterial system may be of serious consequence, depending on the site of arterial obstruction. A foreign body in the left side of the heart that is potentially embolic or one that has embolized to the systemic circulation should be surgically removed without delay. While projectiles in the pulmonary or systemic vascular tree should be removed to prevent ischemia of the involved organ, those adjacent to or embedded within the wall of any of the great arteries should be extracted to prevent subsequent erosion and bleeding.[1] Embolization of thrombi, which may be septic, developing at the site of cardiac injury or subsequent to aneurysm formation, produces the typical clinical consequences, dependent upon the size and termination of the thromboembolus.

Besides the obvious results of either immediate or delayed hemorrhage, a penetrating wound of the great vessels may also result in the formation of a false aneurysm, particularly if the aorta is involved.[15] Subsequent rupture of the aneurysm is then a constant threat. If adjacent large venous and arterial vessels are penetrated, an arteriovenous fistula may develop,[1,29] producing either immediate or latent congestive heart failure (see Chap. 91). Surreptitious heart failure may also result from an iatrogenic arteriovenous fistula produced during intervertebral disk surgery.[30] Traumatic arteriovenous fistulas are occasionally complicated by the development of bacterial endarteritis and endocarditis,[31] providing additional problems in medical and surgical management. Detection and repair of these traumatic vascular lesions should be accomplished as soon as possible.

NONPENETRATING INJURIES

The forces that produce nonpenetrating lesions of the heart and great vessels are of such a nature that external evidence of injury is meager or not detecta-

TABLE 87-2
Nonpenetrating trauma

I Pericardial injury
  A Hemopericardium
  B Rupture or laceration
  C Serofibrinous or suppurative pericarditis
  D Constrictive pericarditis
  E Recurrent pericarditis with effusion
II Myocardial injury
  A Contusion
    1 Anginal syndrome
    2 Aneurysm
    3 Delayed rupture
    4 Thromboembolism
    5 Myocarditis with or without failure
  B Laceration
  C Rupture, including septal rupture
III Coronary artery injury
  A Laceration with or without myocardial infarction
  B Thrombosis with or without myocardial infarction
  C Arteriovenous fistula
IV Valvular injury
  A Laceration, rupture, contusion
  B Papillary muscle or chordae tendineae injury
V Disturbances of rhythm or conduction
VI Great-vessel injury
  A Laceration, rupture
  B Aneurysm formation
  C Thrombotic occlusion

TABLE 87-3
Predominant injury in 546 cases of fatal nonpenetrating cardiac trauma

Predominant type of injury	No. of cases
Myocardial rupture, including septum	353
Myocardial contusion and/or laceration	129
Pericardial laceration	36
Hemopericardium	25
Valvular laceration	1 (6*)
Papillary muscle laceration and/or rupture	1 (23*)
Coronary artery laceration and/or rupture	1 (9*)
Coronary artery thrombosis	0
Total	546

*Combined with other serious cardiac injury.
Source: Modified with permission of the authors and the American Heart Association, Inc., from L. F. Parmley, W. C. Manion, and T. W. Mattingly, Nonpenetrating Traumatic Injury of the Heart, *Circulation*, 18:372, Table 1, 1958.

ble in almost one-third of the traumatized individuals.[1,2] This lack of evidence of chest injury, together with the frequent preoccupation of the physician with the other more obvious injuries, is the most frequent cause of failure to diagnose cardiovascular lesions of this type.

The wide variety of injuries produced by nonpenetrating trauma is summarized in Table 87-2. Although minor insignificant myocardial contusion of the right ventricle is the most frequently occurring lesion, by far the most common fatal lesion is that of myocardial rupture, as has been demonstrated by necropsy study (Table 87-3). Myocardial rupture is extremely difficult to treat successfully because of the rapid demise of the patient, and in fact, very often when traumatic cardiac rupture occurs, it is only one of many severe bodily injuries, any one of which would be fatal.[2] Although rupture of the walls of the ventricular chambers is in most instances not amenable to therapy, there have been reports of successful surgical treatment.[32] Rupture of the atrium or of the interventricular septum may not be rapidly fatal, and surgical repair is often possible.[33,34] In the case of interventricular septal ruptures, surgical repair is accomplished optimally after medical therapy has allowed some stabilization of the hemodynamic changes and healing to take place.[32]

Myocardial contusion is often asymptomatic or its manifestations are masked by symptoms of the usual associated injuries, primarily musculoskeletal. Prior alcohol ingestion, a not uncommon circumstance in automobile victims, may adversely affect the con-

tused heart and lead to rapid deterioration of cardiac function.[35] Often chest pain may appear following a latent period of several hours or days.[36] An anginal syndrome may also be initiated by the contusion[37] but is usually transient unless there is concomitant coronary artery injury or, more likely, antecedent atherosclerotic coronary artery disease. Coronary thrombosis[37,38] may result from nonpenetrating trauma, but this is a rare event[2] and then is usually associated with existing coronary atherosclerotic disease. The rarity is further demonstrated by the fact that in a series of 546 necropsy cases of nonpenetrating cardiac trauma (Table 87-3) not a single instance of coronary thrombosis was found despite instances in which extensive contusion and hemorrhage surrounded a major coronary artery. Electrocardiographic evidence compatible with myocardial infarction may follow myocardial contusion, yet a coronary arteriogram may fail to demonstrate an occlusive lesion.[39] Coronary arteriography has also been used to demonstrate coronary occlusion, presumably on a traumatic basis, in the absence of electrocardiographic evidence diagnostic of myocardial infarction.[40] Laceration of the coronary artery from nonpenetrating injury may occur, producing cardiac tamponade[2] or very rarely a coronary artery fistula.[40a]

Although myocardial contusion is primarily manifest pathologically by hemorrhage within the myocardium, various degrees of necrosis do occur. Usually this is minimal, and healing is complete, with little or no obvious scar or impairment of myocardial function. Nevertheless, large contusions may cause a decrease in cardiac output[40b] and extensive necrosis may occur, leading to rupture, rarely to congestive failure or to the formation of an aneurysm either true or false.[41-43,45] Rupture of a true aneurysm is rare, whereas a false aneurysm is subject to this complication. Other complications from cardiac aneurysms include arrhythmias, congestive heart failure, and mural thrombosis with embolism.[44] Because of these complications their surgical repair is advisable. New posttraumatic ventricular aneurysms, as well as septal defects, can be successfully repaired.[1] Localized areas of necrosis or hemorrhage involving the cardiac conduction system may produce varying degrees of atrioventricular block or any of the different types of intraventricular conduction defects.[2]

Electrocardiographic studies may be the only clinical clue that myocardial contusion has occurred, but the nonspecific ST-T abnormalities produced may be caused by so many different factors, as shown by clinical and experimental studies,[46-48] that their value is not so much that of establishing the diagnosis as it is of altering one to the possibility of cardiac contusion. Similarly, elevated serum enzyme levels may be suggestive of cardiac injury, but these may be elevated by other bodily trauma. Isoenzyme determination, however, such as MB-CPK level, may be of value in differentiating cardiac contusion from other tissue injuries.[49]

When there is more extensive contusion, the electrocardiographic abnormalities may be more persistent, and indeed, changes similar to those produced by myocardial infarction may develop.[50,51] Atrial as well as ventricular arrhythmias of all types[2] may also be produced, and undoubtedly ventricular tachycardia and fibrillation may be the cause of death in some contusive injuries.

Myocardial radioisotope scanning in dogs with experimental contusion of the heart have shown that the areas of injury can be identified.[40b,52] The clinical application of radiocardiography in the detection of myocardial contusion may prove to be of value in identifying the lesions that heretofore have been difficult to detect.

Because of the complications of myocardial contusion, patients with this lesion should be treated by bed rest or restricted activity for several weeks. The propensity of the contused heart to develop arrhythmias and conduction abnormalities indicates the need for electrocardiographic monitoring of the heart rhythm, similar to that employed following myocardial infarction due to coronary atherosclerosis. The increased irritability of the heart must also be taken into consideration when deciding which drugs might be used in the treatment of these traumatized patients. For this reason general anesthesia should be delayed when feasible. When prompt surgical treatment for some other injury is required, the knowledge of the presence of a myocardial contusion should guide the anesthetist in management and selection of an anesthetic agent. Otherwise the treatment is symptomatic, with conventional management of associated abnormalities, such as arrhythmias.

Valvular laceration is an infrequent result of nonpenetrating injury primarily involving AV valves, usually occurring in the presence of severe cardiac trauma causing death.[2] The aortic valve is more commonly involved in the surviving patient, characteristically leading to the rapid development of congestive heart failure secondary to aortic insufficiency,[53] although this course may be delayed[54] and in some patients medical treatment may permit stabilization of the clinical picture prior to surgical correction. Mitral valvular laceration may have somewhat similar severe hemodynamic consequences, but this lesion is seldom encountered clinically. In contrast, tricuspid valve injury may be tolerated for years before surgical correction is required.[55] In addition to the more common complications of congestive failure and arrhythmias, infectious endocarditis may also develop in patients with traumatically injured valves.[56]

Papillary muscle or chordae tendineae rupture and laceration occur more frequently than valvular lacerations (Table 87-3). Myocardial contusion may also result in papillary muscle dysfunction.[57] The patient's outcome depends on whether the structures involved are on the right side of the heart, where the lesion may be well tolerated, or on the left side of the heart, where the high-pressure system leads to serious hemodynamic consequences. The murmurs produced by these lesions are generally typical of valvular insufficiency murmurs, but unusually high pitched diastolic and systolic murmurs of variable intensity may result (Fig. 87-6). Traumatic tricuspid insufficiency may be present despite the absence of any detectable murmur, although a systolic murmur intensified on inspiration is the expected finding.[58] Prompt and correct diagnosis by appropriate hemodynamic and angiographic studies is important, as operative techniques employing extracorporeal circulation and the use of valve prostheses for the

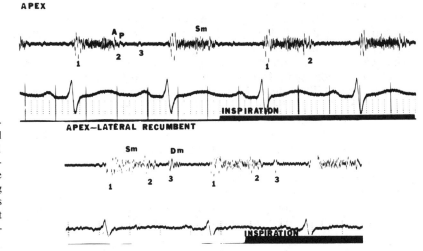

APEX

INSPIRATION

APEX—LATERAL RECUMBENT

INSPIRATION

FIGURE 87-6 Phonocardiogram demonstrating a ventricular diastolic gallop sound (3) and a grade 3 systolic murmur (Sm) and grade 1 diastolic murmur (Dm) in a patient with rupture of the anterior papillary muscle of the mitral valve as a result of nonpenetrating chest trauma. These auscultatory findings first alerted the attending physician to the fact that this patient had a traumatic cardiac injury. *(Courtesy of William F. Nelson, M.D.)*

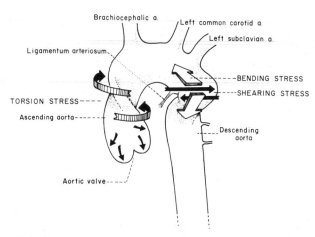

FIGURE 87-7 Diagrammatic illustration of the forces acting upon the aortic wall during rupture of the aorta from blunt trauma. *(Reproduced by permission of the author and publisher; from P. N. Symbas, "Traumatic Injuries of the Heart and Great Vessels," Charles C Thomas, Publisher, Springfield, Ill., 1971, p. 153.)*

surgical corrections of these lesions is now the accepted approach.

Pericardial lesions are common and are clinically similar to those of myocardial contusion, often being overlooked and healing without incident. However, hemopericardium may occur, and if hemorrhage is severe, cardiac tamponade will occur rapidly. When hemopericardium is suspected, echocardiography is an effective way to confirm the diagnosis. If there is a slow oozing of blood, often evoking a pericardial reaction and an associated effusion, tremendous dilatation of the pericardial sac may develop over an extended period of time. Symptoms and signs of traumatic pericarditis are similar to those of pericarditis produced by a wide variety of causes. Also the syndrome of recurrent pericarditis, which is similar to the postmyocardial infarction syndrome, may develop, but this is a less-frequent occurrence than in the penetrating cardiac injuries. Pericardial laceration is usually well tolerated,[60] but herniation of the heart may occur rarely leading to serious consequences and death.[47,59]

Rupture or laceration of the aorta is the most common blunt injury of the great vessels. Rupture, laceration, or avulsion of the great arteries (brachiocephalic, common carotid, and left subclavian) and venae cavae has been rarely observed. Because of a variety of mechanical forces produced by blunt trauma (Fig. 87-7) or deceleration forces combined with anatomic factors, the most frequent sites of rupture of the aorta in this type of injury are the descending aorta just distal to the origin of the left subclavian artery (aortic isthmus) and the ascending aorta just proximal to the origin of the brachiocephalic artery.[61,62] Because of the high association of ascending aortic rupture with severe cardiac injury, the overwhelming majority of patients surviving aortic rupture for a sufficient period of time to receive

definitive surgical correction are those who sustained rupture of the aortic isthmus.[1,61]

Other sites of rupture of the thoracic aorta and rupture of the abdominal aorta are much less common. Displacement of a thoracolumbar vertebra or rib may also be a factor in the causation of aortic rupture under these circumstances. Considering the extent of the lesion, which frequently transects the aorta, it is amazing that at least 15 percent of persons so injured survive—some only a few hours, but others for days, weeks, and even many years.[61] Survival initially is due to the formation of a false aneurysm, the wall of which consists of adventitia, the parietal pleura, and other mediastinal structures. The intactness of these maintains continuity of the circulation.[1]

The common manifestations of traumatic rupture of the aorta are severe chest and midscapular pain, dyspnea, increased pulse amplitude, and hypertension of the upper extremities.[63] However, some patients are surprisingly free of any major symptoms or signs. Hoarseness, evidence of a superior vena cava syndrome, paraplegia, and anuria are less frequent manifestations. Patients with rupture of the aorta, although occasionally without obvious signs of external injury, usually have evident associated injuries of the skeleton, abdominal viscera, or central nervous system. These coexisting injuries may mask the signs of aortic rupture. The signs of paraplegia, commonly due to spinal cord injury; low urine output or anuria, often due to hypovolemia; and chest pain or hemothorax, often due to rib fracture and other thoracic injuries can also be due to aortic rupture.[1] For this reason, any patient who has sustained severe blunt trauma or who has been exposed to major decelerative forces should be suspected of having aortic rupture, particularly if increased pulse amplitude and upper extremity hypertension are present. Chest roentgenography is of considerable diagnostic value in patients with aortic rupture. Widening of the superior mediastinal shadow, disappearance of the aortic knob shadow, depression of the left main bronchus, and displacement of the trachea to the right are common roentgenographic abnormalities (Fig. 87-8). However, other factors including preexisting mediastinal lesions, mediastinal hematoma from rupture of the small mediastinal vessels, and the inability to obtain chest films of good quality in these severely injured patients may be responsible for the presence of the roentgenographic findings suggesting aortic rupture. The delayed appearance of left hemothorax for hours, days, or even months after the traumatic incident should alert one to the possibility of a traumatic aortic aneurysm with impending rupture.[61] The diagnosis of aortic rupture can be definitely established only by aortography, which should be performed immediately if the clinical history, physical examination, and routine chest roentgenograms indicate the possibility of this injury (Fig. 87-8). Surgical treatment can now be effectively provided for these patients and should be carried out, with particular attention to provisions for perfusion of the kidney and spinal cord, as soon as the diagnosis is established.

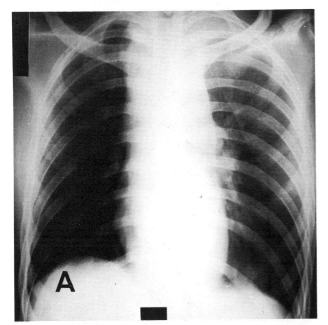

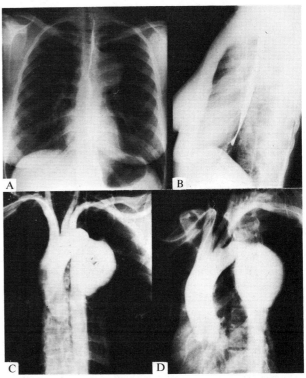

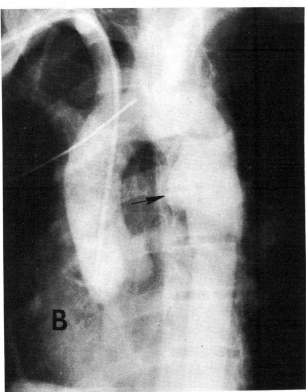

FIGURE 87-8 A. Chest roentgenogram of a young male who shortly before admission was involved in automobile accident. Note the mediastinal widening. *B.* Aortogram the same day showing a false aneurysm distal to the origin of the left subclavian artery and two filling defects, one proximal and one distal to the aneurysm.

FIGURE 87-9 A 20-year-old woman involved in an automobile accident sustained a fracture of a femur and several ribs on the left. No cardiovascular lesion was suspected. She recovered without incident. Posteroanterior and left lateral chest roentgenograms (*A* and *B*) taken for a routine premarital examination 2 years later reveal a density in the area of the aortic knob compatible with traumatic aortic aneurysm. The aneurysm was demonstrated by retrograde aortography (*C* and *D*) to be in the usual location just distal to the left subclavian artery. At the time of surgical correction the aorta was found to be completely transected; the ends of the aorta were separated by 6 cm within the false aneurysm sac.

FIGURE 87-10 Posteroanterior and left lateral chest roentgenograms show a typical traumatic aneurysm just below the left subclavian artery. Note partial calcification of the aneurysm evident in the left lateral view. This 43-year-old man was involved in an automobile accident in 1941, suffering multiple injuries and requiring 6 months' hospitalization. An abnormality was first discovered on the patient's roentgenogram in 1957. The diagnosis of traumatic aortic aneurysm was not made until 1959. By utilizing partial arterial blood bypass from the left atrium to the left femoral artery, the aneurysm was surgically resected, and a Teflon graft was inserted to preserve aortic continuity.

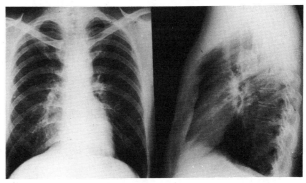

A chronic, false aortic aneurysm may be discovered months or years after the injury[61] (Fig. 87-9) and, in fact, may even be partially calcified (Fig. 87-10). However, rupture of the aneurysm may occur at any time after its formation. Rarely the complications of dissection, peripheral embolization of the thrombus contained in the aneurysm or of a fragment of the vessel wall,[64] the development of bacterial endaortitis,[65] or chronic pseudocoarctation[66] may occur. Because of the relative instability of these aneurysms and the complications as cited, surgical correction is the treatment of choice.

REFERENCES

1 Symbas, P. N.: "Traumatic Injuries of the Heart and Great Vessels," Charles C Thomas, Publisher, Springfield, Ill., 1971, p. 3.

2 Parmley, L. F., Manion, W. C., and Mattingly, T. W.: Nonpenetrating Traumatic Injury of the Heart, *Circulation*, 18:371, 1958.

3 Baldwin, J. J., and Edwards, J. E.: Rupture of Right Ventricle Complicating Closed Chest Cardiac Massage, *Circulation*, 53:562, 1976.

4 Gorlin, R.: Perforations and Other Cardiac Complications: A Cooperative Study on Cardiac Catheterization Performed and Other Cardiac Complications, *Circulation*, 37(suppl. 3):36, 1968.

5 Meyer, J. A., and Millar, K.: Perforation of the Right Ventricle by Electrode Catheters: A Review and Report of Nine Cases, *Ann. Surg.*, 168:1048, 1968.

6 Fitts, C. T., Barnett, T., Webb, C. M., Sexton, J., and Yarbrough, D. R., III: Perforating Wounds of the Heart Caused by Central Venous Catheters, *J. Trauma*, 10:764, 1970.

6a Pace, N. L., and Horton, W.: Indwelling Pulmonary Artery Catheters—Their Relationship to Aseptic Endocardial Vegetations, *JAMA*, 233:893, 1975.

6b Greene, J. J., Fitzwater, J. E., and Clemmer, T. P.: Septic Endocarditis and Indwelling Pulmonary Artery Catheters, *JAMA*, 233:891, 1975.

7 Bloomfield, B. A.: Techniques of Nonsurgical Retrieval of Iatrogenic Foreign Bodies of the Heart, *Am. J. Cardiol.*, 27:538, 1971.

8 Cohn, K. E., Stewart, R. J., Fajardo, L. F., and Hancock, E. W.: Heart Disease Following Radiation, *Medicine*, 46:281, 1967.

9 Morton, D. L., Glancy, D. L., Joseph, W. L., and Adkins, P. C.: Management of Patients with Radiation-induced Pericarditis with Effusion: A Note on the Development of Aortic Regurgitation in Two of Them, *Chest*, 64:291, 1973.

10 Moritz, A. R., and Atkins, J. P.: Cardiac Contusion: An Experimental and Pathologic Study, *AMA Arch. Pathol.*, 25:445, 1938.

11 Samson, P. C.: Battle Wounds and Injuries of the Heart and Pericardium: Experiences in Forward Hospitals, *Ann. Surg.*, 127:1127, 1948.

12 Elkin, D. C.: The Diagnosis and Treatment of Wounds of the Heart, *JAMA*, 111:1750, 1938.

13 Valle, A. R.: War Injuries of the Heart and Mediastinum, *AMA Arch. Surg.*, 70:398, 1955.

14 Warshaw, L. J.: "The Heart in Industry," chap. 15, Hoeber Medical Division, Harper & Row, Publishers, Incorporated, New York, 1960.

15 Parmley, L. F., Mattingly, T. W., and Manion, W. C.: Penetrating Wounds of the Heart and Aorta, *Circulation*, 17:953, 1958.

16 Symbas, P. N., DiOrio, D. A., Tyras, D. H., Ware, R. E., and Hatcher, C. R., Jr.: Penetrating Cardiac Wounds. Significant Residual and Delayed Sequelae. *J. Thorac. Cardiovasc. Surg.*, 66:526, 1973.

17 Isaacs, J. P.: Sixty Penetrating Wounds of the Heart, *Surgery*, 45:696, 1959.

18 Decker, H. R.: Foreign Bodies in the Heart and Pericardium—Should They Be Removed? *J. Thorac. Surg.*, 9:62, 1939.

19 Schechter, D. C., and Gilbert, L.: Injuries of the Heart and Great Vessels due to Pins and Needles, *Thorax*, 24:246, 1969.

20 Sugg, W. L., Rea, W. J., Ecker, R. R., Webb, W. R., Rose, E. F., and Shaw, R. R.: Penetrating Wounds of the Heart: An Analysis of 459 Cases, *J. Thorac. Cardiovasc. Surg.*, 56:531, 1968.

21 Ransdell, H. T., Jr., and Glass, H., Jr.: Gunshot Wounds of the Heart: Review of 20 Cases, *Am. J. Surg.*, 99:788, 1960.

22 Wilkinson, A. H., Jr., Buttram, T. L., Reid, W. A., and Howard, J. M.: Cardiac Injuries: An Evaluation of Immediate and Long Range Results of Treatment, *Ann. Surg.*, 147:347, 1958.

23 Cooley, D. A., Dunn, J. R., Brockman, H. LeR., and DeBakey, M. E.: Treatment of Penetrating Wounds of the Heart: Experimental and Clinical Observations, *Surgery*, 37:882, 1955.

24 Symbas, P. N., Harlaftis, N., and Waldo, W. J.: Penetrating Cardiac Wounds: A Comparison of Different Therapeutic Methods, *Ann. Surg.*, 183:377, 1976.

25 Heitzman, E. J., and Heitzman, G. C.: Myocardial Infarction Following Penetrating Wounds of the Heart, *Am. J. Cardiol.*, 7:283, 1961.

26 Konecke, L. L., Spitzer, S., Mason, D., Kasparian, H., and James, P. M., Jr.: Traumatic Aneurysm of the Left Coronary Artery, *Am. J. Cardiol.*, 27:221, 1971.

27 Bland, E. F., and Beebe, G. W.: Missiles in the Heart: A Twenty-Year Followup Report of World War Cases, *N. Engl. J. Med.*, 274:1039, 1966.

28 Harken, D. E., and Williams, A. C.: Foreign Bodies in, and in Relation to, the Thoracic Blood Vessels and Heart: II. Migratory Foreign Bodies within the Blood Vascular System, *Am. J. Surg.*, 72:80, 1946.

29 Symbas, P. N., Schlant, R. C., Logan, W. D., Jr., Lindsay, J., MacCannell, K. L., and Zakaryia, M.: Traumatic Aorticopulmonary Fistula Complicated by Postoperative Low Cardiac Output Treated with Dopamine, *Ann. Surg.*, 165:614, 1967.

30 Smith, V. M., Hughes, C. W., Sapp, O., Joy, R. J. T., and Mattingly, T. W.: High-Output Circulatory Failure due to Arteriovenous Fistula, *AMA Arch Intern. Med.*, 100:883, 1957.

31 Parmley, L. F., Orbison, J. A., Hughes, C. W., and Mattingly, T. W.: Acquired Arteriovenous Fistulas Complicated by Endarteritis and Endocarditis Lenta due to *Streptococcus faecalis*, *N. Engl. J. Med.*, 250:305, 1954.

32 Trueblood, H. W., Wuerflein, R. D., and Angell, W. W.: Blunt Trauma Rupture of the Heart, *Ann. Surg.*, 177:66, 1973.

33 Cary, F. H., Hurst, J. W., and Arentzen, W. R.: Acquired Interventricular Defect Secondary to Trauma: Report of Four Cases, *N. Engl. J. Med.*, 258, 355, 1958.

34 Rotman, M., Peter, R. H., Sealy, W. C., and Morris, J. J., Jr.: Traumatic Ventricular Septal Defect Secondary to Nonpenetrating Chest Trauma, *Am. J. Med.*, 48:127, 1970.

35 Liedtke, J. A., and DeMuth, W. E.: Effects of Alcohol on Cardiovascular Performance after Experimental Nonpenetrating Chest Trauma, *Am. J. Cardiol.*, 35:243, 1975.

36 Kissane, R. W.: Traumatic Heart Disease: Nonpenetrating Injuries, *Circulation*, 6:421, 1952.

37 Stern, T., Wolf, R. Y., Reichart, B., Harrington, O. B., and Crosby, V. G.: Coronary Artery Occlusion Resulting from Blunt Trauma, *JAMA*, 230:1308, 1974.

38 Levy, H.: Traumatic Coronary Thrombosis with Myocardial Infarction, *AMA Arch. Intern. Med.*, 84:261, 1949.

39 Harthorne, J. W., Kantrowitz, P. A., Dinsmore, R. E., and Sanders, C. A.: Traumatic Myocardial Infarction: Report of a Case with Normal Coronary Angiogram, *Ann. Intern. Med.*, 66:341, 1967.

40 DeMuth, W. E., Jr., and Zinsser, H. F.: Myocardial Contusion, *AMA Arch. Intern. Med.*, 115:434, 1965.

40a Forker, A. D., and Morgan, J. R.: Acquired Coronary Artery Fistula from Nonpenetrating Chest Injury, *JAMA*, 215:289, 1971.

40b Doty, D. B., Anderson, A. E., Rose, E. F., Raymundo, J. G., Chiu, C. L., and Ehrenhaft, J. L.: Cardiac Trauma: Clinical and Experimental Correlations of Myocardial Contusion, *Ann. Surg.,* 180:452, 1974.

41 Silver, G. M., Stampinato, N., Favaloro, R. G., and Groves, L. K.: Ventricular Aneurysm and Blunt Chest Trauma, *Chest,* 63:628, 1973.

42 Killen, D. A., Gobbel, W. G., Jr., France, R., and Vix, V. A.: Post-traumatic Aneurysm of the Left Ventricle, *Circulation,* 39:101, 1969.

43 Singh, R., Nolan, S. P., and Schrank, J. P.: Traumatic Left Ventricular Aneurysm. Two Cases with Normal Coronary Angiograms, *JAMA,* 234:412, 1975.

44 Basta, L. L., Takeshita, A., Theilen, E. O., and Ehren-haft, J. L.: Aneurysmectomy in Treatment of Ventricular and Supra-ventricular Tachyarrhythmias in Patients with Postinfarction and Traumatic Ventricular Aneurysms, *Am. J. Cardiol.,* 32:693, 1973.

45 Barber, H., and Osborn, G. R.: A Fatal Case of Myocardial Contusion, *Br. Heart J.,* 3:127, 1941.

46 Kissane, R. W., Fidler, R. S., and Koons, R. A.: Electrocardiographic Changes Following External Chest Injury to Dogs, *Ann. Intern. Med.,* 11:907, 1937.

47 Louhimo, I.: Heart Injury after Blunt Trauma, *Acta Chir. Scand.,* 1(suppl. 380), 1965.

48 Dolara, A., Morando, P., and Pampaloni, M.: Electrocardiographic Findings in 98 Consecutive Non-penetrating Chest Injuries, *Dis. Chest,* 52:50, 1967.

49 Tonkin, A. M., Lester, R. M., Guthrow, C. E., Roe, C. R., Hackel, D. B., and Wagner, G. S.: Persistence of MB Isoenzyme of Creatine Phosphokinase in the Serum after Minor Iatrogenic Cardiac Trauma, *Circulation,* 51:627, 1975.

50 Jones, F. L., Jr.: Transmural Myocardial Necrosis after Nonpenetrating Cardiac Trauma, *Am. J. Cardiol.,* 26:419, 1970.

51 DeMuth, W. E., Jr., Baue, A. E., and Odom, J. A., Jr.: Contusions of the Heart, *J. Trauma,* 7:443, 1967.

52 Martin, L. G., Larose, J. H., Sybers, R. G., Tyras, D. H., and Symbas, P. N.: Myocardial Perfusion Imaging with ^{99m}Tc-Albumin Microspheres, *Radiology,* 107:367, 1973.

53 Payne, D. D., DeWeese, J. A., Mahoney, E. B., and Murphy, G. W.: Surgical Treatment of Traumatic Rupture of the Normal Aortic Valve, *Ann. Thorac. Surg.,* 17:223, 1974.

54 Case Records of the Massachusetts General Hospital, Case 3-1976, *N. Engl. J. Med.,* 294:152, 1976.

55 Liu, S., Sako, Y., and Alexander, C. S.: Traumatic Tricuspid Insufficiency, *Am. J. Cardiol.,* 26:200, 1970.

56 Morgan, M. G., Glasser, S. P., and Sanusi, I. D.: Bacterial Endocarditis Occurrence on a Traumatically Ruptured Aortic Valve, *JAMA,* 233:810, 1975.

57 Schroeder, J. S., Stinson, E. B., Bieber, C. P., Wexler, L., Shumway, N. E., and Harrison, D. C.: Papillary Muscle Dysfunction Due to Non-penetrating Chest Trauma, Recognition in a Potential Cardiac Donor, *Br. Heart J.,* 34:645, 1972.

58 Marvin, R. F., Schrank, J. P., and Nolan, S. P.: Traumatic Tricuspid Insufficiency, *Am. J. Cardiol.,* 32:723, 1973.

59 Munchow, O. B. G., Carter, R., Vannix, R. S., and Anderson, F. S.: Cardiac Arrest due to Ventricular Herniation: Report of a Case of Two Successful Cardiac Resuscitations, *JAMA,* 173:1350, 1960.

60 Andersen, M., Fredens, M., and Olessen, K. H.: Traumatic Rupture of the Pericardium, *Am. J. Cardiol.,* 27:566, 1971.

61 Parmley, L. F., Mattingly, T. W., Manion, W. C., and Jahnke, E. J., Jr.: Nonpenetrating Traumatic Injury of the Aorta, *Circulation,* 17:1086, 1958.

62 Symbas, P. N., Tyras, D. H., Ware, R. E., and DiOrio, D. A.: Traumatic Rupture of the Aorta, *Ann. Surg.,* 178:6, 1973.

63 Symbas, P. N., Tyras, D. H., Ware, R. E., and Hatcher, C. R., Jr.: Rupture of the Aorta: A Diagnostic Triad, *Ann. Thorac. Surg.,* 15:405, 1973.

64 Gulkin, T. A., and Ashbury, A. K.: Fragment of Great-Vessel Wall Causing Cerebral Embolism, *N. Engl. J. Med.,* 277:751, 1967.

65 Stryker, W. A.: Traumatic Saccular Aneurysms of the Thoracic Aorta, *Am. J. Clin. Pathol.,* 18:152, 1948.

66 Kinley, C. E., and Chandler, B. M.: Traumatic Aneurysm of Thoracic Aorta: A Case Presenting as a Coarctation, *Can. Med. Assoc. J.,* 96:279, 1967.

The Heart and Other Medical Problems

88
The Heart and Collagen Disease

EDWARD R. DORNEY, M.D.

This chapter contains a discussion of the cardiac involvement in that group of diseases referred to as the collagen diseases. The four major members of this group are scleroderma (systemic sclerosis), periarteritis nodosa, lupus erythematosus, and dermatomyositis. They are presented as individual entities, but it should be realized that features of two or more of them may be present in any single patient. These diseases are systemic conditions, and tissues other than the cardiovascular system are usually involved. The reader is referred to standard textbooks of pathology and medicine for detailed descriptions of the noncardiovascular aspects of the disease process.

SCLERODERMA (SYSTEMIC SCLEROSIS)

Weiss et al.[1] first focused attention on the cardiac involvement in scleroderma, and their observations have been confirmed and extended by other authors. The clinical significance of their postmortem findings, however, has been obscured by the simultaneous discovery of severe pulmonary and renal changes, which in themselves could be responsible for pulmonary and systemic hypertension with secondary heart failure.[2,3] In recent years, clinical studies such as that done by Sachner[3] (which incorporates the use of cardiac catheterization, pulmonary and renal function studies, phonocardiography, and autopsy confirmation) have begun to place the problem in its proper perspective.

It is still difficult, therefore, to say clinically how often scleroderma involves the heart, since other occult forms of heart disease may be present in the patient with disseminated sclerosis and may create a false impression that the process has extended to involve the heart. Farmer stated that sclerodermal heart disease was the leading cause of death in his series of 271 cases of disseminated scleroderma followed by the Mayor group, but Oram[2] was able to diagnose sclerodermal heart disease with certainty in only 4 of 21 of his cases, and Sachner[3] in only 3 of 25.

Pathology

Although the endocardium, myocardium, and pericardium may be involved singly or in combination, the myocardium is affected more frequently and seriously than the other two. Since Weiss et al.[1] first called attention to sclerodermal heart disease, many students of the disease have reported replacement of cardiac muscle by connective tissue. This connective tissue seems to be arranged into three basic configurations: (1) there may be only patchy, scarred areas which are not related to coronary vessels; (2) there may be a marked overgrowth of a highly vascular connective tissue which separates the muscle bundles; (3) there may be a massive replacement of cardiac muscle with a nonvascular connective tissue which seems to run parallel to the muscle fibers. These changes have been interpreted as a primary overgrowth of fibrous tissue with a secondary destruction of other myocardial structures.[2] For the most part, this connective tissue has no constant relationship to the coronary arteries and does not contain hemosiderin; the vessels themselves have not been involved. Sachner[3] also mentions an interstitial edema of the cardiac musculature and of the conduction system, and feels, as does Oram,[2] that the patchy fibrotic scars in the myocardium of persons dying with scleroderma need to be interpreted cautiously, since they are nonspecific in nature and may also be seen in patients dying of other diseases. The replacement of cardiac muscle may involve any or all of the chambers of the heart and has been so extensive at times that a gross description of the heart appearing as a "flabby sac" has been recorded. Involvement of the papillary muscles with fibrous replacement has been specifically noted.[1] At times, the fibrotic process in the myocardium has been seen to be confluent with pericardial or endocardial involvement, although the latter is comparatively rare. Bulkley[4] has recently pointed out that both the gross and microscopic muscle changes resemble those described by Herdson[5] and Reichenbach.[6] These changes are commonly found in hearts of patients dying several days after cardiopulmonary bypass and other situations where ischemia and reperfusion have been present. In contrast, James has demonstrated small-vessel involvement throughout the myocardium and particularly in connection with the conduction system and feels that the small-vessel involvement has a direct influence on the myocardial changes.[7]

Oram[2] reported that pericarditis with or without effusion was common in his series, occurring in 66 percent of autopsied cases; Sachner[3] indicated that 14 percent would be a more representative figure. Both agree that constrictive pericarditis with cardiac tamponade has not been seen, although adhesive pericarditis is frequently found at autopsy. Meltzer has reported recurrent pericardial effusions of up to 500 ml with a protein content of 5.9 and 6.8 g/100 ml. Weiss et al.[1] reported a patient with pericardial effusion of 340 ml, with 3.7 g/100 ml protein content. Escudero[8] mentions an effusion of 1,000 ml. The protein content suggests that the fluid is the result of the pathologic process rather than being secondary to congestive heart failure. Myxedema, which could result from sclerodermatous involvement of the thyroid gland and could produce pericardial effusion with a high protein content, has been effectively ruled out in one of Meltzer's cases.

Endocardial involvement is rare. Deformity of the mitral and aortic valves with nodularity of the cusps has been reported by many authors, although with the exception of Roth's[9] case, the lesions probably have been of little clinical significance.[2,3] Biegleman (Case 9) described irregular collagenous thickening of the aortic adventitia with small adventitial arteries showing marked intimal thickening and some containing organized thrombi. This process seems to be similar to that reported by Roth,[9] which also included a ruptrue of an aortic cusp and which to some extent simulated syphilitic aortitis.

Clinical manifestations

There is no pathognomonic sign or symptom of cardiac involvement in diffuse sclerodermatous process, and it is difficult, if not impossible, to make a firm clinical diagnosis. Although cardiac symptoms may appear months or years before skin involvement,[1,2] as a general rule they are not a prominent part of the picture of scleroderma until late in the disease. The average duration of life is 30 months when definite symptoms of myocardial disease appear.[2] This statement does not apply to pericardial disease which may be intermittently symptomatic for long periods of time.[3]

Dyspnea with exertion or at rest is the most common complaint referable to the heart, but in the majority of cases it can be shown to be due to pulmonary fibrosis and hypertension rather than to primary cardiac involvement.

Systolic murmurs at the cardiac apex or base have been reported, but in most cases they are not adequately described. The murmurs may be due to anemia, which occurs in about 30 percent of cases, or to papillary muscle weakness, or in rare cases to true valvular deformity. Chest pain simulating that in coronary artery disease has been reported in 25 percent of cases with no confirmatory findings at postmortem examination. Typical pericardial pain may also occur. The apical impulse may be difficult to palpate in the patients with sclerodermatous involvement of the chest wall. Pulsus paradoxus may be due

to cardiac tamponade or restrictive lung disease. Right ventricular failure may be due to pulmonary hypertension with or without myocardial involvement. In this case, the increase in loudness of the pulmonic component of the second sound or the finding of fixed splitting of the second sound in the absence of right bundle branch block on the electrocardiogram is of some diagnostic help.[3]

Typical angina pectoris with angiographic studies demonstrating normal large coronary arteries has been reported by Traube.[10] He postulated that the slow run-off of the dye seen in these cases was due to vascular resistance within the small nonvisualized vessels. This is particularly interesting in view of Bulkley's[4] suggestion that individuals with the characteristic myocardial findings of progressive systemic sclerosis may also have intermittent ischemia on the basis of Raynaud's phenomenon, and James's[7] findings of diffuse small-vessel disease in these hearts.

The *roentgenogram* of the chest reveals a large cardiac silhouette in about 75 percent of cases[3] but may be entirely normal even in the presence of proved myocardial involvement. The enlargement may be the result of pericardial effusion or myocardial disease; these conditions may be differentiated by observation of the fat line with intensified fluoroscopy or by angiocardiography. The triangular shape of the heart in patients with scleroderma, as described by Weiss,[1] has not proved to be as specific as originally thought. Barium swallow enables one to see a decrease or loss in the primary peristaltic waves in the esophagus.

The *electrocardiographic* findings are entirely nonspecific, and a normal ECG may be seen in a severely involved heart. All degrees of atrioventricular block have been reported.[2,3,8] Right and left bundle branch block are common, as are left and right ventricular hypertrophy.[2,3,8] All varieties of supraventricular and ventricular arrhythmias have been recorded.[2,3,8,9] Tracings which resemble those in myocardial infarction have been seen. Low voltage, which was reported frequently in the earlier literature, is now seldom reported. The voltage is usually low in the standard leads but normal in the precordial leads. When generalized low voltage is present, it may be a clue to the presence of pericaridal fluid. Oram[2] pointed out that the electrocardiographic findings may be definitely helpful in indicating the presence of cardiac involvement when abnormalities are found which cannot be explained by other diagnosable types of heart disease or electrolyte abnormalities in a patient with cutaneous scleroderma.

Catheterization of the right and left sides of the heart and angiocardiography may be needed to ensure a correct evaluation of the cardiac involvement, although these measures are seldom indicated since therapy is not dependent upon the results.

Treatment

There is no specific therapy for sclerodermal heart disease. Some of these patients respond for a time to the usual measures of digitalization, diuretics, and sodium restriction, but there is no treatment to restore destroyed cardiac muscle. Pain of pericardial involvement has been successfully treated with corticosteroids, and it is suggested that similar therapy be tried for pericardial effusion.

PERIARTERITIS NODOSA

Pathology

Periarteritis nodosa is a necrotizing vascular disease of unknown etiology, originally described as occurring along the course of the muscular arteries of the size of the coronaries or hepatic, with some spread to the smaller branches of these vessels but with only occasional involvement of venules. Gross nodularity of the involved vessels, particularly at the point of branching, is seen at autopsy. Arkin[11] divided the pathologic changes of periarteritis nodosa into four stages and presented a clinicopathologic correlation which is valuable in understanding the course of the disease and its response to therapy. The first stage, one of beginning degeneration of the media, occurs in the innermost layer of small vessels without vasa vasorum and in the outer portion of the media near the elastica externa in the larger vessels. This stage may be asymptomatic. The second stage is characterized by spreading of the inflammatory process to involve the whole circumference of the vessel, the adventitia and intima, with aneurysm formation and occlusion of vessels. This stage is associated with high fever and chills and resembles infectious disease. Death may occur from rupture of an aneurysm or infarction of involved organs. Biopsy at this point usually produces a diagnosis. The third stage is characterized by the appearance of granulation tissue, with marked proliferation of the intima. Fever subsides, but death may result from infarction or from ruptured aneurysm. In the fourth or "healed stage," the artery may be unrecognizable because of fibrous replacement of the affected areas; symptoms at this stage are primarily due to lack of blood flow to affected organs. Any or all of these stages may be present at any time in any given patient, and the duration of the stages varies widely with each individual.

Since the time of Arkin's description, involvement of microscopic branches of the vascular system, arteries and veins, without large-vessel involvement or nodule formation has been described. Though the disease seldom involves the pulmonary vessels or the spleen, such involvement is found to be common when the microscopic vessels are primarily affected.[12] Other forms of the disease, with granuloma formation and giant cells, have also been described. This caused much confusion until a classification was proposed by Zeek in 1953. This classification, which has been accepted by many authors in the field,[12-14] divides the necrotizing angitides into five categories: (1) periarteritis nodosa; (2) hypersensitivity angiitis; (3) rheumatic arteritis; (4) allergic granulomatous angiitis; and (5) temporal arteritis.

In the classical periarteritis nodosa, involvement of the major coronary arteries is a common finding and frequently results in myocardial infarction.[12,14,15] Patchy fibrosis in the myocardium is the rule, as is gross enlargement of the left ventricle. The latter is most probably attributable to the combination of myocardial fibrosis and hypertension secondary to renal involvement which occurs in the majority of cases of periarteritis nodosa.[15] Hemorrhage into the pericardial sac, with tamponade and death, has been reported, as has nonspecific inflammatory pericarditis and pericarditis due to uremia.[12] Very little mention has been made of endocardial or valvular involvement. Rupture of a papillary muscle has been reported by Askey.

Biopsy is needed to make a certain antemortem diagnosis, since the clinical picture closely resembles that of the other collagen diseases. Any biopsy made should be taken from areas of active inflammatory disease, such as skin or muscle, since healed areas may be entirely nonspecific.[1] Rose has felt that a blind biopsy of muscle would produce a 50 percent return in the diagnosis, but this feeling is not shared by others.[16] Dahl has suggested testicular biopsy when symptoms or objective evidence of abnormality are present in this tissue and acute skin or muscle involvement is not present. He predicts a 20 percent possibility of diagnosis with testicular biopsy, which is about the same as may be expected from involved skin or muscle sites.

Clinical manifestations

From the clinical standpoint, there is little difference between periarteritis nodosa and hypersensitivity angiitis of the smaller vessels, except that the latter is more often accompanied by pulmonary findings on the roentgenogram. The disease occurs at all ages, from 10 days to 80 years.[12,17] produces fever and multisystem involvement, and may last from weeks to years.[16] Tachycardia is common, even in the absence of fever or heart failure.[15,17] Pericarditis, with friction rub and characteristic pain, occurs but is not common.[15] Pericarditis may also be found secondary to myocardial infarction or uremia. Chest pain of various types has been reported by most authors, but true angina pectoris seems to be rare.[15,17] Classical myocardial infarction occurs, because of periarteritis nodosa, but is not common.[13,15–17] In one series of 41 cases showing myocardial infarction at autopsy, only 3 could be diagnosed clinically.[15] Congestive failure and hypertension are the most prominent clinical findings which are directly related to the heart, and they are the causes of death in the majority of cases.[15,16] Hemoptysis has been reported by Shick.[18] Cardiac arrhythmias, mainly atrial fibrillation and flutter,[13,15,17] have been observed but are not common. Approximately 30 percent of patients will have an apical or basal systolic murmur,[15,17] although little or no valve deformity is reported at postmortem examination, and it is suspected that this murmur is probably due to anemia or to papillary muscle dysfunction.

Roberts[19] and, later, Glanz[20] have reported on periarteritis in infants which resulted in infarction and aneurysm formation. The clinical presentation of Roberts' cases, however, closely resembled the acute mucocutaneous lymph node syndrome, which presents similar changes in the coronary arteries but is now thought to be due to a rickettsial disease.[21]

The *electrocardiogram* usually shows nonspecific T wave changes considered to be secondary to myocardial fibrosis.[14,15] These changes have been noted to be progressive. Myocardial infarction is occasionally seen.[13,15,17] Left ventricular hypertrophy is common. Right and left bundle branch blocks have been reported, as have various degrees of AV block and supraventricular arrhythmias.[13,15,17]

The routine *roentgenogram* of the chest may show left ventricular enlargement or generalized cardiomegaly. Bron et al. have reported angiographic demonstration of multiple visceral aneurysms in the kidney, liver, and spleen when several biopsies had failed to establish a diagnosis of periarteritis nodosa.

Treatment

As with the clinical classification, there is little need to separate periarteritis nodosa from hypersensitivity angiitis for purposes of therapy. All cases of periarteritis with cardiac involvement should be treated with massive adrenocortical steroid therapy. Dosage should be started with 200 to 300 mg hydrocortisone a day or its equivalent.[18] This medication will not interefere with the healing process, nor will it prevent infarction from occlusion of vessels which results from this "healing."[16] It will prevent involvement of additional vessels and will reduce or eliminate pain and toxicity.[16] In cases of refractory heart failure, steroid therapy has resulted in dramatic response somewhat similar to that observed with acute rheumatic myocarditis. Suppressive treatment with steroids should be continued after the disease has been controlled. Unfortunately, although the toxic manifestation of the disease may be brought under control, the long-term prognosis seems little changed,[16] although some authors feel that early diagnosis plus prolonged suppressive therapy may provide long remissions.[18]

LUPUS ERYTHEMATOSUS

Lupus erythematosus, the most common of the collagen diseases, involves the endocardium, myocardium, and pericardium, either singly or in combinations. It is probably the best studied of the members of this group.[22]

Pathology

The most widely known cardiac manifestation of systemic lupus erythematosus is Libman-Sachs endocarditis, which occurs in about 50 percent of cases. This term refers to the verrucous lesions found in the endocardium of patients dying of systemic lupus erythematosus. They were originally described by Libman and Sachs in 1924 but were not recognized as being part of the generalized disease until the dissertation of Klemperer in 1941.[23]

The Libman-Sachs lesions are wartlike in appearance, are dry and granular, and have a pink or tawny color. They may vary from pinhead size to 3 to 4 mm, and may be singular or multiple.[23] These verrucae are composed of degenerating valve tissue which has been extruded beyond the endothelium, and they are accompanied by some fibrosis of the underlying leaflet. The lesions themselves usually contain granular, basophilic masses of cellular debris. The cytoplasm of the cells contains basophilic fragments which make up the characteristic "hematoxylin bodies."[24] They may be formed anywhere on the endocardial surface of the heart but are most common in the angles of the atrioventricular (AV) valves and on the underside of the mitral valve at its base; they may extend on to the chordae tendineae or papillary muscles.[23,24] These lesions are rarely large enough to interfere with the action of the valves.[22,25] Affected valves also may show areas of altered collagen formation not in proximity to these lesions.[24] Generalized involvement of the entire thickness of the heart valves with inflammatory and fibrous changes may also occur.

In a recent autopsy study of 36 corticosteroid-treated patients, Bulkley and Roberts have noted variations in the classical cardiac findings which they attributed to "healing" and prolonged survival by spontaneous means or in combination with the side effects of the corticosteroids.[31] Healing of the Libman-Sachs lesions on the undersurface of the posterior mitral valve leaflet has resulted in binding of the valve leaflet to the mural endocardium with dense, partially calcified, fibrous masses, which has necessitated valve replacement.[31,32] Myocardial infarction due to coronary atherosclerotic disease is now being reported more frequently among such patients than would be expected in a population of similar age and sex distribution.[31,33] The cause of this is not known, but interaction of the disease itself with known metabolic aberrations caused by steroids has been suggested.

The myocardial lesions of systemic lupus erythematosus are primarily due to deposition of fibrinoid material in the septa between the myocardial cells; cellular degeneration is rarely found.[26] In addition the myocardium also participates in the generalized small-vessel changes which were described by Baehr et al. James[27] has described the arteriopathy of vessels which are 0.1 to 1 mm in diameter. The abnormal vessels were located in the conduction system of eight cases selected because of the presence of arrhythmias. These patients showed segmental arteritis and periarteritis with some occlusions of the arterial lumen and small areas of fibrosis distal to the blockage. The findings were particularly prominent in the sinoatrial node, less so in the atrioventricular node. One case of myocardial infarction presumably due to arteritis of the coronary vessels has been reported.[28]

Cardiac enlargement with heart weights up to 750 g is frequently reported and is probably due to a combination of hypertension secondary to renal disease and to small-vessel arteritis as well as to other factors.[22,25,26]

Pericarditis, found in 60 to 70 percent of autopsies, is one of the most common cardiac lesions seen in lupus erythematosus.[22,24,26,29,30] James has described extension of the acute inflammatory process in the pericardium into the sinoatrial node with production of local inflammation, and destruction of the sinus node fibers.[28] Constrictive pericarditis[29] has been reported, as has tamponade due to fluid accumulation.[28,29] The pericardial fluid may be clear or blood, has a high protein content, and may contain the LE factor.[25] Pericardial effusion up to 1,000 ml has been seen.[25] At autopsy, most patients show fibrinoid degeneration and necrosis of the connective tissue of the pericardium, but if the process is inactive at the time of death, there may be only edematous fibrous tissue linking the two layers of the sac together and obliterating the pericardial cavity.[22]

Bacterial endocarditis seems to be more common in the course of systemic lupus erythematosus than in the normal population,[22,24,30] but the lesions are not always seen in association with the Libman-Sachs verrucae. It is probable that the decreased resistance to infection which characterizes this disease, rather than the endocardial change itself, is responsible for the frequency of the endocardial infections and the increasing occurrence of infective pericarditis.[21]

Clinical manifestations

Cardiac manifestations are more prominent in systemic lupus erythematosus than in the other collagen diseases, and may be the presenting symptom.[22,29,30]

Although two-thirds of autopsied patients show pericarditis in one stage or another,[22,24] 30 percent or less have had recognizable symptoms or signs during life.[22,24,25,29] Pericardial involvement may be manifested by a typical pain pattern in the absence of a pericardial rub or electrocardiographic changes, or may be totally asymptomatic and discovered only because of the presence of the three-component friction rub or by the chance finding of the characteristic changes on the electrocardiogram.[25,26,29] Classical findings of cardiac tamponade may occur, and repeated aspiration of the pericardial fluid may be required.[29,30] Pericarditis may be present as an initial manifestation of the disease, and has a tendency to remit and return with no apparent relation to the other activity of the disease.[22,29] Care must be taken not to mistake an early diastolic component of a

pericardial rub for an aortic diastolic murmur. It is possible that some of the aortic diastolic murmurs described during the course of systemic lupus erythematosus for which no explanation is found at postmortem examination may be due to this error.

Systolic and diastolic murmurs at the mitral valve area are frequently reported during the course of systemic lupus erythematosus, but in the majority of cases no acceptable cause is found at autopsy.[22,25,26,29] Acute Libman-Sachs endocarditis has been considered to be the cause of these murmurs, but it is difficult to see how such tiny lesions on an otherwise competent valve could be responsible.[22,25] In many cases the valves are completely normal at autopsy,[22,26,30] but in others they show diffuse thickening and fibrosis. The latter could conceivably produce valvular deficiency. Combinations of anemia, tachycardia, and fever help to explain some of the basal systolic murmurs but not all.[22,30] Brigden has noticed scarring in the papillary muscles in systemic lupus erythematosus,[26] and it is possible that impaired function of this portion of the mitral valve complex is the cause of the mitral regurgitation and its associated murmurs. Diastolic rumbles simulating those of mitral stenosis may be secondary to mitral regurgitation in such cases. This concept would also explain the disappearance of the murmurs with steroid treatment as the myocarditis, papillary muscle dysfunction, and cardiac failure come under control. In several cases brought to autopsy, diastolic murmurs at the apex were found to be due to previous rheumatic heart disease with classical mitral stenosis.[25,29] Aortic diastolic murmurs have been reported by several authors, but here again, the pathologic correlation has been exceedingly poor.[25,29] Hypertension, which is sometimes associated with aortic diastolic murmurs,[26] has been present in some of these cases, while bacterial endocarditis[25,29] and rheumatic heart disease have been found in others. More recently, Bulkley[34] and Paget[32] have reported severe mitral valve insufficiency resulting from "healed" Libman-Sachs endocarditis which has necessitated valve replacement.

Chest pain, common in lupus erythematosus, is usually due to pericarditis or pleuritis,[22,29] but at times it cannot be explained by pathologic changes.[22,29] Coincidental coronary atherosclerosis with angina pectoris and myocardial infarction has also been reported but is not directly related to the primary disease.[29,30]

Congestive heart failure is not a common finding in systemic lupus erythematosus but is reported to occur in 5 to 20 percent of cases.[22,25,29] It is frequently, but not invariably,[26,29] associated with diastolic hypertension secondary to renal disease. Heart failure may be mistakenly diagnosed in the presence of renal failure with edema or pericardial effusion. It has been reported as the ultimate cause of death.[29,30] Tachycardia and gallop rhythm may persist when other signs of failure are not present; they probably indicate active myocarditis.

Surprisingly, in view of the pericarditis and arteritis, arrhythmias are not common and are reported to occur in only 10 percent of cases.[22,25,28-30] Atrial fibrillation and flutter, with various degrees of atrioventricular conduction disturbances, are most often seen.[22,25,28-30] Complete heart block with Stokes-Adams attacks has been reported. James is of the opinion that if continuous monitoring were to be carried out, a higher percentage of arrhythmias and conduction defects would be found.[28]

The *electrocardiogram* is abnormal in most cases of systemic lupus erythematosus at some time during the disease.[22,26] The usual findings are nonspecific ST and T wave changes, low voltage, and the characteristic evolution of the pattern of pericarditis.[22,26,29] Bundle branch block has been reported, as has left ventricular hypertrophy.[29,30] Atrial arrhythmias occur in about 10 percent of cases, and all degrees of AV block have been recorded, although this is not common.[22,25,28-30] Myocardial infarction due to incidental coronary atherosclerosis has also been reported.[30]

The *roentgenogram* of the chest is of no particular help in differential diagnosis but may be of assistance in differentiating cardiac enlargement from pericardial effusion.

Echocardiography may be extremely valuable in lupus erythematosus for demonstrating symptomatic or asymptomatic pericardial involvement. It could also be used for identifying valvular verrucal lesions and for evaluating valve function in the presence of various murmurs.[32,35]

Treatment

The cardiac complications of lupus erythematosus are treated in much the same manner as the remainder of the disease. The usual measures of digitalis, diuretics, and salt restriction are useful in the treatment of congestive failure, but in most cases the addition of prednisone to the regimen will be needed to treat refractory failure.[22,25,26,29] The success of this treatment is presumably due to control of active myocarditis and is similar to the effect of corticosteroids in acute rheumatic fever. Control of hypertension, as outlined elsewhere in this book, is also helpful in the treatment and prevention of congestive failure. Pericardiectomy has been necessary for control of intractable pain or for relief of constrictive pericarditis.[29]

It is interesting to note that while corticosteroid therapy will undoubtedly prolong the life of the individual with systemic lupus erythematosus and will result in healing of the Libman-Sachs lesions, this healing itself may be the cause of valve deformity to the extent of requiring valve replacement.[31,34]

DERMATOMYOSITIS

Dermatomyositis is the least commonly seen, and consequently the least studied and understood, of the collagen diseases. The English language literature contains few good pathologic studies of the heart in this disease, and even less clinicopathologic correlation.[36-39] The scarcity of such information and the diversity of opinions expressed precludes any definitive statement about cardiac involvement in this disease. Most authors concerned with the disease seem to agree that the heart is involved frequently, although in the majority of cases the changes are minimal.[36,38-40]

Pathology

The findings usually described are those of edema between the myocardial fibers, sometimes with lymphocytic infiltration, necrosis, fibrosis, and occasional calcification.[37,41] Cardiac muscle cells have been said to show degeneration atrophy due to primary involvement,[36,38,42] or to pressure atrophy secondary to mucoid degeneration of the connective tissue with pressure on the surrounding muscle cells.[37] Mild and moderate cardiac enlargement may occur.[38,41] One case of calcific pericarditis has been reported.[43] Another report mentions epicardial fibrosis,[41] and still another author mentions "significant pericardial effusion."[39] The myocardial vessels are said not to be affected in adults,[36,43,44] but may be in children.[44] Cor pulmonale with right ventricular hypertrophy secondary to pulmonary hypertension was reported by Goldfischer.[45] Schaumburg[46] has reported the pathologically well documented case of fibrous replacement of the distal third of the bundle of His and left main bundle and sinoatrial node.

Clinical manifestations

Most authors feel that the cardiac involvement causes few if any clinical symptoms.[36,39,41,47] Several, however, have listed cardiac failure as a cause of death, but they provide little clinical or pathologic information.[38,48-50] Murmurs or clinical findings of pericarditis are rarely mentioned.

Schaumburg's case revealed progression through 2:1 AV block, to a combination of left axis deviation and right bundle branch block, and then to complete heart block. A permanent pacemaker was implanted, and the patient did well, but it was noted that 10 months later, when the unit was being replaced because of increased threshold, no spontaneous ventricular activity was present.

The *electrocardiogram* may show ST and T wave changes, which are used as evidence of myocarditis or pericarditis.[39,40,51] Atrial arrhythmias have been reported, as have various degrees of atrioventricular block, including complete heart block. Unfortunately the electrocardiographic findings are usually reported without any clinical or pathologic correlation and, as in the other collagen diseases, could be due to other underlying heart disease as well as to the dermatomyositis.[52]

Treatment

Specific therapy is not available. Heart failure, should it occur, should be treated with usual measures. Little information is available regrading the value of corticosteroids in the treatment of heart disease related to dermatomyositis. Such treatment seems reasonable, however, and should be tried.

REFERENCES

1 Weiss, S., Stead, E., Warren, J., and Bailey, O.: Scleroderma Heart Disease, *Arch. Intern. Med.*, 71:749, 1943.

2 Oram, S., and Stokes, W.: The Heart in Scleroderma, *Br. Heart J.*, 23:243, 1961.

3 Sachner, M., Heinz, E., and Steinberg, A.: The Heart in Scleroderma, *Am. J. Cardiol.*, 17:542, 1966.

4 Bulkley, B., Ridolfi, R., Sayler, W., and Hutchins, G.: Myocardial Lesions of Progressive Systemic Sclerosis, *Circulation*, 53:483, 1976.

5 Herdson, P., Sommers, H., and Jennings, R.: A Comparative Study of the Fine Structure of Normal and Ischemic Dog myocardium with Special Reference to Early Changes Following Temporary Occlusion of a Coronary Artery, *Am. J. Pathol.*, 46:367, 1965.

6 Reichenbach, D., and Benditt, E.: A Response of the Myocardial Cell to Injury, *Arch. Pathol.*, 85:189, 1968.

7 James, T.: Coronary Arteries and Conduction System in Scleroderma Heart Disease, *Circulation*, 50:844, 1974.

8 Escudero, J., and McDevitt, E.: The Electrocardiogram in Scleroderma, *Am. Heart J.*, 56:846, 1958.

9 Roth, L. N., and Kissane, J. M.: Pan Aortitis and Aortic Valvulitis in Progressive Systemic Sclerosis, *Am. J. Clin. Pathol.*, 41:287, 1964.

10 Traube, A., DeMarry, M., Zimmerman, H., and Mascarenhas, E.: Angina Pectoris and Slow Flow Velocity Dye in Coronary Arteries. A New Angiographic Finding, *Am. Heart J.*, 84:66, 1972.

11 Arkin, A.: A Clinical and Pathological Study of Periarteritis Nodosa, *Am. J. Pathol.*, 6:401, 1930.

12 Reidbord, H. E., McCormack, L. J., and O'Duffy, J. D.: Necrotizing Angiitis: II. Findings at Autopsy in Twenty-seven Cases, *Cleve. Clin. Q.*, 32:191, 1965.

13 O'Duffy, J. D., Scherbel, A. L., Reidbord, H. E., and McCormack, L.: Necrotizing Angitis: I. A Clinical Review of Twenty-seven Autopsied Cases, *Cleve. Clin. Q.*, 32:87, 1965.

14 Taubenhaus, M., Eisenstein, B., and Pick, A.: Cardiovascular Manifestations of Collagen Disease, *Circulation*, 12:903, 1955.

15 Holsinger, D., Osmundsen, P., and Edwards, J.: The Heart in Periarteritis Nodosa, *Circulation*, 25:610, 1962.

16 Rose, G.: "Polyarteritis Nodosa—Immunological Diseases," Little, Brown and Company, Boston, 1965, p. 749.

17 Griffith, G., and Vural, I.: Polyarteritis Nodosa, *Circulation*, 3:481, 1951.

18 Shick, R., and Kvole, W.: "Peripheral Vascular Disease," W. B. Saunders Company, Philadelphia, 1962, p. 497.

19 Roberts, F., and Fetterman, G.: Polyarteritis Nodosa in Infancy, *J. Pediatr.*, 63:519, 1963.

20 Glanz, S., Bittner, S. J., Berman, M. A., Olan, T., and Talner, N.: Regression of Coronary-Artery Aneurysms in Infantile Polyarteritis Nodosa, *N. Engl. J. Med.*, 294(17):939, 1976.

21 Kawasaki, T., Kosaki, F., Okawa, S., Shigematsu, I., and Yanagawa, H.; New Infantile Acute Mucocutaneous Lymph Node Syndrome (MLNS) Prevailing in Japan, *Pediatrics*, 54:271, 1974.

22 Dubois, E.: "Lupus Erythematosus," McGraw-Hill Book Company, New York, 1966.

23 Klemperer, P., Pollack, A., and Baehr, G.: Pathology of Disseminated Lupus Erythematosus, *AMA Arch. Pathol.*, 32:569, 1941.

24 Harvey, A., Shulman, L., Tumulty, P., Conley, C., and Schoenrich, E.: Systemic Lupus Erythematosus—A Review of the Literature and Clinical Analyses of 138 Cases, *Medicine*, 33:291, 1954.

25 Shearn, M.: The Heart in Systemic Lupus Erythmatosus, *Am. Heart J.*, 58:452, 1959.

26 Brigden, W., Bywaters, E., Lessof, M., and Ross, I.: The Heart in Systemic Lupus Erythematosus, *Br. Heart J.*, 22:1, 1960.

27 James, T., Rupe, C., and Monto, R.: Pathology of the Cardiac Conduction System in Systemic Lupus Erythematosus, *Ann. Intern. Med.*, 63:402, 1965.

28 Bonfiglio, T., Botti, R., and Hagstrom, J.: Coronary Arteritis, Occlusion, and Myocardial Infarction Due to Lupus Erythematosus, *Am. Heart J.*, 83:153, 1972.

29 Hejtmancik, M., Wright, J., Quint, R., and Jennings, F.: The Cardiovascular Manifestations of Systemic Lupus Erythematosus, *Am. Heart J.*, 68:119, 1964.

30 Kong, T., Kellum, R., and Haserich, J.: Clinical Diagnosis of Cardiac Involvement in Systemic Lupus Erythematosus, *Circulation*, 26:7, 1962.

31 Bulkley, B., and Roberts, W.: The Heart in Systemic Lupus Erythematous and the Changes Induced in It by Corticosteroid Therapy, *Am. J. Med.*, 58:243, 1975.

32 Paget, S., Bulkley, B., Grauer, L., and Seningen, R.: Mitral Valve Disease of Systemic Lupus Erythematosus, *Am. J. Med.*, 59:134, 1975.

33 Meller, J., Conde, C., Deppisch, L., Denoso, E., and Dack, S.: Myocardial Infarction Due to Coronary Atherosclerosis in Three Young Adults with Systemic Lupus Erythematosus, *Am. J. Cardiol.*, 35:309, 1975.

34 Bulkley, B., and Roberts, W.: Systemic Lupus Erythematosus as a Cause of Severe Mitral Regurgitation, *Am. J. Med.*, 35:305, 1975.

35 Maniscalco, B., Felner, J., McCann, J., and Chiapella, J.: Echocardiographic Abnormalities in Systemic Lupus Erythematosus, *Circulation*, 52(suppl. 2):211, 1975.

36 Mendeloff, J.: Myocardial Changes in Dermatomyositis, *N.C. Med. J.*, 15:15, 1954.

37 Wainger, C., and Lever, W.: Dermatomyositis: Report of Three Cases with Postmortem Observations, *Arch. Dermat. Syph.*, 59:196, 1949.

38 O'Leary, P., and Waisman, M.: Dermatomyositis, *Arch. Dermat. Syph.*, 41:1001, 1940.

39 Walton, J., and Adams, R.: "Polymyositis," E. & S. Livingstone, Ltd., Edinburgh, 1958, p. 269.

40 Sheard, C.: Dermatomyositis, *Arch. Intern. Med.*, 88:640, 1951.

41 Kinney, T., and Maher, M.: Dermatomyositis, *Am. J. Pathol.*, 16:561, 1939.

42 Frazer, M.: A Case of Dermatomyositis, *Br. J. Dermatol. Syph.*, 54:265, 1942.

43 Everett, M., and Curtis, A.: Dermatomyositis, *AMA Arch. Intern. Med.*, 100:70, 1957.

44 Banker, B., and Victor, M.: Dermatomyositis, *Medicine*, 45:261, 1966.

45 Goldfischer, J., and Rubin, E.: Dermatomyositis with Pulmonary Lesions, *Ann. Intern. Med.*, 50:194, 1959.

46 Schaumburg, H., Neilson, S., and Yurchak, P.: Heart Block in Polymyositis, *N. Engl. J. Med.*, 284:480, 1971.

47 Pearson, C.: Polymyositis, *Postgrad. Med.*, 31:450, 1962.

48 Marcus, I., and Weinstein, J.: Dermatomyositis, *Ann. Intern. Med.*, 9:406, 1935.

49 Rowland, L.: Muscular Dystrophies, Polymyositis and Other Myopathies, *J. Chronic Dis.*, 8:510, 1958.
50 Stuckey, F.: Dermatomyositis, *Br. J. Dermatol.*, 47:85, 1935.
51 Wedgwood, R., Cook, C., and Cohen, J.: Dermatomyositis, *Pediatrics*, 12:447, 1953.
52 Diessner, G., Howard, F., Winkelmann, R., Lambert, E., and Mulder, D.: Laboratory Tests in Polymyositis, *Arch. Intern. Med.*, 117:757, 1966.

89
The Heart and Obesity

JAMES K. ALEXANDER, M.D.

Other men live to eat, while I eat to live.

SOCRATES[1]

The most striking evidence of circulatory dysfunction in very obese persons is the appearance of congestive heart failure without other apparent cause together with cardiac enlargement and increased heart weight at autopsy, manifestations described as early as 1933.[1a] These observations and the high frequency of cardiorespiratory symptoms in obese subjects have led to clinical investigations demonstrating significant circulatory alterations in very obese subjects.[2] In this chapter are described some of the characteristics of the heart and circulation of very obese subjects weighing 300 lb or more, with body weights ranging from 100 to 300 lb in excess of their ideal weight (Fig. 89-1).

ADIPOSE TISSUE BLOOD FLOW

It is well known from anatomic studies that adipose tissue is a vascular organ and from physiochemical studies that it is metabolically active. Measurements utilizing a variety of direct and indirect methods in both animals and human beings have demonstrated that blood flow to adipose tissue, expressed per unit wet weight, varies ten- to fifteenfold among members of the same species under conditions of rest.[3–5] Changes in adipose tissue mass may result in marked alterations in its composition. When adipose tissue depots increase in size, the fat cells become larger, with greater amounts of lipid, lesser amounts of water and dry residue, and fewer fat cells per unit wet weight. Thus, varying degrees of adiposity may be a major factor in accounting for the wide range of blood flow observed in various adipose tissue depots in animals and in human beings. This is supported by the observation that blood flow per unit wet weight adipose tissue declines with increasing weight in human beings and in animals, reflecting enlargement of the adipose cells.[3,6] Adipose tissue blood flow in human beings at rest, based on several studies utilizing inert gas washout methodology, has averaged about 2 to 3 ml/min/100 g adipose tissue.[7] A variety of factors, including the nutritional state of the individual, neurohumoral mechanisms, and the metabolic state of the tissue, condition adipose tissue flow. For example, in canine subcutaneous adipose tissue, nerve stimulation causes arteriolar vasoconstriction, an effect mimicked by noradrenaline administration and blocked by alpha-adrenergic blockade. Beta-adrenergic agents cause arteriolar and venous dilatation.[8,9] When hypotension is induced by hemorrhage in dogs, subcutaneous adipose tissue blood flow may fall tenfold and oxygen consumption per unit wet weight of tissue, fourfold. The decrement in blood flood in subcutaneous adipose tissue is much greater than that in other organs. This effect is preventable by previous infusion with phenoxybenzamine, which indicates the importance of alpha receptor activity.[10] Reactive hyperemia after ischemia has been observed in the subcutaneous adipose tissue of human beings; it varies with the duration of ischemia.[11]

Recent studies relating adipose tissue blood flow

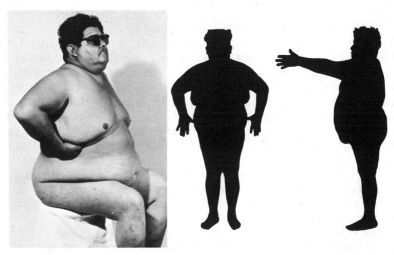

FIGURE 89-1 Sitting and silhouette photographs of a very obese subject representative of the group discussed in this chapter. At the time the picture was taken, the patient weighed 147 kg (325 lb).

to the number and size of fat cells in the adipose tissue depots may have considerable clinical significance. There are two types of adipose tissue mass with obesity: *hyperplastic* with normal or increased cell size, and *hypertrophic* with increased cell size only. The hyperplastic type of obesity implies onset at an early age, that is, less than 5 years of age or from 9 to 13 years of age. Later adult onset is characteristic of hypertrophic obesity.[12] The composition and morphologic characteristics of adipose tissue play a significant role in the regulation of blood flow to this tissue. There is an inverse relationship between blood flow per unit weight of tissue and fat cell size. A positive correlation, on the other hand, has been demonstrated between blood flow per unit weight of tissue and the number of fat cells.[3] Furthermore, by characterizing adipose tissue in terms of fat cell size and number and estimating the blood flow on a *per cell* basis, it has been possible to demonstrate increasing blood flow with increasing fat cell size.[13] This relation between blood flow per adipose tissue cell and adipose cell volume provides a clue to the interpretation of at least two observations of clinical import: First, the increase in adipose tissue blood flow per unit wet tissue weight in human beings following a 3-day fast[6] presumably reflects increasing adipose cell number per unit tissue weight. Second, the significant fall of cardiac output observed in human beings with weight loss[14] appears to reflect marked reduction in adipose tissue cell volume.

HEMODYNAMIC FEATURES

Plasma volume and circulating blood volume are both increased in very obese subjects.[15] Hematocrit tends to be normal or slightly increased. The increase in blood volume is correlated with the amount of excess body weight, reflecting an increase in the size of the vascular bed. When the body weight is 100 kg in excess of ideal, for example, the blood volume is 10 liters, or about twice that predicted for the ideal weight.

Augmentation of blood volume is paralleled by an increment in cardiac output, correlated with the amount of excess body weight.[15] Both cardiac output and body oxygen consumption at rest in extreme obesity may reach levels two or three times that predicted for the ideal weight. Since resting heart rate is normal or only slightly increased, high cardiac output is effected by a large stroke volume. Systemic arteriovenous oxygen difference is usually normal or only slightly widened. Thus, cardiac output increases in proportion to body oxygen consumption, which in turn increases in porportion to body weight. In the absence of heart failure, increases in cardiac output with exercise in very obese subjects are comparable to those in subjects at ideal weight. When the increment in cardiac output with obesity is related to the increment in oxygen consumption of the body in the same way as may be done for exercise, there is a

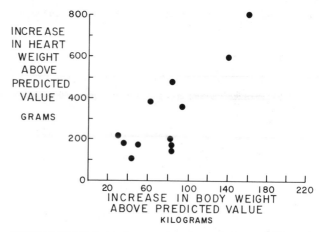

FIGURE 89-2 Relation between increment in heart weight and body weight above predicted values in 12 very obese subjects.

mean increment of 2,270 ml/min in cardiac output per 100-ml increase in body oxygen consumption. This is in contrast to the approximately 900-ml increase in cardiac output per 100-ml increment in body oxygen consumption during exercise.[16] Thus, the circulatory adjustment to excess weight at rest is much less efficient than that during exercise (Fig. 89-2).

Estimates of cardiac work in very obese subjects at rest yield high values, with increases above those levels predicted for ideal weight ranging from 40 to 190 percent. Left ventricular work is also greater than that predicted for ideal body weight, and represents the predominant increment in total cardiac work for three-quarters of these patients.[16]

CARDIAC ANATOMY

As indicated by increases in roentgenographic estimates of transverse cardiac diameter, cardiac enlargement is present in about three-fourths of very obese subjects, with cardiac diameter ranging from 20 to 55 percent above that predicted for ideal weight.[17] These relations obtain in normotensive as well as in hypertensive obese subjects. In obese subjects dying of intercurrent cause without systemic hypertension, coronary, valvular, or other forms of heart disease, increases in heart weight roughly proportional to the increments in body weight are regularly found. Gross and microscopic examination of such hearts indicates that the augmented cardiac weight is due to changes in muscle mass, though fatty infiltration of the myocardium or increased epicardial fat deposition occur in some cases.[18] Increased muscle mass is due to left ventricular hypertrophy, sometimes with right ventricular hypertrophy as well. Isolated or predominant right ventricular hypertrophy has not been observed in these patients. Thus left ventricular hypertrophy is the most specific and significant anatomic alteration in the hearts of very obese subjects (Fig. 89-3).

Although these anatomic changes may be pronounced, electrocardiographic evidences of ventricular hypertrophy are usually absent. Indeed, the amplitude of the spatial QRS vector relating to leads 1, aV_F, and V_2 is usually diminished, though the mean

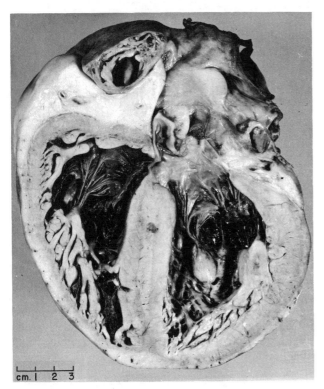

FIGURE 89-3 Heart at autopsy of a man weighing 497 lb who died of cardiac failure at age 42. Cardiac weight has increased to 1,100 g because of biventricular hypertrophy. Thickened left and right ventricular walls measured 25 mm and 10 mm, respectively. Electrocardiogram showed only modest deviation of the mean QRS axis to the right and absence of voltage and other criteria to suggest the severe degree of left ventricular hypertrophy found at necropsy.

frontal plane QRS axis does tend to be more leftward than normal.[19] Failure of the electrocardiogram to reflect myocardial hypertrophy in the grossly obese subject is probably related to the effect of the anatomy of the thorax upon the transmission of electric impulses.

Although mechanisms leading to the development of cardiac hypertrophy in very obese subjects are not well defined, the appreciable increase in the work of the heart must play a significant role. Thus, in some regards the hemodynamic alterations accompanying gross obesity may be similar to those under experimental conditions of prolonged or continuous physical exercise involving chronic left ventricular volume overload. Cardiac hypertrophy may be produced in rats by daily treadmill exercise[20] or by swimming.[21] There is also evidence for cardiac hypertrophy in endurance athletes.[22] However, development of congestive heart failure secondary to prolonged physical exertion in otherwise healthy men or in experimental animals has not been reported; in this respect, the circumstances obtaining with gross obesity differ.

REGIONAL BLOOD FLOW

Cerebral blood flow per unit brain weight in very obese subjects is normal. Since no change in brain weight occurs with the development of obesity, total cerebral flow is also in the normal range.[15] Renal blood flow is low normal or slightly reduced when compared with the predicted flow at ideal body weight in obese subjects, although the kidneys are somewhat larger and heavier than normal.[15] By contrast, splanchnic flow in obesity is high as compared with that at predicted ideal weight. However, the increases in splanchnic flow, ranging up to 800 ml/min in very obese subjects, are by no means sufficient to account for the increments in cardiac output in these same individuals, which reach levels as high as 5 liters/min.[15] Adipose tissue blood flow measurements in extremely obese subjects have not been carried out in sufficient number to draw firm quantitative conclusions. However, the absence of significant changes in organ blood flow indicates that the increment in resting cardiac output with extreme obesity is largely distributed to fat tissue depots. Oxygen consumption, blood volume, and blood flow *per kilogram body weight* are less than in the subject at ideal weight, reflecting a lesser oxygen transport to adipose tissue per unit weight than to the various parenchymal organs.[15] Despite this, in these very obese subjects, fat depots and the blood supply to them are sufficiently large to necessitate a high cardiac output at rest.

HYPERTENSION

Direct and intraarterial pressure measurements indicate that hypertension is common in very obese subjects. Moderate blood pressure elevation (pressure 150/90 mm Hg or higher) is present in about half of these individuals, and severe hypertension (blood pressure greater than 200/120 mm Hg) is present in about 10 percent more. Since approximately 40 percent of very obese people are normotensive, it is apparent that even extreme obesity does not always lead to the development of hypertension. Furthermore, there is no correlation between the level of systemic blood pressure and the amount of excess weight or the total body weight.[17]

Overestimation of the blood pressure by the standard cuff method as the circumference of the arm increases is well documented. However, pressures recorded in the grossly obese are not always overestimated, probably because of variation in configuration of the distribution of adipose tissue in the arms. Comparison of direct intraarterial and indirect standard cuff methods simultaneously in the same arm of very obese subjects yields approximately equivalent values (within 10 mm Hg) in one-third, and overestimations (maximum 30 mm Hg) in the remainder. Use of the larger standard thigh cuff (7 × 14 in.) improves the accuracy of the diastolic determination giving values equivalent to those obtained directly in 50% of subjects.[23] Application of the cuff to the midforearm and auscultation over the radial artery seems to have little usefulness in these subjects, since Korokoff sounds at the radial artery are usually inaudible. However, in instances where the cuff cannot be applied to the upper arm, and Korokoff sounds can be heard over the radial artery, the forearm method may be useful, though it provides information of no greater accuracy than that using the upper arm.[23] Though the indirect cuff method does overestimate blood pressure by no more than 30 mm Hg, direct intraarterial measurement appears to be the only reliable way of determining blood pressure of very obese subjects.[23,24]

Mechanisms responsible for the development of hypertension in very obese people, when it does occur, are poorly understood. There is no evidence to indicate generalized arteriolar luminal narrowing. In most instances, when the pressure gradient across the systemic circulation is related to the cardiac output, a normal value for systemic vascular resistance is found. This comes about as a result of proportional increases in cardiac output and arterial pressure. In normotensive obese subjects, the calculated vascular resistance is actually reduced. Such relations contrast sharply with those obtaining in essential and some other clinical forms of hypertension, where increased vascular resistance is the rule.

CONGESTIVE HEART FAILURE

The pathologic findings of congestive circulatory failure in patients weighing 300 lb or more at the time of death have been well documented. Indeed, cardiac failure frequently appears to play a role in the terminal illness of patients with gross chronic obesity, and clinical manifestations of cardiac failure in these patients have been recorded several years prior to death. The findings at postmortem examination include increased heart weight and left ventricular hypertrophy—sometimes with right ventricular hypertrophy as well—and severe pulmonary and systemic venous congestion.[1,25] Although cardiac failure may eventually take place in patients with long-standing severe obesity, heart catheterization studies indicate that hemodynamic alterations characteristic of a congestive circulatory state may antedate the development of myocardial failure by many years. This congestive state is characterized by high cardiac output and circulating blood volume, elevated left ventricular filling pressure at rest or after increasing venous return by leg raising or exercise, and pulmonary hypertension without a transpulmonary diastolic pressure gradient.[16,26] Studies of left ventricular pressure-volume relationships indicate diminished left ventricular diastolic compliance, presumably reflecting left ventricular hypertrophy.[27] Despite the presence of left ventricular diastolic dysfunction, left ventricular systolic performance may be well maintained for long periods of time, as indicated by normal left ventricular ejection fractions, maximum rate of pressure rise *(dP/dt)*, and cardiac output increment with exercise.[16,26,27]

However, if gross obesity persists for many years, systolic dysfunction of the ventricle follows with exacerbation of the congestive state and development of symptoms secondary to diminished regional blood flow. In some cases, this turn of events appears to be precipitated by rapid weight gain. Longevity over 60 years is not uncommon in these patients, and cardiac failure, once established, does not usually lead to a rapid demise. Increasing somnolence and mental confusion, progressing to terminal coma, characterize the late stages of the clinical picture.[25]

In summary, a current concept of circulatory dysfunction in very obese subjects involves the initial establishment of a high output congestive circulatory state, accompanied by the development of left ventricular hypertrophy and reduced left ventricular compliance. Pulmonary congestion is secondary to increased central and total blood volume, rise in left ventricular filling pressure, and pulmonary venous hypertension at rest or during exercise.[25,26] Progressive ventricular hypertrophy may itself compromise myocardial contractility, and in the face of continuing volume overload, systolic dysfunction of the left ventricle and myocardial insufficiency supervene.

PICKWICKIAN SYNDROME

The Pickwickian or obesity hypoventilation syndrome as originally described involves hypoventilation, somnolence, twitching, cyanosis, periodic respiration, polycythemia, right ventricular hypertrophy, and heart failure.[28] Alveolar hypoventilation develops in only about 10 percent of extremely obese individuals. Actually, the degree of hypercapnea is severe in less than 5 percent, and is not correlated with the amount of excess body weight.[17] Though a diminished ventilatory response to both hypercapnea and hypoxia has been found in very obese patients with hypoventilation, it is not clear whether this respiratory center depression precedes, accompanies, or follows the development of obesity. Reversibility of the hypoventilation and carbon dioxide insensitivity with a persistently reduced response to the hypoxic stimulus may occur following weight reduction.[29] Current hypotheses regarding the pathogenesis of obesity hypoventilation syndrome are that some individuals with inherently low respiratory sensitivity to hypoxia may develop frank hypoventilation when subjected to the increased work of breathing accompanying gross obesity,[29] or that very low chest wall compliance and weakness of inspiratory muscles lead to transient hypercapnea and a vicious cycle of events predisposing to further impairment of pulmonary gas exchange and hypercapnea at rest.[30]

In obese patients with hypoventilation, acidosis, hypoxia, and possibly polycythemia are superimposed upon elevated left ventricular filling pressure, as well as high pulmonary blood volume and flow, to produce an additional component of pulmonary hypertension secondary to vasoconstrictive activity.[26,30] Thus, with the hypoventilation syndrome, there may be a transpulmonary diastolic pressure gradient, in addition to elevation of left ventricular filling pressure. However, isolated right ventricular hypertrophy and failure, initially postulated to be characteristic of the Pickwickian hypoventilation syndrome, must occur rarely, if at all, and has never been documented at autopsy.[31]

WEIGHT REDUCTION AND OTHER THERAPY

It has been established that weight reduction in hypertensive obese patients may be accompanied by a fall in blood pressure, often to normal levels.[14] In some cases, though the patient is still well above ideal weight, significant lowering of blood pressure follows modest weight loss. Also, blood pressure reduction may be effected in obese subjects by sodium restriction alone, without significant change in body weight. In instances of severe hypertension (particularly diastolic) accompanied by funduscopic changes, significant symptoms, compromise of renal function, or clinical evidences of cerebral or cardiac involvement, it seems reasonable to manage the condition much the same way as would be done with essential or any other form of hypertension of this severity. However, in the usual circumstance where the hypertension accompanying obesity is of moderate degree and is primarily systolic, a low-calorie reducing diet may be instituted initially. This dietary regimen is often accompanied by a substantial diuresis, with reduction in both weight and blood pressure in the first several days. If, as weight reduction proceeds, the blood pressure tends to remain elevated, dietary sodium restriction may also be desirable. Persistent hypertension, as the ideal body weight is approached, may be taken as an indication for antihypertensive agents.

The circulatory alterations accompanying extreme obesity are at least partially reversible by weight reduction.[14,26] Substantial weight loss in these individuals results in significant decrements in body oxygen consumption, total and central blood volumes, cardiac output, left ventricular filling pressure, and work of the heart. Reductions in blood volume and cardiac output per kilogram weight loss approximate 30 ml and 30 ml/min, respectively.[32] However, left ventricular filling pressure usually rises abnormally with exercise, suggesting that decreased ventricular compliance and myocardial hypertrophy persist, at least for as long as several months or years, after weight reduction. Additionally, in those subjects with hypoventilation, hypercapnea and hypoxemia may be reversible with weight reduction, further lowering pulmonary artery pressure and reducing or eliminating the transpulmonary diastolic pressure gradient.[26]

Effective long-term therapy of the congestive high output state in obesity necessarily involves weight reduction, though dietary sodium restriction and diuretics may be advantageously employed, particularly in instances where the symptoms are predominantly related to pulmonary congestion. If symptoms are moderately severe or progressive, digitalis may be added to the therapeutic regimen and is also useful in controlling atrial arrhythmias, which occasionally occur. Since the circulatory alterations accompanying obesity may be superimposed on those secondary to coexisting valvular, coronary, or hypertensive heart disease, the therapeutic importance of weight reduction cannot be exaggerated in these circumstances.

REFERENCES

1 "The New Dictionary of Thoughts: A Cyclopedia of Quotations," originally compiled by Tryon Edwards, revised and enlarged by C. N. Catrevas, Jonathan Edwards, and R. E. Browns, Standard Book Company, 1957, p. 754.

1a Smith, H. L., and Willius, F. A.: Adiposity of the Heart, *Arch. Intern. Med.,* 52:911, 1933.

2 Alexander, J. K.: Obesity and the Circulation, *Mod. Concepts Cardiovas. Dis.,* 32:799, 1963.

3 DiGirolamo, M., Skinner, N. S., Jr., Hanley, H. G., and Sachs, R. G.: Relationship of Adipose Tissue Blood Flow to Fat Cell Size and Number, *Am. J. Physiol.,* 220:932, 1971.

4 Heard, J. A., Goodman, H. M., and Grose, S. A.: Blood Flow Rates through Adipose Tissues of Unanesthetized Rats, *Am. J. Physiol.,* 214:263, 1968.

5 Larsen, O. A., Lassen, N. A., and Quaade, F.: Blood Flow through Human Adipose Tissue Determined with Radioactive Xenon, *Acta Physiol. Scand.,* 66:337, 1966.

6 Nielsen, S. L., and Larsen, O. A.: Relationship of Subcutaneous Adipose Tissue Blood Flow to Thickness of Subcutaneous Tissue and Total Body Fat Mass, *Scand. J. Clin. Lab. Invest.,* 31:383, 1973.

7 Nielsen, S. L.: Measurement of Blood Flow in Adipose Tissue from the Washout of Xenon-133 after Atraumatic Labelling, *Acta Physiol. Scand.* 84 (suppl. 2):187, 1972.

8 Fredholm, B. B.: Studies on the Sympathetic Regulation of Circulation and Metabolism in Isolated Canine Subcutaneous Adipose Tissue, *Acta Physiol. Scand.,* 80 (suppl. 354):1, 1970.

9 Ballard, K., Cobb, C. A., and Roswell, S.: Vascular and Lipolytic Responses in Canine Subcutaneous Adipose Tissue Following Infusion of Catecholamines, *Acta Physiol. Scand.,* 81:246, 1971.

10 Kovach, A. G., Rosell, S., Sandar, P., Koltay, E., Kovach, E., and Tomka, N.: Blood Flow, Oxygen Consumption, and Free Fatty Acid Release in Subcutaneous Adipose Tissue during Hemorrhagic Shock in Control and Phenoxybenzamine-treated Dogs, *Circ. Res.,* 26 (suppl. 6):733, 1970.

11 Nielsen, S. L., and Sejrsen, P.: Reactive Hyperemia in Subcutaneous Adipose Tissue in Man, *Acta Physiol. Scand.,* 85:71, 1972.

12 Salans, L., Cushman, S. W., and Weissmann, R. E.: Studies of Human Adipose Tissue. Adipose Cell Size and Number in Nonobese and Obese Patients, *J. Clin. Invest.,* 52:929, 1973.

13 DiGirolamo, M., and Esposito, J.: Adipose Tissue Blood Flow and Cellularity in the Growing Rabbit, *Am. J. Physiol.,* 229:107, 1975.

14 Alexander, J. K., and Peterson, K. L.: Cardiovascular Effects of Weight Reduction, *Circulation,* 45:310, 1972.

15 Alexander, J. K., Dennis, E. W., Smith, W. G., Amad, K. H., Duncan, W. C., and Austin, R. C.: Blood Volume, Cardiac Output and Distribution of Systemic Blood Flow in Extreme Obesity, *Cardiovas. Res. Cent. Bull.,* 1:39, 1962.

16 Alexander, J. K.: Obesity and Cardiac Performance, *Am. J. Cardiol.,* 14:860, 1964.

17 Alexander, J. K., Amad, K. H., and Cole, V. W.: Observations on Some Clinical Features of Extreme Obesity, with Particular Reference to Cardio-respiratory Effects, *Am. J. Med.,* 32:512, 1962.

18 Amad, K. H., Brennan, J. C., and Alexander, J. K.: The Cardiac Pathology of Chronic Exogenous Obesity, *Circulation,* 32:740, 1965.

19 Axelrad, M. A., and Alexander, J. K.: The Electrocardiogram and Cardiac Anatomy in Obesity, *Clin. Res.,* 13:25, 1965.

20 Van Liere, E. J., and Northup, D. W.: Cardiac Hypertrophy Produced by Exercise in Albino and Hooded Rats, *J. Appl. Physiol.,* 11:91, 1957.

21 Shelley, W. B., Code, C. F., and Visscher, M. B.: The Influence of Thyroid, Dinitrophenol, and Swimming on the Glycogen and Phosphocreatine Level of the Rat Heart in Relation to Cardiac Hypertrophy, *Am. J. Physiol.,* 138:652, 1943.

22 Herzkräftigung und echte Herzhypertrophie, durch Sport, *Z. Kreislaufforsch.,* 28:839, 1936.

23 Kvols, L. K., Rohlfing, B. M., and Alexander, J. K.: A Comparison of Intraarterial and Cuff Blood Pressure Measurements in Very Obese Subjects, *Cardiovas. Res. Cent. Bull.,* 7:118, 1969.

24 Blackburn, H., Kihlberg, J., and Brozek, J.: Arm versus Forearm Blood Pressure in Obesity, *Am. Heart J.,* 69:423, 1965.

25 Alexander, J. K., and Pettigrove, J. R.: Obesity and Congestive Heart Failure, *Geriatrics,* 22:101, July 1967.

26 Kaltman, A. J., and Golding, R. M.: Role of Circulatory Congestion in the Cardiorespiratory Failure of Obesity, *Am. J. Med.,* 60:645, 1976.

27 Wilcken, D. E.: Left Ventricular Volume in Man: the Relation to Heart Rate and to End-Diastolic Pressure, *Australas Ann. Med.,* 17 (suppl. 3):195, 1968.

28 Burwell, C. S., Robin, E. D., Whaley, R. D., and Bickelmann, A. G.: Extreme Obesity Associated with Alveolar Hypoventilation—a Pickwickian Syndrome, *Am. J. Med.,* 21:811, 1956.

29 Vogel, J. H. K., Hartley, L. H., Jamieson, G., and Grover, R. F.: Impairment of Ventilatory Response to Hypoxia in Individuals with Obesity and Hypoventilation: A Concept of the Pickwickian Syndrome, *Circulation,* 36 (suppl. 2):258, 1967.

30 Rochester, D. F., and Enson, Y.: Current Concepts in the Pathogenesis of the Obesity-Hypoventilation Syndrome: Mechanical and Circulatory Factors, *Am. J. Med.,* 57:402, 1974.

31 Fisher, R. D.: The Pickwickian Syndrome, *Oklahoma State Med. Assoc. J.,* 56:467, 1963.

32 Alexander, J. K.: Effects of Weight Reduction on the Cardiovascular System, in G. A. Bray, "Obesity in Perspective," DHEW Publication (NIH) 75-708.

90
Athlete's Heart

NANETTE KASS WENGER, M.D., and
CHARLES A. GILBERT, M.D.

The trained endurance athlete has a larger heart, most readily demonstrable by radiologic examination, than his or her nonathletic counterpart. The resting heart rate and heart rate with submaximal exercise are also considerably slower than in sedentary control subjects. This has led to a misunderstanding of the effect of athletic endeavors on the heart. It was previously thought that strenuous exercise was deleterious, causing cardiac dilatation similar to that in heart disease; hence the designation "athletic heart." However, far from demonstrating functional impairment, the myocardium of the endurance-trained athlete has increased pumping capacity and can provide more oxygen to working skeletal muscle at maximal work loads.[1] The high maximal oxygen consumption of well-trained endurance athletes ($\dot{V}_{O_2,max}$ = 4.0 to 5.0 liters/min) is accompanied by a high cardiac output (28 to 40 liters/min); the latter is due largely to an increased stroke volume, as maximal heart rate in athletes is equal to that of nonathletes.[2,3]

In the absence of significant congenital or acquired cardiovascular disease there is little evidence that any exhausting exercise of which a young adult human being is capable imposes any ill effect on the heart. Additionally, strenuous athletic activity, in a trained individual with a normal heart, does not increase the risk of early death or morbidity from cardiovascular disease.[4,5] Certain groups of collegiate "major athletes" have been shown to have a slight decrease in average life expectancy compared with less athletic collegiate groups. Body type may have an important influence in explaining this difference, because the major athletes were heavier and more muscular,[6,7] or postcollege lifestyle and prevalence of coronary risk factors may be important features.

The athletic heart syndrome may be characterized by a history of endurance athletic activities; biventricular cardiac enlargement; a systolic ejection murmur; an S_3; increased stroke volume; increased left ventricular stroke work and cardiac output; sinus bradycardia, often with sinus arrhythmia; recurrent atrial and ventricular arrhythmias; conduction disturbances, particularly a right ventricular conduction delay; and ST-T electrocardiographic changes.[8–10]

PHYSIOLOGIC ADAPTATIONS

Cardiovascular physiologic alterations are most pronounced in the endurance-trained athlete who shows an increase in radiologic heart volume. Speed or strength training causes peripheral muscle hypertrophy with little or no change in x-ray heart volume.[11] Echocardiographic studies of athletes involved in isometric exercise such as wrestling and shot-putting have shown normal left ventricular end-diastolic volume indexes (LVEDVI), but increased left ventricular (LV) wall thickness and LV mass. These results contrast with isotonically trained athletes, i.e., endurance runners or swimmers, who show echocardiographic increases in both LVEDVI and LV mass. Human endurance-trained athletes thus show both cardiac dilatation and hypertrophy.[12–14] Echocardiographic determination of aortic and left atrial dimensions shows no difference between endurance athletes and sedentary controls, but right ventricular dimensions indicate dilatation in the athletes.[13,14]

The cardiac hypertrophy and dilatation due to endurance training is not considered abnormal.[15,16] As noted above, endurance athletes are capable of superior cardiovascular performance, and there is no compelling evidence that their cardiac anatomic alterations adversely affect survival. Whether athletic-induced cardiac hypertrophy and dilatation regresses after training is discontinued has not been completely resolved. There are suggestions from animal models that regression does occur, but further studies are needed both in animals and in human athletes.[17]

Comparison of wild, athletic animals with their nonathletic domesticated counterparts shows that the wild animals have not only increased heart size but also increased myocardial capillary density, increased number of muscle cells per unit of heart mass, and smaller cardiac cells. This myocardial hyperplasia provides a better oxygen supply and utilization for the wild, athletic animal.[18] However, it is not well understood whether the ratio of capillaries to myocardial fibers increases, decreases, or remains the same in athletic-induced cardiac hypertrophy in adult animals or adult humans.[19] Echocardiographic indexes of cardiac contractility, ejection fraction (EF), and velocity of circumferential fiber shortening (Vcf) have shown normal cardiac performance for endurance-trained athletes.[13,14,14a] In animal models of athletic conditioning the functional characteristics of the heart and myocardium studied in vitro are normal; the myocardium of trained rats may have a greater ability to resist hypoxic stress.[20] Some conflicting results, however, have been noted in our own laboratory, and further studies of the effect of endurance training on myocardial contractility at rest and under stress are indicated.[21]

Relative slowing of the heart rate is characteristic of the trained athlete, and the heart rate decreases progressively with training.[22] The mechanism is uncertain but appears related to increased vagal tone. Pharmacologic investigation of the mechanism of the bradycardia using atropine and propranolol suggests that the resting bradycardia with exercise is also related to decreased sympathetic drive.[23] Increased vagal tone in the athlete may, in part, explain occasional arrhythmias, some of which disappear with exercise.

The athlete has an increased stroke volume, both at rest and with exercise, although the athlete and nonathlete have an identical, qualitative hemodynamic pattern of response to exercise.[14,24] The increased stroke volume does not reflect solely the increased diastolic filling time due to bradycardia; after training, subjects with congenital bradycardia did not change their heart rate but increased their stroke volume.

Cardiac catheterization studies show normal filling pressures of the athlete's heart at rest; these pressures increase slightly with exertion. Pressures are normal in the peripheral and pulmonary vascular beds, and there is normal dilatation in response to exercise. Ventricular work per minute is also normal.[9,23,25]

RADIOLOGIC CHANGES

The large heart of the endurance athlete may present problems in the radiologic and electrocardiographic diagnosis of heart disease; it is also of significance in insurance medicine. The cardiac enlargement is accompanied by prominent pulsations observed at fluoroscopy.

ELECTROCARDIOGRAPHIC CHANGES

Resting sinus bradycardia, as slow as 35 beats per minute, may be observed in the well-trained athlete (Fig. 90-1). However, neither the degree of resting

FIGURE 90-1 Trained athlete's electrocardiogram. Sinus bradycardia and increased QRS-T voltage (especially in V₄).

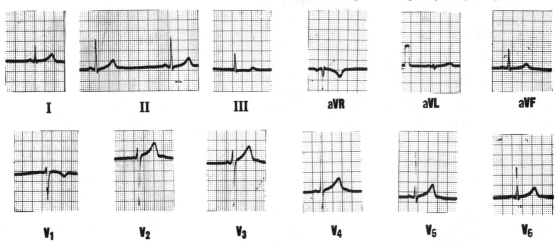

bradycardia, nor the other electrocardiographic findings, nor the heart size is directly related to increased cardiovascular performance ability.[11,26] The trained athlete has increased QRS-complex and T-wave amplitude on the conventional 12-lead electrocardiogram and increased magnitude of all vectorcardiographic forces.[27] There may be a prominent U wave. Possible mechanisms for the increased electromotive force include true myofiber hypertrophy, change in transfer impedance due to decreased distance between the enlarged heart and the recording electrodes, change in length and tension of myocardial fibers, and the effect of decreased subcutaneous fat. It is not surprising, then, that the magnitude of the electrocardiographic forces does not correlate with radiologic estimation of heart size.

The P-Q interval and the QRS duration tend to be at the upper limits of normal in athletes while the $Q-T_c$ interval shows no consistent alteration.[10] Second-degree atrioventricular (AV) block of the Wenckebach type, as well as first-degree AV block, is not infrequently noted in endurance-trained athletes, presumably due to increased vagal tone. Normal AV conduction is usually restored during submaximal exercise.[28] A varying incidence of incomplete right bundle branch block pattern is seen in reported series of athletes.[10]

The athlete's electrocardiogram differs from the electrocardiogram of subjects with left ventricular hypertrophy in that the athlete's T wave is large in amplitude, and frequently a prominent ST vector parallels the T vector in the precordial and inferior leads. The characteristic ST-segment elevation of early repolarization seen in athletes, as well as in sedentary groups, is almost invariably returned to an isoelectric position by exercise.[10] The frequency of electrocardiographic and vectorcardiographic diagnoses of right and left ventricular hypertrophy varies with diagnostic criteria, but is significantly greater in athletes than in the general population.[10,27]

The combination of bradycardia, cardiac enlargement on x-ray, an electrocardiographic pattern of left ventricular diastolic overload, and a left sternal border systolic murmur may also be confused with organic heart disease in the adolescent athlete. It is important that the physician recognize these as normal variants related to training. It has been suggested that the cardiac physiologic adaptation to exercise is now encountered more frequently in the adolescent because of increased emphasis on physical conditioning in the schools.[29]

SUDDEN DEATH IN ATHLETES

Rarely, sudden death may occur in an athlete. A young, seemingly healthy and vigorous individual engaged in performing feats of skill and/or endurance may be dead moments later. Most young athletes who die do so as a result of coronary atherosclerotic heart disease, often with acute myocardial infarction.[30] The terminal event is presumed to be ventricular fibrillation. Autopsy studies also implicate a number of other cardiovascular diseases in sudden death during athletics: acute and chronic myocarditis, cardiac tumors, coarctation of the aorta with aortic rupture, hypoplasia of the aorta and/or coronary arterial tree, congenital coronary artery anomalies, congenital subaortic stenosis, obstructive cardiomyopathy, and valvular aortic stenosis.[31]

Myocardial infarction in the setting of normal coronary arteries has been reported recently in two endurance athletes during exertion. A 44-year-old well-trained Boston marathon runner died after 50 days of coma subsequent to sudden collapse with no heartbeat and extensive transmural anterior myocardial infarction at the 24-mi mark in the 1973 Boston marathon. The ambient temperature was 26°C and the humidity high.[32] A 28-year-old endurance athlete, while training at high altitude (2,000 m), sustained a nontransmural myocardial infarction diagnosed by history, elevated enzymes, and serial electrocardiograms.[33] Coronary arteries examined, respectively, at autopsy and at angiography revealed no significant lesions in either of the two patients. The mechanism(s) of production of myocardial infarction in the setting of anatomically normal coronary arteries is unknown, but markedly increased myocardial oxygen demand (exercise, heat, humidity, catecholamines) in the face of a decreased myocardial oxygen supply (hypoxia, coronary artery spasm, decrease in hemoglobin, shift in oxyhemoglobin dissociation curve) could explain such an event.

Disease of the cardiac conduction system and sinoatrial and atrioventricular node arteries has been implicated in other cases of sudden death during exertion in athletic young subjects.[34-36] James has demonstrated disease of the sinus node in "patched" dalmatian coach hounds, and bundle of His interruption or narrowing in Doberman pinschers and pug dogs, animals with these heritable traits die suddenly.[37]

CARDIOVASCULAR TRAUMA IN ATHLETES

Cardiac contusion[38] and traumatic pericarditis may contribute to the morbidity rates of contact sports (see Chap. 87).

CLINICAL PRECAUTIONS

Subjects engaging in vigorous athletic activities with high risk of developing myocardial infarction by virtue of hypertension, smoking, elevated serum cholesterol levels, and family history of premature coronary artery disease should have periodic medical check-ups with resting and exercise electrocardiograms. Older sportsmen who may not have continued their conditioning programs should use care in returning to athletics or in refereeing.[30] Finally, athletes should be informed of the serious implications and the appropriate actions to take should they develop chest pain, pressure, or undue fatigue before, during, or after sport.

REFERENCES

1 Åstrand, P. O., and Rodahl, K.: "Textbook of Work Physiology," New York, McGraw-Hill Book Company, Inc., 1970, p. 341.

2 Saltin, B., and Åstrand, P. O.: Maximal Oxygen Uptake in Athletes, *J. Appl. Physiol.*, 23:353, 1967.

3 Ekblom, B., and Hermansen, L.: Cardiac Output in Athletes, *J. Appl. Physiol.*, 25:619, 1968.

4 Prout, C.: Life Expectancy of College Oarsmen, *JAMA*, 220:1709, 1972.

5 Karvonen, M. J.: The Relationship of Habitual Physical Activity to Diseases in the Cardiovascular System, in K. Evang and K. L. Anderson (eds.), "Physical Activity in Health and Disease," The Williams & Wilkins Company, Baltimore, 1966, pp. 81–89.

6 Polednak, A. P.: Longevity and Cause of Death among Harvard College Athletes and Their Classmates, *Geriatrics*, 27:53, 1972.

7 Polednak, A. P.: Longevity and Cardiovascular Mortality among Former College Athletes, *Circulation*, 46:649, 1972.

8 Gott, P. H., Roselle, H. A., and Crampton, R. S.: The Athletic Heart Syndrome: Five-Year Cardiac Evaluation of a Champion Athlete, *Arch. Intern. Med.*, 122:340, 1968.

9 Desser, K. B., Benchimol, A., and Schumacher, J. A.: External Pulse and Vectorcardiographic Abnormalities in the Athletic Heart Syndrome, *Chest*, 64:105, 1973.

10 Lichtman, J., O'Rourke, R. A., Klein, A., and Karliner, J. S.: Electrocardiogram of the Athlete: Alterations Simulating Those of Organic Heart Disease, *Arch. Intern. Med.*, 132:763, 1973.

11 Roskamm, H., Reindell, H., and Muller, M.: Heart Size and Ergometrically Tested Endurance of High Achievement Athletes from 9 German Teams, *Z. Kreislaufforsch*, 55:2, 1966.

12 Morganroth, J., Maron, B. J., Henry, W. L., and Epstein, S. E.: Comparative Left Ventricular Dimensions in Trained Athletes, *Ann. Intern. Med.*, 82:521, 1975.

13 Roeske, W. R., O'Rourke, R. A., Klein, A., Leopold, G., and Karliner, J. S.: Non-invasive Evaluation of Ventricular Hypertrophy in Professional Athletes, *Circulation*, 53:286, 1976.

14 Gilbert, C. A., Nutter, D. O., Felner, J. M., Perkins, J. V., Heymsfield, S. B., and Schlant, R. C.: An Echocardiographic Study of Cardiac Dimensions and Function in the Endurance Trained Athlete. *Am. J. Cardiol.* In press.

14a Raskoff, W. J., Goldman, S., and Cohn, K.: The "Athletic Heart:" Prevalence and Physiological Significance of Left Ventricular Enlargement in Distance Runners, *JAMA*, 236:158, 1976.

15 Holmgren, A., and Strandell, T.: The Relationship between Heart Volume, Total Hemoglobin and Physical Working Capacity in Former Athletes, *Acta Med. Scand.*, 163:149, 1959.

16 Pyorala, K., Karvonen, M. J., Taskinen, P., Takkunen, J., and Kyronseppa, H.: Cardiovascular Studies on Former Endurance Athletes, in M. J. Karvonen and A. J. Barry (eds.), "Physical Activity and the Heart," Charles C Thomas, Publisher, Springfield, Ill., 1967, p. 301.

17 Leon, A. S., and Bloor, C. M.: Effects of Exercise and Its Cessation on the Heart and Its Blood Supply, *J. Appl. Physiol.*, 24:485, 1968.

18 Poupa, O., and Rakusan, K.: The Terminal Microcirculatory Bed in the Heart of Athletic and Non-athletic Animals, in K. Evang and K. L. Anderson (eds.), "Physical Activity in Health and Disease," The Williams & Wilkins Company, Baltimore, 1966, pp. 18–29.

19 Honig, C. R., and Bourdeau-Martini, J.: Extravascular Component of Oxygen Transport in Normal and Hypertrophied Hearts with Special Reference to Oxygen Therapy, *Circ. Res.*, 35(suppl. II):II-97, 1974.

20 Scheuer, J.: Physical Training and Intrinsic Cardiac Adaptations, *Circulation*, 47:677, 1973 (editorial).

21 Nutter, D. O., Fuller, E., Watt, E., and Chen, H.: Myocardial Mechanics in Exercise Trained and Detrained Rats, *Fed. Proc.*, 34:461, 1975. (Abstract)

22 Dill, D. B.: Marathoner DeMar: Physiological Studies, *J. Natl. Cancer Inst.*, 35:185, 1965.

23 Frick, M. H.: Coronary Implications of Hemodynamic Changes Caused by Physical Training, *Am. J. Cardiol.*, 22:417, 1968.

24 Marshall, R. J., and Shepherd, J. T.: "Cardiac Function in Health and Disease," W. B. Saunders Company, Philadelphia, 1968, p. 42.

25 Bevegard, S., Holmgren, A., and Jonsson, B.: Circulatory Studies in Well-trained Athletes at Rest and during Heavy Exercise, with Special Reference to Stroke Volume and the Influence of Body Position, *Acta Physiol. Scand.*, 57:26, 1963.

26 Van Ganse, W., Versee, L., Eylenbosch, W., and Vuylsteek, K.: The Electrocardiogram of Athletes: Comparison with Untrained Subjects, *Br. Heart J.*, 32:160, 1970.

27 Arstilla, M., and Koivikko, A.: Electrocardiographic and Vectorcardiographic Signs of Left and Right Ventricular Hypertrophy in Endurance Athletes, *J. Sports Med. Phys. Fitness*, 6:166, 1966.

28 Meytes, I., Kaplinsky, E., Yahini, J. H., Hanne-Paparo, N., and Neufeld, H. N.: Wenckebach AV Block: A Frequent Feature Following Heavy Physical Exercise, *Am. Heart J.*, 90:426, 1975.

29 Marcano, B. A., and Moss, A. J.: Spurious Heart Disease in Athletic Children, *Pediatrics*, 72:664, 1968.

30 Opie, L. H.: Sudden Death and Sport, *Lancet*, 1:263, 1975.

31 Jokl, E., and McClellan, J. T. (eds.): "Exercise and Cardiac Death," vol. 5, "Medicine and Sport," University Park Press, Baltimore, 1971.

32 Green, L. H., Cohen, S. I., and Kurland, G.: Fatal Myocardial Infarction in Marathon Racing, *Ann. Intern. Med.*, 84:704, 1976.

33 Lollgen, H., Just, H. J., and Mathes, P.: Myokardinfarkt bei einem Hochleistungs-Sportler mit Normalin Koronarterien, *Dtsch. Med. Wochenschr.*, 98:620, 1973.

34 James, T. N., Froggartt, P., and Marshall, T. K.: Sudden Death in Young Athletes, *Ann. Intern. Med.*, 67:1013, 1967.

35 James, T. N., Armstrong, R. S., Silverman, J., and Marshall, T. K.: De Subitaneis Mortibus. VI: Two Young Soldiers, *Circulation*, 49:1239, 1974.

36 James, T. N., Marilley, R. J., Jr., and Marriott, H. J. L.: De Subitaneis Mortibus. XI: Young Girl with Palpitations, *Circulation*, 51:743, 1975.

37 James, T. N., Robertson, B. T., Waldo, A. L., and Branch, C. E.: De Subitaneis Mortibus. XV: Hereditary Stenosis of the His Bundle in Pug Dogs, *Circulation*, 52:1152, 1975.

38 Rose, K. D., Stone F., Fuenning, S. I., and Williams, J.: Cardiac Contusion Resulting from "Spearing" in Football, *Arch. Int. Med.*, 118:129, 1966.

91
High Cardiac Output States (Hyperkinetic or Hyperdynamic States)

NOBLE O. FOWLER, M.D.

An operation was decided upon, but for several reasons had to be postponed for a time. The thrill and bruit increased in intensity, and a slight swelling was revealed by palpation. The most mysterious phenomenon connected with the case, one which I have not been able to explain myself, or to obtain a satisfactory reason for from others, was slowing of the heart's beat, when compression of the common femoral was employed. This began to be noticeable after the wound had entirely healed.

HARRIS H. BRANHAM, M.D.,[1] 1890

INTRODUCTION

The disorders discussed in this chapter are those in which the resting cardiac output is increased beyond the normal range in human adults of 2.3 to 3.9 liters/m²/min.[1] The cardiac output may be raised by increasing either the heart rate, the stroke volume, or both. In the pathologic high output states, usually both heart rate and stroke volume are increased. Increase of the heart rate is the principal method of raising the cardiac output during exercise. However, if the cardiac stroke volume during treadmill exercise is compared with that during quiet standing, it is usually found that the cardiac stroke volume is also augmented by exercise.[2] In order to understand the mechanism of an increased resting cardiac output, it is well to consider the several means by which the function of the heart as a pump is controlled.

Braunwald emphasized that the contraction of ventricular muscle is controlled by four major factors.[3]

1 Preload (ventricular end-diastolic fiber tension)
2 Myocardial contractility
3 Afterload
4 Heart rate

Ventricular preload determines the diastolic ventricular wall tension and, thus, by the Frank-Starling mechanism, the ventricular stroke work. Ventricular preload is often estimated from the mean atrial pressure or ventricular end-diastolic pressure. This method is subject to error, since it neglects the effects of changes in ventricular compliance and the effects of alterations in pressure in the pericardial sac or elsewhere in the thorax. Although an important mechanism for altering cardiac output in the heart-lung preparation, variations in cardiac filling pressure are not usually responsible for increasing cardiac output in resting human beings beyond normal values. However, increased preload may contribute to

the high cardiac output occasionally. If the preload is below normal, as is found in shock, cardiac tamponade, or positive-pressure respiration, the cardiac stroke work and output fall. Hence the hyperdynamic states in human beings are not ordinarily explained as a result of increase in atrial or ventricular end-diastolic pressure. In the nonfailing heart, the cardiac output is not limited by the myocardial contractile state, and augmentation of the contractile state, i.e., by digitalis or paired electrical stimulation, does not increase the output of the heart. Hence, although neurohumoral mechanisms are important in controlling the output of the heart, the increased cardiac output of the hyperdynamic states usually does not result from increased cardiac contractility alone. It is of interest that the exercise-induced increase of cardiac output remains almost the same if the heart is denervated or if an increase of circulating catecholamines is prevented. However, if both mechanisms are blocked, maximum exercise tolerance is limited.[4]

In most of the hyperdynamic states, which may be exemplified by anemia or thyrotoxicosis, the increased cardiac output results from a rise in both *heart rate* and *stroke volume,* although the heart rate is seldom greatly above 100 beats per minute. Increase of the heart rate alone does not usually increase the cardiac output. The cardiac output in human beings remains relatively constant when the rate is increased step-wise from 60 to as much as 160 beats per minute by atrial pacing. Hence in the normal human heart the stroke volume declines as the heart rate is increased by pacing or atropine administration.[5] Thus, the increased cardiac output of the hyperdynamic state must depend upon mechanisms in addition to the rise in heart rate.

It is probable that a reduced *afterload* is a major mechanism in many human hyperdynamic states. Left ventricular afterload is defined as the resistance to ejection and further shortening encountered by the contracting muscle fibers at the end of isovolumic systole. Reduced left ventricular afterload may occur when there is peripheral shunting of blood (systemic arteriovenous fistula), central shunting (patent ductus arteriosus), peripheral vasodilatation (thyrotoxicosis), or reduced blood viscosity (anemia). Escobar and associates showed that reduced afterload is important in the increased cardiac output of anemia.[6] Reduction of blood viscosity can be shown to increase the cardiac output in the heart-lung preparation[7] and in intact animals.[8] Restoration of normal mean blood pressure by α-adrenergic agents reduces the elevated cardiac output in people with anemia[9] or thyrotoxicosis,[10] suggesting the importance of reduced ventricular afterload in these two disorders.

Physical findings in the hyperdynamic states

When there is an appreciable increase of the cardiac output at rest, certain physical findings tend to appear. Thyrotoxicosis, liver disease, and severe anemia are by far the commonest clinical disorders associated with an increase of cardiac output at rest, if one excepts pregnancy, fever, and emotional excitement. The physical findings commonly associated with the hyperdynamic state in these disorders may be taken as a model for the physical findings to be expected when the resting cardiac output is increased.

The physical findings in the hyperdynamic states are related to the following areas: the heart rate, the systemic veins, the systemic arteries, the blood pressure, and auscultation of the precordium.

HEART RATE

As already described, the heart rate and stroke volume are each usually increased in the high cardiac output states. Thus one finds, as a rule, an increase in the resting heart rate. However, under most circumstances, the tachycardia is moderate, and the heart rate at rest is likely to be in the range of 85 to 105 beats per minute. Anemic patients with hyperdynamic states usually have a resting heart rate below 100 beats per minute unless there is acute blood loss.[11] In hyperthyroidism, the heart rate is seldom above 110 beats per minute unless there is severe thyrotoxicosis, bordering on thyroid storm, or complicating atrial fibrillation.

SYSTEMIC VEINS

We have stated that the ventricular preload is usually normal in the hyperdynamic states. As a corollary to this statement, we may also state that the systemic venous pressure is normal and that the cervical veins are not abnormally distended unless there is a complicating systemic congestive state with "heart failure." However, the systemic veins may display useful signs of an accelerated circulation. A cervical venous hum, heard over the deep internal jugular veins, more often on the right side, is a common finding in the hyperdynamic states.[12] This continuous murmur with diastolic accentuation can be heard as a normal finding in children in the sitting posture. However, when a cervical venous hum is readily heard in an adult, especially in the recumbent posture, a hyperdynamic state is likely. Uncommonly, there may be a venous hum over the femoral veins, especially in patients with sickle-cell anemia.

SYSTEMIC ARTERIES

The systemic arteries may display signs related to the increased left ventricular stroke volume, to the increased rate of ejection, and to the decreased peripheral resistance. Consequently the pulse tends to be bounding with a quick upstroke. The pulse pressure typically is wide, with a decrease of diastolic pressure and an increase of systolic blood pressure. Pistol-shot sounds and Duroziez's murmur may be heard over the femoral arteries. A systolic bruit may may be heard over the carotid arteries.[13] In the absence of aortic insufficiency or patent ductus arteriosus, or other left-to-right extracardiac shunt, these signs are highly suggestive of an elevated left ventricular stroke volume and, if the heart rate is normal or rapid, of an increased cardiac output. It should be

recalled that the pulse pressure may be high with a normal diastolic pressure where there is increased sclerosis of the thoracic aorta—a finding usually restricted to the elderly. Further, the left ventricular stroke volume may be high but the cardiac output normal or low when there is complete AV block with a slow ventricular rate; this is especially true in congenital complete AV block.

PRECORDIAL AUSCULTATION

The increased rate of ventricular ejection commonly produces turbulence and causes a systolic ejection murmur in the second and third left intercostal spaces. Increased rate of ventricular filling may cause a third heart sound to be audible at the cardiac apex. An apical fourth heart sound is common in thyrotoxicosis if there is sinus rhythm, but its mechanism is uncertain. Diastolic aortic murmurs have been described in occasional patients with severe anemia or thyrotoxicosis but are rare in the absence of associated aortic valvular disease except in uremic patients.[14] Mitral diastolic murmurs are occasionally heard in patients with sickle-cell anemia.

Systemic and pulmonary congestion in the hyperdynamic states

Patients with one of the many high cardiac output states may develop the signs, symptoms, and physiologic evidence of pulmonary or systemic congestion or both. Systemic and pulmonary venous hypertension and water and sodium retention may occur much as in other varieties of cardiac decompensation, even though in these patients the cardiac output, although lower than before the onset of congestion, remains above normal. The appropriate label for the congestive state accompanying the hyperdynamic states is controversial. Eichna suggested that these patients be designated by the term "non-cardiac circulatory congestion"[15] rather than heart failure, since the cardiac output is above normal, and these patients often have little or no response to digitalis. However, since the symptoms and physical findings are similar to those of patients with the more common "low output" congestive failure syndrome, we have used the more common label of congestive failure for the congestive state accompanying the hyperdynamic disorders.

THYROTOXICOSIS

(see also Chap. 93)

Pathologic physiology

There are several considerations in the increased cardiac output associated with thyrotoxicosis. The increased oxygen consumption raises the cardiac output to supply the metabolic needs of the body, yet in many patients there is an increase in cardiac output beyond this requirement. Tachycardia, which is usually found in this disorder, serves to increase the output of the heart while cardiac stroke volume is maintained. In addition, there is often an increased cardiac stroke volume.[16] There are at least three major factors for consideration in the increased cardiac stroke volume of thyrotoxicosis. There is probably a direct action of thyroid hormone upon the heart which causes it to beat more rapidly, even when devoid of adrenergic and cholinergic influences. Increased sensitivity to circulating epinephrine and norepinephrine has been demonstrated in thyrotoxicosis.[17] This tends to increase cardiac stroke volume. However, a recent review concluded that available evidence fails to support the concept of altered sensitivity of the heart in hyperthyroidism to sympathetic nerves or circulating catecholamines. Recent studies of subjects with spontaneous hyperthyroidism demonstrated that β-sympathetic receptor blockade reduced oxygen consumption and heart rate and lengthened the circulation time.[18] However, the left ventricular pre-ejection period and ejection times remained abbreviated, as is characteristic of hyperthyroidism.[19] Similarly administration of reserpine to hyperthyroid patients failed to alter the circulatory dynamics toward normal.[19] Hence the concept that the circulatory effects of thyrotoxicosis are mediated by the sympathetic nervous system was not supported. In thyrotoxicosis there is evidence of decreased peripheral vascular resistance which tends to increase cardiac output.[18] When the systemic vascular resistance was increased in thyrotoxic subjects by infusion of phenylephrine, cardiac output was decreased.[10] This observation suggests that peripheral vasodilatation with decreased left ventricular afterload is important in the increased cardiac output of thyrotoxicosis.

Physical findings

Most patients with thyrotoxicosis have evidence of increased cardiac output without congestive heart failure. Congestive heart failure is said to be uncommon in hyperthyroidism without underlying heart disease unless the patient is in the older age group. It is postulated that most patients who have congestive heart failure with thyrotoxicosis have additional underlying heart disease, but in many instances neither the heart disease nor its nature can be clearly established. In patients under the age of 35 one occasionally observes cardiac decompensation without evident additional heart disease.[16] Most patients with thyrotoxicosis demonstrate the usual physical findings of stare, exophthalmos, enlarged and firm thyroid gland with or without nodule formation, fine tremor of the outstretched hands, warm moist skin of salmon hue, and tachycardia. If the metabolic rate is considerably increased, there is usually a loud cervical venous hum. In this writer's experience, continuous murmurs over the thyroid gland in thyrotoxic patients have almost always been caused by a cervical venous

hum rather than by dilated arteries within the gland. In thyrotoxicosis without heart failure, the cardiac rhythm is usually of normal sinus origin; approximately 10 percent of patients have atrial fibrillation which is often paroxysmal. On the other hand, in patients with heart failure, and here we are referring primarily to the older age groups, atrial fibrillation is found in over 50 percent of instances. There is characteristically an increase of systolic blood pressure with a modest decrease of diastolic pressure, and thus the pulse pressure is increased and the peripheral arterial pulse may be bounding. The heart is usually of normal size, unless there is complicating heart disease or congestive heart failure. The first heart sound is often of increased intensity and may at times suggest an incorrect diagnosis of mitral stenosis. Both presystolic and diastolic apical gallop sounds are common in hyperthyroidism.[20] In older patients with thyrotoxicosis and heart disease, the thyrotoxicosis may be masked; namely, the eye signs may be minimal or absent, and the thyroid enlargement and tachycardia may be inconspicuous. The possibility of thyrotoxic heart disease is often suggested by the observation of atrial fibrillation without obvious cause, some widening of the arterial pulse pressure, and an unusually alert patient with congestive heart failure. It is desirable that studies for thyrotoxicosis be made in patients with unexplained atrial fibrillation. Thyrotoxicosis should be more strongly considered as a possibility in patients with atrial fibrillation whose ventricular rate fails to respond with an adequate decrease with adequate amounts of digitalis. Persistent unexplained sinus tachycardia, especially in elderly patients, should suggest the possibility of thyrotoxicosis. Generalized lymphadenopathy and splenomegaly are found in about 10 percent of instances.

Laboratory data

The diagnosis of thyrotoxicosis can be confirmed by demonstrating an increase in the basal metabolic rate, a serum T_4 level above the normal value, and by a determination of radioactive iodine uptake, which usually considerably exceeds 45 percent in 24 h. Ancillary tests are the triiodothyronine suppression test and the T_3 resin or red blood cell test. The thyroid uptake of radioactive iodine is used less frequently now to diagnose abnormalities of thyroid function; however, suppressibility of uptake with exogenous hormone administration is said to exclude hyperthyroidism.[20a] Measurement of serum free thyroxine level (Murphy Pattee test) may be a more specific test and is less likely to be influenced by iodide administration or oral contraceptive medication.[21] Rarely, hyperthyroidism may be associated with normal serum T_4 (thyroxine) and increased serum T_3 (triiodothyronine) levels.[22] Hemodynamic studies characteristically reveal an increase of the resting cardiac output, and at times an increase of cardiac stroke volume with an arteriovenous oxygen difference decreased below the normal value of 4.5 ± 0.7* ml/100 ml of blood.[18] The circulation time

*Standard deviation.

characteristically is shortened in the absence of heart failure. The heart rate is increased. The central venous pressure and right atrial pressure are normal in the absence of congestive heart failure. When heart failure develops, the circulation time usually lies within the normal arm-to-tongue time of 9 to 16 s measured with Decholin. The cardiac output is lower than before, but usually is still elevated above the normal range.[16]

Diagnosis and treatment

The diagnosis of thyrotoxicosis is based upon the characteristic physical findings and laboratory data. Treatment of younger patients under the age of 25 years usually consists of subtotal thyroidectomy preceded by adequate preparation with the combination of methimazole and Lugol's solution. In older patients, and especially in those with congestive heart failure or recurrent thyrotoxicosis after surgical treatment, the oral administration of radioactive iodine is usually preferred. If there is severe thyrotoxicosis, propranolol may mitigate some of the adverse effects upon the heart until the thyrotoxicosis can be controlled. Guanethidine decreases the cardiac output in induced hyperthyroidism,[23] but it is not generally employed in the therapy of thyrocardiacs. The use of guanethidine may aggravate the manifestations of heart failure in euthyroid patients with cardiac decompensation.[24] Propranolol, a β-adrenergic blocking agent, is often used in dosage of 10 to 40 mg orally four times daily. This agent decreases the heart rate and may decrease the oxygen consumption in thyrotoxic patients, and thus appears useful while awaiting the effects of thyroidectomy or radioactive iodine. However, the pre-ejection period is not affected and the stroke volume remains elevated, and there is some risk of a deleterious effect upon left ventricular function.[25]

BERIBERI HEART DISEASE

Pathologic physiology

Beriberi heart disease is a rare disorder in the United States and is apparently now even less common that it was 20 years ago. Blankenhorn collected 12 cases from 1940 to 1948 at the Cincinnati General Hospital,[26] and Akbarian and associates reported four instances from the Boston City Hospital.[27] In Blankenhorn's study made at a large city general hospital, patients with beriberi heart disease were almost invariably chronic alcoholics. They demonstrated evidence of either (1) peripheral neuritis, with calf tenderness, decreased or absent vibratory sense in the lower extremities, and loss of knee or ankle reflexes, or (2) pellagra, with a red smooth tongue, and perhaps skin changes over the face, neck, upper chest, hands, and elbows. The mechanism of increased cardiac output in beriberi is obscure. Some patients with beriberi have lesions of the sympathetic nuclei[27] which may decrease peripheral arterial resistance, thus increasing cardiac work and leading to congestive failure. In addition, thiamine deficiency interferes with myocardial metabolism of pyruvate to active acetate. Patients with advanced beriberi heart disease display the usual findings of biventricular congestive failure. These findings include elevation of the systemic venous pressure and pulmonary wedge pressure, edema, and hepatic engorgement. Characteristically, there are widening of the arterial pulse pressure and bounding peripheral arterial pulses. Pistol-shot sounds may be heard over the peripheral arteries. The heart is usually dilated, and apical diastolic gallop rhythm is characteristic.

Laboratory data

The electrocardiogram in patients with beriberi heart disease is usually normal except for sinus tachycardia and perhaps minor nonspecific ST-segment and T-wave changes. The circulation time is usually within normal limits. On occasion it is shorter than normal. Hemodynamic studies in patients with heart failure due to beriberi have shown elevations of the right atrial and pulmonary wedge pressures, an increase in cardiac index,[27,28] and a decrease in arteriovenous oxygen difference. These abnormalities can be returned to normal after treatment with thiamine and other vitamins of the B-complex group.

An example of clinical and hemodynamic data in beriberi heart disease is given in the following case description:

> The patient was a 28-year-old barmaid, who was admitted to the Cincinnati General Hospital on 9/18/50. There was a history of alcoholism for 3 years. The diet was considered deficient in bread and meat. She complained of dependent edema and numbness of the hands and legs for 4 days before admission.
>
> On examination, her blood pressure was 150/70 mm Hg. The heart rate was 106 beats per minute; temperature, 99.8°F. The neck veins were abnormally distended. The skin was warm. The heart was enlarged with a ventricular gallop. There were fine rales at the lung bases, and signs of peripheral neuritis were detected.
>
> LABORATORY DATA: Hemoglobin was 10.2 Gm. Arm-to-tongue decholin circulation times were 9.5, 7.5, and 10 sec on three occasions. The electrocardiogram was normal except for very slight decrease of T wave amplitude.

Catheterizations of the right side of the heart

	9/22	11/17	12/29
Pressures, mm Hg			
Right atrium	10	5*	3
Pulmonary artery	36/25(32)	25/8(17)	21/7(14)
Pulmonary wedge	22	8.5	8
Systemic arterial O₂ saturation, percent of capacity	87%	93%	94%
AV O₂ difference, ml/100 ml	3.4	4.5	3.1
Cardiac index, L/min/m²	6.1	4.9	4.5

*Right ventricular end-diastolic pressure.

COMMENT: This patient was first studied 4 days after admission to hospital while still in clinical heart failure. The catheterization data from the right side of the heart were consistent with biventricular failure. There was elevation of both right atrial and pulmonary wedge pressures, and the cardiac output was twice the average normal cardiac index of 3.1 liters/min/m².[24,25] The arteriovenous oxygen difference was decreased. After the patient was treated with rest and thiamine and other vitamins of the B complex, clinical and hemodynamic evidence of congestive heart failure was no longer present when she was studied on 11/17/50 and 12/29/50. The right atrial and pulmonary wedge pressures were normal at the time of the second and third studies. The cardiac output had decreased but remained above the normal range (cardiac index 3.1 ± 0.4* liters/min/m²).

Burwell and Dexter[28] showed that recovery from acute beriberi heart disease was associated with a decrease in cardiac output, heart rate, and oxygen consumption, a return of arteriovenous oxygen difference to normal, and a rise of diastolic blood pressure. Another report described an abnormally great increase in cardiac output with exercise in a patient with beriberi heart disease.[29]

Diagnosis

The criteria for the diagnosis of beriberi heart disease were listed by Blankenhorn.[30] They include a history of a thiamine-deficient diet for 3 months or longer, absence of another cause of heart disease, elevation of systemic venous pressure, edema, enlarged heart, minor electrocardiographic changes, evidence of peripheral neuritis or pellagra, and a response to thiamine with a decrease in heart size, or autopsy findings consistent with the diagnosis. Akbarian and associates reported that elevation of the serum transketolase values was a useful laboratory test.[27] Nutritional cirrhosis is found at autopsy in many instances. At the University of Cincinnati Hospitals, it is doubted that beriberi leads to a specific anatomic form of chronic myocardial disease or intractable congestive failure. In our experience patients with beriberi heart disease either died suddenly in the acute stage or made a complete recovery. However, a recent report described a patient with low output cardiac failure following in the wake of acute beriberi with high output heart failure.[31]

Treatment

These patients should be treated with bed rest. Because there is a tendency to syncope and sudden death, it is important that they receive treatment early. The optimum treatment is thiamine along with the remainder of the vitamin-B complex. Thiamine may be given parenterally in doses of 50 mg daily.

Digitalis has been thought to be of little use[15] but Akbarian and associates showed that ouabain might

be beneficial.[27] Sodium restriction and diuretics are of some value.

ANEMIA

Pathologic physiology

Despite many studies of the mechanism of increased cardiac output in chronic anemia, the exact pathologic physiology is not completely understood. The circulatory effects of anemia were reviewed.[11] Possible factors involved in the elevated cardiac output of anemia, like other hyperdynamic states, include variations in ventricular preload, ventricular contractility, and ventricular afterload. It has been shown that the adrenal glands are not necessary for the increase in cardiac output, nor is the sympathetic nervous system. Blockade of β-adrenergic nerves does not prevent the increase of left ventricular performance with anemia.[6,32] The possibility of an unidentified humoral agent has not been excluded.[6,32] Increased cardiac filling pressure is not essential to the increased cardiac output of acute experimental anemia; thus, increased preload is not likely to be the major factor but may contribute to some degree.[33] Decreased left ventricular afterload seems to be the most important mechanism,[6,32] but the manner in which this decreased peripheral resistance is mediated remains uncertain. Peripheral vasodilatation, arteriovenous shunts, and decreased blood viscosity may be important. Murray and Escobar found that cardiac output did not rise in dogs when blood oxygen transport was reduced without lowering blood viscosity by means of transfusion of red blood cells containing methemoglobin.[34] Fowler and Holmes showed that experimental anemia increased the cardiac output much less when blood viscosity was not allowed to fall.[8] These observations supported the concept that reduction of blood viscosity is an important mechanism in the increased cardiac output of anemia.[34] In patients with chronic anemia, administration of methoxamine decreased the cardiac output an average of 20 percent.[9] This study is consistent with the concept that decreased peripheral resistance is important in the high cardiac output of anemia.[35] Brannon and associates[36] found that the cardiac output was usually not increased by anemia until the hemoglobin is below 7 g/100 ml of blood, or about one-half the normal value. In experimental preparations ventricular function curves were abnormal when the hematocrit was reduced below 24 percent, presumably because coronary blood flow can no longer be increased beyond this point to compensate for the effects of severe anemia.[37] However, Escobar and associates[18] and Fowler and Holmes[32] found improved left ventricular performance in dogs with anemia of this degree. Although angina pectoris may be caused by anemia, it is more likely that anemic patients with angina have associated coronary artery disease[38] than angina caused by anemia alone. Patients who are anemic may develop congestive heart failure. As in thyrotoxicosis, most patients who develop congestive heart failure with anemia have underlying heart disease, and the anemia serves as an aggravating factor which increases the work of the heart.[11] However, with very severe anemia congestive heart failure may occur from anemia alone. This event is uncommon in the United States but apparently is more common in tropical countries. As a rule, it may be said that cardiac enlargement or congestive heart failure caused solely by chronic blood loss anemia is unlikely unless the hemoglobin is below 5 g/100 ml of blood. When anemia results from sickle-cell disease or from thalassemia, cardiac enlargement may occur with lesser degrees of anemia. In sickle-cell anemia this is perhaps a reflection of myocardial and pulmonary arterial disease,[39] and an altered oxyhemoglobin dissociation curve.[40] The increased cardiac output of anemia is produced by both tachycardia and increased cardiac stroke volume. In many patients there is an increase in the systemic arterial pulse pressure. Dyspnea, dependent edema, and reduction in vital capacity may result from anemia alone without added congestive heart failure.[40]

Physical findings

In patients with severe anemia (hemoglobin below 7 g/100 ml of blood) there is pallor of the skin and mucous membranes. Tachycardia is usually present. There is often an increase in systemic arterial pulse pressure which reflects the increase in cardiac stroke volume. The peripheral arterial pulses may be bounding and there may be a Duroziez's sign and pistol-shot sounds over the femoral artery. There may be "capillary" pulsations in the lips and nail beds. Cervical venous hums are common in these patients and were described in the majority of patients receiving hemodialysis for renal failure.[41] Systolic bruits are often found over both carotid arteries.[13] These bruits are usually rather short, occupying little more than the first half of ventricular systole. There is commonly a pulmonary ejection systolic murmur, presumably reflecting the increased blood flow and turbulence in this area. With severe anemia, there may be cardiac dilation with resulting murmurs of mitral and tricuspid insufficiency. Murmurs of aortic insufficiency have been described in patients with severe anemia.[38] This finding is extremely unusual in our experience at the University of Cincinnati Hospitals unless the patient is uremic,[14] where hypertension may be a factor.[42] Anemia may be associated with a vibratory or musical systolic Still's murmur. Patients with sickle-cell anemia may display a wider variety of cardiac murmurs. A diastolic apical murmur may suggest mitral stenosis, and as a rule the diagnosis of mitral stenosis should be made with great caution in patients with sickle-cell anemia. In children with sickle-cell anemia, systolic murmurs are found almost invariably.[43] Most commonly these are loudest in the second left intercostal space and presumably are related to increased pulmonary arterial blood flow.[43] A prominent third heart sound in middiastole is common in sickle-cell anemia. There is a tendency to some exaggeration of the expiratory splitting of the second heart sound,[43] and the auscultatory findings of atrial septal defect may be closely simulated. In sickle-cell anemia, cor pulmonale may develop because of pulmonary arterial thrombosis, but this complication is uncommon.[39]

Laboratory data

In patients with anemia, the circulation time is usually normal or decreased, and this finding may persist during congestive heart failure.[11] Studies made by catheterization of the right side of the heart show an increase of resting cardiac output which is partly the result of tachycardia. There is usually an additional increase of cardiac stroke volume.[44] Graettinger and associates found that in patients with mild anemia (average hemoglobin 9.4 g) the cardiac output was normal at rest, but with exercise it rose more than normal.[44] With maximal treadmill exercise, the peak cardiac output and the exercise level achieved were little affected by anemia, but the oxygen debt was increased.[45] In patients with anemia who develop congestive failure the cardiac output may fall from the peak value but tends to remain above the normal resting value.[44] When studied by echocardiography, adults with sickle-cell anemia had increased left ventricular systolic and diastolic dimensions without evidence of ventricular dysfunction.[45a]

Treatment

The treatment of anemia depends on the underlying cause, whether this be iron deficiency, pernicious anemia, sickle-cell anemia, related to bone marrow replacement, hemolysis, or blood loss. In patients who have anemia associated with congestive heart failure, it may be necessary to correct the anemia before optimal response of the heart failure can occur. It is generally believed that digitalis is of little or no benefit in congestive heart failure accompanied by severe anemia.[15] However, we found that ouabain was effective in anemic heart failure produced in the heart-lung preparation, since it lowered elevated atrial pressures and increased cardiac output.[7] Anemia alone is seldom the cause of heart failure; hence it seems logical to use digitalis when heart failure occurs in an anemic patient. Bed rest, sodium restriction, and diuretics may be desirable. The anemia should be corrected gradually. In chronic anemia,[46] expansion of plasma volume tends to correct total blood volume almost to normal; hence rapid infusion of whole blood in the severely anemic patient may precipitate heart failure with pulmonary edema. When rapid improvement in anemia is necessary, slow infusions of one-half unit of packed red blood cells (125 ml) may be carried out over a period of 3 or 4 h, with careful examination of the patient for dyspnea and auscultation of the lungs for evidence of pulmonary edema. Monitoring of the central venous pressure during transfusion is an added precaution, but it may not necessarily warn of pulmonary edema. Hence monitoring pulmonary wedge pressure with the Swan-Ganz flow-directed catheter technique as a guide to sudden increments of left ventricular diastolic pressure should prove more useful. At times it may be necessary to correct anemia quickly in this way in order to obtain satisfactory improvement in congestive heart failure.

SYSTEMIC ARTERIOVENOUS FISTULA (see also Chap. 104)

Pathologic physiology

The decreased systemic vascular resistance (decreased left ventricular afterload) associated with large systemic arteriovenous fistulas usually evokes an increase of cardiac output to maintain adequate blood pressure and adequate blood supply to the tissues. Increased cardiac output can be demonstrated as a rule only when there is a large fistula which involves a major artery such as the aorta, or such arteries as the subclavian artery, the femoral artery, the common carotid arteries, and the iliac vessels. Multiple small arteriovenous fistulas may cause a rise of cardiac output. Pulmonary arteriovenous fistulas involve the low resistance lesser circulation and seldom, if ever, lead to increased cardiac output, cardiac enlargement, or congestive heart failure. Congenital systemic arteriovenous fistulas are usually not of sufficient size to produce generalized circulatory signs. The mechanism of increased cardiac output in systemic arteriovenous fistula apparently does not involve an increase in cardiac filling pressure. When there is an arteriovenous fistula, arterialized blood from a high pressure artery is shunted into a low pressure vein, thus decreasing the arterial blood flow to the tissue beyond the fistula and increasing the venous pressure distal to the fistula. The venous pressure proximal to the fistula and pressures in the right side of the heart are usually normal unless there is congestive heart failure. As a compensatory mechanism for the low systemic vascular resistance the heart rate and stroke volume increase. The diastolic blood pressure falls, and the cardiac output rises. Obliteration of the arteriovenous fistula by compression results in a fall in cardiac output. There tends to be an increase of plasma volume[47] in patients with systemic arteriovenous fistulas. Catheterization of the right side of the heart in patients with large systemic arteriovenous fistulas reveals increased oxygenation of venous blood at the site of communication.

Intracardiac pressures are ordinarily normal unless congestive heart failure develops.[39] If right-sided heart failure develops, right atrial and peripheral venous pressures rise. The cardiac output is above normal resting levels,[48] and may show a greater than normal increase with mild exercise in the absence of

heart failure. Heart failure may develop in patients with hearts which are apparently otherwise normal.[48] When clinical signs of congestive failure have developed, the cardiac output may fall with exercise;[48] however, we have observed that exercise evoked an above normal increase in cardiac output in such patients when the heart was previously normal. The following description illustrates some of the hemodynamic features of a large systemic arteriovenous fistula:

Catheterization of the right side of the heart

	Rest	Exercise
Pressures, mm Hg		
Right atrium	7	
Pulmonary artery	56/18(31)	64/28(43)
Pulmonary wedge	24	
Systemic arterial O$_2$ saturation,		
percent of capacity	92.5%	94.4%
AV O$_2$ difference, ml/100 ml	3.3	4.4
O$_2$ consumption, ml/min	246	386
Cardiac index, L/min/m^2	4.4	5.1

The patient, a 57-year-old man, was admitted to the hospital because of the symptoms of congestive heart failure which had been present for 4 years. Twenty-two years before admission, he had sustained a gunshot wound of the right supraclavicular area. Physical examination revealed signs of a right subclavian arteriovenous fistula. Hemoglobin was 14.5 g/100 ml blood.

Comment: The cardiac catheterization data were consistent with biventricular failure with an elevated resting cardiac output. Both right atrial and pulmonary wedge pressures were above normal. The cardiac index was well above the normal range of 3.1 ± 0.4 liters/min/m². The increased cardiac output was associated with a narrow arteriovenous oxygen difference. Venous blood proximal to the fistula showed a step-up in oxygen content of 3.4 vol/100 ml blood. With exercise, there was a relatively normal increase of total cardiac output from 7.6 to 8.8 liters/min with an exercise-induced increment of oxygen consumption of 140 ml/min. Such response of cardiac output to exercise would be very unusual for patients with "low output" heart failure.

Physical findings

If the examiner finds an increased systemic arterial pulse pressure when there is no evidence of aortic insufficiency, the possibility of a systemic arteriovenous fistula should be considered. If the patient has had an injury or a surgical operation, careful auscultation should be carried out over that site in order to look for the typical continuous murmur of arteriovenous fistula with a systolic accentuation. Manual compression of the fistula tends to produce slowing of the heart. This response is known as Branham's sign (see quotation at beginning of chapter). We have studied a patient who acquired a large arteriovenous fistula as a complication of nephrectomy. Hepatic arteriovenous fistula was reported in 2 patients with hereditary hemorrhagic telangiectasia,[49,50] and we have studied two similar patients, each of whom had an elevated cardiac output. Patients with large arteriovenous fistulas may develop congestive heart failure. The onset of heart failure may be quite delayed. In one instance a 30-year-old man who was studied at the Cardiac Laboratory of the Cincinnati General

Hospital developed congestive heart failure in 1951, 7 years following a gunshot wound involving the internal iliac artery and vein. In another instance, a 68-year-old patient developed congestive heart failure 57 years after a gunshot wound involving the femoral artery and vein. Presumably, in patients like the latter there is additional underlying heart disease. However, in such patients repair of the fistula may result in the return of heart size and function to normal.

HEPATIC HEMANGIOMATOSIS

This rare condition has been studied by de Lorimer et al.[51] Of 27 patients with hepatic hemangioendothelioma, 23 had cutaneous capillary hemangiomas and all but 2 had heart failure.[51] This lesion acts as an arteriovenous fistula between hepatic artery and veins. The congestive failure responds to hepatic artery ligation. However, in adults hepatic artery ligation might cause fatal hepatic necrosis.

HEMODIALYSIS

Striking increases of cardiac output may be found in patients with subcutaneous arteriovenous fistulas for hemodialysis.[52] Anemia accompanying uremia may contribute to the high cardiac output in such patients.

Diagnosis and treatment

The possibility of a systemic arteriovenous fistula should be considered in all patients who have an increase in systemic arterial pulse pressure with bounding arterial pulses. When there is no obvious cause for heart failure or for a wide arterial pulse pressure, such as aortic insufficiency, patent ductus arteriosus, severe anemia, or thyrotoxicosis, careful auscultation should be carried out over all scars and major arteries. If the characteristic continuous murmur with systolic accentuation is found in an area of trauma or surgical operation, no further studies should be required to establish the diagnosis. When there is doubt, arteriography may be employed to demonstrate the lesion. In some instances the systemic arteriovenous fistula may become infected so that there is endarteritis. This complication in turn may lead to aortic valve involvement with aortic bacterial endocarditis. In dogs with large experimental arteriovenous fistulas, aortic, mitral, or tricuspid endocarditis may develop with or without infection of the fistula. The treatment of a systemic arteriovenous fistula, when it is large enough to produce increased arterial pulse pressure, cardiac enlargement, or congestive heart failure, should be surgical repair or excision of the fistula.

HEPATIC DISEASE

It is known that the resting cardiac output may be increased in patients with liver disease, especially in those with nutritional cirrhosis[53] or infectious hepatitis. The increase in cardiac output in patients with nutritional cirrhosis is usually moderate and occurs in approximately one-third of the patients.[53] The mechanism is uncertain but has been attributed to

increased blood volume, intrahepatic arteriovenous shunts, mesenteric arteriovenous shunts, and defects in inactivation of a circulating vasodilator. Some patients with nutritional cirrhosis have anemia or coexisting beriberi. In a few patients with nutritional cirrhosis or infectious hepatitis, the cardiac output may be considerably elevated and accompanied by the clinical evidence of a bounding pulse and wide pulse pressure. Congestive heart failure may develop,[54] but most patients in this group probably die of hepatic failure before heart failure can develop. One authority has described a cardiac output as high as 15 liters/min, or at least twice the normal, in a patient with infectious hepatitis.[54]

PAGET'S DISEASE OF BONE

In paget's disease of the bone the more common circulatory effects are increased systemic arterial pulse pressure and increased cardiac output.[55] Cor pulmonale and AV block may occasionally occur. In most patients with Paget's disease this is not a prominent finding. Lequime and Denolin found evidence of increased blood flow to limbs involved by Paget's disease, but increase of resting cardiac output was unusual.[56] The cardiac output in patients with extensive bone involvement showed a greater than normal increase with exercise. The increased cardiac output is presumably related to multiple small systemic arteriovenous fistulas in the bones involved by this disorder, especially in the lower extremities. Injection of radioactive albumen microspheres 15 to 30 μ in diameter was made into the femoral arteries of nine patients with Paget's disease of the bone. No evidence of increased AV shunting in the lower extremities was found.[57] The possibility of Paget's disease of the bone as a cause of an increased systemic arterial pulse pressure must be considered in a middle-aged or older patient who has enlargement of the skull, decreased stature, and bowing of the tibias. Radiologic studies of the skull, pelvis, and bones of the lower extremities will usually confirm the diagnosis. As a rule, the serum alkaline phosphatase is increased. Calcitonin therapy may decrease the elevated cardiac output.[58]

HYPERKINETIC HEART SYNDROME

Gorlin and associates[59] described a hyperkinetic syndrome of unknown cause which they found principally in young patients and in those of early middle age. In their report 24 patients were described. The majority of the patients had an increased cardiac output at rest. Others did not but had an increased rate of ventricular ejection. Bounding peripheral pulses were common. Heart failure developed in some patients observed for as long as 16 years. Electrocardiograms usually showed evidence of left ventricular enlargement. Systolic ejection clicks were common. Ejection and apical pansystolic murmurs were found. Gorlin's description of some of these patients is very similar to that of patients who have idiopathic muscular obstruction of the left ventricular outflow tract.[60] The possibility that a common denominator of increased activity of the sympathetic nervous system exists in these two groups of patients must not be overlooked, since β-adrenergic receptor blockade may be of value in therapy.[61]

COR PULMONALE (see Chap. 76)

Studies made by Harvey and associates[62] demonstrated that the resting cardiac output was above normal in some patients with chronic cor pulmonale associated with chronic obstructive airway disease. This finding apparently is most common when the patient has an acute pulmonary infection and may be in part related to acute hypoxia and hypermetabolism associated with fever and infection. In our own experience, and in that of others, increased cardiac output in cor pulmonale associated with obstructive airway disease was not found in the majority of patients.[63] In some a tendency to increased cardiac output may be overcome because the pulmonary vascular resistance is greatly elevated or because heart failure is too advanced. In our study, the cardiac output in patients with cor pulmonale caused by chronic obstructive lung disease was on the average higher during heart failure than in patients with hypertensive or coronary artery disease accompanied by congestive heart failure.[63]

POLYOSTOTIC FIBROUS DYSPLASIA (ALBRIGHT'S SYNDROME)

In patients with polyostotic fibrous dysplasia the cardiac output may be increased above normal. The cardiac index was 3.9 liters/min/m² or greater in 5 of 6 patients studied by McIntosh and associates.[64] The authors thought that anxiety or increased metabolic demands were not responsible. Biopsy material from involved bones showed numerous thin-walled sinusoidal capillaries. The authors postulated that the lesions of polyostotic fibrous dysplasia act as minute arteriovenous fistulas, thus increasing cardiac output by lowering peripheral resistance.

CARCINOID SYNDROME
(see Chap. 78)

The resting cardiac output may be increased in patients with metastatic carcinoid tumors.[65] The patients may have a lowered arteriovenous oxygen difference and decreased peripheral vascular resistance. Serotonin, known to be elaborated by carcinoid tumors, increases myocardial contractility by direct action. It seems likely that the increased cardiac output combined with tricuspid or pulmonary valve deformity, often found in patients with the carcinoid syndrome, may explain the high incidence of heart failure in this disease.

WARM AND HUMID ENVIRONMENT (see Chap. 101)

Burch and associates[66] studied 10 subjects in New Orleans during the summers of 1957 and 1958. The mean of their cardiac outputs when in an air-conditioned ward was 4.0 liters/min. When the subjects were exposed to environmental conditions with the room temperature of 87 to 92°F and relative humidity 58 to 93 percent, the mean cardiac output rose 43 percent to 5.7 liters/min. Calculated ventricular work rose in some subjects, suggesting that an air-conditioned ward may reduce the workload of the heart in some patients with heart disease. Short periods of exposure to dry heat apparently has little effect on cardiac output.[67]

COLD ENVIRONMENT
(see Chap. 101)

In healthy young men exposed to 5°C ambient temperature, cardiac output and total body oxygen consumption were increased.[68] Since the arteriovenous oxygen difference was also increased, the rise of cardiac output can be explained by the increased metabolic demands of the tissues.

RENAL DISEASE

In acute glomerulonephritis, the cardiac output at rest may be normal (in other words, relatively high) when the right atrial pressure is elevated and there are clinical features usually found in heart failure.[69] Some patients have hypervolemia, increased systemic venous pressure, enlargement of the heart, and pulmonary edema. Systemic arterial hypertension is common but is not invariably present. The decreased glomerular filtration and increased aldosterone secretion lead to retention of sodium and water with resultant hypervolemia. Some such patients, when treated with intravenous digoxin, show no decrease of right atrial or venous pressure, no increase of cardiac output, and no sodium or water diuresis.[15] The authors concluded that some patients with edema and increased venous pressure with acute glomerulonephritis do not have heart failure; these patients can be recognized clinically by demonstrating that they have a normal circulation time.

An increase of resting cardiac index, not explained by fever or anemia, may be found in patients with acute renal failure associated with tubular necrosis.[70] With chronic renal failure and anemia, the cardiac output is usually increased.[71] The cardiac output was found to return to normal when the anemia was corrected. Patients undergoing hemodialysis for the treatment of uremia tend to have an elevated cardiac output. In addition to anemia, the shunt used for dialysis and a uremic hypermetabolic state may contribute to the elevated cardiac output.[52]

POLYCYTHEMIA VERA

The cardiac output and cardiac stroke index may be increased in patients with polycythemia vera.[72] The mechanism of increased cardiac output is uncertain but appears to be correlated with the degree of hypervolemia. Right atrial and pulmonary wedge pressures are not increased.

PREGNANCY (see Chap. 92)

During normal pregnancy the cardiac output increases progressively until the seventh or eighth month.[73] The increase averages 30 to 50 percent. Until recently it was believed that the cardiac output declines considerably from its peak elevation during the last 6 weeks of pregnancy. However, the observations responsible for these conclusions were made while the pregnant woman was in the supine position so that the enlarged uterus compromised venous return through the inferior vena cava. When the cardiac output is measured with the pregnant woman lying on her side, the late decline in cardiac output during pregnancy is not observed.[74]

CERTAIN CUTANEOUS DISEASES (see Chap. 13)

A significant increase in the resting cardiac output may occur in patients with "erythrodermic" skin disease.[75] The authors studied 6 patients, 3 with exfoliative dermatitis. Four had distinct increases of cardiac output and of stroke volume. It was believed that increased blood flow to the skin might be at least partly responsible for the elevated cardiac output. Hecht and coworkers confirmed high resting cardiac output in psoriasis and in exfoliative dermatitis and also demonstrated a hyperdynamic state in patients with Kaposi's sarcoma.[76]

OBESITY[77] (see Chap. 89)

In extreme obesity, the cardiac output tends to be increased, but only in proportion to the increased weight and oxygen consumption. The arteriovenous oxygen difference is not decreased.[77]

SYSTEMIC ARTERIAL HYPERTENSION (see Chap. 65)

The resting cardiac index has been found to be elevated in patients with labile hypertension or borderline blood pressure elevation. The cardiac output tends to be higher in those with labile hypertension than in those with established hypertension.[78,79] However, an increased cardiac output may be found in some patients with severe hypertension.[80]

REFERENCES

1 Branham, H. H.: Aneurismal Varix of the Femoral Artery and Vein Following a Gunshot Wound, *Int. J. Surg.,* III:606, 1890.

1a Cournand, A., Riley, R. L., Breed, E. S., Baldwin, E. deF., and Richards, D. W., Jr.: Measurement of Cardiac Output in Man Using the Technique of Catheterization of the Right Auricle or Ventricle, *J. Clin. Invest.,* 24:106, 1945.

2 Wang, Y., Marshall, R. J., and Shepherd, J. T.: The Effect of Changes in Posture and of Graded Exercise on Stroke Volume in Man, *J. Clin. Invest.,* 39:1051, 1960.

3 Braunwald, E.: On the Difference between the Heart's Output and Its Contractile State, *Circulation,* 43:171, 1971 (editorial).

4 Donald, D. E., Ferguson, D. A., and Milburn, S. E.: Effect of Beta-adrenergic Receptor Blockade on Racing Performance of Greyhounds with Normal and with Denervated Hearts, *Circ. Res.,* 22:127, 1968.

5 Stein, E., Damato, A. N., Kosowsky, B. D., Lau, S. H., and Lister, J. W.: The Relation of Heart Rate to Cardiovascular Dynamics: Pacing by Atrial Electrodes, *Circulation,* 33:925, 1966.

6 Escobar, E., Jones, N. L., Rapaport, E., and Murray, J. F.: Ventricular Performance in Acute Normovolemic Anemia and Effects of Beta Blockade, *Am. J. Physiol.,* 211:877, 1966.

7 Fowler, N. O., and Holmes, J. C.: Dextran-Exchange Anemia and Reduction in Blood Viscosity in the Heart-Lung Preparation, *Am. Heart J.,* 68:204, 1964.

8 Fowler, N. O., and Holmes, J. C.: Blood Viscosity and Cardiac Output in Acute Experimental Anemia, *J. Appl. Physiol.,* 39:453, 1975.

9 Duke, M., and Abelmann, W. H.: The Hemodynamic Response to Chronic Anemia, *Circulation,* 39:503, 1969.

10 Theilen, E. O., and Wilson, W. R.: Hemodynamic Effects of Peripheral Vasoconstriction in Normal and Thyrotoxic Subjects, *J. Appl. Physiol.,* 22:207, 1967.

11 Varat, M. A., Adolph, R. J., and Fowler, N. O.: Cardiovascular Effects of Anemia, *Am. Heart J.,* 83:415, 1972.

12 Fowler, N. O., and Gause, R.: The Cervical Venous Hum, *Am. Heart J.,* 67:135, 1964.

13 Fowler, N. O., and Marshall, W. J.: The Supraclavicular Arterial Bruit, *Am. Heart J.,* 69:410, 1965.

14 Matalon, R., Moussalli, A. R. J., Nidus, B. D., et al.: Brief Recording. Functional Aortic Insufficiency: A Feature of Renal Failure, *N. Engl. J. Med.,* 285:1522, 1971.

15 Eichna, L. W., Farber, S. J., Berger, A. R., Rader, B., Smith, W. W., and Albert, R. E.: Non-cardiac Circulatory Congestion Simulating Congestive Heart Failure, *Trans. Assoc. Am. Physicians,* 68:72, 1954.

16 Graettinger, J. S., Muenster, J. J., Selverstone, L. A., and Campbell, J. A.: A Correlation of Clinical and Hemodynamic Studies in Patients with Hyperthyroidism with and without Congestive Heart Failure, *J. Clin. Invest.,* 38:1316, 1959.

17 Levey, G. S.: Catecholamine Sensitivity, Thyroid Hormone, and the Heart, *Am. J. Med.,* 50:413, 1971.

18 Grossman, W., Robin, N. I., Johnson, L. W., Brooks, A. L., Selankow, H. A., and Dexter, L.: The Enhanced Myocardial Contractility of Thyrotoxicosis, *Ann. Intern. Med.,* 74:869, 1971.

19 Amidi, M., Leon, D. F., deGroot, W. J., Kroetz, F. W., and

Leonard, J. J.: Effect of the Thyroid State on Myocardial Contractility and Ventricular Ejection Rate in Man, *Circulation,* 38:229, 1968.

20 Leonard, J. J., and deGroot, W. J.: The Thyroid State and the Cardiovascular System, *Mod. Concepts Cardiovasc. Dis.,* 38:23, 1969.

20a Vagenakis, A. G., and Braverman, L. E.: Thyroid Function Tests—Which One? (editorial). *Ann. Int. Med.,* 84:607, 1976.

21 Sterling, K., Refetoff, S., and Selenkow, H. A.: T₃ Thyrotoxicosis: Thyrotoxicosis Due to Elevated Serum Tri-iodothyronine Levels, *JAMA,* 213:571, 1970.

22 Wahner, H. W., and Gorman, C. A.: Interpretation of Serum Tri-iodothyronine Levels Measured by the Sterling Technique, *N. Engl. J. Med.,* 284:225, 1971.

23 Gaffney, T. E., Braunwald, E., and Kahler, R. L.: Effects of Guanethidine on Tri-iodothyronine-induced Hyperthyroidism in Man, *N. Engl. J. Med.,* 265:16, 1961.

24 Gaffney, T. E., and Braunwald, E.: The Importance of the Adrenergic Nervous System in Support of Circulatory Function in Patients with Congestive Heart Failure, *Am. J. Med.,* 34:320, 1963.

25 Cohen, J.: Correspondence. Beta-adrenergic Blockade in Hyperthyroidism, *N. Engl. J. Med.,* 292:645, 1975.

26 Blankenhorn, M. A.: The Heart in Vitamin Deficiencies, in R. L. Levy (ed.), "Disorders of the Heart and Circulation," Thomas Nelson & Sons, New York, 1949.

27 Akbarian, M. Yankopoulos, N. A., and Abelmann, W. H.: Hemodynamic Studies in Beriberi Heart Disease, *Am. J. Med.,* 41:197, 1966.

28 Burwell, C. S., and Dexter, L.: Beriberi Heart Disease, *Trans. Assoc. Am. Physicians,* 60:59, 1947.

29 Kozam, R. L., Esquerra, O. E., and Smith, J. J.: Cardiovascular Beriberi, *Am. J. Cardiol.,* 30:418, 1972.

30 Blankenhorn, M. A.: Effect of Vitamin Deficiency on the Heart and Circulation, *Circulation,* 11:288, 1955.

31 Robin, E., and Goldschlager, N.: Persistence of Low Cardiac Output after Relief of High Output by Thiamine in a Case of Alcoholic Beriberi and Cardiac Myopathy, *Am. Heart J.,* 80:103, 1970.

32 Fowler, N. O., and Holmes, J. C.: Ventricular Function in Anemia, *J. Appl. Physiol.,* 31:260, 1971.

33 Rodriguez, J. A., Chamarro, G. A., and Rapaport, E. A.: Effect of Isovolemic Anemia on Ventricular Performance at Rest and during Exercise, *J. Appl. Physiol.,* 36:28, 1974.

34 Murray, J. F., and Escobar, E.: Circulatory Effects of Blood Viscosity: Comparison of Methemoglobinemia and Anemia, *J. Appl. Physiol.,* 25:594, 1968.

35 Fowler, N. O.: "Introduction to Panel Discussion: Blood Viscosity Reduction and the Cardiac Output in Anemia (proceedings, international symposium, Cardiovascular Respiratory Effects of Hypoxia)," S. Karger, A. G., Basel, 1966, pp. 248–258.

36 Brannon, E. S., Merrill, A. J., Warren, J. V., and Stead, E. A., Jr.: The Cardiac Output in Patients with Chronic Anemia as Measured by the Technique of Right Atrial Catheterization, *J. Clin. Invest.,* 24:332, 1945.

37 Case, R. B., Berglund, E., and Sarnoff, S. J.: Ventricular Function: VII. Changes in Coronary Resistance and Ventricular Function Resulting from Acutely Induced Anemia and the Effect Thereon of Coronary Stenosis, *Am. J. Med.,* 18:397, 1955.

38 Porter, W. B., and James, G. W., III: The Heart in Anemia, *Circulation,* 8:111, 1953.

39 Leight, L., Snider, T. H., Clifford, G. O., and Hellems, H. K.: Hemodynamic Studies in Sickle Cell Anemia, *Circulation,* 10:653, 1954.

40 Fowler, N. O., Smith, O., and Greenfield, J. C.: Arterial Blood Oxygenation in Sickle Cell Anemia, *Am. J. Med. Sci.,* 234:449, 1957.

41 Danaly, D. T., and Ronan, J. A., Jr.: Cervical Venous Hums in Patients on Chronic Hemodialysis, *N. Engl. J. Med.,* 291:237, 1974.

42 Fowler, N. O., Holmes, J. C., and Spitz, H.: Influence of Acute Hypertension upon Aortic Valve Competence, *J. Appl. Physiol.,* 39:879, 1975.

43 Shubin, H., Kaufman, R., Shapiro, M., and Levinson, D. C.: Cardiovascular Findings in Children with Sickle Cell Anemia, *Am. J. Cardiol.,* 6:875, 1960.

44 Graettinger, J. S., Parsons, R. L., and Campbell, J. A.: A Correlation of Clinical and Hemodynamic Studies in Patients with Mild and Severe Anemia with and without Congestive Failure, *Ann. Intern. Med.,* 58:617, 1963.

45 Mierzwiak, D. S., Mitchell, J. H., and Shapiro, W.: The Effect of Diphenylhydantoin (Dilantin) on Left Ventricular Function in Dogs, *J. Clin. Invest.,* 45:1047, 1966.

45a Gerry, J. L., Baird, M. G., and Fortuin, N. J.: Evaluation of Left Ventricular Function in Patients with Sickle Cell Anemia, *Am. J. Med.,* 60:968, 1976.

46 Duke, M., Herbert, V. D., and Abelmann, W. H.: Hemodynamic Effects of Blood Transfusion in Chronic Anemia, *N. Engl. J. Med.,* 271:975, 1964.

47 Warren, J. V., Nickerson, J. L., and Elkin, D. C.: The Cardiac Output in Patients with Arteriovenous Fistula, *J. Clin. Invest.,* 30:210, 1951.

48 Muenster, J. J., Graettinger, J. S., and Campbell, J. A.: Correlation of Clinical and Hemodynamic Findings in Patients with Systemic Arteriovenous Fistulas, *Circulation,* 20:1079, 1959.

49 Childers, R. W., Ranninger, K., and Rabinowitz, M.: Intrahepatic Arteriovenous Fistula with Pulmonary Vascular Obstruction in Osler-Rendu-Weber Disease, *Am. J. Med.,* 43:304, 1967.

50 Razi, B., Beller, B. M., Ghidoni, J., Linhart, J. W., Talley, R. C., and Urban, E.: Hyperdynamic State Due to Intrahepatic Fistula in Osler-Weber-Rendu Disease, *Am. J. Med.,* 50:809, 1971.

51 deLorimier, A. A., Simpson, E. B., Baum, R. S., and Carlsson, E.: Hepatic Artery Ligation for Hepatic Hemangiomatosis, *N. Engl. J. Med.,* 277:333, 1967.

52 McMillan, R., and Evans, D. B.: Experience with Three Brescia-Cimino Shunts, *Br. Med. J.,* 3:781, 1968.

53 Kowalski, H. J., and Abelmann, W. H.: The Cardiac Output at Rest in Laennec's Cirrhosis, *J. Clin. Invest.,* 32:1025, 1953.

54 Murray, J. F., Dawson, A. M., and Sherlock, S.: Circulatory Changes in Chronic Liver Disease, *Am. J. Med.,* 24:358, 1958.

55 Edholm, O. G., Howarth, S., and McMichael, J.: Heart Failure and Bone Blood Flow in Osteitis Deformans, *Clin. Sci.,* 5:249, 1945.

56 Lequime, J., and Denolin, H.: Circulatory Dynamics in Osteitis Deformans, *Circulation,* 12:215, 1955.

57 Rhodes, B. A., Grayson, N. D., Hamilton, C. R., Jr., White, R. I., Jr., Giargiana, F. A., Jr., and Wagner, H. N., Jr.: Absence of Arteriovenous Shunts in Paget's Disease of Bone, *N. Engl. J. Med.,* 287:686, 1972.

58 Hamilton, C. R., Jr.: Effects of Synthetic Salmon Calcitonin in Patients with Paget's Disease of Bone, *Am. J. Med.,* 56:315, 1974.

59 Gorlin, R.: The Hyperkinetic Heart Syndrome, *JAMA,* 182:823, 1962.

60 Braunwald, E., and Aygen, M. M.: Idiopathic Myocardial Hypertrophy without Congestive Heart Failure or Obstruction to Blood Flow, *Am. J. Med.,* 35:7, 1963.

61 Frolich, E. D.: Beta Adrenergic Blockade in the Circulatory Regulation of Hyperkinetic States, *Am. J. Cardiol.,* 27:195, 1971.

62 Harvey, R. M., Ferrer, M. I., Richards, D. W., and Cournand, A.: Influence of Chronic Pulmonary Disease on the Heart and Circulation, *Am. J. Med.*, 10:719, 1951.

63 Fowler, N. O., Westcott, R. N., Scott, R. C., and Hess, E.: The Cardiac Output in Chronic Cor Pulmonale, *Circulation*, 6:888, 1952.

64 McIntosh, H. D., Miller, D. E., Gleason, W. L., and Goldner, J. L.: The Circulatory Dynamics of Polyostotic Fibrous Dysplasia, *Am. J. Med.*, 32:393, 1962.

65 Schwaber, J. R., and Lukas, D. S.: Hyperkinemia and Cardiac Failure in the Carcinoid Syndrome, *Am. J. Med.*, 32:846, 1962.

66 Burch, G. E., dePasquale, N., Hyman, A., and DeGraff, A. C.: Influence of Tropical Weather on Cardiac Output, Work, and Power of Right and Left Ventricles of Man Resting in Hospital, *AMA Arch. Intern. Med.*, 104:553, 1959.

67 Sancetta, S. M., Kramer, J., and Husni, E.: The Effects of "Dry" Heat on the Circulation of Man: 1. General Hemodynamics, *Am. Heart J.*, 56:212, 1958.

68 Raven, P. B., Niki, I., Dahms, T. E., and Horvath, S. M.: Compensatory Cardiovascular Responses during Environmental Cold Stress, 5°C, *J. Appl. Physiol.*, 29:417, 1970.

69 Farber, S. J.: Physiologic Aspects of Glomerulonephritis, *J. Chronic Dis.*, 5:87, 1957.

70 Agrest, A., and Finkelman, S.: Hemodynamics in Acute Renal Failure: Pathogenesis of Hyperkinetic Circulation, *Am. J. Cardiol.*, 19:213, 1967.

71 Neff, M. S., Kim, K. E., Persoff, M., Onesti, G., and Swartz, C.: Hemodynamics of Uremic Anemia, *Circulation*, 43:876, 1971.

72 Cobb, L. A., Kramer, R. J., and Finch, C. A.: Circulatory Effects of Chronic Hypervolemia in Polycythemia Vera, *J. Clin. Invest.*, 39:1722, 1960.

73 Burwell, C. S., and Metcalfe, J.: "Heart Disease and Pregnancy," Little, Brown and Company, Boston, 1958.

74 Kerr, M. G.: Cardiovascular Dynamics in Pregnancy and Labor, *Br. Med. Bull.*, 24:19, 1968.

75 Voigt, G. C., Kronthal, H. L., and Crounse, R. G.: Cardiac Output in Erythrodermic Skin Disease, *Am. Heart J.*, 72:615, 1966.

76 Hecht, H. H., and (by invitation) Candiolo, B. M., Malkinson, F. D., Nair, K. G., and Saqueton, A. C.: On Cardio-cutaneous Syndromes, *Trans. Assoc. Am. Physicians*, 80:91, 1967.

77 White, R. I., Jr., and Alexander, J. K.: Body Oxygen Consumption and Pulmonary Ventilation in Obese Subjects, *J. Appl. Physiol.*, 20:197, 1965.

78 Conway, J.: Labile Hypertension: The Problem, *Circ. Res.*, 27(suppl. 1):43, 1970.

79 Frolich, E. D., Kozul, V. S., Tourazi, R. C., and Dustan, H. P.: Physiological Comparison of Labile and Essential Hypertension, *Circ. Res.*, 27(suppl. 1):55, 1970.

80 Ibrahim, M. M., Tarazi, R. C., and Dustan, H. P.: Hyperkinetic Heart in Severe Hypertension: A Separate Clinical Hemodynamic Entity, *Am. J. Cardiol.*, 35:667, 1975.

92
The Heart and Pregnancy

JAMES METCALFE, M.D., and
KENT UELAND, M.D.

If disease during pregnancy is to be well managed, the physiological changes of pregnancy must first be known.

C. SIDNEY BURWELL, M.D.,[1] 1958

In order to lay a logical groundwork for discussing the clinical implications of pregnancy with the cardiologist, we will summarize the recognized hemodynamic changes that accompany normal pregnancy.[2]

MATERNAL CIRCULATORY PHYSIOLOGY DURING PREGNANCY

Cardiac output and oxygen consumption

The most profound change which occurs in maternal hemodynamics during pregnancy is an increase in cardiac output. The increase begins early in pregnancy. By the twentieth week of gestation resting maternal cardiac output is at or near its peak, 30 to 40 percent above nonpregnant values. Fig. 92-1 demonstrates this change in a group of normal women studied serially during pregnancy and again 6 weeks postpartum. The increment in cardiac output early in pregnancy is achieved mainly by an increase in stroke volume. Heart rate, in contrast, rises progressively throughout pregnancy, at term reaching a peak about 15 beats per minute above nonpregnant values. So, their increased cardiac output is largely attributable to augmented stroke volume early in pregnancy,

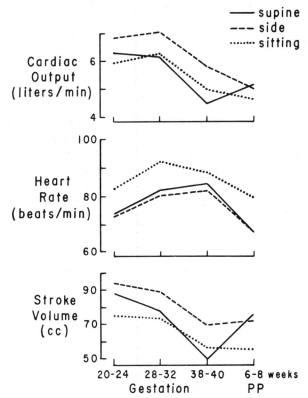

FIGURE 92-1 The effects of time in gestation and of maternal position upon the cardiovascular system of the mother. Data were obtained at three periods during gestation and once postpartum.

but is due increasingly to tachycardia as pregnancy advances and stroke volume declines.

Resting oxygen consumption rises progressively during pregnancy, but proportionately less than cardiac output.[2] Therefore the arteriovenous oxygen difference across the lungs falls, especially early in pregnancy. Near term in the supine position the arteriovenous oxygen difference exceeds nonpregnant values.

The important influence of maternal body position on maternal cardiac output is also illustrated by Fig. 92-1. This influence is most obvious at term and is attributed to obstruction of venous return through the inferior vena cava by the enlarging uterus. Radiographic studies have shown that complete obstruction of the inferior vena cava occurs at term in approximately 90 percent of women when supine. The obstruction is partially relieved when the women assume a lateral recumbent position. In these studies an average rise of 27 percent in resting cardiac output and 31 percent in stroke volume and a 7 percent decline in heart rate occurred when maternal body position changed from supine to lateral recumbent. However, cardiac output declined in all body positions as term approached.

Arterial blood pressure, vascular resistance, and organ blood flow

Despite the increased cardiac output, mean and diastolic arterial blood pressures decline slightly. In other words, a substantial fall in systemic vascular resistance occurs during pregnancy. Burwell likened this phenomenon to the hemodynamic change due to an arteriovenous fistula and postulated that erosion of the maternal vasculature by the invasive trophoblast at the placental site was responsible for the creation of a low-resistance vascular bed in the pregnant uterus.[1]

Subsequent work has demonstrated that the fall in vascular resistance during gestation is not limited to the uterine vasculature. Furthermore, a decrease in peripheral vascular resistance occurs during pregnancy in species where erosion of the uterine vascular bed does not occur during establishment of the placental circulation. It now seems likely that the uterine hyperemia which occurs early in pregnancy can be attributed to ovarian and placental steroid hormones. A small dose of estrogen infused directly into the uterine artery of a nonpregnant sheep produces a major fall in uterine vascular resistance,[3] and the use of oral contraceptives containing both estrogenic and progestational compounds is associated with an increased cardiac output due to an augmentation of stroke volume.[4] In human beings the blood flow to the uterus increases manyfold during pregnancy, from a mean of approximately 15 ml/min at the tenth week to approximately 500 ml/min at term.

Early in gestation, renal blood flow increases to levels 30 percent above those found in nonpregnant subjects. This dramatic increase in renal blood flow

becomes very sensitive to changes in maternal body position as pregnancy progresses[5] and at term, falls to or below nonpregnant levels in the supine woman. Blood flow to the mother's hands increases throughout pregnancy, providing for the increased heat loss necessitated by the metabolic activity of the developing fetus. Engorgement of the breasts begins early in pregnancy with visible dilatation of the overlying veins, probably indicating increased mammary blood flow. Studies of cerebral and hepatic blood flow have been performed, but no change associated with pregnancy has been demonstrated. However, approximately 50 percent of the increment in resting cardiac output at 20 weeks of gestation is still unaccounted for in terms of its distribution to tissues.

There is no measurable increase in pulmonary arterial blood pressure during pregnancy, and calculated values for pulmonary vascular resistance decline. This change in the tone of pulmonary vessels may be important to women with long-standing increases in pulmonary vascular resistance.

Ventricular dynamics

Measurements of systolic time intervals during pregnancy have produced evidence which suggests that the increased stroke volume of early pregnancy is brought about by an increase in the force of ventricular contraction. In a small group of women studied serially during pregnancy and postpartum the ratio of the duration of the pre-ejection period to the ejection phase of ventricular systole was significantly lessened early in pregnancy. The same study[6] showed a significant rise in this ratio after pregnancy, suggesting a physiologic decline in ventricular contractility in the postpartum period. These findings have led us to postulate that changes in the hormonal milieu associated with pregnancy cause an increase in myocardial contractility early in gestation and that withdrawal of these hormones after delivery leads to a temporary depression of ventricular contractility.

Effects of exercise

The increase in maternal cardiac output evoked by mild exercise is greater in pregnancy than that evoked by the same exercise postpartum. This is true even when the exercise is performed on a bicycle ergometer and therefore does not involve weight bearing. The oxygen cost of a standard intensity of exercise on the bicycle ergometer is also greater during pregnancy than postpartum. However, the increment in cardiac output is proportionately greater than the increase in oxygen consumption. This disproportionate increase in cardiac output means that during mild exercise, as well as at rest, arteriovenous oxygen difference is lower during pregnancy (especially early in pregnancy) than it is in the nonpregnant individual. It appears that the maternal heart is called upon to shoulder the major part of the burden of supplying peripheral tissues with the increased oxygen needs of pregnancy while, on the average, the peripheral tissues are not required to extract as much oxygen from their allotted flow of blood. On the other hand, recent studies have demonstrated a significant increase in oxygen debt incurred by mild standard bicycle exercise, raising the possibility that the oxygen supply to some tissues (perhaps including the pregnant uterus) is jeopardized by exercise during pregnancy.[7]

Blood volume and salt and water balance

Another change associated with pregnancy and with important hemodynamic implications is an increase in maternal blood volume.[1] The increment averages 40 percent above nonpregnant values, its magnitude varying with the parity of the mother and with her body composition. The hypervolemia begins early in pregnancy and the increase continues, though at a diminishing rate, until the thirtieth week. Blood volume changes little in the last trimester, and some workers have reported that it falls slightly in the last 10 weeks of pregnancy, probably because their measurements were made in supine subjects.

Although both plasma volume and red blood cell mass increase during pregnancy,[8] plasma volume increases earlier and proportionately more than red blood cell mass (see Fig. 92-2). This leads to relative hemodilution, the so-called physiologic anemia of pregnancy. Recent work suggests that if supplemental iron is taken regularly, this hemodilution does not occur, but the availability of iron for maternal erythropoiesis is so frequently limited that a decline in blood hemoglobin concentration to 11 g/100 ml is commonly observed in normal women[8] at about the thirtieth week of pregnancy. Then plasma volume stops expanding, red blood cell mass continues to rise, and blood hemoglobin concentration increases toward normal.

The blood volume of women with twin pregnancies increases more than that of women with single pregnancies.[9] In experimental animals the same distinction is true, and a greater increase in maternal cardiac output occurs in animals carrying twins than in those with single pregnancies. These data and the finding that in one woman with a twin pregnancy uterine blood flow at term was twice as large as the average in women with single fetuses suggest that twinning imposes a substantially greater load upon the maternal heart than does the production of a single fetus.

FIGURE 92-2 Percentage changes in blood volume, plasma volume, and red blood cell mass during pregnancy. *(Reproduced from D. E. Scott, Anemia in Pregnancy, in R. M. Wynn (ed.), "Obstetrics and Gynecology Annual: 1972," Appleton-Century-Crofts, New York, 1972, with permission of the author and publisher.)*

The increase in plasma volume is associated with profound changes in fluid balance which seem to be mediated by the steroid hormones of pregnancy. Progesterone blocks the action of aldosterone on renal tubular cells[10] and relaxes venous tone.[11] Plasma renin activity increases during normal pregnancy, apparently due in part to estrogens, which stimulate the hepatic production of renin substrate. Thus, both estrogens and progesterone act to promote sodium and water retention during pregnancy.

The distribution of the increased blood volume of pregnancy depends in part on maternal body position. The apparent plasma volume measured by T-1824 is greater in the lateral recumbent position than in supine recumbency when measurements are made late in pregnancy. Studies of central blood volume and right atrial pressure in normal pregnant women have yielded conflicting results, perhaps because of inadequate attention to standardization of body position. Much of the increased blood volume is undoubtedly contained in the enlarged uterine veins and in the venous system below the vena caval compression produced by the gravid uterus.

MATERNAL CIRCULATORY CHANGES ASSOCIATED WITH LABOR, DELIVERY, AND THE PUERPERIUM

Labor and delivery evoke dramatic changes in maternal hemodynamics. As shown in Fig. 92-3, each uterine contraction during labor is associated with an increase in cardiac output. This is attributed to a temporary increase in venous return as uterine contraction squeezes blood out of the uterus. In supine patients cardiac output increases about 25 percent above values between contractions. The transient augmentation of cardiac output is associated with an

FIGURE 92-3 Percentage changes in cardiac output, heart rate, stroke volume, and pulse pressure associated with uterine contractions compared with values obtained between contractions. Studies were made during early labor. *(Reproduced with permission of Grune & Stratton, Inc., from J. Metcalfe and K. Ueland, Maternal Cardiovascular Adjustments to Pregnancy, Prog. Cardiovasc. Dis., 16:363, 1974.)*

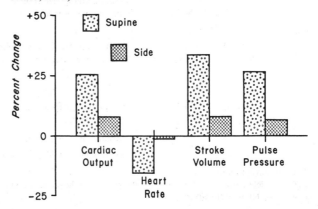

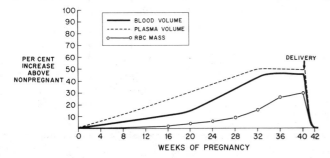

increase in arterial blood pressure and a reflex brady-cardia. The uterine contraction also compresses the distal aorta and the common iliac arteries, causing a redistribution of the maternal cardiac output to the upper portion of the maternal vascular system.[12] These changes are substantially less pronounced in lateral recumbency.

In addition to these intermittent changes, the base-line cardiac output (between contractions) rises progressively during labor, especially during the second stage if local anesthesia is used for delivery. The magnitude of this increase can be lessened by the use of caudal anesthesia.

Immediately after delivery maternal cardiac output rises dramatically, to values approximately 80 percent above those obtaining before labor when delivery is performed under local anesthesia, and about 60 percent above prelabor values when delivery is performed using caudal anesthesia. This increase is attributed to the removal of vena caval compression when the uterus is emptied. A postpartum bradycardia with a heart rate as low as 60 beats per minute is not unusual.

The hemodynamic changes associated with labor can be avoided by cesarean section, and the rise in cardiac output immediately after delivery can be substantially altered,[13] perhaps because cesarean section is associated with substantial blood loss. On the other hand, surgical delivery is accompanied by major hemodynamic alterations. Subarachnoid block, epidural block using an anesthetic solution containing epinephrine, or balanced general anesthe-sia (pentothal, nitrous oxide, oxygen, and succinyl-choline) are all associated with major, although transient, hemodynamic changes. Epidural anesthesia without epinephrine in the anesthetic solution[13] is the most effective of the techniques explored so far in maintaining maternal hemodynamic stability. These findings are summarized in Table 92-1.

Significant hemodynamic changes may be associated with attempts to induce or suppress labor. The injection of hypertonic solutions into the uterus to produce abortion may result in hypervolemia and, if saline is used, hypernatremia. Prostaglandins E2 and F2α are employed as agents for inducing labor, both at term and for therapeutic abortion. Hemodynamic alterations are not observed at the low doses generally recommended.

Ethyl alcohol, administered intravenously in hypertonic concentrations, is sometimes used to avert premature labor. Alcohol itself has important effects on the myocardium, especially in patients with heart disease. Additionally, substantial alterations in fluid balance may occur, especially when prolonged infusion is necessary to maintain uterine quiescence. Ritodrine, isoxsuprine hydrochloride, and other beta-sympathomimetic amines which are sometimes used to stop premature labor have significant cardiovascular effects and should be used with caution in patients with heart disease.

The postpartum increase in maternal cardiac output begins immediately following delivery and amounts to as much as 80 percent above predelivery values, depending upon the type of anesthesia and method of delivery. This dramatic augmentation lasts for less than an hour, but a more sustained increase, averaging 13 percent above nonpregnant values, has been demonstrated to persist for as long as 1 week.

TABLE 92-1

The influence of anesthesia and method of delivery on maternal hemodynamics

No. of patients (ref.)	Type of delivery	Type of anesthesia	Base-line values			During anesthesia			Immediately postdelivery		
			Cardiac output, L/min	Heart rate, beats/min	Stroke volume, ml	Cardiac output, L/min	Heart rate, beats/min	Stroke volume, ml	Cardiac output, L/min	Heart rate, beats/min	Stroke volume, ml
12[40]	Low cervical C-section	Spinal	5.40	90	62	3.56	109	35	8.41	85	106
			Absolute change from base line:			−1.84	19	−27	3.01	−5	43
			Percent change from base line:			−34	21	−44	56	−5	69
17[41]	Low cervical C-section	Pentothal N₂O Succinyl-choline	4.96	96	53	5.29	103	54	6.64	85	79
			Absolute change from base line:			0.33	7	1	1.68	−11	26
			Percent change from base line:			7	7	2	34	−11	49
29[13]	Low cervical C-section	Epidural without epinephrine	6.31	88	73	5.71	93	63	7.53	90	85
			Absolute change from base line:			−0.60	5	−10	1.22	2	12
			Percent change from base line:			−10	6	−14	19	2	16
10[42]	Spontaneous vaginal	Paracervical Pudendal block	5.14	90	59	7.67*	93	83	9.25*	94	102
			Absolute change from base line:			2.53	3	24	4.11	4	43
			Percent change from base line:			49	3	41	80	4	73
13[42]	Spontaneous vaginal	Caudal	5.20	93	59	6.43*	92	72	8.26*	91	91
			Absolute change from base line:			1.23	−1	13	3.06	−1	32
			Percent change from base line:			24	−1	22	59	−1	54

*Legs in stirrups for delivery.

NOTE: All determinations were made with the patients in the supine position. Base-line values were recorded before anesthesia for C-section patients and before labor for vaginal delivery patients.

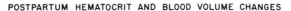

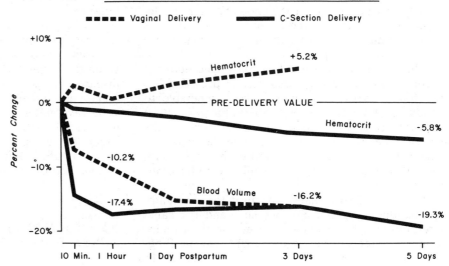

POSTPARTUM HEMATOCRIT AND BLOOD VOLUME CHANGES

▪▪▪▪▪ Vaginal Delivery ▬▬▬ C-Section Delivery

FIGURE 92-4 Serial estimations of blood volume and venous hematocrit in patients undergoing vaginal and cesarean section delivery, expressed as percentage changes from results obtained immediately before delivery. *(Reproduced with permission of Harper & Row, Publishers, Inc., N. Fowler (ed.), from J. Metcalfe and K. Ueland, Heart disease and Pregnancy, in "Cardiac Diagnosis and Treatment," 2d ed., 1976.)*

Bradycardia frequently occurs postpartum and may persist for several days. It is attributed to the rise in cardiac output, the removal at delivery of the low-resistance vascular circuit in the uterus, and the relative hypervolemia which occurs after a normal delivery. Studies of systolic time intervals made several weeks after delivery have shown changes which suggest that ventricular performance is impaired in normal women during the puerperium.[6]

With vaginal delivery approximately 600 cc of blood loss can be expected, and twice that amount is lost on the average with cesarean section. Even the larger loss is well tolerated by most patients because of the hypervolemia associated with pregnancy. As shown in Fig. 92-4, by the third postpartum day the maternal hematocrit increases by an average of 5 percent following a normal vaginal delivery, compared with a 6 percent decline in patients delivered by cesarean section; but the maternal blood volume is similar in both groups.

CLINICAL CORRELATIONS

Patient evaluation

The changes in the maternal circulatory and respiratory systems which occur during pregnancy are sometimes evident to the pregnant woman and her physicians. Hyperventilation occurs normally, both at rest and with exercise, and the work of breathing is increased.[14] Many patients become aware of this change, and some interpret it as dyspnea. Relative tachycardia also occurs, both at rest and with exercise, and other evidence of the hyperdynamic circulation may be detected.

Probably because the heart is displaced by the tumor of pregnancy the apex impulse is more diffuse, and a systolic pulsation along the left sternal border is frequently palpable. The second heart sound may occasionally be palpable in thin-chested women without other evidence of heart disease. Approximately 90 percent of normal pregnant women develop a widely split first sound due to early closure of the mitral valve; 85 percent develop a third heart sound; and 90 percent develop a systolic ejection murmur that usually is heard best high along the left sternal border. These changes become detectable between the twelfth and twentieth weeks of pregnancy; they disappear about 1 week after delivery.[15] Innocent systolic murmurs are most likely to be heard at the third left intercostal space close to the sternum and in the second right intercostal space, but may also be heard at the lower left sternal border. They are typically soft and blowing, short in duration, and unaccompanied by a palpable thrill. The second heart sound is characteristically accentuated during pregnancy. Persistent splitting of the second heart sound is abnormal in pregnancy and raises the possibility of an atrial septal defect: the associated systolic murmur may closely mimic the "flow" murmur of normal pregnancy.

A diastolic murmur originating in the heart almost always indicates organic heart disease, but the normal third sound is often accentuated during pregnancy, and its aftervibrations may be misinterpreted as a diastolic murmur.[15] Confusing extracardiac sounds may also develop, including a systolic bruit from branches of the internal thoracic (mammary) artery. A venous hum originating in the neck may be audible over the precordium, but will disappear when the jugular vein is compressed. A continuous murmur may be audible over the engorged breast of a pregnant woman and more commonly in the lactating breast of a nursing mother. It can be obliterated by pressure with the stethoscope.

The murmurs of mitral and aortic stenosis are typically accentuated by the increased cardiac output of pregnancy, while those of mitral and aortic regurgitation usually decrease in intensity, probably because of the fall in peripheral vascular resistance which normally occurs. The venous pressure is elevated in the lower extremities, and edema of the legs is very common in normal patients if sodium intake is not restricted.

Chest radiographs should be postponed until the second trimester unless disease is suspected. After the first trimester the fetus is less vulnerable to irradiation than early in pregnancy, but not yet so large as to be exposed to the lower edge of the primary beam. The patient should be carefully shielded and the field size limited to the chest. With these precautions the risk is negligible to both mother and fetus.

No characteristic changes occur in the chest radiograph due to pregnancy per se,[16] and the same interpretive criteria should be used for chest radiographs of pregnant and nonpregnant women. Pregnant patients in whom the heart diameter exceeds 110 percent of predicted values should be suspected of heart disease. Lordosis is more common in pregnancy and leads to apparent straightening of the left cardiac border and prominence of the main pulmonary artery segment. If dilatation of the right atrium is detected in the absence of lordosis, an organic cause should be suspected. Occasionally, prominence of the azygos vein is detectable in normal pregnant women; this is apparently due to collateral flow as a result of compression of the inferior vena cava.

Evidence of elevation and rotation of the normal heart may be detectable electrocardiographically during pregnancy. The electrical axis shifts leftward. A Q wave in lead 3 is frequently seen, sometimes persisting until after delivery, but is not accompanied by a Q in aV_F. T_3 is often inverted, but changes in both Q_3 and T_3 revert toward normal with deep inspiration. These changes are attributed to pressure upward from the enlarging uterus.

Echocardiography has added an important tool to our diagnostic armamentarium. Changes due to pregnancy have not been described, so diagnostic criteria are not altered during gestation. The procedure has been particularly helpful in defining disorders of the mitral valve, in detection of idiopathic hypertrophic subaortic stenosis, and in the analysis of cardiomegaly. It may also provide helpful information in the diagnosis of septal defects, pulmonary and aortic stenosis, and tricuspid regurgitation.

Awareness of the normal changes in the maternal cardiovascular system should enable the physician to decide early in pregnancy whether or not a patient has heart disease: a diastolic murmur originating within the heart, an abnormal heart rhythm, or cardiomegaly (general or localized) indicates heart disease. However, soft systolic murmurs of low intensity (grade 1 or 2) are usually not significant in the absence of cardiomegaly or other findings. Particular attention must be paid to other evidence of heart disease, including descriptions of the murmur before pregnancy. In occasional patients, studying the effect of an injection of phenylephrine upon the murmur may be justified. The cardiologist may properly request another opportunity for evaluation after pregnancy, but he should minimize the crippling concern about their heart which many patients date to childbearing.

The *supine hypotensive syndrome* is characterized by recurrent episodes of syncope, apprehension, and hypotension with bradycardia, all occurring only when the patient is supine. It does not indicate heart disease but is due to increased parasympathetic (vagal) activity elicited by obstruction of the inferior vena cava and a resultant large fall in cardiac output in patients with inadequate venous collaterals.[17] Treatment consists of preventing the patient from assuming the supine position and of encouraging venous return by providing elastic support for the legs.

MATERNAL HEART DISEASE AND PREGNANCY

Rheumatic heart disease

Heart disease in women of the childbearing age is usually of rheumatic origin. Of these patients the great majority have mitral stenosis as their sole or predominant valve lesion. Szekely and Snaith[18] found dominant or pure mitral stenosis in 90 percent of 761 patients with rheumatic heart disease in pregnancy. Furthermore, the natural history and physiology of mitral stenosis make it especially dangerous to the young woman during pregnancy. As a result, rheumatic mitral stenosis is the principal nonobstetric cause of death in childbearing.[19]

PATHOPHYSIOLOGY OF RHEUMATIC VALVE DISEASE

The hemodynamic effects of mitral stenosis will be reviewed here only for the sake of continuity in discussion. The primary defect is an obstruction to the blood flow from the left atrium to the left ventricle during diastole. Such an obstruction becomes hemodynamically significant when the valve orifice is diminished to a critical value or when the rate of blood flow through the constricted orifice during diastole increases above a critical value. "Critical" may be defined as that value which leads to an increase of pressure within the left atrium, an increase which is accompanied by pressure changes of similar magnitude in the pulmonary veins and pulmonary capillaries. At some value near 25 mm Hg, pulmonary capillary pressure exceeds the opposing forces of colloid osmotic pressure and lung tissue tension, and transudation of fluid into the alveolar walls and alveoli occurs. Pulmonary congestion may be transient when precipitated by an increased cardiac output due to exercise or the tachycardia of fright or pain, but in pregnancy the hemodynamic effects are persistent and compound, even at rest. The increase in heart rate which accompanies pregnancy is accomplished mainly at the expense of diastolic time per minute, and the diminution in time available for blood to flow from the left atrium to the left ventricle necessitates a higher rate of flow during diastole if cardiac output is to be maintained. In pregnancy the rate of flow is also augmented by the increase in cardiac output which normal pregnancy demands. In the presence of significant mitral stenosis, these increases in flow rate can be accomplished only by an increased pressure within the left atrium, the pulmonary veins, and pulmonary capillaries. It is clear that the circulatory changes which accompany pregnancy will tend to increase pulmonary capillary pressure and distension in women with significant mitral stenosis, thus diminishing their margin of safety from pulmonary transudation and edema. This postulated increase in pulmonary capillary blood volume during pregnancy has been demonstrated in patients with mitral valve lesions.

The pulmonary capillary hypertension, which may lead to pulmonary edema, is due to mechanical obstruction to blood flow in patients with mitral stenosis, and not to myocardial failure. Myocardial failure seldom occurs during pregnancy; patients whose rheumatic lesions are predominantly mitral valve incompetence or aortic stenosis or incompetence rarely experience pulmonary congestion during pregnancy, despite the increased workload upon the left ventricle which pregnancy imposes. Szekely and Snaith[18] have observed two instances of pulmonary edema due to left ventricular failure in their large experience with heart disease and pregnancy: both patients had severe aortic regurgitation, which was complicated in one by hypertensive toxemia and in the other by uncontrollable chorea near term.

Fig. 92-5 shows the changes in cardiac output during pregnancy in women with valve disease, comparing the cardiac output at rest and during bicycle exercise with data from normal women. The results indicate that the hemodynamic response to pregnan-

cy is limited, even in women with functional class II heart disease, especially those with mitral stenosis. This limitation is evident under the stress of exercise during pregnancy. Nevertheless, on the average, cardiac output increases during pregnancy even in women with mitral stenosis, and the increment in cardiac output (and in heart rate) increases the danger of pulmonary congestion and edema. British authors of wide experience[18] emphasize the danger of unanticipated pulmonary edema during pregnancy in young women with a regular heart rhythm and tight mitral stenosis who were unlimited by symptoms before pregnancy and whose pulmonary vascular resistance is usually not greatly increased: episodes of pulmonary edema may occur and recur when the patient is receiving maximum medical treatment. The authors of this chapter have not seen such patients; in our experience pulmonary congestion and edema are predictable upon the basis of an imbalance between cardiac capacity (expressed as an inverse function of mitral valve orifice size) and cardiac demand (the hemodynamic requirements imposed on the maternal heart).

MEDICAL MANAGEMENT

Patients liable to pulmonary edema from mitral stenosis can be identified early in pregnancy by obtaining a careful history of their response to such stresses as exercise, anger, or (most relevant) recent pregnancy. All patients with valve disease should be questioned carefully at each obstetrical visit about the occurrence of dyspnea or orthopnea, hemoptysis, or nighttime cough. A sudden increase in weight, inordinate tachycardia, or evidence of hepatic engorgement should be specifically looked for at each visit. The appearance of rales is a later manifestation of pulmonary congestion and requires immediate hospitalization and therapy: early evidence of pulmonary engorgement can be detected by a fall in vital capacity if careful measurements are made at each visit.

The basis of medical management of the cardiac patient during pregnancy was expressed by Burwell[2]: "We attempt to make a place in the patient's cardiac budget for the expenditures of pregnancy by eliminating equivalent amounts of other expenditures." The principle is to reduce the total cardiac demand of the pregnant women to levels of tolerance within her cardiac capacity. Let us consider first those factors which increase cardiac demand.

Pregnancy itself must head the list in this discussion. Changes in cardiac output and plasma volume during pregnancy can be limited by sodium restriction and the use of diuretics. The use of thiazides should be accompanied by recognition of the possible hazards of potassium depletion, particularly when digitalis is being used concurrently. Furthermore, decreases in blood volume induced by diuretics may accentuate or precipitate postural hypotension. Finally, the fetus may be handicapped by salt and water depletion, and side effects including neo-

FIGURE 92-5 Average values for cardiac output at three stages of gestation and 6 to 8 weeks postpartum in normal women and in women with valve disease. The response to standard bicycle exercise is indicated by the height of each bar. *(Reproduced from Ueland et al., Hemodynamic Responses of Patients with Heart Disease to Pregnancy and Exercise, Am. J. Obstet. Gynecol., 113:47, 1972, with permission of the author and publisher.)*

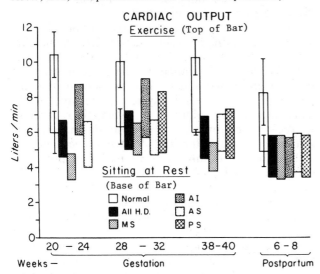

natal jaundice and thrombocytopenia have occurred from the prolonged use of oral diuretics, especially late in pregnancy.[20]

Activity exacts a price in cardiac output and tachycardia. Hours and intensity of rest and sleep should be evaluated, together with hours and intensity of physical activity. Most pregnant cardiac patients need little or no restriction of activity to keep their cardiac demand within safe limits for their cardiac capacity; some need moderate restriction; a few need prolonged hospitalization to survive and succeed in pregnancy. For some patients strict bed rest in the hospital is less restful than carefully regulated ambulation at home.

Infections, especially influenzal pneumonia, impose dangerous burdens upon the heart in pregnancy. Pregnant cardiac patients should be especially protected by being warned to avoid crowds and chilling. Vaccination with a killed influenza vaccine is recommended for all patients with mitral stenosis whose gestational span includes the season of high risk of influenzal infection. Pyelonephritis is more common during pregnancy and the postpartum period than at other times. It should be looked for by repeated "clean catch" cultures throughout pregnancy, and symptoms specifically sought at each visit. Bladder catheterization should be avoided, and proper perineal hygiene should be emphasized.

Women of childbearing age are exposed through their young families to streptococcus infections, and rheumatic fever prophylaxis must be considered. Oral prophylaxis, using penicillin G or sulfadiazine, is recommended in reliable patients. In patients historically unable to establish and maintain good health habits, benzathine penicillin intramuscularly is used monthly. Erythromycin should be substituted for sulfonamides in the last trimester of pregnancy in order to avoid the effect of sulfonamides on bilirubin transport in the newborn.

Disorders of the heartbeat are important to the degree that they interfere with the function of the heart as a pump. In women with mitral stenosis, tachycardia of any type is important. Pregnancy causes a relative sinus tachycardia and increases the susceptibility to paroxysmal atrial tachycardia.[18] In a few women with mitral stenosis, atrial fibrillation begins during pregnancy. The authors attempt reversion in all cases. Quinidine is used during pregnancy, and, in the authors' experience, has not led to obstetric difficulties. Electrically induced cardioversion has been used successfully during pregnancy without precipitating labor and without apparent effect upon the fetus. It is the treatment of choice, especially if evidence of pulmonary congestion appears. Digitalis is used in all pregnant patients with mitral stenosis to minimize tachycardia in case an arrhythmia suddenly develops.

Anemia should be avoided by the use of iron and folic acid supplements. Anemias appearing in the face of iron and folic acid administration are rare and should be investigated promptly so that specific therapy can be instituted at once. If transfusion is necessary, packed red blood cells are preferable to whole blood in patients with pulmonary congestion. All intravenous fluids should be given slowly.

Obesity imposes a cardiac burden; measures should be instituted to curtail excessive weight gain during pregnancy. However, diets aimed at severe weight reduction should not be undertaken during pregnancy.

Anxiety is expensive in terms of heart work. The authors have seen pulmonary edema precipitated by emotional trauma. Less obvious but perhaps more important are the fears of death or disaster, which take their toll over weeks, months, and years. Careful, firm support is more rewarding to the patient and her physician than indecision, conflicting opinions, or scolding.

Pain often accompanies labor and delivery. In patients with mitral stenosis, pain may cause pulmonary congestion, probably on the basis of tachycardia. Avoidance or prompt relief of pain is especially important in these patients.

Hyperthyroidism may coexist with pregnancy, although the clinical diagnosis is more difficult in the face of the normal hypermetabolism of gestation.

Hot and humid environments are poorly tolerated by patients with heart disease because of the primary role of the cardiovascular system in thermal homeostasis. Because of the increased heat loss necessitated by fetal metabolism, pregnant women with heart disease should avoid such climates and should be taught to schedule outside physical activity so as to minimize heat stress.

In the management of patients with heart disease during pregnancy, the obstetrician and cardiologist will recognize that the cardiovascular burden rises early in pregnancy and is maintained at an elevated level until late in gestation. The balance between cardiac capacity and cardiac demand is systematically assessed at each visit. Any sudden gain in weight, or a decrease in vital capacity or in blood hemoglobin concentration, or the development or exacerbation of symptoms of pulmonary congestion is carefully evaluated. Careful attention to these details and rapid response to their implications will usually prevent disabling pulmonary congestion.

For optimum patient care, close communication and understanding between the obstetrician and cardiologist are required. We endorse the statement recently made by Manning[21]: "The problem-oriented record is particularly valuable for patients with complications when several physicians are involved in management." In addition to systematic recording, we recommend that the team—obstetrician, cardiologist, and patient with mitral stenosis—meet together at least once monthly for a discussion of progress, objectives, and plans. A similar meeting 6 weeks postpartum should be held to discuss plans for continued cardiologic supervision.

These, then, are the factors which the authors recognize as important in evaluating the total cardiac burden of the pregnant woman. They are important to the degree that they can be altered to restore a favorable balance of cardiac demand in the patient with heart disease. Less important in the authors' experience are measures for increasing cardiac capacity, such as digitalis. Although the authors employ digitalis in the treatment of pulmonary edema in patients with mitral stenosis, they are not convinced of its efficacy except when it slows the pulse rate. It is, of course, indicated in patients with myocardial failure secondary to acquired or congenital defects.

SURGERY FOR RHEUMATIC VALVE DISEASE

As previously stated, mitral stenosis is the overwhelmingly preponderant cause of pulmonary congestion during the childbearing age. Surgery for mitral stenosis has been employed during pregnancy, but in the opinion of the authors it has a very small part to play. Physicians and surgeons alike would prefer to avoid any and all operations during pregnancy. Surgery should be undertaken only when it is clear that the result desired can be best attained by an operation and the risks are acceptable. At the present time in considering patients for surgery we are guided by the following principles:

1 The most important factor is whether mitral valve surgery will improve the chances for survival of mother and infant through pregnancy and the years subsequent to pregnancy.
2 The safest time for cardiac surgery, judged by mortality rates and subsequent hemodynamic improvement, is the time of greatest cardiac reserve. Pregnancy lowers the cardiac reserve in patients with heart disease.
3 Open heart surgery is often necessary for optimum surgical results. Extracorporeal circulation during pregnancy carries a high fetal mortality rate with a considerable risk of abortion (and its associated physical and psychic trauma) in the postoperative period. Once a decision for surgery is made, the best operation for that patient should be performed. A poor operation is often worse than none at all.
4 Mitral valvulotomy is a palliative rather than a curative procedure.[22,23] The benefits of valvulotomy are often of limited duration. Surgery should be timed for maximum effectiveness and not performed on inadequate or transient evidence. Experience has shown[2] that valvulotomy, even by the best hands, cannot be counted upon to remove the danger of pulmonary congestion in current or subsequent pregnancies. Snaith and Szekely[24] report an 18 percent incidence of heart failure in 45 pregnancies undertaken after mitral valvulotomy.

With these principles in mind, the authors would advise mitral valvulotomy during pregnancy only in the rare patient with disabling mitral stenosis (documented by catheterization of the left side of the heart) whose pulmonary congestion or dangerous hemoptysis persists despite several weeks of intensive medical care under hospital conditions and to whom interruption of pregnancy is not acceptable. The authors believe that the decision for surgery should be made, whenever possible, early in pregnancy and that surgery, in most instances, is not advisable after the sixteenth week, at which time the cardiac burden is already near its peak. Unfortunately, earlier surgery carries a higher risk of teratogenic effects upon the fetus.

It is only by a judicious selection of patients for valvulotomy that we can hope to arrive at the ultimate goal, which is to decrease maternal and fetal mortality rates. Recent experience favors a combined medical and surgical approach. Each patient with symptomatic mitral stenosis should be evaluated early in pregnancy by a cardiac surgeon, a cardiologist, and an obstetrician, and a complete plan for management should be established. Gilchrist[23] achieved a maternal mortality rate of less than 1 percent in 592 patients with heart disease. Mitral valvulotomy was performed eleven times in that series. At the Newcastle General Hospital, Szekely and Snaith[18] achieved an overall maternal mortality rate of 1.6 percent in 761 patients with rheumatic heart disease between 1942 and 1971. Closed mitral valvotomy was performed in twenty-nine patients "seven of whom had only moderate stenosis." Only one of the twenty-nine died postoperatively, and there were only two neonatal deaths in the group.

Open heart surgery has been performed during pregnancy.[24] In one series of 22 patients, only one woman died, but the fetal loss amounted to 33 percent. If open heart surgery is undertaken, a high perfusion rate is essential to maintain adequate fetal oxygenation.

Pregnancy in women with prosthetic heart valves

Patients with valve prostheses require chronic anticoagulation. Oral anticoagulants cross the placenta and expose the fetus to the risk of hemorrhagic and other complications. Therefore, oral anticoagulants should be avoided in the first trimester and again during the last 3 weeks before term, in order to allow the fetal clotting mechanisms to return to normal by the time of delivery. At these times, heparin should be used. Indeed, we prefer to use subcutaneous heparin throughout pregnancy in order to provide maximum safety to both fetus and mother. Should a patient begin labor while receiving oral anticoagulant therapy, the administration of fresh plasma is advised to restore her clotting mechanism to normal, and delivery by cesarean section is suggested in order to minimize the risk of hemorrhagic complications in the infant. Oral anticoagulation can be begun immediately after delivery, but breast-feeding is contraindicated because oral anticoagulants are excreted in the milk.

Anticoagulant action is complicated by the use of salicylates, barbiturates, and some tranquilizers, diuretics, and antibiotics. In addition, the female sex steroids of pregnancy change the clotting factors, and readjustment of anticoagulant dosage is usually required during pregnancy.

Experience with pregnancy in patients with valvular prostheses is limited. Buxbaum[25] analyzed data from 50 pregnancies in 43 patients with prosthetic valves. Only one mother died following cesarean section after a pregnancy complicated by thromboembolism. The fetal mortality rate was 28 percent and was confined to the pregnancies of patients with prosthetic mitral valves. The use of oral anticoagulants was associated with increased risk to the fetus, but omission of anticoagulant treatment increased the danger of systemic embolization to the mother. Again, maximum safety is provided by the use of subcutaneous heparin.

Congenital heart disease

Maternal death is uncommonly associated with pregnancy in patients with most forms of congenital heart disease. In Hibbard's recent summary,[19] maternal deaths associated with all forms of congenital heart disease accounted for only 18 of the total of 77 deaths from heart disease among pregnant women in California during the 9-year period of 1960 to 1968. Of these, at least 5 had pulmonary hypertension, and 10 others had either a ventricular or an atrial septal defect or both: in these 10, the presence of pulmonary hypertension or a right-to-left shunt was not documented.

Surgery for congenital heart disease is seldom necessary during pregnancy for maternal survival; as expressed by Snaith and Szekely,[24] "An urgency to carry out these procedures during pregnancy presents itself uncommonly." Based upon their experience with 372 pregnancies of 125 women with congenital heart disease, Copeland and coworkers[26] reached the conclusion that "the effect of pregnancy in congenital heart disease is not sufficient to indicate cardiac operation in the gravid state." In their extensive series only one patient died (from bacterial endocarditis following a dental extraction). Although multiple reports indicate that surgical correction of congenital defects can be achieved successfully during pregnancy and that even prolonged hypothermia is consistent with fetal survival, reported experience suggests that extracorporeal circulation has been associated with a high incidence of fetal death and deformity. Since current trends in cardiac surgery favor the increased use of open heart techniques and extracorporeal circulation, we consider that careful corrective cardiac surgery is best done under basal conditions which do not obtain during pregnancy.

PULMONARY ARTERIAL HYPERTENSION

Pulmonary arterial hypertension presents a specific hazard during pregnancy. Jones and Howitt[27] reported a maternal mortality rate of 27 percent in patients with Eisenmenger's syndrome, compared with 1.8 percent in patients with uncomplicated shunts at the aortopulmonary, atrial, or ventricular levels. The same authors collected reports of patients with severe pulmonary hypertension in pregnancy from the literature; eight died, a mortality rate of 53 percent. Death occurred most commonly at the time of delivery or during the early puerperium, and the modes of death were essentially similar in both groups of patients: either after syncopal attacks or in associa-

tion with circulatory collapse. Even patients asymptomatic prior to pregnancy are considered to have a high risk of death during pregnancy and in the puerperium. The authors' present working hypothesis concerning the mechanism of death in these patients is that when venous return to the heart is impeded by the pressure of the uterus on the inferior vena cava; by muscular paralysis from spinal anesthesia; or in the postpartum period by pooling of blood in distensible veins surrounded by flaccid muscles of the lower extremities upon the patient's standing upright, right ventricular output is suddenly decreased. In patients with large central shunts this leads to diversion of left ventricular output into the pulmonary circuit and a consequent fall in peripheral cardiac output: in patients without shunts the fall in left ventricular output follows inexorably upon decreased right ventricular output. The decrease in peripheral blood flow leads to syncope: cyanosis is produced by a decrease in peripheral blood flow and is accentuated in patients with shunts by "venoarterial shunting" due to systemic hypotension and by vasoconstriction in the pulmonary circulatory bed secondary to decreased right ventricular output. As evidence for this hypothesis, the authors have observed reversal of the syndrome by elevation of the legs of a patient with a ventricular septal defect who became hypotensive following delivery.

Experience (of the authors and others) with patients with pulmonary hypertension leads to the conviction that every attempt should be made to discourage pregnancy in patients with pulmonary hypertension. Women with a septal defect or a patent ductus arteriosus should have their pulmonary artery pressures measured if they present with pregnancy, and if hypertension is found, interruption should be strongly recommended and performed under the best possible operative conditions. In those who come to term, the principle of management is to encourage venous return and to lower pulmonary vascular resistance during parturition and in the postpartum period. Venous return is encouraged by elevation of the feet and legs, the application of elastic bandages to the legs, prevention of inferior vena cava obstruction by keeping the patient on her side, and avoidance of spinal anesthesia. Measures designed to lower pulmonary vascular resistance include oxygen inhalation. Because of the high risk of pulmonary vascular thrombosis in patients with pulmonary hypertension, anticoagulant therapy both after delivery and after surgery has been recommended.[28]

COARCTATION OF THE AORTA

As pointed out by Snaith and Szekely,[24] an analysis of all published cases of pregnancy complicated by coarctation of the aorta shows a maternal mortality rate of 3.5 percent. Evidently women with coarctation of the aorta (and associated lesions) are subject to significantly greater risks of mortality and morbidity during pregnancy than the general population of the same age. The increased risk of aortic rupture during pregnancy in these patients and in those with Marfan's syndrome has in the past been explained by structural changes in the aortic media, but this finding is now disputed.[29] No logical program for diminishing the risks can be offered in the present state of our knowledge, because aortic dissection may occur at any time in pregnancy and is not avoided by cesarean section.

MARFAN'S SYNDROME

Our experience includes two patients with Marfan's syndrome who suffered sudden aortic dissection, rupture, and death during pregnancy, and we currently regard pregnancy as absolutely contraindicated in patients with this syndrome. There are two theoretical reasons for suspecting that pregnancy may increase the risk of aortic dissection. First, structural changes in the aortic wall have been reported to occur normally during pregnancy. Second, the wide pulse pressure of pregnancy may predispose to aortic dissection. Although propranolol may have undesirable effects on uterine blood flow,[30] we would advise use of this agent throughout pregnancy to diminish pulse pressure in any woman with Marfan's syndrome who refused interruption. The use of propranolol creates problems for the obstetric anesthesiologist which have been discussed by Ostheimer and Alper.[31]

Subacute bacterial endocarditis

Women with organic heart disease are liable to subacute bacterial endocarditis. In a series of 50 cesarean sections performed at the University of Washington School of Medicine, blood cultures were positive in 20 percent of women following delivery of the placenta. Because of the wide diversity of organisms which may be found in the genital tract, a broad spectrum of antibiotic coverage is required. The authors use 600,000 units of procaine penicillin twice daily starting with the onset of labor, together with 1 g of streptomycin daily beginning immediately after delivery. Both antibiotics are continued for 3 days.

Heart disease originating during pregnancy

In addition to the dangers which pregnancy presents to women with preexisting heart disease, complications of pregnancy also may result in disability and death due to cardiovascular involvement in the woman with a previously normal heart. The most common of these accidents is pulmonary embolism from a thrombus in the leg or pelvic veins, but pulmonary embolism from amniotic fluid during labor or from air during attempted abortion may also occur.[19] Aspiration of stomach contents during anesthesia is now infrequent.

The syndrome called peripartal cardiomyopathy[32] is rare. It becomes manifest within 3 months of delivery and is more common in multiparous women, especially those who have delivered twins or whose pregnancy was complicated by toxemia. It is associated with a high mortality rate and a tendency to recur with subsequent pregnancies. Emboli may occur from mural thrombi, and cardiomegaly persists in 50 percent of the survivors. The cause of the syndrome is undetermined, but its geographic distribution suggests protein malnutrition as at least a contributing factor. Based upon the observation that prolongation of the pre-ejection period with a shortened left ventricular ejection time occurs frequently in normal women postpartum, we have suggested that depression of left ventricular function is a common postpartum phenomenon and that peripartal cardiomyopathy is its clinical expression. Successful management requires close liaison between obstetrician and cardiologist and includes prolonged bed rest, treatment of heart failure, and heparin in low doses to lessen the risk of thromboembolism. Future pregnancies carry the risk of recurrence, especially if cardiomegaly persists.

Cardiac arrhythmias

Disturbances of cardiac rhythm are more common during pregnancy[18] even in women without other evidence of heart disease. Atrial and ventricular premature contractions, occasionally occurring in bigemini, and episodes of supraventricular tachycardia are more common during pregnancy than in the nonpregnant state. These disorders can usually be managed by reassurance, but therapeutic intervention is occasionally required in patients with persistent or recurrent supraventricular tachycardia.

Obstetrical considerations

INTERRUPTION OF PREGNANCY

Interruption of pregnancy has historically been of lifesaving importance to many women with heart disease. With increasing medical and surgical skill its use has diminished almost to vanishing. It has important limitations. To some women it is unacceptable on moral grounds, and it threatens the self-confidence of others. After the twelfth week of pregnancy the complication rate of interruption rises sharply, and whenever possible it should be performed before that time. Abortion carries a high risk if performed in a patient with pulmonary congestion, and it does not lead to immediate reversal of the hemodynamic effects of pregnancy.

Interruption of pregnancy is justified, we believe, in a rare patient with mitral stenosis (or other valve lesion) who has clear and persistent pulmonary congestion early in pregnancy despite optimal medical management. Some of these women are candidates for valve surgery or prosthetic replacement, which can be undertaken when the changes of pregnancy have regressed. Subsequently, pregnancy can often be accomplished with a lowered risk of maternal mortality.[22] Interruption of pregnancy is also justified in all women with pulmonary arterial hypertension, in those with Marfan's syndrome, and in women with previously demonstrated peripartal cardiomyopathy, especially if cardiomegaly persists.

Elective sterilization is not advisable in any patient with surgically correctable cardiac disease. Mortensen and Ellsworth[33] studied 62 couples sterilized before the wife's cardiac surgery. Of these, 38 women (61 percent) improved sufficiently so that (in the cited authors' opinion) pregnancy could have been undertaken safely.

MANAGEMENT AT PARTURITION

A term delivery in a well-managed patient offers the best hope of a successful outcome for both mother and child. Term cesarean section is traditionally associated with a high maternal mortality rate in patients with mitral stenosis, but its use should be reevaluated. With vaginal delivery forceps are used to circumvent the "bearing-down" efforts in the second stage of labor, which have marked hemodynamic effects.

Adequate analgesia minimizes the hemodynamic burden of labor, thus reducing the danger of pulmonary edema in women with mitral stenosis. The anesthetic technique which is chosen should depend on the training and competence of the available anesthesiologist. Scopolamine is contraindicated, and atropine should be used in minimal doses and cautiously. In skilled hands caudal analgesia or anesthesia seems at present to be the most desirable method for vaginal delivery, but blood pressure must be monitored constantly and hypotension avoided. The tendency to hypotension can be minimized by proper positioning of the patient, elastic support to the legs, and the use of low concentrations of long-acting local anesthetic solutions. Uterine contraction after delivery is essential for adequate hemostasis; synthetic oxytocin (Pitocin) appears preferable to the natural product in patients with heart disease, because it is uncontaminated by pressor agents. It should be given slowly, intravenously or intramuscularly, to avoid hypotension. Both ergonovine and methylergonovine maleate should be omitted in patients who are in danger of pulmonary congestion.

As previously noted, women with pulmonary arterial hypertension are in danger of sudden death at delivery. An intravenous infusion line should be maintained from the onset of labor, and a cardiologist should be present throughout labor and delivery. Monitoring of the maternal electrocardiogram is essential, and every attempt should be made to maintain and encourage venous return. Cross-matched blood should be close at hand for rapid administration in the event of hypotension.

The supine hypotensive syndrome may occur during cesarean section and may occasionally be responsible for death.[17] In patients with this difficulty cesarean section should be performed while the uterus is mechanically displaced to the left or with the patient tilted onto her left side until the infant is extracted. In all pregnant patients who are subject to sudden death, the possibility of performing a postmortem cesarean section should be recognized.[35]

In women with mitral stenosis, intravenous fluid administration during labor and the postpartum period must be carefully monitored. In a recent discussion of acute pulmonary edema occuring in the postpartum period Mestman and Manning[36] stressed the important of restricting intravenous fluids, especially saline solution, and the judicious use of oxytocin in preventing pulmonary edema during the early postpartum period.[34]

Early ambulation after delivery is encouraged, using carefully fitted elastic support stockings to minimize the dangers of thromboembolism and peripheral pooling of blood.

Heart disease and the fetus

An increased fetal mortality associated with symptomatic maternal heart disease has been demonstrated repeatedly. The fetal mortality rate is insignificantly elevated in mothers with functional class I or II heart disease, but reaches 12 percent (twice the class I rate) in patients of functional class III, and 31 percent in mothers who are symptomatic at rest—i.e., who have class IV heart disease. One mechanism by which maternal heart disease may affect fetal health is suggested by the work of the authors.[37] In contrast to the findings in normal women, the oxygen concentration in mixed venous blood decreases during pregnancy in women with mitral stenosis, even of minimum severity. This is explained by the low cardiac output of these patients in comparison with normal pregnant women. Despite the increased incidence of fetal and neonatal mortality in symptomatic patients with rheumatic heart disease, there is no evidence that the surviving children of such mothers have a higher incidence of congenital deformity.

In women with congenital heart disease who become pregnant, the fetus may suffer both genetic and environmental handicaps in utero. In pregnancies in which one parent had congenital heart disease, there was a 1.8 percent incidence of congenital heart disease in the children. This is six times the "normal" incidence of congenital heart disease. Pregnancies in cyanotic mothers have an extremely high incidence of spontaneous abortion (greater than 60 percent), and live-born children of such mothers are small when contrasted with the offspring of cyanotic fathers. This suggests that the intrauterine environment may be at fault in cyanotic women. The limiting defect is probably an abnormally poor supply of oxygen to the fetus. Copeland and coworkers[26] noted a high fetal loss in patients with congenital heart disease causing cyanosis or accompanied by pulmonary hypertension. In a discussion of a paper by Cannell and Vernon,[38] Dr. Alan C. Barnes of Baltimore reported that in cyanotic mothers with hematocrits greater than 60, 12 pregnancies ended in 10 abortions and 2 premature births. One premature baby died. In cyanotic mothers with hematocrits between 48 and 60, 16 pregnancies yielded 6 abortions, 9 premature infants, and 1 term delivery. Three of these infants died. In cyanotic mothers with hematocrits less than 48, 16 pregnancies resulted in 4 abortions, 11 premature births, and 11 term infants; 2 infants died. This experience gives added weight and urgency to the prompt diagnosis and correction of congenital heart disease early in life, prior to pregnancy.

Long-term management

The responsibility of the physicians who supervise patients with heart disease during pregnancy does not end with the birth of the child. A successfully completed pregnancy offers an optimum opportunity to introduce concepts of long-term planning for maximum health. The desirability of future pregnancies should be discussed, together with the importance of avoiding the risks associated with obesity, anemia, infection, and smoking.

A plan for contraception should be established when indicated. In our opinion, oral contraceptives should be avoided in all patients with organic heart disease because of an increased risk of thromboembolic disease.

At the present time, we consider the intrauterine device (IUD) preferable to oral contraception. Insertion of an IUD should be performed under antibiotic coverage which is maintained for at least 72 h in order to prevent bacteremia and subsequent bacterial endocarditis. As at delivery, a combination of penicillin and streptomycin is used.[39] Because of the reportedly high incidence of low-grade endometritis associated with the IUD, patients are instructed to report vaginal spotting or uterine cramps promptly for evaluation. In patients on anticoagulants the insertion of an IUD may cause uterine bleeding, but that risk appears preferable to estrogen therapy.

A clear and mutually agreeable plan for continuing comprehensive health care should be worked out before the patient leaves the hospital. Except in the case of women with peripartal heart disease, there is no evidence that pregnancy, if survived, affects the long-term prognosis of women with heart disease. It seems likely, however, that proper planning for health maintenance during the years of motherhood will pay dividends in family health of a magnitude at least equal to those achieved by comprehensive care during the months of pregnancy.

REFERENCES

1 Burwell, C. S., and Metcalfe, J.: "Heart Disease and Pregnancy: Physiology and Management," Little, Brown and Company, Boston, 1958.

2 Metcalfe, J., and Ueland, K.: Maternal Cardiovascular Adjustments to Pregnancy, *Prog. Cardiovasc. Dis.*, 16:363, 1974.

3 Resnick, R., Battaglia, F. C., Makowski, E. L., and Meschia, G.: The Effect of Actinomycin-D on Estrogen-induced Uterine Blood Flow, *Gynecol. Invest.*, 5:24, 1974.

4 Walters, W. A. W., and Lim, Y. L.: Cardiovascular Dynamics in Women Receiving Oral Contraceptive Therapy, *Lancet*, 2:879, 1969.

5 Lindheimer, M. D., and Katz, A. I.: Renal Function in Pregnancy, in R. M. Wynn (ed.), "Obstetrics and Gynecology Annual: 1972," Appleton-Century-Crofts, Inc., New York, 1972, p. 139.

6 Burg, J. R., Dodek, A., Kloster, R. E., and Metcalfe, J.: Alterations of Systolic Time Intervals during Pregnancy, *Circulation*, 49:560, 1974.

7 Pernoll, M. L., Metcalfe, J., Schlenker, T. L., Welch, J. E., and Matsumoto, J. A.: Oxygen Consumption at Rest and during Exercise in Pregnancy, *Respir. Physiol.*, 25:285, 1975.

8 Scott, D. E.: Anemia in Pregnancy, in R. M. Wynn (ed.), "Obstetrics and Gynecology Annual: 1972," Appleton-Century-Crofts, Inc., New York, 1972, p. 219.

9 Rovinsky, J. J., and Jaffin, H.: Cardiovascular Hemodynamics in Pregnancy: III. Cardiac Rate, Stroke Volume, Total Peripheral Resistance and Central Blood Volume in Multiple Pregnancy; Synthesis of Results, *Am. J. Obstet. Gynecol.*, 95:787, 1966.

10 Landau, R. L., and Lugibihl, K.: Inhibition of the Sodium-retaining Influence of Aldosterone by Progesterone, *J. Clin. Endocrinol. Metab.*, 18:1237, 1958.

11 Wood, J. E.: The Cardiovascular Effects of Oral Contraceptives, *Mod. Concepts Cardiovasc. Dis.*, 41:37, 1972.

12 Bieniarz, J., Crottogini, J. J., Curuchet, E., Romero-Salinas, G., Yoshida, T., Poseiro, J. J., and Caldeyro-Barcia, R.: Aortocaval Compression by the Uterus in Late Pregnancy: II. An Arteriographic Study, *Am. J. Obstet. Gynecol.*, 100:203, 1968.

13 Ueland, K., Akamatsu, T. J., Eng, M., Bonica, J. J., and Hansen, J. M.: Maternal Cardiovascular Dynamics: VI. Cesarean Section under Epidural Anesthesia without Epinephrine, *Am. J. Obstet. Gynecol.*, 114:775, 1972.

14 Pernoll, M. L., Metcalfe, J., Kovach, P. A., Wachtel, R., and Dunham, M. J.: Ventilation during Rest and Exercise in Pregnancy and Postpartum, *Respir. Physiol.*, 25:295, 1975.

15 Harvey, W. P.: Alterations of the Cardiac Physical Examination in Normal Pregnancy, *Clin. Obstet. Gynecol.*, 18:51, 1975.

16 Turner, A. F.: The Chest Radiograph in Pregnancy, *Clin. Obstet. Gynecol.*, 18:65, 1975.

17 Courtney, L.: Supine Hypotension Syndrome during Caesarean Section, *Br. Med. J.*, 1:797, 1970.

18 Szekely, P., and Snaith, L.: "Heart Disease and Pregnancy," Churchill Livingstone, Edinburgh and London, 1974.

19 Hibbard, L. T.: Maternal Mortality Due to Cardiac Disease, *Clin. Obstet. Gynecol.*, 18:27, 1975.

20 Gray, M. J.: Use and Abuse of Thiazides in Pregnancy, *Clin. Obstet. Gynecol.*, 11:586, 1968.

21 Manning, P. R.: The Problem-oriented Record as a Tool in Management, *Clin. Obstet. Gynecol.*, 18:175, 1975.

22 Wallace, W. A., Harken, D. E., and Ellis, L. B.: Pregnancy Following Closed Mitral Valvuloplasty: A Long-Term Study with Remarks Concerning the Necessity for Careful Cardiac Management, *JAMA*, 217:297, 1971.

23 Gilchrist, A. R.: Cardiological Problems in Young Women: Including Those of Pregnancy and the Puerperium, *Br. Med. J.*, 1:209, 1963.

24 Snaith, L., and Szekely, P.: Cardiovascular Surgery in Relation to Pregnancy, in S. L. Marcus and C. C. Marcus (eds.), "Advances in Obstetrics and Gynecology," vol. I, The Williams & Wilkins Company, Baltimore, 1967, pp. 220–231.

25 Buxbaum, A., Aygen, M. M., Shahin, W., Levy, M. J., and Ekerling, B.: Pregnancy in Patients with Prosthetic Heart Valves, *Chest*, 59:639, 1971.

26 Copeland, W. E., Wooley, C. F., Ryan, J. M., Runco, V., and Levin, H. S.: Pregnancy and Congenital Heart Disease, *Am. J. Obstet. Gynecol.*, 86:107, 1963.

27 Jones, A. M., and Howitt, G.: Eisenmenger Syndrome in Pregnancy, *Br. Med. J.*, 1:1627, 1965.

28 Wilson, G., Galea, E. G., and Blunt, A.: Eisenmenger's Syndrome and Pregnancy, *Med. J. Aust.*, 1:431, 1971.

29 Cavanzo, F. J., and Taylor, H. B.: Effect of Pregnancy on the Human Aorta and Its Relationship to Dissecting Aneurysms, *Am. J. Obstet. Gynecol.*, 105:567, 1969.

30 Ferris, T. F., Stein, J. H., and Kauffman, J.: Uterine Blood

Flow and Uterine Renin Secretion, *J. Clin. Invest.*, 51:2827, 1972.

31 Ostheimer, G. W., and Alper, M. A.: Intrapartum Anesthetic Management of the Pregnant Patient with Heart Disease, *Clin. Obstet. Gynecol.*, 18:81, 1975.

32 Demakis, J. G., and Rahimtoola, S. H.: Peripartum Cardiomyopathy, *Circulation*, 44:964, 1971.

33 Mortensen, J. D., and Ellsworth, H. S.: Pregnancy and Cardiac Surgery, *Circulation*, 28:773, 1963.

34 Hendricks, C. H., and Brenner, W. E.: Cardiovascular Effects of Oxytocic Drugs Used Post Partum, *Am. J. Obstet. Gynecol.*, 108:751, 1970.

35 Weber, C. E.: Postmortem Caesarean Section: Review of the Literature and Case Reports, *Am. J. Obstet. Gynecol.*, 110:158, 1971.

36 Mestman, J. H., and Manning, P. R.: Management of the Postpartum Period, *Clin. Obstet. Gynecol.*, 18:169, 1975.

37 Ueland, K., Novy, M. J., and Metcalfe, J.: Cardiorespiratory Responses to Pregnancy and Exercise in Normal Women and Patients with Heart Disease, *Am. J. Obstet. Gynecol.*, 115:4, 1973.

38 Cannell, D. E., and Vernon, C. P.: Congenital Heart Disease and Pregnancy, *Am. J. Obstet. Gynecol.*, 85:744, 1963.

39 Brenner, P. F., and Mishell, D. R., Jr.: Contraception for the Woman with Significant Cardiac Disease, *Clin. Obstet. Gynecol.*, 18:155, 1975.

40 Ueland, K., Gills, R. E., and Hansen, J.: Maternal Cardiovascular Dynamics; I. Cesarean Section under Subarachnoid Block Anesthesia, *Am. J. Obstet. Gynecol.*, 100:42, 1968.

41 Ueland, K., Hansen, J., Eng, M., Kalappa, R., and Parer, J. T.: Maternal Cardiovascular Dynamics: V. Cesarean Section under Thiopental Nitrous Oxide and Succinylcholine Anesthesia, *Am. J. Obstet. Gynecol.*, 103:8, 1969.

42 Ueland, K., and Hansen, J.: Maternal Cardiovascular Dynamics: III. Labor and Delivery under Local and Caudal Analgesia, *Am. J. Obstet. Gynecol.*, 103:8, 1969.

93

Endocrine and Metabolic Disorders

JAMES H. CHRISTY, M.D., and
STEPHEN D. CLEMENTS, JR., M.D.

I have lately seen three cases of violent and long-continued palpitation in females, in each of which the same peculiarity presented itself, viz., enlargement of the thyroid gland; the size of this gland, at all times considerably greater than natural, was subject to remarkable variations in every one of these patients. When the palpitations were violent, the gland used notably to swell and become distended, having all the appearance of being increased in size, in consequence of an interstitial and sudden effusion of fluid into its substance. The swelling immediately began to subside as the violence of the paroxysm of palpitation decreased, and during the intervals the size of the gland remained stationary. . . . The palpitations have in all lasted considerably more than a year, and with such violence as to be at times exceedingly distressing; and yet there seems no certain grounds for concluding that organic disease of the heart exists. In one, the beating of the heart could be heard during the paroxysm at some distance from the bed—a phenomenon I had never before witnessed, and which strongly excited my attention and curiosity. . . . The enlargement of the thyroid, of which I am now speaking, seems to be essentially different from goiter in not attaining a size at all equal to that observed in the latter disease. Indeed, this enlargement deserves rather the name of hypertrophy.

ROBERT GRAVES, 1835[1]

The cardiovascular system has had a long and honorable guardianship over other organ systems and the body as a whole, but only in recent decades have we begun to realize the intimacy which exists between the heart and the endocrine system.

It is not the purpose of this chapter to give a point by point account of every facet of this fascinating relationship but to highlight those aspects which have clinical applicability, especially in regard to conditions of hormone excess and hormone deficiency.

THE THYROID AND THE HEART

Thyrotoxicosis

The clinical syndrome resulting from excess thyroid hormone is produced in a variety of conditions including diffuse toxic goiter (Graves' disease), nodular toxic goiter (Plummer's disease), toxic adenoma, some stages of Hashimoto's thyroiditis, and excessive exogenous thyroid administration. Long ago Parry, and subsequently Graves, recognized that the cardiovascular manifestations of thyrotoxicosis dominate the clinical picture—tachycardia, bounding pulses, irregular heartbeat, and heart failure; but the precise mechanism by which the cardiovascular abnormalities are produced remains controversial. In many ways the hyperdynamic circulation associated with thyrotoxicosis resembles increased adrenergic activity, and until the past few years, it was thought that the presence of excessive thyroid hormone resulted in increased sensitivity of the heart and other tissues to catecholamines. Another point of controversy has been the question of whether thyrotoxicosis can directly result in heart failure in the absence of some other underlying heart disease. At this point a brief account of what is known about the action of thyroid hormones [thyroxine (T_4) and triiodothyronine (T_3)] is in order.

Cardiovascular pathophysiology

The effects of thyroid hormone on the heart have been studied in animals and in human beings, but the usual difficulties in applying data from animal studies to human physiology obtain. Those actions observed appear to be direct or indirect consequences of (1) increased metabolic rate and oxygen consumption of the heart and other tissues; (2) enhanced inotropic effect on the heart; (3) increased chronotropic effect; and (4) peripheral arteriovenous shunting.

Cardiac catheterization studies[1a] have shown increases in heart rate, stroke volume, cardiac output, mean left ventricular systolic ejection rate, mean left ventricular circumferential shortening rate, left ventricular work, coronary blood flow, and myocardial oxygen consumption. Coronary vascular resistance is decreased but increases after treatment of thyrotoxicosis. Pulmonary blood flow also increases but primarily as a result of increased output from the right side of the heart with no change in the pulmonary vascular resistance. Cardiac work is increased as a consequence of increased myocardial and body metabolism and of the need for increased peripheral blood flow necessitated by augmented peripheral tissue demand for oxygen and dissipation of heat.

In many ways the hyperdynamic circulation of thyrotoxicosis resembles that of increased adrenergic activity, which has given rise to the opinion that the observed hyperactivity may be attributed to either catecholamine excess or increased sensitivity to catecholamines in the thyrotoxic patient. If the former contention were correct, hyperthyroidism would be associated with increased blood levels of epinephrine and norepinephrine and increased catecholamine metabolites in the urine. In point of fact plasma total catecholamines are low, and levels of epinephrine and norepinephrine are normal in the thyrotoxic patient.[2,3] Urinary excretions of norepinephrine and vanillylmandelic acid (VMA) are normal or low.[4,5] Recently the finding of decreased dopamine beta hydroxylase (DBH) in thyrotoxic patients has lent further support to the belief that catecholamine activity is reduced in this disorder.[6,7] The adrenal medulla in experimental animals made thyrotoxic has been shown to have reduced epinephrine content in contrast to increased epinephrine and norepinephrine levels in hypothyroid animals. A similar disparity has been seen in hypothyroid human subjects with regard to plasma catecholamine levels, DBH, and urinary VMA excretion, all of which are increased.[8]

The possibility that thyroid hormones might lead to reduced catecholamine uptake by nervous tissue from the intersynaptic space during sympathetic discharge has been considered as an alternative explanation for the adrenergic aspect of thyrotoxicosis.[8,9] In effect this would leave an excess of catecholamine in the intersynaptic space in the heart and other tissues, thus accounting for many of the sympathomimetic manifestations. The decreased uptake of (3H)-norepinephrine and -epinephrine by the nervous tissues in the thyrotoxic heart together with the observed increased uptake and turnover in hypothyroidism is strongly supportive of this hypothesis. Other factors must be taken into account, however, since thyroid hormones also potentiate the cardiac effects of isoproterenol, a substance which is minimally taken up by nerve endings under normal circumstances.[8] The suggestion has been made that thyroxine could also serve as substrate for tyrosine hydroxylase, an important enzyme in catecholamine biosynthesis, thus increasing neurotransmitter production and sympathetic action.[8,10] Further work must be done to substantiate this as a valid concept. Finally, the question of whether the augmented sympathetic activity of the cardiovascular system in

thyrotoxicosis is due to increased catecholamine sensitivity has yet to be fully answered. As pointed out in a recent review[11] most investigations prior to 1960 strongly supported the role of increased catecholamine sensitivity, but more sophisticated studies since have pointed to a direct action of thyroid hormone as the responsible factor for the inotropic and chronotropic effects on the heart. Certainly compelling evidence against increased catecholamine sensitivity is the finding that both animals and human volunteers made thyrotoxic with thyroxine or triiodothyronine do not show significantly increased response to graded infusions of norepinephrine.[12,13] Moreover, adrenergic blockade therapy does not abolish the increased myocardial contractility or stroke volume in thyrotoxic patients, and in some the heart rate is little affected, thus attesting to an apparently direct effect of thyroid hormone on myocardial contractility and rhythmicity.[11,14] In those situations in which there is apparent increased sensitivity to catecholamines it has been suggested that the effect is mediated through positive sodium balance induced by the thyrotoxic state as evidenced by increased plasma volume and reduced aldosterone secretion rate.[8]

Considering the accumulated evidence to date it now seems that the most plausible explanation for augmented adrenergic activity in thyrotoxicosis is a direct but additive effect of thyroid hormone on the end organs of the sympathoadrenal system, including the heart.

If we accept the premise that thyroxine acts directly on the myocardium, we can look briefly at certain proposed cellular biochemical mechanisms by which it is believed to work.

Biochemical effects of thyroid hormone on the heart[15]

A direct effect of thyroxine on mitochondrial action is suggested by the finding that injection of thyroxine into hypothyroid rats will increase oxygen consumption in isolated mitochondria prepared with ATP but without substrate. Other investigations in vitro have shown that thyroxine acutely increases mitochondrial protein synthesis within minutes, and induces increased numbers and size of mitochondrial units without loss of mitochondrial constituents.

Thyroxine stimulates release of a substance that augments the incorporation of t-RNA–bound amino acids into polypeptides on ribosomes. It also leads to an increase in RNA polymerase activity, followed in several hours by increased RNA synthesis and later by cytoplasmic protein synthesis. The data are suggestive that during the buildup of metabolic response to thyroid hormone the cell is geared to make new respiratory units which in turn provide a higher level of high-energy phosphate bonds.

A possible role of participation by the adenyl cyclase system in the action of thyroid hormone on the heart has not been fully elucidated. On the positive side is the work by Levey and Epstein[16] which demonstrates that thyroxine, catecholamines, and glucagon all stimulate adenyl cyclase in cat ventricular homogenates. The action of thyroxine and glucagon in this regard apparently is not mediated by beta receptor activity since it is not blocked by propranolol. Epinephrine and thyroxine appear to have an additive effect on cyclic AMP accumulation in these preparations, indicating the probable presence of two separate receptors and adenyl cyclase systems for these hormones. The obvious implication is that augmented myocardial contractility produced by thyroid hormone or catecholamines is mediated by cyclic AMP. On the negative side in the argument for a thyroxine–adenyl cyclase–cyclic AMP action on the heart are the findings that myocardial adenyl cyclase is normal and myocardial cyclic AMP levels are not increased in hyperthyroid animals.[17,18]

Heart disease in thyrotoxicosis

The major clinical problems relative to the heart in thyrotoxicosis are cardiac arrhythmias and congestive heart failure. Though we have seen that thyroid hormone exerts a direct effect on the heart, it has long been debated whether either form of cardiac dysfunction could occur in a thyrotoxic patient without underlying heart disease of some other etiology, such as coronary atherosclerosis, hypertension, vasculitis, and the like. This is not difficult to understand in view of the fact that no clear-cut histopathologic lesion is produced in clinical thyrotoxicosis, although induced thyrotoxicosis in animals may produce foci of lymphocytic and eosinophilic infiltration, fibrosis, and fatty infiltration. At autopsy cardiac dilatation and hypertrophy may be seen in patients who have no other heart disease to account for these findings.

In general the incidence of congestive heart failure associated with thyrotoxicosis seems to be greatest in the later decades of life, as might be expected, since the incidence of coronary atherosclerotic heart disease is also increased during this period. Although cardiac dysfunction can be seen in patients without other organic heart disease, it is fair to state that the occurrence of congestive heart failure reflects the presence of some other form of heart disease in the majority of patients. Increased oxygen demand and work load imposed by thyroid excess result in decompensation of an already compromised heart.

CLINICAL MANIFESTATIONS

Even in patients without cardiac dysfunction, cardiovascular manifestations both subjectively and objectively may dominate the clinical picture whether the patient has diffuse or nodular toxic thyroid disease. Palpitations, awareness of rapid heart action, and awareness of abdominal aortic pulsations occasionally accompanied by discomfort in the epigastrium are frequently experienced by the patient. Exertional dyspnea and easy fatigability probably have no relation to cardiovascular involvement but may be confused with cardiopulmonary disease. Inordinate anxiety and apprehension in a patient with shortness of breath due to hyperventilation or fatigue can mimic the symptoms of pulmonary embolism.

Objective clinical findings include sinus tachycardia, full, bounding peripheral, carotid, and aortic pulses of the "water hammer" type, increased systolic blood pressure with wide pulse pressure, brisk and slapping cardiac apical impulse, plethora of the skin, nail bed capillary pulsations, and loud snapping first heart sound. Often a systolic ejection murmur is heard at the base or precordium, reflecting increased flow through the pulmonary artery. A left sternal border systolic scratch (Means-Lermon sign) is infrequently present but is probably due to a dilated hyperdynamic pulmonary artery making contact with the chest wall.

In patients who develop cardiac complications of thyrotoxicosis such as atrial fibrillation, cardiomegaly, or congestive heart failure the usual signs of these disorders are superimposed on the clinical picture outlined above. Actually, a variety of arrhythmias can occur, but most are supraventricular: atrial fibrillation, tachycardia, and flutter and nodal tachycardia. Ventricular arrhythmias would strongly suggest severe underlying heart disease. Paroxysmal arrhythmias are more likely due to thyrotoxicosis per se, whereas chronic arrhythmias usually indicate underlying cardiac disease. Reversion to normal rhythm occurs in over half the patients following restoration of the euthyroid state, and in many patients following institution of adrenergic blockade therapy.

Congestive heart failure can occur abruptly when thyrotoxicosis has a rapid onset in a patient who has some form of preexisting heart disease, but in an otherwise healthy patient it may develop only after years of untreated or ineffectively treated thyrotoxicosis. Heart failure usually responds favorably to treatment of the thyrotoxic state, but persistence of coexisting atrial fibrillation despite effective treatment reduces prognosis considerably.

Most of what has been said thus far pertains to the classic thyrotoxic picture, but there are exceptions which are worthy of comment. The onset of thyrotoxicosis in persons 65 years of age or older may not be heralded by the usual manifestations of adrenergic excess. These patients, who most often have nodular toxic goiter, may present with nothing more than unexplained tachycardia, atrial fibrillation, or heart failure, without heat intolerance, weight loss, tremulousness, or eye signs. They often have proximal muscle atrophy, especially of the lower extremities. The clinical presentation can be overshadowed by an extreme degree of apathy, confusion, or sometimes stupor and semicoma. Another of the exceptions is seen in patients who present with varying degrees of heart block[19]—even complete heart block—in otherwise uncomplicated thyrotoxicosis. The heart block has been attributed to thyroxine-induced inflammatory changes in the atrioventricular node. A third unusual manifestation is the occurrence of hemodynamically severe mitral or tricuspid regurgitation that disappears with adequate antithyroid therapy.[20,21] The mitral regurgitation has been attributed to papillary muscle dysfunction believed to result from relative myocardial hypoxia and the severe tricuspid regurgitation, to left ventricular dysfunction.

RADIOLOGIC MANIFESTATIONS

The radiologic appearance of the heart in thyrotoxicosis is generally normal in the absence of atrial fibrillation or other underlying cardiac disease. Enlargement of the ascending and descending aorta and prominence of the pulmonary artery segment adjacent to the border of the left side of the heart have been reported.[22,23] In more advanced disease, generalized cardiac enlargement may be seen. It has been noted previously that this finding tends to persist after treatment has restored euthyroid function.[23]

ELECTROCARDIOGRAPHIC MANIFESTATIONS

There are no distinctive electrocardiographic features of thyrotoxicosis. Sinus tachycardia at rest and during sleep is generally present. Children who are hyperthyroid rarely have atrial fibrillation,[24] but in adults this is the most common arrhythmia. In addition to atrial fibrillation, paroxysmal atrial tachycardia, nodal tachycardia, and ventricular arrhythmias may be found in the hyperthyroid individual.

As mentioned previously, P-R interval prolongation and even complete heart block have been reported in thyrotoxicosis.[25-27] Also the Wolff-Parkinson-White syndrome has been reported in this disorder.[28] Other findings such as prominent T waves, increased voltage, and changes in Q-T intervals have been mentioned. Many of these changes, of course, may be due to other underlying cardiac disease. The electrocardiographic findings of left ventricular hypertrophy, in the absence of radiographically demonstrable left ventricular enlargement, usually return to normal after therapy for hyperthyroidism.

DIAGNOSIS

The clinical picture, confirmed by an elevated serum thyroxine (T_4) level, is usually sufficient to establish the diagnosis of thyrotoxicosis. Preferably levels of serum T_4 and T_3 should be obtained in the event that "T_3 thyrotoxicosis"[29,30] is the cause of the problem. In such cases T_4 levels are usually normal and could lead to error in diagnosis and management. Quantitative thyroid antibodies, especially if present in high titer, may be of value in establishing the presence of Hashimoto's thyroiditis as the cause of the thyrotoxic state—a situation which would influence considerably plans for definitive therapy. [131]I uptake and scan, while desirable, are necessary only if ^{131}I therapy is contemplated or, in the case of a nonenlarged thyroid gland, to confirm that the gland is the source of the thyrotoxicosis.

TREATMENT

The treatment of uncomplicated thyrotoxicosis has been well delineated and ultimately requires definitive measures—surgery in younger patients (less than 25 years of age) and radioactive iodine in older patients. The exception is Hashimoto's thyroiditis, which needs only temporary treatment with antithyroid drugs or beta blockade until the thyrotoxic phase resolves.

In patients who have cardiac complications—usually atrial fibrillation and/or congestive heart failure—therapeutic considerations are more complex and demand a thorough understanding of all factors which might contribute to the cardiac dysfunction, and steps should be taken to correct any recognized reversible component as soon as the clinical situation permits. From the thyrotoxic standpoint, assuming that a firm diagnosis has been established on clinical or laboratory grounds, the aim of therapy is to reduce the hypermetabolic state and the circulating thyroid hormone level as soon as possible.

The usual measures taken to treat cardiac arrhythmias and heart failure are applicable in thyrotoxic heart disease. Despite the well-known refractoriness of arrhythmias and heart failure to digitalis in thyrotoxic patients, this agent should be used if indicated as in any other patient. It has been shown that digitalis will augment myocardial contractility in thyrotoxic animals to the same degree that it does in normal animals.[31] Larger doses of digitalis than used in the euthyroid patient are required to control the rapid ventricular response to atrial fibrillation, and even then the arrhythmia may not be controlled until adrenergic blockade is utilized or thyroid hormone level is reduced.

While definitive treatment of the thyrotoxicosis is desirable, the immediate goal is to institute therapy that will diminish metabolic demands on the heart and reduce the circulating thyroid hormone level as rapidly as possible. The former can be achieved with any adrenergic blocking agent—reserpine and guanethidine being the time-honored drugs—but in recent years propranolol has become the drug of choice. Depending upon severity of the clinical situation, an oral dose of 40 to 160 mg per day in divided doses can be used in most cases. The peak effect (reduction in adrenergic hyperactivity; slowing of heart rate) occurs within 1 to 2 h of administration, thus allowing one to assess rapidly the efficacy of therapy and to make adjustments in dosage as necessary.[11] Because of a short half-life (approximately 3 h for a given oral dose), any undesirable effects of the drug such as nausea, abdominal cramps, diarrhea, orthostatic hypotension, or worsening of heart failure will dissipate within a short period of time. Once the appropriate dose is established, the patient should be maintained on it until the euthyroid state is reached. A word of caution is necessary in regard to patients who are in severe heart failure. Propranolol is said to have myocardial depressant properties independent of its beta receptor–blocking effect.[11] Obviously this could lead to worsening of heart failure, but with proper monitoring serious trouble can be avoided. Actually, we have not seen this problem arise in a large number of thyrotoxic patients treated with the drug and, to the contrary, have noted improvement in heart failure with slowing of ventricular rate, as well as maintenance of wide pulse pressure, reflecting adequate ventricular performance. This apparently is due to the unabated inotropic effect of excess thyroid hormone. Of much greater danger than the myocardial depressant effect of propranolol is its potentiation of bronchial spasm in asthmatic patients. In that situation compromise of pulmonary ventilation could lead to hypoxia, the consequence of which could be devastating to the patient with thyrotoxicosis and heart disease.

The safest and most efficient way to render the patient euthyroid within a reasonable period of time is to give one of the antithyroid preparations which block biosynthesis of thyroid hormone. Either methimazole in an initial dose of 60 to 80 mg per day or propylthiouracil 400 to 600 mg per day in divided doses can be used. Propylthiouracil has some advantage in that it may have an additional blocking action at the tissue level.[32] Even with these drugs the euthyroid state may not be achieved in less than 3 to 6 weeks, but during this period the patient will be protected from the adrenergic activity of thyrotoxicosis by the concomitant use of adrenergic blockade therapy. When euthyroid function is achieved, the dose of antithyroid drug is reduced to maintenance levels and continued thereafter until a decision regarding definitive treatment is made. In a few individuals euthyroidism is sustained after cessation of antithyroid therapy given for 12 to 18 months, but most will have recurrence of hyperthyroidism under these circumstances.

In the past, stable iodide was used in those situations that demanded more rapid reduction of the circulating thyroid hormone, but recent evidence indicates that iodide may cause a paradoxic worsening of thyrotoxicosis if antithyroid therapy is not given concomitantly.[33] We have not found it necessary to use iodide in the vast majority of patients. In one of our patients with extremely severe thyrotoxicosis and coexisting mitral regurgitation, the T_4 level increased during the administration of inorganic iodide.

Although it is a rare event, thyrotoxic crisis in a patient with heart disease is a medical emergency which requires intensive care, cardiac monitoring, and the intravenous use of beta blockade therapy together with the usual measures for heart failure and arrhythmias. In this condition it is justifiable to give propranolol 1 to 2 mg intravenously initially and to repeat every 4 to 6 h according to need. Reserpine 0.5 to 1.0 mg intramuscularly every 8 h is a reasonable substitute, though its onset of action will be less rapid. The use of corticosteroids is debatable, but in high doses they may have a beneficial effect, especially if the patient is in shock.

In most of the patients with thyrotoxic heart disease definitive treatment will consist of radioactive iodine administration, but it is customary to delay this treatment until several months after antithyroid therapy is begun to allow depletion of thyroid hormone in the gland. This theoretically will prevent the post-^{131}I release of large amounts of thyroid hormone into the blood, thus avoiding a potentially serious insult to the already maligned heart. The only indication for thyroid surgery would be in the patient under 25 years of age whose heart disease had abated or posed no threat under surgical conditions.

Hypothyroidism

For years the status of the heart in the presence of hypothyroidism has been in question. The peripheral edema seen in profound hypothyroidism in the presence of an enlarged cardiac silhouette on radiographic examination is suggestive but not necessarily indicative of cardiac dysfunction. In recent years, more information regarding cardiac function in hypothyroidism suggests that in the absence of other underlying heart disease, cardiac function is appropriate for peripheral tissue demand.

CARDIOVASCULAR PATHOPHYSIOLOGY

In an interesting study by Graettinger et al.[34] hemodynamic data suggest that resting cardiac output in patients who are hypothyroid is significantly reduced. In 12 individuals who were hypothyroid, resting cardiac index varied from 1.35 to 2.19 liters/min/m² as compared to mean control values of 2.92 liters/min/m². Even more important was their finding that with exercise, cardiac output rose appropriately without an abnormal elevation in end-diastolic pressures or pulse rate. This finding contrasts with the response of individuals with cardiac dysfunction who develop high diastolic filling pressures and even pulmonary edema with exercise. The early diastolic dip seen in ventricular pressure recordings of hypothyroid individuals has been thought to be associated with pericardial effusion and perhaps minimal cardiac compression. While pericardial effusion is common, cardiac tamponade is rare. As might be expected, circulation times are classically prolonged.

In vitro studies using cat papillary muscle have shown that thyroid activity in the experimentally induced hypothyroid state modifies the intrinsic myocardial contractility independently of norepinephrine.[31] Increments of change in response to catecholamines are greater than in the hyperthyroid state. Irrespective of the metabolic condition of the preparation (hypothyroid, euthyroid, or hyperthyroid) the maximum generated tension in response to norepinephrine is about the same. The effects of thyroid activity and catecholamines on the heart are additive but not synergistic.

Microscopic findings have been minimal in hypothyroidism. Edematous myocardium with mucopolysaccharide and mucoprotein infiltration in areas of muscle-cell necrosis and fibrinoid degeneration have been reported.[35]

CLINICAL MANIFESTATIONS

Patients with hypothyroidism have symptoms suggestive of, but not necessarily due to, cardiac dysfunction—dyspnea, fatigue, and orthopnea. Objectively, facial and peripheral edema, abnormal venous pulse contours, cardiomegaly, and pleural effusions are commonly seen. Bradycardia is present in most patients, and heart sounds are diminished.

In hypothyroidism, gross congestive heart failure with pulmonary congestion is rare and poorly understood, and a thorough search should be made for other underlying cardiac abnormalities.

Occasionally, a patient with hypothyroidism will experience angina that may actually improve with thyroid hormone treatment.[15] On the other hand, patients with coronary atherosclerotic heart disease may experience angina pectoris as thyroid hormone is begun.

Cardiomegaly frequently is due to pericardial effusion. The effusion sometimes is unique in that a high cholesterol content gives rise to a "gold paint" appearance.[36] Pericardial effusion severe enough to produce tamponade requiring pericardiocentesis is rare.[36–38] Serous effusions of the pericardial, pleural, and peritoneal spaces are probably due to increased capillary permeability.

The association of atherosclerotic heart disease and hypothyroidism has been debated. Some studies indicate increased incidence of coronary narrowing in patients with myxedema.[39] This finding appears to correlate more clearly with the presence of hypertension in these patients. Type III hyperlipoproteinemia is often present in myxedema and may be related to the high frequency of significant atherosclerosis.

RADIOGRAPHIC, ECHOCARDIOGRAPHIC, AND ELECTROCARDIOGRAPHIC MANIFESTATIONS

The chest x-ray shows an enlarged cardiac silhouette with a globular appearance and usually without evidence of pulmonary congestion. Cardiac fluoroscopy shows feeble cardiac action, and pericardial fat lines may be identified on close examination. Echocardiography has special application in the detection of pericardial effusion since it is easily performed and may be the most accurate noninvasive technique for determining the presence of pericardial effusion.[40]

The classic electrocardiographic findings of hypothyroidism are sinus bradycardia and low voltage of all complexes. T-wave abnormalities are common. Arrhythmias and AV block which improve with thyroid hormone therapy[41,42] have been reported in myxedema. The low voltage seen in all complexes frequently is due to pericardial effusion; however, a recent echocardiographic study demonstrated that cardiomegaly on x-ray and low voltage on electrocardiogram were not reliable indicators of pericardial effusion.[40] Of 13 patients with definite cardiomegaly on chest x-ray, only 8 had echocardiographic evidence of effusion; thus other causes of cardiomegaly must have been present. Low voltage was present in half the patients with pericardial effusion and in 5 of 23 who had no effusion. Hence, this finding does not necessarily signify pericardial effusion.

DIAGNOSIS

The clinical picture of hypothyroidism is suggestive of the diagnosis. Confirmation is made by a low serum T_4 level. In primary hypothyroidism, the thyroid-stimulating hormone (TSH) will be elevated, a finding which itself is highly suggestive of hypothyroidism. A low TSH level and low T_4 measurement would suggest hypothalamic-pituitary disease as the cause.

TREATMENT

Thyroxine should be used cautiously in patients with hypothyroidism. Manifestations of underlying heart disease, especially angina pectoris due to coronary atherosclerosis, may be brought out by the effects of added thyroxine. L-Thyroxine beginning with a dose of 0.05 mg/day is used initially, and increments of the same amount can be given every 2 to 3 weeks (or in some cases at much longer intervals) until the optimal metabolic state for that patient is achieved. Usual maintenance doses of L-Thyroxine range from 0.1 to 0.3 mg/day, but this dose range may not be desirable in individuals who have angina pectoris due to coronary atherosclerosis, and an appropriate adjustment should be made. Therapy usually results in disappearance of the edema and restoration of cardiac size, heart rate, output, and contractility to normal.

THE PITUITARY AND THE HEART

Pituitary hypersecretion

The only disorders of pituitary hypersecretion which significantly affect the heart are those related to growth hormone excess (acromegaly) and ACTH excess (Cushing's disease). Because the clinical manifestations of the latter are mainly produced by hypersecretion of cortisol, this disorder will be more appropriately discussed in the section "The Adrenal Cortex and the Heart."

ACROMEGALY

Acromegaly (literally translated "enlargement of the acral parts") results from hypersecretion of growth hormone by pituitary adenoma, usually eosinophile but occasionally chromophobe. The general clinical syndrome is well known and will not be described here. Though heart disease has been described in many patients, the relationship to growth hormone excess is poorly defined.

CARDIOVASCULAR PATHOPHYSIOLOGY

Growth hormone has many metabolic effects, but those which may have bearing on cardiovascular disease in acromegaly are retention of sodium, potassium, nitrogen, and phosphate, and inhibition of the peripheral action of insulin.[43]

Long-term hypersecretion of growth hormone in the adult leads to appositional bone growth, proliferation of the soft tissue, and enlargement of the viscera. The heart like other organs becomes enlarged, but this may not be strictly due to growth hormone excess as there are other abnormalities in acromegaly which contribute to myocardial hypertrophy, such as hypermetabolism, diabetes mellitus, hypertension, and coronary atherosclerosis.

Many do not feel that hypertension is common in acromegaly, but in a recent study by McGuffin and associates[44] hypertension was present in 23 percent of 57 patients and was really the only cardiovascular abnormality which seemed to have significant correlation with plasma growth hormone concentration. The mechanism of hypertension is not clear, but low renin levels have been reported.[45] As stated previously, one of the effects of growth hormone is to promote sodium retention, which may be one explanation for low renin hypertension, but if excessive salt retention were consistently present, all patients with acromegaly should have hypertension, which is not the case.

Atherosclerosis of the coronary arteries and large vessels is commonly found in acromegalic patients and is said to occur prematurely in many cases. The reasons for this are obscure since blood lipids tend to be normal in these patients.[46] Interestingly, in the series reported by McGuffin and associates only 2 of the 57 patients had ischemic heart disease, and of 8 who died only 1, a 75-year-old male, demonstrated severe coronary atherosclerosis.

Diabetes mellitus is present in severe acromegaly due to gluconeogenesis and inhibition of the peripheral action of insulin. The overall incidence of frank diabetes in this disease is about 15 percent, but subclinical glucose intolerance is present in greater than 50 percent of patients. It is possible that these patients may be predisposed to small-vessel disease in the heart and other organs, but the incidence of microangiopathy involving the retina and kidneys has been extremely low.[44]

Cardiomegaly is commonly seen in patients past the fifth decade, occurs in relatively few prior to the fourth decade, and is almost universally present in patients who come to autopsy.[43] If no other cardiovascular problems were present, it would be reasonable to attribute the cardiomegaly simply to the proliferative effects of excessive growth hormone and increased metabolic demands. The frequent coexistence of hypertension, diabetes, and coronary atherosclerosis, however, must be taken into account as contributory factors. In the relatively few patients who have cardiomegaly without the accompaniment of other forms of cardiovascular disease, findings in autopsied cases have revealed nonspecific cardiomyopathy with hypertrophy of muscle bundles and diffuse interstitial myocardial fibrosis.[44] It would seem fair to conclude that the cardiomegaly of acromegaly has no direct relationship to growth hormone but results from the combination of excessive growth hormone and the presence of other cardiovascular disorders, the incidence of which is significantly higher than in the general population.

Of the patients who have significant heart disease and acromegaly, most have cardiac dysfunction or frank congestive heart failure and conduction defects. The heart failure may be the result of malfunc-

tioning hypertrophied myocardial fibers, coronary atherosclerosis with myocardial fibrosis, and systemic hypertension.

CLINICAL CARDIOVASCULAR MANIFESTATIONS

The general features of acromegaly are well known and do not need further comment. Exertional dyspnea is a common complaint and may be related to heart failure or severe kyphoscoliosis. Patients who have coronary atherosclerosis may have angina pectoris, but chest pain may also be related to thoracic vertebral nerve root compression. Weakness and palpitations are frequently present but are not necessarily related to cardiovascular disease.

Systemic arterial hypertension is present in about 25 percent of patients.[44] However, if the adenoma has encroached upon ACTH-secreting cells in the pituitary gland, postural hypotension may develop. Heart disease is most commonly reflected by cardiomegaly and the usual findings of left ventricular failure. Murmurs are nonspecific. Cardiac arrhythmias are present in about one-fourth of patients and most commonly are ventricular premature beats and atrial fibrillation and flutter. Varying degrees of conduction abnormalities can be seen, especially right bundle branch block.[44] In general the severity of cardiovascular disease does not correlate with degree of growth hormone elevation.

The course of the patient with cardiovascular disease is variable and may be one of early death due to myocardial infarction or of unabated congestive heart failure due to cardiomyopathy. With effective treatment for hypertension and heart failure, many will have a nearly normal life span, but some will die of cardiovascular complications before the sixth decade.

DIAGNOSIS

The diagnosis of acromegaly is easily made on clinical grounds and the finding of elevated fasting serum growth hormone levels (above 10 ng/ml) which are not suppressed after a glucose load.

TREATMENT

The hypertension, coronary atherosclerosis, and heart failure of acromegalic patients usually respond to normal therapeutic measures. In one reported case refractory heart failure became easier to manage after rapid reduction of growth hormone levels.[44] In the same study it was brought out that slow reduction in growth hormone does little to alter the course of cardiovascular disease, but most of the patients in that series received pituitary irradiation, which is characteristically associated with slow reduction in plasma growth hormone levels.

At this juncture a point for present and future treatment might be made. Many centers are now capable of performing transsphenoidal removal of pituitary tumors by use of the operating microscope.[47] This procedure results in complete removal of the tumor while sparing most pituitary function present prior to surgery. It achieves immediate reduction in plasma growth hormone levels—a feature that may be crucial in the management, prognosis, and possibly prevention of the cardiovascular complications. Moreover, it has proved to be exceptionally safe and to have acceptably low morbidity and extremely low mortality rates, which makes it a more attractive mode of therapy for high risk patients. For those in whom any kind of surgical procedure is considered dangerous, pituitary irradiation would be the only choice left.

Hypopituitarism

There are basically two types of pituitary insufficiency—anterior and posterior. Anterior gland deficiency is characterized by absent or reduced production and release of growth hormone (GH), thyroid-stimulating hormone (TSH), gonadotropins (LH and FSH), adrenocorticotropin (ACTH), and prolactin (Prl). Posterior pituitary insufficiency is signaled by the deficiency of antidiuretic hormone (ADH). It should be mentioned that for each hormone secreted by the anterior pituitary gland there is a hypothalamic releasing factor or inhibitory factor which regulates the release of the corresponding pituitary hormone. The lesions which lead to insufficiency of either or both areas of pituitary function are hypothalamic, suprasellar, or intrasellar tumors, hemorrhagic necrosis, granulomatous disease, and traumatic injury. Isolated deficiency of any of the hormones is usually hypothalamic in origin.

CARDIOVASCULAR PATHOPHYSIOLOGY

For the most part, involvement of the cardiovascular system in anterior pituitary insufficiency is indirect and mediated through target-organ deficiencies, i.e., TSH—thyroid, ACTH—adrenal cortex, and LH, FSH—gonads. The resulting thyroid deficiency causes the clinical syndrome of myxedema, manifestations of which are usually less severe than in the primary variety. The heart is less subject to development of pericardial effusion, but physiologic alterations are identical to those of primary hypothyroidism. Secondary adrenal insufficiency can lead to atrophy of myocardial fibers just as in the primary disease because of cortisol deficiency. The renin-angiotensin-aldosterone system is intact, preventing total body sodium depletion, but it does not operate as efficiently as normal in the absence of ACTH. Orthostatic drop in blood pressure nevertheless occurs because of deficiency of cortisol, a hormone which is necessary to normal functioning of the sympathetic response to assumption of the upright position.[48] In severe physical stress the lack of cortisol results in shock or secondary adrenal crisis.

Little of cardiovascular consequence occurs with gonadal insufficiency with the possible exception that in the male untreated testosterone deficiency could forestall the onset of coronary atherosclerosis, a point that is more speculative than factual.

Both growth hormone and thyroxine deficiency cause cardiac muscle atrophy in hypophysectomized animals in association with decreased peptide-chain initiation of protein synthesis and increased ribosomal subunits.[49] Replacement of either hormone reverses these changes. The clinical importance of this

phenomenon as applied to human pituitary insufficiency is unknown, though it is tempting to consider its possible role in the postural hypotension of this disorder.

Loss of prolactin reserve has no effect on the cardiovascular system.

Posterior pituitary insufficiency is expressed mainly as loss of ADH reserve, the severity of the defect paralleling the degree of anatomic involvement of the pituitary stalk and hypothalamus. ADH insufficiency causes impairment of urinary concentration without a direct effect on the cardiovascular system. The resulting diabetes insipidus, however, leads to hypovolemia, which with or without the other deficiencies mentioned contributes to hypotension and even shock in decompensated patients.

CLINICAL MANIFESTATIONS

Classic panhypopituitarism (anterior pituitary insufficiency) causes subjective and objective findings of gonadal, thyroid, and adrenal insufficiency, but the expression of any of these defects is generally less severe than in the respective primary target-organ disease. Systemic arterial hypotension, or at least postural hypotension, is the predominant cardiovascular finding. Despite the hypotension the neck and peripheral veins are normally filled, indicating normal plasma volume. In most cases there is no clinical or radiologic evidence of atrophy or enlargement of the heart as there is in primary adrenal insufficiency and primary hypothyroidism, respectively. Pituitary crisis, though rare, may be precipitated by profound physical stress due to infection, trauma, or surgery. The hallmark is shock which is unresponsive to treatment until stress doses of replacement hormones, particularly corticosteroids, are given.

The diabetes insipidus of posterior pituitary or hypothalamic insufficiency is expressed by polyuria and polydipsia with copious quantities of dilute urine excreted each day. Objectively the serum is hypertonic in conjunction with a dilute urine. Although the urinary concentrating defect is equally severe in both isolated ADH insufficiency and combined deficiencies, the diabetes insipidus may not become apparent in panhypopituitarism until cortisol replacement is made. Uncompensated diabetes insipidus in either situation results in a clinical picture of dehydration, poor skin turgor, and hypovolemia with accentuation of hypotension and flattening of the peripheral and neck veins.

DIAGNOSIS

The diagnosis of panhypopituitarism or any component of pituitary insufficiency is made on the basis of the clinical presentation and laboratory data that reflect pituitary-target-organ function, growth hormone, prolactin, and ADH reserve. A detailed description and interpretation of tests referable to pituitary function is beyond the scope of this chapter, and one is referred to standard textbooks of endocrinology for this purpose. Suffice it to say, most of the clinically important deficiencies of pituitary function will be reflected by the same tests as those used for diagnosing target-organ deficiency.

TREATMENT

Management of pituitary insufficiency depends upon the defect(s) identified. Specific target-organ hormones are available as cortisol or analogues, thyroid hormones (synthetic T_4 or T_3) and gonadal hormones (testosterone in the male; estradiol in the female). Growth hormone deficiency except in prepubertal patients requires no replacement. In the case of ADH insufficiency, treatment is dictated by the severity of the problem. Mild cases (or partial ADH insufficiency) require no more than fluid replacement by mouth. If the problem is more severe, vasopressin tannate in oil by injection is required at 48- to 72-h intervals. Recent experience has shown that many patients who formerly required vasopressin can now be treated with clofibrate, which has the unexpected property of stimulating ADH release from partially compromised centers in the hypothalamus.[50]

THE ADRENAL CORTEX AND THE HEART

The primary hormones secreted by the adrenal cortex are glucocorticoids (hydrocortisone or cortisol), mineralocorticoids (aldosterone), and weak androgens (dehydroepiandrosterone and androstenedione). This section will be concerned with those disorders of the adrenal cortex which more closely relate to the cardiovascular system. In this context, discussion will include hyperadrenocorticism (Cushing's syndrome), primary aldosteronism, and primary adrenal insufficiency (Addison's disease). Some lesser known disorders that affect blood pressure will be mentioned briefly.

Cushing's syndrome

GENERAL PATHOPHYSIOLOGY

Hyperadrenocorticism is the inappropriate and excessive production of any or all the hormones of the adrenal cortex. Cushing's syndrome occurs when cortisol excess is present and may be accompanied by varying degrees of increased androgen and mineralocorticoid secretion. The causes are excessive pituitary ACTH secretion (80 percent), adrenocortical adenoma (10 to 15 percent), adrenocortical carcinoma (5 to 10 percent), ectopic ACTH production from oat-cell carcinoma and other malignancies (less than 5 percent), and exogenous glucocorticoids.

In classic Cushing's disease, appropriately termed "pituitary basophilism" by Cushing, the disorder is indeed one arising from the hypothalamic-pituitary system. Whether it occurs as a result of displacement of the normal negative feedback between cortisol, and ACTH or corticotropin-releasing factor to a higher set point, or the presence of an ACTH-

secreting pituitary microadenoma, or a combination of both is uncertain. Recent data[47,51] are supportive of basophilic pituitary microadenoma as the causative lesion, removal of which by transsphenoidal resection results in cure. This does not negate the role of increased corticotropin releasing factor as the initiating mechanism. In any event the result is bilateral adrenocortical hyperplasia with cortisol secretion two to four times the usual amount in a 24-h period and, less consistently, increased weak androgen secretion. Adrenal tumors function autonomously whether benign or malignant and may give rise to any combination of adrenocortical hormone excess. Under these circumstances cortisol production is excessive, pituitary ACTH secretion is inhibited, and the remaining cortex of both adrenal glands is rendered functionally atrophic, providing a differential diagnostic feature. Ectopic ACTH production by malignant tumors causes bilateral adrenocortical hyperplasia of a marked degree, excessive corticosteroid production, and inhibition of pituitary ACTH release.

Cortisol excess at the biologic level leads to protein wasting, increased gluconeogenesis, increased hematopoiesis, increased enzyme activity, increased anti-inflammatory activity, increased renal free water clearance, and facio-cervico-truncal fat accumulation.[52] In addition it has weak mineralocorticoid activity causing sodium retention in exchange for potassium excretion by the renal tubules. Mineralocorticoids normally promote active absorption of sodium in exchange for potassium across certain cell wall membranes, especially the renal tubules, sweat and salivary glands, and intestinal mucosa. Excessive amounts accentuate the normal process, resulting in increased total body sodium and in potassium depletion. The glucocorticoid activity of aldosterone is minimal. Increased androgen secretion causes varying degrees of virilization with amenorrhea in the female but has little effect in males.

Systemic arterial hypertension occurs in about 85 percent of patients with some form of cortisol hypersecretion and in virtually all patients with excessive mineralocorticoid production. It is of interest that only 20 percent of patients with hypercortisolism due to exogenous corticosteroids have hypertension. This may be due to the fact that most of the steroids used in this way are analogues which have negligible mineralocorticoid effect.[53]

The basis for hypertension in hypercortisolism is not clear, but it is suspected that the mineralcorticoid effect of cortisol is the major factor. Another possibility is a vasoconstrictive effect of cortisol due to its potentiation of norepinephrine, but this is strictly conjectural. The hypertension may be quite severe and, if untreated, leads to heart failure, cerebral vascular disease, and even renal failure. Cardiovascular complications were the cause of four to seven deaths in one series of patients.[53] In the same series approximately half of the patients over age 40 had heart failure.

The pathologic consequences of the hypertension of Cushing's syndrome do not differ from those of essential hypertension. The left ventricle is enlarged, the systemic arterioles show medial hypertrophy, and the kidneys show arteriolar nephrosclerosis which may progress to necrotizing arteriolitis if the condition is ineffectively treated. Coronary atherosclerosis and large-vessel arteriosclerosis are believed to be accelerated and are frequently present. This may be related to hypertension, hypercholesterolemia, and diabetes.

CLINICAL MANIFESTATIONS[54]

Cushing's disease is readily identified by the characteristic features of "moon facies," truncal obesity with relatively thin extremities, prominence of the supraclavicular fat pads and cervicodorsal fat pads, paper-thin skin, variable degrees of deeply purple or pink striae, and ecchymoses. It is a relatively uncommon condition which has a predilection for females (4:1) between the ages of 20 and 60 years. Increased incidence is noted during or following pregnancy. Some patients have Addisonian-type pigmentation suggesting high levels of ACTH and/or MSH from the inciting lesion—especially chromophobe adenoma or ACTH-producing malignancy.

Hypertension, as stated, is one of the most consistent findings and in patients with disease of long duration may progress to hypertensive cardiovascular disease. The resulting cardiomegaly and heart failure are reflected by physical findings which are no different from those in other causes of hypertensive cardiovascular disease. Renal failure due to malignant arteriolar nephrosclerosis was not uncommonly seen in the era prior to more effective medical and surgical therapy.

As a general rule, patients with hyperadrenocorticism due to adrenal adenoma or carcinoma have milder clinical features perhaps due to intermittency in the secretion from the tumor. Even milder features are noted in the ectopic ACTH syndromes, despite extremely high cortisol production, because of the general debilitation and wasting caused by the responsible malignancy. The latter cases also have a marked degree of insulin resistance, and these patients are prone to have severe hypertensive vascular disease.

In the untreated patient with Cushing's disease, death due to progressive congestive heart failure, cerebral hemorrhage or thrombosis, or renal failure (all complications of unabated systemic arterial hypertension) can be expected within 5 to 10 years after onset.

DIAGNOSIS[52,55,56]

The diagnosis of hypercortisolism is established by the clinical picture, and confirmation is made by demonstrating nonsuppressibility of the plasma cortisol and urinary 17-hydroxycorticosteroids and 17-ketosteroids to low-dose dexamethasone (0.5 mg every 6 h for 2 days). To further differentiate the source of cortisol excess, response of these parameters to high doses of dexamethasone (2 mg every 6 h for 2 days) and to metyrapone (11β-hydroxylase inhibitor) is measured. Patients who show significant suppresion of the plasma and urinary steroids after high-dose dexamethasone, and a two- to threefold rise in the urinary 17-hydroxysteroids and 17-ketosteroids after metyrapone have Cushing's disease (pituitary ACTH excess). Those who show no response to either maneuver have one of three tumors—adrenal adenoma, carcinoma, or ACTH-producing malignancy—as the source of the syndrome. Patients with Cushing's disease do not usually show enlargement of the sella turcica despite the probable presence of a basophilic microadenoma. A normal chest x-ray will usually but not always rule out an ectopic ACTH source. If adrenal tumor is suspected, selective adrenal arteriography, venography, and venous effluent studies (for cortisol output) will help to localize the responsible lesion—a step that is desirable if not essential for appropriate surgical management.

TREATMENT

If systemic arterial hypertension is present, attempts should be made to control it with appropriate antihypertensives and diuretics (with caution because of excessive potassium excretion) before any definitive surgical treatment for Cushing's syndrome is undertaken. The time-honored approach to Cushing's disease is bilateral adrenalectomy preceded or followed by pituitary irradiation. Adrenal tumors require surgery as indicated by angiographic findings and gross exploration. The ectopic ACTH syndrome carries such a poor prognosis that surgical therapy is usually of no value. Those patients with Cushing's disease who are medically too ill for reasons of heart failure, renal complications, etc., can be treated cautiously with metyrapone, OP'DDD, or aminoglutethemide with or without pituitary irradiation as indicated by the individual circumstance. It is fair to predict that the future approach to Cushing's disease will be transsphenoidal exploration and removal of the responsible microadenoma.

Primary aldosteronism[52,53,57,58]

Primary aldosteronism, first described by Conn in 1955,[57] is a condition produced by excessive and nonsuppressible secretion of aldosterone. It arises from adrenocortical adenoma in the majority of cases (80 percent) and bilateral adrenocortical hyperplasia or nodular hyperplasia in the rest, the incidence of the latter increasing with age of the patient. Adrenocortical carcinoma accounts for less than 1 percent of cases.

PATHOPHYSIOLOGY

Most of the features of the syndrome can be explained on the basis of the effect of aldosterone on electrolyte metabolism as outlined in the previous section. Sodium retention results in increased total body sodium, increased extracellular fluid volume, and suppression of the renin-angiotensin system with low renin secretion. Systemic arterial blood pressure increases and in time the usual features of hypertensive cardiovascular disease may ensue with the exception that malignant hypertension rarely occurs.[52] Myocardial hypertrophy is seen, but heart failure is uncommon. The reason for the hypertension is unknown, but the increased salt retention, increased plasma volume, and excessive sodium in the arteriolar walls are tenable explanations. J. de Champlain et al.[59] have postulated that excessive sodium may inhibit reuptake of norepinephrine by neuronal endings at the motor endplate, leaving an excess of norepinephrine for vasoconstrictive activity. Overt edema does not occur because of an escape phenomenon which allows urinary sodium and water excretion to equal intake after a period of time—a mechanism which may operate through inhibition of proximal tubular sodium by "third factor."[60]

In consequence of potassium wasting, total body potassium depletion leads to hypokalemic alkalosis, muscle weakness and atrophy, electrophysiologic alterations of the myocardium, and kaliopenic nephropathy with loss of urinary concentrating ability. Profound hypokalemia may cause mild to severe disturbances in cardiac conduction and rhythm, even to the point of ventricular fibrillation.[52]

Though not often considered to be of much clinical importance, magnesium wasting by the same mechanism of potassium loss can also contribute to some of the physiologic derangement, and together with profound potassium alkalosis may be responsible for the neuromuscular irritability and tetany observed in a number of patients.

CLINICAL MANIFESTATIONS[58]
Many patients with primary aldosteronism are asymptomatic, depending upon the degree of the potassium depletion. Those who are symptomatic complain of generalized weakness, postural dizziness, paresthesias, polyuria, and polydipsia. Rarely episodic paralysis is noted.

Physical findings are confined primarily to the cardiovascular system with hypertension and sometimes orthostatic drop in blood pressure being the salient features. Hypertensive retinopathy, if present at all, is mild. Cardiomegaly is present in some patients, but rarely is evidence of heart failure seen. In symptomatic patients one may find objective proximal muscle weakness and atrophy and neuromuscular irritability with twitching or frank tetany.

Certainly the most characteristic laboratory finding is hypokalemic alkalosis with potassium levels as low as 2 mEq/liter, but most often in the 3 to 3.5 mEq/liter range. The serum sodium is usually normal or elevated and if the latter, is highly suggestive of primary aldosteronism. Urine specific gravity is usually low and may show persistent alkaline reaction.

DIAGNOSIS[53]
Much has been written of the numerous diagnostic maneuvers available, but the current trend is to demonstrate: (1) unprovoked hypokalemia; (2) inappropriately high 24-h urinary potassium excretion (greater than 30 mEq/24 h); (3) low plasma renin activity after sodium depletion and assumption of the upright position; and (4) nonsuppressibility of plasma aldosterone levels after rapid infusion of saline (2 liters over 4 h). If these criteria are satisfied, a diagnosis of primary aldosteronism is made. The next step is to identify the lesion by adrenal venography and venous effluent studies[61] or, if available, an [131]I-19-iodocholesterol scan.[62]

TREATMENT
Principles of therapy are considered in context of the clinical situation. The main objective is to stop the basic derangement—sodium retention and potassium wasting. This can be achieved by medical means with spironolactone (an aldosterone antagonist) or by surgical removal of the causative lesion. If the patient is less than 50 years of age and one or more adenomas have been identified angiographically, surgery is the treatment of choice. If the patient is older or has suspected bilateral adrenal hyperplasia as determined from angiographic studies and venous effluent aldosterone sampling, medical management is recommended. The difference in therapy is based upon the experience that 20 to 40 percent of patients with bilateral hyperplasia show no significant drop in blood pressure after surgery, reflecting a difference in the pathogenesis of adenoma and hyperplasia.

Mineralocorticoid excess in low renin hypertension

For several years the existence of "low renin essential hypertension" has been recognized and can be seen in 20 to 30 percent of patients with systemic arterial hypertension. Until recently a search for identifiable mineralocorticoid excess has been fruitless, although indirect evidence has indicated its presence (low renin levels after salt depletion; low salivary Na/K ratio). Within the past year, however, Sennett and associates[63] demonstrated beyond any doubt the presence in the urine of these patients of a weak mineralocorticoid, 16β-hydroxydehydroepiandrosterone (one-fortieth the potency of aldosterone), in consistently higher amounts than in the patients with normal renin hypertension and normal controls. The source of this material has not been determined, but an adrenal origin is suspected. Therapeutic implications are uncertain at this time, but an optimistic outlook is warranted.

Primary adrenal insufficiency

We have come a long way since Addison first described the syndrome bearing his name over 120 years ago, but we have done little to improve his description of the clinical presentation. This intriguing disease, once considered sure death, has become attenuated by modern treatment and is no more threat than the ability to obtain replacement medication. It is caused by functional failure of the adrenal cortex which may be due to infection, hemorrhage, trauma, and probably organ-specific autoimmune disease. The most common etiologic factor of several decades ago was tuberculosis, but so-called idiopathic atrophy is now the front-runner. Most evidence points to some type of nonspecific autoimmune disease as the probable cause of this lesion. This is indirectly supported by the fairly common occurrence of other autoimmune diseases in patients with Addison's disease, and the finding of antiadrenal, antithyroidal, and anti-parietal cell antibodies in many of these patients.[64]

PATHOPHYSIOLOGY[52]
The physiologic derangements of this disease are due to insufficiency of cortisol and aldosterone secretion by the adrenal cortex. The alterations produced by cortisol deficiency are increased ACTH and probably MSH secretion by the pituitary, increased insulin sensitivity, hypotension with postural accentuation, decreased hematopoiesis, and decreased muscle activity.

Deficiency of aldosterone results in sodium wasting and potassium retention by the kidney, hypovolemia, and further aggravation of the hypotension of cortisol deficiency. It is probably responsible for the decreased heart size. Although the heart size diminishes in untreated disease, there are no characteristic lesions except for atrophy of myocardial fibers and the presence of hemofuscin (brown pigment).

CLINICAL MANIFESTATIONS
In uncomplicated chronic adrenal insufficiency the picture is one of weakness, lassitude, weight loss, anorexia, abdominal pain, sometimes nausea, vomiting or diarrhea, postural dizziness and/or syncope, and emotional lability. The objective cardiovascular findings most characteristically are chronic systemic arterial hypotension with orthostatic accentuation and small heart. Increased skin pigmentation, either general or localized, involving extensor surfaces of the hands, palmar creases, lips, and buccal membranes, is seen commonly.

Acute decompensation or crisis precipitated by severe physical stress (intercurrent infection, trauma, surgery) or by sudden withdrawal of cortisol therapy results in a classic dramatic picture of severe shock, dehydration, altered levels of consciousness, marked hyponatremia, hyperkalemia, elevated urea nitrogen, and mild to moderate metabolic acidosis.

ELECTROCARDIOGRAPHIC MANIFESTATIONS
The electrocardiographic abnormalities in primary adrenal insufficiency are nonspecific and may be due to intracellular electrolyte imbalance, changes in extracellular fluid volume, diminution of the basal metabolic rate, or anatomic changes in the myocardium.

Bradycardia, low voltage, ST- and T-wave abnormalities, and prolongation of P-R and Q-T intervals have been reported.[65] In Addisonian crisis one may see typical changes of hyperkalemia. Treatment should reverse these changes if other underlying disease is not present.

RADIOLOGIC MANIFESTATIONS
The heart is small in Addison's disease, and the size often corresponds to the severity of the disease. During treatment, heart size approaches normal. A small heart coupled with calcification of adrenal glands suggests Addison's disease.

DIAGNOSIS
A low serum cortisol level (less than 5 μg/100 ml) that fails to increase to greater than 10 μg/100 ml 30 to 60 min after synthetic ACTH (0.25 mg intramuscularly or intravenously) is highly suggestive of the diagnosis. This must be confirmed by ACTH infusion for 48 h (40 units in intravenous drip of saline every 12 h) with monitoring of serum cortisol levels and 24-h urine 17-hydroxycorticosteroid and 17-ketosteroid content. If there is little or no response to this maneuver, primary adrenal insufficiency is confirmed. A partial response (less than twofold rise in the serum or urinary steroids) may suggest secondary adrenal insufficiency, in which case metyrapone stimulation would be in order.

TREATMENT[66]
For uncomplicated adrenal insufficiency, cortisol replacement therapy with hydrocortisone or cortisone acetate is preferable because of their mild mineralocorticoid activity, which together with supplemental salt intake is usually adequate to satisfy both cortisol and sodium needs of the patient. In the adult, hydrocortisone 20 to 30 mg per day in two or three doses with liberal salt intake will usually meet unstressed needs. If the patient continues to show postural hypotension or hyperkalemia, one can add a salt-retaining steroid—9γ-fluorohydrocortisone 0.1 mg to 0.2 mg per day in single or divided doses. This therapy will correct hypotension, bring heart size back to normal, and restore normal sense of well-being, appetite, weight, and strength. The patient must be cautioned to increase cortisol intake to two to three times the usual dose in case of severe stress. If he or she is unable to take medication by mouth, intramuscular hydrocortisone should be given, pending professional consultation.

Acute adrenal crisis demands rapid and efficient action. The patient at the outset of therapy should receive a bolus of hydrocortisone 100 mg intravenously every 6 h while receiving sufficient intravenous fluids to restore blood pressure, plasma volume, and hydration to normal. Vasopressors should be avoided. A useful sign to indicate adequacy of volume repletion is the observation of fullness in the dorsal veins of the feet with the upper half of the body minimally elevated to keep the atrial level above that of the feet. Until volume is fully repleted, these veins will remain collapsed, filling normally when volume becomes adequate.

In the patient going to surgery, supplementary cortisol will be necessary. It is customary to give 50 mg intramuscularly on call to surgery with addition of 50 mg to each liter of intravenous fluid given during surgery. The total dose of steroid received the first 24 h should be approximately 300 mg with gradual decrease over the next 3 to 5 days to maintenance doses. If stressful complications develop following surgery, the patient will need additional corticosteroid coverage as long as the stress is present.

THE ADRENAL MEDULLA AND THE HEART

Pheochromocytoma and related disorders

The clinical syndromes, biochemistry, pharmacology, diagnosis, and treatment of disorders of increased catecholamine production are described in detail elsewhere (Chap. 71). Only the significant effects on the cardiovascular system will be mentioned here.

The major cardiovascular effect of excessive catecholamine release is hypertension. The majority of pheochromocytomas secrete large amounts of norepinephrine and normal to slightly elevated amounts of epinephrine. Norepinephrine, acting upon alpha-adrenergic receptors, causes a rise in both systolic and diastolic blood pressure, and reflexly a decrease in cardiac rate. It also has a minor effect on beta-adrenergic receptors which is brought out when beta-adrenergic blockade is utilized. Epinephrine, working through beta-adrenergic receptors, promotes a rise in systolic pressure, a decrease in diastolic pressure, and an increase in the rate and force of cardiac contraction.[67] The blood pressure and pulse manifestations of pheochromocytomas are variable depending upon the predominant catecholamine secreted by the tumor and the pattern of release (paroxysmal versus constant). A few patients may escape detectable elevations of blood pressure.

For years it has been recognized that one of the most consistent features of patients with catecholamine-secreting tumors is postural hypotension. This interesting paradox is not fully explained but has been attributed to catecholamine-induced decrease in plasma volume and to impaired sympathetic reflexes due to the ganglionic blockade of excessive catecholamines. Probably a combination of these two factors is more correct, since studies from a large series of patients showed that only 2 of 15 patients had a significant decrease in plasma volume in the untreated state.[68] Despite these statistics the frequently present hypovolemia is inferred from the immediate response of post-tumor excision hypotension to volume loading without the addition of vasopressors in many patients.

Cardiac dysfunction and arrhythmias occur in some patients. The cause for these abnormalities stems from a number of factors including the cardiac effects of severe diastolic hypertension (especially if prolonged), biochemical derangement of the myocardium induced by excessive catecholamines, and possibly a direct anatomic effect of catecholamines. High catecholamine concentration may cause defective storage of endogenous amines in the heart[69] and accumulation of high tissue concentration of free fatty acids due to the increased metabolic activity. Either directly or indirectly these may contribute to myocardial lesions which have been seen in human beings and animals. In a penetrating study by Van Vliet and associates[70] it was found that 15 of 26 patients who died with a pheochromocytoma had an active myocarditis, and of these, 11 patients had associated left ventricular failure with pulmonary edema. The myocarditic lesions were characterized by focal degeneration and necrosis of myocardial fibers and foci of histiocytes, plasma cells, and polymorphonuclear leukocytes. A few of the hearts had intimal and medial thickening of the small or medium-sized coronary arteries. To test the hypothesis that the myocarditis might have been directly associated with high catecholamine levels, the same investigators injected norepinephrine into rats and found that the dose which caused death within 72 h in 50 percent of the animals resulted in myocarditic lesions identical to those of the autopsied patients. The surviving animals were sacrificed at periodic intervals and had qualitatively similar but less extensive lesions. Further support of catecholamine-induced myocarditis was cited from studies in other experimental animals and human patients receiving L-norepinephrine therapeutically.

Coronary atherosclerosis is also seen in patients with pheochromocytoma, but it would be difficult indeed to attribute it solely to catecholamine excess since other predisposing factors—hypertension and diabetes—are present in nearly all the patients. The typical features of malignant hypertension can be seen in some patients with untreated disease over a protracted period of time.

DIAGNOSIS

The diagnosis of pheochromocytoma can be established with certainty by the demonstration of elevated 24-h urinary excretion of VMA, total metanephrine, or fractionated catecholamines (epinephrine and norepinephrine) on two separate occasions.

Although controversial, angiographic localization of the lesion with appropriate adrenergic blockade therapy administered prior to or during injection of the contrast medium has proved to be safe and extremely helpful in the positive identification of the tumor(s) in most of the patients we have studied (Fig. 93-1). We would therefore recommend this as the final step of the evaluation prior to surgical treatment.

TREATMENT

Surgery is the only definitve treatment. Presurgical preparation with phenoxybenzamine and propranolol will help avoid the serious complications of cardiac arrhythmias, acute elevations of blood pressure, and

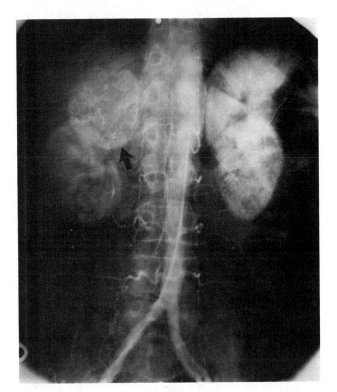

FIGURE 93-1 Aortogram demonstrating a large pheochromocytoma (arrow) in the right suprarenal area.

hypotension at surgery. If the latter occurs, volume loading, not vasopressors, should be used to restore normal blood pressure.

Patients with inoperable lesions (metastatic pheochromocytoma) can be treated with long-term alpha- and beta-adrenergic blockers.

THE PARATHYROID GLANDS AND THE HEART

Hyperparathyroidism

Hyperparathyroidism is the excessive secretion of parathyroid hormone due to parathyroid adenoma, hyperplasia, or rarely carcinoma. The cardiovascular effects of excess parathyroid hormone are mediated through elevated serum calcium levels. More than one-third of patients with hyperparathyroidism and elevated calcium levels are hypertensive[71] and often become normotensive after the lesion has been removed. Hypercalcemia acutely induced by calcium infusion will raise both systolic and diastolic blood pressure, especially in patients with renal failure. In these patients there is close correlation between the increment in serum calcium and blood pressure levels. Other forms of hypercalcemia are also associated with increased blood pressure. The elevation in blood pressure, therefore, seems to be more related to the increased calcium level than to parathyroid hormone per se.

Several theories have been proposed regarding the mechanism of calcium-induced blood pressure changes. These include increased myocardial con-

tractility, increased peripheral vascular resistance, and altered release and/or sensitivity to renin and catecholamines. The bulk of evidence points to increased peripheral vascular resistance as the primary mechanism.[71]

Calcium plays an important role in the initiation of the excitation-contraction sequence in striated and vascular smooth muscle. The rise in intracellular calcium ion concentration counteracts the troponin-tropomyosin inhibition of actomyosinadenosine triphosphatase, and the activated adenosine triphosphatase then causes syneresis of the actomyosin gel. The resulting contractile activity of smooth muscle increases with progressively higher calcium ion concentration, thus making it reasonable to assume that much of the cardiovascular response to hypercalcemia is related to a direct effect of the cation on vascular muscle cells.[71]

Increased cardiac contractility occurs with acute hypercalcemia, but no consistent change in cardiac output has been observed during calcium infusions.[72,73] In light of these findings the hypertension associated with hyperparathyroidism, though inconsistently present, appears to be closely related to blood calcium levels (especially acute elevations) and the presence of renal dysfunction. The complications of hypertensive vascular disease can occur in those patients who have inadequately treated hypertension.

Clinically there is no evidence that the elevated parathormone or calcium levels have a direct adverse effect on cardiac function with the exception that extremely high calcium (greater than 20 mg/100 ml) as seen in hypercalcemic crisis may cause cardiac arrhythmias or arrest. Patients with hypercalcemia may be more predisposed to the complication of digitalis intoxication.

Long-standing hypercalcemia can lead to calcification in the myocardium, large and medium-sized blood vessels, and other soft tissues in the body, but these events appear to be of little clinical consequence.

The electrocardiographic manifestations of hyperparathyroidism are those of hypercalcemia (see section on "Calcium" in this chapter).

DIAGNOSIS AND TREATMENT

The diagnosis of hyperparathyroidism is based upon the findings of elevated blood calcium and parathormone levels and the exclusion of all other causes of hypercalcemia. The only definitive treatment is surgical removal of the responsible parathyroid adenoma or a subtotal resection of hyperplastic glands. Blood pressure will revert to normotensive levels in some but not all hypertensive patients following removal of the parathyroid adenoma.

In the event of acute hypercalcemic crisis, which even in the dehydrated patient may be associated with worsening of hypertension, hydration with sodium-containing fluids and administration of disodium phosphate will effectively reduce the blood calcium to a less dangerous level (less than 14 mg/100 ml).

Hypoparathyroidism

The absolute deficiency of, or insensitivity to, parathyroid hormone results in low serum calcium and high serum phosphate, the cardiovascular manifestations of which are clinically insignificant in most patients. In patients with coexisting heart disease and congestive heart failure, cardiac function improves with restoration of calcium levels to normal, as might be expected from the augmentative effect of calcium on myocardial contractility.

Acutely induced hypocalcemia may be associated with acute reduction in blood pressure or even shock, as occurs in patients treated with chelating agents or rapid intravenous infusion of disodium phosphate.[74] The shock is probably related to acute loss of peripheral vascular tone secondary to acute hypocalcemia, but decreased myocardial contractility may be a factor. Patients with acquired or congenital hypoparathyroidism or other forms of chronic hypocalcemia do not usually have hypotension, probably because of adaptation.

The electrocardiographic manifestations of hypoparathyroidism are those of hypocalcemia (see section on "Calcium" in this chapter).

THE PANCREAS AND THE HEART

Hyperinsulinism

An excess of insulin, whether due to functioning islet-cell adenoma, exogenously administered insulin, or delayed but excessive response to a glucose load (reactive hypoglycemia), has no direct effect on the cardiovascular system. The resulting hypoglycemia, however, sometimes attended by hypokalemia due to rapid cellular uptake of glucose and potassium, triggers a surge of catecholamine release which results in increased cardiac demand, tachycardia, and sometimes arrhythmias. In patients with underlying heart disease, especially that due to coronary atherosclerosis, the increased demand and workload of the heart may lead to relative hypoxia and myocardial infarction.

The electrocardiographic manifestations of acute hypoglycemia include depressed ST-T segment, prolonged Q-T interval, and flattening of the T wave, all of which resemble the effects of hypokalemia, and some of which may be partially corrected by the infusion of potassium chloride. Both supraventricular and ventricular arrhythmias are seen.[75]

That the hypoglycemia-induced electrocardiographic changes are brought about through excessive beta receptor stimulation is supported by a study which showed that propranolol prevents or abolishes the electrocardiographic changes of acutely induced hypoglycemia in normal healthy men.[75] In the same study, it was found that propranolol-treated hypoglycemic subjects also showed a significant rise in systolic and diastolic blood pressure probably as a result of unopposed alpha-adrenergic stimulation. This finding serves as a warning that any hypertensive patient subject to hypoglycemic attacks, whether from endogenous or exogenous insulin, probably should not receive beta blockade therapy.

While the acute hypoglycemia of hyperinsulinism is definitely associated with cardiovascular manifestations, slowly developing or low-grade hypoglycemia is not usually accompanied by cardiovascular or general clinical manifestations of excessive adrenergic activity.

Diabetes mellitus

Severe, premature, symptomatic atherosclerosis is common in patients with diabetes mellitus. Atherosclerotic lesions develop 10 to 12 years earlier than in nondiabetic persons, and atherosclerosis is almost invariably present in patients with diabetes mellitus of over 5 years duration. Among patients with unexplained or premature coronary atherosclerosis, there is an unusually high incidence of preclinical diabetes.[76]

Diabetes mellitus accelerates coronary atherosclerosis more profoundly in women than in men. Coronary atherosclerosis is strikingly increased in diabetic women, including those who are premenopausal, normotensive, and without hyperlipemia.[77] In diabetic patients over age 40, angina pectoris and death from coronary atherosclerosis occur as commonly in women as in men. Coronary atherosclerosis and fatal myocardial infarction occur at least twice as often in diabetic men and three times as frequently in diabetic women as in nondiabetics.

The mortality rate for initial myocardial infarction has been reported by Partamian and Bradley to be 38.0 percent, and the 5-year survival to be 37.8 percent.[78] This has to be compared with general medical service mortality rates of 25 to 35 percent prior to the institution of coronary care units.[79] In the general population, 5-year survival rates following myocardial infarction have been reported to be 49 to 83 percent.[78] There is also an unusually high incidence of painless infarction in individuals with diabetes.[80]

In addition to major-vessel atherosclerosis as an explanation for myocardial disease in diabetes, some have found evidence of small-vessel disease.[81–83] One group reported a small series of patients with diabetes, cardiomyopathy, and diabetic glomerulosclerosis with no major coronary vessel obstruction, but with small-vessel microangiopathy.[81]

A recent study of a large group of patients with congestive heart failure has demonstrated a high incidence of diabetes. It was postulated that some factor such as metabolic or small-vessel disease other than the usual large-vessel disease may be present.[84] Others have not been able to demonstrate these lesions.[85] This area needs more definitive study.

CHAPTER 93 **1749**
ENDOCRINE AND METABOLIC DISORDERS

THE GONADAL HORMONES AND THE HEART

Our notions about the relationship between sex hormones and cardiovascular disorders are derived not from pathologic disorders of gonadal insufficiency or excess, but from observations on sex differences as they relate to onset and complications of coronary artery disease and on the cardiovascular complications of exogenously administered sex steroids.

In general, men are thought to develop coronary atherosclerosis earlier in life and with a greater degree of severity, morbidity, and mortality than women. This has been attributed to protection afforded premenopausal women by estrogen which is lost in postmenopausal life, as the incidence of coronary disease rapidly increases with natural or surgical menopause. The sex difference for onset and severity of coronary atherosclerosis cannot be attributed solely to a protective estrogen effect in women, because in a group of female castrates and a control group of hysterectomy patients there was no difference in incidence of coronary atherosclerotic disease.[86] Moreover, recent data indicate that supraphysiologic doses of estrogen may be associated with an increased incidence of myocardial infarction and thromboembolic disease.[87]

Just as estrogen is said to be protective in the female, testosterone has been implicated as a predisposing factor to coronary atherosclerosis in the male. The data for this are not very convincing except that male castrates appear to have a low incidence of coronary disease. Testosterone administration is associated with increased blood cholesterol, cholesterol/phospholipid ratio, and beta-lipoprotein fraction, whereas physiologic doses of estrogen have the opposite effect. It is convenient but not necessarily valid to relate the preponderance of coronary atherosclerosis in males to sex hormone–related differences in lipid metabolism.

Oral contraceptives and cardiovascular disorders

The era of oral contraception has been one of the most controversial periods in modern medicine. The use of synthetic estrogen and progesterone to suppress ovulation, which is indeed well accomplished, has been associated with an increased incidence of hypertension, diabetes, and thromboembolic disease of the peripheral, cerebral, coronary, and pulmonary circulatory systems in young women.[88] Most of the reports have come from anecdotal or retrospective studies, and even in large populations treated with these agents the majority of women have had no adverse cardiovascular effects.[89] Despite the inconclusive nature of the reports, enough information has been provided to contraindicate the use of oral contraceptives in patients with certain conditions: (1) past or present history of thrombophlebitis and/or pulmo-

nary emboli; (2) hypertension; (3) heart disease with congestive heart failure; (4) pulmonary hypertension; (5) cerebral vascular disease or migraine headaches; and (6) diabetes mellitus. The caution extends even to patients with no personal but a strong family history of the conditions mentioned above.

Occurrence of massive pulmonary embolism in otherwise healthy, nonpredisposed young women using oral contraceptives was among the first observations to call attention to thromboembolic complications associated with these agents. Next came reports of increased cerebral thromboembolic episodes, development or worsening of hypertension, and enhancement of carbohydrate intolerance.

From an epidemiologic point of view the association of hypertension with the oral contraceptives certainly cannot be ignored. In many cases unexplained increased renin and aldosterone levels have been observed, with return to normal after discontinuation of the contraceptive. Boyd et al.[90] in a study of young females who had developed hypertension and/or renal failure while taking oral contraceptives, found angiographic, histologic, and hematologic evidence of microangiopathic hemolytic anemia, the hematologic abnormalities of which completely cleared in all cases together with clinical improvement following cessation of oral contraceptive treatment. In the hypertensive patients without renal but with histologic and angiographic evidence of segmental arteriolar sclerosis there was complete resolution of hypertension after discontinuing hormone therapy. Although renin studies were not done in these patients, the small-vessel disease as described by the authors could provide an explanation for high renin levels seen in patients with oral contraceptive–related hypertension.

Whether or not oral contraceptives deserve the unfavorable publicity they have received remains to be seen. They are said to have certain properties which lead to loss of vascular smooth-muscle tone, as well as venostasis (especially in the lower extremities), increased platelet adhesiveness, increased blood viscosity, and an increase in levels of most of the clotting factors of blood.[91] These properties certainly provide grounds for suspicion, but presence at the scene does not mean they are guilty of the crime. Only carefully controlled prospective studies will resolve the lingering controversy.

ELECTROLYTES AND THE HEART[92,93]

Electrolytes and acid-base abnormalities may exert profound effects on myocardial impulse initiation, conduction, contractility, repolarization, and rhythmicity. Most of the abnormalities are functional rather than anatomic and hence are reversible with correction of the electrolyte derangement. With chronic potassium or magnesium depletion, however, the myocardial degenerative lesions produced by the deficiency may not reverse even with treatment.

Sodium and potassium are the ions chiefly responsible for myocardial electromechanical activity. Myofiber potential is dependent upon the potassium/sodium ratio in the myofiber and/or upon the intracellular-extracellular gradient of these ions. The major effect of potassium is on the resting membrane potential, while sodium influences the action potential. Calcium affects myocardial contractility.

Potassium

Hyperkalemia produces generalized skeletal-muscle weakness and even flaccid paralysis. Before this becomes evident, however, the effects of hyperkalemia on cardiac muscle may result in cardiac arrest and death.

Hyperkalemia lowers the myocardial resting potential and decreases the upstroke velocity and the duration of the myocardial action potential. This decreased rate of ventricular depolarization is evident electrocardiographically as prolongation of both the initial and terminal portions of the QRS complex; there is good correlation between the degree of hyperkalemia and the QRS duration.[92]

The earliest electrocardiographic manifestations of hyperkalemia are peaking of the T waves occurring when plasma potassium concentrations exceed 5.5 mEq/liter. Very tall T waves are not specific for hyperkalemia and may occur in normal individuals with bradycardia but also in various other disorders. When tall T waves are present and hyperkalemia is in question, easily identified U waves are a point against the T waves being due to hyperkalemia. T-wave peaking is almost constant when potassium levels are 7 to 9 mEq/liter of potassium, with T-wave amplitude often exceeding that of the R wave (Fig. 93-2). QRS widening is frequent at potassium levels of 6.5 mEq/liter and is usually diagnostic above 6.7 mEq/liter.

With plasma potassium levels over 7 mEq/liter, slowed atrial conduction is evident electrocardiographically by decreased P-wave amplitude and increased P-wave duration; the P-R interval is prolonged, and atrioventricular conduction is slowed. Atrial excitability is abolished when the serum potassium concentration is greater than 8 to 9 mEq/liter; P waves disappear even though ventricular excitability (QRS complex) is still present[92] (Fig. 93-3).

With advanced hyperkalemia, repolarization begins while some areas of myocardium are still being depolarized; this produces a progressively widened QRS complex which merges with the T wave into a smooth biphasic sine wave. T waves at this point lose their tall, peaked appearance.

Supraventricular tachycardia, ventricular premature beats, or atrial fibrillation may occur, as may sinus arrest with nodal or ventricular escape beats. The ventricular rhythm displays periods of severe irregularity and tachycardia, with and without further QRS aberration. With potassium levels exceeding 10

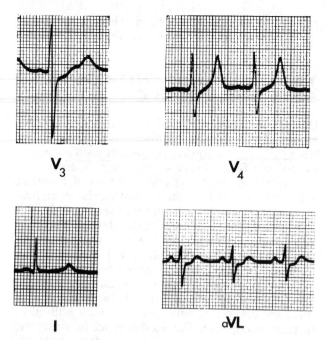

V₃ V₄

I αVL

FIGURE 93-2 Upper left: potassium 1.9 mEq/liter. Upper right: potassium 6.8 mEq/liter. Lower left: calcium 5.3 mg percent. Lower right: calcium 14.7 mg percent.

to 14 mEq/liter, AV dissociation, ventricular fibrillation, or ventricular arrest ensue.

The electrocardiographic changes of hyperkalemia are potentiated by hypocalcemia and hyponatremia. Intravenous administration of saline, bicarbonate, glucose, insulin, or calcium will reverse the electrocardiographic abnormalities of hyperkalemia (Fig. 93-3). The calcium concentration in hyperkalemia may determine the severity of the atrioventricular and intraventricular conduction disturbances as well as the vulnerability to ventricular fibrillation.[92] Hyperkalemia decreases the rate of spontaneous diastolic depolarization of all pacemaker fibers; ectopic pacemakers are more sensitive than the sinoatrial node to this effect of hyperkalemia.

Total body potassium depletion may result from diuretics, inadequate potassium intake, excessive loss with prolonged vomiting and diarrhea, familial periodic paralysis, and, rarely, from renal function loss in chronic nephritis. Therapy of diabetic ketoacidosis may result in hypokalemia, as may treatment with deoxycorticosterone.

Weakness, tachycardia, arrhythmia, hypotension, cardiac dilatation, hypoperistalsis, polyuria, kaliopenic nephropathy, and complicating pyelonephritis are encountered with total body potassium depletion. Electrocardiographic abnormalities constitute the most common cardiovascular manifestation. These manifestations are harder to detect in the presence of myocardial ischemia or infarction and digitalis or quinidine therapy. The anatomic myocardial abnormalities of hypokalemia are described in Chap. 82.

The electrocardiographic changes of hypokalemia are probably due to electrolyte abnormality rather than to degenerative myocardial lesions, as most electrocardiographic alterations are reversed by po-

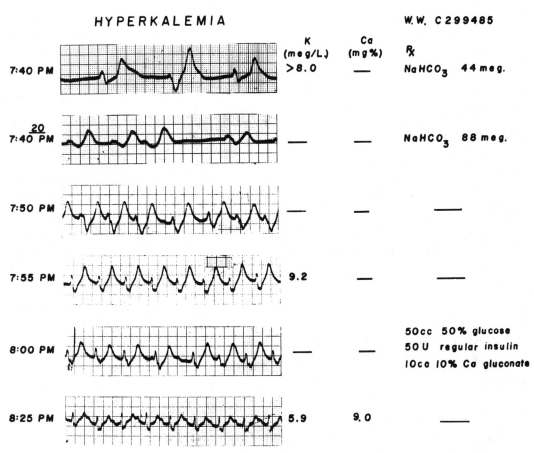

FIGURE 93-3 Progressive resolution of electrocardiographic abnormalities of hyperkalemia with therapy.

tassium administration. Occasional reports, however, fail to relate the electrocardiographic abnormalities of hypokalemia either to a total body potassium deficit or to a low serum potassium concentration.

Hypokalemia impairs myocardial contractility, increases the myocardial action potential duration, and slightly increases resting membrane potential. Slight, diffuse QRS widening is due to generalized slowing of conduction in the ventricular myocardium. The duration of mechanical systole does not change, but the repolarization wave gradually shifts from systole to diastole.[92] With progressive hypokalemia, ST-segment abnormalities, gradual diminution of T-wave amplitude, and increased U-wave amplitude appear; the Q-T interval is not prolonged so long as the T and U waves are separated. T-U fusion produces pseudo Q-T interval prolongation. There may be a slight increase in P-wave amplitude and P-R interval prolongation.

Surawicz found that at serum potassium levels below 2.3 mEq/liter electrocardiographic signs of hypokalemia almost invariably occur[92] (Fig. 93-2). Other investigators describe no correlation between the severity of the hypokalemia and the electrocardiographic abnormalities.[94]

Prominent U waves similar to those of hypokalemia also occur with left ventricular hypertrophy, bradycardia, digitalis, and quinidine therapy. Conversely, unusually tall and narrow U waves simulat-

ing hyperkalemic T waves have been described in hypokalemia.[95]

The prolonged duration of repolarization facilitates ectopic beats. Hypokalemia is commonly associated with supraventricular and ventricular arrhythmias and with disturbances of intraventricular and atrioventricular conduction. These changes occur in most patients with serum potassium levels below 2.6 mEq/liter, even in the absence of heart disease or digitalis therapy. The rhythm disturbances subside with correction of the hypokalemia, but potassium should be administered cautiously, as the potassium-depleted myocardium appears unusually sensitive to sudden increases in potassium concentration. Rapid potassium infusion in animals produces bradycardia and myocardial depression, a potentially lethal combination.[96] Associated hypocalcemia is protective in patients with hypokalemia, whereas hypercalcemia increases the risk of conduction abnormalities and arrhythmias.[92]

Calcium

Hypercalcemia occurs in hyperparathyroidism, multiple myeloma and other malignancies with bone metastasis, sarcoidosis, the milk-alkali syndrome, hypervitaminosis D, and other disorders. Hypercalcemia increases myocardial contractility,[97,98] shortens mechanical ventricular systole, and decreases myocardial automaticity.

The serum calcium level is important in regulating cardiac excitability and myocardial contractility. Calcium probably links myocardial excitation and contraction,[97] regulating the contraction-relaxation cycle. Nayler[99] proposes that most cardioactive drugs act by changing myocardial intracellular calcium concentration, which is the determinant of the state and strength of cardiac relaxation or contraction. Cyclic AMP may mediate the positive inotropic effect of catecholamines by promoting calcium movement across cell membranes.[100]

The electrocardiographic changes of hypercalcemia include short P-R interval and QRS complex prolongation. The typical finding of ST-segment shortening produces a short Q-T interval. The T wave is normal to tall and begins almost immediately after the QRS complex. Shortening of the Q-T interval is almost invariable at a serum calcium level greater than 13 mg/100 ml (Fig. 93-2). Hypercalcemia mimics digitalis both in shortening the Q-T interval and in its toxic manifestations. The decreased conduction velocity and shorter refractory period in hypercalcemia predispose to arrhythmias.

Animal studies demonstrate T-wave changes and AV conduction abnormalities at calcium levels of 15 to 65 mg/100 ml; animals surviving this phase progress to myocardial depression with cardiac arrest at calcium levels of 70 to 190 mg/100 ml. These calcium levels do not occur clinically.

Hypocalcemia occurs in hypoparathyroidism, intestinal malabsorption syndromes, uremia, acute pancreatitis, and vitamin-D deficiency. Hypocalcemia does not usually produce arrhythmias; it depresses myocardial contractility and prolongs mechanical ventricular systole. Mechanical systole is less prolonged than the Q-T interval duration; the P-R interval is shortened, and there is slight diminution of the QRS duration. Hypocalcemic 2:1 atrioventricular block has recently been reported in two neonates; calcium therapy produced reversion to sinus rhythm.[101]

The most common electrocardiographic manifestation of hypocalcemia is Q-T interval prolongation due to ST prolongation with a normal T wave. This contrasts with the Q-U interval prolongation of hypokalemia. Q-T prolongation is common with a serum calcium level below 6 mg/100 ml; the prolongation is proportional to the hypocalcemia and is reversed by calcium infusion (Fig. 93-2).

Hypocalcemia may attenuate the digitalis effect. With combined hypokalemia and hypocalcemia, the electrocardiographic abnormalities are characteristic of hypokalemia and are abolished by administration of potassium rather than calcium.

Animal studies show myofibril degeneration and irreversible depression of myocardial contractility and excitability after perfusion with hypocalcemic solutions. Calcium may be necessary for the morphologic integrity of the myofibril.[102]

Sodium

There is no recognizable electrophysiologic or electrocardiographic effect of altered serum sodium concentration at levels compatible with life. Animal studies show a direct relation between serum sodium level and the upstroke velocity and amplitude of the myocardial action potential.[92]

Magnesium

Magnesium plays a vital coenzyme role in the activation of a wide variety of enzyme systems necessary for normal cellular metabolism. It is especially important in those which are concerned with ATP, oxidative phosphorylation, ribosomal integrity, and DNA synthesis and degradation.[103]

Magnesium deficiency occurs through excessive gastrointestinal or urinary losses without adequate dietary or parenteral replacement. The physiologic effect of magnesium deficiency is increased neuromuscular transmission. Clinically it is manifested by varying degrees of neuromuscular irritability or frank tetany, in some cases progressing to convulsions. There are no distinctive cardiovascular features of acute magnesium depletion, but in experimentally produced chronic magnesium deficiency some definite lesions have been noted. Among these are myocardial necrosis and calcification, lipid deposition in the aorta,[103] and necrotic foci in capillary beds.[104]

Electrocardiographic changes are nonspecific and may resemble those of hypokalemia with ST-T depression and inverted T waves. In digitalis-induced arrhythmias, magnesium may have an ameliorative effect, although one cannot always document hypomagnesemia in these patients. Diuretics can lead to magnesium as well as potassium depletion, and failure of potassium to reverse digitalis-induced arrhythmias in patients receiving diuretics may be a clue to the presence of magnesium depletion.

Hypermagnesemia occurs less commonly than magnesium depletion and is seen primarily in renal failure patients given too much magnesium in therapeutic agents. In this context, seemingly innocent magnesium-containing antacids have lead to hypermagnesemia of a significant degree in a few days, whereas patients with normal renal function rarely, if ever, get this complication.[105] In patients receiving large doses of magnesium sulfate for toxemia of pregnancy there also exists the potential for magnesium intoxication, but serious cardiovascular problems rarely occur from such therapy. Excessive magnesium has a curare-like effect and decreases neuromuscular transmission. Hypotension due to vasodilatation and probably some degree of myocardial depression is often seen when the serum level is greater than 5 mEq/liter, and virtually always is present when the level is greater than 10 mEq/liter. In one case reported recently, shock refractory to all conventional therapy was not reversed until magnesium levels were lowered by peritoneal dialysis.[106]

The electrocardiographic manifestations of hypermagnesemia reflect defects in conduction and repolarization. They are nonspecific, occurring at serum levels of greater than 7 mEq/liter, and consist of prolonged P-R interval, QRS prolongation, increased Q-T interval, and P-wave depression. Theoretically, extremely high magnesium levels (greater than 25 mEq/liter will cause cardiac arrest, but respiratory arrest occurs at lower levels (greater than 15 mEq/liter). The cardiotoxic and other clinical manifestations of hypermagnesemia (depressed deep tendon reflexes, varying degrees of central nervous system depression, nausea, and vomiting) can be reversed with calcium administration or, if necessary, some form of dialysis. In actuality, death that can be attributed solely to hypermagnesemia is rare.

Acidosis and alkalosis

Intracellular pH changes in laboratory animals with acid-base balance derangements may alter myocardial contractility.[107,108] Acidosis depresses myocardial function more profoundly than does alkalosis. Acidosis depresses myocardial contractility, decreases the responsiveness of the heart to epinephrine, and lowers the threshold for ventricular fibrillation.

Electrocardiographic and electrophysiologic changes seen with acidosis and alkalosis do not appear related directly to pH change, but rather to the associated change in potassium and, to a lesser extent, in calcium ion concentration.[109] Changes in oxygen dissociation may also be important. In human beings, electrocardiographic abnormalities cannot be correlated with clinically encountered levels of acidosis and alkalosis (pH 7.3 to 7.64), although these pH changes can produce hemodynamic alterations.[110]

In general, diminished T-wave amplitude is seen with alkalosis and increased T-wave amplitude with acidosis. The "T-P phenomenon" may be an electrocardiographic clue to alkalosis[111] and is characterized by sinus tachycardia with Q-T prolongation and a delayed T wave that is closely followed by the succeeding P wave, or a P wave that begins on the downstroke of the T wave.

REFERENCES

1 Riesman, D.: The Great Irish Clinicians of the Nineteenth Century, *Bull. Johns Hopkins Hosp.,* 24:251–257, 1913.

1a Ueda, H., Sugishita, Y., Nakanishi, A., Ito, L., et al.: Clinical Studies on the Cardiac Performance by Means of Transseptal Left Heart Catheterization: II. Left Ventricular Function in High Output Heart Diseases, Especially in Hyperthyroidism, *Jpn. Heart J.,* 6:396, 1965.

2 Stoffer, S. S., Jiang, N. S., Gorman, C. A., et al.: Plasma Catecholamines in Hypothyroidism and Hyperthyroidism, *J. Clin. Endocrinol. Metab.,* 36:587, 1973.

3 Christensen, N. J.: Increased Levels of Plasma Noradrenalin in Hypothyroidism, *J. Clin. Endocrinol. Metab.,* 35:359, 1972.

4 Harrison, T. S., Siegel, J. H., Wilson, W. S., et al.: Adrenergic Reactivity in Hyperthyroidism, *Arch. Surg.,* 94:396, 1967.

5 Levine, R. J., Oates, J. A., Vendsalu, A., et al.: Studies on the Metabolism of Aromatic Amines in Relation to Altered Thyroid Function in Man, *J. Clin. Endocrinol. Metab.,* 22:1242, 1962.

6 Nishizawa, Y., Hamada, N., Fuju, S., et al.: Serum Dopamine-Beta-Hydroxylase in Thyroid Disorders, *J. Clin.. Endocrinol. Metab.,* 39:599, 1974.

7 Noth, R. H., Spauling, S. W.: Decreased Serum Dopamine-Beta-Hydroxylase in Hyperthyroidism, *J. Clin. Endocrinol, Metab.,* 39:614, 1974.

8 Spaulding, S. W., and Noth, R. H.: Thyroid-Catecholamine Interactions, *Med. Clin. North. Am.,* 59:1123, 1975.

9 Wurtman, R. H., Kopin, I. J., and Axelrod, J.: Thyroid Function and Disposition of Catecholamines, *Endocrinol.,* 73:63, 1963.

10 Dratman, M. B.: On the Mechanism of Action of Thyroxine and Amino Acid Analogue of Tyrosine, *J. Theor. Biol.,* 46:255, 1974.

11 Levey, G. S.: The Heart and Hyperthyroidism; Use of Beta-adrenergic Blocking Drugs, *Med. Clin. North Am.,* 59:1193, 1975.

12 van der Schoot, J. B., and Moran, N. C.: An Experimental Evaluation of the Reputed Influence of Thyroxine on the Cardiovascular Effects of Catecholamines, *J. Pharmacol. Exp. Ther.,* 149:336, 1965.

13 Aoki, V. S., Wilson, W. R., and Theilen, E. O.: Studies of the Reputed Augmentation of the Cardiovascular Effects of Catecholamines in Patients with Spontaneous Hyperthyroidism, *J. Pharmacol. Exp. Ther.,* 181:362, 1967.

14 Grossman, W., Robin, N. I., Johnson, L. W., et al.: The Enhanced Myocardial Contractility of Thyrotoxicosis. Role of the Beta Adrenergic Receptor, *Ann. Intern. Med.,* 74:869, 1971.

15 DeGroot, L. J.: Thyroid and the Heart, *Mayo Clin. Proc.,* 47:864, 1972.

16 Levey, G. S., and Epstein, S. E.: Myocardial Adenyl Cyclase: Activation by Thyroid Hormones and Evidence for Two Adenyl Cyclase Systems, *J. Clin. Invest.,* 48:1663, 1969.

17 Sobel, B. E., Dempsey, P. J., and Cooper, T.: Normal Myocardial Cyclase Activity in Hyperthyroid Cats, *Proc. Soc. Exp. Biol. Med.,* 132:6, 1969.

18 McNeill, J. H., Muschek, L. D., and Brody, T. M: The Effect of Triiodothyronine on Cyclic AMP, Phosporylase, and Adenyl Cyclase in Rat Heart, *Can. J. Physiol. Pharmacol.,* 47:913, 1969.

19 Campus, S., Rappelli, A., Malavasi, A., et al.: Heart Block and Hyperthyroidism, *Arch. Intern. Med.,* 135:1091, 1975.

20 Reynolds, J. L., and Woody, H. B.: Thyrotoxic Mitral Regurgitation, *Am. J. Dis. Child.,* 122:544, 1971.

21 Dougherty, M. J., and Craige, E.: Apathetic Hyperthyroidism Presenting as Tricuspid Regurgitation, *Chest.,* 63:767, 1973.

22 Greenberg, S. U., Rosenkrantz, J. A., and Beranbaum, S. L.: Prominence of the Left Mid-cardiac Segment in Thyrotoxicosis as Visualized by Roentgen Studies, *Am. J. Med. Sci.,* 224:559, 1952.

23 Goodman, N.: Thyrocardiac Disease—Fact or Fancy? *Dis. Chest.,* 49:188, 1966.

24 Pilapil, V. R., and Watson, D. G.: Electrocardiogram in Hyperthyroid Children, *Am. J. Dis. Child.,* 119:245, 1970.

25 Hoffman, I., and Lowery, R. D.: The Electrocardiogram in Thyrotoxicosis, *Am. J. Cardiol.,* 6:893, 1960.

26 Rosenblum, R., and Delman, A. J.: First Degree Heart Block Associated with Thyrotoxicosis, *Arch. Intern. Med.,* 112:488, 1963.

27 Muggia, A. L., Stjernholm, N., and Houle, T.: Complete Heart Block with Thyrotoxic Myocarditis, *N. Engl. J. Med.,* 283:1099, 1970.

28 Shanghir, I. M., and Banerjee, J.: Wolff-Parkinson-White

Syndrome Associated with Thyrotoxicosis, *Am. J. Cardiol.,* 8:431, 1961.

29 Sterling, K., Refetoff, S., and Selenkow, H. A.: T3 Thyrotoxicosis, *JAMA*, 213:571, 1970.

30 Wahner, H. W.: T$_3$ Hyperthyroidism, *Mayo Clin. Proc.,* 47:938, 1972.

31 Buccino, R. A., Spann, J. F., Jr., Pool, P. E., et al.: Influence of the Thyroid State on the Intrinsic Contractile Properties and Energy Stores of the Myocardium, *J. Clin. Invest.,* 46:1669, 1967.

32 Vanderlaan, W. P.: Antithyroid Drugs in Practice, *Mayo Clin. Proc.,* 47:962, 1972.

33 Vagenakis, A. G., Wang, C., Burger, A., et al.: Iodide-induced Thyrotoxicosis in Boston, *N. Engl. J. Med.,* 287:523, 1972.

34 Graettinger, J. L., Meunster, J. J., Checchia, C. S., et al.: Correlation of Clinical and Hemodynamic Studies of Patients with Hypothyroidism, *J. Clin. Invest.,* 37:502, 1958.

35 Douglass, R. C., and Jacobson, S. D.: Pathologic Changes in Adult Myxedema: Survey of 10 Necropsies, *J. Clin. Endocrinol. Metab.,* 17:1354, 1957.

36 Davis, P. J., and Jacobson, S.: Myxedema with Cardiac Tamponade and Pericardial Effusion of "Gold Paint" Appearance, *Arch. Intern. Med.,* 120:615, 1967.

37 Sharma, S. K., and Bordia, A.: Cardiac Tamponade due to Pericardial Effusion in Myxedema, *Indian Heart J.,* 21:210, 1969.

38 Martin, J., and Spathis, G. S.: Case of Myxedema with a Huge Pericardial Effusion and Cardiac Tamponade, *Br. Med. J.,* 2:83, 1965.

39 Steinberg, A. D.: Myxedema and Coronary Artery Disease—A Comparative Autopsy Study, *Ann. Intern. Med.,* 68:388, 1968.

40 Kerber, R. E., and Sherman, B.: Echocardiographic Evaluation of Pericardial Effusion in Myxedema, *Circulation,* 52:823, 1975.

41 Hansen, J. E.: Paroxysmal Ventricular Tachycardia Associated with Myxedema: A Case Report, *Am. Heart J.,* 61:692, 1961.

42 Lee, J. K., and Lewis, J. A.: Myxedema with Complete AV Block and Adams-Stokes Disease Abolished with Thyroid Medication, *Br. Heart J.,* 24:253, 1962.

43 Daughaday, W. H.: The Adenohypophysis, chap. 2, in R. H. Williams (ed.) "Textbook of Endocrinology," W. B. Saunders Company, Philadelphia, 1974.

44 McGuffin, W. L., Sherman, B. M., Roth, J., et al.: Acromegaly and Cardiovascular Disorders: A Prospective Study, *Ann. Intern. Med.,* 81:11, 1974.

45 Cain, J. P., Williams, G. H., and Dluhy, R. G.: Plasma Renin Activity and Aldosterone Secretion in Patients with Acromegaly, *J. Clin. Endocrinol. Metab.,* 34:73, 1972.

46 Aloia, J. F., Roginsky, M. D., and Field, R. A.: Absence of Hyperlipidemia in Acromegaly, *J. Clin. Endocrinol. Metab.,* 35:921, 1972.

47 Hardy, J.: Trans-sphenoidal Microsurgical Removal of Pituitary Microadenoma, *Prog. Neurol. Surg.,* 6:200, 1975.

48 Harrison, T. S., Chawla, R. C., and Wojtalik, R. S.: Steroidal Influences on Catecholamines, *N. Engl. J. Med.,* 279:136, 1968.

49 Morgan, H. E., Hjalmarson, A. C., and Rannels, D. E.: Factors Regulating Atrophy and Growth of the Heart in Hypophysectomized Rates, *Recent Adv. Stud. Cardiac Struct. Metab.,* 3:561, 1973.

50 Moses, A. M., Howanitz, J., van Gamert, M., et al.: Clofibrate-induced Antidiuresis, *J. Clin. Invest.,* 52:535, 1973.

51 Lagerquist, L. G., Meikle, A. W., West, C. D., et al.: Cush-

ing's Disease with Cure by Resection of a Pituitary Adenoma, *Am. J. Med.,* 57:826, 1974.

52 Liddle, G. W.: The Adrenals: The Adrenal Cortex, chap. 5, in R. H. Williams (ed.), "Textbook of Endocrinology," W. B. Saunders Company, Philadelphia, 1974.

53 Kaplan, N. N.: Adrenal Causes of Hypertension, *Arch. Intern. Med.,* 133:1001, 1974.

54 Ross, E. J., Marshall-Jones, P., and Friedman, M.: Cushing's Syndrome: Diagnostic Criteria, *Q. J. Med.,* 35:149, 1966.

55 Liddle, G. W.: Tests of Pituitary-Adrenal Suppressibility in the Diagnosis of Cushing's Syndrome, *J. Clin. Endocrinol. Metab.,* 20:1539, 1960.

56 Weiss, E. R., Rayyis, S. S., Nelson, D. H., et al.: Evaluation of Stimulation and Suppression Tests in the Etiological Diagnosis of Cushing's Syndrome, *Ann. Intern. Med.,* 71:941, 1969.

57 Conn, J. W.: Primary Aldosteronism, A New Clinical Syndrome, *J. Lab. Clin. Med.,* 45:3, 1955.

58 Conn, J. W., Knopf, R. F., and Nesbit, R. M.: Clinical Characteristics of Primary Aldosteronism from an Analysis of 145 Cases, *Am. J. Surg.,* 107:159, 1964.

59 Champlain, J. de, Krakoff, L. R., and Axelrod, J.: Catecholamine Metabolism in Experimental Hypertension in the Rat, *Circ. Res.,* 20:136, 1967.

60 Schrier, R. W., and DeWardener, H. E.: II. Tubular Reabsorption of Sodium Ion: Influence of Factors Other than Localization in Primary Aldosteronism, *N. Engl. J. Med.,* 285:1292, 1971.

61 Horton, R., and Finck, E.: Diagnosis and Localization in Primary Aldosteronism, *Ann. Intern. Med.,* 76:885, 1972.

62 Hogan, M. J., McRae, J., Schambelan, M., et al.: Location of Aldosterone Producing Adenomas with ^{131}I-19-Iodocholesterol, *N. Engl. J. Med.,* 294:410, 1976.

63 Sennett, J. A., Brown, R. D., Island, D. P., et al.: Evidence of a New Mineralocorticoid in Patients with Low-Renin Essential Hypertension, *Circ. Res.* 36(suppl. 1) 37:1-2, 1975.

64 Blizzard, R. M., and Kyle, M.: Studies of the Adrenal Antigens and Antibodies in Addison's Disease, *J. Clin. Invest.,* 42:1653, 1963.

65 Hartog, M., and Joplin, G. F.: Effects of Cortisol Deficiency on the Electrocardiogram, *Br. Med. J.,* 2:275, 1968.

66 Thorn, G. W., and Lauler, D. P.: Clinical Therapeutics of Adrenal Disorders, *Am. J. Med.,* 53:673, 1972.

67 Crago, R. M., Eckholdt, J. W., and Wiswell, J. G.: Pheochromocytoma: Treatment with Alpha and Beta Adrenergic Blocking Drugs, *JAMA,* 202:870, 1967.

68 Sjoerdsma, A., Engelman, K., Waldmann, T. A., et al.: Pheochromocytoma: Current Concepts of Diagnosis and Treatment, *Ann. Intern. Med.,* 65:1302, 1966.

69 Melmon, K. L.: The Adrenals: Catecholamines and the Adrenal Medulla, chap. 5, part II, in R. H. Williams (ed.), "Textbook of Endocrinology," W. B. Saunders Company, Philadelphia, 1974.

70 Van Vliet, P. D., Burchell, H. B., and Titus, J. L.: Focal Myocarditis Associated with Pheochromocytoma, *N. Engl. J. Med.,* 274:1102, 1966.

71 Weidmann, P., Massry, S. G., Coburn, J. W., et al.: Blood Pressure Effects of Acute Hypercalcemia, *Ann. Intern. Med.,* 76:741, 1972.

72 Shiner, P. T., Harris, W. S., and Weissler, A. M.: Effects of Acute Changes in Serum Calcium Levels in the Systolic Time Intervals in Man, *Am. J. Cardiol.,* 24:42, 1969.

73 Sialer, S., McKenna, D. H., Corliss, R. J., et al.: Systemic and Coronary Hemodynamic Effects of Intravenous Administration of Calcium Chloride, *Arch. Int. Pharmacodyn. Ther.,* 169:177, 1967.

74 Shackney, S., and Hasson, J.: Precipitous Fall in Serum Calcium, Hypotension, and Acute Renal Failure after Intravenous Phosphate Therapy for Hypercalcemia, *Ann. Intern. Med.,* 66:906, 1967.

75 Lloyd-Mostyn, R. H., and Oram, S.: Modification by Propran-

olol of Cardiovascular Effects of Induced Hypoglycemia, *Lancet*, 1:1213, 1975.

76 Herman, M. V., and Gorlin, R.: Premature Coronary Artery Disease and the Preclinical Diabetic State, *Am. J. Med.*, 38:481, 1965.

77 Bradley, R. F., and Partamian, J. O.: Coronary Heart Disease in the Diabetic Patient, *Med. Clin. North Am.*, 49:1093, 1965.

78 Partaian, J. O., and Bradley, R. D.: Acute Myocardial Infarction in 258 Cases of Diabetes, *N. Engl. J. Med.*, 273:455, 1965.

79 Brown, K. W. C., and MacMilliam, R. L.: The Effectiveness of the System of Coronary Care in L. E. Meltzer and A. N. Dunning (eds.), "Textbook of Coronary Care," The Charles Press, Philadelphia, 1972.

80 Margolis, J. R., Kannel, W. B., Feinleib, M., et al.: Clinical Features of Unrecognized Myocardial Infarction Silent and Symptomatic, *Am. J. Cardiol.*, 32:1, 1973.

81 Rubler, S., Dulgash, J., Yuceogler, Y. Z., et al.: New Type of Cardiomyopathy Associated with Diabetic Glomerulosclerosis, *Am. J. Cardiol.*, 30:595, 1972.

82 Blumenthal, H. T., Alex, M., and Galbenberg, S.: A Study of Lesions of the Intramural Coronary Artery Branches in Diabetes Mellitus, *Arch. Pathol.*, 70:30, 1960.

83 James, T. N.: Pathology of Small Coronary Arteries, *Am. J. Cardiol.*, 20:679, 1967.

84 Kannel, W. B., Hjortland, N. L., and Castelli, W. P.: Role of Diabetes in Congestive Heart Failure: The Framingham Study, *Am. J. Cardiol.*, 34:29, 1974.

85 Roberts, W. C.: Coronary Arteries in Fatal Acute Myocardial Infarction, *Circulation*, 45:215, 1972.

86 Ritterband, A. B., Jaffee, I. A., Densen, P. M., et al.: Gonadal Function and the Development of Coronary Heart Disease, *Circulation*, 27:237, 1963.

87 The Coronary Drug Project: Initial Findings Leading to Modifications of its Research Protocol, *JAMA*, 214:1303, 1970.

88 Vessey, M. P., and Doll, R.: Investigation of Relation between Use of Oral Contraceptives and Thromboembolic Disease, *Br. Med. J.*, 2:199, 1968.

89 Goldzieher, J. W., and Dozier, T. S.: Oral Contraceptives and Thromboembolism: A Reassessment, *Am. J. Obstet. Gynecol.*, 123:878, 1975.

90 Boyd, W. N., Burden, R. P., and Aber, G. M.: Intrarenal Vascular Changes in Patients Receiving Oestrogen-containing Compounds—A Clinical, Histiological and Angiographic Study, *Q.J. Med.*, 44:415, 1975.

91 Wood, J. E.: The Cardiovascular Effects of Oral Contraceptives, *Mod. Concepts Cardiovasc. Dis.*, 41:37, 1972.

92 Surawicz, B.: Relationship between Electrocardiogram and Electrolytes, *Am. Heart J.*, 73:814, 1967.

93 Lehr, D., Krukowski, M., and Colon, R.: Correlation of Myocardial and Renal Necrosis with Tissue Electrolyte Changes, *JAMA*, 197:105, 1966.

94 Fletcher, G. F., Hurst, J. W., and Schlant, R. C.: Electrocardiographic Changes in Severe Hypokalemia: A Reappraisal, *Am. J. Cardiol.*, 20:628, 1967.

95 Sarma, R. N.: Unusually Tall and Narrow U Waves Simulating Hyperkalemia T Waves: Report of 2 Cases of Hypochloremic Alkalosis with Hypokalemia, *Am. Heart J.*, 70:397, 1965.

96 Surawicz, B., Chlebus, H., and Mazzoleni, A.: Hemodynamic and Electrocardiographic Effects of Hyperpotassemia: Differences in Response to Slow and Rapid Increases in Concentration of Plasma K, *Am. Heart J.*, 73:647, 1967.

97 Harrison, D. C., and Nelson, D.: The Effects of Calcium on Isometric Tension in Isolated Heart Muscle during Coupled Pacing, *Am. Heart J.*, 74:663, 1967.

98 Gilmore, J. P., Daggett, W. N., McDonald, R. H., et al.: Influence of Calcium on Myocardial Potassium Balance, Oxygen Consumption and Performance, *Am. Heart J.*, 75:215, 1968.

99 Nayler, W. G: Calcium Exchange in Cardiac Muscle: A Basic Mechanism of Drug Action, *Am. Heart J.*, 73:379, 1967.

100 Sutherland, E. W., Robinson, G. A., Butcher, R. W.: Some Aspects of the Biological Role of Adenosine-3, 5-Monophosphate (Cyclic AMP), *Circulation*, 37:279, 1968.

101 Griffin, J. H.: Neonatal Hypocalcemia and Complete Heart Block, *Am. J. Dis. Child.*, 110:672, 1965.

102 Weiss, D. L., Surawicz, B., and Rubenstein, I.: Myocardial Lesions of Calcium Deficiency Causing Irreversible Myocardial Failure, *Am. J. Pathol.*, 48:653, 1966.

103 Wacker, W. E. C., and Parisi, A. F.: Magnesium Metabolism, *N. Engl. J. Med.*, 278:658 (Part I), 712 (Part II), 772 (Part III), 1968.

104 Goldsmith, N. F., and Goldsmith, J. R.: Epidemiological Aspects of Magnesium and Calcium Metabolism, *Arch. Environ. Health*, 12:607, 1966.

105 Randall, R. E., Cohen, M. D., Spray, C. C., et al.: Hypermagnesemia in Renal Failure: Etiology and Toxic Manifestations, *Ann. Intern. Med.*, 61:73, 1964.

106 Mordes, J. P., Swartz, R., and Arky, R. A.: Extreme Hypermagnesemia as a Cause of Refractory Hypotension, *Ann. Intern. Med.*, 83:657, 1975.

107 Ng, M. L., Levy, M. N., and Sieske, H. A.: Effects of pH and Carbon Dioxide Tension on Left Ventricular Performance, *Am. J. Physiol.*, 213:115, 1967.

108 Downing, S. E., Talner, N. S., and Gardner, T. H.: Cardiovascular Responses to Metabolic Acidosis, *Am. J. Physiol.*, 208:237, 1965.

109 Cline, R. E., Wallace, A. G., Young, W. G., Jr., et al.: Electrophysiologic Effects of Respiratory and Metabolic Alkalosis on the Heart, *J. Cardiovasc. Surg.*, 52:769, 1966.

110 Reid, J. A., Enson, Y., Harvey, R. M., et al.: The Effect of Variations in Blood pH upon the Electrocardiogram of Man, *Circulation*, 31:369, 1965.

111 Alexander, C. S.: T-P Phenomenon: An Electrocardiographic Clue to Unsuspected Alkalosis, *Arch. Intern. Med.*, 116:220, 1965.

PART VIII

The Heart: Anesthesia and Surgery

94
The Heart and Anesthesia

JOEL A. KAPLAN, M.D., and
JOHN E. STEINHAUS, Ph.D., M.D.

The induction of anesthesia has the primary therapeutic purpose of providing relief of pain and the related therapeutic goals of unconsciousness, amnesia, and skeletal muscle control. Unfortunately, all known anesthetic agents also have adverse actions which impair both respiration and circulation, and consequently a second and equally important purpose of anesthesia is the support and maintenance of the oxygen transport system. As the knowledge of respiratory physiology has expanded and developed, it has become possible to prevent inadequate ventilation during anesthesia to a very large degree. The maintenance of adequate cardiovascular function is a more difficult problem, and consequently it has come to be an increasingly important concern during the administration of anesthetics. In addition, the cardiovascular effects of anesthetic agents have assumed a greater role in recent years because the patients scheduled for anesthesia are older and have more serious diseases of the heart. It is not uncommon to encounter a seriously ill patient in whom difficulty with the resuscitative aspect of anesthesia far outweighs the problem of producing pain relief or muscle control. It is now possible for the anesthesiologist to safely manage patients with severe cardiovascular disease, because of our better understanding of abnormal hemodynamics, cardiovascular monitoring, cardioactive drugs (anesthetics included), and surgical trespass. In fact, diseases which in the past were considered contraindications to surgery, such as coronary artery disease, are today considered primary indications for surgery.

The circulation of the blood is determined by an interrelation of numerous cardiac and vascular factors. Inadequate vasomotor tone or deficient blood volume, reduced due to disease or blood loss, is frequently an important cause of circulatory failure. Poor myocardial function may be related to a conduction disturbance or a depression of myocardial contractility. The cardiovascular system, like many vital-organ systems, has a considerable margin of reserve. Opinions on the cardiac effects of anesthesia have varied from one extreme—that these drugs have no important effect on the heart—to the other—that the heart stops suddenly and somewhat mysteriously (cardiac arrest) under their influence. A more accurate concept, of course, would be that all anesthetic agents produce some alteration of cardiac performance but that the normal cardiovascular system functions adequately over a fairly wide spectrum of drug action.

Changes in cardiovascular function during anesthesia may be due to factors other than the direct effect of anesthetic drugs on the heart. The most important of these factors are changes in ventilation and in the operation of the autonomic nervous system. Almost all anesthetic agents depress ventilation, and if this is not corrected, the resulting hypoxia and hypercapnia will alter cardiac function. Although the changes in heart rate are variable, severe hypoxia will produce an extreme depression of myocardial contractility and acute failure. An increase in blood pressure related to the release of catecholamines commonly occurs during the early phase of hypercapnia. At the same time the increased carbon dioxide, with the consequent acidosis, depresses myocardial contractility and will add to the cardiac depression produced by hypoxia and drugs. Rapid elimination of very high levels of carbon dioxide can produce severe arrhythmias; however, the severe degree of hypercapnia required for this phenomenon is almost never encountered clinically.

Anesthetic agents have complex actions on both the sympathetic and parasympathetic nervous systems. Consequently it is not possible to account for the cardiovascular changes during anesthesia without a careful analysis of their effect on the autonomic nervous system. Most of the commonly used general anesthetics have a direct depressant effect on the heart and peripheral circulation. This cardiovascular depression is antagonized by increased sympathetic stimulation during anesthesia with ether, cyclopropane, fluroxene, ketamine, and possibly with morphine.[1] Therefore, cardiac output is usually normal or elevated with these anesthetic agents. This is in contrast to drugs like halothane which depress the autonomic nervous system and produce a decrease in cardiac output. Catecholamines released during cyclopropane anesthesia appear to be related to the increase in digitalis toxicity observed with this agent; conversely, the increased tolerance to digitalis during halothane anesthesia is related to the low levels of catecholamines.[2,3]

CARDIAC RHYTHM

Cardiac arrhythmias are common in surgical patients. They may occur during operations in patients who otherwise have a normal cardiac rhythm. When continuous electrocardiographic monitoring is used, the incidence of intraoperative arrhythmias may range up to 60 percent.[4] The vast majority of these arrhythmias have little clinical significance and rarely require specific antiarrhythmic treatment. However, the onset of any arrhythmia is a warning of possible physiologic trespass and should initiate an evaluation of the anesthetic and surgical management. Frequently, the arrhythmia will disappear with increased ventilation and lighter anesthesia.

During the anesthesia an imbalance in the autonomic nervous system causes most arrhythmias.

Factors such as hypoxia, hypercarbia, and light anesthesia produce an excess of sympathetic activity. The release of excess catecholamines will produce arrhythmias under anesthesia, especially with the use of cyclopropane and halothane. Early studies with cyclopropane revealed that epinephrine could precipitate both ventricular tachycardia and ventricular fibrillation. Experimental work has shown that epinephrine will produce similar arrhythmias with halothane anesthesia; however, carefully limited dosages of epinephrine in clinical studies did not produce serious arrhythmias in patients anesthetized with this halogenated agent.[5] Other halogenated agents, such as enflurane, methoxyflurane, and fluroxene have a wider margin of safety with exogenous epinephrine administration.[4,6] Stimulation of the parasympathetic nervous system by tracheal intubation, intraabdominal traction, or manipulation of the eye muscles occasionally causes bradycardia and hypotension. These usually respond to the removal of the mechanical stimulation and/or the administration of atropine.

Other causes of cardiac arrhythmias include succinylcholine, which has been found to produce bradycardia and asystole with repeated doses. It is suggested that choline formed from either acetyl- or succinylcholine can sensitize the myocardium to the succeeding doses of the relaxant.[7] This arrhythmia is not frequently encountered in routine anesthesia because of the blocking action of barbiturates commonly employed for induction. Intravenous atropine has also been reported to precipitate severe dysrhythmias. Electrolyte imbalance, especially hypokalemia, in digitalized patients is a common cause of serious arrhythmias. Traction of cerebral structures during intracranial surgery also frequently leads to cardiac arrhythmias. These arrhythmias may be used as warning signs by the neurosurgeon who is exploring the posterior fossa.

A more serious problem in cardiac conduction is found in patients with atrioventricular heart block. The hearts of these patients will tolerate only the mildest depressant action of anesthetic agents. It is very important that preanesthetic medication for these people should include a sufficient dose of atropine to block the vagus, together with the usual measures (sympathomimetic amine or artificial pacemaker) for controlling Stokes-Adams attacks. Anesthetics with minimal cardiac depression, such as nitrous oxide, and with sympathetic stimulation, such as ketamine, are the least hazardous general anesthetic agents for patients in this precarious state.

Prevention and treatment of arrhythmias associated with anesthetics like cyclopropane and halothane have ranged from old drugs such as procaine and barbiturates to new ones like the beta-adrenergic blocking agents. As previously mentioned, ventilation and the reduction of anesthetic concentrations will usually correct this defect so that it will not often be necessary to resort to drug treatment. It should also be noted that spontaneous arrhythmias present in the preanesthetic period commonly disappear with the induction of anesthesia and the maintenance of adequate ventilation. Serious arrhythmias due to disease, mechanical stimulation, or myocardial ische-

mia may require treatment with antiarrhythmia drugs such as propranolol, lidocaine, or procainamide. It should be noted that these drugs may impair cardiac contractility and add to the myocardial depression produced by the anesthetic agent.

There has been a continued interest in lidocaine as an antiarrhythmic agent both for general clinical usage and during anesthesia. Local anesthetics in general have a quinidine-like action, and lidocaine has been used successfully to revert ventricular fibrillation both with and without the use of electroshock.[8] In a dosage of 1 to 2 mg/kg, lidocaine proved to be more effective in controlling ventricular arrhythmias than procainamide, with less depression of myocardial contractility.[9] Increased usage of intravenous lidocaine as an anesthetic supplement makes it important to consider both the antiarrhythmic action and the myocardial depressant action of this agent.

Propranolol, a beta-blocker, has been recommended for controlling serious arrhythmias. There is a suggestion that its effectiveness may be related to its relatively potent local anesthetic activity. The effectiveness of the beta-adrenergic blocker in controlling cardiac arrhythmias during anesthesia must be offset against the hazards of negative inotropism and vagal inhibition.[10]

Drug actions, including both arrhythmia correction and myocardial depression, may be overlooked in the routine use of local anesthetics administered for regional blocks or for topical infiltration anesthesia. These drugs are absorbed systemically, producing high blood concentrations and significant myocardial effects.

MYOCARDIAL CONTRACTILITY

The term *cardiac arrest* has come to be applied to all acute severe depressions of cardiovascular function because of the early belief that the mechanism was similar to the asystole produced by strong vagal stimulation. Although the direct myocardial depressant action of general anesthetic agents has long been recognized, work with the heart-lung preparation[1] and the Walton-Brodie strain gauge[11] has emphasized the importance of this action. It should also be noted that cardiac contractions can become completely ineffective under circumstances in which the pacemaker and conduction remain adequate. The use of electrocardiographic monitors which depend on certain changes in the electric potential represented by the QRS complex may be entirely misleading in these circumstances.

All anesthetic agents decrease the force of myocardial contraction, including the newer agents such as enflurane (Ethrane), which produces a decreased myocardial contractility with increased concentration. A comparison of the degree of myocardial depression produced by various anesthetic agents is very difficult because of the variability of techniques, dosage, and animal species which have been employed. The complexity of the analysis required to determine the effect of anesthetics on myocardial function is thoroughly discussed by Shimosato and Etsten[12] in their comprehensive review of this subject. They emphasize that the effect of anesthetics on myocardial contractility can best be analyzed in terms of preload (end-diastolic ventricular pressure), afterload (mean arterial pressure), and force-velocity relations (inotropic state). A reliable index of myocardial contractility can be obtained from the maximal velocity of shortening (V_{max}). Isolated heart muscle studies of potent inhalation anesthetics indicate that halothane has the most depressant effect and that diethyl ether has the least. If the sympathetic nervous system is functioning as in the ordinary patient, these results are altered. Nevertheless, myocardial depression is apparent with halothane and methoxyflurane, since sympathetic activity is not stimulated. The margin of cardiovascular reserve in most patients is such that the potent agents halothane, cyclopropane, and diethyl ether can be employed with careful management, although serious depression will make it necessary to change the anesthetic agent or technique in some patients. Morphine and fentanyl have been shown to have minimal effects on myocardial contractility, whereas meperidine markedly decreases contractility in cat papillary muscles.[13] Lowenstein showed that 1 mg/kg of morphine given to patients with aortic stenosis actually increased cardiac output.[14] Nitrous oxide has been shown to cause minimal depression of the cardiovascular system by itself; however, when added to morphine, it can cause a significant decrease in cardiac output.[15] Most of the supplements to nitrous oxide anesthesia, such as barbiturates and diazepam, may further decrease cardiac output. The muscle relaxant pancuronium bromide is an exception, and consequently the nitrous oxide–muscle relaxant combination is a very advantageous choice when the myocardium is least able to tolerate depression.

When even minimal myocardial depression should be avoided, another possibility would be the use of local or regional anesthesia. The merit of these techniques would depend upon the amount of drug required and the degree of sympathetic nervous system inhibition produced. Although local anesthetics work their desired effects in a restricted area of the body, they are absorbed systemically. In addition to an antiarrhythmic effect, local anesthetics can depress myocardial contractility to a degree approximating their potency.[16] Total dosage of local anesthetics and rapidity of absorption have been demonstrated to be the critical factors in the production of toxic blood levels of these drugs. In the critically ill patient with serious heart disease, even low concentrations of local anesthetics may cause serious myocardial depression.

INDIRECT CARDIAC EFFECTS

It is difficult to determine the various elements of drug action which are basically responsible for the cardiovascular effects produced by anesthetic agents. In addition to direct action of anesthetic drugs on the heart, Price[1] lists the circulatory actions of anesthetic agents as also being due to reduced metabolic demands of body tissues and their effects on the autonomic nervous system. The reduction of metabolic demand would generally be beneficial and would offset to some degree the direct depressant effects on the heart. The release of catecholamines during diethyl ether anesthesia counteracts the direct myocardial depressant effect of this agent during the lighter levels of anesthesia. The increased level of sympathomimetic amines during cyclopropane anesthesia counteracts myocardial depression and also causes an increase in the level of blood pressure. Halothane lacks this property of releasing catecholamines, and consequently the depression of myocardial contraction is unopposed.

Another factor which makes it difficult to assess the cardiac effects of anesthetic agents accurately is venous return. Cardiac output and even myocardial contractility[12] are dependent upon venous return. Vasomotor paralysis produced by spinal anesthesia can severely depress cardiac output and cause cardiac arrest. Any assessment of the effect of anesthesia on the heart must account for all these factors.

Maintenance of blood pressure becomes an important practical problem in patients with coronary artery disease. Anesthesia for these patients must interfere as little as possible with myocardial metabolism. Decreased morbidity and mortality can only be achieved by avoiding myocardial ischemia, which occurs when the oxygen demand of the myocardium exceeds the oxygen supply. There is a delicate balance between myocardial oxygen supply and demand that must be preserved during anesthesia. Myocardial oxygen supply depends on coronary blood flow and oxygen delivery. Factors that decrease these are hypotension, tachycardia greater than 120 beats per minute, hypoxemia, shift of the hemoglobin dissociation curve to the left, and an increase in blood viscosity. The factors which increase the myocardial oxygen demand are hypertension (increased afterload), tachycardia, increased heart volume (increased preload), and an increased contractility.[17] These four factors can be controlled by continuing preoperative administration of propranolol and by using vasodilators during surgery.[18,19]

PREVENTION AND TREATMENT OF CARDIOVASCULAR DEPRESSION

The preceding discussion would indicate that the cardiovascular changes during anesthesia are complicated and that no simple answer can be supplied for the management of anesthesia in patients who have limited cardiac reserve. Special care is necessary in preoperative preparation regarding the problems of electrolyte levels and blood volume, as well as the treatment of the heart disease. Previous drug therapy must be considered. For example, corticosteroids may be needed in a patient who has been treated with such drugs previously, and the adequacy of digitalization must be considered in the preoperative evaluation and preparation of the patient. Prevention of hypoxia and hypercapnia due to airway difficulties or other problems of ventilation is paramount, since the margin of reserve is narrow. Depression of cardiac output by drugs or hypoxia may reduce arterial oxygenation, which further threatens the adequacy of the supply of oxygen available for the tissues.[20]

No ideal agent or technique exists but certain general principles can be applied in the selection of agents and technique. Local anesthetic techniques produce minimal cardiovascular changes if the dosage is low and vasomotor effects are limited. A subcutaneous dose of procaine, less than 100 mg in the average patient, should produce little cardiovascular effect, whereas 500 mg (50 ml of 1 percent solution) may have substantial systemic effects. Since a patient's tolerance to drugs can be determined only by trial, rapid reversibility is a highly desirable property of an anesthetic agent selected for patients with impaired cardiovascular reserve. In this regard, inhalation agents have a marked advantage over intravenous agents, because the former can be removed by ventilation. Of the various inhalation agents, nitrous oxide and cyclopropane can be removed most rapidly; ether and methoxyflurane (Penthrane) are the slowest, with halothane and enflurane in an intermediate position. On the other hand, intravenous agents provide much smoother inductions, which may be important in certain apprehensive patients.

In patients with marginal blood volumes and in patients who require the maintenance of a stable blood pressure, cyclopropane or ketamine have definite advantages. In these patients halothane and spinal anesthesia are generally the most difficult to manage, while the nitrous oxide and relaxant techniques occupy a middle position. A general anesthetic technique of choice for patients with a severely limited myocardial reserve and in whom muscle relaxation is needed would be nitrous oxide–muscle relaxant–morphine. The use of thiobarbiturate (Pentothal sodium) in patients with heart disease has the limitations of myocardial depression without the reversibility of the inhalation agents. Nevertheless, this agent should not be eliminated from consideration, particularly in those patients in whom ventricular arrhythmias are a major problem. The thiobarbiturate techniques are associated with fewer arrhythmias than the other general anesthetics, and they have particular advantages in providing smooth inductions for anxious, apprehensive patients such as those with a history of myocardial infarctions. Since hypotension is hazardous to these patients, the rate of thiobarbiturate administration must be slow and

the total dosage severely limited. As with all choices the advantages and disadvantages must be carefully weighed. Narcotic-tranquilizer combinations can also be used for a smooth, rapid induction of anesthesia. The most popular are Innovar, which is made up of fentanyl and droperidol, or morphine and diazepam. Both of these techniques produce minimal cardiovascular changes and are associated with few cardiac arrhythmias.

The choice of anesthetic agents is often compromised by surgical requirements, which may exclude the use of explosive agents. As in other medical situations the need for the electrocautery must be *balanced* against the advantages of the explosive anesthetic agent. Mechanical embarrassments of the cardiovascular system are frequently exaggerated in the anesthetized patient because of lack of muscle tone. Particularly serious problems at surgery are frequently caused by the "kidney position," extreme Trendelenburg position, pressure of abdominal packs, traction on thoracic vessels, and sudden movement of the patient such as occurs at the end of the procedure.

The treatment of acute failure of cardiac output, cardiac arrest, should be directed toward the removal of the offending agent or process, if it can be determined. Elimination of the inhalation anesthetic by vigorous ventilation with oxygen both removes the depressant action of the anesthetic and corrects possible hypoxia or hypercarbia. The high concentration of oxygen will aid the severely depressed cardiovascular function in the maintenance of at least minimal oxygen transport to the cells. However, increased intrathoracic pressure decreases venous return and may reduce cardiac output; consequently, care must be exercised with ventilation so that adequate venous return is permitted. Inadequate venous return due to deficient circulating blood volume can be improved by a rapid infusion of balanced salt solution, plasma, or whole blood.

If vasomotor depression is a serious consideration, e.g., with spinal or epidural anesthesia, sympathomimetic amines, ranging in potency from ephedrine to epinephrine and norepinephrine, should be selected for administration according to the degree of cardiovascular depression. Both myocardial stimulation and vasoconstriction may be useful in the severely depressed heart. If circulation is severely depressed, these drugs may be administered by an intracardiac route unless the circulation is effectively reestablished by external cardiac massage. Since irreversible changes occur in the central nervous system with periods of hypoxia over 3 or 4 min, immediate institution of cardiac massage is essential if evidence of adequate circulation cannot be obtained. When cardiac action cannot be readily reestablished, epinephrine and norepinephrine are the most useful drugs. Patients with metabolic derangements or those who have suffered inadequate circulation for a significant period of time will be acidotic and will require treatment with sodium bicarbonate. Although approximation of dosage may be made, a determination of blood pH, P_{CO_2}, and HCO_3 will permit accurate evaluation of the acid-base balance.

Ventricular fibrillation, often associated with cardiac arrest, requires defibrillation. It is important that the myocardium be oxygenated and a normal acid-base balance established. Difficult cases which revert to ventricular fibrillation after electroshock can often be satisfactorily defibrillated with lidocaine, starting with doses of 100 to 200 mg by the intravenous or intracardiac route.

In general, anesthesia introduces some degree of hazard to cardiac function. After a careful appraisal of the patient's general condition and in particular of his cardiovascular status, a physician experienced in the use of anesthetic agents and responsible for their administration should select the anesthetic agent and technique. He will need to weigh carefully the advantages and disadvantages of the alternative techniques, although long experience with a given technique may override the reputed pharmacologic advantages of newer, less well-established methods of anesthetic management. With careful attention to ventilation, dosage, and the pharmacologic properties of these agents, the deleterious effect of these drugs can be reduced so that even a very sick patient will tolerate the necessary operative and diagnostic procedures.

REFERENCES

1 Price, Henry L.: "Circulation during Anesthesia and Operation," Charles C Thomas, Publisher, Springfield, Ill., 1967.
2 Morrow, D. H.: Anesthesia and Digitalis Toxicity: IV, *Anesth. Analg.*, 46:675, 1967.
3 Beller, B. M.: Digitalis and Anesthesia: A Comprehensive Review of the Chemistry, Pharmacology and Clinical Use of the Cardiac Glycosides in Anesthesia, in H. N. Zauder (ed.), "Pharmacology of Adjuvant Drugs," Clinical Anesthesia Series, vol. 10, no. 1, F. A. Davis Company, Philadelphia, 1973.
4 Katz, R. L., and Bigger, J. T.: Cardiac Arrhythmias during Anesthesia and Operation, *Anesthesiology*, 33:193, 1970.
5 Matteo, R. S., Katz, R. L., and Papper, E. M.: The Injection of Epinephrine during General Anesthesia with Halogenated Hydrocarbons and Cyclopropane in Man, *Anesthesiology*, 24:327, 1963.
6 Lippman, M., and Reisner, L. S.: Epinephrine Injection with Enflurane Anesthesia: Incidence of Cardiac Arrhythmias, *Anesth. Analg.*, 53:886, 1974.
7 Schoenstadt, D. A., and Whitcher, C. E.: Observations on the Mechanism of Succinyldicholine-induced Cardiac Arrhythmias, *Anesthesiology*, 24:358, 1963.
8 Carden, N. L., and Steinhaus, J. E.: Lidocaine in Cardiac Resuscitation from Ventricular Fibrillation, *Circ. Res.*, 4:680, 1956.
9 Harrison, D. C., Sprouse, J. H., and Morrow, A. G.: The Antiarrhythmic Properties of Lidocaine and Procaine Amide, *Circulation*, 28:486, 1963.
10 Johnstone, M.: Reflections on Beta-adrenergic Blockade in Anesthetics, *Br. J. Anaesth.*, 42:262, 1970.
11 Brown, J. M.: Anesthesia and the Contractile Force of the Heart, *Anesth. Analg.*, 39:487, 1960.
12 Shimosato, S., and Etsten, B. E.: Effect of Anesthetic Drugs on the Heart: A Critical Review of Myocardial Contractility and its Relationship to Hemodynamics, in L. Fabian (ed.), "A Decade of Clinical Progress," Clinical Anesthesia Series, vol. 7, no. 3, F. A. Davis Company, Philadelphia, 1971.
13 Strauer, B. E.: Contractile Responses to Morphine, Piritramide, Meperidine, and Fentanyl, *Anesthesiology*, 37:304, 1972.
14 Lowenstein, E., Hallowell, P., and Levine, P. H., et al.: Cardiovascular Responses to Large Doses of Intravenous Morphine in Man, *N. Engl. J. Med.*, 281:1389, 1969.
15 McDermott, R. W., and Stanley, T. H.: The Cardiovascular Effects of Low Concentrations of Nitrous Oxide during Morphine Anesthesia, *Anesthesiology*, 41:89, 1974.
16 Stewart, D. M., Rogers, W. P., Mahaffery, J. E., Witherspoon, S., and Woods, E. F.: Effect of Local Anesthetics on the Cardiovascular System of the Dog, *Anesthesiology*, 24:620, 1963.
17 Wynands, J. E., Sheridan, C. A., Batra, M. S., et al.: Coronary Artery Disease, *Anesthesiology*, 33:260, 1970.
18 Kaplan, J. A., Dunbar, R. W., and Jones, E. L.: Nitroglycerin Infusion during Coronary-Artery Surgery, *Anesthesiology*, 45:14, 1976.
19 Kaplan, J. A., Dunbar, R. W., Bland, J. W., et al.: Propranolol and Cardiac Surgery: A Problem for the Anesthesiologist? *Anesth. Analg.*, 54:571, 1975.
20 Kelman, G. R., Nunn, J. F., Prys-Roberts, C., and Greenbaum, R.: The Influence of Cardiac Output on Arterial Oxygenation: A Theoretical Study, *Br. J. Anaesth.*, 39:450, 1967.

95
Surgery in Patients with Heart Disease

A
Medical Management in Noncardiac Surgery

R. BRUCE LOGUE, M.D., and
JOEL A. KAPLAN, M.D.

There are numerous complications involving the cardiovascular system which may occur during surgical treatment or in the postoperative period. These may develop in the presence of a normal cardiovascular system but are more frequent in the presence of heart disease.[1] The incidence and risks associated with such complications are determined by the type and severity of the cardiovascular disease, the magnitude of the surgical procedure, and the expertise of the surgeon, anesthesiologist, and attending physician.

An evaluation of the patient's status prior to surgical treatment may be obtained relatively simply by analyzing the findings gathered from the history, the physical examination, the electrocardiogram, the chest roentgenogram, and the routine examination of the blood and urine. One should determine the following: (1) Is there evidence of heart disease? (2) Is there a history of angina pectoris or myocardial infarction? (3) Is there cardiac enlargement? (4) Are there symptoms or signs of congestive heart failure? (5) Is there significant disturbance of cardiac rhythm such as atrial fibrillation? (6) Is there significant hypertensive disease or postural hypotension? (7) Is there evidence or any symptom of cerebrovascular disease or syncope? (8) Is there evidence of chronic lung disease? (9) Is there a history or evidence of old or recent phlebitis? (10) Has the patient been on antihypertensive or cardiac medication, or has he or she previously received corticosteroids? (11) Is there evidence of kidney disease or prostatic obstruction?

The signs and symptoms associated with heart disease are discussed in Chaps. 12 to 24. Although the details will not be repeated here, a few points deserve emphasis. The history must include a careful search for chest discomfort, dyspnea, palpitation, syncope, cough, hemoptysis, wheezing, cerebral ischemic attacks, and calf pain. The physical examination may give evidence of cerebrovascular disease by the presence of carotid bruits, diminished or absent carotid pulsations, Hollenhorst plaques in the retina, or significant differences in the blood pressure in the arms. Cardiac enlargement is revealed by the presence of a large, sustained apex impulse of left ventricular hypertrophy or the sustained parasternal lift of right ventricular hypertrophy. A visible or audible ventricular diastolic gallop may be the clue to myocardial insufficiency with the need for digitalization. Heart murmurs must be specifically sought for, since the murmurs of mitral stenosis, aortic stenosis, and faint aortic regurgitation are often overlooked. Pulmonary rales may be due to failure of the left side of the heart but are common with chronic lung disease; it is emphasized that failure of the left side of the heart manifested by interstitial edema may be present without rales or ventricular diastolic gallop rhythm and may be detected solely by the roentgenogram. Abnormal venous distension or pulsations may indicate failure of the right side of the heart or pericardial effusion, and pulsus alternans indicates left ventricular myocardial failure. Hepatomegaly without other signs or symptoms is unreliable evidence of heart failure, since it may be due to a hyperesthetic build, to emphysema with depression of the diaphragm, or to intrinsic liver disease. Edema is a late manifestation of congestive heart failure and may be due to noncardiac causes. The rate and rhythm of the heart may furnish evidence of cardiac arrhythmia, such as atrial fibrillation or complete heart block. Prior to surgical treatment one should record the pulses in all extremities and palpate the abdominal aorta for evidence of aneurysm, so that possible embolic or thrombotic complications of

surgical treatment can be evaluated. In the male it is very wise to know the status of the prostate gland prior to surgical treatment.

The electrocardiogram is commonly misused and my give a false sense of security (see Chaps. 23, 28A, and 62E). It may be normal when heart failure is present or when the patient is having life-threatening angina decubitus, and it is commonly normal 6 months or so following myocardial infarction. It gives no indication of the need for digitalis or of when a patient may be optimally digitalized. It may furnish important evidence of overdigitalization, atrioventricular (AV) or bundle branch block, or various cardiac arrhythmias. It may identify prior unsuspected myocardial infarction; some studies indicate that as many as one-third of infarcts were previously unrecognized. It is very important to have a base-line tracing, so that alterations during or after surgical treatment may be evaluated, particularly since myocardial infarction is often unaccompanied by pain, either because infarction occurred during anesthesia or because it was obscured by opiate administration or normal postoperative discomfort. All patients over the age of 40 years should have a preoperative electrocardiogram, as should any patient with signs or symptoms of heart disease. Treadmill exercise tests are very helpful in identifying the presence of ischemic heart disease, in judging its severity, and in bringing into focus symptoms not previously related to the heart by the patient. In selected instances, coronary arteriography may be helpful in demonstrating normal coronary arteries in the patient with a previous diagnosis of coronary disease or in defining the anatomy and extent of coronary artery disease. If disease is present, some information may be obtained regarding prognosis. There may be exceptional instances in which the patient with severe coronary symptoms may require revascularization surgery prior to operation for other disease.

A chest roentgenogram is needed for a complete examination, since interstitial pulmonary edema may be the only clue that heart failure is present (see Chap. 44). The film may reveal cardiac enlargement, a diagnostic cardiac contour, and unsuspected lung and aortic disease. Obviously, when the patient is quite ill, a good film is difficult to obtain and the diagnostic value decreases, but it is still useful.

The routine examination of the blood may reveal anemia, which may require proper diagnosis and treatment prior to surgical treatment. The margin of safety is not as great in patients with cardiovascular disease, and the degrees of anemia ordinarily tolerated by otherwise healthy persons may not be tolerated by patients with heart disease. Postoperative complications are so difficult to predict that it is useful to measure preoperatively the serum concentrations of sodium, potassium, and chloride, and total CO_2 content. All patients taking digitalis or diuretics should have their potassium checked preoperatively. The hematocrit, body weight, levels of serum electrolytes, and output of fluid are all necessary information when intravenous fluid replacement must be continued for a long period of time. Fasting blood sugar and blood urea nitrogen measurements may be needed in the preoperative evaluation of some patients. This especially applies to patients with renal disease, hypertension, or congestive heart failure, and when there is a history of diabetes. Patients with renal disease should have a 24-h creatinine clearance test. Coagulation studies may be required in patients taking Coumadin, heparin, or aspirin.

The routine examination of the urine may reveal albumin, glucose, red blood cell casts, and white blood cell casts. These abnormalities may require therapy prior to an elective operative procedure.

The following discussion highlights the unique features associated with each category of heart disease which influence the evaluation and management of the patient undergoing surgical treatment.

Coronary atherosclerotic heart disease

Coronary atherosclerotic heart disease is the major hazard to the adult over the age of 40. Many studies indicate that the patient with this disease can undergo major surgery with relatively small risk.[2-8] The disease may be asymptomatic and totally unsuspected, but in the overwhelming majority of patients it is recognized by a history of angina pectoris or previous infarction. Unfortunately, the first evidence may be sudden death. Knapp et al.,[9] in a study of 8,984 males over the age of 50, found the following incidence of postoperative coronary occlusion: The incidence of postoperative coronary occlusion was 0.7 percent in the group composed of 8,557 patients who had no preoperative history of coronary disease. The mortality in those who developed coronary occlusion was 18 percent. The incidence of postoperative coronary occlusion was 6 percent in the group composed of 427 patients who had a history of preoperative coronary occlusion. The mortality in those who developed postoperative coronary occlusion was 58 percent. Of patients with a history of preoperative coronary occlusion less than 2 years prior to surgical treatment, 46 percent had a postoperative occlusion. Thus the chances of recurrent infarction are greatly enhanced if the infarction occurs within 24 months. This suggests a factor of selection, since many patients with severe residual disease do not live 2 years in order to undergo surgery. On the other hand, Thompson et al.[10] found no greater mortality in patients having transurethral prostatectomy within 6 months of infarction. The mortality rate of 674 patients undergoing prostatic surgery was 0.74 percent; 131 had coronary disease and the mortality in this group was 0.76 percent.[11] The mortality rate was 4.7 percent in 192 patients. Only 1 of 23 patients receiving an operation within 6 months of prior infarction died. Arkins et al.[12] followed 1,005 patients with coronary atherosclerotic heart disease subjected to operation within 2 months; the mortality rate

was 22.3 percent, or double that of patients in the same age group who had no diagnosis of coronary heart disease. Of 27 patients who had sustained occlusion within 3 months preoperatively, the mortality rate was 40 percent; 10 of 13 patients with transmural infarction died immediately; 1 of 14 with subendocardial infarction died. A total of 55 instances of postoperative myocardial infarction was noted, with a mortality rate of 69 percent.

In a series of 32,877 operations on patients over 30 under general anesthesia, Tarhan found that 422 patients had experienced prior myocardial infarction.[13] During the first postoperative week 6.6 percent of this group experienced another infarction. The incidence of infarction was 37 percent in those operated on within 3 months and 16 percent when operation was performed within 3 to 6 months of the prior attack. The incidence was approximately 4 to 5 percent when the preceding infarction occurred more than 6 months before surgery. The largest percentage of reinfarction, 33 percent, occurred on the third postoperative day, while only 18 percent occurred on the first postoperative day. The mortality rate was 54 percent with 80 percent of deaths occurring within 48 h. Reinfarction was more frequent in surgery in the thorax or the upper part of the abdomen and was independent of the type of anesthesia or the duration of surgery. The incidence of infarction in those without angina or prior infarction was 0.13 percent.

Therefore, the major factors in determining the incidence of reinfarction appear to be (1) the time interval from the myocardial infarction—from Tarhan's recent study,[13] it appears that 6 months is a safe period to wait after a myocardial infarction for elective surgery; (2) the type of infarction—the risk appears to be much greater with a transmural infarction than a subendocardial infarction; (3) complications after the myocardial infarction such as congestive heart failure and arrhythmias; (4) the type of surgery—diagnostic procedures with general anesthesia hold very low risk compared to major surigcal procedures;[15] (5) location of the surgery—thoracic and upper abdominal procedures have higher complication rates than peripheral procedures; (6) skill of the anesthesiologist in dealing with patients with acute cardiovascular disease—the use of modern monitoring equipment, such as the Swan-Ganz catheter, allows the anesthesiologist to evaluate the functions of the heart during surgery much more precisely; (7) recently, use of the intraaortic balloom pump placed before induction of anesthesia in patients with acute myocardial infarctions brought to surgery—a few have survived emergency surgery within days of an acute myocardial infarction using this technique.[16]

The limitations of the electrocardiogram in recognizing postoperative infarction is highlighted by the studies of Mauney et al.[14] who observed 9 deaths due to myocardial infarction without change of the postoperative electrocardiogram, and in only 2 of 9 was there clinical suspicion of infarction. One patient had minimal ischemia and died of myocardial infarction confirmed by autopsy; two additional asymptomatic patients with T-wave inversions were not thought to have myocardial infarcts, but these were documented at postmortem examination. The incidence of myocardial infarction in this study of patients over 50 was 8.8 percent with a mortality of 53 percent. Only 20 of 30 showed diagnostic electrocardiographic changes. The composition of the group studied consisted of 365 patients with no history of myocardial infarction within 2 years and abnormal electrocardiograms as follows:

1 Evidence of old myocardial infarction
2 Bundle branch block
3 Left ventricular hypertrophy or strain
4 ST-T changes of subendocardial injury

The problem of identification of the patient with asymptomatic coronary disease is difficult, since even in the presence of a history of angina pectoris, the electrocardiogram is normal in more than one-half of patients. Furthermore, a documented history of prior myocardial infarction is more reliable than electrocardiographic demonstration of such an event. In a study of 3,000 sudden deaths due to coronary disease there were 775 autopsies.[17] A history of prior infarction correlated with the demonstration of healed infarction in 92 percent of males and 85 percent of females. With no history of prior infarction, evidence of old infarcts was found in 57 percent of males and 49 percent of females. Most subendocardial infarcts produce no electrocardiographic changes, and even when such are present, they generally subside within weeks. In one study of 175 patients with myocardial infarction and only ST-T wave changes, the electrocardiogram returned to normal within 1 year in 54 percent; only 5.6 percent with Q wave abnormalities returned to normal.[18] Often the electrocardiogram may exhibit a pattern compatible with left ventricular hypertrophy. Thus, in a series of 150 autopsied cases, only 75 percent of acute and 20 percent of old infarcts could be diagnosed by the electrocardiogram, and in 50 percent of the old infarcts there was only the pattern of left ventricular hypertrophy.[19] Pruitt et al.[20] emphasized that infarcts are difficult to recognize when they are small, healed, subendocardial infarcts, or if they involve the lateral wall. These authors conclude: "In many instances electrocardiographic diagnosis is more than obscure—it is impossible." With the limitations noted, the electrocardiogram remains the best method of detection of myocardial infarction during surgery or the postoperative period.

The mortality of a myocardial infarction incident to anesthesia and surgery as of this date is more than three times greater than that occurring unrelated to operation and treated in a coronary care unit. These figures are incongruous in view of the reasonably small risk of coronary artery bypass surgery in patients with severe disease and even occasionally in the presence of recent myocardial infarction. The application of the same type of care given the coronary patient in coronary care units would undoubtedly reduce the distressing mortality of myocardial infarction incident to surgery. Thus, constant monitoring of the heart rhythm, control of arrhythmia, early detection and treatment of left-sided heart failure, and careful monitoring of the filling pressures of the heart clincially or by the Swan-Ganz catheter would surely reduce the distressing mortality rate.

Patients with acute cholecystitis, prostatic obstruction, intestinal obstruction, and malignant conditions amenable to surgery fare better with a bolder approach rather than with conservative temporizing.

In assessing the patient's status preoperatively, it is important to elicit a history of angina pectoris, but more important is the determination of whether it has been stable for months or years or whether there has been a recent change in pattern. Does it occur only with strenuous exertion or with mild exercise? Does it occur at rest or nocturnally? Is the discomfort prolonged beyond the usual 3 to 5 min? Does discomfort require repeated doses of nitroglycerin or opiates for relief? With stable angina, the risk of anesthesia and major surgery may vary from 1 to 3 percent, but if it is progressive or occurs at rest, the risk is much greater. With good cardiac reserve and either no angina or stable angina, the risk is enhanced if there has been infarction within 3 months; it is less when infarction has occurred within 3 to 6 months, and it is still less when infarction has occurred a year or more prior to contemplated surgery.

The threshold of angina may be determined by the product of the blood pressure and pulse rate. Sudden increase in either parameter may induce ischemic pain. Adequate sedation and prophylactic nitrites are helpful when given prior to moving the patient to the operative suite. Sublingual isosorbide dinitrate (Isordil) 2.5 to 5.0 mg may be given, or 1 in. of 2 percent nitroglycerin ointment may be applied to the skin, but only if the patient's tolerance to this dose has been established and there is no postural hypotension. Acute rise of pulse and blood pressure may be counteracted by 1 to 2 mg of propranolol given intravenously before anesthesia. During general anesthesia, intravenous doses of 0.25 mg propranolol up to 1 to 2 mg will control tachycardia. Severe hypertension is treated with vasodilator agents such as sodium nitroprusside or nitroglycerin administered by intravenous infusions.[21,21a]

Hypertension

There are no definitive studies which show that mild to moderate essential hypertension appreciably increases the risk of general anesthesia and surgery. Symptomatic or asymptomatic coronary, cerebral, and renal vascular diseases are the major risk factors that place the hypertensive patient in the American Society of Anesthesiologists (ASA) physical status II or III risk categories.[22]

Tarazi has shown that hypertensive patients not taking antihypertensive drugs have a decreased plasma volume. This may be accentuated in those patients on chronic diuretic treatment.[23] This adds to the risk of surgery and anesthesia. The blood pressure should be recorded with the patient standing, in order to detect postural hypotension. When such hypotension is detected, it may be corrected by administration of plasma protein fraction intravenously (Plasmanate) prior to surgery.

The danger of general anesthesia for patients taking reserpine was first reported in 1955.[24,25] This was based on a few individual case reports and the theoretical danger of catecholamine depletion. Since that time, a number of studies have shown that (1) the hypertensive patient, even in the absence of treatment, frequently has marked fluctuation of blood pressure during general anesthesia; and (2) the patient maintained on his or her therapy until surgery has the lowest incidence of both hypotension and hypertension.[26] There is no evidence that discontinuing drug therapy 1 to 2 weeks preoperatively diminishes the likelihood of hypotension or other complications during anesthesia. Preoperative use of antihypertensive agents such as alpha-methyldopa or guanethidine may affect the anesthetic course, but the discontinuation of an effective therapeutic regimen may result in more serious sequelae. If a pressor drug is required during surgery, one with a direct action is preferable in reduced dosage. Most anesthesiologists today look upon the drug-treated hypertensive patient as a good risk candidate for anesthesia.[27]

Hypertensive patients frequently become more hypertensive during surgery and in the postoperative period. Their marked elevations of blood pressure should be controlled acutely to prevent myocardial or cerebral damage. Intraoperatively, sodium nitroprusside (Nipride) (50 mg/500 cc), trimethapan (Arfonad) (500 mg/500 cc), nitroglycerin (8 mg/250 cc), or phentolamine (Regitine) have been used. Postoperatively the intravenous infusion may be continued or therapy changed to intermittent bolus doses of diazoxide (Hyperstat) (250 mg) or regular antihypertensive medication.

Valvular heart disease

Aortic stenosis and insufficiency of severe degree pose a small hazard of sudden death due to ventricular fibrillation. Patients with mild or moderate disease tolerate anesthesia satisfactorily. Those with predominant mitral insufficiency which is well compensated run little increased risk. Those with tight mitral stenosis of class III or IV (New York Heart Association functional classification) may undergo surgical treatment with a slight increase in incidence of pulmonary edema. Even corrective surgical treatment in the form of valvuloplasty in class III patients carries a risk of only 1 to 3 percent. Care to avoid overloading with blood or saline solution during surgical treatment and during the postoperative period is mandatory. Sudden supraventricular arrhythmias in these patients can pose a serious hazard. Patients with valvular heart disease, including Barlow's syndrome, should receive antibiotic prophylaxis to prevent endocarditis. Hypertrophic subaortic stenosis is associated with some increase in risk of sudden death and propranolol (Inderal) should be given before and during surgery.

Congenital heart disease

Patients with congenital heart disease with left-to-right shunts but with good cardiac compensation undergo only a slight increase in risk with anesthesia and surgical treatment. Children with cyanotic congenital heart disease such as tetralogy of Fallot frequently tolerate general anesthesia fairly well. It is critical not to increase the right-to-left shunt by decreasing the afterload with vasodilating anesthetic drugs like enflurane (Ethrane) or halothane (Fluothane) or to increase the pulmonary artery pressure with techniques such as positive end-expiratory pressure. A peripheral vasoconstrictor is occasionally needed in these children to increase the blood pressure and decrease the right-to-left shunt and thus increase the P_{a,O_2}.[28] These patients seem to do very well with the sympathomimetic anesthetic drugs such as ketamine (Ketalar).[29] It is also important to avoid the intravenous injection of any air bubbles with their attendant cerebral or coronary embolization. Patients with congenital heart disease should receive appropriate antibiotics following surgical treatment to minimize the risk of bacterial endocarditis.

Lung disease

Patients with pulmonary disease have an increased anesthetic risk and are subject to postoperative complications. If the patient is able to walk up several flights of stairs without undue dyspnea, there is little anesthetic risk. Those with chronic bronchitis due to smoking have increased bronchial secretions and bronchospasm and are particularly subject to postoperative atelectasis and pneumonia. Hodgkin et al.[30] list the following points in the history and physical to evaluate pulmonary disease: "(1) History of cough, (2) production of sputum, (3) degree of dyspnea, (4) exercise intolerance, (5) smoking, (6) presence of chest pain, (7) coexisting cardiac disease, (8) adequacy of chest expansion, (9) evidence of slowed air flow or forced expiration, (10) use of accessory muscles of respiration with quiet breathing, (11) rales, (12) rhonchi, (13) murmurs." The tests that may indicate unsuitability for anesthesia and surgery, as listed in their paper, are as follows: "(1) Maximum voluntary ventilation or MBC less than 50% of predicted, (2) elevation of P_{a,CO_2}, (3) forced expiratory volume in 1 sec less than 0.50, (4) maximum midexpiratory flow less than 0.6 l/sec., (5) maximum expiratory flow less than 100 l/min., (6) vital capacity less than 1 liter, (7) abnormal EKG, (8) severe hypoxemia with P_{a,O_2} less than 55 mm Hg, (9) failure of improvement after bronchodilator, (1) grossly abnormal xenon ventilation-perfusion scan."

Patients with chronic bronchitis and lung disease should omit smoking for several days (and preferably weeks) prior to surgical treatment. Preoperative preparation of the cardiac patient with chronic lung disease with expectorants, bronchodilators, chest exercises, and the use of aerosol with intermittent positive-pressure breathing may be needed to improve vital capacity and to clear bronchial secretions. Atropine sulfate and scopolamine are usually avoided because of their drying effect on the bronchial mucosa. Preanesthetic medication may induce dangerous respiratory depression in patients with lung disease. For example, serious respiratory depression may occur in patients with emphysema after an average dose of morphine sulfate or barbiturate. Alveolar ventilation is reduced by most anesthetics, positioning on the table, thoracotomy, retained secretions, infections, and bronchospasm. Hypercarbia and hypoxia may occur and predispose to arrhythmia, impaired myocardial contractility, hyperkalemia, and cardiac arrest. Respiration in the patient with chronic obstructive pulmonary disease may be assisted during the postoperative period with an endotracheal tube and a mechanical ventilator. Recently, intermittent mandatory ventilation (IMV) has been shown to be extremely useful in weaning these patients off mechanical ventilation.[31] Pulmonary function should be monitored by serial determinations of arterial blood gases.

Cerebral vascular disease

The major problem in cerebral vascular disease is not hemorrhage but cerebral infarction. Patients should be questioned regarding symptoms of cerebral ischemia; the carotid arteries should be palpated and checked for evidence of carotid bruits. Hollenhorst plaques in the retina should be sought. Postural hypotension should be detected and corrected by volume expansion with plasma protein fraction. Unfortunately, many patients with arteriosclerotic systolic hypertension are given unwarranted and hazardous treatment with chlorothiazide or reserpine derivatives; these agents should be omitted. Anesthesia and surgery, through their effect on the autonomic nervous system, blood volume, position, and cardiac output, may increase hypotension and cerebral vascular accidents. Patients with a history of recurrent attacks of transient cerebral ischemia pose a particular hazard. It is essential to avoid hypovolemia during surgery and in the immediate postoperative period. The elderly person often has bradycardia, which may be spontaneous, associated with disease of the sinus node or AV node with AV block, or related to therapy with drugs such as digitalis, propranolol, or reserpine. Bradycardia may be controlled by atropine (0.5 mg intravenously) or isoproterenol, 1 mg/liter 5 percent glucose intravenously. The drugs should not be given at the same time because of the danger of inducing ventricular tachycardia or ventricular fibrillation. Control of arrhythmia to maintain adequate cerebral perfusion is important.

Congestive heart failure

Compensated congestive heart failure (CHF) may produce a modest increase in risk. The cardiac reserve should be estimated by determining whether the patient is able to carry on normal activities without symptoms of congestive heart failure. If the patient develops dyspnea on walking one block or has paroxysmal nocturnal dyspnea, the operative risk is increased. If he can walk up several flights of steps without symptoms, there is little hazard from the standpoint of congestive heart failure. It is useful to classify the function according to the criteria of the New York Heart Association.[32]

Patients with chronic CHF often exhibit hyponatremia. This hyponatremia is associated with excessive total body sodium content but even more excessive total body water content. In addition they often have a total body deficiency of potassium, frequently despite normal serum potassium levels. Fluid restriction is usually beneficial in management of the hyponatremia. Vigorous diuresis is particularly likely to induce hypokalemia, which may be associated with arrhythmias like those from digitalis intoxication. It is better to take the cardiac patient to surgery with some excess fluid aboard than to attempt reaching "dry weight" by vigorous diuresis. Furthermore, some patients with advanced heart failure have improved cardiac function with increased filling pressure at levels of venous pressure which might ordinarily be considered too high. Patients with chronic congestive failure often have an elevated blood volume, and if this is contracted by excessive diuresis, it may predispose to hypotension when anesthesia is given. A clue to an inadequate volume is postural hypotension.

Lactic acidosis may occur in the setting of poor tissue perfusion secondary to impaired cardiac output. When the pH decreases to 7.10, the myocardial contractility may be reduced by 50 percent. Arrhythmias and AV conduction disturbances occur, and ventricular fibrillation is the common terminal event. An unusually wide anion gap (serum sodium minus the sum of chloride and total CO_2 content) may offer the first clue to the reduced arterial pH. At the bedside a clue may be tachypnea with no evidence of pulmonary edema. It is treated temporarily by intravenous administration of sodium bicarbonate while other efforts are made to improve cardiac output.

Digitalization should be accomplished some days prior to surgery so that a maintenance dose free of toxicity can be established. Digitalis is indicated

1 When there is history of previous congestive heart failure
2 When there is evidence of myocardial insufficiency such as ventricular gallop rhythm, pulsus alternans, pulmonary rales, interstitial edema appearing on the roentgenogram, or abnormal neck vein distension
3 In patients with nocturnal angina
4 In patients with atrial fibrillation or flutter
5 In patients with frequent attacks of atrial or nodal tachycardia

Some authors feel that patients over 60 with an enlarged heart but no symptoms should be digitalized. Braunwald has demonstrated decreased oxygen utilization in patients with enlarged but compensated hearts.[33] There are those who feel that routine preoperative digitalization of the cardiac patient should be avoided.[34] Patients with symptomatic coronary disease have a shocking incidence of areas of impaired myocardial contractility when studied by ventriculography. Such patients are surely at increased risk of developing arrhythmias or heart failure under the stress of anesthesia and surgery. There can be no reasonable objection to digitalization in such patients who have cardiomegaly or any symptoms or signs of dysfunction. In one study 120 patients undergoing open heart surgery were digitalized, and no evidence of toxicity was noted. The authors recommend prophylactic digitalization.[34a] When atrial fibrillation is present, the apical rate should be in the range of 80 at rest and no greater than 100 with mild activity.[35] In cases in which digitalization has been previously carried out, the patient's status should be reviewed to determine whether additional drug is needed or whether the dose should be temporarily omitted or reduced because of evidence of toxicity.

Certain symptoms of underdigitalization may mimic those of overdigitalization: (1) nausea and vomiting due to visceral congestion, and (2) frequent ventricular ectopic beats, bigeminy, or ventricular tachycardia. Toxicity may be evidenced by symptoms but is more often indicated by frequent ventricular premature beats (particularly if multifocal), bigeminy, sinus bradycardia, AV block, interference dissociation, nonparoxysmal nodal tachycardia, or atrial tachycardia with block (see Chaps. 45 and 109). A long rhythm strip showing prominent P waves, such as lead II or V_1, combined with carotid massage may be needed for detection of toxicity. Diuresis with compartmental shifts of sodium, potassium, and other ions may aggravate or precipitate digitalis intoxication.[36] Serum levels of digoxin may be useful where there is questionable evidence of toxicity. Cyclopropane, through mobilization of catecholamines, may decrease tolerance to digitalis, while halothane may increase tolerance. In the postoperative period, fever, atelectasis, or the development of atrial fibrillation may require increased amounts of digitalis. Respiratory alkalosis due to hyperventilation from the use of ventilators may be associated with a shift of potassium from the extracellular to the intracellular compartment and induce digitalis toxicity. The same occurs with metabolic alkalosis from vomiting and gastric or biliary drainage. Postoperative oliguria may be associated with a decreased clearance of creatinine and digitalis. The occurrence of renal failure demands reduction of the maintenance dose by 50 percent. In dogs only 40 percent of the control toxic dose is required to produce ventricular tachycardia if the serum potassium level is lowered to 2 mEq/liter.[35] Furthermore, the animal is more sensitive to digitalis intoxication induced by anoxia and circulatory loading. The myocardial threshold can also be reduced by potassium shift from extracellular to intracellular compartment without any external loss. Thus, digitalis intoxication may follow rapid lowering of potassium by administration of sodium chloride, sodium bicarbonate, glucose, or insulin. When low concentrations of potassium are given in glucose to the patient with hypokalemia, the serum potassium level may fall instead of rising; thus Kunin et al.[37] noted that the serum potassium level failed to rise in 8 and fell in 10 of 21 potassium-depleted patients for periods ranging from 15 to 20 min. Dangerous ventricular arrhythmias were noted in 2 patients. Arrhythmias may also be induced in the potassium-depleted nondigitalized patient. Hypokalemia is treated by 30 to 40 mEq potassium chloride in 500 ml 5 percent glucose intravenously. Rarely, more rapid repletion may require a catheter be placed in the superior vena cava. Careful monitoring of urine flow, serum level of potassium, and the electrocardiogram is required.

Renal disease

Surgery may be carried out even on patients in severe renal failure. The blood pressure may be unstable due to the disease process, hypovolemia or hypervolemia, and drug therapy. Anemia is usual, and transfusion of fresh red blood cells may be given cautiously in the face of oliguria and congestive heart failure. The hyperkalemia may be aggravated by cold blood with its high potassium content. The dose of digitalis may need reduction to 50 percent of the usual dosage in the patient with renal failure. General anesthesia may be safely administered with a variety of agents, but their dosages may have to be reduced. Anesthetic drugs to be avoided include methoxyflurane (Penthrane) and enflurane (Ethrane), due to their renal fluoride ion toxicity; ketamine due to hypertension; and gallamine (Flaxedil) due to its excretion solely by the kidneys. Postoperatively the serum potassium level invariably rises and may require hypertonic glucose and insulin, sodium polystyrene sulfonate (Kayexalate), or peritoneal dialysis.[38] Pericardial tamponade may require installation of insoluble steroids into the pericardial sac or pericardiectomy. Coronary bypass has been done successfully in patients with chronic heart failure.

Arrhythmias, bundle branch block, and heart block

Digitalis should be used to control the ventricular rate in patients with atrial fibrillation or flutter even though the rate may be normal, since undue acceleration may occur during anesthesia. Premature ventricular beats are commonly related to anxiety and require no therapy. If there are frequent premature ventricular beats, lidocaine may be given as a constant infusion during the procedure, using a dose of 1 to 3 mg/min after an initial bolus of 50 to 100 mg. If they are multifocal or if they interrupt the T wave, 0.2 g quinidine sulfate may be given intramuscularly 1 h prior to surgery. The significance of right or left bundle branch block depends on the type and extent of heart disease. Bundle branch block per se does not increase surgical risk.[39] Bundle branch block in persons under the age of 40 may not be associated with any other evidence of cardiac disease. A total of 394 instances of complete right bundle branch block and of 125 cases of complete left bundle branch block were noted in a review of 237,000 electrocardiograms in Air Force personnel under 40. Of those with complete right bundle branch block 97 percent and of those with complete left bundle branch block 89 percent had no obvious evidence of cardiac disease. Follow-up at 10 years showed that 6 percent had developed hypertension while 4 percent had expired. In the group with complete left bundle branch block, 5 percent had developed new evidence of coronary disease, 6 percent had developed hypertension, and 8 percent had died.[40] The presence of right bundle branch block and left anterior hemiblock with or without prolonged P-R interval may increase the risk of development of complete heart block. Prophylactic pacing should be done if there is a history of dizziness or syncope. When complete heart block is present, a temporary transvenous pacemaker is necessary for the safe conduct of surgery and anesthesia; the heart may be paced throughout the surgical procedure and postoperatively for periods of up to a week. The catheter should not be removed until it is clear that normal cardiac pacemakers have been functioning for several days without Stokes-Adams attacks. Procainamide hydrochloride (Pronestyl hydrochloride) and quinidine sulfate are contraindicated for arrhythmias that interrupt complete heart block (see Chap. 46D).

Patients with permanent pacemakers present an increased anesthetic and surgical risk.[41,42] The biggest problem is the use of the electrocautery, which frequently interferes with the pacemaker. This is much more of a problem with demand pacemakers and when the cautery is used within 12 in. of the pacemaker. Improved shielding and newly designed filters in the input circuits of the demand pacemakers have reduced but not eliminated this hazard of the electrocautery. If possible, it is preferable to place the pacemaker on the fixed rate mode during surgery when the cautery is used. The electrodes can also be displaced during thoracic and abdominal surgery with sudden loss of pacing.

General preoperative measures

When corticosteroids have been administered within 6 months, it is well to give prednisone, 40 mg, on the day before surgical treatment and for a few days thereafter. Hydrocortisone 100 mg may be given intramuscularly with the premedication, and 100 mg may be given intravenously during anesthesia if hypotension occurs. Anticoagulants may be continued for dental extractions but should be omitted prior to operations, and the prothrombin time should be at, or close to, normal.

When anemia is so severe that transfusion is needed, it is well to avoid giving whole blood to the patient with congestive heart failure or cardiomegaly, and to use instead packed red blood cells in isotonic glucose. Polycythemia predisposes to thrombosis, and phlebotomy may be helpful in minimizing such complications when the hematocrit is higher than 50 percent. Dehydration should be avoided particularly.

Electrolyte depletion should be corrected prior to surgery. Hypokalemia predisposes to arrhythmias and sensitizes the myocardium to the toxic effects of digitalis. This effect may be aggravated by the intravenous administration of glucose. It is emphasized that this may occur with a normal serum potassium level. Hyponatremia, if associated with a contracted blood volume, will predispose the patient to hypotension during anesthesia.

A prolonged fast should be avoided, and if operation is scheduled late in the day, it is desirable to maintain hydration by intravenous fluids.

It is well to know the response of the patient to opiates prior to preoperative administration. An occasional patient, particularly in the older age group, may develop hypotension or shock from the injection of an opiate. These drugs regularly decrease ventilation and hypoxia, and hypercarbia may ensue. Meperidine hydrochloride (Demerol) should be given with caution to patients with atrial flutter or fibrillation, since an occasional person may experience a sharp rise in ventricular rate because of the anticholinergic action on the conduction tissue.

It is best to avoid narcotics, barbiturates, and scopolamine in premedication for patients over the age of 65, since they may cause hypotension, hypoventilation, agitation, and stupor. Diazepam (Valium) or diphenhydramine (Benadryl) are preferred in this group of patients.

THE MANAGEMENT OF THE CARDIAC PATIENT DURING SURGICAL PROCEDURES

Choice of anesthetic

The choice of anesthesia should be left to the anesthesiologist, whose judgment and experience may dictate the type (see Chap. 94). More important than the type of anesthetic is the knowledgeable anesthesiologist. All anesthetics (1) reduce myocardial contractility, (2) impair ventilation, predisposing to hypoxia and hypercarbia, and (3) affect the autonomic nervous system, either the sympathetic or the parasympathetic branches. These latter effects may reduce arterial and venous tone and produce hypotension. The maintenance of good oxygenation of the myocardium demands a satisfactory diastolic pressure to ensure adequate coronary perfusion. The mean arterial pressure can be reduced by myocardial depression, decreased arterial tone, and reduced venous return incident to venodilatation. The impaired filling of the heart further diminishes cardiac output. Hypotension occurring with induction of the anesthesia may be due to myocardial depression by the anesthetic agent or to its effect on the sympathetic nervous system, impairing normal regulatory vasoconstriction. Adequate blood volume should be restored before induction of anesthesia. If blood volume is still questionable, ketamine may be a preferable induction agent to thiopental (Pentothal) since it supports the blood pressure in these patients.[43,44] Ketamine has given encouraging results in patients with very low cardiac outputs; this drug produces cardiac stimulation with increase in arterial blood pressure.

Though thiopental is excellent for producing a smooth induction in the anxious and excited patient, it does block sympathetic nervous tone and may produce hypotension. In normal doses, it is effective in minimizing arrhythmias, but in excessive doses it may produce myocardial depression and respiratory arrest. Because hypotension is so readily produced by thiopental, the drug must be administered carefully to patients who have coronary atherosclerotic heart disease or cerebral vascular disease.

Oxygenation of the blood is impaired by the reduction of the alveolar ventilation common to all anesthetic agents. This is why most patients under anesthesia have their respirations either assisted or controlled by the anesthesiologist. This is further accentuated by the preoperative administration of opiates and barbiturates and by positioning of the patient on the table.

Muscle relaxants are frequently used during modern anesthesia and require controlled ventilation. Succinylcholine (Anectine) may stimulate the parasympathetic nervous system and produce bradycardia, especially upon repeated doses. d-Tubocurarine (curare) frequently causes hypotension by ganglionic blockade, histamine release, and direct vasodilation. The new muscle relaxant, pancuronium bromide (Pavulon), is now almost routinely used in patients with cardiac diseases. It stimulates the cardiovascular system with a slight increase in heart rate and blood pressure. There is no histamine release or hypotension. The nondepolarizing relaxants (curare and pancuronium) have their effects reversed at the end of surgery by neostigmine (Prostigmine). Atropine is given along with neostigmine to block the muscarinic effect of this drug (salivation, bradycardia, and increased peristalsis).

Local anesthetics are not without some hazard in the patient with heart disease, since in large doses they may be absorbed into the general circulation. When this occurs, there may be an effect on the circulation, including reduction of myocardial contractility and reduction of vasomotor tone. When excessive amounts of local anesthetics are absorbed, they may produce cerebral excitement and convulsions. Because of the propensity to hypotension due to vasodilatation, high spinal anesthesia should not be used in patients with coronary atherosclerotic heart disease, pulmonary hypertension, or marginal blood volume. Should this event occur, there may be a marked reduction of venous return and stroke output which may produce cardiac arrest. Caudal, lumbar epidural, and low spinal anesthesia may be useful in perineal or lower extremity surgery in patients with coronary artery disease.

The advantage of the use of inhalation agents is that their effects can be rapidly reversed by stopping the administration and removing the agent by hyperventilation of the lungs. It is important that high concentrations of oxygen be given in conjunction with these agents. Morphine, in recent years, has become the most commonly used anesthetic agent for patients with decreased left ventricular function. Lowenstein showed that 1 mg/kg of morphine acutally increases cardiac output in patients with aortic stenosis.[45] Administered slowly (5 mg/min), hypotension is not a problem, and morphine causes no myocardial depression. Since morphine by itself does not guarantee amnesia, it is frequently combined with diazepam and/or scopolamine.[45a] Nitrous oxide is also frequently added to the morphine for further amnesia and analgesia. By itself, nitrous oxide causes little myocardial depression.[46] However, with morphine it may be a potent myocardial depressant.[47]

Patients who have coronary artery disease associated with good left ventricular function frequently become hypertensive under light general anesthesia with morphine. They require an agent that depresses their myocardium such as halothane or enflurane. Halothane has minimal effects on total peripheral resistance while enflurane decreases peripheral resistance. These latter two agents have the advantage of being administered by inhalation, and thus they are readily reversible. Halothane frequently causes arrhythmias since it sensitizes the myocardium to both exogenous and endogenous catecholamines. Enflurane is an ether-like drug and stabilizes the myocardium; thus arrhythmias are less common.

Ketamine releases endogenous catecholamines and thus causes an elevation of heart rate, blood pressure, and cardiac output. It is useful in patients with very low cardiac outputs, bradycardia, or pericardial tamponade. It should not be used in patients with critical coronary artery disease since it will markedly increase the myocardial oxygen demand.

Cyclopropane and ether are rarely used in modern anesthesia due to their explosiveness. They should probably not be used in patients with cardiac disease who require extensive electrical monitoring.

Anesthesia with halothane is often accompanied by the development of AV dissociation or various types of arrhythmias. In one series AV dissociation was noted in 13.4 percent of patients, mostly children with eye operations receiving halothane.[48] It is more common in ophthalmic procedures on children, and although it is generally benign, there is the rare danger of cardiac arrest. The vagal-stimulating effects of halothane and eye traction can be counteracted by atropine or retrobulbar lidocaine.

Endotracheal intubation is a time of marked cardiovascular stress. It is frequently associated with hypertension, tachycardia, and various arrhythmias. Endotracheal suction during anesthesia is occasionally associated with arrhythmia; one should aspirate only after a period of hyperventilation with high concentration of oxygen and should limit aspiration to 5 to 10 s. Endotracheal suction should not be done while removing the endotracheal tube, since this will lead to hypoxia, laryngeal reflexes, and laryngospasm. When introducing a suction catheter for removal of secretions, suction should not be applied during the process of introduction, since the removal of oxygen and respiratory gas mixture increases the possibility of hypoxia.

Extreme positions on the table may affect arterial and venous vascular tone. This may decrease adequate filling of the heart, with consequent drop in cardiac output. Such positions are needed for renal operations. With the kidney position, where traction is applied on large vessels, or where pressure has been placed over the abdomen, there may be pooling of blood and the induction of hypotension, either while the patient is in the exaggerated position or at the termination of the procedure. For example, it is not uncommon for hypotension to occur at the termination of the procedure when the patient is suddenly moved on the table or from the table to a stretcher.

The anesthesiologist attempts to maintain the P_{A,O_2}, the P_{CO_2}, and the pH in physiologic range. Hypoxia may be induced by excessive concentrations of the anesthetic agents, obstruction of the airway by the endotracheal tube or by secretions, excessive blood loss, hypovolemia, the development of congestive heart failure, the occurrence of arrhythmia, the development of pulmonary atelectasis, pulmonary embolism, or the development of myocardial ischemia with abrupt drop in strength of myocardial contractility. It is to be noted that hypoxia occurs when no visible cyanosis is present; indeed, the saturation of arterial blood may be reduced to as low as 70 percent before cyanosis may be detected. Warning signs may be a decrease or an increase in the pulse rate, a decrease or an increase in the blood pressure, or arrhythmias. Such signs demand lightening of the anesthetic agent, the administration of a high concentration of oxygen with hyperventilation, and a careful search for helpful remedial factors such as replacement of blood or fluid, or possible improvement in contractility by judicious use of a pressor agent. Carbon dioxide retention may produce respiratory acidosis, which impairs myocardial contractility and predisposes to impaired AV and intraventricular conduction, hyperkalemia, and ventricular fibrillation. Though all anesthetic agents reduce ventilation, this effect may be accentuated with the use of cyclopropane or isoflurane (Forane). Hypercarbia is more likely to occur in the patient with pulmonary insufficiency or following the preoperative administration of opiates. It is affected by positioning on the table, occurrence of secretions in the tracheobronchial tree, inadequate depth or frequency of respirations, the occurrence of pneumothorax, aspiration of gastric contents, pleural effusion, pulmonary infection, abdominal distension, and bronchospasm. It is prevented or corrected by relief of airway obstruction and adequate ventilation of the lungs.

Cardiac arrest

Cardiac arrest associated with anesthesia in the past occurred once in every 3,000 patients. It occurred once in every 1,000 elderly or poor risk patients, and once in 5,000 healthy, good risk patients.[49] Cardiac arrest was reported in 24 cases of a series of 75,556 operations under general anesthesia and 6,115 operations under spinal anesthesia.[50] It was more common in infants less than 1 year of age, developing in 1 out of 700 operations.[51] Normally, warning signs were present before arrest occurred. More often hypoxia was present. Tachycardia, bradycardia, hypotension, acute hypertension, or arrhythmia may precede the cardiac arrest. Hypercarbia may be the major physiologic disturbance. An analysis of 651 deaths at operation in patients over 65 revealed that 115 were due in whole or in part to anesthesia. In 29 the anesthetic agent was thought to be the primary cause, and in 86 it was a contributing cause. There was thus an incidence of 16.1 anesthetic deaths per 100,000 operations, as compared with 3.8 per 10,000 for all ages. The two leading causes of death were (1) aspiration of vomitus and (2) hypoventilation due to neuromuscular blockade.[52] This study was completed prior to 1965. Since then there has been a dramatic improvement in preoperative preparation of patients, anesthetic management, intraoperative monitoring, and postoperative care. Today, intraoperative deaths are quite rare and usually are related to the patient's underlying disease state.

Monitoring

An added margin of safety is afforded by electrocardiographic monitoring of the cardiac rhythm and conduction during surgery. It should be pointed out, however, that the rate, rhythm, and conduction may be normal when there is virtually no cardiac output and cardiac arrest is impending.[53] Thus there is a dissociation between the electrical activity of the heart and its mechanical pumping. This necessitates monitoring of the blood pressure and continuous listening to the heart tones with a chest or esophageal stethoscope. The electroencephalogram may give additional information regarding oxygenation of the brain. For all patients with cardiac disease, a dc defibrillator should be immediately available. In the event of cardiac arrest, prompt cardioversion could be attempted instead of valuable time being lost. Experience in coronary care units indicates that the majority of arrests are due to ventricular fibrillation and that cardiac activity can often be restored within 1 min. If there is no response to a single shock, the usual measures for cardiopulmonary resuscitation must be employed (see Chap. 50). Direct intraarterial monitoring of blood pressure should be undertaken in all patients with severe cardiac or pulmonary disease. This allows continuous blood pressure recording, and the arterial line permits frequent arterial blood gas determinations. The radial artery is usually cannulated percutaneously after checking for adequate collateral ulnar flow. There is minimal morbidity with use of 18- or 20-gauge Teflon catheters.[53a] Central venous pressure is monitored in patients with congestive heart failure undergoing major surgery. The catheter is placed in the superior vena cava either by the internal jugular vein, subclavian vein, or occasionally by an arm vein. This measurement gives the anesthesiologist enormous help in balancing the volume status and function of the patient's heart. It allows him to use the Starling curve to guide fluid therapy. In selected patients, knowledge of the left-sided filling pressure of the heart is needed, and a Swan-Ganz catheter is placed in the patient's pulmonary artery. Cardiac output can easily be measured during surgery by either the indicator dye–dilution technique or by thermodilution techniques. In selected patients, systolic time intervals are measured during surgery to aid in evaluating myocardial contractility.

The frequent measurement of arterial blood gases during surgery has been one of the biggest advances in recent years. Arterial oxygenation can be measured accurately and is extremely useful during major surgery. A falling P_{a,O_2} warns of inadequate inspired oxygen, ventilation-perfusion mismatches, increasing shunting, or decreasing cardiac output. Adequacy of ventilation during anesthesia can be very difficult to judge, but measurement of the P_{a,CO_2} allows easy correction of respiratory acidosis or alkalosis. Metabolic acidosis is common during surgery, and accurate treatment with sodium bicarbonate can be undertaken with frequent determinations of the pH and base excess.

Cardiac arrhythmias
(see also Chap. 46D)

Katz and Bigger [54] in an excellent review point out that arrhythmias are more common (1) in patients with preexisting arrhythmia or heart disease, (2) during intubation, (3) in patients receiving digitalis, and (4) in operations lasting more than 3 h. In general, the occurrence of arrhythmia during anesthesia indicates disturbed physiology; it demands lessening of the anesthesia and an attempt to improve oxygenation and to ensure adequate removal of carbon dioxide. Drugs play only a secondary role and should be used only after measures have been taken to correct hypoxia, hypercapnia, and the effect of disturbance of the autonomic reflexes. Reflex stimulation such as tugging on the mesentery or pleura, spreading ribs, or traction of the heart, great vessels, or pericardium should be discontinued. Thus frequent ventricular premature beats may promptly disappear while one is lightening the load of anesthetic agent, replacing blood or fluid, or counteracting hypotension by elevating the foot of the table to improve venous return. Both atrial and ventricular arrhythmias may respond in the setting of hypotension to the administration of a sympathetic amine such as 0.05 to 0.10 mg phenylephrine hydrochloride (Neo-Synephrine) intravenously. Where the hypotension is due to hypovolemia, the treatment of choice is administration of fluid. Ventricular premature beats or ventricular tachycardia may disappear following lidocaine (Xylocaine), 1 to 2 mg/kg body weight given intravenously. Lidocaine has less tendency to impair myocardial contractility than does procainamide. During anesthesia propranolol in a dose of 0.25 to 0.5 mg every 1 to 3 min up to a total of 2 mg may terminate refractory atrial or ventricular tachycardia. It is particularly useful when digitalis intoxication is suspected and in slowing the ventricular rate with atrial fibrillation. Paroxysmal atrial fibrillation or atrial flutter that does not promptly subside with correction of disturbed physiology may be treated by the administration of an intravenous digitalis preparation such as digoxin. In the undigitalized patient, one may give an initial injection of 0.75 to 1 mg. In the digitalized patient, a single increment of 0.25 mg may result in conversion. Inderal given in increments of 0.5 mg every 3 min for a total dose of 3 to 5 mg may either convert the rhythm or produce slowing of the ventricular rate. If the arrhythmia persists and the ventricular rate is uncontrolled, additional increments of digoxin may be given after 2 h, but the heart rhythm should be monitored with the electrocardiogram to detect evidence of toxicity, such as frequent ventricular ectopic beats, short runs of ventricular tachycardia, paroxysmal atrial tachycardia, or nonparoxysmal nodal tachycardia interrupting the atrial fibrillation. If there is urgent need to correct arrhythmia due to persistent circulatory inadequacy, dc countershock should be used. It is not the treatment of choice, since continuation of precipitating factors may induce recurrence of arrhythmia, necessitating multiple shocks. Quinidine sulfate, 0.2 to 0.4 g intramuscularly followed by 0.2 g at 4-h intervals, may protect against recurrence. An enhanced effect may be produced by propranolol 20 mg given orally every 4 h. Paroxysmal atrial tachycardia may be treated with (1) methoxamine 5 to 10 mg or neostigmine 50 to 100 μg, (2) Tensilon 10 mg, (3) digoxin, or (4) dc countershock.

Acute pulmonary edema

Acute pulmonary edema (see Chaps. 44 and 45) may be treated by elevation of the thorax, tourniquets, intravenously administered opiates, oxygen under positive pressure, 50 mg ethacrynic acid or 40 mg furosemide intravenously (with due regard for subsequent contraction of blood volume), and intravenous digitalization for the undigitalized patient. Reduction in venous pressure by the use of vasodilator therapy has been a great advance in the management of pulmonary edema. Sodium nitroprusside (Nipride), nitroglycerin, trimethaphan, or pentolinium (Ansolysen) may be used by slow intravenous infusion. When pulmonary edema persists in spite of the above treatment, the decrease in venous return produced by sodium nitroprusside, given slowly intravenously until response is obtained or blood pressure begins to fall, may turn the tide. If the pulmonary edema is due to hypervolemia associated with overloading with blood or other fluids, rapid phlebotomy of 300 to 500 ml may produce prompt improvement.

POSTOPERATIVE CARE OF THE CARDIAC PATIENT

In the postoperative care of the cardiac patient it is desirable to obtain (1) blood pressure, (2) pulse, (3) respiratory rate, (4) hourly urine flow, (5) electrolyte status, (6) daily weight, (7) an electrocardiogram when there is an arrhythmia, bradycardia, or tachycardia, (8) repeat electrocardiograms at intervals of several days for the first week of the patient with coronary atherosclerotic heart disease, (9) monitoring of central venous pressure when hypotension occurs until vital signs and urine output are stable, (10) daily chest x-ray, and (11) serum and urine creatinine level determinations if renal insufficiency is suspected.

The immediate problems faced in the postoperative period are (1) respiratory depression due to continued action of anesthetic agents, particularly of those producing neuromuscular blockade, (2) hypovolemia, (3) hypotension due to myocardial depression related to respiratory depression and hypovolemia or because of myocardial ischemia, infarction, or failure.

It is imperative to avoid overloading the circulation of the cardiac patient with fluid; however, this admonition leads the average physician to err on the side of underreplacement, causing the most common problem faced in the postoperative period—hypovolemia. Assessment of hypovolemia is notoriously inaccurate. There is relatively poor correlation between the hematocrit and the blood volume immediately after surgery. Deficits of up to 30 to 40 percent without usual clinical evidence have been noted. In one study there was an average deficit of 900 ml, or 18 percent of preoperative values, despite transfusions during surgery averaging 1,700 ml.[55] The type of procedure influences the extent of fluid loss. Surgery of the abdominal aorta, for example, is accompanied by massive fluid loss. In one study an average replacement of 3,000 ml of Ringer's solution was required during surgery to maintain adequate blood pressure and a urine flow of 100 ml/h.[56] Though blood is conventionally used to replace blood loss, some anesthesiologists use crystalloid (Ringer's lactate) and colloid (plasma protein) solutions for losses of 1 to 1.5 liters. Such solutions avoid problems incident to blood transfusions,[57] but there is some hazard in infusing large volumes of crystalloids, which reduce the osmotic pressure and predispose to pulmonary edema.[57a] Blood loss may be underestimated because of obstruction of chest tubes, organized hematomas in the pleural space, or retroperitoneal bleeding.

The cardiac output and myocardial contractility are dependent on the venous return. The use of a central venous pressure monitor allows a more factual assessment of the need for administration of blood or fluid, but it should be recalled that left ventricular failure may occur with a normal central venous pressure. It should be pointed out that the need for volume replacement at any given level of venous pressure is determined by the response to fluid replacement. Thus in evaluating hypotension due to a low cardiac output with a venous pressure of 10 mm Hg, one might administer 250 ml dextran over a period of 20 to 30 min. If the blood pressure rises, the pulse rate falls, the arrhythmia is corrected, and there is no abnormal increase in central venous pressure, clear evidence is furnished of the need for replacement. If, on the other hand, the venous pressure rises, the blood pressure fails to rise, the pulse rate increases, and perhaps signs of pulmonary congestion occur, it is clear that reduced cardiac filling is not the cause of the reduced cardiac output. This technique is even more important in the postoperative period, when hypovolemia is common. It is essential in this setting that the need for volume replacement not be hidden by the administration of pressor amines to improve myocardial contractility and peripheral resistance. These will simply delay the restoration of normal circulatory dynamics. Where available, the use of a Swan-Ganz catheter to measure the pulmonary capillary pressure may allow more accurate estimation of left-sided heart filling pressures.

In recording blood pressure in shock with high peripheral resistance, it should be recalled that cuff blood pressure readings taken in the arms may give falsely low values because of peripheral constriction; similar changes may be produced by vasoconstrictor drugs when the intraaortic pressure is normal. The unwarranted use of pressor agents in such situations may lead to acute hypertension and heart failure.[58] Rarely, if there is hypovolemia, catecholamine release may produce acute hypertension. Individuals in this state may develop shock with withdrawal of blood or in response to various drugs or anesthesia.[59]

Hypotension and oliguria may be due to (1) hypovolemia, requiring fluid replacement; or (2) myocardial failure, requiring digitalization, diuresis, oxygen, or drugs such as isoproterenol that increase myocardial contractility. It is not always easy to differentiate between hypovolemia and myocardial failure, although the conventional signs of myocardial insufficiency, such as diastolic gallop rhythm, pulmonary rales, and abnormal neck veins, furnish important evidence of heart failure. Dyspnea may not be a complaint until relatively late. Portable x-ray equipment may show interstitial pulmonary edema before other signs of heart failure become manifest. Monitoring central venous pressure is helpful in determining the need for fluid volume replacement, and the response of the venous pressure, blood pressure, pulse, and urine volume to a trial administration of 200 to 250 ml over a 20-min period under the continual direct observation of the physician may serve to differentiate the two conditions. Care is required with central venous catheters to avoid cardiac tamponade, phlebitis, and infection.[60] Though most patients with pulmonary edema due to left ventricular failure have an elevation of the left ventricular end-diastolic pressure, it is possible for this pressure to be normal if there is hypovolemia due to excessive diuresis, excessive sweating, or fluid loss.[61] Thus effective treatment in rare circumstances might require fluid replacement in the presence of persistent x-ray evidence of pulmonary edema, rather than further attempts at diuresis, which may only potentiate shock. Some hearts may require a higher filling pressure than others for optimum contractility according to Starling's principle. The ischemic ventricle may require a filling pressure of 20 to 24 mm Hg for optimum function.[61a] When evidence indicates that hypovolemia is not present and there appears to be an adequate filling pressure, an intravenous diuretic such as 50 mg ethacrynic acid may produce a prompt rise in urine flow, with peak values within an hour. The status of digitalization should be reviewed; if it is satisfactory, a further increase in cardiac output may be obtained through the use of Dopamine 5 to 10 mg/kg/m, intravenously. The speed of administration should be adjusted so that the pulse rate is not unduly accelerated, ectopic rhythms are not stimulated, and urine output increases. Glucagon, 5 to 10 mg, administered intravenously over a period of an hour, may produce a modest increase in cardiac output. Nausea is routine with the drug and may be lessened by prior administration of 5 to 10 mg of prochlorperazine intravenously.

Electrolyte disturbances

The trauma and stress associated with surgery cause secretion of ADH (antidiuretic hormone), which may result in water retention and a drop in the values of the serum electrolytes.[62] The serum osmolality may be reduced, and the body weight may increase. Thus the serum sodium may decrease to 120 to 130 mEq/liter. The total body sodium remains normal; sodium chloride administration is not usually indicated and indeed may be harmful. The changes are self-limited with fluid restriction and usually are spontaneously corrected within a few days. Lithium salts have been reported to rapidly counteract the effects of ADH.[63] Administration of sodium chloride may be needed only when there has been excessive sweating, nausea, vomiting, diarrhea, or losses by gastric suction, or when diuretics have been used in excess. In contrast to ADH-mediated hyponatremia, this variety is associated with clear clinical evidence of sodium depletion manifest clinically by such signs as poor tissue turgor, absent jugular venous pulsations, falling body weight, and resting or postural reductions in blood pressure or increments in heart rate.

When water retention is severe, the serum sodium may decrease to levels of 110 to 115 mEq/liter. Neurologic symptoms such as irritability, confusion, delirium, convulsions, or coma may develop. In the absence of any evidence of congestive heart failure or elevated central venous pressure, treatment may be very cautiously instituted with 200 to 300 ml of 3 percent saline solution intravenously. Other fluids should be restricted to 350 to 500 ml/day plus insensible losses. Potassium replacement is generally required when parenteral fluids are given, unless renal failure is present. When arrhythmias develop in the postoperative period in the digitalized patient, they are often due to myocardial potassium depletion and respond to the administration of potassium chlordie.

Postoperative myocardial infarction

As emphasized earlier, the incidence of postoperative coronary event is small in patients without previous symptoms of coronary disease but occurs in 5 to 6 percent of patients with a history of preoperative coronary atherosclerotic heart disease. A baseline electrocardiogram should be obtained prior to the surgical procedure, and the electrical activity of the heart should be monitored throughout the course of the operative procedure.[64] A precordial V_5 lead should be used in all patients with coronary artery disease.[64a] The monitoring should be continued for several days in patients recognized to be in the high risk group. Myocardial ischemia and cardiac arrhythmias may be recognized with greater facility using this technique. It must be remembered that pain is a symptom in less than half of the cases of postoperative myocardial infarction and that the manifestations are notoriously atypical.[65] In some series one-half of the postoperative infarcts would have been missed without routine postoperative electrocardiograms. An electrocardiogram should be made routinely in the postoperative period in the patient with a prior history of angina pectoris or myocardial infarction, and it is indicated to detect myocardial infarction when any of the following situations are present: (1) unexplained hypotension during or after surgery; (2) development of pulmonary rales, venous distension, or ventricular gallop rhythm; (3) development of an arrhythmia, sinus bradycardia, or sinus tachycardia; (4) complaints of pain or indigestion in the chest, shoulders, back or arms; (5) dyspnea, persistent cough, or wheezing; (6) unexplained syncope. Because changes may occasionally be delayed 7 to 10 days after onset of infarction, serial tracings may be needed if the initial tracing is normal and there is suspicion of myocardial infarction. Elevation of cardiac specific enzymes such as CPK–MB may furnish evidence of myocardial infarction.

Pulmonary infection in the postoperative period may precipitate congestive heart failure. Prompt recognition of and appropriate therapy for this condition are essential. When thoracotomy has been done, significant fever in the first few days suggests atelectasis and infection. Humidification and tracheal suction are generally adequate when combined with chest physiotherapy and intermittent positive-pressure ventilation. Bronchoscopy may rarely be needed. Sinus tachycardia and cardiac arrhythmias refractory to conventional therapy may be associated with atelectasis and may respond to the above measures. Unfortunately, this sequence of events is not generally appreciated.

Phlebothrombosis and pulmonary embolism

Phlebothrombosis of the calf veins may be detected in 30 to 40 percent of patients after general abdominal or hip surgery by ^{125}I-fibrinogen scanning. Only a small number of clots dislodge.[66] The frequency of pulmonary embolism is decreased by early ambulation after surgical treatment. The use of elastic stockings and frequent movement of the lower extremities while the patient is in bed are essential. The overwhelming majority of pulmonary emboli do not produce infarction; thus one does not expect to find pleurisy, hemoptysis, and shadows in the roentgenogram (see Chap. 75). The clinical findings are subtle, and the diagnosis is of necessity imprecise and based on clinical suspicion in most instances. It is worth noting that 50 percent of instances of fatal embolism occur without a prior diagnosis of thromboembolism. One-third of instances of deep-vein thrombi in the calf are silent, and even when local signs are present in one calf, there is an equal chance that a fatal embolus will arise from the opposite leg where no signs are present. The consistency of the normal calf is jelly-like in the relaxed state. Local tenderness and induration precede other findings such as edema, venous distension, and Homans' sign.[66] When leg signs are detected, any symptom or finding in the cardiorespiratory system should be viewed as possibly due to pulmonary embolism. One should institute anticoagulant therapy, rather than wait for the diagnosis to become clearly established. Unfortunately, signs in the legs may not appear until long after embolic episodes, or they may never occur.

Suspicious symptoms of pulmonary embolism are (1) chest pain, (2) unexplained dyspnea, (3) syncope, (4) unexplained bronchospasm,[67] (5) palpitation or consciousness of the heart, (6) atrial arrhythmias, (7) hyperventilation syndrome in an emotionally stable patient, (8) unaccountable anxiety or depression, (9) increase in pulse rate out of proportion to fever, (10) low-grade fever or irregular fever spikes. Johnson et al.[68] emphasize that unexplained atrial flutter may be due to pulmonary embolism. The arterial $P_{a_{O_2}}$ may be decreased below 50.

When roentgenographic changes of pulmonary embolism are present, there may be (1) increased radiolucency of an area of the lung early in the course of the disorder, (2) elevation of a hemidiaphragm, (3) blunting of a costophrenic angle, (4) pleural effusion, (5) irregular mottled density in the lower lobes, (6) dilatation of one of the main branches of the pulmonary artery, (7) later platelike areas of atelectasis, or (8) wedge-shaped densities (these are rare). The lung scan or perfusion scan commonly shows diagnostic changes when the chest film is normal.

Massive pulmonary embolism may be associated with dyspnea, cyanosis, chest pain, shock, fixed splitting of the second sound, right ventricular gallop, acute tricuspid regurgitation, and the ECG pattern of acute cor pulmonale. Recent studies indicate that massive pulmonary embolism may occur without the usual classic clinical picture.[69,70]

Humphries et al.[71] have listed highly suggestive but rare electrocardiographic changes as follows: inverted T wave in leads V_1 through V_4; right bundle block (especially transient); the presence of S_1, Q_3 or S_1, S_2, S_3 (especially transient); right axis deviation; right ventricular hypertrophy; and tall peaked P waves in leads 2, 3, and aV_F. They further list nonspecific but common changes such as: sinus tachycardia; premature beats; ST- and T-wave abnormalities; left axis deviation; low QRS voltage (limb leads); and normal ECG.

Treatment consists of administration of heparin, followed a week later by sodium warfarin (Coumadin) derivatives, which are continued for an arbitrary period of 3 months. Ligation of the vena cava is reserved for patients with repeated embolic episodes who are under good anticoagulant control. Currently, occlusion of the inferior vena cava by use of the "umbrella" is preferred. Embolectomy using partial bypass tecniques should be considered only if shock due to pulmonary embolism does not respond to treatment within an hour. The mortality rate exceeds 50 percent.

Gram-negative sepsis

Surgery of the genitourinary or biliary tract or the presence of an indwelling catheter in the bladder may predispose to septicemia with gram-negative organisms such as *Escherichia coli, Pseudomonas,* or *Aerobacter.* Shock may occur in patients with gram-negative sepsis. This condition may simulate a cerebrovascular accident or myocardial infarction. Blood cultures should be obtained, and use of antibiotics that are effective against common gram-negative organisms should be instituted promptly. The chances of recovery are dependent on early recognition and treatment with drugs such as ampicillin, carbenocillin, and gentamicin. Septic shock in the cardiac patient should be treated by adequate fluid replacement until the central venous pressure reaches 15 cm water or until improvement occurs. A more sensitive indicator may be a rise of the pulmonary arterial pressure. Large volumes of fluid may be required. Isoproterenol hydrochloride (Isuprel) is useful to improve cardiac output, but sympathomimetic drugs that produce peripheral vasoconstriction should be avoided since they may produce further impairment of tissue perfusion. When there is no response to adequate fluid replacement, vasodilators, such as nitroprusside, may be given intravenously. Associated intravascular coagulation may produce clinical hemorrhage and require treatment by heparin. Persistent shock may be accompanied by the development of the "shock lung," characterized by pulmonary congestion, hemorrhage, atelectasis, edema, and capillary thrombi, with subsequent death due to respiratory insufficiency.[72] The use of massive doses of corticosteroids, such as 40 to 60 mg dexamethasone (Decadron) intravenously every 4 to 6 h, may be helpful.[73]

REFERENCES

1 Wessler, S., and Blumgart, H. L.: Management of the Cardiac Patient Requiring Major Surgery, *Circulation,* 23:121, 1961.

2 Kannell, W. B., and Feinleib, M.: Natural History of Angina Pectoris, in the Framingham Study, *Am. J. Cardiol.,* 29:154, 1972.

3 Esten, B. E., Weaver, D. C., Li, T. G., and Friedman, J. B.: Appraisal of the Coronary Patient as an Operative Risk, *N.Y. State J. Med.,* 50:2065, 1964.

4 Etsten, B. E., and Proger, S.: Operative Risk in Patients with Coronary Heart Disease, *JAMA,* 159:845, 1955.

5 Wasserman, F., Bellet, S., and Saicheck, R. P.: Postoperative Myocardial Infarction, *N. Engl. J. Med.,* 252:967, 1955.

6 LaDue, J. S.: Evaluation and Preparation of the Patient with Degenerative Cardiovascular Disease for Major Surgery, *Bull. N.Y. Acad. Med.,* 32:418, 1956.

7 Topkins, M. J., and Artusio, J. F.: Myocardial Infarction and Surgery, *Anesth. Analg.,* 43:716, 1964.

8 Nachlas, M. M., Abrams, S. J., and Goldberg, M. M.: The Influence of Arteriosclerotic Heart Disease on Surgical Risk, *Am. J. Surg.,* 101:447, 1961.

9 Knapp, R. B., Topkins, M. J., and Artusio, J. F.: Occlusion in Anesthesia, *JAMA,* 182:106, 1962.

10 Thompson, G. J., Kelalis, P. P., and Connolly, D. C.: Transurethral Prostatic Resection after Myocardial Infarction, *JAMA,* 182:110, 1962.

11 Erlik, D., Nalero, A., Birkhan, G., and Gersh, I.: Prostatic Surgery and the Cardiovascular Patient, *Br. J. Urol.,* 40:53, 1968.

12 Arkins, R., Smessaert, A. A., and Hicks, R. G.: Mortality and Morbidity in Surgical Patients with Coronary Artery Disease, *JAMA,* 190:485, 1964.

13 Tarhan, S., Moffitt, E. A., Taylor, W. F., and Giuliani, E. R.: Myocardial Infarction after General Anesthesia, *JAMA,* 220: 1451, 1972.

14 Mauney, F. M., Jr., Ebert, P. A., and Sabiston, D. C., Jr.: Postoperative Myocardial Infarction: A Study of Predisposing Factors. Diagnosis and Mortality in a High Risk Group of Surgical Patients, *Ann. Surg.,* 172:497, 1970.

15 Fraser, J. G., Ramachandran, P. R., and Davis, H. S.: Anesthesia and Recent Myocardial Infarction, *JAMA,* 199:96, 1967.

16 Miller, M.: Intra-Aortic Balloon Counterpulsation in a High Risk Cardiac Patient Undergoing Emergency Gastrectomy, *Anesthesiology,* 42:103, 1975.

17 Wikland, B.: Medically Unattended Fatal Cases of Ischaemic Heart Disease in a Defined Population, *Acta Med. Scand.,* 190(suppl. 524), 1971.

18 Burns-Cox, G. J.: Return to Normal of Electrocardiogram after Myocardial Infarction, *Lancet,* 1:1194, 1967.

19 Levine, H. D., and Phillips, E.: An Appraisal of the Newer Electrocardiographic Correlations in One Hundred and Fifty Consecutive Autopsied Cases, *N. Engl. J. Med.,* 245:883, 1951.

20 Pruitt, R. D., Dennis, E. W., and Kincaid, S. A.: The Difficult Electrocardiographic Diagnosis of Myocardial Infarction, *Prog. Cardiovasc. Dis.,* 6:85, 1963.

21 Kaplan, J. A., Dunbar, R. W., and Jones, E. L.: Nitroglycerin Infusion during Coronary Artery Surgery, *Anesthesiology,* 45:14, 1976.

21a Lappas, D. G., Lowenstein, E., Waller, J., Fahmy, N. R., and Daggett, W. M.: Hemodynamic Effects of Nitroprusside Infusion during Coronary Artery Operation in Man, *Circulation,* 54(suppl. 3):4, 1976.

22 Hickle, R. B.: Hypertension, *Anesthesiology,* 33:214, 1970.

23 Terazi, R. C., Frolich, E., and Dustin, H. P.: Plasma Volume in Man with Essential Hypertension, *N. Engl. J. Med.,* 278:762, 1968.

24 Foster, M. W., and Gayle, R. F.: Danger in Combining Reserpine with Electroconvulsive Therapy, *JAMA,* 159:1520, 1955.

25 Alper, M. H., Flacke, W., and Kroger, O.: Pharmacology of Reserpine and Its Implications for Anesthesia, *Anesthesiology,* 24:524, 1963.

26 Ominsky, A. J., and Wollman, H.: Hazards of General Anesthesia in the Reserpined Patient, *Anesthesiology,* 30:443, 1969.

27 Prys-Roberts, C., Meloche, R., and Foex, P.: Studies of Anesthesia in Relation to Hypertension. I: Cardiovascular Responses of Treated and Untreated Patients, *Br. J. Anesth.,* 43:122, 1971.

28 Strong, M. J., Keats, A. S., and Cooley, D. A.: Arterial Gas Tensions under Anesthesia in Tetralogy of Fallot, *Br. J. Anesth.,* 39:427, 1967.

29 Radney, P. A., Arai, T., and Nagashima, H.: Ketamine-Gallamine Anesthesia for Great Vessel Operations in Infants, *Anesth. Analg.,* 53:365, 1974.

30 Hodgkin, J. E., Dines, D. E., and Didier, E. P.: Preoperative Evaluation of the Patient with Pulmonary Disease, *Mayo Clinic Proc.,* 48:114, 1973.

31 Downes, J. B., Klein, E. F., DeSantels, D., et al.: Intermittent Mandatory Ventilation: A New Approach to Weaning Patients from Mechanical Ventilation, *Chest,* 64:331, 1973.

32 Criteria Committee of the New York Heart Association, Inc.: "Nomenclature and Criteria for Diagnosis of Diseases of the Heart and Great Vessels," 7th ed., Little, Brown and Company, Boston, 1973.

33 Braunwald, E., Bloodwell, R. D., Goldberg, L. H., and Morrow, A. G.: Studies on Digitalis: IV. Observations in Man on the Effects of Digitalis on the Contractility of the Non-failing Heart and on Total Vascular Resistance, *J. Clin. Invest.,* 40:52, 1961.

34 Selzer, A., Kelly, J. J., Jr., Cerbode, F., Keith, W. J., Osborn, J. J., and Popper, R. W.: Case Against Routine Use of Digitalis in Patients Undergoing Cardiac Surgery, *JAMA,* 195:549, 1968.

34a Johnson, L. W., Dickstein, R. A., Truehan, C. T., Kane, P., Potts, F. L., Simelyan, H., Well, W. R., and Eich, R. H.: Prophylactic Digitalization for Coronary Artery Bypass Surgery, *Circulation,* 53:819, 1976.

35 Lown, B., and Levine, H. D.: "Atrial Arrhythmias, Digitalis, and Potassium," Landsberger Medical Books, Inc., New York, 1958.

36 Lown, B., Black, H., and Moore, F. D.: Digitalis, Electrolytes, and the Surgical Patient, *Am. J. Cardiol.,* 6:309, 1960.

37 Kunin, A. S., Surawicz, B., and Sims, E. A. H.: Decrease in Serum Potassium Concentrations and Appearance of Cardiac Arrhythmias during Infusion of Potassium with Glucose in Potassium-depleted Patients, *N. Engl. J. Med.,* 266:228, 1967.

38 Lansing, A. M., Leb, D. E., and Berman, L. B.: Cardiovascular Surgery in End-Stage Renal Failure, *JAMA,* 204:682, 1968.

39 Gertler, M. M., Finkle, A. L., Haralson, P. B., and Neidle, E. G.: Cardiovascular Evaluation in Surgery, Operative Risk in Cancer Patients with Bundle Branch Block, *Surg. Gynecol. Obstet.,* 99:441, 1954.

40 Rotman, M., and Trebwasser, J. H.: A Clinical Follow-up Study of Right and Left Bundle Branch Block, *Circulation,* 51:477, 1975.

41 Scott, D. L.: Cardiac Pacemakers as an Anesthetic Problem, *Anesthesia,* 25:87, 1970.

42 Lerner, S. M.: Suppression of a Demand Pacemaker by Transurethral Electrosurgery, *Anesth. Analg.,* 52:704, 1973.

43 Nettle, D. C., Herrin, T. J., and Mullen, J. G.: Ketamine Induction in Poor Risk Patients, *Anesth. Analg.,* 52:59, 1973.

44 Chasapakis, G., Kekis, N., and Sakkalis: Use of Ketamine and Pancuronium for Anesthesia for Patients in Hemorrhagic Shock, *Anesth. Analg.,* 52:282, 1973.

45 Lowenstein, E., Hallowell, P., Levine, P. H., et al.: Cardiovascular Responses to Large Doses of Intravenous Morphine in Man, *N. Engl. J. Med.,* 281:1389, 1969.

45a Lowenstein, E.: Morphine "Anesthesia"—A Perspective, *Anesthesiology,* 35:563, 1971.

46 Eisele, J. H., and Smith, N. T.: Cardiovascular Effects of 40% Nitrous Oxide in Man, *Anesth. Analg.,* 51:956, 1972.

47 McDermott, R. W., and Stanley, T. H.: The Cardiovascular Effect of Low Concentrations of Nitrous Oxide during Morphine Anesthesia, *Anesthesiology,* 41:89, 1974.

48 Reinikainen, N., and Pontinen, P.: Arterioventricular Dissociation during Surgery, *Acta Med. Scand.,* 182(suppl. 2):147, 1967.

49 Stephenson, H. E., Jr., Reid, L. C., and Hinton, H. W.: Some Common Denominators in 1200 Cases of Cardiac Arrest, *Ann. Surg.,* 137:731, 1953.

50 McClure, J. M., Jr., Skardasis, G. M., and Brown, V. J.: Cardiac Arrest in the Operating Room, *Ann. Surg.,* 38:241, 1972.

51 Rackow, H., Salanitre, E., and Green, L. T.: Frequency of Cardiac Arrest Associated with Anesthesia in Infants and Children, *Pediatrics,* 28:697, 1961.

52 Rashad, K. F., Goldman, E. J., Graff, T. D., Berason, D. Q., and Kelley, E. B.: Factors in Geriatric Anesthesia Mortality, *Anesth. Analg.,* 44:462, 1965.

53 Mazzia, V. D. B., Ellis, C. H., Siegel, H., and Hershey, S. G.: The Electrocardiograph as a Monitor of Cardiac Function in the Operating Room, *JAMA,* 198:123, 1966.

53a Bedford, R. F., and Wollman, H.: Complication of Percutaneous Radial-Artery Cannulation, *Anesthesiology,* 38:228, 1973.

54 Katz, R. L., and Bigger, T. J.: Cardiac Arrhythmias during Anesthesia and Operation, *Anesthesiology,* 33:193, 1970.

55 Cartmill, T. B., Ricks, R. K., Garrett, H. E., Williams, J. A., and DeBakey, M. E.: Blood Volume Measurements in Cardiovascular Surgical Patients, *Surg. Gynecol. Obstet.,* 121:1269, 1965.

56 Wheeler, C. G., Thompson, J. E., Kartchner, M. M., Austin, D. J., and Patman, R. D.: Massive Fluid Requirement in Surgery of the Abdominal Aorta, *N. Engl. J. Med.,* 275:320, 1966.

57 Rigor, B., Bosomworth, P., and Rush, B. F., Jr.: Replacement of Operative Blood Loss of More than 1 Liter with Harmann's Solution, *JAMA,* 203, 399, 1968.

57a Stein, L., Bernard, J. J., Morisette, M., Luz, P., Weill, W. H., and Shulin, H.: Pulmonary Edema during Volume Infusion, *Circulation,* 52:483, 1975.

58 Cohn, J. N.: Blood Pressure Measurement in Shock, Mechanism of Inaccuracy in Auscultatory and Palpatory Methods, *JAMA,* 199:972, 1967.

59 Cohn, J. N.: Paroxysmal Hypertension and Hypovolemia, *N. Engl. J. Med.,* 275:643, 1966.

60 Thomas, C. S., Carter, J. W., and Lowder, S. C.: Pericardial Tamponade from Central Venous Catheters, *Arch. Surg.,* 98:217, 1969.

61 Nixon, P. G. F.: Pulmonary Edema with Low Left Ventricular Diastolic Pressure in Acute Myocardial Infarction, *Lancet,* 2:146, 1968.

61a Rackley, C. E., Russell, R. O., Mantle, J. A., and Rogers, W. G.: Modern Approach to the Patient with Acute Myocardial Infarction, *Curr. Probl. Cardiol.,* 1:No. 10, 1977.

62 Barter, F. C., and Scwartz, W. B.: The Syndrome of Inappropriate Secretion of Antidiuretic Hormone, *Am. J. Med.,* 42:790, 1967.

63 White, M. G., and Fetner, C. D., Treatment of the Syndrome of Inappropriate Secretion of Antidiuretic Hormone with Lithium Carbonate, *N. Engl. J. Med.,* 292:390, 1975.

64 Cannard, T. H., Dripps, R. D., Helwig, J., Jr., and Zinsser, H. F.: The Electrocardiogram during Anesthesia and Surgery, *Anesthesiology,* 21:194, 1960.

64a Kaplan, J. A., and King, S. B.: The Precordial Electrocardiographic Lead (V_5) in Patients Who Have Coronary Artery Disease, *Anesthesiology,* 45;570, 1976.

65 Driscoll, A., Hobika, J. H., Etsten, B. E., and Proger, S.: Postoperative Myocardial Infarction, *N. Engl. J. Med.,* 264:633, 1961.

66 Soloff, L. A.: Postoperative Pulmonary Embolism, *Am. J. Cardiol.,* 12:451, 1963.

67 Salem, M. R., Baraka, A., Rattenborg, C. C., and Holaday, D. A.: Bronchospasm: An Early Manifestation of Pulmonary Embolism during and after Anesthesia, *Anesth. Analg.,* 47:103, 1968.

68 Johnson, J. C., Flowers, N. C., and Horan, L.: Unexplained Atrial Flutter: A Frequent Herald of Pulmonary Embolism, *Chest,* 60:29, 1971.

69 Parmley, L. F., Senior, R. M., McKlung, D. H., and Johnston, G. S.: Clinically Deceptive Massive Pulmonary Embolism, *Chest,* 53:15, 1970.

70 Wenger, N., Stein, P. D., and Willis, P., III: Massive Acute Pulmonary Embolism: Deceivingly Non-specific Manifestations, *Am. J. Cardiol.,* 29:296, 1972 (abstract).

71 Humphries, J. O., Bell, W. R., and White, R. I.: Criteria for the Recognition of Pulmonary Emboli, *JAMA,* 235:2011, 1976.

72 Hardaway, R. W., Bredenbery, C. E., and West, R. L.: Intensive Study of Shock and Treatment of Shock in Man, *JAMA,* 199:779, 1967.

73 Christy, J. H.: Treatment of Gram-negative Shock, *Am. J. Med.,* 50:77, 1971.

B

Medical Management in Cardiac Surgery

R. BRUCE LOGUE, M.D.,
PAUL H. ROBINSON, M.D.,
CHARLES R. HATCHER, JR., M.D., and
JOEL A. KAPLAN, M.D.

INTRODUCTION

Many unusual problems occur in the postoperative period after open heart surgery. Most open heart patients have been ill longer than those who undergo the more usual thoracic surgery. Their preoperative status is often precarious because of difficult fluid management and the use of a multiplicity of drugs, including diuretics and digitalis. Frequently there are associated pulmonary problems resulting from prolonged congestive heart failure and pulmonary venous hypertension with or without pulmonary arterial hypertension. The protracted illness of many patients produces psychologic and psychiatric problems. At times the mechanical complexity of open heart surgery is made more difficult by previous thoracic procedures, most commonly mitral commissurotomy.

Control of these various problems is usually not difficult. During the early phase of his or her development or during familiarization with new techniques, the thoracic surgeon experiences a higher incidence of operative and postoperative failures. Thereafter the major morbidity and mortality relate to cardiopulmonary bypass.

Candidates for open heart surgery vary as widely in their age as they do in the complexity of their problems. A detailed evaluation of any individual or particular situation will not be outlined; rather, general principles will be described in regard to (1) the preoperative maintenance and preparation of the patient for open heart surgery, (2) certain specific aspects of the operative management as they relate to postoperative problems, and (3) the postoperative difficulties, their recognition and management. The "medical" complications in the immediate postoperative period are the most important ones determining recovery. In one series of 150 patients medical complications occurred in 71 percent.[1]

It cannot be emphasized too strongly that there is a continued need for constant cooperation and communication among the members of the team caring for the open heart patient. This is especially true of the cardiovascular surgeon, the cardiologist, the hematologist, the anesthesiologist, and the pulmonary therapist.

THE PREOPERATIVE STATUS

General considerations

The optimum state which can be achieved by any particular patient prior to open heart surgery will vary considerably. The cardiac status of most patients who are operated on for congenital problems will be either class I or class II.* This is in marked contrast to those patients who require valvular replacement or coronary bypass surgery because they are in class III or IV. To perform cardiac surgery on patients with valvular or coronary artery disease who are in class II is an error. Surgery is ameliorative, not curative. Mortality and morbidity rates do not justify the theoretical gains of operation in this stage. It is most important that the patient remain as active as possible during the period immediately prior to his

---

*The classification discussed above is based on symptoms only. This method of classifying patients was utilized through the sixth edition of "Nomenclature and Criteria for Diagnosis of Diseases of the Heart and Great Vessels." The new method of classifying the cardiac status of patients utilizes the total assessment of all data and not symptoms alone. This new method of classification began with the seventh edition of "Nomenclature and Criteria for Diagnosis of Diseases of the Heart and Great Vessels" by The Criteria Committee of New York Heart Association, Little, Brown and Company, Boston, 1973.

open heart surgery. Some patients must be kept at bed rest. However, taking a person who is normally up and about and confining him or her to bed, with the consequent development of negative nitrogen balance, decreased plasma volume, weakness, depression, and predisposition to thromboembolism, seems ill-advised.

Some centers in the United States keep their patients in bed for 2 to 3 weeks preoperatively in order to "get them in shape." In the vast majority of patients who are to undergo open heart surgery, careful outpatient management is sufficient. Some of the parameters which are almost automatically taken into consideration should be mentioned. One of these is body weight. Obesity is not only an impediment to good technical surgery but leads to postoperative ventilatory inadequacy and thrombembolic problems. If smoking is discontinued, preferably for a month prior to surgery, there is less difficulty in the postoperative period with secretions and atelectasis. The status of the coronary vessels, kidneys, liver, and hematopoietic system should be evaluated. During the immediate preoperative period the patient should be made familiar with the intensive care unit and especially with the use of the endotracheal tube, positive-pressure breathing apparatus, and techniques of coughing.

Digitalis

Although it is the procedure of some authorities to discontinue digoxin or other cardiac glycosides for from 1 to 5 days preoperatively, we believe that the omission of digitalis preparations the day of surgery is satisfactory. This assumes that there is no evidence of digitalis toxicity. Those who suggest that digitalis be discontinued for a prolonged period preoperatively do so to assure that the arrhythmias occuring in the immediate postoperative period are not digitalis-induced. It seems imprudent and illogical to deny the myocardium the inotropic boost and improved contractility it desperately needs during the crucial period of stressful surgery in order not to have to assess the role of digitalis in postoperative arrhythmias. Digitalization should be accomplished some days prior to surgery in order that a maintenance dose free of toxicity can be established. Digitalis intoxication is not uncommon during the postoperative period when myocardial function is depressed, metabolic demands are increased, varying degrees of renal insufficiency are present, and electrolyte imbalance is frequent.

Patients with compensated congenital heart disease undergoing right ventriculotomy are not digitalized preoperatively. If right ventricular failure occurs postoperatively, digitalization is accomplished at that time.

Diuretics

The two major difficulties encountered with the use of diuretics are (1) potassium depletion and (2) volume depletion. The potassium problem is often unrecognized because the serum potassium level may be within normal limits when total body potassium is depleted.[2] There must be constant cognizance of the fact that most diuretics produce potassium loss and that potassium chloride supplementation is necessary when prolonged therapy is used. Potassium supplementation is not without its difficulties. Spironolactones may produce potassium retention, which may occur in the face of normal renal function but is more likely to develop when there is marginal or deficient renal function. The physician must know the pharmacology of the diuretic agent or run the risk of serious electrolyte disturbance (see Chap. 45).

Some patients do not have to be at their "dry weight" to remain in adequate cardiac compensation. Severe diuresis may produce a decrease in blood volume, with its concomitant deleterious effect on cardiac output. For example, furosemide (Lasix) may reduce the plasma volume 25 percent.[3] Patients in an acute, severe state of diuresis will almost immediately demonstrate the findings of a low cardiac output, manifested by cool, clammy skin, restlessness, and postural hypotension. More characteristically, patients who have undergone diuresis over a long period of time complain of being excessively weak, particularly when they stand. The detection of postural hypotension suggests hypovolemia, and these patients commonly become hypotensive with the administration of opiates or any type of general anesthetic. Blood volume should be restored prior to operation. Although it may seem paradoxic, some patients who remain in congestive heart failure will not improve unless the venous pressure is allowed to remain above normal. It is very important to know the electrolyte status of the patient in the preoperative period and also to know the body weight, not only in the immediate preoperative period but for several weeks, before the operation. Occasional patients may develop dilutional hyponatremia because of inappropriate antidiuretic hormone secretion. This state may exist in the preoperative period and should be corrected by fluid restriction. With a fixed low cardiac output in the class IV cardiac patient who has required vigorous diuresis with contraction of blood volume, tissue perfusion may be sufficiently impaired that lactic acidosis occurs. This may lead to shock and cardiac arrest. Cardiac conduction and cardiac contractility are impaired. An acidotic type of breathing with tachypnea out of proportion to the evidence of pulmonary edema may be present. There may be an anion gap of more than 10. The arterial pH may be severely reduced. Administration of 44 to 132 mEq sodium bicarbonate intravenously may reverse this situation.

Other drugs

The fewer drugs a patient takes, the fewer will be the complications of their administration. Some patients require a wide spectrum of drugs, including the myocardial depressants, quinidine, procainamide (Pronestyl), diphenylhydantoin (Dilantin), and propranolol (Inderal). Propranolol may be safely continued to within 12 to 24 h of both cardiac and noncardiac surgery. Anesthesia can be safely administered to a patient with a stable level of beta-adrenergic blockage.[4,5,5a] Recently 169 patients undergoing cardiac surgery and 73 patients having noncardiac surgery who were taking propranolol (average dose 125 mg/day) were studied. There was no increase in the incidence of hypotension or bradycardia before or after cardiopulmonary bypass. Myocardial contractility as measured by systolic time intervals was normal 24 to 48 h after stopping propranolol therapy. Acute withdrawal of propranolol preoperatively can lead to increasing myocardial ischemia and myocardial infarction. If the drug is to be discontinued preoperatively, it should be tapered instead of being abruptly stopped. Insulin and anticonvulsive therapy should be continued. It is important to question the patient about the use of corticosteroid medication with 6 months of surgery. The patient should also be questioned about the use of antihypertensive medications. These drugs should be continued until the time of surgery, so that the patient is under optimal medical control at the time of anesthesia. It is important that the anesthesiologist know which of these drugs the patient is taking. Anesthetic management can then proceed accordingly and intraoperative hypotension treated with small doses of direct-acting vasopressors. Anticoagulants should be discontinued 48 h prior to surgery, and the prothrombin time should return to normal range. The use of vitamin K should be avoided unless it is necessary to give it to correct the prothrombin time prior to emergency surgery. When possible, aspirin should be omitted 2 weeks prior to surgery because of its antiplatelet effect. Patients should be questioned regarding sensitivity to drugs such as antibiotics, opiates, and sedatives. True allergies to opiates are rare. Patients frequently describe side effects such as nausea and dizziness as allergies to these drugs.

Hematologic status

Although there are a few centers in the United States where special blood studies are not made prior to open heart surgery unless there is a history of bleeding, most institutions carefully analyze the components of blood associated with coagulation and bleeding. The following studies are accomplished: blood group and type, antibody screen, preoperative coagulation survey (coagulation time, plasma prothrombin time, serum prothrombin time, and platelet count), and complete blood count, including hematocrit, hemoglobin, white blood cell count, and differential blood cell count. Coombs' positive antibodies may be detected as a result of various drugs including methyldopa (Aldomet). Patients with cyanotic heart disease have increased platelets and fibrinogen. Those patients who have prolonged congestive heart failure may have a decreased prothrombin time secondary to decreased hepatic perfusion and congestion.

The use of moderate hemodilution and dilute prime mixtures has greatly reduced the amount of blood required for cardiac surgery. Hopefully, these techniques will reduce the stress on our national blood banking resources. Prior to cardiopulmonary bypass, 15 to 20 percent of the patient's blood volume is removed into either CPD (citrate-phosphate-dextrose) or heparinized containers. (See later discussion.) This volume is simultaneously replaced with plasma protein fraction (plasmanate) and crystalloid solution (Ringer's lactate) to maintain stable hemodynamics. Most cardiac patients tolerate this removal of autologous blood surprisingly well. The pump is primed with a combination of normosol, dextran (Rheomacrodex), and 1 unit of whole blood. On bypass with hypothermia, the desired hematocrit is between 20 percent and 30 percent. After bypass the fresh autologous blood is reinfused to obtain the clotting factors and to raise the hematocrit. At the same time, furosemide is given since its greater free water clearance will raise the hematocrit. This use of autologous blood reduces the amount of blood bank products required.[6,7,7b] Open heart surgery in Jehovah's Witnesses has been carried out without the administration of blood; in one series of 42 patients there were only three deaths with a single death being due to anemia.[7a]

THE OPERATIVE PERIOD

Anesthesia

Patients undergoing cardiac surgery experience more anxiety and fear than other surgical patients. There is also a high incidence of postoperative psychoses in cardiac surgical patients.[8] A thorough preoperative discussion of the perioperative period by the anesthesiologist has been shown to be more important than any pharmacologic premedication.[9] The patient should be told what will be done to him using local anesthesia, that he may remember certain parts of the procedure, and that he will wake up in the intensive care unit with an endotracheal tube in place and on a ventilator. This type of discussion relieves the patient of his anxieties of the unknown. A good night's sleep should be ensured by giving either pentobarbitol (Nembutal) 100 mg or flurazepam (Dalmane) 30 mg.

Preoperative medication should also be adequate. The agents selected and doses employed vary with the conditions and diagnosis of the individual patient. The patient should be well sedated without markedly depressing his cardiovascular system and respirations. Close surveillance should accompany the administration of preanesthetic medication. Most adult patients receive morphine (0.1 mg/kg), diazepam (Valium) (5 to 10 mg), and scopolamine (0.3 to 0.6 mg) intramuscularly 1 h before arrival in the operating room.[10] If the patient is seriously ill (for example, most cases of double valve disease) half or less of the usual dose is used. Most pediatric patients receive morphine (0.1 to 0.2 mg/kg) and either atropine or scopolamine (0.02 mg/kg).[11] Barbiturates are avoided due to their negative inotropic effect. Meperidine (Demerol) is avoided because of the occasional rapid tachycardia it produces. Atropine is omitted because of the tachycardia it causes. The advantages of scopolamine over atropine lie in (1) sedation, (2) amnesia, and (3) less tachycardia. However, scopolamine is avoided in the very elderly[10] or the very young.[11] Patients for coronary artery surgery have 2 percent nitroglycerin ointment applied at the time of the premedication and are given nitroglycerin tablets to be used in the preoperative period if chest pain should occur.

For the anesthesiologist to make an intelligent choice of anesthesia, he must thoroughly evaluate the known cardiovascular data of the patient. On the day prior to surgery, the following should be available: (1) a thorough history including the cardiac diagnosis, signs and symptoms of congestive heart failure, weight change, type and frequency of angina, date of prior myocardial infarctions, and any pulmonary diseases; (2) a listing of all medications including the dose and time of the last dose before surgery; (3) laboratory tests including a complete blood count, urine analysis, electrolytes, blood urea nitrogen level, chest x-ray, electrocardiogram, and arterial blood gases—if there is any indication of pulmonary disease, pulmonary function tests should be performed; (4) most importantly, the cardiac catheterization results must be available. A knowledge of valve gradients, chamber pressures, left ventricular function, shunts, pulmonary artery pressure, and location of coronary artery obstruction makes the choice of anesthesia much easier and safer.

The aim of the anesthesiologist is to avoid myocardial depression, ventricular irritability, and an increase in myocardial oxygen demand. Slight degrees of myocardial depression may be catastrophic in the patient with severe valvular heart disease, especially aortic stenosis. However, some myocardial depression may be helpful in patients with coronary ischemia, since it would tend to decrease myocardial oxygen demand.

Large doses of intravenous morphine (0.5 to 3 mg/kg) have been widely used as the primary anesthetic agent in patients undergoing cardiac surgery. Morphine produces no myocardial depression and Lowenstein has shown that cardiac output actually increases in patients with aortic stenosis.[12] Also, there is no potentiation of ventricular irritability, and there is a decrease in vascular resistance and an increase in vascular capacitance.[13] However, morphine by itself will not guarantee amnesia and anesthesia.[14] Therefore, it is usually supplemented with nitrous oxide, diazepam, and scopolamine. Pancuronium bromide (Pavulon) is a new steroidal nondepolarizing muscle relaxant that has been shown to have less adverse effects on the cardiovascular system than previous relaxants.[15] Dimethyl tubocurarine (metocurine) has recently been recommended for muscle relaxation instead of Pavulon, since it produces less tachycardia.[15a]

In patients with good left ventricular function (ejection fraction greater than 0.4, left ventricular end-diastolic pressure less than 12 mm Hg, and no areas of dyskinesia), halothane (Fluothane) or enflurane (Ethrane) are frequently used as the primary or supplementary anesthetic agents. These drugs are especially useful in pediatric patients and certain coronary artery patients. The flammable anesthetics cyclopropane and ether are rarely used in cardiac anesthesia due to the extensive electrical monitoring required by the patients.

In certain clinical situations, circulatory assistance may be instituted prior to induction of anesthesia. For patients with recent myocardial infarction and cardiogenic shock, the intraaortic balloon may be inserted via the femoral artery under local anesthesia and general anesthesia then more safely induced with the aid of counterpulsation. In patients with massive pulmonary embolization, partial cardiopulmonary bypass (using the femoral artery and vein) may be instituted under local anesthesia prior to induction of general anesthesia.[16] Such an approach may make it possible to save patients who might otherwise sustain cardiac arrest when anesthesia is induced, but this practice does have the disadvantage that thoracotomy must be performed after systemic anticoagulation has been obtained.

In recent years, large doses of steroids have been given during open heart surgery. Typical steroid dosage is methylprednisolone (Solumedrol) 30 mg/kg intravenously at the beginning of surgery. The rationale for the use of such large doses of steroids has not been satisfactorily clarified, and theories related to lysosomal stabilization, inotropic effects, effects on anaerobic metabolism, improvement in the microcirculation, and a decrease in cerebral edema have been presented.[17–21]

Monitoring

Extensive cardiovascular monitoring is used in all patients undergoing cardiac surgical procedures. A seven-lead electrocardiogram is used consisting of leads I, II, III, aV_R, aV_L, aV_F, and V_5. The V_5 lead is obtained by placing an electrode under the left nipple and covering it with a waterproof drape out of the surgical field. This lead is especially important in patients with coronary artery disease.[21b] A bifrontal electroencephalogram is also employed in most patients undergoing cardiopulmonary bypass.

Prior to induction of general anesthesia, all patients have arterial and central venous catheters placed using local anesthesia. The radial artery is catheterized percutaneously with an 18- or 20-gauge Teflon catheter after an Allen's test has been performed to assure good collateral ulnar artery flow.[22] The central venous pressure catheter is placed via the right internal jugular vein.[23] Selected patients also have a Swan-Ganz catheter placed percutaneously into their pulmonary artery for measurement of the pulmonary capillary wedge pressure, pulmonary artery pressures, and cardiac output. After cardiopulmonary bypass, all patients with depressed left ventricular function have a left atrial catheter placed for direct measurement of left-sided filling pressures. In certain situations after induction of anesthesia an esophageal phonocardiogram is obtained during surgery so that systolic time intervals can be calculated as an index of myocardial contractility. A Foley catheter is placed in the bladder of all patients, and urine output is recorded at $1/2$-h intervals.

Surgical technique

The type of incision selected for cardiac exposure is usually dictated by the lesion or lesions to be corrected. The vast majority of cardiac surgical procedures are performed through the median sternotomy incision. When the cardiac abnormality can be approached through either a thoracotomy or a median sternotomy, the choice for the incision may be influenced by the status of the patient's pulmonary function or by the suspicion of aortic valvular involvement. If the patient's condition is critical, it may be wise to insert an intraaortic balloon for counterpulsation prior to the induction of general anesthesia. In patients with massive pulmonary embolism or in those undergoing reoperation for certain septic complications of previous cardiovascular surgery, it may be essential to establish partial cardiopulmonary bypass via the femoral artery and vein prior to opening the chest.

The ribs and sternum are spread slowly; if bradycardia secondary to vagal response develops, atropine may be administered. Similar vagal responses may result with the opening of the pericardium. In most instances, the pericardium will be opened widely prior to cannulation; but if a left ventricular aneurysm is present, the pericardium should not be opened widely until cannulation, since the pericardium may be preventing acute myocardial dilatation. Blood pH, P_{a,CO_2}, and P_{a,O_2} readings are performed routinely every $1/2$ h, or as often as conditions dictate. The status of electrolytes has been studied in many patients and shifts in electrolytes may present serious problems. Most commonly a reduction in serum potassium level occurs because of and is exaggerated by an excessive diuresis produced by the bypass. Other factors contributing to hypokalemia are (1) hyperventilation (respiratory alkalosis), (2) lower potassium content of perfusate in hemodilution techniques, and (3) large doses of steroids. Therefore, serum sodium and potassium levels are measured every $1/2$ h during surgery. Frequently, 40 to 100 mEq of potassium chloride are required to maintain the serum potassium level above 4 mEq/liter.

In most instances, venous catheters are placed in the superior and inferior venae cavae via the right atrium, and secured with umbilical tape. If the right side of the heart is not to be opened, it may be simpler to introduce a single large venous pickup into the right atrium via the right atrial appendage. Adequate venous pickup can be achieved through such a catheter with or without occlusion of the pulmonary artery. When the heart is exposed through a left posterolateral thoracotomy, a single venous catheter is placed in the outflow tract of the right ventricle, into the right atrium via the right atrial appendage, or into the pulmonary artery and advanced into the right ventricle. The catheter should be of sufficient size to provide adequate venous pickup; to achieve this, it may be necessary to elevate the operating table to full height.

An arterial input catheter may be placed in either the common femoral vessels or the ascending aorta. The avoidance of a groin incision and the decreased instance of aortic dissection associated with cannulation of the ascending aorta make the ascending aorta the routine site for cannulation in most centers. Personal preference is involved in the site selected for arterial cannulation, but the femoral route should be avoided in elderly patients with aortoiliac occlusive disease. When operating from a left posterolateral thoracotomy, it is convenient to cannulate the descending thoracic aorta, although the femoral vessels should always be available if this incision has been selected.

In aortic and mitral valve surgery, in coronary artery surgery, and in the correction of certain congenital defects, it is often desirable, even mandatory, to insert a left ventricular vent. This catheter is best inserted through the right superior pulmonary vein across the mitral valve and into the left ventricle. In rare circumstances the direct insertion of the catheter into the apex of the left ventricle will be preferred. Gentle suction applied to the vent prevents overdistension of the left ventricle and greatly reduces the risk of air embolism.

With or without the presence of a left ventricular vent it is desirable to aspirate the ascending aorta to remove any air present. Prolonged venting of the ascending aorta is achieved by creating a needle hole at the highest point on the vessel or by using special needles which may be connected to suction. Air ejected from the left ventricle during bypass will remain in the ascending aorta until partial bypass has been resumed. Such air is effectively evacuated by the aortic needle.

It is now an accepted fact that successful surgery may be performed in the heart under conditions of anoxic arrest. However, myocardial preservation is enhanced by the use of local and systemic hypothermia, metabolic drugs, and by intermittent or continuous perfusion of the coronary artery. Ordinarily, periods of total ischemia of the myocardium produced by cross-clamping of the ascending aorta should be limited to approximately 15 min. Uneven cooling of the myocardium may occur if only systemic hypothermia is employed. In addition to the circulation of cool blood by the heart-lung machine, it is wise to provide additional cooling by ice water or slush infused into the pericardium with the head of the table elevated and rotated to the left. The endocardium is cooled by flushing the ventricular cavity(s) with iced saline from time to time throughout the procedure. The advantages of coronary artery perfusion are obvious. There are, however, certain disadvantages associated with coronary artery perfusion. The cannula and other equipment may compromise the operative field to an unbearable extent. The profused myocardium retains muscle tone which makes exposure of the aortic root more difficult, whereas the nonperfused cold heart undergoes a relaxation which enhances surgical exposure. Direct injury to the coronary ostium during coronary artery profusion may produce tear, dissection, or embolism. Overzealous perfusion and high pressure may result in an actual decrease in myocardial functional capacity. If perfusion is maintained at 100 to 150 cc per coronary artery per minute at a mean pressure not exceeding 100 mm Hg, the electrocardiogram attests to satisfactory myocardial oxygenation, and the heart is likely to resume adequate contractions when bypass is discontinued. The work of Hoffman and Buckberg in determining the patterns of coronary blood flow and myocardial oxygenation with various temperatures and functional states is most significant.[23a]

At the present time most cardiac surgeons limit periods of ventricular fibrillation whenever possible, if necessary resorting to the inconvenience of periodic defibrillation during the operative procedure. Other surgeons avoid fibrillation by using cardioplegic solutions which produce asystole and decrease oxygen demand.[23b] Additionally, these studies have provided emphasis on preservation of the endocardium by local hypothermia achieved by ventricular flushing with iced saline and other similar solutions.

Perfusion techniques

Cardiopulmonary bypass has become an established technique. With advanced technology and experience, the equipment and perfusates have been simplified. The use of disposable oxygenators and dilute primes has greatly facilitated the operation of cardiopulmonary bypass. At present, the bubble-type oxygenator is selected by the majority of perfusionists for routine procedures which may be performed in less than 4 h. The membrane oxygenator is used routinely by a few perfusionists, but its greatest present application is for long-term respiratory support. The priming volume of most adult bypass circuits ranges between 1,500 and 2,000 cc. The trend is toward more dilute primes to reduce blood demands and improve tissue perfusion. Hemodilution reduces viscosity, improves microcirculation, and decreases hemolysis. The degree of dilution is limited so as not to reduce the patient's hematocrit below 20 percent. Priming solutions consist of balanced electrolyte solutions, 5 percent dextrose, plasma expanders such as dextran 40, and blood components when indicated. Just prior to bypass 15 to 20 percent of the patient's blood volume may be withdrawn from the inferior caval catheter by gravity into a reservoir and replaced by transfusing prime solution through the arterial cannulas so as to maintain an adequate cardiac output. This homologous blood is transfused postbypass, resulting in improved clotting studies and reduced blood bank demands. The patient's normal fluid balance is usually restored within 5 days postbypass through diuresis. High flow rates in the range of normal cardiac output are desirable. These are normally calculated to be approximately 2.4 liters/m²/min in adults, 2.6 liters/m²/min in children, and 2.8 liters/m²/min in infants.

Hypothermia is employed as an adjunct to perfusion. Direct blood cooling allows for rapid changes in body temperature, which reduces the metabolic rate and oxygen needs of the tissues. With hypothermia the heart can sustain anoxia for various time periods, thus enabling the surgeon to interrupt its blood supply and perform certain procedures such as coronary bypass grafts. Mild hypothermia of 30 to 32°C is utilized for certain congenital procedures such as atrial septal defect and ventricular septal defect closures. Moderate hypothermia of 25 to 28°C is used for procedures which require longer bypass times such as coronary bypass grafts and valve replacements. Profound hypothermia of 15 to 20°C is employed in infant cases which require prolonged periods of total circulatory arrest up to 60 min.

Initially, partial bypass is established by unclamping the caval catheters and allowing gravity drainage from the venae cavae to the heart-lung machine. Total bypass is not achieved until the umbilical tape tourniquets are snug about the catheters within the venae cavae or until the pulmonary artery is occluded. It is necessary for the anesthesiologist to maintain oxygenation during partial bypass, since some pulmonary blood flow is obviously maintained at this time. When there is a marked arteriovenous difference, as is frequently the case in critically ill patients, it is desirable to maintain partial bypass for a somewhat longer period. Such dual oxygenation permits more rapid correction of metabolic derangement.

At the termination of a total bypass, partial bypass is reinstituted and the contribution of the pump oxygenator to cardiac output is progressively decreased. During this interval, right and/or left atrial pressures are monitored carefully. Slight overtransfusion is desirable, and left atrial pressure should be brought to approximately 10 to 20 mm Hg as indicated. In some circumstances it is possible to terminate bypass rather abruptly; in other instances, partial bypass is progressively discontinued over a period of several minutes to several hours. A rare patient would benefit from prolonged assistance to circulation. Techniques that have been employed clinically include the left atrial–aortic bypass pump of DeBakey and the synchronized intraaortic balloon of Kantrowitz. Most patients with valvular heart disease do not present problems of resuscitation at the operating table, but patients with advanced states of disease frequently require diligent postoperative management to assure adequate cardiac output.

Several factors must be considered at the termination of bypass to ensure adequate cardiac output: (1) *Mild overtransfusion:* It is absolutely essential that the vascular bed be filled to the point of tolerance in the critically ill postoperative cardiac patient. Catheters are left in either the right atrium, left atrium, or pulmonary artery for postoperative monitoring of venous pressure. Ordinarily, bypass is terminated with a left atrial pressure of 15± mm Hg and/or a central venous pressure of 10 mm Hg. In situations of low cardiac output the left atrial pressure may be raised to 20+ mm Hg. (2) *Rhythm control:* It is important to provide for cardiac pacing if heart block has developed or if significant bradycardia is present. A single myocardial electrode is inserted routinely in patients undergoing valve replacement or coronary bypass surgery. This is most readily accomplished by means of a unipolar epicardial electrode sutured into either ventricle and led out through the skin at a point well away from the surgical incision and its dressing. This electrode and the reference electrode are then connected to an external pacemaker, and the rate is adjusted to the point of maximal cardiac output. Starr has advocated and emphasized the value of atrial pacing in postoperative patients following valve replacement. (3) *Corticosteroids:* Large doses of corticosteroids provide an inotropic effect and peripheral vasodilatation that may enhance borderline cardiac output and improve organ perfusion. (4) *Drugs:* Almost all patients receive calcium chloride intravenously in a dose of 0.5 to 2 g given over an interval of several minutes. Digitalis may or may not be administered intravenously depending upon cardiac output, rate, and electrolyte concentration. If, at this point, the systolic blood pressure is not maintained above 90 mm Hg, additional volume is administered to raise the left atrial pressure to approximately 20 mm Hg. If inadequate output persists, dopamine (Intropin) is begun at the rate of 5 to 15 μg/kg/min. In the event that inadequate response to dopamine is noted, epinephrine (8 μg/cc) is begun at the rate of 2 to 10 μg/min. If there is reason to suspect beta-adrenergic receptor blockage due to propranolol administration up to the time of surgery, isoproterenol (Isuprel) (4 μg/cc) is the drug of choice and is administered at 2 to 8 μg/min. If these agents are ineffective and the condition of low systemic pressure and elevated left atrial pressure persists, a trial of vasodilator therapy is warranted, and nitroglycerin may be given intravenously at a dosage of 32 to 64 μg/min or intravenous nitroprusside (Nipride) 100 μg/cc may be given at 20 to 40 μg/min.[24–26] We have noted most gratifying responses to both agents. On theoretical grounds nitroglycerin may be a superior drug in patients with coronary artery disease. If cardiac output remains inadequate or if inotropic agents such as epinephrine in a dose of 10 μg or more per minute are required to maintain satisfactory blood pressure for a period of more than 1 to 2 h, the intraaortic balloon should be inserted and placed in operation. Earlier insertion of the intraaortic balloon may be indicated if a known insult to the myocardium has occurred. The counterpulsation decreases the preload and afterload, and also increases coronary diastolic blood flow.[27]

If the systemic blood pressure is higher than normal at the termination of bypass, the anesthetic agent, typically 50 percent nitrous oxide, is turned on, and protamine sulfate may be administered more rapidly than usual. Persistently elevated blood pressure is then managed with intravenous chlorpromazine (Thorazine) 1 to 5 mg or by the intravenous administration of nitroglycerin or nitroprusside in the dosage mentioned above. (5) *Acid-base balance:* The arterial pH, P_{a,CO_2}, P_{a,O_2} are checked before termination of bypass, so that these parameters may be properly adjusted to assure optimal cardiac activity. A slight metabolic alkalosis is preferred at this time to assure maximal effect of catecholamines. Sodium bicarbonate will also tend to increase cardiac output and peripheral perfusion by its vasodilating effect.[28]

Anticoagulation is terminated by the administration of protamine sulfate. The dose of protamine is calculated on the basis of a heparin half-life of 2 h. The calculated remaining heparin is reversed milligram per milligram with protamine. An activated clotting time is performed 10 min after the reversal dose is administered to ensure normal coagulation. Blood is also sent to the coagulation laboratory for confirmation of proper neutralization by the protamine titration test. Additional blood is sent to the laboratory for determination of the prothrombin time, partial thromboplastin time, fibrindex, fibrinolysis, Lee-White clotting time, platelet count, and plasma hemoglobin level. Any abnormalities are promptly treated accordingly.

With satisfactory cardiac activity and adequate hemostasis, wound closure is begun. The thoracotomy is drained with anterior and posterior thoracotomy tubes. The sternotomy is drained by a catheter or catheters placed into the mediastinum, or a pleural space is opened, and both mediastinum and pleural spaces are drained. The pericardium should never be tightly closed. It is frequently left completely open. Some postoperative bleeding will occur with almost all patients; and even with apparently satisfactory tube drainage, liquid and clotted blood may accumulate sufficiently to produce cardiac tamponade. The differentiation of cardiac tamponade from low cardiac output due to other causes is difficult to make, so every effort should be made to see that cardiac tamponade cannot develop. It is desirable to close the pericardium over the right ventricle when this can safely be accomplished, to avoid adherence of the right ventricular myocardium to the sternotomy incision. This is particularly important if a second cardiac procedure will be required at a later date.

Many perfusion operators employ mannitol routinely in the perfusate. Others employ mannitol at the earliest signs of hemoglobinuria. Hemoglobinuria is ordinarily encountered only with prolonged bypass or excessive use of suction equipment or both. The appearance of pigment in the urine should prompt the administration of mannitol or some osmotic diuretic to enhance urine flow. Additional protection should be afforded the kidney in such situations by alkalinization of the urine. Alkalinization of the urine reduces the formation of acid hematin in the presence of hemoglobinuria. It is the acid hematin that is particularly damaging to the distal renal tubule.

POSTOPERATIVE MANAGEMENT

During the first few days following surgery it is essential to have monitoring of the central venous pressure, arterial pressure, arterial blood gases, urine output, daily weight, serial hematocrit readings, frequent estimations of the electrolyte content, and daily chest roentgenograms. An ECG rhythm strip should be taken prior to the administration of digitalis, particularly when repeated doses are given in order to detect signs of intoxication. Constant ECG monitoring is necessary.

Assisted ventilation, controlled ventilation, and intermittent mandatory ventilation (IMV) are valuable techniques to ensure adequate oxygenation in the early postoperative period. It has become common practice to leave an endotracheal tube in place in the early postoperative period until ventilation is adequate. The adequacy of ventilation is determined clinically and by direct measurement of respiratory volumes and blood gases. If prolonged access to the trachea is desirable, the orotracheal tube may be removed and a nasotracheal tube inserted after the clotting mechanism has returned to normal. Placing a nasotracheal tube prior to heparinization or during heparinization may result in a troublesome hemorrhage. The use of an endotracheal tube to avoid tracheostomy in patients with median sternotomy is well conceived. If a tube has been employed for 8 to 10 days and assisted ventilation is still required, it is preferable to convert to tracheostomy, although in special circumstances tubes have been employed successfully for periods of several weeks. The respirator is set to deliver the inspired concentration of oxygen needed to maintain the arterial P_{a,O_2} at about 100 mm Hg. If over 60 percent inspired oxygen is required, positive end-expiratory pressure (PEEP) should be utilized to decrease the risk of oxygen toxicity. Large tidal volumes of 10 to 12 ml/kg should be used at a slow rate of 8 to 10 breaths per minute for best oxygenation and ventilation. Marked respiratory alkalosis should be avoided due to the associated hypokalemia, arrhythmias, and increased oxygen consumption.

Low cardiac output

The cardiac output is impaired for a number of days following cardiopulmonary bypass and can result from a number of problems (see Table 95B-1). A study of 34 patients after open heart surgery revealed cardiac outputs of 2.4 liters/min in 19 patients and of less than 2.0 liters/min in 15 patients. The cause of the low output was unknown in more than one-half the patients. Those with low outputs had a higher mortality rate and more frequent occurrence of the "sudden death" syndrome.[29] A low cardiac output is more common following mitral valve surgery and correction of tetralogy of Fallot than after aortic valve surgery.[30] A low cardiac output is one of the most common immediate complications of open heart surgery. It is recognized on inspection. The

Factors causing low cardiac output

Inadequate intravascular volume
Myocardial infarction
Severe intrinsic heart disease
Acidosis with decreased contractility
Arrhythmia
Improper placement of prosthesis
Unrecognized coronary disease
Tamponade
Pulmonary embolism
Congestive heart failure

skin is cool and often mildly cyanotic; the veins on the dorsum of the hand are constricted or collapsed. The patient may be restless or lethargic. The arterial blood pressure is usually–but not invariably–reduced and the urinary output drops to 30 ml/h or less in the adult. The majority of patients in this group have hypovolemia. The blood volume may be reduced as much as 25 percent within 1 h following bypass and may return to normal within 48 h.[31] If the patient's left atrial pressure is relatively high (up to 20 mm Hg) at termination of bypass, this problem should be minimized.[3] The central venous pressure should be kept above 12 mm Hg during the early hours following operation unless there is excellent stability of the circulation. Because of pericardial effusion, the apparent central venous pressure and the effective transmural pressure may be different. Kirklin has pointed out that the intrapericardial pressure may be as high as 10 mm Hg in the absence of clinical or roentgenographic evidence of significant pericardial fluid.[33] Thus a high filling pressure may be required to maintain adequate cardiac output. The effects over a period of 15 to 30 min of the administration of 250 to 500 ml of blood or plasma protein fraction upon venous pressure, arterial pressure, urine flow, pulse rate, the character of the skin and superficial veins, and the appearance of the patient are more important than any single venous pressure reading. One may expect a loss of 500 to 1,000 ml of blood through the thoracotomy tubes following surgery, and the appearance of signs of a low cardiac output may be delayed for a number of hours. Serial hematocrit readings may help in determining the need for blood or other fluids, but a single value at any given time may not indicate this need.

When large amounts of citrated blood have been given, the ionized calcium level may be depressed, with impairment of cardiac contractility. Calcium chloride, 250 to 500 mg, may be given to improve the contractile force. It should be avoided if there is any question of overdigitalization. Because of the impaired myocardial contractility following total cardiac bypass, the administration of an inotropic agent such as isoproterenol or dopamine by slow intravenous drip may be helpful. When these drugs are used, it is mandatory to maintain an adequate effective circulating blood volume.

Pressor agents to raise the blood pressure should be used only when it is clear that the hypotension does not respond to rapid infusion of blood, dextran, or plasma. It is essential not to hide the need for plasma expansion by the use of pressor agents.[1]

In rare instances there may be decreased cardiac output, arterial hypotension, and cold, dry, cyanotic skin with a high filling pressure. The syndrome is due to increased peripheral vascular resistance and may respond to dilute solutions of nitroprusside, nitroglycerin, or phenoxybenzamine hydrochloride. Hypovolemia is commonly associated with this condition and requires correction.

Hypertension may occur in the previously normotensive patient following bypass and may require an infusion of trimethaphan (Arfonad), sodium nitroprusside, or nitroglycerin.[24-26] Hypertension and tachycardia may also be seen with hypercapnia.

When bypass is carried out with a dilute prime, there may be marked weight gain and sequestration of plasma in the interstitial tissue. When there is mobilization of fluid, hypervolemia may occur in spite of restriction of fluid and increased urine output. In one study the increase in plasma volume averaged 530 ml on the first day, and the rise continued slowly for 5 days. Pulmonary edema and right-sided heart failure occurred in some patients. Treatment consists of administration of conventional diuretic therapy and restriction of fluid.

In most instances a low urinary output is an indication not for osmotic diuretics, but for volume expansion. The oliguria may be due to congestive heart failure and may improve rapidly with intravenous diuretics such as furosemide or ethacrynic acid. It is possible to have shock, alveolar pulmonary edema, and normal left ventricular end-diastolic pressure in the presence of excessive sweating and the administration of diuretics. Pulmonary edema may clear with the improvement of filling pressure of the heart by fluid administration.[36]

Other causes of a low cardiac output include (1) inadequate repair of defects, (2) myocardial factors such as myocardial infarction or coronary embolism with microinfarction,[3] and (3) AV block with slow ventricular rates inadequate to meet the metabolic demands of the postoperative period. Some authors believe that the most common cause of the low cardiac output syndrome is the severity of the intrinsic heart disease.[38] Uncorrected metabolic acidosis from bypass or poor tissue perfusion may reduce myocardial contractility and produce low output.[39-41] Treatment consists of intravenous administration of sodium bicarbonate.

Pericarditis

Some degree of pericardial effusion and/or inflammation invariably follows incision of the pericardium. It is usual to hear a pericardial rub with or without a mediastinal crunch immediately after surgery and for several days thereafter. One must remember, however, that a rub may be produced by the mediastinal drainage tubes. There may or may not be electrocardiographic changes of pericarditis. Pericardial inflammation involving the SA node is an important inciting factor in supraventricular arrhythmias. Such inflammation is one of the common causes of fever after the first few postoperative days. Pericardial effusion due to congestive heart failure or inflammation may increase the size of the cardiac silhouette and make serial assessments of heart size difficult both before and after surgery. Pericardial effusion following incision of the pericardium may respond rapidly to Aldactazide (50 mg spironolactone with 50 mg hydrochlorothiazide) daily for 5 days combined with 40 to 60 mg prednisone daily. Pericardial pain may respond to aspirin or indomethacin (Indocin), but all too often these agents do not adequately control pain, and corticosteroid therapy is then needed. Prednisone is given on a gradual reduction schedule over a period of 3 to 4 weeks. At times there is associated pleural effusion, which may also clear up with corticosteroid therapy. Recurrence of pericarditis weeks or months later is common and may be unassociated with ECG changes, pericardial friction rub, or fever. Recurrences are often overlooked, since pain may be localized to the trapezius region or shoulder and is misdiagnosed as being "muscular" in origin. The diagnosis of recurrent pericarditis after weeks or months is made from the history, since a pericardial rub or electrocardiographic changes are commonly absent. The late occurrence of tamponade has been reported in patients receiving anticoagulants and salicylates after open heart surgery.[42] When patients are receiving anticoagulants, corticosteroids rather than salicylates should be used to control pericardial pain and effusion.

Mediastinal tamponade
(see Chap. 84)

Tamponade may occur whether or not the pericardium is left open or closed at surgery. This serious complication may occur either in the early hours after surgery or days or weeks later. There may be organized clots as well as liquid blood which seal the opening in the pericardium and produce tamponade. This complication is more common in the early postoperative course after removing pacing wires and in the presence of anticoagulation. Its recognition may be difficult since pulsus paradoxus of 10 mm Hg or more, the usual hallmark, may be present due to tubes in the chest, during artificial ventilation, bronchospasm, intubation, myocardial failure, or pneumothorax. Atrial fibrillation or shock may make recognition difficult. Furthermore, the amount of paradox obtained varies with different observers and, of course, with the depth of respiration. There is a range of pulsus paradoxus over which tamponade may be present (8 to 15 mm Hg), but cases have been reported with no significant paradox.[45a] Tamponade

may occur even though no pericardial rub has been previously heard, and no characteristic electrocardiographic changes of pericarditis are present. Occasionally, low amplitude of the complexes may be a clue, although this is absent in the overwhelming majority of patients. Sinus tachycardia is usually present, but there may be atrial fibrillation or flutter incited by inflammation in the area of the SA node. Indeed, early and late atrial arrhythmias should always arouse the suspicion of acute pericarditis. Rarely, we have seen bradycardia at the onset of cardiac tamponade. The differential diagnosis includes (1) low output syndrome, (2) pulmonary embolism, (3) dissecting aneurysm of the aorta, (4) pneumothorax, (5) congestive heart failure, (6) acute myocardial infarction, (7) post-pump perfusion lung, (8) atelectasis, (9) pleural effusion, (10) hemorrhage in the mediastinum, pleura, gastrointestinal tract, or retroperitoneal space, and (11) acute surgical abdomen.

Symptoms of tamponade may vary from restlessness, weakness, dyspnea, increase in respiratory rate, pain in the anterior chest, shoulders, interscapular area, or right upper quadrant. Think of tamponade (1) when there is pain in anterior chest, shoulders, back, and right upper quadrant; (2) when there is sudden deterioration in the postoperative period; (3) with the development of atrial arrhythmias; (4) as a cause of unexplained dyspnea; (5) as a cause of the drop in hematocrit; (6) to explain deterioration of condition within 24 h of removal of epicardial pacing wires; (7) when brisk bleeding from chest tubes in the postoperative period suddenly stops; (8) when there is neck vein distension out of proportion to evidence of heart failure; (9) with widening of the mediastinum or increase in size of heart silhouette over a period of one to several days; (10) when congestive heart failure is suspected, but the chest x-ray does not show the expected congestion of the lungs. Impaired cardiac output may be manifest by cool, clammy skin and oliguria. Abnormal neck vein distension is usually present, but may be difficult to discern in children and adults with short, thick necks. The venous pressure is invariably elevated. It is not widely recognized that the early stage of tamponade may be associated with a blood pressure that is normal or as high as 150 systolic. The pulse pressure may be within normal limits, but as the intrapericardial pressure increases, it becomes narrow. Tamponade, however, should not be excluded in the absence of narrowing to any given level (such as 10 to 15 mm Hg). The inspiratory filling of the right ventricle may produce paradoxic motion of the septum to the left and posteriorly with narrowing of the left ventricular outflow tract, an important factor producing pulsus paradoxus. The x-ray may show new enlargement of the cardiac silhouette, but often no significant change in size can be detected. The echocardiogram may demonstrate pericardial effusion, which is a common finding after open heart operations, but this does not indicate tamponade. A decrease in the E-F slope of the anterior leaflet of the mitral valve has been reported in tamponade but is not diagnostic.[42] Chronic left-sided heart tamponade without elevation of the venous pressure and without pulsus paradoxus but with continued fever for 4 months was reported by Simpkin et al.[43]

CHAPTER 95B **1787**
MEDICAL MANAGEMENT IN CARDIAC SURGERY

We have observed 21 patients with late cardiac tamponade. Of these 19 occurred as a complication of 877 consecutive open heart operations at Emory University Hospital and 2 occurred in patients who were operated on elsewhere.[44]

Tamponade was developed by 5 within 48 h of surgery, while 18 cases occurred after the sixth postoperative day. Of the 18 late cases, less than 50 percent had a blood pressure of 100 diastolic, but 3 were in shock. A decrease of the hematocrit of greater than 5 points over a 72-h period occurred in 8 of 18 patients. Unexplained blood loss in the late postoperative period should lead to the search for tamponade. Widening of the mediastinum was noted in 7 of 15 patients, and clear lung fields tended to differentiate tamponade from heart failure in patients with increasing cardiac silhouette and a low cardiac output state. Mediastinal aspiration was successful in 11 of 15 patients. Since that report, there have been a total of 26 cases of late tamponade observed in 1,300 consecutive operations (2.6 percent) at Emory University Hospital. The seriousness of delayed tamponade in children after open heart surgery was highlighted by 4 deaths in 11 cases collected from the literature.[45]

In questionable cases, bedside catheterization may furnish evidence of tamponade by demonstration of a "pressure plateau" between right atrial, right ventricular diastolic, pulmonary arterial diastolic, and pulmonary wedge pressure similar to that found in constrictive pericarditis.[45a] However, the life-threatening situation may allow no time for confirmational studies.

Treatment consists of increasing the filling pressure by volume loading and isoproterenol 1 to 2 mg/500 cc (2 to 4 µg/cc) to stimulate the myocardium while preparing for pericardiocentesis.[46] Needle aspiration from a subxiphoid approach is carried out using a 14-gauge needle. The inability to obtain fluid by needle pericardiocentesis does not exclude tamponade, and if evidence is compelling, open drainage should be carried out. If the bloody fluid is too thick for aspiration, open drainage may be accomplished at the bedside using intravenous diazepam and opiates or ketamine (Ketalar) and removing stitches and wires from the lower sternum. A drainage tube is left in place, and Prostaphlin is administered for 5 days. Prednisone 40 to 60 mg daily should be used following removal of fluid to lessen the chances of recurrence. The drug is slowly tapered over a period of 3 to 4 weeks. Diuretics may enhance resolution of pericardial and pleural effusions, but due care must be taken to avoid hypokalemia and decrease in ventricular filling pressure.

Arrhythmias

Arrhythmias may be a cause of decreased cardiac output when the ventricular rate is excessively rapid. A listing of common precipitating factors is shown in Table 95B-2. The successful control of arrhythmias

TABLE 95B-2
Precipitating factors in postoperative arrhythmias

Hypoxia
Digitalis intoxication
Hypokalemia
Hypovolemia
Atelectasis
Pericarditis
Pulmonary infection
Pulmonary embolism
Anemia
Hyperoxic alveolopathy
Metabolic acidosis
Metabolic alkalosis
Left-sided heart failure
Hypercarbia
Trauma of ball on septum
Injury to sinus node at operation
Increased levels of catecholamines, either endogenous or exogenous
Myocardial infarction

may depend on correction of the precipitating factors. Atrial fibrillation and, less often, atrial flutter are the most frequent arrhythmias. They are generally best controlled by increasing doses of digoxin by vein, with the addition of 1 to 3 mg propranolol. Often doses that approach toxicity are required. Digoxin may be given in increments of 0.125 to 0.25 mg at intervals of one to several hours until the ventricular rate has been satisfactorily slowed. Ventricular rates of 100 to 120 beats per minute are generally well tolerated, and attempts to produce additional slowing are probably unwise, unless the state of the circulation demands further improvement. Lidocaine (Xylocaine) is contraindicated in atrial flutter since it may increase conduction through the AV node allowing 1:1 conduction. Ventricular tachycardia and ventricular fibrillation may be induced (Fig. 95B-1). This is a particular hazard when atrial fibrillation with aberrant conduction is mistaken for ventricular tachycardia and lidocaine is administered. Frequent ventricular premature beats or ventricular tachycardia may respond to intravenous lidocaine. When shock is present, 1 mg phenylephrine (Neo-Synephrine) intravenously may terminate atrial or ventricular tachycardia. Propranolol's efficacy is attested to by the report that it converted 8 of 13 instances of paroxysmal atrial fibrillation, 4 of 8 instances of atrial flutter, and 3 of 4 instances of frequent ventricular premature beats in the immediate postoperative period.[45] Propranolol may be given intravenously in a dose of 0.5 mg every 4 to 5 min until a total of 3 to 5 mg has been given. Rare instances of cardiac arrest have occurred, even after small doses have been administered. Propranolol may be used in conjunction with digitalis when control of rapid ventricular response in atrial fibrillation is difficult with digitalis alone. It is contraindicated if there is a history of asthma or if pulmonary

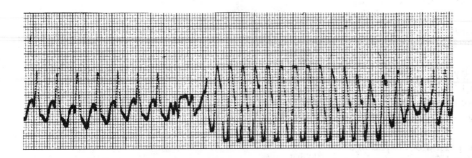

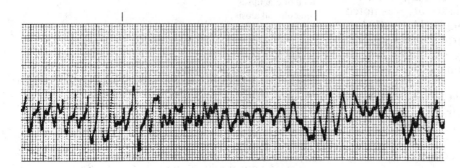

FIGURE 95B-1 W. H., a 63-year-old man, developed atrial flutter with aberrant conduction misinterpreted as ventricular tachycardia—lidocaine produced 1:1 conduction and ventricular fibrillation. The patient was cardioverted and recovered.

edema is present. Bradycardia and AV block may be induced. Propranolol is especially useful when the arrhythmia is thought to be due to digitalis intoxication. There is suggestive evidence of synergistic effect when propranolol is used in conjunction with quinidine in the conversion of atrial fibrillation.[45] Propranolol should be used with great caution since it may produce a low cardiac output with shock or may induce congestive heart failure. When used in conjunction with lidocaine, procainamide, or quinidine, the negative inotropic effects summate with further impairment of the contractile state.

Occasionally dc countershock is needed when the state of the circulation requires prompt conversion. However, dc countershock is generally avoided except when other measures for controlling arrhythmias are ineffective, since there is the small risk of wound dehiscence, and predisposing factors persist, with frequent recurrence of the arrhythmia. The chest should be supported with a tight binder to minimize chances of wound disruption. Diazepam may be used for amnesia in a dose of 5 to 25 mg given intravenously. In the presence of narcotic administration, care should be exercised to avoid respiratory depression.

Later in convalescence, pericarditis may produce atrial arrhythmias because of inflammation in the region of the sinus node. These may respond to conventional therapy but also may subside with administration of steroids. Hypokalemia secondary to the bypass procedure, to diuretics, or to steroids may predispose to arrhythmias. Arrhythmias incident to atelectasis, with its consequent hypoxia and hypercarbia, may not respond until adequate humidification and tracheal suction have been carried out and the arterial blood gases have improved with use of artificial ventilators combined with PEEP. Bronchoscopy is rarely required with modern improvements in respiratory care.

Nursing care

The importance of comprehensive nursing care during the critical postoperative period cannot be overemphasized. The cardiac surgical nurse should be skilled in cardiopulmonary assessment of the patient including the ability to recognize life-threatening arrhythmias and respond appropriately with medications and/or resuscitative measures including defibrillation. An understanding of the various parameters involved in the assessment and their interrelationships is essential in detecting subtle changes or trends in the patient's pressure, heart rate and rhythm, and breath sounds.

The educational program for the cardiac nurse should be continuous and should include content about the pathophysiology of heart disease, fluid and electrolyte balance, pharmacology, respiratory therapy, and electrocardiography. In addition, information about the operation of the various types of pressure modules, ventilatory equipment, and devices to assist in fluid delivery and circulatory management is essential for adequate patient assessment and nursing intervention. The nurse should also be skilled in patient education and work closely with the patient and family during the preoperative and postoperative periods in planning for discharge.

Respiratory care

Hypovolemia, the most significant immediate postoperative hazard, may be accompanied by or quickly replaced by respiratory problems. In addition to those complications common to any operative procedure—atelectasis, inability to cough, inspissated mucus, bronchospasm—there are those specifically resulting from the use of cardiopulmonary bypass and ventilators (oxygen toxicity). Some degree of pulmonary insufficiency is invariably present. Damman et al.[35] list the following causes of respiratory insufficiency:

1 Those that cause alveolar hypoventilation
   a Respiratory depressant drugs
   b Failure to clear anesthetic agents completely
   c Shallow breathing due to incisional pain
   d Circulatory insufficiency with impaired blood flow to the muscles of respiration
2 Faulty pulmonary function with increased respiratory workload
   a Decrease in amount of functioning lung tissue due to retained secretions and atelectasis
   b Compression atelectasis from accumulation of blood in the pericardium or mediastinum and excessively enlarged heart
   c Bronchiolar spasm due to drugs or local trauma
   d Pleural fluid
   e Interstitial or alveolar pulmonary edema
   f Emphysema
   g Acute pulmonary infections
   h Alveolar and capillary thickening resulting from chronic increase in left atrial pressure

Other factors resulting from prolonged bypass may include the interstitial deposition of hemolyzed blood and loss of surfactant with an increase in alveolar surface tension which produces diffuse atelectasis.

Careful management of the respiratory system, with close attention to humidification, periodic overinflation of the lung, elimination of bronchospasm and avoidance of hypoventilation and hyperventilation, with their hazards of acidosis and alkalosis, respectively, must be maintained. In the open heart patient whose arrhythmia-susceptible myocardium is exquisitely sensitive to minimal changes in pH, P_{a,O_2}. and P_{a,CO_2}. such changes occur frequently in the immediate postoperative period. An orotracheal tube is left in place in most patients during the first few hours to 24 h following surgery. With adequate preoperative explanation to the patient regarding its postoperative presence, an endotracheal tube is well tolerated. If ventilation is controlled, the patient may be kept heavily sedated. Frequently, the patient is kept only slightly sedated, so that assisted ventilation and IMV (intermittent mandatory ventilation) may be used. If after 7 to 10 days, it is determined that prolonged ventilatory assistance is required, a tracheostomy may be performed. Today this is rarely required.

Careful monitoring of the adequacy of postoperative ventilation by serial measurements of the arterial P_{a,O_2}. P_{a,CO_2}. pH, and the O_2 concentration in the inspired gases is the only accurate method of assessment. The clinical detection of arterial oxygen desaturation is notoriously poor. The serial measurement of blood gases will establish the ventilation requirement of rate, volume, and oxygen concentration. Oxygen concentration should not exceed 60 percent because of the role of 100 percent oxygen in producing oxygen toxicity.[47] It is frequently possible to maintain adequate arterial oxygenation with lower inspired oxygen if positive end-expiratory pressure is used. This technique leads to an increase in functional residual capacity and a decrease in physiologic venous-arterial shunting. It is not always possible to maintain adequate oxygenation without high concentrations. Furthermore, the concentration of oxygen actually delivered by some machines is not accurate. Hyperoxic alveolopathy may occur after 24 to 36 h of administration of 100 percent oxygen. It is manifested by dyspnea, tachypnea, cyanosis, hypertension, cardiac arrhythmia, and varying amounts of interstitial and alveolar edema. The lungs become stiff, and their compliance is reduced. There may be physiologic right-to-left shunting of blood past collapsed alveoli. Pathologically there may be hyaline membranes, vascular engorgement, interstitial edema, hemorrhage, and changes in the capillary endothelium and alveoli, with proliferation of alveolar lining cells and ultimately fibrosis. Thus pulmonary function may be impaired to some degree over a period of time. Proper humidification plays a very important role in optimum postoperative care. Attempts to assure adequate moisture by bubbling oxygen through water at room temperature are foolhardy and serve mainly to establish a false sense of security. Cascade humidifiers, superheated steam nebulizers, or ultrasonic nebulizers are the only effective instruments for obtaining optimal humidification. Frequent deep endobronchial suctioning to clear inspissated secretions is of primary importance and with improved methods of humidification is very effective.

Fever in the immediate postoperative period is almost always present and may have several causes (see Table 95B-3). It is the common manifestion of atelectasis. Impaired percussion and increased breath sounds over areas of the lungs may be found at a time when the roentgenogram reveals no consolidation. The causes of atelectasis and ventilation and perfusion problems in the postoperative period re-

TABLE 95B-3
Common causes of postoperative fever

Atelectasis
Pleuropericarditis
Hypothalamic injury
Sepsis
Endocarditis
Urinary tract infection
Thrombophlebitis
Drugs
Tissue necrosis
Empyema
Wound infection
Mediastinitis
Pulmonary infarction

main unclear. Some investigators believe that atelectasis due to inadequate production of or decrease of surfactant is a result of improper ventilation during anesthesia. Others have suggested that it is due to enzyme disequilibrium related to oxygen toxicity or that inadequate humidification is the causative factor. Others feel that the inability to cough effectively is of major importance. In addition, the drying effect of respirators coupled with positive-pressure "packing" of secretions further impairs ventilation. Volume ventilators are preferred in some centers because they can be adjusted more accurately to deliver carefully calculated volumes and specifically determined oxygen concentrations. In 65 cases analyzed by Cooperman[48] it was not found that the Engstrom unit was superior to the Bird unit or vice versa. It should be noted that respiratory assistance in the immediate postoperative period can significantly reduce cardiac work, since as much as 50 percent of cardiac output may be used in the work of breathing.[49,50] In the absence of sufficient respiratory support (including proper oxygen administration), hypoventilation, hypoxia, acidosis, and hypercarbia may develop. The consequence of this sequence of events may be hypotension, cardiac arrhythmias, and/or poor tissue perfusion, which lead to cardiovascular collapse.[3,38] Depressed myocardial contractility with decreased myocardial responsiveness to the inotropic effects of catecholamines may be the cause of seriously low cardiac output states.[39-41] Improved ventilation and/or the use of intravenous sodium bicarbonate may be indicated.

Post-perfusion lung[51,52]

Many pathophysiologic mechanisms have been proposed to explain the so-called post-perfusion or "pump" lung.[34] The existence of this complication usually becomes apparent within the first few hours after cardiopulmonary bypass. The inability to wean a patient from the respirator heralds the often rapid and fatally progressive alveolocapillary block syndrome. Care must be taken to distinguish this syndrome from pulmonary edema secondary to left ventricular failure. Alveolar pulmonary edema in the early postoperative period is not common, whereas some degree of interstitial edema is not infrequent. Proper attention to fluid balance, body weight, and central venous pressure and assuring complete or near complete mechanical correction of valvular or shunt defects are probably responsible for the small incidence of pulmonary edema. Overvigorous attempts at volume replacement to improve urinary output in the face of sufficient central venous pressure are most often the causes of pulmonary edema in this setting. Since the post-perfusion lung syndrome may reveal findings similar to those of heart failure, including rales, wheezes, retraction, severe tachypnea, and cyanosis with resultant decreased cardiac output and poor perfusion, a chest roentgenogram is most helpful. The roentgenogram of the post-perfusion lung is characterized by patchy infiltrates.

The length of cardiopulmonary bypass seems to be one of the factors directly proportional to the incidence of pump lung. Experimental evidence in dogs in which the lung was excluded from bypass demonstrated significantly fewer pathologic changes of perivascular hemorrhage and thickened intraalveolar septa. This led Nahas[53] and his associates to postulate that the perfusion itself is the primary cause of the syndrome.[54-56] Others believe that particulate matter in the blood contributes to the syndrome. The use of micropore blood filters may have contributed to the decreased incidence of "pump work." Although the chest roentgenogram is helpful, the inability to wean a patient from the respirator and a need for increased intraalveolar pressure to maintain adequate oxygention establish the diagnosis. The value of corticosteroids in this setting has not been confirmed, but they are used. Continued respiratory support and conscientious pulmonary care are probably more important. If a patient survives 48 to 72 h, he will usually recover, but after 1 to 2 weeks there are occasional deaths due to progressive pulmonary insufficiency secondary to the post-perfusion lung. The patient should be observed closely when respiratory assistance is being reduced, since hypoxia may produce ventricular fibrillation.

Trauma to the phrenic nerve during surgery may result in paresis or paralysis of the diaphragm. This may impair alveolar ventilation and predispose to atelectasis. Often the paralysis is permanent. Hoarseness may persist for months. Disarticulation of ribs incised at surgery may contribute to pulmonary insufficiency, but it more often produces troublesome chest pain for weeks or months.

Electrolyte disturbances

HYPOKALEMIA
Potassium depletion is not uncommon immediately following cardiopulmonary bypass. There is a massive loss of potassium while on cardiopulmonary bypass. Most of the potassium is lost in the urine and recently it has been shown that cardiopulmonary bypass activates the renin-angiotensin-aldosterone system. Occasionally, as much as 100 to 150 mEq of potassium chloride have to be given to the patient while on cardiopulmonary bypass to maintain the serum potassium level over 4.0 mEq/liter. Hypokalemia may also appear in the postoperative period due to reactivation of insulin 2 to 6 h after cardiopulmonary bypass, respiratory or metabolic alkalosis, or diuretics. This hypokalemia plays an important role in precipitating arrhythmias in a digitalized patient. Adequate replacement of potassium is essential.

HYPERKALEMIA
Elevation of the serum potassium level to 6.0 mEq/liter or greater may occur in the first 24 h after surgery at a time when there may be metabolic

acidosis, dimished renal output, hemoglobinuria, multiple transfusions, and accumulation of blood in serous cavities. The serum potassium level should be determined frequently during the first 24 h. Serial ECGs taken at midprecordial leads for evidence of potassium toxicity, such as tenting of the T waves and widening of the QRS complexes, may be helpful. However, these are not reliable as determinations of potassium content. Potassium solutions should be given very slowly intravenously. Cardiac arrest has been noted by the authors after a sudden bolus from the solution in the tubing when infusing sets were changed. This is a particular hazard if concentrated solutions are given through catheters placed in the superior vena cava; two arrests have been reported when 10 million units of potassium penicillin were given rapidly by this route.[58] Cardiac arrest due to ventricular fibrillation occurred in two patients after oral supplements[5] of potassium chloride. Treatment of hyperkalemia consists of administration of sodium bicarbonate, 50 to 150 mEq, and 500 ml 20 percent glucose with 30 units of insulin. This is effective within 30 min. Calcium gluconate 1 to 2 g may also be given slowly intravenously when continued therapy is indicated; sodium polystyrene sulfonate (Kayexalate), orally or by retention enema, may be beneficial. Ordinarily hemodialysis is not required. Hyperkalemia may be rapidly replaced by hypokalemia as urinary output improves.

HYPONATREMIA

Sodium depletion is rare following open heart surgery. When it is present, there has usually been some precipitating factor such as vomiting, intubation, diarrhea, or excessive losses during the diuretic phase of acute tubular necrosis. On the other hand, it is common to find serum sodium concentrations of 130 mEq/liter or less because of overhydration. This may be due to the trauma of surgery and increased secretion of ADH (antidiuretic hormone) or to renal insufficiency. In this setting, the serum osmolarity is reduced, there is weight gain, and the urinary sodium excretion is normal. The serum potassium level may be normal or elevated. When fluids are restricted and diuresis ensues, hypokalemia may occur and produce digitalis toxicity and serious arrhythmias. There is no indication for administration of hypertonic NaCl solutions. This disturbance usually corrects itself spontaneously after a few days.

Water intoxication

When water is retained in excess of electolytes, there may be a decrease of the serum sodium to levels as low as 112 to 115 mEq/liter. Other electrolyte values may be correspondingly low. Because of the selective nature of the blood-brain barrier, water may be retained in the brain out of proportion to sodium. Symptoms such as restlessness, confusion, coma, and convulsions may occur. Treatment consists of restriction of water intake to 300 to 500 ml/day plus insensible loss and the slow intravenous administration of 200 to 300 ml of 3 percent saline solution.

Occasionally, diuresis with furosemide or other diuretics may bring improvement. Mannitol and massive steroid therapy have been used.

Recognition and treatment of congestive heart failure

Congestive heart failure may be difficult to diagnose in the immediate postoperative period. Dyspnea, rales, and tachycardia are usual in these postoperative patients. Abnormal neck vein distension may be obscured because of the increased venomotor tone, use of ventilators, and trauma to the veins incident to monitoring central venous pressure or performing jugular venipuncture for other purposes. There may be abnormal neck vein distension because of pericardial effusion or junctional rhythm. Measurements of central venous pressure may give fallacious results because of use of an improper reference point. An error may be produced if the catheter is not within the thorax, or if there is occlusion of the catheter orifice by the vein wall or blockage by fibrin or clot. Oliguria may be due to hypovolemia or causes other than congestive heart failure. The most reliable means of detecting congestive heart failure is a chest roentgenogram obtained with portable x-ray equipment and demonstrating either interstitial or alveolar pulmonary edema. Interstitial edema is not uncommon but may be confused with intrapulmonary hemorrhage, pneumonia, infarction, or collections of pleural fluid. Alveolar pulmonary edema in the immediate postoperative period is rare. It may be difficult to distinguish the roentgenographic changes due to the post-pump syndrome from pulmonary congestion due to heart failure. In these instances the rapid clearing following administration of 40 to 80 mg of furosemide intravenously furnishes strong evidence of left-sided heart failure. One cannot rely on the existence of the ventricular diastolic gallop rhythm as evidence of left-sided heart failure when the valve leaflets have been replaced by a mitral prosthesis. It is usual for the total body weight to increase 5 to 10 lb after bypass is terminated due to sequestration of fluid. This fluid retention corrects itself after 3 to 4 days. This has been attributed to an increase in the secretion of antidiuretic hormone secondary to surgical trauma and to increased capillary permeability secondary to bypass. Weight gain occurring after the first few days may furnish evidence of heart failure or renal insufficiency.

Because of impaired contractility present in the first 24 to 48 h after operation, a slow intravenous drip of isoproterenol (1 to 2 mg/500 ml of 5 percent dextrose in water) may improve cardiac output. The rate of administration should be adjusted to avoid ectopic beats or excessive ventricular rates (120 beats per minute). Dopamine may also be used. Glucagon, 3 to 5 mg/h given in isotonic glucose, may on occasion improve myocardial contractility, but its action is weak and nausea is frequently produced. Intravenous ethacrynic acid (Edecrin) or furosemide may produce a profound diuresis in a few hours, providing there is adequate renal blood flow. At times diuresis may not occur unless isoproterenol is given concomitantly. Hypovolemia may result from excessive diuresis. In those instances in which excessive fluid administration has resulted in pulmonary edema, phlebotomy may be indicated, with subsequent readministration of packed red blood cells.

In the undigitalized adult, when rapid digitalization is required, an initial dose of 0.75 mg digoxin may be given intravenously with increments of 0.25 mg at intervals of 3 h for two to three additional doses. Caution is used with subsequent therapy to avoid toxicity. Patients with compensated congenital heart disease are not digitalized prior to surgery. Patients requiring right ventriculotomy often have impaired contractility and must be digitalized in the first few days postoperatively because of right ventricular failure. When there is a slow nodal rhythm or AV block due to trauma of surgery, pacing the heart through epicardial wires placed in the atrium or ventricle may improve pump function; they are left in place for a week by which time conduction disturbances have cleared. Rarely, a permanent pacemaker may be required. If such is anticipated, permanent pacing wires may be placed at the time of surgery and used if necessary. A slow rate, at a time when metabolic demands are increased, may be inadequate to prevent heart failure.

Some of the factors responsible for the delayed onset of heart failure are pulmonary embolism, coronary artery embolism, myocardial infarction, pulmonary infection, fibroelastosis occurring in the ventricular myocardium adjacent to a mitral prosthetic ball valve, malpositioned or partially disrupted valves, spontaneous rupture of the endocardium near the base of the papillary muscle, and previously undetected coronary disease. Bacterial endocarditis is a rare cause of heart failure in the early postoperative period. Constrictive pericarditis is a rare cause of predominant right heart failure within a few months following open heart surgery.

Neurologic syndromes

Open heart surgery may be associated with a variety of neurologic disorders such as confusion, coma, postoperative acute toxic phychosis, loss of memory for the immediate postoperative period, cerebral edema, convulsions, embolism to the brain, particulate matter producing hemiplegia, paraplegia, visual disturbances, or spotty brain deficits. Fortunately, the majority clear spontaneously and residual handicaps are infrequent. However, in one study of 417 patients there was a 19.2 percent incidence; there were 21 postoperative deaths, with 11 being associated with the neurologic deficits. Hemiplegia occurred in 36 and coma in 28.[59]

Factors predisposing to neurologic complications

may be listed as long bypass runs, hypotension during pump runs,[60] older age, sleep deprivation, prior neurologic disease, severe atheromatous disease of the aorta or valves, gaseous microembolism,[61] platelet fibrin thrombi, cotton fiber embolism from sponges,[62] etc. Microfilters have reduced but not totally prevented these disorders. Massive doses of penicillin used in the pump solutions have produced seizures; four patients had seizures when 50 million units of penicillin was used.[63]

Drug reactions may contribute to postoperative depression, agitation, or insomnia. Confusion, anxiety, and restlessness may be warning signs of hypoxia. Prompt recognition and immediate corrective measures are mandatory, since cardiac arrest may occur. Morphine and sedatives may hasten this catastropic series of events.

Confusion and toxic psychosis may be due to drugs or to emotional and physical exhaustion in the intensive care unit, where the patient is constantly beset by procedures and examinations that preclude sleep. Blachy[63a] reported that 79 of 278 patients having isolated mitral replacements developed psychoses in the immediate postoperative period. Moving the patient to the more familiar surroundings of a regular hospital room may produce clearing of such psychoses. Psychosis due to steroid administration is rare. Psychosis may be treated by phenothiazines such as Thorazine, 50 mg orally every 4 h. Haldol 2 mg given two or three times daily may benefit the confused patient. When a history of heavy alcohol or barbiturate intake prior to surgery is obtained, these drugs should be administered in the postoperative period to prevent seizures due to withdrawal.

Hematologic problems

Bleeding problems during the immediate postoperative period are usually not the result of inadequate neutralization of heparin, the excessive use of protamine sulfate, the presence of fibrinolysins, or the occurrence of "consumption coagulopathy," but are due to continued oozing or active arterial bleeding. Constant surveillance by the surgeon, hematologist, and cardiologist is necessary to assure prompt and appropriate therapeutic measures. It is occasionally necessary to reopen the chest to identify and control bleeding sites if repeated transfusions do not stabilize the circulation and reduce the rate of blood loss. In the early period of open heart surgery Porter[64] states that even though platelets and other coagulation factors were reduced during extracorporeal circulation, the most common cause of excessive bleeding was inadequate hemostasis. This remains true today.

Despite improvements in oxygenators and shortening of cardiopulmonary bypass time with improved technical abilities, abnormalities in various blood coagulation factors are inevitable.[64-66] To some degree these abnormalities can be minimized by the use of autologous blood transfusions during surgery.

If fibrinolysis of significant degree is demonstrated, epsilon-aminocaproic acid (EACA) therapy is indicated. Some studies suggest that the level of plasminogen activator, the cause of this fibrinolysis, is significantly reduced when EACA is used prophylactically and that postoperative bleeding is similarly decreased.[6] At present EACA is used only when significant fibrinolysis is demonstrated–an uncommon event. Although some hematologists[34] suggest that a careful differentiation must be made between fibrinolysis and consumption coagulopathy (disseminated intravascular coagulation), this abnormality has not been found to cause inordinate hemorrhage. Such a distinction would be of obvious import since use of heparin, which is often employed to treat disseminated intravascular coagulation, might be fatal in fibrinolytic states. Although a few hematologists believe that an anticoagulation or heparin rebound can account for significant postoperative blood loss,[68,69] most authorities do not concur with this opinion. The excessive dose and too rapid administration of protamine sulfate have been implicated in postoperative hemorrhage.[70] Recently we have studied the reduced dose of protamine following cardiopulmonary bypass and found less postoperative bleeding with this regimen.[70a] We reverse only the residual heparin, assuming that heparin has a half-life of 2 h. Care in calculating and injecting protamine coupled with postoperative protamine titration tests eliminate this as a problem.

Isoimmunization on rare occasions may be the cause of massive red blood cell loss in the immediate postoperative period.[71,72] Retyping and transfusion of packed, preferably washed red blood cells are necessary under these circumstances. Lostumbo and associates[73] found that in 45 of 127 patients undergoing open heart surgery, one or more red blood cell antibodies appeared in the postoperative period.

The presence of prosthetic valves with their accompanying hemodynamic turbulence results in red blood cell trauma and decreased red blood cell survival in all cases.[74–77] Malpositioned prostheses, regurgitation around inadequately sutured valves, and regurgitation against Teflon patches[78–80] can result in hemolysis sufficient to produce anemia. Here the urinary iron loss exceeds the absorption capacity of the gastrointestinal tract. Hemolytic anemia may be a problem during convalescence and later. Transfusion of packed red blood cells, large doses of iron, folic acid, and corticosteroids have been used, but persistent severe hemolysis is an indication for replacement of the valve.

Antileukocyte and lymphocytotoxic antibodies have been identified in post-cardiopulmonary bypass patients[81] but are not thought to cause significantly reduced resistance.

Hepatic problems

Kloster and Bristow[82] stated in 1965 that approximately 10 percent of cardiopulmonary bypass patients have elevated serum bilirubin levels at some time in the postoperative period and that 2 percent have overt hepatic failure. Most large series indicate similar incidences.[83–85] In Sanderson's study, no correlation of postoperative jaundice with length of bypass, halothane anesthesia, pH changes, P_{CO_2} levels, or use of vasopressors was found.[83] Of 736 patients, 63 developed serum bilirubin levels greater than 3 mg/100 ml. Of these 73, 59 had bilirubin elevations within the first few days with a peak level occurring at 7 to 10 days and a rapid fall by approximately 2 weeks. There were no deaths in this group, whose SGOT levels were usually between 50 and 150. Of four patients who had late elevations (12 to 14 days), two died and all had very high SGOT levels.

Among a group of 200 patients studied by Rubinson,[85] 24 had hapatitis with jaundice usually occurring approximately 2 months postoperatively. Of these patients 2 had subsequent evidence of chronic hepatic impairment. There was one death from serum hepatitis 35 days postoperatively.

Proposed pathophysiologic mechanisms for early postbypass jaundice include hypoxia, low cardiac output, microembolization, venous cannual obstructions, altered hepatic vein flows, cholestasis, and preexisting marginal hepatic compensation. There are no confirmed hypotheses of a unifactorial etiology. Donor blood seems the most significant source of serum hepatitis. At the present time, a nationwide double-blind study is in progress to determine the efficacy of gamma globulin prophylaxis.

Endocarditis

Sources of contamination and septicemia are common during cardiopulmonary bypass operations and in the postoperative period, although the incidence of endocarditis is small. Kluge et al.[86] found positive blood cultures from the pump in 47 of 66 patients (71 percent), but postoperative blood cultures were sterile. Sites of contamination were repaired areas of myocardium and prostheses prior to wound closure. It was found that 41 percent of urinary catheter tips and 50 percent of intravascular tips yielded a variety of gram-positive and gram-negative organisms and fungi, but there was no case of endocarditis. An interesting study by Yeh of 400 patients revealed positive cultures from 35 of the preoperative pump prime mixtures.[8] Of these patients with positive cultures from the pump prime, all except one had negative blood cultures immediately following surgery. All the patients were placed on procaine penicillin and streptomycin prophylactically. Of 19 patients who had positive postoperative cultures from the pump, only 2 developed endocarditis that was due to the same organism as that cultured from the pump. Intraarterial catheters have been demonstrated to have positive cultures for flavobacillus from stopcocks which had been contaminated by ice used to cool syringes for taking blood gases.[88] A review of 492 patients having indwelling arterial catheters showed no systemic infection; however, 4 percent of 200 requiring cannulas for a longer period of time had positive cultures of the catheter tips.[89] *Pseudomonas* septicemia from contamination of pressure transducers occurring when the sterilizing technique was changed has been observed by the authors. Other sources of infection are suppurative phlebitis of veins, pulmonary infection associated with the use of artificial ventilators, wound infection, and infections of the genitourinary tract. In general, staphylococci and gram-negative organisms are responsible for early infections; however, diphtheroids and fungal infections, while rare, pose especially difficult problems of recognition and cure, since positive cultures are less frequent and large emboli are common in the fungal group. In a series of 45 cases of *Candida* infections, one-half had no fever early, and less than one-half had positive blood cultures in the first month, and the survival rate was only 17 percent.[90] In a review of 35 cases of *Aspergillus* endocarditis, 27 occurred after surgery, 18 being on prosthetic valves; 28 of 34 had negative blood cultures.[91] We believe, however, that this incidence of endocarditis is greater on prosthetic valves that it is on other diseased valves. Wilson et al.[92] noted endocarditis on a prosthetic valve in 45 cases out of 4,706 valves (0.99 percent); 16 (0.35 percent) occurred early, and 29 (0.63 percent) late. *Staphylococcus aureus* (44 percent) and gram-negative bacilli (38 percent) were the most common isolates in the early group, while streptococci viridans (41 percent) and gram-negative bacilli (31 percent) were the most common organisms in the late group. They found that 49 percent survived and the medical therapy was curative in 60 percent, and combined medical and surgical therapy was curative in 40 percent. The mean time of occurrence was 17 days in the early groups and 25 months in the late group. In Starr's series there were no reports of wound sepsis or endocarditis.[93] Similarly in Kloster's review of the medical problems in postoperative open heart patients, no endocarditis was reported.[82] Duvoisin et al.[84] reviewed the late follow-up of 1,355 valve replacements at the Mayo Clinic and found 18 cases involving the aortic valve, 4 involving the mitral valve, and 1 following a multivalvular operation. Roberts' series of 64 patients who died in less than a month after open heart surgery revealed no evidence of infection on the valves, even though a number of the valves were coated with fibrin, and many had clots in the atria and ventricles.[94] On the other hand, endocarditis has been observed in 0.5 percent of 2,288 survivors of open heart surgery.[95] The authors reviewed 97 cases from the literature and reported a mortality of 72 percent.

Renal complications

Renal failure of varying degrees may occur in 6 to 10 percent of patients undergoing cardiopulmonary bypass procedures. The frequency has been reduced with improvements in bypass techniques, apparatus, use of dilute prime solutions containing mannitol, shorter pump runs, and use of bypass assist techniques coming off the pump and in the postoperative period. It may take the form of (1) prerenal azotemia, (2) nonoliguric renal insufficiency with creatinine levels of 2 to 5 mg/ml, or (3) oliguric renal failure with serum creatinine levels above 5 mg/ml.

In one study 150 of 490 patients developed some evidence of renal failure.[96] In 269 the creatinine level did not exceed 2 mg/dl without associated oliguria, and recovery ensued in 4 to 37 days. The creatinine concentration exceeded 5 mg/dl in 21 patients, and 11 were oliguric; 14 died in spite of dialysis from cardiac causes or sepsis. In another study 35 patients out of 500 developed acute renal failure (6 percent), and another 102 had prerenal azotemia, a total of 20.7 percent with some degree of renal dysfunction. The mortality in those with acute renal failure was 88.8 percent.[9] Abel et al.[98] reported that 198 of 507 patients following cardipulmonary bypass developed a blood urea nitrogen level over 50 mg/ml and a creatinine level greater than 30 mg/ml. The mortality in those with normal renal function was 1.6 percent compared to 30.3 percent for those with renal failure. The higher mortality was associated with septicemia, pulmonary insufficiency, gastrointestinal hemorrhage, central nervous system dysfunction, acute electrolyte imbalance causing cardiotoxicity and heart failure due to fluid overload. Yevoah et al.[99] reported some degree of renal failure in 30 percent of 428 patients, but in only 3 percent was renal failure sufficient to cause death. Autopsies of 40 patients dying of all causes showed acute tubular necrosis in 10, renal infarcts in 7, pyogenic abscess in 2, and varying degrees of microembolism. Porter reported 14 percent incidence of renal failure in 21 patients who received no mannitol but only 1 percent in 270 patients who received the drug.[100] Excessive use of mannitol may induce hyperosmolarity, hyponatremia, and pulmonary edema; rarely nephrosis may be induced.[101]

In order to prevent renal complications following open heart surgery, one must be aware of predisposing causes. They are as follows:

1 Preoperative elevation of BUN and creatinine levels
2 Decreased 24-h creatinine clearance
3 Older age
4 Duration of bypass
5 Aortic cross-clamping
6 Total time of operation
7 Postoperative acidosis with pH below 7.25
8 Excessive hemolysis with plasma hemoglobin in excess of 200 mg/100 ml
9 Low urine flow rate (less than 1.8 liters/m²/min)
10 Hypotension prior to or during bypass, or after return to the intensive care unit
11 Occult dissecting aneurysm
12 Atheroembolism to the kidneys
13 Embolism from heart to the kidneys

It should be realized that up to one-third of instances of renal failure may develop without oliguria. Thus, it is essential to monitor the BUN and creatinine levels daily for the first few days following cardiopulmonary bypass. Conversely, oliguria does not of itself indicate renal failure. The most frequent cause of oliguria is inadequate volume replacement, there regularly being sequestration of fluid in the third space, and in addition 500 to 1,000 cc blood loss during the first 12 to 24 h. There may be inadequate replacement of blood and fluid that reduces glomerular filtration and urine flow. Monitoring the left atrial pressure or measuring the wedge pressure by a

Swan-Ganz catheter gives ready evidence of the need for fluid administration. Many sick hearts with decreased compliance require 20 mm Hg filling pressure to maintain an adequate cardiac output and renal blood flow. The measurement of central venous pressure has marked limitations and may give misleading values. It is often wrong to administer a diuretic rather than fluid when urine flow decreases. Diuresis may induce further hypovolemia and compound the problems.

Prerenal azotemia, due either to hypovolemia or impaired cardiac output, may be suspected by spot urine examination revealing 10 mEq of sodium or less. The urine may be concentrated with increase in specific gravity (1.018 to 1.030) and osmolarity. Volume expansion may result in prompt rise in urine output. By contrast, in most patients with acute tubular necrosis, the urine is isosthenuric with specific gravity of 1.010 to 1.015, and the urine sodium is at least 25 mEq/liter, provided the specimen is not collected after a diuretic is given. The urinary/plasma (U/P) osmolarity ratio of 1:1 or less is characteristic of acute tubular necrosis; these patients will not respond to volume expansion, and the response to diuretic therapy is impaired. In prerenal failure the U/P ratio of urea is 20:1, whereas in acute tubular necrosis it is 3:1, rarely exceeding 10:1. In prerenal failure, U/P creatinine ratio is usually 40:1 or more, and less than 10:1 in acute tubular necrosis. Hematin casts, usually considered the hallmark of acute tubular necrosis, are not reliable indexes in patients following cardiopulmonary bypass because of hemolysis and acidification of heme pigments which occur in most patients. Yeh et al. reported albuminuria in 85 percent, gross or microscopic hematuria in 40 percent, and granular casts in 20 percent of patients following cardiopulmonary bypass.

In the postoperative period the most obvious clue that renal function might be diminishing is oliguria or anuria. The significance of oliguria can be determined only with an understanding of the factors known to cause it. Oliguria, defined as urinary output below 400 ml/24 h, may be due to any of the following: (1) physiologic factors (decreased effective plasma volume due to sequestration of fluid in the "third space," increased antidiuretic hormone, increased aldosterone, and decrease in the saluretic or "third factor"); (2) blood and fluid loss (hemorrhage, drainage, diuresis, sweating); (3) low cardiac output syndrome; (4) congestive heart failure; (5) cardiac tamponade; (6) shock of whatever etiology; and (7) renal failure. The latter cause may be regarded as one of two types: (a) functional (decrease in renal blood flow and glomerular filtration rate due to prerenal factors and edema of the kidney without ischemic necrosis) and (b) organic (patchy or diffuse acute tubular necrosis due to renal ischemia).

Salt and water overload is a constant hazard to the patient with renal insufficiency. Peripheral edema, congestion, and hyponatremia may result. When this occurs, fluids must be restricted and protein intake reduced. Fluid restriction to 500 cc plus insensible fluid loss may be needed. Mannitol and furosemide may be repeated at intervals of 4 to 6 h. Monitoring of the serum potassium level and the use of the electrocardiogram to detect hyperkalemia are essential. Electrocardiographic changes of hyperkalemia include sinus arrest with loss of atrial activity and tall tented T waves, best detected in leads V_2 and V_3. The QRS may become prolonged to 0.10 to 0.12 s. This may be treated by giving 50 cc of 50 percent glucose with 50 units insulin intravenously. In addition, 80 to 132 mEq of sodium bicarbonate dissolved in 1 liter of 5 percent glucose in water may be given as follows: One-third of the liter may be given intravenously in the first hour and the remainder may be given intravenously over the next 2 to 5 h to counteract cardiotoxicity. Calcium chloride 10 to 20 cc intravenously is effective. Kayexalate orally or by enema may be administered to lower potassium levels. It is common for the patient to have hypokalemia in the immediate period following a bypass procedure, and due care is needed to replete the potassium by intravenous therapy. Hyperalimentation with amino acids may be helpful during the course of prolonged azotemia. Peritoneal dialysis or hemodialysis with the use of an arteriovenous shunt may be required. Unfortunately, the mortality remains excessively high (65 to 85 percent) in those requiring dialysis. Multisystem disease is common, and death is usually due to septicemia, pulmonary infection, pulmonary insufficiency, renal infection, neurologic complications, or cardiac causes. During the recovery period there may be spontaneous diuresis of up to 2 liters/day, and due care is needed to balance the fluid and electrolytes. Recovery after acute tubular necrosis may continue for 3 to 13 months, and there is commonly some residual degree of renal insufficiency.

Post-pump lymphocytosis

From 1 to 3 months following open heart procedures an occasional patient develops a syndrome consisting of fever, splenomegaly, and lymphocytosis.[102] Most often the clinical setting is one in which bacterial endocarditis is suspect. When infection has been excluded, such patients are diagnosed as having the post-pump or post-perfusion syndrome. Lang[103] has described four patients in whom a significant rise in the complement-fixation antibody to cytomegalovirus (CMV) has been demonstrated. In three of these patients virus was recovered in the blood. Virus was recovered from the urine of all patients. The CMV virus was isolated in five of six patients with the post-pump perfusion syndrome reported by Kantor et al.[104] If the patient's constitutional symptoms are of sufficient magnitude, corticosteroid therapy is indicated. The authors institute prednisone, 10 mg four times a day for 1 to 2 weeks, with a tapering dose scheduled thereafter. Most often a course of therapy covering from 3 to 4 weeks is sufficient. Because of the syndrome's similarity to mononucleosis, a heterophil titer is mandatory. Because of the presence of fever coupled with splenomegaly and lymphocytosis, drug fever must also be considered.

Recurrent pericarditis manifested by fever with or without the presence of a pericardial friction rub may be confused with CMV infection.

Arterial embolism

The major late complication of valve replacement is arterial embolism from thrombi on the prosthetic ring or valve. Obtaining accurate statistics regarding the incidence of such embolization is difficult. Some authors report only those arterial emboli which result in disability or death, while others report those occurring in chronic atrial fibrillation or during sufficient or insufficient anticoagulation.[105] The criteria for determining the adequacy of anticoagulation vary from physician to physician, and the technique of performing the prothrombin time test differs from laboratory to laboratory. Considering these and other problems, statistics regarding arterial embolism are inaccurate, and its incidence is definitely underestimated.

Heparin is ordinarily not used for early postoperative anticoagulation except in certain patients undergoing coronary artery surgery. Warfarin (Coumadin) is started from the second or third postoperative day.[94,106,10] It has been stated that anticoagulation in patients with aortic prostheses does not reduce the incidence of embolization.[91] Most patients with prostheses, whether mitral, aortic, or multiple, or whether in atrial fibrillation or normal rhythm, are, however, on lifelong use of anticoagulants, except where Hancock heterograft valves are used.

In larger series in which patients have been followed at least a year, arterial thromboembolism occurred in more than 25 percent of all cases. In a 6-year follow-up of mitral replacements, 37 percent of those with mitral valve disease and 24 percent of those with multiple valve disease had late emboli, with 2 percent and 3 percent deaths, respectively.[106] Of these patients 50 to 66 percent had no residual disability. Kloster and associates reported that 43 percent of their patients with isolated mitral valve disease and 12 percent with aortic valve disease had emboli in the first 3 months after surgery.[82] Effler and his associates reported 22.6 percent and 5 percent emboli in patients with isolated mitral and aortic valve prostheses, respectively.[108] Akfarion et al. reported thromboembolism in 24 percent of 238 patients with Starr valves, with death in approximately one-fourth of these. In a recent analysis of 1,315 patients, Duvoisin reported that in 228 patients with isolated mitral Starr valves, 22 patients had disabling emboli, 7 of which resulted in death.[84] The introduction of velour-covered valves of the 2300–6300 series has been associated with a decreased incidence of long-term thromboembolism whether or not anticoagulants are used.[109-111] There is an increased incidence of early thromboembolism in the immediate weeks or months following operation. Because of increased gradients the 2300–6300 valves have been replaced by the 2310-6310 series. Current practice suggests that anticoagulation be continued for a period of 6 months with aortic valve and indefinitely for mitral valve prosthesis. Unfortunately, fatal hemorrhage due to anticoagulant therapy still occurs on rare occasions and many surgeons no longer use anticoagulants since the introduction of cloth-covered valves. Beall et al.[112] reported an incidence of 4.5 percent thromboembolism in 202 patients with Teflon-coated disk valves who were followed for 12 to 28 months. Dipyridamole (Persantin) to reduce platelet aggregation has been combined with anticoagulant therapy and has been reported to lessen the incidence of thromboembolism.[113] Further experience is needed to assess this therapy.

The introduction of the Hancock heterograft valve has been associated with a marked reduction of thromboembolism and the need for long-term anticoagulation. We have used this valve at Emory University Hospital for the last several years whenever the cardiac condition permits its use. (See Chap. 60B.) We have not used anticoagulation following the placement of a Hancock aortic valve. We do use anticoagulation following the placement of a Hancock mitral valve when there is chronic atrial fibrillation, giant left atrium, atrial thrombus noted at surgery, or a history of previous systemic embolism. More experience is needed before a final recommendation can be made regarding this subject.

REFERENCES

1 Williams, J. F., Morrow, A. G., and Braunwald, E.: The Incidence and Management of "Medical" Complications following Cardiac Operations, *Circulation*, 32:608, 1965.

2 Lockey, E., Longmore, D. B., Ross, E. N., and Sturridge, M. F.: Potassium and Open-Heart Surgery, *Lancet*, 1:671, 1966.

3 Davidov, M., Kakviatos, N., and Finnerty, F. A.: The Use of Furosemide in Refractory Heart Failure, *Am. Heart J.*, 76: 143, 1968.

4 Kaplan, J. A., Dunbar, R. W., Bland, J. W., et al.: Propranolol and Cardiac Surgery: A Problem for the Anesthesiologist? *Anesth. Analg.*, 54:571, 1975.

5 Kaplan, J. A., and Dunbar, R. W.: Propranolol and Surgical Anesthesia, *Anesth. Analg.*, 55:1, 1976.

5a Jones, E. L., Kaplan, J. A., Dorney, E. R., King, S. B., III, Douglas, J. S., and Hatcher, C. R., Jr.: Propranolol Therapy in Patients Undergoing Myocardial Revascularization, *Am. J. Cardiol.*, 38:696, 1976.

6 Hallowell, P., Land, J. H., Buckley, M. J., et al.: Transfusion of Fresh Autologous Blood in Open-Heart Surgery: A Method of Reducing Blood Bank Requirements, *J. Thorac. Cardiovasc. Surg.*, 64:941, 1972.

7 Lawson, N. W., Ochsner, J. L., Mills, N. L., et al.: The Use of Hemodilution and Fresh Autologous Blood in Open Heart Surgery, *Anesth. Analg.*, 53:672, 1974.

7a Sandiford, F. M., Chiariello, L., Hallman, G. L., and Cooley, D. A.: Aorto-coronary Bypass in Jehovah's Witnesses, *J. Thorac. Cardiovasc. Surg.*, 68:1, 1974.

7b Kaplan, J. A., Cannarella, C., Jones, E. L., Kutner, M. H., Hatcher, C. H., Jr., and Dunbar, R. W.: Autologous Blood Transfusion during Cardiac Surgery—A Re-evaluation of Three Methods, *J. Thorac. Cardiovasc. Surg.* In press.

8 Hazan, S. J.: Psychiatric Complications following Cardiac Surgery, *J. Thorac. Cardiovasc. Surg.*, 51:320, 1966.

9 Egbert, L. D., Battit, G. E., Turndorf, H., et al.: The Value of the Preoperative Visit of the Anesthesiologist, *JAMA*, 185:553, 1963.

10 Adriani, J.: "Appraisal of Current Concepts in Anesthesiology," vol. 3, The C. V. Mosby Company, St. Louis, 1966.

11 Smith, R. M.: "Anesthesia for Infants and Children," The C. V. Mosby Company, St. Louis, 1968.

12 Lowenstein, E., Hallowell, P., and Levine, F.: Cardiovascular Responses to Large Doses of Morphine Sulfate in Man, *N. Engl. J. Med.*, 281:1389, 1969.

13 Henney, R. P., Vasko, J. S., and Brownley, R. K.: The Effects of Morphine on the Resistance and Capacitance Vessels of the Peripheral Circulation, *Am. Heart J.*, 72:242, 1966.

14 Lowenstein, E.: Morphine Anesthesia—A Prospective, *Anesthesiology*, 35:563, 1971.

15 Lyons, S. M., and Clarke, R. S.: A Comparison of Different Drugs for Anesthesia in Cardiac Surgical Patients, *Br. J. Anesthiol.*, 44:575, 1972.

15a Basta, J. W., and Lichtiger, M.: Comparison of Metocurine and Pancuronium-Myocardial Tension-Time Index during Endotracheal Intubation, *Anesthesiology*, 46:366, 1977.

16 Beall, A. C., Jr., and Cooley, D. A.: Use of Cardiopulmonary Bypass for Resuscitation and Treatment of Acute Massive Pulmonary Embolism, *Pacif. Med. Surg.*, 75:67, 1967.

17 Lillehei, R. C., Longerbeam, J. K., Bloch, J. H., and Manax, W. G.: The Nature of Irreversible Shock: Experimental and Clinical Observations, *Ann. Surg.*, 160:682, 1964.

18 Replogle, R. L., Gazzaniga, A. B., and Gross, R. E.: Stabilization of Cellular Lysosome Membrane during Cardiopulmonary Bypass, *Circulation*, 32(suppl. 2):177, 1965.

19 Moses, M. L., Camishion, R. C., Tokunaga, K., Pierussi, L., and Davies, A. L.: Effect of Corticosteroid on the Acidosis of Prolonged Cardiopulmonary Bypass, *Circulation*, 32(suppl. 2):155, 1965.

20 Dietzman, R. H., Manax, W. G., and Lillehei, R. C.: Shock Mechanisms and Therapy, *Can. Anaesth. Soc. J.*, 14:276, 1967.

21 Hardaway, R. M., James, P. M., Anderson, R. W., et al.: Intensive Study and Treatment of Shock in Man, *JAMA*, 199:779, 1967.

21a Kaplan, J. A., and King, S. B.: The Precordial Electrocardiographic Lead (V_5) in Patients Who Have Coronary-Artery Disease, *Anesthesiology*, 45:570, 1976.

22 Greenhow, G. E.: Incorrect Performance of Allen's Test, *Anesthesiology*, 37:356, 1972.

23 Defalque, R. J.: Percutaneous Catheterization of the Internal Jugular Vein, *Anesth. Analg.*, 52:116, 1974.

23 Hoffman, J. I. E., and Buckberg, G. D.: Pathophysiology of Subendocardial Ischemia, *Br. Med. J.*, 1:76, 1975.

23 Nelson, R. L., Goldstein, S. M., McConnell, D. H., Maloney, J. V., and Buckberg, G. D.: Improved Myocardial Performance after Aortic Cross Clamping by Combining Pharmacologic Arrest with Topical Hypothermia, *Circulation*, 54(suppl. 3):11, 1976.

24 Chatterjee, K., Parmley, W. W., and Swan, H. J.: Beneficial Effects of Vasodilating Agents in Severe Mitral Regurgitation, *Circulation*, 48:684, 1973.

25 Dunbar, R. W., Kaplan, J. A., and King, S. B.: Vasodilator Treatment of Heart Failure after Cardiopulmonary Bypass, *Anesth. Analg.*, 54:842, 1975.

26 Brown, D. R., and Sterek, P.: Sodium Nitroprusside Induces Improvement in Cardiac Function in Association with Left Ventricular Failure, *Anesthesiology*, 41:521, 1974.

27 Buckley, M. T., Craver, J. M., Gold, H. K., et al.: Intra-aortic Balloon Pump Assist for Cardiogenic Shock after Cardiopulmonary Bypass, *Circulation*, 47(suppl. 3):90, 1973.

28 Kaplan, J. A., Bush, G. L., Leckey, J. H., et al: Sodium Bicarbonate and Systemic Hemodynamics in Volunteers Anesthetized with Halothane, *Anesthesiology*, 42:550, 1975.

29 Boyd, A. D., Tremblay, R. E., Spencer, F. C., and Bahnson, H. T.: Estimation of Cardiac Output after Intracardiac Surgery with Cardiopulmonary Bypass, *Ann. Surg.*, 150:613, 1959.

30 Kloster, F. E., Bristow, J. D., and Griswold, H. E.: Problems in Mitral and Multiple Valve Replacement, *Prog. Cardiovasc. Dis.*, 7:504, 1965.

31 McClenahan, J. B.: Blood Volume Studies in Cardiac Surgery Patients, *JAMA*, 195:356, 1966.

32 Moffitt, E. A., Sessler, A. D., and Kirklin, J. W.: Postoperative Care in Open-Heart Surgery, *JAMA*, 199:161, 1967.

33 Kirklin, J. W., and Rastelli, G. C.: Low Cardiac Output after Open Intracardiac Operations, *Prog. Cardiovasc. Dis.*, 10:117, 1967.

34 James, P. M., Jr., Gredenberg, C. E., Levitsky, S., Anderson, R. W., Collins, J., and Hardaway, R. M., III: Central Venous Pressure: Its Use and Abuse, in W. W. Oakes, J. F. O'Malley, and J. H. Moyer (eds.), "Pre- and Postoperative Management of the Cardiopulmonary Patient," Grune & Stratton, Inc., New York, 1969.

35 Damman, J. F., Jr., Thung, N., Christlieb, I. I., Littlefield, J. B., and Muller, W. H., Jr.: The Management of the Severely Ill Patient after Open-Heart Surgery, *J. Thorac. Cardiovasc. Surg.*, 45:80, 1963.

36 Nixon, P. G., Jr.: Pulmonary Edema with Low Left Ventricular Diastolic Pressure in Acute Myocardial Infarction, *Lancet*, 2:146, 1968.

37 Morales, A. R., Fine, G., and Taber, R. E.: Cardiac Surgery and Myocardial Necrosis, *Arch. Pathol.*, 83:71, 1967.

38 Mundth, E. D., and Austen, W. G.: Post-operative Intensive Care in the Cardiac Surgical Patient, *Prog. Cardiovasc. Dis.*, 11:229, 1968.

39 Campbell, G. S., Houle, D. B., Crisp, N. W., Jr., Weil, M. H., and Brown, E. B., Jr.: Depressed Response to Intravenous Sympathicomimetic Agents in Humans during Acidosis, *Dis. Chest*, 33:18, 1958.

40 Darby, T. D., Aldinger, E. E., Gadsen, R. H., and Thrower, W. B.: Effects of Metabolic Acidosis on Ventricular Isometric Systolic Tension and the Response to Epinephrine and Levarterenol, *Circ. Res.*, 8:1242, 1960.

41 Clowes, G. H. A., Jr., Sabga, G. A., Konitaxis, A., Tomin, R., Hughes, M., and Simeone, F. A.: Effects of Acidosis on Cardiovascular Function in Surgical Patients, *Ann. Surg.*, 154:524, 1961.

42 D'Cruz, I. A., Cohen, H. C., Prablure, R., and Blick, G.: Diagnosis of Cardiac Tamponade by Echoardiography Changes in Mitral Valve Motion and Ventricular Dimensions with Special Reference to Paradoxical Pulse, *Circulation*, 52:460, 1975.

43 Simpkin, P., Brown, A. H., Erooz, A., and Brainbridge, N. V.: Chronic Left Heart Tamponade, *J. Thorac. Cardiovasc. Surg.*, 65:531, 1973.

44 Douglas, J. S., King, S. B., Hatcher, C. R., Jones, E. L., and Logue, R. B: Late Cardiac Tamponade after Open Heart Surgery: A Problem of Differential Diagnosis, presented at American College of Cardiology, February 11, 1975.

45 Scott, R. A. D., and Drew, C. E.: Delayed Pericardial Effusion with Tamponade after Cardiac Surgery, *Br. Heart J.*, 35:1304, 1973.

45a Weeks, K. R., Chatterjee, K., Block, S., Mattoff, J. M., and Swan, H. J. C.: Bedside Hemodynamic Monitoring, Its Value in the Diagnosis of Tamponade Complicating Cardiac Surgery, *J. Thorac. Cardiovasc. Surg.*, 71:250, 1976.

46 Kaplan, J. A., Bland, J. W., and Dunbar, R. W.: The Perioperative Management of Pericardial Tamponade, *South. Med. J.,* 69:4, 1976.

47 Nash, G., Blennerhassett, J. B., and Pontoppidan, H.: Pulmonary Lesions Associated with Oxygen Therapy and Artificial Ventilation, *N. Engl. J. Med.,* 276:368, 1967.

48 Cooperman, L. H., and Mann, P. E.: Postoperative Respiratory Care: A Review of 65 Consecutive Cases of Open-Heart Surgery on the Mitral Valve, *J. Thorac. Cardiovasc. Surg.,* 53:504, 1967.

49 Bartlett, R. G., Jr., Brubach, H. F., and Specht, H.: Oxygen Cost of Breathing, *J. Appl. Physiol,* 12:413, 1958.

50 Engstrom, C. G., and Norlander, O. P.: A New Method for Analysis of Respiratory Work by Measurement of the Actual Power as a Function of Gas Flow, Pressure, and Time: A Preliminary Report, *Acta Anaesth. Scand.,* 6:49, 1962.

51 Hood, R. M., and Beall, A. C.: Hypoventilation, Hypoxia, and Acidosis Occurring in the Acute Postoperative Period, *J. Thorac. Cardiovasc. Surg.,* 36:729, 1958.

52 Osborn, J. J., Popper, R. W., Kerth, W. J., and Gerbode, F.: Respiratory Insufficiency following Open-Heart Surgery, *Ann. Surg.,* 156:638, 1962.

53 Nahas, R. A., Melrose, D. G., Sykes, M. K., and Robinson, B.: Post-Perfusion Lung Syndrome: Role of Circulatory Excursion, *Lancet,* 2:251, 1965.

54 Rossi, N. P., Shao-Chi Yu, Koepke, Jr., and Spencer, F. C.: Pulmonary Injury from Prolonged Oxygenation with Venous Blood, *Surg. Forum,* 15:277, 1964.

55 Schramel, R., Schmidt, F., Davis, R., Palmisano, D., and Creech, O., Jr.: Pulmonary Lesions Produced by Prolonged Partial Perfusion, *Surgery,* 54:224, 1963.

56 Galletti, P. M., Hopf, M. A., and Brecher, G. A.: Problems Associated with Long-lasting Heart-Lung Bypass, *Trans. Am. Soc. Artif. Intern. Organs,* 6:180, 1960.

57 Hultgren, H. N., Surevson, R., and Metroch, G.: Cardiac Arrest Due to Oral Potassium Administration, *Am. J. Med.,* 58:139, 1975.

58 Camarota, S. J., Weil, M. H., Hamashiro, P. K., and Shubin, Herbert: Cardiac Arrest in the Critically Ill. A Study of Predisposing Causes in 132 Patients, *Circulation,* 44:688, 1971.

59 Branthwaite, M. A.: Neurologic Damage Related to Open Heart Surgery: Clinical Survey, *Thorax,* 27:748, 1972.

60 Stockard, J. J., Bickford, R. G., and Schamble, J. T.: Pressure Dependent Cerebral Ischemia during Cardiopulmonary Bypass, *Neurology,* 23:521, 1973.

61 Gallagher, E. G., and Pearson, D. T.: Ultrasonic Identification of Sources of Gaseous Microemboli during Open Heart Surgery, *Thorax,* 28:295, 1973.

62 Dimmick, J. E., Boue, K. E., Meadows, R. J., and Benzing, G.: Fiber Embolization, A Hazard of Cardiac Surgery and Catheterization, *N. Engl. J. Med.,* 29:625, 1975.

63 Seamans, K. B., Gloot, P., Dobell, A. R. C., and Wyant, J. D.: Pencillin-Induced Seizures during Cardiopulmonary Bypass. A Clinical and Electroencephalographic Study, *N. Engl. J. Med.,* 278:861,

63a Blachy, P. H., and Starr, A.: Post-cardiotomy Delirium, *Am. J. Psychiatry,* 121:371, 1964.

64 Porter, G. A.: Coagulation Problems Associated with Extracorporeal Circulation and Massive Transfusions: Minutes, *Extracorporeal Circ.,* 90:7, 1958.

65 Phillips, L. L., and Malm, J. R.: Coagulation Parameters following Extracorporeal Circulation Using Acid-Citrate-Dextrose Blood Buffered with Tris (hydroxymethyl) Aminomethane, *Transfusion,* 7:185, 1967.

66 Holswade, G. R., Nachman, R. L., and Killip, T.: Thrombocy-

topathies in Patients with Open-Heart Surgery: Preoperative Treatment with Corticosteroids, *Arch. Surg.,* 94:365, 1967.

67 Gans, H., and Krivit, W.: Problems in Hemostasis during Open-Heart Surgery: III. Epsilon Amino Caproic Acid as an Inhibitor of Plasminogen Activator Activity, *Ann. Surg.,* 155:268, 1962.

68 Gollub, S.: Heparin Rebound in Open Heart Surgery, *Surg. Gynecol. Obstet.* 124:337, 1967.

69 Hampers, C. L., Balufox, M. D., and Merrill, J. P.: Anticoagulation Rebound after Hemodialysis, *N. Engl. J. Med.,* 275:776, 1966.

70 Berger, R. L., Ramaswamy, K., and Ryan, T. J.: Reduced Protamine Dosage for Heparin Neutralization in Open-Heart Surgery, *Circulation,* 37(suppl. 2):154, 1968.

70a Guffin, A. N., Dunbar, R. W., Kaplan, J. A., et al.: The Successful Use of a Reduced Dose of Protamine following Cardiopulmonary Bypass, *Anesth. Analg.,* 55:110, 1976.

71 Wallace, J. M., and Henry, J. B.: Isoimmunization after Massive Transfusion for Open Heart Surgery, *Transfusion,* 5:153, 1965.

72 Perkins, H. A., Day, D., and Hill, E.: An Immunologic Basis for Massive Loss of Red Blood Cells after Open-Heart Surgery (Proceedings 9th Congress of International Society of Blood Transfusion, Mexico City, 1962), *Bibl. Haematol.,* 19:97, 1964.

73 Lostumbo, M. M., Holland, P. V., and Schmidt, P. J.: Isoimmunization after Multiple Transfusions, *N. Engl. J. Med.,* 275:141, 1966.

74 Brodeur, M. T. H., Starr, A., Kohler, R. D., and Griswold, H. E.: Red Blood Cell Survival in Patients with Mitral Valvular Disease and Mitral Valve Prostheses, *Circulation,* 33(suppl. 1):140, 1966.

75 Case Records of Massachusetts General Hospital (Case No. 52-1964) (Dr. W. Dameshak, Discussor), *N. Engl. J. Med.,* 271:898, 1964.

76 Ziperovich, S., and Paley, H. W.: Severe Mechanical Hemolytic Anemia Due to Valvular Heart Disease without Prosthesis, *Ann. Intern. Med.,* 65:342, 1966.

77 Westring, D. W.: Aortic Valve Disease and Hemolytic Anemia, *Ann. Intern. Med.,* 65:203, 1966.

78 Sigler, A. T., Forman, E. N., Zinkham, W. H., and Neill, C. A.: Severe Intravascular Hemolysis following Surgical Repair of Endocardial Cushion Defects, *Am. J. Med.,* 35:467, 1963.

79 Verdon, T. A., Jr., Forrester, R. H., and Crosby, W. H.: Hemolytic Anemia after Open-Heart Repair of Ostium-Primum Defects, *N. Engl. J. Med.,* 269:444, 1963.

80 Sears, D. A., and Crosby, W. H.: Intravascular Hemolysis Due to Intracardiac Prosthetic Devices: Diurnal Variations Related to Activity, *Am. J. Med.,* 39:341, 1965.

81 Hattler, B. G., Jr., Young, W. G., Jr., Amos, D. B., Hutchin, P., and MacQueen, M.: White Blood Cell Antibodies: Occurrence in Patients Undergoing Open Heart Surgery, *Arch. Surg.,* 93:741, 1966.

82 Kloster, F. E., Bristow, J. D., and Griswold, H. E.: Problems in Mitral and Multiple Valve Replacement, *Prog. Cardiovasc. Dis.,* 7:504, 1965.

83 Sanderson, R. G., Ellison, J. H. Benson, J. A., and Starr, A.: Jaundice following Open-Heart Surgery, *Ann. Surg.,* 165:217, 1967.

84 Duvoisin, G. E., Wallace, R. B., Ellis, F. H., Jr., Anderson, M. W., and McGoon, D. G.: Late Results of Cardiac-Valve Replacement, *Circulation,* 37(suppl. 2):75, 1968.

85 Rubinson, R. M., Holland, P., Schmidt, P. J., and Morrow, A. G.: Serum Hepatitis after Open-Heart Operations, *J. Thorac. Cardiovasc. Surg.,* 55:575, 1965.

86 Kluge, R. N., Celia, T. M., McLaughlin, J. S., and Hornick, R. B.: Sources of Contamination in Open Heart Surgery, *JAMA,* 230:1415, 1974.

87 Yeh, T. J., Anabtawi, I. N., and Cornett, V. E.: Bacterial Endocarditis following Open-Heart Surgery, *Ann. Thorac. Surg.,* 3:29, 1967.

88 Stamm, W. E., Colella, J. J., Anderson, R. L., and Dixon, R. E.: Indwelling Arterial Catheter as a Source of Nosocomial Bacteremia, an Outbreak Caused by *Fluorobacterium* Species, *N. Engl. J. Med.*, 292:1099, 1975.

89 Gardner, R. N., Schwartz, R., Wong, H. C., et al.: Percutaneous Indwelling Radial Artery Catheters for Monitoring Cardiovascular Fraction: Prospective Study of the Risk of Thromboses and Infection, *N. Engl. J. Med.*, 290:1227, 1974.

90 Seelig, M. S., Speth, C. P., Kozim, P. J., Tovi, E. F., and Tascheljian, C. L.: *Candida* Endocarditis after Cardiac Surgery, *J. Thorac. Catdiovasc. Surg.*, 65:583, 1973.

91 Carrigosa, J., Leuidon, M. E., Lawrence, T., and Kaye, D.: Cure of *Aspergillus ustus* Endocarditis on a Prosthetic Valve, *Arch Intern. Med.*, 133:486, 1974.

92 Wilson, W. R., Janmin, P. D., Davidson, G. K., Guiliani, E. R., Washington, J. A., and Geroci, J. L.: Prosthetic Valve Endocarditis, *Ann. Intern. Med.*, 82:751, 1975.

93 Starr, A., Herr, R. H., and Wood, J. A.: Mitral Replacement: Review of Six Years' Experience, *J. Thorac. Cardiovasc. Surg.*, 54:333, 1967.

94 Roberts, W. C., and Morrow, A. G.: Causes of Early Postoperative Death following Cardiac Valve Replacement: Clinicopathologic Correlations in 64 Patients Studied at Necropsy, *J. Thorac. Cardiovasc. Surg.*, 54:422, 1967.

95 Shafer, R. B., and Hall, W. D.: Bacterial Endocarditis following Open Heart Surgery, *Am. J. Cardiol*, 25:602, 1970.

96 Bhat, H. G., Cluck, M. C., Lowenstein, J., and Baldwin, D. S.: Renal Failure after Open Heart Surgery, *Ann. Intern. Med.*, 84:677, 1976.

97 Brenner, B. M., and Rector, F. C.: "The Kidney II," W. B. Saunders Company, Philadelphia, 1976, p. 821.

98 Abel, R. M., Wick, J., Beck, C. H., Buckley, M. J., and Austen, G.: Renal Dysfunction following Open Heart Operations, *Arch. Surg.*, 108:175, 1974.

99 Yevoah, E. G., Petrie, A., and Tead, J. L.: Acute Renal Failure and Open Heart Surgery, *Br. Med. J.*, 1:415, 1972.

100 Porter, G. A., Kloster, F. E., Herr, R. J., Starr, A., Griswold, H. E., and Kimsey, J.: Renal Complications Associated with Valve Replacement Surgery, *J. Thorac. Cardiovasc. Surg.*, 53:145, 1967.

101 Yeh, T. J., Brackney, E. L., Hall, D. P., and Ellison, R. G.: Renal Complications of Open-Heart Surgery: Predisposing Factors, Prevention and Management, *J. Thorac. Cardiovasc. Surg.*, 47:79, 1964.

102 Wheeler, E. O., Turner, J. D., and Scannell, J. G.: Fever, Splenomegaly, and Atypical Lymphocytes: A Syndrome Observed after Cardiac Surgery Using a Pump Oxygenator, *N. Engl. J. Med.*, 266:454, 1967.

103 Lang, D. J., Scolnick, E. M., and Willerson, J. T.: Association of Cytomegalovirus Infection with the Post-Perfusion Syndrome, *N. Engl. J. Med.*, 278:1147, 1968.

104 Kantor, G. L., and Johnson, B. L.: Cytomegalovirus Infection Associated with Cardiopulmonary Bypass, *Arch. Intern. Med.*, 125:488, 1970.

105 Yeh, T. J., Anabtawa, I. N., Cornett, V. E., and Ellison, R. G.: Influence of Rhythm and Anticoagulation upon the Incidence of Embolization Associated with Starr-Edwards Prostheses, *Circulation,* 35(suppl. 1):77, 1967.

106 Starr, A., Herr, R. H., Wood, J. A.: Mitral Replacement: Review of Six Years' Experience, *J. Thorac. Cardiovasc. Surg.*, 54:333, 1967.

107 Aldridge, H. E., Goldman, B. S., and Bigelow, W. G.: The Course of Patients following Replacement of the Mitral Valve by a Starr-Edwards Prosthesis, *Dis. Chest,* 50:186, 1966.

108 Effler, D. B., Favaloto, R., and Groves, L. K.: Heart Valve Replacement, *Ann. Thorac. Surg.*, 1:4, 1965.

109 Winter, T. Q., Reis, R. L., Glancey, D. L., Roberts, W. C., Epstein, S. E., and Morrow, A. G.: Current Status of the Starr-Edwards Cloth-covered Prosthetic Cardiac Valves, *Circulation,* 45(6)(suppl. 1):14, 1972.

110 Spencer, F. C., Reed, G. E., Clauss, R. H., Tice, D. A., and Reppert, E. H.: Cloth-covered Aortic and Mitral Valve Prostheses, *J. Thorac. Cardiovasc. Surg.*, 59:92, 1970.

111 Hodam, R., Starr, A., Herr, R., and Pierce, W. R.: Early Experience with Cloth-covered Valvular Prostheses, *Ann. Surg.*, 170:471, 1969.

112 Beall, A. C., Jr., G. P., Reul, G. J., and Guinn, G. A.: An Improved Mitral Valve Prosthesis, presented at American College of Cardiology, March, 1972.

113 Sullivan, J. M., Harken, D. F., and Gorlin, R.: Pharmacologic Control of Thromboembolic Complications of Cardiac Valve Replacement, *N. Engl. J. Med.*, 279:576, 1969.

PART IX

The Heart and Emotional Stress

96
Emotional Stress: Cardiovascular Disease and Cardiovascular Symptoms

EDWIN O. WHEELER, M.D., and
DAVID V. SHEEHAN, M.D.

In this paper I propose to consider a form of cardiac malady common among soldiers, but the study of which is equally interesting to the civil practitioner, on account of its intimate bearing on some obscure or doubtful points of pathology. Much of what I am about to say I could duplicate from the experience of private practice; yet I prefer to let this inquiry remain as it was originally conducted on soldiers during our late war. The observations here collected were made on a series of upwards of three hundred cases. That so large a number were examined is thus explained. Shortly after the establishment of military hospitals in our large cities, I was appointed visiting physician to one in Philadelphia, and there I noticed cases of a peculiar form of functional disorder of the heart, to which I gave the name of irritable heart—a name by which the disorder soon became known both within and without the walls of the hospital.

JACOB M. DA COSTA, 1871[70]

Cardiovascular effects of emotions have been evident throughout recorded history. The relation of such phenomena as palpitation, blushing, pallor, and fainting to emotional stress and their increased occurrence in nervous or emotional persons have been well recognized. It has become clear that emotional stimuli may profoundly influence the cardiovascular system through their effects on the system's autonomic nervous control. Sympathetic or adrenergic activity accelerates the heart, elevates the blood pressure, and strengthens the heartbeat, while parasympathetic or cholinergic activity slows the pulse, lowers the blood pressure, and weakens the heartbeat.

Experimental work in human beings and animals has demonstrated that temporary cardiovascular changes can be induced by stimulation of many areas of the brain, but the direction of the effects has varied, depending on the techniques employed, and has often been unpredictable. Thus, stimulation of areas of the hypothalamus has produced effects similar to those of either sympathetic or parasympathetic stimulation.[1,2] Studies of the effects of emotions on human cardiovascular function have produced somewhat variable results, in part because of the use of varying and sometimes inadequate physiologic techniques and in part because of the varying reactions which may be encountered in the same subject at different times. From a number of careful studies, two basic types of cardiovascular response

to acute emotional stress or anxiety have been defined.[3–8]

The usual reaction to emotion-provoking stimuli, such as stressful interviews, mental arithmetic, pre-examination anxiety, criticism, or pain, has been an increase in heart rate, blood pressure, and oxygen consumption with an increase or decrease in cardiac output and total peripheral resistance. Some normal persons respond with a considerable rise in cardiac output and a fall in peripheral resistance, others with a fall in cardiac output and a rise in peripheral resistance, and still others with a small rise in both. Brod[6] points out that there is no basic difference in these reactions. In all instances, emotional stress causes increased vascular resistance in the kidneys, splanchnic area, and skin, and decreased vascular resistance in muscle. The balance of these effects determines the total peripheral resistance. This hemodynamic response is nonspecific and similar to that occurring with muscular exercise aside from the obligatory increase in cardiac output that accompanies physical activity. There is no evidence that the type of response is related to the kind of stimulus which is used.

Another type of hemodynamic response to stress has been observed less frequently and less predictably. It consists of circulatory collapse with a profound fall in heart rate, arterial pressure, and peripheral resistance and a less marked fall in cardiac output.[8,9] This so-called vasodepressor response, or vasovagal syncope, which is familiar to all physicians, has typically been observed just preceding venipuncture (Chap. 47).

The suggestion has been made that specific types of cardiovascular response may follow specific alterations in emotions, or affect.[10–12] Other studies have failed to support these findings.[6–7] It seems probable, however, that there is a quantitative relation between the degree of emotion that is provoked and the magnitude of the cardiovascular response.[6,7,13]

Such studies have been concerned with the transient effects of acute emotional stress. The physiologic effects of prolonged, chronic, or repeated emotional stress have not been adequately studied.

EMOTIONAL STRESS AND CARDIOVASCULAR DISEASE

The obvious relation between emotion and cardiovascular function has led to speculation about, and study of, the possible role of emotions as causative or aggravating factors in cardiovascular disease. Although the significance of such studies has frequently been limited by problems in methodology such as the definition and measurement of "emotional stress" or "personality," the uncritical use of retrospective techniques, and the lack of adequate controls, such problems are now generally recognized, and better techniques are being employed. Such studies continue to support the clinical impression that emotional stress plays an important role in cardiovascular disease.

Hypertension

The fact that transient elevations of blood pressure can be produced by acute emotional stress,[6,7,13] plus the observation that sustained hypertension may develop in later life in persons exhibiting *transient hypertension*,[14] has suggested that emotional stress might play a role in the development of hypertension. *Borderline or labile hypertension* has generally been characterized by an increased cardiac output and a normal or decreased peripheral resistance, in contrast to essential hypertension, where the cardiac output is generally decreased and the peripheral resistance elevated.[15] It has been noted that patients with borderline hypertension who later develop sustained hypertension exhibit the above change in hemodynamics, suggesting that the hemodynamic differences are related to the stage of their disease.[16] Wolf and Wolff[17] noted that the blood pressure increase observed during stressful interviews was the result of a rise in cardiac output and/or peripheral resistance, and that the resistance type occurred more frequently in subjects with repressed hostility and sustained hypertension. However, the work of many others[6,15,16,18] suggests that no sharp separation of hemodynamic responses can be made between subjects with normal blood pressure, with borderline hypertension, or with essential hypertension. Although there seems to be little difference qualitatively between the hemodynamic responses of hypertensive and normal subjects to stress, there is a striking quantitative difference, the responses being greater in magnitude and more prolonged in hypertensive patients. Normotensive individuals with a family history of hypertension as well as persons with labile hypertension have also been found to have exaggerated and prolonged hemodynamic responses to emotional stimuli.[19]

The above observations have suggested that repeated or chronic stress might play a role in the development of essential hypertension. A few studies have been made of large groups of persons exposed to acute stress. In one, 27 percent of soldiers were found to have diastolic pressures above 100 mm Hg 1 to 2 months after combat,[20] while in another 56 percent of 180 persons had diastolic pressures above 95 mm Hg 1 to 2 weeks after the Texas City explosion.[21] The stress in these instances was complex, and no data were presented to indicate that sustained hypertension appeared. A number of studies have attempted to demonstrate a correlation between the onset, the worsening, or the improvement of hypertension and certain events in the life of the patient.[22,23] These studies suffer from being retrospective, anecdotal, and uncontrolled. Although it is evident, both experimentally and clinically, that blood pressure in patients with hypertension is increased by emotional stress, these studies do not

provide evidence that emotional stress alters the course of the disease with regard to morbidity or mortality. Epidemiologic studies of hypertension in various population groups[24] have led to the suggestion that the stress of Western civilization is a factor in hypertension. However, other studies of somewhat similar groups have ascribed the differences in blood pressure to the level of intake of salt in the diet.

Such observations concerning stress and hypertension have led to many attempts to develop a model in animals. A number of these studies lend credence to the belief that emotional stress or psychosocial factors may be an etiologic factor. Hypertension has been produced in a variety of animals including monkeys, rats, and mice by various techniques involving "psychosocial" stress.[25] In some instances sustained hypertension and vascular disease have resulted. The relation of such high blood pressure and such stimuli to hypertension and emotional stress in human beings is yet to be defined.

There has been considerable interest in the use of various "psychologic" techniques in the control of blood pressure. Shapiro et al.[26] studied the effects of operant conditioning, Patel and North[27] used a combination of yoga and biofeedback, while Benson et al.[28] and Stone and DeLeo[29] used versions of transcendental meditation. Both probably produce what Benson has termed the "relaxation response." Krist and Engel,[30] on the other hand, described a technique whereby subjects were taught to lower or raise their blood pressure at will without changes suggesting the relaxation response. The blood pressure responses appeared to be sustained as long as the techniques were practiced. Such techniques may eventually make a contribution to the treatment and understanding of hypertension.

Coronary heart disease

A relation between emotional stress and coronary disease has been postulated for many years but has been difficult to establish. This is not surprising since the cause of coronary disease is likely multifactored, witness the apparent roles of hypertension, hyperlipidemia, cigarette smoking, etc., and since emotional stress is difficult to define and measure. Nonetheless, many studies concerned with such factors as social status, social mobility, educational level, life stress and life change, and behavior patterns, as well as epidemiologic studies of various cultures, have suggested relationships between psychosocial factors and coronary disease.[31]

Rosenman and associates[32] have described a "specific overt behavior pattern" which they label type A and which they believe should be recognized as a risk factor in coronary disease, much as smoking, hypertension, etc., are. This type A individual is described as aggressive, ambitious, competitive, work-oriented, chronically impatient, and preoccupied with deadlines. In several large prospective studies they have been able to identify, on the basis of these characteristics, a group at increased risk of developing coronary heart disease.

A number of studies of populations living under various circumstances have been made; they generally tend to ascribe a low prevalence of coronary disease to a simple, more primitive, or less "stressful" life. A high prevalence of coronary disease is often ascribed to the stress in "civilized" Western countries, although there is little evidence that people in these countries are exposed to more or less stress than those living in less highly developed countries. A number of studies have suggested that persons engaged in "stressful" occupations such as certain types of physicians, dentists, lawyers, and accountants have a high incidence of coronary disease.[31,32] Others have failed to find a relation between executive responsibility or type of industrial occupation and coronary disease.[33,34] Rahe et al.[35] have reported that recent life events such as illness, divorce, financial change, or death of a relative are found to have occurred more frequently in the 6 months immediately preceding a myocardial infarction when compared with the three periods of 6 months prior to that time and the 6 months postmyocardial infarction. Their data suggested that the greater the accumulation of these life events in the 6 months prior to the myocardial infarction, the greater the possibility of sudden death and cardiac arrhythmias with the myocardial infarction. However, these stresses are not specific for coronary disease and may precede other illnesses.

There has been interest in studies showing a rise of serum cholesterol levels at time of emotional stress, as in students prior to examinations[36,37] or tax accountants during the tax season.[32] Whether the observed changes are the result of emotional stress per se or due to other factors such as change in diet, physical activity, sleeping habits, or smoking is not known, but these observations suggest a possible mechanism whereby emotional stress and coronary disease might be connected.

There is abundant evidence that emotional stress may precipitate attacks of angina pectoris. This is not surprising since the hemodynamic responses to exercise and emotional stress are so similar. Emotional reactions involved may vary from intense anger, visible to an onlooker, to carefully concealed stressful thoughts. It is probable that emotional as well as physical stress may precipitate myocardial infarction or fatal arrhythmias in persons with preexisting coronary disease.

The widespread use of coronary care units has led to reassuring and useful observations on (1) the effects of emotional stress in the immediate postinfarction period and (2) the psychologic effects of heart attacks. Despite early reports suggesting a correlation between physicians' rounds and sudden death, prolonged observations in many units have provided no basis for this belief. The majority of patients are reassured by cardiac monitoring and do not find it stressful. Even those who witness a cardiac arrest tend to grasp the most comforting meaning of the event while denying the more threatening aspects.[38,39] Psychiatric complications in the coronary care unit follow different time distributions, with an early peak for anxiety on days 1 and 2, and a later peak for depression on days 3 and 4.[40] Patients who denied the severity of their illness and were optimistic and fearless in the face of it coped better and tended to have lower morbidity and mortality rates after discharge.[41] The greatest psychologic barrier to rehabilitation following myocardial infarction is a depressed mental state which may persist for 6 to 12 months in as many as a third of all patients. This is also reflected in their delay in returning to work and their reduced sexual activity. Supportive discussion and educational groups during convalescence may reduce this morbidity and facilitate early and complete rehabilitation.

Cardiac arrhythmias

Palpitation and tachycardia are among the most widely recognized effects of emotional stress, and perhaps for this reason emotional stress is thought to be a common cause or precipitating factor in cardiac arrhythmias. Stimulation of various parts of the brain or of the autonomic nervous system and the administration of adrenergic or cholinergic drugs have given rise to various arrhythmias.[42] Engel[43] has reviewed a number of anecdotal and retrospective reports of sudden death, many thought to be due to emotionally induced arrhythmia. However, well-documented reports are rare despite the availability of continuous electrocardiographic monitors.

Lown et al.[44] reported psychophysiologic and psychiatric studies on a man with no evidence of heart disease who had two episodes of ventricular fibrillation and numerous ventricular premature beats thought to be associated with emotional stress. In patients with preexisting heart disease, ventricular premature beats have been shown to increase in frequency under stress such as driving an automobile or watching a football game.[45,46] Increases in heart rate and in degree of atrioventricular (AV) block, and frequency of ventricular premature beats have been noted to occur in patients in a coronary care unit following such simple actions as taking the pulse or temperature.[47] The reported effects of sleep on the frequency of ventricular premature beats have been conflicting, one study reporting a decrease during sleep,[48] another no change during wakefulness or varying stages of sleep,[49] and another an increase during rapid-eye-movement sleep.[44] Experiments with dogs[50] and pigs[51] suggest that stress decreases the threshold for ventricular fibrillation induced by electrical stimulation or coronary occlusion.

Thus there is strong evidence that emotional stress can play a role in the precipitation of ventricular arrhythmias in the presence of heart disease and that this results from sympathetic nervous system influences as well as from the more obvious hemodynamic effects. However, it is not so clear that such occurs in the absence of heart disease.

Congestive heart failure

Acute left ventricular failure or pulmonary edema may be precipitated by emotional upsets in persons with preexisting heart disease, through the well-known hemodynamic effects of emotional stress. Although it has been suggested that emotional stress may in some way alter electrolyte and water excretion other than through known hemodynamic changes,[52] this has not been confirmed. The majority of physicians would agree on the benefit of a tranquil existence in patients with myocardial failure. However, psychologic factors such as anxiety, depression, and denial may play important roles in a patient's adherence to a regime of treatment and be major factors in the improvement or worsening of congestive failure.

Electrocardiogram

Electrocardiographic abnormalities have been noted for a number of years in persons with anxiety neurosis, psychoneurosis, and emotional lability.[53–55] In such individuals the abnormalities have usually been limited to inversions of the T waves, most frequently in leads II, III, and aV_F but occasionally involving leads I, aV_L, and V_4, V_5, and V_6. These abnormalities tend to vary from time to time and with factors such as standing, lying down, exercise, hyperventilation, breath holding, and drugs.[56–59] Although such lability of the T waves has generally been reported in anxious patients, it has occasionally been seen in stable, healthy persons. Whether these abnormalities occur more frequently in neurotic persons cannot be ascertained from the literature. Studies comparing the ECGs of persons with anxiety neurosis and of healthy controls have shown no difference in the frequency of T wave abnormalities.[60,61] Whatever the cause of these T wave abnormalities, it is extremely important for physicians to be aware of their existence, since misinterpretation of such findings to a psychoneurotic anxious patient may aggravate his condition.

PSYCHIATRIC DISEASE AND CARDIOVASCULAR SYMPTOMS

Symptoms similar to those of heart disease, such as chest pain, palpitation, shortness of breath, and faintness, are frequently found in certain psychiatric disorders. Patients with such symptoms, with or without heart disease, commonly seek help from an internist or cardiologist. The differentiation of these symptoms from those of heart disease and the proper management of the underlying psychiatric disorder can be one of the most challenging and rewarding problems in cardiology. Correct diagnosis and management may rescue a disabled patient; an incorrect diagnosis of heart disease may aggravate the symptoms and lead to invalidism.

There are two common psychiatric disorders which are frequently confused with heart disease: anxiety neurosis and depressive illness. As many as 20 percent of patients seen in the office practice of cardiology have one of these disorders alone or in conjuction with heart disease. Thus it is important that the internist or cardiologist be well acquainted with these disorders.

Cardiovascular symptoms and anxiety neurosis

DEFINITION

Anxiety neurosis is a syndrome characterized by anxious overconcern extending to panic and frequently associated with somatic symptoms such as palpitations, chest pain, hyperventilation, and tachycardia. The syndrome has appeared under a wide variety of aliases during the past century—usually reflecting the specialty interests or theories of the author observing it. Those labels commonly used include Da Costa's syndrome, neurasthenia, effort syndrome, soldier's heart, irritable heart, cardiac neurosis, neurocirculatory asthenia, anxiety hysteria, anxiety neurosis, and most recently vasoregulatory asthenia and hyperdynamic β-adrenergic circulatory state. An analysis of the symptoms and signs included in these conditions suggests that all are manifestations of the same disorder.[61] Since *anxiety neurosis* is the official American Psychiatric Association (*Diagnostic and Statistical Manual of Mental Disorders*, second edition) term for this syndrome, it will be used in this chapter.

EPIDEMIOLOGY

It is difficult to determine accurately the prevalence of this disorder. Differences in diagnostic criteria and terminology make estimates in the literature difficult to compare. Surveys suggest that approximately 10 percent of patients in cardiology practices and 2 to 5 percent of the normal population are suffering from this disorder.[60–64] Women outnumber men with these symptoms in a ratio of approximately 3:2.[61] Although this is characteristically a disorder of young adults, it may occur at any age from childhood on. The average age of onset is about 25 years. Some (Mendel and Klein[65]) have demonstrated a bimodal distribution through life with a second peak occurring in the age range of 35 to 40 years.

Many investigators have noted the high familial prevalence of anxiety neurosis.[66–68] Slater and Shields[67,68] report that 15 percent of parents and siblings of persons with anxiety neurosis have a similar disorder, compared with 0 to 5 percent of relatives of normal control groups. They found that 50 percent of monozygotic twins of persons with anxiety neuroses had a similar condition. The same trend was found in monozygotic twins reared apart.

In dizygotic twins, the concordance for anxiety neurosis was only 4 percent, while marked anxiety traits were found in 13 percent. Environmental factors and learning, however, still cannot be excluded.

HISTORY

The disorder was first described by A. B. R. Myers[69] in 1870 during the British campaign in India. Jacob Mendes Da Costa,[70] a Philadelphia physician, in 1871 wrote of "a peculiar form of functional disorder of the heart, to which I gave the name irritable heart," in which no evidence could be found of a structural cardiac lesion. He described the case of a Union army private who had suffered this condition through the Civil War. He noted the fluctuations in the intensity of the condition at the time of battles. Subsequently the diagnosis was made frequently during wartime, although the labels used to describe the syndrome changed.[71-74] The stresses of war and the gain to the soldier of getting a medical discharge and disability pension no doubt account for the increased attention the condition has received during wartime.

ETIOLOGY: PSYCHOLOGICAL ASPECTS

Because anxiety neurosis is considered a psychatric disorder, psychologic factors have been implicated at the expense of the physiologic and endogenous aspects in this disorder. Both are undoubtedly important. Since the majority of patients with anxiety neurosis present to internists or cardiologists rather than psychiatrists, they have a special responsibility to diagnose and manage it correctly.

Sometimes it is easy to identify stresses and emotional factors that have aggravated the condition. Indeed it is surprising how often patients will readily volunteer such information when they feel understood and when they find a sympathetic and patient ear to hear them out. A search for life changes and stresses, particularly losses of all kinds, in the weeks and months immediately preceding appearance of the symptoms is often rewarded. The death or loss of a friend or relative, loss of a job, financial loss, and life-threatening stress, like war, are typical examples.

CLINICAL DESCRIPTION

This is a polysymptomatic condition with few objective signs. Although the patient may complain of only two or three symptoms, a careful history will generally uncover a large number of others. The chief complaint, however, dictates which specialist sees the patient. Thus, patients complaining of unsteadiness, dizziness, fainting spells, headaches, heaviness, and paresthesias in their limbs are likely to consult a neurologist, while those with chest pain and tachycardia are likely to consult a cardiologist. The cardiologist is particularly likely to be consulted, because so many of the symptoms fall within his area of expertise. Chest pain, tachycardia, and palpitations are the most common among this cluster. The chest pain of anxiety neurosis must be differentiated from that of ischemic heart disease, pulmonary embolism, pericarditis, etc. It is either a fleeting stabbing pain or a dull aching pressure of prolonged duration. Frequently the patient has experienced both at different times. It is located usually in the left mammary area and only rarely substernally. Tenderness of the chest wall over the affected area is not unusual. This pain may radiate to the axilla, left arm, or into the back and scapular region. It is not associated with exertion and comes on at rest. It may become so severe that it is associated with complaints of breathing difficulties, e.g., "I can't get a full breath." Sighing respiration and even episodes of tachypnea or hyperventilation are not uncommon. It may last from minutes to several hours and as a dull pressure for weeks on end.

Awareness of premature beats and attacks of tachycardia may be accompanied by a fear of impending death or disaster. There may be an intensification of the awareness of the heartbeat, a faint feeling of unreality, hyperventilation, dizzy spell, trembling, perspiration, choking, and an unsteadiness or "giddy sensation" and a need for the patients to support or steady themselves lest the "rubbery" feeling in their legs should cause them to fall. Such patients will often describe phobic situations they avoid, e.g., crowded places, supermarkets, open spaces, elevators, or tunnels, where they are more likely to get these symptoms. They are often fearful of being alone. When the symptoms begin, they may get a sudden urge to flee. They will sit at the back of the church and near theater exits in anticipation of this eventuality. The attack may be followed by a period of exhaustion or demoralization for hours or days and may intensify the phobic avoidance. These anxiety or panic attacks differ from the anxiety normal people experience before giving a public lecture or being in a car accident in that they are more terrifying. Fatigue (neurasthenia) may be experienced even after a full night's sleep. Hypochondriasis and illness phobias are found in almost 70 percent of these patients.

The disorder has no reliable characteristic signs. Brisk tendon reflexes, moist cold palms, tachycardia, and tachypnea are frequently seen. This clinical picture may coexist with heart disease. Some of these symptoms may also occur in other medical disorders like thyrotoxicosis, pheochromocytoma, brucellosis, carcinoid syndrome, Ménière's disease, and even tuberculosis.

LABORATORY FINDINGS

In spite of the prevalence of anxiety neurosis and the considerable attention it has received, little is known of its underlying neurophysiologic and neurochemical processes. However, experimental evidence increasingly implicates a biogenic amine metabolism disturbance especially in the limbic system of the brain. Both the parasympathetic and sympathetic nervous systems mediate many of the bodily symptoms of these patients. Some of the symptoms, e.g., awareness of heart action, can be aggravated by isoproterenol and blocked by the β-adrenergic blocker propranolol.[75,76] Increased β-adrenergic receptor responsiveness may be responsible for some of the symptoms. There is no one physiologic measure or laboratory finding that is useful in this condition.

Although many ECG abnormalities have been reported in this disorder, no characteristic ECG pattern has been found.[60]

Various research studies have found abnormalities in blood lactate,[77,78,79] oxygen consumption,[77,80] palmar skin conductance (sweat gland activity),[81] fingernail capillaries,[82] pulse rate, forearm blood flow, and finger pulse volume,[83] and during muscular work.[77,84,85].

Of special significance are the studies of oxygen consumption and blood lactate production. Patients with anxiety neurosis manifested an excessive rise in blood lactate and a lower oxygen consumption when compared with normal controls in a standard exercise test.[77,78] Cohen and White[84] concluded that these abnormalities supported the hypothesis that these patients had abnormal aerobic metabolism.

Several investigators[79,86] were able to precipitate typical attacks of anxiety in the great majority of these patients, but in only a minority of controls, by giving a standard infusion of sodium lactate. The action of the lactate in lowering the level of ionized calcium may explain this finding. Pitts and McLure[79] were able to prevent the onset of anxiety in almost all these patients by giving them adequate doses of calcium ion. They postulated that causing an increase in lactate production—like a centrally determined overproduction of epinephrine or a disturbance in peripheral metabolic pathways—may lead to the symptoms of anxiety neurosis.

COURSE AND PROGNOSIS

This condition has a chronic relapsing course. Exacerbations and remissions are common. Approximately one-sixth of the patients recover completely and remain symptom-free. One-third remain symptomatic but have no disability. One-third remain symptomatic and are intermittently disabled. The remaining one-sixth are totally disabled.[87] Several studies noted that total disability was more common when the disability was rewarded by a pension, as in the military.[87–89] There is little in the clinical picture that helps in predicting the outcome of the condition. Experience suggests that the degree of environmental stress involved in precipitating and maintaining the disorder, the stability of the patient's personal relationships, the duration of symptoms, and work performance affect the prognosis. These patients have frequently consulted several physicians and psychiatrists for a variety of complaints and have taken many of the psychotropic drugs at one time or another.

In a 20-year follow-up study of these patients in private practice[87] there was no excessive mortality, nor any increase in the prevalence of the conditions often labeled psychosomatic diseases like peptic ulcer, asthma, or ulcerative colitis.

MANAGEMENT

Supportive reassurance and symptom control with drugs are very helpful to the patient even if they are not definitively curative. It is difficult to provide effective reassurance without first excluding other disorders, like ischemic heart disease, hyperthyroidism, thyrotoxicosis, Ménière's disease, and pheochromocytoma, and sharing the clinical and laboratory findings with the patient. This careful exclusion and review is important not only diagnostically but also therapeutically in alleviating the patient's anxiety. Reassurance should also include emphasis on the favorable aspects of the disorder, such as its good prognosis for life expectancy, and, most important, an attempt should be made to identify the psychosocial events that precipitated and aggravate the condition. It is best to avoid ascribing the symptoms to "nerves" or "imagination," as this may alienate the patient and leave him feeling misunderstood.

When the psychosocial precipitants are identified, the specific supportive techniques to be employed become clear. Most patients find that the opportunity to discuss their fears and difficulties with a concerned and sympathetic physician results in a reduction of their anxiety. Indeed many are more comfortable doing this with their internist or cardiologist than with a psychiatrist. If anxiety-provoking external events are identified, it may be possible to manipulate the environment so as to reduce the stressful pressures. Premature or excessive reassurances should be avoided. A patient, sympathetic, and listening posture is most helpful to the patient in reviewing this aspect of the history.

Drugs are a useful adjunct in providing symptom relief. The minor tranquilizers such as chlordiazepoxide (Librium) and diazepam (Valium) are sometimes helpful in dulling the manifestations of anxiety. Not infrequently they are only partially helpful or reduce anxiety for only a few weeks, after which the patient may report feeling more depressed. Barbiturates are best avoided, because these chronically anxious patients easily become physically dependent on them. Flurazepam (Dalmane) and chloral hydrate are more appropriate hypnotics for these patients and may be necessary in acute situations. The major tranquilizers should not be generally prescribed for this class of patient, but should be reserved for the anxiety associated with schizophrenia and other psychotic illness. Indeed they may aggravate rather than relieve the symptoms. The adrenergic blocking agents are helpful in some of these patients, although they are not widely used clinically. One of the authors (Sheehan[89a]) has found that the monoamine oxidase (MAO) inhibitors, phenelzine sulfate (Nardil) 45 to 90 mg/day or imipramine 150 to 250 mg/day, are particularly effective in severe anxiety hysteria. It is best to reserve their use for the more chronically anxious and disabled. At these doses the drugs are maximally effective only after the third week. During the first 2 weeks patients may complain of hypotension and sedation, after which time the drug is well tolerated. With phenelzine, which is somewhat more effective and better tolerated than imipramine, the appropriate dietary and drug restrictions should be rigidly enforced, e.g., avoiding cheese and wine to prevent any hypertensive episodes from this interaction. For this disorder there is no good evidence that intensive psychotherapy or psychoanalysis is any better than simple support, reassurance, drug therapy, and advice about aggravating factors and environmental manipulation.[87] The relaxation techniques of hypnotherapy, behavior therapy, meditation, and biofeedback have been helpful to some patients.[90] In our experience it is the milder cases that benefit from these forms of therapy.

Depressive illness

The cardiologist or internist is likely to see patients with depressive illness because of symptoms mimicking heart disease, because the illness complicates preexisting heart disease, or because depression may result from the treatment of cardiovascular disease. The differentiation from anxiety neurosis is important since depressive illness is less likely than anxiety neurosis to respond to a sympathetic ear, a careful examination, and reassurance, and may require drug therapy, electroconvulsive therapy (ECT), or even hospitalization.

DEFINITION

There is much confusion about the term *depression*, because it is used to refer both to a feeling state and to an illness. As a feeling state, depression is often found in a wide array of illnesses from anxiety neurosis and schizophrenia to anemia. Treatment of the underlying condition usually alleviates the feeling of depression. Depression as an illness is a syndrome of which the feeling of depression is only one element.

Depressive illness is said to cluster into two distinct categories: (1) reactive, neurotic depression and (2) so-called endogenous depression. Reactive, or neurotic, depression is usually a response to psychosocial difficulties, is not transmitted genetically, and is not accompanied by bodily physiologic and biochemical changes such as early morning wakening, psychomotor retardation, and psychotic thought processes. It also responds to supportive psychotherapy but not to drug therapy or ECT. So-called endogenous depression may be reactive to psychosocial stresses, but the resulting depressive illness is more severe and debilitating and responds unpredictably to psychotherapy. It requires more vigorous drug and/or somatic types of therapy like ECT and has a more predictable response to these measures than reactive, neurotic depression has. What follows is a discussion of endogenous depression, since it is this disorder that presents the greatest diagnostic and

management problems for the cardiologist and internist.

CLINICAL DESCRIPTION

Onset Precipitants can usually be identified by a carefully taken history. The loss of loved persons, or possessions, or self-esteem, whether by death, departure, or rejection, are frequent precipitants. It sometimes follows and complicates physical illness like myocardial infarction. It is usually gradual rather than sudden in onset.

Symptoms—subjective experience The central experience is one of empty, gloomy depression, a feeling of hopeless despair, a helplessness to do anything about this feeling state, and consequent feelings of worthlessness and guilt at being a burden to others. Such patients often feel a loneliness and weariness in the presence of others, and every situation appears cheerless and dreary. Insight into the psychologic change may be retained and often intensifies the pain, suffering, self-criticism, and guilt because the sufferers cannot "will" themselves out of these feelings. These patients may feel easily irritated, agitated, and restless with others. They may have difficulty concentrating, feel tired for no reason, and find it difficult to do routine chores and make simple decisions. Crying spells are common. In some cases auditory hallucinations that have an accusatory and denunciatory quality may occur, and hypochondriacal delusions are found, e.g., the persistent belief that they have heart disease or decay in an organ system in spite of adequate reassurance to the contrary. In such cases suicidal ideation is often present.

Physical symptoms Depression is the ubiquitous mimic of physical illness. The cardinal "vegetative" signs of endogenous depression are:

1 Psychomotor retardation—slowness of speech and thought, decreased motor activity, a glum immobile facial expression
2 Loss of appetite and weight
3 Loss of sexual interest and potency
4 Constipation
5 Insomnia, especially early morning wakening and morning agitation

Of these, the last is the most reliable guide and correlates best with the severity of the disorder. These patients may fall asleep at bedtime but toss restlessly and awake at 3 A.M. and are unable to return to sleep. They feel restless and agitated in the early morning; this fades as the day progresses. Palpitation, tachycardia, and "pressure" in the chest are not uncommon.

ETIOLOGY

Once the psychosocial precipitants have elicited depressive illness, it is an autonomous process, carried on independently without regard for external circumstances, probably by a central biochemical vulnerability. The result may be incapacitating and out of proportion to the situation. Current theory proposes that there is a reduction in biogenic amines at functionally important adrenergic receptors in the limbic system of the brain. Recent research[91-92] clearly implicates genetic factors in this biochemical vulnerability.

BIOCHEMICAL AND LABORATORY FINDINGS

There are no laboratory findings at this time that will assist in making the diagnosis of endogenous depression. There have been conflicting and equivocal findings in studies of electrolyte changes, carbohydrate, fat and protein metabolism, and endocrinologic changes. However, the exciting recent research developments in this area may yield useful biochemical measures in the not-too-distant future.

DIFFERENTIAL DIAGNOSIS

Depressive illness may mimic many physical illnesses. Myxedema, myasthenia gravis, and senile dementia are typical examples. For those with cardiovascular symptoms such as palpitations, organic heart disease needs to be ruled out. The cardiologist and internist are likely to see depressive illness as a complication of existing heart disease or a complication of its treatment. It is common after cardiac surgery—usually when the postcardiotomy delirium clears. Antihypertensive drugs, especially reserpine, are particularly likely to precipitate a suicidal depression. They deplete biogenic amines in the limbic system and should be avoided in those with a history of depression.

TREATMENT

Depressive disorders are generally treatable disorders. The first step in management is to evaluate the suicidal potential and, if it is serious, to hospitalize the patient with suitable precautions. If the patient is in the manic (but not the depressive) phase of manic-depressive illness, lithium administration is the most appropriate treatment. This requires careful monitoring, and it is best to refer the patient to a psychiatrist experienced in its administration. It is a potentially dangerous drug and must be used with caution in patients with heart disease.

There is no justification for the use of amphetamines, barbiturates, or psychosurgery in depressive illness. In general, approximately 35 percent of depressed patients will respond to placebo treatment within 3 to 4 weeks (16 percent if chronically and severely depressed, 46 percent if acutely depressed). Seventy percent respond to tricyclic antidepressants within 4 weeks.[93] Of the 30 percent not responding to a tricyclic antidepressant after 4 weeks, half (15 percent) respond to ECT. Of the remainder, some respond to another tricyclic antidepressant or an MAO inhibitor. Supportive psychotherapy and a tricyclic antidepressant are slightly more effective than either alone, especially in preventing relapse.

There are two classes of tricyclic antidepressants. Amitriptyline (Elavil) and its derivatives are very

sedative and used when the depressed patient is agitated or the depression is accompanied by severe insomnia. Imipramine (Tofranil) and its derivative desipramine (Norpramin) are more energizing and used if the depression is retarded, anergic, and accompanied by withdrawal. They are widely and improperly prescribed. It is not generally appreciated that imipramine, desipramine and amitriptyline are not predictably effective as antidepressants in doses of less than 150 mg/day. Yet, physicians persist in prescribing them at 25 mg three times a day orally in the hope of getting some effect. This should be discouraged. These are unpleasant drugs to take, and patients should be advised to expect some subjectively unpleasant effects like dry mouth, hypotension, excessive perspiration, hot flashes, and muscle twitching. Further, these drugs take 3 to 4 weeks at 150 mg/day to have significant antidepressant effect. Advising the patient of these facts avoids disappointment and premature termination of treatment.

CARDIOVASCULAR EFFECTS OF TRICYCLIC ANTIDEPRESSANTS

These drugs have potent cardiovascular effects through their anticholinergic activity, their direct myocardial depressant activity, and their effect on the adrenergic neuron. They may cause cardiac arrhythmias,[94-97] sudden death,[94,98,99] ECG abnormalities,[94,95,96] congestive cardiac failure,[94,100-103] and possibly hyperlipidemia,[94,102] hypertension,[94,104-106] and myocardial infarction.[94] Of these, the most frequent are hypertension and cardiac arrhythmias. These effects are reported to be highest with amitriptyline, lower with imipramine and desipramine, and lowest with doxepin (Sinequan) and the tetracyclic antidepressants, e.g., Ludimoil, which is not yet commercially available in the United States.[94,107-110] The severity of the side effects is considerably greater in those with cardiovascular disease and the elderly. Consequently, they should be used with great caution in such patients. The postural hypotension is worse during the first 4 days and is minimal by the third week. It occurs in approximately two-thirds of patients with cardiovascular disease and one-third of those without cardiovascular disease.[94-100]

A wide variety or rate and rhythm disturbances have been reported in patients on tricyclics. For the most part these include tachycardia (30 percent of patients on amitriptyline, 29 percent of those on doxepin), and reversible T wave alterations. Sudden death was reported in 6 of 52 patients with cardiac disease on tricyclic antidepressants, as compared with none of 53 controls matched for age, sex, diagnosis, and duration of hospital stay.[94,98] Those over 70 years of age are similarly at risk for sudden death.

The tricyclic antidepressants interact with a considerable number of cardiovascular drugs. They antagonize the antihypertensive action of guanethidine and block the vasopressor effect of indirect acting sympathomimetic amines. Any drug with a myocardial depressant action may aggravate the myocardial depressant effect of the tricyclic antidepressants. Awareness of these factors should not lead to a therapeutic "paralysis"—especially in those patients who are severely depressed.

In the majority of studies comparing ECT with tricyclic antidepressants in the treatment of endogenous depressive illness, ECT was more effective in providing relief. In ECT, a charge of 150 to 170 V is delivered to the brain through electrodes placed on the anterior temporal region while the patient is under general anesthesia and deep muscle relaxation (with succinylcholine). A response is usual after six to eight treatments given over a 2-week period. Exceeding 12 to 16 treatments is probably inadvisable. The memory is less disturbed following unilateral ECT, although this effect is not quite as rapid as bilateral ECT. The relapse rate is high (18 to 46 percent after 6 months) unless patients are maintained on antidepressants. Because of the cardiac toxicity of the tricyclic antidepressants, ECT may be the safest and most efficacious treatment for endogenous depression in patients with cardiac disease and in the elderly. However, ECT is contraindicated following recent myocardial infarction, because arrhythmias may occur during the ECT seizure. When the ECG and cardiac enzymes have stabilized following myocardial infarction, ECT may be cautiously administered.

DELIRIUM (ACUTE CONFUSIONAL STATES)

The physician who is managing patients with heart disease should be familiar with the acute confusional states, since they are so commonly seen in acute care units and in the operative cardiac patient. Delirium is confusion plus psychosis. Three to ten percent of coronary care unit patients and fifty to eighty percent of patients after cardiac surgery fall victim to this condition.[38,39] It usually has a rapid onset and an acute fluctuating course. Bonhoeffer (1908) noted the clinical features were similar regardless of etiology. It is a complication of many conditions, notably open heart and eye surgery, use of steroids, psychotropic drug intoxication and withdrawal, use of narcotics, effects of anticholinergic agents, and electrolyte imbalance. Some people are particularly vulnerable, others very resistant to developing delirium. The very young and very old are particularly vulnerable. The delirium rarely lasts more than a few weeks—usually 3 to 6 days. It is generally reversible. It is associated with a higher mortality. It may be replaced by a global or selective dementia. The delirious

material may reflect the patient's conflicts and personality structure.

Although psychodynamic factors and personality organization have been implicated in delirium vulnerability, good controlled experimental evidence is lacking. Cartwright,[111] Cartwright et al.,[112] and Gottschalk et al.[113] found field-dependent people with high anxiety scores were more vulnerable to confusion and hallucinations following both sleep deprivation and administration of anticholinergic drugs (Ditropan). The hallucinations of delirium may result from intrusion of REM mechanisms and dream contents into waking consciousness.[114] Cartwright[111] found that the Ditropan-induced hallucinations were similar in content to the subject's dreams on the night following the drug administration and that the subjects could not differentiate between them. Whether these traits are primary or secondary or dependent on a third independent variable is still unclear.

CLINICAL FEATURES

Observation over time is more helpful diagnostically. Clinical characteristics are not always a reliable guide to diagnosis. They are as follows:

1 Sudden onset usually, although it may be insidious and gradual.
2 Fluctuation of clinical features over 24 h, and often rapidly from moment to moment. Intermittent lucidity may occur and can be misleading diagnostically.
3 Disorientation—at first to time, later to place, and finally to person.
4 Impairment of attention span.
5 Elevation of vital signs; at times, dilatation of pupils.
6 Increasing anxiety, fear, panic, restlessness, and agitation. The patient may become uncooperative, disruptive, and violent or exhibit inappropriate, impulsive, or irrational behavior.
7 Hallucinations are primarily visual and much less frequently auditory, tactile, or olfactory. These are usually dreamlike or nightmarish in quality and content. This is in contrast to schizophrenia, where hallucinations are primarily auditory and the "visual hallucinations" are more frequently perceptual distortions.
8 Delusions and illusions are rarely well organized and rarely persist over time.
9 Memory, comprehension, judgment, abstract thinking ability, ability to calculate, and other intellectual functions may become impaired in severe cases. The impairments are usually transient and reversible. The manner in which the patient does the tests of these functions—with irritability, difficulty, and delay—is more important than the accuracy of the answers.
10 At times, somnolence and lethargy may occur. Stupor, coma, convulsions, slurred speech, ataxia, and deterioration in vital signs appear late and herald death.
11 Amnesia for much of the delirium is common after recovery.
12 Serial EEG's are often helpful diagnostically. They rule out focal lesions. Diffuse slowing of alpha waves parallels closely the reduction in consciousness. This is often an early sign of delirium. The ECG may therefore be used as a reliable indicator of adequacy of treatment. This ECG change does not occur in delirium tremens.

TREATMENT

1 The first step in management is to search for a cause and treat it.

2 Review carefully all medication orders and laboratory data. Special culprits are narcotics, and drugs with anticholinergic properties.

3 Physostigmine will temporarily reverse delirium due to anticholinergic drugs and may be useful diagnostically. Physostigmine has some toxic cardiovascular side effects.[115]

4 Major tranquilizers or high doses of minor tranquilizers may be useful—the evidence is largely anecdotal. Haldol is a better choice than chlorpromazine, which has troublesome cardiovascular side effects.

5 Repeated concrete explanation and reassurance to the delirious patient may be helpful.

6 Avoid restraints where possible. Provide close supervision by others.

7 Adequate sensory stimulation and light at all times is reported anecdotally to be helpful.[116]

REFERENCES

1 Rushmer, R. F., Van Citters, R. L., and Franklin, D. L.: Some Axioma, Popular Notions and Misconceptions regarding Cardiovascular Control, *Circulation,* 27:118, 1963.

2 Ojeman, G. A., and Van Buren, J. M.; Respiratory, Heart Rate and GSR Responses from Human Diencephalon, *Arch. Neurol.,* 16:74, 1967.

3 Grollman, A.: The Effect of Psychic Disturbances on the Cardiac Output, Pulse Rate, Blood Pressure and Oxygen Consumption of Man, *Am. J. Physiol.,* 89:366, 1929.

4 Stead, E. A., Jr., Warren, J. V., Merrill, A. J., and Brannon, E. S.: The Cardiac Output in Male Subjects as Measured by the Technique of Right Atrial Catheterization: Normal Values with Observations on the Effect of Anxiety and Tilting, *J. Clin. Invest.,* 24:326, 1945.

5 Hichan, J. B., Cargill, W. H., and Golden, A.: Cardiovascular Reactions to Emotional Stimuli: Effect on the Cardiac Output, Arteriovenous Oxygen Difference, Arterial Pressure, and Peripheral Resistance, *J. Clin. Invest.,* 27:290, 1948.

6 Brod, J.: Hemodynamic Basis of Acute Pressor Reactions and Hypertension, *Br. Heart J.,* 25:227, 1963.

7 Bodgonoff, M. D., Combs, J. J., Jr., Bryant, G. D. N., and Warren, J. V.: Cardiovascular Responses in Experimentally Induced Alterations of Affect, *Circulation,* 20:353, 1959.

8 Warren, J. V., Brannon, E. S., Stead, E. A., Jr., and Merrill, A. J.: The Effect of Venesection and the Pooling of Blood in the Extremities on the Atrial Pressure and Cardiac Output in Normal Subjects with Observations on Acute Circulatory Collapse in Three Instances, *J. Clin. Invest.,* 24:337, 1945.

9 Ruetz, P. R., Johnson, S. A., Callahan, R., Meade, R. D., and Smith, J. J.: Fainting: A Review of Its Mechanisms and a Study in Blood Donors, *Medicine (Baltimore),* 46:363, 1967.

10 Adsettm, C. A., Schottstaedt, W. W., and Wolf, S. G.: Changes in Coronary Blood Flow and Other Hemodynamic Indicators Induced by Stressful Inverviews, *Psychosom. Med.,* 24:331, 1962.

11 Stevenson, I. P., Duncan, C. H., Flynn, J. T., and Wolf, S: Hypertension as a Reaction Pattern to Stress: Correlation of Circulatory Hemodynamics with Changes in the Attitude of Emotional State, *Am. J. Med. Sci.,* 224:286, 1952.

12 Ax, A. F.: Physiologic Differentiation between Fear and Anger in Humans, *Psychosom. Med.,* 15:443, 1953.

13 Schacter, J.: Pain, Fear and Anger in Hypertensives and Normotensives, *Psychosom. Med.,* 19:17, 1957.

14 Hillman, C. C., Levy, R. L., Stroud, W. D., and White, P. D.: Study of Blood Pressure in Army Officers: Observations Based on an Analysis of the Medical Records of 22,741 Officers of the U.S. Army, *J.A.M.A.,* 125:699, 1944.

15 Julius, S., and Schork, A.: Borderline Hypertension: A Critical Review, *J. Chronic Dis.,* 23:723, 1971.

16 Eich, R. H., Cuddy, R. P., Smulyan, H., and Lyons, R. H.: Hemodynamics in Labile Hypertension: A Follow-up Study, *Circulation,* 34:299, 1966.

17 Wolf, S., and Wolff, H. G.: A Summary of Experimental Evidence Relating Life Stress to the Pathogenesis of Essential Hypertension in Man, in E. Bell (ed.), "Hypertension: A Symposium," The University of Minnesota Press, Minneapolis, 1951, p. 288.

18 Dustan, H. P. Tarazi, R. C., and Bravo, E. L.: Physiologic Characteristics of Hypertension, *Am. J. Med.,* 52:610, 1972.

19 Julius, S., and Conway, J: Hemodynamic Studies in Patients with Broderline Blood Pressure Elevation, *Circulation,* 38:282, 1968.

20 Grahm, J. D. P.: High Blood Pressure after Battle, *Lancet,* 1:239, 1945.

21 Ruskin, A., Beard, D. W., and Schaffer, R. L.: Blast Hypertension: Elevated Arterial Pressure in Victims of the Texas City Disaster, *Am. J. Med.,* 4:228, 1948.

22 Reiser, M. F., Brust, A. A., and Ferris, E. B.: Life Situations, Emotions and Course of Patients with Arterial Hypertension, *Psychosom. Med.,* 13:133, 1951.

23 Moses, L., Daniels, C. E., and Nickerson, J. L.: Psychogenic Factors in Essential Hypertension: Methodology and Preliminary Report, *Psychosom. Med.,* 18:476, 1956.

24 Henry, J. P., and Cassel, J. C.: Psychosocial Factors in Essential Hypertension: Recent Epidemiologic and Animal Experimental Evidence, Am. J. Epidemiol., 90:171, 1969.

25 Reis, D. J., and Doba, N.: The Central Nervous System and Neurogenic Hypertension, *Prog. Cardiovas. Dis.,* 17:51, 1974.

26 Shapiro, D., Tursky, B., and Schwartz, G. E.: Control of Blood Pressure in Man by Operant Conditioning, *Circ. Res.,* 26(suppl. 1):27, 1970.

27 Patel, C., and North, W. R. S.: Randomized Control Trial of Yoga and Biofeedback in Management of Hypertension, *Lancet,* 2:93, 1975.

28 Benson, H., Rosner, B. A., Marzetta, B. R., and Klemchuk, H. M.: Decreased Blood-Pressure in Pharmacologically Treated Hypertensive Patients Who Regularly Elicited the Relaxation Response, *Lancet,* 1:289, 1974.

29 Stone, R. A., and DeLeo, J.: Psychotherapeutic Control of Hypertension, *N. Engl. J. Med.,* 294:80, 1976.

30 Krist, D. A., and Engel, B. T.: Learned Control of Blood Pressure in Patients with High Blood Pressure, *Circulation,* 51:370, 1975.

31 Jenkins, C. D.: Recent Evidence Supporting Psychologic and Social Risk Factors for Coronary Heart Disease, *N. Engl. J. Med.,* 294:987,1033, 1976.

32 Rosenman, R. H., Brand, R. J., Jenkins, C. D., Friedman, M., Straus, R., and Wurin, M.: Coronary Heart Disease in the Western Collaborative Group Study: Final Follow-up Experience of 8½ years, *J.A.M.A.,* 233:872, 1975.

33 Lee, R. E., and Schneider, R. F.: Hypertension and Arteriosclerosis in Executive and Nonexecutive Personnel, *J.A.M.A.,* 167:1447, 1958.

34 Raffle, P. A. B.: Stress as a Factor in Disease, *Lancet,* 2:839, 1959.

35 Rahe, R. H., Bennett, L., Romo, M., Siltanen, P., and Arthur, R. J.: Subjects Recent Life Changes and Coronary Heart Disease in Finland, *Am. J. Psychiat.,* 130:1222, 1973.

36 Thomas, C. B., and Murphy, E. A.: Further Studies on Cholesterol Levels in Johns Hopkins Medical Students: The Effect of Stress at Examinations, *J. Chronic Dis.*, 8:661, 1958.

37 Grundy, S. M., and Griffin, A. C.: Relationship of Periodic Mental Stress to Serum Lipoprotein and Cholesterol Levels, *J.A.M.A.*, 171:1794, 1959.

38 Hackett, T. P., Cassem, E. H., and Wischnic, H. A.: The Coronary Care Unit: An Appraisal of its Psychologic Hazards, *N. Engl. J. Med.*, 279:1365, 1968.

39 Hackett, T. P., and Cassem, E. H.: Psychologic Effect of Acute Coronary Care, in Meltzer and Dunning (eds.), "Textbooks of Coronary Care," Excerpta Medica Monograph, Excerpta Medica, Amsterdam, 1974, p. 443.

40 Cassem, E. H., and Hackett, T. P.: Psychiatric Consultation in a Coronary Care Unit, *Ann. Intern. Med.*, 75:9, 1974.

41 Wihnic, H. A., Hackett, T. P., and Cassem, E. H.: Psychological Hazards of Convalescence following Myocardial Infarction, *J.A.M.A.*, 215:1292, 1971.

42 Hochman, D. H., Mauck, H. P., and Hoff, E. C.: Experimental Neurogenic Arrhythmias, *Bull. N.Y. Acad. Med.*, 43:1097, 1967.

43 Engel, G. L.: Sudden and Rapid Death during Psychological Stress: Folklore or Wisdom? *Ann. Intern. Med.*, 74:771, 1971.

44 Lown, B., Temte, J. V., Reich, P., Saughan, C., Regestein, Q., and Hai, H.: Basis for Recurring Ventricular Fibrillation in the Absence of Coronary Heart Disease and Its Management, *N. Engl. J. Med.*, 294:623, 1976.

45 Bellet, S., Roman, L., Kostis, J., and Slater, A.: Continuous Electrocardiographic Monitoring during Automobile Driving, *Am. J. Cardiol.*, 27:856, 1968.

46 Gazes, P. C., Sovell, B. F., and Dellastratious, J. W.: Continuous Radio-electrocardiographic Monitoring of Football and Basketball Coaches during Games, *Am. Heart J.*, 78:509, 1969.

47 Lynch, J. J., Thomas, S. A., Mills, M. E., Malinow, L., and Katcher, A. H.: The Effects of Human Contact on Cardiac Arrhythmias in Coronary Care Patients, *J. Nerv. Ment. Dis.*, 158:88, 1974.

48 Lown, B., Tychocinski, M. Garfein, A., and Brooks, P.: Sleep and Ventricular Premature Beats, *Circulation*, 48:691, 1973.

49 Smith, R., Johnson, L., Rothfeld, D., Zir, L., and Tharp, B.: Sleep and Cardiac Arrhythmias, *Arch Intern. Med.*, 130:751, 1972.

50 Lown, B., Verrier, R., and Corblan, R.: Psychologic Stress and Threshold for Repetitive Ventricular Response, *Science*, 192:834, 1973.

51 Skinner, J. E., Lie, J. T., and Entman, M. D.: Modification of Ventricular Fibrillation Latency following Coronary Artery Occlusion in the Conscious Pig, *Circulation*, 51:656, 1976.

52 Barnes, R., and Schollstaedt, W. W.: The Relation of Emotional State to Renal Excretion of Water and Electrolytes in Patients with Congestive Heart Failure, *Am. J. Med.*, 29:217, 1960.

53 Graybiel, A., and White, P. D.: Inversion of the T waves in Lead I or II of the Electrocardiogram in Young Individuals with Neurocirculatory Asthenia, with Thyrotoxicosis, in Relation to Certain Infections and following Paroxysmal Ventricular Tachycardia, *Am. Heart J.*, 10:345, 1935.

54 Wendkos, M. H., and Logue, R. B.: Unstable T Waves in Leads II and III in Persons with Neurocirculatory Asthenia, *Am. Heart J.*, 31:711, 1946.

55 Levander-Lindgren, M.: Studies in Neurocirculatory Asthenia (Da Costa's Syndrome): I. Variations with Regard to Symptoms and Some Pathophysiological Signs, *Acta Med. Scand.*, 172:665, 1962.

56 Graybiel, A., Hartwell, A. S., Barrett, J. B., and White, P. D.: The Effect of Exercise and Four Commonly Used Drugs on the Normal Human Electrocardiogram with Particular Reference to T Wave Changes, *J. Clin. Invest.*, 21:409, 1942.

57 Lgung, O.: Alterations in the Electrocardiogram as a Result of Emotionally Stimulated Respiratory Movements, Especially with Reference to the So-called "Fright Electrocardiogram," *Acta Med. Scand.*, 141:221, 1951.

58 Wasserburger, R. H., Siebecker, L. L., Jr., and Lewis, W. C.: The Effect of Hyperventilation on the Normal Adult Electrocardiogram, *Circulation*, 13:850, 1956.

59 White, P. D., Cohen, M. E., and Chapman, W. P.: The Electrocardiogram in Neurocirculatory Asthenia, Anxiety Neurosis, or Effort Syndrome, *Am. Heart J.*, 34:390, 1947.

60 Kannel, W. B., Dawber, T. R., and Cohen, M. E.: The ECG Neurocirculatory Asthenia (Anxiety Neurosis or Neurasthenia): A Study of 203 Neurocirculatory Patients and 757 Healthy Controls in the Framingham Study, *Ann. Intern. Med.*, 49:1351, 1958.

61 Cohen, M. E., White, P. D., and Johnson, R. E.: Neurocirculatory Asthenia, Anxiety Neurosis, or the Effort Syndrome, *Arch. Intern. Med.*, 81:260, 1948.

62 Marks, I., and Lader, M.: Anxiety States: A Review, *J. Nerv. Ment. Dis.*, 156(1):3, 1973.

63 White, P. D., and Jones, T. D.: Heart Disease and Disorders in New England, *Am. Heart J.*, 3:302, 1928.

64 White, P. D.: "Heart Disease," 4th ed., The Macmillan Company, New York, 1956, p. 582.

65 Mendel, J. G. G., and Klein, D. F.: Anxiety Attacks with Subsequent Agoraphobia, *Compr. Psychiatry*, 103:190, 1969.

66 Cohen, M. E., Badal, D., Kilpatrick, A. Reed, E. W., and White, P. D.: The High Familial Prevalence of Neurocirculatory Asthenia (Anxiety Neurosis, Effort Syndrome), *Am. J. Hum. Genet.*, 3:126, 1951.

67 Slater, E., and Shields, J.: Genetical Aspects of Anxiety, in M. H. Lader (ed.), "Studies of Anxiety," Royal Medico-Psychological Association, London, 1969.

68 Shields, J.: "Monozygotic Twins Brought Up Apart and Brought Up Together," Oxford University Press, London, 1962.

69 Myers, A. B. R.: "On the Etiology and Prevalence of Disease of the Heart Among Soldiers," J. Churchill and Sons, London, 1870, p. 22.

70 Da Costa, J. M.: On Irritable Heart: A Clinical Study of a Functional Cardiac Disorder and Its Consequences, *Am. J. Med. Sci.*, 61:17, 1871.

71 Oppenheimer, B. S., Levine, S. A., Morrison, R. A., Rothschild, M. A., St. Lawrence, W., and Wilson F. N.: Report on Neurocirculatory Asthenia and Its Managements, *Milit. Surg.*, 42:409, 1918.

72 Woods, P.: Da Costa's Syndrome (or Effort Syndrome), *Br. Med. J.*, 1:767,805,845, 1941.

73 White, P. D.: The Soldier's Irritable Heart, *J.A.M.A.*, 118:270, 1942.

74 Lewis T.: "Soldiers Heart: Effort Syndrome," Shaw and Sons, Ltd., London, 1940.

75 Frohlich, E. D., Tarazi, R. D., and Dustan, H. P.: Hyperdynamic Beta-Adrenergic Circulatory State: Increased Beat-Receptor Responsiveness, *Arch. Intern. Med.*, 123:1, 1969.

76 Imhof, P., and Brunner, H.: The Treatment of Functional Heart Disorders with Beta-Adrenergic Blocking Agents, *Postgrad. Med.*, 46(suppl):96, 1970.

77 Jones, M., and Mellirsh, V.: A Comparison of the Exercise Response in Various Groups of Neurotic Patients, and a Method or Rapid Determination of Oxygen in Expired Air Using a Catherometer, *Psychosom. Med.*, 1:192, 1946.

78 Cohen, M. D., Consolzaio, R. D., and Johnson, R. E.: Blood Lactate Response During Moderate Exercise in Neurocirculatory Asthenia, Anxiety Neurosis or Effort Syndrome, *J. Clin. Invest.*, 26:339, 1947.

79 Pitts, F. N., Jr., and McLure, J. N., Jr.: Lactate Metabolism in Anxiety Neurosis, *N. Engl. J. Med.*, 277:1329, 1967.

80 Cohen, M. D., Johnson, R. E., Consolazio, F. C., and White, P. D.: Low Oxygen Consumption and Low Ventilatory Efficiency during Exhausting Work in Patients with Neurocirculatory Asthenia, Effort Syndrome, Anxiety Neurosis, *J. Clin. Invest.,* 25:292, 1946.

81 Cohen, M. E.: Studies of Palmar Hand Sweat in Healthy Subjects and in Patients with Neurocirculatory Asthenia (Anxiety Neurosis, Neurasthenia, Effort Syndrome) with a Description of a Simple Method for Its Quantitative Estimation, *Am. J. Med. Sci.,* 220:496, 1950.

82 Cobb, S., Cohen, M. E., and Badal, D. W.: Capillaries of the Nail Fold in Patients with Neurocirculatory Asthenia (Effort Syndrome, Anxiety Neurosis), *Arch. Neurol. Psychiatry,* 56:643, 1946.

83 Lader, M.: The Nature of Anxiety, *Br. J. Psychiatry,* 121:481, 1972.

84 Cohen, M. E., and White, P. D.: Life Situations, Emotions and Neurocirculatory Asthenia (Anxiety Neurosis, Neurasthenia, Effort Syndrome), *Psychosom. Med.,* 13:335, 1951.

85 Holmgren, A., Jonson, B., Levander, M., Linderholm, H., Sjostrand, T., and Strom G.: Low Physical Working Capacity in Suspected Heart Cases Due to Inadequate Adjustment of Peripheral Blood Flow (Vasoregulatory Asthenia), *Acta Med. Scand.,* 159:413, 1957.

86 Kelly, D., Mitchell-Higgs, N., and Sherman, D.: Anxiety and the Effects of Sodium Lactate Assessed Clinically and Physiologically, *Br. J. Psychiatry,* 119:129, 1971.

87 Wheeler, E. O., White, P. D., Reed, E. W., and Cohen, M. E.: Neurocirculatory Asthenia (Anxiety Neurosis, Effort Syndrome, Neurasthenia): A Twenty Year Follow-up Study of 173 Patients, *J.A.M.A.,* 142:878, 1950.

88 Wishaw, R.: A Review of the Physical Condition of 130 Returned Soldiers Suffering from the Effort Syndrome, *Med. J. Aust.,* 2:891, 1939.

89 Bryce, J. C., Wanklin, J. W., and Hobbs, G. E.: Long Term Mortality in Cardiac Neuroses, *Med. Serv. J. Can.,* 17:669, 1961.

89a Sheehan, D. V., Ballenger, J., and Jacobson, G.: Drug Treatment of Endogenous Anxiety with Hysterical, Phobic and Hypochondriacal Symptoms: A Double Blind Placebo Controlled Drug Trial, paper presented to World Congress of Psychiatry, Hawaii, September 1977.

90 Wallace, R. K., and Benson, H.: The Physiology of Meditation, *Sci. Am.,* 226:84, 1972.

91 Cadorety, R. J., Winokur, G., and Clayton, P. J.: Family History Studies: IV. Depressive Disease Types, *Compr. Psychiatry,* 12:148, 1971.

92 Gershon, E., Dunner, D. L., and Goodwin, F. D.: Towards a Biology of Affective Disorders: Genetic Contribution, *Arch. Gen. Psychiatry,* 25:1, 1971.

93 Freedman, A. F., Kaplan, H. I., and Sadock, B. J. (eds.): "Comprehensive Textbook of Psychiatry," 2d ed., The Williams & Wilkins Company, Baltimore, 1975, pp. 1198–1208, 1941–1956, 1969–1976.

94 Jefferson, J. W.: A Review of the Cardiovascular Effects and Toxicity of Tricyclic Antidepressants, *Psychosom. Med.,* 37:160, 1975.

95 Smith, R. B., and Rusbatch, B. J.: Amitriptyline and Heart Block, *Br. Med. J.,* 3:311, 1967.

96 Rasmussen, E. B., and Kristjansen, P.: ECG Changes during Amitriptyline Treatment, *Am. J. Psychiatry,* 119:781, 1963.

97 Moorehead, C. N., and Knox, S. J.: Imipramine Induced Atrial Fibrillation, *Am. J. Psychiatry,* 122:216, 1965.

98 Coull, D. C., Crooks, J., Dingwall-Fordyce, I., et al.: A Method of Monitoring Drugs for Adverse Reactions: II. Amitriptyline and Cardiac Disease, *Eur. J. Clin. Pharmacol.,* 3:51, 1970.

99 Boston Collaborative Drug Surveillance Program: Adverse Reactions to the Tricyclic-Antidepressive Drugs, *Lancet,* 1:529, 1972.

100 Muller, O. F., Goodman, N., and Bellet, S.: The Hypotensive Effect of Imipramine Hydrochloride in Patients with Cardiovascular Disease, *Clin. Pharmacol. Ther.,* 2:300, 1961.

101 Williams, R. B., and Sherter, C.: Cardiac Complications of Tricyclic Antidepressant Therapy, *Ann. Intern. Med.,* 74:395, 1971.

102 Alexander, E. S., and Nino, A.: Cardiovascular Complications in Young Patients Taking Psychotropic Drugs, *Am. Heart J.,* 78:757, 1969.

103 Luke, D. M.: Tricyclic Antidepressants and Heart Disease, *N.Z. Med. J.,* 74:345, 1971.

104 Murray, K. M., and Smith, S. E.: Desipramine and Hypertensive Episodes, *Lancet,* 2:591, 1966.

105 Farman, J. V.: Desipramine and Hypertensive Episodes, *Lancet,* 2:436, 1966.

106 Hessov, I.: Hypertension during Chlorimipramine Therapy, *Br. Med. J.,* 1:406, 1971.

107 Brunner, H., Hedwall, P. R., Meier, M., et al.: Cardiovascular Effects of Preparation CBA 36, 276-Ba and Imipramine, *Agents Actions,* 2:69, 1971.

108 Jefferson, J. W.: Hypotension from Drugs: Incidence, Peril, Prevention, *Dis. Nerv. Syst.,* 35:66, 1974.

109 Pitts, N. F.: The Clinical Evaluation of Doxepin: A New Psychotherapeutic Agent, *Psychosomatics,* 10:164, 1969.

110 Ayd, F. J. (ed.): Maprotiline: An Effective Tetracyclic Antidepressant, *Intern. Drug Ther. Newsletter,* 8:17, 1973.

111 Cartwright, R. D.: Dream and Drug Induced Fantasy Behavior, *Arch. Gen. Psychiatry,* 15:7, 1966.

112 Cartwright, R. D., Monroe, L. J., and Palmer, C.: Individual Differences in Responses to REM Deprivation, *Arch. Gen. Psychiatry,* 16:297, 1967.

113 Gottschalk, L. A., Haer, J., and Bates, D. E.: Changes in Social Alienation, Personal Disorganization, and Cognitive Intellectual Impairment Produced by Sensory Overload, *Arch. Gen. Psychiatry,* 27:351, 1972.

114 Lipowski, Z. J.: Delirium, Clouding of Consciousness and Confusion, *J. Nerv. Ment. Dis.,* 145:227, 1967.

115 Granacher, R. P., and Baldessarini, R. J., Physostigmine, *Arch Gen. Psychiatry,* 32:375, 1975.

116 Weisman, A. D., and Hackett, T. P.: Psychosis after Eye Surgery, *N. Engl. J. Med.,* 258:1284, 1958.

97
Iatrogenic Problems and Heart Disease

J. WILLIS HURST, M.D.

In the last two decades there has been a tremendous growth of interest in electrocardiographic diagnosis and in the number and variety of electrocardiographs in use. In 1914, there was only one instrument of this kind in the state of Michigan and this was not in operation; there were probably no more than a dozen electrocardiographs in the whole of the United States. Now there is one or more in almost every village of any size, and there are comparatively few people who are not in greater danger of having their peace and happiness destroyed by an erroneous diagnosis of cardiac abnormality based on a faulty interpretation

of an electrocardiogram, than of being injured or killed by an atomic bomb.

FRANK WILSON, M.D., 1951*,1

Despite the best intentions of physicians, they may play a role in creating certain problems that may be troublesome to their patients. Such problems may be related to the heart. The term "iatrogenic heart disease"[2-5] is commonly used to describe such a condition. The term is not a good one. First of all, it points an accusing finger solely at the physician. While this is sometimes justified, it is not always justified. Secondly, heart disease may or may not be actually produced in the patient given such a diagnosis. Accordingly, the author has chosen to discuss the matter under a broader heading—iatrogenic problems and heart disease.

Iatrogenic problems related to heart disease can be divided into four groups: (1) problems related to inadequate patient education on the part of the physician; (2) problems produced as a direct result of procedures, drugs, diet, and altered activity; (3) problems resulting from the misinterpretation of symptoms, signs, and laboratory data; (4) problems resulting from the effect of actions, words, and demeanor of a physician on a susceptible patient.

INADEQUATE PATIENT EDUCATION

A patient may be filled with anxiety while he is being transported all over a hospital or as he wanders around in a doctor's office. The anxiety is, at times, produced because no one has explained to him exactly what is to be done to him. For example, strangers may come early in the morning to take the sleepy, upset patient to the proctoscopic room for examination, but he does not know what a proctoscopic examination is.

The problem-oriented record has highlighted this deficit in patient education. Weed recognized the deficiency and made *Patient Education* a visible part of the *Initial Plans* and *Progress Notes* which are written by the physician (Chap. 10).[6] It is incredible to discover at chart audit that *Patient Education* is commonly "delayed" until answers are available. Patient education should imply that the physician explains every element of the work-up as well as the disease he eventually identifies. When this is not done, the patient regards the hospital and doctor's office as being cold, inhumane, and machine-like. When patient education is carried out with skill, the patient will view the hospital and doctor's office in more humane terms. The understanding of this concept will become increasingly important as more allied health workers become involved with patient

care. The problem-oriented record should assist the physician in guiding the work-up and follow-up of the patient. This includes guiding the allied health workers.

EFFECT OF PROCEDURES, DRUGS, DIET, AND ALTERED ACTIVITY

There are no harmless procedures and no harmless drugs available for use in the practice of medicine. Even a recommended change in diet or the alteration of activity may cause problems in some patients. It is highly likely that this will always be true. Accordingly, it is reasonable to expect that new procedures and new drugs of the future will bring new problems.

Procedures

The complications and risks of cardiac surgical procedures are discussed in Chaps. 56, 61, and 62F. Therefore, only a few points will be discussed here. Peripheral emboli may occur during and after aortic and mitral valve surgical procedures. Bacterial endocarditis may develop after intracardiac surgical procedures. Complete heart block may result from closure of an interventricular septal defect. Aortic regurgitation may develop as a complication of surgical treatment for aortic stenosis, and mitral regurgitation may result from the surgical treatment for mitral stenosis. The postmitral commissurotomy and postpericardiotomy syndrome occur in an unpredictable manner. Cardiac tamponade may develop in this setting. Disseminated intravascular coagulation may occur after open heart surgery. Cardiac arrhythmias may occur after thoracotomy and cardiac surgical procedures. Atelectasis may develop after thoracic surgical procedures. Arteritis may occur after correction of coarctation of the aorta. Surgical ligation of the inferior vena cava may lead to persistent edema and venous insufficiency. Cardiac resuscitation utilizing external cardiac compression may produce contusion of the heart, rib and liver fracture, and fat and marrow emboli to the lungs. The use of defibrillators may lead to cardiac arrhythmias and burns of the skin.

Diagnostic procedures are not always innocuous. The complications of these procedures are discussed in detail in Chaps. 28A, 29C, 33, and 36. Cardiac catheterization may precipitate cardiac arrhythmias. For example, all types of tachycardia may develop during the procedure, and complete heart block may develop in patients undergoing catheterization of the right side of the heart who initially have left bundle branch block and in patients undergoing catheterization of the left side of the heart who initially have right bundle branch block. The catheter may penetrate the right or left atrium and produce hemopericardium. Rarely endocarditis may occur as a result of cardiac catheterization. Aortography may cause arterial damage. An arterial puncture may also cause arterial damage and may produce an arteriovenous fistula. Coronary arteriography may precipitate car-

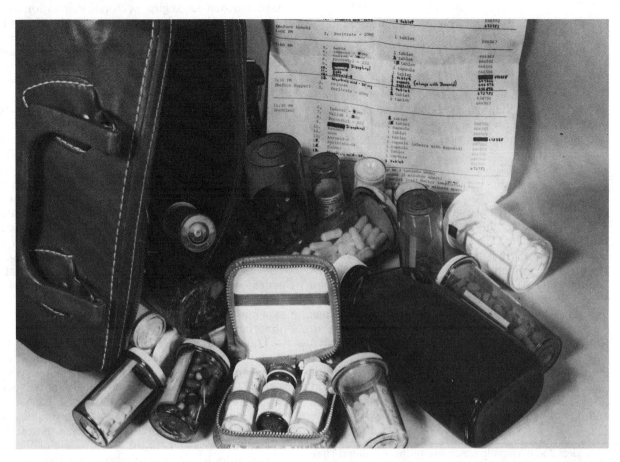

FIGURE 97-1 The drugs shown in this illustration were, believe it or not, all taken by one patient. Note the schedule the patient used so that he never missed a dose. The patient exhibited toxic effects of many of the drugs. It was possible to omit all drugs with enormous benefit.

diac arrhythmia and myocardial infarction. A venipuncture may lead to thrombophlebitis and may even introduce bacteria into the bloodstream.

Drugs

The complications of drug therapy are discussed in detail in Chap. 109. Digitalis may produce anorexia, nausea, diarrhea, and yellow vision. Arrhythmias related to digitalis medication are common. Arrhythmias, especially atrial tachycardia with atrioventricular block, are especially common in patients who receive digitalis and who have a potassium deficit secondary to diuretic therapy. Potassium supplement may not be sufficient to prevent this type of arrhythmia. On the other hand, potassium intoxication may develop when potassium is given in moderate dosage and is continued after a diuretic is no longer effective or has been discontinued. Vigorous diuresis may produce weakness and intravascular clotting. Quinidine sulfate may produce fever, purpura, diarrhea, and cardiac arrhythmias. Procainamide may produce a lupus erythematosus-like picture including pericarditis. Even constrictive pericarditis has been reported to follow the use of this drug.[7] Morphine sulfate may produce nausea, constipation, respiratory depression, and hypotension, and may contribute to atrioventricular block. Norepinephrine may produce

cardiac arrhythmias and necrosis of skin and subcutaneous tissue near the region of intravenous injection or in a distant location. Epinephrine may produce cardiac arrhythmias. Isoproterenol (Isuprel) may produce arrhythmias and hypotension. Antihypertensive drugs including chlorothiazide and ganglionic blocking agents may produce postural hypotension and syncope. Nitroglycerin and digitalis may aggravate angina pectoris in patients with functional hypertrophic subaortic stenosis. Anticoagulants may produce hemorrhage, including hemopericardium, in certain circumstances.

Many patients ingest large numbers of drugs. Sometimes, some of the drugs are not needed, and occasionally one drug is not compatible with another drug. (See Fig. 97-1.)

Diet

A change in diet may produce psychologic problems, electrolyte disturbance, and malnutrition. Frequent determination of serum cholesterol levels in patients on various diets can, at times, lead to much anxiety and unscientific medicine. Fluids administered intravenously may precipitate pulmonary edema.

Altered activity

A recommendation of increased activity may produce cardiac arrhythmias, syncope, angina pectoris, and heart failure, while severe restriction may produce much emotional turmoil, disability, and pulmonary emboli.

Conclusions

This list of problems associated with procedures, drugs, diet, and activity in relation to heart disease is far from complete. The list serves as a background to point out that there is much overlap of what is called "iatrogenic problems" and what is designated as "complications." This is true because the physician is usually in control of the diagnostic work-up and therapy. Since virtually all procedures and all drugs are potentially hazardous, how are physicians to function? If they fail to offer patients corrective surgical treatment, a proper diagnostic work-up, or the proper drug or diet because they are terrified of the possible *complications,* then they will also fail to offer their patients the *benefits* of procedures, drugs, and diet. The problem is solved in two ways:

1 The physicians are obligated to reduce the risk of surgical and diagnostic procedure to the minimum. They do this by assembling the best team that is possible and being cognizant of the complications in order to prevent them if possible. The same approach applies to drug therapy and alterations of the diet. Despite the most careful preparation and execution of a planned program, complications may occur. The obligation of the physician at this point is to recognize the complications and institute the proper therapy when such is available.
2 Physicians must always weigh the risk of what they *do* with the associated complications against the risk of what they *do not do* with the associated complications. They must ask themselves and must answer the following questions: Will the benefit of the surgical procedure with its price—the risk—be worthwhile for the patient as compared with the patient's state without surgical treatment? Will the information gained from a diagnostic procedure be of enough value in the care of the patient to justify the risk involved? Will the potential benefit of drug therapy be worth the risk of drug complications in a certain clinical situation?

MISINTERPRETATION OF SYMPTOMS, SIGNS, AND LABORATORY DATA

The misinterpretation of symptoms, signs, and laboratory data may create iatrogenic problems. Dyspnea due to anxiety or pulmonary disease may be incorrectly attributed to heart disease and treated with digitalis. Chest pain associated with anxiety, gastrointestinal disease, or musculoskeletal disease may be misdiagnosed as angina pectoris. Palpitation due to an occasional ectopic contraction may be disabling to a sensitive patient and thought to be ominous by the physician. Edema of the extremities secondary to obesity or venous insufficiency may be wrongly attributed to congestive heart failure. Episodes of hyperventilation may be diagnosed as acute pulmonary edema. Oral hyperthermia or the normal temperature of a child may be thought to be due to rheumatic fever. A diagnosis of essential hypertension may be made and the patient treated for it simply because the blood pressure is elevated on a single recording. Systolic hypertension may be misinterpreted completely and treatment started for diastolic hypertension. Kinking of the carotid artery may be misdiagnosed as an aneurysm of the artery. Innocent murmurs are very common, are often misinterpreted, and are often attributed to heart disease. This is especially true in children, in pregnant females, when fever is present, and in patients with anemia or thyrotoxicosis. Benign arrhythmias, such as sinus arrhythmia, may be diagnosed as a serious abnormality of cardiac rhythm.

The normal range of the electrocardiogram is wide and is difficult to learn. Many benign ST-T wave "abnormalities" are unfortunately attributed to heart disease. QRS conduction disturbances are frequently misdiagnosed as myocardial infarction. Occasionally myocardial infarction may be correctly diagnosed by electrocardiography but from a tracing that belongs to someone else! Dr. Frank Wilson, one of the great contributors to electrocardiography, wrote the paragraph quoted at the beginning of this chapter in 1951 in order to emphasize his concern that erroneous diagnoses would result from the improper interpretation of the electrocardiogram.

An erroneous diagnosis of cardiac enlargement is often made on examination of the roentgenogram of the chest when the apparent enlargement is really due to a depressed sternum or an epicardial fat pad. The pulmonary artery may be normally prominent when the heart is vertically placed and may be misinterpreted as an abnormality. Elevation of the blood level of the "cardiac enzymes" by noncardiac conditions may be thought to be due to myocardial infarction. The level of the serum cholesterol is often used in a nonscientific manner. The determination of venous pressure and circulation time may be executed poorly, and the results may be no more than the accurate recording of inaccurate data. Cardiac catheterization data may be misinterpreted.

This is a partial list of symptoms, signs, and laboratory data that may be misinterpreted by the physician. Physicians are human, and the problems of medicine are often very complex. Accordingly, even experts acting with great care may misinterpret clinical data.

The conscientious physician is aware of the impact of erroneous diagnosis on his patient. He therefore makes every effort to minimize these problems by careful study and accurate diagnosis, by asking

EFFECT OF ACTIONS, WORDS, AND DEMEANOR OF A PHYSICIAN ON A SUSCEPTIBLE PATIENT[3,5,8]

A patient's visit to a physician's office is an emotional experience for all concerned. The patient is influenced by the physician, the nurse, the technician, the office cleaner, the fellow patients, and the entire environment. The effect of these influences on the patients depends on their emotional status. For example, one patient may be told by the physician that the electrocardiogram is "terrible-looking" and might respond by saying, "It must not mean too much because I feel fine," whereas other patients may become convinced that they have serious heart disease simply because the physician listened to the heart longer than was anticipated. The first patient may remain asymptomatic and return to work. The second type of patient, who may have gone to the physician because of sighing breathing, sticks and stabs of pain near the cardiac apex, palpitation, and exhaustion, may become disabled from the symptoms despite the reassurances of the physician. In the first case, because the patient is emotionally normal, the physician's frightening words cause no great difficulty even though the choice of terms was unwise.[5] In the second case the patient reacts abnormally to a careful examination because he or she was already emotionally disturbed.

Many people, perhaps the majority, have varying degrees of emotional problems. Accordingly, a few comments regarding the emotional makeup of physicians and the emotional makeup of patients are in order.

Physicians may feel insecure and uncertain in their appraisal of a problem. Because of this they hedge in their opinions regarding the problem. The patient who complains of dyspnea and "heart pains" related to anxiety frequently tests the physician. The physician may reassure the patient in many ways, indicating that the blood pressure is normal, the physical examination and electrocardiogram are normal, and "everything seems fine." The patient may seem relieved of worry regarding heart disease and when leaving the office may ask about making a trip, playing golf, etc. When advised to "take it easy," the patient may become firmly convinced that the heart condition is so bad the physician wants to avoid telling the truth. This is a simple and obvious example of "opinion hedging." The physician, of course, may not consciously realize that this has contributed to the patient's anxiety.

Physicians may be extremely concerned that some seriously ill patient may die while under their care. They advise the patient's family of their concern and transmit to them their own anxiety. They may feel protected in that if the family knows how grave the situation is, the physician will not be blamed if the clinical situation deteriorates and death ensues. The physician stands to gain if the patient survives despite the great odds that have been pointed out.

The physician may become frustrated because a difficult medical problem cannot be solved and may transmit this frustration to the patient. A physician may become angry because the patient with emphysema will not stop smoking or the obese patient will not lose weight. Physicians may threaten patients by suggesting that nothing can be done for them if they will not obey the rules.

A patient recovering from a serious illness is frequently very dependent upon the physician. This is as it should be, but at times it is carried to an abnormal degree. If the physician does not recognize this as only one stage of the total rehabilitation process, the patient's progress may remain on a plateau at this level. The insecure physician may have a large number of such patients.

Unless the physicians are aware of the problems that can be caused by thoughtless talk and actions, they may frighten susceptible patients. For example, the physician who whistles or frowns when the blood pressure is noted to be at a high level; who comments that the heart is huge; who uses terms like "floppy valve" or "malignant hypertension"; who says, "you have a time bomb in your chest"; who uses strange words such as organic, physiologic, murmur, skipped beats, systole, or diastole in the presence of the patient; who teaches and points out all findings to students at the bedside; or who threatens patients by saying, "If you don't get your cholesterol down you are going to have a heart attack" is likely to create iatrogenic problems of anxiety in susceptible patients. When this sort of environment prevails, it is likely that many medically unqualified personnel may contribute their own anxiety-provoking statements. For example, the electrocardiographic technician, not wishing to appear unknowing, may answer a query by the patient with frightening statements.

Physical illness is one of the most fear-producing contingencies of modern life. Living has been made secure in many ways, but physical illness remains as the severe threat. Physical illness happens to the individual, yet many other factors influence the patient's response to the illness. Some of these factors are the personality structure of the patient, the family structure, the patient's work, the degree of financial security, and the nature of the illness.

The personality structure of the patient may influence the illness favorably or unfavorably. Some patients exaggerate their illnesses and with minor illnesses become permanent invalids; others minimize their illnesses and deny the existence of real danger. The family influences the course of illness; a family may either exaggerate or minimize the medical problem. At times families bring to the patient stories of friends and neighbors who had a similar illness and had an early demise. These stories intensify the patient's anxieties. In addition to their illnesses, many patients have realistic anxieties about their work and financial security and the degree to which illness will affect their present and future work life. Sometimes these fears are realistic and sometimes they are exaggerated. The nature of the illness has a direct bearing on the degree of anxiety. There is much common knowledge among the general populace about illness today. There is some understanding of the nature of heart disease, but this information and misinformation may either add to or diminish the patient's anxiety.

Most patients pass through a course of illness which may have five phases. In the beginning, there may be *denial* of the illness or the seriousness of the illness.[9] In time this is replaced by *fear* of the illness, which may be considerably exaggerated. This may be followed by a period of regression, clinging, and *dependency* upon the physician and the nursing staff. At times this is followed by *depression* in which the patient has periods of low self-esteem, difficulty in sleeping, loss of appetite, and loss of usual interest in family and friends. This is usually followed by *realistic adaptation* to the illness and the limitations it entails. However, some patients never work through this course. There are some who become anxious about their illnesses and become chronic invalids for the rest of their lives. Physicians must be sensitive to the emotional status of their patients and assist them in working through their difficulties.

The physician has many problems in dealing with patients. The diagnoses must be accurate, and the patients must be taught realistically to take proper care of themselves. If a patient is overly anxious, the physician may stir up anxieties by realistic instruction. On the other hand, if patients deny their illnesses and will not take realistic care of themselves, then the physician must find ways to deal with these denials, without causing undue anxiety.

PREVENTION OF IATROGENIC PROBLEMS

Iatrogenic problems which are the result of the actions, words, and demeanor of a physician in dealing with a susceptible patient may be minimized by considering the following points:

1 The patient education portion of the problem-oriented system must be implemented with devotion and skill.
2 Physicians must be aware of the problem under discussion. They must understand that certain anxious patients will visit them and that the physician's words, actions, and demeanor and the entire environment may enhance a patient's fears, worries, and anxiety.
3 Physicians must know themselves. They cannot manage or prevent anxiety if they do not attempt to analyze their own reactions and emotional makeup.
4 The physician must learn as much as possible about organic disease and try to understand the emotional problems of patients.
5 Physicians must understand the stages of rehabilitation through which a patient may go after having a serious illness. Their job is to lead the patient through the various stages and to establish a healthy and nondependent physician-patient relationship.

REFERENCES

1 Wilson, F.: Foreword, in E. Lepeschkin, "Modern Electrocardiography," vol. 1, The Williams & Wilkins Company, Baltimore, 1951, p. v.
2 Aurbach, A., and Gliebe, P. A.: Iatrogenic Heart Disease: Common Cardiac Neurosis, *J.A.M.A.,* 129:338, 1945.
3 Weinberg, H. B.: Iatrogenic Heart Disease, *Ann. Intern. Med.,* 38:9, 1953.
4 Hart, A. D.: Iatrogenic Cardiac Neurosis: Critique, *J.A.M.A.,* 156:1133, 1954.
5 Wheeler, E. O., Williamson, C. R., and Cohen, M. E.: Heart Scare, Heart Surveys, and Iatrogenic Heart Disease: Emotional and Symptomatological Effects of Suggesting to 162 Adults That They Might Have Heart Disease, *J.A.M.A.,* 167:1096, 1958.
6 Hurst, J. W., and Walker, H. K. (eds.): "The Problem-oriented System," MEDCOM, Inc., New York, May 1972.
7 Sunder, S. K., and Shah, A.: Constrictive Pericarditis in Procainamide-induced Lupus Erythematosus Syndrome, *Am. J. Cardiol.,* 36:961, 1975.
8 Harrison, T. R., and Reeves, T. J.: The Psychologic Management of Patients with Heart Disease, *Am. Heart J.,* 70:136, 1965.
9 Hackett, T. P., Cassem, N. H., and Wishnie, H. A.: The Coronary Care Unit: An Appraisal of Its Psychologic Hazards, *N. Engl. J. Med.,* 279:1365, 1968.

PART X

Environmental Factors Affecting the Heart and Blood Vessels

98
Tobacco and the Cardiovascular System[1-12]

JOSEPH T. DOYLE, M.D.

Warning: The Surgeon General has determined that cigarette smoking is dangerous to your health.

FROM PACK OF AMERICAN CIGARETTES

All toxicologic and pharmacologic studies have shown that the sole physiologically active ingredient of tobacco smoke is nicotine. The possibility that other potent vasoactive substances such as acetaldehyde may be absorbed in pharmacologically significant quantities has not been wholly excluded. Nicotine has no known function in the life of the tobacco plant. It is synthesized in the roots and transported to the leaves. The nicotine content of tobacco varies considerably with regional and climatic factors and can be altered by selective breeding. Although cigar and pipe tobaccos contain considerably larger quantities of nicotine than does cigarette tobacco, their heavy, alkaline smoke is intensely irritating to the respiratory tract and is not usually inhaled. On the other hand, the light, bland smoke of cigarettes is, with practice, readily tolerated by the bronchial tree. Accordingly, nicotine is rapidly and completely absorbed in the lungs by the cigarette smoker, while absorption of nicotine from the buccal mucosa by cigar and pipe smokers and by tobacco chewers is slower and less complete. For all practical purposes, the measurable effects of tobacco smoking relate only to cigarettes and are identical with those produced by equivalent doses of nicotine.

Acquisition of the tobacco habit is clearly related to social, cultural, and psychologic influences. It is universally recognized that, once entrenched, the cigarette habit is difficult to break. There is some evidence that parenterally administered nicotine can induce the same feeling of satiety produced by a cigarette. Some but not all heavy smokers derive complete satisfaction from low-nicotine cigarettes. There is no evidence that nicotine is addicting in the same sense as that applied to narcotics.

The novice smoker commonly experiences the toxic effects of nicotine: giddiness, nausea and vomiting, abdominal cramps, cold sweat, and even vasomotor collapse. These symptoms when unusually severe have, in the past, been incorrectly construed as evidence of sensitivity to tobacco and may, understandably, deter formation of the smoking habit. The veteran smoker does not acquire tolerance to nicotine, inasmuch as all measurable circulatory responses persist without attenuation, but learns to manipulate time-dosage factors so as to avoid poisonous effects. Radioactively labeled nicotine is rapidly degraded after ingestion, but the metabolic pathways are unknown. Approximately 10 percent of ingested nicotine is excreted unchanged. Chronic administration of nicotine to experimental animals produces no demonstrable tissue changes. The possibility of allergic or hypersensitivity reactions to tobacco or its combustion products has been suggested but not convincingly proved.

The pharmacologic and toxic effects of nicotine have been extensively studied in experimental animals for a century and more. The applicability of these observations to human subjects is, however, questionable. Therefore, despite the meagerness of such information, the data to be cited here are based primarily on studies in human beings.

A standard cigarette contains about 20 mg nicotine. Considerable amounts of nicotine are destroyed by heat or dispersed in the side-stream smoke, so that the average, inhaling cigarette smoker absorbs about 2 mg nicotine. Depending on rate of puffing, depth of inhalation, and length of cigarette, the nicotine absorption from a single cigarette in the average adult male is 3 to 6 μg/kg min. The lethal human oral dose of nicotine is estimated to be 1 mg/kg.

In nonsmokers as well as experienced smokers, cigarette smoke and nicotine cause small but consistent increases in heart rate; in systolic, diastolic, and pulse pressures; in cardiac output; and in stroke volume. Noninvasive measurements on human subjects indicate that the inhalation of cigarette smoke is followed by shortening of the isometric period of left ventricular contraction. Skin temperature and blood flow are sharply reduced. Information on muscle blood flow is scanty because of the technical difficulty of measurement. It appears, however, that there is an increase in coronary blood flow after smoking that parallels rises in systemic blood pressure and in left ventricular output. The resultant increase in cardiac work in individuals with overt coronary heart disease is not, however, met by a corresponding augmentation of coronary arterial flow.

No electrocardiographic changes are associated with smoking which cannot be explained by the increase in heart rate. The striking electrocardiographic abnormalities induced by nicotine and tobacco smoke in animals with artificial coronary arterial obstruction have no counterpart in human subjects with coronary disease. Ballistocardiographic abnormalities induced by cigarette smoking are not reproduced by nicotine. The ballistocardiographic cigarette test, after initial enthusiastic acceptance, is no longer regarded as adequate evidence of subclinical coronary heart disease.

The circulatory responses to tobacco smoke in subjects both human and animal are accounted for by the mobilization of epinephrine and norepinephrine from chromaffin tissue in and around blood vessels, from ganglions in the myocardium, and from the adrenal medulla itself. Structures activated by the release of acetylcholine are stimulated by nicotine. Such structures include the central nervous system, notably the chemoreceptors of the carotid and aortic bodies. A "pharmacologic" dose of nicotine produces a blood epinephrine level virtually equivalent to concentrations used therapeutically. In human subjects, urinary epinephrine excretion may increase up to 50 percent after heavy cigarette smoking. In experimental animals, the effect of nicotine can be blocked by ganglioplegics such as hexamethonium. Depletion of the norepinephrine stores of chromaffin cells by reserpine blocks the response to nicotine, an effect with possible therapeutic implications in vasopastic disorders. Stimulation of the posterior pituitary causes measurable antidiuresis, although the amount of pitressin liberated is quite inadequate to produce coronary arterial constriction.

Substantial quantities of free fatty acids are mobilized in the serum of human subjects by their smoking cigarettes or by the injection of nicotine. It has been suggested that high serum concentrations of free fatty acids may interfere with metabolic exchanges across the capillary wall and may induce cardiac dysrhythmias. This metabolic response to sympathetic stimulation can be prevented by ganglionic blockade and is absent in adrenalectomized human subjects. Some data indicate increased serum total-cholesterol levels in heavy cigarette smokers, although other date show no such relation.

An increase in blood sugar has been regularly found in experimental animals after the injection of nicotine, but observations in human beings are contradictory. Oxygen consumption in the human subject, furthermore, is not increased by nicotine or by cigarette smoke. Although blood clotting is not measurably affected by cigarette smoking, there is some evidence that platelet adhesiveness is enhanced. Platelet aggregates could cause ischemic episodes, initiate thrombosis, and thus, according to the Rokitansky-Duguid hypothesis, lead to atheroma formation.

Studies in experimental animals show that the inhalation of cigarette smoke is followed by a significant and prolonged reduction of the threshold for ventricular fibrillation.

Although cigarette smoking is regularly associated with an immediate, although transient, rise in arterial blood pressure, the prognostic significance of this response is unclear. Vascular hyperreactors have an excessive pressor response and a striking reduction in retinal arterial caliber after cigarette smoking, but follow-up observations have not been reported. The sons of hypertensive parents tend to show exaggerated increases in pulse rate, cardiac output, and arterial blood pressure after cigarette smoking, perhaps as a genetic expression. On the other hand, epidemiologic findings are that heavy cigarette smokers tend to have lower blood pressure readings than nonsmokers. No significant differences between smokers and nonsmokers in various male populations are found in the pulse rate, the blood pressure, the response to the cold pressor test, or the response to the inhalation of carbon dioxide. Smokers show no evidence of impaired cardiovascular "fitness" on work tests. On the other hand, young smokers consistently show an increased oxygen debt after moderate exercise which reverts to normal after abstention from smoking. The same impairment is reproduced in nonsmokers by the inhalation of carbon monoxide to carboxyhemoglobin levels typical of smokers. Endurance performance has been shown to be significantly impaired in young male cigarette smokers compared with nonsmokers. Comparable studies on middle-aged populations of heavy smokers are not available.

It seems increasingly probable that carbon monoxide is the chief toxic constituent of cigarette smoke. Heavy cigarette smokers have carboxyhemoglobin concentrations of 2 to 15 percent. Even at low levels, carbon monoxide displaces the oxygen dissociation curve of hemoglobin to the left. In other words, at equivalent oxygen saturations, the partial pressure of oxygen is lower in the presence of carboxyhemoglobin. This peculiarity might assume importance in obstructive disease of the coronary arteries, where an increased myocardial oxygen requirement could not be met by an increase in blood flow. In this situation the secondary compensatory mechanism of further widening of the already large arteriovenous oxygen difference would be impaired. Anoxic damage to the vascular tunics caused by carbon monoxide could, in theory, favor the localization of atheromata and accelerate atherogenesis. Alternatively, mitrochondrial fatty acid synthesis in the arterial wall may be stimulated by an inhibition of oxidation of pyridine nucleotide by carbon monoxide. Animals on an atherogenic diet developed earlier and far more florid fatty arterial lesions when living in high atmospheric concentrations of carbon monoxide than did control animals. The animals exposed to carbon monoxide also become polycythemic. Men with coronary heart disease often have high hemoglobin concentrations and increased blood viscosity, which could impair phasic coronary blood flow. Carbon monoxide has an even greater affinity for myoglobin than for hemoglobin at low oxygen tensions and may thus interfere with oxygen uptake, particularly by the myocardium.

The use of tobacco has been violently condemned on both moral and hygienic grounds virtually from its introduction into Europe, but few scientifically acceptable data on the chronic effects of smoking have been available until recently. "Tobacco angina," so often described by clinicians of a previous generation, has disappeared as the clinical definition of coronary heart disease has become more precise. Since Buerger first described thromboangiitis obliterans in 1908, cigarette smoking has been generally considered to be a primary etiologic factor. On the other hand, Wessler has argued persuasively that Buerger's disease is indistinguishable from the ischemic complications of atherosclerosis, arterial embolization, or thrombosis and is not correlated with the smoking habit. DeBakey and associates imply similar conclusions based on their large clinical experience.

Chronic toxicity studies in animals forced to inhale tobacco smoke have consistently failed to yield evidence of tissue damage. Observations of the long-continued effects of tobacco on human subjects are necessarily descriptive, and the conclusions are inferential. Pearl opined 36 years ago on rather dubious evidence that "the smoking of tobacco is statistically associated with an impairment of life duration, and the amount or degree of this impairment increases as the habitual amount of smoking increases." More recently, Berkson has extended this concept. He holds that tobacco exercises a nonspecific lethal influence on the human organism, since heavy smokers die at an accelerated rate from all causes, most frequently from cardiovascular disease. Large-scale retrospective and prospective studies of the association between the tobacco habit and bronchiogenic carcinoma have been accepted by most physicians and statisticians as clearly inculpating cigarettes. A much more striking although incidental observation has been the large excess of cardiovascular deaths, frequently sudden, in heavy cigarette smokers shown initially in men and subsequently in women. The same trends in mortality as well as in morbidity were first observed prospectively in the pooled data of the Framingham and Albany studies. The risk of cigarette smoking is related to the number of cigarettes smoked daily. The consumption of 20 or more cigarettes daily is associated with a hazard of myocardial infarction up to three times greater than that found in nonsmokers or in cigar or pipe smokers. In common with other coronary risk factors, the hazards of cigarette smoking are attenuated by increasing age. Carefully controlled studies have presented convincing evidence that coronary heart disease found in populations with a low prevalence and incidence of coronary heart disease is explained by the fact that atherosclerosis does not occur at the low serum cholesterol concentration characteristic of such populations. Conversely, in populations highly susceptible to coronary heart disease cigarette smoking contributes powerfully to risk, and the total effect is greater than the sum of the individual contributions of several simultaneously present risk factors. The contribution of cigarette smoking to cerebrovascular disease is far less striking. Cessation of cigarette smoking is associated with reduced mortality, a phenomenon suggested by the Albany-Framingham studies and recently strongly supported by observations made on British physicians who stopped smoking.

Angina pectoris, on the other hand, is no more common in cigarette smokers than in nonsmokers. Similar observations were reported 40 years ago. This striking difference between angina pectoris and other manifestations of coronary heart disease is not easily explained. It is possible that heavy cigarette smoking, despite the absence of supporting experimental evidence, may predispose toward the irreversible ischemic complications of coronary atherosclerosis but may play no role whatsoever in that form of disease manifested only by angina. This is in no way inconsistent with the frequent clinical observation that angina may be precipitated or aggravated by smoking. In support of such a hypothesis is the observation that the risk of myocardial infarction in the ex-cigarette smoker reverts to that of the nonsmoker or of the cigar or pipe smoker, suggesting that the effects of cigarette smoke are acute rather than chronic. The little, if any, increased risk of myocardial infarction in cigar and pipe smokers seems most plausibly explained by the smaller amounts of toxic substances inhaled.

The therapeutic inferences to be derived from these incomplete pharmacologic and epidemiologic observations are necessarily empiric. The acute circulatory responses to smoking are believed to be due to the absorption of nicotine and the resultant mobilization of catecholamines. Heart rate, systolic blood pressure, and cardiac output increase. A narrowed coronary arterial tree may not be able to increase perfusion to sustain the increased myocardial workload, particularly in the presence of carboxyhemoglobin. In contrast, the sharp decrease in blood flow to the extremities is ill tolerated in advanced obliterative vascular disease. Mortality date in both men and women indicate that heavy cigarette smokers die younger and at a more rapid rate than nonsmokers, while morbidity data reveal a threefold greater hazard of myocardial infarction in men who smoke 20 or more cigarettes daily compared with nonsmokers. It is difficult to escape the conclusion that abstention from cigarettes may improve longevity, particularly since morbidity data indicate that former cigarette smokers are at little if any greater risk than nonsmokers or pipe or cigar smokers. Moreover, many, though admittedly anecdotal, observations attest to the amelioration of vasospastic and obliterative vascular diseases of the extremities after the discontinuance of smoking. The Surgeon General's Advisory Committee on Smoking and Health has affirmed repeatedly and emphatically the significance of the association between cigarette smoking and coronary heart disease and has continued to document the evidence which supports this conclusion through the National Clearinghouse for Smoking and Health. The Committee has unequivocally termed cigarette usage the most important of the causes of chronic bronchitis and significantly related to pulmonary emphysema. Both these conditions aggravate heart disease of any type and may cause chronic cor pulmonale. Lastly, the Inter-Society Commission for Heart Disease Resources has recommended that "high priority be given to the elimination of cigarette smoking as a national habit" through restriction of advertising and sales, intensive educational programs, and, indeed, the ultimate elimination of the cigarette industry. Curtailment of advertising and the recent production of low tar–low nicotine cigarettes are encouraging recent developments, however, in view of steadily increasing cigarette sales, particularly to the younger population.

REFERENCES

1 Berkson, J.: Smoking and Cancer of the Lung, *Proc. Staff Meet. Mayo Clin.,* 35:637, 1960.

2 Doyle, J. T., Dawber, T. R., Kannel, W. B., Kinch, S. H., and Kahn, H. A.: The Relationship of Cigarette Smoking to Coronary Heart Disease: The Second Report of the Combined Experience of the Albany, N.Y., and Framingham, Mass., Studies, *J.A.M.A.,* 190:886, 1964.

3 Larson, P. S., Haag, H. B., and Silvette, H.: "Tobacco: Experimental and Clinical Studies," The Williams & Wilkins Company, Baltimore, 1961.

4 Larson, P. S., and Silvette, H.: "Tobacco: Experimental and Clinical Studies, Supplement I," The Williams & Wilkins Company, Baltimore, 1968.

5 Pearl, R.: Tobacco Smoking and Longevity, *Science,* 87:216, 1938.

6 Report of Inter-Society Commission for Heart Disease Resources: Primary Prevention of the Atherosclerotic Diseases, *Circulation,* 42:a-55, 1970.

7 U.S. Public Health Service: Smoking and Health, Report of the Advisory Committee to the Surgeon General of the Public Health Service, Washington, U.S. Department of Health, Education, and Welfare, Public Health Service Publication No. 1103, 1964.

8 U.S. Public Health Service: The Health Consequences of Smoking, U.S. Department of Health, Education, and Welfare, Washington, Public Health Service Publications no. 1696, 1967, revised January 1968; suppl., no. 1696, 1968; no. 1696-2, 1969; no. (HSM) 71-7513, 1971; no. (HSM) 72-6516, 1972; no. (HSM) 73-8704, 1973; no. (CDC) 74-8704, 1974; 1975.

9 Wessler, S., Ming. S., Gurewich, V., and Freiman, D. G.: A Critical Evaluation of Thromboangiitis Obliterans: The Case against Buerger's Disease, *N. Engl. J. Med.,* 262:1149, 1960.

10 World Health Organization: Smoking and Its Effects on Health, Report of a WHO Expert Committee, Geneva, World Health Organization Technical Report Series no. 568, 1975.

11 Wynder, E. L. (ed.): "The Biologic Effects of Tobacco with Emphasis on the Clinical and Experimental Aspects," Little, Brown and Company, Boston, 1955.

12 Wynder, E. L., Hoffman, D., and Gori, G. B. (eds.), "Proceedings of the Third World Conference on Smoking and Health, vol. 1: Modifying the Risk for the Smoker," U.S. Department of Health, Education, and Welfare Publication no. (NIH) 76-1221, 1976.

99
Occupation and Cardiovascular Disease

NANETTE KASS WENGER, M.D.

TOXIC OCCUPATIONAL EXPOSURES

Specific associations of particular occupations with cardiovascular disease relate primarily to toxic occupational exposures.[1] With improved industrial hygiene and with increased automation, toxic occupational exposures are decreasing; however, severe toxicity and death may result from leaks, blowouts, equipment breakdown, etc. Toxic occupational exposures may be classified as physical, biologic, and chemical. Toxic physical exposures include extremes of oxygen pressure, barometric pressure, gravity,

acceleration, noise, temperature, and humidity (see Chaps. 101 and 102). Biologic agents are operative in laboratory-acquired infections or when an individual's work assignments bring him to an endemic area; allergic or hypersensitivity response to injected medications or vaccines may be considered an iatrogenic toxic exposure. A wide variety of chemical agents enter the body by inhalation, by skin absorption, or by ingestion; they produce cardiovascular toxicity by a direct effect on the myocardium, by impairing the oxygen-carrying capacity of the blood, or (as in the case of organic phosphorus insecticides) by cholinesterase inhibition, which is clinically evident as intense parasympathetic stimulation.[1]

Occupational toxic exposures may mimic cardiovascular disease, as exemplified by toxic gases or fumes producing pulmonary edema. This chemical pulmonary edema often occurs after a lag phase and may be associated with substernal pain or discomfort, thus mimicking the presentation of myocardial infarction. Differentiation is important, as morphine administration is contraindicated because of the central nervous system toxicity and respiratory depression also produced by some of these chemicals. Digitalis is generally ineffective. The immediate therapy should include oxygen, bronchodilator drugs, corticosteroid hormones, antibiotics for secondary infection, or tracheostomy as needed.[2]

Additionally, the South American miners who work at high altitudes in the Andes and develop "high-altitude heart disease" may be considered to have occupational heart disease (see Chap. 100). Fire fighters' chronic occupational exposure to carbon monoxide has resulted in maximal allowable blood concentrations of carboxyhemoglobin, even in nonsmoking fire fighters; serum enzyme level changes were interpreted as suggestive of myocardial damage.[3]

An unusual occupational hazard is encountered among persons with coronary atherosclerotic heart disease who work in explosive factories using nitroglycol; this substance is 180 times more volatile than nitroglycerin and is easily absorbed via the lungs and skin. These employees experience angina pectoris during the weekend which disappears upon returning to work; sudden death has also occurred during the weekend, when these individuals were deprived of the vasodilator effect of nitroglycol present during the workweek.[4] Additionally, chest pain and even sudden death have been described as "withdrawal symptoms" in patients without apparent coronary atherosclerotic heart disease after prolonged exposure to nitroglycerin. Exertional and emotional stimuli did not appear to precipitate the pain,[5] and coronary spasm, reversed by nitroglycerin, has been documented by angiography during the withdrawal state.[6] It is suggested that chronic industrial vasodilator exposure or therapy may result in compensatory homeostatic vasoconstriction which persists during nitroglycerin withdrawal, with a resultant cardiac ischemic episode.[7]

CORONARY ATHEROSCLEROTIC HEART DISEASE AND OCCUPATION

A number of studies relate the incidence and severity of clinical coronary atherosclerotic heart disease to differences in occupational activity.[8] Men in sedentary occupations had fatal myocardial infarction at a younger age than those whose occupation involved considerable physical activity; economic status did not seem a significant factor. However, one postmortem study of men who died suddenly of accident or suicide showed comparable coronary atherosclerosis in those engaged in sedentary and in physically active occupations.[9] Obviously, clinically diagnosed coronary atherosclerotic heart disease and that diagnosed at pathologic examination constitute different spectra of disease. In a prospective study of 667 middle-aged London busmen, elevation of systolic blood pressure and serum cholesterol level were the predominant predictive factors for the development of ischemic heart disease; however, the physically active conductors had less symptomatic ischemic heart disease than comparable sedentary drivers.

Farmers, as a group, have a lower than average incidence of coronary heart disease. The requirement of the ability to perform heavy physical work may have been a selecting factor in initially excluding the unfit; alternatively, the activity of farming may exert a prophylactic effect on the manifestations of coronary atherosclerotic heart disease.[10]

Russek[11] considers the emotional stress associated with occupational responsibilities a significant factor in predicting clinical coronary disease; the individuals at high risk are described as aggressive, ambitious, and restless at leisure (see Chap. 96). In addition, low job satisfaction; job pressures, responsibilities, and work overload; and job mobility appear to be associated with an increased incidence of coronary heart disease.

Friedman[12] describes the relation between the "type A personality" and a markedly increased incidence of clinical coronary atherosclerotic heart disease. These individuals have intense ambition, competitive drive, and a sense of urgency; they are constantly preoccupied with deadlines and have a sustained effort to achieve. He suggests that constitutional and personality factors may also influence the selection of an occupation with chronic socioeconomic pressure and emotional trauma.

The relationship of emotional stress to coronary atherosclerosis, as well as to hypertension, remains controversial (see Chaps. 62B, 65, 96). Coronary heart disease had been traditionally thought to occur among persons with heavy responsibility, increased tension, and emotional strain, e.g., executives. Contrary to popular belief, executives and top management personnel have a normal, or possibly reduced, incidence of clinical coronary atherosclerotic heart disease[13] when compared with other sedentary workers. Nevertheless, Friedman[12] described periodic severe occupational stress associated with a rise in serum cholesterol level and an acceleration of the blood coagulation time; the relation to clinical coronary atherosclerotic heart disease is inferential.

Causal relation between occupation and heart disease from the viewpoint of Workmen's Compensation decisions and awards is a different entity. It requires only that the employee be subjected to an unusual or excessive physical or emotional strain in the course of his work, prior to the development of angina pectoris or an acute myocardial infarction. More recently compensation has been awarded both on the basis of ordinary work activity as causally related to heart disease and on the basis that the cumulative physical and mental strain of a lifetime of work may culminate in an acute coronary episode[14] (see Chap. 111). Medical committees[15,15a] properly emphasize that these attitudes often negate efforts to rehabilitate cardiac patients and hamper their employment or reemployment.

There is increasing evidence that regular physical activity militates against the development of clinical coronary atherosclerotic heart disease. An occupational situation may foster or diminish the development of coronary atherosclerotic heart disease by altering coronary risk factors. Comparative studies[16,17] with population groups with similar dietary intake show a greater incidence of ischemic heart disease and myocardial infarction in the sedentary than in the physically active workers. Coronary heart disease occurred more commonly among bus drivers than among conductors on double-deck buses; and more among postal clerks, telephonists, and executives than among the postmen.[17] Postmortem evaluation of coronary atherosclerotic heart disease in middle-aged men dying of noncoronary causes showed no relation between increased physical activity of occupation and coronary artery wall atheroma, some relation between increased physical activity of occupation and lesser occlusion of the coronary artery lumen, and a marked relation between increased physical activity of occupation and less ischemic myocardial fibrosis; physical activity was interpreted as protective against the progression of coronary atherosclerotic heart disease.[17]

HYPERTENSIVE HEART DISEASE AND OCCUPATION

Less comprehensively studied is the relation of occupation to hypertension and hypertensive cardiovascular disease. It was encountered more frequently among employees in the crude oil industry exposed to hydrocarbons and hydrogen sulfide than among administrative workers; noise exposure also seemed a potentiating factor in this study; a pronounced effect of smoking and a hereditary factor were also implicated.[18] Furthermore, there was a subsequent increase in angina pectoris and in fatal and nonfatal myocardial infarction among viscose rayon workers exposed to carbon disulphide, who developed apparent exposure-related hypertension.[19] Another survey showed a higher group prevalence of hypertension among employees subjected to high neuropsychic stress, as compared with manual workers.[20]

OCCUPATION AND VASCULAR HAND TRAUMA

Repeated prolonged occupational hand trauma, as encountered among machinists, welders, plumbers, iron and steel workers, and miners whose use hand-held vibrating tools such as high-frequency pneumatic hammers, chain saws, etc., may result in severe ischemia of the digits (see Chap. 104). This traumatic vasospastic disease was described in 40 percent of a group of lumberjacks,[21] and occurred almost predictably after 3 to 5 years of occupational exposure.

Early changes in the digital arteries, demonstrable by angiography, consist of an exaggeration of the normal vasoconstrictor response; this is potentiated by exposure to cold. Late arterial changes are organic and are characterized by subintimal fibrosis and variable medial hypertrophy of the vessel wall.[22] Symptoms include rest pain, numbness, Raynaud's phenomenon, paresthesias, and coldness. There may be evidence of skin pallor, subcutaneous infarction, nonhealing skin ulceration, cyanosis, absent or diminished pulses, ischemic petechiae, and hypesthesia. Conservative management includes avoidance of further trauma, abstinence from tobacco, and use of vasodilator drugs; sympathectomy, however, may be required.[23]

OCCUPATION AND PREVENTIVE CARDIOLOGY

To the extent that jobs and work environment can be modified to incorporate the elimination or control of coronary risk factors at work, a particular job may be considered "preventive" of coronary atherosclerotic heart disease. This would encompass elimination of smoking on the job; provision of time and facilities for recommended diet in company catering facilities; provision of time and facilities for "exercise breaks" for those in sedentary jobs; and creation of an emotional climate and regulation of work intensity to avoid undue cumulation of stress. The industrial physician can make a significant contribution to the primary prevention of coronary atherosclerotic heart disease by instituting a program of health education and by periodic health screening[24] for the detection of hypertension, electrocardiographic and other evidence of heart abnormalities, and metabolic disorders—diabetes mellitus, hyperuricemia, and lipid abnormalities.

EMPLOYMENT OF THE CARDIAC PATIENT

Many patients with cardiac disease can and should work. However, there are widespread ramifications of the employment or reemployment of the cardiac patient in industry. These relate to the early institution of rehabilitation efforts; selective placement dependent on the patient's type of heart disease and functional capacity; the effects of the work and work environment on the course of his heart disease (see Chaps. 45 and 62E); patient, employer, labor union, and physician education; insurance, law, and Workmen's Compensation decisions; and industry's experience with the cardiac patient as an employee.[15a]

A current statement by the Council on Occupational Health of the American Medical Association deserves emphasis:[25]

Patients with cardiac disease can work. Most patients with cardiac disease should work, usually in gainful employment. Many patients with cardiac disease achieve satisfactory rehabilitation on their own. Many, however, achieve it only by painstaking attention to the varied factors of professionally guided rehabilitation.

The extent of the pathologic symptoms and the apparent limitation of cardiac reserve are often not as important as the emotional factors and the resiliency with which the patient adjusts to his disease.

The physician's alertness, ingenuity, flexibility, and maturity are needed to cope successfully with the variety of factors involved in any individual case. Many forms of assistance are available in the medical profession, in the industrial community, and among the social agencies.

The great number of persons involved makes their successful rehabilitation important to industry, and community and to the nation.

REFERENCES

1 Warshaw, L. J.: "The Heart in Industry," Hoeber Medical Division, Harper & Row, Publishers, Incorporated, New York, 1960, p. 456.

2 Kleinfeld, M.: Acute Pulmonary Edema of Chemical Origin, *Arch. Environ. Health*, 10:942, 1965.

3 Sammons, J. H., and Coleman, R. L.: Firefighters' Occupational Exposure to Carbon Monoxide, *J. Occup. Med.*, 16:543, 1974.

4 Lob, M.: Angine de Poitrine et Carence en Nitroglycol dans les Fabriques d'Explosifs (Angina Pectoris and Nitroglycol Deficiency in Explosive Factories), *Rev. Med. Suisse Romande*, 85:489, 1965.

5 Lund, R. P., Häggendal, J., and Johnsson, G.: Withdrawal Symptoms in Workers Exposed to Nitroglycerine, *Br. J. Ind. Med.*, 25:136, 1968.

6 Klock, J. C.: Nonocclusive Coronary Disease after Chronic Exposure to Nitrates: Evidence for Physiologic Nitrate Dependence, *Am. Heart J.*, 89:510, 1975.

7 Lange, R. L., Reid, M. S., Tresch, D. D., Keelan, M. H., Bernhard, V. M., and Collidge, G.: Nonatheromatous Ischemic Heart Disease Following Withdrawal from Chronic Industrial Nitroglycerin Exposure, *Circulation*, 46:666, 1972.

8 Taylor, H. L.: Occupational Factors in the Study of Coronary Heart Disease and Physical Activity, *Can. Med. Assoc. J.*, 96:825, 1967.

9 Spain, D. M., and Bradess, V. A.: Post Mortem Studies on Coronary Atherosclerosis in One Population Group, *Dis. Chest*, 36:397, 1959.

10 Morris, W. H. M.: The Cardiac on the Farm, in L. J. Warshaw (ed.), "The Heart in Industry," Hoeber Medical Division, Harper & Row, Publishers, Incorporated, New York, 1960, p. 431.

11 Russek, H. I.: Role of Emotional Stress in the Etiology of Clinical Coronary Heart Disease, *Dis. Chest,* 52:1, 1967.

12 Friedman, M.: "Pathogenesis of Coronary Artery Disease," McGraw-Hill Book Company, New York, 1969, p. 75.

13 Hinkle, L. E., Jr., Whitney, L. H., Lehman, E. W., Dunn, J., Benjamin, B., King, R., Plakun, A., and Flehinger, B.: Occupation, Education, and Coronary Heart Disease, *Science,* 161: 238, 1968.

14 Warshaw, L. J.: Heart Cases under Workmen's Compensation Laws, *J. Occup. Med.,* 9:349, 1967.

15 Report of the Committee on the Effect of Strain and Trauma on the Heart and Great Vessels, *Mod. Concepts Cardiovasc. Dis.* 32:793, 1963.

15a American Heart Association: Report of the Committee on Stress, Strain, and Heart Disease, *Circulation,* 55:825A, 1977.

16 Glazunov, I. S., Aronov, D. M., Drombian, Y. G., and Krylova, E. A.: Ischaemic Heart Disease and Occupation, *Cor. Vasa,* 6:274, 1964.

17 Haskell, W. L., and Fox, S. M., III: Exercise and Heart Disease, *Postgrad. Med.,* 44:177, 1968.

18 Geller, L. I., Sakaeva, S. Z., Musina, S. S., Ostrovskaya, R. S., Belomytseva, L. A., Kogan, Ya. D., Lukyanova, I. S., Volkhov, Ya. P., Popova, R. M., and Moskatelnikova, E. V.: (The Prevalence of Cardiovascular Diseases among Some Operators of Crude Oil Industry [On the Role of Occupational Factors in the Development of Affections Implicating the Cardiovascular System]), *Gig. Tr. Prof. Zabol.,* 9:11, 1965.

19 Tolonen, M., Hernberg, S., Nurminen, M., and Tiitola, K.: A Follow-up Study of Coronary Heart Disease in Viscose Rayon Workers Exposed to Carbon Disulphide, *Br. J. Ind. Med.,* 32:1, 1975.

20 Ryvkin, I. A., Maslova, K. K., Tiapina, L. A., and Alpatov, V. V.: The Significance of Employment and Heredity in Hypertensive Disease, *Cor. Vasa,* 8:10, 1966.

21 Pyykkö, I.: The Prevalence and Symptoms of Traumatic Vasospastic Disease among Lumberjacks in Finland. A Field Study, *Work Environ. Health,* 11:118, 1974.

22 Ashe, W. F., and Williams, N.: Occupational Raynaud's. II: Further Studies of This Disorder in Uranium Mine Workers, *Arch. Environ. Health,* 9:425, 1964.

23 Conn, J., Jr., Bergan, J. J., and Bell, J. L.: Hypothenar Hammer Syndrome: Post-traumatic Digital Ischemia, *Surgery,* 68:1122, 1970.

24 Warshaw, L. J.: "The Heart in Industry," Hoeber Medical Division, Harper & Row, Publishers, Incorporated, New York, 1960, p. 167.

25 Employability of Workers Handicapped by Certain Diseases: A Guide for Employers and Physicians, *Arch. Environ. Health,* 17:389, 1968.

100

The Effect of Air Travel and Altitude on the Heart and Circulation

VICTOR F. FROELICHER, JR., M.D.

The cardiovascular problems related to changes in altitude[1-3] are listed in Table 100-1. The cause of these problems can be related either to changes in atmospheric pressure or to decreases in the oxygen content of inhaled air. All these conditions can have more serious consequences in persons with cardiopulmonary diseases. Modern technology, including air travel, rapid transportation up mountains, hyper- and hypobaric chambers, and sports and commercial diving and flying after diving, has made exposure to these atmospheric hazards more common. This emphasizes the need for the development of techniques to screen asymptomatic persons for latent disease.[4] The cardiovascular problems secondary to altitude changes are most commonly encountered during air travel and while vacationing at high altitude.

DECOMPRESSION SICKNESS

Decompression sickness is a medical syndrome resulting from a relative pressure reduction in a surrounding atmosphere after prior equilibration to a higher pressure. The pathophysiology is the evolution of dissolved nitrogen according to Henry's law which forms bubbles in tendons and ligaments and in venous blood. These bubbles have been repeatedly demonstrated in animal models and rarely can be seen in human retinal vessels. Recently, echocardiography has added a new dimension in the evaluation of decompression sickness by enabling the recognition of intracardiac nitrogen bubbles prior to the occurrence of serious symptoms.[5] Symptoms and manifestations include (1) the bends—pruritis and joint, bone, skin, or muscle pain, (2) the chokes—substernal distress, cough, and difficulty breathing, and (3) circulatory and neurologic symptoms—pallor, sweating, nausea, faintness, visual disturbances, paralysis, and/or syncope. Syncope is usually accompanied by bradycardia and hypotension and can proceed to shock. Though pressure changes equivalent to altitudes greater than 18,000 ft are necessary for decompression sickness to occur, the combination of diving followed by a change to altitudes of 4,000 ft or greater can result in decompression sickness.[6] Such pressures can occur in commercial aircraft at high

TABLE 100-1
Cardiovascular problems related to changes in altitude

1 Decompression sickness
2 Acute hypoxia
3 High-altitude pulmonary edema
4 High-altitude cerebral edema
5 Subacute and chronic high-altitude sickness
6 Anemia and hypoxia

altitudes. A 24-h period between diving and flying is required for military aircrew personnel. Decompression sickness can be prevented by avoiding rapid pressure changes or by breathing 100% oxygen prior to drops in atmospheric pressure. The treatment for decompression sickness is rapid recompression, high-pressure oxygen therapy, and the usual support for associated medical complications.

ACUTE HYPOXIA

Acute hypoxia related to altitude changes can be encountered with acute decompression while flying at high altitude or by rapid ascent to altitude. Healthy individuals can tolerate altitudes of 7,000 ft without symptoms of hypoxia, while virtually all have symptoms between 7,000 and 15,000 ft, and altitudes of 23,000 ft or greater are not compatible with life without artificial support. Commercial aircraft cabin pressure is maintained at an oxygen level and atmospheric pressure approximately equivalent to 5,000 ft. Breathing 100% oxygen can avoid hypoxia to about 40,000 ft, but above this, pressurized breathing must be employed to maintain consciousness.[7] The effects of hypoxia are to be separated from those of asphyxia or ischemia, which includes carbon dioxide retention and has more serious effects on the myocardium. Exposure to hypoxia is accompanied by a prompt decrease in arterial oxygen content, an increased breathing rate and ventilatory volume, alkalosis, and an increase in heart rate and cardiac output. The first manifestations of acute hypoxia are neurologic, including visual symptoms, mental confusion, loss of judgment, and later syncope. Increased physical activity at the time of decompression decreases the time to loss of consciousness.[8] The neurologic manifestations of hypoxia are very variable and differ from person to person. Aviators are purposely allowed to become hypoxic during chamber test runs to learn their sensations during hypoxia in order to better enable them to recognize this condition. Initially, the changes associated with the severe oxygen lack are biochemical, potentially reversible, and cause only temporary and functional disturbances. However, irreversible cell death can result especially in susceptible tissues, like nervous tissue, particularly in patients with pulmonary or cardiovascular disease. The electrocardiographic response to a hypoxic stress has been used as a test for the diagnosis of coronary atherosclerotic heart disease. A recent study has demonstrated in great detail the electrocardiographic response of healthy men to simulated altitude.[9] Acute mountain sickness is a form of acute hypoxia which will be discussed later.

HIGH-ALTITUDE PULMONARY EDEMA

High-altitude pulmonary edema is a potentially fatal form of noncardiac pulmonary edema which can occur in unacclimatized persons who ascend to an altitude in excess of 9,000 ft. Exacerbation by physical exertion and cold weather are characteristic. Susceptible persons usually have recurrent episodes with reexposure to altitude. A high-altitude dweller may experience high-altitude pulmonary edema on return to the high altitude after a 2- to 3-week stay at sea level. It is more common in those under 20 years of age than in older persons and more common in males than in females. Probably less than 5 percent of an exposed population are susceptible to high-altitude pulmonary edema, but accurate surveys of its prevalence have not been performed. Cardiac catheterization during hypoxia of men susceptible to high-altitude pulmonary edema has revealed the following: inappropriate pulmonary hypertension, impaired pulmonary oxygen exchange, reduced cardiac output at rest and in response to exercise, and normal capillary wedge pressure.[10,11] Maximal oxygen consumption is decreased in all persons at high altitude and remains decreased for days after exposure to high altitude. Changes in systolic time intervals have suggested a depression of left ventricular function.[12] Symptoms similar to acute mountain sickness (acute hypoxia) including fatigue, headache, weakness, nausea, and anorexia usually are the prodrome. Twelve to twenty-four hours after altitude exposure, shortness of breath, dyspnea on exertion, and cough occur. The signs and symptoms of overt pulmonary edema develop, but at times the differentiation from pneumonia is difficult.[13] Chest x-rays show patchy irregular infiltrates scattered throughout the lungs. The electrocardiogram can show P pulmonale and right axis deviation. Treatment includes bed rest, 100% oxygen, and return to lower altitude. Digitalis is not beneficial. Drug prophylaxis and treatment with furosemide or acetazolamide have been recommended by some investigators, but their use is controversial.

HIGH-ALTITUDE CEREBRAL EDEMA

Neurologic signs and symptoms can predominate during exposure to altitude and appear to be secondary to cerebral edema.[14] Meningitis may be suspected. Permanent neurologic sequelae can ensue if the patient is unconscious for any prolonged period before descent from altitude. The efficacy of treatment with steroids or osmotic agents has not been demonstrated.

NONACUTE MOUNTAIN SICKNESS

A nonacute type of mountain sickness occurs that can be divided into a subacute or mild form and a more severe or chronic form. Mild mountain sickness is characterized by persisting, sometimes incapacitating, symptoms similar to acute mountain sickness and is similar in that it also occurs without pronounced physical findings. Cheyne-Stokes respirations may cause insomnia. Mild mountain sickness is commonly seen in mountaineers but rarely occurs in native mountain dwellers. Persistent anorexia explains the weight loss that occurs in nearly everyone who spends more than 1 week at high altitude. Monge's disease, or the severe form of mountain sickness, is characterized by cyanosis, plethora, clubbing, episodic stupor, and signs of right ventricular failure. Hematocrits as high as 80 percent are common. The electrocardiogram and chest x-ray are consistent with right ventricular overload. The most important diagnostic criterion is the correction of all abnormalities with descent to sea level. Nonacute types of mountain sickness probably are a variety of alveolar hypoventilation occurring at high altitude.

ANEMIA AND HYPOXIA

All types of anemia are potentially serious flight hazards, since anemia acts synergistically with an increase in cabin altitude, respiratory and cardiovascular pathologic conditions, physical exertion, and cabin air pollution in the predisposition to hypoxia.[15] Sickle-cell trait is a potentially life-threatening condition at altitudes.[16] Splenic infarction resulting in surgical removal of the spleen has occurred during high-altitude flying, and sudden death has been reported with exercise at altitudes as low as 4,000 ft in individuals with sickle-cell trait. It is advisable to screen individuals for these blood disorders if they are to be exposed to such conditions.

PREVENTIVE MEASURES FOR TRAVELERS

As previously mentioned, changes in altitude are most commonly encountered during commercial air travel and while vacationing at high altitude. The relationship of these situations to patients with cardiovascular problems can be summarized as follows.

Commercial air travel

Altitude exposure during commercial air travel is limited by cabin pressure which is kept equivalent to altitudes of 5,000 ft or less. With the exception of those with severe pulmonary impairment, air travel does not pose a health problem. Patients with a moderate functional capacity will not have problems with commercial air travel except for those with cyanotic heart disease or severe pulmonary disease. Nonetheless, commercial airlines normally have a source of supplemental oxygen for emergencies.

There are other problems associated with air travel that should be avoided by patients with heart disease. Ample time should be allowed for the patient to arrive at the airport, check in at the ticket counter, walk casually to the takeoff reception room, and

enter the aircraft. This, of course, applies especially to patients with angina pectoris that is precipitated by rushing, walking, and anxiety. Some patients who are severely limited by chest discomfort or dyspnea may require the use of a wheelchair and should make certain that the ramp to enter the plane goes directly from the reception areas to the cabin of the aircraft. Special arrangements must be made for more acutely ill patients, since the transfer may be made directly from the ambulance to the plane cabin. At times, especially if the patient travels just after being discharged from the hospital, the officials of the airline may require the physician's statement that the patient can travel and may ask the patient to sign a document of release. Ill patients should not fly unless it is necessary. At times a physician should travel with the patient. Dr. Willis Hurst's experience with patients with myocardial infarction has shown that certain carefully selected patients with uncomplicated completed infarction can travel by air in 10 to 14 days if all the necessary precautions can be implemented.

It seems wise to advise well patients and even normal subjects to walk about the aircraft several times each hour when the flight is prolonged in an effort to prevent venous stasis, edema, phlebothrombosis, and possibly pulmonary emboli. Dr. Hurst has encountered two patients where such a sequence occurred.

Vacationing at high altitudes

During motorized travel across mountains, a person may be exposed to high altitudes. Highways reaching altitudes of 10,000 ft are not uncommon in mountainous areas. At altitudes above 5,000 ft, patients with heart disease should limit their physical activity. Myocardial hypoxia may be induced in patients with coronary atherosclerotic heart disease at high altitude, and a coronary event can be precipitated by exertion that would not cause a problem at sea level. Angina pectoris exacerbated by exposure to high altitude at times can be controlled by returning to sea level.

REFERENCES

1 Vogel, John H. K. (ed.): "Hypoxia, High Altitude and the Heart" in *Advances in Cardiology,* vol. 5, S. Karger, Basel, 1970.

2 Randel, H. W. (ed.): "Aerospace Medicine," 2d ed. The Williams & Wilkins Company, Baltimore, 1971.

3 Hultgren, H. N., and Lundberg, E.: Medical Problems of High Altitude, *Mod. Concepts Cardiovasc. Dis.,* 31:719, 1962.

4 Froelicher, V. F.: Detection of Asymptomatic Coronary Artery Disease, *Annu. Rev. Med.,* vol. 28:1, 1977.

5 Balldin, U. I., and Borgstrom, P.: Intracardial Bubbles during Decompression to Altitude in Relation to Decompression Sickness in Man, *Aviat. Space Environ. Med.,* 47(2):113, 1976.

6 Davis, J. C.: Decompression Sickness and Air Embolism, in H. E. Stephanson (ed.), "Immediate Care of the Acutely Ill and Injured," chap. 17, The C. V. Mosby Company, St. Louis, 1974.

7 Preston, F. S.: Medical Aspects of Supersonic Travel, *Aviat. Space Environ. Med.,* 46(8):1074, 1975.

8 Busby, D. E., Higgins, E. A., and Funkhouser, G. E.: Effect of Physical Activity of Airline Flight Attendants on Their Time of Useful Consciousness in a Rapid Decompression, *Aviat. Space Environ. Med.*, 47(2):117, 1976.

9 Laciga, P., and Koller, E.: Respiratory, Circulatory, and ECG Changes during Exposure to High Altitude, *J. Appl. Physiol.*, 41(2):159, 1976.

10 Hartley, H.: Effects of High-Altitude Environment on the Cardiovascular System of Man, *J.A.M.A.*, 215:241, 1971.

11 Hultgren, H. N., Grover, R. F., and Hartley, L. H.: Abnormal Circulatory Responses to High Altitude in Subjects with a Previous History of High-Altitude Pulmonary Edema, *Circulation*, 44:759, 1971.

12 Balasubramanian, V., Kaushik, V. S., Manchanda, S. C., and Roy, S. B.: Effects of High Altitude Hypoxia on Left Ventricular Systolic Time Intervals in Man, *Br. Heart J.*, 37:272, 1975.

13 Kleiner, J. P., and Nelson, W. P.: High Altitude Pulmonary Edema, *J.A.M.A.*, 234:491, 1975.

14 Houston, C. S., and Dickinson, J.: Cerebral Form of High-Altitude Illness, *Lancet*, 2:758, 1975.

15 Scott, V.: Anemia and Airline Flight Duties, *Aviat. Space Environ. Med.*, 46:830, 1975.

16 Jones, S. R., Binder, R. A., and Donowho, E. M.: Sudden Death in Sickle-Cell Trait, *N. Engl. J. Med.*, 282:323, 1970.

101
Temperature and Humidity, Radiation, Underwater Environment, Hyperbaric Oxygen, and the Cardiovascular System

CHARLES A. GILBERT, M.D.

Human beings can be exposed to a wide variety of environmental forces. The purpose of this chapter is to highlight the cardiovascular problems created by exposure to a great range of temperature and humidity, radiation, underwater environment, and hyperbaric oxygenation.

HEAT AND HUMIDITY

Patients in mild congestive heart failure may develop acute left ventricular failure in a hot, humid environment.[1,2] Accordingly, the physician caring for such patients must be concerned with the details of climate control and hospital air conditioning.

Knowledge of physiologic changes is helpful in understanding the effects of heat and humidity on the cardiovascular system in both health and disease states. An endogenous (metabolic) or exogenous (direct, or environmental) heat load is dissipated largely by radiation, convection, conduction, and evaporation of sweat from the skin.

Neural information about the thermal state of the body comes from various sources: thermosensitive structures in the central nervous system, other deep body thermosensors, and thermoreceptors in the

skin. These multiple inputs are integrated in the hypothalamus, and control actions are nervously mediated to produce vasomotion and sweating.[3] Local temperatures can modify the blood vessel and sweat gland response to the central thermoregulatory drive.[4,5] In response to a heat load cutaneous vasodilation of both resistance and capacitance vessels is mediated by a withdrawal of sympathetic constrictor impulses. Similarly, sweat rates of up to 1.5 liters/h in healthy volunteers are produced via cholinergic sympathetic fibers to the sweat glands.

With sweating, a proteolytic enzyme diffuses into the surrounding tissue fluids and breaks down the polypeptide bradykinin, which in turn may cause further vasodilatation.

The cardiovascular system undergoes major changes as skin blood flow is increased to accomplish heat delivery from the body core to the periphery. As skin and body core temperature rises, so does the cardiac output and heart rate. Associated with the increase in cardiac output, which in healthy volunteers may reach 6.6 liters/min, there is a reduction in splanchnic, renal, and perhaps nonexercising muscle blood flows of up to 1.2 liters/min. Both the increased cardiac output and the diverted blood flow is directed to the skin, where flow may reach up to 7.9 liters/min for a normal-sized healthy volunteer.[4] Blood volume is diverted away from the central thoracic and splanchnic areas toward the skin where venous pressure and volume increase. Despite the fall in right-sided filling pressures, stroke volume tends to rise during heating, suggesting some positive inotropic stimulation.

Performing physical activity in a warm or hot environment adds even more cardiovascular stress. Heart rate rises markedly and stroke volume falls as a result of the failure of peripheral cutaneous veins to constrict. Central blood volume is reduced, and peak cardiac output, maximal oxygen consumption, and working capacity are also depressed.[4]

Many of the above cardiovascular adjustments observed in healthy subjects exposed to a moderate or severe heat stress also have been documented in cardiac patients with much less heat stress.[6-8] Patients with left ventricular failure, as defined by an elevated pulmonary wedge pressure, have decreased effective renal plasma flow and glomerular filtration rate when exposed to mild heat stress.[7] Patients with pulmonary emphysema subjected to dry heat of 37°C (98°F) have no change in pulmonary artery pressure and an increase in cardiac index. Total pulmonary resistance decreases, but to a lesser degree than in normal patients.[9] Calculated right ventricular work increases in emphysema patients, in contrast to normal individuals, whose right ventricular work decreases.

With the changes in regional blood flow and cardiac output noted above, it is not surprising that as many as 78 percent of compensated congestive heart failure patients in one study developed clinical evidence of overt congestive heart failure when subjected to a hot, humid environment [32°C (90°F), 75% relative humidity].[1] In addition, impaired sweat production in response to thermal stress does occur in patients with congestive heart failure and in those receiving certain pharmacologic agents, i.e., anti-Parkinsonism drugs: benztropine mesylate (Cogentin), atropine, and other anticholinergics; phenothiazines; and antihistamines.[10]

Potassium deficiency may be produced in healthy human beings performing moderate to heavy physical work under hot, humid conditions.[10] Whether potassium deficiency occurs in patients with cardiac diseases who are sedentary or performing mild work in hot, humid climates has not been studied. However, in cardiac patients receiving digitalis under such conditions some caution is needed to prevent hypokalemia.

Therapy and education for the cardiac patient should stress the importance of avoiding physical work or recreational activities during high heat and humidity conditions. Even the sedentary, middle-aged "normal" person should use caution when engaging in vigorous physical activity during warm, humid weather.

COLD

The thermally opposite environment, cold, also offers a unique stress to normal human beings and to patients with cardiac disease. In healthy males exposed without garments to 5°C (41°F) for 2 h, there were significant increases in cardiac output, stroke volume, atrioventricular O_2 difference, mean blood pressure, and heat production compared with control measurements at normal temperature.[11,12] The patient with angina pectoris due to coronary atherosclerotic heart disease will frequently have a worsening of his symptoms in the cold, as Heberden pointed out. The mechanism of production of myocardial ischemia in cold environment is related to an elevated peripheral resistance and higher mean arterial blood pressure at rest and during mild exercise. The "double product," heart rate times blood pressure, an index of myocardial oxygen demand, is therefore increased.[13] Myocardial hypoxia appears to be related to restricted coronary reserve and not to any effect of cold to induce spasm on large or medium-sized coronary arteries.[14] Alterations in coronary blood flow distribution or collateral flow, however, may possibly be involved.[15] Patients with cold-induced angina pectoris should be reminded to take nitroglycerin before stepping out into the cold, and physicians should consider a seasonal increase in beta-adrenergic blocking drugs in such patients.

Physicians treating cardiac patients see hypothermia induced both during surgery and by accidental environmental exposure. Since the development of cardiopulmonary bypass techniques it has no longer been necessary to use moderate hypothermia (28 to 30°C) and cardiac arrest to repair most adult or adolescent valvular or simple congenital lesions. However, several surgical centers have reported good results operating on infants less than 1 year old with congenital heart defects using deep hypothermia (15 to 22°C). These operations have been performed almost uniformly as emergencies on critically ill infants with complex anomalies. Employing surface cooling, limited cardiopulmonary bypass, and 45 to 90 min of cardiac arrest complete corrections have been accomplished in cases of transposition of the great vessels, tetralogy of Fallot, total anomlous venous return, and common atrioventricular canal.[16,17] During hypothermia metabolic activity is reduced markedly but not halted. Neurologic defects have been reported following deep hypothermia and circulatory arrest in infants, but fortunately significant, persistent neurologic damage is unusual.[18] During surface cooling of the infants to 20°C there is a progressive fall in heart rate to 20 percent of control but no ventricular fibrillation, or very little, occurs.[17] This is in contrast to accidental hypothermia where the risk of ventricular fibrillation is high below a temperature of 27 to 30°C.[19,20] Ventricular arrhythmias should be treated with appropriate pharmacologic methods and electrical defibrillation as necessary in cases of accidental hypothermia.

In experimental animals surface cooling to 20°C was associated with an 82 percent decrease in cardiac output and a 40 percent decrease in mean aortic pressure. Stroke volume remained unchanged, and the marked drop in cardiac output was due entirely to diminished heart rate.[17] There are conflicting reports concerning the effect of different levels of hypothermia upon ventricular function.[17,21] Following rewarming, left ventricular pressure, peak aortic flow velocity, and cardiac output returned to control levels in experimental studies.[22] Similar results were seen in a group of accidentally hypothermic, alcoholic patients free of associated disease who suffered no cardiac failure upon rewarming.[23]

Electrocardiographic changes with hypothermia include slowing of the sinus rate and prolongation of all intervals beyond that associated with the sinus bradycardia alone. Atrial and, as noted above, ventricular fibrillation begin at about 27°C. Fine muscle tremor is usually present on the electrocardiogram. A slowly inscribed deflection at the QRS-ST junction, or J point, a frequent but not invariable finding in hypothermic patients, is called the *J wave, Osborn wave,* or *"hypothermic hump"*[24] (see Fig. 101-1). The spatial orientation of the mean vector of this deflection is usually anterior and leftward, making it prominent in the mid- and lateral precordial leads. The J wave is not specific for hypothermia but may be seen in cerebral hemorrhage, cerebral trauma, or other nonhypothermic states.[26]

Accidental hypothermia is seen in winter months or in cold climates in victims of exposure precipitated by old age, debility, alcohol, drug overdose, trauma, or a combination of these. The arguments over passive or active rewarming using surface or core heating (peritoneal lavage, partial bypass with venoarterial pumping) have yet to be resolved. If the core temperature (nasopharyngeal) approaches 25°C, where thermoregulation fails some external heat

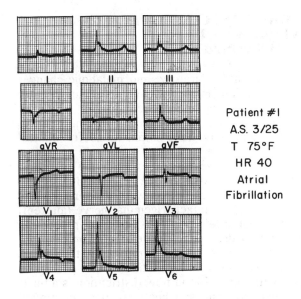

Patient #1

A.S. 3/25

T 75°F

HR 40

Atrial

Fibrillation

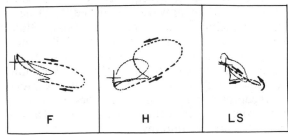

Figure I. Patient #1, A.S. 3/25, Vectorcardiogram

FIGURE 101-1 ECG and vectorcardiogram of accidental hypothermia showing slow ventricular rate, atrial fibrillation, prolonged Q-T interval, and the J wave, or "hypothermic hump." (*Used by permission of authors and publishers, American Journal of Cardiology.*[25])

source is necessary. If the patient is treated in an intensive care unit, active rewarming at a rate of approximately 0.6 to 1°C/h is probably adequate and safe.[23,27]

Caution in drug and fluid therapy is necessary in patients with hypothermia because of delayed detoxification and excretion.[28] Management of accidental hypothermia requires meticulous supportive patient care, which may include fluids, control of blood pH, airway and ventilatory assistance, central venous and systemic arterial pressure monitoring, deep body temperature monitoring, and antibiotics and corticosteroids as needed.

The prognosis of accidental hypothermia is related most firmly to the underlying disease state, if any. In uncomplicated conditions such as alcoholism with no associated disease, recovery can be expected in 94 percent of cases; in patients with other severe disease states such as carcinomatosis, cerebral vascular accidents, and cardiogenic shock mortality approaches 70 to 90 percent.[23]

RADIATION

Heart disease following therapeutic chest irradiation can cause electrocardiographic changes, symptoms of a cardiovascular origin, and death. The syndrome of radiation-induced heart disease (RIHD) has fol-

lowed x-ray treatment for Hodgkin's disease, breast carcinoma, and other thoracic neoplasms. It is important to recognize RIHD because treatment can be efficacious and also because RIHD can mimic a far-advanced neoplasm which might delay or cancel further diagnostic or therapeutic efforts.

Autopsy analysis of cases of RIHD show pericardial thickening, fibrosis, and adhesions with effusion. There may also be pericardial constriction or tamponade.[29] After a variable latent period of months to years the myocardium can show diffuse fibrosis but generally shows no cardiomegaly. However, radiographic enlargement of the pericardial cardiac silhouette is seen and may be due to radiation-induced pericarditis and effusion. The endocardium may demonstrate some patchy fibrosis. The mitral and aortic valves have been reported to be involved producing incompetence and valvular regurgitation.[28,30]

An experimental model of the disease in rabbits studied by both light and electron microscopy showed an initial pancarditis followed by a latent stage with progression to severe pericardial and myocardial lesions.[31] The important lesion of the myocardium occurs in the endothelial cells of capillaries where rupture and occlusion are seen. This results in myocardial ischemia and leads in the late stage to diffuse and progressive fibrosis.[32] A possible human counterpart of acute radiation pancarditis was seen in two healthy nuclear workers who, during separate nuclear criticality excursions, were accidentally exposed to 4,500 and 8,800 rads total body irradiation, respectively. Death occurred within 2 days from intractible cardiovascular shock. At autopsy the heart showed fibrin and polymorphonuclear leukocytes scattered in the myocardium. The dominant lesion, however, was peripheral and organic vascular damage (capillaries and small arteries) underlying the marked fluid transudation, hypotension, and death.[33]

Symptomatic pericardial disease following chest radiation is related to the dose-time factors and to the volume of heart irradiated.[34] The incidence of symptomatic pericardial effusion following 4,000 rads of mantle irradiation over 4 weeks for Hodgkin's disease is 6 to 7 percent.[29,35] Perhaps as many as 20 percent of such patients develop significant (but not necessarily symptomatic) pericardial effusions which resolve spontaneously.[36] However, tamponade and death can occur in patients who develop radiation-induced symptomatic pericardial effusion. The effusion and tamponade usually develop with 12 months of the radiation but may occur as early as 1 month or as late as several years.

Symptoms and signs seen are dyspnea on exertion, fever, chest pain, paradoxic pulse, Kussmaul's sign, hepatomegaly, and rarely a friction rub. Electrocardiograms show low voltage and ST-T wave changes. Echocardiograms are positive for effusion. In symptomatic patients with suggestion of tamponade or constriction cardiac catheterization may show the typical findings of elevated pressures, with a dip and plateau in the right ventricular pressures and a tendency toward equalization of diastolic pressures. A left ventriculogram might show decreased left ventricular function which would suggest myocardial fibrosis simulating constrictive pericarditis.[37] Pericardiocentesis will produce serosanguineous fluid with a high protein content; cytologic examination of the fluid has a poor yield for neoplastic cells. There is usually rapid reaccumulation of the fluid, and pericardiocentesis has limited therapeutic benefit unless it is done immediately prior to surgical pericardiectomy.[30] Large, persistent, but asymptomatic effusions should be followed clinically with chest x-rays, electrocardiograms, and echocardiograms. Surgery is usually recommended for all symptomatic patients and for asymptomatic patients with a 5-cm increase in transverse cardiac diameter who at cardiac catheterization have hemodynamic evidence of tamponade and/or constriction.[30,36] Results of surgery are generally good, but the prognosis remains guarded because of possible late myocardial fibrosis.[29] The role of corticosteroid therapy in the treatment of radiation pericarditis is not clear, although it has been efficacious in certain cases.[38] Patients who do resolve their effusions spontaneously require continued medical observation for late development of constriction.

Radiation-induced pancarditis with myocardial fibrosis, heart failure, and death is probably rare in the usual single-course therapy for Hodgkin's disease. However, carditis can develop in half of retreatment patients who receive at least 6,000 rads in two or more courses.[39]

Associated chemotherapy for treatment of the underlying neoplasm may also potentiate the toxicity and morbidity of RIHD. This chemotherapeutic cardiac toxicity has been suggested for the anthracyclines such as Adriamycin and for the MOPP regimen (Mustargen, Oncovin, procarbazine, and prednisone).[29,39]

The effect of radiation on blood vessels has been noted above in relation to the pathogenesis of myocardial fibrosis in RIHD and also in connection with the pathophysiology of shock and death following large-dose total-body irradiation. There are now several case reports of coronary atherosclerotic heart disease with myocardial infarction following thoracic irradiation.[40] The average age of five such autopsied cases was 26 years (range: 15 to 41 years). The serum cholesterol level, when it could be determined, in three out of five patients tended to be high, i.e., ≥ 200 mg/dl. The effect on coronary arteries of irradiation alone in experimental animals (rabbits, rats, monkeys) is minimal.[41] However, when irradiation is given *with* a high-cholesterol diet, severe coronary atherosclerosis develops. Thus irradiation and hypercholesterolemia appear to act synergistically to produce more atherosclerosis than is produced by either acting alone.

SUBMERSION AND THE UNDERWATER ENVIRONMENT

Cardiovascular, respiratory, and metabolic changes occur when human beings submerge underwater without diving equipment, i.e., in skin diving or breath-hold diving. These changes are important to the diver and may have implications for clinical medicine.

The oxygen-conserving reflex, or diving reflex, has been widely studied in diving animals. Upon submerging immediate cardiac slowing and apnea occurs which requires an intact trigeminal nerve (afferent) and vagus nerve (efferent).[42] As the dive progresses to 30 to 60 s, a delayed response of more pronounced bradycardia occurs with heart rates of 10 to 15 beats per minute associated with an intense peripheral vasoconstriction.[43] Blood flow distribution is adjusted so that the brain and heart receive a continued blood supply while flow is diminished to skeletal muscle, splanchnic, renal, and skin areas.[44] Blood pressure is maintained initially but then falls slowly as the dive is prolonged to minutes. The neural elements of the reflex for these delayed alterations are complex and probably include baroreceptors, chemoreceptors, and mechanoreceptors; the central bulbar cardiovascular "center"; and vagal and alpha-sympathetic efferent outflow.

In human beings, some of the cardiovascular adjustments of the oxygen-conserving reflex are present but in an attenuated form. Sustained apnea at approximately 90 percent of total lung capacity produces a low thoracic transmural pressure, and a negative mean intrathoracic pressure which facilitates diastolic filling and venous return to the heart. By Starling's law of the heart an increased stroke volume and a rise in arterial pressure result. Baroreceptors are stimulated to increase vagal tone, decrease sympathetic tone, or both, resulting in bradycardia.[45] Cutaneous, temperature-sensitive, facial areas, when stimulated by cool water (15 to 25°C) or air (15°C), can produce or augment an apneic bradycardia.[46]

The apneic and cool face-immersion bradycardia can be "masked" by psychologic or conditioned reflex factors and by a physical work rate which is 80 to 100 percent of maximal oxygen consumption.[47] Mild or moderate physical exercise will still allow a bradycardia to develop.

Electrocardiographic changes in human beings with diving and/or breath holding are of a cardioinhibitory type, i.e., sinus bradycardia and sinus arrhythmia, sinus arrest with junctional or ventricular escape, and atrioventricular block. T waves become tall and peaked during both breath holding and diving.[48] As noted above, simple breath holding without submersion can produce bradycardia, arrhythmias, and even syncope.[49] For example, breath holding and face immersion in 0°C water produced runs of ventricular tachycardia in an otherwise healthy 22-year-old student with a history of frequent premature ventricular beats. Patients being given large doses of digitalis for atrial flutter-fibrillation or others susceptible to bradyarrhythmias, such as patients with the "sick sinus" syndrome, may experience syncope from increased atrioventricular block and bradycardia if they take a cold shower or cover the face with a cold washcloth.[50]

The diving reflex, using 2°C face immersion and apnea for 15 to 35 s, has been noted to be useful in certain patients with paroxysmal atrial tachycardia who were unresponsive to carotid sinus massage.[51] While being noninvasive and potentially self-administered, the procedure does carry a risk because of possible unmasking of a ventricular focus and/or prolonged asystole. It should be used with due caution in patients with multifocal premature ventricular contractions, recent myocardial infarction, or susceptibility to ventricular tachycardia or fibrillation.[52] Whether the diving reflex may play a role in the pathogenesis of some cases of sudden death requires more study.

In addition to the diving reflex, other physiologic alterations are important in skin or breath-hold diving. In deeper dives, i.e., 60 to 90 ft, the partial pressure of alveolar carbon dioxide (P_{A,CO_2}) and alveolar oxygen (P_{A,O_2}) rises on descent. Thus in a rapid dive to 66 ft, the P_{A,O_2} will initially be in the range of 300 mm Hg. The P_{A,CO_2}, which could be 70 to 100 mm Hg depending on surface hyperventilation, is usually not over 50 to 60 mm Hg. This is because the P_{A,CO_2} due to the descent to a 66-ft depth exceeds the existing mixed venous CO_2 (P_{V,CO_2}), and CO_2 is quickly transferred from the lungs to the blood.[45,53] The arterial CO_2 (P_{a,CO_2}) rises, and this, plus the small lung volume at 66 ft due to gas compression, makes the diver feel as though the breaking point is quite near. This subjective sensation may be overcome by "willpower," training, and/or a competitive spirit to prolong the dive to 60 to 120 s. During this time, the P_{A,O_2} falls linearly, but the P_{A,CO_2} remains relatively constant at 50 to 60 mm Hg. Finally, because of the progressively smaller lung volume at depth, the low P_{a,O_2}, and the Bohr effect (decreased O_2 saturation with increased P_{a,O_2}, an irresistible breaking point is reached. As the diver ascends and the ambient pressure decreases, the P_{A,O_2} falls so that during the last 10 ft of ascent, values may be as low as 25 to 30 mm Hg. Loss of consciousness will supervene if this low O_2 saturation is produced in arterial blood circulating to the brain. Hypoxia is the chief cause of loss of consciousness with its risk of drowning in underwater swimmers, although CO_2 retention leading to narcosis, and possibly the diving reflex (bradycardia), may also play a role.[45,54,55]

Hyperventilation before breath holding and diving may delay the onset of the breaking point or the urge to breathe. Exercise underwater during breath-hold dives will lower the P_{A,O_2} even more rapidly. Four of twelve subjects who hyperventilated, held their breath, and exercised had low P_{a,O_2} values (33 to 34 mm Hg), normally associated with hemoglobin unsaturation.[56]

Korean diving women (ama) have learned intuitively not to hyperventilate excessively before a dive. They use a method of pursed lips and whistling in a maneuver which limits CO_2 loss and achieves a predive P_{A,CO_2} of 28 mm Hg. They are thereby able to avoid significant hypoxia and resulting loss of consciousness.[57]

Conventional ("hard hat") and scuba (self-contained underwater breathing apparatus) diving produce a wide range of medical and cardiovascular problems and considerations. Barotrauma to the middle ear can cause ruptured eardrum. In cold water, caloric stimulation of the middle ear may cause vertigo, nausea, and disorientation.

During exposure to air at a pressure equivalent to or greater than that encountered at 200 to 300 ft underwater, nitrogen narcosis, or "rapture of the deep," may occur. This is manifest as euphoria and overconfidence, accompanied by dulling of mental ability and difficulty in assimilating facts and in making quick, accurate decisions.

Oxygen toxicity may develop when breathing pure oxygen at depths greater than 25 to 30 ft of seawater.[58-60] Generalized convulsions have occurred from oxygen breathing at even 33 ft of seawater. Prodromal signs of oxygen toxicity, which may occur during underwater exposure, include vertigo, nausea, lip twitching, involuntary tremors, drowsiness and disorientation, acoustic hallucinations, paresthesias, dyspnea, and bradycardia of vagal origin.[61] However, with convulsions, sinus tachycardia and hypertension usually develop. There was no apparent residual neurologic injury in several hundred divers with oxygen toxicity convulsions. The mechanisms of oxygen poisoning are discussed elsewhere.[62,63]

Air embolism may occur in scuba and conventional diving as well as in submarine escape training. As a diver ascends to the surface, lung air expands. If the glottis is inadvertently held closed, the expanding gas may result in interstitial emphysema and air embolism; air probably enters the circulatory system via the pulmonary veins. In experiments with dogs, the critical transpulmonary pressure gradient (intratracheal pressure minus pleural pressure) which produced air embolism was in excess of 60 to 70 mm Hg.[64] Even with proper precautions after diving (controlled rate of ascent, open glottis, and exhalation), air embolism can occur from local pulmonary changes such as broncholiths or bullae.

Decompression sickness, seen during rapid decompression or ascent, occurs when dissolved gas (nitrogen) bubbles are liberated and interfere with the circulation to all organs. This occurs in divers and caisson workers returning to the surface; it may also occur in aviators upon rapid decompression from ground level to high altitude. Severe symptoms of decompression sickness occur in approximately 5 percent of deep-sea divers; careful observance of safety rules would probably lower this to 0.5 to 1.0 percent.[65] Decompression sickness has even been documented in repeated, deep, breath-holding dives when less than 10-min surface intervals were used.[45]

Cardiovascular and cardiorespiratory manifestations of decompression sickness are substernal distress, paroxysmal coughing, tachypnea, asphyxia (chokes), hemoconcentration, and shock from circulatory obstruction. Other signs and symptoms are numbness, weakness, and pains in the extremities (bends); paralysis (staggers); itching and skin rash; and chronic bone lesions. Symptoms usually begin within 1 h after decompression and rarely begin beyond 6 h after decompression. The treatment of decompression sickness is recompression in a treatment facility chamber with subsequent gradual decompression. Attempts by divers to treat themselves by recompression underwater are usually unsuccessful because of the cold and logistics of supply of air tanks.[66] The local United States Coast Guard Rescue Coordination Center can give the location of the nearest treatment facility. During transportation to the chamber and during the last 19 to 20 ft of decompression therapy, breathing 100% oxygen makes nitrogen elimination more rapid. A standard decompression routine in which the diver ascends by steps or pauses may prevent the decompression syndrome by allowing gradual elimination of dissolved nitrogen, preventing the formation of bubbles.[67]

HYPERBARIC OXYGENATION

The medical use of hyperbaric oxygenation is closely related to the diving situation. Oxygen under increased ambient pressure has been used therapeutically since 1956.[68]

Carbon monoxide poisoning represents a clinical situation in which hyperbaric oxygenation (100% oxygen administered under pressure of 2 or 3 atm) has been of value.[69,70] Air embolism is another condition where hyperbaric oxygenation offers a rational and effective therapy.[71]

The use of hyperbaric oxygenation in clostridial infection may occasionally prevent amputation. Whether hyperbaric oxygen alters survival in clostridial myositis is open to question.[72] Malignant tissues appear more sensitive to radiation when exposed to increased concentrations of oxygen; this is the basis for the use of hyperbaric oxygenation in radiation therapy.[73] Patients are irradiated while breathing 100% oxygen under increased ambient pressure; the results of randomized clinical trials have been conflicting.[74]

The use of hyperbaric oxygenation with small-volume cardiopulmonary bypass is of importance in treating critically ill infants with congenital heart defects. The main indication for this use of hyperbaric oxygenation is for palliative procedures in high-risk cases.[69]

Another suggested (although unproved) use for hyperbaric oxygenation is in ischemic disease of the brain, heart, or extremities. Hyperbaric oxygenation in 25 patients with acute cerebrovascular insufficiency produced persistent neurologic improvement in only 2.[75] Hyperbaric oxygenation reduces the incidence of ventricular fibrillation and the volume of ischemic infarct in experimental myocardial infarction.[76] Clinically, however, hyperbaric oxygenation has not impressively increased survival in the treatment of acute myocardial infarction.[77] Hyperbaric oxygenation may be of value in the harvesting and storage of transplantable organs. Perfusion of isolated organs under hypothermic, hyperbaric conditions has permitted their survival and successful transplantation.[69]

The hazards of hyperbaric oxygenation for the patient and attending personnel are considerable: oxygen toxicity; dysbarism, or the bends; barotrauma; and aseptic bone necrosis.[78–80] Furthermore, airway resistance is increased in the hyperbaric environment because of increased gas density. In dyspneic, ill patients who require airway intubation, this procedure decreases airway lumen, increases pulmonary work, and decreases air flow rates. Ambulatory eucapnic patients with pulmonary emphysema tend to develop a progressive hypercapnia during hyperbaric exposure.[81] Finally, the danger of fire or explosion, the high cost of installation, and the special engineering and technical skills needed limit wide applicability of hyperbaric oxygenation.[82,83]

REFERENCES

1 Ansari, A., and Burch, G. E.: Influence of Hot Environment on the Cardiovascular System, *Arch. Intern. Med.*, 123:371, 1969.

2 Burch, G. E., and Giles, T. D.: The Burden of a Hot and Humid Environment on the Heart, *Mod. Concepts Cardiovasc. Dis.*, 39:115, 1970.

3 Hensel, H.: Neural Processes in Thermoregulation, *Physiol. Rev.*, 53:948, 1973.

4 Rowell, L. B.: Human Cardiovascular Adjustments to Exercise and Thermal Stress, *Physiol. Rev.*, 54:75, 1974.

5 Rowell, L. B., Brengelmann, G. L., Detry, J. R., and Wyss, C.: Venomotor Responses to Local and Remote Thermal Stimuli to Skin in Exercising Man, *J. Appl. Physiol.*, 30:72, 1971.

6 Traks, E., and Sancetta, S. M.: The Effects of "Dry" Heat on the Circulation of Man: Splanchnic Hemodynamics, *Am. Heart J.*, 57:438, 1959.

7 Traks, E., and Sancetta, S. M.: The Effects of "Dry" Heat on the Circulation of Man: Renal Hemodynamics, *Am. Heart J.*, 64:235, 1962.

8 Traks, E., and Sancetta, S. M.: The Effects of "Dry" Heat on the Circulation of Man: Cerebral Hemodynamics, *Am. Heart J.*, 70:59, 1965.

9 Traks, E., and Sancetta, S. M.: The Effects of "Dry" Heat on the Circulation of Man: General Hemodynamics in Patients with Chronic Pulmonary Emphysema, *Am. Heart J.*, 61:184, 1961.

10 Knochel, J. P.: Environmental Heat Illness, *Arch. Intern. Med.*, 133:841, 1974.

11 Raven, P. B., Niki, I., Dahms, T. E., and Horvath, S. M.: Compensatory Cardiovascular Responses during an Environmental Cold Stress, 5°C, *J. Appl. Physiol.*, 29:417, 1970.

12 Thauer, R.: Circulatory Adjustments to Climatic Require-

ments, in W. F. Hamilton and P. Dow (eds.), "Handbook of Physiology," sec. 2, "Circulation," vol. 3, American Physiological Society, Washington, D.C., 1965, p. 1921.

13 Epstein, S. E., Stampfer, M., Beiser, G. D., Goldstein, R. E., and Braunwald, E.: Effects of a Reduction in Environmental Temperature on the Circulatory Response to Exercise in Man, *N. Engl. J. Med.*, 280:7, 1969.

14 Neill, W. A., Duncan, D. A., Kloster, F., and Mahler, D. J.: Response of Coronary Circulation to Cutaneous Cold, *Am. J. Med.*, 56:471, 1974.

15 Hattenhauer, M., and Neill, W. A.: The Effect of Cold Air Inhalation on Angina Pectoris and Myocardial Oxygen Supply, *Circulation*, 51:1053, 1975.

16 Barrett-Boyes, B. G., Nicholls, T. T., Brandt, P. W. T., and Neutze, J. M.: Aortic Arch Interruption Associated with Patent Ductus Arteriosus, Ventricular Septal Defect, and Total Anomalous Pulmonary Venous Connection: Total Correction in an 8 Day Old Infant by Means of Profound Hypothermia and Limited Cardiopulmonary Bypass, *J. Thorac. Cardiovasc. Surg.*, 63:367, 1972.

17 Rittenhouse, E. A., Mohri, H., Dillard, D. H., and Merendino, K. A.: Deep Hypothermia in Cardiovascular Surgery, *Ann. Thorac. Surg.*, 17:63, 1974.

18 Brunberg, J. A., Reilly, E. L., and Doty, D. B.: Central Nervous System Consequences in Infants of Cardiac Surgery Using Deep Hypothermia and Circulatory Arrest, *Circulation*, 50(suppl. 2):60, 1974.

19 Lloyd, E. L., and Mitchell, B.: Factors Affecting the Onset of Ventricular Fibrillation in Hypothermia, *Lancet*, 2:1294, 1974.

20 Towne, W. D., Geiss, W. P., Yanes, H. O., and Rahimtoola, S. H.: Intractable Ventricular Fibrillation Associated with Profound Accidental Hypothermia: Successful Treatment with Partial Cardiopulmonary Bypass, *N. Engl. J. Med.*, 287:1135, 1972.

21 Badeer, H. S.: Effect of Hypothermia on the Contractile "Capacity" of the Myocardium, *J. Thorac. Cardiovasc. Surg.* 53:651, 1967.

22 Rittenhouse, E. A., Ito, C. S., Mohri, H., and Merendino, K. A.: Circulatory Dynamics during Surface Induced Deep Hypothermia and after Cardiac Arrest for One Hour, *J. Thorac. Cardiovasc. Surg.*, 61:359, 1971.

23 Weyman, A. E., Greenbaum, D. M., and Grace, W. J.: Accidental Hypothermia in an Alcoholic Population, *Am. J. Med.*, 56:13, 1974.

24 Maclean, D., and Emslie-Smith, D.: The J Loop of the Spatial Vectorcardiogram in Accidental Hypothermia in Man, *Br. Heart J.*, 36:621, 1974.

25 Clements, S. D., and Hurst, J. W.: The Diagnostic Value of the Electrocardiographic Abnormalities Observed in Subjects Accidentally Exposed to Cold, *Am. J. Cardiol.*, 29:729, 1972.

26 Abbott, J. A., and Cheitlin, M. D.: The Nonspecific Camel-Hump Sign, *J.A.M.A.*, 235:413, 1976.

27 Exton-Smith, A. N.: Accidental Hypothermia, *Br. Med. J.*, 4:727, 1973.

28 Blair, E.: "Clinical Hypothermia," McGraw-Hill Book Company, New York, 1964, p. 73.

29 Greenwood, R. D., Rosenthal, A., Cassady, R., Jaffe, N., and Nadas, A. S.: Constrictive Pericarditis in Childhood Due to Mediastinal Irradiation, *Circulation*, 50:1033, 1974.

30 Morton, D. L., Glancy, D. L., Joseph, W. L., and Adkins, P. C.: Management of Patients with Radiation-induced Pericarditis with Effusion: A Note on the Development of Aortic Regurgitation in Two of Them, *Chest*, 64:291, 1973.

31 Fajardo, L. F., and Stewart, J. R.: Experimental Radiation-induced Heart Disease, *Am. J. Pathol.*, 59:299, 1970.

32 Fajardo, L. F., and Stewart, J. R.: Pathogenesis of Radiation-induced Myocardial Fibrosis, *Lab. Invest.*, 29:244, 1973.

33 Fanger, H., and Lushbaugh, C. C.: Radiation Death from Cardiovascular Shock following a Criticality Accident, *Arch. Pathol.*, 83:446, 1967.

34 Stewart, R. J., and Fajardo, L. F.: Dose Response in Human and Experimental Radiation-induced Heart Disease, *Radiology*, 99:408, 1971.

35 Cohn, K. E., Stewart, J. R., Fajardo, L. F., and Hancock, E. W.: Heart Disease following Radiation, *Medicine*, 46:281, 1967.

36 Ruckdeschel, J. C., Chang, P., Martin, R. G., Byhardt, R. W., O'Connell, M. J., Sutherland, J. C., and Wiernik, P. H.: Radiation-related Pericardial Effusions in Patients with Hodgkin's Disease, *Medicine*, 54:245, 1975.

37 Botti, R. E., Driscol, T. E., Pearson, D. H., and Smith, J. C.: Radiation Myocardial Fibrosis Simulating Constrictive Pericarditis, *Cancer*, 22:1254, 1968.

38 Keelan, M. H., Jr., and Rudders, R. A.: Successful Treatment of Radiation Pericarditis with Corticosteroids, *Arch Intern. Med.*, 134:145, 1974.

39 Weinstein, P., Greenwald, E. S., and Grossman, J.: Unusual Cardiac Reaction to Chemotherapy following Mediastinal Irradiation in a Patient with Hodgkin's Disease, *Am. J. Med.*, 60:152, 1976.

40 McReynolds, R. A., Gold, G. L., and Roberts, W. C.: Coronary Heart Disease after Mediastinal Irradiation for Hodgkin's Disease, *Am. J. Med.*, 60:39, 1976.

41 Phillips, S. J., Macken, D. L., and Rugh, R.: Pathologic Sequelae of Acute Cardiac Irradiation in Monkeys, *Am. Heart J.*, 81:528, 1971.

42 Andersen, H. T.: Physiological Adaptations in Diving Vertebrates, *Physiol. Rev.*, 46:212, 1966.

43 Blix, A. S.: The Importance of Asphyxia for the Development of Diving Bradycardia in Ducks, *Acta Physiol. Scand.*, 95:41, 1975.

44 Johansen, K.: Regional Distribution of Circulating Blood during Submersion Asphyxia in the Duck, *Acta Physiol. Scand.*, 62:1, 1964.

45 Paulev, P.-E.: Respiratory and Cardiovascular Effects of Breath-holding, *Acta Physiol. Scand. Suppl.* 324, 1969.

46 Moore, T. O., Lin, Y. C., Lally, D. A., and Hong, S. K.: Effects of Temperature, Immersion, and Ambient Pressure on Human Apneic Bradycardia, *J. Appl. Physiol.*, 33:36, 1972.

47 Paulev, P.-E., and Hansen, H. G.: Cardiac Response to Apnea and Water Immersion during Exercise in Man, *J. Appl. Physiol.*, 33:193, 1972.

48 Olsen, C. R., Fanestil, D. D., and Scholander, P. F.: Some Effects of Breath Holding and Apneic Underwater Diving on the Cardiac Rhythm in Man, *J. Appl. Physiol.*, 17:461, 1962.

49 Lamb, L. E., Dermksian, G., and Sarnoff, C. A.: Significant Cardiac Arrhythmias Induced by Common Respiratory Maneuvers, *Am. J. Cardiol.*, 2:563, 1958.

50 Whayne, T. F., Jr., and Killip, T., III: Simulated Diving in Man: Comparison of Facial Stimuli and Response in Arrhythmia, *J. Appl. Physiol.*, 22:800, 1967.

51 Wildenthal, K., Leshin, S. J., Atkins, J. M., and Skelton, C. L.: The Diving Reflex Used to Treat Paroxysmal Atrial Tachycardia, *Lancet*, 1:12, 1975.

52 Pickering, T., and Bolton-Maggs, P.: Treatment of Paroxysmal Supraventricular Tachycardia, *Lancet*, 1:341, 1975. (Letter.)

53 Mithoefer, J. C.: Breath-holding, in W. F. Hamilton and P. Dow (eds.), "Handbook of Physiology," sec. 3, "Respiration," vol. 2, The Williams & Wilkins Company, Baltimore, 1965, p. 1011.

54 Craig, A. B., Jr.: Underwater Swimming and Loss of Consciousness, *J.A.M.A.*, 176:255, 1961.

55 Bove, A. A., Pierce, A. L., Barrerea, F., Amsbaugh, G. A., and

Lynch, P. R.: Diving Bradycardia as a Factor in Underwater Blackout, *Aerosp. Med.,* 44:245, 1973.

56 Craig, A. B., Jr.: Causes of Loss of Consciousness during Underwater Swimming, *J. Appl. Physiol.,* 16:583, 1961.

57 Hong, S. K., Rahn, H., Kang, D. H., Song, S. H., and Kang, B. S.: Diving Pattern, Long Volumes and Alveolar Gas of the Korean Diving Women (Ama), *J. Appl. Physiol.,* 18:457, 1963.

58 Donald, K. W.: Oxygen Poisoning in Man, I, *Br. Med. J.,* 1:667, 1947.

59 Donald, K. W.: Oxygen Poisoning in Man: II. Signs and Symptoms of Oxygen Poisoning, *Br. Med. J.,* 1:712, 1947.

60 Yarbrough, O. D., Welham, W., Brinton, E. S., and Behnke, A. R.: Symptoms of Oxygen Poisoning and Limits of Tolerance at Rest and at Work, *Res. Rep.* no. 1, U.S. Naval Experimental Diving Unit, Washington, 1947.

61 Daly, W., and Bondurant, J. S.: Effects of Oxygen Breathing on the Heart Rate, Blood Pressure, and Cardiac Index of Normal Men Resting with Reactive Hyperemia and after Atropine, *J. Clin. Invest.,* 41:126, 1962.

62 Haugaard, N.: Cellular Mechanisms of Oxygen Toxicity, *Physiol. Rev.,* 48:311, 1968.

63 Wolfe, W. G., and DeVries, W. C.: Oxygen Toxicity, *Annu. Rev. Med.,* 26:203, 1975.

64 Schaefer, K. E., McNutty, W. P., Jr., Carey, C. R., and Liebow, A. A.: Mechanisms in Development of Interstitial Emphysema and Air Embolism on Decompression from Depth, *J. Appl. Physiol.,* 13:15, 1958.

65 Miles, S.: "Underwater Medicine," 3d ed., J. B. Lippincott Company, Philadelphia, 1969, p. 171.

66 Strauss, R. H., and Prockop, L. D.: Decompression Sickness among Scuba Divers, *J.A.M.A.,* 223:637, 1973.

67 U.S. Navy Diving Manual, Navy Department, NAVSHIPS 0994-001-9010, Washington, D.C., March 1970.

68 Boerema, I.: Operating Room with High Atmospheric Pressure, *Surgery,* 49:291, 1961.

69 Meijne, N. G.: "Hyperbaric Oxygen and Its Clinical Value," Charles C Thomas, Publisher, Springfield, Ill., 1970.

70 Thurston, J.: Hyperbaric Oxygen in Carbon Monoxide Poisoning, *Br. Med. J.,* 4:386, 1968.

71 Baskin, S. E., and Wozniak, R. F.: Hyperbaric Oxygenations in the Treatment of Hemodialysis-Associated Air Embolism, *N. Engl. J. Med.,* 293:184, 1975.

72 Weinstein, L., and Barja, M. A.: Gas Gangrene, *N. Engl. J. Med.,* 289:1129, 1973.

73 Behnke, A. R., and Saltzman, H. R.: Hyperbaric Oxygenation, *N. Engl. J. Med.,* 276:1423, 1967.

74 Oxygen and Radiotherapy, *Br. Med. J.,* 4:125, 1974. (Editorial.)

75 Saltzman, H. A., Anderson, B., Jr., Whalen, R. E., Heyman, A., and Sieker, H. O.: Hyperbaric Oxygen Therapy of Acute Cerebral Vascular Insufficiency, in I. W. Brown, Jr. (ed.), "Proceedings of the Third International Conference on Hyperbaric Medicine," National Research Council Publication 1404, Washington, 1966, p. 440.

76 Trapp, W. G., and Creighton, R.: Experimental Studies of Increased Atmospheric Pressure on Myocardial Ischemia after Coronary Ligation, *J. Thorac. Surg.,* 47:687, 1964.

77 Ashfield, R., and Gavey, C. J.: Severe Acute Myocardial Infarction Treated with Hyperbaric Oxygen, *Postgrad. Med. J.,* 45:648, 1969.

78 Fuson, R. L., Saltzman, H. A., Smith, W. W., Whalen, R. E., Osterhout, S., and Parker, R. T.: Clinical Hyperbaric Oxygenation with Severe Oxygen Toxicity: Report of a Case, *N. Engl. J. Med.,* 273:415, 1965.

79 Anderson, B., Whalen, R. E., and Saltzman, H. A.: Dysbarism among Hyperbaric Personnel, *J.A.M.A.,* 190:1043, 1964.

80 Whalen, R. E., Saltzman, H. A., Holloway, D. H., Jr., McIntosh, H. D., Sieker, H. O., and Brown, I. W. Jr.: Cardiovascular and Blood Gas Responses to Hyperbaric Oxygenation, *Am. J. Cardiol.,* 15:638, 1965.

81 Chusid, E. L., Maher, G. G., Nicogossian, A., Miller, A., Teirstein, A., Bader, R. A., Bader, M. E., and Jacobson, J.: The Effect of a Pressurized Environment (Hyperbaric Chamber) on Pulmonary Emphysema, *Am. J. Med.,* 53:743, 1972.

82 Saltzman, H. A.: Hyperbaric Oxygen in Cardiovascular Disease, *Circulation,* 31:454, 1965.

83 Whalen, R. E., and McIntosh, H. D.: Hyperbaric Oxygenation, *Am. Heart J.,* 69:725, 1965. (Editorial.)

102
Other Environmental Factors and the Cardiovascular System

CHARLES A. GILBERT, M.D.

This chapter is restricted to a discussion of environmental factors influencing the incidence of congenital heart disease. The environmental factors playing a role in the etiology of the other forms of cardiovascular disease are discussed elsewhere. Congenital heart disease is a major public health problem occurring in approximately 6 per 1,000 live births and representing over 50 percent of all heart disease in children.[1] Although etiologic factors have been divided classically into genetic and environmental causes, it is generally accepted that there is an interaction between the two.[2] Lamy et al. summarized their findings in 1,182 cases of congenital heart disease with regard to the relative importance of genetic and nongenetic factors by clinical subgroups (Table 102-1).[3] "Sporadic" should not be equated with "environmental," nor "familial" with "genetic." For example, a nongenetic cause of a familial defect is endemic cretinism due to dietary deficiency in iodine. It should also be remembered that it is the trivial dislocation that ends in congenital malformation, since more serious disturbances interfere with viability.

The following five generalizations applicable to experimental mammalian teratology will bring the subsequent discussion into sharper focus: (1) The activity of a teratogenic agent depends upon the developmental stage at which it is applied to the embryo; (2) because they usually modify specific developmental events, individual teratogens tend to produce characteristic malformation patterns; (3) both the maternal and fetal genotypes modify the response to teratogenic agents; (4) potent teratogenic agents may have little effect on the mother at doses at which they produce malformed offspring; and (5) the production of fetal malformations by teratogenic agents is associated with increased intrauterine mortality.[4] The conclusion that environmental factors must play a major role in the etiology of congenital heart disease offers great hope for eventual prevention and presents a great challenge for investigators

TABLE 102-1
Relative importance of genetic and nongenetic factors in causation of congenital heart disease

	Genetic factors		Nongenetic factors	
Clinical subgroups	Consanguinity	Incidence of congenital heart disease in the sibships	Abnormalities during pregnancy	Frequency of associated malformations
Tetralogy of Fallot	+	+	+ + + +	+ +
Pulmonary valvular stenosis	+ + + +	+ + + +	+	+ +
Patent ductus arteriosus	+ +	+ +	+ + + +	+ +
Interventricular septal defect	+	+	+ + + +	+ +
Atrial septal defect	+ + +	+ +	+ + +	+ + + +

SOURCE: Lamy, De Grouchy, and Schweisguth,[3] reproduced with permission.

to isolate the specific environmental factors responsible. The factors which have been incriminated thus far but which can explain only a fraction of the total number of cases will be divided into three groups: viruses, drugs, and other possible factors.

VIRUSES: RUBELLA, COXSACKIE VIRUSES, AND OTHERS

Rubella (see also Chap. 55)

The original concept espoused by Kreysig in 1814 that environmental factors may play a role in the cause of congenital heart disease was under serious attack in 1941 when Gregg and Swan et al. made their historic observations following a rubella epidemic in Australia.[5,6] For the next 20 years extensive prospective epidemiologic studies were undertaken to assess the risk of serious fetal abnormality following maternal rubella; these investigations were based on clinical information alone, since laboratory confirmation was not possible.[7,8] Studies since the advent of viral isolation and serologic procedures in 1962 have thus far confirmed the estimates arrived at previously.[9] The period of greatest risk is during the first trimester of pregnancy (Fig. 102-1). The variability in frequency of congenital malformations after maternal rubella seen in these prospective studies may be largely due to differences in accuracy of clinical diagnosis of maternal rubella or to biologic changes in the virus leading to greater teratogenicity. Certainly accuracy of clinical diagnosis of rubella during the 1964 epidemic was maximized by the severity of the outbreak, and it is not surprising that higher rates of major malformations were observed. In a prospective study in New York City of 178 cases of maternal rubella resulting in live births of children observed to

age 5, the incidence of children with major malformations was 54.2 percent for cases occurring in the first trimester and 69.2 percent when maternal rubella occurred at 4 to 7 weeks gestation.[10]

The types of congenital heart disease after maternal rubella run the entire gamut, with patent ductus arteriosus and ventricular septal defect heading the list (Table 102-2). Following the 1964 epidemic the additional defect of hypoplasia of the pulmonary artery was recognized.[11] Heart defects are not the most frequent malformation seen in the rubella syndrome infant, but, along with cataracts, they are usually the most common defects identified early. Estimates of the proportion of cases of congenital heart disease due to maternal rubella have been placed at 4 to 6 percent.[12] However, a rubella epidemic such as was experienced in the United States in 1964 can account for a much larger proportion of

FIGURE 102-1 The very small normal risk of bearing a malformed child (about 2.5 percent) is shown by the dotted line. The much greater risk of a malformed child after maternal rubella during the first 16 weeks of pregnancy is within the shaded area but is not known exactly. (*Reproduced with permission of author and publisher from Campbell.*[12])

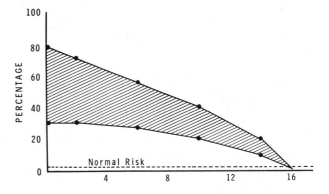

TABLE 102-2
Types of congenital heart disease after maternal rubella

Type	Alone	With other heart defect	Total*	Percentage
Patent ductus ateriosus	74	15	89	58.1
Ventricular septal defect	17	10	27	17.6
Atrial septal defect	9	1	10	6.6
Pulmonary valvular stenosis	4	5	9	5.9
Tetralogy of Fallot	10	1	11	7.2
Other†	5	2	7	4.6
Total*	119	34	153	100.0

*Seventeen cases are included twice, as they had two malfunctions.
†Coarctation, 4 (2 with patent ductus arteriosus); aortic stenosis, 1; transposition, 1; tricuspid atresia, 1.
SOURCE: Modified from Campbell.[12]

cases and greatly distort the observed incidence of congenital heart disease (Fig. 102-2).

The mechanism by which rubella causes its damage to the fetus was studied following the successful isolation of the virus in tissue culture by Weller and Parkman in 1962. Alford et al.[13] first demonstrated direct invasion of the placenta and fetal tissue by the virus and its subsequent excretion in the newborn period.[13] The frequency of virus isolation from therapeutic abortions following first-trimester rubella has been as high as 90 percent in some series.[14] Pathologic lesions in the heart of rubella syndrome babies have been seen and further suggest that direct virus invasion is responsible.[15] Infants with congenital rubella also have persisting antibodies to rubella.[13,16] This latter characteristic makes possible the docu-

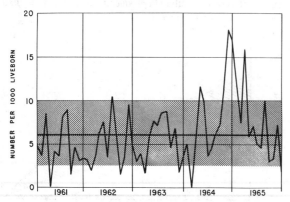

FIGURE 102-2 Incidence of congenital heart disease by month of birth over a 5 year period (1961–1965). Grady Memorial Hospital, Atlanta, Ga. The peak incidence from October 1964 to March 1965 was related to a severe rubella epidemic the previous spring. Checkered area indicates 1 standard deviation.

mentation of congenital rubella in previously unsuspected infants. With the continued and widespread use of the attenuated rubella virus vaccine, it is doubtful that a repeat of the estimated 20,000 cases resulting from the 1964 epidemic in the United States will occur.

Coxsackie viruses

The Coxsackie viruses, especially B_3 and B_4, have been implicated in the etiology of congenital heart disease by demonstration of more frequent serologic evidence of maternal infection during pregnancy in the group who had babies with congenital heart disease than in matched controls.[17,18] This was part of a larger study to determine the role of viruses in congenital anomalies. There was no correlation of congenital heart disease with the other viruses tested, and the Coxsackie viruses did not correlate with any other congenital anomaly noted over a 7-year period with over 9,000 pregnancies under observation. All indications suggest that these infections were larely subclinical. Because of the apparent great frequency of these infections in the young adult population, the Coxsackie viruses may play as important a role as rubella in the overall etiology of congenital heart disease. It is clear, however, that the risk of a deformed infant is much lower after a documented Coxsackie virus infection than after rubella. The estimate for the former is 1.3 percent, which is only twice the estimated occurrence of congenital heart disease in the population at large.

Evidence supporting the cardiotropic properties of the Coxsackie viruses comes from established association with neonatal and adult myocarditis.[19–21] Experimental animal studies also support this group as cardiotropic agents.[22]

Other viruses

The only other established viral teratogen in human beings is cytomegalovirus. Congenital infection with this virus is not associated with congenital heart disease. Rubeola, poliomyelitis, influenza, vaccinia, and variola are all associated with fetal wastage but not with proved fetal survival and malformations.[7]

Mumps virus has been incriminated in endocardial fibroelastosis by some investigators, but this connection has been rather firmly refuted by others.[23,24] The evidence is based on a higher incidence of delayed hypersensitivity to mumps skin test antigen in patients with endocardial fibroelastosis than in controls. Unfortunately, there is no serologic evidence in any of the series of infection with mumps virus. Neither has mumps virus been recovered from patients during postnatal life, and with affected infants there is no maternal history suggesting mumps during pregnancy. In suckling hamsters experimental evidence of a high rate of induction of hydrocephaly resembling the human disease supports the contention that this virus may be teratogenic under certain conditions.

Herpes virus had been cultured from skin lesions present at birth in a 14-month-old girl with chorioretinitis, patent ductus arteriosus, short digits, and growth and developmental retardation.[25] It is possible that further studies will show these viruses to be teratogenic.

Lamy found that women who subsequently had babies with congenital heart disease had twice as many infections during the first trimester of pregnancy as did the controls.[3] This finding encourages continued documentation of maternal infection during this critical period of pregnancy.

DRUGS

Thalidomide

A new chapter of human teratology was written with the discovery that a supposedly harmless sleeping pill, thalidomide (α-N-phthalimidoglutarimide), when taken early in pregnancy, caused a high incidence of phocomelia and other defects, including heart anomalies.[26] Congenital heart defects of no particular type have been associated with approximately 10 percent of the cases. Animal experiments with thalidomide have confirmed that it is capable of causing heart defects. After careful documentation of cases, it appeared that there was a sensitive period from the thirty-fourth to the fiftieth day following the last menstrual period during which time ingestion of the drug in almost any dose resulted in a greater than 50 percent risk of malformation. Temporally the appearance and disappearance of the new syndrome lagged the sale of the drug by one gestation period, and the total amount of drug sold in a country correlated well with the magnitude of that country's phocomelia problem.

Other drugs

The antitumor agents such as Aminopterin, busulfan (Myleran), and cyclophosphamide (Cytoxan) have been incriminated in instances where their ingestion was not associated with abortion.[27] In one case report associated with cyclophosphamide therapy the fetus had a single coronary artery along with absence of all toes.[28]

Diphenylhydantoin (phenytoin), another folic acid antagonist, has been associated with congenital anomalies which include cardiac defects in many reports.[29,30] Other drugs, taken for epilepsy (barbiturates most commonly), seizures, and genetic factors, may also play important roles in the increased incidence of congenital defects in babies born of epileptic mothers receiving diphenylhydantoin. Further epidemiologic and pharmacologic studies are indicated to resolve these relationships.

Oral contraceptive agents, progestogen-estrogen combinations, have been implicated as a possible teratogen in the VACTERL syndrome, involving vertebral, anal, cardiac, tracheoesophageal, renal, and limb birth defects.[31] A high percentage of the VACTERL patients had potential teratogenic exposure during the vulnerable period of embryogenesis, day 15 to day 60. Further confirmation of the birth control pills as possible teratogens will doubtless be sought.[31a]

Lithium and dextroamphetamine are two more drugs which have had isolated reports of fetal congenital cardiac malformations accompanying their use during pregnancy.[32,33]

An almost unlimited number of drugs, including salicylates, have been shown to be teratogenic in animals but with no evidence thus far to incriminate them in human teratology. Although the only drugs contraindicated in pregnancy today are thalidomide, antitumor agents, and steroids, it is probably wise in early pregnancy to take no more drugs than necessary. The most likely source of major breakthroughs in the association of environmental factors with congenital malformations will continue to be the clinician making astute observations at the bedside.

POSSIBLE FACTORS: HYPOXIA, SEASONAL VARIATION, NUTRITION, AND OTHERS

Hypoxia

Initial reports of an unusual incidence of patent ductus arteriosus in patients living above 10,000 ft in Peru have been open to serious question because of incomplete sampling. Studies of babies born at high altitude in this country show a significantly lower mean birth weight but no increase in any anomalies.[34] In mothers giving birth to children with congenital heart disease, a statistically significant greater frequency of smoking has been found than in a control population.[35] Hypoxia is presumed to be the probable mechanism. Studies in experimental animals are convincing that hypoxia and hypercapnia produce congenital cardiac defects.[36]

Seasonal variation

Figure 102-2 shows a seasonal trend of congenital cardiac malformations in children born during the period October 1964 through March 1965. This followed a severe rubella epidemic in the spring of 1964. Other studies show this type of seasonal trend associated with an increased incidence of patent ductus arteriosus temporally attributable to rubella. Still other studies report a definite seasonal trend in patent ductus arteriosus, present in females but not in males and unrelated to rubella incidence.[37] Clusters or trends in heart defect incidence should be carefully examined for possible environmental causes, as they may be the first clue leading to the discovery of new teratogens. This was the case with rubella and thalidomide.

Nutrition

Children of mothers who are chronic alcoholics or are diabetics have been reported to have high incidences of certain congenital malformations which include cardiac defects.[38,39]

Despite numerous animal studies documenting the ability of nutritional deficiency to cause congenital malformation, it is generally conceded that it would be rare indeed for a human being to become so deprived and still be fertile.[41]

Tissue antibodies

Another possible human teratogen is tissue antibodies. Rabbit anti-rat kidney serums produced teratogenic effects in rat offspring in almost 50 percent of the litters.[41] The mechanism of action is not known but could have been due to (1) severe disease in the mother, (2) direct interference with embryonic growth and differentiation, or (3) interference with placental function and permeability (see Chap. 53).

REFERENCES

1 Higgins, I. T. T.: The Epidemiology of Congenital Heart Disease, *J. Chronic Dis.,* 18:699, 1965.

2 Nora, J. J.: Multifactorial Inheritance Hypothesis for the Etiology of Congenital Heart Disease, *Circulation,* 38:604, 1968.

3 Lamy, M., De Grouchy, J., and Schweisguth, O.: Genetic and Non-genetic Factors in the Etiology of Congenital Heart Disease: A Study of 1,188 Cases, *Am. J. Hum. Genet.,* 9:17, 1957.

4 Beck, F., and Lloyd, B.: Embryological Principles of Tetatogenesis, in "Embryopathic Activity of Drugs," Little, Brown and Company, Boston, 1965.

5 Gregg, N. M.: Congenital Cataract following German Measles in Mother, *Trans. Ophthalmol. Soc. Aust.,* 3:35, 1942.

6 Swan, C., Tostevin, A. L., Moore B., Mayo, H., and Black, G. H. B.: Congenital Defects in Infants following Infectious Diseases during Pregnancy, with Special Reference to Relationship between German Measles and Cataract, Deafmutism, Heart Disease, and Microcephaly, and to Period of Pregnancy in Which Occurrence of Rubella Is Followed by Congenital Abnormalities, *Med. J. Aust.,* 2:201, 1943.

7 Manson, M. M., Logan, W. P. D., and Loy, R. M.: "Rubella and Other Virus Infections during Pregnancy," Ministry of Health Reports on Public Health and Medical Subjects, no. 101, Her Majesty's Stationery Office, London, 1960.

8 Lundstrom, R.: Rubella during Pregnancy: A Follow-up Study of Children Born after an Epidemic of Rubella in Sweden, 1951, with Additional Investigations on Prophylaxis and Treatment of Maternal Rubella, *Acta Paediatr. Scand.,* 51(suppl. 133):1, 1962.

9 Butler, N. R., Dudgeon, J. A., Hayes, K., Peckham, C. S. and Wybar, K.: Persistence of Rubella Antibody with and without Embryopathy: A Follow-up Study of Children Exposed to Maternal Rubella, *Br. Med. J.,* 2:1027, 1965.

10 Siegel, M., Fuerst, H. T., and Guinee, V. F.: Rubella Epidemicity and Embryopathy, *Am. J. Dis. Child.,* 121:469, 1971.

11 Tang, J. S., Kauffman, S. L., and Lynfield, J.: Hypoplasia of the Pulmonary Arteries in Infants with Congenital Rubella, *Am. J. Cardiol.,* 27:491, 1971.

12 Campbell, M.: Place of Maternal Rubella in the Aetiology of Congenital Heart Disease, *Br. Med. J.,* 1:691, 1961.

13 Alford, C. A., Jr., Neva, F. A., and Weller, T. H.: Virologic and Serologic Studies on Human Products of Conception after Maternal Rubella, *N. Engl. J. Med.,* 271:1275, 1964.

14 Rawls, W. E., Desmyter, J., and Melnick, J. L.: Serologic Diagnosis and Fetal Involvement in Maternal Rubella, *J.A.M.A.,* 203:627, 1968.

15 Driscoll, S.: Histopathology of Gestational Rubella, *Am. J. Dis. Child.,* 118:49, 1969.

16 Dudgeon, J. A.: Congenital Rubella Pathogenesis and Immunology, *Am. J. Dis. Child.,* 118:35, 1969.

17 Brown, G. C., and Evans, T. N.: Serologic Evidence of Coxsackievirus Etiology of Congenital Heart Disease, *J.A.M.A.,* 199:183, 1967.

18 Brown, G. C., and Karunas, R. S.: Relationship of Congenital Anomalies and Maternal Infection with Selected Enteroviruses, *Am. J. Epidemiol.,* 95:207, 1972.

19 Kibrick, S., and Benirschke, K.: Severe Generalized Disease (Encephalohepatomyocarditis) Occurring in the Newborn Period and Due to Infection with Coxsackie Virus, Group B: Evidence of Intrauterine Infection with This Agent, *Pediatrics,* 22:857, 1958.

20 Burch, G. E., et al.: Interstitial and Coxsackie B Myocarditis in Infants and Children: A Comparative Histologic and Immunofluorescent Study of 50 Autopsied Hearts, *J.A.M.A.,* 203:1, 1968.

21 Grist, N. R., and Bell, E.: A Six Year Study of Coxsackie Virus B Infections in Heart Disease, *J. Hyg. (Camb..),* 73:165, 1974.

22 Burch, G. E., et al.: Experimental Coxsackievirus Endocarditis, *J.A.M.A.,* 196:349, 1966.

23 St. Geme, J. W., Jr., Noren, G. R., and Adams, P., Jr.: Proposed Embryopathic Relation between Mumps Virus and Primary Endocardial Fibroeleastosis, *N. Engl. Med. J.,* 275:339, 1966.

24 Gersony, W. M., Katz, S. L., and Nadas, A. S.: Endocardial Fibroelastosis and Mumps Virus, *Pediatrics,* 37:430, 1966.

25 Montgomery, J. R., Flanders, R. W., and Yow, M. D.: Congenital Anomalies and Herpesvirus Infection, *Am. J. Dis. Child.,* 126:364, 1973.

26 Taussig, H. B.: A Study of the German Outbreak of Phocomelia, *J.A.M.A.,* 180:1106, 1962.

27 Greenberg, L. H., and Tanake, K. R.: Congenital Anomalies Probably Induced by Cyclophosphamide, *J.A.M.A.,* 188:423, 1964.

28 Toledo, T. M., Harper, R. C., and Moser, R. H.: Fetal Effects during Cyclophosphamide and Irradiation Therapy, *Ann. Intern. Med.,* 74:87, 1971.

29 Annegers, J. F., Elveback, L. R., Hauser, W. A., Kurland, L. T.: Do Anticonvulsants Have a Teratogenic Effect? *Arch. Neurol.,* 31:364, 1974.

30 Starrevald-Zimmerman, A. A. E., Vanderkolk, W. J., Elshove, J., and Meinardi, H.: Teratogenicity of Antiepileptic Drugs, *Clin. Neurol. Neurosurg.,* 77:81, 1974.

31 Nora, A. H., and Nora, J. J.: A Syndrome of Multiple Congenital Anomalies Associated with Teratogenic Exposure, *Arch. Environ. Health,* 30:17, 1975.

31a Heinonen, O. P., Slone, D., Monson, R. R., Hook, E. B., and Shapiro, S.: Cardiovascular Birth Defects and Antenatal Exposure to Female Sex Hormones, *N. Eng. J. Med.,* 296:67, 1977.

32 Nora, J. J., Nora, A. H., and Toews, W. H.: Lithium, Ebstein's Anomaly and Other Congenital Heart Defects, *Lancet* 2:594, 1974.

33 Nora, J. J., Vargo, T. A., and Nora, A. H.: Dexamphetamine: A Possible Environmental Trigger in Cardiovascular Malformations, *Lancet,* 1:1290, 1970.

34 Lichey, J. A., Ting, R. Y., Brum, P. D., and Dyar, E.: Studies of Babies Born at High Altitude, *Am. J. Dis. Child.,* 93:666, 1957.

35 Fedrick, J., Alberman, E. D., and Goldstein, H.: Possible Teratogenic Effect of Cigarette Smoking, *Nature,* 231:529, 1971.

36 Haring, Q. M., Patterson, J. R., and Sarche, M. A.: Prenatal Development of the Cardiovascular System in the Chicken, *Arch. Pathol.,* 89:537, 1970.

37 Polani, P. E., and Campbell, M.: Factors in the Causation of Persistent Ductus Arteriosus, *Ann. Hum. Genet.,* 24:343, 1960.

38 Jones, K. L., Smith D. W., Ulleland, C. N., and Streissguth, A.

P.: Pattern of Malformation in Offspring of Chronic Alcoholic Mothers, *Lancet,* 1:1267, 1973.

39 Rowland, T. W., Hubbell, J. P., Jr., and Nadas, A. S.: Congenital Heart Disease in Infants of Diabetic Mothers, *J. Pediatr.,* 83:815, 1973.

40 Warkany, J.: Congenital Malformations Induced by Maternal Dietary Deficiency *Nutr. Rev.,* 13:289, 1955.

41 Brent, R. L., Averich, E., and Drapiewski, V. A.: Production of Congenital Malformation Using Tissue Antibodies: I. Kidney Antisera, *Proc. Soc. Exp. Biol. Med.,* 106:523, 1961.

PART XI

Diseases of the Aorta, Venae Cavae, and Peripheral Arteries and Veins

103
Diseases of the Aorta and Venae Cavae

JOSEPH LINDSAY, JR., M.D.

DISEASES OF THE AORTA

Arteriosclerosis of the aorta

With advancing age, the aorta becomes dilated, elongated, and less elastic. These changes have been attributed to degeneration of the elastic and smooth-muscle fibers of the media. Since this medial degeneration does not encroach upon the lumen, no important clinical manifestations are definitely attributable to it. However, the tortuosity and ectasia of the aorta, commonly seen in radiographs of elderly patients, are at least partly a consequence of it.

A far more important process, atherosclerosis, is an almost inevitable accompaniment of aging in the United States. Intimal deposition of lipid, descriptively labeled "fatty streaks," is observed in early childhood and may be the first manifestation of the process. In young adulthood, distinctly elevated, grayish yellow plaques containing a soft, yellow, porridge-like material are commonly found in the aortic intima. In later life, hemorrhage into these plaques, ulceration, calcification, and the formation of overlying thrombus complete the gross pathologic appearance of aortic atherosclerosis. The media underlying areas of severe intimal disease is weakened.

These changes are most severe in the abdominal aorta distal to the renal arteries, followed in order by the arch and the proximal descending aorta. The ascending aorta, except for the immediate area of the aortic valve, is relatively spared.

Careful radiographic examination of the abdomen will reveal calcification of the aorta or iliac arteries with surprising frequency in asymptomatic individuals. In one epidemiologic study, in 10 percent of men at age 40 and 65 percent at age 64 calcium was detected in the abdominal aorta by means of lateral radiographs. Moreover, nearly 4 percent of these subjects, 60 to 64 years of age, could, on a basis of this examination, be said to have an abdominal aortic aneurysm.[1]

As might be expected from the above description, aortic atherosclerosis is manifest most often as occlusion of or aneurysm of the distal abdominal aorta. In addition, it has recently been noted that embolization of thrombus or of atherosclerotic debris from areas of aortic atherosclerosis may often result in arterial occlusion in the lower extremities.[2]

ARTERIOSCLEROTIC ANEURYSMS

After a review of 633 cases of aortic aneurysm, Kampmeier was able to state in 1938 that "arterio-sclerosis is occasionally thought of as a case of aneurysm."[3] Eighty percent of his cases were attributable to syphilis. In the present day, with the decline of syphilis and the increasing life-span of the population, arteriosclerosis is the most common cause of aortic aneurysm. The vast majority of these aneurysms are located in the abdomen below the renal arteries, but some are located in the thorax.[4]

Destruction of the aortic wall by the atherosclerotic process allows dilatation which may be perpetuated in accordance with the law of Laplace. Eventual rupture seems virtually inevitable. The wall of the aneurysmal sac commonly contains only fibrous tissue, with no recognizable aortic wall. Aneurysms are described as *fusiform* when they are spindle-shaped and as *saccular* if the outpouching occurs with a narrow neck. In some reports, fusiform aneurysms have been labeled saccular when they assume a globular configuration even though a narrow neck is not present. The lumen of an aneurysm is usually filled with laminated thrombus.

Thoracic aneurysms Even though the vast majority of arteriosclerotic aneurysms are abdominal, atherosclerosis is now a more common cause of thoracic aneurysm than syphilis; but unlike syphilitic aneurysms, those of atherosclerotic origin are found more commonly in the arch and descending segments than in the ascending aorta.[5]

Thoracic aneurysm is often a fortuitous radiographic finding, but chest pain, dyspnea, dysphagia, vocal cord paralysis, tracheal deviation or obstruction, and superior vena caval or pulmonary arterial compression may be produced. Hemoptysis, sometimes intermittent for several weeks, may result from erosion of the aneurysm into pulmonary parenchyma.[6] Abdominal aneurysms are sometimes associated. Survival of patients with arteriosclerotic thoracic aortic aneurysms may be somewhat greater than that of their fellows with the abdominal counterpart, but the threat of rupture with thoracic aneurysms is considerable. Diffuse atherosclerotic disease frequently prevents surgical attack.[6,7]

Abdominal aneurysms Abdominal aortic aneurysms, once infrequent and often syphilitic in origin, are now common and almost always due to arteriosclerosis. Whereas the thoracoabdominal portion of the aorta was a frequent location of syphilitic aneurysms, almost all arteriosclerotic abdominal aneurysms lie below the renal arteries (Fig. 103-1).[4]

Clinical features[8] Arteriosclerotic aneurysm is uncommon before age 50, and the typical patient is a man in his seventh or eighth decade.

Most abdominal aortic aneurysms are first detected in the course of an examination for an unrelated, or dubiously related, abdominal symptom. Occasionally, the patient reports for care because he has detected an abdominal mass.

Unless the patient is obese, physical examination will almost always disclose an abdominal mass in the

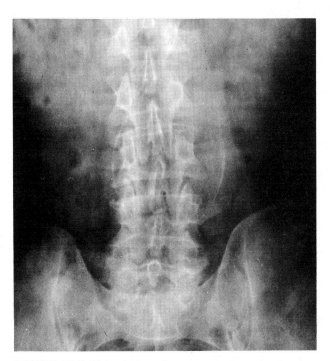

FIGURE 103-1 Abdominal aortic aneurysm. The calcification of the walls of an aneurysm such as this may often be seen on either frontal or lateral projection of the roentgenogram.

periumbilical area or slightly to the left of the midline. If definite expansile movement can be detected, the diagnosis of abdominal aneurysm is reasonably secure. On the other hand, if no pulsations are present or if they seem to be transmitted from the aorta, other causes of abdominal mass must be considered. Bruits may be audible, and femoral pulses are reduced in some patients.

The diagnosis of abdominal aneurysm can be confirmed by anteroposterior and lateral radiographs of the abdomen when characteristic eggshell calcification partially outlines the mass (Fig. 103-1). In some instances aortography provides confirmation or additional information regarding the extent of the aneurysm and the presence or absence of involvement of branch vessels.[9] It may be misleading, however, since the lumen of the aneurysm is characteristically filled with laminated thrombus. Recently the use of ultrasound has proved quite valuable (Fig. 103-2). Not only can the diagnosis be confirmed or denied, but ultrasound may also be valuable in following patients with aneurysms in whom expectant therapy is initially elected. Progressive enlargement of the aneurysm can readily be detected by serial examination.[10] When pain can definitely be attributed to the aneurysm, especially if it is of recent onset, it is likely to herald rupture. A constant midabdominal, lumbar, or pelvic pain, often severe, with a boring quality, found in a patient with a palpable expansile abdominal mass should suggest to the physician the likelihood of expanding abdominal aneurysm and impending rupture.[11]

Rapid exsanguination may result from rupture of the aneurysm into the free peritoneal cavity. Fortunately, more often the rupture is into the retroperitoneal space. Symptoms of abdominal pain and findings of hemorrhagic shock may therefore persist

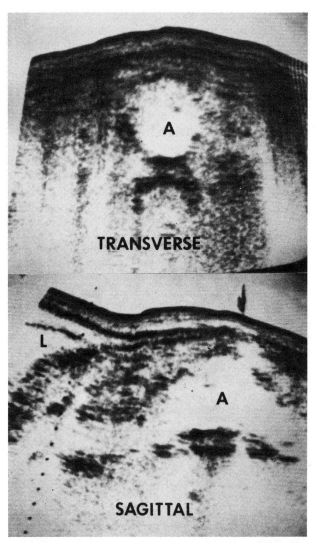

FIGURE 103-2 "B" scan abdominal sonograms in the transverse and sagittal planes are shown. The aortic aneurysm results in an echo-free space (A) in both projections. The triangular echo-free space (L) in the sagittal projection is the liver. The dots at the left of the sagittal projection indicate distances of 1 cm. The aneurysm is thus approximately 5 cm in diameter. *(Courtesy of Dr. T. L. Lawson, Department of Radiology, The George Washington University.)*

for hours or days, allowing the patient to come under medical attention. Occasionally the rupture is locally confined and may present a diagnostic problem of abdominal pain, fever, and evidence of slight to moderate blood loss. Secondary rupture probably always ensues, although there may be a delay of several weeks. Although the risk is great, emergency surgery is called for, since patients with ruptured aneurysm cannot be expected to survive otherwise.[11]

Rarely, secondary bacterial infection may occur on aortic aneurysm, giving rise to fever, leukocytosis, and abdominal pain. It would appear that infection leads to rupture of the aneurysm.[12]

Dramatic clinical syndromes may be produced by abdominal aneurysms. Intestinal obstruction from duodenal compression or peripheral edema from inferior vena caval blockade have rarely been reported, since the mobility of these retroperitoneal structures allow their displacement rather than compression by the aneurysm. Rupture into the duodenum with resulting gastrointestinal bleeding occurs, but aortoduodenal fistulas are more common following graft replacement of the terminal aorta.[13] An aorta-inferior vena caval fistula with a continuous murmur, a high output state, and congestive heart failure follow rupture of the aneurysm into the inferior vena cava.[14] Acute thrombosis of aneurysms occurs rarely, mimicking saddle embolism.[15] Furthermore, it has been shown that embolization of thrombus or atherosclerotic debris from abdominal aneurysms to the lower extremities is relatively frequent.[16]

Treatment Surgical resection of abdominal aneurysms followed by prosthetic graft replacement is now commonplace and is the treatment of choice. A detailed consideration appears in Chap. 107. Rupture of the aneurysm is a major threat to the life of patients with this condition, particularly if the aneurysm is large or symptomatic. Most centers now recommend surgery for any abdominal aneurysm unless life-threatening illness is present or the operative risk is excessive. Some authorities feel that if the aneurysm is small and asymptomatic, the approach may be more conservative.

CHRONIC AORTOILIAC OBSTRUCTION—LERICHE SYNDROME[17,18]

In 1940, Leriche called attention to the symptoms produced by slowly progressive occlusion of the terminal aorta and iliac vessels. Atherosclerotic occlusion of the area of the aortic bifurcation with superimposed thrombosis of the stenotic area is usually found when obstruction is complete. Unlike saddle embolus or sudden thrombosis, the manifestations of ischemia are typically present for months or years before the sufferer seeks medical attention.

Clinical features Men are affected with far greater frequency than women, the highest prevalence being in the fifth, sixth, and seventh decades. Some investigators have felt that, as a group, patients with aortoiliac occlusion are younger than those with arteriosclerosis obliterans of the femoropopliteal arteries.[19]

Pain in the low back, buttocks, or thighs produced by exercise and relieved by brief periods of rest is virtually pathognomonic of aortoiliac occlusion. Claudication may occur in the calf or foot in association with the more proximal distress and may uncommonly be the sole complaint. Asymptomatic aortoiliac occlusion seems to be unusual. Patients commonly report inability to maintain a penile erection if inquiry is made in this regard.

Absence of or marked reduction in the femoral pulses is characteristic. More distal lower-extremity pulses are reduced or absent, and bruits are commonly audible over the femoral arteries and in the midline

of the abdomen near the umbilicus. Low skin temperature, diminished hair growth, atrophy of the skin and subcutaneous tissue, and diminished muscle bulk in the lower extremities are common but not universal findings. Frank gangrene is not frequently encountered, and amputation for ischemia is seldom required.

Differentiation of this disorder from congenital coarctation of the aorta and from aortitis is usually possible on clinical grounds. However, contrast aortography will be needed to define the pathologic anatomy precisely.

A protracted course is usual. Symptoms may be slowly progressive, but about half of these individuals experience periods of accelerated progression of their symptoms. Such periods have been attributed to extension of the aortoiliac thrombosis or to occlusion of collateral vessels.

Chances for survival of persons with Leriche's syndrome appear to be less favorable than those of a control population matched for age and sex, but death rarely results from the aortoiliac disease. It may occasionally be due to occlusion of the renal arteries by proximal extension of the thrombotic process. Coronary heart disease and cerebrovascular disease are frequently present and are largely responsible for the accelerated death rate in these patients.

Treatment Operative attempts at relieving the obstruction are discussed in detail in Chap. 107. The extremely low potential for gangrene or for fatal occlusion of a vital vessel suggests that surgery should be offered only to carefully selected patients, specifically those who have great disability from intermittent claudication but with little or no associated coronary or cerebral vascular disease.

Embolic occlusion of the aortic bifurcation (saddle embolus)[20,21]

Sudden occlusion of the distal aorta by an embolus is an uncommon but dramatic event.

Clinical features The victim almost always complains of moderate or severe pain in the legs and less often, in the abdomen, lumbosacral area, and perineum. Numbness is commonly reported in the ischemic areas. The pulses typically are absent in the legs, although at times faint femoral pulsations may be detected. The legs are cold and pale. Sensory function and motor power are reduced, and total paralysis of both legs is not unusual.

The great majority of emboli large enough to occlude the terminal aorta are thrown off from the heart, almost all in the setting of mitral stenosis and atrial fibrillation or of myocardial infarction. Rarely a severely atherosclerotic aorta may be the origin of the embolus, and infectious endocarditis is also an uncommon source.

Aside from cerebral or visceral sites, it would appear that aortic embolism accounts for about 10 percent of all arterial emboli. Deterline[21] estimates that the aortic bifurcation is the site of 25 percent of the emboli which threaten the viability of the lower extremities. The mortality rate is high, not only because of the severity of the vascular insult, but also because serious underlying heart disease is usually present.

In the proper context, the diagnosis is not difficult, but other causes of sudden aortic bifurcation occlusion must be excluded. Acute aortoiliac thrombosis superimposed on preexisting atherosclerotic disease during severe congestive heart failure or shock may closely simulate saddle embolism.[22] Occlusion of the terminal aorta by medial dissection or by thrombosis following trauma are usually easily identified from the accompanying clinical features.

Saddle emboli in the postoperative period following mitral commissurotomy are of particular note since the symptoms may be masked by the effects of anesthesia or sedation. The femoral pulses should be repeatedly palpated.

Treatment When the diagnosis of saddle embolus is made, the immediate administration of heparin intravenously and extraction of the clot with a balloon catheter are advised, although direct surgical removal of the clot may be necessary (see Chap. 107).

The aorta in Marfan's syndrome and in idiopathic dilatation of the ascending aorta[23-25]

McKusick has termed Marfan's syndrome "a heritable disorder of connective tissue." The full-blown presentation includes arachnodactyly, a high-arched palate, and ectopia of the lenses, as well as skeletal abnormalities and loss of muscle bulk. Cystic medial degeneration of the great vessels, particularly of the ascending aorta, is the hallmark of its cardiovascular manifestations. Mitral regurgitation resulting from myxomatous degeneration of that valve is also frequent.

The changes in the aorta are similar to those labeled *cystic medial necrosis* by Erdheim. The elastic fibers of the media are fragmented, and the resulting clefts are filled with cystic deposits of metachromatic-staining mucoid material. The process is located principally in the ascending aorta, but similar changes are often seen in the pulmonary artery and less commonly in other large arteries or the more distal portions of the aorta (Fig. 103-3).

As a consequence of the weakened aortic wall, dilatation of the ascending aorta, the aortic sinuses, and the valve ring is found. Fusiform aneurysms and aortic regurgitation are produced. Dilatation of the intrapericardial aorta and myxomatous degeneration of the aortic valve leaflets may result in free aortic regurgitation before aneurysmal dilatation of the aortic shadow is visible on the roentgenogram. Areas of limited medical dissection are consistently found within the dilated aorta. More extensive aortic dissection is less frequent.

Strikingly similar abnormalities of the aorta may be observed in patients with none of the skeletal or lenticular abnormalities of the Marfan group. Such patients may present as candidates for surgery because of free aortic regurgitation. The name *idiopathic dilatation of the ascending aorta* has been applied, and disagreement exists as to whether this condition represents a forme fruste of Marfan's syndrome.

Aortic dissection[26-29]

Longitudinal cleavage of the aortic media by a dissecting column of blood has been termed *dissecting aneurysm,* even though aneurysmal dilatation is not invariable (Fig. 103-4). The separation of the layers of the aorta usually does not completely encircle the lumen, but the entire length of the vessel is often involved. The medial cleavage tends to follow the outer, large curve of the aortic wall.

A tear in the aortic intima, communicating with the medial rent, is found most often immediately above the aortic valve, somewhat less commonly just distal to the left subclavian artery, and infrequently in other sites. In 10 percent of autopsied cases, no intimal tear is found. A more distal, or "reentry," intimal tear may also be present.

Symptomatic preexisting aneurysms which are

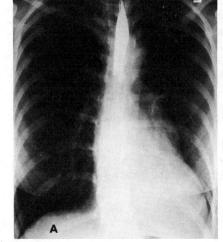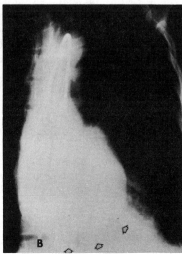

FIGURE 103-3 Dilatation of the ascending aorta and aortic regurgitation in a patient with Marfan's syndrome. Film *A* was thought to show a dilated pulmonary artery, but the aortogram *B* clearly shows the "Florence flask" deformity of the aortic root. The arrows delineate the plane of the aortic valve.

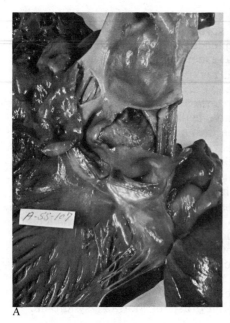
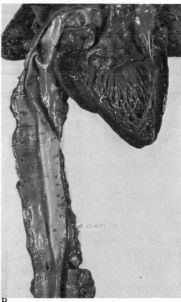

A   B

FIGURE 103-4 Dissecting aortic aneurysm. *A.* The large intimal rent may be seen a few centimeters above the aortic cusps. *B.* The false channel created by the dissecting hematoma is shown. Notice the cleanly sheared layers of aortic media.

undergoing expansion or are leaking sometimes are termed dissecting aneurysms. The present discussion concerns only the specific pathologic entity described in preceding paragraphs. Less precise use of the term *dissecting* results in serious confusion.

A classification of aortic dissection based upon the extent of the process and the location of the intimal tear has proved useful. Those cases which extend from the ascending aorta into the arch and beyond are designated type I (Figs. 103-5, 103-6A, and 103-7). The intimal tear is located just above the aortic valve in most such cases. From 60 to 70 percent of collected cases of aortic dissection are of this variety. Type II includes lesions limited to the ascending aorta. Features of Marfan's syndrome or of idiopathic dilatation of the ascending aorta are frequently seen in this rather small group. Type III (Figs. 103-6B, 103-8, and 103-9) is made up of those aortic dissections which begin distal to the arch vessels and in which an intimal tear is found in the proximal descending aorta. From 20 to 30 percent of cases seem to be of this type. This extremely useful classification does not include small groups of patients in whom no intimal tear is found, or those with an intimal tear within the arch. Nor does it allow inclusion of patients whose dissection involves the ascending aorta but who have an intimal tear located in the descending aorta.

The catastrophic effects of the dissecting process result from occlusion of major branch vessels of the aorta or from external hemorrhage. Death usually follows external rupture into the pericardium or left pleural space. Other sites of external hemorrhage are less common.

Pathogenesis Histologic evidences of medial degeneration in the aortae of patients with this disorder have been noted since the time of Erdheim's description of medial cystic necrosis. Although the lesion appears

to be a marker of medial disease rather than a specific disease process, the presence of such abnormalities has led to the belief that weakening of the aortic media is of great importance in the patho-

FIGURE 103-5 Type I aortic dissection. The features are well shown in this aortogram. The true lumen, well filled with contrast material, is compressed by the medial hematoma. The contrast material can be seen to enter the false channel through the intimal tear above the right coronary artery and to regurgitate into the left ventricle just below the opacified left coronary artery.

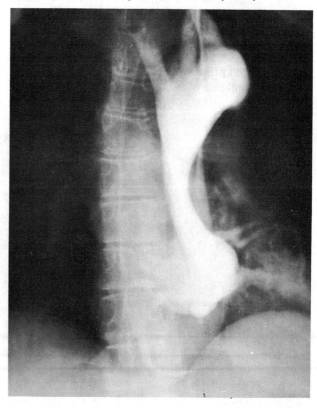

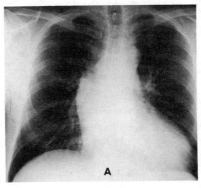
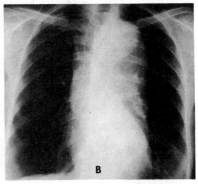

FIGURE 103-6 A. Type I aortic dissection. Characteristic appearance on chest roentgenogram. Note the marked dilatation of the ascending aorta. The aorta may appear normal on the roentgenogram early in the course of aortic dissection. *B.* Type III aortic dissection. In contrast to type I, marked distortion of the aortic arch and dilatation of the descending portions are typical, as seen in this radiograph of a patient with dissection beginning distal to the arch vessels.

genesis of this process.[26,29a] The frequency with which dissecting hematoma is noted in Marfan's syndrome,[25] and in experimental lathyrism,[30] supports this notion.

Forms of medial degeneration other than cystic medial necrosis may also be found in patients with aortic dissection. Braunstein[31] feels that some cases are related to atherosclerosis with secondary medial damage, and believes that once cleavage of the aortic media has begun, it may progress through normal tissue. He, along with Murray and Edwards,[32] feels that the proximal intimal tear is quite important in allowing luminal blood to split the aortic media. Gore and Hirst[28] advocate a more traditional view. They believe that medial weakness leads to hemorrhage from the vasa vasorum and, consequently, formation of an intramural hematoma which splits the medial layers. They reason that the intimal tears are secondary, citing the approximately 10 percent of cases without intimal tear as evidence for their thesis.

Hydraulic stresses on the aortic wall appear to be at least contributing factors to the process. Evidence of systemic hypertension is found in a great many patients with this disorder. The natural occurrence of aortic dissection in certain strains of turkeys prone to such catastrophe may be prevented by the use of drugs to reduce these stresses. Modern drug therapy of patients with dissecting hematoma is based on the premise that propagation of the medial cleavage may be arrested by reduction in the force of pulsatile aortic blood flow and in the mean arterial pressure.[27]

Patients with the greatest degree of medial weakness, such as those with Marfan's syndrome, often have dissection of the aorta, with near-normal blood pressure, while patients with extreme hypertension may indeed have no more medial degeneration than patients of similar age without dissection.[31]

Better understanding of the reasons for an apparent increased frequency of aortic dissection during pregnancy,[26] in certain congenital anomalies of the aorta, particularly coarctation,[26] and in aortic valve disease[33] may provide clues to the factors involved.

It is now agreed that syphilitic aortitis does not protect against aortic dissection, as was previously thought.[26]

Clinical manifestations Dissecting hematoma is not common, but in most large general hospitals several cases are seen each year. Most of the patients with this disorder are between 40 and 70 years old. An earlier age of onset is noted in those with congenital aortic anomalies or Marfan's syndrome. Males are afflicted more often than females.

Unbearable pain, typically abrupt in onset and excruciating from its inception, is the most characteristic clinical feature. A ripping or tearing quality is sometimes reported. When such pain is located in the

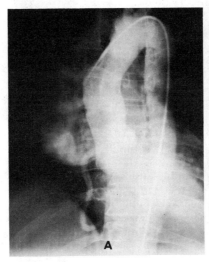
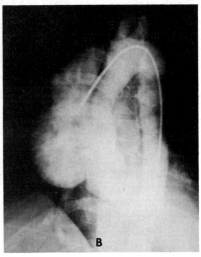

FIGURE 103-7 Serial frames from an aortogram of a patient with type I aortic dissection. Contrast material is seen to fill a tremendously dilated false channel. This accounts for the dilatation of the ascending aorta noted in Fig. 103-6*A.*

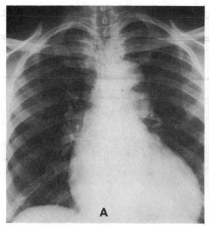
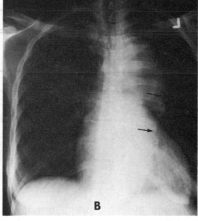

FIGURE 103-8 Aortic dissection, type III. The earlier radiograph (*A*) is that of a patient with severe hypertension. The later radiograph (*B*) was made after aortic dissection had occurred. Note the serial widening and distortion of the descending aorta. Irregularities of the lateral wall (arrows) are also characteristic of this lesion in its early stages.

anterior part of the chest, a characteristic location, myocardial infarction may be simulated. Acute abdominal conditions may be simulated by epigastric or midabdominal pain. Pain may be most severe in the interscapular or lumbar areas from the outset, but more commonly it shifts to these locations after beginning in the thorax. Painless aortic dissection occurs and perhaps is most common in patients with Marfan's syndrome but is not seen exclusively in such patients. Other features of dissecting hematoma are variable, depending particularly on which of the branches of the aorta is compromised by the process.

Sudden occlusion of the iliofemoral or subclavian vessels often may simulate arterial embolism. Anterior chest pain closely followed by arterial occlusion should suggest dissecting aneurysm as well as myocardial infarction with arterial embolism.

Sudden hemiplegia, with or without alteration of consciousness, may reflect occlusion of the cerebral circulation by dissection rather than hypertensive intracerebral hemorrhage or cerebral thrombosis. It is obvious that such patients may not sense pain and may not be able to report it if it has occurred. Ischemia of the spinal cord may produce sudden paraplegia. More commonly, however, limb paralysis is due to ischemia of the peripheral nerves, occurring along with other evidences of circulatory inadequacy in the same limb.

Certain clinical features suggest involvement of the ascending aorta (type I). The appearance of the murmur of aortic regurgitation (the result of loss of support of the aortic leaflets) or of myocardial infarction from occlusion of a coronary artery by the dissecting process is a clue to involvement of the ascending aorta. Evidence of occlusion of the arch vessels, i.e., the loss of radial or carotid pulses or signs of brain infarction, also suggests involvement of the ascending aorta.

Since pain may be the only manifestation of dissecting hematoma, especially when it begins distal to the arch vessels (type III), this diagnosis should be considered in all patients with severe midline thoracic lumbar or abdominal pain. This is particularly true

if a background of hypertension is present. Pulsation of either sternoclavicular joint may occur with other thoracic aneurysms but in the proper setting may be a valuable sign suggesting aortic dissection. Unilateral or bilateral distension of the veins of the neck, shoulder, or anterior part of the chest may reflect compression of thoracic veins by the distorted aorta. Bilateral distension of the neck veins in this disorder may, on the other hand, indicate intrapericardial hemorrhage and tamponade.

FIGURE 103-9 Aortic dissection, type III. A typical aortogram of a patient with aortic dissection beginning distal to the arch vessels. The narrowed true lumen is filled with contrast material and does not occupy the entire aortic shadow. Contrast material can be seen entering the false channel just beyond the left subclavian artery.

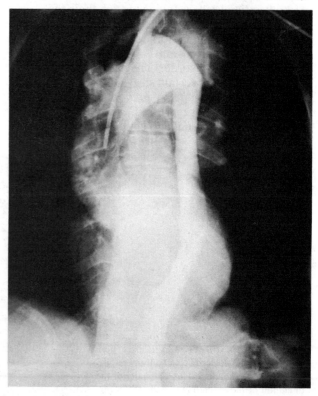

External rupture with hemorrhage into the pericardium, mediastinum, pleural spaces, and, less commonly, peritoneum or retroperitoneal spaces usually abruptly terminates the life of patients with aortic dissection. Those who escape external rupture may succumb to the sequelae of occlusion of a major artery. Patients who survive the acute stage often have developed a distal intimal tear and have formed a "double-barreled" aorta. Aortic leakage manifested by hemothorax or a pericardial friction rub is not always fatal.

Once considered, the diagnosis is often clear from the clinical picture alone and can be confirmed by a widened or distorted aortic contour on a chest radiograph. Progressive widening of the aortic shadow on serial roentgenograms is the most specific sign on plain films. Increase in the distance from intimal calcification to the outer edge of the aortic shadow is a valuable but unusual finding. Unfortunately, because patients with aortic dissection are often gravely ill, the radiographs which can be obtained may be of less than optimum quality.[36]

The electrocardiogram is usually nonspecifically abnormal. Evidence of myocardial infarction is of importance, since cardiac infarction is a relative contraindication to vigorous antihypertensive therapy and also to surgical intervention.

Confirmation of the diagnosis is important for the purpose of prognosis or in preparation for surgical intervention, and aortography should be performed in nearly every instance. Selective injection of contrast material into the aorta through an appropriately positioned catheter is the most sensitive and precise diagnostic method and does not seem to be unduly hazardous.[37]

Prognosis Dissecting aortic aneurysm is highly lethal. In one large series, more than a third of the patients died within the first 48 h. Three-quarters were dead after 2 weeks, and less than 10 percent survived to the end of the first year.[26]

When the dissection begins distal to the arch vessels (type III), there is a much better chance that the patient will survive the acute illness.[34] The early attrition of patients whose dissection involves the ascending aorta is reflected in the greater number with type III dissection who survive long enough to undergo surgery. As has been pointed out, these more favorable cases are actually the less common variety. Assessment of the effectiveness of therapy in this disorder must take into account this quirk in the natural history.

Treatment Supportive treatment of patients with aortic dissection is directed toward pain relief, therapy of heart failure, if present, and transfusion for blood loss, if required.

Advances in modern cardiovascular surgery make possible an attack on any portion of the aorta. The extensive nature of most aortic dissections and the fragility of the aortic media in this disease, especially in the acute phase, have been important obstacles to surgical therapy. In the past the creation of a reentry path, the so-called fenestration procedure, has been employed, but the most favorable results are reported when the intimal tear is resected and the false

channel oversewn at either end of the resection.[27,29] Details of the procedures are described in Chap. 107.

The use of potent drugs to reduce the arterial pressure and the pulsatile forces within the aorta appears to offer an effective mode of medical management of certain patients with aortic dissection. Trimethaphan, nitroprusside, guanethidine, α-methyldopa, parenteral reserpine, and propranolol have been utilized in various regimens. Lowering of the systolic pressure to 100 to 120 mm Hg as quickly as it can be accomplished is the aim of such therapy. Ventricular arrhythmias and oliguria at times force modification of the therapeutic aims.[27,29]

The role of drug therapy vis-à-vis surgery in the acute phase of this disorder has been controversial, but certain principles are now generally accepted. Some patients are seen far from cardiovascular surgical centers; others are prohibitive operative risks by reason of advanced age or of complicating coincident illness. For these, medical management is the choice for initial therapy. On the other hand, leaking dissection, occlusion of a vital artery, or severe heart failure due to aortic regurgitation dictates surgical intervention. When the dissection is limited to the descending aorta, good results with medical management have been reported, and most authorities advocate surgery in such patients only when drug therapy has failed or when complications of the dissection are present.[29] Disappointing results with drug therapy in patients with dissection involving the ascending aorta have led most authors to suggest early operative intervention in all such patients who are suitable candidates.[29]

Some uncertainty exists regarding therapy in patients in the subacute or chronic phase. Recurrent dissection appears to be rare, but expanding saccular aneurysm and progressive aortic regurgitation have been experienced; when these complications occur, operative treatment is indicated. It also seems likely that other selected patients might be best served by operative management in the subacute phase. For example, the outlook for long-term survival appears less favorable for patients in whom the false lumen opacifies during aortography.[38]

Aortitis

BACTERIAL AORTITIS AND MYCOTIC ANEURYSM[12,39,40]
Bacteria may involve the aortic wall directly from contiguous tissue, but more frequently invading organisms are blood-borne. Since the intact aortic intima is quite resistant to bacterial invasion, a previously damaged area almost always provides the site for infection. During septicemia bacteria may also invade the aortic wall through the vasa vasorum.

Aneurysms resulting from damage to the aortic wall by bacterial infection are termed *mycotic aneurysms*. This is a misnomer, since fungus infection is not implicated. Although infectious endocarditis is

the background against which mycotic aneurysms
most often appear, they may result from septicemia
unassociated with endocarditis. In this setting, the
Salmonella group of organisms is particularly noteworthy. Mycotic aneurysms occasionally are found
when no bacteremia is demonstrated. Secondarily
infected arteriosclerotic aortic aneurysms are probably more common than primary mycotic aneurysm of
the aorta.

Direct invasion of the wall of the aorta adjacent to
an aortic valve involved with bacterial endocarditis
may result in valve ring abscess or in rupture of a
sinus of Valsalva.

Spread of tuberculous infection from adjacent
lymph nodes may cause caseous necrosis of the
aortic wall, producing aneurysm, rupture, or both.

SYPHILITIC AORTITIS

Syphilitic involvement of the cardiovascular system,
including the aorta, is discussed in Chap. 85.

NONSPECIFIC AORTITIS[41]

Stenosis or obstruction of the aorta and its branches,
dilatation and aneurysm formation, or aortic regurgitation may be produced by an idiopathic inflammatory process of the aortic wall. This aortitis may be a
lone abnormality or appear in association with rheumatic fever or rheumatoid arthritis, and in such
diverse conditions as scleroderma and Hodgkin's
disease.

A great variety of names have been applied but at
the moment any differences seem a matter of geographic distribution and sex incidence, since distinct
etiologic, pathogenetic, and histologic differences are
not readily apparent. Much of what will follow by
way of description of the clinical and pathologic
features of Takayasu's arteritis can be applied to
these instances of aortopathy.

TAKAYASU'S ARTERITIS[42–44]

This inflammatory disorder of the aorta, of its major
branches, and of the pulmonary artery is named for
the Japanese ophthalmologist who first called attention to the funduscopic findings of the disease. A
striking predilection for young Oriental women is its
most characteristic feature. Because of the frequency with which the brachiocephalic vessels are involved, it has been labeled *pulseless disease* and
aortic arch syndrome.

The cause is unknown. Clinical and serologic data
suggest an "autoimmune" process. Despite a histopathologic resemblance to syphilitic aortitis, serologic and clinical evidence of syphilis is absent. The
morphologic appearance occasionally suggests tuberculous granulomas, but a lack of bacteriologic
evidence is against such a cause.

On histologic examination a panarteritis is found
during active stages of the disease; in late stages
fibrous scarring, intimal proliferation, and thrombosis result in occlusion of the affected vessel.

The origins of the brachiocephalic vessels typically are involved, resulting in the loss of radial and
carotid pulses. The abdominal branches of the aorta
may be affected as well. Aneurysms or acquired
coarctation may result from lesions in the aorta itself.
The pulmonary artery is often found to be involved,
and pulmonary hypertension may be found at catheterization.[45]

Only in the Orient have large series been collected; however, the disorder is found worldwide. Onset
is in the second or third decade in 70 to 80 percent of
cases; however, it has been reported in childhood
and in middle life. Females predominate 8:1 to 9:1
over males.

Constitutional symptoms occur during the early or
"prepulseless" period of the disease. Fever, night
sweats, malaise, weight loss, arthralgia, anemia, nausea, and vomiting are frequently reported. An elevated erythroctye sedimentation rate, anemia, and
serum protein abnormalities are often present, as are
splenomegaly, skin rash, Raynaud's phenomenon,
and occasionally positive serologic tests for lupus
erythematosus or rheumatoid arthritis. It will be
recognized that many features of this disorder reflect
altered immune mechanisms.

Dyspnea, palpitation, angina pectoris, and heart
failure are recorded. Pericarditis has been occasionally observed clinically, but more commonly, healed
pericarditis is noted at autopsy. Aortic regurgitation
may result from a deformed aortic valve or may be
due to dilatation of the aortic root in response to
inflammation of the wall.

Ischemia of the nervous system is commonly
encountered. Syncope, formerly attributed to enhanced carotid sinus sensitivity, more probably reflects cerebral ischemia due to the obstruction of the
brachiocephalic vessels.

The wreathlike anastomoses about the optic disks
to which Takayasu first directed attention are believed to result from ischemia of the retina. Ocular ischemia may also be manifest by transient
loss of vision, cataracts, corneal opacity, and iridial
atrophy.

Fairly typical claudication of the arms and trophic
changes such as perforation of the nasal septum or
ulcerations of the palate, lips, or nose are not uncommon manifestations of obstruction in the brachiocephalic circulation.

Occlusion of the abdominal branches of the aorta
has resulted in bowel infarction and in renovascular
hypertension; however, intermittent claudication due
to aortoiliofemoral obstruction is rather unusual.

Treatment An assessment of the results of therapy is
difficult since the disease typically runs a protracted
course. Some investigators have recommended adre-
nocorticosteroids. Others favor anticoagulation or
immunosuppressive therapy.

GIANT-CELL ARTERITIS[46]

Giant-cell arteritis (temporal arteritis, polymyalgia
rheumatica) may involve the aorta. The histologic
picture of the disorder and its peak incidence in late
life seem to set it apart from other varieties of
aortitis. Like them it may produce occlusion of aortic

arch vessels, aneurysm of the ascending aorta with aortic regurgitation, and dissecting aortic aneurysm.

CHAPTER 103 **1853**
DISEASES OF THE AORTA AND VENAE CAVAE

AORTITIS DUE TO ANKYLOSING SPONDYLITIS (RHEUMATOID SPONDYLITIS)[47]

Among the features of ankylosing spondylitis which allow at least a tentative separation of this disease from rheumatoid arthritis is the occurrence of a rather distinctive inflammatory lesion of the ascending aorta. The histopathologic lesion is not unlike that of syphilis, and, as in syphilis, severe aortic regurgitation may result (see Chap. 85). Unlike syphilis, adventitial thickening extends below the aortic valve to involve the membranous ventricular septum and the base of the mitral valve. When histologic examination is carried out, focal destruction of elastic tissue of the media is seen, but that layer is not thickened as are the intima and adventitia. An obliterative endarteritis of the vasa vasorum may be observed. The aortic root is dilated. The valve cusps are thickened and retracted, and their edges are rolled. The aortic regurgitation which results from these abnormalities may produce life-threatening heart failure.

Such aortitis is more frequent in patients with spondylitis of long duration, in those with peripheral joint complaints in addition to spondylitis, and in patients who have the iritis which accompanies this disorder.

Congenital anomalies of the aorta

Patent ductus arteriosus, coarctation of the aortic isthmus, aortopulmonary window, aneurysm of the aortic sinuses, and anomalies of the aortic arch are considered in the section of this text dealing with congenital heart disease (see Chaps. 53 to 56).

Aortic aneurysm is at times found in patients with congenital aortic stenosis, patent ductus arteriosus, and congenital coarctation. In fact, dissecting aortic aneurysm and spontaneous rupture are significant causes of death in the last of these three conditions.[48,49]

Congenital kinking, so-called pseudocoarctation of the aorta, may present as a mediastinal mass or a systolic murmur, and at times may produce an appreciable reduction or delay in the femoral pulses. True coarctation may be ruled out only by angiography and the demonstration that no pressure difference exists between the upper and lower aortic segments. The abnormality is a sharp downward angulation of the aorta at the attachment of the ligamentum arteriosum.[50,51]

Coarctation of the descending thoracic aorta or of the abdominal aorta is rare. It can be attributed to healed aortitis in some instances but more often seems to be congenital. Such coarctations, either congenital or acquired, may take the form of localized narrowing or of elongated hypoplastic segments.[52-54]

The clinical features of abdominal or thoracoabdominal coarctation are similar to those of the more common variety in that upper-extremity hypertension is present while feeble pulses and hypotension are found in the legs. Attention may be directed to the unusual location of the stenosis by a bruit in the lumbar or umbilical area. Intermittent claudication is more frequent in patients with coarctation of the abdominal aorta than in those patients with the more classic site of narrowing; this is particularly true when the obstruction is distal to the renal arteries. Visceral arteries arising at the site of the constriction may be stenosed, hypoplastic, or thrombosed. Severe hypertension may result from renal ischemia.

Life expectancy in patients with the more distal sites of aortic coarctation is reduced to the same degree as in patients with stenosis of the aortic isthmus. For this reason, surgical correction is considered in most instances.

Trauma to the aorta
(see also Chap. 87)

NONPENETRATING INJURY[55-58]

Traumatic rupture of the aorta occurs most commonly as a result of acceleration-deceleration forces either in a horizontal or vertical plane. Automobile, vehicle-pedestrian, and aircraft accidents account for most of these injuries. The remainder are attributable to falls from great heights or to direct blunt trauma. Surprisingly, a sizable minority of patients will have little or no external evidence of serious thoracic injury.

The most common site of traumatic rupture is just beyond the left subclavian artery at the site of the ligamentum arteriosum. Most authors have felt that the stresses of deceleration are greatest at this point of junction between the relatively fixed aortic arch and the more mobile descending aorta. The ascending aorta just above the aortic valve is the next most common site of traumatic rupture, while the arch area and the abdominal aorta are infrequently damaged by nonpenetrating trauma. Rarely, thrombosis of the abdominal aorta follows blunt trauma.

A triad consisting of increased pulse amplitude and blood pressure in the upper extremities, reduced blood pressure and pulses in the lower extremities, and radiographic evidence of a widened mediastinum is, in the acutely injured patient, virtually diagnostic of aortic rupture. Since surgical intervention may be lifesaving, immediate aortography or exploratory surgery is required.

Though the great majority of patients with such injuries rapidly succumb from exsanguination or from associated trauma, 15 to 20 percent survive the initial insult. Delayed rupture almost invariably occurs, but a few patients are discovered to have aneurysm months or years after the injury. Most of these delayed cases are probably false aneurysms, although it is often difficult to be certain.

Treatment The modern techniques of surgery make resection and graft replacement of the ruptured aorta

possible if exsanguination or associated trauma does
not cause early demise. Many authors advocate
resection of all traumatic aneurysms, but prolonged
survival without surgery has been observed.

PENETRATING INJURY[59,60]

Missile or stab wounds of the aorta usually produce
sudden exsanguination, or if the intrapericardial
aorta is involved, cardiac tamponade. Reports of
diagnosis and repair of such wounds are becoming
more numerous. About 20 percent of one group of
patients with penetrating wounds of the aorta unassociated with injury to the heart survived the initial
insult. False aneurysms or fistulous connections between the aorta and the venae cavae, pulmonary
artery, or heart chambers are occasionally reported
as late sequelae to such wounds. Rarely, during
operations for ruptured intervertebral disk, the aorta
is traumatized. When such trauma is unrecognized,
aortocaval fistula may be a delayed result.

DISEASES OF THE VENAE CAVAE (see also Chap. 108)

Congenital abnormalities of the venae cavae

Congenital abnormalities of the great veins are discussed in Chaps. 53, 55, and 56.

Obstruction of the superior vena cava[61–63]

Occlusion of the superior vena cava produces a
dramatic clinical syndrome, especially if the occlusion develops rapidly (Fig. 103-10). The head, neck,
and arms become edematous. The venous channels
visible over the arms, neck, and thorax are distended
and tortuous because of the necessity for collateral
flow. As a result of venous stasis, the skin of these
areas is dusky. The venous pressure in the upper
extremity is commonly 30 to 50 cm of water. If the

occlusion has occurred rapidly, cerebral edema may
result in headache, somnolence, and convulsions.
The patient may complain of considerable respiratory distress.

Extensive collaterals develop by way of the azy-
gous system, the internal thoracic veins, the lateral
thoracic veins, and the vertebral veins. Connections
with the portal system may develop, producing
"downstream" esophageal varices. Such varices may
involve the entire esophagus or may be atypically
located in the upper or middle segments of that
structure.

Compression of the superior vena cava by a
malignant intrathoracic tumor causes the vast majority of these cases. Bronchogenic carcinoma, especially when located in the right upper lobe, is most
common. Primary mediastinal tumors, lymphomas,
and metastatic lesions are considerably less frequent.
Mediastinal granulomas due to histoplasmosis, or
actinomycosis, idiopathic mediastinal fibrosis, and
aortic aneurysm are among numerous unusual causes. Ascending aortic aneurysm was once a frequent
culprit.

The diagnosis of superior vena caval obstruction
is usually obvious. Radiographic demonstration of
mediastinal widening or of a juxtamediastinal mass
may be helpful in determining the cause. Contrast
venography can be used to demonstrate the site of
blockade and the anatomy of the collaterals. Bronchoscopy will often yield a diagnostic biopsy or
material for cytologic examination. Since the raised
venous pressure is thought to make direct surgical
intervention hazardous, therapy may have to be
undertaken without a definitive diagnosis.

Treatment Therapy usually must be directed toward
the underlying cause. For the majority of patients
with malignant disease, the presence of superior vena
caval obstruction indicates that the lesion is not
resectable. In such patients, the use of diuretics is
advocated to relieve the symptoms rapidly. Subsequent use of chemotherapy and radiotherapy often
will produce a reasonable remission. In the occasional case in which the obstruction is due to an infectious agent, specific therapy may be available. Aortic
aneurysms or benign goiters may be resected surgically. Even if no specific therapy is available, patients whose primary disease is benign usually devel-

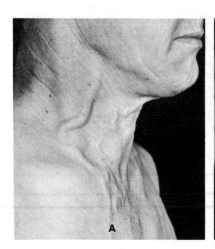
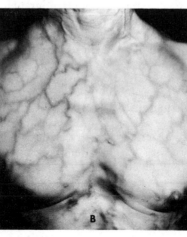

FIGURE 103-10 Superior vena cava obstruction. The dilated veins of the neck, *A*, and
anterior thorax, *B*, form part of the collateral
connections about the obstruction. Photograph
B was exposed with infrared technique. -

op adequate collateral circulation. Surgical attack on the obstruction itself is therefore only rarely advisable.

REFERENCES

1 Schilling, F. J., Christakis, G., Hempel, H. H., and Orbach, A.: The Natural History of Abdominal Aortic and Iliac Atherosclerosis as Detected by Lateral Abdominal Roentgenograms in 2663 Males, *J. Chronic Dis.*, 27:37, 1974.

2 Crane, C.: Atherosclerotic Embolism to Lower Extremities in Arteriosclerosis, *Arch. Surg.*, 94:96, 1967.

3 Kampmeier, R. H.: Saccular Aneurysm of the Thoracic Aorta: A Clinical Study of 633 Cases, *Ann. Intern. Med.*, 12:624, 1938.

4 Blakemore, A. H., and Voorhees, A. B., Jr.: Aneurysm of the Aorta: A Review of 365 Cases. *Angiology*, 5:209, 1954.

5 Joyce, J. W., Fairbairn, J. F., II, Kincaid, O. W., and Juergens, J. L.: Aneurysms of the Thoracic Aorta, *Circulation*, 29:176, 1964.

6 Dillon, M. L., Young, W. G., and Sealy, W. C.: Aneurysms of the Descending Thoracic Aorta, *Ann. Thorac. Surg.*, 3:430, 1967.

7 Ching, C. C., and Hughes, R. K.: Arteriosclerotic Aneurysms of the Thoracic Aorta: Late Stage of a Diffuse Disease, *Am. J. Surg.*, 114:853, 1967.

8 Gore, I., and Hirst, A. E., Jr.: Arteriosclerotic Aneurysms of the Abdominal Aorta: A Review, *Prog. Cardiovasc. Dis.*, 16:113, 1973.

9 Brewster, D. C., Retana, A., Waltman, A. C., and Darling, R. C.: Angiography in the Management of Aneurysms of the Abdominal Aorta, *N. Engl. J. Med.*, 292:822, 1975.

10 Winsberg, F., Cole-Beuglet, C., and Mulder, D. S.: Continuous Ultrasound "B" Scanning of Abdominal Aortic Aneurysms, *Am. J. Roentgenol. Radium Ther. Nucl. Med.*, 121:626, 1974.

11 Dodenhoff, T., and Cox, E. F.: The Acutely Symptomatic Aneurysm: A Surgical Emergency, *Am. Surg.*, 35:691, 1969.

12 Jarrett, F., Darling, R. C., Mundth, E. D., and Austin, W. G.: Experience with Infected Aneurysms of the Abdominal Aorta, *Arch. Surg.*, 110:1281, 1975.

13 Evans, D. M., and Webster, J. H. H.: Spontaneous Aortoduodenal Fistula, *Br. J. Surg.*, 59:368, 1972.

14 Mohr, L. L., and Smith, L. L.: Arteriovenous Fistula from Rupture of Abdominal Aortic Aneurysm, *Arch. Surg.*, 110:806, 1975.

15 Johnson, J. M., Gaspar, M. R., Morris, H. J., and Rosental, J. J.: Sudden and Complete Thrombosis of Aortic and Iliac Aneurysms, *Arch. Surg.*, 108:792, 1974.

16 Lord, J. W., Rossi, G., Daliana, M., Drago, J. R., and Schwartz, A. M.: Unsuspected Abdominal Aortic Aneurysms as the Cause of Peripheral Occlusive Disease, *Ann. Surg.*, 177:767, 1973.

17 Massarelli, J. J., Jr., and Estes, J. E.: Atherosclerotic Occlusion of the Abdominal Aorta and Iliac Arteries: A Study of 105 Patients, *Ann. Intern. Med.*, 47:1125, 1957.

18 Beckwith, R., Huffman, E. R., Eiseman, B., and Blunt, S. G., Jr.: Chronic Aortoiliac Thrombosis, *N. Engl. J. Med.*, 258:721, 1958.

19 Friedman, S. A., Holling, H. E., and Roberts, B.: Etiologic Factors in Aortoiliac and Femoropopliteal Vascular Disease, *N. Engl. J. Med.*, 271:1382, 1964.

20 Schatz, I. J., and Stanley, J. C.: Saddle Embolus of the Aorta, *J.A.M.A.*, 235:1262, 1976.

21 Deterling, R. A.: Acute Arterial Occlusion, *Surg. Clin. North Am.*, 46:587, 1966.

22 Danto, L. A., Fry, W. J., and Kraft, R. O.: Acute Aortic Thrombosis, *Arch. Surg.*, 104:569, 1972.

23 Hirst, A. E., and Gore, I.: Marfan's Syndrome: A Review, *Prog. Cardiovasc. Dis.*, 16:187, 1973.

24 Eisen, S., and Elliott, L. P.: The Roentgenology of Cystic Medial Necrosis of the Ascending Aorta, *Radiol. Clin. North. Am.*, 6:437, 1968.

25 Murdock, J. L., Walker, B. A., Halpern, B. L., Kuzma, J. W., and McKusick, V. A.: Life Expectancy and Causes of Death in the Marfan Syndrome, *N. Engl. J. Med.*, 286:804, 1972.

26 Hirst, A. E., Jr., Johns, V. J., Jr., and Kime, S. W., Jr.: Dissecting Aneurysm of the Aorta: Review of 505 Cases, *Medicine (Baltimore)*, 37:217, 1958.

27 Wheat, M. W., Jr., and Palmer, R. F.: Dissecting Aneurysms of the Aorta, *Curr. Probl. Surg.*, July 1971.

28 Gore, I., and Hirst, A. E., Jr.: Dissecting Aneurysm of the Aorta, *Prog. Cardiovasc. Dis.*, 16:103, 1973.

29 Anagnostopoulos, C. E.: "Acute Aortic Dissections," University Park Press, Baltimore, 1975.

29a Schlatmann, T. J. M., and Becker, A. F.: Pathogenesis of Dissecting Aneurysm of the Aorta, *Am. J. Cardiol.*, 39:21, 1977.

30 Lalich, J. J.: Aortic Aneurysms in Experimental Lathyrism—Contributing Factors, *Arch Pathol.*, 84:528, 1967.

31 Braunstein, H.: Pathogenesis of Dissecting Aneurysm, *Circulation*, 28:1071, 1963.

32 Murray, C. A., and Edwards, J. E.: Spontaneous Laceration of Ascending Aorta, *Circulation*, 47:848, 1973.

33 Fukada, T., Tadavarthy, S. M., and Edwards, J. E.: Dissecting Aneurysm Complicating Aortic Valvular Stenosis, *Circulation*, 53:169, 1976.

34 Lindsay, J., Jr., and Hurst, J. W.: Clinical Features and Prognosis in Dissecting Aneurysm of the Aorta, *Circulation*, 35:880, 1967.

35 Slater, E. E., and DeSanctis, R. W.: The Clinical Recognition of Dissecting Aortic Aneurysm, *Am. J. Med.*, 60:625, 1976.

36 Baron, M. G.: Radiologic Notes in Cardiology: Dissecting Aneurysm of the Aorta, *Circulation*, 43:933, 1971.

37 Beachley, M. C., Ranniger, K., and Roth, F. J.: Roentgenographic Evaluation of Dissecting Aneurysms of the Aorta, *Am. J. Roentgenol. Radium Ther. Nucl. Med.*, 121:617, 1974.

38 Dinsmore, R. E., Willerson, J. T., and Buckley, M. J.: Dissecting Aneurysm of the Aorta: Aortographic Features Affecting Prognosis, *Radiology*, 105:567, 1972.

39 Bennett, D. E.: Primary Mycotic Aneurysms of the Aorta, *Arch. Surg.*, 94:758, 1967.

40 Bennett, D. E., and Cherry, J. K.: Bacterial Infection of Aortic Aneurysms: A Clinico-pathologic Study, *Am. J. Surg.*, 113:321, 1967.

41 Marquis, Y., Richardson, J. B., Ritchie, A. C., and Wigle, E. D.: Idiopathic Medial Aortopathy and Arteriopathy, *Am. J. Med.*, 44:939, 1968.

42 Nakao, K., et al.: Takayasu's Arteritis, *Circulation*, 35:1141, 1967.

43 Vinijchaikul, K.: Primary Arteritis of the Aorta and Main Branches (Takayasu's Arteriopathy), *Am. J. Med.*, 43:15, 1967.

44 Deutsch, V., Wexler, L., Deutsch, H.: Takayasu's Arteritis, *Am. J. Roentgenol. Radium Ther. Nucl. Med.*, 122:13, 1974.

45 Lupi, E., Sanchez, G., Horwitz, S., and Gutierrez, E.: Pulmonary Artery Involvement in Takayasu's Arteritis, *Chest*, 67:69, 1975.

46 Klein, R. G., Hunder, G. G., Stanson, A. W., and Shepps, S. G.: Large Artery Involvement in Giant Cell (Temporal) Arteritis, *Ann. Intern. Med.*, 83:806, 1975.

47 Bulkley, B. H., and Roberts, W. C.: Ankylosing Spondylitis and Aortic Regurgitation, *Circulation*, 43:1014, 1973.

48 Nikaidoh, H., Idriss, F. S., and Riker, W. L.: Aortic Rupture in Children as a Complication of Coarctation of the Aorta, *Arch. Surg.*, 107:838, 1973.

49 Edwards, J. E.: Aneurysms of the Thoracic Aorta Complicating Coarctation, *Circulation*, 43:195, 1973.

50 Hoeffel, J. C., Henry, M., Mentre, B., Louis, J. P., and Pernot, C.: Pseudocoarctation or Congenital Kinking of the Aorta, *Am. Heart J.*, 89:428, 1975.

51 Smyth, P. T., and Edwards, J. E.: Pseudocoarctation, Kinking, or Buckling of the Aorta, *Circulation*, 46:1027, 1972.

52 Onat, T., and Zeren, E.: Coarctation of the Abdominal Aorta: Review of 91 Cases, *Cardiologia (Basel)*, 54:140, 1969.

53 Riemenschneider, T. A., Emmanouilides, G. C., Hirose, F., and Linde, L. M.: Coarctation of the Abdominal Aorta: Report of Three Cases and Review of the Literature, *Pediatrics*, 44:716, 1969.

54 Ben-Shoshan, M., Rossi, N. P., Korns, M. E.: Coarctation of the Abdominal Aorta, *Arch. Pathol.*, 95:221, 1973.

55 Parmley, L. F., Mattingly, T. W., Manion, W. C., and Jahnke, E. J., Jr.: Nonpenetrating Traumatic Injury of the Aorta, *Circulation*, 17:1086, 1958.

56 Symbas, P. N., Tyros, D. H., Ware, R. F., and Diorio, D. A.: Traumatic Rupture of the Aorta, *Ann. Surg.*, 178:6, 1973.

57 Bennett, D. E., and Cherry, J. K.: The Natural History of Traumatic Aneurysms of the Aorta, *Surgery*, 61:516, 1967.

58 Fleming, A. W., and Green, D. C.: Traumatic Aneurysms of the Thoracic Aorta, *Ann. Thorac. Surg.*, 18:91, 1974.

59 Parmley, L. F., Mattingly, T. W., and Manion, W. C.: Penetrating Wounds of the Heart and Aorta, *Circulation*, 17:953, 1958.

60 Symbas, P. N., and Sehdeva, J. S.: Penetrating Wounds of the Thoracic Aorta, *Ann. Surg.*, 171:441, 1970.

61 Banker, V. P., and Maddison, F. E.: Superior Vena Cava Syndrome Secondary to Aortic Disease, *Dis. Chest*, 51:656, 1967.

62 Salsali, M., and Clifton, E. E.: Superior Vena Cava Obstruction with Lung Cancer, *Ann. Thorac. Surg.*, 6:437, 1968.

63 Mahajan, V., Strimlan, V., Van Ordstrand, H. S., and Loop, F. D.: Benign Superior Vena Cava Syndrome, *Chest*, 68:32, 1975.

104
Diseases of the Peripheral Arteries and Veins

JESS R. YOUNG, M.D., and
VICTOR G. de WOLFE, M.D.

DISEASES OF THE PERIPHERAL ARTERIES[1]

Chronic occlusive arterial diseases of the extremities

Peripheral vascular disease is a term that encompasses a wide variety of conditions affecting the arteries, veins, and lymphatic vessels of the extremities. This term, however, often is erroneously used as a synonym for the chronic occlusive arterial diseases, which, taken as a group, are the most frequently encountered conditions affecting the aorta and peripheral arteries. In this section, those diseases that produce chronic ischemia due to organic occlusion of the aorta or peripheral arteries will be discussed.

Other sections will be devoted to acute arterial occlusion and to conditions that produce ischemia as a result of arterial spasm.

ETIOLOGY

Atherosclerosis of the aorta and/or its branches to the extremities (arteriosclerosis obliterans) is the cause of 95 percent of cases of chronic occlusive disease. The etiology and the pathogenesis of coronary atherosclerosis are discussed in Chap. 62B. Although the pathologic characteristics are similar, it is important to remember that, experimentally and clinically, atherosclerosis behaves differently in different vascular beds, and therefore experimental and epidemiologic data pertaining to coronary atherosclerosis may not be strictly applicable to atherosclerosis of the peripheral arteries.

Thromboangiitis obliterans (Buerger's disease), though relatively rare, is the next most common cause for chronic occlusive arterial disease of the extremities. Most authorities agree that the incidence of thromboangiitis obliterans seems to be decreasing,[2] but there are a few who share the opinion of Wessler and colleagues[3] that it is not a separate and distinct clinical entity. When compared with patients with arteriosclerosis obliterans, patients with thromboangiitis obliterans have significantly higher concentrations of the heparin-precipitable fraction of fibrinogen in the blood,[4] and higher values of carboxyhemoglobin probably due to more intensive smoking.[5,6] McPherson and colleagues[7] have shown by follow-up studies that clinically thromboangiitis obliterans and arteriosclerosis obliterans have entirely different prognostic implications. The cause of thromboangiitis obliterans is not definitely known, but the direct relationship to cigarette smoking appears to be indisputable. The arteritis most likely represents a poorly understood sensitivity reaction to tobacco. The disease occurs only in smokers,[8] and cessation of smoking is usually followed by improvement.

Nonspecific arteritis of the aorta and its branches (Takayasu's disease) is a relatively rare cause of chronic occlusive arterial disease in the Western Hemisphere, although it is reported frequently in Japan and other Oriental countries.[9] Typically, the disease affects the subclavian and carotid arteries of young women, but sometimes the descending thoracic and abdominal aorta and its branches are affected,[10] and "acquired coarctation" of the aorta may result. Sclerosing and stenosing aortitis of the lower thoracic and abdominal ampta (middle aoptic syndrome") occurring in children and young women in the tropics is probably related to, if not identical with, the nonspecific arteritis of Takayasu. Immunologic and clinical studies have provided suggestive evidence that Takayasu's arteritis may be an autoimmune disease.[9]

In the United States the syndrome of arterial insufficiency of the upper extremities and the brain occurs with greatest frequency in middle-aged and older people, particularly men. In these cases the cause is usually atherosclerosis, not the nonspecific arteritis that has been described as occurring in young women. The terms *aortic arch syndrome* and

Disorders of collagen (systemic lupus erythematosus, progressive systemic sclerosis (scleroderma), periarteritis nodosa, rheumatoid arthritis, and dermatomyositis[12]) and dysproteinemias (cryoglobulinemia and cryofibrinogenemia) may cause chronic occlusive arterial disease of small arteries with manifestations of ischemia in the fingers or toes, or both.[13]

Occasionally, showers of microemboli arise from atheromatous plaques in the aorta or from aortic, iliac, femoral, or popliteal aneurysms and occlude small digital and cutaneous arteries in the feet and legs, producing ischemic lesions, including ulcers, digital gangrene, ischemic purpura, and livedo reticularis.

It is important to stress that anticoagulant therapy is of no benefit in atheromatous emboli, and may induce a paradoxic response wherein anticoagulants may be the initiating cause of the embolization which will continue until the anticoagulants are stopped.[14]

Patients with homocystinuria frequently have extensive thrombosis of veins and arteries, including the aorta and peripheral arteries, with signs and symptoms of ischemia in the extremities. It is believed that the vascular thrombosis results from sustained, homocystine-induced endothelial injury.[15]

Pachydermoperiostosis (primary hypertrophic osteoarthropathy) is associated with large, cold hands and feet and occasional ischemic ulcers of the fingers or toes. The wrist and foot pulses are reduced or absent. Arteriograms show poor flow with no demonstrable occluded vessels.[16] The cause of this condition is unknown.

The signs and symptoms of chronic occlusive arterial disease are frequently the sequelae to sudden arterial occlusion if the extremity survives the acute insult. Causes of sudden arterial occlusion include arterial embolus, trauma, and simple thrombosis in situ. These are discussed in detail farther on in this chapter, under "Acute Arterial Occlusion of the Extremities" and "Arterial Trauma."

PATHOLOGY

Histopathologic findings in atherosclerosis are well known and are described elsewhere in this book. The lesions in the large and medium-sized vessels supplying the extremities are pathologically similar to those occurring elsewhere in the body, and, characteristically, patients with arteriosclerosis obliterans have a high incidence of atherosclerosis affecting the coronary arteries and the arteries supplying the brain.[17,18] In addition to atherosclerotic lesions in the larger arteries of the extremities, arteriolar and capillary lesions consisting of endothelial proliferation and thickening of the basement membrane in diabetic patients have been described.[19] In a double-blind study Vracko and Strandness[20] could find no difference between diabetic and nondiabetic patients when the areas of the basement membranes of capillaries in abdominal muscles were compared with the total area of the capillaries. Furthermore, in casts made of the vascular lumen of extremities amputated for gangrene, Conrad[21] found that diabetics had more extensive occlusion of calf vessels and less occlusion

in the foot than nondiabetics. There was no increase in small-vessel occlusion in the diabetic limb.

With the use of immunofluorescent techniques it has been shown that in some diabetic patients the small arteries showing endothelial proliferation bind insulin and rabbit anti-human globulin, a reaction suggesting an immunologic basis for the lesions.[22]

The pathologic findings in thromboangiitis obliterans, as described by Buerger in his classic article published in 1908,[23] are usually distinctly different from those of arteriosclerosis obliterans, except in the late stages when old occluding organized thrombus may be seen to fill the lumen of an artery that demonstrates considerable perivascular fibrosis.

In the acute and subacute stages, thromboangiitis obliterans is characterized by an intense inflammatory reaction that, unlike atherosclerosis, involves the veins as well as the arteries. Thromboangiitis obliterans characteristically affects medium-sized and small arteries initially; atherosclerosis usually involves arteries of larger caliber. The visceral arteries rarely are affected by thromboangiitis obliterans, whereas they are commonly the sites of atherosclerosis. Thromboangiitis obliterans is a true panarteritis (or panphlebitis), as all coats of the vessel are affected and the process often extends to the perivascular tissues, leading to fibrosis and scarring that firmly binds together the artery, vein, and nerve. Characteristically, the involvement is segmental, with normal segments interspersed between segments of inflammation. Proliferation of the endothelium and invasion of all three coats by lymphocytes and fibroblasts are common characteristics of this disease. Polymorphonuclear leukocytes are present in the acute stage and for this reason are more likely to be seen in veins, which can be biopsied easily, than in the arteries, which are not usually obtained for microscopic study until the disease has reached the chronic stage. Giant cells may be found both in arteries and in veins during the acute stage. The arterial lumen is compromised by proliferation of the endothelium and invasion of the intima by lymphocytes, but final occlusion is usually the result of thrombus which characteristically is intensely cellular and becomes organized rapidly. Necrosis of the arterial wall does not occur; the internal elastic lamina is preserved, and aneurysm formation as the result of thromboangiitis obliterans is extremely rare. Electron microscopic demonstration of extensive and diffuse degeneration of collagen in the small arteries and lumbar sympathetic ganglions of patients with thromboangiitis obliterans has prompted Peracchia and Vassallo[24] to suggest that this disease should be considered a collagen disorder.

PATHOLOGIC PHYSIOLOGY

The basic pathophysiologic alteration produced by chronic occlusive arterial disease, regardless of its underlying cause, is ischemia of tissues supplied by the obstructed arteries. The severity of the ischemia is dependent not only on the site and extent of the arterial disease but also on the adequacy of the collateral circulation and the metabolic demands of the tissues involved. In general, tissues usually react to prolonged ischemia with atrophy and fibrosis and, ultimately, if ischemia is severe enough, with necrosis.

CLINICAL MANIFESTATIONS

Regardless of the underlying cause, chronic occlusive arterial disease is characterized by (1) subjective symptoms of ischemia such as intermittent claudication, rest pain, and ischemic neuropathy, and (2) objective signs of ischemia, such as absence or diminution of arterial pulsations, pallor of the feet on elevation of affected extremities, rubor of the feet when the extremities are dependent, and various degrees of ischemic changes in the skin. The symptoms and signs that are common to all the chronic occlusive arterial diseases will be discussed first, and those which help to identify the specific cause will be discussed subsequently under "Differential Diagnosis."

Pain is the most frequent presenting complaint of patients with chronic occlusive arterial disease. The characteristics and severity of the pain depend on the extent of the occlusive arterial disease and the tissues involved. Ischemia of muscle produces intermittent claudication; ischemia of nerves produces ischemic neuropathy; ischemia of skin and subcutaneous tissue produces pretrophic pain and the pain of ulceration and gangrene; and ischemia of bone is a contributing factor in the development of painful osteoporosis.

Intermittent claudication is usually the first symptom of chronic occlusive arterial disease and the one that most frequently brings the patient to the physician. The characteristic feature of intermittent claudication is that it occurs when ischemic muscles are active and is relieved promptly by rest. Most frequently it is induced by walking and may be noted in the foot, calf, thigh, or buttock, depending on the site of arterial occlusion.[25] The sensation that occurs with walking may be described as a cramp, "charley horse," numbness, ache, or weakness. Frequently patients will state that it is not a truly painful sensation. Regardless of the description of the discomfort, it occurs only with activity and is relieved promptly (within a few minutes) by rest. It usually forces the person to stop or slow his pace, but it is not necessary for him to sit down to obtain relief. Once the distress has disappeared, the patient may resume walking again, only to be stopped after walking the same distance by the same distress. Patients who have occlusive disease in the subclavian or axillary artery may experience the same type of distress in the muscles of the forearm when engaging in prolonged exercise such as writing, typing, washing windows, painting, or similar types of activity.

Intermittent claudication, or "shin splints (anterior compartment syndrome)," confined to the anterior tibial muscles may occur, usually in young, healthy people, in the absence of chronic occlusive arterial disease.[25a] Presumably this results from pressure as the result of edema or hemorrhage on the active muscles by the fascial sheath which encloses them; capillary circulation is thus compromised. Fasciotomy to decompress the anterior tibial compartment is curative and should be carried out before infarction of the muscles occurs.

Typical intermittent claudication in young men may be caused by intermittent compression, or entrapment, of the popliteal artery by the medial head of the gastrocnemius muscle.[26] In this anomaly the popliteal artery passes medial to or through the medial belly of the muscle and becomes compressed during walking. The pulses are normal at rest. Aneurysm or thrombosis of the artery may result.

The occurrence of pain at rest signifies that ischemia is increasing in severity. Ischemic neuropathy is characterized by severe, lancinating, shooting, or shocklike pains that involve the foot and leg. As is true for other types of ischemic rest pain, pain of ischemic neuropathy is particularly troublesome at night and often requires narcotics for relief.

Pretrophic pain often heralds the onset of necrosis of tissue with ulceration; the pain is steady, boring, and well localized to two or three digits and the adjacent area of the foot, which are most ischemic. It is a demoralizing type of pain that causes insomnia, anorexia, and depression, and forces the patient to hang his foot over the edge of the bed or sleep in a chair in order to obtain relief.

The pain of ulceration and gangrene is similar to, but more severe than, pretrophic pain. It occurs in an area of ulceration or gangrene and, like pretrophic pain, is usually relieved somewhat by placing the involved foot in a dependent position.

It is unlikely that ischemia of bone per se can cause pain and osteoporosis, but it is well recognized that in patients with severe ischemia, osteoporosis often develops in the ischemic extremity. This is probably because of a combination of ischemia and prolonged disuse owing to ischemic pain. The pain of osteoporosis occurs with weight bearing (with or without walking), and tenderness can be elicited by gentle but firm pressure applied to the ischemic foot. This type of pain is similar to that observed in Sudeck's atrophy, which may occur in the presence of normal arterial circulation, and for this reason one may assume that disuse is an important contributing factor to the painful osteoporosis observed in ischemic extremities.

Although chronic occlusive arterial disease can cause pallor or cyanosis and coolness of the skin of the involved extremity, it should be recognized that these are common subjective complaints of neurotic patients; the diagnosis of chronic occlusive arterial disease should never be made on the basis of these complaints unless there are more specific symptoms and other objective findings. The diagnostic significance of these complaints is much greater if the changes in color and temperature are confined to one extremity or to one or two digits of an extremity. Mottled cyanosis (livedo reticularis) of the arms and legs usually is not a sign of chronic occlusive arterial disease. Raynaud's phenomenon may be a symptom

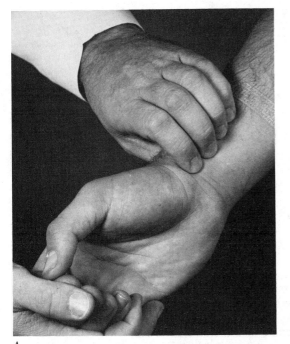

A

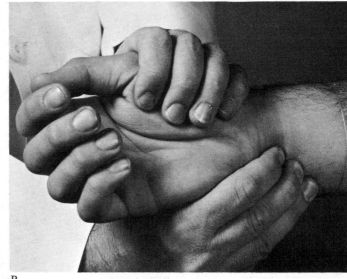

B

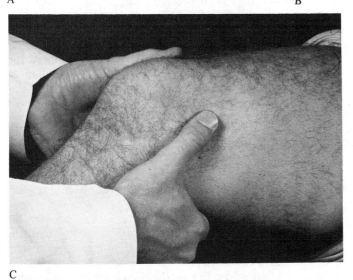

C

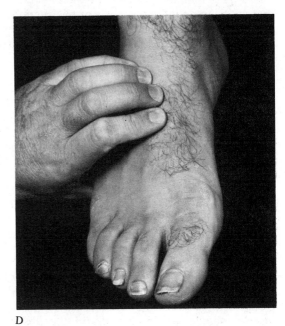

D

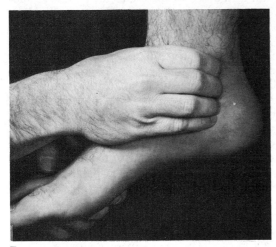

E

FIGURE 104-1 Methods for palpating arteries. *A*. Radial. *B*. Ulnar. *C*. Popliteal. *D*. Dorsalis pedis. *E*. Posterior tibial. Palpation of the aorta and peripheral arteries is the single most important maneuver in the examination of patients for chronic occlusive arterial disease.

of thromboangiitis obliterans when the upper extremities are involved.

When adequate collateral circulation is present, chronic occlusive arterial disease may produce no symptoms, the diagnosis being made on the basis of absence or definite diminution of pulsations in one or more peripheral arteries (exclusive of the dorsalis pedis).

Palpating peripheral pulses is the most important single maneuver in establishing the diagnosis when chronic occlusive arterial disease is suspected (Fig. 104-1). It is perilous to make a diagnosis of chronic occlusive arterial disease when the arterial pulses are all unequivocally normal. On the other hand, the presence of arterial pulsations does not preclude a diagnosis of chronic occlusive arterial disease, for when the occlusion is partial or when complete occlusion involves only a short segment of the termi-

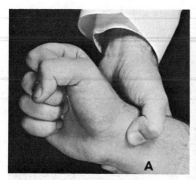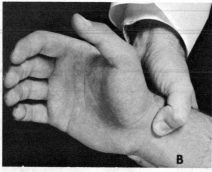

FIGURE 104-2 Radial compression test of Allen, which may be employed to test for patency of the ulnar and radial arteries and the palmar arterial arch. *A.* While the examiner occludes the radial artery, the patient squeezes the blood out of his hand by making a tight fist. *B.* While radial compression is maintained by the examiner, the patient opens his hand. If color does not return to the hand within 3 s, occlusion of the ulnar artery or the ulnar side of the palmar arch is usually present. By compressing the ulnar artery and repeating the maneuver, it is possible to test for patency of the radial artery and the radial side of the palmar arch. Compression tests are more difficult to perform on the foot and give less satisfactory results.

nal aorta or iliac arteries, the distal pulses may be present but dampened. Often pulsations will disappear entirely and bruits may be produced when the patient walks rapidly enough to induce intermittent claudication. Barner and colleagues[27] and Moore and Hall[28] have demonstrated with experimental models that, distal to an inflow stenosis or obstruction, pulse pressure is reduced when blood flow is increased by factors (such as exercise) which lower the resistance in the terminal bed. It is likely that these hemodynamic changes explain the disappearance of arterial pulsations distal to a partial or segmental arterial occlusion in the aortoiliac area when patients are walking.

Arterial pulsations may be unimpaired at the wrist or ankle when the occlusive disease is confined to the palmar or plantar arterial arches or to the digital arteries themselves. It is in such unusual circumstances as this that compression tests (Allen test) (Fig. 104-2) and arteriography are useful to confirm or rule out the diagnosis that has been suggested by the history and other findings. It is equally important to recognize that because of anomalies, in about 5 to 12 percent of normal persons one or both of the dorsalis pedis arteries may be lacking, or may be so anomalously situated that they are not palpable.[29] Hence the diagnosis of chronic occlusive arterial disease should never depend on the absence of dorsalis pedis pulsations alone. On the other hand, an impalpable posterior tibial pulse almost always indicates occlusive arterial disease since congenital absence of this artery is very rare.

A systolic bruit over the abdominal aorta, iliac, or femoral arteries, when the patient has been supine for more than 10 min, usually signifies intimal disease but not necessarily significant occlusion. Conversely, complete occlusion of an artery usually does not produce a bruit. In the absence of an arteriovenous fistula, bruits that have a diastolic component, whether or not they are continuous through the cardiac cycle, usually indicate occlusive arterial disease.[30]

Postural color changes are an indication of the degree of ischemia, and their failure to appear in a setting of diminished or absent pulses indicates occlusive disease compensated for by good collateral circulation. When ischemia is moderate or severe,

hands or feet blanch when they are elevated (elevation pallor) and become excessively red or cyanotic when they are dependent (dependent rubor). Failure of the color to return within 15 s after an ischemic extremity is changed from the elevated to the dependent position is also an indication of moderate to severe ischemia. If the color does not return for 30 s or more after the extremity is brought into the dependent position, ischemia usually is severe.

A delay of more than 15 s in the time required for the veins on the dorsa of the hands or feet to fill after an extremity is changed from the elevated to the dependent position usually indicates ischemia (venous filling test). When the venous system is incompetent, retrograde filling occurs promptly and renders the test invalid. As with the postural color test, a normal response to the venous filling test does not rule out chronic occlusive arterial disease, but in general the longer the time for venous filling, the more severe the ischemia.

Nutritional changes, including loss of hair on the dorsum of the foot and toes, trophic changes of the nails and skin, ulceration, and gangrene, represent end stages of ischemia. Ischemic ulcerations usually occur first at the tips of the digits, around and under the nails, on the interdigital surfaces, or on the heel (Fig. 104-3). Ischemic ulcers may also occur on the lateral and medial sides of the foot overlying the metatarsal heads. Large, indolent, painless ulcers that occur on the plantar surfaces over the metatarsophalangeal joints, usually in callosities, result from infection and neuropathy and are most frequently encountered in diabetic patients (neurotropic ulcer). This type of ulcer is typically associated with a grossly adequate arterial circulation, necessary for the development of the osteomyelitis, or osteopathy which are frequently present. The pathogenesis of the neurotrophic ulcer appears to be related to the neuropathy, which in turn may be caused by microangiopathy in the vasa nervorum.[19,31] Ischemic ulcers are usually small and shallow initially, gradually increasing in size. The base is pale, devoid of granulation tissue, and frequently covered by necrotic debris and crusted exudate (eschar). The rim is indolent, showing no tendency for proliferation and epithelialization of the ulcer. At times the rim is actually necrotic,[31a] and the ulcer spreads peripheral-

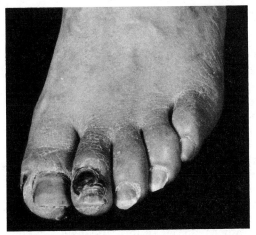

FIGURE 104-3 Ischemic gangrenous ulcer on the dorsum of the second toe of a patient with arteriosclerosis obliterans. Ischemic ulcerations typically occur on toes, whereas stasis ulcers usually occur over or near the malleoli (see Fig. 104-8).

ly in this manner. Stasis ulcers from chronic venous insufficiency tend to occur around the malleoli and lower part of the leg and only rarely occur on the foot and toes. Stasis ulcers are less painful but usually larger than ischemic ulcers, and their bases are filled with luxuriant granulation tissue.[31a] Gangrene is the end stage of chronic occlusive arterial disease. Usually it begins in and around an area of ulceration and at first involves a single digit (Fig. 104-3), from which it spreads to other digits or more proximally onto the foot. If gangrene appears abruptly and involves a large area from the outset, it is virtually certain that trauma and/or sudden arterial occlusion are inciting factors.

DIAGNOSIS

The diagnosis of chronic occlusive arterial disease can be established with certainty in well over 95 percent of cases without the aid of special laboratory procedures. If further information is needed to evaluate the degree of arterial insufficiency, a variety of noninvasive instrumentation is now available, ranging from simple devices to be used in the physician's office to more complicated and expensive instruments suitable only for the vascular laboratory. The use of instrumentation for the evaluation of arterial insufficiency is becoming widespread, technology is rapidly advancing, and more laboratories are appearing. Several of the instruments are simple and accurate, yield reproducible data, and are relatively inexpensive. A comprehensive guideline report, recently updated, has been issued by the Instrumentation Study Group of the Inter-Society Commission on Heart Disease Resources.[32]

The existing instruments are useful for confirming and documenting the arterial insufficiency found by clinical evaluation, for evaluating the patient for sympathectomy, revascularization, or level of amputation, and for following the progress of the patient during a program of conservative therapy or after surgery.

One of the simplest methods for estimating blood flow in the lower extremities is to measure the systolic blood pressure at the levels of the thigh, upper calf, and ankles. These data are helpful in locating the level of the arterial occlusion(s). Systolic pressures are obtained either with a Doppler ultrasound instrument or with a plethysmograph and compared with brachial systolic pressure as an index of the level and extent of the arterial occlusion. The simplicity of the Doppler technique has made it the instrument of choice, particularly since it is suitable for use in the physician's office. Normally, the ankle systolic pressure should be 80 percent or more of the brachial systolic pressure. With mild arterial insufficiency, the ankle pressure is between 50 and 80 percent of the brachial pressure, and with severe arterial insufficiency it is below 50 percent of brachial pressure.[33]

A recently described method of considerable promise is called *ultrasonic arteriography*.[34] This device employs a pulsed Doppler system which is capable of systematically mapping the entire region of an artery where blood is flowing, thus producing a picture which resembles a conventional arteriogram. At the moment this new technique appears to hold promise in the carotid area, the common femoral–profunda femoris artery junction, the superficial femoral artery, and the popliteal artery.

Plain roentgenograms may demonstrate evidence of arterial calcification in some cases of atherosclerotic disease, but this is not necessarily an indication that there is obstruction to blood flow.

Complete angiography (aortography and femoral arteriography) is the only diagnostic method available now which will precisely locate the anatomic disease. It will reveal the site of the occlusion(s), the extent of the disease, and the amount of collateral circulation present. Therefore, it is an essential guide to the vascular surgeon in the evaluation of lesions amenable to surgical repair.

The diagnosis of chronic occlusive arterial disease must be considered whenever a patient mentions pain or discomfort in the extremities. If arterial pulsations are normal in the symptomatic extremity, it is highly unlikely that the pain is due to ischemia. However, serious diagnostic errors may occur if the physician attributes all types of pain to ischemia merely because arterial pulsations are diminished or absent. Chronic occlusive arterial disease is sometimes relatively asymptomatic, and the physician should be aware of the fact that osteoarthritis, peripheral neuropathy, degeneration of lumbar disks, simple muscular pain, and other types of nonischemic pain in the extremities may occur coincidentally with chronic occlusive arterial disease. Accurate diagnosis depends on the correlation of characteristic ischemic pain with the physical findings of occlusive arterial disease already described.

DIFFERENTIAL DIAGNOSIS

Usually the diagnosis of chronic occlusive arterial disease presents less difficulty than the establishment of the specific cause of the arterial obstruction.

Trauma, arterial embolus, and acute arterial thrombosis usually can be ruled out on the basis of the history. Takayasu's disease should be suspected when signs and symptoms of occlusive arterial disease in the upper extremities and/or brain occur in young women. Fever, malaise, weight loss, and elevation of the sedimentation rate of erythrocytes are not uncommon.[9] When the coronary arteries are affected, angina pectoris occurs, and when the renal arteries are affected, hypertension may result. Inflammatory stenosis of the descending thoracic or abdominal aorta can cause intermittent claudication; hypertension may be produced if the stenotic area is above the level of the renal arteries.[10]

Homocystinuria should be suspected when occlusive arterial disease occurs in children or young adults who also have one or more of the following: congenital skeletal abnormalities similar to those in Marfan's syndrome, thrombophlebitis, osteoporosis, mental retardation, ectopia lentis, cutaneous flushing, and evidence of coronary and/or cerebral vascular disease.[15]

Arteritis associated with collagen diseases may cause cutaneous infarcts, ischemic purpura, and digital gangrene with normal arterial pulsations because usually only the small arteries are affected. Evidence of multisystem involvement is a clue to the correct diagnosis. A confusingly similar clinical picture can be caused by atheromatous emboli that lodge not only in the small arteries of the feet and legs but also in small visceral arteries.[14] Compared with patients with arteritis secondary to collagen diseases, patients with atheromatous embolic disease are usually older, are less likely to have fever, and rarely have ischemic lesions in the upper extremities.

A rare, nonvascular cause of intermittent claudication is the cauda equina syndrome in which there is compression on the cauda equina by narrowing of the lumbar canal by spondylosis, a ruptured intervertebral disk, or other cause. The compression causes symptoms of back and leg pain and sensory symptoms and weakness on walking and standing, relieved by rest. The extremity pulses are normal. Diagnosis is by myelography, and the treatment is surgical correction.[35]

Once these uncommon causes of chronic occlusive arterial disease are ruled out, the differential diagnosis between arteriosclerosis obliterans and thromboangiitis obliterans must be made.

When symptoms of chronic occlusive arterial disease appear in persons older than 50 years, the diagnosis is almost certainly arteriosclerosis obliterans. About 80 percent of patients with this disease are men,[36] but the ratio of men to women becomes lower as age increases. The incidence of diabetes among patients with arteriosclerosis obliterans ranges from 20 to 33 percent.[36] A striking feature in patients with arteriosclerosis obliterans is their vulnerability to atherosclerotic disease elsewhere, such as the coronary arteries and the arteries supplying the brain.[17] In the Framingham Study 33 percent of patients with intermittent claudication had cerebrovascular or coronary artery disease.[37] When arteriosclerosis obliterans affects men under the age of 40 years, the differential diagnosis from thromboangiitis obliterans may be particularly difficult. Usually in this age range the lesions of arteriosclerosis appear first in the aortoiliac or femoropopliteal arterial segments, and the first symptom is intermittent claudication of the buttock, thigh, or calf. Pulsations may be diminished or absent in some of the arteries of the upper extremities, but ischemic symptoms of the hands rarely occur as the result of arteriosclerosis obliterans. Hyperlipemia, diabetes, atherosclerosis elsewhere, and roentgenographic evidence of arterial calcification favor the diagnosis of arteriosclerosis obliterans rather than one of thromboangiitis obliterans.

In contrast, thromboangiitis obliterans is predominantly a disease of young men, symptoms usually appearing before the age of 35 years and sometimes before the age of 30 years. Only 1 percent of patients are women. Ninety-nine percent of all patients are or have been heavy users of tobacco, usually cigarettes. Superficial thrombophlebitis, which occurs in about 40 percent of cases, is a helpful diagnostic finding, for its concurrence with arteriosclerosis obliterans is coincidental only and therefore the frequency is low. Lesions of thromboangiitis obliterans characteristically appear first in the tibial arteries, producing intermittent claudication in the arch of the foot or calf. Ischemic symptoms in the upper extremities, especially ulcerations about the fingertips, are strong evidence favoring the diagnosis of thromboangiitis obliterans.

PROGNOSIS

The life expectancy of patients with arteriosclerosis obliterans is compromised because of the high frequency of concomitant atherosclerotic complications in the brain and the heart.[17,37] The occlusive disease in the extremities contributes little if anything to the increased mortality rate. The mortality rate is higher in diabetic patients and in those who have clinical evidence of coexisting cerebral and/or coronary atherosclerosis than in those who do not have these complications.[38] On the other hand, the life expectancy of patients with thromboangiitis obliterans is not appreciably affected by this disease,[7] and this is an important reason for attempting to make a correct differential diagnosis.

Thromboangiitis obliterans is a greater threat to limb survival than is arteriosclerosis obliterans. McPherson and colleagues[7] found that 12.6 percent of patients with thromboangiitis obliterans required amputation of a leg, whereas only 6.4 percent of patients with arteriosclerosis obliterans required major amputation during a 10-year period. In the Framingham experience the amputation rate was 5 percent in a cohort of 125 patients with intermittent claudication over a period of 18 years.[37] For nondiabetic patients with arteriosclerosis obliterans the incidence of major amputation has been reported to range from 4 to 12 percent during follow-up periods of from 5 to 10 years.[39] The incidence of amputation for diabetic patients with arteriosclerosis obliterans ranges from 18 to 34 percent.[17] The prognosis for surviva of an extremity is better when intermittent claudication is the only symptom than when ischemia is severe enough to produce rest pain, ischemic ulcers, and gangrene.[37,39]

Major amputations of upper extremities are almost never necessary for chronic occlusive arterial disease, regardless of the cause.[40]

Arteriosclerosis obliterans is not invariably a progressive disease.[37] Strandness and Stahler[41] used segmental limb pressure to evaluate disease progression, and it occurred in 43 percent of 99 limbs (or 52 percent of 60 patients) during an average 3-year follow-up period. Kuthan et al.[42] made an angiographic follow-up study of 1,196 extremities (705 patients) and found progression in 52 percent of extremities over a period of 6 months to 8 years. Progression was more frequent in extremities of patients 50 years of age or older, extremities of manifest diabetics, and in superficial femoral arteries than in other vessels. Progression was more frequent in arterial segments immediately proximal to occlusions than in those distal, confirming the findings of previous workers.

TREATMENT (see also Chap. 107)

Various surgical methods for revascularizing ischemic limbs have supplemented but have not replaced the more conventional and less glamorous principles of medical management.

Limitations of surgical treatment Surgical treatment of chronic occlusive arterial disease is the subject of another chapter, but it is pertinent to a discussion of medical treatment to consider the limitations and disadvantages of direct arterial surgical procedures. Many patients with severe ischemia who would benefit most from reconstructive operations are not appropriate subjects, because the lesions are too diffuse and involve the branches of the popliteal arteries,[19] making revascularization procedures on the proximal arteries hazardous because runoff is inadequate. Surgical techniques for dealing with segmental occlusive lesions in the tibial arteries are being developed, but they have not been widely used, and results are too preliminary to permit any conclusions.[43,44] Segmental obstructive lesions confined to the aorta, the iliac or femoral arteries, which are technically feasible to remove or bypass frequently cause only intermittent claudication without severe ischemic changes in the skin. Follow-up studies have shown that intermittent claudication usually is not a progressive symptom[37] and does not cause great disability. Consequently only a minority of patients who have operable lesions are subjects for surgical treatment if one uses progressive disability from intermittent claudication as the criterion for operation. Follow-up studies have already been cited[39] which indicate that when intermittent claudication is the only manifestation of ischemia, the survival rate of limbs is extremely good.

Peripheral arteriosclerosis obliterans is not a fatal disease per se; consequently reconstructive arterial operations do not prolong or preserve life. Furthermore they have no beneficial effect on atherogenesis,

either locally or in other arterial beds, and consequently do not ameliorate or prevent atherosclerotic complications in the heart or the brain, or further arterial occlusion in the extremities. Surgical procedures in the aortoiliac region are associated with a mortality rate of approximately 5 percent.[45] As a matter of fact, the immediate mortality rate from this type of operation in some series approaches or even exceeds the 5-year amputation rate that can be expected in the natural course of the disease. In the femoropopliteal area surgical mortality should not exceed 2 percent. The frequency of late failures of synthetic grafts in the femoropopliteal region has been so high that most surgeons no longer advise elective operations for femoropopliteal occlusion. Long-term results with autogenous vein grafts have been much better than those with synthetic prostheses and have renewed the enthusiasm for femoropopliteal bypass operations.[46] However, over two decades of experience have dictated criteria for femoropopliteal surgery which are now rather widely accepted: (1) For symptoms of intermittent claudication alone, surgery should be done only in patients seriously incapacitated and unable to live economically productive lives and who have been tried for at least two months on a program of medical treatment, and (2) surgery is indicated as a limb-salvaging procedure in patients with rest pain, ulceration, or minor gangrene.[47,48]

Sympathectomy Regional sympathectomy is indicated when signs and symptoms of ischemia progress despite adequate medical treatment and revascularization procedures are infeasible or inadvisable. Lumbar sympathectomy does not increase blood flow to muscles and does not relieve intermittent claudication.[49]

Principles of medical management The goals of medical treatment are to stimulate the development of a collateral circulation and to preserve a functional limb; these objectives are accomplished by an exercise program, by prophylactic measures to prevent necrosis of the ischemic skin, by preventing progression of the arterial disease whenever possible, by counteracting the discrepancy between metabolic demands and blood supply of ischemic tissue, by local treatment of ischemic ulcers and gangrene when they are already present, and by relief of ischemic pain.

Prophylaxis There is nothing more important to patients with chronic occlusive arterial disease, regardless of its cause, than careful and detailed instructions concerning the care and hygiene of ischemic extremities. In from 33 to 50 percent of patients who undergo amputation, the initiating factor that led to gangrene was some avoidable injury. It is worthwhile to give each patient with chronic occlusive arterial disease a printed sheet of instructions and to explain them thoroughly. The patient must be warned about the dangers of even minor injuries to ischemic hands or feet. Thermal, chemical, and mechanical trauma should be scrupulously avoided. Only comfortable shoes that do not bind or rub should be worn, and new shoes should be broken in gradually by wearing them about an hour daily. Heat should never be applied directly to ischemic extremities, and the immersion of feet in hot water, a common practice among patients with chronic occlusive arterial disease, is to be strictly condemned. Similarly, exposure to cold temperatures should be avoided unless the patient is warmly attired and the ischemic extremity is adequately protected by proper footwear. Toenails should be cut straight across, and corns, calluses, and bunions should not be trimmed or incised except by physicians or podiatrists who are experienced in the management of ischemic extremities. If the skin is excessively dry and tends to crack or scale, hydrous lanolin or cocoa butter should be applied gently every day. Patent medicines for the treatment of corns, calluses, and athlete's foot should be avoided, for they may contain chemical irritants that can harm the ischemic skin. Adhesive tape or adhesive plasters should not be applied to the skin of ischemic extremities. Dermatophytosis should be treated promptly, since the fissures that are characteristic of this infection can act as the portal of entry for pathogenic bacteria. In the acute stage, dermatophytosis can be treated by soaking the feet for half an hour twice daily in a lukewarm 1:10,000 solution of potassium permanganate. In the subacute stage an ointment or cream containing a reliable fungicide should be applied to the lesions at bedtime, and a powder containing undecylenic acid should be dusted into the shoes before daytime wear.

Methods to prevent progression of arterial disease Tobacco in any form should be forbidden to all patients who have chronic occlusive arterial disease. The close relation between thromboangiitis obliterans and cigarette smoking implicates tobacco as an etiologic agent in this condition, and clinical experience has shown that abstinence from tobacco is the *sine qua non* of treatment, since all other measures usually fail to halt progression of the disease unless the patient abstains totally and permanently from the use of tobacco. Follow-up studies have shown that in both arteriosclerosis obliterans[39] and thromboangiitis obliterans,[7] the incidence of major amputation is greater for patients who continue to smoke than for those who stop smoking. The Framingham Study showed that the occurrence of intermittent claudication was about twice as great among cigarette smokers as among nonsmokers, and the risk tended to increase with the intensity of the habit.[50]

The observed relation between abnormalities of lipid metabolism and atherosclerosis, especially coronary artery disease and arteriosclerosis obliterans,[51] makes it desirable to restrict saturated fat and cholesterol in the diets of patients with arteriosclerosis

obliterans, especially when the serum cholesterol value is elevated. The Atherosclerosis and Epidemiology Study Groups of the Inter-Society Commission on Heart Disease Resources[52] has made the following recommendations for modifications of the diet of persons with atherosclerosis or a marked increase in risk of premature atherosclerotic diseases: (1) adjustment of caloric intake to achieve and maintain optimal weight; (2) reduction of dietary cholesterol to less than 300 mg/day; and (3) substantial reduction of dietary saturated fats, i.e., less than 35 percent of total calories from all fats, with an intake of less than 10 percent of total calories from saturated fats. Unsaturated fats may be used in moderation to replace the portion of saturated fats reduced. If dietary measures fail to reduce the concentration of cholesterol and triglycerides in the serum to reasonably normal levels, lipid-lowering drugs such as clofirate, cholestyramine, dextrothyroxine, and nicotinic acid may be tried. Their effectiveness varies with the type of hyperlipemia present. There is need for further development and evaluation of relatively nontoxic drugs for the lowering of elevated blood lipids. Dietary restrictions are not necessary for patients with thromboangiitis obliterans.

When diabetes is present, it should be adequately controlled to prevent or to ameliorate complications such as infection and neuropathy which add to the problems of the management of arteriosclerosis obliterans.

Methods to increase collateral arterial flow When major arterial trunks are obstructed, any measures that will stimulate development or dilatation of small collateral vessels will increase the arterial blood supply to the ischemic extremity. Although many drugs are advertised as vasodilators, experience has shown that none of them is capable of selectively dilating main arteries or collateral vessels supplying an ischemic extremity.[53,54] When these agents are given in sufficient amounts to cause vasodilatation, the effect is generalized and causes the well-known and predictable physiologic reaction of hypotension, tachycardia, syncope, and even shock. Such a reaction is intolerable and harmful to the patient and of no benefit to an ischemic limb. For these reasons drugs advocated for vasodilatation have no place in the treatment of chronic occlusive arterial disease. Ethyl alcohol (30 to 60 ml whiskey three or four times daily) is an excellent anodyne and sedative, and may be helpful in controlling the pain of the ischemic lesions. It has doubtful significant vasodilating effects. The use of reserpine injected directly into the artery of the affected extremity often works dramatically in vasospastic diseases. Its use in chronic occlusive arterial disease is under study, but the initial results have been disappointing.

A warm environmental temperature tends to promote vasodilatation, whereas exposure to cold may compromise collateral circulation by direct and reflex vasoconstriction. When possible, the hospital room should be maintained at approximately 80°F and the affected limb protected by being wrapped in a blanket or warm, loose, knee-high stocking. Excessive heat, such as that supplied by a heating pad, a hot-water bottle, or a heated foot cradle, causes increased metabolic demands which cannot be met by the already compromised arterial circulation and will increase pain and cause tissue injury; it should be carefully avoided.

During the past 10 years a large bulk of convincing evidence has accumulated which indicates that the most effective treatment for intermittent claudication is physical exercise, particularly walking.[55-59] Maximum walking distances can be at least doubled[59] and often increased severalfold.[55,56] An effective method is to have the patient exercise from 20 to 30 min daily. He should walk to the point of distress, stop, allow the discomfort to disappear, and then walk on again to the point of distress, repeating this exercise for the prescribed period. The resulting decrease in the claudication is often dramatic. Skinner and Strandness[56] have produced evidence to support the theory that exercise increases the collateral circulation, which improves the blood supply to the exercising muscles. Although Alpert et al.[57] demonstrated an increase in calf-muscle blood flow during exercise by the [133]xenon-clearance method, they believe that better coordination of working muscles as well as an increase in number or diameter of collateral vessels is involved in increasing collateral efficiency.

Since the advent of more purified preparations of streptokinase which are less pyrogenic, there has been renewed interest in Europe in the use of this fibrinolytic agent in chronic occlusive arterial disease. Martin and colleagues[60] found streptokinase useful in stenoses of the aorta and common iliac and external iliac arteries and of little use in more distal stenoses. Luminal widening was obtained in 59 percent of common iliac occlusion. On the other hand, Verstraete and coworkers[61] had little success, using a standard dosage scheme, and feel that streptokinase therapy is of limited value in chronic arterial occlusive disease. It is apparent that further work with this agent and other fibrinolytic agents, such as urokinase, is necessary to determine if any material other than fresh clot can be lysed.

At the present time intensive research and large clinical trials are being conducted with agents which influence platelet survival, adhesiveness, and aggregation in both arterial and venous diseases. The role of these agents in chronic occlusive arterial disease has not been elucidated, but perhaps they might be useful as prophylactic agents in the treatment of atheromatous emboli.

A variety of unproved measures have been reported for the treatment of arteriosclerosis obliterans. These include induced hypertension, defibrination with amcrod (Arvin), chelation therapy, and pyridinolcarbamate therapy. None of these attempts at therapy has been shown to be effective, and therefore they are not recommended at this time.

Treatment of ischemic ulcers and gangrene Ischemic ulcers and gangrene are the most feared complications of chronic occlusive arterial disease. Important in the management of these complications are bed rest (with elevation of the head of the bed if edema is not present), relief of pain, eradication of infection, and improvement of the arterial blood supply, if possible. Since ischemic tissues are particularly susceptible to chemical irritants, it is essential to use only bland applications that are not likely to induce more necrosis.

To help eradicate or prevent infection, the affected part may be soaked in a lukewarm solution of 3% boric acid or a mild soap (such as Ivory Snow or Ivory Flakes) or detergent solution (such as Dreft) two or three times daily. The basic principle is to use bland, nonirritating, nonsensitizing solutions. Hexachlorophene should not be used on open ulcers. The temperature of solutions applied to ischemic lesions should never exceed 95°F. A 1:10,000 solution of potassium permanganate may be used to soak the foot when active dermatophytosis is present.

Following soaking, the lesion should be rinsed with clear, lukewarm water, patted dry with a soft towel, and dressed with a clean, dry dressing. A bland nonsensitizing antibiotic ointment, such as erythromycin or gentimycin in a petroleum base, may be used on the ulcer before the dressing is applied.

Cultures of open lesions should be made, and sensitivity studies should be performed on the isolated organisms. Frequently the organisms isolated from ischemic ulcers are multiple, and a dominant organism is difficult to identify. If such an organism is present, appropriate antibiotics are now available to treat most organisms either by mouth or parenterally. During antibiotic treatment the soaks and dressings should be continued.

To remove an adherent, necrotic crust or eschar from an ischemic ulcer, enzymatic debridement has been used, but recently this treatment has been largely abandoned because of local irritation or sensitivity reactions.

In 1967 Pories et al. found patients with arteriosclerosis obliterans to be deficient in zinc, a trace substance, and reported some benefit in symptoms and plethysmographic studies, but not in arteriographic comparisons, in patients treated with zinc.[62] Since that time zinc therapy has been tried for various types of wounds, venous ulcers, and arterial ulcers with inconclusive results.

Relief of pain It is fortunate that intermittent claudication produces only mild and transient discomfort, is relieved promptly by rest, and usually is not a seriously incapacitating symptom. When intermittent claudication becomes a serious handicap and interferes with the earning of a livelihood, arterial reconstructive surgical treatment should be considered.

Management of ischemic rest pain can be one of the most difficult therapeutic problems. Mild ischemic pain can usually be controlled by the judicious use of salicylates. Characteristically, rest pain is worse at night and interferes with sleep. Control of severe rest pain requires use of salicylates in combination with codeine or propoxyphene hydrochloride (Darvon), and not infrequently it is necessary to administer narcotics such as morphine sulfate or levorphanol tartrate (Levo-Dromoran). The latter, in doses of 2 mg every 4 or 6 h with or without chlorpromazine hydrochloride (Thorazine), is particularly helpful, with minimal risk of addiction. Physicians tend to underestimate the severity of ischemic pain and therefore to undertreat it. This is an error, for if uncontrolled, ischemic pain leads to loss of sleep and appetite and may quickly exhaust and demoralize the patient. Furthermore, the pain of ischemia is frequently less severe if the foot is dependent; hence in order to sleep the tortured victim usually resorts to sitting in a chair or dangles the painful limb over the edge of the bed. To avoid this the patient should be told to elevate the head of the bed 6 to 8 in. on blocks (or a suitable substitute). This may keep him sufficiently pain-free to allow him to stay in bed. The physician should not hesitate to use enough narcotic to permit the patient to sleep comfortably in bed. If edema is present due to prolonged dependency, tissue perfusion is further compromised, and the bed should be leveled and the patient given adequate analgesia to relieve his pain.

Individualization of therapy In planning therapy for an individual patient, the stage of the disease and the degree of ischemia must be taken into consideration, for not every patient requires all the forms of treatment outlined in the preceding paragraphs. Every patient with chronic occlusive arterial disease should be admonished to stop smoking and should receive explicit instructions in the proper care and hygiene of ischemic extremities. Beyond this, treatment should be individualized for each patient.

When the only symptom is intermittent claudication and when collateral circulation is good as demonstrated by postural color tests, the patient should be encouraged to walk to tolerance several times daily, and to follow a diet restricted in saturated fat. Routine use of vasodilating drugs for patients in this category is to be deprecated.

Bed rest is indicated for patients with ischemic rest pain, and the head of the bed should be elevated unless edema is present. As stated, relief of pain is extremely important, and narcotics should be given if necessary.

When ulceration and gangrene occur, treatment for these complications should be given as outlined previously, in addition to the measures described in the preceding paragraph.

Direct revascularization procedures are indicated in the following situations: (1) in the patient with incapacitating intermittent claudication whose lesion is in the aortoiliac areas; if the patient is in otherwise good health, a good result is to be expected; (2) in the patient with severe intermittent claudication whose lesion is in the femoropopliteal area but only after a 2- to 3-month trial on a structured walking program; approximately 50 percent of these procedures will fail within 5 years; (3) in the patient who has severe ischemia (rest pain; ischemic ulcers) when possible, as a limb-salvaging procedure.

Amputation When the blood supply to an extremity is reduced to a degree insufficient to support tissue viability, resulting in irreversible gangrene, nonhealing ulcers, or intractable pain, and when reconstructive surgery is not possible, or fails, amputation is indicated. Preservation of the knee, whenever possible, is of great importance in rehabilitation of the amputee.[63] This is especially true in the older patient who may be debilitated and weak, and have poor balance, poor vision, and chronic systemic disease. There are no specific tests available which will determine the lowest possible amputation level at which healing will occur. Burgess and Romano[63] recommend that, unless it is clearly evident that a through-knee or above-knee amputation will be required, the leg should be prepared for both below-knee and above-knee amputations. The final decision as to level can be quickly made once the incision for below-knee amputation is made.

Since the introduction of the immediate postoperative prosthesis by Weiss of Poland at the Sixth International Prosthetics Course in 1963, this method has become widely used, and many workers have reported great success with early healing and early rehabilitation following below-knee amputations. Burgess and Marsden reported successful healing of below-knee amputations in 75 percent of patients amputated following a failed arterial reconstruction and in 83 percent of those who had had no reconstruction, a difference not statistically significant.[64] These impressive results justify the recommendation that when amputation is necessary, a below-knee operation be carried out whenever possible. The enthusiasm for the rigid prosthesis and immediate ambulation has waned somewhat among vascular surgeons because of stump failure, and various modifications of this technique have been advocated. A review of various amputation methods, dressings, and rehabilitation programs has been set forth in the recent comprehensive report of the Amputation Subcommittee of the Inter-Society Commission for Heart Disease Resources.[65] It should be stressed that a trained prosthetic team consisting of a surgeon, a prosthetist, and a psychiatrist is necessary for optimum results.[63] Digital and transmetatarsal amputations are more likely to succeed when ischemia is due to thromboangiitis than when it is due to arteriosclerosis.

Acute arterial occlusion of the extremities

When a major artery to an extremity suddenly becomes occluded, survival of the patient as well as of the limb often depends on prompt and intelligent management.

ETIOLOGY

The two most common causes for sudden occlusion of a peripheral artery are embolization and thrombosis in situ. Emboli originate within the cardiac chambers in approximately 80 to 90 percent of reported cases.[66,67] Rheumatic mitral valvulitis with subsequent enlargement of the left atrium, acute myocardial infarction, and chronic congestive heart failure from any cause predispose to the formation of mural thrombi within the left ventricle or left atrium, which may become detached and lodge as emboli in peripheral arteries. The presence of atrial fibrillation enhances the likelihood of formation of mural thrombus but is not an essential prerequisite. Cardiac surgical procedures such as excision of ventricular aneurysm, valve replacement, and occasionally coronary bypass surgery may be complicated by systemic embolism. Peripheral embolism arising from a valve or the left atrium may occur as a late complication of prosthetic valve replacement. The incidence of embolic phenomena has dropped markedly in recent years as the result of the introduction of less thrombogenic valves and the use of anticoagulants. Recent reports cite an incidence of 5 to 6 percent.[68] Intriguing but rare is the *paradox embolus,* which arises from a venous thrombus and is transported to the peripheral arterial circulation through a septal defect with a right-to-left shunt. Usually one or more previous pulmonary emboli have set the stage for the paradoxic embolus by increasing the blood pressure in the pulmonary circuit and right side of the heart, thereby creating a right-to-left shunt through an otherwise asymptomatic atrial septal defect. The most common peripheral site for lodging of an embolus is the bifurcation of the common femoral artery (45 percent), followed by an iliac artery (19 percent), a popliteal artery (14 percent), the aorta (9 percent), and the axillary and brachial arteries (6 percent).[66] Unusual types of embolism sporadically reported are those of bullets, catheters, other foreign bode consisting of atheromatous debris from a diseased aorta may be responsible for the sudden appearance of small areas of cutaneous gangrene on the feet and toes.[14]

Sudden local thrombosis in an artery usually occurs at the site of an atherosclerotic plaque. Sometimes sudden arterial thrombosis is the first clinical manifestation of peripheral atherosclerosis, but more often it occurs as an unexpected complication of symptomatic arteriosclerosis obliterans.[69] Occasionally acute arterial thrombosis occurs as a complication of thromboangiitis obliterans, polyarteritis nodosum, polycythemia vera, lupus erythematosus, and scleroderma. Thrombosis may occur suddenly in arteries with no intimal disease, presumably because of a hypercoagulable state of the blood, resulting from such abnormal physiologic states as dehydration, anemia, hypotension, stress, or stasis. This type of *primary,* or *simple,* arterial thrombosis may complicate acute infectious diseases, carcinomatosis, chronic ulcerative colitis, congestive heart failure, or any chronic debilitating disease.

The evidence that peripheral arterial thrombosis may occur as the result of the use of oral contraceptives is meager and consists of scattered case reports. More time and further study is necessary to clarify this issue.

Dissecting aneurysm of the abdominal aorta occasionally presents as acute arterial occlusion of one or both of the lower extremities. The rare syndrome of entrapment of the popliteal artery by the medial head of the gastrocnemius muscle, a developmental anomaly of young men, may result in popliteal artery thrombosis.[26] The anterior compartment syndrome or extensive soft-tissue injury to any fascial compartment can result in compression and thrombosis of the arteries contained within the compartment as the result of hemorrhage or edema.[70]

PATHOLOGY

Sudden interruption of blood flow through a major artery to an extremity results in acute ischemia of the tissues supplied by the diseased artery. If adequate collateral circulation is present, recovery without permanent residual is possible. In the absence of collateral circulation, however, ischemia may progress to necrosis and gangrene, with loss of a portion of the extremity. In the majority of cases of sudden arterial occlusion, the involved limb will survive, but residual ischemic changes will have impaired its function. Ischemic neuropathy is a frequent sequela of sudden arterial occlusion, as is intermittent claudication. Necrosis of the muscles in the anterior compartment of the leg (anterior compartment syndrome) is an uncommon but important residual of sudden arterial occlusion, leading to foot drop.[70] When ischemia is severe, venous endothelium is damaged, and the signs and symptoms of ischemic thrombophlebitis appear 2 or 3 days after the acute ischemic insult. When this occurs, the extremity becomes swollen; the resulting pressure on collateral vessels compromises the circulation even further and worsens the prognosis for ultimate recovery.

PATHOLOGIC PHYSIOLOGY

When a major arterial trunk to an extremity becomes occluded, the distal tissues must be nourished by collateral vessels, and the adequacy of the collateral circulation determines the eventual outcome. Initially there is usually reflex arterial spasm involving the main trunk proximal and distal to the site of occlusion as well as the small collateral channels. If the spasm is prolonged, endothelial damage occurs in the arterial tree, favoring deposition of thrombus in collateral channels and thereby diminishing the prospects for recovery. However, when the collateral channels remain patent and are reasonably adequate, it is unlikely that irreversible ischemia will occur. Spontaneous improvement with return of pulsations in major arteries shortly after arterial occlusion may occur through one of two mechanisms:

1 Sudden occlusion of a branch of a main arterial channel can give rise reflexly to spasm in the parent artery for a few minutes or hours, giving the clinical impression that a main arterial trunk has been occluded. When the spasm abates, the major arterial pulses can be felt, and the clinical picture improves rapidly, since occlusion of branch arteries or of one of two paired arteries (such as the anterior and posterior tibial and the radial and ulnar arteries) rarely leads to irreversible ischemia and gangrene. Krause and colleagues[71] have questioned the role of arterial spasm in sudden arterial occlusion.

2 Endogenous fibrinolysin may be responsible for dramatic clinical improvement within the first few minutes or hours after sudden occlusion of major arterial trunks. Lysis may permit fragmentation of a large embolus, the resulting fragments being swept by the bloodstream to more distal sites in the extremity. Arterial pulsations in the large arteries suddenly return, and the extent and severity of ischemia diminish rather abruptly.

CLINICAL MANIFESTATIONS

Diagnosis of sudden arterial occlusion is usually correctly made in the presence of the typical clinical picture characterized by acute onset of pain, coldness, numbness, and hypesthesia of the involved extremity. In half the cases of sudden arterial occlusion, however, pain is not the initial symptom, and the onset is gradual. In 25 percent of cases, pain is entirely absent. In these patients the only symptoms may be numbness and coldness, and sometimes the only clinical manifestation of sudden arterial occlusion may be the abrupt appearance or worsening of intermittent claudication. Paresis is almost never the presenting complaint; if it occurs, it usually appears several hours after other symptoms of ischemia have been present. The sudden onset of ischemic symptoms simultaneously in both lower extremities suggests the possibility of an embolus that has lodged at the bifurcation of the aorta (saddle embolus) or acute aortic thrombosis. The most important physical sign in establishing the diagnosis of sudden arterial occlusion is the absence or severe impairment of pulsations in arteries that were known or were assumed previously to have had palpable pulses. The diagnosis of sudden arterial occlusion of a major arterial trunk is untenable if arterial pulsations are normal throughout the extremity. The acutely ischemic extremity appears pale or cyanotic and is cold and hypesthetic or anesthetic, and the superficial veins are collapsed. In the later stages muscular weakness can sometimes be demonstrated.

DIAGNOSIS

When pain, paresthesia, numbness, and coldness, singly or in various combinations, appear either abruptly or over a period of several hours in an extremity with absent or diminished arterial pulsations, the diagnosis of sudden arterial occlusion should be made. The high frequency of atypical and often undramatic symptoms probably explains the observation that the clinical diagnosis of sudden arterial occlusion is suggested in less than half the patients with this condition. It is advisable routinely to palpate the pulses of any symptomatic extremity. If pulsations are normal, it is safe to assume that symptoms are not due to acute ischemia except in those rare cases when arterial occlusion has occurred distal to the wrists or ankles as in atheromatous embolization or arteritis associated with collagen diseases. In these cases small areas of digital gan-

grene may appear abruptly when all arterial pulsations are normal.

Once the diagnosis of sudden arterial occlusion is established, it is important to determine the level of the occlusion and to differentiate, if possible, between embolus and thrombosis in situ. Emboli usually lodge at bifurcations where the caliber of the artery is suddenly reduced. The site of the occlusion is peripheral to the most distal point at which normal pulsations are noted and proximal to the line at which the temperature of the skin changes from low to normal and to the zone of hypesthesia. Changes in temperature, color, and sensation may be minimal or absent when only one of two paired arteries is involved. When sudden arterial occlusion occurs in the presence of overt heart disease, especially if atrial fibrillation is present, it most likely is due to embolization. Recent myocardial infarction should be considered in every patient with acute arterial occlusion; therefore a careful history and an electrocardiogram should be obtained. When arterial occlusion occurs in the course of chronic occlusive arterial disease and in the absence of overt heart disease, it can usually be attributed to thrombosis in situ. When both these predisposing factors are present or when both are absent, an exact etiologic diagnosis may not be possible, but fortunately medical therapy of the ischemic limb is the same, regardless of whether thrombosis or embolism has caused the ischemia.

DIFFERENTIAL DIAGNOSIS

It is axiomatic that sudden arterial occlusion per se never produces edema, and this is helpful in differentiating this condition from acute thrombophlebitis. The simultaneous disappearance of arterial pulsations and onset of symptoms of ischemia are helpful in differentiating sudden arterial occlusion from osteoarthritis, peripheral neuropathy, lumbar disk protrusion, and other local conditions that cause pain and/or paresthesia in the extremities. When the status of the peripheral pulsations previous to the onset of symptoms is not definitely known, reliance must be placed upon other signs of acute ischemia, such as pallor or cyanosis of the skin, coolness of the involved extremity, and collapse of the superficial veins, and upon specific diagnostic methods such as angiography.

PROGNOSIS

Without treatment acute arterial occlusion (embolism and thrombosis) results in gangrene in about 50 percent of cases.[72] Approximately 40 percent of patients with untreated sudden arterial occlusion die, because most of them are elderly and have serious cardiovascular disease.[72]

Since the advent of effective vascular surgery, it has not been possible to compare the prognosis in patients treated conservatively with those submitted to surgery, because the former have either mild ischemia or are too ill to withstand surgery while the latter have severe ischemia and are reasonable surgical risks. There seems little doubt that since the discovery and use of anticoagulants on a long-term basis the prognosis is better for survival of both life and limb because of the prevention of recurrent thromboembolism.[73] The introduction of the balloon catheter for extraction of thrombi and emboli by Fogarty and Cranley[74] was a revolutionary advance in surgery for acute arterial occlusion. This relatively simple procedure, which can be done under local anesthesia, if necessary, has significantly increased the limb salvage rate and somewhat lowered the mortality rate, although this remains high in all current reported series. In reports since 1970 limb salvage varies from 79 to 95 percent and mortality from 12 to 27 percent.[45,66,67] In spite of the use of anticoagulants and the balloon catheter, mortality remains high, especially in patients who have arteriosclerotic heart disease as the source of the emboli. Embolic occlusion of the aorta or the iliac or common femoral arteries is associated with a high mortality compared with occlusions of the arteries of the upper extremities or below the knees.[66,75] Stallone et al.[75] found the high-operative-risk group to be composed of elderly patients with massive lower extremity ischemia. A study of the mechanism of death in these patients showed a high proportion of pulmonary complications that were believed to be secondary to embolism of platelet-fibrin aggregates and gross thrombi arising from the venous side of the ischemic vascular bed. They recommend exploration of both the artery and the vein during embolectomy and heparinization postoperatively. Although prognosis for limb survival is somewhat worse when sudden arterial occlusion is due to thrombosis than when it is due to embolism,[72] the site of the occlusion has an even greater bearing on the outcome. Prognosis for survival of an upper extremity is far better than that for a lower extremity, and the prognosis for survival of a lower limb is worst when the aorta or common iliac artery is occluded; the prognosis becomes increasingly better as the site of occlusion becomes more distal.[66]

TREATMENT

Embolectomy, thromboendarterectomy, or bypass graft is the treatment of choice if the site of occlusion is proximal to the popliteal artery, if the ischemia is severe, if irreversible ischemic changes have not already taken place, and if the condition of the patient is good enough to make the risks acceptable. Unfortunately most of the patients who have embolic arterial occlusion are victims of serious heart disease, and the risk of embolectomy, even under local anesthesia, is considerable. Surgical treatment for sudden arterial occlusion, which is discussed in another chapter, may be successful after many hours have elapsed.[71]

As soon as the diagnosis of sudden arterial occlusion has been made, heparin sodium should be administered intravenously without delay, unless there are strong contraindications to its use. Even though surgical treatment is being considered, it is advisable to maintain anticoagulation until shortly before the operation is started. If the coagulation time is unduly prolonged, the effect of heparin can be neutralized immediately before operation with protamine sulfate. For prompt anticoagulant effect, aqueous heparin should be administered intravenously (100 units per kilogram of body weight), either by intermittent

injection or by continuous drip, and this dose may be repeated every 4 h. A coumarin anticoagulant can be administered as soon as it is decided that the patient is not to undergo surgical treatment, and the treatment with heparin can be discontinued when the prothrombin time is within the therapeutic range. It should be emphasized that anticoagulant therapy is contraindicated if sudden arterial occlusion is caused by dissecting aneurysm or by atheromatous embolization.[14]

In addition to anticoagulation, relief of pain and of arterial spasm are urgent considerations in the management of sudden arterial occlusion. Narcotics are often needed to relieve pain and should be given in adequate doses as often as necessary. A warm environmental temperature is one of the best measures to relieve arterial spasm, and so the patient should be placed in a room where it is possible to keep the temperature between 80 and 85°F. In addition, it is often advisable to wrap the involved extremity loosely in cotton to preserve body heat and to protect it from trauma.

The blocking of appropriate sympathetic ganglions has been advocated in the treatment of sudden arterial occlusion. This should be done before heparin is administered and should not be repeated while effective anticoagulation is being maintained, because of the danger of bleeding at the sites of injection. Anticoagulation is more important in the management of sudden arterial occlusion than is regional sympathetic denervation, and for this reason anticoagulant drugs should not be withheld for the purpose of blocking sympathetic ganglions safely.

The head of the bed should be elevated on blocks that are 8 or 10 in. high, so that the feet are in a dependent position and the effect of gravity will augment the flow of blood into the ischemic extremity.

Various vasodilator drugs to be used intravenously or directly into the affected artery proximal to the occlusion have been advocated, but there is no evidence that they produce any lasting benefit.

The efficacy of activated fibrinolysin or its activating enzyme (streptokinase) in the treatment of sudden arterial occlusion has not been proved but is being actively investigated and is most promising. If these agents are to be employed, they should be used in addition to conventional anticoagulation therapy, not instead of it. The roles of hyperbaric oxygen and of low-molecular-weight dextran (Rheomacrodex) in the management of sudden arterial occlusion have not been definitively evaluated, but it would appear that the latter holds more promise in the treatment of acute arterial occlusion than in the treatment of chronic occlusive arterial disease.

In patients with systemic arterial emboli a search for the source should be made because recurrence is common. Mitral stenosis and ventricular and arterial aneurysms can be surgically corrected. An attempt can be made to convert atrial fibrillation to normal sinus rhythm. When the source of embolism cannot be eliminated, the patient should be placed on long-term oral anticoagulation therapy in an attempt to prevent future emboli.

There is some evidence that drugs which prevent platelet aggregation, such as aspirin or dipyridamole, may be of value in preventing arterial thrombosis.[76]

Refrigeration of an ischemic extremity is contraindicated as long as there is hope for its survival. When amputation is obviously inevitable but the general condition of the patient makes the procedure hazardous, valuable time can be gained, pain can be relieved, and the absorption of toxins stopped by packing the gangrenous extremity in ice. Refrigeration can be maintained for several days while the patient is being prepared for amputation.

It is worth reemphasizing that elevation of an acutely ischemic extremity and the application of heat to it are contraindicated and may hasten the onset of gangrene.

Arterial trauma

Arterial trauma is an acute surgical emergency. In all injuries, whether penetrating or blunt, including fractures and dislocations, a vascular examination should be performed. Any patient with an obvious or suspected vascular injury who is examined by a physician who is not an expert in this area should be referred immediately to a vascular surgeon or, if none is available, to a general surgeon. This is essential since time is of critical importance. The patient should *not* be observed for possible subsidence of arterial spasm. If an extremity is pulseless, an arteriogram and vascular repair are probably indicated. If the extremity is cold and pale, this is further evidence of severe ischemia. Sensory and motor changes may be misleading because of concomitant nerve injury. Failure to repair an arterial injury may result in the amputation of an extremity which otherwise could be salvaged by arterial reconstruction. If the patient is fortunate enough to escape amputation, delay may result in a false aneurysm, an arteriovenous fistula, or chronic ischemia with intermittent claudication.

The delayed onset of ischemia can result from blunt trauma, especially in those injuries involving a closed compartment, because of the compressive effect of tissue swelling. The patient with such injuries should be continuously and closely observed, because a fasciotomy or fibulectomy to decompress a closed compartment, such as the anterior tibial or posterior tibial compartments in the leg, may avoid severe ischemia, necrosis, and amputation.[77] For details concerning the diagnosis and treatment of vascular injuries, the reader is referred to the literature on vascular surgery.

Iatrogenic arterial injury, especially thrombosis, resulting from brachial or femoral artery catheterization for diagnostic purposes or cardiac bypass operation has become recognized as a definite complication of these procedures and should be routinely looked for following the procedure.[78] The incidence of occlusion following arterial catheterization may seem insignificantly low, but the actual numbers are significant in the light of the number of catheterizations being done. Meaney[79] reports 13 occlusions after 5,000 percutaneous transfemoral arteriograms, an incidence of 0.26 percent.

Catheterization of a brachial artery requires exposure of the artery, the performance of an arteriotomy in order to insert the catheter, and closure of the arterial incision at the end of the procedure. Consequently, there is more trauma to the artery, and the incidence of loss of wrist pulses and ischemia sufficient to require repair is higher than in percutaneous procedures. At the Cleveland Clinic Foundation, of 19,295 retrograde brachial catheterizations done between 1964 and 1970, wrist pulses were absent in 2.7 percent following the procedure. Of these, 58 patients (0.3 percent) required surgical correction.[80] The most current data (July 1976) reveal the thrombosis rate of 2.7 to be the same after 53,000 catheterizations (unpublished statistics). Of these, approximately 25 percent have ischemia sufficiently severe to require surgical repair. It is now the policy to do immediate rather than delayed thrombectomy, especially in young and active patients, because the procedure is simple and highly successful. When done later, more complicated procedures, such as autogenous vein bypass, are usually necessary.[80]

Another more recently recognized cause of arterial injury is that which is self-inflicted by users of drugs. This occurs as a result of accidental injection into an artery or because the arterial route of injection is necessary since all available veins have thrombosed.[81] A less common cause of arterial injury is traumatic occlusion of the superficial palmar arch as a result of using the palm of the hand as a hammer, as in loosening a vise or pounding a hubcap in place, or other types of repeated blunt trauma to the hand (hypothenar hammer syndrome).[1]

Peripheral and visceral arterial aneurysms

Arterial aneurysms may be classified as true aneurysms, false aneurysms, dissecting aneurysms (dissecting hematomas), and arteriovenous aneurysms (arteriovenous fistulas). Aneurysms of the thoracic and abdominal aortae and dissecting aneurysms are discussed in Chap. 103.

TRUE ANEURYSMS

True aneurysms are localized dilatations of arteries which result from atrophy of the media; they may be fusiform or saccular.

Etiology Most arterial aneurysms are arteriosclerotic. Syphilitic aneurysms have seldom been encountered since the advent of penicillin. When they do occur, they are almost always located in the ascending portion or the arch of the thoracic aorta. Mycotic aneurysms are also rare. Trauma sometimes results in true aneurysmal formation, especially in the thoracic aorta, but usually trauma causes false aneurysms rather than true aneurysms. Studies of large series of aneurysms indicated that 75 percent of femoral aneurysms[82] and more than 99 percent of popliteal aneurysms[83] were arteriosclerotic in origin.

Clinical manifestations Arteriosclerotic aneurysms occur predominantly in men, usually after the age of 50 years. They are frequently multiple,[84] so that discovery of one aneurysm should stimulate the search for others.

The most common site for peripheral aneurysms is the popliteal artery. Popliteal aneurysms produce symptoms of acute arterial occlusion if mural thrombus abruptly propagates to occlude the artery or if it gives rise to emboli distally. Popliteal aneurysms also may cause pain in the popliteal region when they become large enough to exert pressure on the medial popliteal nerve and will cause edema and venous distension if the popliteal vein is compressed. The diagnosis usually is made easily by palpating a pulsating, expansile mass in the popliteal space. When thrombosis of the aneurysm has occurred, a firm, nonpulsatile mass may be felt. In doubtful cases, femoral arteriography may be helpful, but usually it is not necessary. Most aneurysms of the femoral artery are easily palpable just above or below the inguinal ligament. Like aneurysms of the popliteal artery, they can suddenly cause signs and symptoms of ischemia in the lower extremity because of acute thrombosis within the aneurysm or embolization of mural thrombi. Aneurysms of the iliac artery usually produce no symptoms until they rupture. Diagnosis can be made by palpating an expansile, pulsatile mass in the abdomen above the inguinal ligament. Aneurysms may also occur in the brachiocephalic (innominate), subclavian, femoral, radial, and ulnar arteries. The appearance of pulsatile masses in these regions is a clue to diagnosis.

Visceral aneurysms are rare and usually asymptomatic until they rupture. Hypertension associated with aneurysms of the renal artery is usually mild unless there is associated occlusive disease of the renal arteries. Hematuria is sometimes the only clue to a renal artery aneurysm (Fig. 104-4). Splenomegaly may be a sign of aneurysm of the splenic artery. The diagnosis may be suggested by plain roentgenograms of the abdomen when circular areas of calcification

are visualized. Visceral aneurysms not containing calcium will cast no shadows on the plain roentgenograms. Aortography has led to greater awareness of visceral aneurysms that sometimes are found incidentally when this procedure is carried out for other diagnostic purposes. Splenic and renal aneurysms are the exception to the rule that aneurysms are usually arteriosclerotic and occur predominantly in men. Stanley and Fry[85] reported that women made up 80 percent of their patients with splenic aneurysms, and the underlying pathologic change was medial degeneration and medial changes thought to be gestational in origin. Nearly 55 percent of patients with large aneurysms of the renal artery were women.[86] Microaneurysms are a consistent pathologic feature of medial fibroplasia of the renal artery, which sometimes causes hypertension in young women.[87] The triad of abdominal pain, gastrointestinal hemorrhage, and jaundice should suggest the diagnosis of aneurysm of the hepatic artery.[88] Epigastric pain (sometimes radiating to the back), nausea, and vomiting are symptoms produced by celiac aneurysms. The diagnosis of visceral artery aneurysms is confirmed by angiography, which is a safe procedure and should be employed whenever abdominal symptoms cannot be satisfactorily explained.[89]

Prognosis Rupture is an uncommon complication of popliteal and femoral aneurysms, but these aneurysms often lead to amputation because of arterial occlusion from thrombosis within the aneurysm or distal embolization. Complications developed in 31 percent of 87 popliteal aneurysms that were initially asymptomatic and were not treated surgically. Complications led to amputation in 3.5 percent of these cases.[83] Complications arising from untreated femoral artery aneurysm led to amputation in 16 percent of 44 patients.[82] Rupture of iliac aneurysms occurred

FIGURE 104-4 Right renal artery aneurysms. *A.* Plain roentgenogram reveals two circular areas of calcification. *B.* Translumbar aortogram demonstrates a saccular aneurysm in a primary branch of the renal artery; the uppermost area of calcification does not opacify with contrast medium, presumably owing to thrombosis within the aneurysm.

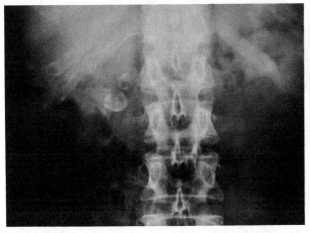

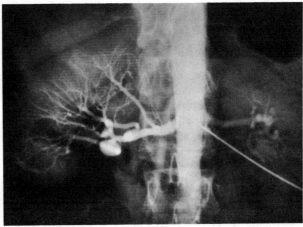

in 16 percent in one series, with an 80 percent mortality rate associated with rupture.[90]

Although there are numerous reports of rupture of aneurysms of the splenic, celiac, and hepatic arteries, it seems reasonable to assume that aneurysms which rupture are more likely to be reported than are asymptomatic aneurysms discovered incidentally. As a matter of fact, most visceral aneurysms are asymptomatic and will escape detection unless they rupture. The true incidence of rupture is, therefore, impossible to determine.

Treatment Surgical extirpation with appropriate arterial reconstruction is the treatment of choice for most aneurysms of peripheral arteries if the patient's condition is good enough to permit operation. Splenic and renal aneurysms are particularly likely to rupture during the third trimester of pregnancy, and for this reason routine resection is recommended only in women of childbearing age. There is insufficient knowledge of the natural history of aneurysms of the celiac and hepatic arteries to justify any statement regarding the necessity for resection of these lesions. In general, the appearance of symptoms heralds the rupture of an aneurysm, and the indication for operation becomes accordingly urgent. Surgical treatment of aneurysms is discussed in Chap. 107.

FALSE ANEURYSMS

False aneurysms result from rupture of true aneurysms or from penetrating trauma to an artery. The clinical manifestations are similar to those of true aneurysm, consisting of an expansile, pulsatile mass. On the basis of clinical history it may be possible to suspect that an aneurysm is false rather than true, but only a pathologic diagnosis can distinguish the two; the distinguishing feature of the false aneurysm is the break in continuity of all three coats of the arterial wall, permitting the extravascular accumulation of blood in adjacent tissues. The wall of the false aneurysmal sac is therefore composed of a mixture of organized blood clot and dense connective tissue. Clinically, the diagnosis and management of false aneurysms are the same as those already described for true aneurysms.

ARTERIOVENOUS ANEURYSMS (ARTERIOVENOUS FISTULAS)

Arteriovenous fistulas are abnormal, direct communications between arteries and veins without the interposition of capillaries. There are two types: acquired and congenital. The hemodynamic effects of peripheral arteriovenous fistulas are discussed in Chap. 91; consequently, only the peripheral manifestations will be described here.

Acquired arteriovenous fistulas Acquired arteriovenous fistulas result from penetrating trauma or from erosion of an arterial aneurysm into the accompanying vein and usually consist of a single communication between an artery and vein that lie in close proximity. If the arteriovenous fistula is near the surface, a pulsatile mass is palpable. The diagnostic features of an arteriovenous fistula are the continuous thrill and bruit over it. Obliteration of the fistula by manual compression of it or its afferent artery is usually followed promptly by a sharp decrease in pulse rate (Branham's bradycardiac sign). The skin overlying an arteriovenous fistula is unusually warm, and, because of increased venous pressure, there may be signs of chronic venous insufficiency, with incompetent varicose veins, in the extremity distal to the fistula. Arterial supply to the extremity may be compromised, and the ipsilateral foot or hand is usually cooler than the opposite normal mate.[91] Ischemic ulcers as well as stasis ulcers may occur on the extremity beyond the fistula.

Arteriography is essential for diagnosis only for those fistulas that are situated so deeply that the pulsatile mass, thrill, and bruit cannot be detected.

The only satisfactory treatment is excision of the fistula, with restoration of arterial continuity whenever possible.

Congenital arteriovenous fistulas Congenital arteriovenous fistulas are usually multiple and involve small cutaneous and subcutaneous arteries and veins. Frequently they are accompanied by prominent birthmarks on the skin of the extremity. Congenital fistulas of this type lead to elongation of the long bones of the affected extremity and thus to a measurable lengthening of the entire limb when compared with the uninvolved companion extremity (Fig. 104-5). In the acquired type, these bony changes do not occur unless the fistula is acquired during the period

FIGURE 104-5 Elongation of the right lower extremity of a 5-year-old boy caused by multiple congenital arteriovenous fistulas.

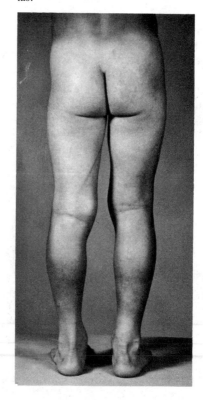

of bone growth. The skin of the extremity harboring congenital arteriovenous fistulas is frequently warmer than the skin of the opposite extremity. Signs of chronic venous insufficiency, including edema, dilated superficial veins, varicosities in atypical locations, and stasis pigmentation with or without stasis ulceration, are frequently associated with congenital arteriovenous fistulas because of increased venous pressure. Because the fistulas are small and multiple, thrills and bruits are seldom detected, and there are no localized pulsatile masses.

Arteriography is sometimes helpful in establishing the diagnosis of congenital arteriovenous fistulas. Congenital arteriovenous fistulas have been classified as microfistulous (in which the arteriovenous communications cannot be demonstrated by angiography) and macrofistulous (in which the communications are readily demonstrable).[92] An increased oxygen content of the venous blood from the involved limb as compared with that of the opposite limb is a pathognomonic sign of arteriovenous fistula.

Treatment of congenital arteriovenous fistulas is not satisfactory, since usually it is impossible to eradicate the numerous small abnormal arteriovenous communications.[92] Ligation of arterial branches that lead to the fistulas may give partial relief. The use of an elastic bandage or stocking is advisable to prevent edema and the other complications of chronic venous insufficiency.

Arteriospastic diseases

Acrocyanosis, livedo reticularis, and Raynaud's phenomenon result from spasm of small arteries and arterioles in the skin and subcutaneous tissues without actual organic occlusion. Although they usually occur separately, two of these conditions and sometimes all three may occur concomitantly.

ETIOLOGY

The cause of arteriospasm, which is the common denominator of these three conditions, is unknown. Patients with Raynaud's phenomenon or primary Raynaud's disease have, on the average, significantly smaller total and capillary blood flow in the fingers, in both warm and cold environments, than do normal subjects.[93,94] Concentrations of epinephrine and norepinephrine in venous blood coming from the hands of patients with Raynaud's phenomenon are not greater than those found in normal subjects. Mendlowitz and Naftchi[95] found no evidence of increased sensitivity to the vasoconstricting action of norepinephrine in patients with Raynaud's disease and concluded that in some patients with this condition an increased vasomotor tone is responsible, while in others there is intrinsic vascular disease with normal vasomotor responses. Increased blood viscosity and red blood cell aggregation have been found in patients with Raynaud's phenomenon.[96]

CLINICAL MANIFESTATIONS

Typically, the arteriospastic disorders affect young women who are nervous, easily fatigued, emotionally labile, and often unmarried. The clinical manifestations are localized to the skin of the extremities and

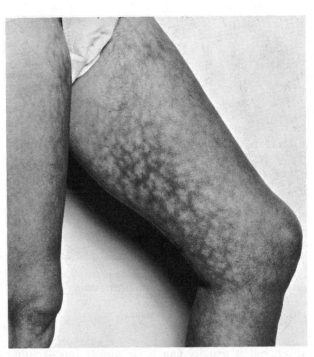

FIGURE 104-6 Mottled, reticulated cyanosis of livedo reticularis involving the thigh and to a lesser extent the leg. *(From R. W. Gifford, Jr., Arteriospastic Disorders of the Extremities, Circulation, 27:970, 1963. Reproduced by permission of the American Heart Association, Inc.)*

are characterized by changes in color and temperature. The location, appearance, and duration of the color changes are important in making a differential diagnosis of the arteriospastic disorders.[97] In addition to the typical color changes of the skin, the hands and feet may be chronically cold and often tend to perspire excessively.

Acrocyanosis is the rarest and most innocuous of the arteriospastic disorders. The arteriospasm is persistent and is confined to the hands and/or feet; as a result they are chronically cyanotic. The cyanosis tends to be less severe in a warm environment, but it usually does not disappear entirely and is a source of embarrassment to the patients, who are usually young women. Major arterial pulsations are always palpable, although at times it is necessary to have the patient in a warm environment to demonstrate them. The absence of clubbing and of cyanosis elsewhere, as well as the lack of heart murmurs and of other signs of heart disease, serves to distinguish this benign condition from cyanotic heart disease. The prognosis is excellent, inasmuch as gangrene and other complications of ischemia never occur.

Livedo reticularis, a common condition, is characterized by mottled or reticulated cyanotic discoloration of the skin (Fig. 104-6). Livedo reticularis not only involves the hands and feet but may extend onto the arms and legs and, in some cases, is apparent on the buttocks and the trunk. The reticulated, or fishnet, pattern of cyanosis is more notable when the patients are in a cold environment or are emotionally

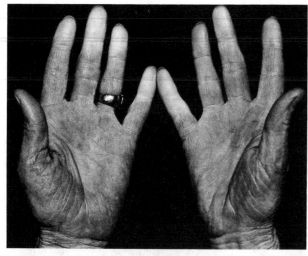

FIGURE 104-7 Pallor phase of Raynaud's phenomenon involving the fingers. *(From R. W. Gifford, Jr., Arteriospastic Disorders of the Extremities, Circulation, 27:970, 1963. Reproduced by permission of the American Heart Association, Inc.)*

TABLE 104-1

Causes of secondary Raynaud's phenomenon: Conditions to be ruled out before diagnosis of Raynaud's disease (primary Raynaud's phenomenon) can be made

1 Occlusive arterial disease
  a Arteriosclerosis obliterans (10% of patients demonstrate Raynaud's phenomenon)
  b Thromboangiitis obliterans (30% of patients demonstrate Raynaud's phenomenon)
2 Systemic diseases
  a Systemic scleroderma
  b Rheumatoid arthritis
  c Systemic lupus erythematosus
  d Periarteritis nodosa
3 Trauma
  a Pneumatic tools
  b Raynaud's phenomenon in typists and pianists
  c Occupational occlusive arterial disease of the hand (mechanics, butchers, creamery workers, gynecologists, farmers, plumbers, etc.)
4 Occupational acro-osteolysis (Raynaud's phenomenon and osteolysis of distal phalanges of fingers in workmen involved in vinyl chloride polymerization process; it is probably the result of a combination of chemical and physical insults and personal idiosyncrasy)
5 Neurogenic lesions
  a Thoracic outlet syndromes (scalenus anticus syndrome, hyperabduction syndrome, costoclavicular syndrome)
  b Diseases of nervous system (multiple sclerosis, peripheral neuropathy, transverse myelitis, syringomyelia, hemiplegia, myelodysplasia, causalgia, and spinal cord tumors)
6 Intoxication
  a Lead
  b Arsenic
  c Ergot
7 Drug ingestion (ergotamine preparations, methysergide, propranolol)
8 Abnormalities of blood
  a Cryoglobulins
  b Macroglobulins
  c Cold agglutinins
9 Late result of cold injury
  a Trench foot
  b Immersion foot
  c Frostbite
10 Primary pulmonary hypertension
11 Occult carcinoma

upset, but it usually can be demonstrated to some degree at all times. Cutis marmorata is simply intermittent livedo reticularis that appears only when the patient is in a cool environment and disappears when he is warm. Livedo reticularis usually does not cause pain unless ischemic ulceration of the skin occurs. Pulsations are normal in the peripheral arteries, provided that the patient is in a warm environment. Livedo reticularis may be primary, in which case it exists in the absence of any underlying or causative disease, or it may be secondary to such conditions as systemic lupus erythematosus, periarteritis nodosa, cryoglobulinemia, or cholesterol embolization from an abdominal aortic aneurysm. Primary, or idiopathic, livedo reticularis infrequently leads to complications and is usually only cosmetically objectionable to the patient. Secondary or symptomatic livedo reticularis sometimes results in ischemic ulcerations at the tips of the digits or in the malleolar areas. The ischemic ulcerations resulting from livedo reticularis may be difficult to heal, but amputation is seldom, if ever, necessary.

Raynaud's phenomenon is characterized by intermittent changes in color of the skin of the fingers and/or toes (Fig. 104-7). The change in color persists for only a few minutes at a time. Rarely is the entire hand or foot affected, and often only one or two digits at a time are involved. Typically the affected digits turn dead white (pallor phase), after which they become cyanotic (cyanotic phase). Before normal color returns to the affected parts, they may become excessively hyperemic (rubor phase) because of reactive vasodilatation. Raynaud's phenomenon can occur without the rubor phase, but pallor and/or cyanosis must be present before the diagnosis of Raynaud's phenomenon is tenable. The color changes of Raynaud's phenomenon are usually induced by exposure of the affected extremity or the entire body

to a cool or cold environment. Occasionally the typical color changes occur when the patient is emotionally upset, and sometimes they occur for no obvious reason.

Raynaud's phenomenon is often secondary to some disease or condition that may not be clinically obvious at the time when the vasospastic phenomena first appear. Some of the diseases or conditions that may manifest Raynaud's phenomenon as a symptom are listed in Table 104-1. Among the most common causes of secondary Raynaud's phenomenon are rheumatoid arthritis, systemic lupus erythematosus, and systemic scleroderma. Indications that Raynaud's phenomenon may be secondary to some underlying disease include onset after the age of 50 years, especially in men; unilateral Raynaud's phenomenon, especially when confined to one or two digits; rapid progression to ulceration shortly after onset of symptoms; extensive ulceration or gangrene; and presence of fever, systemic symptoms, anemia, and elevation of sedimentation rate of erythrocytes. When one or more of the peripheral arterial pulses are reduced in amplitude or are not palpable in the symptomatic extremity or when Allen's compression test is positive (Fig. 104-2), the physician should suspect that Raynaud's phenomenon is secondary to chronic occlusive arterial disease, such as arteriosclerosis obliterans, thromboangiitis obliterans, or chronic occupational trauma of the hand.[97]

The diagnosis of primary Raynaud's phenomenon, or Raynaud's disease, cannot be made until the diseases and conditions listed in Table 104-1 have been ruled out. Allen and Brown[98] proposed the following criteria for establishing the diagnosis of primary Raynaud's disease: (1) episodes of Raynaud's phenomenon excited by cold or emotion; (2) bilaterality of Raynaud's phenomenon; (3) absence of gangrene or, if present, its limitation to minimal grades of cutaneous gangrene; (4) presence of normal pulsations in the palpable arteries; (5) absence of any other primary disease that might be causal (see Table 104-1); and (6) duration of symptoms for at least 2 years (to permit any occult underlying disease to become manifest).

Extensive gangrene does not occur as a complication of Raynaud's disease, and major amputations never are necessary. In a large series of patients with Raynaud's disease, fewer than 30 percent had complications and less than 1 percent required amputation of one or more phalanges.[99] The chief complications are sclerodactylia, which refers to sclerodermatous changes that remain confined to the skin of the digits (in contradistinction to progressive involvement of systemic scleroderma), and trophic changes, such as ulceration, superficial necrosis, scarring, and fissuring of the tips of the digits, or chronic paronychia.

The prognosis for patients with secondary Raynaud's phenomenon depends on the underlying disease and may be quite dismal in regard to survival and cutaneous necrosis. The importance and difficulties of correct differential diagnosis are illustrated by the fact that of 220 patients with systemic scleroderma, 81 percent had Raynaud's phenomenon as a symptom, and in 32 percent it was the initial manifestation.[100] Nearly 50 percent of these patients were dead after an average follow-up period of 9 years, and 40 percent of them had trophic ulcerations of their fingers as a result of their disease. On the other hand, of 307 women with primary Raynaud's disease whose progress was followed for an average period of 12 years after the diagnosis was established, only 12 died, and none of the deaths was due to Raynaud's disease.[99] In less than 10 percent of these patients ischemic ulcerations of the fingers developed during the period of follow-up.

TREATMENT

Most patients with acrocyanosis, livedo reticularis, or Raynaud's disease require no specific treatment other than reassurance that the condition is benign and will not lead to major amputation, as so many of them fear. They should be advised to avoid unnecessary exposure to cold and to wear warm clothing as well as gloves whenever they go out in cool or cold weather. They should avoid defrosting refrigerators. Patients with Raynaud's disease should avoid mechanical and chemical trauma as much as possible. Repeated exposure of the hands to water and detergents leads to drying and fissuring of the skin. Patients with Raynaud's disease should be advised to apply an emollient such as lanolin to the fingers at least twice daily, oftener if the hands are exposed to water and detergents. These precautions are not so necessary for patients with acrocyanosis and livedo reticularis, since dryness and fissuring of the skin are less likely to occur in these conditions.

Vasodilating drugs are not necessary routinely in the management of any of these diseases. If symptoms are unusually severe, phenoxybenzamine hydrochloride (Dibenzyline) may be administered in doses of 0.01 or 0.02 g three or four times daily. Often the side effects of vasodilating drugs are more troublesome than the disease itself. If phenoxybenzamine hydrochloride is not well tolerated, cyclandelate (Cyclospasmol) may be administered in doses of 0.1 or 0.2 g three or four times daily. Reserpine in doses of 0.5 or 1.0 mg injected directly into the brachial artery has been reported to give relief from symptoms of Raynaud's disease for a few days to several months in some patients.[101] Reserpine may also be given orally in doses of 1 mg daily.

Sympathectomy may be beneficial in all these conditions. Since acrocyanosis is primarily a cosmetic defect that never leads to complications, sympathectomy is seldom if ever advisable. When livedo reticularis is complicated by ischemic ulcerations, sympathectomy may be helpful in healing them and keeping them healed. Sympathectomy should be advised for patients with Raynaud's disease when conservative measures fail to prevent or to control ischemic ulcerations at the tips of the digits. Experience has shown that less than 25 percent of patients with Raynaud's disease require sympathectomy and that it is beneficial in about two-thirds of the patients who have this operation.[102] The results are much better in the lower extremities than in the upper, where the disease is usually much more severe. Sympathectomy for secondary Raynaud's phenomenon has yielded such poor results that it should be recommended only in unusual circumstances.[102]

Treatment of ischemic ulcerations secondary to livedo reticularis or Raynaud's disease is similar to that already discussed for ulcerations secondary to chronic occlusive arterial disease. The affected part should be soaked in a lukewarm saturated solution of boric acid for $1/2$ h three or four times daily. Appropriate antibiotics should be given systemically after cultures of the ulcers have been made and sensitivities determined. Local applications of a 1% solution or ointment of neomycin sulfate may be helpful in eradicating organisms resistant to the usual antibiotics. When ischemic ulcerations are present, the patient should not be permitted to use the involved hand until after it has healed.

Erythermalgia (erythromelalgia)

Erythermalgia is among the rarest of the syndromes included under the general term peripheral vascular disease. In contrast to the arteriospastic diseases, the primary fault in erythermalgia appears to be excessive vasodilatation, occurring in the hands and/or feet.

ETIOLOGY

The mechanisms and pathogenesis are poorly understood. During the attacks of pain that characterize this syndrome, the arteries of the involved part are dilated, but it appears that the pain is related more to skin temperature than to increased blood flow per se.[103]

CLINICAL MANIFESTATIONS

In approximately 60 percent of patients erythermalgia exists as a primary disease; in the others it is a symptom of other diseases, notably polycythemia vera and hypertension.[104] Erythermalgia may precede other clinical manifestations of polycythemia vera by as much as 16 years.[105] In contrast to primary erythermalgia, which affects men more often than women and may occur at any age, the secondary form affects the sexes equally and occurs almost invariably after the age of 40 years. In primary erythermalgia the distress tends to be more severe, to involve a larger area of the extremity, and to be symmetric in distribution more often than in the secondary type.[104]

DIAGNOSIS

Clinically erythermalgia is characterized by paroxysms of burning pain in the hands and/or more often the feet. During the painful paroxysms, the parts are red and objectively as well as subjectively warm. Relief is obtained by exposing the affected extremities to cold air or by immersing them in cold water. It must be emphasized that erythermalgia is an extremely rare condition, although many people complain of burning pain of the hands or feet. In differentiating between erythermalgia and burning paresthesia of the extremities, which may imitate erythermalgia, the important finding is the presence or absence of *objective* warmth of the affected part during the episodes of pain. In most cases of burning paresthetic pain, as well as in patients with angiokeratoma corporis diffusum (Fabry's disease) who frequently complain of burning pain in the extremities, the affected part is actually cool.

In establishing the diagnosis of erythermalgia, studies of skin temperatures are essential. By using thermocouples on the digits it is possible to establish a *critical* skin temperature, which usually is in the range of 32 to 36°C. When the temperature of the skin is above this critical level, the patient experiences the burning pain; when it is below this level, the pain is absent or rapidly subsides. Burning pain due to other causes is not so definitely related to a critical skin temperature.

TREATMENT

Patients learn from experience to avoid warm environmental temperatures and to wear perforated shoes or sandals. Treatment should be directed to the underlying disease when erythermalgia is secondary. Salicylates are helpful in controlling the symptoms of either the primary or secondary type of erythermalgia. For reasons that are not apparent, one dose of aspirin (0.65 g) may prevent attacks of pain for several days in some cases. When the pain is resistant to salicylates, ephedrine sulfate (0.024 g) may be administered three or four times daily. Methysergide maleate (Sansert), 0.002 to 0.008 g daily, has been reported to relieve the symptoms of primary erythermalgia.

Cold injury

In addition to the arteriospastic diseases that are aggravated but not necessarily caused by exposure to cold temperatures, there is a group of conditions that can be attributed directly to cold exposure.

Exposure to cold may result in freezing of tissue (frostbite) or in injury without actual freezing (pernio syndromes, immersion foot, trench foot, or mild frostbite). Relatively short exposure to subfreezing temperatures is responsible for freezing injuries; the colder the temperature, the shorter the exposure necessary to produce tissue damage. Relatively prolonged exposure (usually several days) to dampness and cold above the freezing point is necessary for production of immersion foot or trench foot. Although chronic pernio is classified as a nonfreezing injury, exposure to cold need not be prolonged, since patients affected with this syndrome seem to manifest unusual susceptibility to cold.

Freezing of extracellular fluid results in hypertonicity of the extracellular compartment, and this in turn leads to dehydration and destruction of cells.[106] Contributing to tissue destruction is sludging and actual coagulation of blood in the arteries, veins, and capillaries of the exposed parts. The mechanism of tissue damage in nonfreezing cold injury is not so well understood; it may simply be a slow metabolic strangling due to reduced blood flow and direct inhibiting effect of the cold on metabolic processes and exchange of metabolites.[106,107]

NONFREEZING INJURY

Chronic pernio is characterized clinically by the development of superficial ulcers that occur in crops over the lower third of the leg and on the ankles, feet, and toes. They begin as small erythematous papules or nodules, which then break down into superficial ulcers with a hemorrhagic base surrounded by a violaceous border. Healing ordinarily is spontaneous in from 3 to 5 weeks, leaving pigmented and often depressed scars, but new lesions may appear as the older ones heal. The lesions result from actual necrosis of the skin, because of a combination of spasm and endothelial proliferation of the arterioles and small arteries. The lesions appear after exposure to cold, although the temperature need not be excessively low nor the exposure prolonged. Apparently individual hypersusceptibility to cold is a major factor. Although at first the lesions occur during the winter months only, in some cases the relation to the seasons may be less pronounced as time goes on. Protection from cold is the most important facet of treatment. When ulcers occur, the patient should be put to bed and treated with applications of local dressings of a saturated solution of boric acid. Vasodilating drugs such as phenoxybenzamine or cyclandelate are sometimes helpful. Sympathectomy may be necessary in intractable cases.

Immobility in the dependent position and dampness are important contributing factors in the development of trench foot and immersion foot, which are characterized by three clinical stages: During the initial stage of exposure the feet become edematous and painful. Later, hypesthesia or even anesthesia may supervene. Violaceous ulcers similar to those of chronic pernio may appear. The second stage occurs after the patient has been removed from the cold and placed in a warm environment. Reactive hyperemia occurs, and the foot becomes red and warm. Swelling increases unless the foot is elevated. Hyperesthesia and burning, throbbing pain are characteristic. Arterial pulsations are full and bounding, and hemorrhagic blebs, infarcts in the skin, ulcers, and even superficial gangrene may appear. Following this phase, which lasts for several days or weeks, the chronic phase of arterial spasm and ischemia appears. The extremities are chronically cold, cyanotic, and hyperhydrotic. Secondary Raynaud's phenomenon may occur; when severe, this chronic stage may greatly handicap the patient, because even mild degrees of cold produce distressing paresthesia and pain.

The use of proper footwear to keep the feet dry and warm will prevent this syndrome or will minimize the chronic disability from it. During the period of exposure it is important to elevate the feet as often as possible to reduce edema. In the hyperemic stage the legs should be elevated and kept at room temperature. Local and systemic measures to prevent infection or to combat it if it is present are indicated. Treatment of the chronic arteriospastic, ischemic phase frequently is ineffective. Protection of the feet from cold is important, as is abstinence from tobacco. Vasodilating drugs, mild heat, light massage, and sympathectomy have been helpful in some cases.

As a result of the Vietnam conflict, a new syndrome of "warm-water-immersion foot" has been described in combat soldiers in warm environmental temperatures who went for several days without being able to dry their feet. The feet became white, wrinkled, and so painful that walking was difficult if not impossible. No permanent disability resulted. Insulated boots have failed to protect volunteers from developing symptoms when the feet were kept immersed in water for prolonged periods,[108] whereas a protective silicone grease applied to the skin has been an effective prophylactic measure.[109]

Acute pernio (acute chilblains) is similar to, and sometimes indistinguishable from, first-degree frost-

bite. Although the inciting exposure is usually to subfreezing temperatures, it is doubtful that the tissues are actually frozen, and hence these two conditions are properly included with the nonfreezing cold injuries. During or immediately after exposure, the exposed parts, usually the hands, nose, ears, or shins, become bluish red and slightly swollen, and they burn or itch. The injured part is susceptible to infection; treatment consists of immediate warming to room temperature and prevention of infection by protection of the inflamed skin with sterile dressings and administration of antibiotics.

FREEZING INJURY
Frostbite may be classified according to the degree of severity: (1) First-degree frostbite has been discussed in the previous paragraph, since it is unlikely that actual freezing of tissue occurs in the mild form. (2) Second-degree frostbite is characterized by the formation of blebs, or vesicles, in the skin of the region affected. (3) Third-degree frostbite results in necrosis of subcutaneous tissue. (4) Fourth-degree frostbite results in gangrene with loss of an extremity or portion of an extremity. The extent of tissue loss is directly related to the depth of temperature and duration of cold exposure.[110] Contact with metal or wetness enhances tissue loss for any given temperature and duration of exposure. Alcoholism and emotional instability are important predisposing factors to frostbite, but these factors do not influence the extent of tissue destruction.[110] Initially, the affected part appears pale or waxy yellow; it is objectively anesthetic, but frequently is subjectively pruritic. Affected parts frequently remain hypersensitive to cold for long periods after the initial insult, and secondary Raynaud's phenomenon may appear. Frostbite is best treated by rapid thawing.[111] Preferably the part should be immersed in a water bath at a temperature not exceeding 105°F for at least 20 min or until all tissues show flushing to the distal nailbed and volar pad. Hexachlorophene may be added to the bath to prevent infection. After thawing, the injured part should be thoroughly but gently cleansed with a mild soap and water. Since infection is the greatest danger during the recovery phase, strict isolation and aseptic nursing care should be carried out until the blebs have dried. The blebs should be allowed to remain intact, since they protect the denuded underlying surface from bacterial invasion. A whirlpool bath using water at body temperature has been helpful at this stage. Vasodilating drugs and anticoagulants have not been consistently beneficial. It has been reported that sympathectomy performed promptly during the acute phase hastens resolution of skin lesions and minimizes the frequency and severity of late sequelae.[112] An experiment using rabbits has shown that intravenous administration of low-molecular-weight dextran (M.W.40,000) immediately after a standardized cold injury reduced the area of necrosis compared with that observed in

control animals.[113] Sympathectomy, however, was more effective than dextran. Gangrene from cold injury often is superficial and frequently appears to be worse than it actually is. For this reason decision about amputation should be postponed for several weeks until the true extent of necrosis can be adequately evaluated.

DISEASES OF VEINS

Thrombophlebitis

In the past, there has been some confusion in the use of the terms phlebitis, phlebothrombosis, and thrombophlebitis. *Phlebitis* would indicate inflammation of a vein with no accompanying thrombus. However, phlebitis cannot exist very long without inciting thrombus formation on the inflamed endothelium. *Phlebothrombosis* would indicate a venous thrombosis with no inflammation in the vein wall. Some inflammatory reaction of the venous intima usually does occur, however, even though it is so minimal that it cannot be detected clinically. Consequently the term *thrombophlebitis,* which indicates the existence of both thrombosis and inflammation, is preferable to the others, although from the standpoint of pathogenesis and clinical behavior it should be recognized that thrombosis is the most common initiating factor.

ETIOLOGY

In most patients, venous thrombosis arises during the course of another illness. Stasis, hypercoagulability, and injury of the endothelium of the vein are the most important factors in the etiology of thrombophlebitis. Venous stasis is an important factor in postoperative, postpartum, and varicose thrombophlebitis as well as in the thrombophlebitis which complicates prolonged bed rest for any chronic illness, congestive failure, or trauma. Hypercoagulability of the blood may play a major role in thrombophlebitis associated with malignant disease and blood dyscrasias, as well as in idiopathic thrombophlebitis. Endothelial injury appears to be the predominant factor in thrombophlebitis associated with thromboangiitis obliterans (Buerger's disease), in septic thrombophlebitis, and in thrombophlebitis resulting from direct trauma to veins, including intravenous injections and indwelling catheters.

It is likely that multiple etiologic factors are present in most patients with thrombophlebitis. For example, direct trauma to veins (endothelial injury) and release of tissue thromboplastin (hypercoagulability) at the time of laparotomy may combine with prolonged bed rest, inadequate hydration, and hypotension following surgical treatment (venous stasis) to produce postoperative thrombophlebitis. It should not be forgotten, however, that the majority of venous thromboses occur in patients with medical disease, including myocardial infarction, chronic congestive heart failure, cancer, and ulcerative colitis.

Clinical and autopsy studies indicate an almost linear increase of thrombophlebitis with increasing age. Again this association is probably related to multiple factors such as decreased mobility, slow return to ambulation after bed rest, dilatation of the veins of the lower limbs that would produce venous stasis, and a higher association of cancer and heart disease.

The controversy regarding the relation of oral contraceptive drugs and thromboembolic phenomena, both venous and arterial, as well as other medical aspects of oral contraceptives is summarized in a review by Elgee.[114] The statistical evidence suggests that oral contraceptive agents, especially those containing estrogen, increase the risk of thromboembolic problems. However, a review of prospective and retrospective studies by Drill[115] found no increase in thromboembolic complications when oral contraceptives were used. In view of these and other conflicting reports, it would seem reasonable at present to follow the advice of the Food and Drug Administration which states that oral contraceptives are contraindicated in "patients with thrombophlebitis, thromboembolic disorders, cerebral vascular disease, myocardial infarction or coronary thrombosis, or with a past history of these conditions."

PATHOLOGY

Hume, Sevitt, and Thomas[116] emphasize the point that available evidence suggests that venous thrombi, unlike arterial thrombi, probably develop on normal endothelium. They postulate a pathogenesis whose key is the local generation of thrombin, with its dual ability to aggregate platelets and to transform fibrinogen into fibrin. They believe that the coagulation process starts in the valve cusps, where local venous stasis allows the accumulation of activated clotting factors which would otherwise be removed from the circulation. The resultant generation of thrombin, combined with a local silting of platelets, causes a platelet thrombus to form. This grows by local deposition of successive layers of fibrin and aggregated platelets. When this propagating thrombus occludes the vein, retrograde thrombosis occurs in a manner similar to the clotting of blood in a test tube.

Wessler et al.[117] have also stressed the therapeutic importance of differentiating the red fibrin thrombus of venous thrombi from the white platelet thrombus of arterial thrombi. Conventional anticoagulant therapy should be of value in red thrombi, but are of little use in white thrombi.

Histologically, numerous red blood cells trapped in a fibrin mesh may dominate the picture, but the layering phenomenon characterizes most venous thrombi. The layering consists of red blood cell masses, laminated between seams of fibrin, leukocytes, and platelets. Organization can also be seen at the points of attachment of the thrombus to the vein intima. If the underlying process is thromboangiitis obliterans, a very extensive panphlebitis will be found with cellular infiltration and fibroblastic proliferation involving the thrombus, the vein wall, and the perivenous tissues.

The greater the inflammatory reaction of the vein, the sooner the thrombus will become securely attached to the intimal surface and the less will be the chance for embolization. Only the "tail" of the fresh thrombus is likely to become detached and give rise to pulmonary embolism. If it does not become detached, however, it will usually undergo lysis or become organized and firmly adherent within 24 to 48 h after its formation, thus markedly reducing the risk of embolization. However, propagation of organized or organizing thrombi may occur, giving rise to another loosely attached tail that once again places the patient in jeopardy of pulmonary embolism.

The term *chronic thrombophlebitis* is a misnomer, since healing inevitably takes place once the acute inflammatory reaction has subsided. Recanalization of the organized thrombus usually occurs, restoring patency of the lumen within a period of a few weeks.

PATHOLOGIC PHYSIOLOGY
Because of the abundant collateral venous channels, there is usually little functional disturbance as a result of thrombophlebitis unless major venous trunks, such as the iliofemoral, axillary, or subclavian veins are completely occluded by thrombus. When these major veins are obstructed, there is passive congestion with elevation of venous pressure distally in the involved limb. This causes cyanosis and visible distension of veins. Although the limb becomes swollen, there initially is no pitting edema, since the swelling results almost entirely from the

increased intravascular volume. Eventually the increased venous and capillary pressure leads to increased transudation of fluid into the extravascular compartment, with the formation of pitting edema. Usually arterial blood supply is unaffected. In the rare instance of massive iliofemoral thrombophlebitis (phlegmasia cerulea dolens), a mechanical arterial insufficiency results because of the complete obstruction of the venous tree. With this unusual exception, thrombophlebitis does not lead to tissue necrosis.

CLINICAL MANIFESTATIONS
The clinical findings in thrombophlebitis vary with the site and extent of the venous involvement. From the standpoint of clinical behavior, prognosis, and therapy it is helpful to consider superficial thrombophlebitis and deep thrombophlebitis separately (Table 104-2).

Superficial thrombophlebitis Since the thrombus in superficial thrombophlebitis is in a superficial subcutaneous vein, it can be seen and felt, making the diagnosis easy in most patients. A tender, indurated cord that extends for various distances can be felt along the vein. During the acute stage, redness, local heat, and tenderness are prominent features.

TABLE 104-2
Summary of clinical characteristics of thrombophlebitis

Clinical classification	Usual causes	Usual location	Clinical findings	Edema of extremities	Embolization	Chronic venous insufficiency
Superficial	Varicose veins Direct trauma I.V. injections Thromboangiitis obliterans Malignant disease Blood dyscrasias Idiopathic	Saphenous veins and their tributaries Forearm	Tender, red, inflamed induration along course of subcutaneous vein (visible and palpable)	Almost never	Almost never	Almost never
Deep: Small veins and	Postoperative Pre- and postpartum Direct or distant trauma Congestive heart failure Prolonged bed rest Acute febrile disease Sepsis Debilitating disease Malignant disease Blood dyscrasias	Soleal Posterior tibial, other deep calf veins Popliteal Pelvic (see text)	Tenderness to deep pressure Induration of overlying muscle Minimal or no venous distension	Occasional	Always a threat	Usually not
Major venous trunks	Systemic lupus erythematosus Pressure of tumors on veins Oral contraceptive (anovulatory) drugs(?) Idiopathic	Femoral Iliac Inferior or superior vena cava Axillary Subclavian	Swelling Cyanosis Venous distension of limb with mild to moderate pain Tenderness over involved vein (groin or axilla)	Usual	Always a threat	Frequently

The thrombus usually remains palpable for several days or weeks after the inflammatory component subsides. Fever is minimal or absent, and there is no systemic reaction. Most importantly, no generalized edema of the extremity should occur. The most common cause of superficial thrombophlebitis in the arm is intravenous injection of irritating solutions. The most common cause in the legs is thrombophlebitis involving varicose veins. The unexplained appearance of superficial thrombophlebitis in a young man would suggest the possibility of thromboangiitis obliterans. In the middle-aged or older person, superficial thrombophlebitis, especially if it is of the recurrent type, should suggest occult malignancy. Superficial thrombophlebitis involving longitudinal veins of the anterolateral aspect of the thorax (including the breasts in women) is a benign condition that has been given the eponym of *Mondor's disease.*

Differential diagnosis of superficial thrombophlebitis includes all types of inflammatory nodular lesions of the extremities. These include erythema nodosum, erythema induratum, nodular vasculitis, periarteritis nodosa, chronic pernio, and nonsuppurative panniculitis. Usually these lesions are globular, and some of them eventually ulcerate. Typically, the lesion of superficial thrombophlebitis is linear, not globular, extends along the course of a subcutaneous vein, and does not ulcerate. In questionable cases however, biopsy is necessary.

Deep thrombophlebitis It must be emphasized that deep thrombophlebitis of the calf often goes unrecognized clinically simply because of the paucity of signs and symptoms. For this reason, a presumptive diagnosis of deep calf thrombophlebitis should be made whenever a patient complains of swelling, pain, or tenderness in the calf after operation, trauma, or childbirth, or during the course of any severe debilitating illness. The diagnosis is more certain if the signs and symptoms are unilateral. Since many collateral channels are present, edema and venous distension rarely result from calf thrombophlebitis, although the calf muscles may be somewhat indurated. Local calf tenderness may be the first positive sign. Typically, the tenderness is elicited more consistently by fingertip compression into the belly of the calf muscles in an anteroposterior direction. Homans' sign (pain in the calf induced by forcible dorsiflexion of the foot) is not a reliable diagnostic aid since it is absent in about half of patients with phlebographic evidence of venous thrombosis and is present in many conditions other than venous thrombosis.

When deep thrombophlebitis occurs in a major venous trunk such as the iliofemoral, axillary, or subclavian veins, a typical clinical picture usually results because of the passive congestion of the extremity. The entire extremity over a period of several hours becomes swollen and mildly to moderately painful and has a reddish cyanotic hue. The skin is warm, superficial veins are distended, and there is tenderness along the course of the involved vein in the groin or axilla. When iliofemoral thrombophlebitis results from extension of calf thrombophlebitis, the calf and popliteal space are tender also. Temperature rarely exceeds 101°F and is usually lower. There may be moderate malaise. Chills should not be present. Subclavian thrombophlebitis may result from unusual use of the arms, especially involving work overhead (effort thrombophlebitis), or from direct trauma to the extremity. Iliofemoral thrombophlebitis is usually a postoperative, postpartum, or posttraumatic complication. When the inferior vena cava is involved, both legs are swollen and cyanotic. If one or both renal veins also become obstructed, the nephrotic syndrome may occur. When the superior vena cava is obstructed, both upper extremities as well as the face and neck become swollen and cyanotic. For a detailed discussion of thrombosis and/or obstruction of the inferior and superior vena cava, see Chap. 103.

Phlegmasia cerulea dolens is an unusually extensive thrombosis of the iliofemoral vein and most of its tributaries. This usually occurs abruptly with sudden, massive swelling and intense cyanosis of the extremity. Shock may result from trapping of blood in the swollen extremity. Gangrene may ensue when the massive venous thrombosis mechanically blocks the flow of blood to the extremity.

In the differential diagnosis of iliofemoral and axillary-subclavian thrombophlebitis, acute cellulitis, lymphangitis, and lymphedema should be considered. Lymphedema usually appears gradually and progresses slowly, so that for the first few weeks or months edema occurs on the dorsum of the foot and around the ankle during the day and disappears at night. Only later in the course of the disease is the entire extremity swollen. There is no accompanying venous distension, no evidence of inflammation, no discoloration, and no elevation of venous pressure. Cellulitis and lymphangitis are usually accompanied by a higher temperature (103°F or higher) and a more profound systemic reaction (chills, nausea, vomiting, and malaise) than is iliofemoral or axillary-subclavian thrombophlebitis. The extremity may become swollen rather abruptly in both thrombophlebitis and cellulitis, but in cellulitis the skin is erythematous and not cyanotic, there is more local heat in the involved extremity, red streaks of lymphangitis may be present, and regional lymph nodes may be enlarged and tender. Iliofemoral thrombophlebitis is sometimes confused with sudden arterial occlusion. Pain accompanying sudden arterial occlusion is usually more prominent and more severe than that produced by iliofemoral thrombophlebitis. In addition, other distinguishing features in arterial occlusion include absence of edema, absence of arterial pulsations, coolness and pallor of the skin, collapsed superficial veins, and various degrees of hypesthesia.

When thrombophlebitis recurs without obvious cause, the physician should exclude occult malignancy (often in the lung, female genital tract, or pancreas), blood dyscrasias, and systemic lupus erythematosus before making the diagnosis of idiopathic recurrent thrombophlebitis.

Thrombophlebitis involving pelvic veins occurs after childbirth and following operative procedures on the pelvic viscera. Except for low-grade fever, symptoms are absent unless pulmonary embolism occurs or unless the thrombus extends to the common iliac vein to produce the clinical findings of iliofemoral thrombophlebitis already described. Although asymptomatic pelvic thrombophlebitis may be the source of some postpartum and postoperative pulmonary emboli that occur in the absence of signs of peripheral thrombophlebitis, the majority of such emboli probably arise in the calf veins. The advent of antibiotics has sharply reduced the incidence of septic thrombophlebitis that rather commonly occurred in the uterine venous plexus after induced abortions or as a complication of parturition.

DIAGNOSTIC AIDS

When the clinical diagnosis of deep thrombophlebitis is uncertain, several procedures are available to help clarify the situation. The technique of phlebography was revived in this country by DeWeese and Rogoff[118] and is still one of the most valuable procedures in detecting venous thrombi. In the experience of most workers, embolism has not occurred as a result of phlebography, thrombosis resulting from the injection of contrast material is uncommon, and local complications such as cellulitis are minimal. Premedication and slower injection can decrease the pain accompanying the pressure distension of the veins during the intravenous administration of the contrast medium. Limitations of this procedure include inadequate visualization of the soleal venous sinuses, the anterior tibial veins, the profunda femoris system, and the iliofemoral system. These limitations can be minimized by using modifications on the original techniques such as those suggested by Athanasoulis.[119]

Localization of propagating venous thrombi by injecting ^{125}I-fibrinogen is a very sensitive screening method for venous thrombi in the legs. Limitations of this method include the fact that it is not reliable when hematomas or healing wounds are present in the extremity, it is unable to detect venous thromboses in the upper femoral and iliac regions, it cannot differentiate superficial from deep phlebitis, and there is a slight chance of inducing hepatitis since fibrinogen requires preparation from pooled plasma.

The Doppler-effect flowmeter has been described in detail by Strandness[120] and others, and appears to provide useful evidence of patency of the accessible veins such as femoral, popliteal, or posterior tibial. However, it does not detect clot when only tributary veins are involved and when patent collateral veins are present. Error may also arise from improper positioning of the probe or by emptying the veins by gravity or a compression bandage. It seems most useful as a screening procedure, particularly in recent thromboses involving the femoral vein.

The technique of impedance phlebography has been extensively studied and reported by Wheeler[121] and others. This is a noninvasive method of monitoring changes in blood volume which normally occur with deep breathing, but which are diminished in patients with venous thrombosis. This is a promising method with good correlation with phlebography. The best results reported to date with regard to

both sensitivity and specificity are by Cranley and associates[122] with their phleborheographic technique. It is hoped that other investigators will apply this method and report their results.

Other methods including blood tests, thermography, and measurements of venous pressure have less clinical usefulness at the present.

COMPLICATIONS

The major complications of thrombophlebitis are pulmonary embolism, chronic venous insufficiency, and postphlebitic neurosis.

The most feared, because of its lethal potentialities, is pulmonary embolism. The manifestations of pulmonary embolism are discussed in Chap. 75. It is worth noting that many cases of fatal embolism are not associated with clinical evidence of thrombosis in the extremities. Borgström and associates[123] totaled the figures from a number of published series and found that thrombosis was not clinically apparent in 71.6 percent of 1,477 fatal cases of embolism. Mavor and Galloway[124] reported that the legs were without evidence of thrombosis in 46 out of 119 patients with pulmonary embolism. It seems reasonable to conclude that at least half of the cases of fatal embolism occur in patients without clinically evident venous thrombosis. In addition there must be many nonfatal and subclinical pulmonary embolic episodes in the large number of patients in whom venous thrombi are present but not suspected.

Chronic venous insufficiency, a common sequela of deep thrombophlebitis, will be discussed subsequently.

Postphlebitis neurosis is often iatrogenically induced. Most patients in whom this complication develops are apprehensive women who have been kept in bed for unnecessarily long periods for treatment of thrombophlebitis and who, through careless statements or implications on the part of physicians, nurses, or friends, acquire the misconception that their veins harbor "clots" which may suddenly break loose and "go to the heart or brain." The involved extremity remains inordinately painful and tender, and the patients refuse to bear weight on it or walk normally. Successful treatment depends on the physician's ability to convince the patient that the danger of embolism is no longer present and to outline a program of progressive rehabilitation.

PROPHYLAXIS

Prophylactic measures include avoidance of blood loss, shock, and dehydration during surgery, and early ambulation postoperatively. Also helpful are leg exercises, the use of elastic stockings, and elevation of the foot of the bed 15° above horizontal following surgery. A clinical trial of electrical stimulation of the calf during surgery by Doran and White[125] resulted in an impressive decrease in thrombosis in the stimulated leg. This finding was confirmed by Rosenberg and Pollock[126] and others. The use of intermittent pneumatic compression with inflatable boots to prevent deep venous thrombosis has also produced encouraging results.[127]

The evidence that low-dose heparin (5,000 units subcutaneously every 8 to 12 h) can prevent deep venous thrombosis in most postoperative patients without producing excessive bleeding is irrefutable, as shown in a review of several studies by Hirsh and Genton.[128] The fact that this regimen also reduces death from pulmonary embolism was documented by an international multicenter trial reported by Kakkar.[129] This form of prophylaxis can now be recommended in "high risk" patients who are at bed rest for any reason or who are undergoing major surgery. Those patients who are predisposed to the development of thrombophlebitis would include those with a history of venous thrombosis and pulmonary embolism, and especially those who have evidence of chronic venous insufficiency or varicose veins, elderly patients, obese patients, patients with carcinoma, women on birth-control pills, and patients who are bedridden with a stroke, fractured hip, myocardial infarction, or congestive heart failure. Surgical procedures that particularly predispose to the development of postoperative thrombophlebitis include splenectomy, pelvic operations, extensive intestinal resections for carcinoma, and prosthetic hip replacements.

Oral anticoagulants can be given to prevent thrombophlebitis. In the surgical patient, therapy should be started 2 to 3 days prior to operation, strict laboratory control is mandatory, and the risk of hemorrhage is always present.

The ability to prevent the initial platelet nidus, on which a large clot eventually develops, is an exciting area for investigation. The studies reviewed by Clagett and Salzman[130] indicate that while dextran and hydroxychloroquine sulfate seem to be effective in preventing venous thromboembolism, dipyridamole is ineffective, and the results with aspirin are controversial.

TREATMENT

Bed rest with elevation of the involved extremity is usually advisable until tenderness subsides, but only in unusual circumstances should the patient be kept in bed for more than 7 to 10 days. Warm, moist packs are helpful in alleviating pain and hastening resolution of the inflammatory process. Salicylates are usually all that is necessary to relieve pain in the first 2 or 3 days, but occasionally propoxyphene hydrochloride (Darvon) (0.032 to 0.065 g every 4 to 6 h) or codeine sulfate (0.032 to 0.065 g every 4 to 6 h) may be necessary. If pain is severe, phenylbutazone (Butazolidin) (0.1 g four times daily for 3 to 5 days) is remarkably effective in relieving pain and hastening the resolution of the inflammatory reaction.

Anticoagulant drugs are seldom indicated for the treatment of superficial thrombophlebitis. They are used if thrombosis progresses proximally in spite of treatment, or if the involved segment is near the deep venous system at the groin. In the latter situation, surgical interruption of the long saphenous vein at its junction with the femoral vein should be seriously considered. Anticoagulant drugs should be employed in the management of deep thrombophlebitis unless urgent contraindications are present. Their usefulness in preventing fatal pulmonary embolism has been convincingly proved. Heparin sodium should be given intravenously (5,000 units) as soon as the diagnosis of deep venous thrombosis is made, and should be continued either intravenously or subcutaneously until the patient is fully ambulatory (a minimum of 5 to 7 days). The total daily dose of heparin sodium is 500 units per kilogram, and can be given either by intravenous drip, by intermittent intravenous injection every 4 h, or by intermittent subcutaneous injection every 6 to 12 h. The heparin is tapered and stopped prior to the patient's discharge. Most clinicians believe that a subsequent 3- to 4-month course of oral anticoagulants is also necessary.

The effectiveness of fibrinolysin (Thrombolysin) or its activator, streptokinase, in the management of thrombophlebitis has not been established, nor has adequate laboratory control of its administration been defined. For these reasons, and because of the high cost of these preparations and the high incidence of side effects, this type of treatment is not recommended for routine use.

If edema is present or appears when the patient becomes ambulatory, elastic stockings or elastic bandages should be applied whenever the patient is out of bed. The use of elastic support may be discontinued whenever the extremity remains free of edema without it. However, if edema is present, adequate elastic support is the most important measure to prevent chronic venous insufficiency.

Inferior vena caval interruption should be considered only when pulmonary embolism occurs in spite of adequate anticoagulant treatment or when anticoagulation is absolutely contraindicated for a patient with a deep thrombophlebitis or a pulmonary embolus. The application of a serrated Teflon clip seems less likely to produce late sequelae of venous insufficiency and is associated with a lower operative mortality than is inferior vena caval ligation.[131] If the patient is considered to be a poor surgical risk for inferior vena caval clipping, the transvenous insertion of an umbrella filter[132] may be considered (see Chap. 108).

Claims that thrombectomy in the management of iliofemoral thrombophlebitis may reduce the frequency and severity of late complications of chronic venous insufficiency have not been substantiated. However, this procedure has reduced the morbidity and mortality associated with phlegmasia cerulea dolens (see Chap. 108).

Varicose veins

Varicose veins, or dilated veins, are commonly encountered in clinical practice. They range in severity from the innocuous but sometimes cosmetically objectionable dilatation of superficial cutaneous veins to the huge, serpiginous dilatation of the long saphenous vein that renders it functionally incompetent and leads to venous stasis and insufficiency. Only rarely are varicose veins found in the upper extremities, and when they do occur in this location, they almost always signify the presence of a congenital vascular anomaly or an acquired arteriovenous fistula.

ETIOLOGY

Varicose veins may be primary or secondary. Primary varicose veins appear without antecedent thrombophlebitis and are presumably the result of a congenital weakness of the veins that becomes manifest at puberty or later in life, often during pregnancy. The familial incidence of varicose veins is striking and is evidence of an inherited defect, although this has never been conclusively demonstrated. In addition to pregnancy, obesity and occupations that entail prolonged standing predispose to development of varicose veins.

Secondary varicose veins usually result from previous deep thrombophlebitis with resulting insufficiency of the deep venous system; rarer causes include acquired or congenital arteriovenous fistulas and extrinsic pressure on the inferior vena cava or iliofemoral veins.

PATHOLOGY

Characteristically, varicose veins, whether primary or secondary, are dilated and elongated. The thickness of the wall varies considerably, but in general it is thicker than normal as a result of an increase in fibrous connective tissue. There are usually also hypertrophy of the muscular coat and increase in thickness of the intima. As the veins dilate, the valves become incompetent and atrophy.

With the exception of the hemorrhoidal plexus, the most commonly involved veins are the greater and lesser saphenous and their tributaries.

PATHOLOGIC PHYSIOLOGY

Venous stasis results when valves in varicose veins are rendered incompetent. The increased venous pressure is transmitted to the capillary bed, promoting the formation of edema, the deposition of hemosiderin, and the proliferation of subcutaneous fibrous tissue. These changes are considered more in detail farther on under "Chronic Venous Insufficiency." Normally, venous pressure in the lower extremities decreases during walking when veins are competent. In the presence of incompetent varicose veins, however, there is less than the normal decrease in venous pressure during walking; thus the capillaries around the ankles are subjected to higher than normal pressures during physical activity.

CLINICAL MANIFESTATIONS

Primary varicose veins are almost always bilateral, although they may not appear simultaneously in both extremities. Varicosities of this type appear without antecedent history of thrombophlebitis or other predisposing cause. Women frequently notice them for the first time during pregnancy. Secondary varicose veins on the other hand are not infrequently unilateral, since usually they are the result of deep venous insufficiency from previous iliofemoral thrombophlebitis. The history of previous thrombophlebitis and chronic swelling of the involved extremity are clues that varicose veins are secondary. When varicose veins are present at birth or appear early in life or when they occur in the upper extremity, congenital arteriovenous fistula should be suspected.

Usually varicose veins produce minimal or no symptoms. Hypersensitive patients, especially women, complain of a variety of bizarre pains that are usually located in the varices. When venous insufficiency is present, diffuse dull aching in the leg after prolonged standing or walking is a common complaint. This is usually relieved by a period of elevation of the legs. If the deep veins are competent, orthostatic edema and stasis pigmentation of the ankles and lower legs are usually minimal or absent.

SPECIAL EXAMINATIONS FOR VENOUS COMPETENCY

Varicose veins are not necessarily incompetent, for in some cases the varicosities may be so localized that they do not interfere with function of the valves. For this reason incompetency of the veins should be established before surgical intervention is considered. The course of the vein can be traced by firmly compressing it with one hand while the fingertips of the other hand feel for the impact above and below the area of compression. If the impulse can be felt for a distance of 20 cm above or below the compression, the vein is usually incompetent. By the application of tourniquets at various levels in the thigh and leg and the observation of the direction and rapidity of filling of superficial veins after the leg has been placed in a dependent position following elevation, it is possible to locate incompetent perforating veins and to determine whether the greater and lesser saphenous veins are incompetent.[134]

COMPLICATIONS

The most frequent complication of incompetent varicose veins is venous insufficiency manifested by chronic edema, pigmentation, induration, and sometimes ulceration of the lower part of the legs and ankles. This complication is more likely to occur when deep venous insufficiency is also present; it is discussed below, under "Chronic Venous Insufficiency."

Thrombophlebitis may occur in varicose veins either spontaneously or following trauma, surgical procedures, or parturition. It may occur repeatedly for no apparent reason. Pulmonary embolism from thrombophlebitis in superficial varices is rare.

Rupture of varicose veins with massive bleeding is

extremely uncommon, although many patients secretly or otherwise harbor a fear of it.

TREATMENT

Reassurance is the only treatment necessary for patients with dilated cutaneous capillaries. This is also true for patients with minor and localized varicose veins without incompetency of the saphenous systems.

Adequate elastic support in the form of bandages or stockings should be recommended if the saphenous veins are extensively incompetent and especially if edema occurs when the patient is standing. When the deep veins are also incompetent, to prevent accumulation of edema a heavier support is required than when only the superficial veins are involved. Proper elastic support, faithfully worn, will prevent the complications of venous insufficiency in most cases and obviate the need for surgical intervention.

Injections of sclerosing solutions may be helpful if only short segments of small tributary veins are involved. Large and extensive varicosities cannot be successfully treated in this manner, for ultimately the thrombus so induced recanalizes. Injection therapy is sometimes useful in conjunction with surgical stripping when small varicose veins remain after the main channels have been eradicated.

Operation becomes necessary whenever signs and symptoms of chronic venous insufficiency, including stasis ulcer, cannot be controlled by elastic support or the patient refuses to wear the support faithfully. Recurrent thrombophlebitis in varicose veins is another indication for operation, and in some cases it may be justifiable to operate on varicose veins for cosmetic reasons only. It must be remembered that many patients with varicose veins can get along without symptoms or complications for many years with no treatment whatsoever. Stripping of the entire vein as well as careful dissection and evulsion of its incompetent tributaries and resection of all incompetent perforating veins constitute the procedure of choice when surgical intervention becomes necessary. The late results of extensive stripping operations are much superior to those of simple ligation and injection.

Cellulitis and lymphangitis, serious systemic diseases, acute thrombophlebitis in deep veins, and arterial insufficiency are contraindications to surgical treatment of varicose veins. Deep venous insufficiency is not a contraindication to stripping superficial veins that are incompetent. However, the patient with deep venous insufficiency should understand before operation that he must continue to wear adequate elastic support after operation, whereas most patients who have competent deep veins can eventually discard the elastic support after the successful stripping of the incompetent varicose veins.

Chronic venous insufficiency

Chronic venous insufficiency is the end result of incompetency of the valves of damaged veins. Most frequently it occurs in the lower extremity following iliofemoral thrombophlebitis with resulting destruction of the valves. Occasionally incompetency of the saphenous system will lead to chronic venous insufficiency even through the deep veins are competent. Rarely, chronic venous insufficiency occurs in the upper extremity following axillary-subclavian thrombophlebitis.

PATHOLOGY

Chronic venous insufficiency is characterized by edema and induration of the subcutaneous tissues around the malleoli and in the lower third or more of the leg. The foot is seldom involved to any appreciable degree unless for some reason shoes are not worn regularly. Chronic edema of the subcutaneous tissue leads to fibrosis, inflammation, and induration (chronic stasis cellulitis). The cellulitis is usually a sterile inflammation. The characteristic brownish pigmentation of the distal third of the leg and the malleolar areas is due to deposition of melanin and hemosiderin. The latter comes from disintegration of erythrocytes that reach the subcutaneous tissues when capillaries rupture. Not infrequently ulcers occur spontaneously or following trauma, and these are characteristically located in the malleolar areas, usually on the internal side (Fig. 104-8). Weeping, eczematoid dermatitis is a frequent occurrence.

PATHOLOGIC PHYSIOLOGY

The basic fault is incompetence of the valves of the deep or superficial veins or of both, with incompetency of the perforating veins at the ankle. Under these circumstances the usual decrease in venous pressure that results from walking no longer occurs, and consequently the venous capillaries of the lower extremities are subjected to pressures that equal the height of a column of blood extending from the right

FIGURE 104-8 Chronic venous insufficiency with typical pigmentation and stasis ulceration overlying the internal malleolus.

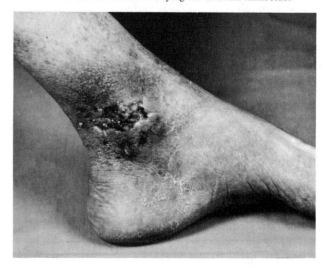

atrium to the level of the malleoli, whether the patient is walking or standing still. This inevitably leads to increased transudation of fluid into the extravascular compartment, with formation of edema.

CLINICAL MANIFESTATIONS
Chronic venous insufficiency presents a characteristic clinical picture.

Often only one leg is involved, and it is chronically swollen; the skin and subcutaneous tissue around and above the malleoli are indurated and firm, and the entire area has a typical brownish pigmentation.

Usually a history of iliofemoral thrombophlebitis can be elicited. Occasionally this diagnosis has not been made previously to the patient's knowledge, but the patient can date the onset of swelling from childbirth, operation, or major trauma. Sometimes the chronic swelling does not appear for several years or months after the episode of thrombophlebitis. Chronic venous insufficiency may result from incompetent varicose veins of the long saphenous system without deep venous incompetency, but this is unusual. Incompetency of the long or short saphenous vein or of both can usually be demonstrated in patients who have chronic venous insufficiency, but in the majority of cases this is secondary to deep insufficiency.

Stasis or varicose ulcers usually occur after chronic venous insufficiency is well established and the pigmentation and chronic induration have already occurred (Fig. 104-8). The ulcers are rarely very painful, and although they are frequently infected, it is obvious that granulation tissue is abundant unless arterial circulation is also impaired. The ulcers usually occur in the area of, or just above, the internal malleolus. Rarely they occur on the foot or toes; often in such circumstances it can be demonstrated that the patients wear slippers or go barefoot instead of using shoes regularly.

Early in the course of chronic venous insufficiency, before induration and pigmentation have occurred, lymphedema must be ruled out. Lymphedema usually occurs in adolescent girls or young women, and there is no history of preceding thrombophlebitis, nor can incompetency of superficial veins be demonstrated. Recording of venous pressure at the ankle during walking is helpful in particularly difficult cases. The venous pressure will decrease when patients with lymphedema walk, since the venous system is competent, whereas the venous pressure will not change when patients with incompetent veins walk. Phlebography can be done if the diagnosis is still in doubt.

PROPHYLAXIS
Chronic venous insufficiency can usually be prevented if patients with acute femoral or iliofemoral thrombophlebitis wear an adequate elastic support on the involved leg below the knee as soon as they begin to ambulate. The elastic support, whether it be a stocking or wrap-around bandage, should be strong enough and should be applied firmly enough to

prevent the accumulation of edema when the patient is upright. It should be worn whenever the patient is up and around, but it can be removed when the patient is recumbent. The use of the support can be omitted for 1 day every 3 or 4 months to see if edema recurs and can be discontinued whenever the leg remains free of edema. It is a clinical impression that prompt treatment of acute iliofemoral thrombophlebitis with heparin and elevation of the extremity reduces the frequency and severity of chronic venous insufficiency.

TREATMENT
Once chronic venous insufficiency is well developed, the patient must use an adequate elastic support for the rest of his life, if he is to avoid disability from recurrent ulcerations and eczematoid dermatitis. If edema is prominent, the patient should be put to bed with the leg elevated in order to reduce the swelling as much as possible. Following this, the leg should be fitted with a good elastic support that will prevent reaccumulation of edema when the patient is ambulatory. Rubber-reinforced elastic bandages usually provide excellent support, but their daily application is a nuisance. If elastic stockings are to be used, they must be constructed well enough to offer the necessary support, and they must be fitted to measurement after the leg is free of edema.

Ulcers of chronic venous insufficiency (stasis ulcers) are best treated by bed rest with the involved extremity elevated. Continuous application of dressings moistened with isotonic saline solution or saturated solution of boric acid will help to eliminate infection and stimulate granulation. If specific pathogens are isolated from the ulcers, appropriate antibiotics can be applied locally in the form of solution or ointment, or given systemically if cellulitis or fever is present. If the ulcer is small and if spending 2 or 3 weeks in bed is economically inconvenient for the patient, repeated application of a modified Unna's paste dressing (Domepast) from the distal metatarsal level to the knee often permits healing while the patient remains ambulatory. A sterile dry-gauze dressing and a foam rubber pad are placed over the ulcer before applying the paste dressing. If the ulcers are large, healing can be hastened by applying skin grafts after the base of the ulcer has become clean and covered with healthy granulation tissue. Stasis ulcers usually heal remarkably rapidly, provided that arterial blood supply is normal. It sometimes becomes necessary to excise incompetent perforating or superficial veins that lead to an area of recurrent or recalcitrant stasis ulceration. If indurated cellulitis is far advanced to the point that subcutaneous tissue has a woody consistency, it is often difficult to prevent recurrent ulceration in spite of adequate elastic support. When this occurs, wide excision of the indurated area followed by application of skin grafts is indicated. When stasis ulcers have healed, recurrence can usually be prevented by applying, under a rubber-reinforced elastic bandage, a foam rubber pad to the pigmented ulcer-bearing region around and above the internal malleolus.

Eczematoid dermatitis (stasis eczema) may be particularly difficult to manage, since the intense pruritus incites scratching, which in turn aggravates and spreads the dermatitis. Patients with active eczematoid dermatitis should be put to bed with the extremity elevated. Continuous application of packs moistened with a 0.5% solution of aluminum subacetate (Burow's solution) or Wescodyne solution, 3%, is the treatment of choice when the involved skin is wet and oozing. In the subacute stage a corticosteroid cream or an ointment containing 3% Ichthyol in zinc oxide often prevents pruritus and promotes healing.

Patients with chronic venous insufficiency should be instructed carefully about the adverse effect of gravity on venous circulation; they should be encouraged to elevate their legs on footstools or hassocks when sitting and should be warned to avoid trauma to the skin of the ulcer-bearing areas. The importance of wearing elastic supports must be stressed.

REFERENCES

1 Fairbairn, J. F., II, Juergens, J. L., and Spittell, J. A., Jr.: "Allen-Barker-Hines Peripheral Vascular Diseases," 4th ed., W. B. Saunders Company, Philadelphia, 1972.

2 Tibell, B.: Peripheral Arterial Insufficiency: An Epidemiological Study of 2,243 Hospital Admissions Caused by Arteriosclerosis Obliterans, Diabetes Mellitus, Thromboangiitis Obliterans and Arterial Embolism, Acta Orthop. Scand. Suppl., 139, 1971.

3 Wessler, S.: Buerger's Disease Revisited, Surg. Clin. North Am., 49:703, 1969.

4 Craven, J. L., and Cotton, R. C.: Haemotologic Differences between Thromboangiitis Obliterans and Atherosclerosis, Br. J. Surg., 54:862, 1967.

5 Kjeldsen, K., and Moses, M.: Buerger's Disease in Israel: Investigations on Carboxyhemoglobin and Serum Cholesterol Levels after Smoking, Acta Chir. Scand., 135:495, 1969.

6 Wald, N., Howard, S., Smith, P. G., and Kjeldsen, K.: Association between Atherosclerotic Disease and Carboxyhaemoglobin Levels in Tobacco Smokers, Br. Med. J., 1:761, 1973.

7 McPherson, J. R., Juergens, J. L., and Gifford, R. W., Jr.: Thromboangiitis Obliterans and Arteriosclerosis Obliterans: Clinical and Prognostic Differences, Ann. Intern. Med., 59:288, 1963.

8 Correlli, F.: Buerger's Disease: Cigarette Smoker Disease May Always Be Cured by Medical Therapy, J. Cardiovasc. Surg. (Torino), 14:28, 1973.

9 Nakao, K., Ikeda, M., Kimata, S., Niitani, H., Miyahara, M., Ishima, Z., Hashiba, K., Takeda, Y., Ozawa, T., Matsushita, S., and Kuramochi, M.: Takayasu's Arteritis: Clinical Report of Eighty-four Cases and Immunological Studies of Seven Cases, Circulation, 35:1141, 1967.

10 Lande, A., and Rossi, P.: The Value of Total Aortography in the Diagnosis of Takayasu's Arteritis, Radiology, 114:287, 1975.

11 Ochsner, J. L., and Hewitt, R. L.: Aortic Arch Syndrome (Brachiocephalic Ischemia), Dis. Chest, 52:69, 1967.

12 DePalma, R. G., Moskowitz, R. W., and Holden, W. D.: Peripheral Ischemia and Collagen Disease, Arch. Surg., 105:313, 1972.

13 Hardy, J. D., Conn, J. H., and Fain, W. R.: Nonatherosclerotic Occlusive Lesions of Small Arteries, Surgery, 57:1, 1965.

14 Holdveen-Geronimus, M., and Merriam, J. C., Jr.: Cholesterol Embolization: From Pathological Curiosity to Clinical Entity, Circulation, 35:946, 1967.

15 Harker, L. A., Slichter, S. J., Scott, C. R., and Ross, R.: Homocystinemia: Vascular Injury and Arterial Thrombosis, N. Engl. J. Med., 291:537, 1974.

16 Kerleer, R. E., and Vogl, A.: Pachydermoperiostosis: Peripheral Circulatory Studies, Arch Intern. Med., 132:245, 1973.

17 Little, J. M., Petritsi-Jones, D., Sylotra, P., Williams, R., and Kerr, C.: A Survey of Amputations for Degenerative Vascular Disease, Med. J. Aust., 1:329, 1973.

18 Nielsen, J.: Arteriosclerosis Obliterans of the Lower Extremities in Non-diabetic Men: Survival and Causes of Death, Dan. Med. Bull., 22:10, 1975.

19 Marble, A.: Angiopathy in Diabetes: An Unsolved Problem, Diabetes, 16:825, 1967.

20 Vracko, R., and Strandness, D. E., Jr.: Basal Lamina of Abdominal Skeletal Muscle Capillaries in Diabetics and Nondiabetics, Circulation, 35:690, 1967.

21 Conrad, M. C.: Large and Small Artery Occlusion in Diabetics and Nondiabetics with Severe Vascular Disease, Circulation, 36:83, 1967.

22 Blumenthal, H. T., Berns, A. W., Goldenberg, S., and Lowenstein, P. W.: Etiologic Considerations in Peripheral Vascular Diseases of the Lower Extremity with Special Reference to Diabetes Mellitus, Circulation, 33:98, 1966.

23 Buerger, L.: Thromboangiitis Obliterans: A Study of the Vascular Lesions Leading to Presenile Spontaneous Gangrene, Am. J. Med. Sci., 135:567, 1908.

24 Peracchia, C., and Vassallo, C.: Alterations in Collagen in the Arteries of Thromboangiitic Patients, Angiology, 17:451, 1966.

25 DeWolfe, V. G., and Beven, E. G.: Arteriosclerosis Obliterans in the Lower Extremities: Correlation of Clinical and Angiographic Findings, Cardiovasc. Clin., 3:65, 1971.

25a Kennelly, B. N., and Blumberg, L.: Bilateral Anterior Tibial Claudication: Report of Two Cases in which the Patients Were Cured by Bilateral Fasciotomy, J.A.M.A., 203:487, 1968.

26 Darling, R. C., Buckley, C. J., Abbott, W. M., and Raines, J. K.: Intermittent Claudication in Young Athletes: Popliteal Entrapment Syndrome, J. Trauma, 14:543, 1974.

27 Barner, H. B., Kauer, G. C., Willman, V. L., and Hanlon, C. R.: Clinical Documentation of the Hemodynamics of the Disappearing Pulse, Arch. Surg., 97:341, 1968.

28 Moore, W. J., and Hall, A. D.: Unrecognized Aortoiliac Stenosis, Arch. Surg., 103:633, 1971.

29 Barnhorst, D. A., and Barner, H. B.: Prevalence of Congenitally Absent Pedal Pulses, N. Engl. J. Med., 278:264, 1968.

30 Baker, J. D., Del Banco, T. L., Price, J. B., Rogers, W. M., Salomon, P. F., and McAllister, F. F.: Experimental Study of Murmurs in Stenotic Arteries, Surgery, 59:88, 1966.

31 Friedman, S. A., and Rakow, R. B.: Osseous Lesions of the Foot in Diabetic Neuropathy, Diabetes, 20:302, 1971.

31a Roenigk, H. H., Jr., and Young, J. R.: "Leg Ulcers," Harper and Row, Publishers, Inc., Hagerstown, Maryland, 1975.

32 Bergan, J. J., Darling, R. C., deWolfe, V. G., Raines, J. K., Strandness, D. E., and Yao, J. S. T., Report of the Inter-Society Commission for Heart Disease Resources: Medical Instrumentation in Peripheral Vascular Disease, Circulation, 54:A-1, 1976.

33 Carter, S. A.: Clinical Measurement of Systolic Pressures in Limbs with Arterial Occlusive Disease, J.A.M.A., 207:1869, 1969.

34 Strandness, D. E., and Sumner, D. S.: Applications of Ultrasound to the Study of Arteriosclerosis Obliterans, *Angiology*, 26:187, 1975.

35 Snyder, E. N., Mulfinger, G. L., and Lambert, R. W.: Claudication Caused by Compression of the Cauda Equina, *Am. J. Surg.*, 130:172, 1975.

36 Hines, E. A., Jr., and Barker, N. W.: Arteriosclerosis Obliterans: A Clinical and Pathologic Study, *Am. J. Med. Sci.*, 200:717, 1940.

37 Kannel, W. B., and Shurtleff, D.: The Natural History of Arteriosclerosis Obliterans, *Cardiovasc. Clin.*, 3:37, 1971.

38 Kannel, W. B., Skinner, J. J., Jr., Schwartz, M. J., and Sturlleff, M. J.: Intermittent Claudication: Incidence in the Framingham Study, *Circulation*, 41:875, 1970.

39 Juergens, J. L., Barker, N. W., and Hines, E. A., Jr.: Arteriosclerosis Obliterans: Review of 520 Cases with Special Reference to Pathogenic and Prognostic Factors, *Circulation*, 21:188, 1960.

40 Dale, W. A., and Lewis, M. R.: Management of Ischemia of the Hand and Fingers, *Surgery*, 67:62, 1970.

41 Strandness, D. E., and Stahler, C.: Arteriosclerosis Obliterans: Manner and Rate of Progression, *J.A.M.A.*, 196:1, 1966.

42 Kuthan, F., Burkhaltar, A., Baitsch, R., Luden, H., and Wedmer, L. K.: Development of Occlusive Arterial Disease in Lower Limbs and Angiographic Follow-up of 705 Medical Patients, *Arch. Surg.*, 103:545, 1971.

43 Bernhard, V. M., Ashmore, C. S., Rodgers, R. E., and Evans, W. E.: Operative Blood Flow in Femoral-Popliteal and Femoral-Tibial Grafts for Lower Extremity Ischemia, *Arch. Surg.*, 103:595, 1971.

44 Noon, G. P., Diethrich, E. B., Richardson, W. P., and DeBakey, M. E.: Distal Tibial Arterial Bypass: Analysis of 91 Cases, *Arch. Surg.*, 99:770, 1969.

45 DeWeese, J. A., Blaisdell, F. W., Foster, J. H., Garrett, H. E., and deWolfe, V. G.: Report of the Inter-Society Commission for Heart Disease Resources, Optimum Resources for Vascular Surgery, *Circulation*, 53:A-39, 1976.

46 Lye, C. R., Sumner, D. S., and Strandness, D. E.: The Effects of Femoropopliteal Vein Graft Failure on Limb Function, *Ann. Surg.*, 183:38, 1976.

47 Baddeley, R. M., Ashton, F., Slaney, G., and Barnes, A. D.: Late Results of Autogenous Vein Bypass Grafts in Femoropopliteal Arterial Occlusion, *Br. Med. J.*, 1:653, 1970.

48 Stoney, R. J., James, D. R., and Wylie, E. J.: Surgery for Femoropopliteal Atherosclerosis, *Arch. Surg.*, 103:548, 1971.

49 Szilagyi, D. E., Smith, R. F., Scerpella, J. R., and Hoffman, K.: Lumbar Sympathectomy: Current Role in the Treatment of Arteriosclerotic Occlusive Disease, *Arch. Surg.*, 95:753, 1967.

50 Kannel, W. B., and Shurtleff, D.: The Framingham Study: Cigarettes and the Development of Intermittent Claudication, *Geriatrics*, 28:61, 1973.

51 Leren, P., and Haabrekke, O.: Blood Lipids in Patients with Arteriosclerosis Obliterans of the Lower Limbs, *Acta Med. Scand.*, 180:511, 1971.

52 Stamler, J., and Lilienfeld, A. M.: Report of Inter-Society Commission on Heart Disease Resources: Primary Prevention of the Atherosclerotic Diseases, *Circulation*, 42:A55, 1970. Revised, 1972.

53 Coffman, J. O., and Mannick, J. A.: Failure of Vasodilator Drugs in Arteriosclerosis Obliterans, *Ann. Intern Med.*, 76:35, 1972.

54 Hansteen, V., and Lorentsen, E.: Vasodilator Drugs in the Treatment of Peripheral Arterial Insufficiency, *Acta Med. Scand. Suppl.*, 556:9, 1974.

55 Skinner, J. S., and Strandness, D. E.: Exercise and Intermittent Claudication: I. Effect of Repetition and Intensity of Exercise, *Circulation*, 36:15, 1967.

56 Skinner, J. S., and Strandness, D. E.: Exercise and Intermittent Claudication: II. Effect of Physical Training, *Circulation*, 36:23, 1967.

57 Alpert, J. S., Larsen, O., and Lassen, N. A.: Exercise and Intermittent Claudication, *Circulation*, 39:353, 1969.

58 Zetterquest, S.: Effect of Active Training on Nutritive Blood Flow in Exercising Ischemic Legs, *Scand. J. Clin. Lab. Invest.*, 25:101, 1970.

59 Ericsson, B., Haeger, K., and Kindell, S. E.: Effect of Physical Training on Intermittent Claudication, *Angiology*, 21:188, 1970.

60 Martin, M., Schoop, W., and Zeitler, E.: Strepokinase in Chronic Arterial Occlusive Disease, *J.A.M.A.*, 211:1169, 1970.

61 Verstraete, M., Vermulen, J., and Donati, M. B.: The Effect of Streptokinase Infusion on Chronic Arterial Occlusions and Stenoses, *Ann. Intern. Med.*, 74:377, 1971.

62 Pories, W. J., Rob, C. G., Smith, J. L., Henzel, J. H., and Strain, W. H.: "The Treatment of Atherosclerosis with Zinc Sulfate," (paper presented at Military Medicine Section, A.M.A. convention, Atlantic City, N.J., June 1967),

63 Burgess, E. M., and Romano, R. L.: The Management of Lower Extremity Amputees Using Immediate Postsurgical Prosthesis, *Clin. Orthop.*, 57:137, 1968.

64 Burgess, E. M., and Marsden, F. W.: Major Lower Extremity Amputations following Arterial Reconstruction, *Arch. Surg.*, 198:655, 1974.

65 Lippmann, H. I., and Corcoran, P. J.: Report of the Inter-Society Commission for Heart Disease Resources: Optimal Resources for Amputation Programs: A Hospital Planning Guide, *Circulation*, 55:A-1, 1977.

66 Thompson, J. E., Sider, L., Raub, P. S., Austin, D. I., and Patman, R. D.: Arterial Embolectomy: A 20 Year Experience with 163 Cases, *Surgery*, 67:212, 1970.

67 Hight, D. W., Telney, N. L., and Couch, N. P.: Changing Clinical Trends in Patients with Peripheral Arterial Emboli, *Surgery*, 79:172, 1976.

68 Bonchek, L. I., and Starr, A.: Ball Valve Prosthesis: A Current Appraisal of Late Results, *Am. J. Cardiol.*, 35:843, 1975.

69 deWolfe, V. G., Humphries, A. W., Young, J. R., and LeFevre, F. A.: A Comparison of the Natural History of Arteriosclerosis Obliterans with the Results of Arterial Reconstruction, *Heart Bull.*, 12:101, 1963.

70 Patman, R. D., and Thompson, J. E.: Fasciotomy in Peripheral Vascular Surgery, *Arch. Surg.*, 101:663, 1970.

71 Krause, R. J., Cranley, J. J., Strasser, E. S., Hafner, C. D., and Fogarty, T. J.: Further Experience with a New Embolectomy Catheter, *Surgery*, 59:81, 1966.

72 McKechnie, R. E., and Allen, E. V.: Sudden Occlusion of Arteries of the Extremities: A Study of 100 Cases of Embolism and Thrombosis, *Surg. Gynecol. Obstet.*, 63:231, 1936.

73 Young, J. R., Humphries, A. W., deWolfe, V. G., and LeFevre, F. A.: Peripheral Arterial Embolism, *J.A.M.A.*, 185:621, 1963.

74 Fogarty, T. J., and Cranley, J. J.: Catheter Technic for Embolectomy, *Ann. Surg.*, 161:325, 1965.

75 Stallone, R. J., Blaisdell, F. W., Cofferata, H. T., and Levin, S. M.: Analysis of Morbidity and Mortality from Arterial Embolectomy, *Surgery*, 65:207, 1969.

76 Mustard, J., and Packham, H.: Platelet Aggregation and Platelet Release Reaction in Thromboembolism, *J. Can. Med. Assoc.*, 103:859, 1970.

77 Lord, R. S. A., and Irani, C. N.: Assessment of Arterial Injury in Limb Trauma, *J. Trauma*, 14:1042, 1974.

78 Rich, N. M., Hobson, R. W., II, and Feddi, C. W.: Vascular Trauma Secondary to Diagnostic and Therapeutic Procedures, *Am. J. Surg.*, 128:715, 1974.

79 Meaney, T. F.: Percutaneous Femoral Angiography, in T. F. Meany, A. F. Lalli, and R. J. Alfidi: "Complications and Legal Implications of Radiologic Special Procedures," chap. 2, The C. V. Mosby Company, St. Louis, 1973, p. 15.

80 Beven E. G.: Surgical Treatment of Angiographic Complications, in T. F. Meany, A. F. Lalli, and R. J. Alfidi: "Complications and Legal Implications of Radiologic Special Procedures," chap. 5, The C. V. Mosby Company, St. Louis, 1973, p. 63.

81 Maxwell, T. M., Olcott, C., IV, and Blaisdell, F. W.: Vascular Complications of Drug Abuse, Arch. Surg., 105:875, 1972.

82 Pappas, G., Janes, J. M., Bernatz, P. E., and Schirger, A.: Femoral Aneurysms: Review of Surgical Management, J.A. M.A., 190:489, 1964.

83 Wychulis, A. R., Spittell, J. A., and Wallace, R. B.: Popliteal Aneurysms, Surgery, 68:942, 1970.

84 Dent, T., Lindenauer, S., Ernst, C., and Fry, W.: Multiple Arteriosclerotic Arterial Aneurysms, Arch. Surg., 105:338, 1972.

85 Stanley, J., and Fry, W.: Pathogenesis and Clinical Significance of Splenic Artery Aneurysms, Surgery, 76:898, 1974.

86 Stanley, J., Rhodes, E., Gewertz, B., Chang, C., Walter, J., and Fry, W.: Renal Artery Aneurysms: Significance of Macroaneurysms Exclusive of Dissections and Fibrodysplastic Mural Dilations, Arch. Surg., 110:1327, 1975.

87 Harrison, E. G., Jr. and McCormack, L. J.: Pathologic Classification of Renal Arterial Disease in Renovascular Hypertension, Mayo Clin. Proc., 46:161, 1971.

88 Stanley, J., Thompson, N., and Fry, W.: Splanchnic Artery Aneurysms, Arch. Surg., 101:689, 1970.

89 Meaney, T. F., Buonocore, E., and Alfidi, R. J.: Arteriographic Clues to Intra-abdominal Disease, Heart Bull., 17:34, 1968.

90 Markowitz, A. M., and Norman, J. C.: Aneurysms of the Iliac Artery, Ann. Surg., 154:777, 1961.

91 Fee, H., Jr., and Golding, A.: Lower Extremity Ischemia after Femoral Arteriovenous Bovine Shunts, Ann. Surg., 183:42, 1976.

92 Szilagyi, D. E., Elliott, J. P., DeRusso, F. J., and Smith, R. F.: Peripheral Congenital Arteriovenous Fistulas, Surgery, 57:61, 1965.

93 Coffman, J. D., and Cohen, A. S.: Total and Capillary Fingertip Blood Flow in Raynaud's Phenomenon, N. Engl. J. Med., 285:259, 1971.

94 Willerson, J. T., Thompson, R. H., Hookman, P., Herdt, J., and Decker, J. L.: Reserpine in Raynaud's Disease and Phenomenon, Ann. Intern. Med., 72:17, 1970.

95 Mendlowitz, M., and Naftchi, N.: The Digital Circulation in Raynaud's Disease, Am. J. Cardiol., 4:580, 1959.

96 Tietjen, G., Chein, S., Leroy, E., Gavras, I., Gavras, H., and Gump. F.: Blood Viscosity, Plasma Proteins, and Raynaud's Syndrome, Arch. Surg., 110:1343, 1975.

97 Gifford, R. W., Jr.: The Arteriospastic Diseases: Clinical Significance and Management, Cardiovasc. Clin., 3:1, 1971.

98 Allen, E. V., and Brown, G. E.: Raynaud's Disease Affecting Men, Ann. Intern. Med., 5:1384, 1932.

99 Gifford, R. W., Jr. and Hines, E. A., Jr.: Raynaud's Disease among Women and Girls, Circulation, 16:1012, 1957.

100 Farmer, R. G., Gifford, R. W., Jr., and Hines, E. A., Jr.: Prognostic Significance of Raynaud's Phenomenon and Other Clinical Characteristics of Systemic Scleroderma, Circulation, 21:1088, 1960.

101 Tindall, J., Whalen, R., and Burton, E., Jr.: Medical Uses of Intra-arterial Injections of Reserpine, Arch Dermatol., 110:233, 1974.

102 Gifford, R. W., Jr., Hines, E. A., Jr., and Craig, W. McK.: Sympathectomy for Raynaud's Phenomenon: Follow-up

Study of 70 Women with Raynaud's Disease and 54 Women with Secondary Raynaud's Phenomenon, Circulation, 17:5, 1958.

103 Burbank, M. K., Spittell, J. A., Jr., and Fairbairn, J. F., II: Familial Erythromelalgia: Genetic and Physiologic Observations, J. Lab. Clin. Med., 68:861, 1968 (abstract).

104 Babb, R. R., Alarcon-Segovia, D., and Fairbairn, J. F., II: Erythermalgia: Review of 51 Cases, Circulation, 29:136, 1964.

105 Alarcon-Segovia, D., Babb, R. R., Fairbairn, J. F., II, and Hagedorn, A. B.: Erythermalgia: A Clue to the Early Diagnosis of Myeloproliferative Disorders, Arch. Intern. Med., 117:511, 1966.

106 Merryman, H. T.: Tissue Freezing and Local Cold Injury, Physiol. Rev., 37:233, 1957.

107 Montgomery, H.: Experimental Immersion Foot: Review of Physiopathology, Physiol. Rev., 34:127, 1954.

108 Taplin, D., Zaias, N., and Blank, H.: The Role of Temperature in Tropical Immersion Foot Syndrome, J.A.M.A., 202:546, 1967.

109 Buckels, L. J., Gill, K. A., Jr., and Anderson, G. T.: Prophylaxis of Warm-Water-Immersion Foot, J.A.M.A., 200:681, 1967.

110 Knize, D. M., Weatherley-White, R. C. A., Paton, B. C., and Owens, J. C.: Prognostic Factors in the Management of Frostbite, J. Trauma, 9:749, 1969.

111 Mills, W., Jr.: Frostbite, Alaska Med., 15:26, 1973.

112 Shumacker, H. B., and Kilman, J. W.: Sympathectomy in the Treatment of Frostbite, Arch Surg., 89:575, 1964.

113 Goodhead, B.: The Comparative Valve of Low Molecular Weight Dextran and Sympathectomy in the Treatment of Experimental Frost-Bite, Br. J. Surg., 53:1060, 1966.

114 Elgee, N.: Medical Aspects of Oral Contraceptives, Ann. Intern. Med., 72:409, 1970.

115 Drill, V.: Oral Contraceptives and Thromboembolic Disease, J.A.M.A., 219:583, 1972.

116 Hume, M., Sevitt, S., and Thomas, D.: "Venous Thrombosis and Pulmonary Embolism," Harvard University Press, Cambridge, Mass., 1970.

117 Wessler, S., Alexander, B., Beall, A., deWolfe, V. G., and Miale, J.: Prevention and Early Detection of Thromboembolic Disease, Circulation, 41:A-31, 1970.

118 DeWeese, J., and Rogoff, S.: Phlebographic Patterns of Acute Deep Venous Thrombosis of the Leg, Surgery, 53:99, 1963.

119 Athanasoulis, C.: Phlebography for the Diagnosis of Deep Leg Vein Thrombosis, in J. Frantantoni and S. Wessler (eds.), "Prophylactic Therapy of Deep Vein Thrombosis and Pulmonary Embolism," DHEW Publication (NIH) 76-866, 1975, p. 62.

120 Strandness, D., Jr.: Ultrasound and Plethysmography in the Diagnosis of Acute Venous Thrombosis, in J. Frantantoni and S. Wessler (eds.), "Prophylactic Therapy of Deep Vein Thrombosis and Pulmonary Embolism," DHEW Publication (NIH) 76-866, 1975, p. 100.

121 Wheeler, H., O'Donnell, J., Anderson, F., Jr., and Benedict, K.: Occlusive Impedance Phlebography: A Diagnostic Procedure for Venous Thrombosis and Pulmonary Embolism, Prog. Cardiovasc. Dis., 12:199, 1974.

122 Cranely, J., Canos, A., Sull, W., and Gross, A.: Phleborheographic Technique for Diagnosing Deep Venous Thrombosis of the Lower Extremities, Surg. Gynecol. Obstet., 141:331, 1975.

123 Borgström, S., Greitz, T., van der Linden, W., Molin, J., and Rudics, I.: Ascending Phlebography in Fresh Thrombosis of the Lower Limb, Am. J. Roentgenol. Radium Ther. Nucl. Med., 94:207, 1965.

124 Mavor, G. E., and Galloway, J. M. D.: The Ilio-femoral Venous Segment as a Source of Pulmonary Emboli, Lancet, 1:871, 1967.

125 Doran, F. S. A., and White, H. M.: A Demonstration that the Risk of Post-operative Deep Venous Thrombosis is Reduced

by Stimulating the Calf Muscles Electrically during the Operation, *Br. J. Surg.,* 54:686, 1967.

126 Rosenberg, I., and Pollock, A.: A Comparison of Mechanical and Chemical Methods of Prevention of Post-operative Venous Thrombosis, *Br. Med. J.,* 1:358, 1974.

127 Collins, R.: Physical Methods of Prophylaxis against Deep Vein Thrombosis, in J. Frantantoni and S. Wessler (eds.), in "Prophylactic Therapy of Deep Vein Thrombosis and Pulmonary Embolism," DHEW Publication (NIH) 76-866, 1975, p. 158.

128 Hirsh, J., and Genton, E.: Low-Dose Heparin Prophylaxis for Venous Thromboembolism, in J. Frantantoni and S. Wessler (eds.), "Prophylactic Therapy of Deep Vein Thrombosis and Pulmonary Embolism," DHEW Publication (NIH) 76-866, 1975, p. 183.

129 Kakkar, V.: Prevention of Fatal Pulmonary Embolism by Low Doses of Heparin, *Lancet,* 2:45, 1975.

130 Clagett, G., and Salzman, E.: Prevention of Venous Thromboembolism, *Prog. Cardiovasc. Dis.,* 17:345, 1975.

131 Adams, J. Feingold, B., and De Weese, J: Comparative Evaluation of Ligation and Partial Interruption of the Inferior Vena Cava, *Arch. Surg.,* 103:272, 1971.

132 Mobin-Uddin, K., Utley, J., and Bryant, L.: The Inferior Vena Cava Umbrella Filter, *Prog. Cardiovasc. Dis.,* 17:391, 1975.

133 Brockman, S., and Vasko, J.: Phlegmasia Cerulea Dolens, *Surg. Gynecol. Obstet.,* 121:1, 1965.

134 Lofgren, E.: Present-day Indications for Surgical Treatment of Varicose Veins, *Mayo Clin. Proc.,* 41:515, 1966.

105
Cerebral Vascular Disease and Neurologic Manifestations of Cardiovascular Disease

HERBERT R. KARP, M.D.

Neurologic signs and symptoms are often seen as a prominent manifestation of diseases of the cardiovascular system. The correct interpretation of these neurologic findings frequently provides the clinician with important clues as to the nature and extent of the primary disease process. It is the purpose of this chapter to discuss the major cardiovascular diseases in which the nervous system may be significantly involved and to relate the neurologic manifestation to the pathophysiology of the underlying cardiovascular disease.

In many of the diseases to be discussed the involvement of the nervous system is mediated by the cerebral vessels. The neurologic deficit which results from such involvement usually can be related to a lesion in the distribution of a particular cerebral vessel. This focal, vascular nature of the neurologic deficit, its sudden onset, and the clinical setting in which it occurs constitute the major clinical features of the diseases of the cerebral vessels. Therefore, in order to recognize the manifestations of the diseases affecting these vessels, it is essential to have an understanding of the territory of supply of the principal arteries and the nature of the neurologic deficit

produced by ischemia in their distribution. An outline of these anatomic relations is given in Table 105-13.

NEUROLOGIC MANIFESTATIONS OF MYOCARDIAL AND VALVULAR DISEASE

The most frequent neurologic manifestation of disease of the heart or its valves is cerebral embolization. The clinical presentation of cerebral embolism is dominated by the sudden onset of a focal neurologic deficit. Although there are usually no premonitory symptoms such as those seen in cerebral thrombosis, Wells[1] calls attention to the fact that such symptoms occasionally do occur in patients with cerebral emboli. Headache is the most common prodromal complaint and is thought to be due to stretching and distortion of the artery as the embolic particle first becomes lodged in a proximal segment. Perhaps as the vessel dilates, the embolus becomes dislodged, only to occlude the more distal branches and produce a persistent neurologic deficit. Often the headache clears as the neurologic deficit appears. Other patients experience more focal prodromal symptoms, suggesting either multiple emboli in the same vascular distribution or an embolus advancing from a proximal segment in which collateral vessels can compensate for the occlusion to more distal segments where the available collateral flow is inadequate to prevent ischemia. Such premonitory symptoms are rare, and the interval between them and the onset of the neurologic deficit is often so short that one is unable to institute any therapy which might modify the subsequent ischemia.

The nature of the focal neurologic deficit is of course dependent on the vessel which is occluded and the extent of the ischemia which follows. Any cerebral vessel may be involved; reliable figures as to the distribution of cerebral emboli are not available.

Cerebral emboli occur, in decreasing order of frequency, in the territory of the middle cerebral artery, the posterior cerebral artery, the superficial branches of the vertebral artery, particularly involving the inferior surfaces of the cerebellum, and least frequently in the territory of the anterior cerebral artery and the vessels supplying the more medial aspects of the brainstem. Although there is no predilection for the right or left side of the brain, one is impressed by the frequency with which recurrent emboli in a given patient are seen to involve one side to the almost complete exclusion of the other. As most emboli are small, it then follows that very frequently the smaller distal arborizations are occluded, often leading to ischemia in the terminal distribution of the arteries. Consequently, discrete neurologic deficit such as an isolated aphasia, weakness or sensory loss limited to one hand, or a homonymous visual defect without other neurologic findings may result. The incidence of seizures as early or late sequelae is greater in embolic than in thrombotic occlusion of cerebral arteries, related in part to the higher incidence of small cortical infarctions in cerebral embolism.[2]

Arterial embolization can be encountered in any myocardial or valvular disease in which there is a thrombus in the left side of the heart. The major causes of the formation of intracardiac thrombi are rheumatic heart disease, atherosclerotic heart disease, and bacterial endocarditis. Less frequent cardiac sources of emboli include endocardial fibroelastosis, thyrotoxic heart disease with atrial fibrillation, cardiac myxoma, idiopathic myocarditis, and prolapse of the mitral valve. In patients under the age of 50, the most frequent cause of cerebral embolization is rheumatic heart disease, particulary in association with either chronic atrial fibrillation, mitral valvular disease, or both.

In the age group over 50 the incidence of cerebral embolism of cardiac origin is highest in patients with arteriosclerotic heart disease. The likelihood of left ventricular thrombus formation and peripheral embolization is greatest in the acute stages of myocardial infarction, especially in infarctions which involve a large area of myocardium, and in infarction of the anterior wall of the left ventricle. Cerebral emboli occurring in the later stages of myocardial infarction are usually associated with a ventricular aneurysm. Coexisting aortic valvular disease appears not to influence mural thrombus formation except insofar as it increases the probability of congestive heart failure.[3] Atrial fibrillation due to arteriosclerotic heart disease, as in rheumatic heart disease, predisposes to left atrial thrombi. Mitral stenosis in the absence of atrial fibrillation may also lead to left atrial thrombus formation and cerebral embolus.[4]

The immediate treatment of cerebral embolism is based primarily on anticoagulant therapy. The embolus can be removed surgically only if it is lodged in an accessible portion of the cervical arteries. The objective of anticoagulant therapy in patients with cerebral embolus is to prevent repeated emboli rather than to affect the existing embolic infarction. Uncontrolled, retrospective studies present data which suggest a statistical advantage in the immediate use of anticoagulants.[5,6] Whereas cerebral thrombosis results in a pale infarction, cerebral embolization may produce either pale or hemorrhagic infarction (Fig. 105-1).[7] In view of the frequency with which hemorrhagic infarction is seen in cerebral embolism, the decision to use anticoagulants should take into consideration the risk of increasing the amount of hemorrhage in the cerebral infarct. In experimental embolic infarction in dogs, Whisnant et al.[8] have shown higher morbidity and mortality in animals receiving anticoagulants immediately after infarction, because of an increase in the hemorrhagic component of the cerebral infarct. When anticoagulation was delayed 36 to 48 h after the infarction, there was no significant difference in clinical and pathologic findings between the treated and control groups. Though a similar deleteri-

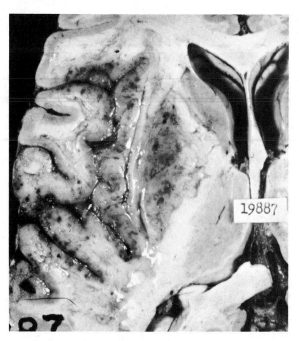

FIGURE 105-1 Hemorrhagic infarction resulting from embolic occlusion of the middle cerebral artery. Note the relative preservation of neural architecture and the predominance of hemorrhage in the depths of the sulci and deep gray matter.

ous effect has not been firmly documented in human beings, the author's practice is to regard an increase in the extent of hemorrhage as a potential risk and to use a slower-acting anticoagulant, such as bishydroxycoumarin or oral warfarin, rather than more rapidly acting forms, such as heparin or intravenously administered warfarin.

The prophylactic aspects of the treatment of cerebral embolism consist of long-term anticoagulant therapy, prophylaxis for bacterial endocarditis, the surgical correction of the lesions predisposing to the formation of thrombi of the left side of the heart, and the proper management of cardiac arrhythmias.

Of all cardiac states predisposing to cerebral embolism, endocarditis shows the greatest likelihood of leading to cerebral embolic lesions. The neurologic findings in bacterial endocarditis are usually the same as those seen in other forms of cerebral embolization. Focal signs may be quite discrete. Because of multiple embolization by small particles, the patient may exhibit signs of diffuse cerebral involvement such as agitated confusion (delirium) or depressed consciousness. Some may have signs of meningitis only. Focal signs, when present, may be quite discrete. Mycotic cerebral aneurysms can result in intracranial bleeding with the characteristics of either intracerebral or primary subarachnoid hemorrhage. When the infective organism is a pyogenic one, such as *Staphylococcus,* an episode of cerebral embolism followed by progressive worsening of the neurologic deficit and increasing intracranial pressure suggests a cerebral abscess.

The treatment of the cerebral complications of bacterial endocarditis is primarily directed at the eradication of the bacterial infection. The occasional occurrence of an episode of brain embolism after the bloodstream is sterile raises the question of the concomitant use of anticoagulants, particularly in the later phases of therapy. Most of the recorded instances of catastrophic intracranial hemorrhage attributed to anticoagulant therapy in bacterial endocarditis occurred in the preantibiotic era, when the sulfonamide drugs were the only available antimicrobial agent. This suggests that continuing infection was as significant a factor as the anticoagulants in the production of the hemorrhage. In spite of this possibility, it is still generally held that anticoagulants are contraindicated in either early or late phases of the treatment of bacterial endocarditis.

Nonbacterial thrombotic endocarditis in association with cancer or other debilitating diseases, frequently referred to as *marantic endocarditis,* has been regarded as a rare cause of pheripheral embolization. This condition has been shown to be a more frequent cause of cerebral embolism than had been previously suspected. Barron et al.[9] presented autopsy data from a hospital with a large service for the treatment of terminal cases of malignant neoplasm. These workers found that 85 percent of the cases of nonbacterial thrombotic endocarditis were associated with cancer, vegetations of the cardiac valves accounting for 10 percent of all the autopsied cases of cerebral emboli. MacDonald and Robbins,[10] in an analysis of 18,486 cases, found 78 instances of nonbacterial thrombotic endocarditis, 14 percent of which had resulted in arterial emboli. Clinically, there was a frequent association with thrombophlebitis. Thus, the acute onset of a focal neurologic deficit in a patient with suspected or known cancer seen in association with thrombophlebitis should suggest cerebral embolization from nonbacterial thrombotic endocarditis. The recognition of this clinical picture is important in preventing the erroneous diagnosis of cerebral metastasis, since an otherwise operable neoplasm may not receive adequate treatment because of the inaccurate conclusion that the cerebral symptoms indicate that the lesion has become disseminated. Occasionally cerebral embolism may be the first evidence of neoplasm.

The nonembolic neurologic aspects of myocardial and valvular disease consist primarily of alterations of consciousness and are discussed in Chaps. 60B and 62E.

NEUROLOGIC COMPLICATIONS OF CARDIAC SURGERY

Central nervous system emboli constitute a significant complication of cardiac surgery. Valvulotomy for the correction of mitral stenosis, whether transatrial or transventricular, carries the risk of peripheral embolization either by calcific valve fragments or as a result of accidental dislodgment of thrombotic material in the left atrium. Wood, quoted in a personal communication by Emanuel,[11] states that in mitral stenosis uncomplicated by valve calcification the risk of arterial embolization at operation is between 5 and 8 percent. However, when stenosis is accompanied by incompetence and calcification of the valve, the risk of emboli increases to 13 percent. In open heart

surgical procedures employing extracorporeal circulation, the risk of cerebral embolization is theoretically greater than it is with closed procedures. Here, along with embolization by calcium plaques, there are the added hazards of air emboli as well as systemic emboli by thrombi, silicon, and fat. In an excellent review of this subject, Allen[12] reports an incidence of 18 embolic episodes in 500 cases of bypass surgical procedures performed at the Vancouver General Hospital. Air emboli were the most frequently encountered, occurring most often in the repair of mitral and aortic valves and to a lesser degree during the closure of atrial septal defects of the ostium secundum and primum types. Calcium emboli were seen in calcific lesions of the aortic or mitral valves. Thrombotic emboli were less frequent and were usually encountered during active attempts to remove a left atrial thrombus rather than resulting from accidental dislodgment at the time of operation. Thrombotic emboli were also seen in resection of postinfarction myocardial aneurysms in which friable thrombi were dislodged during the resection of the aneurysmal sac. Silicon emboli, though infrequent, may be seen in systems using a defoaming agent and are more likely to occur during procedures requiring high-volume perfusion over an extended period during which the silicon may be washed from the oxygenator into the arterial system.

The neurologic manifestations of central nervous system emboli in association with cardiac surgery are highly variable.[13] The early manifestations, such as slowness to respond after anesthesia, persistently depressed consciousness, or generalized seizures in the absence of focal neurologic signs, suggest a general disorder and are likely to be due to air, silicon, fat emboli, or hypoxia. An intermediate group also thought to be due to air or silicon is characterized by a normal response for the first 12 to 24 h followed by depressed consciousness and frequently by generalized seizures. The third clinical picture is dominated by focal signs (either focal neurologic deficits or focal seizures) with or without impaired consciousness and is seen immediately postoperatively. This picture is more likely to be due to calcific or thrombotic emboli. Focal central nervous system manifestations appearing 48 h after an operation or later are most likely due to embolization from thrombi forming on operative suture lines.

Comparatively little has been written about fat embolization during cardiotomy and cardiopulmonary bypass. Caguin and Carter,[14] reporting on 93 bypass operations, noted an occasional patient who exhibited a wide variety of vague neurologic signs and symptoms, usually appearing between the third and seventh postoperative days. The neurologic features ranged form mild confusion and amnesia to a picture resembling delirium tremens which responded to sedation. Focal signs were minimal, and all patients recovered without apparent residual deficits. Petechiae were not encountered in any patients. None of the patients developing delirium gave a

TABLE 105-1
Clinical features of embolic complications of cardiac surgical treatment

Time of onset	Clinical findings	Probable type of emboli
Immediate or 12–24 h postoperatively	Failure to respond after surgical treatment; persistently depressed consciousness; possibly generalized seizures; no focal signs	Air, fat, silicon, or hypoxia (generalized petechiae and hematuria favor silicon or fat)
	Prominent focal signs; neurologic defect and/or focal seizures	Calcific fragments or intracardiac thrombi
Delayed—48 h or later postoperatively	Prominent focal signs	Thrombotic from thrombi on suture lines
	Confusion, stupor, delirium tremens-like picture usually without focal signs; significant lipuria	Fat

history of significant alcohol consumption. Although hypoxia could not be ruled out, the electroencephalograms done during the operation were normal in all patients, and none had undue respiratory symptoms. Because of the similarity of these symptoms to those seen in some patients with multiple fractures, fat embolization was suspected as a cause. Subsequently, evidence of fat embolization was looked for routinely, and significant lipuria was found in 10 to 45 patients, 8 of whom demonstrated these neurologic events. Fat globules were demonstrated in the cerebrospinal fluid of one patient who also had lesions in his retinal arterioles consistent with fat emboli. There was no correlation with the type of thoracotomy, the surgical procedure, or the duration of the bypass.

The writers noted that the symptoms seem to have occurred only in patients in whom the blood overflowed from the cardiac chambers into the pericardial sac or the pleural space and was then returned to the bypass circuit via the coronary suction apparatus. Fat globules could be seen on the surface of the blood pooled in these cavities. Sudan III stains on the pooled blood were positive, whereas venous blood drawn simultaneously was negative for free fat. This suggests that the source of the fat was the marrow of the ribs and sternum or other surfaces cut during the operative procedure. In subsequent operations on 56 patients, recirculation of the blood in the pericardial sac was avoided if possible. In one patient in whom technical problems necessitated return of pericardial blood, neurologic signs and severe lipuria developed. In two others mild lipuria developed without neurologic findings. These patients differ in some respects from those with fat embolization after trauma reported by Sevitt,[15] who emphasizes a characteristic petechial rash over the anterior part of the chest and shoulders as a prominent and reliable sign. Sevitt also regards the examination of the urine to be unreliable, though he apparently examined only random specimens rather than 24-h pooled specimens as done in Caguin's study.

There is no explanation for the delayed appearance of the neurologic symptoms in these cases. The close relation between the appearance of lipuria and the development of neurologic symptoms in Caguin's cases favors fat embolization as being the primary pathogenetic factor. Fromm[16] regards a "free interval" of 12 to 48 h between the trauma and the onset of cerebral symptoms as characteristic of cerebral fat embolization. This time sequence is reminiscent of the biphasic course seen in patients with carbon monoxide intoxication and other forms of hypoxia as reported by Plum et al.[17] These patients recovered from the initial episode with little or no disturbance in brain function, only to experience the onset of progressive deterioration as they resumed activity. The author and others have seen a similar sequence of events in patients following successful cardiac resuscitation.

A classification of the neurologic complications of open heart surgical procedure with cardiopulmonary bypass is presented in Table 105-1. This classification, although incomplete, provides the clinician with a reasonable basis for establishing the source of emboli associated with open heart surgical procedures. The problem is compounded by such factors as unrecognized fat emboli, hypoxia, hemoconcentration, and hypoglycemia possibly related to the use of stored, whole blood. Similarly, the neuropathologic data on autopsy cases are frequently incomplete because of failure to use appropriate histologic techniques, as silicon and fat emboli are dissolved by the usual solvents used in routine histologic preparation.

The study by Brierly[18] provides excellent clinicopathologic correlation in 11 patients who died after open heart surgical operation. These patients include two in whom cardiopulmonary bypass was not used but in whom there was deliberate circulatory arrest under mild hypothermia, and nine patients in whom cardiopulmonary bypass with a pump oxygenator was used along with mild hypothermia. The predominant pathologic lesions were multifocal, perivascular, irregular areas of ischemic changes involving the cortex and underlying white matter, seen predominantly in the dependent portions of the brain (posterior portion of the middle cerebral artery territory, occipital lobes, and cerebellum). These lesions had neither the histologic features nor the distribution characteristic of diffuse cerebral anoxia. Brierly postulates that these lesions are due either to severely reduced cerebral blood flow or to air embolism. The predominance of lesions in the posterior portions of the brain suggests that a gravitational pooling may have occurred in this region in patients lying in the supine position. The resulting congestion of the dependent portion of the vascular bed might delay the resumption of normal pulsatile blood flow when normal cardiac function is resumed and thus might lead to ischemia.

NEUROLOGIC COMPLICATIONS OF CONGENITAL HEART DISEASE

Tyler and Clark[19,20] reviewed the neurologic complications of congenital heart disease and found evidence of neurologic involvement in 25 percent of 1,875 patients of the cardiac clinic at the Harriett Lane Home of the Johns Hopkins Hospital. Those patients with congenital heart disease in whom the major physiologic defect was decreased pulmonary flow or transposition (e.g., tetralogy of Fallot, truncus arteriosus with decreased flow) had a high incidence of episodic loss of consciousness. This clinical picture consists of loss of consciousness lasting from minutes to 2 to 3 h, characteristically brought on by increased physical activity and preceded in most patients by severe cyanosis and dyspnea. On the basis of the history of cyanosis and dyspnea preceding the loss of consciousness or convulsions, the writers conclude that these episodes are caused by a sudden shift of hemodynamics in which more venous blood enters the systemic circulation. In this study there were 27 cases of cerebral abscess, all occurring in patients with cardiac defects which allowed the passage of venous blood directly into systemic circulation, bypassing the pulmonary circuit. Abscesses were significantly more frequent in patients with tetralogy of Fallot (1.4 percent), transposition (1.7 percent), and septal defects (0.7 percent). No abscesses were seen in association with patent ductus arteriosus. No cerebral abscesses were found in patients under 2 years of age. Mental retardation was seen in patients with a variety of cardiac malformations and was related to associated developmental abnormalities of the brain rather than to the severity of the cardiac lesion.

Cerebrovascular accidents were more frequent in patients with transposition of the great vessels, tricuspid atresia, and other forms of congenital heart disease which produced a high degree of cyanosis and hypoxia in the first 2 years of life. The majority of cerebrovascular accidents (74 percent) occurred in the first 20 months of life, decreasing in frequency up to age 6 and then recurring in the midteens. On postmortem examination all infarctions were in the distribution of the middle cerebral arteries, but an actual thrombosis was found in only 3 of the 14 autopsied cases. No patient had a proved source of emboli. Determinations of red blood cell count and oxygen saturation at the time of the cerebrovascular accident suggest to these writers that in the younger group hypoxia is a major factor in the pathogenesis of cerebral lesions, whereas in the older group polycythemia appears to be of greater pathogenetic importance. The frequency with which these events were associated with acute illness suggests that fever and dehydration were contributing factors.

NEUROLOGIC MANIFESTATIONS OF ATHEROSCLEROSIS

The principal mechanisms by which atherosclerosis affects the nervous system are (1) direct involvement of the intracranial arteries, (2) stenosis or occlusion of the cervicobrachial arteries, and (3) embolization of the cerebral vessels from atheromatous deposits in the thoracic aorta and the cervical arteries. The cerebroarterial circulation is involved by atherosclerosis in a manner that tends to parallel the atherosclerotic process in other systemic arteries. The earliest and most frequently involved segment is the proximal internal carotid and the carotid sinus. The common carotid artery may be involved but to a much lesser degree. Significant narrowing of the cervical portion of the vertebral artery is less than that seen in the carotid and tends to be concentrated in its proximal 2 cm. Examinations of the entire length of the vertebral arteries have shown atheromatous changes to be more widely distributed, in many instances bearing a relation to distortion of the vessel by osteoarthritis of the cervical spine.[21]

Maximum involvement of the intracranial arteries is seen at the carotid siphon, at the trifurcation of the internal carotid, at the first bifurcation of the middle cerebral artery, in the basilar artery at its bifurcation, at the proximal segment of the posterior cerebral artery as it passes around the cerebral peduncles, and at the anterior cerebral artery in its course over the genu of the corpus callosum. Hypertension and diabetes increase the severity of the atherosclerotic process in both the extra- and intracranial arteries and the perforating branches originating from the main stem of the middle cerebral, basilar, and posterior cerebral arteries.

In 100 consecutive autopsies of patients over the age of 50 years, Martin et al.[22] found 40 percent of the cases to have stenosis of at least one major cervical artery to a degree of 50 percent or greater. However, only 17 of these 40 patients had symptoms of cerebral ischemia during life. The only significant difference between the symptomatic and asymptomatic patients was a greater degree of atherosclerosis of

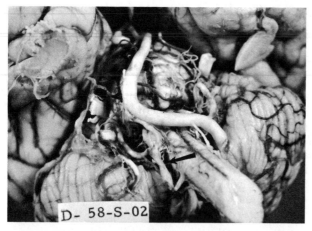

FIGURE 105-2 Anomalous vertebral-basilar artery system with
an atretic right vertebral artery (arrow). The patient had recurrent
transient ischemic attacks in the distribution of the vertebral
artery.

the intracranial arteries in the symptomatic group.
There was also a close relation between atherosclerosis of the cervical arteries and coronary artery
disease, both tending to reach their maximum extent
in the same age group. The peak incidence of significant atherosclerosis of the intracranial arteries occurred some 10 years later. These data suggest that
although a large segment of the population over 50
has significant atherosclerosis of the cervical arteries, most of these cases are asymptomatic. The
occurrence of symptoms of ischemia depends on
other factors, one of which is concomitant involvement of the intracranial arteries. Other recognized
factors predisposing to symptoms of ischemia include anemia, hypoxia, hemoconcentration, decreased perfusion pressure (on the basis of decreased
arterial pressure, increased venous pressure, or increased intracranial pressure), and inadequacy of
collateral channels due to congenital variations in the
distribution and size of the major cerebral arteries
(Fig. 105-2).

The clinical features of atherosclerosis of the
cerebral vessels with thrombosis are quite varied.
However, there are signs and symptoms which can
be of assistance in arriving at a diagnosis of cerebral
thrombosis. The clinical manifestations may develop
in one of several forms. There may be a stuttering
progression, with the full deficit appearing over several hours or even days, or severe paralysis may clear
within hours or a day, only to be followed by
persistent paralysis.

Many patients with cerebral thrombosis have a
history of one or more transient episodes of neurologic deficit that preceded the accomplished infarction. Such episodes do not precede intracranial hemorrhage and are uncommon in cerebral embolism.
These episodes, referred to as *transient ischemic
attacks* (TIA), consist of recurrent, transient episodes of neurologic dysfunction. They may be considered a reversible fragment of the stroke which

TABLE 105-2

**Common signs and symptoms of transient ischemic attacks in the
distribution of the internal carotid artery system**

Unilateral weakness and numbness on side opposite involved vessel

Aphasia (when dominant hemisphere is involved)

Monocular blindness on side of involved vessel

Reduced pulsations in carotid artery

Reduced central retinal artery pressure

Neck or cranial bruit

may ultimately follow. Onset is usually sudden, most
often when the patient is active, and the attack may
last from a few seconds to several hours. The attack
usually ends as suddenly as it began, clearing up
without significant residual deficit. The successive
attacks are usually of the same pattern, although
somewhat different in detail. The clinical manifestations are related to the area of ischemia and are
always in a vascular pattern.

In the carotid system the episodes commonly take
the form of unilateral numbness and weakness of the
side of the body opposite the involved vessel. Monocular blindness and associated symptoms that affect the opposite side of the body are virtually
pathognomonic of involvement of the carotid artery
on the same side as the blindness. Diminished or
absent pulsations in the carotid artery in the neck,
reduced retinal artery pressure, and a bruit over the
carotid artery or the orbit suggest narrowing or
occlusion of the carotid artery. These features are
summarized in Table 105-2.

The characteristic features in the vertebral-basilar
system are summarized in Table 105-3.

In differential diagnosis the following conditions
must be considered: cerebral seizures, Ménière's
syndrome and other forms of aural vertigo, paralytic
migraine, Stokes-Adams attacks and hyperactive carotid sinus reflexes, and cerebral embolism.

The differentiation of cerebral seizures is outlined
in Table 105-4. Although motor convulsions do not
occur in transient ischemic attacks, patients may
frequently report feelings of distortion or contortion
of the extremities. Paralysis is, of course, frequent in
transient ischemic attacks. Paralysis may also occur
in seizures but always follows a frank motor convulsion. Sensory seizures are much more difficult to
differentiate from transient ischemic attacks. As a

TABLE 105-3

**Common signs and symptoms of transient ischemic attacks involving
the vertebral-basilar artery system**

Weakness, numbness of one or both sides of the body

"Crossed symptoms" such as one side of the face and the
opposite body half

Dizziness

Diplopia

Partial or complete blindness

Dysarthria or speechlessness

Dysphagia

Staggering

Peculiar head and face sensations

Hiccuping

"Apparent" unconsciousness

Drop attacks

TABLE 105-4
Differential diagnosis of cerebral seizures and transient ischemic attacks

Symptoms	Seizures	TIA
Frank motor convulsion	+	−
Paralysis as only manifestation	−	+
Numbness, paresthesias, scintillating scotoma, sensory march	+	+
Associated phenomena, such as monocular blindness, diplopia, dizziness	−	+
Unconsciousness, incontinence, residual drowsiness, myalgia	+	−

TABLE 105-6
Differential diagnosis of "paralytic" migraine and transient ischemic attacks

Symptoms	Paralytic migraine	TIA
Visual, sensory, motor phenomena	+	+
Headache	+	−
History beginning in early life	+	−

rule, the sensory march in cerebral seizure is extremely rapid, whereas in transient ischemic attack the rate of spread is slower, extending over a period of several minutes.

Dizziness is one of the most frequent neurologic symptoms in the older age group and poses a difficult diagnostic problem. There are no characteristics of the dizziness itself which make it possible to determine whether the complaint is of aural origin or whether it represents a manifestation of brainstem ischemia. Only by careful search for signs of disturbance of function of other structures that are innervated by the brainstem can this differentiation be made (Table 105-5).

Differential diagnosis between "paralytic" migraine and transient ischemic attack is difficult, because focal sensory or motor phenomena with attendant headache of a vascular nature may be seen in both conditions. Scintillating scotoma is frequent in migraine, whereas the visual symptom in transient ischemic attack is a negative one. It is not at all unusual for patients with the full migraine syndrome in early life to have an asymptomatic period followed in later life by the occurrence of the prodromas without headache.[23] Thus a history of such symptoms from early life suggests migraine (Table 105-6).

If only one episode of transient neurologic disturbance has occurred, it is virtually impossible to differentiate between cerebral embolism and transient ischemic attack. When there have been several attacks of similar character the most likely diagnosis is transient ischemic attack, since it would be highly unlikely that successive showers of embolic particles would always find their way to the same cerebral vessel.

Stokes-Adams attacks and hyperactive carotid sinus reflexes as a rule produce syncopal symptoms and are not associated with focal sensory or motor disturbances. If the reduction in cardiac output is

TABLE 105-5
Differential diagnosis of Ménière's syndrome and transient ischemic attacks

Symptoms	Ménière's syndrome	TIA
Dizziness	+	+
Dizziness, tinnitus, deafness in "isolation"	+	−
Other evidence of brainstem involvement, such as diplopia, facial numbness, and dysarthria	−	+

prolonged, seizures may be seen. Most often the seizures under these circumstances consist of bilateral extensor regidity and opisthotonus (see Chap. 47).

The pathophysiology of transient ischemic attacks remains obscure. Whatever their exact mechanism, they are closely related to cerebral atherosclerosis. The observed effect of anticoagulants of reducing the frequency of attacks, the finding in some patients of fibrin or cholesterol emboli in the retinal arterioles during an attack, and the arteriographic evidence of ulcerated plaque of the cervical arteries in many patients with transient ischemic attacks all suggest that in some instances recurrent emboli from cervical arterial atheroma may precipitate the episodes. On the other hand, the stereotyped nature of successive attacks could be explained only by embolic particles entering the same arterial segment. Although this could happen on the basis of the pattern of arterial flow in a given patient, it seems statistically unlikely. An alternative explanation is based on the supposition that the area of brain from which the symptoms arise is one in which collateral blood flow is marginal, being adequate only under basal conditions. The added limitations imposed by stenosis of the cervical arteries and other factors such as a minimal reduction in blood pressure or a mild degree of hypoxia might then be sufficient to render the area ischemic. This theory is more compatible with the stereotyped nature of the recurrent attacks but is less tenable when one considers how infrequently transient ischemic attacks can be precipitated in these patients by artificially inducing hypotension or hypoxia. An association between cardiac arrhythmia and transient ischemic attacks has been noted,[24] but the report deals with patients with diffuse rather than focal neurologic symptoms.[24]

Though it is true that many patients with cerebral thrombosis do have an antecedent history of transient ischemic attacks, it does not necessarily follow that these episodes invariably lead to a cerebral infarction with persistent neurologic deficit. In fact, observations of patients with transient ischemic attacks have shown that the majority did not develop cerebral infarction within the 2- to 3-year observation period (Table 105-10).[25] In a study in Rochester, Minnesota, extending over 14 years 36 percent of 198 patients with transient ischemic attacks had a subsequent stroke. The risk of stroke was 16.5 times higher than in the general population.[26] These data suggest

that there may be a group of patients in whom
transient ischemic attacks do not portend an impending stroke. However, in the absence of clinical criteria by which to recognize this group, it remains
important to regard transient ischemic attacks as
"warning episodes," in order that appropriate diagnostic procedures and therapy may be instituted
before a permanent neurologic deficit occurs. In the
absence of effective means of modifying the process
of atherosclerosis, the treatment of transient ischemic attacks and other forms of arherosclerosis is
twofold: (1) the use of anticoagulants or antiplatelet
agents and (2) surgical excision or bypass of obstructions of the cervicobrachial portion of the cerebral
circulation. The role of anticoagulant drugs has not
been established. Earlier reports suggested that this
form of therapy in patients with transient ischemic
attacks reduced the number and frequency of attacks
and postponed or prevented cerebral infarction. It
was also held that anticoagulants favorably influenced the course of an advancing cerebral thrombosis. Results of several controlled, cooperative studies
of the effects of anticoagulant drugs have failed to
demonstrate any statistically significant reduction of
either the incidence of cerebral infarction or the
mortality rate in patients with transient ischemic
attacks.[27,28] There was, however, a reduction in the
number of ischemic attacks, this effect being most
prominent in the first 3 to 4 months of the observation period. The benefit of anticoagulants in patients
with advancing thrombosis is often offset by the high
incidence of hemorrhagic complication in the treated
group. Studies conclusively demonstrated that there
is no advantage in the use of anticoagulant drugs in
the accomplished cerebral infarction.[27,29] Whisnant et
al.[30] examined the clinical course of treated and
untreated patients during the first 12 months of
illness and concluded that the most beneficial effect
of anticoagulant therapy is in the first 2 months
following onset of transient ischemic attacks.

In a controlled trial of aspirin in cerebral infarction, analysis of the first 6 months of follow-up
revealed a reduction in the frequency of transient
ischemic attacks. This effect was most apparent in
patients with multiple transient ischemic attacks and
in whom there was a carotid lesion appropriate to the
transient ischemic attack symptom. There was no
protection from a completed stroke due to cerebral
infarction.[30a]

The published results of surgery in the treatment
of carotid artery extracranial cerebrovascular disease vary, but most centers agree that the best results
are seen in patients with transient ischemic

TABLE 105-7
Neurologic risk factors

Progressing deficit
Deficit less than 24 h duration
Frequent daily TIA
Multiple cerebral infarctions

TABLE 105-8
Angiographic risk factors

Occlusion of opposite internal carotid artery (ICA)
Stenosis of ICA in region of siphon
Extensive involvement of vessel to be operated on (linear,
  above and below bifurcation)
Bifurcation at level of C-2
Evidence of soft thrombosis and ulceration

attacks.[31–33] Surgery in patients with an acute stroke
or established chronic strokes is not beneficial, and in
fact has been shown in many instances to be harmful.[34]

The objectives of management of arteriosclerotic
cerebrovascular disease are to prevent the development of a stroke or to limit the extent of the
neurologic deficit. Thus, patients with transient ischemic attacks in the distribution of the carotid
artery without neurologic deficit or those with an
accomplished infarction followed by functional recovery with only a minimal residual deficit should be
considered for arteriography in an attempt to demonstrate a surgically accessible lesion. Carotid bruits,
decreased retinal artery pressure, or retinal emboli in
such patients are absolute indications for arteriography. Sundt et al.[67] have defined medical, arteriographic, and neurologic factors which increase the
risk of arteriography and surgery. These are summarized in Tables 105-7 to 105-9.

OTHER FORMS OF CERVICOBRACHIAL CIRCULATION DISEASE WITH CEREBRAL SYMPTOMS

Other forms of disease of the cervical and brachial
arteries producing cerebral symptoms include kinking of the carotid arteries, obstruction of the brachiocephalic or subclavian arteries, and the various forms
of the aortic arch syndrome. Kinking of the cervical
arteries has been attributed to the effects of hypertension and atherosclerosis or the persistence of fetal
configuration of the carotid artery. Examples of kinking have been found in every decade from the first to
the ninth, frequently without relation to hypertension
or atherosclerosis. Metz et al.[36] found no greater
incidence of cerebral manifestation in patients with
severe kinking when compared with patients of similar age without this abnormality. They were able to
produce vague cerebral symptoms in 4 of 24 patients

TABLE 105-9
Medical risk factors

Angina pectoris
Myocardial infarction during previous 6 months
Congestive heart failure
B.P. greater than 180/110
Chronic obstructive pulmonary disease
Patient over 70 years
Obesity

TABLE 105-10
Prognosis of untreated transient ischemic attacks (24- to 41-month follow-up)

	Patients with TIA	Patients developing cerebral infarction	Deaths from cerebral infarction	Deaths from other causes
PHS cooperative study[27]	20	4	1	1
VA cooperative study[28]	15	0	0	0
David and Heyman[35]	8	3	3	1
Total	43	7	4	2

by rotation of the neck. In spite of the lack of firm clinical correlation, one is justified in carefully considering the surgical excision of an area of kinking in a patient who clearly has recurrent cerebrovascular episodes related to turning of the neck and in whom no other adequate cause can be demonstrated.

Fibromuscular dysplasia (FMD) is a disease of unknown cause affecting small to medium-size arteries including the cervicobrachial vessels. In many instances, FMD of the cerebral vessels is asymptomatic, but it has been seen in patients with a variety of symptoms including positional cerebral ischemia, transient ischemic attacks, cerebral infarction, arteriovenous malformations, and berry aneurysms. Though it is likely that in some cases FMD is directly related to the neurologic symptoms, in others coexisting vascular disease has been thought responsible for the cerebral symptoms.[37]

Occlusion or stenosis of the subclavian or brachiocephalic artery can lead to symptoms which in most instances are referable to the vertebral-basilar artery. This condition should be considered when there is a significant difference in the blood pressure in each arm or a bruit which is maximal over the supraclavicular area. Occasionally symptoms may be precipitated by exercise of the homolateral arm leading to retrograde collateral flow to the arm at the expense of the vertebral-basilar system. This syndrome has been called the *subclavian steal*[38] syndrome (Fig. 105-3).

Cerebral symptoms are frequently seen in the various forms of the aortic arch syndrome, in which there is obliteration of the large arteries arising from the convexity of the aorta. Causes of such involvement include atherosclerosis, syphilitic aortitis, Takayasu's arteritis of young females, trauma, neoplasm, and congenital malformation. The neurologic manifestations are dependent on the relative degree of involvement of the major vessels and may include findings such as those described in conjunction with the carotid or vertebral-basilar arteries. The cerebral manifestations of aortic dissection are discussed in Chap. 103.

The association between coarctation of the aorta and aneurysms of the intracranial arteries is well known. Reifenstein et al.[39] found that subarachnoid hemorrhage from a berry aneurysm accounted for 10.6 percent of deaths in their series of cases. In addition they report three cases of cerebral embolism

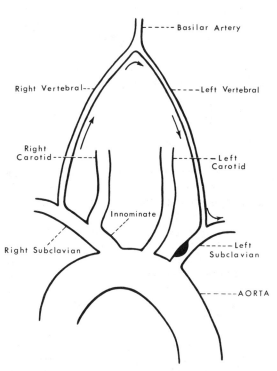

FIGURE 105-3 Retrograde flow in the left vertebral artery bypassing a stenotic area in the left subclavian artery, as seen in the subclavian steal syndrome.

from bacterial endocarditis arising from associated congenital valvular malformation.

AORTIC DISEASE INVOLVING THE SPINAL CORD

The spinal cord is frequently cited as being that portion of the central nervous system less likely to be affected by vascular disease. This statement is in general valid with regard to atherosclerotic involvement of the intrinsic arteries of the cord. However, the spinal cord may be significantly involved in several types of aortic disease. The most familiar of these is dissecting aortic aneurysm, in which the spinal cord may be rendered ischemic by virtue of the dissection occluding the ostia of the intercostal and lumbar arteries. Occlusion of the abdominal aorta by atherosclerosis or embolus may lead to dysfunction of the spinal cord. Infarction of the spinal cord may also be seen as a manifestation of aortic disease which has otherwise been asymptomatic.[40] Disturbance of spinal cord function of a vascular nature is also seen as a sequel to the insertion of an aortic graft.[41]

Coarctation of the aorta may affect the spinal cord as a result of hypertrophy of the anterior spinal artery as it participates in the collateral circulation to the trunk and lower limbs. Such hypertrophy may lead to the formation of a false aneurysm which can act as an extramedullary compressive lesion.[42]

HYPERTENSION AND THE NERVOUS SYSTEM

The major central nervous system manifestations of hypertension are (1) spontaneous intracerebral hemorrhage, (2) hypertensive encephalopathy, and (3) cerebral atherosclerosis as modified and accelerated by hypertension.

The spontaneous or hypertensive intracerebral hemorrhage is one of the most frequent nervous system concomitants of hypertension. It occurs almost without exception in patients who have significant and persistent elevation of blood pressure or who have evidence of hypertension in the past as manifested by changes in the retinal arterioles, cardiomegaly, left ventricular hypertrophy pattern on ECG, etc. The hemorrhages arise in one of several sites: the putamen, the thalamus and subthalamic region, the external capsule, the tegmentum of the pons, or the cerebellum. These areas have in common the fact that they are in the distribution of the short, penetrating arteries which originate from major arterial trunks and pass immediately into cerebral substance. The hemorrhage appears to originate within deep nuclear masses, e.g., the putamen, the thalamus, or the dentate nucleus of the cerebellum, and then dissect through and compress surrounding white matter.

Using the putaminal hemorrhage as the paradigm of a hypertensive intracerebral hemorrhage, the clinical events are as follows: The onset is abrupt, usually while the patient is active, and is not preceded by recurrent prodromal symptoms such as are seen in cerebral thrombosis. The patient usually complains of an abnormal head sensation, which is frequently, though not invariably, a severe headache. Initially there may be no localizing signs, but as the adjacent internal capsule is compressed, a contralateral hemiparesis and sensory deficit develop. As the process extends anteriorly, there may be paralysis or weakness of gaze to the opposite side, often with the eyes conjugately deviated to the side of the hemorrhage. If the dominant hemisphere is involved, there may be aphasia; in the nondominant hemisphere, the syndrome of apractagnosia may be seen. Gradually, the hemiparesis worsens, and the patient becomes more stuporous. In its severest forms the hemorrhage ruptures into the lateral ventricle. The involved hemisphere is shifted medially under the tentorium, producing compression of the hemolateral third nerve, the earliest manifestation of which may be a fluctuation of size of the pupil. As the midbrain is compressed further, coma deepens and bilateral signs appear. Respiration becomes irregular, and there is decerebrate posturing with fixed miotic pupils and death in a few hours. It is to be emphasized, however, that not all cases take this form. An estimated 10 to 15 percent of patients survive, sometimes with amazing return of neurologic function (Fig. 105-4). Others survive for 5 to 10 days, gradually losing ground each day, reflecting either slow

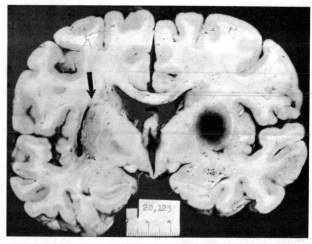

FIGURE 105-4 Nonfatal hypertensive intracerebral hemorrhage. Slit hemorrhage in the left putamen and external capsule (arrow) is the residuum of an episode that occurred 12 months previously. Ball hemorrhage on the right is of 2 days' duration. The patient died of a hemorrhage in the tegmentum of the pons.

continued bleeding or progressive swelling of the brain in response to the original bleeding. Though it was previously believed that coma was invariably seen when the blood entered the ventricular system, there are well-documented cases of patients with grossly bloody cerebrospinal fluid and massive hemiplegia and hemisensory deficits who are sufficiently alert to respond to commands. The most difficult problem in differential diagnosis is posed by the patient who has a massive intracerebral hemorrhage which does not extend into the ventricular system and who, as a consequence, does not have blood in the cerebrospinal fluid. In general, however, a safe clinical rule is that a massive hemiplegia with a well-preserved state of consciousness speaks in favor of occlusive rather than hemorrhagic disease.

The general criteria in Table 105-11 based on those originally proposed by Fisher[43,44] are useful in establishing the clinical diagnosis of hypertensive intracerebral hemorrhage.

The clinical differentiation as to the site of hemorrhage can be made using the following summary:

1 Putaminal hemorrhage. Contralateral hemiparesis usually extensive; hemianopsia *usually* present, but sensory loss *always* present. Cortical signs such as aphasia or

TABLE 105-11
Criteria helpful in establishing the clinical diagnosis of hypertensive intracerebral hemorrhage

Hypertension or corollary evidence of hypertension present
Recurrent prodromal attacks not seen
Onset during activity rather than in sleep
Severe unilateral headache at onset
Moderately rapid progression of neurologic deficit which may extend beyond the distribution of a given cerebral artery
Rapid progression to coma
Absence of rapid fluctuation in clinical course or reversal of signs and symptoms
Displacement of pineal gland early in the episode
Blood in the cerebrospinal fluid in most instances
Probably no late rebleeding from the same site

apractagnosia if patient sufficiently alert to permit examination; deepening coma along with other evidence of brainstem compression as late event.

2 Thalamic hemorrhage. Extensive contralateral sensory loss—hemiplegia may be of lesser degree; prominent ocular signs primarily involving vertical gaze with eyes deviated downward and medially; contralateral hemianopsia; brainstem compression and coma if the process is extensive.

3 Cerebellar hemorrhage. Onset, if sufficiently slow, with ataxia and inability to maintain upright position; frank motor paralysis not present; conjugate paralysis of gaze to side of hemorrhage and/or ipsilateral peripheral facial weakness from extension into, or compression of, the pons. Coma usually rapid; if patient survives, may have late appearance of raised intracranial pressure secondary to compression of fourth ventricle or cerebral aqueduct.

4 Pontine hemorrhage. Usually produces coma in minutes; bilateral signs present initially; pupils characteristically miotic and unreactive; frequently total paralysis of conjugate eye movement; decerebrate rigidity early—may disappear as condition worsens.

The immediate treatment of intracerebral hemorrhages consists of intensive nursing care, constant medical supervision, and prevention of pulmonary complications. Adrenocortical steroids and osmotic diuretics such as mannitol have been used with apparent benefit in an attempt to control cerebral edema. Surgical evacuation of putaminal and thalamic hemorrhages has been tried with varying results. McKissock et al.[45] compared conservative and surgical therapy in a controlled study of 180 unselected cases of primary intracerebral hemorrhages and found that formal craniotomy within 3 days offered no advantage over conservative management as outlined above. There is no comparable study of patients operated upon in the later stages of the hemorrhage.

The hemorrhage within the cerebellum acts as an extraaxial compressive mass (Fig. 105-5). Evacuation of the hematoma is frequently lifesaving in what is otherwise a highly lethal condition.[46,47] The diagnosis can frequently be made clinically, and the surgical evacuation should be carried out as soon as possible.

The association between intracerebral hemorrhage and hypertension has been recognized for over a century, but the basic pathogenesis of these lesions has not yet been elucidated. Russell, using a radiographic technique, has reported the results of a survey of changes in the small arteries in brains from elderly normotensive and hypertensive subjects without intracerebral hemorrhage.[48] The smaller penetrating arteries showed an increase in thickness of the wall and a narrowing of the lumen. In addition, Russell demonstrated miliary aneurysms arising from these small vessels. The aneurysms were more numerous in the hypertensive group and were located most commonly in the basal ganglions and thalamus. He concludes from his findings that the combination of age and hypertension produces degenerative changes in the muscular and elastic coats of the small penetrating arteries; these changes lead to the formation of multiple miliary aneurysms. The aneurysms frequently showed evidence of minor hemorrhage,

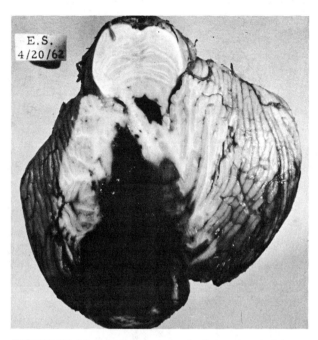

FIGURE 105-5 Spontaneous hypertensive hemorrhage in left lobe of cerebellum with compression of pons and fourth ventricle. Note the superficial location and accessibility of the bulk of the hemorrhage.

suggesting that at some point in their development, perhaps before the stage of intimal thickening, there is a potential for massive hemorrhages.

The term *hypertensive encephalopathy* has been erroneously applied to virtually any form of neurologic illness occurring in a patient with hypertension. More correctly, hypertensive encephalopathy designates a specific clinical entity appearing in an acute or subacute manner in a patient with hypertension and is characterized by headache, impaired consciousness, convulsions, and evidence of elevated intracranial pressure. Focal neurologic findings are rare and when present are frequently the result of other forms of cerebrovascular disease, such as cerebral thrombosis or embolus. Impaired renal function and congestive heart failure may also be present. Another frequent, though not invariable, feature of hypertensive encephalopathy is improvement of the neurologic status when the blood pressure is lowered. The neuropathologic findings are brain swelling and, in severe cases, hemorrhages of petechial or larger size (Fig. 105-6). Microscopically, the smaller arteries show fibrinoid degeneration, occasionally with frank necrosis. These vessels are surrounded by areas of fibrin deposition and small aggregations of glial cells which have been referred to as microinfarcts. Gross areas of infarction are infrequent and are usually related to incidental vascular disease. The clinical and pathologic aspects of hypertensive encephalopathy have been reproduced by Byrom[49] in experimental hypertension in the rat. He presents evidence that the clinical events are related to widespread vascular spasm, which leads to

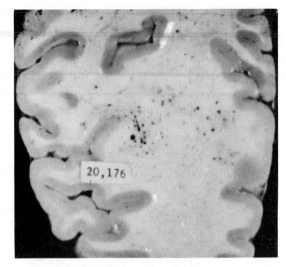

FIGURE 105-6 Hypertensive encephalopathy demonstrating cerebral edema and multiple petechial hemorrhages.

transient disturbances of function, progressing in more severe instances to increased capillary permeability with focal edema and local necrosis of both the arterial wall and the tissue supplied by the involved vessel. Furthermore, he was able to reduce or abolish the arterial spasm by lowering the blood pressure.

As previously mentioned in the discussion of atherosclerosis of the brain, hypertension not only accelerates the atheromatous process at the usual sites but also predisposes the smaller penetrating arteries to the development of atheromatous changes. These changes in vessels which supply deep medial structures lead to multiple small lacunar infarcts in the deep gray and white matter. Such lesions in the cerebral hemispheres are most numerous in the region of the basal ganglions and internal capsule and produce a clinical picture characterized by bilateral pyramidal tract signs with rigidity and increased reflexes. The patient's gait is one of small mincing steps (*marche à petit pas*). There is also evidence of pseudobulbar palsy, emotional lability, and varying degrees of dementia.[50,51] This picture has been erroneously referred to as arteriosclerotic parkinsonism. Lesions in the median and paramedian area of the brainstem are less frequent but may produce predominantly motor signs or defects in medial gaze (internuclear ophthalmoplegia, frequently unilateral).

The relation between lacunar infarction and hypertension has been confirmed by Fisher[52] in a review of 1,042 adults whose brains were examined at autopsy. In this study occlusion of the smaller penetrating arteries was found in six of the seven cases in which the search was undertaken. Serial sections of brain in areas of lacunas have demonstrated that the lacunas occur distal to obliterated aneurysmal dilatations of the penetrating vessels.[53]

It is obvious from a consideration of the relation of the brain to chronic elevation of blood pressure

that it is to the patient's advantage to detect significant hypertension early and control it as effectively as possible. However, there is considerable controversy regarding the use of antihypertensive therapy once clinically apparent cerebrovascular disease is present. In the management of the acute hypertensive intracerebral hemorrhage, there is no evidence that lowering of blood pressure has any favorable effect on prognosis for survival or recovery of function. In a patient with evidence of cerebral atherosclerosis, the dangers of inadvertent, drastic lowering of blood pressure outweigh any postulated benefit of antihypertensive therapy on vascular changes which are by this time fixed. Evidence to the contrary is presented by Marshall[54] in a study of patients with nonembolic cerebral infarction with diastolic blood pressures of 110 mm Hg or higher. The aim was to reduce the blood pressure to 100 to 110 mm Hg (an estimated mean reduction of 19.4 mm in men and 18.7 mm in women) rather than to a level considered desirable in a young patient with severe hypertension. In this series, using a wide variety of antihypertensive drugs, there was no instance of transient ischemic episodes appearing after therapy was begun, nor were cerebrovascular incidents precipitated by unusually low blood pressures. Marshall concludes that there was a significant reduction in the incidence of further cerebrovascular accidents in the treated group. The beneficial effect was more significant in men than in women. In the author's experience, reduction of blood pressure to the degree reported in Marshall's series can frequently be achieved by simple measures such as weight reduction, sodium restriction, mild sedation, and the use of thiazide diuretics, thus sparing the patient the potential hazards of medication which might predispose to the development of orthostatic hypotension.

Epidemiologic studies have conclusively demonstrated that hypertension is the most consistent risk factor predisposing to both ischemic and hemorrhagic strokes.[55] Though there are questions regarding the vigorous treatment of hypertension once symptoms of cerebrovascular disease are present, there are strong arguments to support the early detection and therapy of hypertension as a preventive measure.

MISCELLANEOUS CONDITIONS AFFECTING NERVOUS SYSTEM AND VESSELS

The inflammatory vasculitis of periarteritis nodosa tends to involve small and medium-sized arteries and produces neurologic symptoms in approximately one-third of the cases. The most frequent neurologic manifestation is mononeuropathy multiplex. Involvement of the central nervous system is less common and may result in focal neurologic deficits or seizures as a result of thrombosis of small arteries. Subarachnoid hemorrhage or intracerebral hemorrhage is said to occur in rare instances. Lupus erythematosus involves small arteries and may be associated with polyneuropathy or a wide variety of central nervous system manifestations, such as dementia, seizures, and focal neurologic deficits. Involvement of the nervous system in scleroderma and dermatomyositis is less frequent and usually consists of a perpheral neuropathy.[56,57] Giant-cell arteritis (temporal arteritis) may, in addition to blindness, be associated with ocular palsies[58] or focal neurologic deficits which result from the involvement of larger arteries, such as the carotid or vertebral artery, and their major branches.[59]

Involvement of the central nervous system in rheumatic fever is most frequently the result of cerebral embolism. Changes in cerebral vessels and brain parenchyma have been described as related to rheumatic fever, but their pathologic and clinical significance is still open to question. Acute (Sydenham's) chorea and chorea gravidarum are well-recognized neurologic accompaniments of rheumatic fever. The pathogenesis of chorea in rheumatic fever is still undetermined, and there is no recognized cerebral lesion to account for this syndrome.

Cardiac abnormalities, predominently arrhythmias, have been described in various acute central nervous system diseases. Electrocardiographic changes consisting of atrial and ventricular arrhythmias, alterations in the configuration of the QRS complex, lengthening of the Q-T interval, abnormalities of T waves, and changes in the S-T segment have been reported in patients with subarachnoid hemorrhage. Many of the electrocardiographic changes have simulated myocardial ischemia and infarction. In a study of cases of subarachnoid hemorrhage, Cropp and Manning[60] found such changes in a large proportion of their patients. Four of the five autopsied cases had abnormal electrocardiograms, two simulating an acute myocardial infarction. All five cases had normal coronary arteries. In the majority of the cases the site of intracranial hemorrhage was in the anterior fossa near the orbital surfaces of the frontal lobes, the area considered to be the cortical representation of the vagus nerve. Weintraub and McHenry[61] have summarized the current literature dealing with cardiac abnormalities and subarachnoid hemorrhage. Grossman[62] reported an accelerating ventricular tachycardia in a patient with an aneurysm at the bifurcation of the basilar artery. The arrhythmia was refracted through various forms of therapy including procainamide (Pronestyl), propranolol, and atropine sulfate administration. The arrhythmia disappeared 15 min after injection of 1% lidocaine (Xylocaine) into the left stellate ganglion. This form of therapy was suggested by the fact that the changes in the Q-T interval and the T wave configuration were quite similar to those described in dogs with stimulation of the left stellate ganglion. It is of interest to note that prior to the local injection the patient had not responded to 600 mg lidocaine given intravenously, suggesting that the effect was caused by the left stellate ganglion block rather than by the direct effect of absorbed lidocaine on the ventricle.

In a prospective study of patients selected solely on the basis of the diagnosis of one of the major types of muscular dystrophy, Perloff, de Leon, and O'Doherty[63] correlated the history and physical signs of the muscular disease with various cardiopulmonary findings. They studied electrocardiograms, vectorcardiograms, phonocardiograms, roentgenograns, serum enzyme levels, pulmonary ventilatory function, and hemodynamics. A summary of their observations is presented in Table 105-12.

The myocardial lesions consist of multiple areas of scarring, which tend to divide the muscle fibers into fasciculi of various sizes. Individual muscle fibers may show vasuolization and fragmentation.[64]

James[65] reported the morphologic changes in the heart of a patient with progressive muscular dystrophy who died following acute onset of atrial flutter.

TABLE 105-12
Summary of observations of the four types of dystrophy

	Duchenne's	Limb girdle	Benign Duchenne's or limb girdle with pseudohypertrophy	Fascioscapular humeral
Sex	M	M = F	M or F	M = F
Age of onset	5 yr	2d decade	Probably early 2d decade	Adolescence
Common mode of inheritance	X-linked recessive	Autosomal recessive	Autosomal or X-linked recessive	Autosomal dominant
Pseudohypertrophy	Characteristic marked	Occasional mild	Characteristic moderate	Rare
Rate of progression	Rapid	Moderate but variable	Moderate	Insidious
Serum enzyme elevations	High	Moderate	Moderate	Mild to moderate
Cardiomyopathy:				
Overt	Common	Uncommon	May be common	Rare
Occult	Very common	May be common	May be common	Uncommon
Physical signs	Atrial and 3d heart sounds	Atrial and 3d heart sounds	Atrial and 3d heart sounds	Atrial and 3d heart sounds
ECG signs	Very common	Uncommon	May be common	Rare
Type of ECG	Specific	Variable	Variable	Variable
X-rays signs	Uncommon	Uncommon	May be overt	Rare
Thoracic deformity	Marked	Moderate	Moderate	Moderate

SOURCE: Perloff, de Leon, and O'Doherty,[63] by permission of the author and the American Heart Association, Inc.

There was degeneration of fibers in the sinus node, with noninflammatory degeneration of the arteries supplying both the sinus node and the atrioventricular node. The arteriopathy was said to resemble that seen in the larger vessels in Marfan's syndrome and in three patients with primary pulmonary hypertension.

Recently two families with 37 males were described as having a remarkably stereotyped neuromuscular disease affecting distal leg and proximal arm musculature, which in every instance was associated with cardiac dysfunction. The onset is proximal weakness of the arms in the first decade of life. Within several years there is weakness in distal leg musculature. There is progression during the second decade, followed by stabilization. Pseudohypertrophy is absent. Facial involvement is minimal, and reflexes are markedly reduced to absent. Sensation is normal. The resultant neuromuscular disability is relatively mild but there is shortening of the Achilles tendon, fixed contractures in flexion at the elbow, and marked limitations of neck flexion. Muscle enzymes are moderately elevated. Electromyography, nerve conduction velocities, and muscle biopsies show predominantly myopathy in the proximal muscles and neuropathy distally. Inheritance is by a sex-linked recessive pattern. The characteristic cardiac syndrome consists of varying degrees of atrial arrhythmia, often progressing to permanent atrial paralysis, and profound bradycardia requiring a pacemaker. Sudden death in young adulthood has been frequent. Two of the reported patients had cerebral emboli. No patients had clinical neuromuscular disease without the electrocardiographic atrial disease. The early recognition of the neuromuscular syndrome can lead to genetic counseling and appropriate lifesaving cardiac therapy.[66]

TABLE 105-13
Distribution of major cerebral arteries; neurologic deficit produced by ischemia in their territory of supply

I Anterior (carotid) circulation.
  A Internal carotid artery.
    1 Supplies:
      a The optic nerve and retina via the ophthalmic artery.
      b Major portion of the cerebral hemispheres via the anterior and middle cerebral arteries.
    2 Signs and symptoms of ischemia:
      a Homolateral blindness.
      b Contralateral motor and/or sensory manifestations, usually referable to the distribution of the middle cerebral artery. May have evidence of involvement of anterior cerebral artery territory as well.
  B Middle cerebral artery. (Lesions in superficial distribution can result in discrete deficit due to the fact that representation of various regions of the body is over a large area of brain. In contrast, lesions in the deep branches may produce widespread neurologic deficit since descending and ascending tracts are in a compact bundle in the internal capsule.)
    1 Superficial (cortical) branches.
      a Supply lateral surface of cerebral hemisphere except

for frontal pole and strip along the superomedial aspect. This area includes centers for contraversive head and eye movements, cortical sensory and motor representation, and major part of optic radiations. In hemisphere dominant for speech it includes those regions concerned with the sensory and motor aspects of language. In nondominant hemisphere it includes the regions concerned with spatial orientation and body image.
      b Signs and symptoms of ischemia (all or part of the following):
        (1) Either hemisphere.
          (a) Motor and/or sensory impairment of opposite side of the body affecting the arm and face more than the leg.
          (b) Contralateral homonymous visual field defect.
          (c) Impairment of conjugate gaze to the opposite side.
        (2) Additional findings dependent on the hemisphere involved.
          (a) Dominant hemisphere: (i) motor and/or sensory aphasia; (ii) Gerstmann's syndrome (inability to recognize and use fingers, defects in calculating and writing, right-left disorientation); (iii) perseveration.
          (b) Nondominant hemisphere: (i) apractognosia (denial of neurologic deficit, neglect of opposite body half, dressing apraxia, loss of topographic memory); (ii) motor impersistence.
    2 Deep branches.
      a Supply basal ganglions, posterior limb of internal capsule, and corona radiata.
      b Signs and symptoms of ischemia:
        (1) Motor and sensory impairment of contralateral face, arm, and leg. Deficit may be purely motor.
        (2) No detectable signs of dysfunction of basal ganglions.
        (3) No visual field loss.
        (4) Occasionally aphasia, the basis of which remains unexplained.
  C Anterior cerebral artery. (Aphasia and visual field loss not usually seen. Infrequently involved in occlusive disease probably because of cross vascularization and anastomosis by way of anterior communicating artery. Therefore, findings referable to anterior cerebral artery suggest stenosis or occlusion in internal carotid artery *or* a cause other than ischemia.)
    1 Superficial branches.
      a Supply the anterior four-fifths of the medial surface of the cerebral hemisphere, medial part of the orbital surface of the frontal lobe, the frontal poles, and the majority of the corpus callosum. This includes areas of cortical representation of leg, bladder, and shoulder girdle.
      b Signs and symptoms of ischemia:
        (1) Unilateral lesion.
          (a) Motor and/or sensory loss of contralateral leg and, to a lesser extent, shoulder, with face and distal upper extremity frequently spared.
          (b) Prominent grasp and sucking reflexes.
          (c) Apraxia (inability to use a limb to execute movements even though there is no significant weakness, sensory loss, or incoordination).
        (2) Bilateral involvement.
          (a) Quadriparesis with limbs in flexion.
          (b) Akinetic mutism (lack of spontaneous movement or speech).
          (c) Profound mental changes.
          (d) Gait apraxia.
    2 Deep branches. Syndrome of ischemia in distribution of penetrating branches of anterior cerebral artery has not been recognized clinically.

II Posterior (vertebral-basilar) circulation.

  A Vertebral and basilar arteries. Supply medulla and pons which contain cranial nerve nuclei in association with major ascending and descending tracts. Also supply cerebellar hemispheres, their nuclei and tracts. [Lesions in distribution of these vessels characterized by involvement of one or more cranial nerve nuclei, cerebellar incoordination, and motor and sensory findings which may involve both sides of body in asymmetric or "crossed" distribution, i.e., one side of face and opposite body half. Localization of brainstem lesions in longitudinal axis (segmental level) is determined on basis of involved cranial nerve; e.g., ophthalmoplegia (third and fourth cranial nerves) indicates midbrain lesion; paralysis of muscles of mastication (motor, fifth), a midpontine lesion; peripheral-type facial paralysis (seventh), a lesion at the pontomedullary junction; palatal paralysis and dysphagia (nucleus ambiguus, ninth and tenth), midmedullary lesion; paralysis of tongue (twelfth), low-medullary lesion.]

    1 Superficial (lateral) branches.

      a Supply cerebellum and lateral portion of pons and medulla.

      b Signs and symptoms of ischemia:

        (1) Incoordination, particularly in lesions affecting the medulla.

        (2) Impaired pain and temperature sensation over same side of face and opposite body half.

        (3) Disturbed sympathetic function on the same side (Horner's syndrome).

        (4) Involvement of visceral and branchial motor nuclei (fifth, seventh, ninth, tenth, eleventh cranial nerves), along with special sensory nuclei (eighth).

        (5) Does not produce corticospinal tract signs or impairment of proprioception and light touch to body.

    2 Deep (median) branches.

      a Supply median and paramedian regions of medulla and pons.

      b Signs and symptoms of ischemia:

        (1) Involvement of somatic motor nuclei (third, fourth, sixth, twelfth cranial nerves).

        (2) Paralysis of medial gaze with sparing of other functions of third nerve. Due to involvement of medial longitudinal fasciculus (internuclear ophthalmoplegia).

        (3) Weakness of opposite body half due to involvement of descending motor fibers.

        (4) May have impaired light-touch and proprioception on opposite body half with sparing of pain and temperature (involvement of medial lemniscus).

  B Posterior cerebral artery.

    1 Cortical branches.

      a Supply inferior and medial surface of temporal lobe and the entire occipital lobe including the visual cortex.

      b Signs and symptoms of ischemia:

        (1) Unilateral.

          (a) May have only contralateral homonymous visual field deficit, frequently with macular sparing.

          (b) On dominant hemisphere may have difficulty reading or other disturbances of higher level of integration of visual image.

        (2) Bilateral.

          (a) Cortical blindness (blindness with intact pupillary reflex to light, no optic atrophy, and frequently denial of blindness).

          (b) Profound memory deficit (bilateral involvement of hippocampal formation of temporal lobes).

    2 Deep branches.

      a Supply midbrain subthalamic nucleus, cerebral peduncles, third nerve nucleus, reticular formation, thalamus including the lateral geniculate bodies, i.e., sensory or "optic" thalamus.

      b Signs and symptoms of ischemia:

        (1) Thalamic syndrome (Dejerine-Roussy)—loss of all sensory modalities from opposite body half, including vision—frequently followed by severe spontaneous pain. Motor loss mild or absent.

        (2) Weber's syndrome—homolateral third nerve paralysis and contralateral paralysis of face, arm, and leg.

        (3) Hemichorea of contralateral limbs.

        (4) Peduncular hallucinosis—visual hallucinations, usually vivid, colorful scenes. Not alarming to patient.

        (5) Extensive infarction can lead to quadriplegia and profound coma.

REFERENCES

1 Wells, C. E.: Premonitory Symptoms of Cerebral Embolism, *Arch. Neurol.*, 5:490, 1961.

2 Dodge, P. R., Richardson, E. P., Jr., and Victor, M.: Recurrent Convulsive Seizures as a Sequel to Cerebral Infarction: A Clinical and Pathological Study, *Brain,* 77:610, 1959.

3 Kumpfe, C. W., and Bean, W. B.: Aortic Stenosis: A Study of the Clinical and Pathologic Aspects of 107 Proved Cases, *Medicine (Baltimore),* 27:139, 1948.

4 Kane, W. C., and Aronson, S. M.: Cardiac Disorders Predisposing to Embolic Stroke, *Stroke,* 1:164, 1970.

5 Wells, C. E.: Cerebral Embolism: Natural History, Prognostic Signs and Effects of Anticoagulation, *A.M.A. Arch. Neurol. Psychiatr.,* 81:667, 1959.

6 Carter, A. B.: The Immediate Treatment of Cerebral Embolism, *Q. J. Med.* (n.s.) 26:335, 1957.

7 Fisher, C. M., and Adams, R. D.: Observation on Brain Hemorrhage with Special Reference to the Mechanism of Hemorrhagic Infarction, *J. Neuropathol. Exp. Neurol.,* 10:92, 1950.

8 Whisnant, J. P., Milikan, C. H., Sayre, G. P., and Wakim, K. G.: Effect of Anticoagulants on Experimental Cerebral Infarction: Clinical Implications, *Circulation,* 20:56, 1959.

9 Barron, K. D., Siqueira, E., and Hirano, A.: Cerebral Embolism Caused by Nonbacterial Thrombotic Endocartis, *Neurology,* 10:391, 1960.

10 MacDonald, R. A., and Robbins, S. L.: The Significance of Nonbacterial Thrombotic Endocarditis: An Autopsy and Clinical Study of 78 Cases, *Ann. Intern. Med.,* 46:255, 1957.

11 Emanuel, R.: Valvotomy in Mitral Stenosis with Extreme Pulmonary Vascular Resistance, *Br. Heart J.,* 25:119, 1963.

12 Allen, P.: Central Nervous System Emboli in Open Heart Surgery, *Can. J. Surg.,* 6:332, 1963.

13 Gillman, S.: Cerebral Disorders after Open Heart Operation, *N. Engl. J. Med.,* 272:489, 1965.

14 Caguin, F., and Carter, M. G.: Fat Embolization with Cardiotomy with the Use of Cardiopulmonary Bypass, *J. Thorac. Cardiovasc. Surg.,* 5:665, 1963.

15 Sevitt, S.: The Significance and Classification of Fat Embolism, *Lancet,* 2:825, 1960.

16 Fromm, von Hartnut: Sur Differentialdiagnose und Prognose der cerebralen Fettembolie, *Nervenarzt,* 33:430, 1962.

17 Plum, F., Posner, J. B., and Hain, R. F.: Delayed Neurological Deterioration after Anoxia, *Arch. Intern. Med.,* 110:18, 1962.

18 Brierly, J. B.: Neuropathologic Findings in Patients Dying after Open-Heart Surgery, *Thorax,* 18:291, 1963.

19 Tyler, H. R., and Clark, D. B.: Incidence of Neurological Complication in Congenital Heart Disease, *A.M.A. Arch. Neurol. Psychiatr.,* 77:17, 1957.

20 Tyler, H. R., and Clark, D. B.: Cerebrovascular Accidents in Patients with Congenital Heart Disease, *A.M.A. Arch. Neurol. Psychiatr.*, 77:438, 1957.

21 Yates, P. O., and Hutchinson, E. C.: The Role of Stenosis of the Extracranial Cerebral Arteries, *Med. Res. Counc. Spec. Rep. Ser. (Lond.)*, no. 300, 1961.

22 Martin, M. J., Whisnant, J. P., and Sayre, G. P.: Occlusive Vascular Disease in the Extracranial Cerebral Circulation, *Arch. Neurol.*, 3:530, 1960.

23 Aring, C. D.: The Migrainous Scintillating Scotoma, *J.A.M.A.*, 220:519, 1972.

24 Walter, P. F., Reid, S. D., and Wenger, N. K.: Transient Cerebral Ischemia due to Arrhythmia, *Ann. Intern. Med.*, 72:471, 1970.

25 Patterson, J. L., and Heyman, A.: Cerebral Vascular Insufficiency, *Disease-A-Month,* July 1963.

26 Whisnant, J. P., Matsumoto, N., and Elveback, L. R.: Transient Cerebral Ischemic Attacks in a Community, *Mayo Clin. Proc.*, 48:194, 1973.

27 Baker, R. N., Broward, J. A., Fang, H. C. Fisher, C. M., Groch, S. N., Heyman, A., Karp, H. R., McDevitt, E., Schwartz, W., and Toole, J. F.: Anticoagulant Therapy in Cerebral Infarction: Report on Cooperative Study, *Neurology,* 12:828, 1962.

28 Baker, R. N.: An Evaluation of Anticoagulant Therapy in the Treatment of Cerebrovascular Disease: Report of the Veterans Administration Cooperative Study of Atherosclerosis, Neurology Section, *Neurology,* 11(suppl.):132, 1961.

29 Millikan, C. H.: Reassessment of Anticoagulant Therapy in Various Types of Occlusive Cerebrovascular Disease, *Stroke,* 2:201, 1971.

30 Whisnant, J. P., Matsumato, N., and Elveback, L. R.: The Effect of Anticoagulant Therapy on the Prognosis of Patients with Transient Cerebral Ischemic Attacks in a Community, Rochester, Minnesota, 1955 through 1969, *Mayo Clin. Proc.*, 48:844, 1973.

30a Fields, W. S., Lemak, N. A., Franbowski, R. F., and Hardy, R. J.: Controlled Trial of Aspirin in Cerebral Ischemia, *Stroke,* 8:301, 1977.

31 Wylie, E. J., and Ehrenfeld, W. K.: "Extracranial Occlusive Cerebrovascular Disease: Diagnosis and Management," W. B. Sanders Company, Philadelphia, 1970.

32 DeWeese, A. A., Rob, C. G., Satron, R., Marsh, D. O., Joynt, R. J., Summers, D. G., and Nichols, C.: Results of Carotid Endarterectomies for Transient Ischemic Attacks: Five Years Later, *Ann. Surg.*, 178:25, 1973.

33 Lawson, L. J., in E. C. Hutchison and E. J. Acheson, "Strokes: Natural History, Pathology and Surgical Treatment," W. B. Saunders Company, Philadelphia, 1975, p. 237.

34 Bauer, R. B., Meyer, J. S., Fields, W. S., Remington, R., McDonald, N. C., and Calvan, P.: Joint Study of Extracranial Arterial Occlusion: Progress Report of Controlled Study of Long-Term Survival with or without Operation, *J.A.M.A.*, 208:509, 1969.

35 David, N. J., and Heyman, A.: Factors Influencing the Prognosis of Cerebral Thrombosis and Infarction due to Atherosclerosis, *J. Chronic Dis.*, 11:394, 1960.

36 Metz, H., Murray-Leslie, R. M., Bannister, R. G., Bull, J., and Marshall, J.: Kinking of the Internal Carotid Artery in Relation to Cerebrovascular Disease, *Lancet,* 1:424, 1961.

37 Sandok, B. A., Houser, O. W., Baker, H. L., Jr., and Holley, K. E.: Fibromuscular Dysplasia: Neurologic Disorders Associated with Diseases Involving the Great Vessels in the Neck, *Arch. Neurol.*, 23:462, 1971.

38 Reivich, M., Holling, H. E., Roberts, B., and Toole, J. F.: Reversal of Blood Flow through the Vertebral Artery and Its Effect on the Cerebral Circulation, *N. Engl. J. Med.*, 265:878, 1961.

39 Reifenstein, G. H., Levine, S. A., and Gross, R. E.: Coarctation of the Aorta, *Am. Heart J.*, 33:146, 1947.

40 Herrick, M. K., and Mills, P. E., Jr.: Infarction of Spinal Cord: Two Cases of Selective Gray Matter Involvement Secondary to Asymptomatic Aortic Disease, *Arch. Neurol.*, 24:228, 1971.

41 Hogan, E. L., and Romanoul, F. C. A.: Spinal Cord Infarction Occurring during Insertion of Aortic Graft, *Neurology,* 16:67, 1966.

42 Blackwood, W., McMenemy, W. H., Meyer, A., Norman, R. M., and Russell, D. S.: Vascular Disease of the Central Nervous System, in "Greenfield's Neuropathology," The Williams & Wilkins Company, Baltimore, 1963, p. 133.

43 Fisher, C. M.: Clinical Syndromes in Cerebral Hemorrhage, in W. S. Fields (ed.), "Pathogenesis and Treatment of Cerebrovascular Disease," Charles C Thomas, Publisher, Springfield, Ill., 1961, p. 318.

44 Fisher, C. M.: The Pathology of Intracerebral Hemorrhage, in W. S. Fields (ed.), "Pathogenesis and Treatment of Cerebrovascular Disease," Charles C Thomas, Publisher, Springfield, Ill., 1961, p. 318.

45 McKissock, W., Richardson, A., and Taylor, J.: Primary Intracerebral Hemorrhage: A Controlled Trial of Surgical and Conservative Treatment in 180 Unselected Cases, *Lancet,* 1:221, 1961.

46 Fisher, C. M., Picard, E. H., Polak, A., Dalal, P., and Ojemann, R. G.: Acute Hypertensive Cerebellar Hemorrhage: Diagnosis and Surgical Treatment, *J. Nerv. Ment. Dis.*, 140:38, 1965.

47 McKissock, W., Richardson, A., and Walsh, L.: Spontaneous Cerebellar Hemorrhage: A Study of 34 Consecutive Cases Treated Surgically, *Brain,* 83:1, 1960.

48 Russell, R. W. R.: Observation on Intracerebral Aneurysms, *Brain,* 86:425, 1963.

49 Byrom. F. B.: The Pathogenesis of Hypertensive Encephalopathy and Its Relation to the Malignant Phase of Hypertension: Experimental Evidence from the Hypertensive Rat, *Lancet,* 2:201, 1954.

50 Fisher, C. M.: Dementia in Cerebral Vascular Disease, in R. G. Siekert and J. P. Whisnant (eds.), "Cerebral Vascular Diseases," Grune & Stratton, Inc., New York, 1968, p. 232.

51 Karp, H. R.: Dementia in Cerebrovascular Disease and Other Systemic Illnesses, *Cur. Concepts Cerebrovasc. Dis.-Stroke,* vol. 7, no. 3, 1972.

52 Fisher, C. M.: Lacunes: Small, Deep Cerebral Infarcts, *Neurology,* 15:774, 1965.

53 Fisher, C. M.: Personal communication.

54 Marshall, J.: A Trial of Long Term Hypotensive Therapy in Cerebrovascular Disease, *Lancet,* 1:10, 1964.

55 Heyman, A., Karp, H. R., Heyden, S., Bartel, A., Cassel, J. C., Tyroler, H. A., and Hames, C. G.: Cerebrovascular Disease in the Biracial Population of Evans County, Georgia, *Arch. Intern. Med.*, 128:949, 1971.

56 Kibler, R. F., and Rose, F. C.: Peripheral Neuropathy in the "Collagen Diseases": A Case of Scleroderma Neuropathy, *Br. Med. J.*, 1:1781, 1960.

57 Johnson, R. T., and Richardson, E. P.: The Neurologic Manifestations of Systemic Lupus Erythematosus: A Clinicopathological Study of 24 Cases and Review of the Literature, *Medicine,* 47:337, 1968.

58 Ferber, C. M.: Ocular Palsy in Temporal Arteritis, *Minn. Med.,* 42:1258, 1959.

59 Hollenhorst, R. W., Brown, J. R., Wagener, H. P., and Shick, R. M.: Neurologic Aspects of Temporal Arteritis, *Neurology,* 10:490, 1960.

60 Cropp, G. J., and Manning, G. W.: Electrocardiographic Changes Simulating Myocardial Ischemia and Infarction Associated with Spontaneous Intracranial Hemorrhage, *Circulation,* 22:25, 1960.

61 Weintraub, B. M., and McHenry, L. C., Jr.: Cardiac Abnormalities in Subarachnoid Hemorrhage: A Resumé, *Stroke*, 5:384, 1974.

62 Grossman, M. A.: Cardiac Arrhythmias in Acute Central Nervous System Disease: Successful Management with Stellate Ganglion Block, *Arch. Intern. Med.*, 136:203, 1976.

63 Perloff, J., de Leon, A., and O'Doherty, D.: The Cardiomyopathy of Progressive Muscular Dystrophy, *Circulation*, 33:625, 1966.

64 Nothacker, W. G., and Netsky, M. G.: Myocardial Lesions in Progressive Muscular Dystrophy, *A.M.A. Arch. Pathol.*, 50: 578, 1950.

65 James, T. N.: Observations on the Cardiovascular Involvement, Including the Cardiac Conduction System, in Progressive Muscular Dystrophy, *Am. Heart J.*, 63:48, 1962.

66 Waters, D. D., Nutter, D. O., Hopkins, L. C., and Dorney, E. R.: Cardiac Features of an Unusual X-linked Humeroperoneal Neuromuscular Disease, *N. Engl. J. Med.*, 293:1017, 1975.

67 Sandt, T. M., Sandok, B. A., and Whisnant, J. P.: Carotid Endarterectomy: Complications and Pre-operative Assessment of Risk, *Mayo Clin. Proc.*, 50:301, 1975.

106

Vascular Disease of the Digestive System[1]

JOHN T. GALAMBOS, M.D., and
W. SCOTT BROOKS, JR., M.D.

Clinically informative and safe methods for the study of the vasculature of the abdominal viscera were recently reviewed.[2] The wider application of these roentgenographic techniques will no doubt increase the frequency of recognized mesenteric vascular disease. Unfortunately, reliable methods are not available for the measurement of total, let alone regional, blood flow of the gastrointestinal tract, although promising techniques have been suggested. Solutions of many clinical problems are awaiting the development of such methods as could be used safely in clinically ill human beings.

The difficulty in obtaining reliable measurements lies in the anatomy of the blood supply to the intestine. There are three major arterial inflows, each of which can vary independently of the others; and the intestine has a venous outflow, the portal vein, which is not only difficult to reach for repeated samples, but also carries significant amounts of blood from the spleen. Even if total intestinal blood flow could be measured with reasonable accuracy, its interpretation would be difficult. The distribution of the arterial inflow among the mucosal, the muscular, and the other supportive structures still needs to be determined. Intestinal blood flow studies done in experimental animals are difficult to relate to human beings because of species variations; moreover they frequently show confusing and conflicting data.

Clinically, vascular diseases of the intestine may be grouped into six categories: (1) a catastrophic event due to acute occlusion of a major splanchnic artery or vein; (2) transient abdominal ischemic attack; (3) recurrent mesenteric ischemia due to gradual narrowing and occlusion of the splanchnic arteries; (4) systemic vascular diseases affecting the splanchnic vessels which may simulate the symptoms of recurrent mesenteric ischemia; (5) intestinal infarction without recognizable mesenteric vascular occlusion (nonocclusive mesenteric ischemia); and (6) other types of vascular lesions.

ACUTE OCCLUSION OF A MAJOR SPLANCHNIC VESSEL

Complete occlusion of a mesenteric artery may be associated with three types of clinical responses: (1) a dramatic abdominal crisis, (2) a difficult diagnostic problem of an abdominal disease, in which pain is usually an outstanding feature, and (3) no symptoms at all.

Occlusion of the mesenteric artery in a patient was first reported in 1843.[3] Virchow in 1847 attributed the thrombosis of this vessel to arterial inflammation.[4] In 1875 Litten reviewed the reported clinical experience with mesenteric arterial occlusion,[5] and in the same year Faber gave the first description of embolization of the mesenteric artery. In 1913 Trotter published a review of 350 cases,[6] and by 1964 Laufman et al. found over 800 articles dealing with mesenteric vascular occlusion.[7]

Acute occlusion of the superior mesenteric artery or vein is a sudden, catastrophic, usually fatal event due to ischemia and gangrene of the intestine. The clinical signs and symptoms of bowel ischemia are not clear-cut, but are best categorized at the time of initial presentation in a restless patient with obvious, severe abdominal pain and yet a relatively normal abdominal examination. Leukocytosis, hemoconcentration, and elevated amylase level may contribute to the diagnosis.[8] Abdominal embolus should be suspected in a patient with previous embolus or atrial fibrillation. In this setting arteriography should be performed as quickly as possible, as this is the only definitive diagnostic procedure short of laparotomy to identify the problems prior to infarction.

Whether acute intestinal ischemia is caused by embolus or by sudden thrombosis, the lesion precipitates an extremely complex alteration of the normal physiology. This includes massive plasma volume depletion combined with severe metabolic acidosis and bacterial invasion of the bowel, the peritoneum, and the bloodstream. These catastrophic events are usually seen in patients who have another serious cardiovascular disease already. It is not surprising, therefore, that the survival figures have not improved much during the last two decades.

The urgency of making a diagnosis of mesenteric artery embolism cannot be stressed too strongly. When the clinical setting makes such an event likely and angiography confirms the suspicion, the surgical removal of the embolus should be attempted. If the condition is left untreated, the mortality rate is 100 percent. Successful surgical cures have been reported following embolic obstruction of the splanchnic branches of the aorta. Perdue performed successful mesenteric embolectomies and reestablished adequate intestinal blood flow in 7 to 15 operations.[9] However, 5 of the 7 patients subsequently died as a result of their underlying disease; 2 of the patients survived.

Embolic occlusion of the celiac axis is rare. Because of efficient collateral circulation through the marginal artery, embolus to the inferior mesenteric artery usually does not result in bowel necrosis if the superior mesenteric artery is patent.

Atheromatous embolization of the splanchnic arteries has also been reported. This usually causes gastrointestinal ulcerations and bleeding.[10] Embolic occlusion of the smaller branches of the mesenteric arteries may cause no bowel ischemia unless progressive thrombosis involves the arcades, where the usually rich anastomoses do not exist. Mesenteric arterial occlusion may be associated with vasospasm because splanchnic nerve block appears to be helpful in reversing the ischemic changes of the bowel.

The clinical picture of bowel ischemia and necrosis due to mesenteric arterial thrombosis is sometimes indistinguishable from that caused by mesenteric venous occlusion. The abdominal pain associated with mesenteric venous occlusion tends to occur over several days, becoming progressively more severe. The distinction from arterial thrombosis must be made by angiographic criteria indicating the absence of arterial occlusion with arterial spasm and prolonged staining of the arterial wall. Clemett and Chang have described a characteristic small-bowel pattern of edematous submucosa with long transition zones at either end in venous obstruction.[11]

Portal or mesenteric venous thrombosis causes hemorrhagic necrosis of the intestine unless the rate of occlusion is slow enough to allow the development of adequate collaterals. Early diagnosis and resection of necrotic bowel are essential for survival in the acute case. Anticoagulants may be helpful in preventing infarction.[8]

Surgical ligation of the portal vein in human beings is feasible. It results in transient engorgement of the intestine and fall of the blood pressure. The catastrophic events which follow the sudden thrombosis of the portal vein in human beings are most likely due to the simultaneous thrombosis of the mesenteric and splenic veins, which, as a rule, accompanies spontaneous portal vein thrombosis. Gradual occlusion of the portal veins results in portal hypertension.

Hepatic vein occlusion may involve either the major or the small hepatic veins. It may be due to a primary lesion of the vein itself, it may be associated with polycythemia, or it may be secondary to infection or tumor. The venocclusive disease of hepatic venules is secondary to Senecio or Crotalaria toxicity.[12] Shock, for whatever reason, may result in massive hemorrhagic necrosis of the liver along the distribution of the efferent veins.

Congestive heart failure with or without recognizable pulmonary emboli may cause intermittent jaundice. Although heart failure is associated occasionally with hepatic anoxia and centrilobular necrosis, cardiac cirrhosis is uncommon, seen only in longstanding heart failure.

TRANSIENT INTESTINAL ISCHEMIC ATTACK

Occlusion of branches of the inferior mesenteric artery results in transient ischemia of a portion of the colon (ischemic colitis).[13] The collateral circulation usually remains adequate to maintain viability of the bowel wall, but reduction of the blood flow causes ischemic changes in the mucosa. As the colon is rich in bacteria, such areas of mucosal ischemia are rapidly converted to colitis.

The patients who have been recognized to have transient intestinal ischemic attack are usually over 45 years of age, and most of them are in the sixth or seventh decade of their lives. The onset of symptoms is usually acute. Abdominal pain may be constant or cramping. It is usually localized in the lower part of the abdomen or in the left side of the abdomen. The onset of pain may be accompanied by an urge to defecate. The patient may have nausea and vomiting; often there is occult blood in the stool, or bright red blood and blood clots are passed rectally. Fever and leukocytosis are common. The splenic flexure and the descending colon are the most frequently involved portions of the colon. One reason for this is that the marginal artery is the major collateral channel between the superior and inferior mesenteric systems. Occlusion of this artery will delay the development of adequate collateral blood supply to the splenic flexure. In the experience of the authors, an occlusion of a branch of a mesenteric artery was documented by angiography (Fig. 106-1). This patient was similar to one described by Coligado and Fleshler, who showed that the ischemic lesion of the splenic flexure is associated with occlusion of small arterial branches inside the bowel wall and ulceration of the mucosa.[13] It is possible that obstruction of a branch of the inferior mesenteric artery may be missed if angiograms are not performed in time. Williams and Wittenberg[14] point out that the clinical course for the patient with ischemic colitis is not correlated with the presence of occlusion on the angiogram, which may not be noted even if the procedure is done within the first 24 h. Their assessment is that arteriography is not essential to clinical management of this syndrome.

Barium enema may show mass lesion or mucosal edema manifested by a pseudotumor or "thumbprinting" (Fig. 106-2A).[15] The ischemia usually leads to destruction and ulceration of the mucosa which may be indistinguishable from idiopathic ulcerative colitis. Healing may lead to stricture formation (Fig. 106-2B). It is likely, however, that occlusion of a

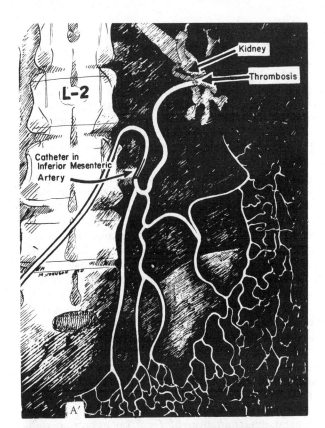

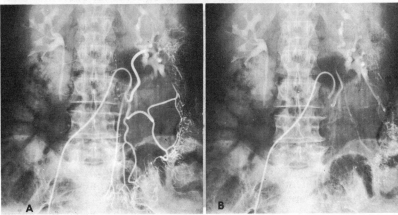

FIGURE 106-1 Selective inferior mesenteric arteriogram. The most proximal branch of the inferior mesenteric artery is occluded just prior to its bifurcation. (The occlusion overlies the opacified left renal pelvis.) Ischemia of the splenic flexure and proximal descending colon was due to the lack of adequate collateral blood flow through Riolan's arc from the superior mesenteric artery. A. Note the increased density and wider diameter of the occluded branch of the inferior mesenteric artery. The landmarks of this roentgenogram are accentuated in the illustration (A'). Note the extensive anastomosis among the branches of the inferior mesenteric artery after the tertiary bifurcations. Such an extensive anastomotic network also characterizes the branches of the superior mesenteric artery. B. The thrombosed vessel remained opacified during the venous phase when none of the normal arterial branches contained visible contrast material.

mesenteric artery or one of its branches comes more often without intestinal infarction than with it. When ischemic injury does occur, resection of the ischemic colon may be required if signs of peritoneal inflammation develop. More often the lesion is self-limited and will heal without a permanent defect; consequently, immediate surgery is not required.

The superior mesenteric artery branches may also be involved in transient ischemic attacks. Either embolic or thrombotic occlusion of a small branch of the mesenteric artery has been associated with ulceration of the small-intestinal mucosa and subsequent stricture formation.

Wolf and Marshak emphasized that not all the components of the bowel wall are equally sensitive to interference with their blood supply.[16] The mucosa may be destroyed by a degree of ischemia which is not sufficient to inflict persistent or permanent injury in the muscular coat or the supportive connective tissue elements of the intestinal wall. Nevertheless,

FIGURE 106-2 A. Barium enema shows "thumbprinting" of the splenic flexure after the proximal branch of the inferior mesenteric artery became suddenly occluded (see Fig. 106-1). B. Eight days later a repeat barium enema shows only stricture formation.

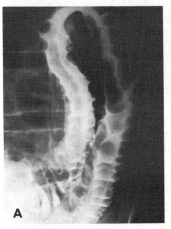
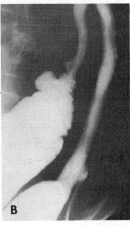

development of ulceration in the mucosa itself may lead to stricture formation in the small bowel.

Localized, transient mucosal ischemia in the small bowel can also produce a mass formation with a pseudotumor appearance, which has been described in the colon. These lesions may heal without perforation or necrosis or may progress to smaller or larger strictures. It is possible that vascular lesions are responsible for small-intestinal stricutres which have been attributed to enteric-coated potassium chloride, as these lesions may be noted independent of potassium ingestion.

RECURRENT MESENTERIC ISCHEMIA DUE TO GRADUAL NARROWING AND OCCLUSION OF SPLANCHNIC ARTERIES

The symptoms of recurrent mesenteric ischemia have been recognized by clinicians for a long time and were described at the turn of the century in the German literature.[17] In the American literature these symptoms were first described in 1921 by Klein, who suggested the term "mesenteric intermittent ischemia."[18] In the same year, Davis compared mesenteric ischemic pain with that of angina pectoris or claudication of the legs.[19] The term "angina" was corrupted to describe these symptoms because of an assumed etiologic similarity with angina pectoris and the association of this term with ischemia. This is a misuse of terms, because angina refers to "strangling" and denotes pressure or tightness, while mesenteric ischemia often induces sharp, cramping pain; nitroglycerin may be harmful.

Clinical findings

The classic symptom of recurrent mesenteric ischemia is postprandial pain. It may begin soon after the completion of a meal or may be delayed as long as an hour or two. Most patients begin to have pain within 30 min. The pain is usually poorly localized. Sometimes it is periumbilical, and it may radiate to the back. The pain is usually intense; it may be constant and gnawing, but usually it is colicky in nature. Some patients may also develop abdominal distension, bloating, and nausea. The pain may subside gradually within 30 to 60 min, but more often it lasts for several hours. There is no medication which can consistenly prevent or ameliorate the pain of recurrent mesenteric ischemia. Specifically, nitroglycerin is of no therapeutic value; indeed, by reducing aortic pressure, it may be expected to decrease splanchnic perfusion even further and may accentuate bowel ischemia.

Some patients are able to control their pain by eating small amounts at one time. In most patients, however, the size of the meal is not related to the severity of their symptoms. Any solid or liquid food can precipitate pain. The food → pain sequence eventually conditions the patient to avoid eating. Consequently, weight loss may become an outstanding problem.

It should be emphasized that the symptoms of recurrent mesenteric ischemia are not specific and vary considerably from patient to patient.[20] Physical examination usually shows nonspecific abdominal tenderness. The most significant diagnostic finding is a bruit heard in the epigastrium or middle part of the abdomen. The patient should be turned during auscultation because the bruit may change as the position of the mesentery shifts. A bruit has been present in 19 of the 21 patients studied by Rob.[21] It must be stressed that a bruit in the abdomen may arise from sources other than narrowing of the splanchnic arteries or, in spite of the vascular narrowing, the patient's symptoms may be due to some other cause. Atherosclerosis of the aorta may be present without similar lesions in its visceral branches.[22]

Laboratory examinations may demonstrate excessive fecal fat loss. Recurrent ischemia damages the intestinal mucosal function and structure. The resulting malabsorption undoubtedly contributes to weight loss. The patients usually do not give a history of steatorrhea because their food intake is too small to permit development of this symptom. Unwillingness to eat fatty food because of fear of pain makes the chemical determination of fecal fat excretion difficult to interpret.

Biopsy of the small intestine may be helpful. Abnormal small-bowel histology was documented in three of four patients with steatorrhea and was associated with depressed intestinal disaccharidase activity and a flat lactose tolerance curve. Malabsorption has also been described by Heard and coworkers, whose review suggested a 26 percent incidence of steatorrhea among patients with recurrent mesenteric ischemia.[23]

Occult blood in the stool is a frequent finding. The source of gastrointestinal bleeding is not known. Conventional barium x-rays of the intestine as a rule are unremarkable.

Recurrent mesenteric ischemia is suspected on the basis of the clinical findings, but the diagnosis must be correlated and the extent of the arterial disease must be defined by angiography. Aortography with lateral exposures is of aid in identifying lesions at the orifice of the vessels (Figs. 106-3 and 106-4). The occlusive lesion commonly involves the ostium or the proximal 2 cm of the main arterial trunk.[20] It may involve a proximal segment of the artery without occluding the orifice (Fig. 106-5). When narrowing involves a longer, more distal segment, selective angiography of the suspected vessels may give superior diagnostic information. During operation, decreased or absent pulsations of the involved vessels and their branches may be easily overlooked, and the correct diagnosis missed unless these arteries are deliberately palpated.

The angiographic findings should be interpreted with caution. Postprandial abdominal pain in an older patient may not be due to mesenteric ischemia although the angiogram shows atherosclerotic narrowing of the splanchnic vessels. A large, collateral, meandering vessel has been demonstrated by aortog-

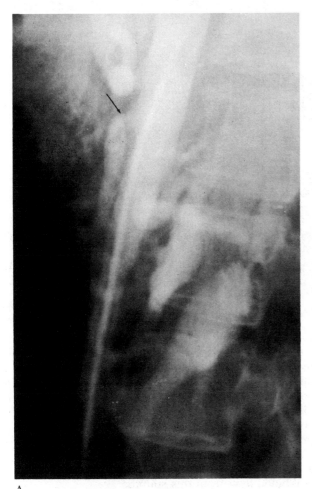

A

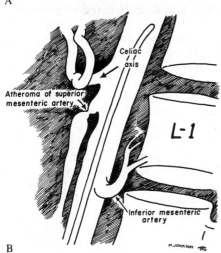

B

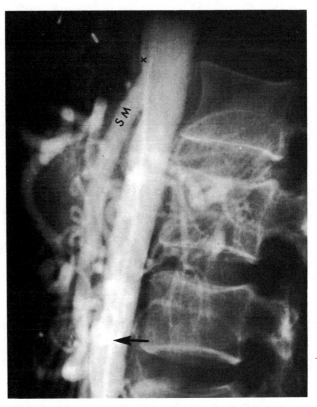

FIGURE 106-4 Recurrent mesenteric ischemia. The lateral aortogram shows a completely occluded celiac axis, X, a large superior mesenteric artery, SM, and a large meandering artery which came from the inferior mesenteric artery. The origin of the latter is marked by the large black arrow. *(Courtesy of Dr. Garland Perdue.)*

FIGURE 106-3 A. Lateral abdominal aortogram. The plastic radiopaque catheter is seen in the aorta with its tip in front of the twelfth thoracic vertebra (T-12). A narrowing is seen in the superior mesenteric artery at 1 cm from its aortic ostium. *B.* An atheromatous plaque was found in this location at subsequent surgical treatment. A selective superior mesenteric arteriogram was also performed in this patient. The area of narrowing was not detected by this selective angiogram, because the positioning of the catheter tip permitted the injection of contrast material across the narrowed portion without detection of the lesion in the proximal 1 cm of the artery.

raphy as an incidental finding (Fig. 106-6). Furthermore, collateral vessels may be seen on selective or superior mesenteric angiograms even in the absence of narrowing or occlusion of the splanchnic arteries (Fig. 106-7).

Pathogenesis and natural history

Recurrent mesenteric ischemia is not recognized commonly. It has been seen in 0.002 to 0.3 percent of patients admitted to a hospital.[24] Yet severe atheromatous narrowing of the superior mesenteric artery has been reported to occur in 37 to 40 percent of unselected patients in two series of autopsies and in 77 percent of patients whose mesenteric arterial system was injected at autopsy.[25]

Reiner and his associates in their postmortem injection studies found some correlation between atherosclerotic narrowing of the orifices of the splanchnic arteries and generalized atherosclerosis elsewhere.[25] However, these investigators were not able to document a good correlation between the degree of atherosclerosis in these splanchnic arteries and ischemic lesions of the bowel. On the other hand, a quantitative relation was suggested by Dick et al.[20] These investigators found that a reduction of the

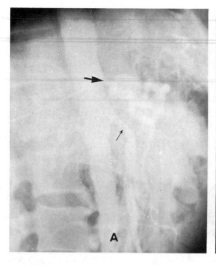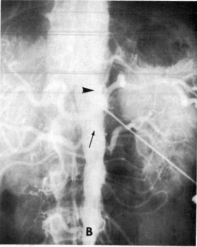

FIGURE 106-5 Recurrent mesenteric ischemia. The lateral, *A,* and anteroposterior, *B,* aortograms show narrowing of the origin of the celiac axis (large arrow) and of a proximal segment of the superior mesenteric artery (small arrow). The inferior mesenteric artery is absent. The proximal segment of the right renal artery is stenosed. The distal aorta shows severe atherosclerosis. *(Courtesy of Dr. Garland Perdue.)*

total cross-sectional area of the celiac and superior and inferior mesenteric arteries to less than two-thirds of normal was required before symptoms of ischemia appeared.

Recurrent mesenteric ischemia is always characterized by involvement of the superior mesenteric artery with gradual occlusion.[22] A potentially extensive collateral circulation exists between the branches of the celiac axis and the superior and inferior mesenteric arteries. Collateral circulation between these three major branches usually becomes adequate to compensate for the narrowing or occlusion of one or two of the splanchnic arteries. The potential of adequate collateral circulation is so great that both the inferior mesenteric and the celiac arteries have been ligated in human beings without incident. Therefore, narrowing or occlusion of at least two of the three major visceral branches of the abdominal aorta is required to produce clinically significant symptomatic bowel ischemia.[21,26]

The efficiency of the mesenteric collateral circulation is exemplified by those cases in which celiac and superior mesenteric arteries are occluded and the entire abdominal viscera are supplied by a meandering inferior mesenteric artery (Fig. 106-6). Other unnamed branches of the aorta may also contribute to visceral blood flow. The inferior phrenic and internal iliac arteries supplied the entire bowel in a patient with recurrent mesenteric ischemia. This type of anastomosis must have existed in the patient described by Chiene in 1869.[27] This patient had no symptoms of mesenteric ischemia; yet he had complete occlusion of the celiac artery and the superior and inferior mesenteric arteries. Indeed, adequate blood supply was provided to the abdominal viscera in a patient whose aorta was occluded from the diaphragm to the renal arteries (so that both the celiac axis and the superior mesenteric artery were occluded) and whose distal aorta and inferior mesenteric artery were filled by the lumbar arteries.[21]

Adequate, although precarious, blood flow may be delivered to the splanchnic circulation through col

laterals when both the celiac axis and the superior mesenteric arteries are occluded. If the large, meandering collateral artery is used for construction of an aortoiliac bypass without consideration for visceral blood flow, an aortoiliac steal is induced that leads to bowel ischemia and necrosis. The ligation of the inferior mesenteric artery during left colectomy or during resection of an aortic aneurysm may result in mesenteric ischemia if the bowel depends on collateral blood flow from this source.[28]

Dunphy suggested in 1936 that recurrent mesenteric ischemia may be compared with intermittent claudication of the legs and should be considered as a prodromal symptom of fatal mesenteric thrombosis.[29] Fry and Kraft described 20 patients between 36 and 82 years of age who died with acute mesenteric artery thrombosis and bowel infarction following a period of recurrent mesenteric ischemia.[30] The symptoms in these patients lasted for variable periods; the extremes were as short as 3 weeks in 1 and as long as 24 months in 2 of the 20 patients. Others have made similar observations.[22] We have seen 18 patients with recurrent mesenteric ischemia. Of these patients 12 developed fatal mesenteric artery thrombosis. The duration of their symptoms ranged from 2 weeks to 2 years, but was less than 6 months in 9 of the 12 cases. We successfully operated upon 5 of the 18 patients, and 1 declined surgery after 9 months of symptoms.

When congenital abnormalities prevent the development of the usual collateral circulation, then only moderate atheromatous narrowing of a splanchnic artery may cause symptoms of mesenteric ischemia. Recurrent mesenteric ischemia of 9 months' duration progressed to massive bowel necrosis in a 40-year-old woman during pregnancy.[31] In two cases thrombosis of the celiac artery resulted in recurrent mesenteric ischemia and terminated by necrosis of both the liver and the bowel in 3 weeks and 6 months, respectively. Coarctation of the abdomenal aorta on occasion involves the celiac and mesenteric arteries bur rarely causes recurrent mesenteric ischemia.

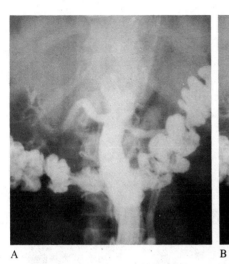
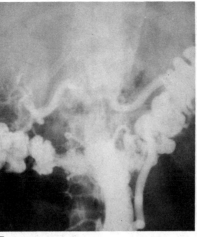
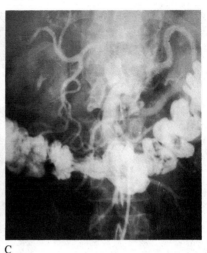

A B C

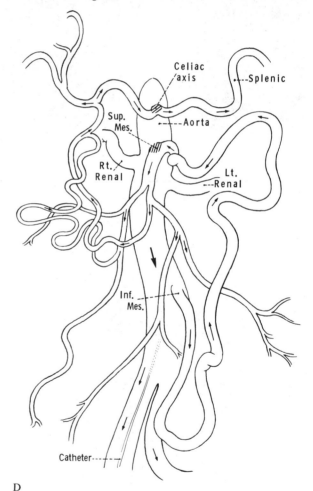

D

FIGURE 106-6 Meandering artery. The catheter was introduced into the aorta from the right femoral artery and was injected at the level of the twelfth thoracic vertebra (T-12). The composite drawing describes the direction of blood flow. The three illustrations represent exposure 3, 7, and 14 s after the injection of contrast material. Barium is in the transverse colon. *A.* 3 s: opacification of the aorta and renal, iliac, and inferior mesenteric arteries is seen. A large, meandering artery has begun to opacify. The orifices of both the celiac axis and the superior mesenteric arteries are occluded. *B.* 7 s: the meandering artery is completely visualized now; from it the contrast material enters the superior mesenteric artery. *C.* 14 s: the branches of the superior mesenteric artery have become well opacified. The contrast material goes from the superior mesenteric artery to the hepatic artery through the pancreaticoduodenal artery. From the hepatic, it goes in two directions: into the celiac and splenic and also into the right and left hepatic arteries. *D.* A drawing of the vasculature, based on *A,* *B,* and *C,* indicating the direction of the blood flow. The orifices of both the celiac and superior mesenteric arteries are occluded. Blood flows from the inferior mesenteric → meandering → superior mesenteric and tributaries → gastroduodenal → hepatic → celiac and tributaries. The patient did not have symptoms of mesenteric ischemia. *(Courtesy of Dr. Garland Perdue.)*

Contrary to the prevailing concept, stenosis of a single artery has been blamed for recurrent mesenteric ischemia in the absence of congenital vascular defects. Bircher and coworkers reported arteriosclerotic involvment of the superior mesenteric artery alone in four patients who were successfully operated upon for recurrent mesenteric ischemia.[22]

Compression of the celiac axis by a fibrous band was claimed to be the cause of recurrent mesenteric ischemia in several reports. A 40-year-old man who had steatorrhea, lactose malabsorption and intestinal lactase deficiency, and 8.5 percent Bromsulphalein (BSP) retention at 45 min was operated on for recurrent mesenteric ischemia. Both the steatorrhea and BSP retention improved postoperatively. Morris et al.[32] operated on 31 patients for recurrent mesenteric ischemia of whom 6 had only compression of the celiac axis. Marable et al. operated on 30 patients with celiac axis compression.[33]

Whether the compression of the celiac axis is due to the celiac plexus or to the anterior decussating fibers of the aortic hiatus of the diaphragm is a moot question.[33] It seems important, however, that Drapanaas saw such a lesion during angiography in 90 of 692 patients (13 percent) during a period of 4 years.[34] All these patients had other reasons for their symptoms than celiac artery compression. In one of these

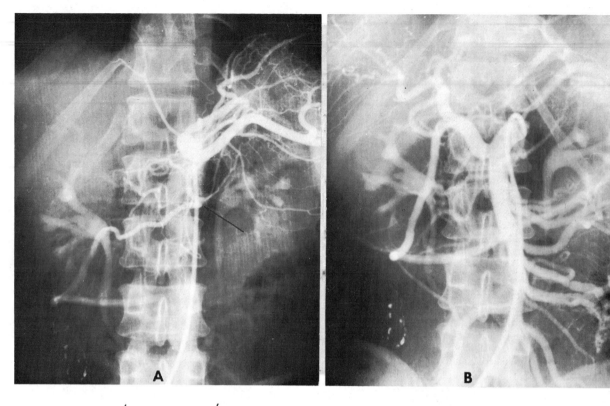

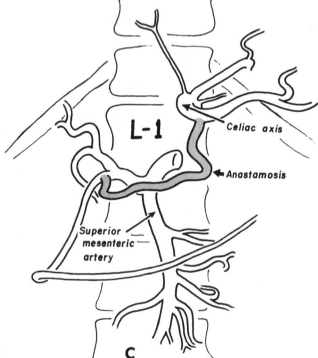

FIGURE 106-7 A large anastomotic vessel between the celiac axis and superior mesenteric artery. Such readily demonstrable anastomosis occurs so frequently that it is considered normal. *A.* Selective celiac arteriogram. The splenic and left gastric arteries are opacified, but the hepatic artery is not seen. A large artery pursues a tortuous course, traveling down over the first lumbar vetebra (L-1) medially from the catheter, which is in the aorta; it crosses to the right of the spine at the L-1-L-2 interspace and over the top of L-2 and turns sharply down over the right ureteropelvic junction; after a sharp turn to the right it crosses over L-3 as the right gastroepiploic artery. Note the characteristic course of this vessel to the right of the spine, and compare it with that seen in *B.* *B.* Selective superior mesenteric arteriogram. The x-ray tube was moved caudally for this exposure from that seen in *A.* The most proximal branch of the superior mesenteric artery is the hepatic artery. Note that the first branch of the hepatic artery runs the same characteristic course as that shown in *A* and ends at the right gastroepiploic artery. The density of this artery is less than that of the hepatic distal to the bifurcation, because the radiopaque contrast material was diluted with blood entering from the collateral vessel of the celiac artery. This collateral artery across the spine did not opacify, confirming that the direction of flow was from the celiac toward the superior mescenteric arterial system. *C.* A composite drawing of *A* and *B* illustrating the large collateral artery connecting the celiac with the superior mesenteric arterial system, which is a normal variation.

patients the compression of the celiac axis was surgically corrected. Postoperative angiogram demonstrated the disappearance of the previously noted large collaterals, as well as relief of the celiac compression. This patient, however, continued to have the same abdominal complaints. Furthermore, spon-

taneous remission of abdominal distress may occur in such patients. Evans, in reviewing the follow-up of 59 patients with the celiac compression syndrome, urged a skeptical and cautious approach to these patients as long-term follow-up did not bear out the initial good results noted.[35]

One must interpret with great caution vague and unexplained abdominal symptoms with celiac artery stenosis. When the narrowing of the celiac axis is demonstrated by selective celiac angiography rather than by lateral aortography, the appearance of stenosis may be due to an artifact. While the finding of an epigastric bruit most commonly does represent celiac compression,[36] the majority of these lesions are asymptomatic.[37]

An interesting relation between renal vascular hypertension and narrowing of the superior mesenteric artery has been described by Schwartz.[38] He reported 10 patients with renal artery lesions or with intrinsic renal disease who were known to be normotensive before the obstruction of their superior mesenteric artery. These patients became hypertensive thereafter. The data suggested that the superior mesenteric artery insufficiency itself does not affect blood pressure but may predispose to hypertension in the presence of renal abnormality.

Therapy

There are only a few reported series in the literature on the successful surgical therapy of recurrent mesenteric ischemia due to atheromatous occlusion of the splanchnic vessels. By 1966, the Houston group successfully treated 25 patients.[32] Bircher et al. performed 9 successive elective revascularizations of mesenteric vessels.[22] Watt et al. obtained good clinical and laboratory results in 3 of 4 operations.[39] In addition to these, only isolated case reports have been published.

The principle of surgical therapy is to establish blood flow in the superior mesenteric artery. Correction of flow in the celiac or inferior mesenteric arteries is not essential to give relief, but may provide the additional safeguard against furture ischemia. A bypass of the atheromatous, occluded vessel is preferred by some authorities, but thromboendarterectomy is advocated by others. If viability of the intestine is in doubt, a "second look" in 24 h is advocated. Postoperative malabsorption may persist.

Celiac axis compression can be relieved by resecting the compressing fibrous band with or without removal of the celiac ganglion.

SYSTEMIC VASCULAR DISEASE AFFECTING THE SPLANCHNIC ARTERIES

The symptoms of recurrent mesenteric ischemia may be caused by involvement of the splanchnic arteries in a generalized vascular disease. The symptoms are indistinguishable from those caused by atheromatous occlusion.

Visceral involvement with thromboangiitis obliterans has been well documented, although this lesion may be difficult to differentiate from arteriosclerosis.[22] The small inflammatory reaction in the ileum caused by this vascular lesion may be confused with early regional enteritis.[22]

Periarteritis nodosa involves the gastrointestinal tract in about half the patients with this disease. The most common manifestation is abdominal pain.[22] Indeed, the splanchnic arteries may be the only ones so affected. The segmental destruction of the arteriolar wall associated with small aneurysmal dilatation and ischemia may result in focal ulcerations or, at times, perforation of the viscera. Gastrointestinal bleeding may occur, but it is rarely severe. Although involvement of hepatic or cystic arterial radicals is common, only an occasional patient develops clinical manifestations of liver disease before the terminal episode. Periarteritis may produce hepatic infarctions. In some patients with periarteritis nodosa, the hepatic lesions dominate the clinical picture; such patients are usually suspected to have primary liver disease.

In patients with lupus erythematosus, small-vessel involvement of the abdominal viscera may be associated with abdominal symptoms severe enough to simulate an acute surgical condition. The abdominal catastrophe may be associated with vasculitis in the bowel or in the pancreas. The peritoneum may be involved, with polyserositis simulating peritonitis. Illeus involving the duodenum and/or the jejunum may be seen. Abdominal pain on occasion has been the presenting symptom of acute rheumatic fever. At operation, mesenteric lymphadenitis, peritoneal hyperemia, and an increased amount of peritoneal fluid were found. Arteritis with fibrinoid changes and with perivascular inflammation involving medium and small peripheral arteries and arterioles has been described in this disease in the visceral vessels. An arteritis was observed on rectal biopsies in some patients with rheumatoid arthritis. Ulceration of the intestine due to necrotizing arteritis has been described in malignant hypertension.

The gastrointestinal tract may be involved with angiomas in either of two forms: (1) the hereditary hemorrhagic telangiectasia, with or without cutaneous or nasopharyngeal involvement, or (2) angiomas associated with hypertrophy of one or both limbs. Osler in 1901 noted liver involvement when he first described this entity.[40] Since then, other investigators also have described hepatic lesions due to telangiectasias. In some cases arteriovenous shunting may cause epigastric bruit and hepatic coma. Angiomas may be the source of occult gastrointestinal bleeding which may be severe and is often recurrent.[41] An angiographic study was performed on 20 patients who had hemorrhagic hereditary telangiectasia. All but 2 patients had marked arteriovenous shunting within the liver; multiple arteriovenous anastomoses were demonstrated in the pancreas, spleen, small bowel, and the visceral vessels of the mesentery. It seems that angiodysplasia within the abdominal viscera is a consistent and integral part of hemorrhagic hereditary telangiectasia.

Pseudoxanthoma elasticum is commonly associated with vascular lesions. These vascular lesions may occur in the mesentery and in the pancreas and may be associated with massive gastrointestinal hemorrhage.[42]

Exclusive vascular involvement of the abdominal viscera is more conspicuous in primary than in secondary amyloidosis.[43] In 16 of 47 patients with hepatic amyloidosis, the amyloid was deposited exclusively in the blood vessels. In 4 of these cases, the involvement was confined exclusively to the hepatic arterioles. In an extensive review of primary amyloidosis, vascular involvement of the gastrointestinal tract was found in 70 percent of cases, and the liver was involved in 35 percent of the cases.

Since 1941, 19 cases of an unusual progressive arterial occlusive disease have been reported.[44] Degos' disease involves medium and small arteries by subendothelial fibrosis. Vascular occlusions most commonly involve the skin and gastrointestinal tract. The disease was seen in 17 men and 2 women from the age of 14 to 59 years. Eleven of the nineteen were 30 years old or younger. The appearance of grayish pink papules of a few millimeters in size heralds the disease. These ischemic lesions develop in crops. Abdominal pain, diarrhea, malabsorption, and weight loss are noticed weeks or months later. Perforation of the intestine is the rule. The disease may progress slowly, lasting 6 to 9 years, or it may be fulminant, lasting for a few months only.

INTESTINAL INFARCTION WITHOUT RECOGNIZABLE VASCULAR OCCLUSION (NONOCCLUSIVE INFARCTION)

Ischemic necrosis of the bowel without demonstrable mesenteric arterial occlusion was first described by Penner and Bernhein in 1939.[45] They reported 40 patients who developed enterocolitis after surgery. The same disease was described by Kleckner et al. in 1952 as pseudomembranous enterocolitis in 14 patients who were not operated upon.[46] Since then, numerous reports have described this syndrome.[47,48] The hemorrhagic mucosal necrosis may develop anywhere in the gastrointestinal tract except the esophagus. The distribution of the lesions is not related to the distribution of the mesenteric arteries. The lesions involve patchy areas of the mucosa and affect shorter or longer segments of the colon. Aortic insufficiency was said to predispose to massive infarction of the intestine. The mild lesion is characterized by congestion and the severe one by hemorrhage of the mucosa and submucosa. Edema and thickening of the entire bowel wall may develop, progressing to extensive or multiple infarctions. Small, superficial ulcerations may be seen in a third of the cases, but membranous exudate is less commonly found. Emphysema of the submucosa and proximal dilata-

tion of the bowel have been described. No vascular occlusion was detectable at autopsy.

The association of this lesion with elderly, chronically ill patients was noted over 20 years ago and has been repeatedly confirmed. Hemorrhagic enterocolitis is almost always secondary to another serious clinical illness. Shock may or may not precede the onset of this syndrome. Digitalis, pressor amines, hypotensive or diuretic drugs, and anticoagulants have been given to patients before the onset of this complication.[49] The abdominal symptoms are relatively mild and nonspecific. The onset is usually sudden, and the pain may be cramping and poorly localized; some patients have recurrent postprandial pain for several days. The patient may have nausea, vomiting, bloody diarrhea, or any combination of these complaints. Gastrointestinal bleeding may be severe. Among 673 autopsies Kane et al. found 25 cases of massive gastrointestinal hemorrhage.[50] Abdominal tenderness may or may not be marked and may be difficult to interpret because of recent surgery. Laboratory findings are of little help. Albuminuria was a constant finding among 31 patients, and progressive azotemia was also described.

Hemorrhagic enterocolitis may last from 1 to 12 days and may be the main or a major contributory cause of death. The mortality rate is very high, but recovery may occur. Occasionally, recurrent attacks are seen.

The pathogenesis of ischemic infarction, necrosis, and gangrene of the bowels has been attributed to reduction of blood flow without demonstrable organic occlusion of the vessel leading to the injured bowel. Shock is not required for the precipitation of this type of bowel ischemia; and conversely, shock usually is not followed by hemorrhagic enterocolitis. It is generally accepted that splanchnic blood flow is readily sacrificed when cardiac output is needed elsewhere. This splanchnic vasomotor reflex depends on alpha-adrenergic vasoconstrictors and may be similar to the "diving reflex" in ducks.

Other pathogenetic mechanisms were also considered. The production of hemorrhagic enterocolitis was attributed to a bacterium. Clostridia or staphylococci were cultured from some of the affected intestines. Furthermore, intraarterial injection of Forssman antiserum produced intestinal infarction simulating this lesion. Gazes and coworkers suggested that digitalization-induced splanchnic venous stasis is the cause of hemorrhagic necrosis of the bowel mucosa, at least in some cases.[49] Levinsky and coworkers have reproduced mesenteric vasoconstriction in the dog with an experimentally stenosed artery by means of infusing digoxin. This effect was reversed by glucagon.[51]

The diagnosis of hemorrhagic enterocolitis most commonly is established at autopsy. At times it is an unrecognized terminal event. When suspected, it is difficult to differentiate clinically from mesenteric vascular occlusion. Aortography can demonstrate the patency of the splanchnic arteries, and selective mesenteric angiography can demonstrate the patency of mesenteric veins.

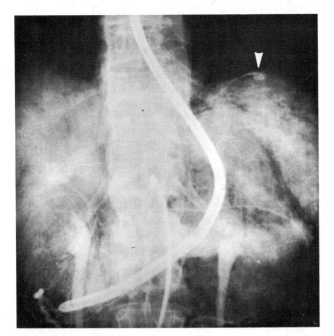

FIGURE 106-8 Bleeding gastric ulcer. Selective celiac angiogram, capillary phase. The arrow shows the bleeding site high in the fundus. Contrast material has accumulated outside the vascular bed and is spreading over the mucosa toward the cardia. A deflated Sengstaken-Blakemore tube is seen in the stomach. On clinical grounds the patient was thought to have had bleeding from varices. At surgery a bleeding peptic ulcer was found high in the fundus, confirming the the angiographic diagnosis.

Hemorrhagic necrosis of the intestinal mucosa should be suspected in all elderly patients with congestive heart failure in whom abdominal pain appears during or after severe stress, such as cardiac decompensation, myocardial or pulmonary infarction, or infection; or in debilitated patients during postoperative convalescence. If bloody diarrhea and shock develop, the diagnosis must always be considered in such a clinical setting.

There is no satisfactory treatment of hemorrhagic enterocolitis. Surgery should not be performed if bowel resection can possibly be avoided. Therapy is based on the principles of supportive care. Treatment is to be directed to the precipitating cause. Patients may require massive expansion of the circulating blood volume which is lost in the intestinal lumen. Correction of splanchnic vasoconstriction with phenoxybenzamine or with a similar alpha-adrenergic blocker should be attempted. Epidural block has also been utilized.[47] The use of these drugs expands the capacity of the vascular bed, and corresponding rapid expansion of the blood volume is essential. Because of the danger of circulatory overload, the central venous pressure should be constantly monitored. Massive antibiotic therapy for the control of septicemia and anti-gas-gangrene serum directed against *Clostridium welchii* have also been recommended. In general, the treatment is similar to that of gram-negative sepsis.

OTHER TYPES OF VASCULAR LESIONS

Postoperative mesenteric arteritis

Some patients develop necrotizing splanchnic arteritis after successful operative correction of the coarctation of the aorta.[52] This process usually affects the branches of the superior mesenteric artery. In its full-blown form, arteritis leads to bowel ischemia, ulceration, and gangrene. This lesion developed most commonly in children between 8 and 12 years of age. The symptoms usually begin between the third and tenth postoperative days; if left untreated, the condition progresses rapidly to gangrene of the intestine, peritonitis, and death. This syndrome should be suspected in patients whose blood pressure begins to rise instead of decreasing to normal after surgery. The increase of diastolic pressure exceeds that of the systolic pressure, resulting in a narrowed pulse pressure. These patients have increasingly severe abdominal pain and leukocytosis. The development of the full-blown syndrome can be prevented by prompt and effective antihypertensive therapy with a combination of Apresoline (hydralazine) and reserpine.

FIGURE 106-9 Bleeding duodenal diverticulum. *A.* Superior mesenteric angiogram. The proximal segment of the superior mesenteric artery is dilated. Contrast material accumulated outside the artery (▽)—left of the patient's second lumbar vertebra (L-2). The arteries leading into this area are more prominent than were expected. *B.* Barium-contrast small-bowel series. Some barium is left in the stomach, and the entire small intestine is well filled. In the fourth portion of the duodenum a diverticulum is visible (▽)—just left of the patient's second lumbar vertebra (L-2). This is the same area where the accumulation of contrast material was seen on the superior mesenteric angiogram.

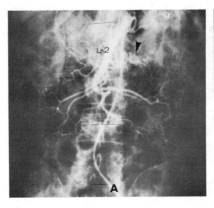
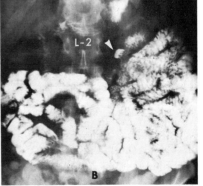

REFERENCES

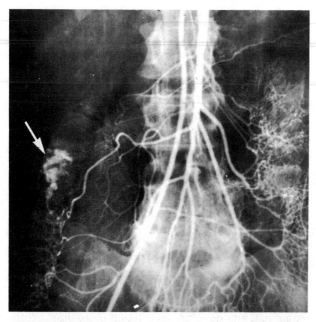

FIGURE 106-10 Bleeding diverticulum in the ascending colon. Inferior mesenteric angiogram 2 s after injection. The contrast material has already accumulated in the lumen of the ascending colon (↓). This indicated vigorous active bleeding. At the time of operation, the entire colon was filled with blood, and the bleeding site was not readily apparent.

Aneurysms of the visceral arteries

The splanchnic arteries occasionally develop aneurysms. These involve the splenic artery in 40 percent of the cases, the hepatic artery in 25 percent, the superior mesenteric artery in 20 percent, and the smaller branches in 15 percent. Gastrointestinal bleeding, jaundice, or abdominal pain may complicate aneurysms of the hepatic artery. By 1966, there were only 170 reported cases in the literature. Aneurysms of the visceral arteries are often asymptomatic and remain unsuspected clinically until their rupture. Such unsuspected aneurysms of the splenic artery have a tendency to rupture during pregnancy. Aneurysms of the splenic or hepatic artery may be associated with familial hemorrhagic telangiectasias.[53]

Of the splanchnic arteries, the superior mesenteric artery is the one which is involved most commonly with mycotic aneurysms. Rob et al. reported that of 138 mycotic aneurysms, 28 involved the superior mesenteric artery.[54]

Erosion

Another dramatic vascular lesion is the development of a communication with the gastrointestinal tract. A discussion of gastrointestinal bleeding is not within the scope of this brief review. Suffice it to mention that the bleeding site can be documented by selective abdominal angiography (Figs. 106-8 to 106-10).

1 Boley, S. J., Schwartz, S. S., and Williams, L. F., Jr. (eds.): "Vascular Disorders of the Intestine," Appleton Century Crofts, New York, 1971.

2 Sybers, R. G., and Galambos, J. T.: Angiography in Diseases of the G.I. Tract, in G. B. J. Glass (ed.), "Progress in Gastroenterology," Grune & Stratton, Inc., New York, 1968.

3 Tiedemann, F.: "Von der Verengung und Schliessung der Pulsadern in Krankheiten," K. Groos, Heidelberg and Leipzig, 1843.

4 Virchow, R. L. K.: Ueber die Akute Entzundung der Arterien, *Arch. Pathol. Anat.*, 1:272, 1847.

5 Litten, M.: Ueber die Folgen des Verschlusses ier Arteria Mesaraica Superior, *Arch. Pathol. Anat.*, 63:289, 1875.

6 Trotter, L. B. C.: "Embolism and Thrombosis of Mesenteric Vessels," Cambridge University Press, New York, 1913.

7 Laufman, H., Nora, P. F., and Mittelpunkt, A. I.: Mesenteric Blood Vessels: Advances in Surgery and Physiology, *Arch. Surg.*, 88:1021, 1964.

8 Skinner, D. B., Zarins, C. K., and Moossa, A. R.: Mesenteric Vascular Disease, *Am. J. Surg.*, 128:835, 1974.

9 Perdue, G. D., Jr., and Smith, R. B., III: Intestinal Ischemia Due to Mesenteric Arterial Disease, *Am. Surg.*, 36:152, 1972.

10 Taylor, N. S., Guelt, B., and Lebowich, R. J.: Atheromatous Embolization: A Cause of Gastric Ulcers and Small Bowel Necrosis, *Gastroenterology*, 47:97, 1964.

11 Clemmett, A. R., and Chang, J.: The Radiologic Diagnosis of Spontaneous Mesenteric Venous Thrombosis, *Am. J. Dig. Dis.*, 63:209, 1975.

12 Bras, G., Berry, D. M., and Gyorgy, P.: Plants as Etiological Factors in Veno-occlusive Disease of the Liver, *Lancet*, 1:960, 1957.

13 Coligado, E. Y., and Fleshler, B.: Reversible Vascular Occlusion of the Colon, *Radiology*, 89:432, 1967.

14 Williams, L. F., and Wittenberg, J.: Ischemic Colitis: A Useful Clinical Diagnosis, But Is It Ischemic? *Ann. Surg.*, 182:439, 1975.

15 Boley, S. J., Schwartz, S., Lash, J., and Sternhill, V.: Reversible Vascular Occlusion of the Colon, *Surg. Gynecol. Obstet.*, 116:53, 1961.

16 Wolf, B. S., and Marshak, R. H.: Segmental Infarction of the Small Bowel, *Radiology*, 66:702, 1956.

17 Schnitzler, F.: Zur Symptomatik des Darmarterienverschlusses, *Wien. Med. Wochenschr.*, 11 & 12:506, 1901.

18 Klein, E.: Embolism and Thrombosis of the Superior Mesenteric Artery, *Surg. Gynecol. Obstet.*, 33:385, 1921.

19 Davis, B. B.: Thrombosis and Embolism of the Mesenteric Vessels, *Nebr. State Med. J.*, 6:101, 1921.

20 Dick, A. P., Graff, R., Gregg, D. McC., Peters, N., and Sarner, M.: An Arteriographic Study of Mesenteric Arterial Disease, *Gut*, 8:206, 1967.

21 Rob, C.: Surgical Diseases of the Celiac and Mesenteric Arteries, *Arch. Surg.*, 93:21, 1966.

22 Bircher, J., Bartholomew, L. G., Cain, J. C., and Adson, M. A.: Syndrome of Intestinal Arterial Insufficiency ("Abdominal Angina"), *Arch. Intern. Med.*, 117:362, 1966.

23 Heard, G., Jefferies, J. D., and Peters, D. K.: Chronic Intestinal Ischaemia: Successful Aorta/Superior Mesenteric Bypass, *Lancet*, 2:975, 1963.

24 Jackson, B. B.: "Occlusion of the Superior Mesenteric Artery," Charles C Thomas, Publisher, Springfield, Ill., 1963, p. 6.

25 Reiner, L., Jimenez, F. A., and Rodriguez, F. L.: Atherosclerosis in the Mesenteric Circulation: Observations and Correlations with Aortic and Coronary Atherosclerosis, *Am. Heart J.*, 66:200, 1963.

26 Ranniger, K., and Saldino, R. N.: Abdominal Angiography, in "Current Problems in Surgery," Year Book Medical Publishers, Inc., Chicago, March 1968.

27 Chiene, J.: Complete Obliteration of Coeliac and Mesenteric Arteries, *J. Anat. Physiol.*, 3:65, 1869.

28 Gonzalez, L. L., and Jaffe, M. S.: Mesenteric Arterial Insufficiency Following Abdominal Aortic Resection, *Arch. Surg.*, 93:10, 1966.

29 Dunphy, J. E.: Abdominal Pain of Vascular Origin, *Am. J. Med. Sci.*, 192:109, 1936.

30 Fry, W. O., and Kraft, R. O.: Visceral Angina, *Surg. Gynecol. Obstet.*, 117:417, 1963.

31 Kempers, R. D., and Bartholomew, L. F.: Intestinal Angina Associated with Pregnancy, *Am. J. Obstet. Gynecol.*, 90:882, 1964.

32 Morris, G. C., Jr., DeBakey, M. E., and Bernhard, V.: Abdominal Angina, *Surg. Clin. North Am.*, 46:919, 1966.

33 Marable, S. A., Kaplan, M. F., Beman, F. M., and Molnar, W.: Celiac Compression Syndrome, *Am. J. Surg.*, ll5:97, 1968.

34 Drapanas, T.: in Discussion of Celiac Compression Syndrome by S. A. Marable, M. F. Kaplan, F. M. Beman, and W. Molnar, *Am. J. Surg.*, 115:101, 1968.

35 Evans, W. E.: Long-Term Evaluation of the Celiac Band Syndrome, *Surgery*, 76:867, 1974.

36 McLoughlin, M. J., Colapinto, R. F., and Hobbs, B. B.: Abdominal Bruits: Clinical and Angiographic Correlation, *JAMA*, 232:1238, 1975.

37 McLoughlin, M. J., Colapinto, R. F., and Hobbs, B. B.: Correlating Abdominal Bruits with Angiographic Findings, *JAMA*, 234:916, 1975.

38 Schwartz, D. T.: Relation of Superior Mesenteric Artery Obstruction to Renal Hypertension: A Review of 56 Cases, *N. Engl. J. Med.*, 272:1318, 1965.

39 Watt, J. K., Watson, W. C., and Haase, S.: Chronic Intestinal Ischaemia, *Br. Med. J.*, 3:199, 1967.

40 Osler, W.: On Multiple Hemorrhagic Telangiectases with Recurring Hemorrhages, *Q. J. Med.*, 1:53, 1901.

41 Bean, W. B.: "Vascular Spiders and Related Lesions of the Skin," Charles C Thomas, Publisher, Springfield, Ill., 1958, p. 132.

42 Whitecomb, F. F., and Brown, C. H.: Pseudoxanthoma Elasticum, *Ann. Intern. Med.*, 56:834, 1962.

43 Levine, R. A.: Amyloid Disease of the Liver, *Am. J. Med.*, 33:349, 1962.

44 Strole, W. E., Clark, W. H., and Isselbacher, K. J.: Progressive Arterial Occlusive Disease (Kohlmeier-Degos): A Frequently Fatal Cutaneosystemic Disorder, *N. Engl. J. Med.*, 276:195, 1967.

45 Penner, A., and Bernheim, A. I.: Acute Postoperative Enterocolitis: A Study on the Pathologic Nature of Shock, *AMA Arch. Pathol.*, 27:966, 1939.

46 Kleckner, M. S., Jr., Bargen, J. A., and Baggenstoss, A. H.: Pseudomembranous Enterocolitis: Clinicopathologic Study of 14 cases in Which the Disease Was Not Preceded by an Operation, *Gastroenterology*, 21:212, 1952.

47 Habboushe, F., Wallace, H. W., Nusbaum, M., Baum, S., Dratch, P., and Blakemore, W. S.: Nonocclusive Mesenteric Vascular Insufficiency, *Ann. Surg.*, 180:819, 1974.

48 Ottinger, L. W.: Nonocclusive Mesenteric Infarction, *Surg. Clin. North Am.*, 54:689, 1974.

49 Gazes, P. C., Holmes, C. R., Moseley, V., and Pratt-Thomas, N. R.: Acute Hemorrhage and Necrosis of Intestines Associated with Digitalization, *Circulation*, 23:358, 1961.

50 Kane, J. M., Meyer, K. A., and Kozoll, D. D.: Anatomical Approach to Problem of Massive Gastrointestinal Hemorrhage, *Arch. Surg.*, 70:570, 1955.

51 Levinsky, R. A., Lewis, R. M., Bynum, T. E., and Hanley, H. G.: Digoxin Induced Intestinal Vasoconstriction: The Effects of Proximal Arterial Stenosis and Glucagon Administration, *Circulation*, 52:130, 1975.

52 Benson, W. R., and Sealy, W. C.: Arterial Necrosis Following Resection of Coarctation of Aorta, *Lab. Invest.*, 5:359, 1956.

53 Schuster, N. H.: Familial Hemorrhagic Telangiectasia Associated with Multiple Aneurysms of Splenic Artery, *J. Pathol. Bacteriol.*, 144:39, 1937.

54 Rob, C. G., Goadby, H. K., and McSweeny, R. R.: Mycotic Aneurysm, *St. Thomas' Rep.*, 5:44, 1953.

107
Surgical Treatment of Diseases of the Aorta and Major Arteries

MICHAEL E. DEBAKEY, M.D.,
ARTHUR C. BEALL, JR., M.D., and
KENNETH L. MATTOX, M.D.

Although Galen in *Methodus Medendi* 6, Chap. 1, did not approve of physicians who discuss the precise meaning of medical terms, for it is more important to examine the nature of things than the meanings of words; nevertheless, since names are bestowed by wise men, as was believed by Cratylus, Heraclitus, and the Pythagoreans, and they are a means of conveying the ideas of speakers or writers to hearers or readers and they arouse in us the images of things; my decision is that we must, to begin with, declare what the ancients, who had the final verdict and the right to give names to things, thought about the derivation of *aneurysma*.

GIOVANNI MARIA LANCISI, 1745[1]

Arterial diseases, especially those of arteriosclerotic origin, have consistently ranked among the most common ailments of the Western world and now account for more deaths than all other diseases combined. Although the cause of most of these diseases remains undetermined, great progress has been made in recent years toward a better understanding of their nature and better methods for their treatment. This striking progress has been influenced by a number of factors, the most important being (1) the development of relatively safe and readily applied methods of angiography, which by providing roentgenographic visualization of the arterial tree permit precise delineation of the location and extent of the diseased area as well as its hemodynamic disturbances;[1a] and (2) the development of highly successful methods of vascular surgical procedures including the use of vascular replacements which may be applied to correct both the pathologic and hemodynamic disturbances of the lesion.[2]

Still another important factor responsible for this progress has been the great intensification of experimental and clinical investigations in this field of endeavor. As a consequence of these studies and surgical experience, certain conceptual changes have evolved concerning diseases of the aorta and major arteries that provide the basis for rational and more effective therapy. Most important among these changes has been the emphasis placed upon the anatomic-pathologic characteristics of the lesion itself and its hemodynamic effects, rather than upon its causation. The concept has thus evolved that regardless of cause the lesion in many forms of aortic and arterial disease may be well localized and segmental in nature, with a relatively normal patent proximal and distal arterial bed. The great significance of this idea lies in the fact that it provides the basis for corrective surgical therapy designed to eliminate the pathologic and hemodynamic disturbance of the lesion and to restore normal circulation.[2]

To achieve this objective, four basic principles of surgical therapy may be employed: excision with graft replacement, the bypass procedure, thromboendarterectomy, and patch angioplasty. The application of each of these procedures or, in some instances, their combined use is dependent on the nature, location, and extent of the lesion.

Most, if not all, arterial diseases may be classified in two major categories: aneurysms and occlusive lesions. The lesions in both categories may be of congenital, acquired, or traumatic origin, but from a practical therapeutic standpoint their etiologic considerations are much less significant than their nature and location or the hemodynamic disturbances that they produce. The most significant facts about aneurysms of the aorta, for example, are (1) that all types if untreated have the same ultimately disabling and even fatal course, and (2) that they may be cured by the same surgical techniques. Actually, aneurysms and occlusive lesions may have the same basic cause, arteriosclerosis being the most common cause of both.

ANEURYSMS

Aneurysm is a word derived from the Greek *aneurynein,* meaning "to widen or dilate"; it refers to a hollow tumor or sac directly connected with the lumen of an artery and filled with liquid or coagulated blood. Aneurysms may be classified in numerous ways, according to the nature and cause of the lesion. For our purposes, however, we shall classify them morphologically as sacciform, fusiform, and dissecting; subsequently they will be classified by locations.

Sacciform aneurysms are pouchlike, with a relatively narrow neck constituting the orifice from the side of the artery to which the sac is connected. Fusiform aneurysms are more spindle-shaped and involve the entire circumference of the parent artery. Dissecting aneurysms are a marked entity and will be dealt with separately.

Once an aneurysmal lesion has formed, through weakening and destruction of the media, it tends to

progress and to produce serious and ultimately lethal complications from compression of surrounding structures or from rupture, with possibly fatal hemorrhage. In the past, treatment of aneurysm of the aorta was directed toward obliteration of the aneurysm by inducing thrombosis within the lesion or by reinforcing the wall to forestall perforation. Such procedures proved to be inadequate and may now be considered obsolete. The only effective treatment consists of obliteration or preferably extirpation of the aneurysm, with restoration of normal aortic continuity and function. This may be accomplished by one of several methods, depending on the type and location of the lesion. In sacciform aneurysms, for example, it may be possible to apply an occluding clamp across the relatively narrow neck of the lesion and in this way to perform tangential excision of the aneurysm, with repair by lateral aortorrhaphy or patch graft angioplasty. In fusiform aneurysms the entire segment of aorta involved by the aneurysm must be removed and replaced by a graft. A flexible, knitted or woven, seamless Dacron tube has been proved to be the most satisfactory vascular replacement in such cases.[3] Under some circumstances it is preferable to obliterate a fusiform aneurysm by endoaneurysmorrhaphy and to restore circulation by means of a bypass graft attached end-to-side above and below the obliterated segment.

The site and extent of the aneurysmal lesion also have great influence on operability and method of operation. Aneurysms of the aorta and major arteries may accordingly be classified usefully by their location as follows (Fig. 107-1):

1 Aneurysms of the aortic arch (Fig. 107-1*A* and *B*)
2 Aneurysms of the descending thoracic aorta (Fig. 107-1*C*)
3 Aneurysms of the thoracoabdominal segment of aorta (Fig. 107-1*D*)
4 Aneurysms of the abdominal aorta distal to the renal arteries (Fig. 107-1*E*)
5 Aneurysms of the major peripheral arteries (Fig. 107-1*F* and *G*)

The risk of operation may be considered greatest in the first category and least in the last two, because in applying surgical treatment, circulation is necessarily arrested temporarily through the segment to be resected and replaced with a graft. The potentially hazardous consequences of this procedure are (1) increased vascular resistance, with left ventricular strain, and (2) possible ischemic damage to the tissues distal to the occlusion. These problems assume significance for the first three categories only, since temporary arrest of aortic circulation below the renal arteries is well tolerated (Fig. 107-2).

Several methods have been devised to overcome problems arising from temporary arrest of aortic circulation. For aneurysms involving the ascending aorta, cardiopulmonary bypass with the pump oxygenator is used, and each coronary artery is perfused individually (Fig. 107-3*A*). When the transverse portion of the aortic arch containing origins of the brachiocephalic vessels is involved, extracorporeal

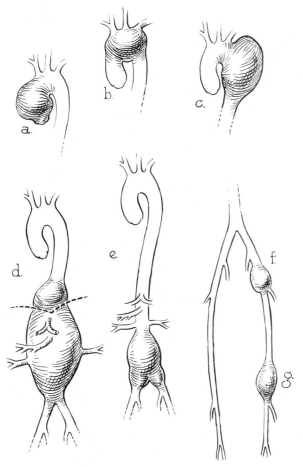

FIGURE 107-1 Most frequent sites of aneurysms of the aorta and major arteries. *A.* Fusiform aneurysm of the ascending aorta. *B.* Fusiform aneurysm of the aortic arch involving the brachiocephalic, carotid, and subclavian arteries. *C.* Fusiform aneurysm of the descending portion of the aortic arch. *D.* Large fusiform thoracoabdominal aneurysm involving the celiac, superior mesenteric, and renal arteries. *E.* Fusiform aneurysm of the abdominal aorta and iliac arteries. *F.* Fusiform aneurysm of the femoral artery. *G.* Fusiform aneurysm of the popliteal artery.

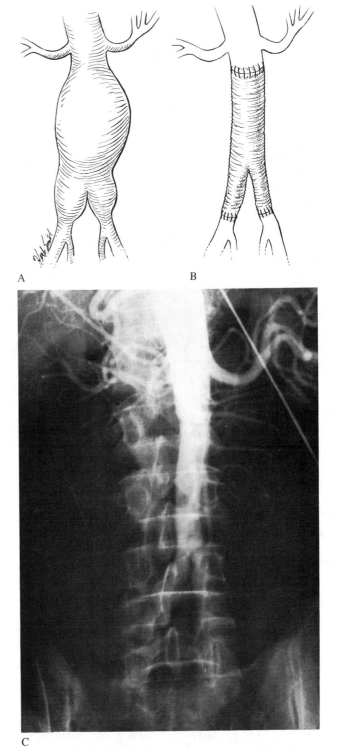

FIGURE 107-2 *A.* Characteristic type of arteriosclerotic aneurysm of the abdominal aorta arising just below the origin of the renal arteries, treated by (*B*) resection and replacement with a bifurcation Dacron graft. *C.* Aortogram, made 5 years after operation, showing the restoration of normal circulation.

perfusion of the brain also is necessary (Fig. 107-3*B*).[4] For aneurysms arising distal to the origin of the left common carotid artery and those involving the descending thoracic aorta, the pump-bypass method traditionally has been employed, with oxygenated blood removed from the left atrium and pumped proximally via the common femoral artery (Figs. 107-3*C* and 107-5).[5,6] Aneurysms involving the thoracoabdominal segment of the aorta are bypassed by the use of Dacron tubes progressively sewn into place in such a manner as to minimize ischemia to the abdominal viscera (Fig. 107-4).[8]

At the Baylor College of Medicine, the described methods of surgical treatment have been used in more than 8,000 patients, and analysis of the results is most encouraging. The risk of operation varies in accordance with a number of factors, particularly the type and location of the lesion, the presence or absence of rupture, heart disease, or hypertension, and the patient's age. The total operative mortality

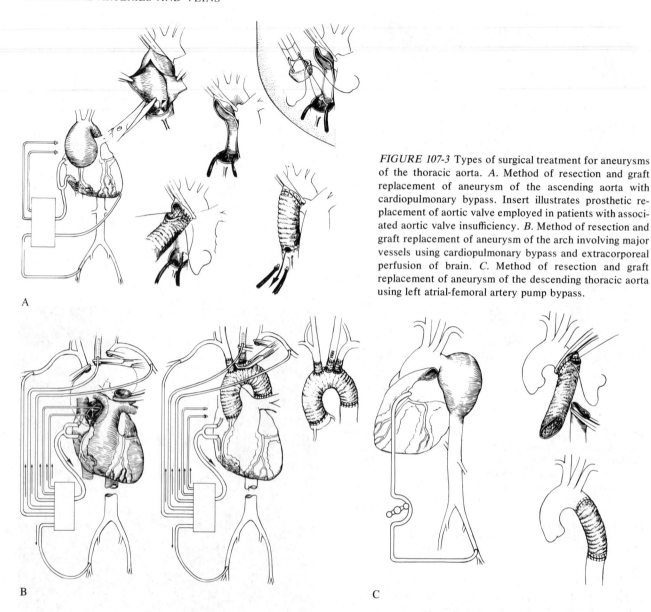

FIGURE 107-3 Types of surgical treatment for aneurysms of the thoracic aorta. *A*. Method of resection and graft replacement of aneurysm of the ascending aorta with cardiopulmonary bypass. Insert illustrates prosthetic replacement of aortic valve employed in patients with associated aortic valve insufficiency. *B*. Method of resection and graft replacement of aneurysm of the arch involving major vessels using cardiopulmonary bypass and extracorporeal perfusion of brain. *C*. Method of resection and graft replacement of aneurysm of the descending thoracic aorta using left atrial-femoral artery pump bypass.

rate for aneurysms of the descending thoracic aorta (Fig. 107-5) is about 15 percent, but for aneurysms of the abdominal aorta it is less than 5 percent. Rupture is very significant, the operative mortality rate for ruptured aneurysms of the abdominal aorta being about 33 percent. For nonruptured aneurysms it is less than 4 percent. The influence of heart disease may be illustrated by the fact that the operative mortality rate for aneurysms of the abdominal aorta in patients with heart disease is 13 percent, whereas in patients without heart disease it is less than 2 percent.

Follow-up studies on these patients for periods of more than 20 years provide evidence of maintenance of good results with long-term survival. The 5- to 10-year survival rate, for example, for patients operated on for aneurysms of the abdominal aorta closely

parallels that for comparable age groups in the normal population.[9]

Dissecting aneurysm

Dissecting aneurysm of the aorta is a distinct clinical and pathologic entity characterized by hemorrhagic intramural separation of the medial layer of the aortic wall, usually communicating with the normal lumen by an intimal tear. The cause is unknown, but the underlying predominant lesion appears to be degeneration of the elements of the media in the form of cystic medionecrosis. Certain factors have been considered to have a causal relation to dissecting aneurysm owing to their frequent association with its occurrence. These include Marfan's syndrome, pregnancy, hypertension, coarctation, and idiopathic

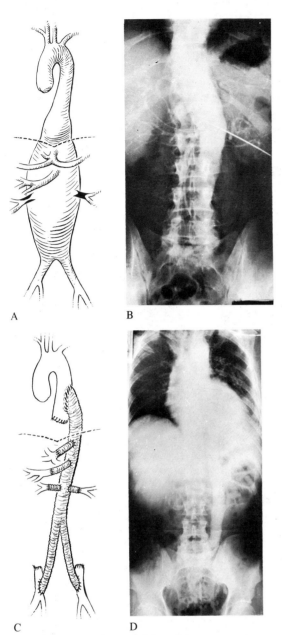

FIGURE 107-4 Drawing (*A*) and aortogram (*B*) showing the extent of a large fusiform aneurysm involving the lower segment of the descending thoracic aorta and the entire abdominal aorta associated with occlusive lesions involving the origin of both renal arteries and producing incomplete occlusion of the right renal and complete occlusion of the left renal artery in a 38-year-old white man with manifestations of severe hypertension and abdominal pain. *C*. Method of surgical treatment consisting of resection of the aneurysm and replacement with a Dacron graft. *D*. Postoperative aortogram showing restoration of normal circulation through a Dacron graft to the lower extremities, as well as to both renal arteries and the celiac and superior mesenteric arteries. The patient was able to resume normal activities after the operation.

kyphoscoliosis. Men are affected about twice as often as women, with the highest age incidence in the fourth to seventh decades. The prognosis in untreated cases is extremely grave, with a fatal termination in about half the cases within the first 24 h after onset, and in about three-fourths of the cases within the first week after onset.

On the basis of both anatomic and pathologic patterns of the lesions and their respective methods of surgical treatment, dissecting aneurysms may be classified into three basic types, as follows (Fig. 107-6): type I, in which the dissecting process arises in the ascending aorta and extends distally, often into the abdominal aorta; type II, in which the dissecting process is limited to the ascending aorta and is characterized by a transverse tear in the intima just above the aortic valves; and type III, in which the dissecting process arises in the descending thoracic aorta at, or just distal to, the origin of the left subclavian artery and extends distally for a varying distance, sometimes being limited to the descending thoracic aorta but more often extending into the abdominal aorta (Fig. 107-7).[10]

Surgical treatment for type I aneurysms consists of transection of the ascending aorta using cardiopulmonary bypass; obliteration of the false lumen by approximation of the inner and outer walls of the dissecting process with a continuous suture proximally and distally; and end-to-end anastomosis of the transected aorta (Fig. 107-6). In instances in which this method of direct repair is inapplicable, it may be necessary to resect the proximal segment and restore vascular continuity by means of a Dacron patch or tube graft. In many cases aortic valve incompetence is encountered, secondary to loss of commissural support of the valve leaflets. This is usually corrected by suture approximation of the inner and outer layers of the dissecting process, with resultant resuspension of the valve, although in some instances prosthetic valve replacement is required.

Surgical treatment for type II aneurysms consists essentially of resection and graft replacement of the entire ascending aorta using cardiopulmonary bypass (Fig. 107-6). Aortic valve incompetence is more often encountered in this type than in type I and is less frequently amendable to reparative techniques, because of the more chronic nature of the dissecting process in most instances. Under such circumstances prosthetic replacement of the aortic valve usually is performed concomitantly with graft replacement of the ascending aorta.

Surgical treatment for type III aneurysms consists in resection of the descending thoracic aorta above the level of the origin of the dissecting process (usually at, or just below, the origin of the left subclavian artery); obliteration of the distal false passage by suture closure of the inner and outer layers; and replacement of the excised segment with an aortic graft (Figs. 107-6 and 107-7).

Analysis of experience with more than 475 cases treated at Baylor College of Medicine in which these methods of surgical treatment have been applied reveals gratifying results, with an operative mortality rate of about 20 percent. Follow-up observations extending over more than 20 years reveal maintenance of good functional activity.

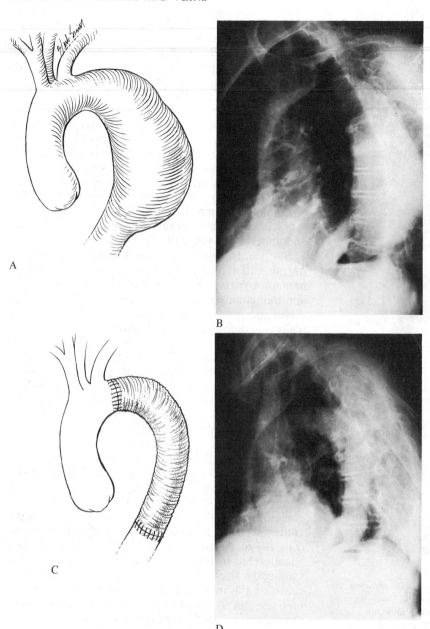

FIGURE 107-5 Drawing (*A*) and preoperative aortogram (*B*) showing a large fusiform aneurysm of the descending aorta in a 67-year-old white woman. *C*. Method of surgical treatment consisting of resection of an aneurysm and replacement with a Dacron graft. *D*. Postoperative aortogram made 5 years after operation shows restoration of normal aortic continuity and function.

OCCLUSIVE LESIONS

Occlusive lesions of the aorta and major arteries may be of congenital or acquired origin. The former are represented largely by coarctation and the latter predominantly by arteriosclerosis or atherosclerosis, although in a small proportion of cases they may be due to nonspecific forms of arteritis or to embolic phenomenons. Acquired forms of arterial occlusive lesions are by far the most common. Except for those associated with embolic episodes, their characteristic patterns of involvement and manifestations of arterial insufficiency may be classified into two subgroups: (1) lesions involving the major branches of the aortic arch, (2) lesions involving the visceral branches of the abdominal aorta, and (3) lesions involving the terminal abdominal aorta and its major branches (Fig. 107-8).

Coarctation of the aorta

Coarctation of the aorta is a congenital disease characterized by narrowing or complete obstruction of the aortic lumen usually occurring in the distal segment of the aortic arch but occasionally in the descending thoracic or abdominal aorta.

The most satisfactory classification of the forms of coarctation is based on two factors: (1) relation of the coarctation to the ductus arteriosus (preductile or postductile), and (2) patency of the ductus arteriosus.

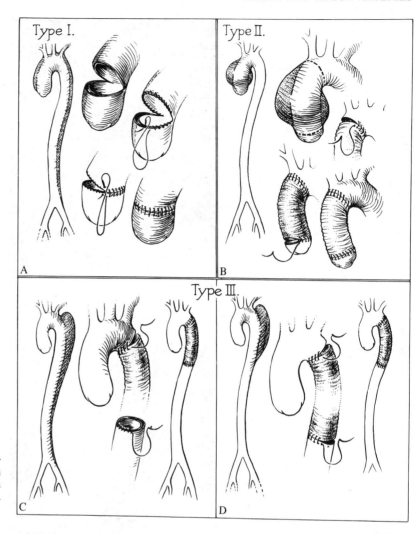

FIGURE 107-6 Surgical classification of dissecting aneurysms of the aorta based on anatomic and pathologic patterns of the lesions and their respective methods of surgical treatment.

The coarctation is usually located close to, and just distal to, the aortic insertion of the ligamentum arteriosum. Occasionally the areas of narrowing may lie more proximally to involve the segment between the left common carotid and left subclavian arteries, or they may be located in the distal portion of the descending thoracic aorta, extending down to involve even the upper segment of the abdominal aorta.

Other congenital anomalies involving the cardiovascular system are associated with coarctation in a significant proportion of cases. Patent ductus arteriosus, for instance, occurs in about 15 percent of patients surviving to adulthood. Other associated anomalies include aortic valve deformity, interventricular or interatrial septal defects, mitral valve deformity, pulmonary stenosis, and subendocardial fibroelastosis.

Most cases of coarctation, particularly of the postductile type, may be treated by surgical removal of the coarcted segment, with restoration of aortic continuity by end-to-end anastomosis. Occasionally, wedge resection laterally with direct repair is a satisfactory precedure for young patients with very short isthmic coarctations. This type of suture repair is similar to end-to-end anastomosis except that the posteromedial wall of the aorta in the stenotic area is not resected and forms one segment of the aortic wall opposite the suture line. In cases associated with aneurysm formation or in which a longer segment is involved, it may be necessary to replace the resected portion with a graft. Graft repair mimimizes necessary dissection of the distal aortic segment, since a suitable curved vascular clamp may be used to control this segment and exclude the origin of the intercostal vessels. Occasionally, particularly in older or poor risk patients, the preferred method of treatment consists of insertion of a bypass graft (Fig. 107-9).

Results of surgical treatment are gratifying, with low mortality and morbidity rates. Symptoms are

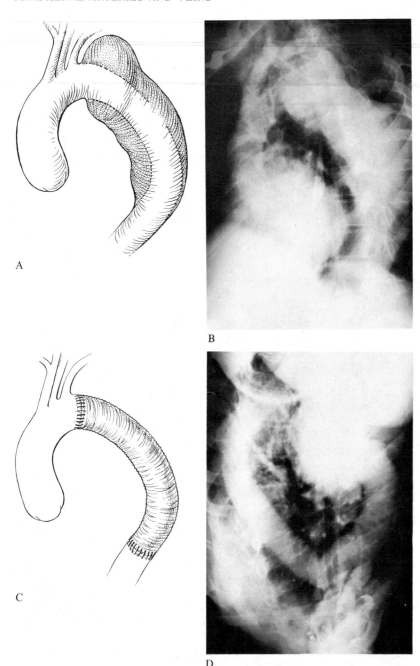

A

B

C

D

FIGURE 107-7 Drawing (*A*) and preoperative aortogram (*B*) showing extensive dissecting aneurysm arising just distal to the left subclavian artery and involving the entire descending thoracic aorta in a 54-year-old white man. *C.* Operative procedure consisting of resection of a dissecting aneurysm and replacement with a Dacron graft. *D.* Postoperative aortogram showing restoration of normal continuity and function of the thoracic aorta.

usually relieved, and blood pressure in the extremities is restored to normal levels.[11]

Arterial emboli

Peripheral arterial emboli usually are associated with atherosclerotic or rheumatic heart disease. They may originate from within the left atrium in the presence of atrial fibrillation, from the ventricular endocardial surface following myocardial infarction, or from the mitral or aortic valve in association with valvular heart disease. Embolization usually is associated with a change in heart rate or rhythm, and diagnosis

and localization of the embolus often are possible on the basis of clinical findings alone. Occasionally, arteriography is helpful in exact localization (Fig. 107-10*A* and *B*).

Delay in embolectomy may result in varying degrees of distal thrombosis; the embolus should be removed surgically as soon as is feasible. The artery first is exposed in the region of the proximal extent of the embolus, and the embolus is extracted through a small arteriotomy. Fogarty catheters then are passed proximally and distally, their balloons are inflated, and they are withdrawn, thus ensuring against retained embolic material. A second arteriotomy rarely

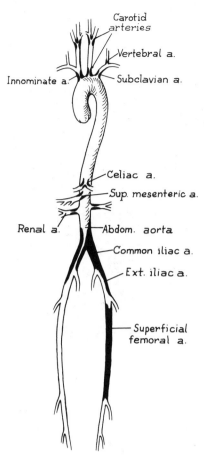

FIGURE 107-8 Typical patterns of location and extent of occlusive disease of the aorta and its major branches.

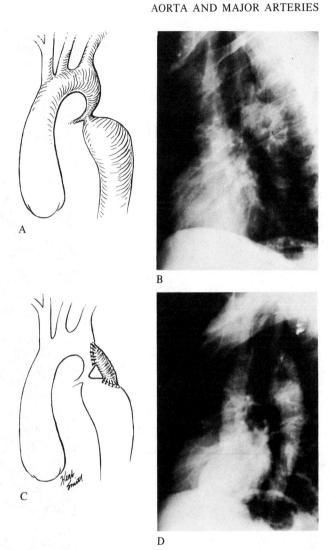

FIGURE 107-9 Drawing (A) and preoperative aortogram (B) showing typical coarctation of the aorta in a 36-year-old white man. C. Application of the bypass principle employing a Dacron graft attached by end-to-side anastomosis to the left subclavian artery above and to the descending thoracic aorta below the coarcted segment. D. Postoperative aortogram showing restoration of normal aortic circulation through the bypass graft. The patient remained asymptomatic after the operation, with normal blood pressure in both upper and lower extremities.

is necessary if the Fogarty catheters are employed properly. Dilute heparin solution usually is placed into the vessel proximally and distally during arteriotomy repair, and the vessel is again flushed proximally and distally prior to completion of repair.[12] In patients with peripheral arterial embolization secondary to rheumatic heart disease with mitral stenosis, concomitant definitive valve surgical treatment should be considered at the same time as embolectomy.

Lesions involving major branches of the aortic arch

These lesions may be classified as proximal or distal. Proximal occlusive lesions are located near the origin of the brachiocephalic, left common carotid, and left subclavian arties (Fig. 107-11). These lesions may produce complete or incomplete occlusion and are usually multiple, but they are predominantly segmental in nature and therefore operable. Characteristic sites of involvement in the distal form are the vertebral arteries at their origin from the subclavian arteries, the common carotid arteries at their bifurcation, and the internal carotid arteries at their origin (Fig. 107-12). In this type of case also, the occlusive process may be complete or incomplete and is often multiple. Incomplete occlusions are usually segmental and therefore operable, whereas complete occlusions of long duration are rarely amenable to surgical repair. Depending on the location and extent of the lesion, the clinical manifestations vary considerably, the proximal type being associated with symptoms of ischemia of the cerebrum and upper extremities and the distal type with episodes of cerebrovascular insufficiency which may be transient, progressive, or apoplectic in nature. Arteriography is mandatory to establish the diagnosis with certainty and to determine the precise location and extent of the occlusive lesions in order to facilitate application of proper surgical treatment.

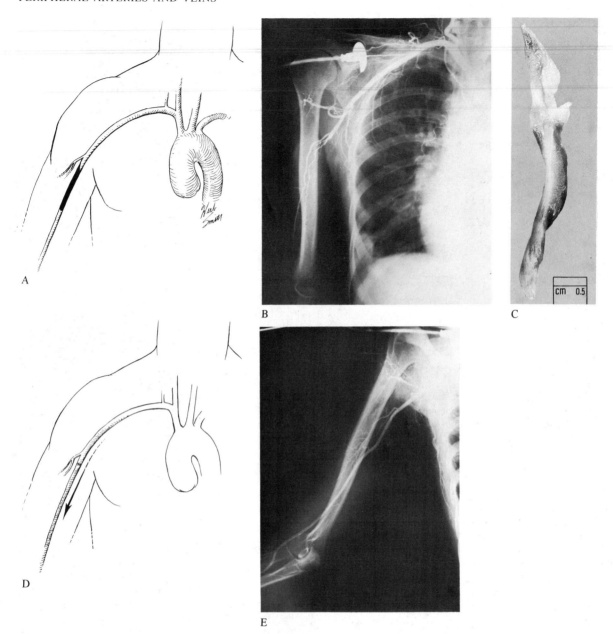

FIGURE 107-10 Right brachial artery embolism following myocardial infarction. *A.* Location of an embolus. *B.* Right subclavian
arteriogram demonstrating occlusion of the brachial artery at the
junction of the upper and middle thirds. *C.* Embolus following
removal. *D.* Completed operation. *E.* Right subclavian arteriogram
following an operation demonstrating patency of brachial artery.

Lesions involving visceral branches of abdominal aorta

This category includes lesions which produce (1)
abdominal or intestinal angina or (2) renovascular
hypertension. The occlusive lesions in group 1 are
located in the celiac axis and superior mesenteric
artery near their origins from the aorta and are
usually caused by atherosclerosis. They may be
complete or incomplete but are usually well localized
and segmental in nature and therefore are surgically
correctible. These lesions, producing the syndrome
of abdominal or intestinal angina, are characterized
by manifestations of abdominal pain occurring after
meals, disturbances in bowel rhythm and function,
bulky stools, nutritional disturbances, and weight
loss. Lumbar aortography, performed in the lateral
position rather than in the usual prone position, is
essential to establish the diagnosis and to determine
proper surgical treatment.

Occlusive lesions in group 2 involve the renal
arteries. In this group also the occlusive process
tends to be fairly well localized in the main renal
artery, usually near its origin from the aorta (Fig.
107-13). In the great majority of cases the lesion is

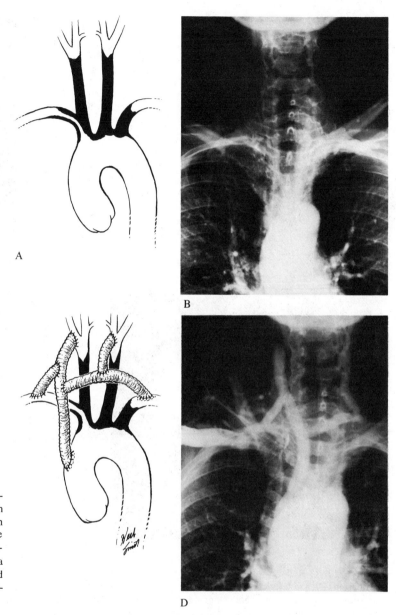

FIGURE 107-11 Drawing (*A*) and preoperative arteriogram (*B*) showing complete occlusion of both carotid and subclavian arteries and partial occlusion of the brachiocephalic artery in a 46-year-old white woman. *C.* Operative procedure employed, consisting of Dacron bypass grafts from the ascending aorta to the brachiocephalic, both common carotid, and the subclavian arteries. *D.* Postoperative arteriogram showing restoration of normal circulation.

atherosclerotic, but occasionally, most often in young women, the pathologic features of the lesion may be described as fibromuscular hyperplasia. Apparently, no distinctive clinical features in history or physical examination distinguish this type of renovascular hypertension from essential hypertension, and the definitive diagnosis of this form can be established only by means of properly performed aortography.

Lesions involving terminal abdominal aorta and its major branches

There are two main groups: proximal (or aortoiliac) occlusions and distal (or femoropopliteal) occlusions.

Variation in the nature, extent, and pathologic features of the occlusive process is often encountered. In general, however, proximal lesions with complete occlusion tend to be well localized to the terminal abdominal aorta and bifurcation and the common iliac arteries, whereas those with incomplete occlusion are more frequently associated with occlusive disease of the superficial femoral arteries (Figs. 107-14 and 107-15). Combinations of both proximal and distal types of involvement are not uncommon (Fig. 107-15). The distal forms of occlusion seem to be more often associated with diffuse involvement, particularly when diabetes is also present.[13]

No matter how extensive the pattern of occlusive disease, effective therapy most often depends on the presence of a patent distal arterial bed, particularly in

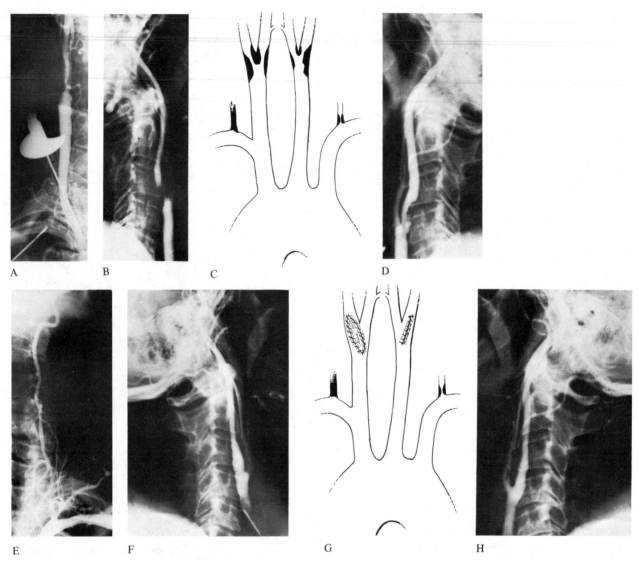

FIGURE 107-12 Right carotid arteriograms (*A, B*), left carotid arteriogram (*D*), and left vertebral arteriogram (*E*) in a 67-year-old man with partial occlusion of both common carotid arteries at the bifurcation, involving the origin of internal and external carotid arteries and with complete occlusion of the right vertebral and severe stenosis of the left vertebral arteries, producing severe manifestations of cerebrovascular insufficiency, as depicted in (*C*) Operative procedure consists of endarterectomy with patch graft angioplasty in the right carotid and endarterectomy with primary closure in the left carotid (*G*). Postoperative right (*F*) and left (*H*) arteriograms made 2 years after operation demonstrate restoration of normal blood flow. The patient has remained asymptomatic.

cases involving segments and branches of the popliteal artery. For this reason arteriographic visualization of the aortoiliac and femoropopliteal arterial circulation is absolutely essential. The diagnosis can usually be made from clinical manifestations or arterial insufficiency of the lower extemities, and with experience one can even be fairly sure of the location and pattern of the occlusive process, but in order to determine the proper surgical procedure to employ, it is necessary to ascertain precisely by arteriography the full extent and location of the occlusive process.

Experience with these major categories of arterial occlusive disease has disclosed that they may occur in various combinations in the same patient (Figs. 107-14 to 107-16). This should not be unexpected, since the predominant underlying pathologic lesion in these forms of occlusive disease is atherosclerosis, which has a predilection for involving and blocking the origin or bifurcations of major arteries. Patients have been observed who have such combinations of the three major categories as cerebrovascular insufficiency with renovascular hypertension or with arterial insufficiency of the lower patterns may also be associated with aneurysms of the aorta or major arteries.

Four basic principles of surgical therapy have been developed for occlusive diseases: thromboendarterectomy, excision with graft replacement, bypass graft, and patch graft angioplasty. The applica-

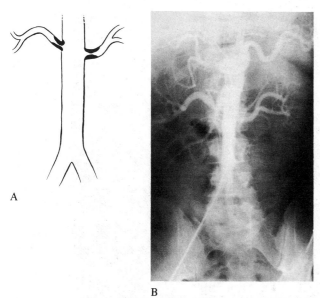

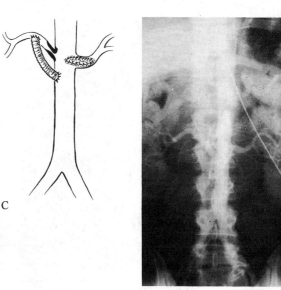

B

D

FIGURE 107-13 Drawing (*A*) and preoperative aortogram (*B*) showing well-localized and severe stenotic lesions involving both renal arteries at their origin in a 46-year-old white man with manifestations of severe hypertension (blood pressure 220/130 mm Hg). *C.* Method of surgical treatment consisting of insertion of a Dacron bypass graft from the abdominal aorta to the right renal artery distal to the occlusive lesion, and endarterectomy and patch graft angioplasty of the left renal artery. Postoperative aortogram (*D*) shows restoration of normal circulation to both renal arteries.

FIGURE 107-14 Drawing (*A*) and aortogram (*B*) showing complete occlusion of the abdominal aorta arising at the level of the renal arteries and extending down to involve the bifurcation and both common iliac arteries. Well-localized stenotic lesions involve the origin of both renal arteries in this 61-year-old white man who had severe manifestations of intermittent claudication of the lower extermities and hypertension (blood pressure 230/130 mm Hg). *C.* Operative procedure employed in this patient consisting of excision of abdominal aorta and replacement with a Dacron bifurcation graft, with bypass to both renal arteries distal to the occlusive lesion and to both external iliac arteries distal to the occlusive process. *D.* Aortogram made 2 years after operation shows restoration of normal circulation through a graft to both arteries and to the lower extremities. The patient's blood pressure at this time was 120/80 mm Hg, and he was completely relieved of his previous symptoms of intermittent claudication.

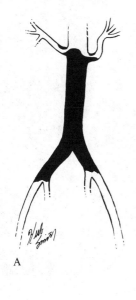

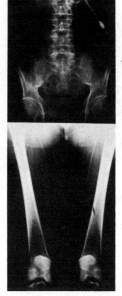

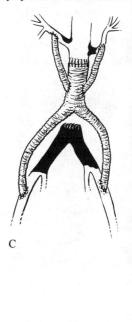

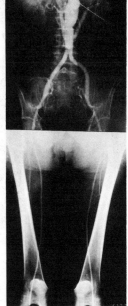

A

B

C

D

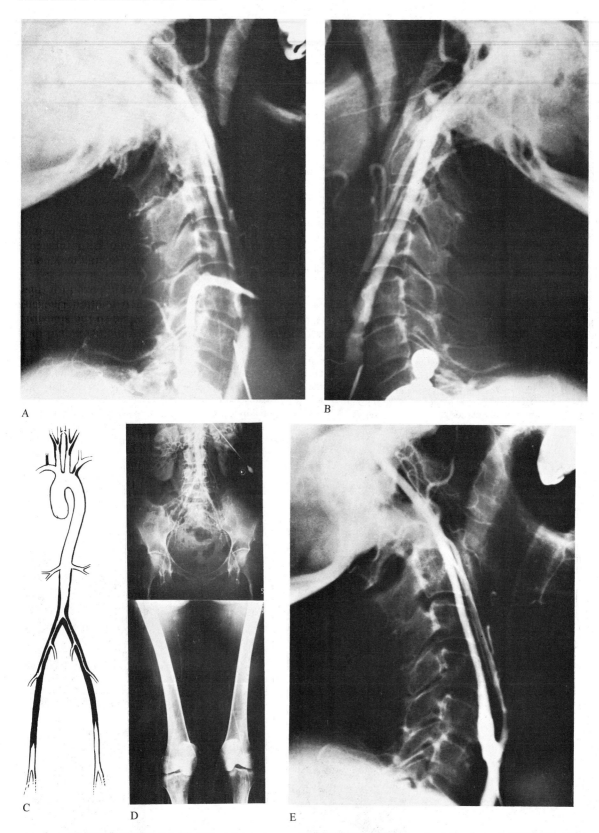

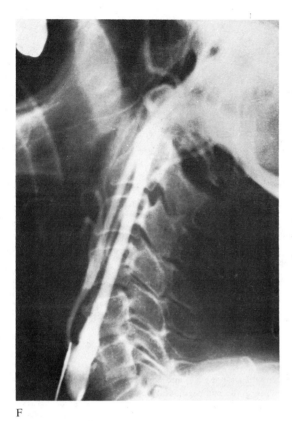

F

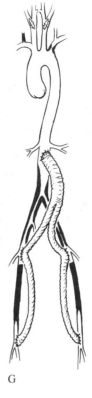

G

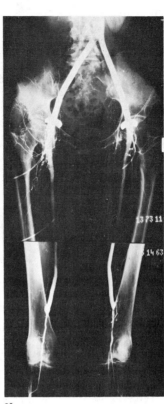

H

FIGURE 107-15 Location and extent of multiple segmental occlusive lesions of atherosclerotic origin (*C*) in 60-year-old white woman with manifestations of cerebrovascular insufficiency indicative primarily of basilar artery insufficiency and severe intermittent claudication of the lower extremities. Preoperative right carotid (*A*) and left carotid (*B*) arteriograms showing well-localized segmental occlusive lesions of the internal carotid arteries near their origins. There was complete occlusion of the right vertebral artery and marked stenosis of the left subclavian artery. *D.* Preoperative lumbar aortogram showing extensive incomplete occlusive disease of the lower abdominal aorta and common iliac arteries and bilateral complete segmental occlusive lesions of superficial femoral arteries. *G.* Operative procedures employed. Right (*E*) and left (*F*) carotid arteriograms and aortogram (*H*) made 3 years after operation, showing restoration of normal circulation.

tion of each of these procedures, and in some instances their combined use, is dependent on a number of factors, including particularly the nature, extent, and site of involvement of the occlusive lesions.

Lesions located in the internal carotid and vertebral arteries are treated by endarterectomy and patch graft angioplasty (Fig. 107-12). The involved arterial segment is exposed, and temporary arterial clamps are placed proximally and distally. A longitudinal incision is made through the involved segment, and the diseased intima is removed by dissection through a well-defined cleavage plane. The arterial incision is then closed by inserting a patch graft, the edges of which are sutured circumferentially to the arterial wound edges.[14]

Occlusions of the great vessels arising from the aortic arch are preferably treated by end-to-side bypass graft, because lesions at this level are usually more extensive and involve long segments of vessel (Fig. 107-11). The proximal end of the graft is attached to the side of the ascending aorta, and the distal end (or ends) of the graft is attached to the patent arterial segments in the neck or supraclavicular region distal to the occlusion. The ascending aorta is exposed through a second or third right anterior intercostal incision. Using a partial occlusion clamp and end-to-side anastomosis, the proximal end of the graft is attached to the aorta. The patent distal arterial segments are exposed through separate incisions in the neck and supraclavicular regions. The other end of the graft is drawn retrosternally through a tunnel made by blunt dessection and attached to the side of the patent distal segment. In the presence of multiple occlusions, the appropriate limbs are attached to the side of this graft in the neck, and the other ends of the limbs are attached to the sides of the other patent arterial segments. Knitted Dacron Velour tubes 6 to 8 mm in diameter are used for this purpose.[14]

Operation in cases of abdominal angina may consist of endarterectomy, excision and graft replacement, or bypass graft, the latter procedure being preferable in most instances. The abdominal aorta is exposed between the renal and the common iliac

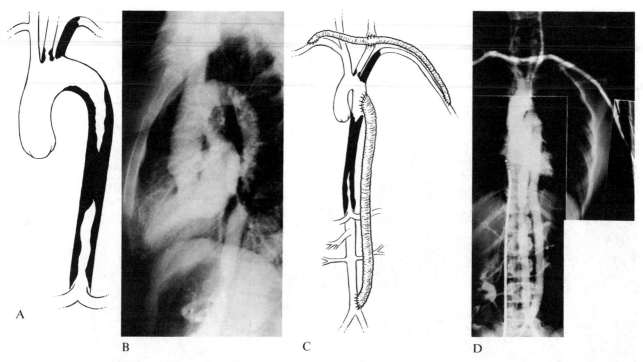

A

B

C

D

FIGURE 107-16 Drawing (A) and aortogram (B) made preoperatively showing extensive segmental occlusive disease producing severe stenosis of the left common carotid artery at its origin and complete occlusion of the left subclavian artery and descending thoracic aorta in a 23-year-old white woman with manifestations of cerebrovascular insufficiency, including dizziness, headache, syncope, and transient aphasia, intermittent claudication of the left upper extremity and both lower extremities, and hypertension. A blood pressure of 170/60 could be obtained only in the right upper extremity. The occlusive process in this condition, which has been termed *pulseless disease*, or *Takayasu's disease*, is a nonspecific arteritis of undetermined cause. C. Operative procedure employed in this patient consisting of application of the bypass principle. A Dacron graft was attached first by end-to-side anastomosis to the right subclavian artery, then by side-to-side anastomosis to the left common carotid artery, and finally by end-to-side anastomosis to the left axillary artery. Another Dacron graft was attached by end-to-side anastomoses to the descending thoracic aorta above and to the abdominal aorta below the occluded segment. D. Aortogram made almost 1 year after operation, showing restoration of normal circulation through bypass grafts.

arteries. The proximal end of the graft is attached to the side of the abdominal aorta in this region, and the other end of the graft is carried behind the transverse mesocolon and stomach and sutured to the side of the normal hepatic or splenic artery. Since the trifurcation of the celiac artery usually is uninvolved by the occlusive process, attachment of the graft to the hepatic or splenic artery provides complete revascularization of the celiac distribution. One end of a second tube is sutured to the side of the graft, and the other end is carried through a tunnel in the small-bowel mesentery under the duodenum and attached to the side of the superior mesenteric artery distal to the site of the occlusive lesion. Knitted Dacron Velour tubes 8 mm in diameter are employed in most instances.[15]

Treatment for renovascular hypertension is directed toward correction of renal ischemia. Well-localized lesions may be treated by endarterectomy and patch graft angioplasty. For more extensive segmental lesions the end-to-side bypass principle is preferred. The proximal end of an 8-mm Dacron Velour graft is attached to the abdominal aorta below the origin of the renal arteries, and the distal end of the graft is attached to the side of the renal artery distal to the obstruction (Figs. 107-13 and 107-14). Bifurcation grafts are, of course, required in the treatment of bilateral lesions when this method is employed. The bypass graft method has been found particularly effective in restoring normal circulation to both the kidneys and the lower extremities in patients with combined lesions of the aorta, iliac arteries, and renal arteries. The proximal end of the renal artery graft is attached to the side of the aortic

segment of the aortoiliac bypass graft in these cases. Reconstructive operation is impossible in a small number of cases because of both location and extent of the disease. Nephrectomy or partial nephrectomy may be required in these cases.[16]

In cases of aortoiliac occlusion the method of reconstruction is selected at the time of operation on the basis of the extent of the disease and the characteristics of the outer layers of the arterial wall. Thromboendarterectomy is employed when the occlusive process is well confined to the intima of the distal aorta and common iliac arteries. This operation is performed through separate longitudinal incisions placed in the common iliac arteries and the aorta, exposing both the proximal and distal extent of the lesion. The proper cleavage plane between the diseased intima and more normal outer layers is entered, and the occlusive process is removed using sharp and blunt dissection. In larger vessels vascular continuity is restored by simple closure of the arterial incisions. In smaller vessels, to avoid arterial constriction, the incisions are closed by inserting patch grafts made of knitted Dacron fabric, the edges of which are sutured circumferentially to the arterial wound edges by simple over-and-over suture.

Excision and graft replacement are employed when the occlusive process is associated with destructive changes of the entire vessel wall (Fig. 107-14). This procedure consists simply of excising the involved segment and replacing it with a bifurcation Dacron graft. The aortic end of the graft is attached to the proximal cut end of the aorta. Afterward the end of one iliac limb of the graft and then the other is attached to the distal end of the appropriate common or external iliac or femoral artery.

In cases in which the external iliac arteries are involved, the entire aortoiliac segment must be considered. The end-to-side bypass graft procedure, using a flexible knitted Dacron graft, is the preferable treatment. One end of the graft is attached to the side of the uninvolved abdominal aorta above the obstruction, and the other end of the graft is drawn through a tunnel made behind the peritoneum and attached to the side of the distal patent segment, either in the external iliac artery or in the common femoral artery opposite the origin of the deep femoral artery in the groin (Fig. 107-15).[17]

The type of procedure employed for occlusive lesions involving the superficial femoral and popliteal arteries depends on the location and extent of occlusion. Lesions localized to a short segment of vessel, 15 cm or less, are well suited to endarterectomy and patch graft angioplasty. The involved segment of artery is exposed, and temporary occluding clamps are placed across the uninvolved vessel above and below the obstruction, as well as on all branches arising from the occluded segment. A longitudinal incision is made through the region of obstruction, and under direct vision the diseased intima is removed both from the main central channel and from the orifices of the arterial branches arising from this segment. The arterial incision is then closed by inserting a patch graft with simple sutures.[18]

More extensive lesions are usually treated by the end-to-side bypass graft technique (Fig. 107-15). Through a small incision in the groin one end of an 8-mm Dacron Velour graft is attached by simply over-and-over suture to the side of the common femoral artery, and the other end of the graft is drawn through a subcutaneous tunnel made by blunt dissection into a second incision employed to expose the distal patent segment, usually located in the popliteal artery. This end of the graft is then sutured to the side of the distal patent segment. By temporarily releasing the proximal clamp before the latter anastomosis is completed, blood is allowed to flow through the graft momentarily to flush out thrombi

which may have formed in the graft during its insertion.

Analysis of experience with these methods of therapy at the Baylor College of Medicine in more than 10,000 patients with arterial occlusive disease reveals highly gratifying results. Although the incidence of successful results is not uniform in the various categories of occlusive disease because of the differences in location, nature, and extent of involvement of the occlusive process, the figures for successful restoration of normal circulation range from about 80 percent to more than 95 percent of cases treated. In patients with occlusive disease of the major branches of the aortic arch, for example, successful restoration of normal circulation was obtained in about 85 percent of those with distal occlusions and in virtually all those with proximal occlusions. Similarly, in patients with renovascular hypertension, successful restoration of normal circulation and normotension was obtained in 80 percent of our cases. Even better results were obtained in the category involving the terminal abdominal aorta and its major branches, normal circulation being successfully restored in 97 percent of patients with aortoiliac occlusions and in 90 percent of those with femoropopliteal occlusions. Follow-up observations in these patients extending over 20 years have provided evidence of maintenance of good long-term results with a relatively low recurrence rate of about 5 percent in the proximal type of occlusion and about 20 percent in the distal form.

REFERENCES

1 Lancisi, G. M.: "Aneurysms: The Latin Text of De Aneurysmatibus," revised with translation and notes by Wilmer C. Wright, The Macmillan Company, New York, 1952.

1a Beall, A. C., Jr., Lewis, J. M., Weibel, J., Crawford, E. S., and DeBakey, M. E.: Angiographic Evaluation of the Vascular Surgery Patient, *Surg. Clin. North Am.*, 46:843, 1966.

2 DeBakey, M. E.: Basic Concepts of Therapy in Arterial Disease, *JAMA*, 186:484, 1963.

3 Jordan, G. L., Jr., DeBakey, M. E., O'Neal, R. M., and Halpert, B.: Vascular Replacements and Suture Materials, *Surg. Clin. North Am.*, 46:831, 1966.

4 DeBakey, M. E., Beall, A. C., Jr., Cooley, D. A., Crawford, E. S., Morris, G. C., Jr., and Garrett, H. E.: Resection and Graft Replacement of Aneurysms Involving the Transverse Arch of the Aorta, *Surg. Clin. North Am.*, 46:1057, 1966.

5 Bloodwell, R. D., Hallman, G. L., Beall, A. C., Jr., Cooley, D. A., and DeBakey, M. E.: Aneurysms of the Descending Thoracic Aorta: Surgical Considerations, *Surg. Clin. North Am.*, 46:901, 1966.

6 Liddicoat, J. E., Dekassy, S. M., Rubio, P. A., Noon, G. P., and DeBakey, M. E.: Ascending Aortic Aneurysms—A Review of 100 Consecutive Cases, *Circulation*, 52(suppl. 1):202, 1975.

7 Crawford, E. S., and Rubio, P. A.: Reappraisal of Adjuncts to Avoid Ischemia in the Treatment of Aneurysms of Descending Thoracic Aorta, *J. Thorac. Cardiovasc. Surg.*, 66:693, 1973.

8 DeBakey, M. E., Crawford, E. S., Garrett, H. E., Beall, A. C., Jr., and Howell, J. F.: Surgical Considerations in the Treatment of Aneurysms of the Thoraco-abdominal Aorta, *Ann. Surg.*, 162:650, 1965.

9 DeBakey, M. E., Crawford, E. S., Cooley, D. A., Morris, G. C.,
Jr., Royster, T. S., and Abbott, W. P.: Aneurysm of the
Abdominal Aorta: Analysis of Graft Replacement Therapy
One to Eleven Years after Operation, *Ann. Surg.*, 160:622,
1964.

10 DeBakey, M. E., Beall, A. C., Jr., Cooley, D. A., Crawford, E.
S., Morris, G. C., Jr., Garrett, H. E., and Howell, J. F.:
Dissecting Aneurysms of the Aorta, *Surg. Clin. North Am.*,
46:1045, 1966.

11 Morris, G. C., Jr., Cooley, D. A., DeBakey, M. E., and
Crawford, E. S.: Coarctation of the Aorta with Particular
Emphasis upon Improved Techniques of Surgical Repair, *J.
Thorac. Cardiovasc. Surg.*, 40:705, 1960.

12 Hallman, G. L., Billig, D. M., Beall, A. C., Jr., and Cooley, D.
A.: Surgical Considerations in Arterial Embolism, *Surg. Clin.
North Am.*, 46:1013, 1966.

13 Liddicoat, J. E., Bekassy, S. M., Dang, M. H., and DeBakey,
M. E.: Complete Occlusion of the Infrarenal Abdominal Aorta:
Management and Results in 64 Patients, *Surgery*, 77:467,
1975.

14 DeBakey, M. E., Crawford, E. S., Cooley, D. A., Morris, G. C.,
Jr., Garrett, H. E., and Fields, W. S.: Cerebral Arterial Insufficiency: One to 11-Year Results Following Arterial Reconstructive Operation, *Ann. Surg.*, 161:921, 1965.

15 Morris, G. C., Jr., DeBakey, M. E., and Bernhard, V.: Abdominal Angina, *Aurg. Clin. North Am.*, 46:919, 1966.

16 Morris, G. C., Jr., DeBakey, M. E., Crawford, E. S., Cooley, D.
A., and Zanger, L. C. C.: Late Results of Surgical Treatment in
Renovascular Hypertension, *Surg. Gynecol. Obstet.*, 122:1255,
1966.

17 DeBakey, M. E., Cooley, D. A., Morris, G. C., Jr., Crawford,
E. S., Beall, A. C., Jr., and Diethrich, E. B.: Surgery of
Acquired Cardiovascular Disease, in W. H. Cole and R. M.
Zollinger (eds.), "Textbook of Surgery," 9th ed., Appleton-
Century-Crofts, Inc., New York, 1970, p. 972.

18 Crawford, E. S., Garrett, H. E., DeBakey, M. E., and Howell,
J. F.: Occlusive Disease of the Femoral Artery and Its Branches, *Surg. Clin. North Am.*, 46:991, 1966.

108
Surgical Treatment of Diseases of the Venous System

ARTHUR C. BEALL, JR., M.D.,
KENNETH L. MATTOX, M.D., and
MICHAEL E. DEBAKEY, M.D.

Though advances in arterial reconstructive surgery
recently have progressed at a phenomenal rate, most
diseases of the venous system continue partially or
completely to elude surgical correction. Operative
techniques employed successfully in the arterial system, where blood flow at high pressure is dependent
on cardiac action, have found little application in the
venous system, where propulsion of blood at low
pressure is brought about by the combined action of
valves within the lumen and external muscular compression. Techniques for the repair of incompetent
venous valves have been proposed,[10] and autogenous

as well as synthetic material has been suggested as a
venous substitute.[2,8] However, in the past, such
techniques have not met with long-term success.
Even if early thrombosis is prevented by meticulous
surgical technique and vigorous use of anticoagulants, most venous grafts are doomed to late fibrous
tissue occlusion because of the low-pressure system
involved. In a few diseases of the venous system,
however, surgical therapy may be quite helpful and
occasionally lifesaving.

VARICOSE VEINS

Varicosities of the saphenous system may occur
primarily or secondarily to involvement of the deep
venous system. When varicose veins occur primarily
and are associated with symptoms, surgical extirpation may prove helpful. When they develop secondarily to deep venous insufficiency, surgical therapy
is far less applicable. However, judiciously applied
operative intervention occasionally may be indicated
even in this latter category of varicose veins, especially if they are associated with skin ulceration.
Techniques of surgical therapy for varicose veins
now have become rather standardized and are described in detail in most textbooks of surgery.[4] In
many instances, however, varicose veins can be
controlled adequately by well-fitted elastic supports
and avoidance of prolonged ambulation.

THROMBOSIS OF THE DEEP VENOUS SYSTEM

A precise knowledge of the causes and pathogenesis
of deep venous thrombosis is lacking. Little has been
added to Virchow's original hypothesis that damage
to the vessel wall, increased coagulability of the
blood, and stasis of the venous circulation are the
basic mechanisms involved in venous thrombus formation. Predisposing factors in the development of
venous thrombosis include congestive heart failure,
trauma, immobility, surgical procedures, pregnancy,
polycythemia, malignant tumors, and varicose veins.

Complications of deep venous thrombosis can be
divided into those occurring acutely and those of the
postphlebitic state. During the acute phase signs and
symptoms may vary from almost total absence
(phlebothrombosis) to the acute fulminating illness
seen with phlegmasia cerulea dolens. In the former
category dangers of pulmonary embolism always
exist, whereas the massive reaction associated with
iliofemoral thrombosis in the latter category may
progress from loss of a portion of the extremity to
death of the patient. With subsidence of the acute
phase of deep venous thrombosis, varying degrees of
recannulation occur, but the patient frequently is left
with chronic venous insufficiency and numerous
postphlebitic sequelae.

Anticoagulant therapy has been used extensively
in patients with deep venous thrombosis and in many
instances probably has resulted in functional salvage
of varying portions of the deep venous system. In
recent years considerable interest has developed in

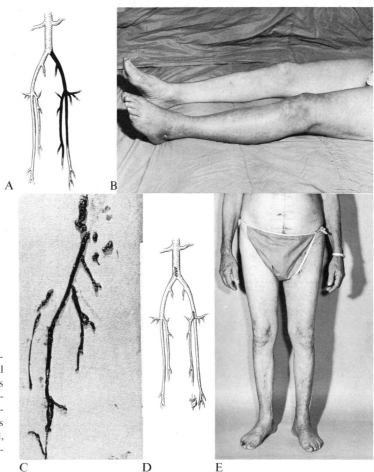

FIGURE 108-1 Iliofemoral thrombectomy for phlegmasia cerulea dolens. *A.* Location and extent of iliofemoral thrombosis. *B.* Patient with left iliofemoral thrombosis demonstrating a swollen, cyanotic leg. *C.* Thrombi removed at operation. *D.* Completed operation with inferior vena cava and left common femoral venotomies repaired. *E.* Patient prior to discharge from the hospital, demonstrating normal appearance of the left leg following iliofemoral thrombectomy.

A   B   C   D   E

direct surgical removal of the venous thrombus through single or multiple venotomies, particularly in the acutely ill patient with phlegmasia cerulea dolens. With increasing experience these techniques have been applied successfully to patients with lesser degrees of deep venous thrombosis in an effort to prevent development of chronic venous insufficiency.[9]

Operative techniques employed are not unlike those used for embolectomy in the arterial system. Venography often is helpful in determining the location and extent of venous thrombosis, thereby aiding in planning the surgical approach. The common femoral vein first is exposed through the incision in the groin, and in many instances complete extirpation of the thrombus is possible through this incision alone. When involvement is more extensive, as in patients with phlegmasia cerulea dolens secondary to iliofemoral thrombosis, an abdominal incision also may be necessary in order to expose the inferior vena cava and allow complete removal of the thrombus while preventing possible pulmonary embolization (Fig. 108-1). However, recently developed techniques employing Fogarty catheters inserted through both groins under local anesthesia now allow prevention of pulmonary embolism without the necessity of directly exposing the inferior vena cava during ilio-

femoral thrombectomy (Fig. 108-2).[7] During such procedures heparinization has been helpful in preventing recurrence of thrombosis, and many investigators advise continued anticoagulation for a period of days to weeks. Results of these procedures have been encouraging, and with the passage of time operative intervention probably will be employed in an increasing number of patients with deep venous thrombosis.

PULMONARY EMBOLISM

Even less clearly understood than other diseases of the venous system, and often with far more devastating results, is pulmonary embolism. Although numerous historical and statistical reviews of venous thromboembolic phenomena have done much to increase recognition of these occurrences, few conditions in medicine have been subjected to so much analysis with so little elucidation. Not only is the cause unknown, the true incidence in doubt, and the diagnosis frequently questionable, but methods of treatment are highly arguable.[5]

Most pulmonary emboli are small, and treatment is aimed toward prevention of further embolic episodes. The patient is put to bed with the legs wrapped

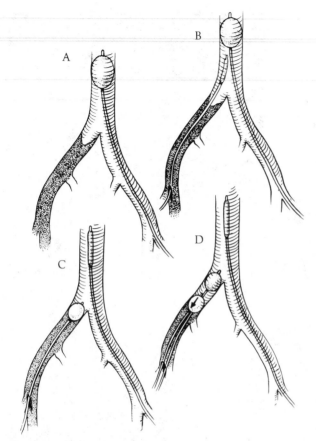

FIGURE 108-2 Technique of iliofemoral thrombectomy employing Fogarty catheters through groin incisions. *A.* Catheter passed into inferior vena cava through saphenous vein on uninvolved side and balloon inflated to prevent pulmonary embolization. *B.* Catheter then passed up involved side, and, *C,* balloon inflated and pulled back into common iliac vein, allowing deflation of inferior vena caval balloon. *D.* Second catheter used for proximal thrombectomy, following which both catheters were removed, distal thrombectomy performed with single catheter, and venotomy repaired.

and elevated, and most physicians place heavy reliance on anticoagulation therapy. Evaluation of the use of fibrinolytic agents, such as urokinase, in patients with pulmonary embolism still is in progress. When these measures are unsuccessful in preventing further pulmonary emboli, some form of venous ligation should be considered, either alone or in conjunction with anticoagulant therapy. Ligation of the superficial femoral veins for prevention of fatal pulmonary embolism has been used extensively; however, most surgeons now believe that ligation at this level is inadequate. Thrombus formation often has extended proximally beyond the femoral vessels, or emboli have originated in the pelvic or prostatic venous plexuses, and higher ligation is required.

When venous interruption is indicated in patients with pulmonary embolism, it should be done at the level of the inferior vena cava.[13] Occurrence of

venous insufficiency following inferior vena cava ligation varies greatly and depends to a great extent on the underlying disease rather than on vena cava ligation per se. In an effort to avoid unfavorable sequelae of inferior vena cava ligation, several ingenious procedures have been devised to prevent fatal pulmonary embolism without permanent interruption of blood flow. These include insertion of a "filter" into the inferior vena cava with small sutures (Fig. 108-3),[6] the use of suture techniques to partition the inferior vena cava into several channels large enough to allow flow of blood but small enough to prevent passage of pulmonary emboli of significant size (Fig. 108-3),[14] and the use of a serrated Teflon clip to accomplish similar partitioning (Fig. 108-3).[12] These modifications of vena cava ligation are relatively new, and additional experience is necessary to evaluate accurately whether they are superior to ligation.

Recently, Mobin-Uddin and his associates have developed an ingenious method of vena cava interruption.[15] It uses an "umbrella" composed of heparinized Silastic bonded to stainless-steel spokes. The umbrella may produce complete occlusion of the inferior vena cava or may be of the sieve type, thereby permitting the filtering of clots without interrupting blood flow. It is folded into a capsule which is attached to a specially designed catheter containing an obturator. The capsule is inserted into the right internal jugular vein and guided under fluoroscopic visualization to a point in the inferior vena cava which is below the renal veins. The umbrella is ejected from the capsule and opened, the spokes penetrating the walls of the vessel. This device has been used in patients who are too ill for a surgical procedure. It is now being used more extensively in several medical centers, and the indications and complications of this procedure should be apparent in the near future.

In some patients with pulmonary embolism the magnitude of obstruction to pulmonary arterial flow precludes long-term survival. Although death in such a patient occasionally is almost instantaneous, the majority live for varying periods of time following embolization. For these patients Trendelenburg advocated immediate embolectomy, but because of numerous technical difficulties this procedure never became popular. Development of the pump oxygenator for temporary cardiopulmonary bypass and widespread use of this technique provided a logical means of pulmonary embolectomy under more favorable circumstances, and successful surgical treatment of acute massive pulmonary embolism using temporary cardiopulmonary bypass was reported from Baylor University College of Medicine, Houston, Texas, in 1961.[3] Subsequently, the feasibility and advantages of such a technique of pulmonary embolectomy have been demonstrated on numerous occasions.[11]

Though diagnosis of acute massive pulmonary embolism usually can be made on clinical grounds alone, definitive diagnosis by pulmonary angiography is mandatory prior to pulmonary embolectomy (Fig. 108-4*A* and *B*). Under extenuating circumstances, sufficient time may be gained for such a definitive

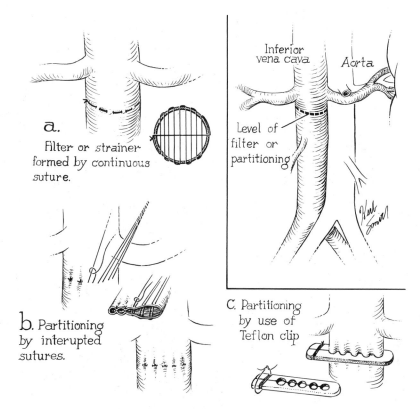

a.
Filter or strainer formed by continuous suture.

b. Partitioning by interupted sutures.

Inferior vena cava   Aorta

Level of filter or partitioning

C. Partitioning by use of Teflon clip

FIGURE 108-3 Operative procedures designed to prevent passage of pulmonary emboli of significant size through inferior vena cava without complete interruption of blood flow.

diagnostic study by institution of partial cardiopulmonary bypass, cannulating the femoral vein and artery under local anesthesia (Fig. 108-5A). This technique of partial cardiopulmonary bypass also is applicable for resuscitation, while preparations are made for pulmonary embolectomy.

The technique of pulmonary embolectomy employing cardiopulmonary bypass is not complicated

and is facilitated by immediate availability of cardiopulmonary bypass using disposable plastic oxygenators primed with 5% dextrose in distilled water. General endotracheal anesthesia with only minimal amounts of depressant drugs should be used. A median sternotomy incision provides excellent exposure of the main pulmonary artery. If partial cardiopulmonary bypass previously has been necessary for

FIGURE 108-4 Patient with acute massive pulmonary embolism. A. Pulmonary arteriogram prior to operation, showing the right side of the heart distended, almost no opacification of pulmonary arterial tree, and minimal amounts of contrast material passing through the lesser circulation into the aorta. B. Numerous thrombi removed at operation.

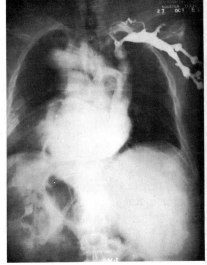

A

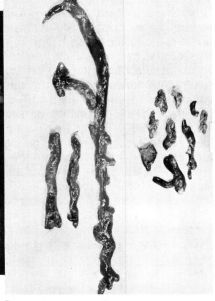

B

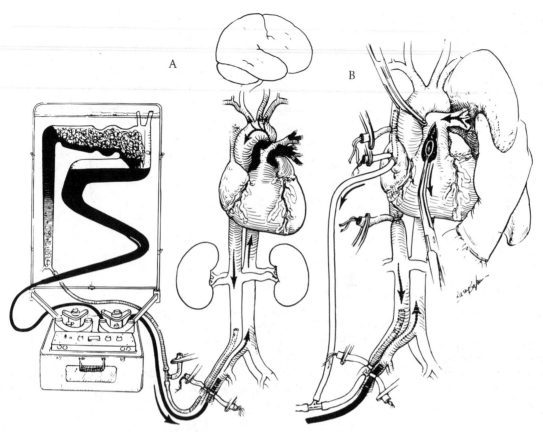

FIGURE 108-5 Technique of pulmonary embolectomy using cardiopulmonary bypass. *A.* Partial cardiopulmonary bypass cannulating femoral artery and vein under local anesthesia for resuscitation. *B.* Partial converted to total cardiopulmonary bypass for definitive embolectomy.

resuscitation, this is converted to total bypass by cannulation of the superior vena cava (Fig. 108-5*B*). Otherwise, standard cannulation for total cardiopulmonary bypass is employed. A longitudinal arteriotomy is made in the anterior wall of the main pulmonary artery, extending almost to its bifurcation, and accessible embolic material is extracted. Both pleural spaces then are entered, and the lungs are vigorously compressed toward the hilus until only liquid blood is obtained. During this maneuver, suction and curved sponge forceps are used to extract emboli once they have been dislodged from the peripheral postions of the pulmonary arterial tree into the main pulmonary arteries. On completion of embolectomy, the pulmonary arteriotomy is repaired, and cardiopulmonary bypass is discontinued once the patient's own cardiorespiratory system is able to maintain satisfactory function.[1]

Increasing experience with pulmonary embolectomy using cardiopulmonary bypass has demonstrated clearly that many lives which would otherwise be lost may be salvaged by an aggressive surgical approach. Pulmonary embolectomy by this technique should be considered in the management of every patient with pulmonary embolism in order that it may be available for those who will require such a procedure for survival and in order that the indications for pulmonary embolectomy may be defined further. Additional improvements in the technical aspect of pulmonary embolectomy are foreseeable, and extensions of the procedure into other areas of pulmonary embolism should be forthcoming.[11]

REFERENCES

1 Beall, A. C., Jr., Fred, H. L., and Cooley, D. A.: Pulmonary Embolism, *Curr. Probl. Surg.,* 1:1, 1964.

2 Chiu, C. J., Terzis, J., and MacRae, M. L.: Replacement of Superior Vena Cava with the Spiral Composite Vein Graft, *Ann. Thorac. Surg.,* 17:555, 1974.

3 Cooley, D. A., Beall, A. C., Jr., and Alexander, J. K.: Acute Massive Pulmonary Embolism: Successful Surgical Treatment Using Temporary Cardiopulmonary Bypass, *J.A.M.A.,* 177: 283, 1961.

4 Cole, W. H., and Zollinger, R. M.: "Textbook of Surgery," 9th ed., Appleton Century Crofts, New York, 1970.

5 DeBakey, M. E.: A Critical Evaluation of the Problem of Thromboembolism, *Surg. Gynecol. Obstet.,* 98:1, 1954.

6 DeWeese, M. S., and Hunter, D. C., Jr.: A Vena Cava Filter for the Prevention of Pulmonary Embolism: A Five-Year Clinical Experience, *Arch. Surg.,* 86:852, 1963.

7 Fogarty, T. J., Cranley, J. J., Krause, R. J., Strasser, E. S., and Hafner, C. D.: Surgical Management of Phlegmasia Cerulea Dolens, *Arch. Surg.,* 86:256, 1963.

8 Fujiwara, Y., Cohn, L. H., Adams, D., and Collins, J. J.: Use of Cortex Grafts for Replacement of the Superior and Inferior Venae Cavae, *J. Thorac. Cardiovasc. Surg.*, 67:774, 1974.

9 Haller, J. A., Jr.: Thrombectomy for Deep Thrombophlebitis of the Leg, *N. Engl. J. Med.*, 267:65, 1962.

10 Kistner, R. L.: Surgical Repair of the Incompetent Femoral Vein Valve, *Arch. Surg.*, 110:1336, 1975.

11 Mattox, K. L., and Beall, A. C., Jr.: Resuscitation of the Moribund Patient Utilizing Portable Cardiopulmonary Bypass, *Ann. Thorac. Surg.*, 22:436, 1976.

12 Miles, R. M., Chappel, F., and Renner, O.: A Partially Occluding Vena Cava Clip for Prevention of Pulmonary Embolism, *Am. Surg.*, 30:40, 1964.

13 Ochsner, A.: Indications for and Results of Inferior Vena Caval Ligation for Thromboembolic Disease, *Postgrad. Med.*, 27:193, 1960.

14 Spencer, F. C., Quattlebaum, J. K., Jr., Sharp, E. H., and Jude, J. R.: Plication of the Inferior Vena Cava for Pulmonary Embolism: A Report of 20 Cases, *Ann. Surg.*, 155:827, 1962.

15 Mobin-Uddin, K., McLean, R., Bolooki, H., and Jude, J. R.: Caval Interruption for Prevention of Pulmonary Embolism, *Arch. Surg.*, 99:711, 1969.

PART XII

Pharmacology of Drugs Used in the Treatment of Cardiovascular Disease

109
Pharmocology of Cardiovascular Drugs

A
Introduction

YEN-YAU HSIEH, M.D.,
MORTON F. ARNSDORF, M.D., and
LEON I. GOLDBERG, M.D., Ph.D.

The indications and directions for the use of many cardiovascular drugs have been described in many chapters of this book. This chapter is designed to supplement the previous presentations and is concerned primarily with a few of the more important agents. The actions of drugs that act primarily on the heart and circulation are emphasized. Diuretics are discussed in Chap. 45.

CLINICAL PHARMACOKINETICS

The term *pharmacokinetics* denotes the absorption, distribution, metabolism, and excretion of drugs.[1] After administration of a drug orally, intramuscularly, intravenously, or through other routes, the percentage of the administered dose entering the systemic circulation in an unchanged form is known as its *bioavailability*.[2] Once entering the systemic circulation, the action and fate of a drug are affected by the extent of serum or plasma protein binding, and the route and rate of biotransformation and elimination. Only the unbound, or free, drug diffuses through capillary walls, reaches receptors and other sites of drug action, and is subject to elimination from the body. The unbound fraction is in equilibrium with the protein-bound fraction in the plasma as well as with the fraction bound to the tissues.[3-5]

A two-compartment open model is frequently used to describe human pharmacokinetics of drugs. In this simplified scheme, the central compartment consists of the intravascular space, together with the highly perfused organs such as heart, lungs, liver, kidneys, and endocrine glands. The peripheral compartment includes less perfused tissues, such as muscle, skin, and body fat, into which drugs enter more slowly.[4,5]

The total apparent volume of distribution (Vd) of a drug is an expression of its distribution through body fluid compartments and its uptake by tissues. It is calculated by the equation $Vd = D/C_0$, where D is the intravenous dose and C_0 the extrapolated plasma drug concentration at time zero. Wide distribution and extensive tissue uptake result in an apparent volume of distribution much larger than the actual volume of the body.[4,5] Vasoconstriction, as might occur in shock, is an example of a condition which would reduce the apparent volume of distribution.

The transfer of a drug between two compartments most commonly follows first-order kinetics; that is, a constant fraction of the pool is transferred per unit of time. When the transfer requires an enzyme system with a limited capacity, first-order kinetics are involved only when the drug load is less than the maximal capacity of the enzyme system. With saturation of the capacity by a large dose, transfer involves zero-order kinetics; that is, a fixed amount of drug independent of the concentration in the compartment is transferred per unit of time.[4,5]

The elimination of a drug is determined by plasma protein binding, volume of distribution, function(s) of the organ(s) responsible for biotransformation and/or excretion (or secretion), and in some cases also by the size of doses (zero-order kinetics),[5] blood flow (drugs with rapid clearance),[6] urine pH,[5] and concurrent drug therapy.[7] The plasma half-time (or half-life), $T^{1/2}$, is defined as the time interval required for the plasma drug concentration to decrease by one-half.

The time course of the plasma concentration of a drug fitting the two-compartment open model and following first-order kinetics is biexponential. The initial rapid fall in the plasma concentration is due to distribution, with a distribution phase half-time designated as $T^{1/2}\alpha$. The elimination phase half-time, $T^{1/2}\beta$, is the commonly described half-time of a drug[4,5] and, unless specified, it will be the $T^{1/2}$ used in Chaps. 109B to D. Detailed explanations and mathematical interpretations of pharmacokinetic principles are given in several references.[4,5] It is important that the reader understand the following concepts: (1) The $T^{1/2}$ of a drug with zero-order kinetics becomes longer with increase in dose, while the $T^{1/2}$ of a drug with first-order kinetics is independent of dose; (2) during constant-rate intravenous infusion or multiple-dose administration with dosage intervals equal to or shorter than the plasma $T^{1/2}$, the steady-state serum or plasma concentration is approximately 97 percent, achieved after five cycles of $T^{1/2}$.[4,5]

REFERENCES

1 Notari, R. E.: "Biopharmaceutics and Pharmacokinetics. An Introduction," Marcel Dekker, Inc., New York, 1975.

2 Koch-Weser, J.: Bioavailability of Drugs, *N. Engl. J. Med.,* 291:233,503, 1974.

3 Koch-Weser, J., and Sellers, E. M.: Binding of Drugs to Serum Albumin, *N. Engl. J. Med.,* 294:311,526, 1976.

4 Greenblatt, D. J., and Koch-Weser, J.: Clinical Pharmacokinetics, *N. Engl. J. Med.,* 293:702,964, 1975.

5 Rowland, M.: Drug Administration and Regimens, in K. L. Melmon and H. F. Morrelli (eds.), "Clinical Pharmacology: Basic Principles in Therapeutics," The Macmillan Company, New York, 1972, p. 21.

6 Nies, A. S., Shand, D. G., and Branch, R. A.: Hemodynamic Drug Interactions, *Cardiovasc. Clin.*, 62:43, 1974.

7 Koch-Weser, J.: Drug Interactions in Cardiovascular Therapy, *Am. Heart J.*, 90:93, 1975.

B
Antiarrhythmic Agents

MORTON F. ARNSDORF, M.D.,
AND YEN-YAU HSIEH, M.D.

Cardiac arrhythmias remain a major public health threat in the United States, and the use of antiarrhythmic agents is a strict challenge to the practicing physician. Despite the rapidly increasing electrophysiologic literature in the last 20 years regarding arrhythmogenesis and the mechanisms of antiarrhythmic drug action, the relevance of this work for the clinician has been somewhat limited. We feel that an electrophysiologically sound and clinically useful classification of antiarrhythmic agents is needed that fulfills the following requirements: (1) It should be based on drug-induced alterations in basic membrane properties (i.e., ionic currents and membrane conductances); (2) it should correlate with clinical realities; and (3) it should serve as a rational guide to

therapy including initial indications, bioelectrical complications, and combination therapy.

We are employing a modification of the classification suggested by Arnsdorf[1] which is summarized in Table 109B-1. The suggested antiarrhythmic mechanisms are based on present and admittedly incomplete knowledge. Since its initial appearance, the classification has required revision and certainly will continue to do so. Nevertheless, we feel this classification most nearly fulfills the above requirements, and we have found it to serve as a useful conceptual framework for the clinician.

BASIC ELECTROPHYSIOLOGY RELEVANT TO THE PHARMACOLOGY OF CARDIOVASCULAR DRUGS

The passive and active properties of the cardiac membrane have been recently reviewed.[2-7] A certain background, however, is required for the clinician to deal with the pharmacology of cardiovascular drugs. The following is a brief review with emphasis on certain approximations. The intracellular potassium concentration $[K^+]_i$ exceeds the extracellular, $[K^+]_o$,

TABLE 109B-1
Electrophysiologic classification of antiarrhythmic drugs based on alterations in membrane ionic conductances

Electrophysiologic group	Representative drugs	Postulated antiarrhythmic mechanisms
I	Procainamide Quinidine ? Disopyramide phosphate	Act primarily by decreasing g_m,* particularly g_{Na}. May decrease I_{si}. Indirect effects on autonomic nervous system.
II	Lidocaine Phenytoin (DPH)	Mechanism 1: Lidocaine increases g_K in Purkinje and ventricular, but not atrial, tissue. Evidence that DPH increases g_K is inferential. Mechanism 2: Both may decrease g_{Na}, particularly in depolarized tissue and in the presence of elevated $[K^+]_o$, and may influence g_{Na} reactivation kinetics. Effect on g_{Na} is dose-related. DPH has effects on central nervous system.
III	Propranolol Tolamolol (UK 6558-01) Alprenolol	Primary mechanism is β-adrenergic receptor blockade. Group I and perhaps II (mechanism 1) direct membrane effects are potentially important. May suppress I_{si}-dependent membrane activity.
IV	Bretylium tosylate	Act primarily by antiadrenergic action. Little significant direct membrane effect.
V	Verapamil	Directly affects channel carrying I_{si}. Effective against the slow response. Suppresses automaticity in fast cardiac fiber through unknown mechanism.
VI	Cardiac glycosides	In "therapeutic" concentrations, the effects are primarily autonomically mediated with direct membrane action probably minor. In "toxic" concentrations, may induce or enhance I_{ti} (see Chap. 109C).

*g_m, membrane conductance; g_{Na}, membrane sodium conductance; g_K, membrane potassium conductance; I_{si}, the slow inward current; I_{ti}, the transient inward current. See electrophysiologic discussions in text of this chapter and chap. 109C for details.
SOURCE: Modified from the classification of Arnsdorf.[1]

the reverse holding for $[Na^+]$ and $[Ca^{2+}]$. These concentration differences (or more properly activities) across a selectively permeable membrane produce an electropotential difference. The downhill chemical gradients cause K^+ to leak outward and both Na^+ and Ca^{2+} inward. Energy-requiring uphill ionic pumps maintain the normal ionic distribution. The membrane is selectively permeable to different ionic species which pass through "channels" or "pores" controlled by "gates" that open and close in response to the transmembrane voltage (V_m) and/or time. It follows then, that the flow of a given ionic species depends both on a driving force which is the electrochemical gradient (i.e., $V_m - E_i$ is the equilibrium potential for a given ionic species) and the ease with which the ions flow through the membrane channels (the membrane conductance, g_m, which is the reciprocal of the membrane resistance). Although nine separate ionic currents have been described, we will consider only K^+, Na^+, and two others. One current, carried primarily by Ca^{2+}, has been termed the slow inward current (I_{si}). The second has been termed the transient inward current, I_{ti}, and the ionic species is uncertain but probably includes both Na^+ and Ca^{2+} through a channel different from that of I_{si}.

Given this background, three approximations can be made that are useful conceptually:

Approximation 1: The net ionic current is determined by a balance between these several currents and their determinants. The contribution of the various ionic currents can be represented by the biologic statement of Ohm's law with the realization that this is a linear statement of essentially nonlinear situations. The nonlinearities can be included in the conductance term:

$$I_i = g_K(V_m - E_K) + g_{Na}(V_m - E_{Na})$$
$$+ g_{si}(V_m - E_{si})g_{ti}(V_m - E_{ti}) + g_x(V_m - E_x)$$

where the abbreviations are as previously noted and x represents other ionic species that are not specifically defined.

Approximation 2: I_i is determined not only by the equation given in approximation 1 but by other passive resistance-capacitance (RC) properties of the membrane not included in the conductance terms.[2,7]

Approximation 3: Inward positive currents (primarily I_{Na}, I_{si}, and I_{ti}) *depolarize* the membrane (i.e., make V_m less negative); outward positive currents (several potassium currents) *repolarize* the membrane. These currents are modified by factors considered in approximations 1 and 2.

Cardiac tissue with I_{Na}-dependent depolarization ("fast" cardiac fibers)

Figure 109B-1 depicts the action potential of a so-called fast cardiac fiber. At the resting transmembrane voltage (V_r), membrane g_K predominates, and as a result V_r approximates E_K at about −95 mV. If the cell spontaneously depolarizes or is depolarized

by a current, g_m in the subthreshold potential range is determined primarily by the voltage-dependent component of K^+ conductance (g_{K1}). As the membrane is further depolarized to about −60 mV, the threshold voltage for regenerative depolarization (V_{th}) is approached. Should a critical amount of membrane be raised above threshold providing local circuit current sufficient to overcome the repolarizing effects of adjacent tissue (the so-called liminal length[8]), a marked increase in g_{Na} occurs that far outweighs the influence of other membrane conductances. Sodium ions rush through open channels into the cell, resulting in the rapid depolarization phase of the action potential (phase 0) with the spike of the action potential approaching E_{Na} at about +40 mV. Phase 0 is completed in a few milliseconds. Adjacent tissue is raised above threshold, and a regenerative response develops.

Attempts have been made to measure I_{Na} directly in heart muscle, but the initial capacitative current and the difficulty in maintaining voltage control of membrane by voltage clamping have interfered with these efforts.[2,9] As a result, strength-duration curves[10,11] and the maximal rate of rise of phase 0 of the action potential ($\dot{V}_{max}$) have been used[12] as indirect measures of g_{Na}. Membrane sodium conductance (g_{Na}) is modified by fast voltage-dependent activation (m) and slower inactivation (h) variables. Conceptually, these can be considered "on" and "off" gates within the Na^+ membrane channel. The extent to which these on and off gates are opened or closed determines the availability of the sodium system. Estimates of the voltage-dependent magnitude of h can be made by plotting $\dot{V}_{max}$ versus V_m either using voltage or current clamp presteps or as part of "membrane responsiveness" studies. Experimentally, membrane responsiveness is defined by the curve relating $\dot{V}_{max}$ to the V_m at which the membrane is activated during and subsequent to phase 3 repolarization. This leads to our next three approximations:

Approximation 4: At a steady low V_m (i.e., less negative than the normal V_r for the fast fiber), g_{Na} is decreased for several reasons including imcomplete activation of the m variable (the on gate is not fully open), a reduced value of h (the off gate is partially closed), a decreased driving force ($V_m - E_{Na}$ is less than normal), and alterations in other factors such as cable properties and liminal length. V_r can be made less negative by a variety of interventions including drugs, injury, hyperkalemia, and the like.

Approximation 5: Inactivation of the sodium system generally leads to a *decreased* conduction velocity, although the determinants of conduction velocity are complex.[2-7,13,14] The conduction velocity in the fast cardiac fiber normally is 0.5 to 4.0 m/s.

Approximation 6: Restoration of V_m toward normal usually reverses g_{Na} inactivation and increases conduction velocity.

Repolarization is also regenerative. Phase 1 repolarization depends both on g_{Na} inactivation, and in Purkinje fibers on the activation of an inward negative current which has been termed the *positive*

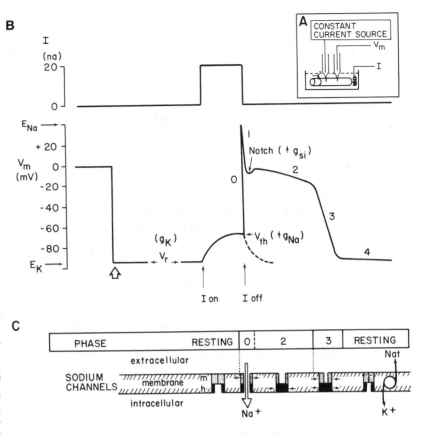

FIGURE 109B-1 A. Two microelectrodes are impaled in a strand of cardiac Purkinje fiber: one for measuring the intracellular voltage, the other for injecting current intracellularly. The external electrode in the tissue bath serves as the zero reference against which the intracellular voltage is measured, permitting assessment of the transmembrane voltage (V_m). The bath is kept at virtual ground using an operational amplifier which also produces a voltage signal proportional to the current collected by the bath ground. *B.* The resultant current (I) and V_m changes are depicted diagrammatically. Before the microelectrode is inserted into the cell, V_m is zero. With impalement of the Purkinje strand (white arrow), V_m suddenly becomes -95 mV which is the resting transmembrane voltage (V_r). Since membrane conductance in the quiescent fiber is determined primarily by potassium conductance (g_K), V_r in the normal fiber at physiologic extracellular potassium concentrations approximates the potassium equilibrium potential (E_K). Depolarizing current is injected intracellularly (I_{on}), and V_m is shifted from V_r toward threshold (V_{th}). If V_{th} is attained and the liminal length requirements are met, an action potential is elicited, and the spike of the action potential approaches the sodium equilibrium potential (E_{Na}). If not, V_m decays exponentially after current offset (I_{off}) as indicated by the interrupted line. The various phases of the action potential are indicated (0,1,2,3,4), as are the relevant membrane conductances (g_K, g_{Na}, g_{si}), the significance of which is discussed in the text. *C.* The positions of the "on" (*m*, activation variable) and "off" (*h*, inactivation variable) gates in the sodium channel at different phases in the cardiac cycle are diagrammatically shown. In general, at a low V_m (i.e., less negative than the normal V_r), the on gate is not fully open, the off gate is partially or completely closed,

and the driving force of Na^+ is decreased (i.e., $V_m - E_{Na}$ is less than at V_r) resulting in varying degrees of sodium system "inactivation" and usually a decreased conduction velocity. The horizontal arrows next to the gates show the direction of gate movement in time. During phase 3 repolarization, the off gate begins to open but does not open fully until, in most cases, after the termination of the action potential. See text for a detailed discussion.

dynamic current and attributed to Cl^-. Following phase 1, a second inward current turns on that is carried primarily by Ca^{2+} and to a lesser extent by Na^+ through a channel distinct from that used by the rapid transient inward I_{Na}. Because its kinetics are slow compared with that of the rapid sodium system, this has been termed the *slow inward current* (I_{si}). I_{si} helps maintain the plateau (phase 2), and its inactivation, as well as the activation of other repolarizing outward K^+ currents, causes the membrane to return to its resting level (phase 3). Reactivation of the sodium system occurs progressively during phase 3.

Automaticity in these fibers results from a changing balance between the inward depolarizing and outward repolarizing positive currents. The relationship is complex, but the following is a useful approximation:

Approximation 7: The background inward depolarizing current is carried primarily by Na^+ and to a smaller extent by Ca^{2+}, the contribution of the latter presumably in-

creasing as V_m becomes less negative. The opposing outward currents are the voltage-dependent I_{K1}, which decreases as V_m becomes less negative, and I_{K2}, which decreases with time after repolarization. The time-dependent decrease in I_{K2} initiates the alterations in the other currents. Together these changes result in a progressively increasing net depolarizing inward current and phase 4 depolarization. The rate of the spontaneous pacemaker depends on the various determinants of the maximum diastolic transmembrane voltage, the slope of phase 4, and the threshold for regenerative depolarization. If diastolic depolarization is rapid, phase 0 will be I_{Na}-dependent; if diastolic depolarization is slow, the sodium system may be partially or completely inactivated, and phase 0 may become I_{si}-dependent.

Fibers that normally have such electrophysiologic properties include working and specialized atrial tissues, the Purkinje fibers of the specialized infranodal conduction system, and ventricular muscle. The rapid depolarization of atrial and ventricular tissues is represented by the P and the QRS waves, respectively, of the ECG (electrocardiogram), with the T wave reflecting repolarization of the ventricular mass. The action potential duration of the ventricular mass is reflected in the Q-T interval. U waves may represent repolarization of the smaller Purkinje mass.

Cardiac tissue with I_{si}-dependent depolarization ("slow" cardiac fibers)

Recently, the role of the so-called slow cardiac fiber and the slow response in cardiac electrophysiology has been receiving increasing attention.[4,15-17] Depolarization in these fibers is dependent on I_{si} rather than I_{Na}. I_{si} is carried largely by Ca^{2+} and to a lesser extent by Na^+ through a channel distinct from that of rapid I_{Na} in terms of voltage dependence and time dependence and response to alterations in ionic milieu and in terms of response to chemical blocking agents, catecholamines, and drugs.[4] These slow cardiac fibers are characterized by the following:

Approximation 8: They usually have a lower V_r (about -60 mV), a slower $\dot{V}_{max}$, and a very slow conduction velocity of 0.01 to 0.1 m/s. Reactivation is also slow and is not complete until long after a return to V_r. Slow fibers demonstrate automatic and repetitive activity presumably reflecting a balance between I_{si} and outward K^+ currents.

Fibers of this type are found normally in the sinoatrial (SA) and atrioventricular (AV) nodes. Injury or disease can depolarize a fast cardiac fiber, and, for the reasons discussed above, inactivate the sodium system (approximation 4). Under these conditions the fiber may be converted into an I_{si}-dependent slow-response fiber.

Cardiac tissue with I_{ti}-influenced depolarization

I_{ti} is an inward positive depolarizing current that differs from I_{si} in terms of its voltage dependence.[18,19] It is normally quite small but can be enhanced significantly by digitalis. This current is considered in detail under "Cardiac Glycosides" in Chap. 109C.

THEORIES OF ARRHYTHMOGENESIS

Theories of arrhythmogenesis have been recently reviewed in terms of automaticity, impulse propagation, and excitability.[13,20-24] The inferential links between basic membrane observations and the clinical situation remain problematic, but this type of classification is conceptually useful.[20]

Normal automaticity has already been discussed (approximations 7 and 8). One or several of the components determining the maximum diastolic transmembrane voltage, the slope of phase 4, and the liminal length (including V_{th}) can be altered by ions, autonomic mediators, ischemia, hypoxia, drugs, and the like. As mentioned, I_{Na}-dependent fibers can be converted to I_{si}-dependent fibers.[4] Unusual oscillatory, sustained nondriven rhythmic, and triggered sustained rhythmic activity which may well be I_{si}-dependent have been described in isolated cardiac tissues of both the experimental animal and the human being.[4,11,25-27] Recently, digitalis has been found to enhance an inward current (I_{ti}) that is carried through a channel distinct from I_{si}.[18,19] As discussed in the section on the cardiac glycosides, I_{ti} may underlie the arrhythmogenic effects of cardiac glycosides.

Alterations of impulse propagation may lead to unidirectional block and reentry (Figure 109B-2). Although the term *reentry* has been criticized recently,[4] it will be retained in this discussion since it is both a familiar and a useful concept. Experimentally and clinically, reentry may result in a single premature depolarization or in reentrant rhythms both in supraventricular and ventricular tissues.[28-36] Inactivation of I_{Na}- or I_{si}-dependent depolarization can sufficiently decrease conduction velocity so as to permit the previously excited tissue in the reentrant circuit time to recover its excitability. Varying degrees of cellular electrotonic uncoupling may also affect the conduction velocity. Although the heart has innumerable potential reentrant loops, the normally rapid conduction velocity and the hierarchy of refractory periods are protective.[4,22-25,35]

To these mechanisms might be added the concept of altered cardiac "excitability" which does not fall conveniently into either of the other categories.[2,10,11] Although the term cardiac "excitability" has a certain intuitive meaning (i.e., the ease with which cardiac cells can be made to depolarize regeneratively in a normal or abnormal manner), quantitative electrophysiologic definition of the term has remained a strict challenge. Electrophysiologic studies using microelectrode techniques recently have defined several of the component passive and active membrane events relevant to cardiac excitability,[8,10,11] but the basic membrane alterations underlying certain widely used and frequently cited measures of cardiac excitability, in particular the "multiple response" or "fibrillation" threshold, remain poorly understood.[20,36a,b] Quite possibly, some of the unusual I_{si}-dependent membrane activity, particularly triggered sustained rhythmic activity,[4,17,25,26] should be considered altered excitability as well as abnormal automaticity. Such sustained membrane activity may underlie the repetitive depolarizations induced by electrical stimuli in animals and human beings.[6,13] The possible relationship between such repetitive membrane activity and the "vulnerable" period of the T wave, the so-called malignant PVC (premature ventricular contraction) that falls on the T wave (R on T phenomenon), and the resistance of the resultant ventricular arrhythmias to the usual antiarrhythmic drugs is intriguing.[37,37a,38]

A. NORMAL

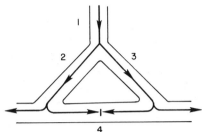

B. UNIDIRECTIONAL BLOCK WITH REENTRY

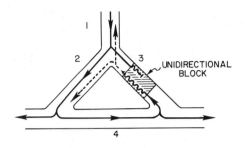

C. PRODUCTION OF BIDIRECTIONAL BLOCK

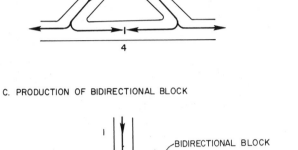

BIDIRECTIONAL BLOCK

I PA QUINIDINE
II LIDO, DPH (Mechanism 2)
III PROPRANOLOL
V VERAPAMIL (Slow Response)
VI DIGITALIS (SAN, Atrium, AVN)

D. ABOLITION OF UNIDIRECTIONAL BLOCK

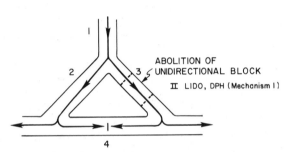

ABOLITION OF
UNIDIRECTIONAL BLOCK

II LIDO, DPH (Mechanism 1)

FIGURE 109B-2 Postulated effects of antiarrhythmic agents on reentry. *A.* Normally an impulse travels from the central Purkinje (1) down the two branches (2 and 3) and activates the ventricular tissue (4). *B.* As a result of ischemia or other injury, a segment with unidirectional block and slow retrograde conduction is established in one limb of the Purkinje branches (3). The impulse descending from the central Purkinje branch is blocked proximally by the area of unidirectional block, but traverses the other limb (2) normally and enters the ventricular tissue resulting in a normal QRS complex on the surface ECG. From the ventricular tissue, it may penetrate the depressed limb distally and conduct in a retrograde fashion to the bifurcation. As indicated by the interrupted lines, if the bifurcation and limb 2 have recovered their excitability, the impulse may reenter this pathway, once more reaching the ventricular tissue, this time resulting in a premature ventricular depolarization. It may even travel in a retrograde manner up the central Purkinje branch. The success or failure of reentry, then, depends on the length of the functionally isolated depressed segment, the conduction velocity both within the depressed segment and in the "normal" tissue that is to be reactivated, the refractoriness or reactivation kinetics of previously excited tissue in the circuit, and other passive and active membrane properties of the depressed and "normal" tissue. Conceivably, not only a reentrant beat but also a reentrant rhythm can be established by such circus movement. The circuit may be anatomic or functional, involving supraventricular, junctional, and/or ventricular tissue. The segment with unidirectional block may be a normally I_{si}-dependent tissue such as is found in the SA and AV nodes or may be diseased tissue. *C.* The reentrant loop is abolished by the conversion of unidirectional to bidirectional block. Groups I and V (slow response) act in this manner as may group II through mechanism 2 (i.e., depression of g_{Na}; see text) and group III. Group VI, the cardiac glycosides, may act in this manner, particularly when the SA node, atrium, and/or the AV node are part of the reentrant loop. Alterations in refractoriness at the bifurcation or elsewhere in the circuit may prevent reexcitation, and this may be important, particularly in group I antiarrhythmic action. *D.* The conditions for reentry are eliminated by the abolition of the area of unidirectional block. The group II drugs may accomplish this by increasing g_K, repolarizing the membrane, and improving conduction velocity (mechanism 1: see text for details).

GROUP I ANTIARRHYTHMIC AGENTS

Electrophysiologic effects

Group I includes quinidine and procainamide. The electrophysiologic effects of quinidine and procainamide have been the subject of recent reviews.[39,40] Group I drugs decrease membrane conductance, particularly g_{Na}, in working and specialized atrial tissue, in Purkinje fibers, and in ventricular muscle as assessed by the indirect measures of $\dot{V}_{max}$, membrane responsiveness, action potential amplitude, and strength-duration curves.[11,41-48] Quinidine makes the g_{Na}-dependent V_{th} less negative[43]; procainamide makes V_{th} less negative and results in more time being required to produce the current, charge, and liminal length depolarization necessary to attain threshold.[11] The group I effect on I_{si} is less clear: Hordof et al. found procainamide to have little effect on I_{si}-dependent action potentials,[49] while Arnsdorf observed triggered sustained rhythmic activity at low V_m to be suppressed by procainamide.[25] The voltage-dependent membrane potassium conductance, g_{K1}, is either little affected[47] or actually decreased by procainamide.[11] Group I drugs delay repolarization, prolonging both the effective refractory period (ERP) and the action potential duration (APD), with the ratio of the change in APD to ERP ($\Delta APD/\Delta ERP$) less than 1, which would shorten the interval during which premature depolarizations with a low membrane activation voltage and a slow conduction velocity (approximations 4 and 5) could be induced.[40]

The decreased conduction velocity produced by the group I drugs is thought to be mediated by depression of normal g_{Na} (approximations 4 and 5), at times perhaps by a conversion of an I_{Na}-dependent to an I_{si}-dependent response (approximation 8), or even by suppressing I_{si}. A drug-induced depression of conduction velocity would tend to convert an area of unidirectional block to one of bidirectional block, thereby interrupting the circuit (Fig. 109B-2C). Giardina and Bigger showed in human beings that the coupling interval of reentrant premature beats increased as a function of procainamide plasma levels.[50] This would be anticipated if the coupling interval were an indirect measure of the reentrant circuit time and if increasing concentrations of the drug produced progressively increasing conduction delay through the depressed segment. Prolongation of the ERP in tissues that need to be reexcited in the reentrant circuit may render them refractory to depolarization.[40] Procainamide may suppress automaticity by decreasing the depolarizing background inward current and by making V_{th} less negative.[11] Presumably, quinidine has a similar action. The effect of group I drugs on cellular electrotonic coupling is uncertain.

In the innervated heart, the sinus rate may increase after quinidine therapy because of reflex sympathetic activity induced by the drug's hypotensive effect. The antiadrenergic and anticholinergic activities of quinidine may further modify the sinus rate.[40,51,52] Procainamide may increase the sinus rate through an anticholinergic effect.[40] The anticholinergic activity of quinidine and procainamide may counteract the direct lengthening effect on the ERP of the AV node. The balance of direct and indirect effects, therefore, may depress AV nodal conduction, enhance it, or leave it unchanged. The ERP of the accessory pathway of the Wolff-Parkinson-White syndrome is prolonged by quinidine and procainamide and, in diseased pathways, ajmaline.[53a,b]

Group I drugs may be arrhythmogenic as well as antiarrhythmic. Procainamide alters both passive RC (resistance-capacitance) and active generator membrane properties, the balance between the two determining whether the tissue will be more or less excitable.[11] Group I drugs may depolarize the resting membrane, enhance automaticity, and perhaps establish situations conducive to reentry by depressing conduction velocity and altering refractoriness.[40] Procainamide may inhibit normal phase 3 regenerative repolarization and stabilize the membrane at the plateau.[25] The normal sodium system is inactivated at this low V_m, conduction velocity is reduced (approximations 4 and 5), and the conditions conducive to unidirectional block with reentry are created. On the other hand, these drugs conceivably could increase conduction velocity by suppressing phase 4 depolarization, permitting membrane activation from a more negative V_m, at which point there is less inactivation of the sodium system (approximation 6).[40,54,55]

An increased $[K^+]_o$ would further inactivate the sodium system and potentiate the g_{Na}-dependent actions of the group I agents. It has been suggested that disopyramide phospate, 17-MCAA (ajmaline), amiodarone, aprindine, and propranolol be considered members of the same group due to their "quinidine-like" effect.[56] For the reasons discussed below, propranolol has been included under a separate category, and too little is known about the electrophysiologic mechanisms of the others to classify them with certainty.

The bioelectric complications of group I would be expected to be those of conduction disturbances and asystole. These drugs produce AV conduction delay in the tissues having I_{Na}-dependent action potentials, particularly the Purkinje fibers of the infranodal specialized conduction system and the ventricular muscle. This would be reflected in prolongation of the His-ventricular (HV) conduction time,[57-59a] in QRS prolongation,[60-61] and in the development of bundle branch block and complete heart block.[60] The QRS duration has been shown to be a function of plasma quinidine levels.[61] QRS widening of 35 to 50 percent mandates discontinuation of the drug. The balance between direct and indirect drug effects on conduction in the atrium, AV node, and infranodal tissue will determine the length of the P-R interval.

Complete heart block may be complicated by the antiautomatic effect of these drugs with suppression of subsidiary pacemakers and resultant asystole. The $Q-T_c$ prolongation caused by group I drugs is expected given the known effects on APD.

The relationship between ST-segment mapping and the direct membrane effects of the group I drugs is uncertain, but these drugs could affect one or several determinants of net systolic or diastolic ionic flow included in the equation in approximation 1.[61a]

Other pharmacologic actions

Quinidine and procainamide depress myocardial contractility.[40,51] As mentioned before, these drugs may reduce I_{si}, which appears to play a role in activation of contraction. Quinidine decreases peripheral vascular resistance by direct vasodilation and by indirect α-adrenergic blockade, and the intravenous injection of procainamide also causes vasodilation.[40,51]

Pharmacokinetics (Table 109B-2)

QUINIDINE

Quinidine is 95 percent absorbed after oral ingestion, and 60 to 80 percent is bound to plasma protein. The peak plasma level following a single oral dose occurs in 1 to 2 h. The chief metabolic fate is hepatic hydroxylation, which results in the loss of antiar-

TABLE 109B-2
Administration, metabolism, and excretion of antiarrhythmic agents (groups I to III)

	Group I		Group II		Group III
	Quinidine	Procainamide	Lidocaine	Phenytoin (DPH)	Propranolol
Route	Oral, I.M.	Oral, I.V., I.M.[b]	I.V., I.M.[i]	Oral, I.V., I.M.[k]	Oral, I.V.
Oral:					
Total/day	1.2–3.2 g	1.0–4.0 g	. . . .	300–1,000 mg	40–320$^+$ mg (oral)
Frequency	q 4–6 h	q 4–6 h	. . . .	Divided	q 4–6 h
GI absorption	90–100%	75–95%	. . . .	57–85%	90% or more
Intravenous:					
Initial	Not advised (hypotension)	100 mg q 5 min to 1 g total^{c-e}	1–2 mg/kg q. 3–5 min. to 200–300 mg total	50–100 mg q 5 min to 1 g total^m	Not over 1.0 mg q 10 min to 5 mg total^p
Maintenance	. . . .	20–80 μg/kg/min ($\simeq$ 1.5–5.0 mg/min)	20–50 μg/kg/min ($\simeq$ 1–4.0 mg/min)	Intermittent by dividing daily dose^n	Intermittent by dividing daily dose
Plasma level:					
Single oral dose, peak	1–2 h	0.5–1.5 h	. . . .	6–12 h	1–4 h
Chronic oral dose, plateau	2–3 days	3 days	. . . .	6–7 days	2–4 days
Effective plasma concentration, μg/ml	2.0–6.0	4.0–8.0	1.5–5.0	10.0–18.0	0.04–0.1
Protein binding	60–80%	15%	60–70%	70 to 95%	90–95%
Metabolism:					
Site	Liver	Liver, plasma	Liver^j	Liver^o	Liver, kidney
Mechanism	Hydroxylation	Major acetylation to NAPA (hepatic) Minor hydrolysis (plasma)	Deethylation Hydrolysis	Hydroxylation	Complex with many steps with numerous metabolites
Renal excretion:					
Unmetabolized	10%	40–70%	<10%	<5%	<5%
Unmetabolized + metabolized	95%	90% NAPA (active)^f	90%	$\simeq$50% (lacks activity of DPH itself)	90% with active metabolites
Elimination:					
Plasma half-time	5–7 h^a	2–3.5 h^{a,h}	8–17 min after initial I.V. ($T\frac{1}{2}_\alpha$) 87–108 min after tissue loading ($T\frac{1}{2}_\beta$)	16–20 h	2.0–3.5 h

^{a}Caution in hepatic disease; prolonged absorption after oral administration may increase the $T\frac{1}{2}_\beta$.
^{b}I.M. erratic.
^{c}I.V. bolus of > 100 mg often leads to hypotension.
^{d}More rapid administration may be used with caution (see text).
^{e}Monitor conduction (ECG) and B.P.
^{f}NAPA 70% potency of potency of procainamide.
^{g}q 4 h p.o. may result in low plasma levels at 5–6 h.
^{h}Caution in CHF (congestive heart failure), hepatic, and renal disease. T½ of NAPA twice that of procainamide.
^{i}200 mg I.M.$\rightarrow$ [2.4 μg/ml]$_{pl}$ at 30 min.
^{j}Caution in CHF, hepatic disease. Phenobarbital, etc., increase metabolism (see text).
^{k}I.M. erratic and not advised.
^{l}High doses p.o. for loading, not maintenance (see text).
^{m}I.V. bolus of > 100 mg often leads to hypotension.
^{n}Diluent pH 11.0$\rightarrow$ pain and phlebitis with continuous I.V.
^{o}Bishydroxycoumarin, etc., decrease metabolism; phenobarbital, etc., increase metabolism (see text).
^{p}Lower doses preferred for I.V. use due to side effects. On occasion up to 10 mg total may be administered (see text). I.V. use requires extreme caution with ECG and B.P. monitoring.
^{q}Active metabolites need to be considered.
NOTE: These recommendations for drug use are general guidelines and may require modification in light of the clinical situation.

rhythmic activity. Elimination may be notably impaired in patients with abnormal hepatic function. The normal plasma half-time ($T^{1/2}$) is between 5 and 7 h.[62–64a] The $T^{1/2}$ may be 11 h or more after oral administration, perhaps reflecting distortion due to prolonged drug absorption.[64a] Only 10 percent appears unchanged in the urine, and if the rather specific double extraction method is used to determine quinidine concentrations, neither quinidine elimination nor the plasma $T^{1/2}$ is significantly altered in patients with renal dysfunction or congestive heart failure.[65] Since only a small fraction of quinidine is excreted unchanged in the urine, the effect of pH on urinary excretion is significant only in the presence of high drug concentrations. Aciduria augments and alkaluria diminishes urinary quinidine excretion.[66] Quinidine effect and toxicity are little affected by changes in plasma protein binding because of its large volume of distribution.[67]

PROCAINAMIDE

Procainamide is 75 to 95 percent absorbed following an oral dose, and only 15 percent is bound to plasma proteins. The plasma level after an oral dose peaks within 1 h in the normal subject, but may be delayed up to 5 h in patients with cardiac disease.[68,69] The plasma concentration peaks within 25 min of an intramuscular injection.[68] Procainamide undergoes major hepatic acetylation and minor plasma hydrolysis with 40 to 67 percent excreted unchanged in the urine. The elimination of procainamide is dependent both on the glomerular filtration rate and active renal tubular secretion.[68–70] The major metabolite of procainamide is N-acetylprocainamide (NAPA), which has an antiarrhythmic potency 70 percent that of the parent compound.[71–73]

Procainamide's plasma $T^{1/2}$ depends on cardiac, renal, and hepatic function, being 2.9 ± 0.5 h normally, 5.5 ± 0.9 h in the cardiac patient,[72] and up to 16 h in the presence of severe renal failure.[74] The percentage appearing unchanged in the urine varies from 40 to 70 percent, which in turn depends on the rate of acetylation and renal excretion. The rate of acetylation to NAPA is genetically determined. It should be remembered that NAPA has a $T^{1/2}$ twice that of procainamide.[71] Whether procainamide is metabolized by a bimodally distributed enzyme system is not yet certain.[74a]

Since a greater portion of procainamide is excreted in the urine in the active form than quinidine and since procainamide is a weak base, it would be expected that elimination might be affected by acid-base disturbances and by changes in the urinary pH. The renal clearance of procainamide, however, is not significantly altered by acid or alkali loading.[70]

Adverse reactions

The most common adverse effects of quinidine are diarrhea, nausea, and vomiting. Idiosyncratic and hypersensitive reactions may follow quinidine ad-

ministration. Tinnitus, hearing impairment, vertigo, visual disturbances, diplopia, photophobia, confusion, skin rashes, headaches, fever, angioedema, abdominal pain, an immune response thrombocytopenia, and granulomatous hepatitis have been reported.[40,75,76] Quinidine intoxication may include cinchonism, hypotension, myocardial depression, failure to respond to artificial pacemaking, syncope, ventricular tachycardia and fibrillation, disturbances of impulse conduction, and asystole[51,77] (see bioelectric complications under "Electrophysiologic Effects" above).

Procainamide also causes gastrointestinal problems. Other adverse effects include a skin rash, fever, flushing, a bitter taste, mental depression, psychosis, giddiness, fever, headache, hallucinations, convulsions, and agranulocytosis.[40,60,75] Seventy-five percent of patients on long-term therapy will develop serologic abnormalities such as positive antinuclear antibodies. A third of these patients will be afflicted with one or more lupus erythematosus-like symptoms of fever, arthralgia, myalgia, skin rash, pleuritic chest pain, pericarditis, and rarely pericardial tamponade or even constrictive pericarditis.[75,78,79] Generally, the kidney is spared, and discontinuation of the drug abolishes the syndrome. Digital vasculitis, Raynaud's phenomenon, and Sjögren's syndrome have been attributed to this drug.[60] Many of the bioelectric complications have been discussed (see "Electrophysiologic Effects" above), but include conduction disturbances, pacemaker suppression and asystole, ventricular tachycardia, ventricular fibrillation, and the failure to respond to artificial pacemaking.[80,81] Heart failure and hypotension may also be induced or enhanced by the negative inotropic effects of procainamide.

Drug interactions

Antacids may delay the absorption of quinidine, but are unlikely to cause incomplete absorption.[67] Phenobarbital and phenytoin, however, may reduce the plasma $T^{1/2}$ of quinidine by 50 percent.[82] Quinidine may potentiate the neuromuscular blocking effect and ventilatory depression of patients receiving tubocurarine, succinylcholine, or decamethonium. The anticoagulant effect of warfarin is augmented by quinidine.[67] Procainamide has no interaction with oral anticoagulants.[67] Concurrent use with acetazolamide may decrease the elimination of procainamide.[83] Increased plasma or serum [K^+] generally will enhance the g_{Na}-dependent electrophysiologic effects of both drugs.[56]

Clinical use

Group I drugs are effective against supraventricular and ventricular arrhythmias, whether caused by enhanced automaticity or reentry[40,50,56,58,60,84] (see Table 109B-3). The clinical indications and the method of treatment have been considered in earlier chapters and elsewhere,[1,37a,40,50,60,84] but a few comments are needed here.

If a group I drug is appropriate in the treatment of supraventricular arrhythmias, additional AV nodal

TABLE 109B-3
Clinical effectiveness of antiarrhythmic agents (groups I to III)

	Group I		Group II		Group III
	Quinidine	Procainamide	Phenytoin	Lidocaine	Propranolol
Supraventricular:					
Premature atrial contractions	1*	1	3	4	3
Paroxysmal atrial tachycardia	2†	2	3	4	2
Atrial flutter	2	2	4	4	2–3‡
Atrial fibrillation:					
Conversion	1†	1	4	4	2–3†
Maintenance	1†	1	4	4	2–3
Junctional premature contractions and tachycardia	2	2	4	4	4
Ventricular:					
Ventricular premature contractions	2	1	1–2	1	2
Tachycardia	3	1	1–2	1	2
Digitalis-induced arrhythmias					
Supraventricular and ventricular	3§	3§	1	1	2§

*Response: 1 = excellent; 2 = good; 3 = fair; 4 = poor.
†The use of digitalis or propranolol to depress conduction through the AV node may be required to control the ventricular response to the atrial tachyarrhythmia.
‡Propranolol effectively decreases the ventricular response to atrial flutter and fibrillation by decreasing conduction through the AV node, but is of little value in the direct conversion of these arrhythmias to a sinus mechanism.
§Although effective in suppressing digitalis-induced arrhythmias, these drugs may themselves produce problems of conduction which combined with their antiautomatic effects may eventuate in AV dissociation and asystole.

blockade with digitalis or propranolol may be required. The reason is that supraventricular arrhythmias such as atrial fibrillation often change to atrial flutter or a rapid atrial tachycardia. Group I drugs may slow the flutter or tachycardia rate and enhance AV nodal conduction, resulting in a potentially catastrophic ventricular response (see Fig. 207 in Katz and Pick, Clinical Electrocardiography: The Arrhythmias[85]). Quinidine, and to a lesser extent procainamide, are favored for maintenance therapy after the reversion of atrial flutter or fibrillation to sinus rhythm.[60,86–89] Given the high recurrence rate of these atrial arrhythmias,[86] maintenance therapy must include consideration that a recurrence may be associated with a rapid ventricular response and that prophylactic inhibition of the AV node with digitalis or propranolol is usually required. AV nodal blockage with digitalis or propranolol in the presence of preexisting AV nodal disease, however, may produce complete AV block, and the risk of the group I drugs in such a situation would be suppression of subsidiary pacemakers and asystole. In the presence of fascicular or bundle branch conduction disturbances, the group I drugs may produce complete infranodal heart block, may suppress lower pacemakers, and may result in asystole. If a group I drug is needed in such a situation, the use of a prophylactic artificial pacemaker may be indicated. It has been said that quinidine may be more effective than procainamide in the treatment of supraventricular arrhythmias, but the drugs are probably equally effective in appropriate doses.[60] Some 10 to 15 percent of patients in atrial fibrillation will revert to normal sinus rhythm on "maintenance" doses of quinidine.[90] The literature disagrees as to whether pretreatment with group I drugs before dc (direct current) electroversion and subsequent drug maintenance is clinically beneficial in maintaining the normal sinus mechanism, and careful patient selection is necessary.[86–90]

Patient selection for the treatment of ventricular arrhythmias is problematic.[37,37a] Intravenously administered procainamide is extremely effective in the emergency treatment of ventricular arrhythmias.[50] Procainamide is generally used after lidocaine has been found ineffective. Quinidine should not be given intravenously due to its profound hypotensive effects. Proper patient selection in the chronic administration of these drugs for the prevention of ventricular arrhythmias is of importance, given the high incidence of side effects and adverse reactions to the group I agents. Many clinicians favor quinidine over procainamide for chronic maintenance since the latter drug has a shorter duration of action and is associated with the lupus erythematosus-like syndrome in a high percentage of patients.[72,75,78,79] The group I drugs may in themselves produce further conduction problems which, combined with their antiautomatic effects, may eventuate in AV dissociation and asystole. The group I agents may be useful against arrhythmias associated with the Wolff-Parkinson-White syndrome.[53a,b]

The therapeutic plasma concentration of quinidine ranges from 2 to 6 μg/ml.[40,51] A 200-mg dose of quinidine sulfate has been suggested by some authors as a test dose for idiosyncratic or hypersensitivity reactions. The usual maintenance dose is 200 to 400 mg every 6 h. Quinidine gluconate, which contains 62 mg anhydrous quinidine per 100 mg as compared to

82 mg anhydrous quinidine per 100 mg for quinidine sulfate, is available as a long-acting preparation.

For the emergency treatment of life-threatening quinidine intoxication, intravenously administered sodium bicarbonate or sodium lactate may be used to decrease the extracellular potassium concentration and to increase plasma protein binding. In the presence of myocardial depression and hypotension, β-adrenergic sympathomimetic amines may be administered to counteract the toxic quinidine effect.[40]

The therapeutic plasma concentration of procainamide ranges from 4 to 8 μg/ml.[40,50,80,84] Procainamide can be administered quite safely according to the method of Giardina and Bigger by giving 100 mg intravenously every 5 min until a therapeutic effect is achieved, an adverse action results, or a total dose of 1,000 mg is attained.[50,84] Up to 50 mg/min to a total of 1 g may be given, although the risk of hypotension is greater with this rate of infusion.[91] The blood pressure and ECG must be monitored with each dose. The maintenance intravenous dose is 20 to 80 μg/kg/min ($\approx$1.5 to 5.0 mg/min). Orally, 1 to 4 g in divided doses (every 4 h) is the usual maintenance range. The interval between the discontinuation of intravenously administered procainamide and the initiation of oral therapy must be properly spaced to avoid toxic effects.[60,68]

The dosage schedules of quinidine may require adjustment in patients with hepatic dysfunction; of procainamide, in those with hepatic or renal dysfunction (see "Pharmacokinetics" above). Both drugs should be used cautiously in patients with severe heart failure due to their negative inotropic actions.

Quinidine and procainamide are contraindicated in patients with a history of idiosyncratic or hypersensitivity reactions to the drugs. For reasons already mentioned, they may be contraindicated in the presence of high-degree infranodal AV block without an artificial pacemaker and are not recommended in the treatment of arrhythmias resulting from digitalis intoxication. Idiopathic or drug-induced (phenothiazines, tricyclic antidepressants, etc.) prolongation of the Q-T interval is a relative contraindication. It has been said that the administration of quinidine in the presence of PVCs with unusually short coupling intervals may increase the risk of the R on T phenomenon.[40]

GROUP II
ANTIARRHYTHMIC AGENTS

Electrophysiologic effects

Lidocaine and phenytoin (diphenylhydantoin, DPH) have been separated from quinidine and procainamide in several classifications for both clinical and electrophysiologic reasons.[1,60,92–94] Recent work suggests lidocaine and DPH may be more dissimilar than originally supposed.[95,96] The electrophysiologic similarities, however, seem to include mechanism 1, the ability to increase membrane potassium conductance (g_K) and/or mechanism 2, the ability, under certain conditions, to decrease sodium conductance (g_{Na}). The net effect of the drug seems to result from a balance between these two factors which, in turn, is influenced by the condition of the membrane, the milieu, and the drug concentration.

MECHANISM 1

Lidocaine has been shown to increase membrane g_K (primarily g_{K1}) as assessed both by electrophysiologic and ^{42}K flux measurements in Purkinje fibers and ventricular muscle.[10,97–99] Lidocaine is presumed to suppress automaticity by enhancing the repolarizing outward current in the subthreshold potential range which would decrease the slope of phase 4 and might make the maximum diastolic transmembrane voltage more negative (approximations 3 and 7). Lidocaine has little effect on conduction velocity in normal Purkinje fibers, but may increase it in tissue injured due to stretch[25,100] or hypoxia (Arnsdorf, unpublished observations). In Purkinje fibers depolarized by injury, lidocaine, by increasing g_K, causes V_r to approach its normal value.[10,25,100] It should be recalled that membrane depolarization inactivates g_{Na}, which, in turn, leads to a decreased conduction velocity (approximations 4 and 5). Repolarization mediated by a lidocaine-induced increase in g_K (approximations 1 and 3) decreases the inactivation of g_{Na}, thereby increasing conduction velocity (approximation 6). An I_{Na}-dependent fast cardiac fiber may be converted into an I_{si}-dependent slow cardiac fiber by injury, and lidocaine might be able to return it to its I_{Na}-dependency by repolarizing the membrane. In fibers showing triggered sustained rhythmic activity at a low V_m that presumably is I_{si}-mediated, lidocaine enhances the regenerative repolarization process by increasing g_K, thereby allowing the membrane to return to a more nearly normal V_r.[25] In these several instances, conduction velocity would increase, favoring the abolition of the area of unidirectional block (Fig. 109B-2D). Lidocaine decreases the ERP and APD to a greater extent in tissues with an initially long rather than a short ERP and APD duration.[95] ΔAPD/ΔERP is less than 1. These actions might eliminate the unidirectional block of early premature impulses. Lidocaine may decrease excitability as manifested by an upward shift in the strength-duration curve, an action mediated by an increase in the subthreshold g_K without affecting the g_{Na}-dependent term V_{th},[10] a mechanism quite distinct from that of procainamide.[11]

The cellular basis of DPH action is rather poorly defined, and its inclusion with lidocaine in group II is tentative. The evidence that DPH increases g_K is inferential, based on changes in V_r and APD.[101–103] In the presence of an increased K+ driving force (i.e., $V_m - E_K$ is significantly greater than zero) such as in hypokalemia or injury, DPH may increase both V_r and $\dot{V}_{max}$, decrease the APD, and presumably increase the conduction velocity in atrial and Purkinje fibers[101,102,104,106] (approximation 6), which, as in the case of lidocaine, would be expected if the drug increased g_K (approximations 1 and 3). DPH decreases both the ERP and APD, the latter being more greatly affected. This might permit premature impulses to conduct with greater facility, favoring abolition of unidirectional block and reentry (Fig. 109B-2D). The slope of phase 4 depolarization may be decreased due to the increase in g_K, the membrane activation voltage in late diastole may be more negative than before, and conduction may be facilitated.

MECHANISM 2

The effect of lidocaine on g_{Na} has been assessed by the determination of $\dot{V}_{max}$, membrane responsiveness, and strength-duration curves. The results differ, with some studies showing lidocaine to have little effect on g_{Na},[100,107,108] while others show lidocaine to depress g_{Na} significantly in atrial[105] and Purkinje[109] tissues. The elegant voltage-clamp studies in Purkinje fiber by Weld and Bigger[110] clarified some of these results, showing that the drug may reduce $\dot{V}_{max}$ at high drug concentrations, in depolarized tissue, and at $[K^+]_0$ above 3.0 mmol. Lidocaine also decreases the reactivation kinetics of the sodium system.[48,110] Recently, evidence has been presented that lidocaine may not hyperpolize and improve conduction in cardiac cells which have a V_r decreased due to ischemia or infarction.[111,112] In any event, a depression in $\dot{V}_{max}$ would tend to abolish the reentrant circuit by establishing bidirectional block within the injured segment (Fig. 109B-2C), and, in a sense, this could be considered a group I action. DPH also depresses the indirect measures of g_{Na} at high concentrations or at $[K^+]_0$ greater than 4 to 5 mmol.[96]

Other electrophysiologic effects

Lidocaine has little effect on autonomic tone.[113] A case of sinus standstill following lidocaine administration has been reported.[114] Lidocaine has no consistent effect on the sinus rate, SA node recovery time, and atrial refractoriness in patients with the "sick sinus" syndrome.[115] In contrast to Purkinje and ventricular tissues, lidocaine does not enhance ^{42}K flux in atrial tissues,[99] which is of interest in view of its relative ineffectiveness against atrial arrhythmias. DPH exerts a depressant action on the sympathetic centers in the central nervous system although the peripheral hypotensive effect may induce sympathetic discharge.[96,113,116] Neither drug dramatically affects AV nodal transmission, although DPH may somewhat facilitate it. The effect of group II drugs on cellular electrotonic coupling is uncertain. The actions of lidocaine in ischemic and hypoxic tissue, however, could be explained in terms of alterations in intercellular conductivity, but the hypothesis remains to be tested experimentally.

In view of the electrophysiologic findings, the relative lack of *bioelectric complications* clinically on the ECG and in His bundle studies from either lidocaine[117,118] or DPH[119–121] is not suprising. The cases of alleged lidocaine-induced complete heart block prior to 1974 have been disputed,[118] but two cases since then have been reported that seem secondary to infranodal block.[122] DPH may actually eliminate functional bundle branch block.[119–121] The relationship between the direct membrane effects of these drugs and ST-segment mapping is uncertain.[61a] Repolarization of tissue depolarized due to injury with resultant "normalization" of the action potential, however, might be expected to decrease areas of electromotive differences, thereby decreasing the magnitude of ST-segment elevations or depressions. Several determinants of systolic and diastolic ionic flow indicated in the equation in approximation 1 could be affected by the group II drugs.[61a]

Both lidocaine and DPH are efficacious against digitalis-induced arrhythmias. Whether lidocaine has effects other than the direct membrane actions is unknown. DPH not only has direct effects but may reverse the digitalis-induced intracellular K^+ loss and Na^+ accumulation by stimulating the Na^+-K^+ pump,[123,124] although this effect has been challenged.[96] Possibly, the effects of DPH on the central nervous system contribute to its antiarrhythmic activity in digitalis toxicity.[96]

Other pharmacologic actions

Lidocaine and DPH have some negative inotropic effects[89,90,125–127] but less than the group I drugs. The diseased heart is more sensitive to the negative inotropic and hypotensive effects of both agents. DPH is insoluble in water, and its solvent consists of 40% propylene glycol and 10% ethyl alcohol with the pH adjusted to 11. The solvent may produce electrophysiologic effects opposite to those of DPH,[101] and intravenous administration causes disturbances of cardiac rhythm, hypotension, and alterations of the ECG.[128]

Pharmacokinetics (Table 109B-2)

LIDOCAINE

After a single intravenous injection, lidocaine is rapidly distributed to well-perfused tissues with a $T^{1/2}\alpha$ of 8 to 17 min. This phase is responsible for the 15- to 20-min duration of the antiarrhythmic effect after a bolus injection. The elimination phase $T^{1/2}$ ranges from 87 to 108 min, a figure that must be remembered after tissue loading takes place.[125,129] Lidocaine is rapidly biotransformed by the hepatic microsomal oxidases to monoethylglycinexylidide and xylidide. The hepatic metabolism is sensitive to hemodynamic alteration and susceptible to enzyme-inducing or enzyme-inhibiting agents. The drug is 70 percent bound to protein. Less than 10 percent is excreted unchanged in the urine.[125,129]

PHENYTOIN (DPH)

In contrast to quinidine, procainamide, and lidocaine, which are weak bases, DPH is a weak acid with a pK_a of 8.3. Absorption after oral ingestion is slow and variable, and may be incomplete with significant differences in bioavailability ranging from 57 to 85 percent depending on the pharmaceutical preparation.[130,131] The plasma protein binding varies from 70 to 95 percent. DPH is mainly hydroxylated by hepatic microsomal enzymes to *p*-hydroxyphenylhydantoin with less than 5 percent excreted unchanged in the urine.[130]

With a daily dose of 10 mg/kg or at a plasma concentration below 10 µg/ml, a fixed percentage of the total body store is eliminated per unit of time (first-order kinetics). With larger daily doses or higher plasma concentrations, the capacity of the hepatic metabolizing enzyme is saturated, and a fixed amount of the drug is eliminated per unit of time (zero-order kinetics), and the plasma $T^{1/2}$ is prolonged with increasing dose.[96] The mean plasma $T^{1/2}$ of a single 300-mg dose is 17 ± 1.5 h. On continued therapy with the same daily dose for 2 weeks, the $T^{1/2}$ is prolonged to 19 ± 1.5 h.[131] The rate of biotransformation and elimination is dependent not only on dose but also on a genetic factor.[96]

Adverse reactions

The most common adverse effects of lidocaine are symptoms of neurotoxicity including dizziness, drowsiness, euphoria, dysarthria, and blurred vision. More severe intoxication may lead to dyspnea, muscular fasciculation, convulsions, and respiratory arrest. These toxic manifestations may develop in the face of low plasma lidocaine concentrations but a high level of its metabolites.[129] Myocardial depression may occur with excessive doses in patients with acute myocardial infarctions. Rare effects include conversion of 2:1 to 1:1 AV conduction during atrial flutter, sinus arrest, AV block, and death.[95]

DPH may lead to blurred vision, dizziness, vertigo, nausea, nystagmus, ataxia, other cerebellar signs, and drowsiness. Hypotension may occur when a single bolus of 300 mg is given or when the cumulative intravenous dose of 500 mg is approached. Rarely, sinus bradycardia, sinus arrest, profound hypotension, and ventricular fibrillation have been reported.[96,132,134] Chronic DPH therapy may lead to the development of skin reactions, megaloblastic anemia, a lymphoma-like syndrome, and gingival hyperplasia.[75,96] The offspring of epileptic women receiving DPH during pregnancy have a higher incidence of congenital malformations.[133]

Drug interactions

Phenobarbital increases and isoniazid, as well as chloramphenicol, decreases lidocaine biotransformation by altering the hepatic microsomal enzymatic activity. Propranolol and norepinephrine retard and both isoproterenol and glucagon enhance lidocaine disposition through hemodynamic interactions.[125,129] The hepatic biotransformation of DPH is accelerated by barbiturates and other enzyme-inducing drugs and is inhibited by aminosalicylate, bishydroxycoumarin, chloramphenicol, disulfiram, isoniazid, methylphenidate, phenylbutazone, and others. DPH accelerates coumarin metabolism.[67,96]

Clinical use

Clinically, the group II drugs are effective against both automatic and reentrant ventricular arrhythmias but are relatively ineffective against supraventricular arrhythmias (Table 109B-3).[58,95,96,134] These group II drugs are the most effective against both experimental and clinical digitalis-induced arrhythmias which may involve changes both in cellular ionic concentrations as mediated by the Na^+-K^+ pump and central mechanisms[95,96] (see "Electrophysiologic Effects" above). Pretreatment with lidocaine or DPH before dc electroversion should be considered in the heavily digitalized patient.[86,87]

Because of its efficacy and relative safety lidocaine is the drug of choice in the emergency treatment of ventricular arrhythmias. Some 8 percent of ventricular arrhythmias treated in the coronary care unit do not respond to lidocaine.[135] Those occurring during the first hour after myocardial infarction or PVCs falling on the "vulnerable" phase of the T wave are most resistant to therapy.[136] Lidocaine is not particularly effective against atrial or AV junctional arrhythmias. Lidocaine may be useful in the treatment of arrhythmias associated with the Wolff-Parkinson-White syndrome, presumably by depressing conduction in the anomalous pathway.[137]

Clinically effective antiarrhythmic plasma concentrations of lidocaine range from 1.5 to 5.0 µg/ml. Lidocaine is usually administered by giving an initial intravenous bolus of 1 to 2 mg/kg followed by a constant infusion at a rate of 20 to 50 µg/kg/min ($\approx$1.5 to 4.0 mg/min).[125] It may also be given as repeated boluses of 1 mg/kg at 10- to 20-min intervals. Cumulative doses over 300 mg/h should be avoided.[125] Whenever an acute increase of lidocaine plasma concentration is required during constant rate infusion, a bolus injection of 25 mg or less should be added by titration every 15 min in addition to increasing the infusion rate. A change in the infusion rate alone requires 5 to 8 h to reach a new steady state.

In the presence of a moderately reduced cardiac output or shock, the dose should be reduced to 0.75 mg/kg for bolus injections and 20 µg/kg/min or less for continuous infusion. Congestive heart failure may lead to a decreased hepatic blood flow, and normally "therapeutic" doses may become "toxic." Lidocaine may not need to be discontinued due to its central nervous system toxicity; all that may be required is a downward adjustment in the drug dosage. An intramuscular injection of 250 mg lidocaine reaches a plasma concentration of 1 µg/ml or greater within 5 to 10 min and about 2.5 µg/ml at 30 min, and is maintained for 2 h except in the presence of shock.[125] Interest remains high in the development of an oral form of lidocaine, but none is currently available for general clinical use.

DPH is effective against digitalis-induced atrial arrhythmias but is essentially ineffective against other atrial arrhythmias. Junctional tachycardias do not respond well to DPH. DPH is effective against ventricular arrhythmias but has few advantages over either lidocaine or procainamide except perhaps in the presence of digitalis excess.[138] It has been suggested that DPH may counter the central nervous system toxicity of lidocaine,[75] but a high incidence of central nervous system side effects in patients on combined lidocaine and DPH therapy has been reported.[139]

The therapeutic plasma level of DPH is between 10 and 18 μg/ml with toxic symptoms developing in the range of 20 μg/ml.[134] For the emergency treatment of ventricular arrhythmias, DPH may be given intravenously in boluses of 50 to 100 mg every 5 min until a therapeutic effect is attained, an adverse reaction observed, or a total dose of 1,000 mg administered. Frequently, the borderline between a "therapeutic" and "toxic" dose is manifested by the appearance of slight nystagmus.[134] A maintenance dose of 300 to 500 mg/day may be given intravenously or orally in divided doses. DPH should not be given as a continuous infusion, because the alkaline solution may cause thrombophlebitis. Intramuscular injection of DPH results in erratic absorption and may cause tissue necrosis and sterile abscess formation.

Oral DPH administration with a dose of 300 to 500 mg/day takes 5 to 15 days to reach an effective therapeutic plasma concentration. An initial loading dose, therefore, is required to obtain a more rapid therapeutic effect. For an effect within 24 h, 1,000 mg should be given on day 1, followed by 500 mg on days 2 and 3, and then the maintenance dose.[134] Divided doses should be used when more than 300 mg is given daily.

GROUP III ANTIARRHYTHMIC AGENTS

Electrophysiologic effects

The pharmacology of β-adrenergic receptor stimulation and blockage is complex, and the reader is referred to recent reviews[140–143a] and to Chap. 109D concerning the β-adrenergic receptor blockers. As antiarrhythmic agents, the drugs in this group may have membrane effects that are either direct or indirect. The latter are mediated through the β-receptor blockade. The consensus is that β-receptor blockade is the primary antiarrhythmic mechanism, and this is the reason a separate category has been reserved for these agents. On the other hand, as Wit and his coworkers emphasize, the direct membrane effects are probably quite important as antiarrhythmic mechanisms.[141]

Propranolol, the prototype for group III, combines both group I and perhaps group II direct membrane effects with β-receptor adrenergic blockade. Propranolol has a group I direct membrane effect in that it depresses g_{Na} in atrial, Purkinje, and ventricular muscle.[143–145] ^{22}Na flux studies showed propranolol to inhibit sodium entry into the cell in a manner similar to that of quinidine.[146] Electrophysiologic studies in Purkinje fibers suggest propranolol may have a group II effect by increasing g_K.[147] ^{42}K flux studies in cat papillary muscle, however, indicate propranolol decreases K$^+$ efflux, increases K$^+$ influx, and increases

total K$^+$ content.[146] Propranolol may accelerate repolarization and shorten the APD of Purkinje fibers, particularly at the site with the longest APD. The ERP is shortened, but not as much as the APD. Repolarization of atrial and ventricular fibers is also accelerated, but to a lesser degree.[139–141] The direct membrane effects of propranolol occur at drug concentrations higher than those for β-adrenergic receptor blockade in normal tissue, but little information is available concerning direct membrane effects in diseased tissue. Tolamolol (UK-6558-01), however, is a relatively cardioselective β-adrenergic receptor blocker that immediately suppresses presumably I_{si}-dependent triggered sustained rhythmic activity in isolated Purkinje fibers superfused with drug concentrations equivalent to clinically effective antiarrhythmic plasma levels.[25]

β-Adrenergic *stimulation* increases the slope of phase 4 depolarization by means of several postulated mechanisms, including $\dot{V}_{max}$ of phase 0, and the action potential amplitude of fast I_{Na}-dependent cells, thereby enhancing automaticity and increasing conduction velocity.[141] β-Adrenergic stimulation shortens the functional and effective refractory period of the AV node and accelerates AV nodal conduction. In depolarized tissue, whether due to injury or an increased $[K^+]_0$, the sodium system is inactivated (approximation 4). In this situation, β-adrenergic sympathomimetic amines induce I_{si}-dependent action potentials and the slow response.[4,142] Triggered repetitive membrane activity, also thought to be I_{si}-dependent, is induced or enhanced by the catecholamines in the simian mitral valve.[149]

Propranolol, by inducing β-adrenergic receptor blockade, would antagonize the electrophysiologic effects of β-adrenergic stimulation. Propranolol slows sinus automaticity, increases the effective refractory period of atrial and AV nodal tissue, but has little effect on atrial and infranodal Purkinje conduction. Clinically, propranolol prolongs the P-R interval by its action on the AV node, increasing the A-H but not the H-V interval.[148,150,151] A drug-induced high degree of AV nodal block must be avoided since the drug may suppress subsidiary pacemakers and eventuate in asystole.

It has been suggested that propranolol may reduce ischemic injury as assessed by ST-segment mapping in patients with acute myocardial infarction,[152–154] and there is experimental evidence to support this interpretation.[155] On the other hand, these results must be viewed with caution, since the multiple direct and indirect electrophysiologic effects of propranolol could modify both systolic and diastolic injury currents without affecting the actual area of infarction (see the equation in approximation 1).[61a]

Pharmacokinetics (Table 109B-2)

Details are considered in Chap. 109D, but important aspects are summarized in Table 109B-2.

Clinical use

As seen in Table 109B-3, the clinical indications for propranolol seem to be a combination of groups I and II. It is effective against both automatic and reentrant arrhythmias.[143,148,156] Although of limited value in directly converting atrial flutter or fibrillation to a normal sinus rhythm, the drug effectively decreases the ventricular response by depressing AV nodal conduction. The decreased ventricular response may improve the hemodynamic status and favor reversion of the arrhythmia to a sinus mechanism. The drug is of use in controlling the ventricular response to atrial fibrillation in the presence of thyrotoxicosis. The effect of propranolol on AV nodal conduction must always be considered in the presence of AV nodal disease, or when used in combination with other drugs, such as digitalis, which also inhibit conduction through the AV node. Propranolol is quite effective against reentrant paroxysmal supraventricular tachycardia, presumably by interfering with the AV nodal segment of the reentrant loop, by decreasing or eliminating the echo zone, or at least by decreasing the rate of the tachyarrhythmia.[157] In some patients echo zones may develop after the drug is administered.[137] Propranolol is effective against arrhythmias associated with increased sympathetic activity, the use of cyclopropane or halothane anesthesia, tricyclic antidepressant therapy, the Wolff-Parkinson-White syndrome, and the prolonged Q-T interval syndrome.[140–143a,158] Although effective against digitalis-induced arrhythmias, it is generally not used for fear of producing SA or AV block. When given for the tachycardia in a patient with a pheochromocytoma, an α-adrenergic blocking agent, such as phenoxybenzamine or phentolamine should be given prior to the initiation of propranolol. This is necessary to prevent a further elevation of blood pressure which may occur following the abolition of vasodilatation by β-adrenergic blockade.[158] Alprenolol and practolol may be useful in the prevention of sudden death.[159,160] The efficacy of propranolol against sudden death in the patient with chronic ventricular arrhythmia awaits clinical testing.

In general, propranolol is not the drug of choice for the acute termination of arrhythmias, but it may be tried if the first-line drugs fail. The intravenous administration of propranolol may precipitate acute heart failure, intensive bronchospasm, life-threatening hypotension, and cardiac arrest. If this route of administration is deemed necessary, Shand suggests the drug should be given in increments of 0.1 to 0.2 mg not exceeding 1 mg in 10 min or a total of 5 to 10 mg.[158] Frequently, larger doses are given intravenously; 1-mg doses have been suggested.[161] The oral dose varies widely and ranges from 40 to 320 mg/day or more in divided doses. The effect of a single (perhaps 320+mg) oral dose peaks in 1 to 4 h. Therapy is usually started with a daily dose of 40 mg followed by increments until the response is achieved, an adverse reaction occurs, or a total daily dose of 320 mg has been reached.[158] The plasma $T^{1/2}$ is 2.0 to 3.5 h. The metabolism is complex with active metabolites (see Chap. 109D), and appropriate plasma assays are useful in selecting an appropriate regimen.

Propranolol is frequently used in combination with digitalis, quinidine, or procainamide for the treatment and prevention of various kinds of arrhythmias. The potential for additive toxicity, particularly hypotension and heart failure, in these situations is real. Additional clinically useful pharmacologic properties of propranolol are considered in Chap. 109D.

Precautions and contraindications

Propranolol is contraindicated in patients with significant heart failure, bronchial asthma, chronic obstructive pulmonary disease, "sick sinus" syndrome, and high-grade AV nodal block without an artificial pacemaker except under rigidly controlled conditions. It must be used cautiously in patients with diabetes mellitus and peripheral vascular disease. Propranolol is subject to drug interactions and may require dose adjustment in patients with changing hemodynamics[158,162] (see Chap. 109D). The sudden withdrawal of propranolol may precipitate angina pectoris, serious arrhythmias, and acute myocardial infarction, and, in nonurgent situations, should be accomplished over a period of at least 2 weeks.[158,163]

GROUP IV ANTIARRHYTHMIC AGENTS

Bretylium tosylate, the prototype of group IV, has minimal direct membrane effects and is thought to act primarily by its antiadrenergic actions.[164,165] It has been used against ventricular arrhythmias,[166–167a] but only limitedly. Bretylium initially causes the release of norepinephrine from sympathetic nerve endings, and may enhance automaticity.[94,165]

GROUP V ANTIARRHYTHMIC AGENTS

Electrophysiologic effects

Verapamil is the prototype for group V and directly blocks the slow inward channel, thereby decreasing I_{si}.[2,4,168] Verapamil can suppress automaticity in fibers in which g_{Na} has been inactivated by depolarization and in fibers superfused with Na^+-free, Ca^{2+}-rich solutions.[4,168,169] Automaticity can be decreased in fast cardiac fibers, but the mechanism is yet uncertain.[168] The drug does not affect $\dot{V}_{max}$, membrane responsiveness, and action potential amplitude in normal Purkinje fibers, suggesting little effect on g_{Na}.[168,169] It does reduce conduction velocity in depolarized tissue and may interrupt reentrant circuits dependent on the slow response by producing bidirectional block (Fig. 109B-2*C*).[4,168] Triggered and spontaneous nondriven rhythmic activity that occurs at low transmembrane voltages in the simian mitral valve and in atrial specialized fibers can be suppressed by verapamil.[168]

Verapamil can suppress SA nodal activity and sinus node recovery time after overdrive suppression is increased 10 to 15 percent.[165] The decrease in heart rate is not blocked by atropine, suggesting that this is a direct effect.[170] Verapamil depresses the AV nodal action potential and conduction velocity[168] and prolongs the A-H interval.[171]

Pathologic studies in dogs suggest that verapamil may limit cardiac necrosis after coronary occlusion which, in turn, could influence the electrophysiologic characteristics of the myocardium.[171a]

Clinical use

What little is known about the pharmacokinetics of verapamil has been recently summarized.[168] At the time of writing, verapamil is not available for clinical use in the United States. The few available clinical studies suggest the drug is most useful against supraventricular tachyarrhythmias, particularly in the control of the ventricular response to atrial fibrillation and flutter, and in the reversion of reentrant paroxysmal supraventricular tachycardia and junctional tachycardia to normal sinus rhythm.[160,168,172,173] This would be anticipated since the SA and AV nodes have I_{si}-dependent action potentials, control of the ventricular response in atrial fibrillation and flutter is at the level of the AV node, and reentrant paroxysmal supraventricular and junctional tachycardias are thought to use a portion of the AV node in the reentrant pathway.[4,22,23,31–35,168] The drug has had mixed success in treating premature ventricular beats and paroxysmal ventricular tachycardia.[172,173] Controlled studies are needed to find out whether verapamil is effective against "malignant" PVCs and primary ventricular fibrillation. The question as to whether repetitive sustained arrhythmias following a PVC falling on the "vulnerable" period of the T wave involve an I_{si}-dependent mechanism has been discussed earlier. Verapamil seems to have little effect on conduction through the anomalous pathway in the Wolff-Parkinson-White syndrome.[173,174] Heng et al. suggest that verapamil does not lead to serious post-dc electroversion arrhythmias.[173]

Although verapamil has a negative inotropic effect, the drug is said not to decrease cardiac output in patients with cardiac disease[175] and is thought by Heng et al. to be safer when given by slow intravenous injection than β-adrenergic blocking agents.[173] Transient, mild decreases in blood pressure are frequently observed.[164,165,166,172–179] Hypotension, bradycardia, and asystole have been reported,[169,171,176,177] but most of these patients had been on β-adrenergic blockers before receiving verapamil. The drug does not alter ventilatory function in asthmatic patients.[180] Verapamil must be used with extreme caution in patients with SA or AV nodal dysfunction, and, if needed, consideration should be given to the insertion of an artificial ventricular pacemaker. The

majority of patients in the series by Schamroth et al.[172] and Heng et al.[173] were on digitalis, and the additive effects verapamil and digitalis may have on the SA and AV nodes must be appreciated.

GROUP VI ANTIARRHYTHMIC AGENTS

Due to their unique electrophysiologic agents, the cardiac glycosides should be considered a separate group of antiarrhythmic drugs. These agents have both direct and indirect effects on cardiac electrophysiology. The topic is considered in Chap. 109C, under "Cardiac Glycosides."

COMMENTS ON SINGLE, ALTERNATIVE, AND COMBINATION ANTIARRHYTHMIC DRUG THERAPY

Several groups have considered this topic recently, advising great caution in the use of the antiarrhythmic agents.[1,37a,75,94] Antiarrhythmic therapy, like all therapy, is initiated with the hope of improving the patient's medical condition. The "failure" of the initially chosen antiarrhythmic agent frequently leads to the selection of alternative drugs, or, at times, to the use of drug combinations that may have selective and/or additive actions.

The "failure" of an initial antiarrhythmic drug may result from inappropriate drug selection, inadequate dose, single or multiple arrhythmogenic mechanisms that may respond to one but not another drug or to a combination of drugs, a resistant arrhythmogenic mechanism, and complicating factors such as acid-base abnormalities, electrolyte imbalance, associated drug therapy and toxicity, the severity of cardiac disease, or coexistent disease in other organ systems. The relationship between the central nervous system and cardiac arrhythmias is only beginning to be understood.[181]

An often difficult problem is making a precise electrocardiographic diagnosis. Frequently, the use of manuevers (Valsalva, exercise, etc.), drugs (atropine, edrophonium, verapamil, etc.), special electrocardiographic techniques (high-speed recording, double standardization, multichannel simultaneous recordings, special leads, esophageal electrograms, and intracavitary electrograms), and other procedures (phonocardiography, pulse recordings, apex cardiography, echocardiography, pacing studies, tape monitoring, etc.) may be required in establishing the correct diagnosis.

The natural history of a given cardiac arrhythmia and the ability of drugs to favorably influence the natural history must be considered. The prognostic gravity of ventricular arrhythmias, for example, may depend more on the associated cardiac disease than on the frequency or configuration of the abnormal ventricular beats.[37,37a] Whether the usual antiarrhythmic agents are effective in maintaining normal sinus rhythm after dc electroversion in supraventricular arrhythmias,[86] against ventricular arrhythmias immediately following acute myocardial infarction during the "prehospital" and early hospital phases, and against sudden death in the patient with chronic ventricular arrhythmias[37,37a,75,159,160a-c] are questions that have not yet been satisfactorily answered. This is of particular importance given the significant toxicity of the available antiarrhythmic agents. In life-threatening supraventricular and ventricular arrhythmias, dc electroversion may be the therapy of choice, often in combination with antiarrhythmic drugs.[86] At times, electrical pacing may be used with an antiarrhythmic drug[75] and, as has been mentioned above, the use of an artificial ventricular pacemaker frequently needs to be considered before an antiarrhythmic agent is administered. Once the decision to use an antiarrhythmic drug is made, clinical endpoints must be defined, appropriate doses given, pharmacokinetics considered in terms of achieving a therapeutic plasma level and drug clearance, and bioelectric as well as other complications anticipated.

Specific antiarrhythmic drug failures may result from the existence of single or multiple arrhythmogenic mechanisms that may or may not respond to one another or several drugs. Since it is usually impossible to define the arrhythmogenic mechanism with certainty clinically, therapy is basically empirical. Empirical therapy, however, can be guided from the philosophy included in the proposed classification of antiarrhythmic agents. Since drug failure may represent the inappropriate drug action for a given arrhythmogenic mechanism, *alternative therapy, as a rule, should employ a drug from a different antiarrhythmic group.* The exception to this statement might be in digitalis-induced arrhythmias where lidocaine (group II), if unsuccessful, should be followed by DPH (also group II), since the latter possesses some unique central nervous system effects.

Drug failure may reflect the coexistence of multiple treatable arrhythmogenic mechanisms. Examples might be a reentrant paroxysmal superventricular tachycardia initiated by an atrial premature depolarization with each mechanism requiring selective drug action, or the initial enhancement of ventricular automaticity caused by a bretylium-induced release of catecholamines which may require suppression with an antiautomatic drug such as lidocaine. Empirically, Mason et al.[94] and Bigger and Giardina[75] have had clinical success with several drug combinations including quinidine and propranolol against supraventricular arrhythmias; DPH and procainamide against arrhythmias complicated by functional conduction disturbances; various combinations of procainamide, lidocaine, propranolol, and bretylium against resistant ventricular arrhythmias; and digital-

is used in various combinations with one or several of the other antiarrhythmic agents. Note that each drug in a clinically useful combination comes *from a different electrophysiologic group* in the proposed classification.

Currently untreatable arrhythmogenic mechanisms may be involved. Normal and abnormal I_{si} responses, as discussed above, are frequently resistant to the standard antiarrhythmic drugs. The distinctive electrophysiologic actions of verapamil (group V) and its clinical efficacy suggest that heretofore untreatable arrhythmias may be responsive to this new family of drugs. Little is known about the I_{ti} current in digitalis intoxication (see Chap. 109C, under "Cardiac Glycosides"), but definition of underlying electrophysiologic mechanisms may well lead to the development of appropriate drugs to be used selectively.

Frequently, arrhythmias are best countered by means other than specific antiarrhythmic agents. Antiarrhythmic drugs tend to be less effective in the presence of acid-base abnormalities, hypoxia, and electrolyte imbalance. The potential interaction of other drugs must be considered, since they may have direct or indirect cardiac effects or may interfere with the metabolism of antiarrhythmic drugs, thus complicating therapy. Coexistent renal and hepatic disease may influence pharmacokinetics. Congestive heart failure itself may decrease hepatic blood flow, rendering a normally therapeutic dose toxic. This problem is often encountered with lidocaine, and both the maintenance of an effective antiarrhythmic plasma level and the avoidance of toxicity may be accomplished simply by decreasing the dosage. Other organ system disease (pulmonary, gastrointestinal, hematologic, etc.) may also complicate therapy. The undesirable as well as the desirable effects of antiarrhythmic drugs may also be additive. Many of the potentially additive bioelectric and hemodynamic effects have already been discussed which may actually worsen rather than alleviate cardiac arrhythmias. At times, surgical intervention may be the appropriate antiarrhythmic therapy.[181-187] As has been mentioned, dc electroversion frequently is the antiarrhythmic intervention of choice. The direct and indirect electrophysiologic changes caused by the dc electroshock, including pacemaker depression, enhanced excitability, AV conduction disturbances, and the like, must be considered[188] in light of the clinical setting and drug use.

Clinical discretion and a firm knowledge of the natural history of arrhythmias, then, is a necessity for deciding when to use an antiarrhythmic drug. Clinical understanding of pharmacokinetics, electrophysiology, and bioelectric and other complications is required for the rational use of these agents. Clinical vigilance is mandatory in order to benefit rather than harm the patient.

REFERENCES

1 Arnsdorf, M. F.: Electrophysiologic Properties of Antidysrhythmic Drugs as a Rational Basis for Therapy, *Med. Clin. North Am.,* 60:213, 1976.

2 Trautwein, W.: Membrane Currents in Cardiac Muscle Fibers, *Physiol. Rev.,* 53:793, 1973.

3 Rosen, M. R., Wit, A. L., and Hoffman, B. F.: Electrophysiology and Pharmacology of Cardiac Arrhythmias: I. Cellular Electrophysiology of the Mammalian Heart, *Am. Heart J.,* 88:380, 1974.

4 Cranefield, P. F.: "The Slow Response and Cardiac Arrhythmias in The Conduction of the Cardiac Impulse," Futura Publishing Company, Mt. Kisco, N.Y., 1975.

5 Noble, D.: "The Initiation of the Heart Beat," Clarendon Press, Oxford, 1975.

6 Jack, J. J. B., Noble, D., and Tsien, R. W.: Electric Current Flow in Excitable Cells, Clarendon Press, Oxford, 1975.

7 Fozzard, H. A.: Cardiac Muscle: Excitability and Passive Electrical Properties, *Prog. Cardiovasc. Dis.,* 14:343, 1977.

8 Fozzard, H. A., and Schoenberg, M.: Strength-Duration Curves in Cardiac Purkinje Fibers: Effects of Liminal Length and Charge Distribution, *J. Physiol. (London),* 226:618, 1972.

9 Fozzard, H. A., and Beeler, G. W., Jr.: The Voltage Clamp and Cardiac Electrophysiology, *Circ. Res.,* 37:403, 1975.

10 Arnsdorf, M. F., and Bigger, J. T., Jr.: The Effect of Lidocaine on Components of Excitability in Long Mammalian Cardiac Purkinje Fibers, *J. Pharmacol. Exp. Ther.,* 195:206, 1975.

11 Arnsdorf, M. F., and Bigger, J. T., Jr.: The Effect of Procaine Amide on Components of Excitability in Long Mammalian Cardiac Purkinje Fibers, *Circ. Res.,* 38:115, 1976.

12 Weidmann, S.: The Effect of Cardiac Membrane Potential on the Rapid Availability of the Sodium-carrying System, *J. Physiol. (London),* 127:213, 1955.

13 Bigger, J. R., Jr.: Electrical Properties of Cardiac Muscle and Possible Causes of Cardiac Arrhythmias, in L. Dreifus and W. Likoff (eds.), "Cardiac Arrhythmias," Grune & Stratton, Inc., New York, 1973.

14 Schoenberg, M., Dominguez, G., and Fozzard, H. A.: Effect of Diameter on Membrane Capacity and Conductance of Sheep Cardiac Purkinje Fibers, *J. Gen. Physiol.,* 65:441, 1975.

15 Zipes, D. P., Besch, H. R., and Watanabe, A. M.: Role of the Slow Current in Cardiac Electrophysiology, *Circulation,* 51:761, 1975.

16 Zipes, D. P.: Recent Observations Supporting the Role of Slow Current in Cardiac Electrophysiology, in H. J. J. Wellens, K. I. Lie, and M. F. Janse (eds.), "The Conduction System of the Heart: Structure, Function, and Clinical Implications," Lea & Febiger, Philadelphia, 1976, p. 85.

17 Wit, A. L., Wiggins, J. R., and Cranefield, P. F.: Some Effects of Electrical Stimulation on Impulse Initiation in Cardiac Fibers: Its Relevance for the Determination of the Mechanisms of Clinical Cardiac Arrhythmias, in H. J. J. Wellens, K. I. Lie, and M. F. Janse (eds.), "The Conduction System of the Heart: Structure, Function, and Clinical Implications," Lea & Febiger, Philadelphia, 1976, p. 163.

18 Lederer, W. J., and Tsien, R. W.: Transient Inward Current Underlying Arrhythmogenic Effects of Cardiotonic Steroids in Purkinje Fibers, *J. Physiol. (London),* 263:73, 1976.

19 Ferrier, G. R.: Digitalis Arrhythmias: Role of Oscillatory Afterpotentials, *Progr. Cardiovasc. Dis.,* 19:459, 1977.

20 Arnsdorf, M. F.: Membrane Factors in Arrhythmogenesis: Concepts and Definitions, *Prog. Cardiovasc. Dis.,* 19:413, 1977.

21 Wit, A. L., Rosen, M. R., and Hoffman, B. F.: Electrophysiology and Pharmacology of Cardiac Arrhythmias: II. Relationship of Normal and Abnormal Electrical Activity of Cardiac Fibers to the Genesis of Arrhythmias, part A, Automaticity, *Am. Heart J.,* 88:515-524, 1974.

22 Wit, A. L., Rosen, M. R., and Hoffman, B. F.: Electrophysiology and Pharmacology of Cardiac Arrhythmias: II. Relationship of Normal and Abnormal Electrical Activity of Cardiac Fibers to the Genesis of Arrhythmias, part B, Reentry, sec. I, *Am. Heart J.,* 88:664, 1974.

23 Wit, A. L., Rosen, M. R., and Hoffman, B. F.: Electrophysiology and Pharmacology of Cardiac Arrhythmias: II. Relationship of Normal and Abnormal Electrical Activity of Cardiac Fibers to the Genesis of Arrhythmias, part B, Reentry, sec. II, *Am. Heart J.,* 88:798, 1974.

24 Hoffman, B. R., Rosen, M. R., and Wit, A. L.: Electrophysiology and Pharmacology of Cardiac Arrhythmias: III. The Causes and Treatment of Cardiac Arrhythmias, part A, *Am. Heart J.,* 89:115, 1975.

25 Arnsdorf, M. F.: The Effect of Antiarrhythmic Drugs on Triggered Sustained Rhythmic Activity in Cardiac Purkinje Fibers, *J. Pharmacol. Exp. Ther.,* in press.

26 Arnsdorf, M. F., and Friedlander, I.: The Electrophysiologic Effects of Tolamolol (UK-6558-01) on the Passive Membrane Properties of Mammalian Cardiac Purkinje Fibers, *J. Pharmacol. Exp. Ther.,* 199:601, 1976.

27 Hauswirth, O., Noble, D., and Tsien, R. W.: The Mechanism of Oscillatory Activity at Low Membrane Potentials in Cardiac Purkinje Fibres, *J. Physiol. (London),* 200:255, 1969.

28 Singer, D. H., Ten Eick, R. E., and De Boer, A. A.: Electrophysiologic Correlates of Human Atrial Tachyarrhythmias, in L. Dreifus and W. Likoff (eds.), "Cardiac Arrhythmias," Grune & Stratton, Inc., New York, 1973, p. 97.

29 Wit, A. L., Hoffman, B. F., and Cranefield, P. F.: Slow Conduction and Reentry in the Ventricular Conducting System: I. Return Extrasystoles in Canine Purkinje Fibers, *Circ. Res.,* 30:1, 1972.

30 Wit, A. L., Cranefield, P. F., and Hoffman, B. F.: Slow Conduction and Reentry in the Ventricular Conducting System: II. Single and Sustained Circus movement in Networks of Canine and Bovine Purkinje Fibers, *Circ. Res.,* 30:11, 1972.

31 Wit, A. L., Goldreyer, B. N., and Damato, A. N.: An In Vitro Model of Paroxysmal Supraventricular Tachycardia, *Circulation,* 43:862, 1971.

32 Wit, A. L., and Cranefield, P. F.: Effect of Verapamil on the Sinoatrial and Atrioventricular Nodes of the Rabbit and the Mechanism by Which It Arrests Reentrant Atrioventricular Nodal Tachycardia, *Circ. Res.,* 35:413, 1974.

33 Bigger, J. T., Jr., and Goldreyer, B. N.: The Mechanism of Supraventricular Tachycardia, *Circulation,* 42:673, 1970.

34 Goldreyer, B. N., and Bigger, J. T., Jr.: Site of Reentry in Paroxysmal Supraventricular Tachycardia in Man, *Circulation,* 43:15, 1971.

35 Myerburg, R. J., Gelband, H., and Hoffman, B. F.: Functional Characteristics of the Gating Mechanism in the Canine A-V Conducting System, *Circ. Res.,* 28:136, 1971.

36 Rytand, D. A.: The Circus Movement (Entrapped Circuit Wave) Hypothesis and Atrial Flutter, *Ann. Intern. Med.,* 65:127, 1966.

36a Harumi, K., Owens, J., Burgess, M. J., and Abildskov, J. A.: Relationship of Ventricular Excitability Characteristics to Ventricular Arrhythmias in Dogs, *Circ. Res.,* 35:464, 1974.

36b Tamargo, J., Moe, B., and Moe, G. K.: Interaction of Sequential Stimuli Applied during the Relative Refractory Period in Relation to Determination of Fibrillation Threshold in the Canine Ventricle, *Circ. Res.,* 37:534, 1975.

37 Moss, A. J., and Akiyama, T.: Prognostic Significance of Ventricular Premature Beats, *Cardiovasc. Clin.* 6:274, 1974.

37a Bigger J. T., Jr., Dresdale, R. J., Heissenbuttel, R. H., Weld, F. M., and Wit, A. L.: Ventricular Arrhythmias in Ischemic Heart Disease: Mechanism, Prevalence Significance, and Management, *Progr. Cardiovasc. Dis.,* 19:255, 1977.

38 Epstein, S. E., Beiser, G. D., Rosing, D. R., Talano, J. V., and Karsh, R. B.: Experimental Acute Myocardial Infarction, *Circulation,* 47:446, 1973.

39 Bassett, A. L., and Wit, A. L.: Recent Advances in Electro-

physiology of Antiarrhythmic Drugs, *Prog. Drug Res.*, 17:34, 1973.

40 Hoffman, B. F., Rosen, M. F., and Wit, A. L.: Electrophysiology and Pharmacology of Cardiac Arrhythmias: VII. Cardiac Effects of Quinidine and Procainamide, part A, *Am. Heart J.*, 89:804, 1975; part B, *Am. Heart J.*, 90:117, 1975.

41 Weidmann, S. L.: Effects of Calcium ions and Local Anesthetics on Electrical Properties of Purkinje Fibers, *J. Physiol. (London)*, 129:568, 1955.

42 Johnson, E. A.: The Effects of Quinidine, Procaine Amide and Pyrilamine on the Membrane Resting and Action Potential of Guinea Pig Ventricular Muscle Fibers, *J. Pharmacol. Exp. Ther.*, 117:237, 1956.

43 Hoffman, B. F.: The Action of Quinidine and Procaine Amide on Single Fibers of Dog Ventricle and Specialized Conducting System, *An. Acad. Bras. Cienc.* 29:365, 1957.

44 Vaughan Williams, E. M.: Mode of Action of Quinidine in Isolated Rabbit Atria Interpreted from Intracellular Records, *Br. J. Pharmacol.*, 13:276, 1958.

45 Rosen, M. R., Gelband, H., and Hoffman, B. F.: Canine Electrocardiographic and Cardiac Electrophysiologic Changes Induced by Procaine Amide, *Circulation*, 46:528, 1972.

46 Rosen, M. R., Merker, C., Gelband, H., and Hoffman, B. F.: Effects of Procaine Amide on the Electrophysiologic Properties of the Canine Ventricular Conducting System, *J. Pharmacol. Exp. Ther.*, 185:438, 1973.

47 Weld, F. M., and Bigger, J. T., Jr.: Effect of Procaine Amide on Membrane Conductance of Cardiac Purkinje Fibers, *Circulation*, 46(suppl. 2):39, 1972. (Abstract.)

48 Chen, C. M., Gettes, L. S., and Katzung, B. G.: Effect of Lidocaine and Quinidine on Steady-State Characteristics and Recovery Kinetics of $(dV/dt)_{max}$ in Guinea Pig Ventricular Myocardium, *Circ. Res.*, 37:20, 1975.

49 Hordof, A., Edie, R., Malm, J., and Rosen, M.: Effects of Procaine Amide and Verapamil on Electrophysiologic Properties of Human Atrial Tissues, *Pediatr. Res.*, 9:267, 1975.

50 Giardina, E. G., and Bigger, J. T., Jr.: Procaine Amide against Reentrant Ventricular Arrhythmias: Lengthening of R-V Intervals of Coupled Ventricular Premature Depolarizations as an Insight into the Mechanisms of Action of Procaine Amide, *Circulation*, 48:959, 1973.

51 Moe, G. K., and Abildskov, J. A.: Antiarrhythmic Drugs, in L. S. Goodman and A. Gilman (eds.), "The Pharmacological Basis of Therapeutics," 5th ed., The Macmillan Company, New York, 1975, p. 683.

52 Schmid, P. G., Nelson, L. D., Mark, A. L., et al.: Inhibition of Adrenergic Vasoconstriction by Quinidine, *J. Pharmacol. Exp. Ther.*, 188:124, 1974.

53 Wellens, H. J. J., and Durrer, D.: Effect of Procaine Amide, Quinidine, and Ajmaline in the Wolff-Parkinson-White Syndrome, *Circulation*, 50:115, 1974.

53a Chiale, P. A., Przbylski, J., Halpern, M. S., Lazzari, J. O., Elizari, M. V., and Rosenbaum, M. B.: Comparative Effects of Ajmaline on Intermittent Bundle Branch Block and the Wolff-Parkinson-White Syndrome, *Am. J. Cardiol.*, 39:651, 1977.

53b Sellers, T. D., Jr., Campbell, R. W., Bashore, T. M., and Gallagher, J. J.: Effects of Procainamide and Quinidine Sulfate in the Wolff-Parkinson-White Syndrome, *Circulation*, 55:15, 1977.

54 Singer, D. H., Strauss, H. C., and Hoffman, B. F.: Biphasic Effects of Procaine Amide on Cardiac Conduction, *Bull. N.Y. Acad. Med.*, 43:1994, 1967.

55 Singer, D. H., and Ten Eick, R. E.: Pharmacology of Cardiac Arrhythmias, *Prog. Cardiovasc. Dis.*, 11:488, 1969.

56 Dreifus, L. S., Watanabe, Y., Dreifus, H. N., and De Aze-

vedo, I.: The Effect of Antiarrhythmic Agents on Impulse Formation and Impulse Conduction, in H. J. J. Wellens, K. E. Lie, and M. J. Janse (eds.), "The Conduction System of the Heart: Structure, Function, and Clinical Implications," Lea & Febiger, Philadelphia, 1976, p. 182.

57 Josephson, M. E., Seides, S. F., Batsford, W. P., Weisfogel, G. M., Akhtar, M., Caracta, A. R., Lau, S. H., and Damato, A. N.: The Electrophysiological Effects of Intramuscular Quinidine on the Atrioventricular Conducting System in Man, *Am. Heart J.*, 87:55, 1974.

58 Josephson, M. E., Caracta, A. R., Ricciuti, M. A., Lau, S. H., and Damato, A. N.: Electrophysiologic Properties of Procainamide in Man, *Am. J. Cardiol.*, 33:96, 1974.

59 Scheinman, M. M., Weiss, A. N., Shafton, E., Benowitz, N., and Rowland, M.: Electrophysiologic Effects of Procaine Amide in Patients with Intraventricular Conduction Delay, *Circulation*, 49:522, 1974.

59a Mason, J. W., Winkle, R. A., Rider, A. K., Stinson, E. B., and Harrison, D. C.: The Electrophysiologic Effects of Quinidine in the Transplanted Human Heart, *J. Clin. Invest.*, 59:481, 1977.

60 Bigger, J. T., Jr., and Heissenbuttel, R. H.: The Use of Procaine Amide and Lidocaine in the Treatment of Cardiac Arrhythmias, *Prog. Cardiovasc. Dis.*, 11:515, 1969.

61 Heissenbuttel, R. H., and Bigger, J. T., Jr.: The Effect of Oral Quinidine on Intraventricular Conduction in Man: Correlation of Plasma Quinidine with Changes in QRS Duration, *Am. Heart J.*, 80:792, 1970.

61a Holland, R. P., and Arnsdorf, M. F.: Solid Angle Theory and The Electrogram: Physiologic and Quantitative Interpretation, *Progr. Cardiovasc. Dis.*, 19:431, 1977.

62 Winkle, R. A., Glantz, S. A., and Harrison, D. C.: Pharmacologic Therapy of Ventricular Arrhythmias, *Am. J. Cardiol.*, 36:629, 1975.

63 Ueda, C. T., Hirschfeld, D. S., Scheinman, M. M., et al.: Disposition Kinetics of Quinidine, *Clin. Pharmacol. Ther.*, 19:30, 1976.

64 Kessler, K. M.: Individualization of Dosage of Antiarrhythmic Drugs, *Med. Clin. North Am.*, 58:1019, 1974.

64a Conrad, K. A., Molk, B. L., Chidsey, C. A.: Pharmacokinetic Studies of Quinidine in Patient with Arrhythmias, *Circulation*, 55:1, 1977.

65 Kessler, K. M., Lowenthal, D. T., Warner, H., et al.: Quinidine Elimination in Patients with Congestive Heart Failure or Poor Renal Function, *N. Engl. J. Med.*, 290:706, 1974.

66 Gerhardt, R. E., Knouss, R. F., Thyrum, P. T., et al.: Quinidine Excretion in Aciduria and Alkaluria, *Ann. Intern. Med.*, 71:927, 1969.

67 Koch-Weser, J.: Drug Interactions in Cardiovascular Therapy, *Am. Heart J.*, 90:93, 1975.

68 Koch-Weser, J., and Klein, S. W.: Procainamide Dosage Schedules, Plasma Concentrations and Clinical Effects, *J.A.M.A.*, 215:1454, 1971.

69 Craffner, C., Johnsson, G., and Sjörgren, J.: Pharmacokinetics of Procainamide Intravenously and Orally as Conventional and Slow Release Tablets, *Clin. Pharmacol. Ther.*, 17:414, 1975.

70 Galeazzi, R. L., Sheiner, L. B., Lock, T., and Benet, L. S.: The Renal Elimination of Procainamide, *Clin. Pharmacol. Ther.*, 19:55, 1976.

71 Elson, J., Strong, J. M., Lee, W. K., et al.: Antiarrhythmic Potency of *N*-Acetylprocainamide, *Clin. Pharmacol. Ther.*, 17:134, 1975.

72 Giardina, E. V., Dreyfuss, J., Bigger, J. T., et al.: Metabolism of Procainamide in Normal and Cardiac Subjects, *Clin. Pharmacol. Ther.*, 19:339, 1976.

73 Strong, J. M., Dutcher, J. S., Lee, W. K., et al.: Absolute Bioavailability in Man of *N*-Acetylprocainamide Determined by a Novel Stable Isotope Method, *Clin. Pharmacol. Ther.*, 18:613, 1975.

74 Gibson, T. P., Lowenthal, D. T., Nelson, H. A., and Briggs, W. A.: Elimination of Procainamide in End Stage Renal Failure, *Clin. Pharmacol. Ther.*, 17:321, 1975.

74a Giardina, E. G. V., Stein, R. M., and Bigger, J. T., Jr.: The Relationship between the Metabolism of Procainamide and Sulfamethazine, *Circulation*, 55:388, 1977.

75 Bigger, J. T., Jr., and Giardina, E. G. V.: Rational Use of Antiarrhythmic Drugs Alone and in Combination, *Cardiovasc. Clin.*, 6(2):103, 1974.

76 Ghajek, T., Lehrer, B., Geltner, D., and Levij, I. S.: Quinidine-induced Granulomatous Hepatitis, *Ann. Intern. Med.*, 81:774, 1974.

77 Kerr, F., Kenoyer, G., and Bilitch, M.: Quinidine Overdose, Neurological and Cardiovascular Toxicity in a Normal Person, *Br. Heart J.*, 33:629, 1971.

78 Kosowsky, B. D., Taylor, J., Lown, B., and Ritchie, R. F.: Long Term Use of Procainamide following Acute Myocardial Infarction, *Circulation*, 47:1204, 1973.

79 Sunder, S. K., and Shah, A.: Constrictive Pericarditis in Procainamide-induced Lupus Erythematosus Syndrome, *Am. J. Cardiol.*, 36:960, 1975.

80 Villalba-Pimentel, L., Epstein, L. M., Sellers, E. M., et al.: Survival after Massive Procainamide Ingestion, *Am. J. Cardiol.*, 32:727, 1973.

81 Gay, R. J., and Brown, D. F.: Pacemaker Failure Due to Procainamide Toxicity, *Am. J. Cardiol.*, 34:728, 1974.

82 Data, J. L., Wilkinson, G. R., and Nies, A. S.: Interaction of Quinidine with Anticonvulsant Drugs, *N. Engl. J. Med.*, 294:699, 1976.

83 Weily, H. S., and Genton, E.: Pharmacokinetics of Procainamide, *Arch. Intern. Med.*, 130:366, 1972.

84 Giardina, E. G. V., Heissenbuttel, R. H., and Bigger, J. T., Jr.: Intermittent Intravenous Procainamide to Treat Ventricular Arrhythmias: Correlation of Plasma Concentrations with Effects on Arrhythmia, Electrocardiogram and Blood Pressure, *Ann. Intern. Med.*, 7:183, 1973.

85 Katz, L., and Pick, A.: "Clinical Electrocardiography: The Arrhythmias," Lea & Febiger, Philadelphia, 1956.

86 Resnekov, L.: Drug Therapy before and after the Electroversion of Cardiac Dysrhythmias, *Prog. Cardiovasc. Dis.*, 16:531, 1974.

87 Wagner, G. S., and McIntosh, H. D.: The Use of Drugs in Achieving Successful DC Cardioversion, *Prog. Cardiovas. Dis.*, 11:431, 1969.

88 Ross, M., and Lown, B.: Use of Quinidine in Cardioversion, *Am. J. Cardiol.*, 19:234, 1967.

89 Morris, J. J., Kong, Y., North, W. C., and McIntosh, H. D.: Experience with Cardioversion of Atrial Fibrillation and Flutter, *Am. J. Cardiol.*, 14:94, 1964.

90 Hurst, J. W., Paulk, E. A., Proctor, H. D., and Schlant, R. C.: Management of Patients with Atrial Fibrillation, *Am. J. Med.*, 37:728, 1964.

91 Kayden, H. J.: Antiarrhythmic Drugs: VI. Clinical Use of Procaineamide, *Am. Heart J.*, 70:567, 1965.

92 Hoffman, B. F., and Bigger, J. T., Jr.: Antiarrhythmic Drugs, in J. R. DiPalma (ed.), "Drill's Pharmacology in Medicine," 4th ed., McGraw-Hill Book Company, New York, 1971.

93 Rosen, M. R., and Hoffman, B. F.: Mechanisms of Action of Antiarrhythmic Drugs, *Circ. Res.*, 37:1, 1973.

94 Mason, D., Amsterdam, E., Massumi, R., Mansour, E., Hughes, J., and Zelis, R.: Combined Actions of Antiarrhythmic Drugs: Electrophysiologic and Therapeutic Considerations, in L. Dreifus and W. Likoff (eds.), "Cardiac Arrhythmias," Grune & Stratton, Inc., New York, 1973, p. 531.

95 Rosen, M. R., Hoffman, B. F., and Wit, A. L.: Electrophysiology and Pharmacology of Cardiac Arrhythmias: V. Cardiac Antiarrhythmic Effects of Lidocaine, 89:526, 1975.

96 Wit, A. L., Rosen, M. R., and Hoffman, B. F.: Electrophysiology and Pharmacology of Cardiac Arrhythmias: VIII. Cardiac Effects of Diphenylhydantoin, part A, *Am. Heart J.*, 90:265, 1975; part B, *Am. Heart J.*, 90:397, 1975.

97 Arnsdorf, M. F., Bigger, J. T., Jr.: Effect of Lidocaine Hydrochloride on Membrane Conductance in Mammalian Cardiac Purkinje Fibers, *J. Clin. Invest.*, 51:2252, 1972.

98 Weld, F. M., and Bigger, J. T., Jr.: The Effect of Lidocaine on Diastolic Transmembrane Currents Determining Pacemaker Depolarization in Cardiac Purkinje Fibers, *Circ. Res.*, 38:203, 1976.

99 Kabela, E.: The Effect of Lidocaine on Potassium Efflux from Various Tissues of Dog Heart, *J. Pharmacol. Exp.*, 184:611, 1973.

100 Bigger, J. T., Jr., and Mandel, W.: The Effect of Lidocaine on Conduction in Canine Purkinje Fibers and at the Ventricular Muscle–Purkinje Fiber Junction, *J. Pharmacol. Exp. Ther.*, 172:239, 1970.

101 Bigger, J. T., Jr., Bassett, A. L., and Hoffman, B. F.: Electrophysiological Effects of Diphenylhydantoin on Canine Purkinje Fibers, *Circ. Res.*, 22:221, 1968.

102 Strauss, H. C., Bigger, J. T., Jr., Bassett, A. L., and Hoffman, B. F.: Action of Diphenylhydantoin on the Electrical Properties of Isolated Rabbit and Canine Atria, *Circ. Res.*, 23:463, 1968.

103 Bigger, J. T., Jr.: Antiarrhythmic Drugs in Ischemic Heart Disease, *Hosp. Pract.*, 7:69, 1972.

104 Jensen, R. A., and Katzung, B. G.: Electrophysiological Actions of Diphenylhydantoin on Rabbit Atria: Dependence on Stimulation Frequency, Potassium and Sodium, *Circ. Res.*, 28:17, 1970.

105 Singh, B. N., and Vaughan Williams, E. M.: Effect of Altering Potassium Concentration on the Action of Lidocaine and Diphenylhydantoin on Rabbit Atrial and Ventricular Muscle, *Circ. Res.*, 29:286, 1971.

106 Bassett, A. L., Bigger, J. T., Jr., and Hoffman, B. F.: "Protective" Action of Diphenylhydantoin on Canine Purkinje Fibers During Hypoxia, *J. Pharmacol. Exp. Ther.*, 173:336, 1970.

107 Bigger, J. T., Jr., and Mandel, W.: The Effect of Lidocaine on the Electrophysiological Properties of Ventricular Muscle and Purkinje Fibers, *J. Clin. Invest.*, 49:63, 1970.

108 Davis, L. D., and Temte, J. V.: Electrophysiological Actions of Lidocaine on Canine Ventricular Muscle and Purkinje Fibers, *Circ. Res.*, 24:639, 1969.

109 Rosen, M. R., Merker, C., and Pippenger, C.: The Effects of Lidocaine on the Canine ECG and Electrophysiologic Properties of Purkinje Fibers, *Am. Heart J.*, 91:191, 1976.

110 Weld, F. M., and Bigger, J. T., Jr.: Effect of Lidocaine on the Early Inward Transient Current in Sheep Cardiac Purkinje Fibers, *Circ. Res.*, 37:630, 1975.

111 Lazzara, R., El-Sherif, N., Befeler, B., and Scherlag, B. J.: Lidocaine Action on Depressed Cardiac Cells, *Circulation*, 52(suppl. 2):85, 1975. (Abstract.)

112 Sasyniuk, B. I., and Kus, T.: Comparison of the Effects of Lidocaine on Electrophysiological Properties of Normal Purkinje Fibers and Those Surviving Acute Myocardial Infarction, *Fed. Proc.*, 33:476, 1974.

113 Evans, D. E., and Gillis, R. A.: Effect of Diphenylhydantoin and Lidocaine on Cardiac Arrhythmias Induced by Hypothalamic Stimulation, *J. Pharmacol. Exp. Ther.*, 191:506, 1974.

114 Chang, T. O., Wadhwa, K.: Sinus Standstill following Intravenous Lidocaine Administration, *J.A.M.A.*, 223:1973.

115 Roos, J. C., and Dunning, A. J.: Effects of Lidocaine on Impulse Formation and Conduction Defects in Man, *Am. Heart J.*, 89:686, 1975.

116 Gillis, R. A., McClellan, J. R., Sauer, T. S., and Standaert, F.

G.: Depression of Cardiac Sympathetic Nerve Activity by Diphenylhydantoin, *J. Pharmacol. Exp. Ther.*, 173:599, 1971.

117 Josephson, M. E., Caracta, A. R., Lau, S. H., Gallagher, J. J., and Damato, A. N.: Effects of Lidocaine on Refractory Periods in Man, *Am. Heart J.*, 84:778, 1972.

118 Kunkel, F., Rowland, M., and Scheinman, M. M.: The Electrophysiologic Effects of Lidocaine in Patients with Intraventricular Conduction Defects, *Circulation*, 49:894, 1974.

119 Damato, A. N.: Diphenylhydantoin: Pharmacological and Clinical Use, *Prog. Cardiovasc. Dis.*, 12:1, 1969.

120 Bissett, J. K., DeSoyza, N. D. B., Kane, J. J., and Doherty, J. E.: Effect of Diphenylhydantoin on Induced Aberrant Conduction, *J. Electrocardiol.*, 7:65, 1974.

121 Haiat, R., Chapelle, M., Benaim, R., Witchitz, S., and Chiche, P.: Effect of Diphenylhydantoin on Intraventricular Conduction Disturbance: Report of a Case, *J. Electrocardiol.*, 5:197, 1972.

122 Gupta, P. K., Lichstein, E., and Dhadda, K. D.: Lidocaine-induced Heart Block in Patients with Bundle Branch Block, *Am. J. Cardiol.*, 33:487, 1974.

123 Helfant, R. H., Ricciutti, M. A., Scherlag, B. J., and Damato, A. N.: Effect of Diphenylhydantoin Sodium (Dilantin) on Myocardial A-V Potassium Difference, *Am. J. Physiol.*, 214:880, 1968.

124 Bashkin, S. I., Dotta, S., and Marks, B. H.: The Effects of Diphenylhydantoin and Potassium on the Biological Activity of Ouabain in the Guinea Pig Heart, *Br. J. Pharmacol.*, 47:85, 1973.

125 Collinsworth, K. A., Kalman, S. M., and Harrison, D. C.: The Clinical Pharmacology of Lidocaine as an Antiarrhythmic Drug, *Circulation*, 50:1217, 1974.

126 Rowe, G. G., McKenna, D. H., Sailer, S., and Corliss, R. J.: Systemic and Coronary Hemodynamic Effects of Diphenylhydantoin, *Am. J. Med. Sci.*, 254:534, 1967.

127 Lieberson, A. D., Schumacher, R. R., Childress, R. H., et al.: Effect of Diphenylhydantoin on Left Ventricular Function in Patients with Heart Disease, *Circulation*, 36:692, 1967.

128 Louis, S., Kutt, H., and McDowell, F.: The Cardiocirculatory Changes Caused by Intravenous Dilantin and Its Solvent, *Am. Heart J.*, 74:523, 1967.

129 Benowitz, N. L.: Clinical Applications of the Pharmacokinetics of Lidocaine, *Cardiovas. Clin.*, 6(2):77, 1974.

130 Woodbury, D. M., and Fingle, E.: Drugs Effective in the Therapy of Epilepsies, in L. S. Goodman and A. Gilman (eds.), "The Pharmacological Basis of Therapeutics," 5th. ed., The Macmillan Company, New York, 1975, p. 204.

131 Gugler, R., Manion, C. V., and Azarnoff, D. L.: Phenytoin: Pharmacokinetics and Bioavailability, *Clin. Pharmacol. Ther.*, 19:135, 1976.

132 Gellerman, G. L., and Martinez, C.: Fatal Ventricular Fibrillation following Intravenous Sodium Diphenylhydantoin Therapy, *J.A.M.A.*, 200:337, 1967.

133 Monson, R. R., Rosenberg, L., Hartz, S. C., et al.: Diphenylhydantoin and Selected Congential Malformation, *N. Engl. J. Med.*, 289:1049, 1973.

134 Bigger, J. T., Jr., Schmidt, D. H., and Kutt, H.: Relationship between the Plasma Level of Diphenylhydantoin Sodium and Its Cardiac Antiarrhythmic Effects, *Circulation*, 38:363, 1968.

135 Alderman, E. L., Kerber, R. E., and Harrison, D. C.: Evaluation of Lidocaine Resistance in Man Using Intermittent Large Dose Infusion Techniques, *Am. J. Cardiol.*, 34:342, 1974.

136 Pantridge, J. F., and Geddes, J. S.: Primary Ventricular Fibrillation, *Eur. J. Cardiol.*, 1:335, 1974.

137 Rosen, K. M., Barwolf, C., Eshani, A., and Rahimtoola, S. H.: Effects of Lidocaine and Propranolol on the Normal and

Anomalous Pathways in Patients with Preexcitation, *Am. J. Cardiol.*, 30:801, 1972.

138 Karlsson, E.: Procainamide and Phenytoin: Comparative Study of Their Antiarrhythmic Effects at Apparent Therapeutic Plasma Levels, *Br. Heart J.*, 37:731, 1975.

139 Karlsson, E., Collste, P., and Rawlins, M. D.: Plasma Levels of Lidocaine during Combined Treatment with Phenytoin and Procainamide, *Eur. J. Clin. Pharmacol.*, 7:455, 1974.

140 Wit, A. L., Hoffman, B. F., and Rosen, M. R.: Electrophysiology and Pharmacology of Cardiac Arrhythmias: IX. Cardiac Electrophysiologic Effects of Beta Adrenergic Receptor Stimulation and Blockade, part A, *Am. Heart J.*, 90:521, 1975.

141 Wit, A. L., Hoffman, B. F., and Rosen, M. R.: Electrophysiology and Pharmacology of Cardiac Arrhythmias: IX. Cardiac Electrophysiologic Effects of Beta Adrenergic Receptor Stimulation and Blockade, part B, *Am Heart J.*, 90:665, 1975.

142 Wit, A. L., Hoffman, B. F., and Rosen, M. R.: Electrophysiology and Pharmacology of Cardiac Arrhythmias: IX. Cardiac Electrophysiologic Effects of Beta Adrenergic Receptor Stimulation and Blockade, part C, *Am. Heart J.*, 90:795, 1975.

143 Abrams, W. B., and Davies, R. O.: The Antiarrhythmic Mechanisms of Beta-adrenergic Blocking Agents, in L. S. Dreifus and W. Likoff, (eds.), "Cardiac Arrhythmias," Grune & Stratton, Inc., New York, 1973, p. 517.

143a Conolly, M. E., Kersting, F., and Dollery, C.: The Clinical Pharmacology of Beta-Adrenoceptor Blocking Drugs, *Progr. Cardiovasc. Dis.*, 19:203, 1976.

144 Davis, L. D., and Temte, J. V.: Effects of Propranolol on the Transmembrane Potentials of Ventricular Muscle and Purkinje Fibers of the Dog, *Circ. Res.*, 22:661, 1968.

145 Tarr, M., Luckstead, E. F., Jurewicz, P. A., and Haas, H. G.: Effect of Propranolol on the Fast Inward Sodium Current in Frog Atrial Muscle, *J. Pharmoacol. Exp. Ther.*, 184:599, 1973.

146 Choi, S. J., Roberts, J., and Kelliher, G. J.: The Effect of Propranolol and Quinidine on ^{22}Na- and ^{42}K- Exchange in the Cat Papillary Muscle, *Eur. J. Pharmacol.*, 20:20, 1972.

147 Stagg, A. L., Wallace, A. G.: The Effect of Propranolol on Membrane Conductance in Canine Cardiac Purkinje Fibers, *Circulation*, 50(suppl. 3):145, 1974. (Abstract.)

148 Seides, S. F., Josephson, M. E., Batsford, W. P., Weisfogel, G. M., Lau, S. H., and Damato, A. N.: The Electrophysiology of Propranolol in Man, *Am. Heart J.*, 88:733, 1974.

149 Wit, A. L., and Cranefield, P. F.: Triggered Activity in Cardiac Muscle Fibers of the Simian Mitral Valve, *Circ. Res.*, 38:85, 1976.

150 Berkowitz, W. D., Wit, A. L., Lau, S. H., Steiner, C., and Damato, A. N.: The Effects of Propranolol on Cardiac Conduction, *Circulation*, 40:855, 1969.

151 Smithen, C. S., Balcon, R., and Sowton, E.: Use of Bundle of His Potentials to Assess Changes in Atrioventricular Conduction Produced by a Series of Beta-Adrenergic Blocking Agents, *Br. Heart J.*, 33:955, 1971.

152 Pelides, L. J., Reid, D. S., Thomas, P., and Shillinford, J. P.: Inhibition by β-blockade of the ST Segment Elevation after Acute Myocardial Infarction in Man, *Cardiovasc. Res.*, 6:255, 1972.

153 Solo, H. K., Leinbach, R. C., and Maroko, P. R.: Reduction of Myocardial Injury in Patients with Acute Infarction by Propranolol, *Circulation*, 48(suppl. 3):33, 1974. (Abstract.)

154 Maroko, P. R., and Braunwald, E.: Effects of Metabolic and Pharmacologic Interventions on Myocardial Infarct Size following Coronary Occlusion, in E. Braunwald (ed.), Protection of the Ischemic Myocardium: V. Assessment of Interventions Designed to Reduce Myocardial Infarct Size following Coronary Occlusion, *Circulation*, 53(suppl. 1):162, 1976.

155 Maroko, P. R., Kjehshiis, J. K., Sobel, B. E., Wantanabe, Y.,

et al.: Factors influencing Infarct Size following Experimental Coronary Occlusions, *Circulation*, 43:67, 1971.

156 Gettes, L. W.: Beta-adrenergic Blocking Drugs in the Treatment of Cardiac Arrhythmias, *Cardiovasc. Clin.*, 2:211, 1970.

157 Wu, D., Denes, P., Dhingra, R., et al.: The Effect of Propranolol on Induction of A-V Nodal Reentrant Paroxysmal Tachycardia, *Circulation*, 50:665, 1974.

158 Shand, D. G.: Drug Therapy: Propranolol, *N. Engl. J. Med.*, 293:280, 1975.

159 Wilhelmson, C., Vedin, J. A., Wilhelsen, L., Tibblin, G., and Werkö, L.: Reduction of Sudden Deaths after Myocardial Infarction by Treatment with Alprenolol, *Lancet*, 2:1157, 1974.

160 A Multicentre International Study: Improvement in Prognosis of Myocardial Infarction by Long-Term Beta-Adrenoreceptor Blockade Using Practolol, *Br. Med., J.*, 3:735, 1975.

160a Moss, A. J., DeCamilla, J. J., Davis, H. P., and Bayer, L.: Clinical Significance of Ventricular Ectopic Beats in the Posthospital Phase of Myocardial Infarction, *Am. J. Cardiol.*, 39:635, 1977.

160b Lown, B., and Graboys, T. B.: Management of Patients with Malignant Ventricular Arrhythmias, *Am. J. Cardiol.*, 39:910, 1977.

160c Fasola, A., Noble, R. J., and Zipes, D. P.: Treatment of Recurrent Ventricular Tachycardia and Fibrillation with Aprindine, *Am. J. Cardiol.*, 39:903, 1977.

161 National Conference Steering Committee: Standards for Cardiopulmonary Resuscitation (CPR) and Emergency Cardiac Care (ECC), *J.A.M.A.*, 227:837, 1974.

162 Nies, A. S., and Shand, D. G.: Clinical Pharmacology of Propranolol, *Circulation*, 52:6, 1975.

163 Alderman, E. L., Coltart, D. J., Wettach, G. E., and Harrison, D. C.: Coronary Artery Syndrome after Sudden Propranolol Withdrawal, *Ann. Intern. Med.*, 81:624, 1974.

164 Wit, A. L., Steiner, C., and Damato, A. N.: Electrophysiologic Effects of Bretylium Tosylate on Single Fibers of the Canine Specialized Conducting System and Ventricle, *J. Pharmacol. Exp. Ther.*, 173:334, 1970.

165 Bigger, J. T., Jr., and Jaffe, C.: The Effect of Bretylium Tosylate on the Electrophysiologic Properties of Ventricular Muscle and Purkinje Fibers, *Am. J. Cardiol.*, 27:82, 1971.

166 Bacaner, M.: Quantitative Comparison of Bretylium with Other Antifibrillatory Drugs, *Am. J. Cardiol.*, 21:504, 1968.

167 Bacaner, M. R.: Treatment of Ventricular Fibrillation and Other Acute Arrhythmias with Bretylium Tosylate, *Am. J. Cardiol.*, 21:530, 1968.

167a Holder, A. A., Sniderman, A. D., Fraser, G., and Fallen, E. L.: Experience with Bretylium Tosylate by a Cardiac Arrest Team, *Circulation*, 55:541, 1977.

168 Rosen, M. R., Wit, A. L., and Hoffman, B. F.: Electrophysiology and Pharmacology of Cardiac Arrhythmias: VI. Cardiac Effects of Verapamil, *Am. Heart J.*, 89:665, 1975.

169 Cranefield, P. F., Aronson, R. S., and Wit, A. L.: Effect of Verapamil on the Normal Action Potential and on a Calcium-dependent Slow Response of Canine Cardiac Purkinje Fibers, *Circ. Res.*, 34:204, 1974.

170 Singh, B. N., Vaughan Williams, E. M.: Fourth Class of Antidysrhythmic Action? Effect of Verapamil on Ouabain Toxicity, on Atrial and Ventricular Intracellular Potentials and on Other Features of Cardiac Function, *Cardiovasc. Res.*, 6:109, 1972.

171 Husaini, M. H., Kvasnicka, J., Ryden, L., and Holmberg, S.: Action of Verapamil in Sinus Node, Atrioventricular and Intraventricular Conduction, *Br. Heart J.*, 35:734, 1973.

171a Reimer, K. A., Lowe, J. E., and Jennings, R. B.: Effect of the Calcium Antagonist Verapamil on Necrosis Following Temporary Coronary Artery Occlusion in Dogs, *Circulation*, 55:581, 1977.

172 Schamroth, L., Krikler, D. M., and Garret, C.: Immediate Effects of Intravenous Verapamil in Cardiac Arrhythmias, *Br. Med. J.*, 1:660, 1972.

173 Heng, M. K., Singh, B. N., Roche, A. H. G., Norris, R. M., and Mercer, C. J.: Effects of Intravenous Verapamil on Cardiac Arrhythmias and on the Electrocardiogram, *Am. Heart J.*, 90:487, 1975.

174 Spurrell, R. A., Krikler, D. M., and Sowton, G. E.: The Effects of Verapamil on the Electrophysiological Properties of the Anomalous Atrioventricular Connexions in Wolff-Parkinson-White Syndrome, *Br. Heart J.*, 36:256, 1974.

175 Singh, B. N., and Roche, A. G. H.: Hemodynamic Effects of Intravenous Verapamil in Patients with Cardiac Disease, quoted in Heng et al., Effects of Intravenous Verapamil on Cardiac Arrhythmias and on the Electrocardiogram, *Am. Heart J.*, 90:487, 1975.

176 Donnelly, G. L., and Scamps, P.: Intravenous Verapamil in Cardiac Arrhythmias, *Aust. N.Z. J. Med.*, 3:63, 1973.

177 Benaim, M. E.: Asystole after Verapamil, *Br. Med. J.*, 21:169, 1972.

178 Boothby, C. B., Garrard, C. S., and Pickering, D.: Intravenous Verapamil in Cardiac arrhythmias, *Br. Med. J.*, 2:349, 1972.

179 Sacks, H., and Kennelly, B. M.: Verapamil in Cardiac Arrhythmias, *Br. Med. J.*, 2:716, 1972.

180 Hills, E. A.: Effects of Verapamil on Airways Resistance in Patients with Bronchial Asthma, *Br. J. Clin. Pract.*, 24:116, 1970.

181 Lown, B., Verrier, R. L., and Rabinowitz, S. H.: Neural and Psychological Mechanisms and the Problem of Sudden Cardiac Death, *Am. J. Cardiol.*, 39:890, 1977.

181a Estes, E. H., Jr., and Izlar, H. L., Jr.: Recurrent Ventricular Tachycardia: A Case Successfully Treated by Bilateral Cardiac Sympathectomy, *Am. J. Med.*, 31:493, 1961.

182 Ecker, R. R., Mullins, D. V., Grammer, J. C., et al.: Control of Intractable Ventricular Tachycardia by Coronary Revascularization, *Circulation*, 44:666, 1971.

183 Graham, A. F., Miller, D. C., Stinson, E. B., et al.: Surgical Treatment of Refractory Life-threatening Ventricular Tachycardia, *Am. J. Cardiol.*, 32:909, 1973.

184 Winkle, R. A., Alderman, E. L., Fitzgerald, J. W., and Harrison, D. C.: Treatment of Recurrent Symptomatic Ventricular Tachycardia, *Ann. Intern. Med.*, 85:1, 1976.

185 Dreifus, L. S., Nichols, H., Morse, D., Wantanabe, Y., and Truex, R.: Control of Recurrent Tachycardia of Wolff-Parkinson-White Syndrome by Surgical Ligature of the A-V Bundle, *Circulation*, 38:1030, 1968.

186 Sealy, W. C., and Wallace, A. G.: Surgical Treatment of Wolff-Parkinson-White Syndrome, *J. Thorac. Cardiovasc. Surg.*, 68:757, 1974.

187 Wallace, A. G., Sealy, W. C., Gallagher, I., Svenson, R. H., Strauss, H. C., and Kasell, J.: Surgical Correction of Anomalous Left Ventricular Preexcitation: Wolff-Parkinson-White (Type A), *Circulation*, 49:206, 1974.

188 Arnsdorf, M. F., Rothbaum, D. A., and Childers, R. W.: The Effect of Direct Current Countershock on Atrial and Ventricular Properties and Myocardial Potassium Efflux in the Thoracotomised Dog, *Cardiovasc. Res.*, in press.

C
Cardiac Glycosides, Theophylline, Morphine, and Vasodilators

YEN-YAU HSIEH, M.D.,

LEON I. GOLDBERG, M.D., Ph.D., and

MORTON F. ARNSDORF, M.D.

CARDIAC GLYCOSIDES

Cardiac glycosides are found in a large number of plants. The most commonly used preparations are obtained from *Digitalis purpurea* (digitoxin, gitalin, digitalis leaf, U.S.P.), *D. lanata* (lanatoside C, digoxin), and *Strophanthus gratus* (strophanthin, ouabain). In addition, cardiac glycosides are present in the venom from skin glands of toads; these glycosides contain a six-membered lactone ring.[1-3]

All cardioactive glycosides have two major constituents: an aglycone (genin), a steroid structure to which is attached either a five- or six-membered lactone ring, and several sugar molecules (three for commonly used digitoxin, digoxin, and lanatoside C). The aglycone is essential for the pharmacologic activity, while the particular sugar attached to the aglycone determines the water solubility, cell permeability, and potency of the glycosides.[1-3]

Increased myocardial contractility (increased contractile force, positive inotropic effect)[1-4]

The positive inotropic effect is due to direct action of cardiac glycosides on myocardial cells and can be demonstrated in the denervated heart, the heart devoid of catecholamines,[4a] and the failing as well as the nonfailing heart.[5]

The mechanism responsible for the postitive inotropic action of cardiac glycosides has not been fully defined. Calcium ions apparently play a central role. Many interesting studies have demonstrated the effects of cardiac glycosides on Ca^{2+} flux as well as on the uptake and release of Ca^{2+} from subcellular structures. The relation between this effect and positive inotropism, however, has not been definitely established.[6-8] In this regard, data have been presented suggesting that the positive inotropic effect and the inhibition of Na^+,K^+-ATPase may be independent phenomena.[9]

Autonomic nervous system actions[10-12]

Recent studies with the denervated human heart have confirmed previous observations in animals indicating that the indirect actions of digitalis on the sympathetic and parasympathetic nervous system influence its pharmacologic actions. Digitalis augments vagal activity by both central stimulation of the vagus nerve and by sensitization of cardiac cells to the action of acetylcholine. The effects of cardiac glycosides on the sympathetic nervous system is more complex. Low doses of digitalis increase the sensitivity of carotid sinus baroreceptors, thus enhancing vagal tone and reducing sympathetic activity. Large doses of digitalis increase central sympathetic outflow and may release endogenous catecholamines.

Electrophysiologic effects

Although great effort has been devoted to investigating the cardiac effects of digitalis, at many points the inferential links between basic cellular theory and the situation in vivo are quite tenuous. This results from gaps in our basic biochemical and electrophysiologic knowledge, the balance at any given time between the multiple direct and indirect effects of digitalis, and the presence of modifying factors. In the isolated preparation, it is often unclear whether an observed action is "therapeutic" or "toxic." For the sake of convenience, the electrophysiologic effects will be divided into therapeutic and toxic, but the distinction is often uncertain.

THERAPEUTIC

Sinoatrial (SA) node The direct effect of digitalis in therapeutic concentrations on the SA node is minimal.[11,12] The slowing of sinus rate by digitalis in the innervated heart is mainly mediated through vagal effect and withdrawal of sympathetic tone. The latter effect is especially prominent in the failing heart after hemodynamic improvement. Reduced response to adrenergic stimulation may also play a role.[4,5,10-12]

Atrial tissues The direct effects of digitalis on atrial myocardial and specialized conducting cells include a less negative resting transmembrane voltage (V_r), a decreased maximal rate of rise of phase 0 of the I_{Na}-dependent action potential ($\dot{V}_{max}$), depressed conduction velocity, and a prolonged effective refractory period (ERP). Whether these effects occur at therapeutic or toxic concentrations is uncertain. The drug-induced vagotonia and increased "sensitivity" of atrial tissues to acetylcholine may have counterbalancing effects.[13] Acetylcholine increases membrane potassium conductance.[14] An increase in the repolarizing outward K^+ current would make V_r more negative if the tissue had been initially depolarized by injury or as a result of the direct digitalis effect. This, in turn, would decrease sodium inactivation, resulting in a more rapid $\dot{V}_{max}$ and conduction velocity. The net result may be no significant changes, or a shortening in ERP and enhancement of intraatrial conduction.[13] This effect is responsible for the clinically observed increase in atrial rate in patients with atrial flutter or fibrillation after digitalization. In addition, vagal stimulation may enhance temporal dispersion in atrial repolarization, thereby favoring the development of atrial fibrillation or conversion of atrial flutter to fibrillation.[10,15] In the denervated, transplanted heart, digitalis tends to convert atrial flutter to sinus rhythm; in the innervated heart, atrial fibrillation may be reverted to sinus rhythm.[11,12] In one study of 14 patients with the "sick sinus" syndrome, therapeutic doses of digitalis shorten the SA recovery time and prolong the atrio-His interval without significantly affecting the sinus rate.[16]

Atrioventricular node Digitalis impedes conduction through the atrioventricular (AV) node. This results from a drug-induced decrease in conduction velocity and a prolongation in both the effective and functional refractory periods. Since these actions occur at drug concentrations having little effect on the AV node action potential, the primary mechanism seems to be an alteration in autonomic activity.[17] In the denervated, transplanted heart, therapeutic digitalis concentrations cause only insignificant prolongation of the effective and functional refractory periods.[18] At high concentrations, digitalis may decrease $\dot{V}_{max}$, make the maximum diastolic transmembrane voltage less negative, induce a time-dependent prolongation of the refractory period, and further depress conduction.[13]

Anomalous atrioventricular pathways Although digitalis prolongs the ERP of normal AV node conduction, it shortens the ERP in the anomalous AV pathways. Administration of digitalis to patients with the Wolff-Parkinson-White syndrome may preferentially facilitate conduction through the anomalous pathway, resulting in potentially catastrophic ventricular response during atrial fibrillation.[19,20]

Purkinje fibers and ventricular muscle Digitalis in low concentrations appears to decrease membrane K^+ conductance, resulting in a small and somewhat variable prolongation of the voltage-time course of repolarization. Prolonged perfusion or higher concentrations increase membrane K^+ conductance and accelerate repolarization.[21] The latter effect has recently been considered a toxic rather than a therapeutic effect.[13] The refractoriness of His-Purkinje conduction is not altered by therapeutic doses of digitalis.[22] Rosen et al. correlated the electrophysiologic changes in isolated canine Purkinje fibers superfused with blood obtained from an intact dog with the electrocardiographic changes recorded in that dog during the course of ouabain administration.[23] They found that the prolongation of the action potential duration in the isolated Purkinje fiber correlated with the relevant electrocardiographic ST-T wave changes.

TOXIC

Automaticity Enhanced automaticity, nondriven rhythmic activity, oscillations, and other unusual membrane phenomena have been observed in isolated atrial, Purkinje, and ventricular preparations exposed to high concentrations of digitalis.[13,24-27] Nondriven activity and oscillations of this type have been termed low-amplitude potentials, enhanced diastolic depolarizations, transient depolarizations, after hyperpolarizations, and after depolarizations. Four mechanisms have been inferred on the basis of studies in Purkinje fibers: (1) Aronson et al. suggested that ouabain enhances automatic activity by decreasing the magnitude of the outward repolarizing current, I_{K_2} (for the meaning of this and subsequent currents, see Chap. 109B), without affecting its voltage dependence for activation[28]; (2) Isenberg and Trautwein found ouabain reduced the time-dependent outward current which they attributed to a blockade of electrogenic sodium pumping[29]; (3) alterations in slow inward current, I_{si}, have been suggested by Cranefield[27]; and (4) digitalis induces or enhances a depolarizing transient inward current, I_{ti}.[24]

Digitalis does not seem to affect I_{si},[24,30] except perhaps indirectly by increasing intracellular calcium ion concentrations, $[Ca^{2+}]_i$. Intracellular uncoupling and steady contracture as manifestations of digitalis toxicity have been attributed to an increased $[Ca^{2+}]_i$.[31,32]

Recent voltage clamp studies indicated that enhanced automaticity after digitalis administration is dominated by I_{ti}.[24,25] The ionic mechanism of this current is unclear. This current normally is absent or very small in preparations not exposed to digitalis, and, on the basis of kinetic studies, is quite distinct from I_{K_2} and differs from I_{si} in its voltage dependence.[24] Digitalis-induced transient depolarizations may reflect phasic I_{ti} activity.

The contrasting properties of I_{K_2} may explain, in part, the differences between automatic activity not related to digitalis and digitalis-induced transient depolarizations after repetitive drive. Repetitive stimulation depresses automaticity of the first type probably by activation of electrogenic sodium transport or extracellular potassium accumulation,[13,33] which in the intact animal or human being would be analogous to "overdrive suppression." In contrast, digitalis-induced acceleration of spontaneous activity may follow repetitive depolarization.[26,34-36] In the isolated preparation, the amplitude of the transient depolarizations are increased by driving the preparations more rapidly.[36] Of interest is that successive depolarizations additively induce I_{ti}.[24]

Alterations in impulse propagation In toxic concentrations, digitalis makes V_r less negative, decreases $\dot{V}_{max}$ as well as the action potential amplitude, and slows conduction velocity.[13] Rosen et al. investigated Purkinje fiber properties as the isolated preparation was bathed in blood from an electrocardiographically monitored dog.[23] During ouabain infusion, they found their indices of sodium conductance ($\dot{V}_{max}$ and action potential amplitude) to be severely depressed at the time ventricular tachyarrhythmias appeared on the ECG. The situation conducive to reentry existed, but enhanced automaticity of the type described above may also have been present. Moreover, enhanced automaticity in itself may depolarize segments of cardiac tissue, thereby increasing the liability to decreased conduction velocity, unidirectional block, and reentry.

Indirect effects The autonomic effects of digitalis have already been discussed. The vagal and antiadrenergic effects may further suppress sinus pacemaker activity and decrease AV nodal conduction at the same time that the direct toxic effects of digitalis are present. On the other hand, it has been demonstrated in animals that large doses of digitalis excite the central nervous system, resulting in enhanced sympathetic outflow and cardiac arrhythmias.[11] Catecholamines are known to enhance I_{si},[27] and it is interesting to speculate whether catecholamines may influence I_{ti} as well. Acid-base imbalance, hypoxia, electrolyte disturbances, and the like also have arrhythmogenic potential and may facilitate the appearance of digitalis-induced electrophysiologic toxicity.

Digitalis and potassium Hypokalemia facilitates and hyperkalemia suppresses digitalis-induced arrhythmias. Increasing extracellular potassium ion concentrations, $[K^+]_o$, has several effects, including the direct suppression of slow diastolic depolarization,[37] an increase in membrane K^+ conductance,[38,39] a decrease in excitability,[39] and an increase in the capacity of the membrane to transport K^+ and Na^+.[37] These direct cellular effects of increased $[K^+]_o$ might be expected to counteract the "toxic" effects of digitalis.

Effects on blood vessels

ARTERIES

Direct injection of cardiac glycosides into perfused arteries produces vasoconstriction.[40] This vasoconstriction may explain in part the increase in blood pressure which sometimes occurs following intravenous administration of large doses of cardiac glycosides to experimental animals and human beings.[41,42] Studies in human beings during cardiopulmonary bypass procedures have shown that the arterial vasoconstriction is an immediate and transient phenomenon in contrast to the slowly developing and prolonged positive inotropic effects.[5] Vasoconstriction with possible increase in left ventricular end-diastolic pressure is most likely to occur after rapid intravenous injection of cardiac glycosides.[42,43] Mesenteric blood flow is decreased after administration of digitalis to patients without heart failure.[44] In patients with congestive heart failure, mesenteric blood flow may remain unchanged or even decrease despite hemodynamic improvement by digitalis.[45] Vasocon-

striction has been observed in coronary arteries of dogs,[46] but the clinical occurrence and significance of coronary vasoconstriction are difficult to determine.

VEINS

Effects of digitalis on the venous system has been the subject of considerable controversy. Plethysmographic techniques have shown that venous constriction is produced in normal subjects by cardiac glycosides.[47] In patients with congestive heart failure, however, cardiac glycosides produce venous dilation because of decreased sympathetic activity resulting from improvements in hemodynamic status.[4]

Studies in the dog have demonstrated that cardiac glycosides cause constriction of the hepatic vein with resulting pooling of blood in the splanchnic regions,[48] and there is a possibility that this effect also occurs in the human being.[49] Investigations during cardiopulmonary bypass have also demonstrated an increase in the capacity of the vascular system after administration of cardiac glycosides.[50] However, the site of the venous dilation has not been determined.

Effects of cardiac glycosides on the intact heart and circulation

Cardiac glycosides increase cardiac output in most patients with congestive heart failure.[47,51,52] In contrast, the cardiac output of normal subjects usually either does not change or may even decrease after administration of cardiac glycosides, despite an increase in myocardial contractility. This apparent paradox is related to the effects of cardiac glycosides to reduce heart rate, increase peripheral vascular resistance, and reduce venous return in normal subjects.[4,6,47]

Although the positive inotropic effects of cardiac glycosides increase myocardial oxygen requirements, myocardial oxygen consumption of the failing heart may be reduced because of the secondary effects of reduction in heart size, ventricular filling pressure, heart rate, and peripheral vascular resistance.[4,6,53,54]

Electrocardiographic changes of digitalization

The earliest and most frequently observed ECG changes of digitalization consist of a sagging or depressed ST segment along with either an inversion of the initial portion of the T wave or lowering of the amplitude of the T wave. Except in lead aV_R the ST segment has an appearance of downward concavity or straight line. In the absence of hypokalemia, the amplitude of the U wave may be increased, resulting in what may appear to be "notched" T waves.[55] This notching may give the appearance of a prolonged Q-T interval, while in reality the interval is actually decreased. The Q-T interval is shortened because digitalis abbreviates the duration of the ventricular muscle action potential and its refractory period.[55a] The P-R interval may be prolonged late in the course of digitalization but seldom exceeds 0.25 s except in the presence of preexisting pathology of the AV conduction system. The ST-T wave changes may appear as early as 2 to 4 h following digitalization and may not disappear for 2 to 4 weeks after the drug has been discontinued.[55]

The "secondary" type of T wave change may occur in the heavily digitalized patients, but the symmetrically inverted T waves never result from digitalis effect alone.[55] Digitalis may produce false positive ST-T wave changes in patients performing the exercise test.[56]

The ST-T wave changes described above appear to have no correlation with the occurrence of digitalis toxicity or therapeutic effect.[55] However, marked ST segment sagging associated with variable degrees of P-R interval prolongation or with prominent reduction of T wave amplitude tends to reflect high serum digitalis concentrations.[57,58]

Specific glycosides

DIGITOXIN

Digitoxin, a nonpolar, lipid-soluble compound, is rapidly and completely absorbed from the gastrointestinal tract under normal conditions.[6,59,60] However, absorption may be incomplete in the presence of congestive heart failure and various malabsorption states.[61,62] The relative bioavailability as tested on two commercial preparations showed no statistical difference, but a significant difference in peak plasma levels did exist.[63]

Digitoxin is 97 percent bound to plasma protein,[64] with 26 percent entering the enterohepatic circulation.[59] Peak plasma concentration is reached within $^1/_2$ to 3 h after oral intake. Distribution is almost complete at 6 h.[64] The plasma concentration has no definite correlation to age, but is correlated to body weight.[62] Deposition in fetal tissue may occur since digitoxin is able to cross the placental barrier.[65]

Approximately 10 percent of the body pool of digitoxin is eliminated daily. The major metabolic pathway of digitoxin is cleavage of the side chain to yield the cardioactive, but less potent, digitoxigenin bisdigitoxoside, digitoxigenin monodigitoxoside, and digitoxigenin. Further degradation of digitoxigenin to epidigitoxigenin and the alternative metabolic product, dihydrodigitoxin, causes marked loss of activity.[59,64,66–68] About 8 percent of a dose is β-hydroxylated at C-12 to digoxin by the hepatic microsomal enzymes. Only a small amount (8 percent each) is excreted unchanged in urine and feces. Between 60 and 80 percent of the total dose is excreted in urine as the metabolites and in the unchanged form over a period of 3 weeks.[69,70] A recent study revealed excretion of 22 percent in urine and 13 percent in feces within 8 days, with 60 percent of the amount excreted in urine found as the parent compound.[70a]

The elimination of digitoxin follows first-order kinetics.[61,66] The plasma half-life ($T^1/_2$) determined by the double isotope dilution method ranges from 4.4 to 5.9 days, with a mean of 4.8 days.[64] Measurement made by the modified ^{86}Rb uptake inhibition technique, which measures the total biologic activity of digitoxin and its active metabolites, reveals a plasma $T^1/_2$ of 8.1 days, with a range varying between 5.9 to 11.3 days.[61]

DIGOXIN

Digoxin (12-β-hydroxydigitoxin), is a water-soluble, polar compound because of the presence of a hydroxyl group at the C-12 position. Unlike digitoxin, digoxin is incompletely absorbed from the gastrointestinal tract, and wide variations in absorption rate and bioavailability have been demonstrated in different pharmaceutical preparations. Digoxin solution is better absorbed than the conventional tablet. However, there is little difference between the solution and recently developed tablets which have dissolution rates faster than 70 percent at 1 h because of the limiting factor of uptake by the intestinal mucosa.[69,71,72]

The absolute bioavailability of currently marketed digoxin solutions ranges between 65 to 85 percent.[72] The relative bioavailability of conventional tablets ranges from 47 to 77 percent of that of solutions, with a mean of 62 percent.[71] The bioavailability of both digoxin tablets and solutions has been improved recently by altering the formulation. A new preparation consisting of encapsulated solution may yield a bioavailability approaching that obtained by the intravenous route.[72]

After oral administration of conventional digoxin tablets, plasma concentrations are detectable within 30 min, maximum levels occur between 30 and 60 min, and a plateau is observed within 6 h.[73] Postprandial ingestion of digoxin tablets delay the peak time for an average of 45 min without significantly affecting the total bioavailability and peak plasma concentration. Digoxin elixir is not influenced by food.[74] The pharmacologic effects of digoxin occur 15 to 30 min after intravenous injection and reach a peak within 1 to 5 h.[3]

The plasma protein binding of digoxin is 25 percent or less.[75,76] Only 6.8 percent of the administered dose enters the enterohepatic circulation.[77] Fifteen percent is biotransformed to the cardioactive digoxigenin and its monodigitoxosides and bisdigitoxosides, and a small amount of the relatively inactive epidigoxigenin and dihydrodigoxin.[68–70,78] Eighty percent is eliminated through the kidney with 98 percent of that percentage in the unchanged form. The remaining 20 percent is excreted by the biliary-fecal route, half being the parent compound.

Digoxin is eliminated mainly by glomerular filtration; thus renal digoxin clearance should be related to endogenous creatinine clearance.[69] However, recent studies have demonstrated that renal digoxin clearance is greater than inulin clearance[79] and correlates better with urea clearance than with creatinine clearance.[80] Therefore, the possibility of renal tubular secretion and reabsorption has been raised.[79,80] At high urine flow rate (greater than 1.5 ml/min) the renal excretion of digoxin is independent of urine flow,[81] while at low urine flow rate (less than 1 ml/min) it is proportionally related to urine output.[80]

The plasma $T^{1/2}$ of digoxin ranges between 33 and 44 h.[69,82,83] The volume of distribution at steady-state (Vd_{ss}) ranges from 420 to 1,026 liters, with a mean of 590 liters.[82] The blood concentration of digoxin is higher and the $T^{1/2}$ longer in the elderly subject because of smaller muscle mass and diminished renal excretion.[84] The blood digoxin concentration of overweight, obese patients given the usual dose of digoxin is not different from that of subjects with normal weight, because adipose tissue binds little digoxin.[85]

Clinical uses

HEART FAILURE

Digitalis is indicated in all forms of heart failure but is most effective in those due to hypertensive, rheumatic, or congenital heart diseases without primary myocardial disease. It is also effective in treating heart failure of chronic ischemic heart disease. Digitalis is relatively ineffective in the treatment of heart failure associated with high cardiac output, such as thyrotoxicosis, anemia, arteriovenous fistula, beriberi heart disease, and acute glomerulonephritis. Heart failure due to obstructive lesions such as mitral or aortic stenosis with sinus rhythm or due to cardiomyopathy responds poorly to digitalis therapy.[4,86,87] Digitalis must be used with caution in patients with idiopathic hypertrophic subaortic stenosis complicated with heart failure, since it may increase the obstructive gradient.[87a]

CARDIAC ARRHYTHMIAS

Digitalis alone, or in combination with other antiarrhythmic drugs, is very useful for the treatment and prevention of paroxysmal supraventricular tachycardia.[88,89] It is also indicated in treating atrial fibrillation or flutter with rapid ventricular rate. Chronic atrial fibrillation or flutter is seldom reverted to sinus rhythm, but the ventricular rate may be reduced by increased concealed conduction into the AV node, decreased conduction velocity, and prolonged ERP of the AV node[3,13] (see also Chap. 109-B).

DIGITALIS BLOOD LEVELS AND PRINCIPLES OF DIGITALIZATION

Radioimmunoassays of digoxin and digitoxin are now widely used in clinical cardiology. The assay is of value in determining prior digitalization and compliance, and for assessing digitalis arrhythmias. Its use as a guide for the therapeutic effect of cardiac glycosides is controversial.[90,91] Although therapeutic serum or plasma concentrations of digitoxin are usually considered to range between 14 and 26 ng/ml and those of digoxin between 0.8 and 1.6 ng/ml,[3,69,87,92,93] there is considerable overlap between therapeutic and toxic levels.[92,94,95] Although some studies[96,97] showed rather consistent serum/atrial digoxin ratio (1:24) and serum/papillary muscle digoxin ratio (1:67), other reports demonstrated no simple relationship[98] or no significant correlation.[99] In the presence of myocardial ischemia, the serum digoxin concentration may not reflect the myocardial digoxin content.[100]

Other problems of assay methods require caution. First, a survey of 11 commercial digoxin radioimmunoassay kits revealed wide variations in precision and accuracy.[101] Second, the specificity of digoxin antiserum is not perfect; cross reactivity with digitoxin, spironolactone, and steroid hormones may occur.[102]

The recommended doses of digitalis found in textbooks and monographs vary considerably.[103] The data given here are to provide the reader with a starting point with the understanding that the data may be subject to modification in individuals receiving different pharmaceutical preparations and in variable clinical situations.

The administration of digitalis has been traditionally divided into rapid and slow methods. Rapid digitalization may be achieved by administering a loading dose, e.g., 0.5 to 1.0 mg digoxin given intravenously or 1.0 to 1.5 mg orally, in suitably divided doses and at appropriate intervals, depending on the urgency of clinical situations. A common practice is to give one-half of the loading dose initially and the remainder divided into two equal doses with 6-h intervals. This mode of administration is frequently used to treat severe congestive heart failure or paroxysmal supraventricular tachycardia. Slow digitalization may be started by giving an oral maintenance dose of 0.125 to 0.5 mg (usually 0.25 mg) digoxin without a loading dose. A steady state is reached after 7 days (five cycles of $T^{1/2}$). Slow digitalization, while requiring more time for optimal therapeutic effect, incurs less risk of digitalis intoxication. The average oral loading and maintenance doses of digitoxin are 1.2 to 1.6 mg and 0.05 to 0.2 mg, respectively.[3] Due to the long $T^{1/2}$ of digitoxin, slow digitalization without a loading dose is not practical.

Intramuscular injection of digoxin is not recommended, because it is erratically absorbed from the injection site and produces intense pain and local tissue necrosis. In some cases, elevation of serum creatine phosphokinase levels occur.[104,105]

Special problems in the use of cardiac glycosides

RENAL FAILURE

The absorption of digitoxin is not altered in patients with renal failure. Due to qualitative and quantitative changes in plasma protein binding, enhanced hydroxylation to digoxin and increased biliary-fecal elimination, the total plasma digitoxin concentration is decreased, the unbound fraction is increased, and the $T^{1/2}$ remains unchanged or shortened in uremic patients, despite decreased renal excretion of digitoxin and its metabolites. The apparent volume of distribution is slightly, but insignificantly, decreased.[64,69,106,107]

The plasma digoxin concentration is elevated in azotemic patients due to decreased apparent volume of distribution and impaired renal elimination. The $T^{1/2}$ varies from 1.5 to 5.2 days, depending on the degree of renal damage. The nonrenal elimination of digoxin is not increased in the presence of renal failure.[6,69,83,108]

The pharmacologic effects of digitalis may be modified by electrolyte (hyperkalemia and hypocalcemia) and acid-base disturbances of uremia (see below). Hemodialysis or peritoneal dialysis can rapidly correct these abnormalities but does not effectively alter the tissue digitalis concentrations. Because of these problems, the use of digitalis in uremic patients is complex. The appropriate use of digitalis in uremic patients is difficult, and the choice of digoxin or digitoxin must be made on an individual basis.[6,69,86,109] However, since most physicians are more familiar with digoxin than digitoxin, there appears to be no advantage in switching to the relatively unfamiliar digitoxin in a complicated, difficult situation.

The size of the loading dose and the time to achieve full digitalization must also be determined on the basis of clinical urgency and estimations of changes in apparent volume of distribution, electrolyte and acid-base disturbances, and the degree of impairment in renal function. The maintenance dose of digoxin may be approximated according to the following formulas:[87]

$$\text{Percent daily loss in males} = 11.6 + \frac{20}{C}$$

$$\text{Percent daily loss in females} = 12.6 + \frac{16}{C}$$

$$\text{Percent daily loss} = 14 + \frac{C_{Cr}}{5}$$

where C indicates stable serum creatinine concentration in milligrams per 100 milliliters and C_{Cr} the creatinine clearance in milliliters per minute.

ACUTE MYOCARDIAL INFARCTION

The use of digitalis in the presence of acute myocardial infarction is controversial. An investigation suggested that there is no increased arrhythmogenic effect of digitalis in patients with acute myocardial infarction.[110] On the other hand, animal experiments demonstrated that digitalis is unevenly distributed in the infarcted myocardium and the dose of digitalis required to produce ventricular fibrillation is decreased.[111] Another concern based on studies in dogs is that digitalis, because of its positive inotropic effect, may increase the infarct size of the nonfailing heart.[112]

Clinical investigations have shown that the decreased cardiac output occurring in patients with heart failure or shock complicating acute myocardial infarction is not increased by digitalis.[42,113–115] However, other parameters of left ventricular function such as left ventricular end-diastolic pressure, pre-ejection period, left ventricular stroke work, and peak left ventricular *dp/dt* may demonstrate improvement.[115] Accordingly, there may still be rationale for using digitalis to treat heart failure or cardiogenic shock in patients with acute myocardial infarction, especially in the presence of high ventricular filling pressure unresponsive to diuretic therapy.[4,116] It is important to recognize that rapid digitalization may increase afterload due to peripheral vasoconstriction.[42,43]

ELECTRIC CARDIOVERSION

Ventricular tachyarrhythmias may be induced after cardioversion in a heavily digitalized patient because of decreased threshold for the development of ventricular arrhythmias, especially in the presence of hypokalemia or rapid lowering of serum potassium level.[117] In nonurgent situations, the serum potassium concentration should be maintained at normal value and digoxin discontinued for 1 day and digitoxin for 2 days before performing a synchronized cardioversion.[118] The energy used should be started from 10 W/s (joules) and increased by 5 to 10 W/s, up to 200 W/s.[119] In cases of ventricular fibrillation, cardioversion may be started from 200 W/s, and larger increments may be necessary. When emergency situations require immediate cardioversion in digitalized patients, intravenous injection of 50 to 100 mg lidocaine, 100 mg phenytoin, or 100 mg procainamide prior to cardioversion has been recommended.[118] However, the possibility of suppressing postcardioversion automaticity and conduction should be considered.

CARDIOPULMONARY BYPASS

Serum digoxin levels fall during bypass and return to pre-bypass level within 2 h after discontinuing the procedure. The plasma concentration may overshoot the pre-bypass level within 24 h after surgery, probably due to depressed renal clearance. Concurrent hypokalemia and hypomagnesemia may sensitize the heart and precipitate the occurrence of digitalis intoxication, especially in recently digitalized patients.[120–122] The incidence of this complication may be decreased by avoiding initiation of digitalization during the week prior to operation, by discontinuing digitalis 24 h before operation, and by carefully resuming an adjusted maintenance dose of digitalis at least 12 h after the discontinuation of bypass.[120–123]

GENERAL ANESTHESIA

Alteration of autonomic tone and the electrolyte and acid-base disturbances secondary to hypo- or hyperventilation associated with general anesthesia are arrhythmogenic, and may sensitize the heart to digitalis and induce arrhythmias. Use of cyclopropane in a digitalized patient may result in the development of arrhythmias, possibly due to elevated plasma catecholamine levels.[123]

HEPATOBILIARY DISEASES

In the presence of a biliary fistula, the plasma $T^{1/2}$ of digitoxin is shortened by approximately 50 percent[124]; digoxin is not affected.[77] The disposition of digitoxin and digoxin is not significantly altered in patients with parenchymal liver damage or biliary obstruction.[125-127]

ALTERED THYROID STATUS

The elimination of digitoxin is accelerated in the hyperthyroid state and normal or decreased in hypothyroidism.[86,128] Serum digitoxin or digoxin concentrations tend to be lower in hyperthyroid and higher in hypothyroid patients than in patients with normal thyroid function. Increased sensitivity to digitalis-induced arrhythmias in myxedematous patients and resistance to the therapeutic effects of digitalis in hyperthyroidism are well-described clinical phenomena.[86,128,129]

PULMONARY HEART DISEASE (CHRONIC COR PULMONALE)

The positive inotropic effect and disposition of digitalis in patients with chronic cor pulmonale is not significantly different from those in other cardiac patients. The observed digitalis sensitivity in this situation may be attributed to (1) hypoxia and hypercapnia and (2) acid-base and electrolyte disturbances. Because of the primary lung disease, the response to digitalization may not be obvious and satisfactory; therefore, the possibility of overdigitalization must be kept in mind.[55,86,130]

MALABSORPTION SYNDROME

The gastrointestinal absorption of digitoxin and digoxin is impaired in patients with malabsorption syndrome. However, since bile salts and pancreatic secretion are not required for digoxin absorption, it is not affected in patients with pancreatic insufficiency. Moreover, the absorption of digoxin may be improved by giving the patient digoxin in alcohol solution instead of the tablet form.[62,131,132] The bioavailability of oral digoxin is not impaired in obese patients who underwent jejunoileal bypass surgery.[132a]

Drug interactions

ELECTROLYTE IMBALANCE

Studies in animals have demonstrated that hyperkalemia inhibits myocardial binding of digitalis and protects against digitalis intoxication.[133] Whether the positive inotropic effect is decreased[133] or not affected[134] by hyperkalemia is controversial. Clinically, hypokalemia sensitizes the heart to digitalis intoxication.[55,92,93] The positive inotropic and arrhythmogenic effects of digitalis are augmented by hypercalcemia.[55,87,135] In animal experiments, low extracellular Na^+ concentrations delay the onset of digitalis toxicity, but do not antagonize an established toxic manifestation.[136] Hypomagnesemia increases myocardial uptake of digoxin and sensitizes the heart to digitalis effects. Magnesium sulfate has been shown to sup-

press digitalis-induced arrhythmias unresponsive to potassium therapy.[137,138] One proposed explanation of this phenomenon is that magnesium salts may activate the Mg^{2+}-dependent Na^+,K^+-ATPase.[139] Magnesium also inhibits K^+ efflux, decreases intracellular Ca^{2+}, and causes autonomic blockade by interfering with the action of calcium.[140,141]

SYMPATHOMIMETIC AMINES AND RESERPINE

Sympathomimetic amines with β-adrenergic activity potentiate the digitalis-induced increase in automaticity of Purkinje fibers.[142] Conversely, near-toxic doses of digitalis sensitize the ventricle to the effect of adrenergic stimulation.[143] Ventricular tachyarrhythmias have been described after administration of reserpine to digitalized patients. Both release of catecholamines and potentiation of vagal tone by reserpine have been implicated.[144,145] In contrast, depletion of catecholamine stores by pretreatment with reserpine has been shown to reduce digitalis-induced ventricular arrhythmias in animals.[143]

AGENTS AFFECTING GASTROINTESTINAL MOTILITY

Metoclopramide, a drug which increases gastrointestinal motility, has been found to interfere with intestinal absorption of conventional digoxin tablets. In contrast, propantheline, which decreases gastrointestinal motility, lengthens the effective absorption time and increases the plasma digoxin concentrations.[146]

ANION EXCHANGE RESINS

Both cholestyramine and colestipol bind digoxin and digitoxin, thereby interfering with intestinal absorption. In addition, because of a greater portion of the body pool of digitoxin entering enterohepatic circulation, cholestyramine shortens the $T^{1/2}$ of digitoxin and enhances dissipation of its pharmacologic effects.[147,148]

HEPATIC MICROSOMAL ENZYME INDUCERS

Phenobarbital, phenylbutazone, and phenytoin increase β-hydroxylation of digitoxin, resulting in decreased plasma concentration and shortened plasma $T^{1/2}$. The effect resulting from competition on plasma protein binding is not conspicuous.[149]

DIURETICS

Chronic diuretic therapy or acute massive diuresis may cause hypokalemia and/or hypomagnesemia and thus lower the threshold for digitalis-induced arrhythmias.

Digitalis intoxication

Optimal digitalization is difficult to achieve because of lack of definite endpoints. Indeed, the proper dose of digitalis may vary not only from patient to patient but even within the same patient. This difficulty is reflected by the fact that digitalis intoxication is one of the most common adverse drug reactions, occurring in an estimate of 4 to 35 percent (average 20 percent) of digitalized patients. On the other hand, perhaps 11 to 36 percent are underdigitalized.[93]

The risk of digitalis intoxication is increased in the elderly with organic heart disease, and in patients with hypokalemia, renal failure, acute hypoxia, pulmonary disease, and acid-base disturbances.[6,55,86,92]

The most serious consequence of digitalis intoxication is cardiac arrhythmias. These bioelectric complications of digitalis can be anticipated from its known electrophysiologic effects. Combined manifestations of altered automaticity and impulse propagation are not uncommon. Digitalis may enhance automaticity in any pacemaker tissue and facilitate reentry at various parts of the heart, with atrial, junctional, and ventricular tachyarrhythmias as frequent manifestations of digitalis excess. However, the arrhythmias are rarely specific, and the diagnosis of digitalis intoxication cannot be made with any degree of assurance from the ECG alone.[55,55a]

Premature ventricular beats (PVBs) are probably the most common, but at the same time the least specific, manifestation of digitalis toxicity. Ventricular bigeminy with fixed coupling interval but varying QRS morphologic features, PVBs associated with depression of conduction, or other ectopic rhythms in a digitalized patient are highly suggestive of digitalis intoxication.[55a] Severe intoxication leads to the development of ventricular tachycardia, bidirectional ventricular tachycardia, and ventricular fibrillation, which are notoriously resistant to the usual antiarrhythmic drugs and to electric cardioversion. These serious arrhythmias may be induced by carotid sinus stimulation in a patient with digitalis toxicity.[55] Moreover, the likelihood of ventricular fibrillation following electric depolarization increases markedly in the setting of digitalis toxicity.[118]

Paroxysmal atrial tachycardia with AV block (usually 2:1) is a manifestation of combined altered automaticity and impulse propagation. Atrial fibrillation occurring during the course of digitalization is not uncommon and has been attributed to digitalis toxicity, especially when associated with ventricular arrhythmias or extremely slow ventricular rate.[151,152] However, lone atrial fibrillation is not a common manifestation of digitalis intoxication.[55]

Sinus bradycardia, nonparoxysmal junctional tachycardia, AV dissociation, and Mobitz type I AV block are frequently seen in patients with digitalis intoxication, but may be due to other causes. SA block, sinus arrest, and complete AV block may occur with severe intoxication.[55,55a] In the diseased heart, digitalis intoxication tends to produce tachyarrhythmias, while in the normal heart, it is more likely to induce AV block.[13,55,153,154] Digitalis-induced AV block is usually intranodal and may be associated with accelerated junctional rhythm. Stokes-Adams syndrome therefore rarely occurs as a manifestation of digitalis intoxication.[13,151,152]

The cardiac function frequently deteriorates with digitalis intoxication.[55] Fatigue and anorexia are early and common extracardiac symptoms of digitalis intoxication. They are followed by nausea and vomiting. Other, less common symptoms include distorted color vision, insomnia, headache, diarrhea, abdominal pain, depression, scotomas, and confusion.[55,92,155] Hyperkalemia may occur in severely intoxicated patients.[153,154]

The first step in treating digitalis intoxication is the withdrawal of digitalis. In the absence of life-threatening arrhythmia the symptoms of digitalis intoxication usually subside after discontinuing digitalis therapy if the patient is treated with digoxin; more slowly, with digitoxin. Rhythm disturbances that impair cardiac performance or carry the risk of cardiac arrest should be treated actively under ECG monitoring. Precipitating or contributing factors such as hypoxia, inappropriate ventilation, or electrolyte and acid-base disturbances must be removed or corrected, if possible.

In the absence of renal failure and hyperkalemia, potassium chloride, 20 to 40 mEq in 500 ml of 5% dextrose solution, may be infused at a rate of 20 mEq/h under careful ECG monitoring. Due to inhibition of Na^+,K^+-ATPase by digitalis, the infused K^+ may not enter the intracellular space easily. As a result, hyperkalemia may occur after administration of relatively small doses of potassium chloride. Rapid increase in the serum potassium level should be avoided because of the hazard of precipitating conduction disturbances. Infusion of potassium salt is contraindicated in the presence of conduction disturbances or renal failure.[55,152,156,157]

If the administration of potassium chloride alone fails to suppress the digitalis arrhythmias and the patient is hypomagnesemic without renal failure, the slow intravenous injection of 5 to 10 ml of 10% magnesium sulfate solution may be tried.[137,158]

The group II antiarrhythmic agents are most effective against digitalis-induced arrhythmias (see Chap. 109B). Lidocaine is the drug of choice to suppress ventricular arrhythmias not controlled by electrolyte therapy. Phenytoin may be tried if lidocaine yields unsatisfactory results. Phenytoin may be used to treat digitalis-induced atrial tachycardia with or without AV block, but is not effective for atrial fibrillation or flutter.[152,156,157] It should be recalled that digitalis-induced supraventricular tachycardia may not require aggressive therapy if it does not seriously jeopardize hemodynamics or endanger life.

Propranolol (group III antiarrhythmic agent) is effective in treating digitalis-induced supraventricular and ventricular arrhythmias but is usually not used for this purpose because of potential hazard of further depressing AV nodal conduction and impairing myocardial contractility.[156,157]

Although ventricular pacing has been successfully used in suppressing digitalis-induced tachyarrhythmias in animals[159] and human beings,[160] this mode of therapy may be hazardous because the threshold for spontaneous repetitive ventricular responses to pacemaker stimuli is lowered in the presence of digitalis intoxication. Furthermore, overdrive pacing may accelerate rather than suppress digitalis-induced ventricular tachyarrhythmias.[13,26,34–36,156] (See "Automaticity" under toxic "Electrophysiologic Effects" above.) Electric cardioversion may be carefully used to treat life-threatening tachyarrhythmias refractory to pharmacologic therapy.[117–119]

Atropine may be used to treat symptomatic sinus bradycardia, SA block, sinus arrest, Mobitz type I block, or complete AV block. Temporary artificial pacing may be required in patients with symptomatic bradyarrhythmias unresponsive to atropine therapy.[55,152,155–157]

The administration of steroid-binding resins such as cholestyramine or colestipol has been used to increase the elimination of digitoxin.[147,148] More recently, a patient with severe digoxin intoxication was successfully treated with purified Fab fragments of bovine digoxin-specific antibodies.[154] Dialysis is not effective in treating digitalis intoxication.[86]

Other adverse effects

Hypersensitivity to digitalis is rare. Thrombocytopenia has been reported but rarely. Occasional patients may experience anginal attack after digitalization. Gynecomastia in men and estrogen-like activity in vaginal smears of postmenopausal women are not uncommon in chronic digitalis therapy. Elevated serum estrogen levels and lowered luteinizing hormone and testosterone levels have been found in patients receiving digoxin therapy for more than 2 years.[3,6,161–163]

Contraindications and precautions in the use of digitalis

Digitalis is contraindicated in patients with digitalis intoxication, hypersensitivity, and uncomplicated idiopathic hypertrophic subaortic stenosis (IHSS). However, digitalis may be used to control the ventricular rate of persistent atrial fibrillation and to treat heart failure in patients with IHSS.[164]

Digitalis must be used with caution in patients with AV block or sick sinus syndrome.[166] Clearly its use in such patients carries the risk of increasing block and cardiac asystole,[165,167] and the prophylactic use of an artificial pacemaker may need to be considered.

Digitalis is contraindicated in patients with complete AV block with a history of Stokes-Adams syndrome.[165] The administration of digitalis to patients with the Wolff-Parkinson-White syndrome may lead to preferential conduction through the anomalous pathway. In the presence of atrial fibrillation the ventricular response may be very rapid, and rarely ventricular fibrillation results.[19,20] Digitalis toxicity may develop during hemodialysis or peritoneal dialysis because of an acute lowering of serum potassium levels without a concomitant decrease in myocardial digitalis concentrations.[86]

The intravenous injection of calcium salts should not be given to a digitalized patient. Digitalis is a mesenteric vasoconstrictor and should be avoided or used with great caution in patients with compromised mesenteric circulation.[44] In patients with compromised oxygen supply or poor ventricular function, rapid intravenous injection of loading doses of digitalis should be avoided.[42,43]

Digitalis should be used cautiously in patients with risk factors prone to the development of digitalis intoxication as discussed previously. Special problems of digitalis have been considered earlier in this section.

THEOPHYLLINE ETHYLENEDIAMINE (AMINOPHYLLINE)

Aminophylline and other xanthine derivatives inhibit phosphodiesterase, which results in an increased intracellular concentration of cyclic AMP (adenosine monophosphate).[168] Aminophylline increases myocardial contractility and the heart rate.[169] The positive inotropic effect is thought to be primarily responsible for the increased cardiac output and decreased right atrial pressure observed following intravenous administration in patients with congestive heart failure.[170] The increase in cardiac output is of relatively short duration (20 to 30 min).

Aminophylline has a direct vasodilating effect on arteries and veins.[171] This action may contribute to its efficacy in the treatment of patients with congestive heart failure. Aminophylline dilates the coronary arteries,[172] the clinical significance of which is uncertain. Aminophylline is a potent bronchodilator and may be useful in relaxing the bronchial spasm which frequently accompanies cardiac dyspnea.[171] Aminophylline promotes diuresis because it increases renal blood flow and glomerular filtration rate and because it directly inhibits the renal tubular reabsorption of sodium.[173] The central nervous system actions of aminophylline can revert the periodic breathing of Cheyne-Stokes respiration to a more normal pattern.[171]

Aminophylline is absorbed erratically after oral ingestion. The drug is absorbed more reliably rectally. Approximately 20 percent is bound to plasma protein. About 90 percent of aminophylline is biotransformed in the liver. The plasma $T^{1/2}$ ranges from 3.0 to 9.5 h, with a mean of 4.5 h. The $T^{1/2}$ may be prolonged in patients with hepatic dysfunction and congestive heart failure.[174,175] Therapeutic plasma concentrations of theophylline have been calculated with respect to improvement in ventilatory function and range from 10 to 20 μg/ml.[174–176] The usual intravenous dose of aminophylline is 250 mg diluted in glucose solution. The drug should be injected slowly over a period of 10 to 15 min to avoid toxicity. A total daily dose of 1,000 mg or less seldom produces toxicity.[175] Direct injection of aminophylline into the central venous pressure line should be avoided.[177] Toxicity and adverse reactions most commonly occur when the plasma level exceeds 15 μg/ml or when the drug is injected rapidly. The most serious toxic effects are cardiac arrhythmias, hypotension, and convulsions. Nausea, vomiting, and abdominal distress are common adverse effects when aminophylline is taken orally.[174,176–178]

MORPHINE

There are two principal indications for the use of morphine in cardiovascular diseases: (1) for relief of pain and anxiety and (2) for the treatment of cardiac asthma and acute pulmonary edema.

The central nervous system actions of morphine that produce analgesia, sedation, and respiratory depression have been extensively reviewed.[179] The mechanism responsible for the beneficial cardiac effects is most likely vasodilation in the arterial and venous beds, which leads to decreased peripheral resistance and to peripheral venous pooling.[180–182] A combination of the central nervous system and vascular effects together reduce oxygen consumption and pulmonary congestion.[182,183]

Although large doses of morphine may depress myocardial contractility, therapeutic doses have little effect.[184] If the blood volume is increased or adequate to meet the drug-induced increase in vascular capacitance, cardiac output may increase. On the other hand, low cardiac output and hypotension may occur in the presence of hypovolemia.[185] Hypotension is most prominent in the erect position, but it can occur in patients in the supine position.[186] Morphine may increase vagal activity centrally and may also activate the sympathoadrenal system.[187,188] Accordingly, the heart rate will vary according to the dominant autonomic influence. Occasional patients develop severe bradycardia which may be countered with atropine.[189]

The usual dose of morphine is 5 to 10 mg administered by intramuscular or subcutaneous injections. Intravenous administration is recommended for patients with impaired peripheral circulation or for those with pulmonary edema to avoid delayed absorption from subcutaneous sites.[179]

Due regard should be paid to the possible deterioration of cardiorespiratory function in the critically ill and in those patients with preexistent pulmonary disease. The most serious adverse effect of morphine is respiratory depression.[180] Hypercapnia increases respiratory effort. Morphine may depress hypercapnia-dependent respiratory drive. Morphine may induce bronchoconstriction, particularly in asthmatic patients, perhaps by causing histamine release.[190] Nausea and vomiting are frequent adverse effects. Hypotension is also commonly seen and must be differentiated from shock in patients with myocardial infarction. Other side effects include constipation, urinary retention, and paradoxic excitation rather than sedation.[180] A feature of morphine

pharmacology that should never be forgotten is addiction.

Morphine is contraindicated in the patient with chronic obstructive pulmonary disease or respiratory depression. Mechanical ventilatory support should be available if necessary. Death after morphine administration to patients with chronic cor pulmonale has been reported. Morphine should be used with great caution in patients with limited ventilatory reserve, such as those with kyphoscoliosis or severe obesity.[179,180]

The respiratory and central nervous system depression produced by morphine and related narcotics may be antagonized by naloxone. Despite claims to the contrary, respiratory depression and hypotension occur with all potent narcotics. A less effective narcotic, pentazocaine (Talwin) exhibits different peripheral vascular effects than morphine in that vasoconstriction rather than vasodilation may occur.[191,192]

NITRATES AND SODIUM NITROPRUSSIDE

Cardiovascular effects

Organic nitrates and sodium nitroprusside cause vasodilation in both arterial and venous vacular beds by direct relaxation of the vascular smooth muscle.[193] This results in venous pooling, a reduction of peripheral vascular resistance, and a decrease in both ventricular filling pressure and ventricular volume. As a result, the blood pressure is lowered, myocardial oxygen consumption is decreased, and the ventricular function of an ischemic or overloaded heart may be improved. Reflex sympathetic activity, induced by hypotension, may lead to a faster heart rate and increased myocardial contractility which will tend to offset the hypotension and reduction in myocardial oxygen consumption.[194–197] There is no convincing evidence that either nitroprusside or organic nitrates exert a direct positive inotropic effect on the myocardium.[193,195]

Repeated investigations in experimental animals and human beings have demonstrated that the organic nitrates dilate coronary vessels.[198,199] There is no good evidence, however, that they cause vasodilation in diseased coronary vessels in preference to other vessels. In fact, no consistent increase in myocardial blood flow follows the administration of organic nitrates.[200,201] On the contrary, the drug-induced decrease in systemic blood pressure may decrease the coronary perfusion pressure, which, in turn, may lower the coronary blood flow. The relief of angina pectoris appears to be related more to the reduction of myocardial oxygen consumption secondary to arterial and venous vasodilating actions[193,200,202] than to an increase in coronary blood flow.

Nitroglycerin (glyceryl trinitrate) and other organic nitrates

Nitroglycerin appears to produce more vasodilation in venous than in arterial vascular beds. Most studies have demonstrated a greater decrease in ventricular filling pressure than in peripheral resistance.[203-205] Oral ingestion of nitroglycerin and other oral nitrates has limited bioavailability because of rapid hepatic biotransformation.[206] Organic nitrates are rapidly absorbed from the oral mucosa and exert pronounced effects when administered by sublingual or buccal routes. Nitroglycerin acts within 1 to 2 min and usually lasts less than 1 h.[207-209] Nitroglycerin is also absorbed through the skin, and nitroglycerin ointment is an effective treatment for angina pectoris.[209,209a]

The usual sublingual dose of nitroglycerin is from 0.3 to 0.6 mg. When the drug is used prophylactically to prevent anticipated attacks of angina, it should be taken about 3 min before exertion.[193,207]

Conventional nitroglycerin tablets lose potency on storage, especially when the tablets are in contact with cotton, paper, or plastics.[210,211] When stored in a tightly capped amber glass bottle in the refrigerator, their potency may be maintained for approximately 5 months. On the other hand, when kept in a pillbox by the patient, they may deteriorate within a week.[211] The absence of a burning sensation on sublingual administration should alert the patient to the possibility that the drug has lost potency. Several currently marketed preparations with modified formulation have improved the stability of nitroglycerin.

Adverse effects

Headache is the most common adverse effect produced by organic nitrates which results from dilation of the cerebral vessels. After repeated use of the drug, the symptom usually becomes less troublesome. In some patients, severe hypotension may occur with either fast or slow heart rate.[193,211a] The patient should be warned of these adverse effects and should take the first tablet in the presence of the physician. The organic nitrates increase intracranial pressure, and therefore, are contraindicated in patients with increased intracranial pressure. The possibility of precipitating glaucoma has been mentioned, but is not well established.[193] Traditionally, the use of nitroglycerin has not been recommended in acute myocardial infarction. Recently, however, it has been used experimentally for the treatment of heart failure or shock complicating acute myocardial infarction.[203-205]

Isosorbide dinitrate is useful when it is chewed or used sublingually (see Chap. 62E).

Numerous organic nitrates including isosorbide dinitrate and pentaerythritol tetranitrate have been promoted for sustained action after oral administration.[212] Although large doses of these agents have been shown to exert hemodynamic effects after oral administration, repeated controlled studies have not shown them to be more effective in preventing angina than a placebo.[213] The action of sublingual isosorbide dinitrate is similar to that of nitroglycerin. The duration of action of oral or buccal isosorbide may be prolonged 3 to 5 h in patients with congestive heart failure.[214a,214b]

Sodium nitroprusside

Sodium nitroprusside acts on both arterioles and venules but appears to exert a more potent arteriolar effect than nitroglycerin.[196,205] Sodium nitroprusside is administered intravenously. Its onset of action is within 1 min, and the effect dissipates within 3 to 5 min.[215] The drug, therefore, must be continuously infused. At the time of writing the only approved indication for sodium nitroprusside is in the treatment of severe or malignant hypertension (see Chap. 73). More recently, however, it has become widely used experimentally as a part of the treatment of heart failure and low output states after cardiac surgery.[194-197,215-218] It is also being studied as a means of decreasing afterload in patients with acute myocardial infarction.[216]

When used for the treatment of heart failure or other low output states, the ECG, intraarterial pressure, pulmonary capillary wedge pressure (as an indirect measurement of left ventricular filling pressure), and preferably also cardiac output should be monitored. The drug should be administered by constant-rate infusion pump, beginning at a rate of 0.5 μg/kg/min with an increment of 0.5 to 1 μg/kg/min every 5 to 20 min depending upon the change of blood pressure and response of the patient. The maximal rate should not exceed 8 μg/kg/min. Several studies have demonstrated that nitroprusside increases cardiac output in patients with elevated left ventricular filling pressure, usually above 25 to 30 mm Hg, and markedly increases peripheral vascular resistance.[195,217] Responders generally show a significant lowering of ventricular filling pressure, mean pulmonary artery pressure, and peripheral vascular resistance, as well as a slight lowering of mean arterial pressure without a significant change in heart rate.[195,217,218] The reduction of afterload is more important than the reduction of preload in increasing cardiac output.[194] The infusion rate should be reduced or discontinued if there is excessive lowering of blood pressure or increase in heart rate.

Acute adverse effects of nitroprusside include hypotension and tachycardia. Intracranial pressure is increased by nitroprusside.[219] A case of methemoglobinemia following nitroprusside infusion has been reported.[220] Chronic toxic effects of nitroprusside due to accumulation of the major metabolite thiocyanate include fatigue, nausea, anorexia, disorientation, psychotic behavior, and muscle spasm. These symptoms begin to appear at plasma thiocyanate levels of 5 to 10 mg/100 ml with fatalities reported to have occurred at levels exceeding 20 mg/100 ml. Thiocyanate is eliminated mainly through the kidney with a $T^{1/2}$ of about 7 days.[197] Therefore, the plasma thiocyanate level should be monitored when prolonged infusion of nitroprusside is used in patients with poor renal function.

1 Fisch, C., and Surawicz, B. (eds.): "Digitalis," Grune & Stratton, Inc., New York, 1969.

2 Walton, R. P., and Gazes, P. C.: Cardiac Glycosides: II. Pharmacology and Clinical Use, in J. R. DiPalma (ed.), "Drill's Pharmacology in Medicine," 4th ed., McGraw-Hill Book Company, New York, 1971, p. 780.

3 Moe, G. K., and Farah, A. E.: Digitalis and Allied Cardiac Glycosides, in L. S. Goodman, and A. Gilman (eds.), "The Pharmacological Basis of Therapeutics," 5th ed., The Macmillan Company, New York, 1975, p. 653.

4 Mason, D. T.: Digitalis Pharmocology and Therapeutics: Recent Advances, *Ann. Intern. Med.*, 80:520, 1974.

4a Spann, J. F., Jr., Sonnenblick, E. H., Cooper, T., Chidsey, C. A., Willman, V. L., and Braunwald, E.: Digitalis: XIV. Influence of Cardiac Norepinephrine Stores on the Response of Isolated Heart Muscle to Digitalis, *Circ. Res.*, 19:326, 1966.

5 Braunwald, E., Bloodwell, R. D., Goldberg, L. I., and Morrow, A. G.: Studies on Digitalis: IV. Observations in Man on the Effects of Digitalis Preparations on the Contractility of the Non-failing Heart and on Total Vascular Resistance, *J. Clin. Invest.*, 40:52, 1961.

6 Smith, T. W., and Haber, E.: Digitalis, *N. Engl. J. Med.*, 289:945, 1010, 1063, 1125, 1973.

7 Schwartz, A., Lindenmayer, G. E., and Allen, J. C.: The Sodium-Potassium Adenosine Triphosphatase: Pharmacological, Physiological and Biochemical Aspects, *Pharmacol. Rev.*, 27:3, 1975.

8 Fozzard, H. A.: Heart: Excitation-Contraction Coupling, *Ann. Rev. Physiol.*, 39:201, 1977.

9 Rhee, H. M., Dutta, S., and Marks, B. H.: Cardiac Na,K-ATPase Activity during Inotropic and Toxic Actions of Ouabain, *Eur. J. Pharmacol.*, 37:141, 1976.

10 Moe, G. K., and Han, J.: Digitalis and the Autonomic Nervous System, in C. Fisch, and B. Surawicz (eds.), "Digitalis," Grune & Stratton, Inc., New York, 1969, p. 110.

11 Gillis, R. A., Pearle, D. L., and Levitt, B.: Digitalis: A Neuroexcitatory Drug, *Circulation*, 52:739, 1975, (Editorial).

12 Leachman, R. D., Cokkinos, D. V. P., Cabrera, R., Leatherman, L. L., and Rochelle, D. G.: Response of the Transplanted, Denervated Human Heart to Cardiovascular Drugs, *Am. J. Cardiol.*, 27:272, 1971.

13 Rosen, M. R., Wit, A. L., and Hoffman, B. F.: Electrophysiology and Pharmacology of Cardiac Arrhythmias: IV. Cardiac Antiarrhythmic and Toxic Effects of Digitalis, *Am. Heart J.*, 89:391, 1975.

14 Fozzard, H. A., and Sleator, W.: Membrane Ionic Conductances during Rest and Activity in Guinea Pig Atrial Muscle, *Am. J. Physiol.*, 212:945, 1967.

15 Abildskov, J. A.: The Nervous System and Cardiac Arrhythmias, *Circulation*, 51/52 (suppl. 3):116, 1975.

16 Engel, T. R., and Schaal, S. F.: Digitalis in the Sick Sinus Syndrome: The Effect of Digitalis on Sinoatrial Automaticity and Atrioventricular Conduction, *Circulation*, 48:1201, 1973.

17 Toda, N., and West, T. C.: The Action of Ouabain on the Function of the Atrioventricular Node in Rabbits, *J. Parmacol. Exp. Ther.*, 169:287, 1969.

18 Goodman, D. J., Rossen, R. M., Cannon, D. S., Dider, A. K., and Harrison, D. C.: Effect of Digoxin on Atrioventricular Conduction: Studies in Patients with and without Cardiac Autonomic Innervation, *Circulation*, 51:251, 1975.

19 Wellens, H. J., and Durrer, D.: Effect of Digitalis on A-V Conduction and Circus Movement Tachycardia in Patients with Wolff-Parkinson-White Syndrome, *Circulation*, 47:1229, 1973.

20 Dreifus, L. S., Haiat, R., Watanabe, Y., Arriaga, J., and Reitman, N.: Ventricular Fibrillation: A Possible Mechanism of Sudden Death in Patients with Wolff-Parkinson-White Syndrome, *Circulation*, 43:520, 1971.

21 Kassebaum, D. C.: Electrophysiological Effects of Strophanthin on the Heart, *J. Pharmacol. Exp. Ther.*, 140:329, 1963.

22 Przybyla, A. G., Paulay, K. L., Stein, E., and Damato, A. N.: Effects of Digoxin on A-V Conduction Pathways in Man, *Am. J. Cardiol.*, 33:344, 1974.

23 Rosen, M. R., Gelband, H., and Hoffman, B. F.: Correlation between Effects of Ouabain on the Canine Electrocardiogram and Transmembrane Potentials in Isolated Purkinje Fibers, *Circulation*, 47:65, 1973.

24 Lederer, W. J., and Tsien, R. W.: Transient Inward Current Underlying Arrhythmogenic Effects of Cardiotonic Steroids in Purkinje Fibers, *J. Physiol. (Lond.)*, 263:73, 1976.

25 Ferrier, G. R.: Digitalis Arrhythmias: Roles of Oscillatory Afterpotentials, *Prog. Cardiovasc. Dis.*, 19:459, 1977.

26 Davis, L. D.: Effect of Changes in Cycle Length on Diastolic Depolarization Produced by Ouabain in Canine Purkinje Fibers, *Circ. Res.*, 32:206, 1973.

27 Cranefield, P. F.: "The Conduction of the Cardiac Impulse: The Slow Response and Cardiac Arrhythmias," Futura Publishing Company, Mt. Kisco, N.Y., 1975.

28 Aronson, R. S., Gelles, J. M., and Hoffman, B. F.: Effect of Ouabain on the Current Underlying Spontaneous Diastolic Depolarization in Cardiac Purkinje Fibers, *Nature [New Biol.]*, 245:118, 1973.

29 Isenberg, G., and Trautwein, W.: The Effect of Dihydro-Ouabain and Lithium Ions on the Outward Current in Cardiac Purkinje Fibers, *Pfluegers Arch.*, 350:41, 1974.

30 McDonald, T. F., Nawrath, H., and Tautwein, W.: Membrane Currents and Tension in Cat Ventricular Muscle Treated with Cardiac Glycosides, *Circ. Res.*, 37:674, 1975.

31 De Mello, W. C.: Effect of Intracellular Injection of Calcium and Strontium on Cell Communication in Heart, *J. Physiol. (Lond.)*, 250:231, 1975.

32 Winegrad, R.: Electrical Uncoupling in Mammalian Heart Muscle Induced by Cardiac Glycosides, *Experientia (Basel)*, 31:715, 1975.

33 Vassalle, M.: Electrogenic Suppression of Automaticity in Sheep and Dog Purkinje Fibers, *Circ. Res.*, 27:361, 1970.

34 Ferrier, G. R., Saunders, J. H., and Mendez, C.: A Cellular Mechanism for the Generation of Ventricular Arrhythmias by Acetylstrophanthidin, *Circ. Res.*, 32:600, 1973.

35 Hagemeijer, F., and Lown, B.: Effect of Heart Rate on Electrically Induced Repetitive Ventricular Responses in the Digitalized Dog, *Circ. Res.*, 27:333, 1970.

36 Ferrier, G. R.: The Effects of Tension on Acetylstrophanthidin-induced Transient Depolarizations and after Contractions in Canine Myocardial and Purkinje Tissues, *Circ. Res.*, 38:156, 1976.

37 Hoffman, B. F.: Effects of Digitalis on Electrical Activity of Cardiac Membranes, in B. H. Marks and A. M. Weissler (eds.), "Basic and Clinical Parmacology of Digitalis," Charles C Thomas, Publisher, Springfield, Ill., 1972, p. 118.

38 Vassale, M.: Analysis of Cardiac Pacemaker Potential Using "Voltage-Clamp" Technique, *Am. J. Physiol.*, 210:1335, 1966.

39 Dominguez, G., and Fozzard, H. A.: Influence of Extracellular K^+ Concentration on Cable Properties and Excitability of Sheep Cardiac Purkinje Fibers, *Circ. Res.*, 26:565, 1970.

40 Ross, J., Jr., Waldhausen, J. A., and Braunwald, E.: Studies on Digitalis I: Direct Effects on Peripheral Vascular Resistance, *J. Clin. Invest.*, 39:930, 1960.

41 Williams, M. H., Jr., Zohman, L. R., and Ratner, A. C.: Hemodynamic Effects of Cardiac Glycosides on Normal Human Subjects during Rest and Exercise, *J. Appl. Physiol.*, 13:417, 1958.

42 Balcon, R., Hoy, J., and Sowton, E.: Haemodynamic Effects of Rapid Digitalization following Acute Myocardial Infarction, *Br. Heart J.,* 30:373, 1968.

43 Cohn, J. N., Tristani, F. E., and Khatri, I. M.: Cardiac and Peripheral Vascular Effects of Digitalis in Cardiogenic Shock, *Am. Heart J.,* 78:318, 1969.

44 Bynum, T. E., and Jacobson, E. D.: Shock, Intestinal Ischemia, and Digitalis, *Circ. Shock,* 2:235, 1975. (Editorial.)

45 Ferrer, M. I., Bradley, S. E., Wheeler, H. O., Enson, Y., Preisig, R., and Harvey, R. M.: The Effect of Digoxin in the Splanchnic Circulation in Ventricular Failure, *Circulation,* 32:524, 1965.

46 Vatner, S. F., Higgisn, C. B., Franklin, D., and Braunwald, E.: Effects of a Cardiac Glycoside on Coronary and Systemic Dynamics in Conscious Dogs, *Circ. Res.,* 28:470, 1971.

47 Mason, D. T., and Braunwald, E.: Studies on Digitalis: X. Effects of Ouabain on Forearm Vascular Resistance and Venous Tone in Normal Subjects and in Patients in Heart Failure, *J. Clin. Invest.,* 43:532, 1964.

48 Taintner, M. L., and Dock, W.: Further Observations on the Circulatory Actions of Digitalis and Strophanthus with Special Reference to the Liver, and Comparisons with Histamine and Epinephrine, *J. Clin. Invest.,* 8:485, 1930.

49 Baschieri, L., Ricci, P. D., Mazzuoli, G. F., and Vassale, M.: Studi su la portata epatica nell'uomo: Modificazioni de flusso epatico da digitale, *Cuore Circolaz,* 41:103, 1957.

50 Ross, J., Jr., Braunwald, E., and Waldhausen, J. A.: Studies on Digitalis: II. Extracardiac Effects on Venous Return and on the Capacity of the Peripheral Vascular Bed, *J. Clin. Invest.,* 39:937, 1960.

51 Stead, E. A., Jr., Warren, J. V., and Brannon, E. S.: Effect of Lanatoside C on the Circulation of Patients with Congestive Failure, *Arch. Intern. Med.,* 81:282, 1948.

52 Harvey, R. M., Ferrer, M. I., Cathcart, R. T., Richards, D. W., Jr., and Cournand, A.: Some Effects of Digoxin upon Heart and Circulation in Man: Digoxin in Left Ventricular Failure, *Am. J. Med.,* 7:439, 1949.

53 Covell, J. W., Braunwald, E., Ross, J., Jr., and Sonnenblick, E. H.: Studies on Digitalis: XVI. Effects on Myocardial Oxygen Consumption, *J. Clin. Invest.,* 45:1535, 1966.

54 Sonnenblick, E. H., Ross, J., Jr., and Braunwald, E.: Oxygen Consumption of the Heart: Newer Concepts of Its Multifactoral Determination, *Am. J. Cardiol.,* 22:328, 1968.

55 Chung, E. K.: "Digitalis Intoxication," The Williams & Wilkins Company, Baltimore, 1969, p. 161.

55a Fisch, C., Zipes, D. P., and Noble, R. J.: Digitalis Toxicity, Mechanism and Recognition, *Prog. Cardiol.,* 4:37, 1975.

56 Linhart, J. W., Lows, J. G., and Satinsky, J. D.: Maximum Treadmill Exercise Electrocardiography in Female Patients, *Circulation,* 50:1173, 1974.

57 Bentley, J. D., Burnett, G. H., Gonklin, R. W., and Wassenburger, R. H.: Clinical Application of Serum Digitoxin Levels: A Simplified Plasma Determination, *Circulation,* 41:67, 1970.

58 Joubert, P., Kroening, B., and Weintraub, M.: Serial Serum Digoxin Concentrations and Quantitative Electrocardiographic Changes, *Clin. Pharmacol. Ther.,* 18:757, 1975.

59 Okita, G. T.: Species Differences in Duration of Action of Cardiac Glycosides, *Fed. Proc.,* 26:1125, 1967.

60 Beerman, B., Hellström, K., and Rosen, A.: Fate of Orally Administered ³H-Digitoxin in Man with Special Reference to the Absorption, *Circulation,* 43:852, 1971.

61 Rassmussen, K., Jervell, J., and Storstein, O.: Clinical Use of a Bioassay of Serum Digitoxin Activity, *Eur. J. Clin. Pharmacol.,* 3:236, 1971.

62 Gjerdum, K.: Digitoxin Studies: Serum Concentration during Digitalization, Maintenance Therapy and Withdrawal: Estimation of Proper Maintenance Dose, *Acta Med. Scand.,* 191:25, 1972.

63 Stoll, R. G., Christensen, M. S., Sakmar, E., Blair, D., and Wagner, J. G.: Determination of Bioavailability of Digitoxin Using the Radioimmunassay Procedure, *J. Pharm. Sci.,* 62: 1615, 1973.

64 Lukas, D. S.: Some Aspects of the Distribution and Disposition of Digitoxin in Man, *Ann. N.Y. Acad. Sci.,* 179:338, 1971.

65 Okita, G. T., Plotz, M. D., and Davis, M. E.: Placenta Transfer of Radioactive Digitoxin in Pregnant Women and Its Fetal Disposition, *Circ. Res.,* 4:376, 1956.

66 Storstein, L.: Studies on Digitalis: I. Renal Excretion of Digitoxin and Its Cardioactive Metabolites, *Clin. Pharmacol. Ther.,* 16:14, 1974.

67 Sorstein, L.: Studies on Digitalis: VIII. Digitoxin Metabolism on a Maintenance Regimen and after a Single Dose, *Clin. Pharmacol. Ther.,* 21:125, 1977.

68 Luchi, R. J., and Gruber, J. W.: Unusually Large Digitalis Requirements: A Study of Altered Digoxin Metabolism, *Am. J. Med.,* 45:322, 1968.

69 Doherty, J. E.: Digitalis Glycosides: Pharmacokinetics and Their Clinical Implications, *Ann. Intern. Med.,* 79:229, 1973.

70 Okita, G. T.: Distribution, Disposition and Excretion of Digitalis Glycosides, in C. Fisch and B. Surarwicz (eds.), "Digitalis," Grune & Stratton, Inc., New York, 1969, p. 13.

70a Vöringer, H. F., and Rietbrook, N.: Metabolism and Excretion of Digitoxin in Man, *Clin. Pharmacol. Ther.,* 16:796, 1974.

71 Lindenbaum, J.: Bioavailability of Digoxin Tablets, *Pharmacol. Rev.,* 25:229, 1973.

72 Mallis, G. I., Schmidt, D. H., and Lindenbaum, J.: Superior Bioavailability of Digoxin Solution in Capsules, *Clin. Pharmacol. Ther.,* 18:761, 1975.

73 White, R. J., Chamberlain, D. A., Howard, M., and Smith, T. W.: Plasma Concentrations of Digoxin after Oral Administration in the Fasting and Postprandial State, *Br. Med., J.,* 1:380, 1971.

74 Greenblatt, D. J., Duhme, D. W., Kosch-Weser, J., and Smith, T. W.: Bioavailability of Digoxin Tablets and Elixir in the Fasting and Postprandial States, *Clin. Pharmacol. Ther.,* 16:444, 1974.

75 Ohnhaus, E. E., Sprung, P., and Dettli, L.: Protein Binding of Digoxin in Human Serum, *Eur. J. Clin. Pharmacol.,* 5:34, 1972.

76 Doherty, J. E., and Hall, W. H.: Tritiated Digoxin: XV. Serum Protein Binding in Human Subjects, *Am. J. Cardiol.,* 28:326, 1971.

77 Doherty, J. E., Flanigan, W. J., Murphy, M. L., Bulloch, R. T., Dalrymple, G. L., Beard, O. W., and Perkins, W. H.: Tritiated Digoxin: XIV. Enterohepatic Circulation, Absorption, and Excretion Studies in Human Volunteers, *Circulation,* 42:867, 1970.

78 Abshagen, U., Rennekamp, H., Kuchler, R., and Rietbrock, N.: Formation and Disposition of Bis- and Mono-Glycosides after Administration of ³H-4′′′-Methyl-Digoxin to Man, *Eur. J. Clin. Pharmacol.,* 7:177, 1974.

79 Steiness, E.: Renal Tubular Secretion of Digoxin, *Circulation,* 50:103, 1974.

80 Halkin, H., Sheiner, L. B., Peck, C. C., and Melmon, K. L.: Determinants of the Renal Clearance of Digoxin, *Clin. Pharmacol. Ther.,* 17:385, 1975.

81 Bisset, J. K., Doherty, J. E., Flanigan, W. L., and Dalrymple, G. V.: Tritiated Digoxin: XIX. Turnover Studies in Diabetes Insipidus, *Am. J. Cardiol.,* 31:327, 1973.

82 Koup, J. R., Greenblatt, D. J., Jusko, W. J., Smith, T. W., and Koch-Weser, J.: Pharmacokinetics of Digoxin in Normal Subjects after Intravenous Bolus and Infusion Doses, *J. Pharmacokinet. Biopharm.,* 3:181, 1975.

83 Doherty, J. E., Bissett, J. K., Kane, J. J., de Soyza, N., Murphy, M. L., Flanigan, W. J., and Dalrymple, G. V.: Tritiated Digoxin: Studies in Renal Disease in Human Subjects, *Int. J. Clin. Pharmacol. Biopharm.*, 12:89, 1975.

84 Ewy, G. A., Kapadia, G. G., Yao, L., Lullin, M., and Marcus, F. I.: Digoxin Metabolism in the Elderly, *Circulation*, 39:449, 1969.

85 Ewy, G. A., Groves, B. M., Ball, M. F., Nimo, L., Jackson, B., and Marcus, F.: Digoxin Metabolism in Obesity, *Circulation*, 44:810, 1971.

86 Doherty, J. E.: The Clinical Pharmacology of Digitalis Glycosides: A Review, *Am. J. Med. Sci.*, 255:382, 1968.

87 Smith, T. W.: Drug Therapy: Digitalis Glycosides, *N. Engl. J. Med.*, 288:719,942, 1973.

87a Spodick, D. H.: Hypertrophic Obstructive Cardiomyopathy of the Left Ventricle, *Cardiovasc. Clin.*, 4(1):133, 1972.

88 Wu, D., Wyndham, C., Amat-Y-Leon, F., Denes, P., Dhingra, R. C., and Rosen, K. M.: The Effects of Ouabain on Induction of Atrioventricular Nodal Re-entrant Paroxysmal Supraventricular Tachycardia, *Circulation*, 52:201, 1975.

89 Wellens, H. J. J., Düren, D. R., Liem, K. L., and Lie, K. I.: Effect of Digitalis in Patients with Paroxysmal Atrioventricular Tachycardia, *Circulation*, 52:779, 1975.

90 Carliner, N. H., Gilbert, C. A., Pruitt, A. W., and Goldberg, L. I.: Effects of Maintenance Digoxin Therapy on Systolic Time Intervals and Serum Digoxin Concentrations, *Circulation*, 50:94, 1974.

91 Ingelfinger, J. A., and Goldman, P.: The Serum Digitalis Concentration: Does It Diagnose Digitalis Toxicity? *N. Engl. J. Med.*, 294:867, 1976.

92 Beller, G. A., Smith, T. W., Abelmann, W. H., Haber, E., and Hood, W. B.: Digitalis Intoxication: A Prospective Clinical Study with Serum Level Correlation, *N. Engl. J. Med.*, 284:989, 1971.

93 Smith, T. W.: Digitalis Toxicity: Epidemiology and Clinical Use of Serum Concentration Measurements, *Am. J. Med.*, 58:470, 1975.

94 Evered, D. C., and Chapman, C.: Plasma Digoxin Concentrations and Digoxin Toxicity in Hospital Patients, *Br. Heart J.*, 33:540, 1971.

95 Fogelman, A. M., La Mont, J. T., Finkelstein, S., and Rado, E.: Fallibility of Plasma Digoxin in Differentiating Toxic from Non-toxic Patients, *Lancet*, 2:727, 1971.

96 Güllner, H-G., Stinson, E. B., Harrison, D. C., and Kalman, S. M.: Correlation of Serum Concentrations with Heart Concentrations of Digoxin in Human Subjects, *Circulation*, 50:653, 1974.

97 Härtel, G., Kyllönen, K., Merikallio, E., Ojala, K., Manninen, V., and Reissell, P.: Human Serum and Myocardial Digoxin, *Clin. Pharmacol. Ther.*, 19:153, 1976.

98 Coltart, D. J., Howard, M., and Chamberlain, D.: Myocardial and Skeletal Muscle Concentrations of Digoxin in Patients on Long-Term Therapy, *Br. Med. J.*, 2:318, 1972.

99 Jusko, W. J., and Weintraub, M.: Myocardial Distribution of Digoxin and Renal Function, *Clin. Pharmacol. Ther.*, 16:449, 1974.

100 Coltart, D. J., Güllner, H. G., Billingham, M., Goldman, R. H., Stinson, E. B., Kalman, S. M., and Harrison, D. C.: Physiological Distribution of Digoxin in Human Heart, *Br. Med. J.*, 4:733, 1974.

101 Kubasic, N. P., Brody, B. B., and Barold, S. S.: Problems in Measurement of Serum Digoxin by Commercially Available Radioimmunoassay Kits, *Am. J. Cardiol.*, 36:975, 1975.

102 Phillips, A. P.: The Improvement of Specificity of Radioimmunoassay, *Clin. Chim. Acta*, 44:333, 1973.

103 Chiou, W. L.: Potential Problems in Digoxin Therapy Due to Variations in Recommended Dosage Regimens, *J. Clin. Pharmacol.*, 15:272, 1975.

104 Greenblatt, D. J., Duhme, D. W., and Koch-Weser, J.: Pain and CPK Elevation after Intramuscular Digoxin, *N. Engl. J. Med.*, 288:689, 1973.

105 Steiness, E., Svensen, O., and Rasmussen, F.: Plasma Digoxin after Parenteral Administration: Local Digoxin after Intramuscular Injection, *Clin. Pharmacol. Ther.*, 16:430, 1974.

106 Storstein, L.: Studies on Digitalis: II. The Influence of Impaired Renal Function on the Renal Excretion of Digitoxin and Its Cardioactive Metabolites, *Clin. Pharmacol. Ther.*, 16:25, 1974.

107 Shoeman, D. W., and Azarnoff, D. D.: The Alteration of Plasma Proteins in Uremia as Related in Their Ability to Bind Digitoxin and Diphenylhydantoin, *Pharmacology*, 7:169, 1972.

108 Koup, J. R., Jusko, W. J., Elwood, C. M., and Kohli, R. K.: Digoxin Pharmacokinetics: Role of Renal Failure in Dosage Regiment Design, *Clin. Pharmacol. Ther.*, 18:9, 1975.

109 Lukas, D. S.: Of Toads and Flowers, *Circulation*, 46:1, 1972. (Editorial.)

110 Lown, B., Klein, M. D., Barr, I., Hagemeijer, F., Kosowsky, B. D., and Garrison, H.: Sensitivity to Digitalis Drugs in Acute Myocardial Infarction, *Am. J. Cardiol.*, 30:388, 1972.

111 Thompson, A. J., Hargis, J., Murphy, M. L., and Doherty, J. E.: Tritiated Digoxin: XX. Tissue Distribution in Experimental Myocardial Infarction, *Am. Heart J.*, 88:319, 1974.

112 Maroko, P. R., and Braunwald, E.: Effects of Metabolic and Pharmacologic Interventions on Myocardial Infarct Size following Coronary Occlusion, *Circulation*, 53(suppl. 1):162, 1976.

113 Hodges, M., Friesinger, C. G., Riggins, R. C. K., and Dagenais, G. R.: Effects of Intravenously Administered Digoxin on Mild Left Ventricular Failure in Acute Myocardial Infarction in Man, *Am. J. Cardiol.*, 29:749, 1972.

114 Ratshin, R. A., Rackley, C. E., and Russel, R. O.: Hemodynamic Evaluation of Left Ventricular Function in Shock Complicating Myocardial Infarction, *Circulation*, 45:127, 1972.

115 Rahimtoola, S. H., Sinno, Z., Chuguimia, R., Loeb, H. S., Rosen, K. M., and Gunnar, R. M.: Impaired Left Ventricular Function in Acute Myocardial Infarction, *N. Engl. J. Med.*, 287:527, 1972.

116 Karliner, J. S., and Braunwald, E.: Present Status of Digitalis Treatment of Acute Myocardial Infarction, *Circulation*, 45: 891, 1972.

117 Lown, B., and Wittenberg, S.: Cardioversion and Digitalis: III. Effect of Change in Serum Potassium Concentration, *Am. J. Cardiol.*, 21:513, 1968.

118 Resnekov, L.: Drug Therapy before and after the Electroversion of Cardiac Dysrhythmias, *Prog. Cardiovasc. Dis.*, 16:531, 1974.

119 Hagemeijer, F., and van Houwe, E.: Titrated Energy Cardioversion of Patients on Digitalis, *Br. Heart J.*, 37:1303, 1975.

120 Coltart, D. J., Chamberlain, D. A., Howard, M. R., Kettlewell, M. G., Mercer, J. L., and Smith, T. W.: Bypass on Plasma Digoxin Concentrations, *Br. Heart J.*, 33:334, 1971.

121 Morrison, J., and Killip, T.: Serum Digitalis and Arrhythmias in Patients Undergoing Cardiopulmonary Bypass, *Circulation*, 47:341, 1973.

122 Krasula, R. W., Hastreiter, A. R., Levistsky, S., Yanagi, R., and Soyka, L. F.: Digoxin Levels during Cardiopulmonary Bypass in Children, *Circulation*, 49:1047, 1974.

123 Beller, B. M.: Digitalis and Anesthesia: A Comprehensive Review of the Chemistry, Pharmacology, and Clinical Use of the Cardiac Glycosides in Anesthesia, *Clin. Anesth.*, 10(1): 143, 1973.

124 Storstein, L.: Studies on Digitalis: III. Biliary Excretion and

Enterohepatic Circulation of Digitoxin and Its Cardioactive Metabolites, *Clin. Pharmacol. Ther.*, 17:313, 1975.

125 Marcus, F. I., and Kapadia, G. G.: The Metabolism of Tritiated Digoxin in Cirrhotic Patients, *Gastroenterology*, 47:517, 1964.

126 Lahrtz, H. G., Reinhold, H. M., and van Zwieten, P. A.: Serumkonzentration und Ausscheidung von ³H-digitoxin bein Menschen unter normalen und pathologischen Bedingungen, *Klin. Wochenschr.*, 47:695, 1969.

127 Zilly, W., Richter, E., and Rietbrock, N.: Pharmacokinetics and Metabolism of Digoxin and β-Methyldigoxin-12-α-³H in Patients with Acute Hepatitis, *Clin. Pharmacol. Ther.*, 17:302, 1975.

128 Eichenbusch, W., Lahrtz, H.-G., Seppelt, U., and van Zwieten, P. A.: Serum Concentration and Urinary Excretion of ³H-Ouabain and ³H-digitoxin in Patients Suffering from Hyperthyroidism or Hypothyroidism, *Klin. Wochenschr.*, 48:270, 1970.

129 Butler, V. P., and Lindenbaum, J.: Serum Digitalis Measurement in the Assessment of Digitalis Resistance and Sensitivity, *Am. J. Med.*, 58:460, 1975.

130 Malovang, R. J., and Koerner, S. K.: Acute Respiratory Insufficiency and Cor Pulmonale, *Am. Heart J.*, 88:251, 1974.

131 Heizer, W. D., Smith, T. W., and Goldfinger, S. E.: Absorption of Digoxin in Patients with Malabsorption Syndrome, *N. Engl. J. Med.*, 285:257, 1971.

132 Hall, W. H., and Doherty, J. E.: Trititated Digoxin: XXII. Absorption and Excretion in Malabsorption Syndrome, *Am. J. Med.*, 56:437, 1974.

132a Marcus, F. I., Quinn, E. J., Horton, H., Shannon, J., Pippin, S., Stafford, M., and Zukoski, C.: The Effect of Jejunoileal Bypass on the Pharmacokinetics of Digoxin in Man, *Circulation*, 55:537, 1977.

133 Goldman, R. H., Deutscher, R. N., Schweizer, E., and Harrison, D. C.: Effect of a Pharmacologic Dose of Digoxin on Inotropy in Hyper- and Normokalemic Dogs, *Am. J. Physiol.*, 223:1438, 1972.

134 Williams, J. F., Jr., Klocke, F. J., and Braunwald, E.: Studies on Digitalis: XIII. A Comparison of the Effects on Potassium on the Inotropic and Arrhythmic Producing Actions of Ouabain, *J. Clin. Invest.*, 45:346, 1966.

135 Ferrier, G. R., and Moe, G. K.: Effect of Calcium on Acetylstrophanthidin Induced Transient Depolarization in Canine Purkinje Tissue, *Circ. Res.*, 33:508, 1973.

136 Toda, N., and West, T. C.: Modification by Sodium and Calcium of the Cardiotoxicity Induced by Ouabain, *J. Pharmacol. Exp. Ther.*, 154:239, 1966.

137 Beller, G. A., Hood, W. B., and Smith, T. W.: Correlation of Serum Magnesium Level and Cardiac Digitalis Intoxication, *Am. J. Cardiol.*, 33:225, 1974.

138 Goldman, R. H., Kleiger, R. E., Schweizer, E., and Harrison, D. C.: The Effect on Myocardial ³H-Digoxin of Magnesium Deficiency, *Proc. Soc. Exp. Biol. Med.*, 136:747, 1971.

139 Seller, R. H.: The Role of Magnesium in Digitalis Toxicity, *Am. Heart J.*, 82:551, 1971.

140 Specter, M. J., Schweizer, E., and Goldman, R. H.: Studies on Magnesium's Mechanism of Action in Digitalis-induced Arrhythmias, *Circulation*, 52:1001, 1975.

141 Shine, K. I., and Douglas, A. M.: Magnesium Effect on Ionic Exchange and Mechanical Function in the Rat Ventricle, *Am. J. Physiol.*, 227:317, 1974.

142 Tse, W. W., and Han, J.: Interaction of Epinephrine and Ouabain on Automaticity of Purkinje Fibers, *Circ. Res.*, 34:777, 1974.

143 Pearle, D. L., and Gillis, R. A.: Effect of Digitalis on Response of the Ventricular Pacemaker to Sympathetic Neural Stimulation and Isoproterenol, *Am. J. Cardiol.*, 34:704, 1974.

144 Dick, H. L. H., McCowley, E. L., and Fisher, W. A.: Reserpine-Digitalis Toxicity, *Arch. Intern., Med.*, 109:503, 1962.

145 Lown, B., Ehrlich, L., Lysschultz, B., and Blake, J.: Effect of Digitalis in Patients Receiving Reserpine, *Circulation*, 24:1185, 1961.

146 Manninen, V., Apajalahti, A., Melin, J., and Karesoja, M.: Altered Absorption of Digoxin in Patients Given Propantheline and Metoclopramide, *Lancet*, 1:398, 1973.

147 Bazzano, G., and Bazzano, G. S.: Digitalis Intoxication Treated with a New Steroid-binding Resin, *JAMA*, 220:828, 1972.

148 Caldwell, J. H., Bush, C. A., and Greenberger, N. J.: Interruption of the Enterohepatic Circulation of Digitoxin by Cholestyramine: II. Effect on Metabolic Disposition of Tritium-labelled Digitoxin and Cardiac Systolic Time Intervals in Man, *J. Clin. Invest.*, 50:2638, 1971.

149 Solomon, H. M., and Abram, W. B.: Interaction between Digitoxin and Other Drugs in Man, *Am. Heart J.*, 83:277, 1972.

150 Taylor, S. A., Rawlins, M. D., and Smith S. E.: Spironolactone: A Weak Enzyme Inducer in Man, *J. Pharm. Pharmacol.*, 24:578, 1972.

151 Schwartz, L. S., and Schwartz, S. P.: Adams-Stokes Syndrome during Atrial Fibrillation with A-V block: Observations on Toxic Reactions to Digitalis, *Am. J. Cardiol.*, 14:483, 1964.

152 Rios, J. C., Dziok, C. A., and Ali, N. A.: Digitalis-induced Arrhythmias: Recognition and Management, *Cardiovasc. Clin.*, 2(2):262, 1972.

153 Smith, T. W., and Willerson, J. T.: Suicidal and Accidental Digoxin Ingestion, *Circulation*, 44:29, 1971.

154 Smith, T. W., Haber, E., Yeatman, L., and Buttler, V. P.: Reversal of Advanced Digoxin Intoxication with Fab Fragments of Digoxin-specific Antibodies, *N. Engl. J. Med.*, 294:797, 1976.

155 Lely, A. H., and van Enter, C. H. J.: Large-Scale Digitoxin Intoxication, *Br. Med. J.*, 3:737, 1970.

156 Fisch, C., and Knoebel, S. B.: Recognition and Therapy of Digitalis Toxicity, *Prog. Cardiovasc. Dis.*, 13:71, 1970.

157 Ewy, G. A., Marcus, F. I., Fillmore, S. J., and Mathews, N. P.: Digitalis Intoxication: Diagnosis, Management and Prevention, *Cardiovasc. Clin.*, 6(2):153, 1974.

158 Ghani, M. F., and Smith, J. R.: The Effectiveness of Magnesium Chloride in the Treatment of Ventricular Tachyarrhythmias Due to Digitalis Intoxication, *Am. Heart J.*, 88:621, 1974.

159 Zelis, R., Mason, D. T., Spann, J. F., Jr., and Braunwald, E.: Effects of Ventricular Stimulation and Potassium Administration on Digitalis-induced arrhythmias, *Am. J. Cardiol.*, 25:428, 1970.

160 Beller, B. M., Kotler, M. N., and Collens, R.: The Use of Ventricular Pacing for Suppression of Ectopic Ventricular Activity, *Am. J. Cardiol.*, 25:467, 1970.

161 LeWinn, E. B.: Gynecomastia during Digitalis Therapy, *N. Engl. J. Med.*, 248:316, 1953.

162 Navab, A., Koss, L. G., and LaDue, J. S.: Estrogen-like Activity of Digitalis, *JAMA*, 194:142, 1965.

163 Stoffer, S. S., Hynes, K. M., Jiang, N. S., and Ryan, R. J.: Digoxin and Abnormal Serum Hormone Levels, *JAMA*, 225:1643, 1973.

164 Duca, P., and Brest, A. N.: Indications, Contraindications and Nonindications for Digitalis Therapy, *Cardiovasc. Clin.* 6(2):131, 1974.

165 Schwartz, L. S., and Schwartz, S. P.: The Effects of Digitalis Bodies on Patients with Heart Block and Congestive Heart Failure, *Prog. Cardiovasc. Dis.*, 6:366, 1964.

166 Kaplan, B. M., Langendorf, R., Lev, M., and Pick, A.: Tachycardia-Bradycardia Syndrome (So-called "Sick Sinus Syndrome"), *Am. J. Cardiol.*, 31:497, 1973.

167 Rubenstein, J. J., Schulman, C. L., Yurchak, P. M., and DeSanctis, R. W.: Clinical Spectrum of the Sick Sinus Syndrome, *Circulation*, 46:5, 1972.

168 Sutherland, E. W., Robinson, G. A., and Butcher, R. W.: Some Aspects of the Biological Role of Adenosine 3',5'-Monophosphate (Cyclic AMP), *Circulation*, 37:279, 1968.

169 Darby, T. D., Sprouse, J. H., and Walton, R. P.: Evaluation of Sympathetic Reflex Effects on the Inotropic Action of Nitroglycerin, Quinidine, Papaverine, Aminophylline and Isoproterenol, *J. Pharmacol. Exp. Ther.*, 122:386, 1958.

170 Howarth, S., McMichael, J., and Sharpey-Shafer, E. P.: The Circulatory Action of Theophylline Ethylene Diamine, *Clin. Sci.*, 6:125, 1947.

171 Ritchie, J. M.: Central Nervous System Stimulants: The Xanthines, in L. S. Goodman and A. Gilman (eds.), "The Pharmacological Basis of Therapeutics," 5th ed., The Macmillan Company, New York, 1975, p. 367.

172 Maxwell, G. M., White, D. H., Jr., Crampton, C. W., Rowe, G. G., and Castillo, C. A.: Effects of Intravenous Aminophylline upon Coronary Hemodynamics and Myocardial O_2 and CO_2 Metabolism in Normal and Diseased Hearts, *Circulation*, 18:757, 1958.

173 Pitts, R. F.: "The Physiological Basis of Diuretic Therapy," Charles C. Thomas, Publisher, Springfield, Ill., 1959.

174 Piafsky, K., and Ogilivie, R. I.: Drug Therapy: Dosage of Theophylline in Bronchial Asthma, *N. Engl. J. Med.*, 292:1218, 1975.

175 Jenne, J. W., Wyze, E., Rood, F. S., and MacDonald, F. M.: Pharmacokinetics of Theophylline, *Clin. Pharmacol. Ther.*, 13:349, 1972.

176 Zwillich, C. W., Sutton, F. D., Neff, T. A., Cohn, W. M., Matthay, R. A., and Weinberger, M. M.: Theophylline Induced Seizures in Adults, *Ann. Intern. Med.*, 82:784, 1975.

177 Camarata, S. J., Weil, M. H., Hanashiro, P. K., and Shubin, H.: Cardiac Arrest in the Critically Ill: I. A Study of Predisposing Causes in 132 Patients, *Circulation*, 44:688, 1971.

178 Jacobs, M. H., and Senior, R. M.: Theophylline Toxicity Due to Impaired Theophylline Degradation, *Am. Rev. Respir. Dis.*, 110:342, 1974.

179 Murphree, H. B.: Clinical Pharmacology of Potent Analgesics, *Clin. Pharmacol. Ther.*, 3:473, 1962.

180 Eckenhoff, J. E., and Oech, S. R.: The Effects of Narcotics and Antagonists upon Respiration and Circulation in Man: A Review, *Clin. Pharmacol. Ther.*, 1:483, 1960.

181 Jaffe, J. H., and Martin, W. R.: Narcotic Analgesics and Antagonists, in L. S. Goodman and A. Gilman (eds.), "The Pharmacological Basis of Therapeutics," 5th ed., The Macmillan Company, New York, 1975, p. 245.

182 Ward, J. M., McGrath, P. L., and Wei, J. V.: Effects of Morphine on the Peripheral Vascular Response to Sympathetic Stimulation, *Am. J. Cardiol.*, 29:659, 1972.

183 Ramirez, A., and Abelmann, W. H.: Current Concepts: Cardiac Decompensation, *N. Engl. J. Med.*, 290:499, 1974.

184 Kirshna, G., and Paradise, R. R.: Effects of Morphine on Isolated Human Atrial Muscle, *Anesthesiology*, 40:147, 1974.

185 Lowenstein, E., Hallowell, P., Levine, F. H., Daggett, W. M., Austen, W. G., and Laver, M. B.: Cardiovascular Response to Large Dose of Intravenous Morphine in Man, *N. Engl. J. Med.*, 281:1389, 1969.

186 Thomas, M., Malcrona, R., Fillmore, S., and Shillingford, J.: Haemodynamic Effects of Morphine in Patients with Acute Myocardial Infarction, *Br. Heart J.*, 27:863, 1965.

187 Walker, J. F., Hoff, H. E., Huggins, R. A., and Deavers, S.: Influence of Morphine on Central Control of Respiration and Circulation in the Dog, *Arch. Int. Pharmacodyn. Ther.*, 170:216, 1967.

188 Vasko, J. S., Hennery, R. P., Brawley, R. K., Oldham, H. N., and Morrow, A. G.: Effects of Morphine on Ventricular Function and Myocardial Contractile Force, *Am. J. Physiol.*, 210:329, 1966.

189 Rees, H. A.: The Effect of Opiates in Acute Myocardial Infarction, in L. E. Meltzer and A. L. Dunning (eds.), "Textbook of Coronary Care," Exerpta Medica, Amsterdam, 1972, p. 512.

190 Paton, W. D. M.: Histamine Release by Compounds of Simple Chemical Structure, *Pharmacol. Rev.*, 9:269, 1957.

191 Lal, S., and Savidge, R. S.: Cardiovascular and Respiratory Effects of Morphine and Pentazocine in Patients with Myocardial Infarction, *Lancet*, 1:379, 1969.

192 Scott, M. E., and Orr, R.: Effects of Diamorphine, Methadone, Morphine, and Pentazocine in Patients with Suspected Acute Myocardial Infarction, *Lancet*, 1:1065, 1969.

193 Nickerson, M.: Vasodilator Drugs, in L. S. Goodman and A. Gilman (eds.), "The Pharmacological Basis of Therapeutics," 5th ed., The Macmillan Company, New York, 1975, p. 727.

194 Cohn, J. N.: Vasodilatory Therapy for Heart Failure: The Influence of Impedance in Left Ventricular Performance, *Circulation*, 48:5, 1973.

195 Chatterjee, K., and Parmley, W. W.: The Role of Vasodilator Therapy in Heart Failure, *Prog. Cardiovasc. Dis.*, 19:301, 1977.

196 Stinson, E. B., Holloway, E. L., Derby, G., Oyer, D. E., Hollingworth, J., Griepp, R. B., and Harrison, D. C.: Comparative Hemodynamic Responses to Chlorpromazine, Nitroprusside, Nitroglycerin, and Trimethaphan Immediately after Open Heart Operations, *Circulation*, 51/52 (suppl. 1):26, 1975.

197 Palmer, R. F., and Lasseter, K. C.: Sodium Nitroprusside, *N. Engl. J. Med.*, 292:294, 1975.

198 West, J. W., and Guzman, S. V.: Coronary Dilatation and Constriction Visualized by Selective Arteriography, *Circ. Res.*, 7:527, 1959.

199 Likoff, W., Kasparian, H., Lehman, J. S., and Segal, B. L.: Evaluation of "Coronary Vasodilators" by Coronary Arteriography, *Am. J. Cardiol.*, 13:7, 1964.

200 Berstein, L., Friesinger, G. C., Lichtlen, P. R., and Ross, R. S.: The Effect of Nitroglycerin on the Systemic and Coronary Circulation in Man and Dogs: Myocardial Blood Flow Measurement with Xenon[133], *Circulation*, 33:107, 1966.

201 Horwitz, L. D., Gorlin, R., Taylor, W. J., and Kemp, H. G.: Effects of Nitroglycerin on Regional Myocardial Blood Flow in Coronary Artery Disease, *J. Clin. Invest.*, 50:1578, 1971.

202 Aronow, W. S.: Medical Treatment of Angina Pectoris: III. Pharmacology of Sublingual Nitrates as Antianginal Drugs, *Am. Heart J.*, 84:273, 1972.

203 Flaherty, J. T., Reid, P. R., Kelly, D. T., Taylor, D. R., Weisfeldt, M. L., and Pitt, B.: Intravenous Nitroglycerin in Acute Myocardial Infarction, *Circulation*, 51:132, 1975.

204 Williams, D. O., Amsterdam, E. A., and Mason, D. T.: Hemodynamic Effects of Nitroglycerin in Acute Myocardial Infarction: Decrease in Ventricular Preload at the Expense of Cardiac Output, *Circulation*, 51:421, 1975.

205 Armstrong, P. W., Walker, D. C., Burton, J. R., and Parker, J. O.: Vasodilator Therapy in Acute Myocardial Infarction: A Comparison of Sodium Nitroprusside and Nitroglycerin, *Circulation*, 52:1118, 1975.

206 Needleman, P., Lang, S., and Johnson, E. M., Jr.: Relationship between Biotransformation and Rational Angina Pectoris Therapy, *J. Pharmacol. Exp. Ther.*, 181:489, 1972.

207 Aronow, W. S.: The Medical Treatment of Angina Pectoris:

IV. Nitroglycerin as an Antianginal Drug, *Am. Heart J.,* 84:415, 1972.

208 Horwitz, L. D., Herman, M. V., and Gorlin, R.: Clinical Response to Nitroglycerin as a Diagnostic Test for Coronary Artery Disease, *Am. J. Cardiol.,* 29:149, 1972.

209 Goldstein, R. E., and Epstein, S. E.: Nitrates in the Prophylactic Treatment of Angina Pectoris, *Circulation,* 48:917, 1973.

209a Parker, J. O., Augustine, R. J., Burton, J. R., West, R. O., and Armstrong, P. W.: Effect of Nitroglycerin Ointment on the Clinical and Hemodynamic Response to Exercise, *Am. J. Cardiol.,* 38:162, 1976.

210 Fusari, S. A.: Nitroglycerin Sublingual Tablets: II. Preparations and Stability of a New, Stabilized, Molded Nitroglycerin, *J. Pharm. Sci.,* 62:2012, 1973.

211 Mayer, G. A.: Instability of Nitroglycerin Tablets, *Can. Med. Assoc. J.,* 110:788, 1974.

211a Come, P. C., and Pitt, B.: Nitroglycerin-induced Severe Hypotension and Bradycardia in Patients with Acute Myocardial Infarction, *Circulation,* 54:624, 1976.

212 Russek, H. I.: Therapeutic Role of Coronary Vasodilators: Glyceryl Trinitrate, Isosorbide Dinitrate, and Pentaerythritol Tetranitrate, *Am. J. Med. Sci.,* 252:9, 1966.

213 Aronow, W. S.: The Medical Treatment of Angina Pectoris: V. Long-acting Nitrates as Antianginal Drugs, *Am. Heart J.,* 84:567, 1972.

214 Goldstein, R., Rosing, D., Redwood, P., Beiser, G. D., and Epstein, S. E.: Clinical and Circulatory Effects of Isosorbide Dinitrate, *Circulation,* 43:629, 1971.

214a Mikulic, E., Franciosa, J. A., and Cohn, J. N.: Comparative Hemodynamic Effects of Chewable Isosorbide Dinitrate and Nitroglycerin in Patients with Congestive Heart Failure, *Circulation,* 52:477, 1975.

214b Bussmann, W. D., Lonner, J., and Kaltenbach, M.: Orally Administered Isosorbide Dinitrate in Patients with and without Ventricular Failure due to Acute Myocardial Infarction, *Am. J. Cardiol.,* 39:91, 1977.

215 Tourville, J.: Drug Evaluation Data: Sodium Nitroprusside, *Drug Intell. Clin. Pharm.,* 9:361, 1975.

216 Franciosa, J. A., Guiha, N. H., Limas, C. J., Rodriguera, E. R., and Cohn, J. N.: Improved Left Ventricular Function during Nitroprusside Infusion in Acute Myocardial Infarction, *Lancet,* 1:650, 1972.

217 Lukes, S. A., Romero, C. A., Jr., and Resnekov, L.: Hemodynamic Effects of Sodium Nitroprusside in 21 Subjects with Congestive Heart Failure: Documentation of Responders and Nonresponders. (Submitted for publication.)

218 Miller, R. R., Vismara, L. A., Zelis, R., Amsterdam, E. A., and Mason, D. T.: Clinical Use of Sodium Nitroprusside in Chronic Ischemic Heart Disease, *Circulation,* 51:328, 1975.

219 Turner, J. M., Powell, D., Robert, M. G., and McDowall, D. G.: The Effects of Sodium Nitroprusside on Intracranial Pressure and Autoregulation, in N. Lundberg, U. Ponten, and M. Brock (eds.), "Intracranial Pressure II," Springer-Verlag New York, Inc., 1975, p. 345.

220 Bower, P. J., and Peterson, J. N.: Methemoglobinemia after Sodium Nitroprusside Therapy, *N. Engl. J. Med.,* 293:865, 1976.

D

Drugs Acting on the Autonomic Nervous System

LEON I. GOLDBERG, M.D., Ph.D., and
YEN-YAU HSIEH, M.D.

SYMPATHOMIMETIC AMINES

Classification

The ability of sympathomimetic amines to produce excitatory and inhibitory effects in various organ systems suggested to Ahlquist[1] that these amines could be classified into two types, α and β. According to this concept, vasoconstriction produced by sympathomimetic amines is the result of action of the amines on α-adrenergic receptors; vasodilatation and cardiac stimulation are considered to be produced by action on β-adrenergic receptors. More recently, β-adrenergic receptors have been subdivided; the receptors in the heart are termed β_1 and those in the smooth muscle, β_2.[2,3]

Sympathomimetic amines may also be classified according to whether they act directly on the adrenergic receptors or act indirectly by causing release of norepinephrine from storage sites in the sympathetic nerves. Table 109D-1 lists several sympathomimetic amines and describes the types of actions they exhibit in usual clinical doses.

Cardiac actions[4-6]

Sympathomimetic amines acting on β_1-adrenergic receptors increase myocardial contractility. This effect may be due to direct action on the receptor or may take place indirectly by the release of norepinephrine from sympathetic nerve storage sites. Norepinephrine (Levophed), epinephrine, isoproterenol (Isuprel), and the newly synthesized sympathomimetic amine dobutamine[7] produce their cardiac effects by direct action on β_1-adrenergic receptors. Dopamine (Intropin) causes cardiac stimulation by approximately equal direct and indirect actions.[8] The longer-acting mephentermine (Wyamine) and metaraminol (Aramine) are primarily indirect-acting amines.

Other cardiac responses resulting from stimulation of β_1-adrenergic receptors are increased heart rate by action on the sinoatrial (SA) node, enhanced conduction through the atrioventricular (AV) node, and increased ectopic activity. The increase in ectopic activity is particularly evident in the presence of cyclopropane anesthesia and hypoxia (see group III antiarrhythmic drugs in Chap. 109B).

The biochemical basis for the cardiac actions of sympathomimetic amines is being extensively investigated. It was once thought that the positive inotropic action of catecholamines was the result of activation of phosphorylase, but there is good evidence for dissociating these phenomena.[9,10] Current interest is centered on the action of sympathomimetic amines

TABLE 109D-1
Effects of several sympathomimetic amines on heart and blood vessels

Amine	Effect on heart	Effect on blood vessels
Norepinephrine (Levophed)	Beta	Alpha
Epinephrine (Adrenalin)	Beta	Alpha Beta
Metaraminol (Aramine)*	Beta	Alpha
Mephentermine (Wyamine)*	Beta	Alpha
Ephedrine*	Beta	Alpha
Methamphetamine* (Methedrine)	Beta	Alpha
Isoproterenol (Isuprel)	Beta	Beta
Methoxamine (Vasoxyl)	0	Alpha
Phenylephrine (Neo-Synephrine)	±	Alpha
Dopamine	Beta	Alpha (most peripheral blood vessels) Nonadrenergic (vasodilatation —renal and mesenteric vessels)

*Acts totally or predominately by release of norepinephrine (indirect).

to stimulate the enzyme adenylate cyclase which results in increased intracellular content of cyclic adenosine monophosphate (cAMP).[10] An unanswered question with proponents on both sides is whether the elevation of intracellular cAMP is necessary for demonstration of cardiac effects.[10] As with cardiac glycosides the ultimate requirement for the action of sympathomimetic amines appears to be an increase in intracellular calcium, and, indeed, there is substantial evidence demonstrating increased calcium flux after catecholamines.[11] However, the subject is still controversial.[10,12]

Peripheral vascular effects

Sympathomimetic amines may either constrict or dilate blood vessels. All the amines in Table 109D-1 in clinical doses can constrict blood vessels with the exception of isoproterenol, which has only vasodilating (β2-adrenergic) actions.

The amines differ considerably in their effects on various vascular beds. Certain amines will constrict one vascular bed and dilate another. As an example of such dual action, epinephrine dilates the blood vessels in skeletal muscles and simultaneously constricts skin and renal arterioles. It is important to be aware of this dual action because renal arteriolar constriction produced by epinephrine may result in reduction of renal blood flow even though total peripheral vascular resistance is decreased.

Dopamine also exerts a biphasic effect on the peripheral vasculature. In small doses, dopamine decreases peripheral vascular resistance because of renal and mesenteric vasodilation resulting from action on specific dopamine receptors. In higher doses, dopamine also causes vasoconstriction which

occurs primarily in the blood vessels of the skeletal muscle. As the dose is further elevated, vasoconstriction predominates and peripheral vascular resistance increases.[8] Dobutamine has much weaker α-adrenergic action than norepinephrine and weaker β2-adrenergic actions than isoproterenol. Thus dobutamine has the potential of exerting β1 actions with minimal peripheral effects.[7,13] Dobutamine differs, however, from dopamine in that it does not act on dopamine receptors to cause renal and mesenteric vasodilation.[13,14] Effects of sympathomimetic amines on coronary arteries are difficult to evaluate and are more closely related to their influence on myocardial contractility, heart rate, and systemic pressure than to their direct action on coronary vascular receptors.

Effect on the intact circulation

The effects of sympathomimetic amines on cardiac output and heart rate depend on their relative cardiac and peripheral actions. Potent vasoconstrictor drugs such as norepinephrine may not increase cardiac output despite a positive inotropic effect because of increase in peripheral vascular resistance (thereby increasing blood pressure) with reflex reduction in heart rate. At the other extreme, isoproterenol markedly increases cardiac output directly by augmenting myocardial contractility, increasing heart rate, and reducing afterload, and indirectly by inducing reflex sympathetic cardiac stimulation resulting from baroreceptor response to vasodilation. Dopamine and dobutamine exert hemodynamic effects intermediate between norepinephrine and isoproterenol. Dobutamine and dopamine produce less tachycardia than isoproterenol because of less reflex cardiac stimulation; other mechanism may also be involved.[8,15]

Indications

TREATMENT OF SHOCK[15-19]

Sympathomimetic amines are probably the most widely used drugs in the treatment of shock. The objective of such therapy is to increase the flow of blood to vital organs. This can be accomplished with sympathomimetic amines by increasing myocardial contractility, by maintaining adequate perfusing pressure, by decreasing resistance in blood vessels supplying the vital organs, or by a combination of these actions. Obviously the benefits obtained in an individual patient will depend not only on the pharmacologic actions of a sympathomimetic amine but also on whether the expected actions of the amine will take place in the patient in shock. In general, patients in shock due to myocardial infarction are more resistant to therapy with sympathomimetic amines and other means than are patients with septic shock (see Chap. 48). It is usually impossible to predict the action of sympathomimetic amines in the individual patient. Accordingly, therapy must be initiated on a trial basis, and the physician must be prepared to alter therapy if the patient's condition is not improved. Before discussing advantages and disadvantages of the various sympathomimetic amines it should be stressed that the drugs should be used only after plasma and blood volume deficits have been corrected. Abnormal serum electrolyte and arterial blood gas levels should be improved, and hemodynamically significant arrhythmias should be treated. If possible, the ECG should be constantly monitored; cardiac output, direct arterial blood pressure, pulmonary capillary wedge pressure (as a reflection of left ventricular filling pressure), arterial blood gas, and urine flow rate (by means of a bladder catheter) should be measured periodically.

The initial choice of a sympathomimetic amine will depend on whether a potent vasoconstrictor agent is required to elevate blood pressure for adequate perfusion of the heart and brain or whether time is available to institute therapy with an agent that has fewer or no vasoconstrictor properties. If elevation of blood pressure is imperative, therapy probably should be started with norepinephrine. This drug is most reliable for elevating blood pressure because of its potent vasoconstrictor and myocardial stimulating actions. Infusion of norepinephrine should be discontinued as soon as possible, or the treatment should be changed to less vasoconstricting drugs to prevent initiation of a vicious cycle caused by the profound vasoconstriction (see "α-Adrenergic Blocking Agents" below).

Because of the ability of dopamine to increase cardiac output, dilate renal and mesenteric blood vessels, and constrict skeletal muscle vasculature, this amine has become widely used for treatment of shock.[8,15,20,21] Isoproterenol, formerly a drug of choice, is now considered inappropriate for treatment of most patients with acute myocardial infarction complicated with shock,[22] although it may have some use in patients with septic shock.[23] Isoproterenol decreases peripheral vascular resistance because of β_2-adrenergic vasodilation primarily in the skeletal

muscles, and any increase in blood pressure would have to be the result of increased cardiac output. The danger in the use of isoproterenol is that blood pressure may be further decreased by vasodilation and perfusion of the brain and heart may be compromised. Isoproterenol is particularly dangerous in the patient with myocardial ischemia because of the combined effects of tachycardia and decreased coronary perfusion.

Use of sympathomimetic amine with only or predominately α-adrenergic vasoconstricting properties such as methoxamine (Vasoxyl) or phenylephrine (Neo-Synephrine) may be detrimental to patients in shock, especially to those with myocardial insufficiency.[24,25]

HEART BLOCK[26]

Sympathomimetic amines with cardiac stimulating actions are used to increase the rate of junctional and ventricular pacemakers and improve AV conduction in patients with heart block. Isoproterenol is most commonly used for this purpose; epinephrine and ephedrine have also been employed.

PAROXYSMAL ATRIAL TACHYCARDIA[26]

Sympathomimetic amines are sometimes used to treat resistant cases of paroxysmal atrial tachycardia by elevating the blood pressure and thereby stimulating vagal inhibitory reflexes. The amines without cardiac stimulating effects, phenylephrine and methoxamine, would appear to be most suitable for this purpose.

LOW OUTPUT STATE FOLLOWING CARDIAC SURGERY

Dopamine is being extensively used for treatment of low output syndromes during and after cardiac surgery. Many investigators have demonstrated increases in cardiac output and urine flow.[20,27,28] Figure 109D-1 illustrates the use of dopamine in such a patient.[20] Isoproterenol and dobutamine have also been tried.[15,28]

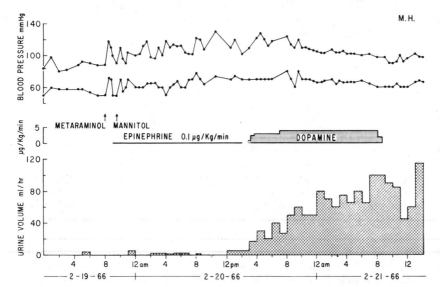

FIGURE 109D-1 Use of dopamine in the treatment of shock. A prosthetic mitral valve was inserted 8 h before the period shown. The administration of epinephrine was associated with oliguria; the subsequent administration of dopamine was associated with a diuresis in spite of a fall in the systemic blood pressure. (From MacCannell, McNay, Meyer, and Goldberg,[20] by permission of the authors and publisher.)

CONGESTIVE HEART FAILURE

Although sympathomimetic amines can increase myocardial contractility as much as, or more than, digitalis, they have been used previously only for treatment of acute cardiac failure. Intravenous infusion of dopamine, however, increases sodium excretion of patients with congestive heart failure, suggesting that an oral dopamine-like amine may be useful in the treatment of chronic congestive heart failure.[8,15,29–31]

Adverse effects

Most adverse effects of sympathomimetic amines are extensions of their basic pharmacologic actions. Cardiac arrhythmias may be produced both by direct cardiac actions of sympathomimetic amines and by increased peripheral vascular resistance.[8,23] Ischemic damage to the heart, liver, kidney, extremities, and other organs has been blamed on the action of sympathomimetic amines.[32–34] Prolonged infusion of sympathomimetic amines with vasoconstrictor properties may cause a vicious cycle requiring ever-increasing amounts of drug to maintain blood pressure.[35,36] Extravasation of norepinephrine, metaraminol, and dopamine can cause ischemic necrosis and sloughing of tissues. This danger can be minimized by administering the agents through polyethylene catheters inserted well into the vein and by local administration of phentolamine in the event of extravasation.

β-ADRENERGIC BLOCKING AGENTS

β-Adrenergic blocking agents specifically antagonize the action of sympathomimetic amines and the responses of sympathetic stimulation at β-adrenergic receptor sites.[37,38] These drugs are competitive antagonists of the receptor; thus, their effects can be overcome by administration of higher doses of β-adrenergic agonists. A large number of β-adrenergic blocking agents have been synthesized, and the different compounds vary with respect to absolute potency, duration of action, intrinsic sympathomimetic activity, membrane depressant action, and cardiac selectivity.[39,40] Propranolol is the only β-adrenergic blocking agent available in the United States, but others are currently under investigation and may be released in the near future.

Effects on cardiovascular function

The effects of β-adrenergic antagonists on cardiac function in the intact animal and the human being depends upon the degree of sympathomimetic drive present at the time of drug administration. For example, only slight reductions of heart rate and cardiac index occur in normal subjects in a supine position when sympathetic activity is at minimum.[41,42] Greater reductions of cardiac index and left ventricular work occur in normal subjects in the standing position.[43] β-Adrenergic blocking agents attenuate but do not

completely block the circulatory response to exercise indicating that the sympathetic nervous system is active during exercise.[43,44]

Of more importance clinically is the fact that β-adrenergic blocking agents may prevent catecholamine-induced increase in cardiac contractility and heart rate in patients with heart disease. The reduction in cardiac function in heart failure is evident both hemodynamically and by impairment of the ability of the patient to excrete sodium.[45,46] Currently the cardiac actions of β-adrenergic blocking agents are thought to be due mainly to β-adrenergic blockade[39]; however, a direct membrane action cannot be completely ruled out.[47,48]

The peripheral vascular effects of β-adrenergic blocking agents is complex. Vascular β-adrenergic receptors are not considered to be important in most physiologic states. Nevertheless, administration of propranolol may increase peripheral vascular resistance,[49–51] and peripheral vascular insufficiency precipitated by propranolol has been reported.[52–54] Peripheral vascular resistance has been found to be decreased 4 weeks after continued therapy, presumably because of a central mechanism.[51]

β-Adrenergic blocking agents lower blood pressure both because of reduced cardiac output[50,54] and because of decreased peripheral resistance.[55–57] Suppression of plasma renin activity may contribute in part to the antihypertensive effect, but is not essential and does not operate in every responsive patient.[51] (The antihypertensive actions of β-adrenergic blocking agents are discussed in detail in Chap. 73.)

Propranolol

Propranolol is a racemic mixture of equal parts of d- and l-propranolol. d-Propranolol has no β-adrenergic activity but retains membrane depressant effects. l-Propranolol has both effects. Neither isomer exhibits intrinsic sympathomimetic activity.[39,58] (The electrophysiologic effects of propranolol are discussed in Chap. 109B.)

PHARMACOKINETICS OF PROPRANOLOL

Propranolol is rapidly and completely absorbed from the gastrointestinal tract. However, because of extremely high hepatic extraction, estimated to range from 50 to 80 percent, very little of the free compound enters the circulation after oral administration (presystemic, or first-pass, effect). Variations in hepatic metabolism cause differences in plasma drug concentration among individuals which may be 20-fold. Propranolol is 90 to 95 percent bound to plasma protein. Several metabolites are produced after oral administration; a major metabolite, 4-hydroxypropranolol, is equipotent to propranolol as an antiarrhythmic agent but has a shorter half-life ($T_{1/2}$).[59]

A single oral dose of propranolol of less than 30 mg has a plasma $T_{1/2}$ of 2 to 3 h in normal subjects. With larger doses and on chronic therapy the $T_{1/2}$

may increase from 3 to 6 h and result in increased plasma drug concentrations. Unlike other drugs, decreased plasma protein binding lengthens the $T^{1/2}$ instead of shortening it because of the rapid hepatic clearance. The plasma $T^{1/2}$ of propranolol may be prolonged to as much as 35 h in patients with cirrhosis of the liver. The $T^{1/2}$ is relatively not prolonged in patients with impaired renal function, and in some cases it may be shortened.[59] After administration of propranolol for at least 4 weeks, in doses up to 300 mg/day, the effects of β-adrenergic blockade were found to dissipate within 18 h after acute withdrawal.[60]

TREATMENT OF ANGINA PECTORIS

Propranolol is an effective agent for the treatment of angina pectoris. The usual daily dose ranges from 160 to 320 mg. The drug is usually administered every 6 h before meals and at bedtime.[58,59,61]

The antianginal effect of propranolol is due to reduction of myocardial oxygen consumption resulting from slowed heart rate, lowered blood pressure, and diminished myocardial contractility. Although increase in heart size may occur with augmentation of myocardial oxygen consumption, the usual net effect is reduction of myocardial oxygen consumption.[58,62] Accordingly, myocardial lactate extraction is usually increased in spite of the decrease in coronary blood flow.[39,63]

Abrupt withdrawal of propranolol had caused exacerbation of angina and acute myocardial infarction in patients with angina pectoris.[64–65] Accordingly, the patient should be cautioned against interruption or sudden cessation of therapy. After chronic administration the dosage should be gradually reduced over a period of weeks and the patient should be carefully monitored.[65] Propranolol is also used to treat symptomatic patients with idiopathic hypertrophic subaortic stenosis[66] or thyrotoxicosis.[67]

Propranolol is usually started at a dose of 10 to 20 mg three or four times daily. The dose should be gradually increased at 3- to 7-day intervals until optimum response is obtained. If the heart rate is reduced to 55 beats per minute with the patient in the standing position, the dose should not be increased further, or may require reduction.

CONTRAINDICATION AND ADVERSE EFFECTS

Propranolol is contraindicated in (1) bronchial asthma, (2) allergic rhinitis during the pollen season, (3) sinus bradycardia and AV block, (4) cardiogenic shock, (5) right ventricular failure secondary to pulmonary hypertension, (6) congestive heart failure unless the failure is secondary to a tachyarrhythmia treatable with propranolol, (7) patients receiving anesthetics that produce myocardial depression such as chloroform and ether, (8) patients on adrenergic-augmenting psychotropic drugs [including mono-

amine oxidase (MAO) inhibitors], and during the 2-week withdrawal period from such drugs.

In addition to these contraindications, propranolol must be used with extreme caution in patients with either frank or incipient congestive heart failure. Caution also must be used in patients susceptible to hypoglycemia, because propranolol may prevent the appearance of premonitory signs and symptoms of acute hypoglycemia.[39] A number of other adverse reactions have been reported, including nausea, vomiting, light-headedness, mild diarrhea, constipation, and mental depression.[68]

Other β-adrenergic blocking agents

A major therapeutic goal has been to develop β-adrenergic blocking agents which specifically antagonize $β_1$-adrenergic receptors. Such a compound would be less likely to precipitate bronchial asthma which is caused by blockade of bronchial $β_2$-adrenergic receptors. One drug, practolol,[40] with more selective $β_1$-antagonism than propranolol, has been widely used outside the United States in the past. Unfortunately, practolol produced a series of severe and unusual adverse effects including sclerosing peritonitis,[69] cutaneous and ocular reactions,[70] and a lupus erythematosus-like syndrome.[71] As a result, it has been withdrawn from the market. Fortunately, other $β_1$-antagonists have been synthesized,[39] and they may eventually become available for clinical use.

α-ADRENERGIC BLOCKING AGENTS[72,73]

α-Adrenergic blocking agents specifically block the action of sympathomimetic amines and sympathetic activity on α-adrenergic receptors. Many drugs exert a weak α-adrenergic blocking action, but only phentolamine (Regitine) and phenoxybenzamine (Dibenzyline) are used primarily because of this property. Phentolamine is a competitive antagonist and has a relatively transient action. Other effects produced by phentolamine include "histamine-like" vasodilation and "sympathomimetic" cardiac stimulation. Phenoxybenzamine is a noncompetitive antagonist with a prolonged action. The use of phentolamine and phenoxybenzamine for the diagnosis and treatment of pheochromocytoma is outlined in Chap. 71. These drugs also have been investigated for many years for their use in the treatment of shock but are still not approved for this purpose.

The basis for the use of α-adrenergic blocking agents in the treatment of shock is the blockade of arteriolar and venular constriction produced by excessive sympathetic activity and adrenal discharge occurring in the shock state. Vasoconstriction increases capillary pressure and tissue anoxia, which results in loss of plasma volume and the perpetuation of a vicious cycle. When α-adrenergic blocking agents are administered, the excessive vasoconstriction is blocked and the cycle interrupted. After administration of α-adrenergic blocking agents, it is frequently possible to administer additional plasma expanders without elevating venous pressure.

Extreme caution must be exercised when these drugs are used, since the block of the vasoconstriction could result in hypotension, especially in the hypovolemic patient. The physician must be prepared to rapidly expand the plasma volume and, if this is not successful, to administer norepinephrine or metaraminol. α-Adrenergic blocking agents have been used with norepinephrine[74] or dopamine[19,20] to block vasoconstriction without affecting cardiac stimulation.

ATROPINE

Atropine and other cholinergic agents are used in the treatment of certain arrhythmias and conduction defects because of their ability to block the cardiac actions of the vagus nerve. Because of this vagal blocking action, atropine increases the rate of the SA node and the speed of conduction through the AV node.[75,76] Accordingly it has application in treating severe sinus bradycardia and partial AV block when they are due to increased vagal tone. Paradoxically, small doses of atropine have been found to cause bradycardia and delayed AV transmission, presumably by central nervous system stimulation of the vagus. Thus, if bradycardia or AV dissociation occurs, a larger dose should be administered.[76–78]

Indiscriminate use of atropine in patients with acute myocardial infarction has been discouraged recently. The "malignant forms" of premature ventricular beat (PVB) are not effectively suppressed by increasing heart rate with atropine.[79] On the other hand, the augmented myocardial oxygen consumption resulting from cardiac acceleration may increase myocardial damage and mortality rate.[79,80] However, when low cardiac output is due to excessive vagal tone and its resulting bradycardia, cautious use of atropine may be lifesaving.[81,82] Another use of atropine is to reduce the gastrointestinal and potentially dangerous vagal effects of morphine.

In order to avoid bradycardia, atropine should be given by intravenous injection at doses between 0.5 and 1.0 mg. Onset of action begins about 25 s after injection and reaches a peak in 2 to 3 min. The injection may be repeated every 5 to 10 min until a therapeutic effect is obtained, adverse effect appears, or a total dose of 2 to 3 mg has been given.[76,83] The principal adverse effects of atropine are related to cholinergic block. They include dryness of mouth and skin, constipation, dilation of pupils, paralysis of accommodation, exacerbation of glaucoma, and dysuria.[83] AV dissociation and junctional rhythm may occur.[77,84] Ventricular tachycardia and fibrillation have been reported rarely.[85]

With large doses and in sensitive individuals, excessive tachycardia and marked central nervous system stimulation may occur, with hallucinations and hyperpyrexia.[83] Preliminary studies suggest that methylscopolamine bromide, which does not cross blood-brain barrier, may be as effective as atropine without causing central nervous system excitation.[84]

REFERENCES

1 Ahlquist, R. P.: A Study of Adrenotropic Receptors, *Am. J. Physiol.*, 153:586, 1948.

2 Lands, A. M., Arnold, A., McAuliff, J. P., Luduena, F. P., and Brown, T. G., Jr.: Differentiation of Receptor Systems Activated by Sympathomimetic Amines, *Nature*, 214:597, 1967.

3 Lefkowitz, R. J.: Selectivity in a Beta-adrenergic Responses: Clinical Implications, *Circulation*, 49:783, 1974.

4 Goldberg, L. I., Cotten, M. deV., Darby, T. D., and Howell, E. V.: Comparative Heart Contractile Force Effects of Equipressor Doses of Several Sympathomimetic Amines, *J. Pharmacol. Exp. Ther.*, 108:177, 1953.

5 Brewster, W. R., Jr., Osgood, P. F., Isaacs, J. P., and Goldberg, L. I.: Hemodynamic Effects of Pressor Amine (Methoxamine) with Predominant Vasoconstrictor Activity, *Circ. Res.*, 8:980, 1960.

6 Goldberg, L. I., Bloodwell, R. D., Braunwald, E., and Morrow, A. G.: The Direct Effects of Norepinephrine, Epinephrine, and Methoxamine on Myocardial Contractile Force in Man, *Circulation*, 22:1125, 1960.

7 Tuttle, R. R., and Mills, J.: Dobutamine: Development of a New Catecholamine to Selectively Increase Cardiac Contractility, *Circ. Res.*, 36:185, 1975.

8 Goldberg, L. I.: Cardiovascular and Renal Actions of Dopamine: Potential Clinical Applications, *Pharmacol. Rev.*, 24:1, 1972.

9 Moran, N. C.: Neurohumoral Agents: A Pharmacological Analysis of the Actions of Catecholamines upon the Heart, in S. A. Briller and H. L. Conn, Jr. (eds.), "The Myocardial Cell," University of Pennsylvania Press, Philadelphia, 1966, p. 331.

10 Sobel, B. E., and Mayer, S. E.: Cyclic Adenosine Monophosphate and Cardiac Contractility, *Circ. Res.*, 32:407, 1973.

11 Entman, M. L., Levey, G. S., and Epstein, S. E.: Mechanism of Action of Epinephrine and Glucagon on the Canine Heart: Evidence for Increase in Sarcotubular Calcium Stores Mediated by Cyclic 3',5'-AMP, *Circ. Res.*, 25:429, 1969.

12 Sulakhe, P. V., and Dhalla, N. S.: Excitation-Contraction Coupling in Heart: III. Evidence against the Involvement of Adenosine 3',5'-Monophosphate in Calcium Transport by Sarcotubular Vesicles of Canine Myocardium, *Mol. Pharmacol.*, 6:659, 1970.

13 Robie, N. W., Nutter, D. C., Moddy, C., and McNay, J. L.: In Vivo Analysis of Adrenergic Receptor Activity of Dobutamine, *Circ. Res.*, 34:663, 1974.

14 Robie, N. W., and Goldberg, L. I.: Comparative Systemic and Regional Hemodynamic Effects of Dopamine and Dobutamine, *Am. Heart J.*, 90:340, 1975.

15 Goldberg, L. I., Hsieh, Y. Y., and Resnekov, L.: Newer Catecholamine for Treatment of Heart Failure and Shock: An Update on Dopamine and a First Look at Dobutamine, *Prog. Cardiovasc. Dis.*, 19:327, 1977.

16 Smith, N. T., and Carbascio, A. N.: Use and Misuse of Pressor Agents, *Anesthesiology*, 33:58, 1970.

17 Goldberg, L. I., and Talley, R. C.: Current Therapy of Shock, in G. Stollerman (ed.), "Advances in Internal Medicine," Year Book Medical Publishers, Inc., Chicago, 1971, p. 363.

18 Goldberg, L. I.: The Treatment of Cardiogenic Shock: VI. The Search for an Ideal Drug, *Am. Heart J.*, 75:416, 1968.

19 Goldberg, L. I., Talley, R. C., and McNay, J. L.: The Potential Role of Dopamine in the Treatment of Shock, *Prog. Cardiovasc. Dis.*, 12:40, 1969.

20 MacCannell, K. L., McNay, J. L., Meyer, M. B., and Goldberg, L. I.: Dopamine in the Treatment of Hypotension and Shock, *N. Engl. J. Med.,* 275:1389, 1966.

21 Talley, R. C., Goldberg, L. I., Johnson, C. E., and McNay, J. L.: A Hemodynamic Comparison of Dopamine and Isoproterenol in Patients in Shock, *Circulation,* 39:361, 1969.

22 Gunnar, R. M., Loeb, H. S., Pietras, R. J., and Tobin, J. R., Jr.: Ineffectiveness of Isoproterenol in Shock Due to Acute Myocardial Infarction, *J.A.M.A.,* 202:1124, 1967.

23 Winslow, E. J., Loeb, H. S., Rahimtoola, S. H., Kamath, S., and Gunnar, R. M.: Hemodynamic Studies and Results of Therapy in 50 Patients with Bacteremic Shock, *Am. J. Med.,* 54:421, 1973.

24 Gunnar, R. M., Cruz, A., Boswell, J., Coe, B. S., Pietras, R. J., and Tobin J. R.: Myocardial Infarction with Shock: Hemodynamic Studies and Results of Therapy, *Circulation,* 33:753, 1966.

25 Brown, R. S., Carey, J. S., Mohr, P. A., Monson, D. O., and Shoemaker, W. C.: Comparative Evaluation of Sympathomimetic Amines in Clinical Shock, *Circulation,* 34:260, 1966.

26 Bellet, S.: Clinical Pharmacology of Antiarrhythmic Drugs, *Clin. Pharmacol. Ther.,* 2:345, 1961.

27 Rosenblum, R., and Frieden, J.: Intravenous Dopamine in the Treatment of Myocardial Dysfunction after Open Heart Surgery, *Am. Heart J.,* 83:743, 1972.

28 Holloway, E. L., Stinson, E. B., Derby, G. C., and Harrison, D. C.: Actions of Drugs in Patients Early after Cardiac Surgery: I. Comparison of Isoproterenol and Dopamine, *Am. J. Cardiol.,* 35:656, 1975.

29 Goldberg, L. I., McDonald, R. H., Jr., and Zimmerman, A. M.: Sodium Diuresis Produced by Dopamine in Patients with Congestive Heart Failure, *N. Engl. J. Med.,* 269:1060, 1963.

30 McDonald, R. H., Jr., Goldberg, L. I., McNay, J. L., and Tuttle, E. P., Jr.: Effects of Dopamine in Man: Augmentation of Sodium Excretion, Glomerular Filtration Rate and Renal Plasma Flow, *J. Clin. Invest.,* 43:1116, 1964.

31 Goldberg, L. I.: The Use of Sympathomimetic Amines in the Treatment of Heart Failure, *Am. J. Cardiol.,* 22:177, 1968.

32 Whitaker, A. N., and McKay, D. G.: Disseminated Intravascular Coagulation in Rabbits by Intravenous Infusion of Epinephrine, *Fed. Proc.,* 27:2, 1968.

33 Rosenblum, I., Wohl, A., and Stein, A. A.: Studies in Cardiac Necrosis: II. Cardiovascular Effects of Sympathomimetic Amines Producing Cardiac Lesions, *Toxicol. Appl. Pharmacol.,* 7:9, 1965.

34 Haft, J. I.: Cardiovascular Injury Induced by Sympathetic Catecholamines, *Prog. Cardiovasc. Dis.,* 17:73, 1974.

35 Botticelli, J. T., Tsagaris, T. J., and Lange, R. L.: Mechanisms of Pressor Amine Dependence, *Am. J. Cardiol.,* 16:847, 1965.

36 Moss, A. J., Vittands, I., and Schenk, E. A.: Cardiovascular Effects of Sustained Norepinephrine Infusion: I. Hemodynamics, *Circ. Res.,* 18:596, 1966.

37 Powell, C. E., and Slater, I. H.: Blocking of Inhibitory Adrenergic Receptors by a Dichloro Analog of Isoproterenol, *J. Pharmacol. Exp. Ther.,* 122:480, 1958.

38 Moran, N. C., and Perkins, M. E.: Adrenergic Blockade of the Mammalian Heart by a Dichloro Analog of Isoproterenol, *J. Pharmacol. Exp. Ther.,* 124:223, 1958.

39 Conolly, M., Kersting, F., and Dollery, C. T.: The Clinical Pharmacology of Beta-Adrenoceptor-Blocking Drugs, *Prog. Cardiovasc. Dis.,* 19:203, 1976.

40 Barret, A. M.: The Pharmacology of Practolol, *Postgrad. Med. J.,* 47(suppl.):7, 1971.

41 Harrison, D. C., Braunwald, E., Glick, G., Mason, D. T., Chidsey, C. A., and Ross, J., Jr.: Effects of Beta Adrenergic Blockade on the Circulation, with Particular Reference to Observations in Patients with Hypertrophic Subaortic Stenosis, *Circulation,* 29:186, 1964.

42 Sonnenblick, E. M., Braunwald, E., Williams, J. F., Jr., and Click, G.: Effects of Exercise on Myocardial Force-Velocity Relations in Intact Unanesthetized Man: Relative Role of Changes in Heart Rate, Sympathetic Activity and Ventricular Dimensions, *J. Clin. Invest.,* 44:2051, 1965.

43 Epstein, S. E., Robinson, B. F., Kahler, R. L., and Braunwald, E.: Effects of Beta-Adrenergic Blockade on the Cardiac Response to Maximal and Submaximal Exercise in Man, *J. Clin. Invest.,* 44:1745, 1966.

44 Donald, D. E., Ferguson, D. A., and Milburn, S. E.: Effect of Beta-Adrenergic Blockade on Racing Performance of Greyhounds with Normal and with Denervated Hearts, *Circ. Res.,* 22:127, 1968.

45 Gaffney, T. E., and Braunwald, E.: Importance of the Adrenergic Nervous System in the Support of Circulatory Function in Patients with Congestive Heart Failure, *Am. J. Med.,* 34:420, 1963.

46 Epstein, S. E., and Braunwald, E.: The Effect of Beta-Adrenergic Blockade on Patterns of Sodium Excretion: Studies in Normal Subjects and in Patients with Heart Disease, *Ann. Intern. Med.,* 65:20, 1966.

47 Rahn, K. H., and Ockenga, T.: Über die Beiziehungen zwischen den β-adrenolytischen Wirkungen und dem Einfluss auf Herzfrequenz und Herzminutenvolumen von β-Receptoren blockierenden Substanzen, *Klin. Wochenschr.,* 45:1087, 1967.

48 Ekelund, L. G., Melcher, A., and Oroe, L.: Central Haemodynamic Effects in Man of Intravenous *d*-Alprenolol during Rest and Exercise, *Eur. J. Clin. Pharmacol.,* 3:198, 1971.

49 MacDonald, H. R., Sapru, R. P., Taylor, S. H., and Donald K. W.: Effect of Intravenous Propranolol on the Systemic Circulatory Response to Sustained Hand Grip, *Am. J. Cardiol.,* 18:333, 1966.

50 Frohlich, E. D., Tarazi, R. C., Dustan, H. P., and Page, I. H.: The Paradox of β-Adrenergic Blockade in Hypertension, *Circulation,* 37:417, 1968.

51 Bühler, F. R., Burkart, F., Lütold, B. E., Küng, M., Marbet, G., and Pfisterer, M.: Antihypertensive Beta Blocking Actions Related to Renin and Age: A Pharmacologic Tool to Identify Pathogenetic Mechanisms in Essential Hypertension, *Am. J. Cardiol.,* 36:653, 1972.

52 Tarazi, R. C., and Dustan, H.P.: Beta Adrenergic Blockade in Hypertension, *Am. J. Cardiol.,* 29:633, 1972.

53 Zacharias, F. J., Cowen, K. J., Presst, J., Vickers, J., and Wall, B. G.: Propranolol in Hypertension: A Study of Long-Term Therapy, 1964–1970, *Am. Heart J.,* 83:755, 1972.

54 Simpson, F. O.: β-Adrenergic Receptor Blocking Drugs in Hypertension, *Drugs,* 7:85, 1974.

55 Dollery, C. T., Lewis, P. J., Myers, M. G., and Reid, J. L.: Mechanism of the Early Pressure Effect of Centrally Administered Propranolol in the Conscious Rabbit, *Br. J. Pharmacol.,* 48:343p, 1973.

56 Srivastava, R. K., Kulshrestha, V. K., Battista, A., Sing, N., and Bhargava, K. P.: Central Cardiovascular Effects of Intracerebroventricular Propranolol, *Eur. J. Pharmacol.,* 21:222, 1973.

57 Garvey, H. L., and Ram, N.: Centrally Induced Hypotensive Effects of β-Adrenergic Blocking Drugs, *Eur. J. Pharmacol.,* 33:283, 1975.

58 Prichard, B. N. C.: β-Adrenergic Receptor Blocking Drugs in Angina Pectoris, *Drugs,* 7:55, 1974.

59 Nies, A. S., and Shand, D. G.: Clinical Pharmacology of Propranolol, *Circulation,* 52:6, 1975.

60 Romagnoli, A., and Keats, A. S.: Plasma and Atrial Propranolol after Preoperative Withdrawal, *Circulation,* 52:1123, 1975.

61 Heatherington, D. J., Comerford, M. B., Myberg, G., and Besterman, E. M. M.: Comparison of Two Adrenergic Beta-

Blocking Agents, Alprenolol and Propranolol, in Treatment of Angina Pectoris, *Br. Heart J.,* 35:320, 1973.

62 Sowton, E., and Hamer, J.: Hemodynamic Changes after Beta Adrenergic Blockade, *Am. J. Cardiol.,* 18:317, 1966.

63 Wolfson, S., and Gorlin, R.: Cardiovascular Pharmacology of Propranolol in Man, *Circulation,* 40:501, 1969.

64 Alderman, E. L., Coltart, D. J., Wettach, G. E., and Harrison, D. C.: Coronary Artery Syndromes after Sudden Propranolol Withdrawal, *Ann. Intern. Med.,* 81:625, 1974.

64a Miller, R. R., Olson, H. C., Amsterdam, E. A., and Dean, M. T.: Propranolol-withdrawal Rebound Phenomenon, *N. Eng. J. Med.,* 293:416, 1975.

65 Shand, D. G.: Drug Therapy: Propranolol, *N. Engl. J. Med.,* 293:280, 1975.

66 Hubner, P. J. B., Ziady, G. M., Lane, G. K., Hardarson, T., Scales, B., Oakley, C. M., and Goodwin, J. F.: Double-blind Trial of Propranolol and Practolol in Hypertrophic Cardiomyopathy, *Br. Heart J.,* 35:1116, 1973.

67 Turner, P.: β-Adrenergic Receptor Blocking Drugs in Hyperthyroidism, *Drugs,* 7:48, 1974.

68 Greenblatt, D. J., and Koch-Weser, J.: Adverse Reactions to Propranolol in Hospital Medical Patients: A Report from the Boston Collaborative Drug Surveillance Program, *Am. Heart J.,* 86:478, 1973.

69 Brown, P., Baddeley, H., Read, A. E., Davies, J. D., and McGary, J.: Sclerosing Peritonitis: An Unusual Reaction to a β-Adrenergic Blocking Drug (Practolol), *Lancet,* 2:1477, 1974.

70 Felix, R. H., Ive, F. A., and Dahl, M. G. C.: Cutaneous and Ocular Reactions to Practolol, *Br. Med., J.,* 4:321, 1974.

71 Raftery, E. B., and Denaman, A. M.: Systemic Lupus Erythematosus Syndrome Induced by Practolol, *Br. Med. J.,* 2:452, 1973.

72 Nickerson, M.: Blockade of the Actions of Adrenaline and Noradrenaline, *Pharmacol. Rev.,* 11:443, 1959.

73 Nickerson, M.: Drug Therapy of Shock, in K. D. Bock (ed.), "Shock: Pathogenesis and Therapy, An International Symposium (Ciba)," Springer-Verlag OHG, Berlin, 1962, p. 356.

74 Wilson, R. F.: Combined Use of Norepinephrine and Dibenzyline in Clinical Shock, *Surg. Forum,* 15:30, 1964.

75 Akhtar, M., Damato, A. N., Batsford, W. P., Caracta, A. R.,

Ruskin, J. N., Weisfogel, G. M., and Lau, S. H.: Induction of Atrioventricular Nodal Reentrant Tachycardia after Atropine, *Am. J. Cardiol.,* 36:286, 1975.

76 Das, G., Talmers, F. N., and Weissler, A. M.: New Observations on the Effects of Atropine on the Sinoatrial and Atrioventricular Nodes in Man, *Am. J. Cardiol.,* 36:281, 1975.

77 Averill, K. H., and Lamb, L. E.: Less Commonly Recognized Actions of Atropine on Cardiac Rhythm, *Am. J. Med. Sci.,* 237:304, 1959.

78 Kosowsky, S. D., Stein, E., Lau, S. H., Lister, J. W., Hoft, J. I., and Damato, A. N.: A Comparison of the Hemodynamic Effects of Tachycardia Produced by Atrial Pacing and Atropine, *Am. Heart J.,* 72:594, 1966.

79 Epstein, S. E., Goldstein, R. E., Redwood, D. R., Kent, K. M., and Smith, E. R.: The Early Phase of Acute Myocardial Infarction: Pharmacologic Aspects of Therapy, *Ann. Intern. Med.,* 78:918, 1973.

80 Knoebel, S. B., McHenry, P. L., Phillips, J. F., and Widlausky, S.: Atropine-induced Cardioacceleration and Myocardial Blood Flow in Subjects with and without Coronary Artery Diseases, *Am. J. Cardiol.,* 33:327, 1974.

81 Webb, S. W., Adgey, A. A. J., and Pantridge, J. F.: Autonomic Disturbance at Onset of Acute Myocardial Infarction, *Br. Med. J.,* 3:89, 1972.

82 Warren, J. V., and Lewis, R. P.: Beneficial Effects of Atropine in the Prehospital Phase of Coronary Care, *Am. J. Cardiol.,* 37:68, 1976.

83 Greenblatt, D. J., and Shader, R. I.: Anticholinergics, *N. Engl. J. Med.,* 288:1215, 1973.

84 Neeld, J. B., Jr., Allen, A. T., III, Coleman, E., Frederickson, E. L., and Goldberg, L. I.: Cardiac Rate and Rhythm Changes with Atropine and Methscopolamine, *Clin. Pharmacol. Ther.,* 17:290, 1975.

85 Massumi, R. A., Mason, D. T., Amsterdam, R. A., DeMaria, A., Miller, R. R., Scheinman, M. M., and Zelis, R.: Ventricular Fibrillation and Tachycardia after Intravenous Atropine for Treatment of Bradycardia, *N. Engl. J. Med.,* 287:336, 1972.

PART XIII

Medicolegal and Insurance Problems Related to Cardiovascular Disease

110
Insurance Problems in Heart Disease

ROYAL S. SCHAAF, M.D.

On the whole, this text tends to be glacier-like in its rate of change, reflecting, of course, the granite stability of the insurance industry.

ROYAL S. SCHAAF, M.D., 1976[1]

There are two main problems related to heart disease and insurance. First, there is the clinical task of detection, diagnosis, and estimation of the severity of any disease or impairments present in each applicant for insurance. Here, clinicians and insurance underwriters are on common ground. Second, and inseparable from the first for insurace purposes, is evaluation of the applicant's long-term prognosis, and it is here that misunderstandings sometimes arise. Many a physician has been astonished to find that a patient he has treated or an applicant he has examined has been charged an increased premium for some condition that the physician regards as of little or no clinical importance.

Why do these differences of opinion arise? For one thing, when a clinician considers the prognosis of a disease entity, he is thinking of a relatively short time—usually not more than 5 or 10 years. Possibilities of accident, additional disease, or a great advance in treatment of the patient's current disease make speculation on the future of the individual unprofitable. An insurance company, however, must take into consideration a much longer period of time, since its contracts often run for 50 years or more. To do this, a company must make predictions based on statistical studies on its own policyholders or on large, multicompany experience like the *Impairment Study, 1951,*[1a] made by the Society of Actuaries. In such studies the measuring rod is the mortality experienced on standard lives—that is, on individuals without any detectable impairments who were issued insurance at standard premium rates. The mortality rates obtained from these standard lives are applied, age by age and year by year, to whatever group of impaired lives is being studied, to get the "expected deaths"—that is, the number of deaths that would have been expected among the members of the impaired group if they had had no impairment. The number of deaths that actually occurred among the impaired lives is then divided by the number of expected deaths to give a mortality ratio. If, for example, in a particular impairment, 50 deaths are expected and actually 75 occur, the mortality ratio is 150 percent. Conversely, if only 45 deaths take place where 50 are expected, the mortality ratio is 90 percent, i.e., lower than standard, a preferred group of risks. The mortality ratio thus arrived at is the

basis for calculating the premiums needed to cover the impairment under consideration.

In all fairness, every insurance group must pay its own way. Policyholders who are considered impaired risks and have been charged an extra premium must, as a group, live up to the life expectancy assumed for them, and this may be a long time indeed. Table 110-1 shows the number of years that applicants with various degrees of impairment would have to live, on the average, for their premiums to be sufficient.

It should be emphasized that these figures are averages. Some persons in each rating group must live much longer than the average to offset those in the same group who die early. Further, as medical progress continues, these life expectancy figures will doubtless have to be revised upward.

A mortality ratio of 150 percent may represent only one or two extra deaths a year out of each 1,000 persons insured. For purposes of clinical statistics an increase of 0.1 or 0.2 percent in the annual death rate would be virtually imperceptible and certainly not reason enough to justify alarming a patient. Yet for this small increase in mortality an insurance company must charge an additional premium if it is to cover its claims.

It would be a simple matter actuarially to work out a premium which, varying of course with age and provided everyone took the insurance, would be enough to insure the entire population without regard to physical health or prospects, including the coronary patient, the cancer patient, and the victim of central nervous system disease. Clearly these three groups are the types of people who need insurance the most. Unfortunately, their situation is like that of the man who seeks to buy fire insurance when his house is already in flames. Insurance is designed to help people protect themselves against hazards which are possible in the future but which are not yet in being in the individual. Few people enjoying good health would be willing to pay the very high premiums necessary to cover all, taxing themselves for the benefit of others for whom they bear no personal responsibility. On the other hand, those knowing or believing themselves shortly to die would bend every effort to purchase a maximum amount of insurance. In this way the claims would rise, the premium

TABLE 110-1
Life expectancy for various degrees of impairment (in years)

Age at issue	Standard, 100%	Impairment, %				
		150	200	300	400	500
0	71	67	64	60	55	50
10	62	58	55	51	47	43
20	52	49	46	42	38	34
30	43	39	36	33	30	27
40	33	30	27	24	21	18
50	24	22	19	16	14	12
60	17	15	12	10	8	7

receipts decrease, and the company trying such a program quickly go under.

Only a system of compulsory inclusion of the healthy with the sick could make a uniform premium plan work, and this is unacceptable to the great majority. Therefore, it becomes necessary to place a very high rating on some policies and to exclude some persons altogether from coverage. Still, the numbers involved are relatively small. Despite all the possible impairments and combinations of impairments to which mankind is heir, slightly over 90 percent of all life insurance policies are issued at standard rates, about 5 percent receive some substandard rating, and only about 3 percent of all applications are rejected.

Another way of looking at mortality ratios is illustrated by Table 110-2. These figures indicate that of 1,000 men who are standard risks at age 35, only 25 are expected to die over the next 10 years from all causes (disease, accident, suicide); 975 will still be alive at age 45. Even if a group of 35-year-old men have an impairment that gives them a mortality ratio of 500 percent, out of 1,000 such there would still be 830 alive 10 years later. In other words there would be an 83 percent survival rate. Most clinicians would feel that such a survival rate is little short of ordinary "normal health" in comparison with really serious disease. Yet for insurance purposes the premiums required to cover a mortality ratio of 500 percent are so high that as a practical matter few persons are willing to pay them.

A second cause for misunderstanding between clinician and medical underwriter is a difference in viewpoint. The attention of the attending physician is centered on his patients as individuals, and when adverse action has been taken on one of them by an insurance company, he tends to recall the people he has known with the same impairment who have lived far into old age. Insurance companies see these long-lived individuals, too. There are some in every impaired group, and without them the average future lifetime would be less (and the premium more) than it is. Still, the insurance company must be concerned with the performance of the entire group, the short-lived as well as the long-lived. It is impossible to foresee which individuals will live long and which will die early; this is why people buy insurance. But with large groups of individuals it is possible to predict mortality with sufficient accuracy to cover the death claims; that is why insurance companies can exist.

There is a widespread impression that insurance companies are living in the past, basing their premiums on old statistics with high death rates that have long since become obsolete. This is not true. It is true that the companies take their past experience as a starting point, but they restudy their data at frequent intervals, and if it appears resonable to assume that a more favorable mortality may be expected in the future, they modify their calculations accordingly. When a modification of existing tables will no longer produce equity among policyholders, a new mortality table is prepared.

A similar procedure is followed on individual medical impairments to bring the companies' action in line with current medical thought. Insurance companies must be wary of accepting too completely the early rosy clinical reports of new therapeutic measures, many of which later prove to have been overoptimistic, but they do not wait years for supporting statistical evidence. For example, well before recent statistical evidence[2] appeared to support such action, ratings for hypertension were reduced where modern treatment persistently lowered blood pressure levels. It must be remembered, however, that the latest techniques in diagnosis and treatment, used first in the big cities and medical centers, require time to attain widespread use and to lower appreciably the general mortality.

Moreover, old statistics are not always so out of date as one might suppose. Though spectacular progress has been made clinically in some fields, in others little has been accomplished. Table 110-3 shows comparative results of two large multicompany studies on heart murmurs: the *Impairment Study, 1951,*

TABLE 110-2
Proportion of men aged 35 years surviving 10 years at various mortality ratios

Mortality percentage	Proportion surviving 10 years
Standard	0.975
150	0.961
200	0.945
300	0.915
400	0.875
500	0.830

TABLE 110-3
Comparative results of two impairment studies of mortality ratios for certain heart murmurs

Description of heart murmur	1951 study, %	1929 study, %
Systolic pulmonary, not transmitted	107	102
Systolic at apex, inconstant, not transmitted	111	104
Systolic at apex, constant, not transmitted	139	156
Systolic at apex, constant, transmitted to left	220	224
Systolic at apex, constant, transmitted to left, with history of rheumatic fever or chorea	267	332
Systolic at apex, constant, transmitted to left, with history of streptococcal infection	263	181
Systolic aortic, constant, not transmitted	191	131
Systolic aortic, constant, transmitted upward	491	257

NOTE: This table illustrates the fact that, despite general medical progress, old statistics may still give a substantially accurate prediction of current mortality experience and in some instances may be even more favorable than current experience.

covering the period from 1935 to 1950, and the *Medical Impairment Study, 1929,* covering the period from 1908 to 1928.[3] If one is inclined to feel that we are doing so much better now than we were doing in 1935 to 1950 and that all statistics for that period are outmoded, it would be well to reflect that in 1945 we might have thought we were doing greatly better than in 1908 to 1928, but the mortality ratios on some murmurs are virtually the same and on others are actually higher. In each of these studies, moreover, the impaired lives were being measured by the standard mortality rates that were then current. This automatically takes into account the improvement in the general mortality among people living under the same social and economic conditions and in the same era of medicine as the impaired group that is being studied. Impaired groups whose mortality ratios have remained essentially unchanged over the years have done no better than to improve in the same proportion as the standard mortality. Those whose mortality ratios are higher than before have shown less than the general improvement. As might be expected, the increased mortality observed in the classifications in Table 110-3 was preponderantly of cardiovascular causes.

An insurance classification like the one in Table 110-3, in which heart murmurs are classified according to the description of the murmur, may seem inadequate to a clinician. The evaluation of symptoms and physical signs is often difficult and in clinical practice may require extensive study and a considerable period of observation. This is now and should properly remain within the province of the practicing physician. The insurance classification must be based on the findings that are available on all applicants from the insurance examination, which is, because of factors of convenience, cost, and the unwillingness of applicants to undergo extensive study for insurance purposes, less searching than a clinician's diagnostic study. Of course, when such a study has already been made for clinical purposes, the company will usually try to obtain it from the attending physician and give it full weight in the underwriting decision.

An insurance company action may sometimes appear overly conservative to the clinician for another reason. If the diagnosis is obscure, the company is at a disadvantage as compared with the clinician. The latter can, in such a case, await developments and defer his opinion until the situation becomes clearer. The company, however, must make its decision at the moment, either to decline the application or to enter into a contract that cannot be changed later except in favor of the insured. If subsequent developments show that the company has overestimated the risk, it can reduce the premium and often does. But if it has underestimated the risk, it cannot increase the premium or refuse to accept a premium tendered by the policyholder.

Insurance is a business, of course, but it is also a public trust. Whenever an insurance company accepts an applicant for insurance, it is backing its judgment with money—other people's money. Policyholders place their money in the company's hands, not for speculative purposes or even for "a businessman's risk," but to guarantee funds to their families after their deaths. The company is required to invest these funds in certain types of high-quality securities that are specified by law. It must show equal conservatism in selecting its risks, a conservatism always tempered, however, by the competition of over 1,000 other life insurance companies and by the reluctance, natural to any enterprise, to cause ill will and alarm in its clients by unfavorable action.

UNDERWRITING CARDIOVASCULAR IMPAIRMENTS

It is not practical in a single chapter to discuss the underwriting aspects of the full range of cardiovascular impairments. Attention instead will be directed to some of the conditions most frequently encountered in clinical and insurance medicine, illustrating more specifically the way the underwriting approach to individuals must differ from the clinical. Unless otherwise indicated, the figures appearing hereafter derive from the *Impairment Study, 1951.* The material for this study was contributed by a group of companies whose business makes up 70 percent of the insurance in force in the United States and Canada. Overall, the study covered a total of 725,000 policies, of which 18,000 ended in death during the observation period. It is interesting to look first at the experience with persons giving a family history of two or more parents or siblings known to have or have had cardiovascular-renal disease under the age of 60. Table 110-4 summarizes this experience in almost 15,000 applicants giving such a history.

The number of lives involved minimizes the possibility that these ratios reflect chance fluctuation. Although the increased mortality is not great, it is nonetheless significant as compared with standard ratios. It must be pointed out that these individuals, aside from their family history, were standard risks, in no case presenting any other impairment requiring a rating.

TABLE 110-4
Family history* of cardiovascular-renal disease

Age at issue	Actual deaths	Expected deaths	Mortality ratio, %
15–29	42	31	136
30–39	140	101	139
40–49	298	190	157
50–64	251	196	128
15–64	731	518	141

*Two or more patients under age 60. When there are two or more deaths due to cardiovascular-renal disease before the age of 60 in the parents and siblings of an individual, there will be a small but significant increase in mortality ratio.

CONGENITAL HEART DISEASE

No insurance statistics are available on long-term prognosis of congenital heart disease, because until recently no cases were accepted, and the policies issued over the past two decades on relatively mild types and degrees of congenital impairment have not been in force long enough to develop a reliable insurance experience. Enough has been said, however, about the relatively low mortality ratios and long survival periods associated with even highly rated insurance, especially among young persons, to make it evident that the majority of persons with congenital cardiac anomalies are uninsurable. This is especially true, of course, of those with cyanotic heart disease, in which large numbers of the victims may not even survive to adulthood, but in acyanotic anomalies, as well, the frequency of onset of serious complications in early or middle life leads to mortality ratios beyond the scope of insurance coverage in most cases.

Adults with certain types of acyanotic congenital heart disease that have not been or cannot be treated surgically constitute a more favorable group for possible insurance consideration than do children having similar defects. This is for the obvious reason that by simply surviving to age 20 or over, the adults give proof of a lesser degree of severity of impairment or of greater ability to tolerate their disease, or both. Here, when the diagnosis is definite (as proved by catheterization or angiocardiography or as diagnosed clinically by a qualified cardiologist), when there is no significant cardiac enlargement, and when the electrocardiogram is normal or nearly so, many companies may be willing to make a substandard insurance offer. Defects in this category include interventricular septal defects, congenital pulmonic or subaortic stenosis, and asymmetric septal hypertrophy responsive to treatment.

Rapid advance in recent years in the techniques and capabilities of cardiovascular surgical treatment is apparently achieving results which may greatly improve the long-range outlook for both morbidity and mortality in congenital cardiac anomalies. Pending the passage of a significant number of years, however, and the accumulation of clinical experience with patients who have had surgical correction of these anomalies, insurance medicine will have to maintain a conservative and strictly experimental approach to these surgically treated cases. At present two extracardiac procedures can be considered as established successes for insurance purposes. Most companies would be willing to accept a person with corrected patent ductus arteriosus. There is a tendency to take more favorable action when the surgical procedure has been carried out early in the patient's life, and when both ligation and division of the ductus rather than ligation alone have been done. Correction of a coarctation of the aorta, preferably without use of a graft, is also acceptable in many instances after passage of a year or so following operation to give assurance of good healing of the anastomosis and persistent reduction of the blood pressure. Again,

TABLE 110-5
Acute articular rheumatism: one attack within 5 years of application

Age at issue	Actual deaths	Expected deaths	Mortality ratio, %
15–29	27	15	182
30–39	26	20	127
40–49	26	28	92
50–64	30	21	142
15–64	109	84	129

patients operated on below age 20 are considered probably more favorable. Many companies are accepting persons with corrected interatrial and interventricular septal defects, usually after a waiting period following surgical treatment. More complicated and daring surgical approaches to heart disease, including fracture and cutting techniques for stenosed valves, may qualify for substandard insurance where other features are favorable. An occasional venturesome company will even make experimental offers in the 1,000 to 2,000 percent mortality range to some individuals with prosthetic heart valves.

In summary, insurance medicine approaches the long-term prognosis of untreated or surgically treated congenital cardiac anomalies slowly and cautiously, but the rapid progress in the clinical handling of such cases gives promise of increasingly optimistic insurance action in the future.

RHEUMATIC FEVER WITHOUT RESIDUAL MURMUR

From the clinical viewpoint, both the incidence and severity of rheumatic fever have been decreasing in recent decades, and it is gratifying to find that actuarially the experience with acute rheumatic fever is also favorable, as evidenced by Tables 110-5 and 110-6. In both categories, acute rheumatic fever without complications occurring within 5 years of application and over 5 years prior to application, the mortality ratios are low enough to justify standard issue in most cases. The exceptions are persons still within a year or two of rheumatic activity. Here a small substandard rating is necessary to cover the

TABLE 110-6
Acute articular rheumatism: one attack over 5 years before application

Age at issue	Actual deaths	Expected deaths	Mortality ratio, %
15–29	29	28	102
30–39	85	64	134
40–49	106	103	102
50–64	103	82	126
15–64	323	277	116

TABLE 110-7
Inconstant apical systolic murmurs

Age at issue	Actual deaths	Expected deaths	Mortality ratio, %
15-29	27	24	110
30–39	41	41	101
40–49	67	54	125
50–64	41	40	103
15–64	176	159	111

occasional patient in whom a cardiac murmur develops only after a latent period following the active inflammatory disease.

SYSTOLIC HEART MURMURS, INCLUDING RHEUMATIC

For practical purposes it is impossible to have every applicant with a heart murmur examined by a cardiologist. Instead, most heart murmurs are detected, described, and diagnosed by physicians who have not had extensive training in cardiac auscultation. As a result, in many cases confusion and even contradiction may still remain when the insurance examination has been completed, whether by a single examining physician or with an alternate heart examination by another physician. Largely offsetting this relative lack of full and accurate cardiac evaluation, however, is the fact that the broad groups in which acceptable heart murmurs may be placed are relatively few and the numbers of lives in each group large, so that a certain range of diagnostic uncertainty can be included in each group without materially affecting the overall long-range experience.

The first categories for consideration are the localized apical systolic murmurs, inconstant or constant, as summarized in Tables 110-7 and 110-8. These figures, based on 7,500 and 10,000 lives respectively, show a generally favorable mortality rate except for persons in the younger groups with a constant murmur. Probably here a few cases of unrecognized rheumatic or other organic disease have led to the very few extra deaths required to give a substantial boost to the mortality ratio at ages 15 to 29.

When the apical systolic murmur is constant and also transmitted to the left or is specifically diag-

TABLE 110-8
Constant, localized apical systolic murmurs

Age at issue	Actual deaths	Expected deaths	Mortality ratio, %
15–29	52	31	170
30–39	60	43	141
40–49	87	65	134
50–64	70	56	126
15–64	269	195	139

TABLE 110-9
Apical systolic murmurs, constant, transmitted to the left

Age of issue	Actual deaths	Expected deaths	Mortality ratio, %
15–29	188	58	325
30–39	178	78	226
40–49	248	118	210
50–64	120	79	152
15–64	734	333	220

nosed as mitral regurgitation, the mortality ratios are sharply increased, as seen in Table 110-9, covering almost 19,000 lives. When, in addition to being constant and transmitted to the left or diagnosed as mitral regurgitation, the murmur is accompanied by a history of rheumatic fever or chorea or by a history of tonsilitis or other streptococcal infection (not definitely known to have been followed by rheumatic fever or chorea), the mortality ratios climb another significant distance, from 220 percent of Table 110-9 to 267 and 263 percent, respectively (Table 110-3). Most constant, transmitted apical systolic murmurs are of moderate to loud intensity and of harsh or musical quality. However, for underwriting purposes, if a suggestive or definite history of rheumatic fever is present, even the soft, or blowing, apical systolic murmurs, which on auscultation may sound physiologic, may be expected over the long run to entail distinctly higher than standard mortality rates and hence require a substandard rating. If cardiac hypertrophy is present, especially as proved by x-ray, or if the electrocardiogram is abnormal in association with an organic apical systolic murmur, the mortality ratios rise beyond the usual insurable range.

The experience with basal systolic murmurs at the pulmonary area, not transmitted, supports their clinical reputation for being physiologic and harmless (Table 110-10).

Basal systolic murmurs at the aortic area, not transmitted, are distinctly more significant, however, and when the aortic systolic murmur is transmitted as well, the mortality ratio approaches the limit of insurability. The number of deaths in these two categories is too small to justify breakdown by ages, because isolated aortic systolic murmurs are not common and most aortic murmurs occur in combination with other clinical features which make the applicant uninsurable. Composite Table 110-11 summarizes the mortality experience of both groups of aortic systolic murmurs.

TABLE 110-10
Localized pulmonary systolic murmurs

Age at issue	Actual deaths	Expected deaths	Mortality ratio, %
15–29	30	30	100
30–39	54	42	129
40–49	26	27	97
50–64	8	11	71
15–64	118	110	107

NOTE: Clinically physiologic pulmonary systolic murmurs are compatible with standard mortality rates.

TABLE 110-11
Aortic systolic murmurs (age at issue 15 to 64)

Murmur	Mortality ratio, %
Not transmitted	191
Transmitted upward	491

NOTE: Even localized aortic systolic murmurs show almost twice the standard mortality rate, and organic aortic systolic murmurs have a mortality ratio of five times standard.

In general summary, systolic heart murmurs having the characteristics identifying them clinically as organic are not compatible with standard mortality rates, even though roentgenogram and electrocardiogram may currently be normal, and especially not when there is a history of rheumatic fever or streptococcal infection. Diastolic heart murmurs have long been known to carry greater hazard than systolic murmurs as a class, and persons with diastolic murmurs were generally considered uninsurable. In recent years, however, many companies have issued highly rated insurance to adults with diastolic murmurs whose heart size has been normal as seen by x-ray and who do not have a history or signs of cardiac failure. Insured cases remain too few and the period of observation still too short to provide reliable experience.

CORONARY ARTERY DISEASE

Despite its prominent position among the causes of death at the present time, coronary artery disease is not an area on which life insurance experience can throw much light. Again the reason for this is that the mortality is known to be so high that until recent years no company would knowingly issue insurance to an applicant giving a history or showing clinical evidence of a coronary episode or angina pectoris. As with diastolic murmurs, a number of companies have lately been issuing policies to selected coronary patients on a very highly rated, experimental basis, but as yet too few policies have been accepted and have remained in force long enough to build up adequate experience. It is well recognized that a very significant proportion of persons surviving a first myocardial infarction will succumb to their disease within 5 years, after which the still-surviving members of the group will die at a fairly steady rate, with some living into old age. Consequently, in offering insurance to certain selected persons with coronary artery disease, in addition to providing a moderately high substandard permanent rating, underwriters require a very substantial temporary extra premium for the first 5 or 6 years after a coronary episode to cover the high claim rate in these early policy years. A review of 1,551 disability claims due to myocardial infarction illustrates the marked shortening of life expectancy in these cases (see Table 110-12).[4] Finally, despite insufficient experience, a few companies are responding to the popularity of coronary bypass surgery by making high substandard experimental

TABLE 110-12
Average life expectancy after myocardial infarction

Age at onset	Expectancy after infarction, yr	Normal expectancy, yr
30–39	11.5	33.4
40–49	10.5	25.2
50–60	8.5	17.8

offers in relatively favorable cases a year or more after surgery.

ELECTROCARDIOGRAPHY

Electrocardiographic experience on insured lives is sketchy and difficult to evaluate. Most people are insured without benefit of any electrocardiographic study whatever, past or present, and in those cases where tracings may be available, complete details of clinical history and current status are not assured, which makes useful follow-up difficult. Althoug underwriters in many instances are now making insurance offers to persons with various types of electrocardiographic abnormalities, these actions for the most part must be taken on a cautious, judgment basis; one should weigh especially the degree to which any particular abnormality may reflect the possible presence of coronary artery disease. The recently clarified hemiblocks are facets of this problem.

One area of electrocardiographic evaluation in which there tends to be a divergence between clinical and insurance judgments is that of T wave changes appearing in otherwise normal tracings taken on persons having no history or clinical evidence of cardiac or related impairments. Transient T wave changes can be brought about in many people by a number of everyday physiologic actions. As a result, when a clinician encounters a person in whom the only objective finding is a T wave change, the clinician rightly takes an optimistic view and either makes no mention of the finding to the patient or gives assurance that it is not a cause for alarm, leaving it to follow-up examinations at later dates to determine whether the finding has long-range significance. Needless to say, the patient is sorely taken aback if an insurance company on the basis of the same electrocardiogram finds it necessary to apply a rating or to decline. Someone must be making a mistake! In an effort to quantitate the qualitative judgment that persons with even isolated T wave changes often are not standard risks, in 1955 the Prudential Insurance Company undertook a study of the problem based on its own employees. A file was available of about 22,000 electrocardiograms taken in the Employee Health Service since 1933, with full details of all the illnesses, physical examinations, and laboratory studies of each individual on whom a

MEDICOLEGAL AND INSURANCE PROBLEMS
RELATED TO CARDIOVASCULAR DISEASE

TABLE 110-13
Analysis by groups of men, ages 40 to 69, with electrocardiograms showing T wave changes

Group	No.	Deaths	Percentage of actual to expected deaths	Deaths from cardiovascular causes, %	Total number subsequently developing coronary occlusion, %
1955 study:					
Normal	1,388	75	84	47	3.2
Minor T wave changes	273	29	163	65.5	10.6
Major T wave changes	43	7	302	71.4	16.3
Previous coronary history	112	40	526	95	
1961 study:					
Normal	1,805	145	78	36	6
Minor T wave changes	422	65	166	49	12

NOTE: Even minor T wave abnormalities, unaccompanied by any other electrocardiographic or clinical abnormality, show a significant increase in mortality ratio and in subsequent incidence of coronary occlusion. The period of follow-up observation in these cases averaged about 7 years.

tracing had been taken. The marked job stability of Prudential personnel, together with retirement and death benefit records, made follow-up relatively easy and complete.

Among all the persons in the file, selections were restricted to the men between the ages of 40 and 69, when coronary disease is considered to be most prevalent. From these men four groups were further selected. The normal group was composed of individuals who had normal electrocardiograms and who appeared normal clinically, with no evidence of organic disease, cardiac or otherwise. Blood pressure readings were consistently below 150/90 in all cases. Contrasting with the normal and serving only as a basis for comparison with the groups being studied were 112 persons who had had a coronary occlusion and survived the acute episode by at least 60 days. In these men the coronary disease was uncomplicated by diabetes, hypertension, valvular heart disease, or any other organic impairment. The remaining two groups were those whose electrocardiograms were normal at all times except for showing slight, or minor, T wave changes (flat or disproportionately low in relation to the QRS) and those showing marked, or major, T wave changes (diphasic or inverted where one would normally expect an upright T wave). Again, only those men were included who had normal clinical findings and case histories, excluding even those with seemingly irrelevant disease such as peptic ulcer or tuberculosis. Table 110-13 shows the results of this study, together with a second one carried out in 1961.[5]

From these figures, certain conclusions seem valid. Although the electrocardiogram may be of very little prognostic value in the individual case, groups of individuals showing T wave changes, even though slight, will show a higher mortality rate. There will be more cardiovascular disease in such groups than in groups not showing similar T wave changes. Isolated major T wave changes are rare in clinically normal people but when found carry a sharply raised mortality ratio. (There were, of course, hundreds of examples of major T wave changes in the file, but almost always in association with obvious organic disease.) The more pronounced the isolated T wave changes, the greater the possibility that they indicate cardiovascular disease, and it is against this possibility that increases in premium rates are required. Further-

TABLE 110-14
Mortality ratios of men, ages 30 to 39, observation period 1935-1954

Systolic pressures	Diastolic pressures, %					
	48–67	68–82	83–87	88–92	93–97	98–102
98–127	45	88	116	120	(113)	—
128–137	99	113	134	160	240	—
138–147	(121)	140	176	221	249	277
148–157	—	171	246	201	261	498
158–167	—	—	—	(292)	(439)	—

NOTE: Dashes indicate groups in which the number of deaths was less than 10. Parentheses indicate groups in which the number of deaths was between 10 and 34. Altogether there were 20,383 deaths in the 30-to-39 age group and 22,850 deaths in the 50-to-59 age group.

Clinically mild to insignificant blood pressure readings may give highly significant mortality experience, especially in younger men.

TABLE 110-15
Mortality ratios of men, ages 50 to 59, observation period 1935-1954

Systolic pressures	Diastolic pressures, %					
	48–67	68–82	83–87	88–92	93–97	98–102
98–127	73	83	97	107	—	—
128–137	109	107	116	112	163	(162)
138–147	165	142	145	153	199	201
148–157	(245)	158	193	195	208	196
158–167	—	202	201	219	270	336

NOTE: Dashes indicate groups in which the number of deaths was less than 10. Parentheses indicate groups in which the number of deaths was between 10 and 34. Altogether there were 20,383 deaths in the 30-to-39 age group and 22,850 deaths in the 50-to-59 age group.

Clinically mild to insignificant blood pressure readings may give highly significant mortality experience, especially in younger men.

more, since the persons in this study were clinically normal, it can reasonably be inferred that if an applicant for life insurance should show other evidence of cardiovascular disease, such as hypertension or a murmur, the T wave changes, even though slight, may take on even greater significance.

In 1961 a second study was completed on all clinically normal men in the file, ages 40 to 69, having normal electrocardiograms or showing isolated minor T wave changes. The figures fell closely in line with the earlier study, as shown in the lower part of Table 110-13.

Decision as to whether a T wave is normal or slightly or markedly abnormal is often difficult and may have to be made arbitrarily. However, to the extent that some way might be found to remove borderline instances from a particular group, the remainder of the group may be expected to show a corresponding increase in mortality ratio, and vice versa. Further, the observed mortalities of 84 to 78 percent in the normal employees in these studies fall distinctly below the standard (100 percent) mortality of insured lives in general. Accordingly, it is probable that a somewhat higher mortality ratio for isolated T wave changes may occur among the population at large than was observed in this sheltered population.

Insurance statistics do not yet clarify the underwriting significance of the W-P-W (Wolff-Parkinson-White) syndrome, although preliminary figures suggest no great mortality increase. Pending longer experience with more cases, underwriters currently accept the W-P-W anomaly without tachycardia at standard or with a low rating, the younger cases receiving the more favorable action. With a history of paroxysmal tachycardia, individuals with W-P-W syndrome receive slightly higher ratings, again increasing with age.

BLOOD PRESSURE

Blood pressure is a subject on which insurance companies have accumulated a vast experience, which can only be touched on here. In general, as might be predicted clinically, the evidence shows that for any given systolic pressure, the mortality ratio rises as the diastolic pressure rises. Correspondingly,

TABLE 110-16
Average blood pressures, males

Ages	Systolic	Diastolic
15–19	117	71
20–24	119	73
25–29	121	75
30–34	122	76
35–39	123	77
40–44	124	78
45–49	126	78
50–54	128	79
55–59	130	79
60–64	132	80

NOTE: Average blood pressure remains relatively low at least up to age 65.

for any given diastolic pressure, the mortality ratio rises as the systolic pressure rises. For this reason it is not possible to give a single specific reading indicating the limit between normal and elevated readings. What is arresting to anyone accustomed to the clinical approach to blood pressure elevation is the evidence that even mild elevations of systolic or diastolic blood pressure, or both, are accompanied by significant rises in mortality ratios. Indeed, by the time an individual exhibits blood pressure readings high enough to call for close follow-up or treatment clinically, he may already be near or beyond the limits of insurability. In other words, a clinically "mild" or "moderate" blood pressure elevation may be "severe" for insurance purposes.

The most recent major blood pressure review from the insurance viewpoint is the *Build and Blood Pressure Study, 1959,*[6] made by the Society of Actuaries. In the blood pressure section of this study there were 3,900,000 entrants, with 102,000 deaths, with an average duration of exposure of little over 7 years. Tables 110-14 and 110-15 give an indication of the experience developed. In each table builds are normal, and no other significant impairments are involved.

For the same blood pressure readings, mortality ratios are higher among the younger men. Female experience, not quoted here, is more favorable than male. These features should be borne in mind in attempting to compare clinical hypertensive series with insurance mortality tables. Since the insured lives on which insurance mortality tables are built tend to be about 90 percent male and clinical hypertensive series tend to have a preponderance of female lives, it is not always possible to make meaningful comparisons between the two.

A final point of interest is how low average blood pressues are, as shown for males of various ages in the figures in Table 110-16 based on 235,000 males, a representative sample taken from the larger study. The best mortality ratios are experienced with pressures even lower than these averages.

REFERENCES

1 Personal communication, Apr. 14, 1976.

1a Society of Acturaries: "Impairment Study, 1951," New York, 1954.

2 Freis, E. D.: Effect of Treatment on Morbidity and Mortality in Hypertension, *Trans. Assoc. Life Ins. Med. Dir. Am.,* 54:113, 1970.

3 Actuarial Society of America and Association of Life Insurance Medical Directors: "Medical Impairment Study, 1929," New York, 1931.

4 Waldron, F. A., and Constable, W. P.: Myocardial Infarction: A Mortality Study, *Trans. Assoc. Life Ins. Med. Dir. Am.,* 34:69, 1950.

5 Kiessling, C. E., Schaaf, R. S., and Lyle, A. M.: A Re-evaluation of the T-Wave Changes in the Electrocardiograms of Otherwise Normal People, *Trans. Assoc. Life Ins. Med. Dir. Am.,* 45:70, 1961.

6 Society of Acturaries: "Build and Blood Pressure Study, 1959," Chicago, 1959.

111
The Heart and the Law

OGLESBY PAUL, M.D.

It is reasonable to expect that situations will arise in which the inevitable hazards of ordinary life will be claimed to have accelerated a degenerative disease, such as coronary atherosclerosis, to a point of disability or death sooner than would have been projected. Where such a stress can be shown to be related to the act of an individual or corporation, there may be the basis for legal redress.

HOWARD B. SPRAGUE, M.D., 1966[1]

There is ample evidence that in our modern society, so characterized by litigation, problems involving heart disease frequently are presented to industrial commissions, courts of law, and insurance and pension bodies. This is not remarkable in view of the importance of cardiovascular disease as a cause of death, the fact that many persons with such disease are actually employed, the expansion of many forms of social insurance, and the increasing disposition of patients and their families to seek legal action in instances of alleged injury, illness, or death.

VARIETIES OF LEGAL INVOLVEMENT

Legal considerations may arise in a variety of settings. In one situation, there may be a question of benefits claimed for a heart attack under an accident insurance policy or a question of double indemnity under an accidental injury provision in a life insurance policy. In another situation, the issue may involve an automobile accident subsequent to which a heart attack occurred, with claims of a causal relation between the two. Also, there may be legal action arising from death from a cardiac cause of an employee on or off the job, with an attempt to identify the fatal event as an accident or injury arising out of employment. Yet another instance may be provided by an attempt to recover disability payments for a heart condition under a disability benefits law or an attempt to obtain retirement benefits under a retirement statute or company retirement plan. There may also be legal action in the courts by a patient or the family of a patient asserting that the physicians, nurses, and hospitals had not exercised appropriate judgment and knowledge in the diagnosis and treatment of a cardiac disorder.

WORKMEN'S COMPENSATION

Workmen's compensation, which has been described as the grandfather of all the health insurance programs, is the largest field of coinvolvement of heart disease and the law. Workmen's compensation was first introduced in central Europe in the mid-1800s, the first English law was introduced in 1897, and the first United States law in 1911. As each of the states adopted the system over the next 35 years, claims relating to heart disease became relatively frequent and in some areas increased steadily in number. Thus, Hellmuth et al.[2] noted that in Wisconsin from 1953–1954 to 1961–1962, the number of cardiac claims rose from 78 to 106, although Bergy and Sparkman[3] indicated that in the state of Washington a similar rise was not seen. Bergy and Sparkman also noted, as have others, that cardiac claims are mostly from manifestations of atherosclerosis: of 431 claims, 68 percent were given a diagnosis of myocardial infarction, 10 percent had acute coronary insufficiency, 6.7 percent involved an acute arrhythmia, and only 1 percent involved cardiac trauma.

OCCUPATIONAL CARDIOVASCULAR DISEASE

Compensation for occupational cardiovascular disease has been introduced by statute in approximately 18 states.[4] Such statutes have been written to provide that in the absence of adequate rebuttal, the development of a cardiovascular disorder is presumed to be the result of the occupation peculiar to the categories of employees defined by law. The chief categories have been civil service employees such as firemen and policemen, but other occupational groups have also been included. Such legislation has been without proper scientific evidence that any of these occupations is truly more prone to injure or unfavorably affect the cardiovascular system than any other occupation, and the motivation for these laws appears to have been political.

DEFINITION OF AN ACCIDENT OR INJURY

The definition of an accident or injury within the meaning of workmen's compensation laws has undergone change over the past 50 and more years. For example, in Illinois in 1919, in a case involving an aortic rupture during heavy work, the Supreme Court of Illinois (288 Ill., Sup. p. 87) ruled that "if an injury can be traceable to a definite time, place and cause, and the injury occurs in the course of employment, the injury is accidental within the meaning of the act and the obligation to provide and pay compensation arises."[5] However, in 1944, in a case involving the onset of atrial fibrillation at work, the court ruled (386 Ill. Sup. 11) that undue exertion which aggravates a preexisting heart condition constitutes an accidental injury within the meaning of the Workmen's Compensation Act.[5] Further, in 1950, the same court ruled (404 Ill, Sup. p. 487), in the case of a fireman who died while fighting a fire, that the exertion, even though involving the regular duties of the job, could be considered as precipitating a heart attack, which was accepted as an accident under the meaning of the Workmen's Compensation Act.[5]

Such a legal interpretation regarding usual exertion was at variance with the Report of the Medical-Pathological Subcommittee of the Committee on the Effect of Strain and Trauma on the Heart and Great Vessels of the American Heart Association issued in 1962,[6] which stated that "heart failure either of the congestive type (with acute dilatation or rhythm disturbance), or of the coronary insufficiency type (with angina pectoris or other evidence of myocardial ischemia or sudden death), or of the myocardial infarction type (with or without survival), shall be considered related to physical or emotional exertion only if the heart failure occurs during the actual period of stress clearly unusual for the individual involved."

As stated by Dalenberg,[4] the problem of usual versus unusual exertion has arisen in more than 30 states. He believed that 12 states in 1970 were following the rule that only unusual exertion could give rise to a compensable heart attack. However, 20 or more states would grant compensation when the evidence indicated that the activity involved in the cardiac problem was merely usual for the individual. This kind of reasoning harks back to a milestone decision in Great Britain[4] in 1910 *(Clover, Clayton & Co. v. Hughes)* which involved a worker whose aortic aneurysm ruptured in the course of his ordinary daily work. The majority decision in favor of the plaintiff put forward the test question: "Was it the disease that did it, or did the work he was doing help in any material degree?"

Today, it is clear in cases brought before industrial commissions and courts that compensation for a cardiovascular episode is often awarded both without regard to clear evidence of preexisting disease and without regard to unusual exertion, and if there is a reasonable probability that aggravation or precipitation of a cardiovascular condition may have been attributable to the short- or long-term effects of exertion during employment.

Trauma to the heart is, as noted, a relatively rare basis for claims. As reported by Teare and Bowen,[7] such trauma may include penetrating injury with puncture or laceration of the myocardium or its vessels and nonpenetrating injury including contusion of the heart, rupture of the heart, arrhythmias, electrocardiographic changes, and myocardial infarction. Today, steering-wheel automobile accidents are a common cause of such injury.

White and Smith[8] cited six cases of direct trauma representative of what may be encountered when the cause-and-effect relation is clear legally. One was that of a 6-year-old girl run over by the wheel of a car, a rupture of both ventricles resulting. A second instance was that of a 56-year-old man who died 4 months after a blow to his abdomen and presumably his chest, the autopsy showing an irregular rupture of the wall of the right ventricle. The third case was that of a 49-year-old man who experienced a steering-wheel injury and died 6 days later with contusions and a laceration of the myocardium without rupture. The fourth example was that of a 16-year-old boy who suffered a bullet wound of the heart and survived. The fifth case represented a stab wound in a 23-year-old man resulting in a division of the left anterior descending coronary artery leading to tamponade—a condition corrected surgically. The final case was that of a 24-year-old seaman involved in an automobile accident leading to rupture of the anterior papillary muscle of the left ventricle and death.

They also mention that less obvious but nevertheless related to physical effort or trauma may be aortic valve rupture and rupture of the chordae tendineae of the mitral valve. Rupture of the aorta in automobile and other accidents and traumatic injury to the other great vessels may also be encountered.

The temporal coincidence of the alleged trauma and the appearance of manifestations of injury is crucial in establishing a convincing causal relation. When an asymptomatic period of many days or weeks or months has elapsed between the alleged trauma and the onset of cardiac complaints, it is difficult to reason that a trauma was the cause of the heart disease.

The roles of mental strain and of emotion are more difficult to define satisfactorily. There are few areas in medicine in which more widely divergent views are held. Few awards have been made by the courts in cardiac cases solely on the basis of mental stress or emotional shock. This has been especially true of alleged long-term mental and emotional strain, but less true where a single identifiable event has been cited. Most awards have been based upon the presumed joint influence of physical and mental factors aggravating or precipitating a cardiovascular episode.

Those who decry the looseness of the scientific evidence relating mental strain and emotions to coronary disease in particular must recognize that the scientific literature contains numerous statements by presumed authorities linking these processes, and such statements are available for quotation in the courts by lawyers and professional witnesses. Thus, there are such comments as "Emotion, although more difficult to define and describe than physical effort, is in fact better established than the latter as a causative factor . . ."[7] Sagall and Reed[9] list six reputable scientific investigators who had published up to 1967 statements linking emotional stress to coronary disease, and since that time others have added further scientific comments. However, a great many cardiologists would subscribe to the statement by Friedberg[10] that "in no area of pathogenesis of coronary heart disease is there more loose talk, more articulation of half-truths, more casual dismissal of observations which do not fit the proposed concept, more lack of precise definition and more unawareness of the meaning of scientific controls than in the reports on the purported relation of emotion to coronary heart disease." At present, it would seem fair to conclude that scientific support for a causative or aggravating role of mental strain, tension, and emotion in the production of cardiovascular disease leading to disability or death is still tenuous. This does not preclude relatively rare apparent association of unusual emotion with a fatal cardiac episode as in the famous case of John Hunter, who in 1793 had an attack of angina during a violent dispute at a meeting of the board of St. George's Hospital, causing him to cease speaking, following which he went into an adjoining room and died in a matter of minutes.

MALPRACTICE AND THE CARDIOVASCULAR SYSTEM

Although the diagnosis and management of heart disease has not evidently presented the opportunities for litigation involving alleged malpractice which have been encountered in certain other specialties such as orthopedic surgery, malpractice suits relating to cardiovascular problems have increased in recent years. A charge of professional negligence includes four crucial elements, namely, the obligation of the defendant to conform to a certain standard of conduct, failure of the defendant to fulfill that obligation, damage suffered by the plaintiff, and evidence that the damage was the consequence of the conduct of the defendant. Particular legal problems conforming to these critical elements have of course been encountered in emergency room situations. Here often it is stated that the patient presented with complaints

which were not typical of a heart attack or, if typical, were misinterpreted or ignored, and that the patient received no or allegedly inappropriate treatment and not long afterward dropped dead on the street or at home. Not only the physician but also emergency room nurses and the hospital have been sued in such cases. The existence of such suits has constituted yet another reason for employing experienced staff in emergency rooms, and for leaning over backward to observe suspect myocardial infarction cases for 24 to 48 h. Other suits have alleged such errors as failure by a physician to forbid moderately heavy work [*Krusilla v. United States* (1961)],[11] failure to compare an old and a recent electrocardiogram [*Blackwell v. Southern Florida Sanitarium and Hospital Corporation, et al.* (1965)],[12] and failure to use commonly accepted doses of cardiac drugs [*Norton v. Argonaut Insurance Co, La.,* (1962)].[13]

THE PATIENT WITH HEART DISEASE AS A WITNESS OR DEFENDANT

Physicians are commonly asked to excuse a patient with heart disease from appearing as a witness or a defendant in a court of law, on the basis that the appearance might cause the patient to become gravely ill or even to die. Such an excuse is especially sought for those with a history of previous myocardial infarction. No one can deny that the necessity for providing testimony and for answering questions may be very unpleasant and emotion provoking—particularly for those who are defendants. A prolonged trial may also be very fatiguing. However, to excuse everyone with heart disease from participation in such exercises of our legal system is to do a disservice to society. It should indeed be the exception when a person with cardiovascular disease is considered by a physician too ill to appear either as a witness or defendant. Such exceptions may include the presence of a recent myocardial infarction (within 2 months for an uncomplicated infarction), or incapacitating angina appearing very frequently on minimal or no effort or emotion, or serious congestive heart failure. It is often wise merely to defer court appearance until an acute episode is over. It may also be prudent for the physician to indicate to the court limitations on the amount of time to be devoted to interrogation each day. Rarely, the presence of a physician or nurse in the courtroom may be advised for the protection of the best interests of defendant, prosecution, and the physician himself. At times, a deposition only may be sufficient and may be taken in the home or office or hospital room of the witness or defendant; but such depositions are not considered adequate for all legal purposes. Further, the physician who acts in such difficult and important matters is well advised often to request that a second physician should also provide advice in a given case.

Finally, because of the implications of such advice on the life and welfare of one or more involved persons, the physicians serving as expert consultants to the court, defense, or prosecution must be comfortable with their own qualifications as experts. It is embarrassing for a physician to have his or her recommendations considered invalid because of lack of evidence of adequate training and experience in the field of cardiology.

THE PHYSICIAN AS AN EXPERT WITNESS IN CARDIAC CASES

While there is much that has been written regarding the physician as a witness, it may be wise to mention a few caveats particularly relevant to the field of heart disease. Physicians acting as expert witnesses should, as mentioned above, undertake such a role only if their qualifications in cardiology are solid in terms of training and years of experience. Frequently, the physician will be posed with a long hypothetical question modeled after the exact events and findings in the case at issue. Therefore, the physician must be provided with an exhaustive review of all pertinent documents, including, for careful scrutiny, all notes in hospital or other records made by attending physicians and house staff, all notes by nurses, and all laboratory reports. The physician must be sure to know how to interpret any x-rays, electrocardiograms, and biochemical tests made available. A physician who does not feel comfortable in interpretating special laboratory findings such as echocardiograms should rely on the report provided in the record and indicate that the findings in question are not in the physician's own area of expertise. Physicians who are expert witnesses are also well advised to be able to quote from one or more authoritative books or articles relating to the particular issue at hand and must not be disturbed if asked about their familiarity with a report or other reference which they have never heard of. Judges and juries are more impressed with the honesty and reliability of an expert witness who does not pretend to see all and know all than with the testimony of one who professes an encyclopedic knowledge.

REFERENCES

1 Sprague, H. B.: Medicolegal Aspects of Heart Disease, in J. W. Hurst and R. B. Logue (eds.), "The Heart: Arteries and Veins," McGraw-Hill Book Company, New York, 1966, p. 1184.

2 Hellmuth, G. A., Rodey, G., Johannsen, W. J., and Belknap, E. L.: Work and Heart Disease in Wisconsin, *J.A.M.A.*, 198:127, 1966.

3 Bergy, G. G., and Sparkman, D. R.: Analysis of Experience in Workmen's Compensation for Heart Cases, *Circulation*, 33:461, 1966.

4 Dalenberg, R. V. R.: Coronary Heart Disease and the Law, *Mod. Concepts Cardiovasc. Dis.*, 42:29, 1973.

5 Greenfield, I. M.: Workmen's Compensation and the Cardiac, in *Proc. 14th Heart-in-Industry Conf., Chicago, Apr. 19, 1967*, Chicago Heart Association, 1967, p. 8.

6 Report of the Committee on the Effect of Strain and Trauma on the Heart and Great Vessels, *Circulation*, 26:612, 1962.

7 Teare, R. D., and Bowen, D. A. L.: Medico-legal Aspects of Heart Disease, *Practitioner*, 196:247, 1966.

8 White, P. D., and Smith, H. W.: Scientific Proof in Respect to Injuries of the Heart, *North Carolina Law Rev.*, 24:107, 1946.

9 Sagall, E. L., and Reed, B. C.: "The Heart and the Law," The MacMillan Company, New York, 1968, p. 622.

10 Friedberg, C. K.: "Diseases of the Heart," 3d ed., W. B. Saunders Company, Philadelphia, 1966, p. 651.

11 *Krusilla v. United States*, 287 F. 2d 34 (1961).

12 *Blackwell v. Southern Florida Sanitarium and Hospital Corporation, et al.*, 174 So. 2d 45 (1965).

13 *Norton v. Argonaut Insurance Co., La.*, 144 So. 2d 249 (1962).

PART XIV

Errors Made in the Recognition and Treatment of Heart Disease

Common Mistakes Made in Practice

PETER C. GAZES, M.D., and
R. BRUCE LOGUE, M.D.

> To make no mistakes is not in the power of man; but from their errors and mistakes the wise and good learn wisdom for the future.
>
> PLUTARCH[1]

The best of people may make mistakes. The following discussion points out some of the mistakes which are made in the recognition and treatment of heart disease. They may have already been mentioned but are repeated here since they represent important precautions. Reviewing them, it is hoped, will help prevent such errors in the future.

CORONARY ATHEROSCLEROSIS

The concept that the history is the essential feature in the clinical diagnosis of angina pectoris was established by Heberden[1a] in 1768, and this is essentially unchanged today. The examiner should not merely ask the patient if he has chest pain, for often he denies this. Pain to most individuals is sharp, and this is not the type usually associated with angina. Anginal distress is usually described as burning, a tight sensation, heaviness, aching, or a pressing sensation. Although classically the distress is located in the retrosternal area with radiation to the neck, jaw, or arms, often it occurs in only a segment of this distribution such as only in the chest, only in the jaw or neck, only in the left arm or right arm, or only in the elbows or wrists. Origin of the discomfort in these segments, other than the chest, is often very suggestive of angina, since there are very few conditions which affect these areas. In some patients dyspnea or weakness may be the only symptom. The discomfort is usually brought on by increased cardiac work such as is associated with exertion or excitement and is relieved by rest. It does not remain constant over several hours or days. Coronary arteriography has taught us that the history is more classic than atypical. The public is more aware of heart disease, and they can mimic the typical symptoms. However, these patients will often state that their attacks last continuously for days, which would be most unusual unless infarction has occurred. Nitroglycerin is of limited value as a diagnostic test since it can also give relief in other conditions. However, if there is a typical history of angina with relief within 3 min after nitroglycerin, correlation with obstructive lesions of the coronary arteries has been reported in 90 percent of patients.[2]

Anxiety state with hyperventilation may produce tightness in the chest on exercise or abnormal electrocardiographic changes including false positive exercise tests. One should not fail to hyperventilate patients with atypical symptoms and electrocardiographic changes. Reproduction of the symptoms may indicate the correct diagnosis.

The physical examination often is nonrevealing. The fact that a patient has cardiomegaly or any other evidence of heart disease does not mean that the chest pain necessarily is cardiac in origin. Observation of the patient during an episode of discomfort may at times reveal some physical clues such as S_3 or S_4 gallops, abnormal chest pulsations, or a murmur of the late apical systolic papillary muscle dysfunction type with or without a preceding click.

The resting electrocardiogram is normal in 60 to 70 percent of patients and offers virtually no help in the diagnosis of angina. Even if it is abnormal, this may not be due to ischemic heart disease. Abnormal degrees of axis deviation, bundle branch blocks, and T wave changes cause the greatest problems. The interpreter lacking clinical and laboratory data should mention these and state that they are nonspecific. The term is vague and annoying to some, but it is preferable to use it rather than label a person as having coronary disease from the findings detected in the tracing alone. Levine[3] has listed 67 causes for T wave changes.

Master's two-step test is seldom used today because it frequently produces an inadequate heart rate. Ninety percent of maximum (near-maximal) or maximal exercise on the treadmill or bicycle ergometer are now popular as diagnostic aids. Positive exercise stress tests (Master's, near-maximal, and maximal) are associated with a high incidence of coronary artery disease.[4] Depressed downsloping ST segments appearing in the first 3 min of exercise and those persisting 8 min in recovery were associated with 90 percent prevalence of two- to three-vessel or main left coronary disease.[4a] Tracings should be followed at least up to 8 minutes after exercise, for changes may not develop for several minutes. There are great differences of opinion among interpreters of exercise stress tests. In fact, interpreters are guilty of reading the same exercise stress test on the same patient differently on different occasions. False positive tests can occur with digitalis therapy or reducing pills containing digitalis, hypokalemia, systolic click-murmur syndrome, the Wolff-Parkinson-White syndrome,[5] valvular heart disease, and autonomic changes. A positive exercise test in women is of little value in predicting the presence of significant coronary disease.[5a] Interpretation is difficult in the presence of an old myocardial infarction, left ventricular hypertrophy, or left bundle branch block. Suspicious tests are even more confusing and should be evaluated in conjunction with other findings. Finally, it is very important to remember that a negative stress test (even maximal) does not exclude coronary artery disease. It may be more appropriate to describe the changes that occur during or after exercise rather than stating the test is positive, negative, or suspicious.

Nitroglycerin remains the drug of choice for acute anginal attacks, and it usually relieves the pain within 3 min. The psychoneurotic patient often will not obtain relief until after 15 min or longer, which indicates that the pain was probably not angina. Nitroglycerin is not specific for angina. It can relieve spasm in some gastrointestinal disorders such as esophageal spasm or colic due to gallstones. Failure to respond to nitroglycerin does not exclude angina; it may indicate severe ischemia, nonischemic origin of discomfort, or impotent nitroglycerin. Occasionally, angina worsens with the use of nitroglycerin, suggesting that the cause of this angina may be severe aortic stenosis or idiopathic hypertrophic subaortic stenosis or that the chest discomfort is due to other disorders such as the systolic click-murmur syndrome.

Propranolol can be expected to cause sinus bradycardia, which is not an indication for discontinuing or reducing the dosage of the drug unless the heart rate drops below 55 beats per minute. However, it is contraindicated in severe heart failure, asthma, or atrioventricular (AV) heart block. The drug should be omitted prior to coronary arteriography, anesthesia, and surgery. Recently, it has been noted that sudden withdrawal of the drug may precipitate arrhythmias, increasing angina or infarction.[6,7] It has been observed in rare instances to precipitate Prinzmetal-type angina due to spasm of the coronary arteries. The drug may be decreased the day before bypass surgery and omitted the night before. (See Chap. 62E.) The indications for bypass coronary surgery are changing rapidly as more information is becoming available regarding the natural history of specific coronary syndromes and anatomical lesions and as the surgical mortality approaches 0.5 to 1.5 percent. (See Chap. 26E.) We must be alert to the rapid changes that are occurring in this field.

Myocardial infarction may present with a classic history, and yet there may be no physical abnormalities or electrocardiographic changes. Electrocardiographic changes may take several days to appear; therefore, serial tracings should be obtained. There are also many other conditions which can give electrocardiographic changes (in addition to ST-T changes there may be Q waves) that simulate those of an infarction, such as brain lesions, myocarditis, tumors of the heart, Wolff-Parkinson-White syndrome, pulmonary embolism, hypokalemia, and muscular dystrophy. Therefore, knowledge of the patient is of the utmost importance. Evolutionary electrocardiographic changes of an acute myocardial infarction can be obscured by many factors, especially cardiac drugs, old myocardial infarctions, repeated episodes of coronary insufficiency, and development of a ventricular aneurysm. The tracings do not provide much information about functional recovery and should not be the determinant for the speed of mobilization of the patient or the duration of hospitalization. It is hazardous to predict the outcome on the basis of the electrocardiogram. Infarctions can be localized by the interpreter, but to designate an infarction as small or massive by an electrocardiogram is misleading. A patient with a clinically severe infarction may have a tracing that is equivocal, borderline, or even normal. Emphasis should be placed on the clinical setting and not on the electrocardiogram alone. A patient with chest pain should not be delayed at home in order for a tracing to be obtained, nor should admission to the coronary care unit depend on the presence or absence of electrocardiographic findings. Unfortunately, during the early hours after the onset of myocardial infarction when the patient is most susceptible to primary ventricular fibrillation, the electrocardiogram may be normal.

After an infarction, the tracing can return to normal. In a study of 480 consecutive coronary arteriograms, 21 patients were found with normal resting electrocardiograms associated with complete or nearly complete occlusion of one or more major coronary vessels.[8] Another study noted disappearance of the electrocardiographic features of necrosis in 12 percent of 775 patients with healed infarction.[9] It may be that viable muscle surrounds the scarred area, or the infarction may have occurred in an area not contributing to the genesis of the electrocardiogram.[10] Less than half of old infarcts demonstrated at autopsy can be detected by electrocardiography, and 20 percent of acute infarcts may show no diagnostic changes during life. Changes of prior infarction commonly obscure abnormalities due to acute myocardial infarction or may show a pattern of left ventricular hypertrophy.[11]

Cardiac enzymes may remain normal if there is a small area of myocardial necrosis, and, conversely, elevations may be due to such a host of extracardiac factors as to cause confusion. For example, liver disease or even congestion can cause elevation of the serum transaminase, and skeletal muscle reaction after a hypodermic injection can cause elevation of the creatine phosphokinase (CPK) level. Isoenzymes as MB (metabolite) fraction of CPK or the flipped ratio of LDH_1 to LDH_2 (LDH_1 levels higher than LDH_2) are more specific for myocardial infarction than total levels of CPK and LDH (lactic dehydrogenase).[12] At times an infarction may present with a Stokes-Adams attack, with pulmonary edema, with cerebral vascular accident, or during anesthesia, obscuring chest pain. Also occasionally electrocardiographic changes of a previous infarction can be present, though the patient cannot recall an attack.

Too many patients with acute myocardial infarctions still do not reach a hospital as soon as they should. Once there, they should be treated in coronary care units. The greatest advantages of treatment in such units are prevention, early recognition, and prompt treatment of life-threatening complications,

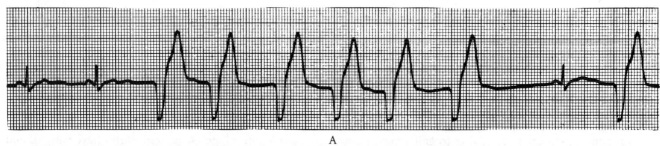

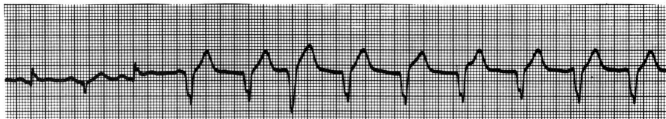

A

B

FIGURE 112-1 Idioventricular tachycardia in two patients (*A* and *B*). Lidocaine in each case produced longer runs of idioventricular rhythm with slower rates. Increasing the sinus rhythm with atropine abolished the arrhythmia. *(From P. C. Gazes, Treatment of Acute Myocardial Infarction, Postgrad. Med., 48:168, 1970, by permission.)*

especially the arrhythmias. As yet there is no full agreement about the use of antiarrhythmic drugs prophylactically in cases of acute myocardial infarctions presenting with a regular sinus rhythm. However, there have been reports indicating benefits with lidocaine.[13,14]

Individuals in charge of coronary care units should be well versed in arrhythmias. Errors in recognition of the types of arrhythmia can cause problems in therapy. Figure 112-1 was misinterpreted as slow ventricular tachycardia and treated with lidocaine, which only aggravated the accelerated

idioventricular rhythm. Electrocardiographic interpreters must be aware of artifacts which will cause confusion in diagnosis and therapy. Figure 112-2 produced considerable discussion among members of our house staff. This, appearing at first as a major ventricular arrhythmia, on close inspection was recognized as an artifact superimposed on a regular sinus rhythm.

Monitoring patients with acute myocardial infarctions is especially important during the first 48 h when the peak incidence of ventricular fibrillation occurs. Lidocaine is very helpful in preventing and treating ventricular arrhythmias, but not all ventricular premature beats or ventricular tachyarrhythmias respond to this drug; some respond to procainamide and not to lidocaine. Since an infusion with lidocaine takes up to 6 h to reach a therapeutic level, several intermittent doses of lidocaine may be necessary

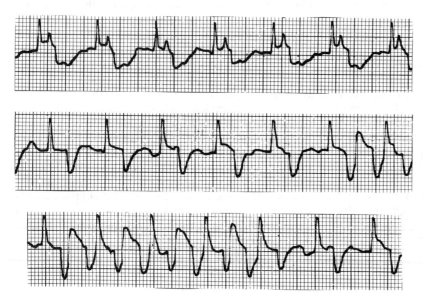

FIGURE 112-2 Continuous tracing from magnetic tape in the axis of the second lumbar vertebra (L-2). Bizarre tracing on the monitor is due to artifacts. The upright complexes with cycle length 0.64 s are the normal complexes preceded by P waves. Subsequent tracings without the artifacts were similar to these in configuration and rate.

during this period for recurrent ventricular arrhythmias.[15] If hypotension is present, tachyarrhythmias may revert with elevation of the blood pressure by phenylephrine or norepinephrine. Exceptionally, atrial flutter or ventricular tachycardia will not respond to dc countershock. Lidocaine is not generally helpful in the treatment of supraventricular arrhythmia and on occasion may produce excessive ventricular rates from acceleration of AV conduction.

Propranolol may terminate attacks of ventricular tachycardia and prevent recurrent ventricular tachycardia and ventricular fibrillation at times when the usual gamut of antiarrhythmic drugs has been ineffective. When arrhythmias are persistent or recurrent, one should not forget the importance of hypoxia and changes in pH in their production. Oxygen delivered by a tight-fitting face mask may be beneficial, but at times the use of an endotracheal tube and controlled ventilation may be required.[16] Quinidine, procainamide, propranolol, and to a lesser extent diphenylhydantoin and lidocaine decrease myocardial contractility, and if large doses are required, decreased cardiac output and hypotension may ensue. Bradycardia and hypotension are not infrequent during the first hour of onset of chest pain, occurring in 30 percent of inferior and 18 percent of anterior infarctions in one series of 284 patients.[17] Both may be aggravated by morphine administration. One should not forget the value of elevation of the legs when bradycardia and hypotension are present.

The use of atropine in sinus bradycardia is debatable since it may produce sinus tachycardia which may precipitate serious ventricular arrhythmias. If the rate is below 50 or the bradycardia is complicated by either ventricular arrhythmias or hypotension, atropine should be given.[18,19] A recent study has shown that atropine in doses lower than 0.4 mg may produce a paradoxic slowing of the rate.[20] Therefore, one should start with higher doses but should not exceed a total dose of 2.5 mg within $2\frac{1}{2}$ h.

Relief of pain is important since continued pain predisposes to arrhythmia and shock; however, decreased alveolar ventilation with increased right-to-left shunting and decrease in arterial P_{O_2} is the price one accepts when opiates are given. A decrease in frequency and depth of respiration has been cited as a factor in the production of focal atelectasis and ventilation-perfusion abnormalities, and so patients should be encouraged to take periodic deep breaths.

A temporary pervenous demand pacing catheter may be indicated in acute myocardial infarction with:

1 Persistent bradycardia and hypotension
2 Inferior infarction with second- or third-degree AV block and hypotension, ventricular arrhythmia, or heart failure[21]
3 Inferior infarction with third-degree AV block and a ventricular rate below 50, especially if perfusion is inadequate
4 Anterior infarction with bifascicular block, i.e., right bundle branch block with left anterior or posterior hemiblock, acute onset of right or left bundle branch block,[21a] bundle branch block with first-degree AV block, or alternating right and left bundle branch block
5 Mobitz type II block

It should be recalled that there is significant incidence of ventricular tachycardia with insertion of the pacemaker or from competition of a malfunctioning demand pacemaker. One cannot always derive satisfactory and dependable pacing, because of catheter displacement or the contact with infarcted tissue. In most hospitals patients must be transported to a distant fluoroscopy room, and while only a short period may be required for insertion of a catheter, occasionally 1 or 2 h may be required. AV block associated with inferior infarction is due to ischemia of the AV node and is generally reversible, whereas AV block associated with anterior infarction is generally due to necrosis of the bundle of His and its fascicles and is generally associated with extensive infarction of the septum and paraseptal area. The block may be permanent and the likelihood of death may remain high in spite of pacing.[22] If recovery ensues from the acute episode, permanent pacing may be required,[23,24] although one study concluded that generally this is not required.[25]

A mild sedative is often necessary, but many sedatives, such as phenobarbital, may induce enzymes which metabolize coumarin anticoagulants, reducing their effect on the prothrombin time.[26] Thus, if phenobarbital is discontinued and the anticoagulant is continued, hemorrhage may occur because of the slowed metabolism of the anticoagulant.

Cardiogenic shock should be differentiated from hypotension. Often the blood pressure may drop below 90 mm Hg, and yet the patient is warm and has adequate urinary output. The patient in shock is usually cold and clammy, and the urine output is less than 0.5 ml/min. It is an error to overlook hypovolemia in the presence of cardiogenic shock, since this may be an important treatable factor. Challenge with 200-ml increments of dextran over a period of 10 to 15 min may reverse shock. Parameters to watch are pulse and respiratory rate, urine flow, and development or extension of pulmonary congestion, as well as the blood pressure and skin perfusion. Since the advent of treating preload and afterload especially with vasodilator drugs such as sodium nitroprusside, it is important that hemodynamic data be available. Therefore, prior to such therapy a Swan-Ganz catheter[27] should be inserted to measure the pulmonary wedge or pulmonary artery end-diastolic pressures, which in the absence of pulmonary vascular disease or mitral valve block represent left ventricular filling pressure. The central venous pressure (reflecting right ventricular filling) may be normal and yet the pulmonary wedge pressure may be near pulmonary edema levels.

In spite of recent controversy among investigators, many physicians still use anticoagulants routinely in acute myocardial infarction. Anticoagulants are given to lessen thromboembolism. The frequency of the latter problem is highlighted by the demonstration of a 39 percent incidence of thrombosis of the calf veins during the acute phase of myocardial infarction using radioactive fibrinogen.[28,29] Two recent retrospective studies showed a reduction of hospital mortality from acute myocardial infarction by anticoagulant therapy.[30,31] A collaborative study[32] in which our group participated showed a higher survival rate and fewer bleeding complications among patients given warfarin alone than among those receiving heparin or warfarin and heparin. Data are not yet available as to the value of low-dose heparin in acute myocardial infarction.[32a]

Left ventricular failure of varying degree occurs in the overwhelming majority of patients during the first week after onset of infarction. One should not expect dyspnea until heart failure is advanced. Left-sided heart failure may occur with a heart of normal size, with normal pulse rate, in the absence of ventricular gallops, and in the presence of a normal central venous pressure. Rales are often an early physical finding, but these may be absent when the x-ray shows clear-cut interstitial edema. While a portable chest x-ray has limitations, it may demonstrate early evidence of left ventricular failure. One should note the following:

1 Dilatation of upper lobe vessels due to increasing shunting of blood
2 Loss of normal sharp definition of hilar arteries and veins (haze)
3 Increased interstitial density of lungs with ultimate prominence of small vessels in the outer areas of the lung
4 Confluent areas of edema

Less often one may note thickening of the interlobar fissures by fluid, Kerley A and B lines, dilatation of the right descending branch of the pulmonary artery, and mild pleural effusions. One should not confuse the changes with pneumonia, pulmonary infarction, pneumonitis, or pulmonary fibrosis. McHugh et al.[33] report that x-ray changes correlate reasonably well with hemodynamic changes except when the following conditions are present:

1 Preclinical edema
2 Posttherapeutic lag of the pattern of pulmonary edema
3 Severe hypoxia

However, there may be abnormal elevation of the wedge pressure in the absence of x-ray changes. There is not general agreement on the treatment of early left-sided heart failure by digitalis, but all agree on its use in the presence of well-marked congestive heart failure. Many prefer diuretic therapy; however, there is real danger of impairing ventricular function by excessive decrease in filling pressure. It is obvious that the ischemic and infarcted left ventricle shows marked decrease in compliance, and a high filling pressure may be required for optimal pumping efficiency. Thus some patients do better in face of continued interstitial edema if it is not progressive than they would if an inappropriate decrease in the pulmonary volume and left ventricular filling pressure were risked by diuretic therapy. The optimal pulmonary capillary wedge pressure to sustain cardiac output is usually between 14 and 18 mm Hg. In the absence of pressure monitoring of the pulmonary arterial and wedge pressures, one must exhibit good clinical judgment based on trial-and-error response to diuretics and challenge with small amounts of dextran or isotonic glucose. Recently, vasodilator therapy (sodium nitroprusside, and nitrates) has been used for pump failure depending on the measured hemodynamic data. However, some have used such therapy in the absence of a Swan-Ganz catheter. Parameters used are 10- to 20-mm reduction of the systolic pressure with avoidance of hypotension and the increase in urine output. Persistent ventricular dysfunction is still present in the majority of patients in the third week after onset of myocardial infarction, and severe dysfunction may be one factor predisposing to late cardiac arrest.

One should suspect pulmonary embolism if a patient has periods of hypotension, tachypnea, tachycardia, and fever and not wait for pulmonary findings or evidence of thrombophlebitis or phlebothrombosis prior to institution of heparin therapy. It has only recently been recognized that massive pulmonary embolism can occur in the absence of dyspnea, cyanosis, or hypotension.[34] The demonstration of reduced arterial P_{02} below 55 mm Hg and the use of lung scan is helpful in the diagnosis.

Heart murmurs can occur in myocardial infarction because of papillary muscle dysfunction, papillary muscle rupture, rupture of the interventricular septum, and rarely rupture of the chordae tendineae. Rupture of the septum produces a pansystolic murmur and thrill along the left lower sternal border; it is occasionally maximal farther toward the apex and may be confused with the murmur of papillary muscle dysfunction. Rupture of a papillary muscle is less often associated with a thrill. Since the advent of bypass grafts for the treatment of coronary atherosclerosis, such patients, if doing poorly, should have heart catheterization and be considered for replacement of the mitral valve or repair of a ruptured septum. If feasible, vein graft bypass surgery should be performed at the same time. External rupture of the ventricle is suggested by bradycardia followed by electromechanical dissociation with absent blood pressure and venous distension in the presence of an unchanged electrocardiogram. Tented T waves may be noted occasionally. Prompt recognition, pericardial drainage, and immediate repair without use of bypass may be lifesaving. Erroneous diagnosis of both systolic and diastolic murmurs may be made in the presence of pericarditis.

Postmyocardial infarction syndrome (Dressler's syndrome) is a recurrent febrile illness with pericarditis, pleuritis, and pneumonitis and should not be mistaken for pulmonary embolism or recurrent myocardial infarction.

Early ambulation is encouraged for patients with acute myocardial infarction. If there are no complications, chair rest is allowed in 2 to 3 days with immediate use of a portable commode; in 1 week bathroom privileges are given and walking in the room is allowed.

During the hospital stay, patient and family should

be given a clear understanding of the disease, and it should be emphasized that the patient can usually return to his or her former occupation and activities. Often patients think they will be totally disabled, and if this impression is given, convincing them later that they can return to work may be very difficult.

There are many conditions which are misdiagnosed as coronary artery disease. Often patients with angina will have more discomfort in the recumbent position, and the symptoms may be mistakenly attributed to the common asymptomatic sliding hiatus hernia noted by x-ray study. Symptoms produced by coronary disease and gallbladder disease are frequently noted in the same patient. Unfortunately, cholecystectomy may aid but not cure the angina. A patient with coronary disease may also have pain in the jaw or teeth and have unnecessary dental extractions.

Early fever and friction rub are more suggestive of pericarditis than a myocardial infarction. This is especially important when there is only transient ST elevation or minor T wave changes. Dissecting aneurysm should be considered if there is persistent hypertension in the presence of severe tearing chest pain, development of aortic insufficiency, loss or decrease of peripheral pulses, pulsating sternoclavicular joint, and minor ST-T changes.

CONGENITAL HEART DISEASE

The color and texture of the skin may give the first clue to cardiovascular disease. Cyanosis of the skin and mucous membranes should suggest congenital heart disease in the child and pulmonary disease in the adult.

A hoarse voice may indicate congenital heart disease or mitral valve disease. These conditions can dilate the pulmonary artery, causing pressure on the left recurrent laryngeal nerve and producing hoarseness. Hoarseness also may be a symptom of an aortic arch aneurysm.

On examining the chest, one should always palpate the right and left sides for dextrocardia. Dextrocardia with situs inversus is often innocuous, but isolated dextrocardia may be associated with serious congenital heart disease.

An emphysematous-appearing chest or anterior bowing in the area of the manubrium sterni, especially in a child, suggests pulmonary hypertension such as that occurring with a ventricular septal defect.[35] This is an important clue in a patient with a balanced shunt and no heart murmur.

Chest deformities such as pectus excavatum and the straight-back syndrome may produce cardiac findings that simulate congenital heart lesions.[36] Often such patients have an innocent short systolic ejection murmur associated with a normal widely split second heart sound over the pulmonic area.

Polydactyly and variation in the shape and size of the fingers, toes, or their joints may be associated with congenital heart disease.[37]

A patient with big shoulders and arms and small legs may have coarctation of the aorta. Blood pressure should be checked routinely in both arms and legs.

Errors are numerous in evaluation of heart murmurs. Attention to the character of the carotid pulse, second heart sound, heart size, history of duration of murmur, and other information gained from the history, physical examination, electrocardiogram, and x-ray may serve to indicate the presence or absence of organic disease.

Many infants with congenital heart disease have no murmurs at birth or during the early weeks of life. Small muscular interventricular septal defects frequently close, especially during the first few years of life, but even up to adult life. The common short, basal systolic murmur, usually localized to the second and third left interspaces, may be physiologic or due to an organic lesion. Listening carefully to the second sound and for ejection sounds may give the clue to the diagnosis. Fixed splitting of the second sound occurs with atrial septal defects; however, it may be detected in a small number of children with normal hearts.[38] This also can occur with mild valvular pulmonary stenosis, but often associated with this lesion is a pulmonary ejection sound that precedes the murmur. Mild aortic valvular stenosis will not alter the second sound but may give an aortic ejection sound, best heard at the apex. If the second sound is normally split with inspiration and there are no ejection sounds, then the murmur can be considered a physiologic systolic pulmonary murmur, especially if it is accentuated with inspiration and associated with a normal heart size. The increase in intensity during periods of excitement, fever, or anemia should not cause concern as to a possible organic cause. It is a fallacy to think that innocent murmurs decrease or disappear after exercise. An increase in cardiac output due to any cause will usually increase the intensity of all murmurs. Ejection sounds are often mistaken for the first heart sound, especially if the first heart sound which precedes it is very faint. The ejection sound also has to be differentiated from an S_4 gallop. An aortic ejection sound, usually best heard at the apex, may be the clue to the presence of a bicuspid valve, even though there is no murmur or just a faint one. Bacterial endocarditis can occur on such a valve. In addition, such a valve is the most common cause of calcific aortic stenosis in adults.[39] The precordial murmur of Still may be confused with an organic murmur. It occurs in young children, is vibratory, occasionally musical, ejection in type, and maximal in the parasternal area in the fourth and fifth intercostal spaces.

Organic murmurs are likely to be associated with abnormalities of the carotid pulse, second heart sound, cardiac enlargement, abnormal electrocardiogram, or x-ray. All diastolic and pansystolic murmurs are due to organic disease. Systolic ejection murmurs at the base or apex may or may not be attributable to disease. Apical clicks usually associated with late systolic murmurs due to prolapse of a large, redundant, thickened, and voluminous posterior leaflet or both leaflets of the mitral valve may not be accompanied by other abnormalities. Studies have shown that disease of supporting structures of the mitral valve allow the slack chordae to snap with varying degrees of prolapse of the valve leaflets.[40] The apical systolic murmur may either appear or be accentuated in the standing position or by the administration of Neo-Synephrine or amyl nitrite. In the past, such findings were not attributable to intracardiac disease, and while they usually are not hemodynamically significant, they may be associated with chest pain, palpitation, electrocardiographic changes such as ST-T abnormalities in the inferolateral leads, and susceptibility to bacterial endocarditis. Chest pain and arrhythmias are common complaints and may respond to propranolol therapy. Click-murmurs may occur in addition to other types of heart disease such as rheumatic heart disease, ischemic heart disease, or papillary muscle dysfunction. The syndrome may be familial and is not uncommon with secundum atrial septal defects. The echocardiogram may be normal in the presence of a click without associated murmurs.

Many normal children have a venous hum, heard best on the right side of the neck, that can be confused with a patent ductus arteriosus if it is transmitted to the chest. The venous hum will vary with rotation of the patient's head, and usually disappears when the patient is recumbent or when light pressure is applied over the neck veins. A patent ductus arteriosus most often produces a continuous murmur, heard best in the second left intercostal space just adjacent to the sternum. When it is heard maximally lower than this area, we should consider a ruptured sinus of Valsalva, coronary arteriovenous fistula, anomalous coronary artery, coarctations of the pulmonary arteries, persistent truncus arteriosus, aortopulmonary fistula, or a pseudotruncus arteriosus. The murmur of a ductus arteriosus in infants may be only systolic and not continuous. When pulmonary hypertension occurs, the murmur may even disappear.

Coarctation of the aorta is often associated with a congenital bicuspid aortic valve with aortic insufficiency or aortic stenosis.[41]

A flow diastolic rumbling murmur at the apex may be associated with moderate or large, but not small, left-to-right shunts as occur with a patent ductus arteriosus, ventricular septal defect, or atrial septal defect. This murmur can be confused with that of organic mitral stenosis. Seldom do diastolic flow murmurs produce a thrill.

There is usually no systolic thrill with an uncomplicated atrial septal defect. If a thrill is present in the pulmonary area in a patient with an atrial septal defect, associated pulmonic stenosis is often present. Bacterial endocarditis is uncommon in atrial septal defects. However, prophylactic antibiotics should be given as with other types of congenital heart lesions.

Endocardial cushion defects, usually the complete form (atrioventricularis communis), are often associated with Down's syndrome (mongolism), and a patent ductus arteriosus with the rubella syndrome.

Supravalvular aortic stenosis may give an unusual elfin facies with fullness of the lower lips and cheeks, prominence of the chin and nose, and strabismus. Mental retardation is often present. In the presence of signs of aortic stenosis, the diagnosis of supravalvular aortic stenosis should be suspected if the blood pressure is significantly greater in the right than in the left upper extremity.[42]

Idiopathic hypertrophic muscular subaortic stenosis (IHSS)[43] may give only a faint, short, ejection-type systolic murmur along the left sternal border or apex, or it may be absent until adolescence. It may be misdiagnosed as functional. It may be accentuated by the Valsalva maneuver, amyl nitrite, or isoproterenol (Isuprel) administration. One should suspect IHSS when the patient has a heart murmur and an electrocardiogram simulating a myocardial infarction. Such patients may have angina or atypical chest pain, and because of prominent Q waves in the inferior or lateral precordial leads due to septal hypertrophy, a false diagnosis of an infarction may be made and the murmur considered to be due to papillary muscle dysfunction. On occasion the murmur of IHSS may be confused with that of mitral regurgitation or a ventricular septal defect. Post-extrasystolic decrease of the carotid pulse pressure is noteworthy in patients with IHSS and obstruction to left ventricular outflow. The echocardiogram may show diagnostic changes.

Severe pulmonic stenosis may be associated with hypertelorism and a "moon" facies. A giant a wave in the venous pulse is also a helpful clue. Tetralogy of Fallot does not give a prominent a wave, since the right and left ventricular pressures are equal; congestive heart failure does not usually occur with this condition. Often these patients are digitalized unnecessarily because of attacks of tachypnea, increasing cyanosis, and exertional dyspnea, and at times because of hypoxic spells, syncope, and convulsions. These attacks may respond to propranolol. Twenty-five percent of patients with tetralogy of Fallot have a right aortic arch that may produce right sternoclavicular joint pulsation.

Patients with cyanotic congenital heart disease should be suspected of having brain abscess if they have headaches, fever, and leukocytosis. Convulsions and hemiparesis may develop.

A relative anemia may cause an accentuation of symptoms in the cyanotic infant. A moderately high incidence of pheochromocytoma has been noted in cyanotic congenital heart disease.[44]

Tricuspid atresia should always be thought of when a cyanotic patient has left ventricular hypertrophy.

Patients with mild cyanosis, arrhythmias, multiple heart sounds, and occasionally Wolff-Parkinson-White syndrome may have Ebstein's anomaly. Infrequently such patients can survive to late adulthood.

Complete transposition of the great vessels should be suspected if a patient has cyanosis, no murmur, and congestive failure in the first month of life.

Truncus arteriosus should be considered if there is mild cyanosis, a continuous murmur, or the murmur of aortic insufficiency and the clinical features of a large left-to-right shunt.

Double outlet of the right ventricle clinically may resemble a ventricular septal defect. Careful study of the right and left ventricles by angiocardiography should be made, since closure of the septal defect will produce death.

Many congenital heart lesions are seen in adulthood because they have been overlooked in the earlier years or are inoperable or had palliative procedures in childhood. Often these simulate acquired heart disease, especially the valvular types or a cardiomyopathy. The most common congenital lesions encountered in adults are atrial and ventricular septal defects, patent ductus arteriosus, valvular or subvalvular aortic stenosis, coarctation of the aorta, tetralogy of Fallot, and the Eisenmenger syndrome. Often attention is drawn to these because of arrhythmias, heart failure, or endocarditis. The chest x-ray may give the first clue to the lesion's being a congenital one because of the appearance of the heart and pulmonary vasculature. Atrial septal defect may be mistaken for mitral stenosis; coarctation of the aorta, for systemic hypertension because the blood pressure was not checked in the legs; and cyanotic lesions, for chronic lung disease.

RHEUMATIC HEART DISEASE

Acute rheumatic fever seldom occurs outside the age limits of 2 to 25 years. The Jones criteria for diagnosis of rheumatic fever have been very important in directing attention to this disease. However, these on occasion are inadequate, since certain of the minor criteria are almost prerequisite for making a diagnosis; e.g., fever is a minor criterion, and yet it is essential for the diagnosis. Likewise, the sedimentation rate and antistreptococcal test (minor criteria) are important adjuncts to diagnosis. The presence of two major criteria, or one major and two minor, is considered highly diagnostic. Yet we must realize that the combined findings of polyarthritis, fever, and elevated sedimentation rate (one major and two minor criteria) are rather weak indicators, since these can occur with many conditions, such as rheumatoid arthritis and streptococcal arthritis. Also, the P-Q (P-R) interval prolongation is very nonspecific. Subcutaneous nodules and erythema marginatum, though rare, are very specific. Rheumatic nodules develop on the extensor surface of the elbows or on any bony prominence, and they vary in size from the diameter of a pinhead to about 2 cm, and the skin moves over them freely. Erythema marginatum is confined primarily to the trunk and arms and does not affect the face. These lesions are evanescent and can recur long after the acute phase of rheumatic fever has subsided.

Carditis is a most important criterion with many pitfalls in its recognition. Murmurs in children are often misinterpreted. Young children often have a short early systolic or midsystolic vibratory murmur, heard best between the sternum and apex, and teenagers often have a short ejection, at times scratchy, systolic murmur in the pulmonary area. Rheumatic fever is often erroneously suspected in children with a history of sore throat, largely because of the presence of these functional murmurs. Errors can be avoided by the knowledge that the common significant murmur of acute rheumatic fever is apical and pansystolic, irrespective of intensity. Persistent heart failure with mitral regurgitation and active rheumatic carditis may require mitral valve replacement.

Systolic murmurs in the region of the outflow tract or the aortic area are not generally due to acute rheumatic fever. Systolic bruit from the carotid, subclavian, or brachiocephalic artery may radiate to the upper part of the chest and cause further confusion. These bruits are often heard in normal children and young adults with a hyperkinetic circulation.

Mitral stenosis may be wrongly diagnosed because of a middiastolic rumble at the apex, often heard in patients with large left-to-right shunts such as are associated with atrial or ventricular septal defects, a patent ductus arteriosus, severe anemia, or left ventricular enlargement from any cause. A broad physiologic third heart sound at the apex may also be confused with a diastolic rumble. An opening snap is frequently confused with a widely split second sound or an S_3 gallop. This also can be confused with the physiologic third heart sound heard often in the normal child. An opening snap is usually higher-pitched and closer to the second sound than a gallop or physiologic third heart sound and is heard best at the upper or lower left sternal border, particularly with the patient in the standing position.

A loud first sound may be the clue to mitral stenosis when no rumble is audible, especially in the presence of atrial fibrillation. In advanced stages of mitral stenosis with increased pulmonary arterial pressure, chronic pulmonary infections and fibrosis develop which may lead to a misdiagnosis of chronic asthmatic bronchitis. Acute pulmonary edema may obscure the murmur of mitral stenosis. Atrial fibrillation and systemic embolization demand careful evaluation for mitral stenosis. Tight mitral stenosis may be present even though there is a loud apical systolic murmur.

The loud pansystolic murmur of relative tricuspid insufficiency may be mistaken as due to mitral insufficiency; as a result the patient may be denied the benefit of closed commissurotomy. Snycope in the presence of mitral stenosis should suggest a ball valve thrombus. If a patient has a variable mitral diastolic murmur, scratchy systolic murmur, fever, and arthralgias, a left atrial myxoma should be suspected rather than bacterial endocarditis or acute rheumatic fever. Patients with severe uncomplicated mitral or aortic regurgitation usually give a history of acute rheumatic fever. If such a history is not given, one must think of fibromyxomatous changes in the valve (the floppy valve syndrome).

In the long-term care of the patient with documented rheumatic fever, the appearance of the murmur of aortic insufficiency in the absence of other findings does not necessarily indicate recurrent rheumatic fever or bacterial endocarditis. It is more likely that the newly discovered murmur may have been previously overlooked, particularly if detected by an examiner other than the original physician. The appearance of a functional murmur of aortic insufficiency in the patient with chronic renal failure may be due to a combination of fluid overload, anemia, and hypertension. This finding should not deny such a patient chronic hemodialysis or transplantation for fear that he has organic valvular disease. Also, in such a patient, a diastolic component of a pericardial rub may simulate aortic insufficiency. The murmur of aortic insufficiency may decrease in intensity when there is a decrease in peripheral vascular resistance as with exercise or during pregnancy with the placenta acting as an arteriovenous fistula. A thrill may be associated with aortic insufficiency if there is prolapse, eversion, or perforation of leaflets.

Changing intensity of murmurs at the apex over a period of time may be due to rheumatic fever, bacterial endocarditis, papillary muscle dysfunction, or rupture of chordae tendineae.[45] Loud pansystolic murmurs may decrease remarkably or disappear in the patient with cardiomyopathy when congestive heart failure is controlled. One may mistakenly search for another cause of heart failure in the patient with aortic insufficiency and advanced congestive failure because of a relatively normal diastolic pressure. This is related to a damping effect on the murmur by the markedly elevated end-diastolic pressure in the left ventricle. In some patients with severe aortic stenosis and acute congestive heart failure, the classic murmur may lessen in intensity or even be inaudible, and the cause may be overlooked. The murmur may be obscured in the presence of acute pulmonary edema.

The development of mitral regurgitation between annual examinations, particularly in the middle-aged male, in the absence of usual causes such as rheumatic fever, bacterial endocarditis, cardiomyopathy, or ischemic heart disease, suggests the possibility of ruptured chordae tendineae.

The length of a murmur is often more indicative of the severity of a lesion than its intensity. A very loud murmur may be due to a very small lesion, and a faint murmur may be associated with a severe lesion.

Pericarditis is unusual as the sole evidence of rheumatic carditis and is usually associated with pancarditis. Pericardial effusion at times may mask the endocarditis. The murmur of mitral or aortic insufficiency may become audible only after the effusion subsides.

Streptococcal pharyngitis should be treated with penicillin for 10 days or with a single injection of benzathine penicillin. Dental procedures such as filling, cleaning, root canal work, bridgework, and extraction can result in bacteremia. Bacteremia also can occur in many other procedures such as surgery of the genitourinary or intestinal tract, urethral catheterization, cystoscopy, and tonsillectomy, or in pregnancy. Patients with rheumatic heart disease undergoing such procedures should have subacute bacterial endocarditis (SBE) prophylaxis. Rheumatic fever prophylaxis (antistreptococcal) should not be confused with prophylaxis against bacterial endocarditis, which requires extra antibiotic protection.

The diagnosis of recurrent rheumatic fever is often difficult. The adult with known rheumatic heart disease and fever more likely has bacterial endocarditis than another attack of acute rheumatic fever. Treatment for bacterial endocarditis may be indicated even in the presence of negative blood cultures.

HYPERTENSION

The blood pressure should be checked routinely in both arms and legs so that one does not overlook coarctation of the aorta or a dissecting aneurysm. The standard 12-cm cuff can indicate an erroneously high blood pressure in arms with a large diameter and too low pressure in persons with thin arms. The same cuff will give a pressure in the legs 30 mm Hg or more higher than in the arms. A cuff of about 16 cm is preferable for the legs. The width of the cuff should be about 20 percent greater than the diameter of the extremity.[46] In the obese, it may be more accurate to place the cuff on the forearm and listen over the radial artery.

Certain selected patients with hypertension should have extensive studies prior to treatment to exclude renovascular disease, intrinsic renal disease, primary aldosteronism, and pheochromocytoma. (The indications for such a workup are discussed in Chap. 68.) A family history of hypertension suggests that essential hypertension is most likely. Hypokalemia, polydipsia, muscle weakness, and metabolic alkalosis suggest primary aldosteronism. Episodes of sweating, palpitation, hyperglycemia, and postural hypotension in the presence of hypertension may be the clues to a pheochromocytoma. Accelerated hypertension with an abdominal bruit and a unilateral small kidney suggests a renal origin for the hypertension. The hypertension may be associated with Cushing's syndrome if there is central obesity, buffalo hump, and thin skin.

The association of essential hypertension with low, normal, or high plasma renin activity under conditions that normally stimulate renin release is probably important but not yet clarified.

A patient may have hypertensive heart disease yet have normal blood pressure. This is often seen at the stage when the patient has marked left ventricular enlargement and heart failure. Such patients today may be mistakenly classified as having a primary cardiomyopathy rather than the end stage of hypertensive heart disease. As a general rule, however, early heart failure due to hypertension does not develop with diastolic pressures lower than 110 mm Hg.

It is best in certain instances (even though the Framingham data have shown that systolic pressure is closely related to the pathologic and clinical consequences of hypertension) not to aggressively treat the systolic hypertension of the elderly, for cerebral ischemic attacks may be precipitated.

BACTERIAL ENDOCARDITIS

Unexplained fever for more than a week or 10 days in the patient with congenital rheumatic heart disease or with a significant heart murmur from any cause should be considered to be due to bacterial endocarditis until proved otherwise.[47] Classic findings such as organic heart murmur, fever, petechiae, splenomegaly, peripheral emboli, and positive blood cultures present no problem, but one should be aware of the atypical presentations. Among these are metastatic septic endophthalmitis, mycotic aneurysm, sterile meningitis, neurologic syndromes, hematuria, gastrointestinal hemorrhage due to a ruptured mycotic aneurysm, renal failure, severe musculoskeletal backache, thrombophlebitis, recurrent bacterial pneumonia, congestive heart failure, pericarditis, and large-vessel embolism; also atypical is the patient on a hemodialysis program. Clubbing is a rare and late finding, and splinter hemorrhages are not diagnostic of the disease because of their nonspecificity.

Bacterial endocarditis should be considered in any patient with multisystem involvement. A heart murmur may be absent initially in *Staphylococcus aureus* or enterococcal endocarditis. The portal of entry may give the clue to the type of organism involved. Infection by enterococci rather than by gram-negative organisms is much more likely after urinary tract instrumentation, or in females after abortion or delivery. *Streptococcus viridans* infections occur frequently after dental procedures and staphylococcal, gram-negative bacterial and fungal infections occur in drug addicts and after open heart surgery. Blood cultures may be sterile in fungal endocarditis after open heart surgery, particularly in the first month of onset. Arteriosclerotic heart disease may more often be the etiologic factor in older people rather than rheumatic or congenital heart disease. Persistent bacteremia with no obvious focus of infection suggests endothelial surface involvement.

It is an error not to provide appropriate prophylactic antibiotic therapy for dental work or surgery in patients with valvular or congenital heart disease and those with mitral regurgitation due to prolapse of the posterior mitral leaflet. Endocarditis most frequently occurs on mild lesions such as mild mitral or aortic insufficiency rather than a severly damaged valve. It rarely occurs in a patient with mitral stenosis and in the presence of atrial fibrillation. The most common underlying congenital lesions are ventricular septal defect, patent ductus arteriosus, bicuspid aortic valve, and pulmonary stenosis. It rarely occurs in a patient with atrial septal defect. Tetralogy of Fallot is the most common cyanotic lesion involved. With such lesions one should suspect bacterial endocarditis in the presence of unexplained fever, anemia, embolism, or malaise. Antibiotics should not be administered until blood cultures are obtained. Penicillin remains the therapy of choice for most infec-

tions. Even when blood cultures remain sterile, it may be necessary to continue a course of the therapy if the clinical evidence of endocarditis is strong and if the response to therapy is that expected for endocarditis. The recurrence of fever during treatment may not indicate that the choice of antibiotic is not satisfactory but may suggest drug fever, phlebitis, embolism, or valve ring abscess.

One cannot exclude endocarditis in the absence of murmurs, since infection may be superimposed on a bicuspid aortic valve, or, as often happens with acute infections on the tricuspid or mitral valve, there may be a delay before a murmur is detectable, or the murmur may appear to be insignificant. Although involvement of the aortic and mitral valves is more common, tricuspid valve endocarditis is seen with increasing frequency in narcotic addicts, and the first signs may be septic embolism to the lung. Murmurs due to acute tricuspid regurgitation may be soft decrescendo of grade 1 or 2 of six grades of intensity, loudest at the lower left parasternal area. Prominent right-sided S_4 gallop may be associated.[48] Changing murmurs, splenomegaly, petechiae, and clubbing of the fingers are infrequent during the early course of endocarditis, and their absence is worthless in excluding the diagnosis.

The clinical picture of infective endocarditis can be confused with many other disease states that give somewhat similar findings. Left atrial myxoma can produce changing murmurs, emboli, and fever. Acute rheumatic fever, especially if the patient has had known prior rheumatic heart disease, and fever after cardiac surgery probably present the most difficult problems to differentiate from infectious endocarditis. The presence of acute pericarditis would be more in favor of acute rheumatic fever. At times when the blood cultures are negative, the differential may depend on a therapeutic trial. If the patient fails to respond to antibiotic therapy and promptly responds to salicylates, then acute rheumatic fever is most likely. After open heart surgery if fever persists beyond 10 days, the patient should be investigated for bacterial endocarditis, even though pericarditis is a more likely cause.

Laboratory studies are very important for diagnosis and following therapy in patients with endocarditis. Aerobic and anaerobic blood cultures should be taken from different sites. Three sets of cultures (six bottles) should be obtained, and 5 ml blood should be used for each 30- to 50-ml medium. Bacteremia is usually persistent when present; blood cultures should be obtained over 2- to 3-h periods, and then antibiotic therapy begun based on clinical judgment until the culture results are known. Tube dilution sensitivity studies are superior to routine disk sensitivity studies, which do not distinguish bactericidal from bacteriostatic activity and do not separate the more sensitive from the resistant organisms. Tube dilution and serum dilution studies are necessary for guidance of effective therapy. A serologic test is required for the diagnosis of Q fever endocarditis.

Surgical therapy is indicated if the patient does not respond to antibiotic therapy or is deteriorating, namely because of intractable failure, and has a correctable lesion.

In the preantibiotic era, infection was the most common cause of death in patients with endocarditis, but now with antibiotics available, congestive heart failure is the most common cause.

Fungous endocarditis is becoming more frequent because of prolonged antibiotic therapy, intravascular portal of entry, and cardiac valve abnormalities requiring prosthetic valves. Most endocarditis in drug addicts is bacterial, but there is an increased incidence of fungous endocarditis in such patients. The aortic valve is usually involved, and almost all cases are due to *Candida albicans*. During intravenous therapy for bacterial endocarditis, there is an increased incidence of superinfection with *Candida*. Blood cultures are often positive for *Candida* but not for endocarditis due to other fungi. Because of the bulk of the vegetative mass on the valve, changing heart murmurs should suggest fungous endocarditis. Fungous involvement of prosthetic valves usually requires reoperation for cure. Amphotericin B is the usual treatment for fungous endocarditis and is arbitrarily given for 10 weeks. Nausea, vomiting, and nephrotoxicity may prevent adequate therapy. 5-Fluorocytosine may prove effective against fungous infections at less toxicity than amphotericin B.

Thrombophlebitis, diabetes mellitus, chronic obstructive lung disease, prolonged antibiotic therapy, and corticosteroid therapy are commonly noted in patients who develop anaerobic endocarditis.

Nonbacterial thrombotic endocarditis (marantic endocarditis) may be significant or associated with thromboembolic episodes, and may mimic the clinical findings of bacterial endocarditis.

PERICARDIAL DISEASE

Pericarditis rather than myocardial infarction should be considered when fever and a pericardial rub occur early in the individual with chest pain. Pericardial (typically precordial or neck) pain is often aggravated by deep inspiration, sneezing, coughing, or rotating the trunk. In some cases no rub or electrocardiographic changes develop. Acute pericarditis may be painless.

Many patients are miserable because of pericarditis and are denied relief because of reluctance of the physician to diagnose the disorder in the absence of full-blown findings. The absence of ancillary findings is more common with recurrent pericarditis. When pericarditis follows myocardial infarction, the symptoms may be wrongly attributed to ischemic disease, especially if no friction rub is heard.

At times patients present with generalized enlargement of the cardiac silhouette and no other striking evidence of pericarditis. An erroneous diagnosis of myocarditis or cardiomyopathy may be entertained. Pericardial effusion may be demonstrated by usual techniques (especially echocardiography) or a short course of steroids and diuretics. A therapeutic trial of steroids and diuretics for 1 week may indicate the pericardial origin by dramatic shrinkage of the cardiac silhouette. The ventricular diastolic component of a pericardial rub may exactly mimic the murmur of aortic insufficiency, and when there is only a systolic component of a rub, mitral or tricuspid valve insufficiency may be suspected. The transient nature of the sounds clearly indicates their pericardial origin. A pericardial friction rub may be audible even when there is a large effusion. The apical impulse is often absent and the precordium quiet, but a palpable apical impulse does not exclude pericardial effusion.

Cardiac tamponade is related to the rapidity of fluid accumulation and the distensibility of the pericardium rather than the quantity. Sudden accumulation of less than 100 ml can produce tamponade. Cardiac tamponade (most often due to infection, trauma, or neoplastic disease), a life-threatening situation, may be overlooked since symptoms may be referred to other organ systems with complaints such as weakness, dizziness, nausea, vomiting, or abdominal pain or fullness. Abnormal distension of the neck veins and pulsus paradoxus may alert the physician to the correct diagnosis. One should check for pulsus paradoxus by using the blood pressure cuff. The examiner should note whether the sounds disappear during inspiration as the cuff pressure is reduced a few millimeters at a time from the top systolic level. If this occurs for 10 mm Hg or more, it may indicate pericardial effusion or, less often, constriction. However, it also may be present in myocardial disease and in airway obstructive lung disease. The neck veins may aid in differentiating pericardial disease from airway obstruction when pulsus paradoxus is present. The neck veins fill on inspiration or become further distended in pericardial disease and collapse in airway obstruction. Finally, one should not confuse an enlarged cardiac silhouette after intrapericardial surgery as due to myocardial dilatation, since varying amounts of pericardial effusion may add to the size and some weeks may pass before fluid is reabsorbed.

Occasionally a pericardial friction rub can produce a thrill. Most often when this occurs the pericarditis is due to uremia. Atrial fibrillation is present in about one-fourth of patients with chronic pericarditis because of the thickened pericardium being contiguous to the sinoatrial (SA) node. In such patients, one should place tuberculosis or neoplastic disease high on the list of possibilities. Atrial arrhythmias may also occur during the course of acute pericarditis. In a study of 100 consecutive patients with acute pericarditis only seven arrhythmias, all atrial, occurred and these only in patients with other evidence of heart disease such as myocardial, valvular, or coronary disease.[49]

Constrictive pericarditis should always be considered whenever a patient with chronic right-sided failure survives over 5 years. The Framingham study showed that the probability of death within 5 years from the onset of heart failure due to hypertension, coronary artery disease, or rheumatic heart disease was 62 percent for men and 42 percent for women.[50] The heart may be moderately enlarged with constrictive pericarditis.

Constriction in the AV groove can produce murmurs of mitral or tricuspid stenosis, and such patients often are misdiagnosed as having rheumatic heart disease. This is compounded by the fact that atrial fibrillation is often present and the diastolic knock sound is mistaken for an opening snap. The diastolic knock may be accentuated by squatting. In addition, when the neck veins are overlooked, these patients are often mistakenly followed as having cirrhosis of the liver.

Acute pericarditis may be the first manifestation of such systemic diseases as rheumatoid arthritis or lupus erythematosus. That such drugs as procainamide and hydralazine can produce pericarditis should not be overlooked. After radiation therapy, acute pericarditis, chronic effusion, or even constriction can occur. Often such cases are missed because the history of radiation therapy was not noted.

COR PULMONALE

Pulmonary emboli producing acute or chronic cor pulmonale are often overlooked because one waits for evidence of phlebitis, hemoptysis, chest pain, or lung x-ray findings. Pulmonary infarction occurs in only about 10 percent of patients with pulmonary emboli. In the proper setting, such as after an operation, if a patient has periods of unexplained fever, sinus tachycardia, or arrhythmias, tachypnea, hypotension, confusion, or apprehension, therapy should be initiated for pulmonary embolism. Dilatation of the proximal pulmonary arteries with distal narrowing may be the radiologic clue to thromboembolic pulmonary hypertension.

Electrocardiographic changes occur in only 30 percent of patients and are more reliably diagnostic if the changes are transient. Wacker's triad of an elevated lactic dehydrogenase (LDH) level, a normal serum glutamic oxaloacetic transaminase (SGOT) level, and an elevated serum bilirubin level has been found to be of little value in differentiating pulmonary embolism and infarction from other entities. An abnormal lung scan, especially in the presence of a normal chest x-ray, favors pulmonary embolism. Likewise, a negative lung scan and a normal arterial P_{O_2} are good evidence against a pulmonary embolism.

Since right ventricular hypertrophy is difficult to detect clinically, cor pulmonale may not be recognized until heart failure develops. In addition, chronic airway obstruction with emphysema can produce cough, dyspnea, orthopnea, peripheral edema due to venous stasis, and a palpable liver due to a low diaphragm simulating heart failure. Distended neck veins may be the only clue confirming the presence of heart failure. The venous pressure level may be difficult to determine because of fluctuation produced from the great variation in intrapleural pressure due to respiratory effort. Retrograde filling will aid in recognizing true elevation of venous pressure. Cheyne-Stokes respiration is rarely seen with CO_2

retention, and hydrothorax from heart failure due to chronic airway obstruction is rare.

In addition to masking failure of the right side of the heart, emphysema often presents findings suggestive of left ventricular failure. The problem is further accentuated when aging changes in the thoracic cage ("senile emphysema") and associated failure of the left side of the heart must be differentiated from chronic airway obstructive lung disease. Orthopnea, paroxysmal nocturnal dyspnea, pulsus alternans, and frothy sputum, especially with very little wheezing, are features which suggest left-sided heart failure, whereas repeated bouts of bronchitis and progressive dyspnea for many years suggest pulmonary disease. A palpable apical impulse, S_3 gallop, and pulsus alternans favor the diagnosis of left ventricular failure.

Patients with chronic airway obstruction may have a paradoxic pulse. Because of this, differentiation from pericardial effusion with tamponade or constrictive pericarditis may be a problem since all these conditions may cause distended neck veins, hepatomegaly, diminished heart sounds, and low electrocardiographic voltage. The patient with known chronic airway obstruction also may develop pericardial effusion or constriction from another associated condition, thus causing further confusion.

Though right atrial and right ventricular hypertrophy aid in the diagnosis of cor pulmonale, it must be recognized that even in well-advanced cases the electrocardiogram may be normal.

Digitalis toxicity frequently occurs in the management of chronic airway obstruction because it is increased in an attempt to control edema and dyspnea (which often are due to the lung disease) and to slow the sinus tachycardia. The heart rate is often rapid not only because of heart failure but also as a result of hypoxia. Also the action of digitalis may be obscured because of the hyperkalemia often noted with respiratory acidosis. With reversal of the respiratory acidisis, sudden hypokalemia and systemic alkalosis may develop with concomitant digitalis toxicity.

CARDIOMYOPATHIES

During the past several years many patients without evidence of the usual forms of heart diseases have been found to have diseases of the heart muscle. The causes of many of these cardiomyopathies remain obscure. These patients often tolerate congestive failure for many more years than the usual cardiac problems such as those due to hypertension, coronary artery disease, or valvular disease. Some of these can be related to one of many systemic diseases such as sarcoidosis or rheumatoid arthritis. Sarcoid involvement of the heart should be considered highly likely if the patient is black, is under age 40, and has ventricular arrhythmias or heart block. Pericarditis and aortic valve involvement are the most common findings in patients with rheumatoid arthritis. Skeletal deformities may be the clue to mucopolysaccharidosis (Hunter-Hurler's syndrome) or Marfan's syndrome. The Duchenne type of muscular dystrophy with cardiac involvement may present with an electrocardiogram simulating an old anterolateral infarction.

Myocardial infiltration frequently occurs in patients with leukemia and rarely in Hodgkin's disease. The cardiac findings of sickle-cell anemia can mimic rheumatic heart disease.[51] A hyperdynamic circulation, cardiomegaly, murmurs, and signs of pulmonary hypertension may be detected in patients with sickle-cell anemia. An apical systolic murmur and a middiastolic rumble often mimic rheumatic mitral disease, and a sickle-cell crisis may simulate acute rheumatic fever.

Hypersensitive reactions to drugs such as penicillin may produce cardiac changes. Many drugs and chemicals, such as phenothiazine tranquilizers and antidepressant drugs, can affect the myocardium.

Ischemic cardiomyopathy without prior angina or infarction and nondiagnostic electrocardiographic changes may occur more frequently in diabetics and the elderly and can be detected by coronary arteriography.

CONGESTIVE HEART FAILURE

Heart failure is not a diagnosis, and its cause should be diligently sought. Heart failure does not directly cause symptoms, but does produce abnormalities on physical examination. Symptoms occur when the heart's compensatory mechanisms fail and congestion develops in the lungs, liver, and kidneys. Careful examination of the heart, arteries, and veins may reveal abnormalities of myocardial dysfunction.

Cardiovascular findings of myocardial dysfunction, such as cardiomegaly, S_3 or S_4 gallop, paradoxic splitting of the second sound, pulsus alternans, and deep jugular vein pulsation in the position 45° from the horizontal, often occur prior to secondary congestive phenomena as noted in the lungs, liver, kidneys, or tissues. As congestion increases, the deep jugular vein pulsations ascend and may reach the earlobes. The pulsations become less visible when the veins are tensely distended from the very high venous pressure of congestive heart failure or pericardial constriction. Eventually, the external jugular veins become visible. Obstruction of the superior vena cava or the brachiocephalic veins may produce unilateral or bilateral venous distension without pulsations. Unilateral left venous distension can occur because of compression of the brachiocephalic vein against the sternum by an atherosclerotic aorta. Even though cardiomegaly is usually a prerequisite to heart failure, the heart can be of normal size in acute myocardial infarction, cor pulmonale, acute renal failure, constrictive pericarditis, mitral stenosis, and

acute infection of the valves or myocardium. Heart failure can be diagnosed from the history, physical examination, and chest x-ray without highly technical studies. X-ray is usually the most reliable method of detecting cardiomegaly. However, at times concentric hypertrophy may not be evident on x-ray and yet can be detected clinically or in the electrocardiogram. Electrocardiograms do not aid in the detection of heart failure, though they may be helpful in the diagnosis of its cause.

The symptoms of left ventricular failure can be overt or occult. Even though dyspnea is an important complaint, it must be evaluated carefully, for on first questioning many patients with normal hearts complain of shortness of breath. Often their complaint is not dyspnea but inability to get enough air, described as a slow, deep, sighing respiration. Cough may be an early finding of left-sided heart failure, especially when it clears in the sitting position, whereas with lung disease it may persist. Left-sided heart failure may produce insomnia due to Cheyne-Stokes respiration with the patient restless during the hyperpneic phase. Nocturnal angina may be a manifestation of heart failure.

Rales are not specific for heart failure and can be due to a variety of bronchorespiratory diseases. Rales are usually present in pulmonary congestion secondary to increased pulmonary venous pressure, but may be absent in interstitial edema when fluid has not extravasated into the alveoli. This can be detected by x-ray. Wheezing is most often associated with bronchitis, but can be caused by the bronchial edema of heart failure. Differentiation from bronchitis can be made when the apex impulse is palpable or when gallops, pulsus alternans, or x-ray changes are present. Monitoring of central venous pressure may cause confusion since left ventricular failure is commonly present with normal values. The central venous pressure reflects right ventricular function and may be elevated in some instances of diaphragmatic infarction when the pulmonary artery pressures are normal. The use of the Swan-Ganz catheter to measure the pulmonary artery and wedge pressures may help in selected cases of left ventricular failure. Its use may allow one to obtain a more optimal filling pressure of the noncompliant left ventricle.

Paroxysmal nocturnal dyspnea may occur for months prior to a diagnosis of heart failure. If the patient is not seen during an attack, the lungs later may be clear.

Symptoms of right-sided heart failure occur relatively late. Water retention may be first noted because of weight gain or nocturia rather than pitting edema, which becomes manifest only after retention of about 10 lb of fluid.

Pleural effusion is more common in the right pleural cavity in association with right-sided heart failure. However, it can occur with left-sided heart failure, as the pleural venous drainage is into both the pulmonary and systemic veins. The fluid is nonhemorrhagic unless associated with or due to pulmonary infarction.

Hepatomegaly is not considered to be present unless the distance between its flat, percussed upper edge and palpable lower edge is more than 11 cm.

Right-sided heart failure is often misdiagnosed because the liver is palpable (due to a low diaphragm) and edema due to venous stasis is present. Upper right quadrant tenderness may be mistaken for hepatitis or cholecystitis rather than rapid distension of the liver from heart failure.

Peripheral edema is most unusual in heart failure unless cardiomegaly, hepatomegaly, and neck vein distension are present. Peripheral edema is commonly due to obesity, venous stasis, varicosities and other venous diseases, hormonal administration, menopause, and psychogenic, hepatic, and renal disease. Patients are often digitalized and given diuretics when the edema is noncardiac. Even normal persons can lose up to 3 lb in weight when given a diuretic.

The most common cause of refractory heart failure is pulmonary embolism, but other causes may be overlooked, such as electrolyte imbalance, infections, anemia, surgically correctable lesions, and hyperthyroidism. Mitral stenosis as a cause of heart failure may be overlooked particularly in the older person, and the possibility of corrective surgery may be denied the patient.[52] Often the murmur of mitral stenosis is missed if the patient is examined during an episode of pulmonary edema.

The trial-and-error method of giving digitalis was used for many years. Recent pharmacokinetic data and methods for measuring cardiac glycoside blood levels have given a more specific method of prescribing digitalis with less chance of toxicity. Former recommendations for dosage were too high. In addition, digitalis should be prescribed according to lean body weight rather than total weight. Therapeutic levels of digoxin usually range between 0.8 and 1.6 ng/ml, possible toxicity levels are between 1.6 and 3.0 ng/ml, and probable toxicity levels are greater than 3.0 ng/ml. A review of several studies showed that it was impossible to determine digitalis toxicity on the basis of the serum level alone any more accurately than could have been done on clinical grounds.[53] Larger doses may be necessary for supraventricular arrhythmias in order to achieve the proper chronotrophic effect, and in such cases the serum levels may be higher than 3 ng/ml without evidence of toxicity. Blood sampling should be taken at least 6 to 8 h after a dose of digoxin has been given to allow time for tissue distribution and equilibrium in the blood and in the myocardium. The radioimmunoassay method for digitalis levels may give low readings if the patient has received isotopes such as radioactive iodine uptake test. Laboratory results should be considered along with the clinical data. Heart rate cannot be used in gauging digitalis dosage unless atrial fibrillation is present. Larger doses of digitalis are usually required in atrial flutter to block the AV node as compared with doses for atrial fibrillation.

The electrocardiogram cannot be used as a guide to optimal dosage. At therapeutic levels of digitalis some patients have ST depression and/or T wave inversion which do not correlate with the loading dose, toxic effects, or need for digitalis. Maintenance dose of digoxin depends on renal function.

Digitalis should be given cautiously to the following: patients with severe heart disease, elderly patients, and patients with hyperthyroidism with atrial fibrillation, mitral stenosis with a normal sinus rhythm, acute myocardial infarction, high output failures as with anemia, renal insufficiency, and electrolyte imbalance. Certain preparations such as reserpine, calcium, and propranolol can increase sensitivity to digitalis; others, such as cholestyramine, kaopectate, or aluminum and magnesium hydroxides (Maalox), may increase resistance to digitalis. Hypertrophic subaortic stenosis, Wolff-Parkinson-White syndrome, and constrictive pericarditis are relative contraindications to the use of digitalis.

When restricted activity, digitalis, and low salt intake can control heart failure, diuretics should be withheld. The potassium-sparing diuretics such as spironolactone (Aldactone) and triamterene (Dyrenium) should be used with caution in the presence of renal diseases and with excessive intake of foods or salt substitutes with large amounts of potassium, because hyperkalemia can develop. In addition, they should not be prescribed with potassium supplements.

ELECTROCARDIOGRAPHIC FINDINGS

Left axis deviation recently has assumed increased importance. A deviation of more than $-30°$ to the left is abnormal. This abnormality is most often due to block or delay in the left anterosuperior fascicle of the left bundle (left anterior hemiblock) and can be caused by many conditions such as coronary artery disease, left ventricular hypertrophy, congenital heart disease, and very commonly fibrosis of the conducting system.[54,55] Rarely this degree of axis shift is due to an abnormal anatomic position of the heart.

Right axis deviation of $+120°$ or more is abnormal. This may be due to right ventricular hypertrophy, chronic lung disease, or a block or delay in the posteroinferior fascicle of the left bundle (left posterior hemiblock), may appear transiently with a pulmonary embolism, or may be factitious due to reversal of the right and left arm leads.

Left bundle branch block may be due to significant cardiac disorders, and the prognosis depends on the associated type of disease[56]; however, it may be found in the young individual in the absence of detectable disease. Right bundle branch block occurs more often than left bundle branch block either as an isolated congenital anomaly or asymptomatically without other evidence of heart disease. Complete right or left bundle branch block in persons under age 40 may be unassociated with other evidence of cardiovascular disease in up to 90 percent. The prognosis of bundle branch block is determined by the presence or absence and the degree of associated cardiovascular disease.[57] Moore and his colleagues have presented evidence that the incomplete right bundle branch block pattern may be due to a heritable focal hypertrophy of the right ventricle and not caused by delayed conduction within the right bundle branch.[58]

The identification of left ventricular hypertrophy by the electrocardiogram is not simple, because many criteria are used.[59,60] Highly sensitive criteria produce overdiagnosis.

The term *nonspecific T waves* is vague but should be used rather than labeling a person as having organic disease, especially coronary artery disease. As noted earlier in this chapter, Levine[3] has listed 67 causes for T wave changes which can be due to physiologic, hemodynamic, or metabolic factors. These T wave changes should be considered in conjunction with other findings.

Exercise stress tests, as mentioned previously, are difficult to interpret, may be false positive, and even if negative do not exclude coronary artery disease.

Early repolarization,[61] often noted in blacks, can simulate a current of injury as seen with acute pericarditis or myocardial infarction. Tuberculous pericarditis seldom presents with a current of injury, because it occurs insidiously and is more often first detected in the evolving stage.

Many lesions can give electrocardiographic findings which simulate myocardial infarction, such as myocarditis, brain lesions, tumors of the heart, Wolff-Parkinson-White syndrome, idiopathic hypertrophic subaortic stenosis, or muscular dystrophy. Left bundle branch block can obscure the electrocardiographic findings of myocardial infarction. An infarction may be present although the tracings are normal, or later they can return to normal.[8,9] One should not predict the outcome of a patient's condition on the basis of the electrocardiogram.

The ST depression produced by digitalis is not due to a toxic effect and does not correlate with the amount of digitalis that should be given as a loading or maintenance dose.

Electrical alternation is less common than pulsus alternans, and in addition to left ventricular dysfunction it can be seen with pericardial effusion, hypertension, digitalis intoxication, and other conditions. The electrocardiogram may give the first clue to an electrolyte disturbance.

The electrocardiogram of dextrocardia should not be confused with reversal of the right and left arm leads.

The electrocardiogram can at times give some idea about the hemodynamic state. For example, a patient with congenital valvular aortic stenosis and a normal T wave in lead V_6 probably has a small left ventricular aortic pressure gradient as compared with a patient with a flattened or inverted T wave.

ARRHYTHMIAS

Premature beats are very common even in many persons without other evidence of heart disease.

Even though recent epidemiologic studies suggest that ventricular premature beats occurring after age 30 may be associated with an increased risk of coronary artery disease and sudden death,[62] the practicing physician realizes that these are extremely common in individuals with normal hearts and it may be unwise to treat the usual types of premature ventricular beats unrelated to tachyarrhythmias.

Idioventricular rhythm at a rate of 60 to 100 beats per minute occurs often in the presence of an inferior infarction, is usually transient, and produces no complications.[63] At times it may coexist with paroxysmal ventricular tachycardia.[63a]

Atrial fibrillation can be seen in patients with apparently normal hearts, but atrial flutter is more often associated with organic heart disease. Atrial flutter in the absence of prior evidence of heart disease suggests pulmonary embolism.[64] Quinidine should not be used initially for atrial flutter, since it may enhance AV conduction through its vagolytic effect and thus increase the ventricular rate. Paroxysmal atrial fibrillation may be precipitated by social drinking. Sudden regular ventricular rhythm in the presence of atrial fibrillation should suggest third-degree AV block if the rate is below 50 beats per minute or AV dissociation with nonparoxysmal junction tachycardia if the ventricular rate is between 70 and 130 beats per minute. Often such patients are passed off as having a regular sinus rhythm, whereas actually they are overdigitalized.

Ventricular tachycardia can be diagnosed by electrocardiogram with certainty in only 50 percent of instances, for it is often impossible to distinguish it from a supraventricular tachycardia with aberrant conduction or bundle branch block.

Chronic third-degree AV block is more commonly due to bilateral bundle branch block rather than a block in the AV node. Degenerative or fibrotic changes in the bundles appear to be very common causes of third-degree AV block. Stokes-Adams attacks are the main indication for a permanent cardiac pacemaker. AV block or SA block is a diagnostic feature. However, frequently between attacks a regular sinus rhythm is noted, and one must search in routine or monitored tracings for other electrocardiographic clues. The following changes suggest that the attacks may be cardiac in origin: different degrees of AV block, bifascicular block (right bundle branch block with left hemiblocks), right or left bundle branch block with first-degree AV block, left axis (about $-60°$) or right axis (about $+120°$), SA block or sinus arrest, marked sinus bradycardia or slow junctional rhythm, and a hypersensitive carotid sinus.

The Wenckebach groupings are very important. In the typical Wenckebach structure the QRS complexes approach each other as the P-R interval lengthens until a sinus beat is not conducted. The interval with the nonconducted QRS complex is less than twice the preceding R-R interval. In addition, this latter interval is less than the R-R interval after the nonconducted QRS complex. If only two beats are conducted prior to the nonconducted QRS, then a 3:2 block (three atrial and two ventricular complexes) is produced. This gives a Wenckebach block grouping

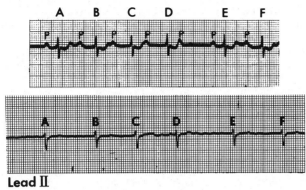

Lead II

FIGURE 112-3 Wenckebach AV node block. Top tracing shows the typical Wenckebach structure. The QRS complexes approach each other as the P-R interval lengthens until a sinus beat is not conducted. The interval DE with the nonconducted QRS complex is less than twice the preceding R-R interval CD. In addition, interval CD is less than the R-R interval EF after the concoducted QRS complex. Lower tracing shows atrial fibrillation with Wenckebach AV node block. Even though P waves are not seen, the grouping of QRS complexes indicates a Wenckebach AV block (QRS complexes approach each other, DE is less than 2 CD, and EF is greater than CD). *(From Peter C. Gazes, "Clinical Cardiology," copyright 1975 by Year Book Medical Publishers, Inc., Chicago. Used by permission.)*

of QRS complexes in pairs (pseudobigeminy) followed by a pause. Knowing these two groupings, one can suspect Wenckebach block even if the P waves are not visible, as with atrial fibrillation (Figs. 112-3 and 112-4). Often in such cases the Wenckebach block is passed off as atrial fibrillation with a satisfactory ventricular response. In addition, Wenckebach block of the SA node can be recognized and not missed as sinus arrhythmia. The QRS groupings are the same for SA node Wenckebach block, but the P-R interval does not change as it does in the AV types. A clue to the cardiac cause of syncope due to complete heart block is the presence of a prolonged Q-T interval with deeply inverted T waves that may be detected for several days following an attack. Permanent pacemakers should be considered for patients who have Stokes-Adams attacks, or without such attacks if heart block is present with a ventricular rate below 40 beats per minute, widened QRS complexes, heart failure, angina, cerebral insufficiency, or renal insufficiency. Pacemakers are also used for patients with drug-resistant tacharrhythmias and for patients with tachybradyarrhythmias that cannot be controlled with drugs.

Nonparoxysmal junctional tachycardia with AV dissociation should not be confused with third-degree AV block. In the former, the ventricular rate from the junctional focus is more rapid than the sinus rhythm which activates the atria. In addition, there is a retrograde AV block to the atria, but the sinus node at the slower rate may at times conduct antegrade and capture the ventricles if they are nonrefractory. This form of junctional tachycardia commonly occurs with digitalis toxicity.

Most tachycardias in the presence of the Wolff-Parkinson-White syndrome have impulses descending toward the ventricles by way of the normal His

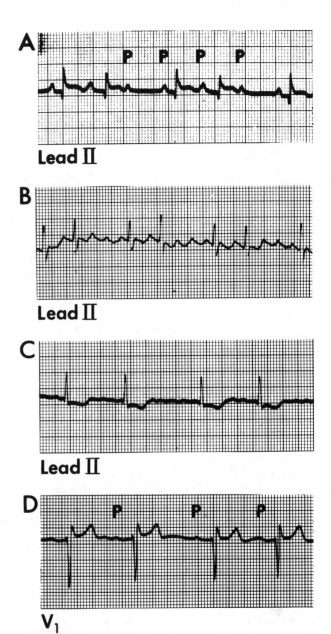

FIGURE 112-4 SA and AV node Wenckebach block with 3:2 block. These are characterized by the QRS complexes occurring in pairs followed by a pause. *A.* Sinus rhythm with 3:2 AV node Wenckebach block (three atrial and two ventricular complexes). *B.* Atrial flutter with 3:2 AV node Wenckebach block. *C.* Atrial fibrillation with 3:2 AV node Wenckebach block. *D.* Sinus rhythm with 3:2 SA Wenckebach block. *(From Peter C. Gazes, "Clinical Cardiology," copyright 1975 by Year Book Medical Publishers, Inc., Chicago. Used by permission.)*

bundle and returning to the atria via the anomalous pathway, thus giving rise to normal QRS complexes. However, atrial fibrillation bombards the AV node, producing concealed conduction; thus antegrade conduction is more often by way of the anomalous bundle. In such cases, the QRS complexes will be those of the Wolff-Parkinson-White type, and this arrhythmia may simulate ventricular tachycardia.

REFERENCES

1 Edwards, T. (ed.): "The New Dictionary of Thoughts: A Cyclopedia of Quotations," revised and enlarged by C. N. Catrevas, J. Edwards, and R. E. Browns, Standard Book Company, 1957, p. 181.

1a Heberden, W.: Some Account of a Disorder of the Heart, *Med. Trans. R. Coll. Physicians,* 2:59, 1772.

2 Horwitz, L. Q., Herman, M. V., and Gorlin, R.: Clinical Responses to Nitroglycerin as a Diagnostic Test for Coronary Artery Disease, *Am. J. Cardiol.,* 29:149, 1972.

3 Levine, H. D.: Non-Specificity of the Electrocardiogram Associated with Coronary Artery Disease, *Am. J. Med.,* 15:344, 1953.

4 Mattingly, T. W.: The Post-Exercise Electrocardiogram, *Am. J. Cardiol.,* 9:395, 1962.

4a Goldschlager, N. Selzer, A., and Cohn, K.: Treadmill Stress Tests as Indicators of Presence and Severity of Coronary Artery Disease; *Ann. Intern. Med.,* 85:277, 1976.

5 Gazes, P. C.: False-Positive Exercise Test in the Presence of the Wolff-Parkinson-White Syndrome, *Am. Heart J.,* 78:13, 1969.

5a Sketch, M. H., Mohiuddin, S. M., Lynch, J. D., Zencka, A. E., and Runco, V.: Significant Sex Differences in the Correlation of Electrocardiographic Exercise Testing and Coronary Arteriograms, *Am. J. Cardiol.,* 36:169, 1975.

6 Alderman, E. L., Coltart, D. J., Wettach, G. E., and Harrison, D. C.: Coronary Artery Syndrome after Sudden Propranolol Withdrawal, *Ann. Intern. Med.,* 81:625, 1974.

7 Miller, R. R., Olson, H. G., Amsterdam, E. A., and Mason, D. T.: Propranolol-Withdrawal Rebound Phenomenon: Exacerbation of Coronary Event after Abrupt Cessation of Antianginal Therapy, *N. Engl. J. Med.,* 293:416, 1975.

8 Martinez-Rios, M. A., Bruto DaCosta, B. C., Cecena-Seldner, F. A., and Gensini, G. G.: Normal Electrocardiogram in the Presence of Severe Coronary Artery Disease, *Am. J. Cardiol.,* 25:320, 1970.

9 Kalbfleish, M. M., Shadakharappa, K. S., and Conrad, L. L.: Disappearance of the Q Deflection following Myocardial Infarction, *Am. Heart J.,* 76:196, 1968.

10 Sodi-Pollares, D., Bisteni, A., and Cisneros, F.: Reliability of the Electrocardiogram in Diagnosis of Myocardial Infarction, in W. Likoff and J. Moyer (eds.), "Coronary Heart Disease," Grune & Stratton, Inc., New York, 1963, p. 278.

11 Levine, H. D., and Phillips, E.: An Appraisal of the Newer Electrocardiography: Correlations in One Hundred and Fifty Consecutive Autopsied Cases, *N. Engl. J. Med.,* 245:833, 1951.

12 Galen, R. S., Reiffel, J. A., and Gambino, S. R.: Diagnosis of Acute Myocardial Infarction: Relative Efficiency of Serum Enzymes and Isoenzyme Measurements, *J.A.M.A.,* 232:145, 1975.

13 Lie, K. I., Wellens, H. J., vanCapelle, F. J., and Durrer, D.: Lidocaine in the Prevention of Primary Ventricular Fibrillation: A Double-blind, Randomized Study of 212 Consecutive Patients, *N. Engl. J. Med.,* 291:1324, 1974.

14 Valentine, P. A., Frew, J. L., Mashford, M. L., and Sloman, J. G.: Lidocaine in the Prevention of Sudden Death in the Pre-Hospital Phase of Acute Infarction: A Double-blind Study, *N. Engl. J. Med.,* 291:1327, 1974.

15 Bigger, J. T.: Pharmacologic and Clinical Control of Antiarrhythmic Drugs, *Am. J. Med.,* 58:479, 1975.

16 Ayers, S. M., and Grace, W. J.: Inappropriate Ventilation and Hypoxemia as Causes of Cardiac Arrhythmias, *Am. J. Med.,* 416:495, 1969.

17 Adgey, A. A. J., Geddes, J. S., Webb, S. W., Allen, J. D., James, R. G. G., Zaidi, S. A., and Pantridge, J. F.: Acute Phase of Myocardial Infarction, *Lancet,* 2:501, 1971.

18 Warren, J. V., and Lewis, R. P.: Beneficial Effects of Atropine in the Pre-Hospital Phase of Coronary Care, *Am. J. Cardiol.,* 37:68, 1976.

19 Scheinman, M. M., Thorburn, D., and Abbott, J. A.: Use of Atropine in Patients with Acute Myocardial Infarction and Sinus Bradycardia, *Circulation,* 52:627, 1975.

20 Das, G., Talmers, F. N., and Weissler, A. M.: New Observations on the Effects of Atropine on the Sinoatrial and Atrioventricular Nodes in Man, *Am. J. Cardiol.,* 36:281, 1975.

21 Rotman, M., Wagner, G. S., and Waugh, R. A.: Significance of High Degree Atrioventricular Block in Acute Posterior Myocardial Infarction, *Circulation,* 47:257, 1973.

21a Furman S.: Cardiac Pacing and Pacemakers: I. Indications for Pacing Bradyarrhythmias, *Am. Heart J.,* 93:523, 1977.

22 Kostuk, W. J., and Beanlands, D. S.: Complete Heart Block Associated with Acute Myocardial Infarction, *Am. J. Cardiol.,* 26:380, 1971.

23 Mullins, C. B., and Atkins, J. M.: Prognoses and Management of Ventricular Conduction Blocks in Acute Myocardial Infarction, *Mod. Concepts Cardiovasc. Dis.,* 45:129, 1976.

24 Waugh, R. A., Wagner, G. S., Haney, T. L., Rosati, R. A., and Morris, J. J., Jr.: Immediate and Remote Prognostic Significance of Fascicular Block during Acute Myocardial Infarction, *Circulation,* 47:765, 1973.

25 Waters, D. D., and Mizgala, H. F.: Long-Term Prognosis of Patients with Incomplete Bilateral Bundle Branch Block Complicating Acute Myocardial Infarction: Role of Cardiac Pacing, *Am. J. Cardiol.,* 34:1, 1974.

26 Cucinel, S. A., Connez, A. H., Sansur, M. S., and Burns, J. J.: Drug Interactions in Man: I. Lowering Effect of Phenobarbital on Plasma Levels of Bishydroxycourmarin (Dicumarol) and Diphenylhydantoin (Dilantin), *Clin. Pharmacol. Ther.,* 6:420, 1965.

27 Swan, H. J. C.: Balloon Flotation Catheters: Their Use in Hemodynamic Monitoring in Clinical Practice, *J.A.M.A.,* 233:865, 1975.

28 Cristal, N., Stern, J., Ronen, M., Silverman, C., Ho, W., and Bartov, E.: Identifying Patients at Risk for Thromboembolism. Use of ^{125}I-labeled Fibrinogen in Patients with Acute Myocardial Infarction, *J.A.M.A.,* 236:2755, 1976.

29 Wray, R., Maurer, B., and Shillingford, J.: Prophylactic Anticoagulant Therapy in the Prevention of Calf-Vein Thrombosis after Myocardial Infarction, *N. Engl. J. Med.,* 288:815, 1973.

30 Modan, B., Shani, M., Schor, S., and Modan, M.: Reduction of Hospital Mortality from Acute Myocardial Infarction by Anticoagulant Therapy, *N. Engl. J. Med.,* 292:1359, 1975.

31 Tonascia, J., Gordis, L., and Schmerler, H.: Retrospective Evidence Favoring Use of Anticoagulants for Myocardial Infarction, *N. Engl. J. Med.,* 292:1362, 1975.

32 Collaborative Study at 13 Hospitals: Sodium Heparin vs. Sodium Warfarin in Acute Myocardial Infarction, *J.A.M.A.,* 189:555, 1964.

32a Wessler, S.: Heparin as an Antithrombotic Agent, *J.A.M.A.,* 236:389, 1976.

33 McHugh, T. J., Forrester, J. S., Adler, L., Zion, D., and Swan, H. J.: Pulmonary Vascular Congestion in Acute Myocardial Infarction: Hemodynamic and Radiologic Correlations, *Ann. Intern. Med.,* 76:29, 1972.

34 Wenger, N. K., Stein, P. D., and Willis, P. W., III: Massive Acute Pulmonary Embolism: Deceivingly Nonspecific Manifestations, *Am. J. Cardkiol.,* 29:296, 1972.

35 Arosemena, E., Elliott, T. P., and Eliot, R. S.: Chest Deformity in Adults with Congenital Heart Disease, *Am. J. Cardiol.,* 20:303, 1967.

36 Gooch, A. S., Maranhao, V., and Goldberg, H.: The Straight Thoracic Spine in Cardiac Diagnosis, *Am. Heart J.,* 74:595, 1967.

37 Silverman, M. E., and Hurst, J. W.: The Hand and the Heart, *Am. J. Cardiol.,* 22:718, 1968.

38 Ehlers, K. H., Engle, M. A., Farnworth, P. B., and Levin, A. R.: Wide Splitting of the Second Heart Sound without Demonstable Heart Disease, *Am. J. Cardiol.,* 23:690, 1969.

39 Roberts, W. C.: Anatomically Isolated Aortic Valvular Disease: The Case against It Being of Rheumatic Etiology, *Am. J. Med.,* 49:151, 1970.

40 Barlow, J. B., Bosman, C. K., Pocock, W. A., and Marchand, P.: Late Systolic Murmurs and Non-Ejection ("Mid-late") Systolic Clicks: An Analysis of 90 Patients, *Br. Heart J.,* 30:203, 1968.

41 Edwards, J. E.: Congenital Biscuspid Aortic Valve, *Circulation,* 23:485, 1961.

42 Myers, A. R., and Willis, P. W., III: Clinical Spectrum of Supravalvular Aortic Stenosis, *Arch. Intern. Med.,* 118:552, 1966.

43 Braunwald, E., Lambrew, C. T., Rockoff, S. D., Ross, J., Jr., and Morrow, A. G.: Idiopathic Hypertrophic Subaortic Stenosis: Description of the Disease Based upon Analysis of 64 Patients, *Circulation,* 29(suppl. 4):1, 1964.

44 Folger, G. M., et al.: Cyanotic Malformations of the Heart with Pheochromocytoma, *Circulation,* 29:750, 1964.

45 Ronan, J. A., Steelman, R. B., DeLeon, A. C., Waters, T. J., Perloff, J. D., and Harvey, W. P.: The Clinical Diagnosis of Acute Severe Mitral Insufficiency, *Am. J. Cardiol.,* 27:284, 1971.

46 Burch, G. E., and DePasquale, N. P.: "Primer of Clinical Management of Blood Pressure," The C. V. Mosby Company, St. Louis, 1962.

47 Friedberg, C.: "Diseases of the Heart," 2d ed., W. B. Saunders Company, Philadelphia, 1956.

48 Rios, J. C., Massumi, R. A., Bressman, W. T., and Sarin, R. K.: Ausculatatory Features of Acute Tricuspid Regurgitation, *Am. J. Cardiol.,* 23:4, 1969.

49 Spodick, D. H.: Arrhythmias During Acute Pericarditis: A Prospective Study of 100 Consecutive Cases, *J.A.M.A.,* 235:39, 1976.

50 McKee, P. A., Castelli, W. P., McNamara, P. M., and Kannel, W. B.: The Natural History of Congestive Heart Failure: The Framingham Study, *N. Engl. J. Med.,* 285:1441, 1971.

51 Lindsay, J., Jr., Meshel, J. C., and Patterson, R. H.: The Cardiovascular Manifestations of Sickle Cell Disease, *Arch. Intern. Med.,* 133:643, 1974.

52 Myers, J. W., and Horley, C. J.: "Silent" Mitral Stenosis: Diagnostic Problems, Particularly in the Elderly Patient, *Heart Bull.,* 20:30, 1971.

53 Ingelfinger, J. A., and Goldman, P.: The Serum Digitalis Concentration: Does It Diagnose Digitalis Toxicity? *N. Engl. J. Med.,* 294:867, 1976.

54 Rosenbaum, M. B., Elizari, M. V., Lazzari, J. O., Nau, G. J., Levi, R. J., and Halpern, M. S.: Intraventricular Trifascicular Blocks, *Am. Heart J.,* 78:450, 1969.

55 Lev, M.: Pathology of Bundle Branch Block, *Heart Bull.,* 16:107, 1967.

56 Beach, T. B., Gracey, J. G., Peter, R. H., and Gruenwald, P. W.: Benign Left Bundle Branch Block, *Ann. Intern. Med.,* 70:273, 1969.

57 Rotman, M., and Triebwasser, J. H.: A Clinical and Follow-up Study of Right and Left Bundle Branch Block, *Circulation,* 51:477, 1975.

58 Moore, E. N., Boineau, J. P., and Patterson, D. F.: Incomplete Right Bundle Branch Block: An Electrocardiographic Enigma and Possible Misnomer, *Circulation,* 44:678, 1971.

59 Baxley, W. A., Dodge, H. T., and Sandler, H.: A Quantitative Angiocardiographic Study of Left Ventricular Hypertrophy and the Electrocardiogram, *Circulation,* 37:509, 1968.

60 Romhilt, D. W., and Estes, E. H., Jr.: A Pointsure System for the ECG Diagnosis of Left Ventricular Hypertrophy, *Am. Heart J.,* 75:752, 1968.

61 Goldman, M. J.: RS-T Segment Elevation in Mid and Left Precordial Leads as Normal Variant, *Am. Heart J.,* 46:817, 1953.

62 Chiang, B. N., Perlman, L. V., Ostrander, L. P., Jr., and Epstein, F. H.: Relationship of Premature Systoles to the Coronary Heart Disease and Sudden Death in the Tecumseh Epidemiologic Study, *Ann. Intern. Med.,* 70:1159, 1969.

63 Schamroth, L.: Idioventricular Tachycardia, *Dis. Chest,* 56:466, 1969.

63a Talbot, S., and Greaves, M.: Association of Ventricular Extrasystoles and Ventricular Tachycardia with Idioventricular Rhythm, *Br. Heart J.,* 38:457, 1976.

64 Johnson, J. C., Flowers, N. C., and Horan, L. J.: Unexplained Atrial Flutter: A Frequent Herald of Pulmonary Embolism, *Chest,* 60:29, 1971.

INDEX

INDEX

Page references in **boldface** indicate major areas of descriptions and information. More than one number is shown in **boldface** when the discussions are presented from a different point of view.

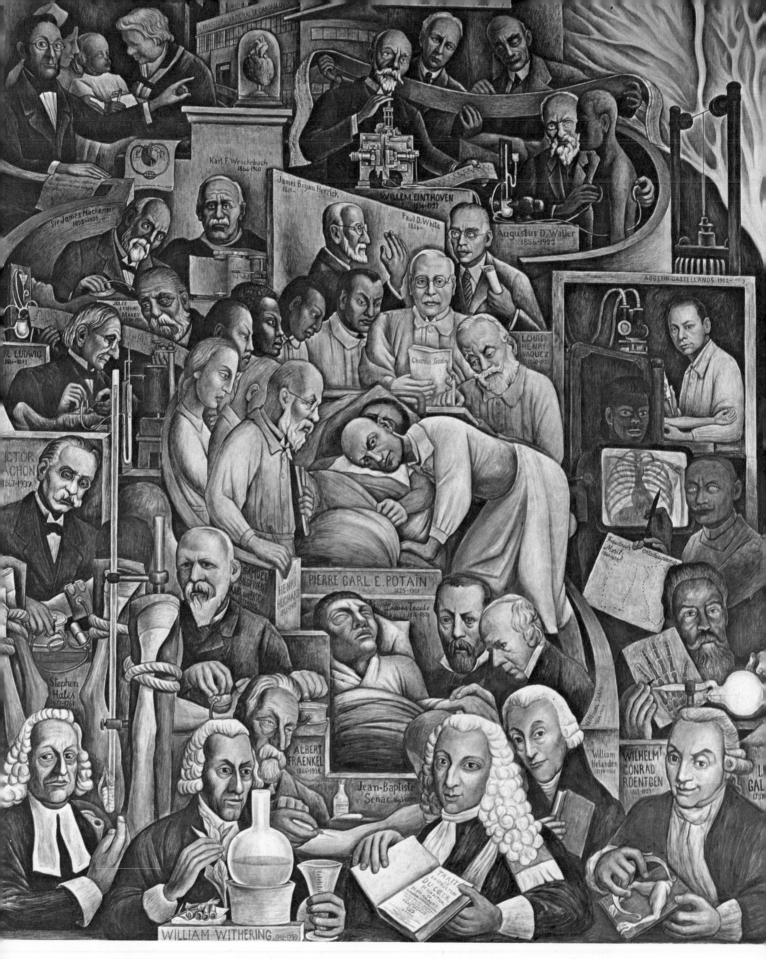

DIEGO RIVERA   "The History of Cardiological Doctrines" 1946

National Institute of Cardiology   Mexico D.F.